Pediatric Primary Care

A Handbook for Nurse Practitioners

2nd Edition

Catherine E. Burns, PhD, RN, CPNP, FAAN
Professor
Primary Health Care Nurse Practitioner Specialty
Oregon Health Sciences University School of Nursing
Portland, Oregon

Margaret A. Brady, PhD, RN, CPNP
Professor
California State University Long Beach Department of Nursing
Pediatric Nurse Practitioner, Miller Children's Hospital
Long Beach, California

Ardys M. Dunn, PhD, RN, PNP
Associate Professor
University of Portland School of Nursing
Portland, Oregon

Nancy Barber Starr, MS, RNC, CPNP
Pediatric Nurse Practitioner
Aurora Pediatric Associates
Aurora, Colorado

W.B. SAUNDERS COMPANY
A Harcourt Health Sciences Company
Philadelphia • London • New York • St. Louis • Sydney • Toronto

W.B. SAUNDERS COMPANY
A Harcourt Health Sciences Company

The Curtis Center
Independence Square West
Philadelphia, Pennsylvania 19106

Library of Congress Cataloging-in-Publication Data

Pediatric primary care: a handbook for nurse practitioners / Catherine E. Burns—2nd ed.

p. ; cm.

Includes bibliographical references and index.

ISBN 0–7216–8062–3

1. Pediatric nursing—Handbooks, manuals, etc. 2. Ambulatory medical care for children—Handbooks, manuals, etc. I. Burns, Catherine E.
[DNLM: 1. Pediatrics—United States. 2. Primary Health Care—United States. WS 100 P3658 2000]

RJ245 .P43 2000 618.91—dc21

DNLM/DLC 99–047085

Editor-in-Chief: Sally Schrefer

Acquisitions Editor: Barbara Nelson Cullen

Developmental Editor: Kara L. Johnson

Manuscript Editor: Mary C. Reinwald

Production Manager: Denise LeMelledo

Illustration Specialist: Lisa Lambert

PEDIATRIC PRIMARY CARE: A Handbook for Nurse Practitioners   ISBN 0-7216-8062-3

Printed in the United States of America.

Last digit is the print number: 9   8   7   6   5   4   3   2

This book is dedicated to the infants, children, adolescents,
and their families about whom the book was written,
wishing them health, loving support,
and happiness,
the real goals of this book.

CONTRIBUTORS

Jean Betschart, MSN, MN, CPNP, CDE
Adjunct Faculty, Department of Health Promotion and Development, University of Pittsburgh School of Nursing; Pediatric Nurse Practitioner, Department of Diabetes, Endocrinology, and Metabolism, Children's Hospital of Pittsburgh, Pittsburgh, Pennsylvania
    Endocrine and Metabolic Diseases

Patricia Billings, RN, MPH, CPNP
Physicians Center, Twin Falls, Idaho
    Developmental Management of School-Age Children

Catherine Blosser, CPNP
Pediatric Nurse Practitioner, Multnomah County Health Department, Portland, Oregon

Margaret A. Brady, PhD, RN, CPNP
Professor, California State University Long Beach, Department of Nursing, Pediatric Nurse Practitioner, Miller Children's Hospital, Long Beach, California
    Role Relationships; Introduction to Disease and Pain Management; Infectious Diseases; Atopic Disorders and Rheumatic Diseases; Respiratory Disorders; Musculoskeletal Disorders; Common Injuries

Jeanette M. Broering, MS, RN, MPH, CPNP
Director, Data Quality Assurance, Urology Outcomes Research Group, Department of Urology, University of California, San Francisco, San Francisco, California
    Sexuality

Catherine E. Burns, PhD, RN, CPNP, FAAN
Professor, Primary Health Care Nurse Practitioner Specialty, Oregon Health Sciences University School of Nursing, Portland, Oregon
    Child Health Status in the United States; Child Assessment in Pediatric Primary Care; Developmental Management of School-Age Children; Introduction to Health Promotion; Activities and Sports for Children and Adolescents; Sleep and Rest; Cognitive-Perceptual Patterns; Neurological Disorders; Musculoskeletal Disorders; Genetic Disorders; Environmental Health Issues; Appendix C: Normal Laboratory Values; Appendix D: Healthy People 2010 Objectives: Draft for Public Comment; Child and Adolescent Focused Objectives

Melanie A. Canady, MSN, RN, CPNP
Adjunct Clinical Faculty, East Carolina University, Greenville; Certified Pediatric Nurse Practitioner, Partners in Pediatric Healthcare, Craven County Health Department-Child Health Clinic, New Bern, North Carolina
    Appendix A: Medications

Jeffrey A. Dean, DDS, MSD
Associate Professor of Pediatric Dentistry and Orthodontics, Director of Advanced Education Program in Pediatric Dentistry, Indiana University School of Dentistry; Active Staff Member, Riley Hospital for Children, Indianapolis, Indiana
    Dental and Oral Diseases

Barbara Jones Deloian, PhD, RN, CPNP
Assistant Professor, Adjunct, University of Colorado Health Sciences Center School of Nursing; Pediatric Nurse Practitioner, Program Evaluator, Child Development Unit/ Nursing Research, The Children's Hospital, Denver, Colorado
    Developmental Management in Pediatric Primary Care; Developmental Management of Infants

Ardys M. Dunn, PhD, RN, PNP
Associate Professor, University of Portland School of Nursing, Portland, Oregon
    Health Perception and Health Management Pattern; Nutrition; Elimination Pattern; Sexuality; Values and Beliefs; Environmental Health Issues; Appendix B: Growth Grids

Connie Evers, MS, RD, LD
Portland, Oregon
    Nutrition

Judith W. Fisher, RN, FNP, MHS
Multnomah County Health Department, School-Based Clinics, Portland, Oregon
    Developmental Management of Adolescents

Jan Freitas-Nichols, MSN, RN, CPNP
Primary Faculty, School of Nursing; Director of Children's Services, Doernbecher Children's Hospital, Oregon Health Sciences University, Portland, Oregon
    Cardiovascular Disorders

Mark H. Goodman, MD
Adjunct Professor of Nursing, California State University, Long Beach, Long Beach, California; Associate Clinical Professor of Pediatrics, University of California, Irvine, College of Medicine, Irvine, California; Attending Physician, Miller Children's Hospital, Long Beach, California
    Infectious Diseases; Respiratory Disorders

Steven Goodstein, MS, MT (ASCP)
Assistant Professor, Oregon Health Sciences University, Portland, Oregon
    Appendix C: Normal Laboratory Values

Pamela J. Hellings, PhD, RN, CPNP
Professor and Chair, Department of Primary Care, Oregon Health Sciences University School of Nursing, Portland, Oregon
    Breastfeeding

Gail M. Houck, PhD, RN
Associate Professor, Division of Children, Adolescents, and Families School of Nursing, Oregon Health Sciences University School of Nursing, Portland, Oregon
    Coping and Stress Tolerance

Sheila M. Kodadek
Oregon Health Sciences University School of Nursing, Portland, Oregon
    Family Assessment in Pediatric Primary Care

Margaret MacDonald, EdD, RN, CPNP
Pediatric Nurse Practitioner, Multnomah County Health Department, Portland, Oregon
    Cultural Perspectives for Primary Health Care; Eye Problems

Diane F. Montgomery, MSN, RN, CPNP
Assistant Professor of Pediatrics, University of Texas-Houston Medical School, Houston, Texas
    Perinatal Conditions

Mary A. Murphy, PhD, RN, CPNP
Instructor, Department of Pediatrics and Clinical Associate Professor, University of Colorado Health Sciences Center School of Nursing, Denver, Colorado
    Developmental Management of Toddlers and Preschoolers

Deborah K. Parks, MSN, RN, PNP
Associate Professor of Pediatrics and Director, Division of Nurse Practitioners, University of Texas-Houston Medical School, Houston, Texas
Perinatal Conditions

Ann M. Petersen-Smith, MS, RN, CPNP
Clinical Faculty, University of Colorado Health Sciences Center; Clinical Faculty, Regis University; Pediatric Nurse Practitioner, Emergency Department, The Children's Hospital, Denver, Colorado
Ear Disorders; Gastrointestinal Disorders

Charles Poland II, DDS
Associate Professor, Pediatric Dentistry, Indiana University School of Dentistry; Private Practice, Pediatric Dentistry, Indianapolis, Indiana
Dental and Oral Diseases

Kathleen C. Shelton, MN, RN, CPNP
Examiner, CARES (Child Abuse Response and Evaluation Services) Northwest, Portland, Oregon
Cognitive-Perceptual Patterns

Nancy Barber Starr, MS, RNC, CPNP
Pediatric Nurse Practitioner, Aurora Pediatric Associates, Aurora, Colorado
Self-Perception; Eye Problems; Genitourinary Disorders; Gynecological Conditions; Dermatological Diseases

Martha K. Swartz, MS, RN, CS, PNP
Associate Professor, Yale University School of Nursing; Pediatric Nurse Practitioner, Yale-New Haven Hospital, New Haven, Connecticut
Hematological Diseases

Linda Wildey
Adjunct Clinical Faculty, University of Cincinnati, College of Nursing and Health; Associate Director of Training, Division of Adolescent Medicine, Children's Hospital Medical Center, Cincinnati, Ohio
Developmental Management of Adolescents

Robert J. Yetman, MD
Professor and Director, Division of Community and General Pediatrics, University of Texas-Houston Medical School, Houston, Texas
Perinatal Conditions

We are delighted to introduce the second edition of *Pediatric Primary Care: A Handbook for Nurse Practitioners.* As with the first edition, this book is designed for advanced practice nurses serving the primary health-care needs of infants, children, and adolescents. Pediatric nurse practitioners (PNPs) and family nurse practitioners are anticipated to be our primary audience, but pediatric clinical nurse specialists, community health nurses, pediatric ambulatory care nurses, school nurses, and other primary care providers should also find the book to be a valuable resource. Our goal has been to provide a textbook for nurse practitioner students as well as a handbook for clinicians. Feedback from our readers over the past several years indicates that we achieved our goal: both students and experienced clinicians find it to be a key resource for their work and study.

Each of the authors brings a special perspective to the subject of pediatric primary health care: nurse practitioner educators, practicing PNPs, and a PNP working in and teaching community health. Each author has unique areas of expertise—development, nursing theory, cultural competence, as well as extensive experience with a variety of health-care problems. A number of other specialists have been invited to contribute to the work. Some have continued from the first edition, whereas others are new.

ORGANIZATION OF THE BOOK

After four introductory chapters that discuss child health issues and assessment of children in the context of their families and cultures, the book is organized into three major sections—Development, Functional Health Patterns, and Diseases. Conceptually, this format follows Burns' taxonomy of diagnoses for use by pediatric nurse practitioners (Burns, 1993).

Some new features of the second edition that we are excited about include:

- Color figures of some important ear, skin, and dental pathologies to help with diagnosis
- A new chapter on Environmental Health Issues for Children, an area of increasing concern and interest for pediatric clinicians
- A new chapter on Complementary Therapies for children
- More tables to facilitate differential diagnosis of related conditions or conditions that have some common elements
- More tables to summarize management strategies for common conditions
- Resource boxes at the end of chapters that now include websites as well as organizations and printed materials that may be useful for clinicians and their clients
- Improved formatting of the text to make it even easier to read
- A related Pocket Reference book that includes many of the tables and summarizes key information for busy clinicians

Of course, every chapter has been updated to bring the most current information available to the reader.

We have maintained key features that have made the first edition so successful:

- An assessment chapter that emphasizes a holistic approach, including identification of both medical and nursing problems

- Attention to family and cultural factors
- Emphasis on prevention as well as management of problems from the PNP's point of view and scope of practice
- Explicit reference to *Healthy People 2000* and preliminary 2010 Gudelines (United States [US] Department of Health and Human Services [DHHS], 1990 and 1998), *Guidelines for Adolescent Preventive Services (GAPS)* (Elster & Kuznets, 1994), standards of nursing care for children, and practice guidelines from the US Preventive Services Task Force, the American Academy of Pediatrics and others
- Introduction of key concepts and foundations for care in a narrative format followed by identification and management of diagnoses discussed using an outline format
- Organization of information into tables and appendices for quick access and efficient use by working nurse practitioners and nurses
- Selection of common medical and nursing diagnoses that are managed by primary care providers in practice

It is assumed that the reader has a baccalaureate degree in nursing and advanced course work in physiology, child development, health assessment, pharmacology, and family systems. Thus, this book guides clinical application of concepts important to the nursing specialty, primary health care of children and their families.

INTRODUCTORY SECTION

The first chapter in this section begins with a review of the major morbidity and mortality statistics highlighting the health problems of children in the United States. The chapter then identifies the important goals for health care of children and describes several sets of current guidelines and standards designed to safeguard primary care of the nation's children. Working with managed care organizations is discussed. Chapter Two presents the health assessment of the child, including both history and physical examination data. The chapter uses a model that supports identification and management of

Development, Functional Health Patterns, and Disease problems. The third and fourth chapters highlight important family and cultural components of care to be incorporated into the assessment and management plans for all clients.

DEVELOPMENT SECTION

The development section includes five chapters—an introduction to development for primary care, and chapters on infants, toddlers and preschoolers, school age children, and adolescents. Each chapter begins with a review of the major developmental theories used to understand children in the particular age group. The assessment of developmental needs of children in primary care is then reviewed. Topics for discussion with parents are outlined. Finally, several important developmental issues for each age group are discussed from a problem-oriented perspective. Application of principles of child development to primary care is the key feature for these chapters.

FUNCTIONAL HEALTH PATTERNS SECTION

Functional Health Patterns (Gordon, 1987) serve as the organizational framework of this section. There are 11 patterns that are common to people of all cultures and ages. The first seven chapters provide a platform for discussing health promotion through the various components of healthy living—health maintenance, nutrition, elimination, sleep, activity, and exercise. The remaining functional health pattern chapters are more psychosocial in nature—self-perception, role relationships, coping/stress tolerance, cognitive/perceptual patterns, sexuality, and values/beliefs. In all chapters, foundations of psychology and the basic sciences are first introduced and then applied to common problems of children. Common North American Nursing Diagnosis Association (NANDA) nursing diagnoses related to the respective health pattern are identified. Current standards and recommendations for care related to the area are stated. Normative behaviors are discussed and the assessment process is reviewed. Common management strategies with which the clinician should be familiar are identified. Finally, common problems of each pattern are presented with the aid of a problem-oriented framework. There is a special chapter on breastfeeding and the activities chapter focuses on sports participation issues.

DISEASES SECTION

The Diseases section of the book is organized with a chapter for each of the main components of the *International Classification of Diseases,* 22 chapters in all. This section begins with a chapter introducing approaches to diseases and their management. Next, the infectious diseases chapter reviews key communicable diseases and includes a comprehensive subsection on immunizations. A major set of chapters focus on principal body systems, with additional chapters devoted to neonatology, genetics, and uncomplicated trauma. An environmental health chapter has been added. Finally, a new chapter on complementary therapies promotes PNPs' knowledge about many of the strategies families may be using. Following the same format throughout, standards and guidelines for care are highlighted, the physiological and assessment parameters are discussed, management strategies are identified, and management of common problems is explained in a problem-oriented format. Each disease or condition is explained as follows:

- Description
- Etiology and incidence
- Clinical findings
  - ○ History
  - ○ Physical examination
  - ○ Laboratory and other studies
- Differential diagnosis
- Management
- Complications
- Preventive and patient education measures

Tables highlight and summarize differential diagnoses, management, and other pertinent information. The scope of practice of the nurse practitioner is always kept in mind with appropriate referral and consultation points identi-

fied. At the end of many chapters, useful resources, such as national organizations for various disorders, are listed.

APPENDICES

The appendices include sections on growth, laboratory data, and common drugs used in pediatric primary care settings. The appendices are designed for easy access to reference data.

SUMMARY

This book is written by and for NPs interested in the primary health care of children. It provides a comprehensive resource for students and serves as a reference for practicing clinicians. The book is conceptually organized around domains of interest to PNPs—development, functional health patterns related to health maintenance and psychosocial well-being of children and their families, and diseases of children that require intervention, monitoring, and/or referral. The book uses a problem-oriented focus consistent with the education of PNPs and has been written using the latest standards and guidelines available. Content is consistent with the major recommendations for primary care of children in the United States. We are delighted to bring forward a second edition of this needed resource for nurse practitioners who work with and for children.

Catherine E. Burns, PhD, RN, CPNP, FAAN
Margaret A. Brady, PhD, RN, CPNP
Ardys M. Dunn, PhD, RN, PNP
Nancy Barber Starr, MS, RN, CPNP

REFERENCES

Burns C: Using a comprehensive taxonomy of diagnoses to describe the practice of pediatric nurse practitioners: Findings of a field study. J Pediatr Health Care 7:115-121, 1993.
Elster A, Kuznets N: AMA Guidelines for Adolescent Preventive Services (GAPS). Baltimore: Williams & Wilkins, 1994.
Gordon M: Nursing Diagnosis: Process and Application. McGraw-Hill, 1987.

US Department of Health and Human Services: Healthy People 2000: National Health Promotion and Disease Prevention Objectives for the Year 2000. Washington, DC, US Government Printing Office, 1990.

US Department of Health and Human Services: Healthy People 2010: National Health Promotion and Disease Prevention Objectives for the Year 2010. Draft Copy for Comments. Washington, DC, US Government Printing Office.

ACKNOWLEDGMENTS

A book of this size and complexity could never have been completed without considerable help—the work of the contributors who researched, wrote, and revised; the consultation and review of experts in various specialties who critiqued drafts and provided important perspectives and guidance; and the essential technical support from those who managed the production of the manuscript and the final product. Another kind of help came from family and friends who offered unending support and encouragement for the duration of the project. We are indebted to so many people and want to say thanks to them all. The following are some of the many people we want to acknowledge.

CONTRIBUTORS TO THE FIRST EDITION:

These people were instrumental in helping us to develop the first edition of the book. Although they are not authors in this edition, their ideas and work have contributed greatly to our work, and we are deeply indebted to them.

Natalie Cheffer, MN, CPNP—the endocrine chapter
Donna L.O.K. Ching, MN, RN, CPNP–the laboratory values appendix
Amy Feldman, MSN, RN, CPNP, IBCLC—the breastfeeding chapter
Joel H. Berg, DDS, MS, and Kenneth Jones, DDS—the dental chapter
Julie Novak, DNSc, PhD, RN, CPNP—the cardiology chapter
Sandra Symes, MSN, RN, CPNP—the perinatal conditions chapter

EXPERT CONSULTANTS:

Cheryl L.N. Aldridge, MN, RN, CPNP
Dallas, Texas

Cheryl Alto, RD
Portland, Oregon

Patricia Reiter Becker, MS, RN, CS
Philadelphia, Pennsylvania

Catherine Blosser, PNP
Portland, Oregon

Doreen E. Brock, BSN, MBA
Beaumont, Texas

Leslie Capin, MD
Aurora, Colorado

James Chesnutt, MD
Portland, Oregon

Patricia Clinton, PhD, RN, ARNP
Iowa City, Iowa

Sandra L. Elvik, MS, RN, CPNP
Torrance, California

Mehmet Ertem, MD
New Haven, Connecticut

Nan M. Gaylord, RN, MSN, MA, CPNP, CSNP
Knoxville, Tennessee

Terea Giannetta, RN, MSN, CPNP
Fresno, California

Peggy Gilbertson, RN, MPH, CPNP
Mankato, Minnesota

Freeman Ginsburg, MD
Aurora, Colorado

Janice A. Goertz, RN, CPNP, BS
Portage, Michigan

James Harris, MD
Aurora, Colorado

Amy Heneghan, MD
New Haven, Connecticut

Cynthia Hobbie, MPH, RN, CPNP
St. Paul, Minnesota

Chris M. Kucinkas, RN, MA, CPNP
Corpus Christi, Texas

Michael Kurtz, MD
Aurora, Colorado

Paula Levin, MD
Aurora, Colorado

Vickers R. Myers, RN, BSN, MSN, CPNP
Denver, Colorado

Mark H. Pearlman, MD
Aurora, Colorado

Ann Peterson-Smith, MS, RN, CPNP
Aurora, Colorado

Margo Salisbury, MS, RN, WHCNP
Portland, Oregon

Jane S. Sherborne, MS, PNP
Houston, Texas

Lee Thompson, MD
Aurora, Colorado

TECHNICAL SUPPORT:

Amy Dunnavant
Portland, Oregon

We are especially indebted to Catherine Blosser, PNP, Portland, Oregon, who provided us with uncounted hours of library and resource help, good cheer, and advice from a practicing PNP.

FAMILY AND FRIENDS:

Jerry Burns, Jennifer and Jill, and other family and friends of Catherine Burns

Marvin, Malcolm, and Philip Dunn, and other family and friends of Ardys Dunn

Mary, Martha, Greg, and Katie, and other family and friends of Margaret Brady

Jon and Jonah Starr, my APA colleagues, and in memory of John T. Barber, and APA colleagues of Nancy Barber Starr

NOTICE

Nursing is an ever-changing field. Standard safety precautions must be followed, but as new research and clinical experience broaden our knowledge, changes in treatment and drug therapy become necessary or appropriate. Readers are advised to check the product information currently provided by the manufacturer of each drug to be administered to verify the recommended dose, the method and duration of administration, and contraindications. It is the responsibility of the treating licensed prescriber, relying on experience and knowledge of the patient, to determine dosages and the best treatment for the patient. Neither the Publisher nor the editors assumes any responsibility for any injury and/or damage to persons or property.

THE PUBLISHER

CONTENTS

Color Section follows page xxxii.

UNIT 2

Management of Development   77

U N I T **3**

Approaches to Health
Management in Pediatric
Primary Care 187

UNIT 4

Approaches to Disease Management 543

CHAPTER 23

Introduction to Disease and Pain Management 545

Margaret A. Brady

CHAPTER 24

Infectious Diseases 561

Mark H. Goodman and Margaret A. Brady

CHAPTER **25**

**Atopic Disorders and
Rheumatic Diseases   625**

Margaret A. Brady

CHAPTER **26**

**Endocrine and Metabolic
Diseases   662**

Jean Betschart

CHAPTER **27**

Hematological Diseases   689

Martha K. Swartz

CHAPTER **28**

Neurological Disorders   *714*

Catherine E. Burns

CHAPTER **29**

Eye Problems   *744*

Margaret MacDonald and
Nancy Barber Starr

CHAPTER **30**

Ear Disorders   *783*

Ann M. Petersen-Smith

CHAPTER **33**

Gastrointestinal Disorders   892

Ann M. Petersen-Smith

CHAPTER **34**

Dental and Oral Diseases   937

Charles Poland II and Jeffrey A. Dean

CHAPTER **35**

Genitourinary Disorders   974

Nancy Barber Starr

CHAPTER **38**

Musculoskeletal Disorders   1134

Catherine E. Burns and Margaret A. Brady

CHAPTER **39**

Perinatal Conditions   1172

*Deborah K. Parks, Diane F. Montgomery,
and Robert J. Yetman*

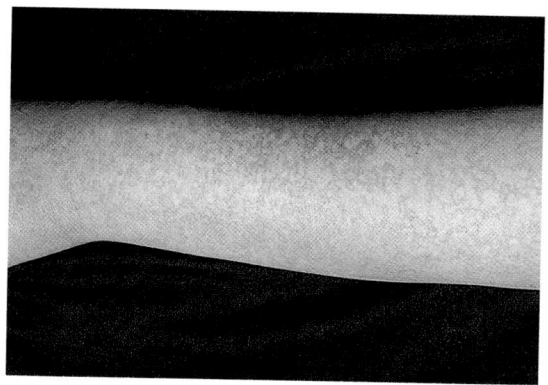

COLOR FIGURE 1
Erythema infectiosum ("fifth disease") with reticulate, lace-like eruption of erythema infectiosum. (From Callen JP, Greer KE, Paller AS: Color Atlas of Dermatology, 2nd ed. Philadelphia, WB Saunders, 2000, p 49.)

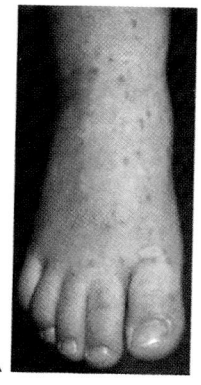 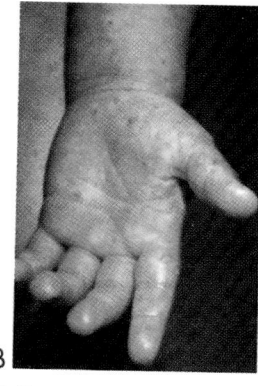

A   B

COLOR FIGURE 2
Lesions on the feet (A) and hands (B) in hand-foot-and-mouth disease. (From Aly R, Maibach H: Atlas of Infections of the Skin. Philadelphia, WB Saunders, 1999, p 240.)

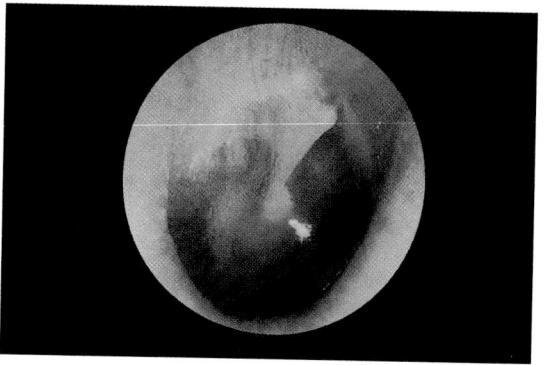

COLOR FIGURE 3
Normal right tympanic membrane. (Photograph courtesy of Sylvan Stool, MD, The Children's Hospital, Denver, CO.)

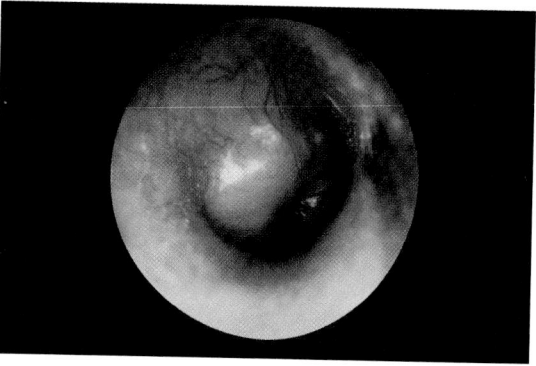

COLOR FIGURE 4
Acute otitis media of the right ear. (Photograph courtesy of Sylvan Stool, MD, The Children's Hospital, Denver, CO.)

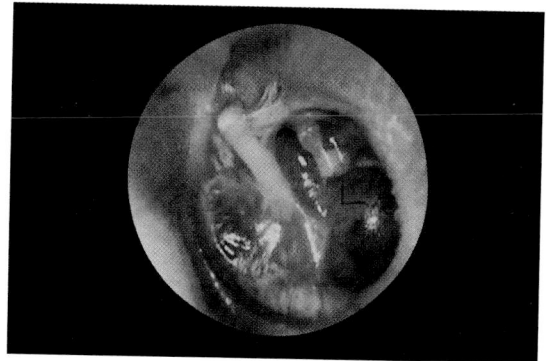

COLOR FIGURE 5
Left ear with posterior retraction. (Photograph courtesy of Sylvan Stool, MD, The Children's Hospital, Denver, CO.)

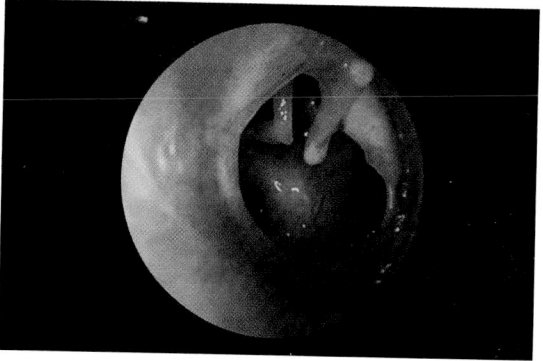

COLOR FIGURE 6
Near total perforation of the right ear. (Photograph courtesy of Sylvan Stool, MD, The Children's Hospital, Denver, CO.)

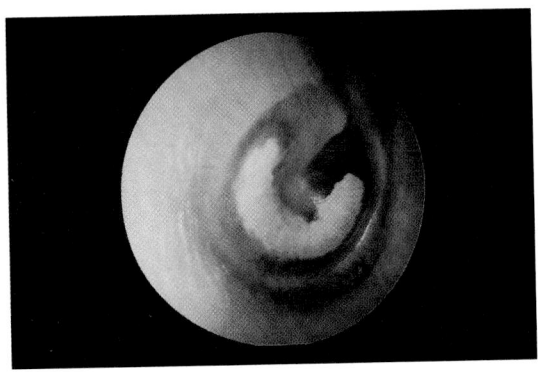

COLOR FIGURE 7
Tympanosclerosis of the right ear. (Photograph courtesy of Sylvan Stool, MD, The Children's Hospital, Denver, CO.)

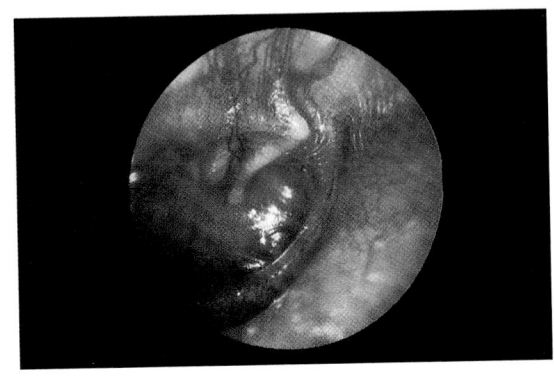

COLOR FIGURE 8
Severely retracted, opaque right tympanic membrane in otitis media with effusion. (From Bluestone CD, Klein JO: Otitis Media in Infants and Children, 2nd ed. Philadelphia, WB Saunders, 1995.)

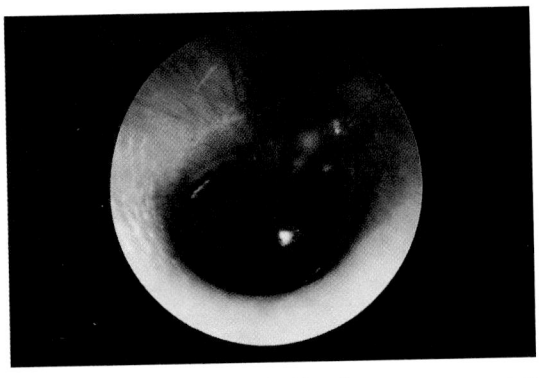

COLOR FIGURE 9
Serous effusion (note bubbles and air-fluid level). (Photograph courtesy of Sylvan Stool, MD, The Children's Hospital, Denver, CO.)

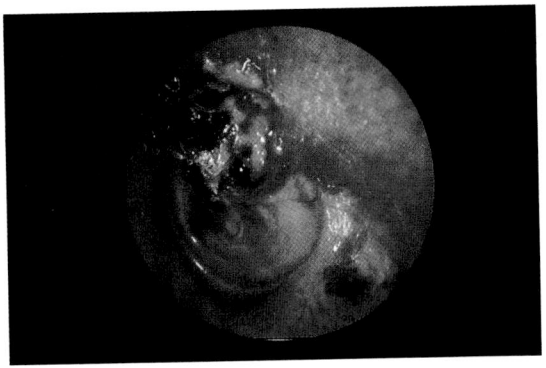

COLOR FIGURE 10
Cholesteatoma of the left ear. (Photograph courtesy of Sylvan Stool, MD, The Children's Hospital, Denver, CO.)

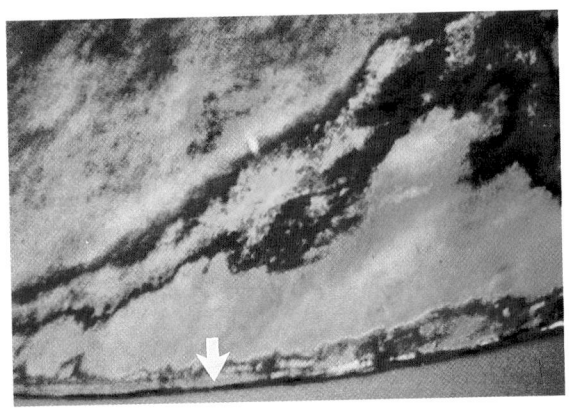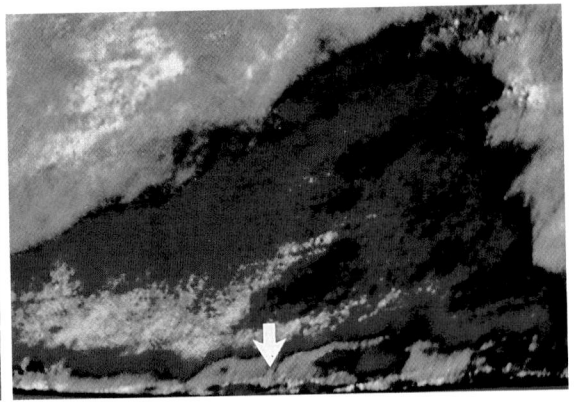

COLOR FIGURE 11
Photomicrographs of subsurface carious lesions. *Left,* Demineralized carious lesion. *Right,* Remineralized subsurface carious lesion. Note intact enamel surface layer. (Photograph courtesy of Charles Poland, DDS.)

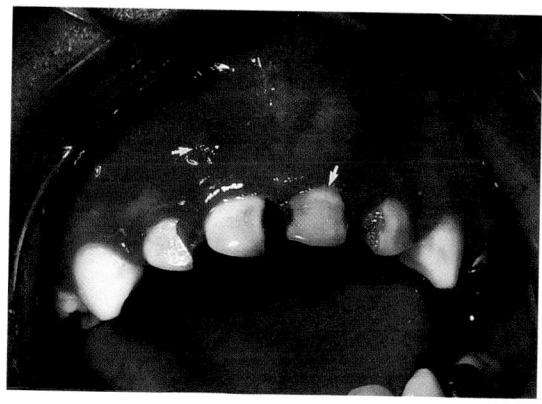

COLOR FIGURE 12
Early childhood caries. Classic appearance of demineralized cervical enamel adjacent to decayed areas. Draining sinus tract (parulis) and edematous red gingival margin (gingivitis) are evident. (Photograph courtesy of Charles Poland, DDS.)

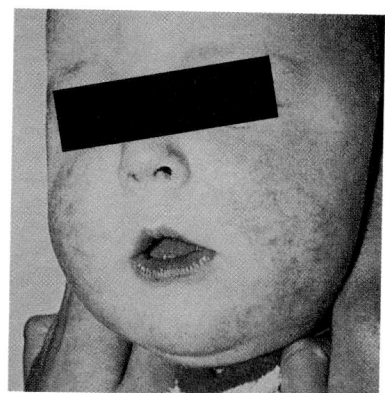

COLOR FIGURE 13
Facial plaques of acute infantile atopic dermatitis. (Photograph courtesy of Peggy Vernon, RN, MA, CPNP, Aurora/Parker Skin Care Center, CO.)

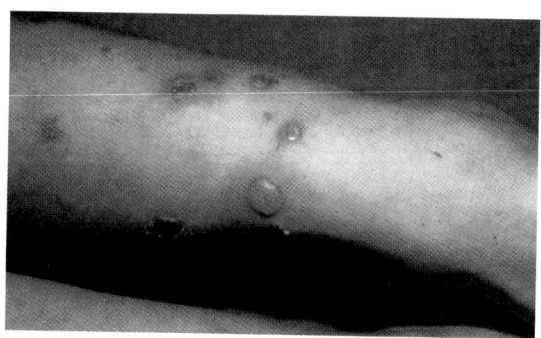

COLOR FIGURE 14
Bullous impetigo on the legs with several lesions in different stages. (From Aly R, Maibach H: Atlas of Infections of the Skin. Philadelphia, WB Saunders, 1999, p 117.)

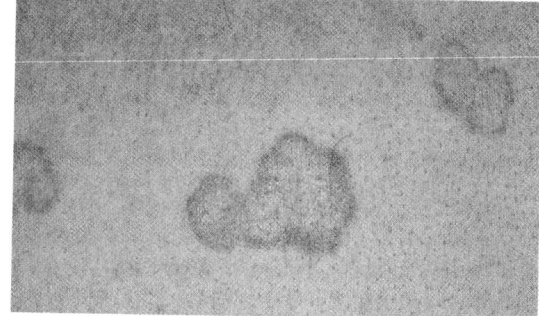

COLOR FIGURE 15
Tinea corporis. Lesions are annular with a raised inflammatory edge and central clearing. (From Aly R, Maibach H: Atlas of Infections of the Skin. Philadelphia, WB Saunders, 1999, p 23.)

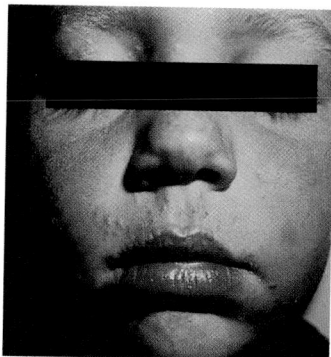

COLOR FIGURE 16
Oral herpes simplex infection in a preschooler. (Photograph courtesy of Peggy Vernon, RN, MA, CPNP, Aurora/Parker Skin Care Center, CO.)

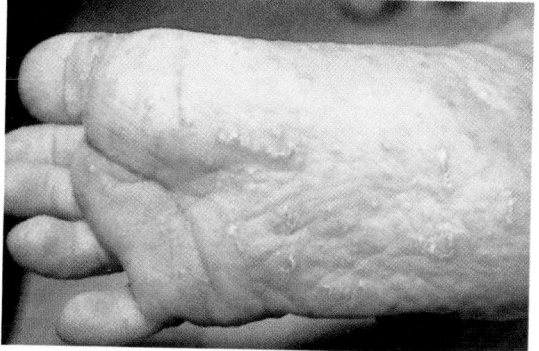

COLOR FIGURE 17
Scabies in an infant with multiple burrows and pustules on soles. (From Aly R, Maibach H: Atlas of Infections of the Skin. Philadelphia, WB Saunders, 1999, p 176.)

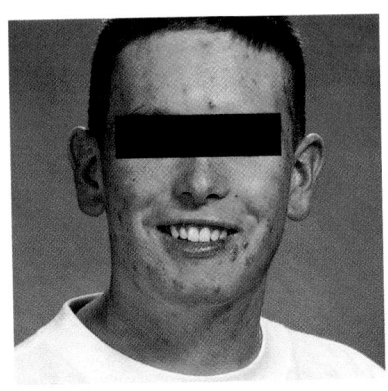

COLOR FIGURE 18
An adolescent with acne vulgaris. (Photograph courtesy of Peggy Vernon, RN, MA, CPNP, Aurora/Parker Skin Care Center, CO.)

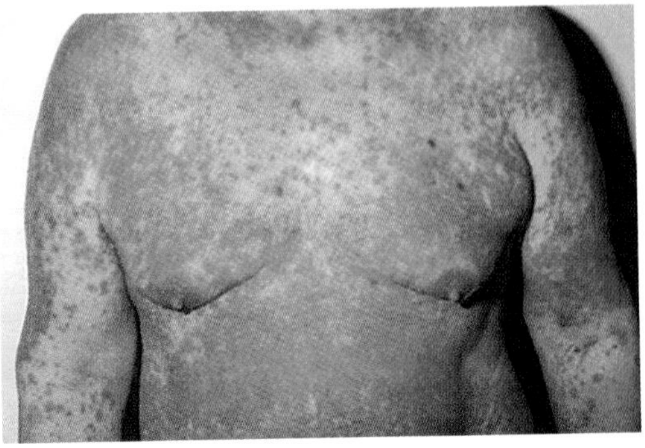

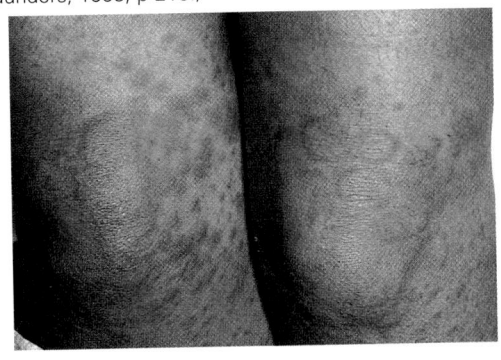

COLOR FIGURE 19
Allergic drug eruption is an erythematous and symmetric rash, usually generalized. (From Lookingbill DP, Marks JG: Principles of Dermatology, 2nd ed. Philadelphia, WB Saunders, 1993, p 218.)

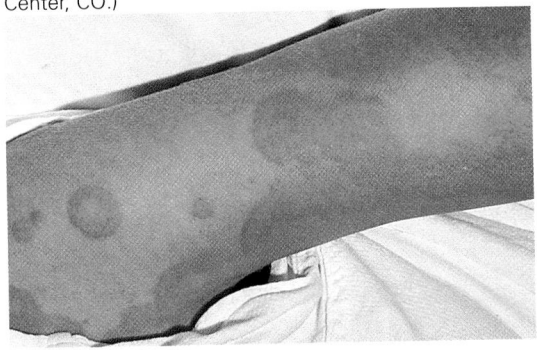

COLOR FIGURE 20
Urticaria. (Photograph courtesy of Frank Parker, MD, Oregon Health Sciences University, Portland, OR.)

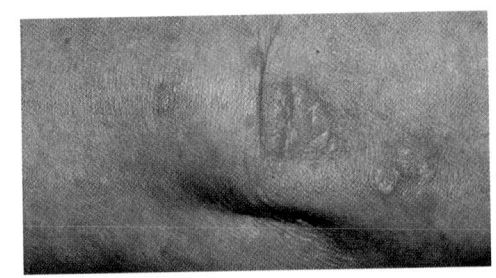

COLOR FIGURE 21
Erythema multiforme secondary to herpes simplex. (From Arndt KA, Wintroub BU, Robinson JK, et al: Primary Care Dermatology. Philadelphia, WB Saunders, 1997.)

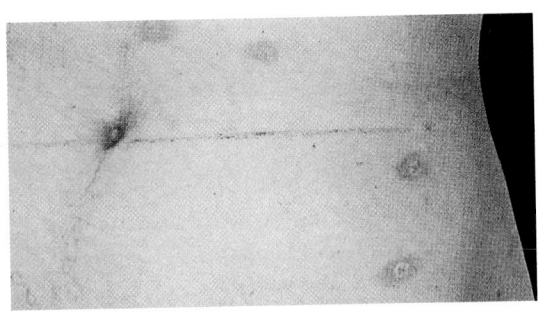

COLOR FIGURE 22
Pityriasis rosea. (Photograph courtesy of Peggy Vernon, RN, MA, CPNP, Aurora/Parker Skin Care Center, CO.)

COLOR FIGURE 23
Plaque-like erythematous lesions of psoriasis. (From Aly R, Maibach H: Atlas of Infections of the Skin. Philadelphia, WB Saunders, 1999, p 239.)

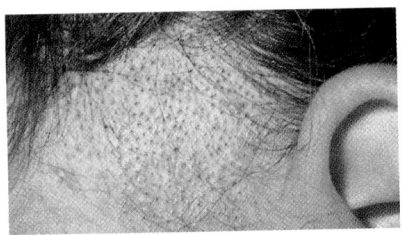

COLOR FIGURE 24
Tinea capitis showing a black dot variety with minimal inflammation. (From Aly R, Maibach H: Atlas of Infections of the Skin. Philadelphia, WB Saunders, 1999, p 20.)

Pediatric Primary Care Foundations

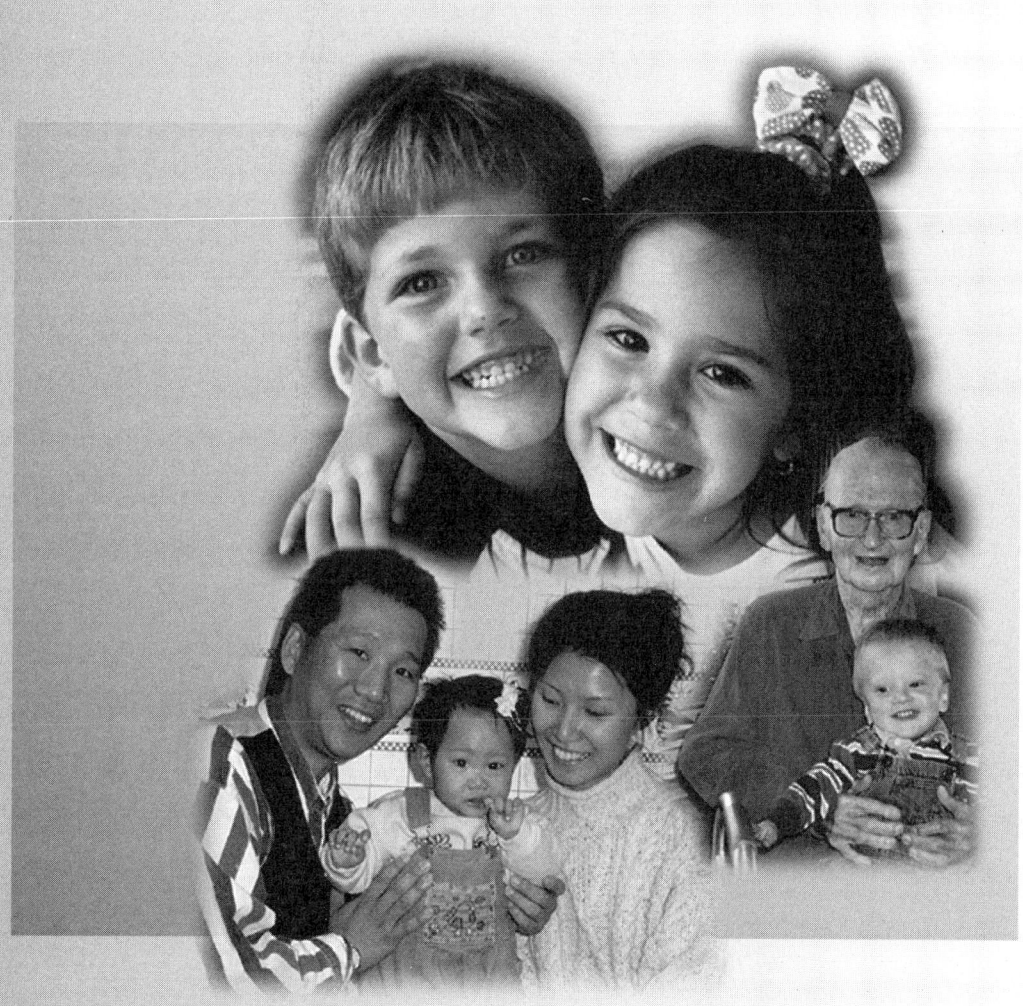

CHAPTER 1

Child Health Status in the United States

Catherine E. Burns

INTRODUCTION

America's children represent the future of the country. Society has given the families of those children responsibility for raising them in loving and stable homes in the belief that nurtured, healthy children will be productive citizens and leaders for coming generations. Far too many children, however, are growing up without the benefits of families with adequate resources. Millions of children grow up hungry, neglected, abused, living in unsafe environments, and receiving inadequate education. The nation's commitment to children should involve providing for them directly, as well as ensuring opportunities for families to be successful in their child-rearing efforts. Primary health care providers have unique opportunities to be involved with families and children as they work to solve the problems of living to achieve and maintain hopeful, fulfilled lives.

This book describes the health of children and their families, their development, their health problems, and their health care. This chapter presents the status of children's health in America. Standards and guidelines for health care of children are identified because they represent the goals to be achieved. Finally, the role of the nurse practitioner (NP) in the delivery of health care is defined. Children need to be healthy if they are to achieve their maximum potential as productive, happy people.

CHILD HEALTH STATUS IN AMERICA

In 1996, 83 million children through age 21 represented 31.5% of the total population (US Department of Health & Human Services, 1997). A variety of indicators are used to measure the health status of children in the United States: low birth weight rates, infant mortality rate, child death rate, teen death rate, and teen birth rate. Other indicators may include the violent crime arrest rate, percentage of teens who are high school dropouts, and the percentage of children who live in poverty or live in single-parent households. A variety of these indicators are discussed in this book. If healthcare providers are to substantially influence the health of children, they need to understand child health risks and primary sources of disease and death among children. Furthermore, the government and major professional organizations have established goals for health care and guidelines to provide preventive care efficiently and effectively. Providers need to adopt these goals for their own practices.

Infant Mortality

The 1997 infant death rate fell to an all-time low of 7.1 per 1000 live births (Births, 1998). In the *Healthy People 2000: National Health*

Promotion and Disease Prevention Objectives for the Year 2000 (US Department of Health and Human Services, 1990), the goal for the year 2000 is 7 per 1000 live births. Despite the good news of 1997, some striking disparities can be noted. Infant mortality rates continue to be different for blacks and whites, with black infants 2.6 times more likely to die than white babies (Births, 1998) (see Fig. 1-1). In 1995, infants of black mothers were 4.5 times more likely to die of low birth weight and short gestation than were infants of white mothers (MacDorman & Atkinson, 1998). Both short gestation and low birth weight are considered to be preventable conditions. Infants born into poor families are 50% more likely to die than children born into families with incomes above the poverty line (Annie E. Casey Foundation, 1997). See Figures 1-2 and 1-3 for leading causes of neonatal and infant mortality.

In 1993, the United States ranked 25th in infant mortality, behind such places as Greece, Belgium, Spain, and Israel (US Department of Health and Human Services, 1997). Sudden infant death syndrome remains an important cause of mortality in infants up to 1 year of age, although the death rates have dropped

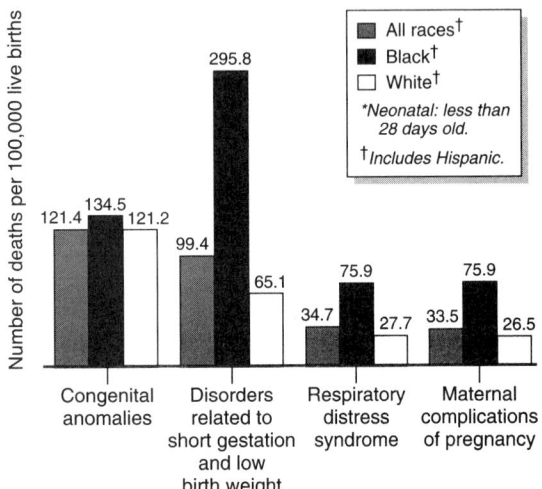

FIGURE 1-2
Leading causes of neonatal* mortality: 1995. (From US Department of Health & Human Services [1997]. Child Health USA 96–97, p 20.)

significantly with the emphasis on infants sleeping on their backs.

Injury (both unintentional and intentional) death rates of infants between 1986 and 1992 resulted from homicides (27%), suffocation (19%), other unintentional injuries (16%), motor vehicle accidents (13%), and choking, drowning, and fire each at 8% (Baker et al., 1996).

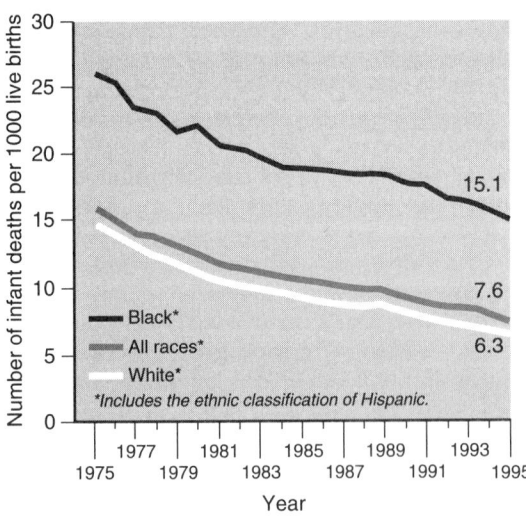

FIGURE 1-1
US Infant mortality rates by race of mother: 1975–1995. (From US Department of Health & Human Services [1997]. Child Health USA 96–97, p 19.)

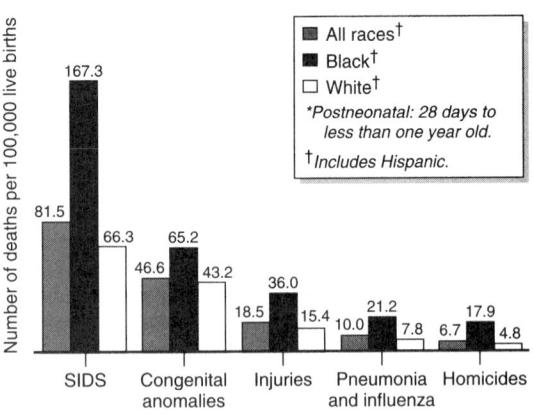

FIGURE 1-3
Leading causes of postneonatal* mortality: 1995. (From US Department of Health & Human Services [1997]. Child Health USA 96–97, p 20.)

Births

In 1996, 7.4% of all live births had low birth weight (less than 2,500 g or 5.5 lb). The proportion of low birth weight babies has not changed significantly since the 1970s. Infants with a low birth weight have a 6 times higher risk of death before their first birthday and those weighing less than 1500 g have an 89 times higher risk than do babies having a normal birth weight (Ventura et al., 1998).

Teen birth rates are important to assess because teen childbearing diminishes the opportunities of both child and mother. Generally, teen mothers younger than 18 years are unmarried and have not completed high school. A child born to a teen mother is 10 times more likely to live in poverty at 8 to 12 years of age (Annie E. Casey Foundation, 1997). The birth rate for teenagers declined in 1996, falling 4%. In 1996, the live birth rate for teens aged 10 to 14 was 1.2 per 1000, 33.8 per 1000 for those 15 to 17 years, and 86.0 per 1000 for those 18 to 19 years old. For 15- to 19-year-olds, Hispanic teens had higher birth rates than did blacks or whites. Among teens of Hispanic origin (Mexican, Puerto Rican, Cuban, and Central and South American) aged 15 to 19 years, rates were highest for Mexican teens (120.7 per 1000). In all age groups, black teen mothers had a significantly higher birth rate than did whites. Asian–Pacific Islanders had the lowest teen birth rates (24.6 per 1000). Teen birth rates also varied considerably by state, with New Hampshire the lowest and the District of Columbia and Guam the highest. Declines in birth rates between 1991 and 1996 ranged from 6% to 29% (Ventura et al., 1998).

Injuries are also important to assess in pediatric populations because they account for so much of the total mortality and morbidity statistics for children. Injuries are classified as unintentional (such as burns and falls) or intentional (homicides and suicides). Unintentional injuries to young infants are most often due to burns, drowning, and falls. Poisonings are added to the list when infants gain mobility (Rivara & Aitken, 1998). See Table 1-1 for leading causes of death in children and adolescents.

Child Mortality

The child death rate for children aged 1 to 14 years was at its lowest rate ever in 1994—29 deaths per 100,000 children (Annie E. Casey Foundation, 1997). More than 40% of those deaths came as a result of unintentional injuries, almost half of which were from motor vehicle accidents. The number of homicides rose by 35.9% between 1980 and 1992 (Baker et al., 1996). As with infants, the overall child death rate in 1997 was higher for black children—

T A B L E 1-1

Leading Causes of Death in Children and Adolescents, 1995

RANK	AGE 1–4 yr	(%)	AGE 5–14 yr	(%)	AGE 15–19 yr	(%)
1	Injury	14.5	Injury	9.3	Unintentional injury	36
	MVA	5.2	MVA	5.4		
	Drowning	3.4	Drowning	1.1		
	Fires/burns	2.8	Fires/burns	0.8		
2	Congenital anomaly	4.4	Malignant neoplasm	2.7	Firearms—homicide	15.6
3	Malignant neoplasm	3.1	Homicide	1.5	Firearms—suicide	7.0
4	Homicide	2.9	Congenital anomaly	1.2	Malignant neoplasm	3.8
5	Heart disease	1.6	Suicide	0.9	Heart disease	2.2
					Drowning	2.2
6	HIV/AIDS	1.3	Heart disease	0.8	Congenital anomaly	1.4

AIDS = acquired immunodeficiency syndrome; HIV = human immunodeficiency virus; MVA = motor vehicle accident.

US Department of Health & Human Services, Bureau of Maternal & Child Health: Child Health USA 96–97. Washington, DC, US Department of Health & Human Services, 1997.

54.5 deaths per 100,000 black children aged 1 to 4 years as compared with 31.0 deaths per 100,000 white children of the same age (Centers for Disease Control and Prevention, 1998c). The death rates decreased in 43 states between 1986 and 1992 but rose in 7 states (Rivara & Aitken, 1998).

Unintentional injuries, primarily those resulting from motor vehicle collisions, remain the major cause of death in childhood and are responsible for 75% of injury deaths. Intentional injuries, including homicide and suicide, cause the other 25% of injury deaths. Pedestrian accidents are most common among 5- to 9-year-olds, followed by 1- to 4-year olds. Bicycle deaths occur most commonly among males 5 to 19 years of age, primarily from head injuries.

In 1995, among children aged 1 to 4 years, homicide was the fourth leading cause of death. Among 5- to 14-year-olds, homicide was the third leading cause of death and suicide was fifth. Of all the childhood homicides reported by 26 countries in 1995, 73% were among US children. Suicide among the same 26 countries accounted for 599 deaths; about 54% were US children. Firearms were involved in 55% of the homicides and 20% of the suicides. The firearm-related homicide rate in the United States was almost 16 times higher than that of the remaining 25 countries combined (Centers for Disease Control and Prevention, 1997). Deaths from injuries and violence far exceed those from cancer or congenital anomalies for children in the United States.

Child Health and Morbidity

From the 1992–1994 National Health Interview Survey of 99,513 children, it was estimated that 6.5% of children younger than 18 years, or almost 4.4 million children, have one or more chronic conditions that result in limitation of activities. These chronic conditions range from asthma to heart defects, cerebral palsy, cystic fibrosis, mental retardation, and other severe problems. Chronic conditions are more prevalent among older children, boys, and black children. Poor children also had more disabilities than nonpoor children. On average, children with disabilities missed daily activities for slightly more than 2 weeks per year, or an estimated 66 million restricted days annually for the total group (Newacheck & Halfon, 1998).

In an earlier paper, Newacheck and Taylor (1992) estimated that 31% of US children had chronic health conditions. Twenty percent experienced only mild conditions, 9% experienced moderately severe conditions, and only 2% were severely affected. The severely affected group spent an average of 10 days in bed and missed 11 days of school annually. These children used medical services more heavily, with 16 physician contacts per year and 16% hospitalized in the previous year. This 2% of children accounted for 33% of all hospital days for chronic conditions. Thirty-five percent of children with diabetes, 19% of children with epilepsy and seizures, and 12% of children with cerebral palsy had been hospitalized in the past year (Newacheck & Taylor, 1992). It is estimated that 12 to 15% of US children suffer from mental and emotional disorders.

The most frequent childhood unintentional injuries are classified by type: pedestrian injuries, bicycle-related injuries, and motor vehicle occupant injuries. Intentional injuries result primarily from firearms (Rivara & Aitken, 1998).

Adolescent Mortality

Adolescent (15 to 19 years old) death rates decreased 13% from 1985 to 1991. However, shifts have been noted in the causes of mortality, with decreases in motor vehicle fatalities (41% of adolescent deaths in 1992) but dramatic increases in interpersonal violence deaths (29% in 1992). Although white teens died primarily in motor vehicle accidents, black teens were more than twice as likely to be murdered. Homicide is the leading cause of death for black males, who are eight times more likely to die of this cause than white males of the same age (Sells & Blum, 1996). The good news was a 20% decline in this rate in 1995, the first in a decade (Children's Defense Fund, 1998). Among teens, more die of violence than disease (Ginsburg, 1997). See Table 1–1 for further adolescent death information.

In 1995, white suicide rates continued to be much higher than rates for other racial groups. Black youth suicide rates, although still lower than the rates for whites, increased substantially. Among high school youth, black and white teen suicide rates became equal in 1995. Firearms were the predominant method of suicide for black teens, followed by strangulation. The rates increased most for youth in the South. Risk factors for all youths included hopelessness, depression, family history of suicide, impulsive/aggressive behavior, social isolation, previous suicide attempt, and easy access to alcohol, drugs, and lethal weapons (Centers for Disease Control, 1998c).

Approximately 21% of child abuse victims were adolescents aged 13 to 18 years (US Department of Health & Human Services, 1997).

Teens aged 15 to 19 accounted for 44% of all the childhood motor vehicle deaths in 1992. However, 78% of all unintentional injury deaths just of teens were due to motor vehicle accidents. More occurred at night and in rural areas. Between 1979 and 1992, motor vehicle death rates for individuals aged 15 to 24 years decreased by 38%, and alcohol-related traffic fatalities decreased by 33% between 1987 and 1992. However, teens involved in fatal crashes are still more likely to be intoxicated than those in any other age group (Sells & Blum, 1996).

Adolescent Health

Education has always been a key predictor for health and life outcomes. Despite the importance of education, about 30% of Hispanic teens dropped out of school, whereas 12% of black and 9% of white adolescents aged 16 to 24 years had dropped out of school before high school graduation (US Department of Health & Human Services, 1997). In 1994, the percentage of adolescents in the United States not in school, working, in the military, or defining themselves as homemakers ranged from 4% in Connecticut to 17% in West Virginia (Annie E. Casey Foundation, 1997). The juvenile violent crime arrest rates increased 70% from 1986 to 1991 but decreased some in 1995 and 1996 (a 12% drop). Again, good news—arrest rates for black children for homicide decreased 24% in 1995 (Children's Defense Fund, 1998).

In 1997, smoking cigarettes had risen for the sixth year in a row among high school students surveyed with the Youth Risk Behavior survey. Thirty-four percent of high school seniors re-

ported that they had smoked in the 30 days before being surveyed. Rates have increased among all socioeconomic groups, those going to college and those not, in all regions of the country, and among all racial and gender groups, although whites smoked somewhat more than blacks or Hispanics. The overall prevalence rates for lifetime, current, and frequent cigarette use were 70.2%, 36.4%, and 16.7%. The overall prevalence rate for all types of tobacco use (cigarettes, smokeless, and cigars) was 42.7% (Centers for Disease Control and Prevention, 1998b).

Substance abuse, including alcohol, marijuana, and cocaine use, decreased from 10.9% in 1995 to 9% in 1996. Alcohol rates decreased more than marijuana or cocaine rates did. Heroin and hallucinogen rates were increasing in 1996 (US Department of Health & Human Services, 1997). See Figure 1-4 for the prevalence of drug use among adolescents.

Adolescent injuries are most commonly due to motor vehicles or firearm-related homicide or suicide (Rivara & Aitken, 1998).

AIDS AND SEXUALLY TRANSMITTED DISEASES

The number of acquired immunodeficiency syndrome (AIDS) cases reported among adolescents and young adults has risen steadily since 1981. Human immunodeficiency virus (HIV) in-

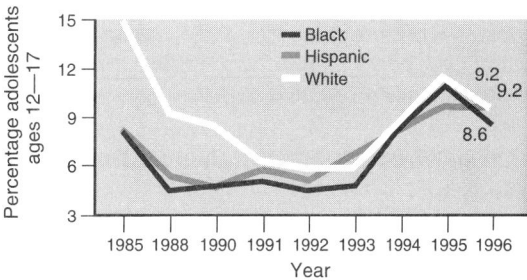

Illicit drugs include marijuana or hashish, cocaine (including crack), inhalants, hallucinogens (including PCP and LSD), heroin, or any prescription-type psychotherapeutic used nonmedically.

FIGURE 1-4
Long-term trends in 30-day prevalence of use of any illicit* drug among adolescents aged 12 to 17 by race/ethnicity, 1985–1996. (From US Department of Health & Human Services. Child Health USA 96–97 [1997], p 42.)

fection/AIDS has been the sixth leading cause of death among 15- to 24-year-olds since 1989. It is also the sixth leading cause of death among 1- to 4-year-olds (Leslie et al., 1998). White adolescents represent 34% of those cases, 62% of whom were exposed through blood transfusions or clotting factor for hemophilia. Forty-six percent of adolescent AIDS cases were among black non-Hispanics, most often through male-to-male sexual contact. Thirty-seven percent of adolescent AIDS cases were among females, most often acquired through heterosexual contact (US Department of Health & Human Services, 1997). In New York City in 1993, HIV-related illness was the leading cause of death for Hispanic children 1 to 4 years of age and the second leading cause of death for black children of the same age (Annunziato & Frenkel, 1993). Thankfully, HIV rates for newborns dropped 43% from 1992 to 1996 nationwide with the provision of zidovudine (AZT) to infected pregnant women (Children's Defense Fund, 1998).

Gonorrhea in 1996 decreased to half the rate in 1973 among 15- to 19-year-olds. Syphilis rates for the same age group decreased by one third during that time (Children's Defense Fund, 1998).

Immunizations

The US government monitors immunization levels across the country through the National Immunization Survey. The survey covers children aged 19 to 35 months. About 69% of children were immunized in 1997, up from fewer than 60% in 1992 (Centers for Disease Control and Prevention, 1998a).

Social Factors Influencing Child Health

Currently, more than 25% of America's children live in single-parent households, a percentage that has doubled in the last 10 years. Almost 1 million children are affected by divorce each year, and almost 11 million mothers with pre-school-aged children work outside the home. In 1996, 62% of all mothers with preschool children worked outside the home (US Department of Health & Human Services, 1997).

In 1979, only 17% of children were poor. By the end of 1996, 20.5% of children in America were poor. They were 81% more likely to be poor than adults were that year (Children's Defense Fund, 1998). The elderly have improved their economic status, whereas children have become more impoverished. Today, children are twice as likely as the elderly to be poor (Annie E. Casey Foundation, 1993; US Department of Health & Human Services, 1997). The poverty rate for Hispanic children was 40.3%, whereas 39.9% of black, 19.5% of Asian or Pacific Islander, and 16.3% of white children were poor (Children's Defense Fund, 1998). Reading (1997) cited other data showing that 33% of all American children lived in poverty. Sixty percent are white, 33% live in suburbs, 33% live in families with married parents, and 67% live in working families (Children's Defense Fund, 1998).

Children in poverty have higher mortality rates, poorer health at birth, poorer growth, and more physical morbidity from respiratory infections, gastrointestinal infections, wheezing, failure to thrive, anemia, asthma, dental caries, otitis media, and visual loss. They also have higher accident rates and more psychological and developmental disorders (Reading, 1997).

Access to Health Care

The health status of black and low-income children is worse than that of other children, and they receive the fewest health services of all children. About 25% of all US children are enrolled in Medicaid programs. Another 10 million or more children are uninsured (Leslie et al., 1998). Seventy percent of the Americans added to the lists of uninsured in 1996 were children (Children's Defense Fund, 1998).

Changes in the health-care delivery system in the United States could improve this situation. The fact that so many children have no insurance certainly indicates a need for change. Poverty as a principal factor for mortality of children and adolescents follows a social gradient for all conditions except cancer (Reading, 1997). In 1997 the government enacted the Children's Health Insurance Program (CHIP), which may significantly increase the number of children with health insurance.

Access to care is a function of insurance coverage, as well as a function of the area in which one lives. Nearly 43 million people, almost half of them women of childbearing age and children, lived in underserved areas. These settings included both rural and inner-city areas with shortages of physicians and clinics (Children's Defense Fund, 1992).

These statistics are depressing. However, they indicate where the emphasis should be placed to improve the health of our children: injury prevention, including motor vehicle accidents, homicides, and suicides; HIV prevention; immunizations; prenatal care; and access-to-care issues.

Managed Care Effects on Child Health

The health of US children is significantly affected by the health care delivery system in the place where they live. Managed care is becoming the predominant health care system in most states. This system was developed in response to excessive, uncontrolled costs of health care. Employers and the government have supported the development of managed care through cost-conscious insurance plans. The main features of managed health care plans include

- Strong incentives for members to obtain care only from selected providers and hospitals that are part of the plan
- Control of access to specialty care, diagnostic tests, and hospitalization
- Shared financial risk among doctors, the health plan, and other health professionals through capitated payments or bonuses and penalties

Whereas the main problem of fee-for-service care was excessive charges, the main problem of managed care is underprovision of needed services.

These plans were designed to meet the health needs of working adults. However, in many states, Medicaid clients are also enrolled in managed care plans. Furthermore, children are being enrolled in managed care plans at a higher rate than adults (The David and Lucile Packard Foundation, 1998).

Because the health care needs of children are unique, managed care plans need to create benefits packages that meet children's needs. These benefits packages include preventive health care, immunizations, anticipatory guidance, psychosocial counseling, and access to prompt care for acute illnesses. Pediatric specialists need to receive fair reimbursement rates to provide care for children with chronic or disabling conditions. Care needs to be coordinated between the home, managed care organization, school, day care, and other service providers. Parents need to be involved in decisions made about their child's health care. Managed care organizations should be accountable for the health care of enrollees and rewarded for improving the health of their pediatric population (The David and Lucile Packard Foundation, 1998).

Health care outcomes are hard to measure. Evidenced-based care offering guidance to clinicians for many common conditions and health maintenance has been shown to improve care. Individual clinicians need to be involved with regular quality-of-care reviews and contribute to the criteria by which care is evaluated. Patient and family satisfaction is also important to assess regularly; they must be viewed as partners in the health care plan. A variety of evidence-based guidelines for the health care of children are identified later in this chapter.

▬▬ HEALTH, HEALTH PROMOTION, DISEASE PREVENTION, AND PRIMARY CARE DEFINITIONS

Health, Health Promotion, and Disease Prevention

The American Nurses' Association defines health as "a dynamic state of being in which the developmental and behavioral potential of an individual is realized to the fullest extent possible" (American Nurses' Association, 1980; Broering, 1993). The process of achieving one's optimal potential is influenced by systems both within and outside the individual, including biological, cognitive, and emotional systems within the person, as well as the social, economic, and political systems of family, community, race, culture, and country.

Health promotion focuses on moving individuals to actualize their full potential, whereas disease prevention focuses on stabilizing the human organism to resist disease. Health promotion depends on active participation by the client to develop and maintain a lifestyle that maximizes well-being. It cannot be achieved solely by the activities of the primary health care provider, although that person is essential to identify risks, help the individual develop a health promotion plan, offer support and motivation for changing health behavior, and evaluate progress over time. Health promotion activities may also occur at the family, community, and society levels and be guided by primary care providers and health experts who design interventions helpful to groups of people. Fluoride supplementation in water supplies, laws requiring seat belt use, community health fairs, and regulations related to the content of school lunches and clean air standards are examples of broader efforts to promote health and prevent disease.

Primary Care

Primary care includes the following elements: first-contact care, comprehensive care, coordinated or integrated care, and care that is longitudinal rather than episodic. First-contact care is the extent to which a patient contacts the source of care whenever that person perceives a new need for care. Comprehensive means that it includes all the health problems of the individual. Coordination of care entails a health-care provider's ability to provide for continuity of information within that provider's practice setting, as well as coordinating specialists' care on behalf of the child and family. Providing longitudinal care refers to the extent to which a provider serves as a source of care over time regardless of the presence of a particular type of problem (US Congress, Office of Technology Assessment, 1991).

A somewhat more recent definition that is widely cited reads as follows:

> *Primary care is the* provision of *integrated, accessible health care services by clinicians* who are *accountable* for addressing a large *majority of personal health care needs,* developing *a sustained partnership with patients,* and practicing in the *context of family and community.*
>
> —*Institute of Medicine, Committee on the Future of Primary Care, 1994.*

Primary care must be incorporated into the health-care delivery system as a basic tenet; availability of primary care services for all children and families is essential. Primary health care, including minor acute and chronic illness and well-child care, may be provided in traditional offices and clinics but may also be found in settings such as the workplace, schools, churches, child care centers, and mobile units. Primary care should also be incorporated into the work of tertiary care centers—that is, children with serious illnesses also need primary care. Primary care providers include some physicians (internal medicine, family practice, pediatrics, and sometimes obstetrics/gynecology), NPs, and physician assistants.

NATIONAL HEALTH GOALS

In 1990, under the leadership of Dr. Louis Sullivan, then Secretary of Health and Human Services, national health promotion and disease prevention objectives were released in a report called *Healthy People 2000: National Health Promotion and Disease Prevention Objectives for the Year 2000* (US Department of Health & Human Services, 1990). To meet these goals, 298 specific measurable objectives were identified. Almost 100 of these goals related to health status, risk reduction, and service and protection of infants and children. Objectives for the nation for 2010 are under development as this book is being published. They are to be released in 2000 and will continue to focus on most of the same themes as did the first set. It is important for primary care providers to understand these goals because they influence practice guidelines and allocation of federal and state resources. They should guide health care decisions and patient education for all patients. If the statistical trends are to be modified to reduce morbidity and mortality, health supervision must become more efficient and effective. The traditional health care of the past is insufficient given the current needs. National goals are intended to provide direction for changes in the health care delivery system, most of which must occur in the primary health care arena.

Clinical Preventive Services: Health Supervision as a Component of Primary Care

Clinical preventive services can be viewed as evidence-based care guidelines. These services include screening tests, immunizations, and preventive counseling—all areas of expertise for NPs. They are designed as cost-effective means to achieve the national goals. NPs should be familiar with several sets of guidelines for providing clinical preventive services. The American Academy of Pediatrics (AAP) guidelines for health supervision are incorporated into *Bright Futures: National Guidelines for Health Supervision of Infants, Children, and Adolescents*, a book from the Bureau of Maternal and Child Health (US Department of Health & Human Services, 1994). A variation is found in the AAP's own publication *Guidelines for Health Supervision III* (American Academy of Pediatrics, 1997). These guidelines provide information for conducting health promotion visits from infancy through adolescence. A summary of health promotion assessments and interventions for each age group is presented in Figure 1-5. AAP recommendations are incorporated throughout this text.

AMA Guidelines for Adolescent Preventive Services (GAPS) (Elster & Kuznets, 1994) provides another set of guidelines developed by experts on adolescence under the sponsorship of the American Medical Association (AMA). Their 24 recommendations are summarized in Table 1-2. The rationale and suggested interventions found in GAPS are also incorporated into this text. It is recommended that primary care providers be familiar with both the *Bright Futures* and *GAPS* guidelines.

Another widely accepted publication is the *Clinician's Handbook of Preventive Services* (1998), prepared by the US Preventive Services Task Force. This book rigorously reviews evidence for 169 interventions to prevent 60 different illnesses and conditions across the life span.

Barriers to the Use of Clinical Preventive Services Guidelines

Griffith (1993) identified a variety of barriers to the provision of clinical preventive services by all primary care providers: uncertainty about the guidelines, lack of reimbursement, lack of time, limited patient education efforts associated with lack of commitment to facilitate behavior changes, lack of office system organization, clinician attitudes more focused on acute care than prevention, and less feedback from patients and the agency about the effects of preventive care. In other words, primary care providers cannot blame low immunization rates just on access-to-care issues on the patient side of the equation!

It is hoped that health care initiatives will continue to reduce the financial barriers to child health care. Recommended clinical preventive services should be included in the essential benefits packages of all insurance plans. The barriers related to clinician attitudes, motivation, and office systems are harder to eliminate, but if the health of our nation's children and adults is to improve, they must be addressed.

The Putting Prevention into Practice (PPIP) program is designed to assist clinicians to implement the *Clinician's Handbook of Preventive Services* recommendations. Unlike the *Bright Futures* and *GAPS* standards, the PPIP program offers strategies for patients, providers, and office systems to increase the likelihood that the recommendations will indeed be followed. PPIP's *Child Health Guide* and *Personal Health Guide* (for adults) are passport-size, patient-held records that also provide information about the recommended services. The *Clinician's Handbook of Clinical Preventive Services* (US Public Health Service, 1998), is a manual of 62 chapters, each including steps to delivery of a service, recommendations from major authorities, and provider resources. Finally, the office materials include chart flow sheets to track the clinical preventive services status of clients, prevention prescription pads to contract with patients for behavioral

T A B L E 1-2

American Medical Association Guidelines for Adolescent Preventive Services

I. Recommendations for delivery of health services

Recommendation 1: From ages 11 to 21, all adolescents should have an annual routine health visit.

Visits should address biomedical and psychosocial aspects of health with a preventive focus. A complete physical examination should be performed during three of these visits—11–14 years, 15–17 years, and 18–21 years—unless more frequent examinations are warranted by clinical signs or symptoms.

Recommendation 2: Preventive services should be age and developmentally appropriate and sensitive to individual and sociocultural differences.

Recommendation 3: Physicians should establish office policies regarding confidential care for adolescents and how parents will be involved in that care. These policies should be made clear to adolescents and their parents.

II. Recommendations for health guidance

Recommendation 4: Parents or other adult caregivers of adolescents should receive health guidance at least once during early adolescence, middle adolescence, and late adolescence.

Normative adolescent development (physical, sexual, and emotional), signs and symptoms of disease and emotional stress, parenting behavior that promotes healthy adolescent adjustment, benefits of discussing health-related behavior with their adolescents, planning family activities, and acting as a role model should be discussed with parents or caregivers.

Caregivers or parents should be advised of methods for helping their adolescents avoid potentially harmful behavior such as monitoring and managing the use of motor vehicles, avoiding weapons in the home, removing weapons and potentially lethal medications from homes of adolescents with suicidal intent, and monitoring social and recreational activities to restrict sexual behavior and tobacco, alcohol, and other drug use.

Recommendation 5: All adolescents should receive health guidance annually to promote a better understanding of their physical growth, psychosocial and psychosexual development, and the importance of becoming actively involved in decisions about their health care.

Recommendation 6: All adolescents should receive health guidance annually to promote the reduction of injuries, including avoidance of the use of alcohol or drugs while operating motor vehicles or where impaired judgment may lead to injury, and the use of safety devices, including safety belts, helmets, and appropriate sports protective devices.

Recommendation 7: All adolescents should receive health guidance annually about dietary habits, including the benefits of a healthy diet and ways to achieve a healthy diet and safe weight management.

Recommendation 8: All adolescents should receive health guidance annually about the benefits of exercise and should be encouraged to engage in safe exercise regularly.

Recommendation 9: All adolescents should receive health guidance annually regarding responsible sexual behavior, including abstinence. Latex condoms to prevent STDs and appropriate methods of birth control should be made available with instructions on how to use them effectively. Counseling should include effectiveness of abstinence; HIV transmission, dangers, and prevention by latex condoms; and sensible sexual behavior for those who are not sexually active, as well as for those who are using condoms and birth control appropriately.

Recommendation 10: All adolescents should receive health guidance to promote avoidance of tobacco, alcohol, abusable substances, and anabolic steroids.

TABLE 1-2 *Continued*

American Medical Association Guidelines for Adolescent Preventive Services

III. Recommendations for screening

    Recommendation 11: All adolescents should be screened annually for hypertension according to the National Heart, Lung, and Blood Institute Second Task Force on Blood Pressure Control in Children.

    Recommendation 12: Selected adolescents should be screened to determine their risk for hyperlipidemia and adult coronary disease, as per the protocol developed by the Expert Panel on Blood Cholesterol Levels in Children and Adolescents. High-risk adolescents include those with serum cholesterol levels greater than 240 mg/dl who are older than 19 years and those with an unknown family history or parents or grandparents with coronary artery disease.

    Recommendation 13: All adolescents should be screened annually for eating disorders and obesity by determining weight and stature and asking about body image and dieting patterns.

    Recommendation 14: All adolescents should be asked annually about their use of tobacco products, including cigarettes and smokeless tobacco.

    A pattern of use and a cessation plan should be provided to those who use tobacco.

    Recommendation 15: All adolescents should be asked annually about the use of alcohol and other abusable substances and their use of over-the-counter or prescription drugs for nonmedical purposes, including anabolic steroids.

    Recommendation 16: All adolescents should be asked annually about involvement in sexual behavior that may result in unintended pregnancy and STDs, including HIV infection.

    Recommendation 17: Sexually active adolescents should be screened for STDs.

    Recommendation 18: Adolescents at risk for HIV infection should be offered confidential HIV screening with the ELISA and confirmatory tests.

    Risk factors include intravenous drug use, STD infection, residence in a high-prevalence area, more than one sexual partner in the past 6 months, exchange of sex for drugs or money, male gender and engaging in sex with another male, or a sexual partner at risk for HIV infection.

    Recommendation 19: Female adolescents who are sexually active or any female 18 years or older should be screened annually for cervical cancer by use of a Papanicolaou test.

    Recommendation 20: All adolescents should be asked annually about behavior or emotions that indicate recurrent or severe depression or a risk of suicide.

    Recommendation 21: All adolescents should be asked annually about a history of emotional, physical, or sexual abuse.

    Recommendation 22: All adolescents should be asked annually about learning or school problems.

    Recommendation 23: Adolescents should receive a tuberculin skin test if they have been exposed to active tuberculosis, have lived in a homeless shelter, have been incarcerated, have lived in or come from an area with a high prevalence of tuberculosis, or are currently working in a health-care setting.

IV. Recommendations for immunizations

    Recommendation 24: All adolescents should receive prophylactic immunizations according to the guidelines established by the federally convened Advisory Committee on Immunization Practices.

ELISA = enzyme-linked immunosorbent assay; HIV = human immunodeficiency virus; STD = sexually transmitted disease.

From Elster A, Kuznets N: AMA Guidelines for Adolescent and Preventive Services (GAPS). Baltimore, Williams & Wilkins, 1994.

RECOMMENDATIONS FOR PREVENTIVE PEDIATRIC HEALTH CARE

Committee on Practice and Ambulatory Medicine

Each child and family is unique; therefore, these Recommendations for Preventive Pediatric Health Care are designed for the care of children who are receiving competent parenting, have no manifestations of any important health problems, and are growing and developing in satisfactory fashion. Additional visits may become necessary if circumstances suggest variations from normal.

These guidelines represent a consensus by the Committee on Practice and Ambulatory Medicine in consultation with national committees and sections of the American Academy of Pediatrics. The Committee emphasizes the great importance of continuity of care in comprehensive health supervision and the need to avoid fragmentation of care.

A prenatal visit is recommended for parents who are at high risk, for first-time parents, and for those who request a conference. The prenatal visit should include anticipatory guidance and pertinent medical history. Every infant should have a newborn evaluation after birth.

AGE[1]	NEWBORN[1]	2-4d[2]	By1mo	2mo	4mo	6mo	9mo	12mo	15mo	18mo	24mo	3y	4y	5y	6y	8y	10y	11y	12y	13y	14y	15y	16y	17y	18y	19y	20y	21y
HISTORY																												
Initial/Interval	•	•	•	•	•	•	•	•	•	•	•	•	•	•	•	•	•	•	•	•	•	•	•	•	•	•	•	•
MEASUREMENTS																												
Height and Weight	•	•	•	•	•	•	•	•	•	•	•	•	•	•	•	•	•	•	•	•	•	•	•	•	•	•	•	•
Head Circumference	•	•	•	•	•	•	•	•	•	•	•																	
Blood Pressure												•	•	•	•	•	•	•	•	•	•	•	•	•	•	•	•	•
SENSORY SCREENING																												
Vision	S	S	S	S	S	S	S	S	S	S	S	O[5]	O	O	S	S	O	O	S	S	S	S	S	S	O	S	S	S
Hearing[6]	S/O	S	S	S	S	S	S	S	S	S	S	O	O	O	S	S	O	O	S	S	S	S	S	S	O	S	S	S
DEVELOPMENTAL/ BEHAVIORAL ASSESSMENT[7]	•	•	•	•	•	•	•	•	•	•	•	•	•	•	•	•	•	•	•	•	•	•	•	•	•	•	•	•
PHYSICAL EXAMINATION[8]	•	•	•	•	•	•	•	•	•	•	•	•	•	•	•	•	•	•	•	•	•	•	•	•	•	•	•	•
PROCEDURES – GENERAL[9]																												
Hereditary/Metabolic Screening[10]																												
Immunization[11]																												
Lead Screening[12]							•																					
Hematocrit or Hemoglobin[13]																												
Urinalysis[14]													•		•													
PROCEDURES – PATIENTS AT RISK																												
Tuberculin Test[15]																												
Cholesterol Screening[16]																		*	*	*	*	*	*	*	*	*	*	*
STD Screening[17]																		*	*	*	*	*	*	*	*	*	*	*
Pelvic Exam[18]																		*	*	*	*	*	*	*	18	*	*	*
ANTICIPATORY GUIDANCE[19]	•	•	•	•	•	•	•	•	•	•	•	•	•	•	•	•	•	•	•	•	•	•	•	•	•	•	•	•
Injury Prevention[20]																												
INITIAL DENTAL REFERRAL[21]																												

INFANCY[3] — EARLY CHILDHOOD[3] — MIDDLE CHILDHOOD[3] — ADOLESCENCE[3]

1. Breastfeeding encouraged and instruction and support offered.
2. For newborns discharged in less than 48 hours after delivery.
3. Developmental, psychosocial, and chronic disease issues for children and adolescents may require frequent counseling and treatment visits separate from preventive care visits.
4. If a child comes under care for the first time at any point on the schedule, or if any items are not accomplished at the suggested age, the schedule should be brought up to date at the earliest possible time.
5. If the patient is uncooperative, rescreen within six months.
6. Some experts recommend objective appraisal of hearing in the newborn period. The Joint Committee on Infant Hearing has identified patients at significant risk for hearing loss. All children meeting these criteria should be objectively screened. See the Joint Committee on Infant Hearing 1994 Position Statement.
7. By history and appropriate physical examination; if suspicious, by specific objective developmental testing.
8. At each visit, a complete physical examination is essential, with infant totally unclothed, older child undressed and suitably draped.
9. These may be modified, depending upon entry point into schedule and individual need.
10. Metabolic screening (eg, thyroid, hemoglobinopathies, PKU, galactosemia) should be done according to state law.
11. Schedule(s) per the Committee on Infectious Diseases, published periodically in Pediatrics. Every visit should be an opportunity to update and complete a child's immunizations.
12. Blood lead screen per AAP statement "Lead Poisoning: From Screening to Primary Prevention" (1993).
13. All menstruating adolescents should be screened.
14. Conduct dipstick urinalysis for leukocytes for male and female adolescents.
15. TB testing per AAP statement "Screening for Tuberculosis in Infants and Children" (1994). Testing should be done upon recognition of high risk factors. If results are negative but high risk situation continues, testing should be repeated on an annual basis.
16. Cholesterol screening for high risk patients per AAP "Statement on Cholesterol" (1992). If family history cannot be ascertained and other risk factors are present, screening should be at the discretion of the physician.
17. All sexually active patients should be screened for sexually transmitted diseases (STDs).
18. All sexually active females should have a pelvic examination. A pelvic examination and routine pap smear should be offered as part of preventive health maintenance between the ages of 18 and 21 years.
19. Appropriate discussion and counseling should be an integral part of each visit for care.
20. From birth to age 12, refer to AAP's injury prevention program (TIPP[R]) as described in "A Guide to Safety Counseling in Office Practice" (1994).
21. Earlier initial dental evaluations may be appropriate for some children. Subsequent examinations as prescribed by dentist.

Key: • = to be performed   * = to be performed for patients at risk   S = subjective, by history   O = objective, by history   ◯ = objective, by a standard testing method   ↔ = the range during which a service may be provided, with the dot indicating the preferred age.

NB: Special chemical, immunologic, and endocrine testing is usually carried out upon specific indications. Testing other than newborn (eg, inborn errors of metabolism, sickle disease, etc.) is discretionary with the physician.

The recommendations in this publication do not indicate an exclusive course of treatment or serve as a standard of medical care. Variations, taking into account individual circumstances, may be appropriate.

FIGURE 1-5
Recommendations for preventive pediatric health care. Committee on Practice and Ambulatory Medicine.
(Used with permission of the American Academy of Pediatrics.)

changes, reminder postcards, chart stickers and Post-it notes to remind providers of needed services, and posters for waiting and examining rooms with age-specific timelines for delivery of services.

Clinical preventive services guidelines need to be part of the practice of every primary health care provider. Whether the clinician chooses the PPIP program, the *Bright Futures* guidelines, the *GAPS* recommendations, or all three, one should select and define the standard of care for practice. The clinical setting is designed to support delivery of those services by incorporating the guidelines into the plan of care for every patient whether sick or well. One goal of sick care should always be to move the patient back into the health promotion arena, thereby providing appropriate health promotion services even to sick patients. For instance, recommendations for providing immunizations are much more flexible than they were several years ago. In many cases, immunizations should be given to patients coming for illness visits.

Health promotion work with patients and families needs to be individualized. Cultural diversity, family values and lifestyles, and economics are all important factors to consider in helping families plan for their health. Health promotion care also needs to be viewed as a longitudinal process. Planning must be done across visits. Families need to understand the plan over time and whether they are on target with their health promotion activities (e.g., the status of immunization series completion, the next immunizations required, and the time at which they should be given). Continuity of care should be viewed over time. Continuity should also be viewed across health and human services centers. In other words, care provided by a variety of professionals (including social workers, therapists, teachers, physicians, nurses, and others) across agencies and time should be integrated and "seamless."

NURSE PRACTITIONERS WORKING IN MANAGED CARE SETTINGS

Child health care has changed considerably over the past 20 years. Financing and organiza-

tion of services have changed to a system of managed care. The number of child visits to primary care providers has increased 22% since 1979, whereas the average patient age decreased from 6.7 years to 5.7 years. The ethnic diversity of clients has increased, with a greater proportion of visits by Hispanics and Asians. Shifts in the frequencies with which some common conditions are diagnosed and treated have also been observed. Counseling has apparently increased in primary care visits (Ferris et al., 1998).

NPs as well as physicians are expected to be efficient, effective providers. Unlike physicians, NPs are expected to provide more health teaching and bring a more holistic perspective to their analysis of patient and family problems. NPs manage health as well as illness. The problem-oriented model for care, which is a theme of this book, is found in Chapter 2. It includes assessment and management of diseases, daily living problems (functional health problems), and developmental problems. Community-based care is another theme for NP practice that is less emphasized in this book but nonetheless important. Despite the pleasures of working with children, the problems NPs face, such as juggling the expectations of employers and managed care payers vs. the needs and expectations of their patients and families, make providing care stressful for many. Unfortunately, much of their work becomes invisible when billed under physician names. With the current system of 85% reimbursement to NPs as direct providers under Medicaid and Medicare, many are reluctant to take the penalty of loss of revenue for their practice to be acknowledged as providers in their own right. Utilization of clinical preventive services guidelines, working with auxiliary personnel to eliminate the nonprofessional tasks of the day, and working toward clerical personnel management of paperwork for reimbursement and referrals will increase efficiency. Generation of data about the effectiveness of NP services as well as their economic value to a practice will continue to be important to NP viability as providers of the future. Patient and family satisfaction with NPs can have important effects on the system as it shifts to meet consumer demands; one must remember that employers as well as employees

TABLE 1-3

Region X Nursing Network Child Health Standards

NUTRITION/METABOLIC GOALS

Newborn	The newborn's nutrition contributes to growth and wellness
1 mo to 3 yr	The child's nutrition promotes growth and wellness
School age	The school-age child's nutrition promotes growth and wellness
Adolescent	The adolescent develops nutrition patterns that contribute to physical growth, individual needs, and lifelong health

ELIMINATION

Newborn	The newborn's elimination pattern is normal for a healthy newborn
1 mo to 3 yr	The child's elimination pattern is normal for a healthy child
School age	The school-age child's elimination pattern is normal for a healthy child
Adolescent	The adolescent's elimination pattern is normal for a healthy adolescent

SLEEP/REST PATTERN

Newborn	The newborn's sleep, rest, and relaxation contribute to health, growth, and development
1 mo to 3 yr, school age	The child's sleep, rest, and relaxation promote health, growth, and development
Adolescent	The adolescent's sleep/rest/relaxation pattern promotes optimal cognitive, physical, and emotional functioning

ACTIVITY/EXERCISE PATTERN

Newborn, 1 mo to 3 yr	The child's play and activities are appropriate for age
School age	The child's exercise and activity levels are appropriate to maintain optimal health outcomes
Adolescent	The adolescent's activity/exercise patterns promote physical and emotional health

COGNITIVE/PERCEPTUAL PATTERN

Newborn, 1 mo to 3 yr, school age	The child's cognitive-perceptual development is appropriate for age
Adolescent	The adolescent's cognitive-perceptual development is within normal limits

HEALTH PERCEPTION/HEALTH MANAGEMENT PATTERN

Newborn, 1 mo to 3 yr	The newborn's environment promotes positive health behavior
School age	The child's environment promotes an awareness of and participation in positive health behavior
Adolescent	The adolescent exhibits positive behavior to achieve and maintain health

SELF-CONCEPT/SELF-PERCEPTION PATTERN

Newborn	The newborn's environment promotes development of self-respect
1 mo to 3 yr, school age	The child sees self in a positive way and is aware of personal competence
Adolescent	The adolescent demonstrates a positive self-image while moving through the stages of adolescence

ROLES/RELATIONSHIPS PATTERN

Newborn	The newborn's environment promotes roles and relationships appropriate for age within the family and other social environments
1 mo to 3 yr, school age	The child's behavior shows that the child has developed roles and relationships within the family and the social environment appropriate for age and the developmental situation
Adolescent	The adolescent establishes and maintains role/relationship patterns that promote accomplishment of developmental task and socialization needs

T A B L E 1-3 *Continued*

Region X Nursing Network Child Health Standards

SEXUALITY/REPRODUCTIVE PATTERN

Newborn	The child develops age-appropriate sexuality
1 mo to 3 yr, school age	The child has age-appropriate sexuality
Adolescent	The adolescent demonstrates age-appropriate sexuality and feels positive about personal sexuality

COPING/STRESS TOLERANCE PATTERN

Newborn, 1 mo to 3 yr	The newborn copes and tolerates stress in a way that promotes health, growth, and development
School age	The child's coping patterns promote health, growth, and development
Adolescent	The adolescent develops and demonstrates patterns of coping and stress reduction that promote optimal physical and emotional health

VALUES/BELIEF PATTERN

Newborn	The newborn's values are a source of strength and hope and promote health
1 mo to 3 yr, school age	The child is developing values that are a source of strength and hope and promote health
Adolescent	The adolescent's emerging value system provides a source of strength, hope, stability, and well-being

From Region X Nursing Standards Board: Nursing Standards for Prenatal and Child Health. Seattle, University of Washington, 1998.

are the current consumers of health care insurance plans.

NURSING STANDARDS FOR CHILD HEALTH CARE

The national health goals and various clinical preventive services guidelines presented to this point represent public health and medical viewpoints of optimal child health care. NPs are first and foremost nurses, so it is also appropriate to present community health nursing standards for child health care. A set of standards, developed in 1989 and revised in 1998 under the leadership of Barnard at the University of Washington (Region X Nursing Standards Board, 1998), are organized around the nursing functional health patterns of Gordon (1987). They work well for this text because the functional health patterns framework serves to organize the chapters in Unit II of this book. The revised standards are summarized in Table 1-3.

SUMMARY

It must be understood that much of the work of NPs and other primary health care providers is in the realm of common illness management and coordination of care for children with serious and chronic illnesses. However, the real long-term positive impact of primary health care occurs when health-promoting activities are provided to patients and their families in such a way that they are participants in, not recipients of, their health care. Health for children as they grow is essential because it helps them cope in an increasingly complex world and achieve their dreams.

REFERENCES

American Academy of Pediatrics: Guidelines for Health Supervision III. Elk Grove Village, IL, American Academy of Pediatrics, 1997.
American Academy of Pediatrics: Recommendations for preventive pediatric health care. Committee on Practice and Ambulatory Medicine. Pediatrics 96:373-374, 1995.
American Nurses' Association: Nursing: A Social Policy

Statement. Kansas City, MO, American Nurses' Association, 1980.

Annie E. Casey Foundation Center for the Study of Social Policy: Kids Count Data Book. Washington, DC, Annie E. Casey Foundation, 1997.

Annie E. Casey Foundation Center for the Study of Social Policy: Kids Count Data Book. Washington, DC, Annie E. Casey Foundation, 1993.

Annunziato P, Frenkel L: The epidemiology of pediatric HIV-1 infection. Pediatr Ann 22:401–405, 1993.

Baker S, Fingerhut L, Higgins L, et al: Injury to Children and Teenagers: State by State Mortality Facts. Baltimore, Johns Hopkins Center for Injury Research and Policy, 1996.

Births, marriages, divorces, and deaths for November 1997. Mon Vital Stat Rep 46:11, 1998.

Broering J: The adolescent, health, and society: Commentary from the perspective of nursing. *In* Millstein SG, Petersen AC, Nightingale EO (eds): Promoting the Health of Adolescents: New Directions for the Twenty-First Century. New York, Oxford University Press, 1993, pp 151–157.

Centers for Disease Control and Prevention: National, state, and urban area vaccination coverage levels among children aged 19-35 months—United States, 1997. MMWR Morb Mortal Wkly Rep 47:547–555, 1998a.

Centers for Disease Control and Prevention: Tobacco use among high school students—United States, 1997. MMWR Morb Mortal Wkly Rep 47:229–235, 1998b.

Centers for Disease Control and Prevention: Suicide among black youth—United States, 1980–1995. MMWR Morb Mortal Wkly Rep 47:193–196, 1998c.

Centers for Disease Control and Prevention: Rates of homicide, suicide, and firearm-related death among children—26 industrialized countries. MMWR Morb Mortal Wkly Rep 46:101–105, 1997.

Children's Defense Fund: The State of America's Children: Yearbook 1998. Washington, DC, Children's Defense Fund, 1998.

Children's Defense Fund: The Health of America's Children 1992: Maternal and Child Health Data Book. Washington, DC, Children's Defense Fund, 1992.

Elster A, Kuznets N: AMA Guidelines for Adolescent Preventive Services (GAPS). Baltimore, Williams & Wilkins, 1994.

Ferris T, Saglam D, Stafford R, et al: Changes in the daily practice of primary care for children. Arch Pediatr Adolesc Med 152:227–233, 1998.

Ginsburg K: Guiding adolescents away from violence. Contemp Pediatr 14:101–111, 1997.

Gordon M: Nursing Diagnosis: Process and Application. New York, McGraw-Hill, 1987.

Griffith H: Needed—a strong nursing position on preventive services. Image 15:360, 1993.

Institute of Medicine, Committee on the Future of Primary Care: Defining Primary Care: An Interim Report. Washington, DC, Division of Health Care Services, 1994.

Leslie L, Sarah R, Palfrey J: Child health care in changing times. Pediatrics 101:746–752, 1998.

MacDorman MF, Atkinson JO: Infant mortality statistics from the linked birth/infant death data set—1995 period data. Mon Vital Stat Rep 46(suppl 2):S1–22, 1998.

Newacheck P, Halfon N: Prevalence and impact of disabling chronic conditions in childhood. Am J Public Health 88:610–617, 1998.

Newacheck P, Taylor W: Childhood chronic illness: Prevalence, severity, and impact. Am J Public Health 82:364–371, 1992.

Reading R: Poverty and the health of children and adolescents. Arch Dis Child 76:463–467, 1997.

Region X Nursing Standards Board: Nursing Standards for Prenatal and Child Health. Seattle, University of Washington, 1998.

Rivara F, Aitken M: Prevention of injuries to children and adolescents. Adv Pediatr 45:37–71, 1998.

Sells W, Blum R: Morbidity and mortality among US adolescents: An overview of data and trends. Am J Public Health 86:513–519, 1996.

The David and Lucile Packard Foundation: Children and managed health care. The Future of Children 8(2):1998.

US Congress, Office of Technology Assessment: Adolescent Health. Vol 1: Summary and Policy Options (OTA-H-468). Washington, DC, Office of Technology Assessment, 1991.

US Department of Health & Human Services: Healthy People 2000: National Health Promotion and Disease Prevention Objectives for the Year 2000. Publication (PHS) 91-50212. Washington, DC, US Government Printing Office, 1990.

US Department of Health & Human Services, Bureau of Maternal and Child Health: Bright Futures: National Guidelines for Health Supervision of Infants, Children, and Adolescents. Washington, DC, US Department of Health & Human Services, 1994.

US Department of Health & Human Services, Bureau of Maternal and Child Health: Child Health USA '96–'97. Washington, DC, Department of Health & Human Services, 1997.

US Public Health Service: Clinician's Handbook of Preventive Services, 2nd ed. McLean, VA, International Medical Publishers, 1998.

Ventura SJ, Martin JA, Curtin SC, et al: Report of final natality statistics, 1996. Mon Vital Stat Rep 46(11 suppl):S1–99, 1998.

CHAPTER 2

Child Assessment in Pediatric Primary Care

Catherine E. Burns

INTRODUCTION

A careful, complete, and thoughtful assessment of the child's health status is absolutely essential to provide excellent primary health care. This assessment is based on knowledge of child development, family structure and functions, culture, anatomy and physiology, pathophysiology, pharmacology, health care delivery systems, communities, and standards of primary health care for children. The assessment must also be viewed through the lens of the provider's experience to allow the provider to modify perceptions and validate data on the basis of previous work. When providers analyze patient care situations, they are engaged in critical thinking. This chapter cannot teach critical thinking, nor does it teach physical assessment. Rather, it provides frameworks for gathering data to facilitate expert decision making. It is assumed that the reader already knows how to do a complete physical examination and has some experience working with children and families in health care settings. It is also assumed that nurse practitioners (NPs) have the requisite knowledge in the areas just listed.

An important corollary to health assessment is the skill to communicate information obtained both in oral and in written forms. A record of the care given must always be written to communicate the provider's logical thinking based on data obtained. This record is im-portant because it provides information for later care, as well as serves as a communication link with other providers. In addition, the written record documents the quality of care provided. Verbal communication of health care information is also essential. The words must paint a picture of the child and family for the reader (e.g., a consultant). Knowledge of the classic format used by other health care providers is important. Using that same format or one that is closely related facilitates efficient communication about patient problems.

This chapter provides the basic framework for health assessment of children. In-depth assessments related to specific topics are included in later chapters.

THE ASSESSMENT MODEL

When analyzing patient problems, most NPs are comfortable with classification of diseases using the following categories of the *International Classification of Diseases*, 9th revised edition, *Clinical Modification* (ICD-9-CM) (U.S. Department of Health and Human Services, 1981): infectious, endocrine, nutritional, metabolic, immunological, respiratory, cardiovascular, musculoskeletal, gastrointestinal, genitourinary, neurological, and so on. NPs consistently record the disease diagnoses they make for problems in these body systems. One reason that

NPs use this classification system so easily is that the classic health history format used drives decision making into these categories. This classic health history format includes the following (Table 2-1):

- Chief complaint (C/C)
- History of the present illness (HPI)
- Past medical history (PMH)
- Review of systems (ROS)

T A B L E 2-1

The Classic Health History

    I. Patient identifying information: Name, birth date, sex, address, record number, and name of historian, along with relationship to the patient stated
    II. Chief complaint
    III. History of present illness
    IV. Past medical history
      A. Prenatal, natal, postnatal
      B. Past illnesses
      C. Allergies
      D. Accidents
      E. Hospitalizations
      F. Immunization history
      G. Nutrition history
      H. Growth
      I. Development
    V. Review of systems: As in Table 2–3, except add the following
      A. Psychological—colic, breath holding, thumb sucking, head banging, fears, tics, behavior disorders, temper tantrums, nail biting, hair pulling, masturbation. Adjustment to home, school, neighborhood. Temperament—activity level, predictability, moods, intensity of reactions, adaptability, initial responses, distractibility. Sleep—amount, habits, problems
    VI. Family history
    VII. Socioeconomic
      A. Occupations of father and mother
      B. Time spent with child by parents, activities together
      C. Finances—adequacy
      D. Persons in the home
      E. House or apartment living arrangements
      F. General relationship of family members
      G. Community support systems—friends, church, agencies involved with family

- Family history (FH)
- Socioeconomic history (SE)

The classic medical history is written to expand on the chief complaint, which is generally a physical problem. Issues such as nutrition, development, and activities of daily living are included, primarily as they relate to various diseases. The system works well and has generally been taught to physicians and NPs. The system fails, however, to provide a framework for integrating nursing aspects of NP work into the problem list and management plan. Without that framework, NPs may fail to clearly identify and document the unique contributions they make as nurses providing primary health care. Without that identification, the special aspects of their work with patients remain invisible.

An alternative model is offered in this chapter that integrates the nursing and medical aspects of NP work conceptually and clinically. This assessment model (Burns, 1991a, 1992) is based on the assumption that patient problems can be grouped into three distinct domains: developmental problems, functional health problems, and diseases.

The problems that children bring to NPs in primary care are organized into an integrated taxonomy or classification list of medical and nursing diagnoses sorted by the three domains, which form a framework for analysis of the problems (Table 2-2).

Developmental Problems

This domain includes the long-term issues of development and maturation over the life span. In pediatrics, developmental issues are prominent. Missing a developmental problem plus failing to plan for its management is as serious as missing diabetes mellitus or a dislocated hip. Problems of either type can affect the child's entire future if not remedied or managed to minimize the effects. Because no good taxonomy of developmental problems is available for NPs to use, the lists of problems here are short. Generally, NPs assess gross motor, fine motor, speech and language, cognitive, and social and adaptive areas.

Text continued on page 25

T A B L E 2-2

Integrated Classification System of Diagnoses for Use by Nurse Practitioners

DOMAIN I. DEVELOPMENT DIAGNOSES
Cognitive development
  Cognitive delay
  Learning disorder
Language development
  Language delay
  Speech delay
Motor development
  Gross motor delay
  Fine motor delay
Social development
  Social development delay
  Attachment failure

DOMAIN II. FUNCTIONAL HEALTH DIAGNOSES
Health perception/health management pattern
  Adjustment impaired
  Health maintenance alteration
  Health-seeking behavior
  Home maintenance management impaired
  Home care resources inadequate
  Knowledge deficits
  Noncompliance
  Risk of injury—suffocation/poisoning/trauma/aspiration
  Self-care deficits, dressing/toileting/hygiene
  Skill deficit
  Therapeutic regimen management ineffective—individual/family
  Decisional conflict
Nutritional-metabolic pattern
  Anorexia
  Anorexia nervosa
  Breastfeeding ineffective/interrupted/effective
  Bulimia
  Colic
  Infant feeding pattern ineffective
  Nausea
  Nutrition alterations less than/greater than body requirements
  Swallowing impaired
Elimination pattern
  Constipation
  Encopresis
  Enuresis
  Incontinence, bowel/urinary
Activity/exercise pattern
  Activity intolerance
  Diversional activities deficit
  Fatigue
  Physical mobility impaired
Sleep pattern
  Sleep pattern disturbance

Table continued on following page

T A B L E 2-2

Integrated Classification System of Diagnoses for Use by Nurse Practitioners *Continued*

DOMAIN II. FUNCTIONAL HEALTH DIAGNOSES *Continued*

Cognitive/perceptual pattern
  Attention deficit disorder
  Disorganized infant behavior
  Memory impaired
  Potential for enhanced organized infant behavior
  Sensory-perceptual alteration
      Blind
      Deaf
  Self-perception/self-concept pattern
  Depression
  Body image disturbance
  Self-esteem disturbance, chronic/situational
  Personal identity disturbance
Role relationships pattern
  Abuse
  Caregiver role strain
  Communication impaired—verbal
  Family coping ineffective, disabling/compromised/potential for growth
  Family process alteration
  Family process alteration: alcoholism
  Loneliness, risk for
  Parenting alteration
  Parental role conflict
  Risk of alteration in parent/infant/child attachment
  Role performance alteration
  Social interaction impaired
  Social isolation
Sexuality pattern
  Pregnancy
  Sexual dysfunction
  Sexual pattern alteration
Coping/stress tolerance pattern
  Anxiety
  Comfort alteration
  Coping individual ineffective/defensive
  Fear
  Pain/chronic pain
  Post-trauma response
  Rape-trauma response
  Self-mutilation risk
  Grieving, anticipatory/dysfunctional
  Hopelessness
  Ineffective denial
  Powerlessness
  Substance misuse
  Violence potential, self/others
Values/beliefs pattern
  Potential for enhanced spiritual well-being
  Spiritual distress

T A B L E 2-2

Integrated Classification System of Diagnoses for Use by Nurse Practitioners *Continued*

DOMAIN III. PEDIATRIC DISEASE DIAGNOSES
Infectious diseases
  Candidiasis
  Chickenpox
  Diarrhea
  Giardiasis
  Gonorrhea
  Herpes simplex
  Infection, potential for
  Influenza
  Parasites
  Roseola
  Scabies
  Tuberculosis
  Viral hepatitis
  Viral warts
Endocrine, nutritional, metabolic, and immune diseases
  Fluid volume excess
  Fluid volume deficit
  Food allergy
  Thyroid disorders
  Diabetes mellitus
  Immune deficiency disease
Diseases of blood and blood-forming organs
  Anemias
  Jaundice
  Leukemia
Neurological/sense organ diseases
  Central nervous system
    Epilepsy/seizures
    Cerebral palsy
  Eye
    Amblyopia
    Conjunctivitis
    Dacryocystitis
    Myopia
    Strabismus
  Ear
    Otitis externa
    Otitis media
    Serous otitis
Circulatory system diseases
  Cardiac output decreased
  Congenital heart disease
Respiratory system disease
  Acute nasopharyngitis
  Airway clearance ineffective
  Allergic rhinitis

Table continued on following page

T A B L E 2-2

Integrated Classification System of Diagnoses for Use by Nurse Practitioners Continued

DOMAIN III. PEDIATRIC DISEASE DIAGNOSES *Continued*
  Asthma
  Bronchiolitis
  Croup
  Pharyngitis
  Pneumonia
  Tonsillitis
Digestive system diseases
  Acute abdomen
  Constipation (not encopresis)
  Diarrhea
  Hernia
  Swallowing impaired
  Vomiting
Dental disorders
  Caries
  Dentition impairment
  Malocclusion
  Oral mucous membrane alteration
Genitourinary system disorders
  Adhesions
  Cryptorchidism
  Hydrocele
  Hypospadias
  Incontinence
  Urinary tract infection
  Urinary elimination alteration
  Urinary retention
  Menstrual disorder
  Vaginitis
Skin diseases
  Acne
  Atopic dermatitis
  Cellulitis
  Contact dermatitis
  Folliculitis
  Impetigo
  Nevus
  Seborrhea
  Urticaria
Musculoskeletal diseases
  Developmental dislocated hip
  Genu varum/valgum
  Internal tibial torsion
  Lordosis
  Metatarsus adductus
  Osgood-Schlatter disease
  Scoliosis

T A B L E 2-2

Integrated Classification System of Diagnoses for Use by Nurse Practitioners *Continued*

DOMAIN III. PEDIATRIC DISEASE DIAGNOSES *Continued*

Symptoms/signs/ill-defined conditions
   Hypotonia
   Jaundice
   Lack of physiological maturity
   Temperature alteration—hypothermia, hyperthermia
Injury and poisoning
   Abrasion
   Bee sting
   Burn
   Contusion
   Corneal abrasion
   Fracture
   Insect bites
   Sprain/strain
   Injury, high risk for

Adapted from Burns C: Development and content validity testing of a comprehensive classification of diagnoses for use by pediatric nurse practitioners. *Nurs Diagn* 2:93–104, 1991.

Functional Health Problems

Functional health problems are derived from Gordon's functional health patterns (Gordon, 1987). These patterns provide a way of thinking about the problems that nurses have always managed independently. They represent the universal health behavior patterns of all humans, no matter what their culture, sex, age, or economic status. Gordon's 11 patterns include health beliefs and behavior, nutrition, elimination, activity, sleep, role relationships, coping, self-perception, cognitive/perceptual, sexuality, and values/beliefs. Nursing's primary mission is management of these problems to maximize a person's health. In hospital settings, nurses help patients eat or receive nutrition, facilitate sleep, promote coping with illness, and maximize activity (even if only rolling a comatose patient over). In primary care, NPs are also concerned about these issues, although their management strategies differ with the nature and complexity of the problems.

Labels for the problems from this domain are derived primarily from the North American Nursing Diagnosis Association (NANDA) (NANDA, 1996) taxonomy terms. This system is the nursing profession's effort to classify the phenomena of concern for the profession. The NANDA taxonomy is expanded and updated every 2 years. It was first developed in the 1980s and thus represents a taxonomy in its early stages, as compared, for instance, with the taxonomy for disease diagnoses. To illustrate, *consumption*, a disease diagnosis of the 1800s, is now replaced with *tuberculosis*. Although the NANDA system includes physiological responses to illnesses, generally these diagnoses are of less interest to NPs because NPs treat illnesses directly with the medical model.

Diseases

Diseases are conditions assessed and managed at the tissue or organ level of analysis. The diagnoses found in this domain generally come from the ICD-9-CM, as well as some physiological diagnoses from NANDA. Otitis media, streptococcal pharyngitis, and appendicitis are examples of disease diagnoses. It is not expected that NPs use nursing diagnosis language for traditional disease diagnoses. For example, "seborrheic dermatitis" would not be called "alteration in skin integrity."

The *International Classification of Diseases* has been under development for more than 100 years and is designed to represent the phenomena of concern to physicians. It is broad and mature in scope. It represents physiological problems of patients extremely well but does not include labels, or rubrics, for the behavioral, social, and developmental problems that NPs also manage. The ICD-9-CM listings are recognized by many insurance carriers for billing purposes and, as such, have become the "currency" for much health care delivery in the United States, whereas the NANDA nursing diagnoses have not yet achieved that recognition. Fortunately, many diagnoses similar to those in the NANDA classification can be found in the medical listings, thus facilitating reimbursement for nursing aspects of NP work.

Problem Interactions

The concept of interactions of problems across domains is important to understand. For instance, iron deficiency anemia can be considered a disease if looked at from the effects of lack of iron on heme production, red blood cells, oxygen transport, and cellular metabolism. The NP can diagnose this disease and prescribe an iron supplement to manage the problem at this physiological level. However, if the problem is found to be related to a lack of iron in the diet, the NP can choose to intervene at the daily living–nutrition level, call the problem "nutrition: less than body requirements for iron," and teach the family how to increase the selection of iron-rich foods for the table. Iron deficiency has also been shown to cause developmental delays. If a goal for the visit is to provide additional support in the school setting, a developmental problem would be diagnosed (Fig. 2–1).

A particular domain can also serve as the context for the problem in another area. For instance, Down syndrome, a chromosomal disorder, can be the etiology or context for a cognitive development problem. If the intervention is for cognition, a developmental problem of cognitive delay is listed. Content issues for which the NP is planning interventions are the diagnoses. The contextual issues are not the diagnoses.

The most important point to remember is that interventions must be based on or derived from diagnoses. A situation should never arise in which the NP intervenes without explicit

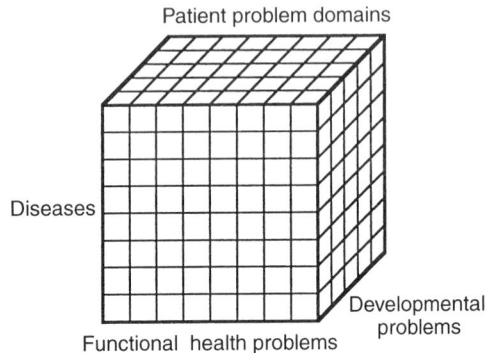

F I G U R E 2–1
Patient Problem Domains. Development and content validity testing of a comprehensive classification of diagnoses for use by pediatric nurse practitioners. (Adapted from Burns C: Nurs Diagn 2:93–104, 1991. Reprinted with permission, Nursecom Inc.)

reasons for doing so. The reasons are stated as diagnoses, either actual or potential, and enumerated in the problem list. The preventive work (i.e., to avoid potential problems) done by NPs also needs to be identified. The diagnoses, as well as the interventions, need to be recorded.

THE DATABASE

The Child Health History

It is said that 80% of diagnoses are made on the basis of the history. The physical examination only provides a view of the situation as it is at the moment. It is often a cloudy picture because the body frequently responds similarly to different assaults. It is the history of the problem—its onset, duration, progress, associated symptoms, meaning, and effects on daily living—that brings the health care provider to an understanding in sufficient depth to choose appropriate management. Functional health and developmental problems present the same issues for the provider. A thorough, thoughtful history is essential.

THE ENVIRONMENT FOR DATA COLLECTION

Primary health care is delivered in many settings, not just examination rooms in outpatient clinics. Wherever the patient and the family are to be cared for, privacy must be ensured. People should have places to sit down, and the room in which the examination is conducted should be well lighted and allow the patient to lie down comfortably. The examiner must be able to work comfortably too. The environment needs to be safe, given the developmental ages of the children to be cared for, and should present an atmosphere of warmth and welcome.

The health care provider should sit down during the history to make data collection a conversation, to equalize the status of clients and examiner, and to help clients feel that they have time to talk. Sitting also helps the provider conserve energy for a busy day.

For young children, the conversation time gives them the opportunity to become familiar with the examiner and setting, which is essential for cooperation when needed. Remember that young children are learning the "script" for health care visits. The visit should help them learn a script that is understandable and not too stressful. When the script is to be varied, alert them of the change with cues and explanations for the new experiences of this visit and the likelihood that the new script will be repeated at future visits. All those in the room need to be addressed at one time or another. Health care is a family event in pediatrics.

For adolescents, the history can be started with the parents and teen together; however, they need to then separate, with the NP getting information from the parents and then the teen independently.

THE INITIAL (COMPLETE) HEALTH HISTORY

Data can be collected verbally, through record review, via written forms completed by the family, or through a combination of these methods. It might not be practical for data to be fully collected on the first visit; rather, the collection can be staged according to the visit priorities. When time with patients is limited, it is common to ask new families to come early for their first appointment to complete a written history before meeting the NP. Notation of any missing data should be made so that further

baseline data can be collected at the next visit. The complete format is listed later in the chapter and should be *mastered* so that it becomes core to the provider's approach to all patient situations. If data are omitted, the omissions should be by choice, not by an error committed through haste, distraction, ignorance, or habit.

The model used in this book integrates the classic medical history with a functional health patterns approach that leads to identification of problems specific to the three domains. It uses a basic problem-oriented format that begins with subjective data (the history), moves to objective data (the physical examination, laboratory, and test data), then lists the problems by domain identified through the subjective and objective data, and finally, plans care, problem by problem (Table 2-3). The items listed under topics are meant to serve as suggestions. The history needs to be individualized.

The adolescent history needs special modification because their health care needs and risks are different, because they are so different developmentally from infants and young children, and because they are interviewed directly. See Table 2-4 for a modification of the initial health history for adolescents.

Patient Identifying Information

Data here are standard to medical records: date, name, medical record number, birth date, sex, address, phone number, and names of other family members. The information about the informant is designed to give the reader a sense of the probability that the history is accurate and complete and from a knowledgeable source.

The Database—Subjective Information

CONTEXTUAL INFORMATION. The intent of this section is to identify family, day care, school, work, or community agency factors that need to be considered in planning care.

- People in the home.
- Home environment description: Apartment, home, or farm? Fenced yard or unsafe neighborhood?

Text continued on page 33

T A B L E 2-3

Problem-Oriented Health Record for Nurse Practitioners with Consideration of Disease, Daily Living, and Development Domains

I. PRELIMINARY INFORMATION

Date:
Name:
Birth date:
Record no:
Corrected age for preterm infant younger than
   2 yr:
Caregiver's name:
Address:
Phone:
Informant, relationship to patient, reliability as
   historian:

Referral source:

II. DATABASE: SUBJECTIVE INFORMATION

  A. Contextual information
   1. Family/household profile
       People in the home:
       Home environment description:
       Family care issues (time, energy,
          needs of other family members,
          emotional stresses):
       Family structure issues (marital
          status):
       Family financial issues:
   2. School/employment:
   3. Agencies involved:
  B. Chief complaint (number each one and then
      record the subjective history for each, ac-
      cording to number)
   1. Concerns:
   2. Present problem history:
  C. Disease history database
   1. Medical history
       Prenatal:
       Perinatal—birth weight, length, head
          circumference:
       Past diseases profile:
       Current health problems:

DIAGNOSIS	DATE	PROVIDER	CURRENT STATUS
1.			
2.			
3.			

       Operations/hospitalizations:
       Injuries:
       Allergies:
       Growth:
       Immunizations:
       Medication:

   2. Review of systems
       General:
       Skin:
       Head:
       EENT:
       Respiratory:
       Cardiovascular:
       GU:
       GI:
       MS:
       Neurological:
       Endocrine:
       Hematological:
   3. Family history of diseases
       Mother and father (age, health):
       Mother's pregnancy history:
       Familial diseases:
       Genogram if appropriate:
  D. Daily living problems database
   1. Health maintenance/health perceptions
       Primary care provider:
          Last visit:
       Dentist:
          Last visit:
       Knowledge and skills for caregiving
          (self-care):
       Safety measures
          Car:
          Smoke alarm:
          Occupational:
          Guns locked:
          Other:
       Home and health management/
          resource issues:
   2. Nutrition
       Diet—breakfast, lunch, dinner:
       Supplements:
       Feeding strategies/patterns:
       Restrictions—calories, other:
   3. Activities
       Amount and type of activities:
       Play:
       Limitations/equipment:
   4. Sleep
       Number of hours:
       Disturbances:
   5. Elimination habits
       Urinary:
       Bowel:

Problem-Oriented Health Record for Nurse Practitioners with Consideration of Disease, Daily Living, and Development Domains *Continued*

    6. Role relationships
        Family patterns:
        Parenting patterns:
        Peers/social support:
        Communication
          Verbal:
          Nonverbal:
    7. Coping/temperament and discipline
        Substance abuse—alcohol, drugs, tobacco:
    8. Cognitive/perceptual problems
        Cognitive disturbances:
        Hearing deficit:
        Vision deficit:
        Kinesthetic disturbances:
    9. Self-perception/self-concept
        Role identity:
        Self-concept, self-esteem, body image:
  10. Sexual and menstrual patterns:
  11. Values and beliefs/religious patterns:
E. Developmental issues/problems database
    1. Motor development
        Gross motor development—past milestones and current skills:
        Fine motor development—past milestones and current skills:
    2. Language development—past milestones and current skills:
    3. Cognitive development—past milestones and current skills:
    4. Social development—past milestones and current skills:
    5. Development test scores:

III. DATABASE: OBJECTIVE INFORMATION
  A. Physical examination

Age:	Sex:	Height:	Weight:
HC:	BP:	TPR:	

    1. General appearance:
    2. Skin:
    3. Head:
    4. Eyes:
    5. Ears:
    6. Nose:
    7. Mouth:

    8. Neck:
    9. Chest/breasts:
  10. Lungs:
  11. Heart:
  12. Abdomen:
  13. Genitalia:
  14. Anus/rectum:
  15. MS:
  16. Neurological
    Motor
      Tone:
      Strength:
    Reflexes:
    Cranial nerves:
    Responsiveness:
    Extraneous movements:
    Gait/position:
    Cerebellar, including coordination, balance, nystagmus:
    Primitive reflexes (sensory function):
  B. Screening/laboratory data:
    1. Hct:
    2. Hearing:
    3. Vision:
    4. TB:
    5. Metabolic/newborn screens:
    6. Other:
  C. Data from other disciplines—Physical therapy, occupational therapy, speech therapy, audiology, social work, physician, other:

IV. PROBLEM LIST (USE CLASSIFICATION LIST FOR DIAGNOSES)
  Include all chief complaints and problems identified by the nurse practitioner.
  Categorize all problems identified according to the following groups:
  Diseases
  Daily living problems
  Developmental problems

V. PLAN
  For each problem, describe plans according to diagnostic, therapeutic, and/or educational activities:
  A. Disease problems
  B. Daily living problems
  C. Developmental problems
  D. Disposition/return appointments

BP = blood pressure; EENT = ear, eye, nose, throat; GI = gastrointestinal; GU = genitourinary; HC = head circumference; Hct = hematocrit; MS = musculoskeletal; TB = tuberculosis; TPR = temperature, pulse, respiration. From Burns C: A new assessment model and tool for nurse practitioners. *J Pediatr Health Care* 6:76–79, 1992.

T A B L E 2-4

Problem-Oriented History for Adolescents

I. DATABASE—SUBJECTIVE INFORMATION

A. Contextual information
   1. With whom do you live?
   2. In the past year, have there been any changes in your immediate family such as
      Marriage, separation, divorce
      Serious illness or injury
      Loss of job
      Move/change of address
      Change of school
      Births, deaths
      Other
   3. What languages are spoken in your home?
B. Chief complaint
C. Past medical history
   1. In the past year, have you had any injury or illness that made you miss school or cut down on activities, or that required medical care?
   2. Have you been hospitalized in the past year?
   3. Do you have any illnesses or medical conditions?
   4. Are you taking any medications?
   5. Have you been exposed to tuberculosis in the past year?
   6. Have you stayed overnight in a homeless shelter, jail, or detention center in the past year?
   7. Girls only: Have you had a period? Date of last one
D. Review of systems
   1. Do you have any concerns about
      Height/weight
      Blood pressure
      Headaches/migraines
      Eyes/vision
      Hearing/ears/earaches
      Nose
      Frequent colds
      Mouth/teeth (Frequency of tooth brushing, flossing)
      Neck/back
      Chest pain
      Coughing/wheezing
      Breasts
      Heart
      Stomach
      Nausea/vomiting
      Diarrhea/constipation
      Skin (rash, acne, sore, use of sunscreen)
      Muscle or joint pain
      Frequent or painful urination
      Sexual organs/genitals
      Menstruation/periods
      Future plans/job
      Physical or sexual abuse
      Masturbation
      Cancer or dying
      Other (explain)

II. FUNCTIONAL HEALTH DATABASE

A. Health maintenance/health perception
   1. Do you usually wear a helmet for rollerblade, bicycle, skateboard, motorcycle, or all-terrain vehicle use?
   2. Do you usually wear a seat belt when riding in a car, truck, or van?
   3. In the past year, have you been in a car when the driver has been drinking or using drugs?
   4. Do you use electric tools or heavy equipment at work or home?
   5. Do you have questions or concerns about avoiding accidents or injuries?
B. Nutrition
   1. Do you eat from the four food groups almost every day?
   2. Do you have any diet/food/appetite concerns?
   3. Are you eating in secret?
   4. Are you satisfied with your eating patterns?
   5. Do you prefer a change in your current weight?
   6. Have you tried to lose weight or control weight by vomiting, taking diet pills or laxatives, or starving yourself?
   7. Do you have concerns about your weight?
C. Activities
   1. Do you watch television or play video games more than 2 hours per day?
   2. Are you involved with exercises that make you sweat and breathe hard at least three times per week?
   3. What do you do after school?
   4. Do you have physical problems that limit your exercise?
   5. Do you have questions or concerns about exercise or physical activity?
D. Sleep
   1. Do you have trouble sleeping?
   2. Do you have trouble with tiredness?
E. Elimination habits
   1. Do you sometimes wet the bed?

T A B L E 2-4

Problem-Oriented History for Adolescents *Continued*

II. FUNCTIONAL HEALTH DATABASE *Continued*

F. Role relationships

1. Do you have at least one friend you really like and feel you can talk to?
2. Do parents or guardian usually listen to you and take your feelings seriously?
3. Do you and your parents or guardian do things together on a regular basis such as eating meals, attending religious activities, performing chores or errands, playing sports, or watching television?
4. Is there a lot of tension or conflict in your home?
5. Do you have questions or concerns about family or friends?

G. Coping/temperament and discipline

1. Alcohol

In the past year, did you or friends get drunk or very high on alcoholic beverages?

Have you ever consumed alcohol and then done any of the following: driven a vehicle, gone swimming or boating, gotten in a fight, used tools or equipment, done something you later regretted?

In the past year, have you ridden in a car driven by someone who was drinking or using drugs?

Have you been criticized or gotten in trouble because of drinking?

Do you have any questions or concerns about alcohol?

2. Drugs

Do you or your friends ever use marijuana or street drugs?

Some drugs can be bought at a store without a doctor's prescription. Do you ever use nonprescription drugs to get to sleep, stay awake, calm down, or get high?

Have you ever used steroids without a doctor telling you to do so?

Do you have any questions or concerns about drugs or drug use?

3. Tobacco

Do you or your friends ever smoke cigarettes or use smokeless tobacco?

Does anyone you live with smoke cigarettes or use smokeless tobacco?

Do you have any questions or concerns about cigarettes or other tobacco products?

4. Emotions

Have you had fun during the past 2 weeks?

In general, are you happy with the way things are going for you these days?

During the past few weeks, have you often felt sad or down with nothing to look forward to?

Have you ever seriously thought about killing yourself, made a plan to kill yourself, or actually tried to kill yourself?

Do you think counseling would help you or someone in your family?

Do you have any questions or concerns about physical, sexual, or emotional abuse?

5. Weapons/violence

Do you or does anyone you live with have a gun, rifle, shotgun, or other firearm in your home?

In the past year, have you ever carried a gun, knife, razorblade, club, or other weapon?

Have you been in a physical fight during the past 3 months?

Are guns or violence a problem in your neighborhood?

When you are angry, do you ever get violent?

Do you have any questions or concerns about violence or your safety?

H. Cognitive/perceptual problems

In general, do you like school? Why?

Are your grades this year better or worse than the year before? What are your usual grades?

Have you ever had to repeat a grade in school?

Do you cut classes or skip school?

How many days of school have you missed this year?

Have you ever been suspended or dropped out of school?

Do you have any questions or concerns about school or your learning?

Table continued on following page

Problem-Oriented History for Adolescents Continued

II. FUNCTIONAL HEALTH DATABASE *Continued*
  I. Self-perception/self-concept
     1. Do you have any concerns about the size or shape of your body or your physical appearance?
     2. What do you like about yourself?
     3. What do you do best?
     4. If you could, what would you change about your life or yourself?
  J. Sexual and menstrual
     1. Do you date?
     2. Do you or your friends have sexual intercourse?
     3. Do you think you might be gay, lesbian, homosexual, or bisexual?
     4. Have you ever been told that you have a sexually transmitted disease such as gonorrhea, genital herpes, chlamydia, trichomonas, syphilis, hepatitis, genital warts, AIDS, or HIV infection?
     5. Do you have any questions or concerns about sex or relationships?
     6. Are you worried about getting pregnant (girls) or do you worry about getting someone pregnant (boys)?
     7. Have you ever been forced to do something sexual that you didn't want to do?
     8. Do you practice abstinence?
     9. Do you want information or supplies to prevent pregnancy or sexually transmitted diseases, including HIV?
  K. Values and beliefs/religious
     1. Are you involved with any religious groups or activities on a regular basis?

III. DEVELOPMENT DATABASE
Throughout the history, listen for data that allow you to assess the following areas (see Developmental Management of Adolescents, Chapter 9):
  A. Motor development
     1. All teens should be active and skilled in a variety of physical activities and sports.
     2. Fine motor development should also be mature. Special arts/crafts or occupational activities may be learned.
  B. Cognitive development
     1. Early adolescents are still concrete and generally present rather than future oriented. Questions can be answered quite literally.
     2. Middle adolescents can use and understand if-then statements. They are able to understand long-term consequences and think of the future. They might challenge many ideas and rules with their newfound skills in logic and reasoning.
     3. Late adolescents are able to consider options before making decisions, engage in sophisticated moral reasoning, and use principles to guide their decisions.
  C. Social development
     1. Early adolescents are egocentric in thinking. They can vacillate between childish and mature behavior, especially around their parents. Their peers are usually of the same sex. Group activities are the norm.
     2. Middle adolescents are concerned with their identity within society and less concerned with their sexual identity unless they are struggling with recognizing their homosexuality. They tend to distance themselves from parents, spend less time at home, and increasingly challenge parental control. Cliques or friends prevail, with only a few close friends. Physical intimacy can occur during this stage, and romantic partners are common.
     3. Late adolescents have distanced themselves from parents and then re-established relationships with family on a new basis of independence. Romantic, emotional intimacy appears.
  D. School/vocational development
     1. Early adolescents are usually adjusting to the expectations of middle school. Setting priorities and completing homework independently can be a challenge. Future goals are often unrealistic and change frequently.
     2. Middle adolescents are entering high school and beginning to develop an awareness that their performance in school will affect their future options for work and/or college. They do not usually have specific ideas about future vocations in mind.
     3. Late adolescents are making decisions about vocations, college, working, or entering the military.

Adapted from American Medical Association, Department of Adolescent Health: *Guidelines for Adolescent Preventive Services (GAPS) User's Manual.* Chicago, American Medical Association, 1994; other sources.

- Family care issues: Primary caregiver? Who helps? What stresses are faced by the caregiver? Do other family members require more attention than the patient? Is the caregiver well both physically and emotionally?
- Family structure issues: Is this a two-parent family, a single-parent family, or a foster home? Are divorced parents dividing caregiving, and what is the meaning of the family structure for the child? How much time do parents and the child spend in the home together, given job, school, and other obligations? Is this a latchkey child?
- Family financial issues: Health insurance? Money for basic necessities? Does the child have an allowance or access to money? What are the sources of money—jobs or welfare? Are financial issues causing family stress?
- School/employment: Where does the child go for day care, school, or work (if an adolescent)? What is the quality of the setting?
- Agencies involved: What other community agencies know this child or family?
- What resources and family support systems are being used and with what success?

CHIEF COMPLAINT AND HISTORY OF PRESENT PROBLEM

- Concerns: What brings the child to the clinic today? The chief complaint is a brief statement of the problem and its duration. Remember that new concerns can arise at any point during the visit. Agendas can be hidden or unconscious. The chief complaint or complaints can involve disease, the functional health pattern, or development.
- Present problem history: For each concern, a chronological description should be made that includes onset, duration, characteristics or symptoms, exposure to illnesses or other causative factors, similar problems in other family members or neighbors, previous episodes of similar illnesses or symptoms, previous diagnostic measures, pertinent negative data, things that have been tried in attempts to manage the concern and their success, and the meaning of the concern for the family and child.

DISEASE DOMAIN DATABASE

1. Past medical history:
   - Prenatal: Planned pregnancy? When did prenatal care begin? What was the mother's health during pregnancy? Drugs, alcohol, and tobacco use? Illnesses and medications? Weight gain? Accidents?
   - Perinatal: Where was the baby born and who delivered the infant? Duration and process of labor? Vaginal or cesarean delivery and process? Anesthesia? Infant response to labor and delivery (breathing, crying)—resuscitation needed? Apgar scores? Birth weight, length, and head circumference? Gestational age? Neonatal course: Infections or other health problems, physiological stabilization, feeding, responsiveness? Jaundice? Weight at discharge? Hospital duration? Neonatal follow-up over the first few weeks?
   - Past diseases profile: What health problems has the child experienced, and what have the outcomes been? Who has provided care? Infectious diseases?
   - Other current health problems (not related to the chief complaint): What problems does the child have now? What was the date of onset? Who is the principal care provider for each problem, and what is the current status (e.g., medications, awaiting surgery, problem in remission)?
   - Operations/hospitalizations: Has the child been hospitalized for any reason? Why, when, where, outcomes? Response to hospitalization? Problems resolved?
   - Injuries: What significant injuries has the child experienced? What care was needed, and does the child currently have any sequelae? How often is the emergency department used?
   - Allergies: Allergies to foods, medications, or environmental factors? How are the allergies manifested? What care is given?
   - Growth: What has the child's growth pattern been? (Always plot growth data on a growth grid to assess progress.) Is the child similar in size to peers? Are clothing sizes changing? Has growth been a worry for the child or family?

- Immunizations and laboratory tests: Obtain a record with dates for all immunizations received in the past. Reactions? Blood tests and screening tests?
- Medications: Is the child taking any medications? What? Why? How much? Responses to the medication?

2. Review of systems: Remember that this section documents the *history* of body systems, not the physical assessment findings.
   - General: Is the child considered to be well, happy, and developing normally?
   - Skin: History of birthmarks, lesions, or skin conditions?
   - Head: Head trauma? Head growth—microcephaly, macrocephaly? Headaches?
   - Eyes, ears, nose, throat: Vision and eye problems? Hearing and ear problems? Nose—discharge or bleeding episodes, breathing interference? Throat problems or infections?
   - Respiratory: Breathing problems? Respiratory infections? Blue spells? Cough?
   - Cardiovascular: Heart murmur history? Cyanosis? Blood pressure problems? Activity intolerance? Syncope?
   - Gastrointestinal: Infections, diarrhea, constipation, vomiting, or reflux? Structural problems? Anal itching or fissures? Stomachaches?
   - Genitourinary: Infections, discharges? Structural problems? Stream appearance? Frequency or burning?
   - Gynecological: Menstrual history? Vaginal discharge or bleeding? Itching?
   - Musculoskeletal: Movement or structural problems? Broken bones or joint sprains? Joint inflammation?
   - Neurological: Seizures? Movement disorders? Tremors? Tics? Loss-of-consciousness episodes?
   - Endocrine: Problems with growth or pubescence?
   - Hematological: Anemia history or symptoms? Blood transfusions? Bleeding disorders?
   - Dentition: Number of teeth and eruption pattern? Dental trauma? Dental care? Use of fluoride? Teeth brushing? Toothaches?

3. Family history of diseases:
   - Mother and father: Ages and health history.

- Mother's pregnancy history: Number of pregnancies, births, status of offspring.
- Familial diseases: Age, sex, and health status of each family member. Familial and communicable diseases such as diabetes, epilepsy, tuberculosis, hypertension or heart disease, cancer, sickle cell anemia, birth defects, known genetic disorders?
- Genogram: Draw out a genogram of the family members, including sex, age, and health status of each member. (See Chapters 3 and 41 for genogram notations.)

FUNCTIONAL HEALTH DOMAIN DATABASE. The questions in this section are organized by functional health patterns and relate to the nursing diagnoses for each pattern.

1. Health maintenance/health perceptions: All people take steps to influence and protect their health. These choices include selection of health care providers, use of safety devices, learning how to take care of one's self, and daily care of the body. Nursing diagnoses can include health-seeking behavior, altered health maintenance, or noncompliance to a preventive or adaptive health care regimen. Usual data include
   - Usual primary care provider—last visit?
   - Dentist—last visit?
   - Child's self-care or caregiver needs for more knowledge of caregiving?
   - Health care recommendations that the family chooses not to follow?
   - Safety measures used. Car seats or seat belts? Smoke and carbon monoxide alarms? Window screens? Home safety measures? Firearms in the home? Ipecac available?
   - Routine health promotion regimens?
   - Home and health management resource issues for the chronically ill or handicapped child? Home nursing? Equipment needs? Transportation needs?

2. Nutrition: Quality and quantity of the daily diet and the processes of feeding and swallowing. Data to support diagnoses such as nutrition less than or greater than body requirements, anorexia, bulimia, impaired swallowing, and the breastfeeding diagnoses would be found in this section.
   - Daily diet—breakfast, lunch, and dinner?

- Supplements/vitamins?
- Feeding patterns—meal times and snack times? Feeding strategies? Self-feeding skills? Breastfeeding and bottle-feeding issues?
- Nutritional restrictions—calories, other?
- Satisfaction with weight?
- Difficulties chewing or swallowing?

3. Activities: Physical mobility as well as the diversional and occupational activities of daily life should be described here.
   - Amount, timing, and types of physical activities?
   - Television time?
   - Reading time?
   - Play opportunities and activities in which the child engages?
   - Sports, organized activities, and hobbies of older children and adolescents?
   - Activity limitations caused by health problems?
   - Special equipment used or needed to support mobility?

4. Sleep: Sleep and rest patterns are described here. Hours? Disturbances for the child or family? Sleep aids? Sleep position for infants.

5. Elimination: Problems of elimination can be analyzed at the physiological level of the genitourinary or gastrointestinal systems or in terms of daily living patterns. Enuresis and encopresis are daily living problems (bowel and bladder habits) that fall in this area. Physiologically, the child is well but the elimination habits are not functioning well.
   - Urinary patterns: Bed wetting? Toilet training? Voiding schedule?
   - Bowel patterns: Constipation or soiling? Stooling patterns? Toilet training?

6. Role relationships: Role relationships include family relationships and relationships with peers and friends in the community. Both family and individual diagnoses need to be considered here. Family coping, family process alteration, parenting alteration, abuse, and social interaction or isolation can be addressed.
   - Family interactions: Between parents? Parents and children? With other family members?
   - Parenting style and activities?

- Peers/social supports for the child and family? Special adults in the child's life?
- Communication with and by the child: Verbal? Nonverbal?

7. Coping/temperament and discipline used: People select and use a variety of coping strategies in their daily lives. Temperament is also important to understand child behavior and likely responses to the environment. The discipline strategies used are important to identify. Anxiety, fear, hopelessness, grief, powerlessness, substance abuse, pain, and potential for violence might be identified nursing diagnoses.
   - Stressors for the child and family? Losses?
   - Coping strategies of the child and caregivers?
   - Use of alcohol or drugs?
   - Temperament characteristics of the child and the "fit" with other family members?
   - Problem behavior, discipline strategies used and their outcomes?

8. Cognitive/perceptual: Cognitive or perceptual problems are identified here. Attention deficit disorder is an example. Also, when hearing, vision, tactile, or taste senses are impaired, the functional health problems are identified here and adaptations needed to cope with the impairment considered.
   - Hearing or vision problems?
   - Attention problems?
   - Adaptations made at home and school to assist the child, especially for problems of comprehension.

9. Self-perception/self-concept: Personal role identity, body image, and self-esteem are issues to be identified here.
   - Satisfaction with self?
   - Feelings of depression?

10. Sexual: All people have sexuality issues that affect their lives. Within their sexual preferences and habits, problems are identified when these patterns are interrupted or viewed as problematic by the client or family. Pregnancy, viewed from the psychosocial perspective, is also identified here.
    - Sexual habits?
    - Sexual relationships?
    - Development of sexual identity?

11. Values and beliefs/religion: In this last section, the NP explores religious patterns and

personal values and beliefs that affect functional health patterns and health.
- Involvement with church?
- Religious rituals?
- Sense of alienation?
- Values the family wants to impart to their children?

DEVELOPMENT DOMAIN DATABASE. The levels of motor, language, cognitive, and social development are assessed and documented in this area. Both past milestones and current functioning are important. Sometimes, developmental tests are administered to provide data in this area.

- Motor landmarks—sitting, standing, walking, and so on
- Language landmarks—words, sentences, intelligibility, understanding
- Personal and social—play, attachment, self-care, peer relationships
- Scholastic grade and progress

After the history is completed, the physical examination is conducted and the results recorded. Laboratory or other tests are also obtained. The problem list is derived from the history and physical examination data.

THE INTERVAL HISTORY

The complete history should need to be completed only once for new patients. After that, for routine scheduled health maintenance visits, the history is updated only from the last contact to the present. The format remains the same as for the complete history; however, questions are modified to verify that the situations are as they were in the past or to add new information. All areas of the history should be assessed.

THE EPISODIC HISTORY

Many times, patients come for help with specific problems. The history includes the chief complaint and history of present illness sections of the complete history. The framework for dealing with these problems is as follows, with each symptom dealt with in chronological sequence:

Symptom Analysis:
1. Onset—initial and episodic. Date and time, sudden or gradual, setting
2. Location—local, radiation, generalized, superficial, or deep
3. Duration
4. Characteristics and course
   - Symptom quality: Nature of symptoms
   - Symptom quantity: Severity, frequency, volume, number, size or extent, degree of functional impairment
   - Course: Continuous or intermittent, pattern of variation
5. Activating (precipitating) and aggravating factors
6. Relieving factors and patient's reactions to symptoms
7. Tests and treatment: What, when, where, who, and results, including complications and sequelae

Even though the patient comes in for a specific problem, always ask some screening questions that tap into the other domains of the history—disease, daily living, and/or developmental. At visits for minor illnesses, health promotion and disease prevention issues should be considered, as well as the problem at hand. The potential for giving immunizations should be considered at every visit.

The Physical Examination and Laboratory and Other Studies

THE PHYSICAL EXAMINATION

The physical examination is conducted next (although younger children might do better with developmental testing preceding the physical examination). Height, weight, head circumference, and vital signs are recorded here also. Principal findings that the NP is expected to identify are presented in the following list. Screening hearing and vision tests, as well as laboratory data and data from other disciplines, are included as other types of objective information.

1. General appearance: Ill or well, distressed, alert, cooperative, body build. Reaction to parents. Characteristic position, movements, nutrition, developmental appearance as contrasted with the stated age.

2. Skin: Color—pigmentation, cyanosis, jaundice, carotenemia, erythema, pallor. Vascular—visible veins, arteries. Eruptions, petechiae, ecchymosis, hives, rashes. Nodules. Texture, scaling, striae, scars. Sweat, edema, turgor. Subcutaneous tissue. Distribution and color of hair. Nail appearance.

3. Lymph nodes: Occipital, postauricular, cervical, parotid, submaxillary, sublingual, axillary, epitrochlear, inguinal. Size, mobility, tenderness, heat.

4. Head: Position, shape, sutures, fontanels. Size—circumference, microcephaly, macrocephaly, hydrocephaly. Facial paralysis, twitching.

5. Eyes: Vision, visual fields. Blinking. Position—exophthalmos, enophthalmos, hypertelorism, hypotelorism. Movements—strabismus, extraocular movements, nystagmus. Ptosis, eyelids, sclera, conjunctivae. Lesions—styes, chalazion. Corneas, corneal reflex. Discharge. Pupils, accommodation, iris. Retina, red reflex, fundus.

6. Ears: Anomalies. Position. Discharge. Tenderness. Canals. Drums—redness, light reflex, landmarks, bulging or retraction, perforation, mobility. Mastoid, nodes. Hearing. Vestibular function.

7. Nose: Shape. Alae nasi, flaring. Mucosa, secretions, bleeding, airway. Septum. Polyps, tumors.

8. Mouth: Odor. Teeth—number, edges, occlusion, caries, formation, color. Gums—discoloration, bleeding. Buccal mucosa, tongue—coating, color, tremor. Palate—cleft, arch. Tonsils—size, color, exudate. Pharynx—appearance, color, lesions.

9. Neck: Size. Anomalies—webbing, edema, nodes, masses. Sternocleidomastoids. Trachea. Thyroid. Vessels. Neurological—opisthotonos, Brudzinski's sign. Motion—head drop, tilting, nodding, range of motion.

10. Chest: Shape—circumference, symmetry, Harrison's groove. Movement—flaring, expansion, abdominal/thoracic breathing, intercostal retractions.

11. Breasts: Tanner stage of development, symmetry, redness, heat, tenderness, lumps. Gynecomastia.

12. Lungs: Respiration—type, rate, dyspnea. Exercise tolerance. Cough, hemoptysis, sputum. Palpation—masses, tenderness, fremitus. Percussion—dullness, hyperresonance, diaphragm. Auscultation—breath sounds, crackles (rales), rubs, rhonchi, wheezes, vocal resonance, peristalsis.

13. Cardiovascular/heart: Blood pressure and pulse rate.
    • Inspection: Vascularity, bulging, impulse. Distress, cyanosis, edema, clubbing, pulsations, venous distention.
    • Palpation: Femoral pulses, point of maximal impulse, thrill.
    • Percussion: Location, size.
    • Auscultation: First and second heart sounds, rhythm, split, third heart sound, gallop, friction rub, venous hum, murmurs.

14. Abdomen:
    • Inspection: Shape, distention, transillumination. Umbilicus, diastasis rectus, veins. Peristaltic, gastric waves.
    • Palpation: Superficial or deep tenderness, rebound. Spleen, liver, masses, kidneys, bladder, uterus.
    • Percussion: Masses, fluid, flatus.
    • Auscultation: Bowel sounds, bruits.

15. Genitalia: Discharge, foreign body. Tags. Labia, adhesions, vagina, clitoris. Penis—hypospadias, epispadias, phimosis. Meatus, scrotum, testes, hydrocele, hernia. Cremasteric reflex. Tanner's staging. Vaginal, bimanual examination for teenage girls. (Pelvic examination observations are discussed further in the gynecology chapter.)

16. Anus and rectum: Buttocks, fistula, fissure, prolapse, polyps, hemorrhoids, rashes. Rectal—rectum, fistula, megacolon, masses, prostate, uterus, tenderness. Sensation.

17. Musculoskeletal: Anomalies, length, clubbing, pain, tenderness, temperature, swelling, shape.
    • Gait: Stance, balance, limp. Feet.
    • Spine: Tufts of hair, dimples, masses, spina bifida, tenderness, mobility, scoliosis.
    • Posture: Lordosis, kyphosis.
    • Joints: Heat, tenderness, mobility, swelling, effusion.

• Muscles: Development, pain, tone, spasm, paralysis, rigidity, contractures, atrophy.
18. Nervous system:
   • General impression, abilities, responsiveness, position, spontaneous movements, play activity.
   • Development.
   • State of consciousness, irritability, seizure activity.
   • Gait, stance, limp, ataxia. Coordination, Romberg's sign.
   • Tremors, twitching, choreiform movements, athetosis, spasticity, paralysis, flaccidity.
   • Reflexes: Superficial, deep tendon, clonus, Chvostek's sign.
   • Primitive reflexes: Moro, tonic neck, Babinski, grasp, suck. Thumb position.
   • Sensation: Hyperesthesia, paresthesia, temperature, touch. Stereognosis.
   • Cranial nerves I to XII.
   • Hearing and vision.

OTHER DATA

LABORATORY AND RADIOGRAPHIC DATA. Record hearing, vision, hematocrit or other blood test, lead, urinalysis, newborn screening tests, tuberculosis screening.

DEVELOPMENTAL AND/OR PSYCHOLOGICAL TEST SCORES. Scores need to be recorded and considered when problems are being identified.

DATA FROM OTHER DISCIPLINES. Summarize social work, nutrition, physical therapy, occupational therapy, medical specialist, speech pathology, education, and other reports.

Creating the Problem List

The problem list is derived from analysis of the subjective and objective data collected. Differential diagnosis is the mental process used to derive the problems listed. To use this process, the clinician considers all the possible diagnoses for the problems presented by the patient. Then the factors that support or rule out each of the various options considered are analyzed. The best fit of subjective and objective data with the possible diagnoses is the goal. If further data are needed to confirm a diagnosis, collection of these data is incorporated into the plan. For example, the differential diagnoses for coryza (a runny nose) include, among others, allergic rhinitis, upper respiratory infection, and a foreign body in the nose. The NP uses data about related symptoms (e.g., itchy eyes, a sore throat, systemic symptoms, and/or bilateral or unilateral drainage from the nostrils) to choose which diagnosis best fits the child's picture. That analysis for fit is the diagnostic reasoning process.

Functional health problems and developmental problems are also subject to the notion of differential diagnosis. For example, a child who is not sleeping well might be fearful, a trained night feeder, or experiencing episodes of obstructive sleep apnea. The interventions for each problem are quite different. Thus the NP must use the differential diagnosis process to identify the problem or problems at hand. If care is planned or given, a problem must be listed. Likewise, a problem should *never* be listed on the problem list that is not supported by subjective and objective data found and recorded in the database. "Rule out" should not be listed as a diagnosis. The diagnosis would be the unexplained symptom, e.g., "dysuria" or "dysuria, r/o urinary tract infection."

Creating the Management Plan

A plan must be developed for every identified problem. It is helpful to consider *diagnostic, therapeutic,* and *educational* interventions for every problem listed. Of course, not every problem requires work in all three areas, but they should be considered. The management activities are listed in the record. The plan should always include a recommendation for the next visit and what is to be done at that visit in an attempt to move the patient into health maintenance rather than only episodic visits. In the same way as the problem list must be consistent with the data at hand, plans should *never* be made for problems that are not listed in the problem list. In other words, the plan is internally consistent with the data and diagnoses.

Validating Data Collection

Data collection for clinical practice, just as for research, needs to be as reliable and valid as possible. To assist with reliability, consider the following techniques (Burns, 1991b):

TEST-RETEST

Ask the question again later. Take a blood pressure reading twice. Look for the physical finding a second time a bit later.

INTERRATER RELIABILITY

Ask someone else to listen, palpate, and so on for the same finding. Does someone else get the same answer to the same question you asked?

INTERNAL CONSISTENCY

Look for a logical consistency to the findings you are getting. If something is out of sync, question it. For example, do the height points on the graph line up, or is one badly off the trajectory? If it is, consider a measuring error before looking for a significant health problem that has altered growth. Does the history support the physical findings? Does the story keep changing?

Algorithms, protocols, and flow sheets can improve the consistency and reliability of the data collected, especially when several staff members are involved with the data for a given patient.

To assess the validity, or meaning, of data collected, the provider should consider sources of error:

- Do the cumulative data fit and support a given diagnosis? If not, perhaps the diagnosis was inadequate or an error in data collection, sequencing, or interpretation occurred.
- Was the diagnosis made on the basis of one isolated finding or a cluster? For instance, diagnosing pneumonia after hearing a cough and diagnosing failure to thrive with one growth measurement are mono-operation bias errors.
- Sometimes two problems occur with overlapping findings. One problem might be missed while the other is pursued.
- The patient might change the data provided because of stress or worry about the outcomes of the assessment visit. Both findings and their meaning to patients need to be explored with the patient and family.
- Provider expectations can also threaten accurate diagnosing.
- Were cues missed or questions unasked?
- Data are often compared with specific criteria (e.g., heights and weights for age are known, developmental milestones are established, laboratory norms are set for children of different ages). Which test has been used? What is its specificity and sensitivity? Is the right criterion being used?
- Clinicians constantly need to attend to age, sex, race, culture, and other issues when they consider data. Is it likely for a white child to have sickle cell disease? What diagnoses should one consider when a teenage girl has abdominal pain, as opposed to the diagnoses possible for a boy of the same age?

▩ SUMMARY

The assessment of a child and family is the basis for all the primary care work that NPs do. The knowledge and skills needed for accurate, comprehensive, individualized care are considerable and will develop over time. Data collection begins with collection of a health history. A physical examination and laboratory and developmental testing data are added to the historical data. From the total database, the clinician develops a list of diagnoses and a plan of care for each. Errors either in data collection or in analysis can result in diagnostic errors, which always need to be minimized.

REFERENCES

American Medical Association, Department of Adolescent Health: Guidelines for Adolescent Preventive Services (GAPS) User's Manual. Chicago, American Medical Association, 1994.

Burns C: Development and content validity testing of a comprehensive classification of diagnoses for use by pediatric nurse practitioners. Nurs Diagn 2:93–104, 1991a.

Burns C: Parallels between research and diagnosis: The reliability and validity issues of clinical practice. Nurs Pract 16:42–50, 1991b.

Burns C: A new assessment model and tool for nurse practitioners. J Pediatr Health Care 6:73–81, 1992a.

Burns C: Using a comprehensive taxonomy of diagnoses to describe the practice of pediatric nurse practitioners: Findings of a field study. J Pediatr Health Care 7:115–121, 1992b.

Gordon M: Nursing Diagnosis: Process and Application. New York, McGraw-Hill, 1987.

North American Nursing Diagnosis Association: NANDA Nursing Diagnoses: Definitions and Classification 1997–98. Philadelphia, North American Nursing Diagnosis Association, 1996.

US Department of Health and Human Services: International Classification of Diseases, 9th rev ed, Clinical Modification. DHHS Publication No. PHS 80-1260. Washington, DC, US Government Printing Office, 1981.

CHAPTER 3

Family Assessment in Pediatric Primary Care

Sheila M. Kodadek

INTRODUCTION

Family-centered, community-based primary care for children is recognized as the best possible practice model for providing health-care services to children and their families. Nurse practitioners (NPs) perhaps understand this point better than any other group of primary care providers, but they, like their colleagues, face significant challenges in implementing family-centered care. At minimum, family-centered care is perceived as time consuming. In addition, families are still too often viewed from a pathology-based model borrowed from psychiatry and psychology, and primary care providers often report feeling inadequate to the task of working with the complex and often stressed families they meet in their practices (Wells & Stein, 1999).

However daunting the perceived barriers to family-centered care, investing in family assessment and management is essential in contemporary pediatric primary care practice. Duffy (1988) wrote over a decade ago that understanding family health promotion begins with understanding family dynamics. Research has repeatedly demonstrated that a mother's level of education, her beliefs and attitudes about health, and her own health practices have a significant influence on the health status of her children. As fathers have increasingly become involved in their children's health care, questions about relationships between characteristics of fathers and family health behavior are being raised. It is not surprising that parents who believe that they can improve their health status by practicing health promotion behavior tend to raise children who share similar beliefs.

Research has provided us with definitive evidence that children, from birth through adolescence, need nurturing time and attention from the significant adults in their lives (Gunnar, 1998; Resnick et al., 1997). These significant adults most often are the child's birth or adoptive parents, but they may also be grandparents, extended family members, or foster parents. Evidence is strong that when children are raised without this consistent, affectionate attention and without sensitive interactions with a caring adult, the results can be devastating for both the child and society (Gunnar et al., 1996; Nachmias et al., 1996; Perry & Pollard, 1998). In contrast, when a parent or another significant adult responds consistently and sensitively to a child's needs, such as a need to play, to eat, to sleep, to be comforted, or to be left alone, the child is likely to grow up competent to initiate and build strong, nurturing relationships (Gunnar, 1998; Resnick et al., 1997).

Histories of physical or emotional neglect alone have increasingly been associated with children and adolescents who are withdrawn, anxious, and socially isolated (Ogawa et al., 1997; Perry & Pollard, 1998). Although inadequate or poor parenting is linked in the literature to factors such as poverty, substance abuse, and minimal education, contemporary research suggests that a poor "fit" between a child and a significant adult can occur in any family, including those in which the adults are well educated, socially competent, and economically successful (Perry & Pollard, 1998). For example, parents who value competition and athletic success may be a good parenting fit for their daughter who is star of her soccer team. However, they may not be able to connect with their younger son, who prefers reading to sports and who avoids competition in all forms.

This chapter begins with the assumption that families are central to and inseparable from the health of children. It is based on a family health promotion framework that assumes that the vast majority of family members are competent, want to do what is best for their children, and desire to be active participants in their children's health care. It describes characteristics of expert nursing practice with families. Finally, this chapter presents an approach to family assessment that can be incorporated with relative ease into a busy primary care practice.

BACKGROUND

It is said that three families are present in every primary care encounter: the family of the patient, the family of the NP, and the "family" of the practice, agency, or unit. The health- and illness-related beliefs, values, and behavior of each of these families have a significant potential to influence the outcome of the encounter.

Research evidence links expert nursing practice in a variety of settings and specialties with knowledge and skills in family nursing, particularly because such nursing practice reflects an appreciation of the complex interactions linking the health status of individuals with their families (Chesla, 1996; Kitzman et al., 1997; Olds et al., 1997). Family nursing practice is based on the assumption that families are influential in how an individual defines health. Families also teach behaviors used to promote health and prevent disease and manage illnesses and healing. These assumptions go far beyond the

biological contribution made through blood ties within families and equally far beyond the limited view of families as convenient (or unavoidable) caregivers.

The importance of family can be seen more readily in delivery of primary care to children than to adults. In general, pediatric NPs encounter far more family members in the course of their practice than do adult primary care providers. A child is usually accompanied by a family member who, at minimum, is legally responsible for the child's welfare. As stated earlier, children are dependent on their families "to create a nurturing environment to assure physical survival and personal development" (Terkelsen, 1980). In turn, NPs are dependent on families, primarily on parents, to accomplish health-related goals for children. Entering into a true partnership with parents, with NPs as expert consultants, sets the stage for optimal pediatric health care.

Expert nursing practice that honors the family's critical roles in a child's health outcomes is characterized by the following: recognition and validation of the family's primary position in a child's world; provision of perspective, knowledge, and skills to families; facilitation of access of family members to ill or suffering members; assistance for family members who need to emotionally reconnect with ill or suffering members; and assistance for families to mobilize their healing capacities when needed (Chesla, 1996). This level of expert care is possible when NPs have knowledge of normal family development and family systems, are aware of their own participation in systems, and incorporate systematic family assessment in their practice.

THE ASSESSMENT MODEL

Family assessment in primary care practice with children requires attention to family structure, family life cycle stage, family functioning, and social network. In other words, a basic family assessment addresses characteristics of the family, transitions that the family is experiencing, how family members interact and get things done, what they believe and value, and how they interact with the community.

It is important to recognize that NPs' own definitions of family and healthy family functioning are culturally and temporally bound, determine who is and who is not family, and can profoundly affect assessment, treatment, and outcomes. NPs might find it useful to periodically examine their own assumptions and beliefs regarding families and use the knowledge gained to foster increased sensitivity and openness to the rich diversity that their clients present.

Legal definitions of family usually address bonds of blood, marriage, and adoption. A significant number of contemporary families do not fit such restrictive definitions. To address this reality, Whall (1986) defined family as "a self-identified group of two or more individuals whose association is characterized by special terms, who may or may not be related by blood lines or law, but who function in such a way that they consider themselves to be a family." Wherever NPs' personal definitions might fall on a continuum of inclusiveness, it is imperative that they know and understand the implications of that definition in practice.

Many family assessment models and tools can be used in primary care practice. The following is a baseline assessment model that provides NPs with essential data on which to build a management plan. It is tailored for a relatively busy practice, can be done in stages across visits, and invites additional data entries to update the family database over time.

Family Structure and Roles

Assessment of a family's structure and roles includes the composition of the family or household, demographic data, intergenerational data, and information about family roles. Implicit in the data is the way the family defines itself (i.e., who the family says is "family") and how the family gets its work done.

Family Life Cycle

Family life cycle assessment includes data on the present family life cycle stage (such as a family with young children), family life cycle transitions or developmental crises (such as serious illness of a frail, elderly grandparent), and

family life cycle events that are untimely or "out of sync" (such as the terminal illness of a young wife and mother).

Family Functioning

Healthy family functioning should result in what Terkelsen (1980) called the "good-enough family." Families have both strengths and limitations, but the majority of families are able to meet most of their members' needs most of the time. This is a hopeful stance, one that allows for the less than perfect family to feel successful and empowered.

Characteristics of healthy family functioning have been identified by a number of researchers, and lists differ. For example, deChesnay (1986) used an extensive research literature review to identify healthy families as those characterized by open communication, mutual respect and support, differentiation, shared problem solving, shared decision making, flexibility, and enhancement of personal growth of members. Additions to that list might include a sense of play and humor (Curran, 1983), a shared spiritual value system (Curran, 1983; Lewis et al., 1976; Stinnett et al., 1979), and a shared value of service to others (Curran, 1983).

Family Social Network

The family's social network includes those persons, activities, agencies, and institutions that have the potential to support, harm, or drain energy from the family. Assessing the family's relationships with extended family, friends, and the community provides information on which to base recommendations and further assessment.

FAMILY DATABASE

Genograms and Ecomaps

The construction of genograms and ecomaps, two approaches to developing a family database, is described in the following sections. Neither requires the purchase of standardized assessment tools, and both can be updated over time, a characteristic making them valuable to NPs in understanding patterns in children and families. Together, the genogram and ecomap assist NPs in assessing family structure and roles, life cycle transitions, family functioning, and social networks in a relatively quick and efficient manner. Both have the advantage of providing a means for interacting with children and their family members in a focused, non-threatening way around potentially complex and difficult issues. Both also are inherently appealing to families. They help families see themselves in new ways and provide ways for families to be partners in their own diagnosis and management.

Clinicians who use genograms and ecomaps in their practice frequently come to the conclusion that the tools are as useful for intervention as they are for assessment. In addition, nurse clinicians working with children find that including the children in the construction and updating of genograms and ecomaps helps children be active in their own care, as well as provides data on family interactions (Visscher & Clore, 1992).

GENOGRAMS

Genograms are sociometric, paper-and-pencil tools used to depict a family's composition and history across generations (Fig. 3–1). Although not essential, computer programs to facilitate genogram data management have become available in recent years and can be easily included in computerized patient records. These programs have made updating genogram data easy and efficient. Genograms are appealing to clinicians because they provide graphic representations of complex family data; they allow clinicians to map family structure clearly and to update the picture as it emerges; they are an efficient clinical summary; they make it easier for clinicians to keep in mind family members, patterns, and events that may have recurring significance in a family's ongoing care; they help clinicians think systematically about how events and relationships in their clients' lives are related to patterns of health and illness; and they are a subjective, interpretive tool with which the clinician can generate tentative hypotheses for further systematic evaluation

(Like et al., 1988; McGoldrick & Gerson, 1985; Rogers & Cohn, 1987; Visscher & Clore, 1992).

Priorities for organizing genogram data for clinical use rely less on formal blood and legal links and more on repetitive symptoms and relationships or functioning patterns seen across the family or over generations. Genograms highlight coincidences of dates, such as deaths and symptoms, and the impact of change and untimely life cycle transitions (McGoldrick & Gerson, 1985).

Genograms are meant to be a part of a general health assessment. They are most effective when constructed during an initial visit with children and their families and then revised as new information becomes available.

The NP begins by drawing a basic family tree, with the family members present guiding identification of family members. Because the primary purpose of using a genogram in primary care is not to trace genetic lines, the use of symbols to indicate relationships can be less rigorous. In fact, it can be more informative and useful to learn who is living in a household than who is related by blood or birth.

Conventional symbols used in genograms can be seen in Figure 3–1. Again, the purpose of the family genogram is primarily psychosocial, and symbols that speak eloquently to legal and blood lines may be perceived as offensive to both parents and children. For example, use of solid lines to connect birth children to parents and broken lines to connect adopted children to parents may be precise but may also suggest parent–child relationship differences that do not exist. In practice, it is more informative and respectful to let the family decide how to indicate relationships.

As mentioned earlier, it is clinically useful to identify members of the current household in which children live. This objective can be met by drawing a circle around the members of the genogram who currently live together; for example, the circle may include parents and three children, or it may include one of two parents, two of three children, and a grandparent. It is also useful to include at least three generations of the family.

Health history information, including serious medical, behavioral, and emotional problems, can be noted on the genogram; examples in-

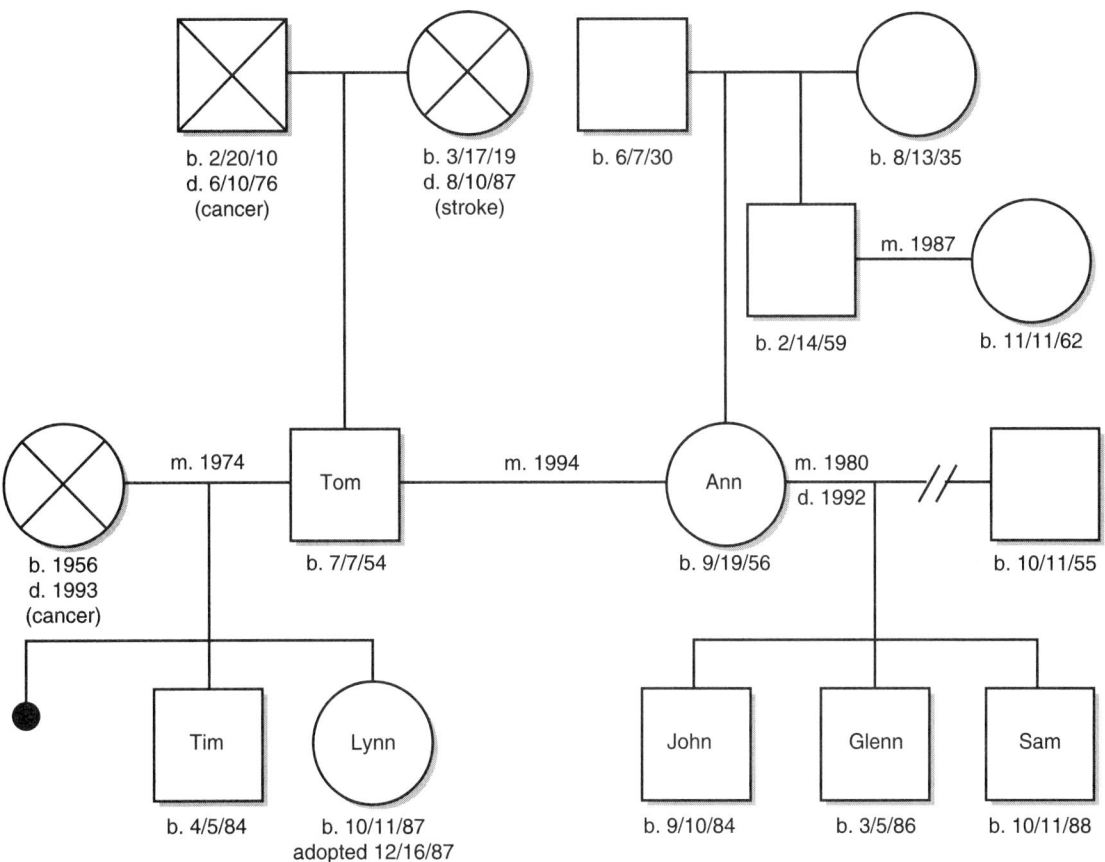

FIGURE 3-1
A three-generational genogram

clude drug or alcohol problems, serious problems with the law, and causes of death. Likewise, family information that is significant to the health of the child can be included, such as ethnic background, language spoken in the home, education of parents, occupations, religious affiliation, major family moves, and current location of family members. Significant others who live with or are important to the family should be included, including family friends, foster parents, and baby sitters. In some cases, the significant other is a family pet.

Practical pointers include using pencil instead of pen, leaving space at the bottom of the page for notes, and including a key to notations or unusual symbols. It also is useful to provide child patients with their own paper and pencils or crayons to use while conducting

the interview; they might even draw a picture of their family for you.

The genogram interview can begin with an open question, such as "Tell me about your family." It can be addressed to children, to parents, or to both. As the genogram is being constructed, questions can be used to elicit information about family functioning. McGoldrick and Gerson (1985) suggest the following order of questions; the specific questions are suggestions only and are not exhaustive.

Chief Problem and the Immediate Family

Family Composition and Structure
Who is in your family?
Who currently lives with you and your child?

If the relationships are not clear: How are you related to the members of your household?

If divorce or separation is involved: Where does the child's other parent live? What are the custody and visitation agreements? How often does the child see or hear from the other parent?

Who in your family was involved in the decision to come here today?

If a health-related problem is involved:
How do other members of your family see this problem?
With whom will you discuss today's visit when you go home?

Current Family Situation

An understanding of the current family situation is helpful, especially if a significant time period has elapsed since the child and family were last seen. Understanding changes that the family is facing and where they are in the family life cycle is also important:

Have there been any major stresses in your family since your last visit?
Have there been any changes in your family since your last visit?
What, if any, changes do you anticipate in the near future?

Extended Family Context

The following questions suggest a way to begin to collect data about extended family members. This information may not seem relevant to parents or children, but patterns that can have an impact on children's health often do not become evident until this kind of intergenerational mapping is done. This more extensive mapping of a family may be used when the clinical picture includes conflicting information or when the effectiveness of a prevention activity is a concern. For example, knowing that both the mother and grandmother of the young adolescent in your office became pregnant at 14 and dropped out of high school may be helpful in deciding how to best use a brief visit.

It would help me to help your child if I knew more about your child's grandpar-

ents, aunts, uncles, and other relatives. Let's begin with your mother's family.
When was your mother born? Where? Who were her parents?
Who was in her family while she was growing up?
Is she living? (If yes) Where does she live now? How often do you have contact with her? (If no) When did she die? What was the cause of death?
How did she meet your father? When were they married (if applicable)? (And so on.)

Demographic Data

Demographic data include dates of birth, death, adoption, marriage, separation, divorce, significant illness, and major family events; culture/ethnicity; religion; education; and occupations. The NP can probe for more information about specific data as they appear to be significant in a given situation. For example, faith and strength of adherence to a specific religion may have an unexpected impact on care decisions for a child. Disagreement about adherence within a family may result in mixed messages and uneven follow-through with a treatment plan.

Historical Perspective

Knowledge of the timing and repetition of significant family events or behavior may be helpful. For example, adolescent pregnancy, alcohol abuse, dropping out of high school, and suicide may be patterns of behavior in a family's intergenerational history.

If gaps in data become evident, they need to be explored. It is also helpful to keep in mind events external to the family that may have influenced family choices. For example, the years of conflict in Vietnam interrupted many life plans, with effects seen in the present generation. Immigration, voluntary or forced, can have an impact on family health status. Natural disasters such as floods, hurricanes, and droughts have changed family histories and the health status of family members.

Family Relationships and Roles

In developing the database, NPs can begin to probe for family relationships and roles. For example, understanding how parents make decisions and solve problems can be useful in helping parents improve health promotion practices. Examples of questions that can lead to an increased appreciation for a specific family include the following:

How would you describe your parenting style? How does it compare with your partner's?

Who in your family is responsible for monitoring your children's health?

What does your family enjoy most about this child?

What are some of the things you do together as a family? How often?

How do you generally make important decisions in your family?

To whom does your child tend to tell problems and concerns?

How do family members show their support for one another?

How well do you think your family adapts to change?

How does your family nurture the interests and talents of each individual family member?

To whom do you go for advice about being a good parent? Why do you go to that person?

How do you deal with unwanted advice from family members about raising your child(ren)?

In summary, genograms provide clinicians with data about family structure, life cycle fit, pattern repeating across generations, life experiences, and relational patterns (Like et al., 1988; McGoldrick & Gerson, 1985).

Targeted Assessments

Families come with a variety of issues, some of which are related to the composition and structure of the family. Family-related issues may have the potential to influence the health and well-being of children and adolescents in significant ways. Although much about family assessment remains constant across families, it is useful to pay attention to some of the unique potential family variations.

WORKING PARENTS AND CHILD CARE. When a single parent works outside the home or both parents in a two-parent family work outside the home, specific considerations involve all members of the family. The following are examples of questions to help parents explore the interface between work and home.

What tensions do you anticipate (or are you experiencing) to be associated with balancing work and home?

What child care arrangements have you made? How satisfactory are they? What would you change if you could?

How do you manage care for a child who is ill on a workday?

MULTIPLE BIRTHS. A family faced with caring for newborn twins, triplets, or more, even while delighted, can be quickly overwhelmed by the responsibility and amount of work involved. Assessing parents' level of fatigue, ability to seek and accept support, and plans for ongoing care is useful to both the NP and the parents.

Have things gone as you expected with the babies?

When you have questions about their care, whom do you ask?

Have you had help from your partner? Family members? Friends?

How are your babies similar? How do they differ from one another?

How have you managed those times that happen to all new parents when you feel overwhelmed?

How have the babies' sibling(s) responded to them?

FAMILIES WITH A PREMATURE INFANT. Low birth weight and premature infants present special issues for new parents. There may be an extended time between the birth of the child and being able to bring the child home. Concerns about the child's physiological vulnerability may arise. Almost certainly, costs and time commitments around the care of the infant will be increased. Parents may have similar concerns to those of parents of a full-term newborn, but their fears and anxieties about being responsible for a seemingly fragile newborn may be close to overwhelming.

Similar to the situation of a multiple birth,

exploring who is caring for the child and who is helping the parents is a priority.

BLENDED FAMILIES. A blended family is one in which two adults create a reorganized family by joining together with their children from previous relationships. Although this term usually refers to families created by remarriage after divorce, it is also used to describe families created by remarriage after the death of spouses. Assessing how the children are coping with the significant changes in their lives can help both the NP and the parents direct their attention.

Have things gone as you expected they would in your new family?

How is each child coping with the new family?

How do their responses vary with their ages and developmental levels?

How has their child care or school situation changed and how have they responded?

What do the parents identify as the most significant loss for each child in the blended family? The most significant benefit?

How are the relationships between parents (including stepparent) and children?

How are the relationships among the stepsiblings?

How are the parents handling discipline issues?

SINGLE-PARENT FAMILIES. Single-parent families are relatively common in the United States today. Although the vast majority of single parents are women, fathers are increasingly raising their children in single-parent homes. Today, single parents may be adolescents enrolled in welfare programs or company executives with live-in nannies. Understanding the family context is essential.

Single parents across socioeconomic parameters do share the burden of raising a child alone. Even with help, the weight of responsibility is felt. Questions probing how the parent is managing as a single parent can be useful. Examples include the following:

What is the best thing about being your child's only parent?

What is most challenging for you about being a single parent?

How do you get the support you need as a parent?

What would most help you raise your child at this point in time?

ADOLESCENT PARENTS. Adolescents who become parents generally face the problems inherent when a major role is assumed before the adolescent is developmentally ready. Adolescent parents have developmental needs of their own, and not infrequently their needs are in conflict with those of their children. In addition, children of adolescent mothers are more likely than children of older mothers to have a low birth weight, to have ongoing health problems during childhood, to grow up in homes without fathers, and to be raised in poverty or near poverty. Questions that can help get a picture of the family in which a child will be raised include exploring the adolescent parent's own support system, attitudes toward parenting, and source of parenting advice. In addition, it is helpful to understand the adolescent's school status, child care arrangements, financial situation, and plans for the future.

GAY/LESBIAN PARENT FAMILIES. Gay and lesbian parents face the problems of all parents, with an added concern about societal attitudes and behavior that add stress to their lives and the lives of their children. These parents generally need support in raising their children to deal with beliefs and attitudes that may include isolation and teasing. Assessing the ability of these families to find and use community support is important, as is exploring their ideas about how they will prepare their children to handle curiosity, possible negative responses, and the experience of "being different."

ADOPTIVE PARENT FAMILIES. Adoptive parents come in every variety, married couples, single parents, gay and lesbian parents, grandparents or other extended family members, and so on. Assessment of these families includes asking about the legal status of the adoption, the timing of the adoption in the child's life, arrangements regarding involvement of the birth parents or other family members, decisions about how and when to tell the child about being adopted, and potential health concerns related to the birth parents or family, if known.

FOSTER PARENT FAMILIES. Children in foster

care are usually in some form of protective custody. These children, first and foremost, are at risk for deep-seated feelings of insecurity, loss, and anger. Assessment of these families includes exploration of the child's history that resulted in foster family placement, identification of health issues that precipitated or resulted from separation from the birth parents, and evaluation of the foster parent.

ECOMAP

Ecomaps are similar to genograms in their inherent and deceptive simplicity (Fig. 3-2). Ecomaps depict, in a clear and dynamic way, "the major systems that are a part of the family's life and the nature of the family's relationship with the various systems" (Hartman, 1978). Mapping of family relationships within and outside family boundaries highlights the nature of those relationships, their potential for support, conflicts in the relationships, and areas of current or potential strain and stress.

As with genograms, all that is needed is a piece of paper and a pencil. A large circle representing the family boundary is drawn in the center of the paper; smaller circles representing different parts of the environment (individuals, organizations and institutions, hobbies, work, and so on) are drawn around the large circle.

Inside the large circle, a genogram depiction of the family members in the household is drawn. Family members are then asked to label the smaller circles with those people, places, and activities, whether enjoyable, stressful, or both, that make up their world. Examples of labels include extended family members, friends, work, school, band practice, church or synagogue, camping, exercise, and health care.

Connections between individual family members or the family as a whole and the smaller circles are then drawn. Coded lines and brief descriptions are used to indicate the strength and quality of the relationships. Common codes for the lines include

- A solid line for a strong connection, with one to three additional lines added to indicate increasing degree of strength
- A broken line for a tenuous connection or relationship

- Hatch marks over a solid line for a stressful or conflicted relationship

Direction of the flow of energy, resources, or interest can be indicated by drawing arrows along the connecting lines. An example is a family with three children, one of whom loves school and does well (three solid lines with arrows pointing from school to the child), one of whom is an indifferent student but likes the social aspect of school (a dotted line with no arrows), and one who has serious academic problems and dreads going to school each morning (a solid line with hatch marks and arrows pointing from the child to school) (see Fig. 3-2).

Sometimes the whole family is connected to an activity, and the energy flow is similar for all members. For example, a family might identify a particular family friend as supportive. In other cases, the experience differs across family members. For example, family vacations may be positive for all members of the family except adolescents, who would prefer to stay home near their friends. A scarcity of connections outside the household suggests isolation and may be a problem if the family needs significant support during a crisis. A sheet full of circles may indicate a family overcommitted and overwhelmed by activities and responsibilities.

In summary, ecomaps provide both additional data about a family's social network and potential for social support. They also provide a way of validating information from the genogram interview, especially around family relationships and roles.

Selected Family Assessment Tools

The process of constructing a genogram and ecomap results in a fairly complete picture of the family's composition, social network, and family functioning. However, at times additional information is needed. The following assessment models and tools offer NPs other resources that are clinically relevant and reasonably efficient. In addition, the tools have research evidence of reliability and validity supporting their use in practice.

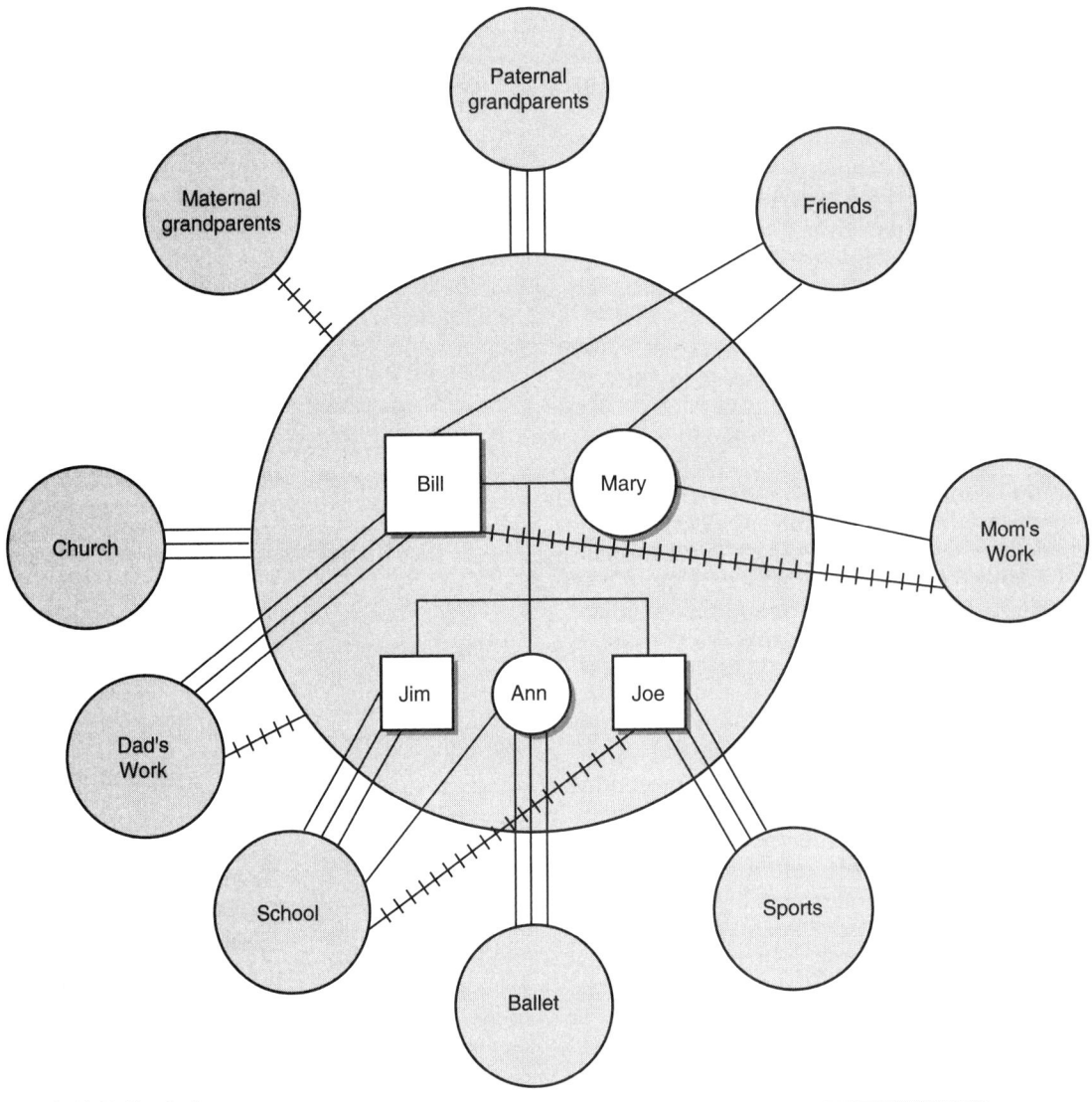

F I G U R E 3–2
Ecomap showing family with three children. Ecomaps can provide additional data.

COMPREHENSIVE FAMILY ASSESSMENT MODELS

These models provide ways to organize family assessment material. They can provide NPs with a database characterized by both breadth and depth.

- Calgary Family Assessment Model (CFAM) (Wright & Leahey, 1994)

- Family Health Assessment Form (Friedman, 1986)

FAMILY ASSESSMENT SCREENING TOOL

- Family Apgar (Smilkstein, 1978)

This screening tool is quick to administer (5 minutes) and provides an overview assessment of family functioning.

FAMILY FUNCTIONING TOOLS

These tools vary in length and complexity, but all are easy to score and provide NPs with in-depth data about family functioning.

- Family Adaptability and Cohesion Evaluation Scale (FACES III) (Olson et al., 1985) (Source: Family Social Sciences, University of Minnesota, 290 McNeal Hall, St Paul, MN 55108)
- Family Environment Scale (FES) (Moos, 1974)
- Feetham Family Functioning Survey (FFFS) (Feetham & Humerick, 1982)

FAMILY STRESS AND COPING TOOLS

These tools provide NPs with information about how families define and manage stress. They can be used to help families self-diagnose their strengths and identify areas needing modification.

- Assessing Adolescent Stress: Adolescent-Family Inventory of Life Events and Changes (A-FILE) (Olson et al., 1982) (Source: Family Social Sciences, University of Minnesota, 290 McNeal Hall, St Paul, MN 55108)
- Family Inventory of Life Events (FILE) (McCubbin & Patterson, 1983) (Source: McCubbin HI, Thompson AI: Family assessment inventories for research and practice. *In* Family Stress and Coping Project. Madison, WI, University of Wisconsin, 1987)
- Family Coping Strategies (F-COPES) (Olson et al., 1979) (Source: McCubbin HI, Thompson AI: Family assessment inventories for research and practice. *In* Family Stress and Coping Project. Madison, WI, University of Wisconsin, 1987)

Creating the Problem List

The problem list is derived from data collected during the family assessment. Similar to the child health assessment process, NPs working with family members identify possible family issues and problems and weigh them against what they know is occurring within the family

at that time. If further data are needed, time should be designated to explore the area of concern in more detail.

Creating the Management Plan

Again, similar to the child health assessment, a plan should be developed in collaboration with family members for every identified problem or issue. Management plans should be written in the record and evaluated at the next visit.

Research suggests that few, if any, adequately functioning families seek professional help for normal transitions in the life cycle (Olson et al., 1989). Requests for assistance with parenting, routine family caregiving, or other normative stressors can be met in the context of primary care practice. Education and supportive counseling can be done with a variety of strategies, including listening with empathy; normalizing when appropriate; providing individualized anticipatory guidance; offering suggestions of books, videos, and audiotapes; and referring to community support groups when appropriate and available.

Family conferences are a useful strategy for NPs when a pattern of recurring problems can be observed or when the family would clearly benefit from a group educational session. Family conferences are also essential at times of significant family stress or transition, including the onset of chronic illness, serious acute illness, significant psychosocial issues, lifestyle problems, terminal illness, and death.

Long-term management of significant family problems, problems that exceed a family's ability to adapt, or problems that exceed an NP's skills, time, or resources require referral for family therapy or counseling. Findings of family violence, chemical dependency, chronic depression or anxiety, or child neglect or maltreatment require a referral and, in some cases, a report to appropriate authorities. A list of family therapists and counselors is useful to have available for families in or near crisis. Families that are not functioning optimally but whose members are not endangered may need time to recognize their need for assistance.

NPs who use a family perspective in their practice do not need every possible bit of information about a family, nor do they need to interact with all family members. Incorporating a sensitivity to family issues in health care recommendations can be a major contribution to a family's well-being, even if the only person with whom NPs communicate is a worried parent.

REFERENCES

Chesla C: Reconciling technological and family care in critical-care nursing. Image 28:199-203, 1996.

Curran D: Traits of a Healthy Family. New York, Ballantine, 1983.

deChesnay M: Promoting healthy family functioning in acute care units. J Pediatr Nurs 1:96-101, 1986.

Duffy ME: Health promotion in the family: Current findings and directives for nursing research. J Adv Nurs 13:109-117, 1988.

Feetham SL, Humerick SS: The Feetham Family Functioning Survey. *In* Humerick SS (ed): Analysis of Current Assessment Strategies in the Health Care of Young Children and Childbearing Families. E Norwalk, CT, Appleton-Century-Crofts, 1982, pp 268-359.

Friedman MM: Family Nursing: Theory and Assessment, 2nd ed. E Norwalk, CT, Appleton-Century-Crofts, 1986.

Gunnar MR: Quality of early care and buffering of neuroendocrine stress reactions: Potential effects on the developing human brain. Prev Med 27:209-211, 1998.

Gunnar MR, Brodersen L, Nachmias M, et al: Stress reactivity and attachment security. Dev Psychobiol 29:191-204, 1996.

Hartman A: Diagrammatic assessment of family relationships. Social Casework 59:465-476, 1978.

Kitzman H, Olds DL, Henderson CR Jr, et al: Effect of prenatal and infancy home visitation by nurses on pregnancy outcomes, childhood injuries, and repeated childbearing. JAMA 278:644-652, 1997.

Lewis JM, Beavers WR, Gossett JT, et al: No Single Thread: Psychological Health in Family Systems. New York, Brunner/Mazel, 1976.

Like RC, Rogers J, McGoldrick M: Reading and interpreting genograms: A systematic approach. J Fam Pract 28:407-412, 1988.

McCubbin HI, Patterson JM: Stress: The family inventory of life events. *In* Fillsinger EE (ed): Marriage and Family Assessment: A Sourcebook for Family Therapy. Beverly Hills, CA, Sage, 1983, pp 275-298.

McGoldrick M, Gerson R: Genograms in Family Assessment. New York, Norton, 1985.

Moos R: Family Environment Scales. Palo Alto, CA, Consulting Psychologists Press, 1974.

Nachmias M, Gunnar M, Mangelsdorf S, et al: Behavioral

inhibition and stress reactivity: The moderating role of attachment security. Child Dev 67:508-522, 1996.

Ogawa JR, Sroufe LA, Weinfield NS, et al: Development and the fragmented self: Longitudinal study of dissociative symptomatology in a nonclinical sample. Dev Psychopathol 9:855-879, 1997.

Olds DL, Eckenrode J, Henderson CR, et al: Long term effects of home visitation on maternal life course and child abuse and neglect: Fifteen year follow-up of a randomized trial. JAMA 278:637-643, 1997.

Olson DH, McCubbin HI, Barnes H, et al: Families: What Makes Them Work. Beverly Hills, CA, Sage, 1989.

Olson D, McCubbin HI, Barnes H, et al: Family Inventories. St Paul, MN, University of Minnesota, 1982.

Olson DH, Portner J, Lavee Y: FACES III. St Paul, MN, Family Social Sciences, University of Minnesota, 1985.

Olson DH, Sprenkle DH, Russell CS: Circumplex model of marital and family systems I: Cohesion and adaptability dimensions, family types, and clinical applications. Fam Process 18:3-28, 1979.

Perry BD, Pollard R: Homeostasis, stress, trauma, and adaptation: A neurodevelopmental view of childhood trauma. Child Adolesc Psychiatr Clin N Am 7:33-51, 1998.

Resnick MD, Bearman PS, Blum RW, et al: Protecting adolescents from harm: Findings from the National Longitudinal Study on Adolescent Health. JAMA 278:823-832, 1997.

Roberts RN, Magrab PR: Psychologists' role in a family-centered approach to practice, training and research with young children. Am Psychol 46:144-148, 1991.

Rogers JC, Cohn P: Impact of a screening family genogram on first encounters in primary care. Fam Pract 4:291-301, 1987.

Smilkstein G: The family APGAR: A proposal for a family function test and its use by physicians. J Fam Pract 6:1231-1239, 1978.

Stinnett N, Chesser B, DeFrain J (eds): Building Family Strengths: Blueprints for Action. Lincoln, NE, University of Nebraska, 1979.

Terkelsen KG: Toward a theory of the family life cycle. *In* Carter EA, McGoldrick M (eds): The Family Life Cycle: A Framework for Family Theory. New York, Gardner, 1980, pp 21-52.

Visscher EM, Clore ER: The genogram: A strategy for assessment. J Pediatr Health Care 6:361-367, 1992.

Wells RD, Stein MT: Special families. *In* Dixon SD, Stein MT (eds): Encounters With Children: Pediatric Behavior and Development, 3rd ed. St Louis, MO, CV Mosby, 1999, pp 501-523.

Whall AL: The family as the unit of care in nursing: A historical review. Public Health Nurs 3:240-249, 1986.

Wright LM, Leahey M: Nurses and Families: A Guide to Family Assessment and Intervention, 2nd ed. Philadelphia, FA Davis, 1994.

CHAPTER 4

Cultural Perspectives for Primary Health Care

Margaret MacDonald

▤ INTRODUCTION

The Concept of Culture

The word culture has acquired multiple meanings and connotations. Today, the term is used in three distinct ways:

1. To describe a general human condition that is universal
2. To distinguish a particular group in society that shares a collection of unique characteristics and customs (usually based on ethnicity, religion, or race)
3. To denote a regional metaethnic entity, such as referring to an individual as an American or a westerner.

The ancient scholar Cicero borrowed the Latin term *cultura,* meaning care or cultivation, to describe philosophy as the *cultura animi,* or cultivation of the mind. In the Middle Ages, German philosophers referred to culture *(kultur)* as a lifestyle dedicated to the cultivation of mental and spiritual capacities as a means of achieving an enlightened, sensitized, humane state of being. Therefore, an individual with a highly developed sense of style and an aesthetic appreciation of the finer things (i.e., art, music, literature) was considered a "cultured" person. By the 16th century, the term culture had taken on yet another meaning, coming to denote or differentiate the customs and institutions of specific ethnic and religious entities.

The term ethnicity is now used to identify a group of people within a society who share common traits and customs. Ethnicity differs from race; the latter classifies humans according to specific physical characteristics (e.g., pigmentation, facial features) (Henderson & Primeaux, 1981). However, members of ethnic or racial groups do not necessarily share a common cultural heritage.

A common denominator in any application of the term culture lies in the realization that culture is represented in every aspect of an individual's life. The most widely accepted contemporary definition of culture comes from the work of Edward Tylor (1958): "Culture is that complex whole which includes knowledge, belief, art, law, custom, and any other capabilities and habits acquired by man as a member of a society."

Cultural Socialization

Culture influences everything humans as members of social groups do, use, produce, know, and believe in. The elements of culture form a consistent and integrated framework that serves as a blueprint for living for each member of a social group. Attitudes regarding health, wellness, disease, and disability are an intricate part of this blueprint. The elements of culture are transmitted from one generation to another through a complicated process of social interaction. This socialization process shapes a child's reality; through it, children learn how to perceive the world, the prevailing problem-solving ideology, and the rules that define behavior. The concept of self (identity) and the roles played in society are culturally dependent (Berger & Luckmann, 1966). The acquisition of the capabilities necessary to function in a given culture is facilitated by the long period of dependency that humans have before reaching physical and social maturity (Erikson, 1964).

A number of social and legal institutions influence and support cultural socialization, including the family, school, peer groups, and the media.

FAMILY

The first socializing force an individual encounters is the family. A powerful primary group, the family exposes the child to a set of values in the context of intensely personal relationships as well as material and psychological support. The family molds and influences behavior through mechanisms of social control, such as guilt and shame. Universally employed within cultural groups, these mechanisms influence the development of the self-concept and facilitate conformity to the prevailing standards and codes of behavior.

Each culture possesses its own values, attitudes, and practices with regard to families and child rearing, providing care and guidance in culturally prescribed ways. Children learn what they need to know to care for themselves and to assume the roles necessary to participate as members of families, schools, churches, and communities. As they become familiar with the patterns of behavior dictated by their culture, children develop distinctive personalities, thoughts, and feelings.

SCHOOL

The school plays a primary role in molding the child to the prevailing culture. It functions to expand the child's socialization beyond the narrow boundaries of the family and to instill a sense of collective identity and commitment to the society as a whole. School serves as a model for much of the adult social world. It lays the groundwork for developing methods for negotiating one's way within the institutions of adult society (e.g., workplace, politics, organized recreation).

PEER GROUP

Peer groups also play a powerful role in socializing children to their culture. Peer groups place children in a position of social equality unlike the socially inferior position that they may experience at home or school.

MEDIA

Television, radio, magazines, newspapers, and films have an enormous influence on the cultural socialization of children, especially in contemporary America. As an audience, Americans are conditioned to receive mass culture passively via these vehicles. Through the media, the child is exposed to a wide array of values, many of which may conflict with those of the family and the school. A number of authorities have expressed concern about the negative effect this exposure has on personality and cognitive and moral development (Gadow & Sprafkin, 1989).

SUBCULTURAL AFFILIATIONS

In a complex society, children may be exposed to a number of subcultural groups that further shape their cultural identity. In addition to ethnicity or race, individuals may have one or more subcultural affiliations based on social class, religion, occupation, or socioeconomic status. The family provides the child with initial exposure to such affiliations, the importance of which varies from family to family.

Meeting the social expectations of various subcultures can be a source of considerable stress in complex societies. An individual or group that straddles two or more cultures and attempts to embrace more than one set of values is termed bicultural. These individuals or groups are at risk for the loss of their native cultural characteristics through cultural assimilation or acculturation.

Characteristics of Culture

There are five key characteristics of culture. These are summarized in Table 4-1.

Cultural Identity: Dominant and Minority Groups

Every society, however diverse or heterogeneous, possesses a distinct cultural identity that

T A B L E 4-1

Characteristics of Culture

CHARACTERISTIC	IMPORTANCE
1. Culture is universal, but no two cultures are alike	• Social groups have their own ways of seeing, doing, making things, and keeping traditions
2. Culture is learned through socialization	• All humans are socialized to a culture and participate in a culture
3. Culture is stable yet dynamic	• Customs, beliefs, and practices gradually change over time to meet the needs of the social group • Acculturation results when individuals learn characteristics of a new culture; usually, they also lose the characteristics of their native culture
4. Culture is symbolic	• Language is the method of categorizing, transmitting, and interpreting culture; language assists with the acculturation process • A culture uses artifacts (e.g., clothing, jewelry) to communicate among members of the social group • Nonverbal language is integral to communication
5. Culture meets the needs of the social group	• The culture helps meet biological needs • The culture provides a framework of values and beliefs that gives the social group integrity and meaning

is an expression of its dominant group. The dominant group frequently is the largest proportion of a population in a given society, but this is not always the case. Regardless of size, the culture of the dominant group characterizes the lifestyle and collective consciousness of the community, and functions as the guardian and sustainer of the controlling value system and the prime allocator of rewards. A minority group within a society, on the other hand, shares racial, religious, or ethnic characteristics that differ from those of the dominant group.

Cultural embeddedness refers to the extent to which individuals identify with a given cultural framework and incorporate its traditions and customs into their daily life and decision-making. Many factors influence this, including level of education, socioeconomic status, country of origin of individuals or their ancestors, exposure to other cultures, lifestyle (e.g., urban vs. rural), length of stay in the host country, and the exact region of the host country in which individuals grew up, reside, or both.

The cultural identity of individuals who emigrate as children or who are born in the host country is likely to be very different from that of adult émigrés, owing to exposure to the socialization forces of the dominant culture.

Characteristics (e.g., skin color, religion) that set a minority group apart from the dominant group may result in collective discrimination within the society. Ethnocentrism and racism create and perpetuate the distinctions of dominant and minority groups. Ethnocentrism is the belief that one's own ethnic culture or subculture is superior to all others (Friedman, 1990). Racism is the assumption of inherent racial superiority or inferiority with consequent discrimination.

▨ PROVIDING CULTURALLY SENSITIVE CARE

According to the United States (US) Bureau of the Census (1990), by 2030, people of color will represent more than half of the population in the United States. The changes in immigration patterns in the last decade alone are reflected in the ever-increasing diversity of cultures that we experience on a daily basis. As the economies of nations become more global and advanced transportation and communication systems facilitate ease of access, interdependence between countries and their peoples will continue to increase (Porter & Samovar, 1997). Thus, nurse practitioners (NPs) will need to prepare themselves to provide culturally sensitive care.

Culturally sensitive care, according to Chrisman (1991), is based on three interrelated principles: knowledge, respect, and negotiation.

- NPs must be knowledgeable of the tendencies or possibilities that may exist with regard to world views, customs, values, and traditions of the dominant culture and the minority cultures of the families they serve.
- NPs must show respect for an individual's cultural beliefs.
- NPs must be willing to negotiate different approaches in developing a therapeutic plan.

Incorporation of these principles—knowledge, respect, and negotiation—facilitates the development of a therapeutic relationship grounded in trust as well as effective, high-quality care outcomes.

Recognizing Culture Shock

The process of emigrating—leaving one's homeland to settle in a different country—presents the individual and the family with many challenges. Changes in diet, exposure to unfamiliar environmental hazards, and lack of appropriate immunity may threaten physical health. In addition, considerable energy is required to interpret and respond to the unfamiliar behavior and symbols individuals encounter on a daily basis as they attempt to meet basic and complex needs in the absence of familiar resources. The feelings of helplessness and exhaustion that may ensue are part of the phenomenon known as culture shock (Leininger, 1988, 1990).

The degree of culture shock that is experienced depends on many variables, including social status, personality characteristics, age, occupation, availability of support systems, language familiarity, general state of health, and the extent of cultural differences between the home and host countries.

Culture shock impacts the physical, emotional, and psychological well-being of every member of the family, and may take many months to overcome. In the presence of healthcare providers, patients and perhaps their family members as well, who are experiencing culture shock, may appear inappropriately complacent or over-reactive. Rather than being noncompliant or uncooperative, they may, in reality, be overwhelmed and exhausted.

NPs who care for clients and families from culturally diverse backgrounds frequently experience culture shock too. Lack of knowledge of differences in cultural practices, beliefs, and values can result in feelings of helplessness, frustration, and inadequacy for everyone involved in the helping relationship. NPs can reduce their own culture shock and that of their clients by learning about the different cultural groups they encounter and recognizing the signs of culture shock in their clients and themselves.

Developing Cultural Competence

Cultural competence requires recognition of culture as a distinctive way of life, specific to a particular group but not necessarily related to ethnicity or race. Tremendous intraethnic diversity may exist in life perspective, values, problem-solving strategies, and customs among individual members of dominant and minority groups. Thus, one can expect to see variations within as well as between cultures. Culture viewed from this perspective becomes a value-free concept. Cultural competence requires:

- An awareness of the cultural foundations of the health care system in which one lives and works. In the United States, for example, the health care system is designed by and for a specific population group that holds an activistic, rational-mastery, future-oriented approach to life. When people who have different modes of thought and different ways of dealing with time are expected to function in a social system tailored primarily to a single cultural entity, conflicts are inevitable. Providers who possess an understanding of the nature of the system, their own culture's health values and practices, and the health values and practices of the families they serve can defuse some of this conflict (Niederhauser, 1989). Delivering care in a nonjudgmental manner that demonstrates recognition and respect of ethnic and cultural differences does not call for NPs to abdicate their own standards. Rather, NPs should think in terms of the context within which those standards exist.

- Development of a partnership with the family that is rooted in basic trust and dedicated to maintaining or restoring health. Every plan of management for a given patient should be based on a culturally sensitive assessment of the individual (Friedman, 1990; Giger & Davidhizar, 1995).
- Knowledge of cultural variation. This provides insight into views of health and sickness, but the NP must view cultural characteristics as a continuum, *recognizing that not all individuals from the same social group have the same characteristics.*

Intraethnic variations must be anticipated and incorporated into the plan of care for a truly individualized approach. Attempting to fit a family or individual into any preconceived cultural framework is not a manifestation of cultural sensitivity—it is stereotyping. The distinction between individualizing care based on cultural characteristics and stereotyping is a fine one. Stereotyping and cross-cultural comparisons are to be avoided because they interfere with the development of basic trust and threaten the success of the therapeutic relationship and the plan of care.

Communicating Cultural Sensitivity

Whether the provider is dealing with a patient and family who appear to be a part of the dominant culture or of a minority group, the following guidelines create an environment of recognition and respect that facilitate the development of trust (Niederhauser, 1989).

APPROPRIATE USE OF NAME

In general, a good way to begin a visit is to use the family's surname when addressing the parent or parents, or ask what they prefer to be called. Regardless of the culture, it is best not to assume that it is acceptable to call an adult (particularly one who is older than the provider) by his or her first name. All family members who accompany the child should be acknowledged. For some cultural groups, the presence of numerous family members represents an expression of respect and caring for children and their parents. When family elders are present, they should be included in all conversations and decision-making that take place regarding the child.

DISCOVERING PERSPECTIVES ON HEALTH PROBLEMS

The NP must be willing to question the dominant cultural belief that the biomedical model is the only effective way of providing health care. Problem-solving approaches vary throughout the world; everyone does not solve problems in the linear, cause-and-effect way that is the tradition of the dominant culture in the United States. Insisting that patients and their families deal with their problems from this perspective only is not helpful in cross-cultural situations and will very likely interfere with the success of the management plan.

Identifying beliefs about causative factors and relief measures can provide insight, help the NP make an accurate diagnosis, and lay the groundwork for a mutually agreed on treatment plan that works because the family understands it. Table 4–2 provides assessment areas to help identify the family's perspectives on health problems (Jackson, 1993; Torres, 1993). When developing the plan, incorporate culture-related practices whenever possible and appropriate (Pachter, 1994, 1997).

TIME AND SPATIAL PERSPECTIVES

TIME. Just as problems are perceived differently among peoples, so too are the concepts of time and space. Some cultures view time as steady, predictable, and mobile. It is always

T A B L E 4-2

Identifying Family Perspectives on Health Areas

* What is the problem called?
* What does the family believe is happening and why?
* What aspects of the problem are important to the family?
* Why do you think the problem started when it did?
* What do you think the problem does?
* How severe is the problem?
* What treatment should the patient receive?
* What results do you hope for?
* What do you fear most about the illness?
* How has the problem affected the family?
* What are the family's goals for health care?
* How can the problem be avoided in the future?
* What relief measures have been tried?
* Who has been consulted for help (besides dominant culture health care providers)?
* What has helped in the past?

Includes some items from Kleinman A: The Illness Narratives: Suffering, Healing, and the Human Condition. New York, Basic Books, 1988.

moving forward, and the impressions of past, present, and future are distinct.

For others, the reality of time exists only in relation to the present occurrence of events. There is no such thing as early or late. The future is less important than the present, and problems of daily survival take priority over far-reaching goals. An understanding of these differences can aid the provider in looking at failed treatment plans from a different and less judgmental perspective.

SPACE. Human beings seek to maintain a certain spatial distance from others. This desire for control over a certain amount of personal space is known as territoriality, and while it varies from one individual to another, Watson (1980) found a correlation between personal space requirements and culture. Three dimensions or zones of spatial distancing are recognized: the intimate zone allows close proximity and is reserved for family members and those in the roles of caregiver, comforter, and protector; the personal zone provides more spatial distance between individuals and is reserved for friends and close acquaintances; the public zone is the spatial distance expected between coworkers and individuals in business encounters.

The degree of territoriality and the amount of space considered appropriate in each zone varies from one individual to another and is influenced by gender, age, and situation, as well as culture. Failure to recognize and respect an individual's personal space needs may be interpreted as a threatening invasion of personal space or a lack of caring and compassion, depending on the situation.

Most people are not consciously aware of their personal space requirements and the variables that influence spatial distance. Nonverbal cues, such as turning to avoid direct face-to-face contact or stepping back, are indications that an individual needs more personal space (Giger & Davidhizar, 1995). The tendency to move closer, lean forward, and maintain direct eye contact for sustained periods indicates the need for less spatial distance. Awareness of territoriality and appropriate response to cues received with regard to the spatial needs of an individual client or family enhance the development of a satisfactory client-provider relationship.

INDIVIDUALISM VS. COLLECTIVISM

On the continuum of tendencies or possibilities within a given culture are the characteristics of collectivism and individualism. In cultures that value individualism highly, individual interests, values, and needs take precedence over those of the community; individual goals are considered more important than collective goals; and children are socialized to autonomy and independent decision-making. Among these cultural groups, caring for oneself and one's immediate family takes priority over the larger community and society as a whole (Gudykunst & Ting-Toomey, 1988).

At the other end of the continuum is a commitment to collectivism. In collectivist cultures, social norms supersede individual initiatives, and greater value is placed on the interests or the good of the community. Consensus is stressed in decision-making in collectivist cultures and individual members attend to their own needs and aspirations only after first attending to the concerns of the group.

Awareness of the value that a given cultural group tends to place on individualism vs. collectivism enhances communication. Verbal and nonverbal communication in highly individualistic cultures is characterized by spontaneity, independence, and relatively few rules. Conversely, within highly collectivistic cultures, communication that closely follows the norms and rules of the group is expected and encouraged. Nonverbal communication is directed toward group solidarity and harmony and is respective of social status. Among these cultures, avoidance strategies and face-saving displays are common.

CONTEXT

Context is a characteristic of culture that influences how verbal and nonverbal communications are constructed and delivered, as well as the recipient's perception and response. Cultural groups can be classified as high context or low context. A cultural group in which members send and receive verbal and nonverbal messages according to well-defined rules is referred to as high context. Among these group, the context of the message (e.g., the situation in which the communication takes place, the status of the speaker, and the nonverbal aspects of the message) is more significant than what is actually said. As a result of the emphasis on context, individuals from high-context cultures tend to be less direct in their verbal statements and very sensitive to nonverbal and situational cues.

In low-context cultures, the emphasis is on the content of the verbal message. Few rules are observed in communicating and the status of the speaker is of little significance. Verbal communication is direct, explicit, and nonverbal, and situational cues are not as significant as in high-context cultures.

According to Gervais (1996), context lends structure to communication, influencing not just how individuals interpret messages but how they respond to them. This can help people cope with the sensory overload that contributes to culture shock.

Awareness of context is invaluable in communicating with individuals and families. In encounters with clients who engage in highly contextual communication, the client may speak very little and be highly sensitive to the NP's body language and situational cues. Reliance on validation and clarification techniques, as well as less explicit or direct verbal messages, promotes a therapeutic relationship with these clients (Porter & Samovar, 1997).

The NP should be very direct and explicit in verbal communication with clients from low-context cultures, recognizing that they may not pick up on situational and nonverbal cues.

CULTURALLY SENSITIVE COMMUNICATION TECHNIQUES

Reliance on an interrogative approach (asking questions) may be viewed by some as intrusive, thus interfering with the development of a trusting relationship. The NP should be sensitive to signs of discomfort, such as evasive answers or visible uneasiness, and switch from asking questions to making gentle declarative statements based on observations and information already acquired.

Extensive note taking in the family's presence can also cause uneasiness. If this occurs, the NP should stop the note taking and listen more intently—but never with continuous, unbroken eye contact. Follow the parent's lead with regard to eye contact. Among some cultures and in different regions across the United States, consistent eye contact can be perceived as threatening or rude. In others, breaking eye contact frequently may be interpreted as a sign of disrespect or boredom. If family elders are present, they should be included in obtaining the history and developing the treatment plan.

In general, a low tone of voice helps to calm anxious patients and parents. The provider should also resist the temptation to talk fast. Focus on the parent first, and ask permission before touching the infant or young child. This shows respect for the parent and can also have a calming effect on the patient.

CULTURALLY SENSITIVE PATIENT EDUCATION

It is incorrect to assume that all clients and their families appreciate and benefit from patient education material. Although members of low-context cultures may seek and appreciate written educational material, it may be overwhelming for members of high-context cultures who are trying to interpret a myriad of nonverbal and situational cues as well as the verbal message associated with the visit. The best approach is to make clients aware of the written educational material that is available and let them know they may take it if they wish to do so.

Any instructions for home management should be written in simple terms in the client's native language, and educational efforts should be directed toward any elder family members present, and fathers as well as mothers. Abbreviations should be avoided, and all written material should be reviewed with the patient, parent, or both, with the help of an interpreter when necessary.

Do not assume that all parents can read English or their own native language. However, assessing literacy must be done indirectly and with sensitivity with most people, because illiteracy is a source of shame among some peoples.

Out of respect for the authority of the practitioner, the parent or patient may not wish to ask questions or request clarification, so the NP should encourage questions and check frequently for understanding. (Caudle, 1993; Torres, 1993).

USING AN INTERPRETER

The importance of using a qualified interpreter cannot be overemphasized. Interpreters who are familiar with the culture as well as the language are especially helpful, as they are likely to be more sensitive to the nonverbal cues inherent in a patient's presentation of the complaint. When family members or unqualified persons are relied on to translate what is being said, patient confidentiality, as well as provider and family understanding, can be jeopardized.

The qualified interpreter stands or sits behind the provider so as not to interfere with eye contact between the patient, the parent, and the provider. In some instances, the interpreter can even stand or sit behind a screen if privacy is an issue. The interpreter should make

an effort to translate the dialogue as closely and accurately as possible for both parties. When a provider's yes or no question results in a lengthy response, the interpreter must ensure that the provider is apprised of the whole statement, including any seemingly unrelated data.

The interpreter facilitates the process of explaining the pathophysiology of a health problem, instructions for home management, and assessment of the patient and parental level of knowledge and understanding of what is being said. It is helpful if the interpreter can write instructions for the family in their language and review them again before the family leaves.

It is especially difficult to convey emotion through verbal translation, and this component of communication may be lost or diminished when interpreters are used. This should not be perceived as lack of concern on the part of the patient or family. In addition, language barriers can arise even among people who speak the same language, and communication patterns differ among subcultures and from one region of a country to another (Grasska & McFarland, 1982).

▓▓ CULTURES IN AMERICAN SOCIETY

Introduction

The population of the United States consists of numerous ethnic groups, races, and subcultures. It may be broken down into the dominant white middle class and a number of minority groups, including African Americans, Hispanic Americans, Asian Americans, and Native Americans, and two rapidly growing population groups, Russian Americans and Arab Americans. According to the 1990 census report, 78% of the US population is white, 11.7% is African American, 6.4% is Hispanic American, 1.5% is Asian American, 0.6% is Native American, and 1.8% are Russian American and Arab American.

The dominant group providing cultural identity in American society is the white middle class. This group is composed primarily of second-, third-, and fourth-generation Americans. Judeo-Christian values and a linear, problem-solving paradigm provide the foundation of the value system of American society and the institutions that support and sustain it.

As a collective, Americans have an activistic, rational-mastery, future-oriented approach to life. Their basic world view is one of optimism, progress, and upward mobility. The pace of life is fast, and people tend to be consumer-oriented and materialistic. Work is taken seriously and valued highly, especially when it is pleasurable and fulfilling as opposed to being just a means to survival.

Currently, a community-oriented, other-directed philosophy is gaining prominence, which is a departure from the revered entrepreneurial spirit credited with launching American democracy. There is also more emphasis on collective, as opposed to individual, accomplishment.

As in many other societies around the world, within the United States there is a long-held tradition of male dominance or patriarchy. However, as educational standards of women have increased, traditional ideas about male dominance have been questioned. As a result of disdain for the inequality inherent in patriarchy, American society is experiencing significant social upheaval with regard to traditional male and female roles.

It is difficult to describe the contemporary American family. Traditionally characterized by geographical and economic mobility, the quality of the family experience is being modified by changing work patterns, a spiraling divorce rate, increased potential for financial uncertainty, and adolescent pregnancy. Although the nuclear family has been and continues to be considered the mainstay of American society, this notion is changing as the single-parent household becomes more common.

Values related to child rearing and parenting vary with socioeconomic status, but there is considerable overlap from one level to another regardless of ethnic heritage.

As in other societies, minority groups in America do not always share the cognitive and normative elements of the dominant culture. When members of minority groups find their cultural values and life views in conflict with those of either the dominant group or the minority group, considerable tension can result.

Ethnic, cultural, and racial characteristics are influenced by many factors, including educational level, occupation, social class, socioeconomic level, religion, immigration status, country of origin, length of residency in the United States, and degree of acculturation. Notions of health and illness are particularly influenced by these factors. Table 4–3 outlines different cultural contexts that the NP may encounter.

Cultural Perspectives of the Major US Population Groups

In this section, perceptions of health and illness specific to the major population groups in the United States are explored. The discussion focuses on the shared tendencies within specific cultural frameworks that may influence these perceptions. Individuals accept, reject, or modify these tendencies as they grow and live as members of a given society; thus one can expect to see variations within as well as between these population groups. The effects of poverty and homelessness, two growing trends in America, are also explored.

WHITE MIDDLE-CLASS AMERICANS

Cultural Identity

The ethnicity of the white middle-class population in America is an expression of the old melting pot adage: it is a blend of European cultures. The American white middle class, presently the dominant cultural group in America, maintains a strong work ethic. Work has traditionally been a major life focus, especially for men, and is expected to be pleasurable and fulfilling as well as to provide a means of survival. In two-parent families, both parents are frequently employed in an effort to maintain the middle-class lifestyle.

Historically, entrepreneurism and individualism have been highly valued by the American white middle class. Increasing emphasis on community and a more collectivistic approach has taken hold in recent years.

Family Structure

Some white middle-class American children live in an extended family arrangement, but this

TABLE 4-3

Contextual Communication

PARAMETER OF CULTURAL DIVERSITY	BEHAVIOR OBSERVED	IMPLICATIONS FOR PATIENT–PROVIDER COMMUNICATION
HEALTH PERSPECTIVE	Western biomedical alternative modalities	• Emphasize, negotiate, and provide a rationale for why patient should comply • Explore with client ways he or she can best meet the regimen
TIME	Future-oriented Present-oriented Cycle-oriented	• Client may be late for appointments • Client may fail to use prescribed medications • Client may have a fatalistic attitude → noncompliance
SPACE	Close: 1½ ft Distant: 3 ft Client may move away from the provider or get in provider's face Client may refuse to establish eye contact	Provider needs to be aware of behavioral anomalies: • May not be attempting to avoid contact; don't get defensive • Reflects patient need for more space; ensure space
INDIVIDUALISM VS. COLLECTIVISM	Individualistic: • Focus is on self Collectivistic: • Many family members are included in patient care • Client may defer to provider as authority	• Clarify who makes health care decisions • Include appropriate individuals in planning care • Provide positive reinforcement for efforts to foster health • Encourage active participation in decision-making
HIGH CONTEXT VS. LOW CONTEXT	High context: • Many rules for communication • Sensitivity to nonverbal cues Low context: • Emphasis on content • Few rules should be established for nonverbal communication	• With high-context clients, watch nonverbal cues • With low-context clients, be very clear in verbal communication

is not the norm. Rather, these children are likely to come from a nuclear family. However, single-parent families are increasing and, with this change, the family's middle-class lifestyle may be threatened. In divorce cases, joint custody arrangements are gaining in popularity. These arrangements have the potential to threaten the continuity of care and raise specific emotional and adjustment issues for the children involved in such families.

Because parents often work outside the home, many children are in the care of nonfam-ily members during the day, or they may come home from school and be alone for some portion of the afternoon before their parents return from work.

Time and Spatial Perspectives

Future oriented and time conscious, this group has a fast-paced day-to-day life. Waiting for long periods to see a health care provider can be a source of considerable frustration and interfere with the development of a trusting relationship.

White middle-class Americans tend to have considerable territoriality needs, preferring a large degree of personal space. Tactile contact is limited to the intimate and personal zones.

Health Perspectives

This group is generally well educated and may view health as more than just the absence of disease. Although they are somewhat knowledgeable about germ theory and the multifactorial nature of illness, poor health may nevertheless be viewed by some as divine punishment.

There is general comfort with concepts of primary prevention, such as immunizations and well child care, and confidence in professionals and their scientific expertise. Optimism oriented to action and a tendency to look to the future characterize this group and facilitate compliance with restorative and preventive health-care measures. Sickness in a child puts considerable strain on parents employed outside the home.

Language and Communication Style

The primary language of white middle-class American society is English, but in keeping with the multiethnic nature of American society, numerous other languages may be spoken, requiring the services of qualified interpreters. In addition, variations in English are not uncommon from one region of the country to another.

The communication style generally demonstrated by the white middle class is characterized as low context. Thus, the emphasis is placed primarily on the verbal message. There are few rules for communication, and there may be little awareness of nonverbal and situational cues.

A client in this group may prefer to stand or sit some distance from the provider when talking. It is acceptable to touch a young patient without necessarily asking the parent's permission beforehand, but before doing so the NP should wash his or her hands in the parent's presence. Although families may appear to reveal themselves easily, privacy and patient confidentiality are extremely important.

Risk Factors

In caring for the white middle-class child, the NP should be alert to signs of stress that may be present because of a fast-paced lifestyle and reduced family time. A busy lifestyle can interfere with the preparation of nutritious meals and eating together as a family. The result is overconsumption of fast food and junk food as well as a loss of valuable family time for socialization. Emphasis should be placed on good nutrition; stress management; exercise; limiting exposure to the media, especially television; and fostering regular, positive family interactions.

Adolescents should be taught self-assessment measures, including self-testicular and self-breast examination, because cancer rates are significant in the white race. Pregnancy and human immunodeficiency virus (HIV) risk evaluation are important aspects of preventive care as well.

AFRICAN AMERICANS

Cultural Identity

Cultural identity among African Americans in the United States today is diverse because of increasing assimilation to the values of the dominant group, specifically by the large and growing African American middle class. Factors such as social class, age, sex roles, socialization patterns, and individual life experiences all contribute to the diversity that presently exists within the African American culture in America.

In spite of the assimilation of the African American middle class into the dominant culture, there is a separate and distinct black identity that is based on shared experiences and reinforced not only by close proximity and interactions with others but also by the racism that persists in American society.

The average African American, along with members of other minority groups, deals on a daily basis with situations that cause social anxiety. These ever-present tensions have the potential to negatively influence the development of self-esteem in the growing child. The African American church and the black consciousness movement that began in the 1960s have been instrumental in fostering a collective sense of pride and racial solidarity.

These social movements have fostered the development of strength and resilience among African Americans, enhancing adaptation to cultural demands despite pervasive social, political, and economic discrimination.

Family Structure

More than half of all African American children live in female-headed households. Although a distinct middle class has emerged, the median income of African American families remains much lower than that of white families. Many African American families must rely on government assistance for survival. In 1995, 41.5% of black children younger than 18 years of age lived below the federal poverty level (US Public Health Service, 1998).

Extended family configurations are common in the African American culture, and strong kinship bonds are influential in preserving the collective identity of the culture. Survival and oneness of being or group unity and togetherness are expressed in the concept of a domestic circle of kinfolk who support and help one another.

Time and Spatial Perspectives

The middle-class African American is future oriented and time conscious. Low-income African Americans tend, on the other hand, to be present oriented as they focus more on day-to-day survival needs.

As with all cultural characteristics in every population group, territoriality needs vary among African Americans. Those who have experienced considerable racial prejudice and hostility may demonstrate greater territoriality needs and avoid direct or prolonged eye contact in encounters with authority figures of the dominant cultural group.

Although members of this group are comfortable with touch in the intimate and personal zones, the formality associated with the client-provider relationship may preclude it.

Health Perspectives

The tendency to view life as a process rather than a state, with no separation of mind and body, is a remnant of African tribal philosophy that prevails today among many African Americans. Health may be defined as being in harmony with nature; thus, disease results from disharmony. Illness may be considered preventable by cleanliness, a nutritious diet, and proper rest. A family might believe that their child's sickness is due to nature's forces, evil influences, or spiritual punishment (Bloch, 1976). Home remedies in the forms of herbs, oils, powders, tokens, and rituals are sometimes used, especially among poor African American families who originate in the rural South.

Middle-class African Americans tend to have their health care needs met in the private sector, or they use county health department clinics for health maintenance and acute illness. Among the indigent, the emergency room is frequently the port of entry to the health care system, at which point health care problems are likely to be complicated and serious. This delay in seeking care is partly the result of a time orientation that focuses on the present. For the poor, the struggle for day-to-day survival hinders long-range planning; thus, a proactive approach to health in the form of health maintenance may not be commonly seen.

Language and Communication Styles

In approaching the African American family, the primary care provider should ask the parent what he or she would like to be called. Many African American patients and their family members speak a highly stylized form of English called Black English. Politeness and respect for the values of modesty and privacy lay the groundwork for the development of a trusting relationship. A modicum of formality may be seen in communication with the health care provider, and nonverbal and situational cues are important.

When a plan of management is being formulated, better compliance may be achieved if ranges or approximations rather than specific times are given for medications and treatments. If the health care provider explains the benefits of a proactive approach and uses examples of how others have benefited, the understanding of information and instructions given may be enhanced. Discussions of prognosis or matters of a serious nature may be better received if the spatial proximity between the provider and the client is reduced and communication is less explicit.

Risk Factors

According to the National Vital Statistics System of the Centers for Disease Control (US Department of Health & Human Services, 1990), the infant mortality rate among the African American population group is twice that of the white population. Sickle cell disease is prevalent among African American children, and they are at risk for lead poisoning as a result of environmental exposure. Hypertension among adolescents should be closely monitored, and nutritional counseling is advised. In many black families, the traditional diet of pork, cabbage, rice, greens, and black-eyed peas has been replaced by a fast-food diet that is high in fat and calories and low in nutrients.

Among low-income African American families, overcrowding, substandard housing, poor sanitation systems, improper nutrition, lack of supervision, and violence place children at great risk for death and disability. The homicide rate for adolescents and young men is seven times higher than that of white adolescents and young men. Just as the tobacco companies are targeting Hispanic adolescents with their marketing campaigns, they are also designing their advertising to appeal to African American youth.

Pregnancy is on the rise among African American adolescents nationwide, and with unprotected sexual intercourse, the risk of HIV transmission increases. These health issues should be addressed whenever an African American child or adolescent is seen for any reason.

HISPANICS

Cultural Identity

The Hispanic ethnic group is America's fastest growing minority. Approximately 40% are younger than 20 years of age and about one third of these children live in poverty. In 1990, 49.8% had a high school diploma or higher education (Zambrana & Dorrington, 1998). The term Hispanic refers to Puerto Ricans, Cubans, Mexicans and Chicanos, Spanish, Central Americans, and South Americans. Although diversity exists among the various cultures of this population group, many similarities in customs, traditions, values, and social institutions (family, community, and church) can be found. Hispanic families encountered in America may be American citizens, permanent residents, undocumented aliens, or seasonal or migrant farm workers.

Hispanic cultures tend to value collectivism: social norms supersede individual initiative and consensus is stressed in decision-making.

As the Hispanic population group rapidly becomes the largest minority group in America, a distinct Hispanic middle class is emerging and assimilating many of the characteristics of the dominant cultural group.

Family Structure

Hispanic Americans are intensely proud of their heritage, music, and food, and the hub of Hispanic culture is often the family home. Great emphasis may be placed on the importance of interpersonal relationships; families tend to be large, extended, and close. Children are highly regarded, especially male children, and may be encouraged to be independent and assertive as long as such behavior is congruent with family goals. Obedience to authorities, especially elders, is a common expectation. Food may be a significant socializing force for the Hispanic group.

Time and Spatial Perspectives

Traditionally oriented to the present, the Hispanic concept of time is changing to a more future-oriented perspective among those who are achieving higher socioeconomic status and assimilating the values of the dominant culture. Personal interaction among many Hispanic Americans is still considered more important than time.

Watson (1980) found that members of Hispanic cultures demonstrate close proximity in spatial distancing. In addition, tactile contact is frequent among family members and acquaintances.

Health Perspectives

Although perspectives may vary among the varied Hispanic groups, many Hispanics consider that good health is a gift from God, and that illness can be prevented through prayers and devotions along with hard work, good food, and proper behavior (Marsh & Hentges, 1988). In gathering a history, the NP might learn that the child's illness is thought to be caused by divine punishment, supernatural forces (witchcraft), an internal imbalance in body humors (hot-cold theory), or a dislocation of internal organs (Carr, 1990; Caudle, 1993).

As with other minority groups in America, the Hispanic peoples may not take full advantage of health services, particularly preventive care (Munoz, 1988). Some families are ineligible for health care services. Forty percent had no health insurance in 1992 (Reddy, 1995). When a child is seen, it is more likely to be in response to an acute problem than for preventive health care. A number of interrelated factors are thought to be responsible for this, including a different world view and concept of time, as well as discrimination and language barriers. Regardless of the actual reason for seeing a child, immunizations should be updated whenever possible, and dental screening or referrals should be made as necessary.

It is not unusual for a sick child to have been seen by a folk healer _(curandero),_ spiritualist _(espiritualista),_ or herbalist _(yerbero)_ before the assistance of a western practitioner is sought. Over-the-counter as well as home (folk) remedies are commonly employed by members of the Hispanic population, regardless of their socioeconomic and educational levels, as methods of maintaining and restoring health (Gonzalez-Swafford & Gutierrez, 1988). Management plans that incorporate folk remedies, such as prayers, rituals, herbs, massage, and general laying on of hands, along with western practices, are likely to be the most satisfying and successful. Caution should be exercised, however, in allowing concurrent use of some herbs and western medicines, because they can be toxic (Carr, 1990). If, in the course of gathering a history, the NP learns that potentially harmful folk remedies, such as lead tetroxide or dried rattlesnake, are being used, an effort should be made to educate the family and discourage this behavior.

Language and Communication Styles

Communication in Hispanic cultures is highly contextual. The status of the speaker is significant, and nonverbal and situational cues are important.

The predominant language of the Hispanic culture is Spanish, so the non–Spanish-speaking provider may require the services of an interpreter. Almost 25% of Hispanics live in linguistically isolated families (Zambrana & Dorrington, 1998). Even with interpretive assistance, the NP should be prepared for regional dialects or one of the Indian languages. Even if young children in the family speak English, they should not be relied on to translate information. Out of respect for the parents, arrangements for an interpreter should be made. Home-care instructions should be demonstrated whenever possible, as well as written down and explained verbally.

When addressing adult Hispanic family members, the primary care provider should use their surnames unless otherwise instructed. Modesty, privacy, and politeness are highly valued, even for children, and should be respected. It is advisable to request permission of the parent before examining a child. Some individuals believe that admiring a child without touching him or her may cause a magical illness (characterized by fever, diarrhea, and vomiting) called _mal ojo_ or evil eye.

If elderly family members accompany the client and parent to an appointment, they should be acknowledged and encouraged to participate in the visit.

Risk Factors

In caring for the Hispanic child, the NP should be alert to the potential for illness stemming from lack of access to preventive health and dental care. Deficiencies in calcium and riboflavin are common because of low intake of dairy products. The tendency to breastfeed children well into the third year reduces the danger of bone weakness and deformity secondary to calcium deficiency. Anticipatory guidance should include information about the relationships between a diet high in sweets and dental caries; lack of proper immunizations and communicable disease; and starchy diets and lifelong obesity with its myriad complications.

Adolescents, especially those who are struggling to be assimilated, need guidance in acquiring positive attitudes with regard to individual and collective identity. Adolescent pregnancy rates are high among this group because family planning is not widely practiced; however, family planning is becoming more acceptable. The NP may still encounter reluctance on the part of Hispanic Americans to use family planning methods that require the touching of one's own genitals. In addition, the risk of HIV transmission is significant because of the low use of condoms. Tobacco use is also on the rise among all teens. About 34% of Hispanic teens reported smoking in 1997 (Centers for Disease Control and Prevention, 1998).

ASIAN AMERICANS

Cultural Identity

The Asian American segment of the population in the United States is actually composed of five distinct ethnic groups: Chinese, Japanese, Korean, Vietnamese, and Pacific Islander. The United States also has many Southeast Asian refugee groups, including Hmong, Khmer, Lao, Mien, and others. Although there is considerable diversity among these ethnic groups, they have some common characteristics rooted in Chinese traditions. In general, the world view of the Asian cultures emphasizes the preservation of harmony with nature, filial piety, consideration of others' rights and feelings, and deference to authority (Char, 1981; Chow, 1976; Bliatout, 1998). Asian Americans tend to be achievement oriented. Education is highly valued, and work is taken seriously.

The Asian cultures are traditionally highly collectivistic; social norms supersede individual initiative and cooperation is the norm. Among Asian Americans who have assimilated the values of the dominant culture, greater emphasis on autonomy and individual goals may be seen.

Family Structure

Asian Americans tend to be family-centered. Whereas once extended families were the norm, today's Asian American families tend to be nuclear, with two working parents. Households tend to be male-dominated, and male children may be valued over female children. Devotion and loyalty to the family are expected of all members, and the needs of the family may take precedence over those of the individual. Children are loved and cared for and, in return, are expected to respect and honor the wishes of elders (Bliatout, 1998).

Time and Spatial Perspectives

A high degree of assimilation to the dominant culture has occurred among many Asian Americans, accompanied by a change in their concept of time. Traditionally oriented to the past, many Asian Americans consider time to be valuable and have become increasingly future oriented.

Territoriality needs among Asian Americans tend to be modest, and tactile expressions vary intraethnically. Touch may be rarely seen, however, in the public zone.

Health Perspectives

Asian Americans' attitudes regarding health have been greatly affected by personal experiences and exposure to the dominant culture. Traditionally, health has been defined as a balance of the positive and negative forces found in nature. Illness may be thought to occur when there is disharmony, resulting in an imbalance in these forces, which are referred to as yin and yang. Evil spirits may also cause illness (Bliatout, 1998). Many environmental elements, such as wind and water, are thought to possess negative or positive properties that can affect health and illness. Certain foods and home remedies may be relied on to restore balance (Chow, 1976). Shamans, massage therapists, herbalists, acupuncturists, and others may be consulted. Today, many Asian Americans attribute illness to germ theory or a combination of traditional and modern theories.

Members of Asian cultures, especially newly

arrived immigrants and women of older generations, may experience problems in accessing the health care system because of language barriers. Intensely private, Asian American patients and their family members might be reluctant to disclose personal and family information with a stranger. Because open expression of emotions may be considered unacceptable, affect and responses can be misinterpreted.

Where and how care is accessed by Asian Americans is greatly influenced by individual socioeconomic status. Members of the large Asian American middle class in America access care in the private sector, whereas those in the lower socioeconomic groups may seek care at county health clinics and public hospitals.

Language and Communication Styles

Many rules govern communication among members of the Asian cultures. Verbal communication is formal, and nonverbal and situational cues are very important. In addition, the status and age of the speaker are significant.

In approaching the Asian American family, politeness is paramount. Parents should be addressed by their surnames. Ethnic heritage should not be assumed or guessed at; rather, the family should be asked what their ethnic heritage is. The NP should follow the family's cues with regard to formality and directness in verbal communication.

Out of respect for authority, the Asian American parents or patients may not admit to the health care provider that they do not understand something the health care provider has explained, and they may not ask questions. To be certain that the diagnosis and management plan are understood, avoid questions that require a yes or no response and encourage parent and patient to repeat any instructions that are given.

Among those who possess traditional beliefs regarding health and illness, the goal of therapy in caring for the sick Asian American child is to restore balance. Under these circumstances, collaboration with the family and incorporation of traditional foods, herbs, and folk remedies into the management plan foster a trusting relationship and facilitate compliance.

Risk Factors

Intolerance to dairy products is not uncommon among Asian Americans, especially children. Adherents to traditional ways may breastfeed their children into the fourth or fifth year. Middle-class Asian Americans who have assimilated the diet and lifestyle of the dominant middle class in America experience health problems reflective of these changes. Among low-income Asian Americans and new immigrants, tuberculosis, dental caries, and malnutrition are seen.

NATIVE AMERICANS

Cultural Identity

There is considerable cultural diversity among the Native American minority group, as evidenced by the existence of more than 200 different tribes, each with its own language and cultural identity. Although traditionally many Native Americans have resided on federally mandated reservations, more and more have moved to urban areas, mainstreaming into general society with varying degrees of difficulty (Buehler, 1993; van Breda, 1989).

Despite assimilation to the dominant culture, many Native Americans continue to value their ancestors' world view, which emphasizes living in harmony with nature and protecting the earth by taking only what is needed to live. Emotional attachments to the land and nature may be strong, whereas accumulation of material goods and exploitation of resources for material gain may be discouraged. Much emphasis may be placed on teaching children to be sensitive to the environment and collectively oriented in establishing goals and making decisions.

Family Structure

Native American families on the reservations have traditionally been large and extended, with several generations living in a single household. Elders may be greatly revered, and grandparents frequently participate extensively in raising the grandchildren. Qualities such as autonomy, self-initiation, and cooperation are highly valued, whereas competitive behavior is discouraged. Among those who reside in urban environments across the country, nuclear families and single parent families are becoming more commonplace.

Time and Spatial Perspectives

Native Americans tend to live for the present but with a reverence for the past. In some tribal languages, in fact, there is no noun for time and no past or future verb tenses. Traditional homes may not have clocks, and individuals may not wear wristwatches.

Native Americans tend to have moderate territoriality needs. Because Native Americans are intensely private, acquaintances are not invited into the family's intimate zone until a strong sense of trust has developed.

Perspectives on Health

Native Americans often hold traditional tribal beliefs relating to health and illness. Thus, illness may be thought to be due to lack of harmony, imbalance, or a manifestation of bad thoughts or unresolved anger (Buehler, 1993). Folk cures and healers may be relied on first or in conjunction with health care providers. Many foods, events, and substances have symbolic value.

Language and Communication Style

Communication in Native American cultures is highly contextual. There are many rules associated with encoding and decoding messages, and the rank of the speaker is very significant.

In communicating with a Native American, the NP should not rush, never interrupt, and remain sensitive to nonverbal and situational cues. The patient may be accompanied by several adult members of the family, all of whom are expected to participate in the encounter. A short period of silence after each member speaks is customary. The tendency to avoid prolonged eye contact should not be interpreted as rudeness or lack of interest or motivation; rather, it is a demonstration of respect. A gentle declarative style of interviewing, as opposed to a questioning style, better facilitates the development of a trusting relationship. For example, one can say "There has been no change in the baby's appetite with this runny nose" rather than "Has the baby been eating as usual?"

Because Native Americans may view time from a different perspective, they may be late for appointments or miss medication doses. It is helpful to speak in terms of approximate times ("Take this medication in the afternoon") or relate instructions to other events ("Give the baby the medicine before you sit down to dinner"). Compliance is enhanced if management plans incorporate tribal rituals and remedies with a Western approach.

Risk Factors

Alcoholism and poverty play major roles in the health problems experienced by this population group (van Breda, 1989). Native American infants had the second highest mortality rate in 1995 (Centers for Disease Control and Prevention, 1995). Families are generally poor, and they have poor housing and low levels of education. Families are likely to seek health care for their children for complex problems rather than prevention and maintenance. Malnutrition, gastroenteritis, severe infections, tuberculosis, and the effects of maternal alcohol consumption are commonly seen among Native American children. Accidental trauma and poisoning, suicide, and homicide, as well as an increased incidence of developmental, behavioral, and emotional disorders, also afflict this population (US Department of Health & Human Services, 1990).

ARAB AMERICANS

Cultural Identity

Arab Americans speak Arabic and are usually of Semitic origin. The term refers to natives of many countries of the Middle East, including Armenia, Palestine, Egypt, Iran, Iraq, Jordan, Lebanon, Saudi Arabia, Syria, Yemen, and several other countries. The Lebanese were the largest group in the 1990 US census (310,000). A diverse group in terms of socioeconomic status and education, there are approximately 1 million Arab Americans with permanent residency status living in the United States (US Department of Commerce, 1990). Many work in professional and semiprofessional jobs.

Primarily urban dwellers, Middle Easterners have been migrating to the United States since 1875. In the last 35 years, the rate of immigration among Middle Eastern peoples to North America has increased as a result of political instability and wars in their homelands. Although Middle Easterners vary ethnically, they share a core of common values and behaviors related to family affiliation, time and space orientation, interactional style, and attitudes toward health and illness (Lipson & Meleis, 1983).

Family Structure

Two distinct circles of affiliation exist in Middle Eastern culture: an inner circle of family members and close friends who share intense devotion to one another, and an outer circle of acquaintances and strangers. The family is the most influential social institution in Middle Eastern culture (Rugh, 1984). The structure of the family tends to be patriarchal; decision-making by the family's male elders is highly contextual and devoted to the good of the family as a group. In addition, the Middle Eastern family is likely to have an extended configuration; members who do not live together frequently live in close proximity to one another and have daily contact. It is common for children to live with their parents until they marry and for them to maintain close contact afterwards (Lipson & Meleis, 1983).

Outside the inner circle of the family, relationships develop very slowly and are shrouded in mistrust until the outsider is accepted. Ritual courtesy may be extended to strangers with offers of hospitality that are not intended to be taken literally.

Time and Spatial Perspectives

Traditionally, the Middle Eastern cultures are oriented to the present; punctuality is not as important as it is in the United States. Highly assimilated Arab Americans, however, may reflect the perspectives of the dominant majority in punctuality and orientation to the future.

Watson's (1980) studies of cultural variations in territoriality needs revealed that persons of Middle Eastern background demonstrated low spatial distancing requirements, preferring to stand approximately two to three feet apart during conversation.

Health Perspective

Intraethnic variations are reflected in the multiple disease etiologies recognized by members of the Arab American culture. Germ theory, the concept of the evil eye, humoral theory, and the will of God may be encountered. Amulets may be worn or esfame seed burned to ward off the evil eye, which is inspired by another's jealousy of an individual's good fortune. In general, Western medicine is greatly respected, and an Arab American family may seek out the services of the top person in a given specialty. Commonly, however, the family's lay referral system (consisting of family, friends, neighbors, and others) is accessed before professional advice is sought (May, 1992).

Language and Communication Style

Traditionally, communication in Middle Eastern cultures is highly contextual. As a result, verbal communication may be less direct, and awareness of nonverbal and situational cues is essential. There are many rules governing verbal and nonverbal communication, and the age and educational level of the speaker are significant. The Middle Eastern individual may seek close proximity when communicating, and a speech pattern involving repetition may be employed when emphasis is desired (Hall, 1976). The tendency of members of the dominant majority culture to immediately get down to the business at hand may be offensive to Middle Easterners, as their custom requires the establishment of the relationship first (Meleis & LaFever, 1984). Touch as a component of communication is frequently engaged in, and friends and family are embraced on arriving and leaving.

Numerous family members may accompany the child to a health care appointment, especially if the appointment is for an acute or chronic illness. All family members should be acknowledged, and any elder family members present should be included in decision-making related to the treatment plan (Meleis, 1981).

Sexual topics and issues relating to family planning may be considered extremely private matters among those of Middle Eastern descent (Meleis & Sorrell, 1981). As a result, Arab Americans may shun the services of a male provider when seeking care for health issues relating to female sexual activity and reproduction.

Risk Factors

In many Middle Eastern families preventive care and family planning may be unfamiliar concepts, as they connote planning ahead, which may be perceived as defying God's will (Giger & Davidhizar, 1995). As a result, conditions that may be discovered in the early stages through routine screening may be missed.

Assimilation of the norms and customs of the dominant culture brings the same risks to health as seen in other groups who consume highly processed food on a regular basis and live a fast-paced lifestyle.

RUSSIAN AMERICANS

Cultural Identity

In 1990, there were approximately 2 million former citizens of the Soviet Union living in the United States (US Department of Commerce, Bureau of Census, 1990). The term Russian Americans refers to immigrants and refugees from the 15 republics that once comprised the Soviet Union, including Russia (the largest and most heavily populated region), Georgia, Belarus, Estonia, Ukraine, Azerbaijan, and Kazakhstan. Those with refugee status are primarily Jews granted political asylum in the United States in response to ever-increasing anti-Semitism in their homeland (US Department of Justice, 1992). Since 1990, approximately 50,000 Russians have emigrated to the United States annually, primarily in family groups.

Under the Soviet political structure, advanced education, including vocational training programs and university studies, was free and readily accessible; therefore, it is common for immigrants and refugees from the former Soviet Union to be either well educated, to have a viable trade, or both. Russian Americans tend to value education highly, seeing it as a means to prosperity and self-fulfillment for themselves and their children.

In spite of the emphasis on collectivism inherent in the Soviet cultural ideology, many Russian Americans are avidly individualistic and possess a strong work ethic. To work hard for a better future for themselves and their families is a strong cultural ideal.

Primarily urban dwellers, Russian Americans are likely to be found in large North American cities in communities of Russian Americans who emigrated earlier. Many of these communities provide transition assistance in the form of work training and career guidance programs, English language classes, and social activities.

Religious expression of any kind was prohibited under the Soviet regime. As a result, many Russian Americans (with the exception of those who are Jewish) have had little exposure to organized religion. Since glasnost and perestroika, however, there has been a remarkable resurgence in the Eastern Orthodox religion in Russia and among Russian American immigrants in North America. Among Jewish Russian American refugees, many have found it possible to practice their faith openly for the first time in their lives.

Family Structure

The concept of the family is very important in the Russian culture. For many years, Soviet policy required that Russian families emigrate as a unit. As a result, many Russian Americans live in extended, multigenerational family configurations.

Russian American families tend to be patriarchal; the paternal figure, with input from his wife and the family elders, establishes family priorities and makes decisions. Children are greatly valued, and, although they tend to be cared for by the female members of the family, fathers frequently spend a significant amount of time with their children, even when they are very young.

Time and Spatial Perspectives

Time perspective varies among members of the Russian American population. While there is a considerable reverence for history and past experience, many, especially those who are well educated, have a future orientation. Many Russian Americans consider it bad manners to fail to keep a scheduled appointment or to be late for an appointment.

Russian Americans generally do not have significant territoriality needs; it is not unusual for friends to maintain little spatial distance when they talk and to embrace when they meet.

Language and Communication Style

Most Russian American immigrants speak Russian. Elderly Russians of Jewish heritage may also speak Yiddish, but their children typically do not. Many Russian Americans studied French, German, or English in Russia but had little opportunity to practice with native speakers. Priority is placed on becoming proficient in English as quickly as possible. It is not unusual for young children in Russian American families to understand Russian when they hear it but respond in English.

Russian Americans may communicate on two different levels: With strangers and acquaintances (the public zone), communication tends to be formal and reserved, with very little gesturing. In public places, a Russian American may avoid eye contact and assume a tight, low posture. Communication in the intimate zone (generally reserved for family and close friends) is characterized by embracing, kissing, touching, and gesturing. A handshake connotes a binding agreement. Regardless of the zone in which an encounter takes place, communication is highly contextual.

Health Care Perspectives

Under the Soviet government, health care services, although free, were frequently limited in scope and continuity. Since the demise of the communist regime, health care has become even more difficult to access in Russia. As a result, Russian Americans may be reluctant to seek health care services and have low expectations of the American health care system.

When a child arrives for an appointment with the NP, especially for an acute or chronic illness, he or she may be accompanied by both parents as well as elder family members. The NP should acknowledge elders and parents equally and involve all in the development of the treatment plan.

Many Russian Americans expect the provider–patient relationship to be an authoritarian one. They expect the NP to be serious, formal, and reserved, and they may not ask questions or engage in informal dialogue because it is considered disrespectful to do so.

As with other cultural groups, it is best to use the family name when addressing adult family members; a married woman, however, may have a different surname from her children because of the custom of retaining one's maiden name and using it exclusively in a business or professional context.

Russian Americans may occasionally use folk or home remedies before, or in addition to, seeking professional advice. Incorporating these practices into the treatment regimen, if it is safe to do so, promotes the development of a trusting relationship and enhances compliance.

Risk Factors

According to Duncan (1996), the health-care system in the Soviet Union placed little emphasis on promoting a healthful lifestyle. As a result, it is anticipated that the effects of heavy tobacco and alcohol use, poor dietary intake, crowded living conditions, and environmental pollution will be reflected for many years to come in the health care needs of Russian immigrants.

Russian immigrant families, therefore, may have little experience with preventive health care practices beyond the most basic screening measures. Education efforts that focus on preventive care (e.g., screening measures, immunizations, family planning, and exercise) will help to reduce the potential for illness and accidental injury. In addition, eating nutritious foods for optimal growth and development (especially fresh fruits and vegetables) and understanding the dangers of tobacco exposure should be emphasized.

Just as in any other newly arrived group of individuals, Russian immigrants may experience anxiety and disorientation as they pursue their activities of daily living in the United States.

Having always lived and worked in an authoritarian, highly regimented, bureaucratic society, the multiple choices encountered on a daily basis in a fast-paced, free society may be stressful. The NP should be alert to evidence of culture shock and stress in patients and parents.

POOR AMERICANS

Cultural Identity

Huston, McLoyd, and Coll (1994) define poverty as inadequate resources to meet daily living needs. According to the US Bureau of the Census (1990), more than 35 million people, including 6 million children younger than 15 years of age, live below the poverty line at any point in time. Almost 12 million more survive just barely above the poverty line, and the number goes up every year.

In America, higher proportions of African Americans, Native Americans, and Hispanics are poor. When such households are headed by a woman (an increasingly common phenomenon), the poverty is more severe. The gender and ethnic characteristics associated with poverty reinforce racist and sexist attitudes, compounding the social stigma. Research studies document that poor Americans have a strong work ethic, but lack of incentives prevents them from securing and maintaining employment (Mason, 1981).

Family Structure

Indigent families live in urban and rural areas, in areas of the country that have had a strong subculture of poverty for generations, and in places where affluence is the norm. Thus, they are described as a subculture that transcends ethnic and regional boundaries because they possess their own material and nonmaterial qualities and characteristics that tend to be passed down from generation to generation.

Every year, more poor families in America slip into homelessness. Single mothers with two or three children are, in fact, the fastest growing segment of the homeless population. Runaway adolescents form another significant homeless group; they come primarily from minority groups and troubled families and are at risk of becoming involved in prostitution, substance abuse, and violent activities (Wiecha et al., 1991).

Time and Spatial Perspectives

Poor people tend to be oriented to the present in the gratification of needs, especially in the concrete, physical realm. Problems of survival may take precedence over planning for future goals. A wide range of territoriality needs may be seen.

Health Perspectives

A fatalistic view of life is common among the poor, and health tends to be defined in terms of the ability to work. The poor may believe that events such as illness are not preventable. They are more inclined to seek relief from a folk healer or by use of home remedies rather than from a health care professional in part because of difficulty in understanding a health care system that is an expression of the dominant class's value assumptions. When they do seek care, they may reluctantly go to county health department clinics or emergency facilities, often with conditions that are advanced or complicated.

Language and Communication Style

Developing a therapeutic relationship grounded in basic trust can be a challenge for the primary care provider who is working with the poor and the homeless populations. As a rule, these groups do not participate in the larger society and possess a general attitude of hostility and mistrust of bureaucratic authority figures. This attitude, combined with the feelings of helplessness, dependence, and inferiority that characterize poverty, necessitates a slow, deliberate approach by the primary care provider. Everything should be explained and diagrammed, if possible, because literacy levels vary and the individual may be embarrassed to admit illiteracy.

Risk Factors

Poverty is particularly hard on children. Childhood is typically not valued among the poor, and children may be expected to assume responsibility for younger siblings and household chores at an early age. Predisposed to harsh discipline at home and violence on the streets, poor children also have a high rate of injuries caused by accidents. The infant mortality rate is higher among the poor, and health statistics show that children who survive infancy to live below the poverty line are at risk for a myriad of health problems, including frequent infections, dental caries, gum disease, nutritional anemia, mental retardation, lead poisoning, emotional and behavioral problems, learning disabilities, and vision and speech impairments. Poor health and poor nutrition have a profound impact on school readiness and the educability of children (Pollitt, 1994).

The health problems associated with poverty are compounded by homelessness. Unsanitary living conditions, low immunization rates, erratic schooling and health care services, poor nutrition, and the emotional trauma associated with a transient lifestyle contribute to the pervasive feelings of helplessness, isolation, and desperation these children experience (Alperstein & Arnstein, 1988).

CONCLUSION

Every day, the United States becomes more culturally diverse. This diversity brings with it many challenges for health care providers. As a factor in the commitment to serve that is shared by primary care providers, the development of cultural sensitivity facilitates the delivery of quality care that is culturally competent.

REFERENCES

Alperstein G, Arnstein E: Homeless children: A challenge for pediatricians. Pediatr Clin North Am 35:1413–1425, 1988.

Berger P, Luckmann T: The Social Construction of Reality. New York, Doubleday, 1966.

Bliatout B: Some aspects of Southeast Asian-American traditional health beliefs and practices. Paper presented at Oregon Health Sciences University, School of Nursing, 2/24/98.

Buehler J: Nursing in rural Native-American communities. Nurs Clin North Am 28:211–217, 1993.

Carr S: Understanding Latino folk medicines. Nurseweek 17:23, Sept 1990.

Caudle P: Providing culturally sensitive care to Hispanic clients. Nurs Pract 18:40–50, 1993.

Centers for Disease Control and Prevention: Infant mortality statistics from the linked birth/infant data set—1995 period data. Mon Vital Stat Rep 46(suppl 2), Feb 26, 1995.

Centers for Disease Control and Prevention: Tobacco use among high school students–United States, 1997. MMWR Morb Mortal Wkly Rep 47, Apr 3, 1998.

Char EL: The Chinese American. In Clark AL (ed): Culture and Childrearing. Philadelphia, FA Davis, 1981.

Children's Defense Fund: The State of America's Children, 1992: Leave No Child Behind. Washington, DC, Children's Defense Fund, 1992.

Chow E: Cultural health traditions. In Branch MF, Paxon PP, (eds): Providing Safe Nursing Care for Ethnic People of Color. New York, Appleton-Century-Crofts, 1976.

Chrisman NJ: Cultural systems. In McCorkle R, Grant M, Frank-Stromborg M, et al (eds): Cancer Nursing: A Comprehensive Textbook. Philadelphia, WB Saunders, 1991, pp. 45–54.

Duncan L: Health practices among Russian and Ukrainian immigrants. J Commun Health Nurs 13:129–137, 1996.

Erikson E: Childhood and Society. New York, Norton, 1964.

Friedman MM: Transcultural family nursing: Application to Latino and black families. J Pediatr Nurs 5:214–222, 1990.

Gadow K, Sprafkin J: Field experiments of television violence with children: Evidence for an environmental hazard? Pediatrics, 83:399–405, 1989.

Gervais KG: Providing culturally competent health care to Hmong patients. Minn Med 79:49–51, 1996.

Giger JN, Davidhizar RE: Transcultural nursing: Assessment and Intervention. St. Louis, Mosby, 1995.

Gonzalez-Swafford MJ, Gutierrez MG: Ethno-medical beliefs and practices of Mexican-Americans. Nurs Pract Nov/Dec, 1988, pp 29–34.

Grasska MA, McFarland T: Overcoming the language barrier: Problems and solutions. Am J Nurs 82:1376–1379, 1982.

Gudykunst WB, Ting-Toomey S: Culture and Interpersonal Communication. Thousand Oaks, CA: Sage, 1988.

Hall ET: Beyond Culture. New York, Doubleday, 1976.

Henderson G, Primeaux M: Transcultural Health Care. Menlo Park, CA, Addison-Wesley, 1981.

Huston AE, McLoyd VC, Coll CG: Children and poverty: Issues in contemporary research. Child Dev 65:275, 1994.

Jackson L: Understanding, eliciting, and negotiating clients' multicultural health beliefs. Nurse Pract 18:30–43, 1993.

Kleinman A: The Illness Narratives: Suffering, Healing, and the Human Condition. New York, Basic Books, 1988.

Leininger MM: The significance of cultural concepts in nursing. J Transcultural Nurs 2:52–59, 1990.

Leininger MM: Leininger's theory of nursing: Cultural care diversity and universality. Nurs Sci Q 1:152–160, 1988.

Lipson JG, Meleis AI: Issues in the health care of Middle Eastern patients. West J Med 139:854–861, 1983.

Marsh WW, Hentges K: Mexican folk remedies and conventional care. Am Fam Phys 37:257–262, 1988.

Mason D: Perspectives on poverty. Image 13:82–85, 1981.

May KM: Middle-Eastern immigrant parents' social networks and help-seeking for child health care. J Adv Nurs 17:905–912, 1992.

Meleis AI: The Arab-American in the health care system. Am J Nurs June 81:1180-1183, 1981.

Meleis AI, LaFever CW: The Arab-American and psychiatric care. Perspect Psychiatr Care 22:72-76; 85-86, 1984.

Meleis AI, Sorrell L: Arab-American women and their birth experiences. Am J Matern Child Nurs 6:171-176, 1981.

Munoz E: Care for the Hispanic poor: A growing segment of American society. JAMA 260:2711-2712, 1988.

Niederhauser VP: Health care of immigrant children: Incorporating culture into practice. Pediatr Nurs 15:569-574, 1989.

Pachter LM: Culture and clinical care: Folk illness beliefs and behaviors and their implications for health care delivery. JAMA 271:690-694, 1994.

Pachter LM: Practicing culturally sensitive pediatrics. Contemp Pediatr 14:139-146, 1997.

Pollitt E: Poverty and child development: Relevance of research in developing countries to the United States. Child Dev 65:283-295, 1994.

Porter RE, Samovar LA: Intercultural Communication: A Reader, 8th ed. Belmont, CA: Wadsworth, 1997.

Reddy M: Statistical Record of Hispanic-Americans, 2nd ed. New York, Gale Research, Inc., 1995.

Rugh AB: Family in Contemporary Egypt. Syracuse, NY, Syracuse University Press, 1984.

Torres S: Cultural sensitivity: A must for today's primary care provider. Adv Nurse Pract 1:16-18, 1993.

Tylor E: Primitive Culture: Researches into the Mythology, Philosophy, Religion, Art, and Custom. Vol 1: London, John Murray, 1958.

US Department of Commerce, Bureau of the Census: Current populations: Reports, Divisions, and States. Washington, DC, US Department of Commerce, Bureau of the Census, 1988.

US Department of Commerce, Bureau of the Census: 1990 Census of Population. Washington, DC, U.S. Department of Commerce, Bureau of the Census, 1990.

US Department of Health and Human Services: Healthy People 2000. Washington, DC, 1990.

US Department of Justice, Immigration, and Naturalization Service: Immigration from the former Soviet Union, 1989-1991. Washington, DC, Government Printing Office, 1992.

US Public Health Service: Child Health USA 96-97. US Public Service, Bureau of Maternal and Child Health, 1998.

van Breda A: Health issues facing Native-American children. Pediatr Nurs 15:575-577, 1989.

Watson OM: Proxemic Behavior: A Cross-Cultural Study. The Hague, Netherlands, Mouton, 1980.

Wiecha JL, Dwyer JT, Dunn-Strohecker M: Nutrition and health service needs among the homeless. Public Health Rep 106:365-374, 1991.

Zambrana R, Dorrington C: Economic and social vulnerability of Latino children and families by subgroup: Implications for child welfare. Child Welfare 77:5-27, 1998.

Management of Development

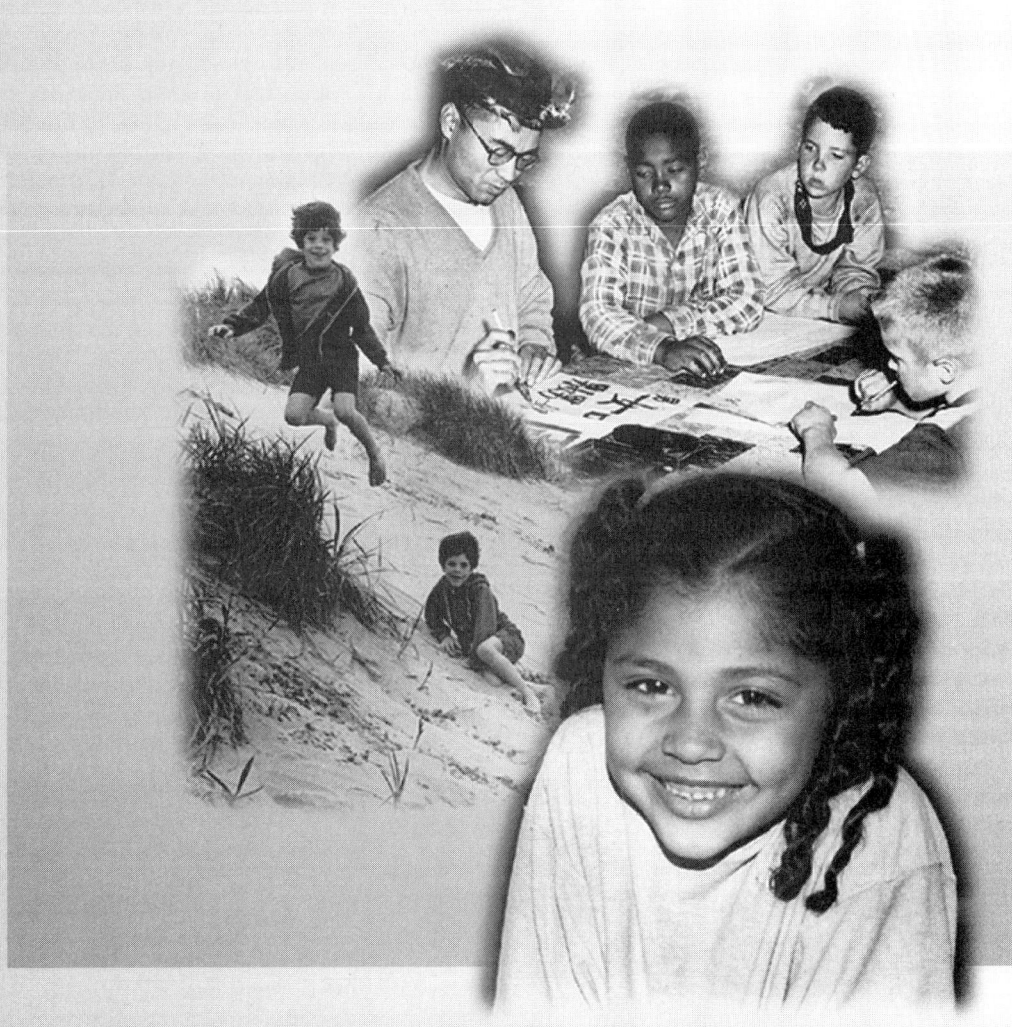

CHAPTER 5

Developmental Management in Pediatric Primary Care

Barbara Jones Deloian

INTRODUCTION

Primary care providers have a responsibility to monitor children's overall physical and psychosocial development and to provide anticipatory guidance to families as children grow. This requires a strong background in child development and a knowledge of clinical strategies that will help parents better understand their child's development. Nurse practitioners (NPs) who work with parents and their children share in the parents' pride as their child accomplishes a new developmental task. NPs assist parents to understand the challenges that new accomplishments create and how parents may best handle these challenges. Modern approaches to managing children's well-being today differ dramatically from those that prevailed at the turn of the last century, when health supervision consisted of a brief examination to detect communicable or contagious diseases. As the 21st century begins, significant social, economic, and demographic changes continue to influence the American family and affect children's health. Children's health supervision must take a broader approach than would be necessary only for detection of disease.

The *Diagnostic and Statistical Manual for Primary Care (DSM-PC), Child and Adolescent Version* (Wolraich et al., 1996) has been published to establish a more comprehensive description of the physical and psychosocial developmental concerns of childhood and adolescence. The pediatric primary care provider must have a sound knowledge of these developmental issues. The next four chapters of this unit review developmental theories, describe normal patterns of development, and recommend anticipatory guidance for families based on the unique characteristics of parents and children.

The concept of developmental surveillance as described by Dworkin (1989) provides the framework for this discussion:

> Surveillance encompasses all primary care activities related to the monitoring of the development of children. It includes obtaining a relevant developmental history, making accurate and informative observations of children, and eliciting and attending to parental concerns. Emphasis is placed on monitoring development within the context of the child's overall well-being rather than viewing development in isolation during a testing session.

Developmental Surveillance

Developmental surveillance involves more than asking developmental questions, completing a developmental screening checklist, asking how a child is doing in school, or completing a school physical examination. The developmental surveillance model is based on several basic assumptions about development, such as those outlined by Dixon and Stein (1992). These assumptions include the following:

- Development is a self-fueling, ongoing process that requires physical and emotional energy.
- Development occurs in stages and is dynamic and interactional.
- Development is influenced by the child and his or her environment.
- Development occurs in "spurts and lulls." Periods of disorganization, disharmony, and turbulence are usually followed by periods of harmony, balance, and organization as new skills are integrated.
- All areas of development are interrelated.

Providing supportive care for children through developmental surveillance also involves certain beliefs. These include the following:

1. Children are generally healthy and have adaptive capabilities. Therefore, the goal of the NP is to maintain health rather than solely to resolve problems.
2. Individual differences among children are reflected in developmental variations. These arise, in part, from the unique characteristics of families, cultures, and social circumstances. Individual developmental variations and positive adaptations should be appreciated and facilitated.
3. Children and families have the capacity to learn and grow from their limitations when interventions are based on their abilities.
4. Preventive health care for children includes developmentally supportive mental health care.
5. The goal of anticipatory guidance is to increase parenting skills, confidence, and competence in problem solving. Quick, pat answers to complex parenting issues do not facilitate parental growth.
6. Because the family is changing, it is important to expand an understanding of the roles of significant adults in a child's life.

The practitioner-family relationship can be a powerful tool to guide family members' management of their child's temperament, behavior, and development. It also can benefit parental efficacy through building parental confidence and competency. The benefit of establishing a long-term, continuous relationship with a child and family cannot be overestimated.

Developmental Principles

The study of developmental theories reveals a fascinating array of ideas about how children progress from infancy through adolescence, providing many perspectives on children's growth and development. NPs need to continue to stay abreast of changing ideas of child development and appreciate new developmental theories relating to children. Developmental theories are based on various cultures, personalities, environmental issues, philosophical beliefs, and investigative methods. Thus, when using a developmental perspective in practice, the NP should understand how the theory was developed and how it may relate to a particular family and child.

Developmental theories provide guidelines for understanding the unfolding of the child's behavior, personality, and physical abilities. Therefore, it is necessary to combine several theories to understand the child as a whole person. Development is a lifelong, dynamic process. Achievement of changes in one phase sets the stage for the next phase. Development is also a dynamic and reciprocal process that occurs between the child's internal and external environment.

Key principles are often used to understand concepts of development. Exactly how these principles are manifested in a particular child depends on the child's genetic background as well as personality and environment.

PRINCIPLE 1. Growth and development are orderly and sequential. Although children differ in rates and timing of developmental changes, they generally follow certain predictable stages or phases. Specific examples include the rapid growth during the first year of life, progress toward independence throughout childhood, and the unfolding of secondary sex characteristics during adolescence.

PRINCIPLE 2. The pace of growth and development is specific for each child. Developmental changes vary considerably for each child. Some children demonstrate early skill in motor coordination, others in language acquisition. These changes represent the uniqueness of each child.

PRINCIPLE 3. Development occurs in a cephalocaudal direction. An example of this principle is seen as infants develop increasing motor coordination, gaining head control before sitting and walking.

PRINCIPLE 4. Development occurs in a proximodistal direction. Similarly, developmental progress is seen in controlled movements that occur near the midline of the body first, such as rolling over. Eventually, distal coordination of the hands, such as mastery of the pincer grasp, occurs.

PRINCIPLE 5. Growth and development become increasingly integrated. Behavior that is often taken for granted, such as self-feeding, occurs as a result of numerous small changes and skills acquired by the child. Simple skills and behaviors are integrated into more complex behaviors as the child grows and develops.

PRINCIPLE 6. Developmental abilities become increasingly differentiated. As a result of increasing experience and maturation, children's behaviors and responses to internal and external cues become more differentiated. The infant's crying and body movements in response to hunger cues are different from the toddler's walking to the refrigerator in response to the same cues.

PRINCIPLE 7. Growth and development are affected by the child's internal and external environment. Opportunities for play, societal norms, cultural values, family traditions, and family beliefs all influence the development of children. Similarly, children influence their environment to achieve desired experiences and opportunities.

PRINCIPLE 8. Certain periods are critical during growth and development. Critical periods are defined as points of time when developmental advances occur more readily than they do at other times. The occurrence of congenital anomalies when the fetus is exposed to certain viruses during fetal growth is one example.

PRINCIPLE 9. Growth and development are continual processes influenced by many factors. Development is a dynamic process, often without smooth transitions. Phases of development are marked by periods of change, growth, and plateaus of stability. Attempts to predict and control the developmental process often emphasize the individual nature of development and the numerous individual factors that influence developmental outcomes.

DEVELOPMENTAL THEORIES

Ethology: Animal Studies

The study of animal behavior has led to some theoretical assumptions that assist in the study of child development. These include four major propositions on the concepts of bonding, altruism, social intelligence, and dominant and submissive behavior. Bonding is of interest here. Bowlby (1969) first generalized theories developed about animal behavior to bonding for humans. This was followed by Klaus and Kennel's (1976) work, which emphasized the importance of early mother–infant contact and resulted in changes in hospital rooming-in care. Ainsworth and colleagues (1971) continued to examine the elements of early attachment and separation in child development and personality.

Maturational Theories: Developmental Milestones

Early theories about human behavior set the stage for studies in child development. The religious and cultural beliefs based on the sinful and obstinate child that derive from Puritan beliefs can be seen currently in strict child-rearing practices. Rousseau's descriptions in 1762 of the natural, innately good growth of the child, if not misled by a "corrupt social environment," provided the foundation for maturational theories. Gesell (1940) is credited with the term *maturation* in reference to the orderly, sequential developmental changes that occur over time. He also described cycles of behavior that correspond to certain chronological ages. His work resulted in the chronological growth and development norms for motor, affective, linguistic, and social domains that are now used to assess developmental progress.

Lewin's (1936) work provided the identification of growth principles and the currently acknowledged stages, including infancy, early childhood, and adolescence. He also provided an understanding of the play and decision-making phases that children go through.

Havighurst's (1953) work, a summation of ideas from many theorists, popularized the concept of developmental tasks described as "successful achievement which leads to . . . happiness and to success with later tasks, while failure leads to unhappiness in the individual, disapproval by society, and difficulty with later tasks."

Cognitive-Structural Theories: Language and Thought

Cognitive–structural theories examine the ways in which children think, reason, and use language. Their primary premise is based on assumptions of maturation of the central nervous system and children's interactions with their environment. Individual differences are ascribed to genetic endowment and environmental influences.

Jean Piaget's observations provide an understanding of children's cognitive development and their perception and use of the world around them. Piaget described how children actively use their life experiences, incorporating them into their own mental and physical being over time. He emphasized how children modify themselves depending on their environmental experiences and their stage-related level of competencies. Piaget described four stages of cognitive development (Table 5-1).

SENSORIMOTOR STAGE (BIRTH TO 2 YEARS). At this stage, children learn about the world through their actions and sensory and motor movements. Key concepts that are assimilated during this period include perception of object permanence, spatial relationships, causality, use of instruments, and combination of objects. The child's framework for learning is the self, and there is little cognitive connection to objects outside the self.

PREOPERATIONAL STAGE (2 TO 7 YEARS). Children next attempt to make sense of the world and reality. However, this is based on their own *egocentric* perspective and is accomplished through certain mental operations that are linked to concrete objects. Children at this stage are not able to understand cause and effect. Therefore, their reasoning is often flawed. Children are able to begin to use *semiotic functioning*, or the use of one thing to represent another. *Intuitive reasoning* emerges toward the end of this stage, but reasoning continues to be connected to the concrete reality of the here and now.

CONCRETE OPERATIONAL STAGE (7 TO 12 YEARS). Children are able finally to use symbols to represent concrete objects (here and now) and perform mental operations in their head. This process involves cognitive skills required to organize experiences and classify increasingly complex information. Most schoolwork requires functioning at this level with *flexibility of thought, declining egocentrism, logical reasoning, and greater social cognition.*

FORMAL OPERATIONAL STAGE (13 YEARS THROUGH ADULTHOOD). At this stage, children begin to think abstractly and to imagine different solutions to problems and different outcomes. During this stage, adolescents begin to develop increased awareness of degrees of illness as well as personal control of one's health. Renewed egocentrism may be noted early in this stage as a result of lack of differentiation between what others are thinking and one's own thoughts. This egocentric thinking eventually gives way to appreciation of differences in judgment between the adolescent and other individuals, societies, and cultures, and becomes the basis of an adolescent's ability to think about politics, law, and society in terms of abstract principles and benefits rather than focusing only on the punitive aspects of societal laws.

Piaget's work was expanded by theorists such as Flavell (1977) and Siegler and colleagues (1973), who looked at specific intellectual capabilities via the information processing model, which included concepts of attention, perception, memory, and inferencing. The information processing model provides initial understanding of how mental activity leads progressively to more sophisticated ways of handling information.

Kohlberg (1969) provided a theoretical focus on moral development and socialization, emphasizing the process by which children learn the expectations and norms of their society and culture (see Table 5-1). His work primarily involved male participants, whereas much of Piaget's work was formulated from observations of his own children.

Gilligan (1982) suggested that female thoughts and actions involve significantly different objectives and goals. Additional criticism has been expressed that early theorists' work lacked experimental support, especially related to different cultural and socioeconomic settings. More research is being conducted to validate and test developmental theories, especially to gain a better understanding of the learning mechanisms of children who have visual or motor compromises and need special interventions.

Fowler's (1981) theory described the spiritual dimension of human life, or the development of faith. This theory addressed the process by which humans develop meaning for daily life. Faith is described as the structure that people use to build their lives. Fowler emphasized that achieving the stages is not due to intelligence but, rather, occurs through valuing, thinking, and interacting with others.

Psychoanalytical Theories

PERSONALITY AND EMOTIONS

Factors that influence the emotional and psychological behavior of an individual have been studied by psychodynamic theorists. Personality includes the characteristics of temperament and motivation and concepts related to self-esteem and self-concept. Sigmund Freud (1938) was one of the most influential theorists in this area. He sought to find links between the conscious mind and the body through the unconscious mind (see Table 5-1). Some of his most significant contributions were his descriptions of the interactions of id, ego, and superego (Thomas, 1985).

Anna Freud continued the work of her father, focusing particularly on children. It was through her studies that the implications of psychoanalysis for raising normal children were developed. She believed that psychoanalytical theory could help parents gain "insight into the potential harm done to young children during the critical years of their development by the manner in which their needs, drives, wishes, and emotional dependencies are met" (Freud, 1974).

Erikson (1964) also expanded Freud's theories, describing the stages of the individual through the life span (see Table 5-1). Each stage presents problems that the individual seeks to master. Erikson believed that if problems were not resolved, they would be revisited again at future stages.

Sullivan (1964) emphasized the importance of self-concept and the environmental influences that modulate it. He defined the most crucial cultural environment as the home and the parent. Progression toward mature relationships is based on communication skills and the integration of social experiences.

Mahler and colleagues (1975) analyzed the development of an infant's evolving independence through study of the mother-infant dyad. Three phases of development were proposed, including autism, symbiosis, and separation–individuation. These phases account for the gradually increasing awareness of the infant's sense of self and others. The *autistic phase* refers to the period between 3 and 5 weeks of age when the infant has no concept of self but is working, physiologically, to achieve homeostasis in the extrauterine world. The second phase, *symbiosis*, refers to a period of undifferentiation or fusion with the mother in which infant and mother form a dual unity. *Separation–individuation* occurs as the infant becomes more mobile and is characterized by a steady increase in awareness of the separateness of the self and the other. A growing awareness occurs by 4 to 5 months of age, when the infant demonstrates a specific, preferential smile in response to the mother. *Differentiation*, a subphase of separation–individuation, occurs at about 6 to 7 months of age, when the infant uses visual and tactile exploration of the mother or caregiver. *Practicing*, a second subphase of separation–individuation, occurs as the infant explores movement toward more autonomous functions. Transitional objects, such as blankets or toys, make separation from the mother easier and help the infant establish familiarity with a broader segment of the world. The infant may move back and forth from the mother for emotional refueling. During this

T A B L E 5-1
Comparison of Early Developmental Theorists

AGE	FREUD	KOHLBERG		PIAGET		ERIKSON	
		Stages	Stages/Substages	Characteristics		Psychological Crisis	Themes
0–12 mo	Oral stage	"Amoral" preconventional level	1: Punishment and obedience	Sensorimotor stage 1. Reflexive stage: 0–1 mo	Innate infant reflexes	Trust vs. mistrust	To get; to give in return
				2. Primary circular stage: 1–4 mo	Repetitive responses		
				3. Secondary circular stage: 4–8 mo	Outward-directed behaviors		
				4. Coordination of secondary circular stage: 8–12 mo	Object permanence and goal-directed behaviors		
12–18 mo				5. Tertiary circular reactions stage: 2–18 mo	Causality and object permanence through several steps	Autonomy vs. shame	To hold on; to let go
18–36 mo	Anal stage	Stages 1–2 conventional level	2: Instrumental realistic orientation	6. Mental combinations stage: 18–24 mo	Memory used for problem solving		
3–6 yr	Oedipal stage	Stages 1–3	3: Interpersonal acceptance of "nice" girl and "good" boy social concept	Preoperational stage 1. Preconceptual stage: 2–4 yr	Increased use of symbols, especially language; representational thought, egocentrism, assimilation, and symbolic play	Initiative vs. guilt	To make things, to play

Age	(Freud) stage	(Kohlberg) stages	(Kohlberg) orientation	(Piaget) stage	Cognitive/social description	(Erikson) conflict	Goal
				2. Intuitive stage: 4–7 yr	Increased symbolic functioning, language, decreasing egocentricity, imitation of reality		
6–11 yr	Latency stage	Stages 2–5	4: The "law and order" orientation 5: Social contract, and utilitarian orientation	Concrete operational stage	Flexible thought: understands rules of reversibility and deconcentration, conservation, and identity. Declining egocentrism: ability to understand another's perspective. Logical reasoning: understands concepts of relation, ordering, conservation; able to classify objects. Social cognition: improved sense of equality and justice	Industry vs. inferiority	To make things; to complete
12–17 yr	Adolescence (Oedipus complex)	Stages 4–6	6: Universal ethical principle orientation	Formal operational stage	Development of logical thinking, the ability to work with abstract ideas; able to synthesize and integrate concepts into larger schemes	Identity vs. role confusion	To be oneself; to share being oneself or not being oneself
17–30 yr	Young adult	Stages 4–6		Formal operational stage		Intimacy vs. isolation	To lose and find oneself in another

practice period, weaning may be easier because the natural tendency for exploration and separation is occurring. *Rapprochement*, a third subphase of the separation–individuation phase, occurring at 14 to 24 months, accounts for the child's use of the mother as an extension of self. Shyness with strangers and adverse reactions to separations may be due to a growing sense of vulnerability. A final subphase, *consolidation* (occurring at 24 to 36 months), is demonstrated as the infant is able to separate from the mother without extreme anxiety. Symbolic play emerges, and the child is better able to delay gratification of needs.

Infant attachment within the context of separation and connectedness has been explored by contemporary theorists Stern (1985), Emde and Buchsbaum (1990), and Rogoff (1990). They propose that infants develop a sense of self through the experience of the infant–caregiver relationship. The quality and consistency of relationships help them develop an affective, or emotional, sense of self. The early beginnings of the sense of self are based on three biological principles: self-regulation, social fittedness, and affective monitoring (Emde, 1988). Infants with attachment security and a sense of connectedness are more likely to explore and be autonomous. This is called an internal working model, guiding the individual in later attachments. Rogoff's (1990) work defines the idea of intersubjectivity, that is, shared meaning or shared purpose between individuals. The parent guides the infant in connecting with others and experiencing mutuality. According to these theories, the major influences on infant development are social interactions and engagement of infants with their parents and objects in their world.

Behavioral Theories: Human

ACTIONS AND INTERACTIONS

Behaviorism is the study of the general laws of human behavior. Behaviorism focuses on the present and the ways that the environment influences human behavior. Skinner's view of child development focused on learning controlled through classic operant conditioning. Behavior modification therapy is largely based on this theory. Bandura's social learning theory

looked at imitation and modeling as a means of learning, emphasizing the social variables involved (Mott, 1990; Thomas, 1985). Bijou and Baer (1965) responded to critics who faulted behaviorism's view of the child as a passive object. They expressed the notion that children's responses to environmental stimuli are dependent on their genetic structure and personal history (Thomas, 1985).

Humanistic Theories: Innermost Self

Maslow (1971), Buhler and Allen (1972), and Mahrer (1978) are the best known humanistic theorists. They focus on development throughout the life span. Maslow's (1971) hierarchy of needs included physiological, safety, belongingness and love, esteem, and self-actualization needs. He differentiated deficiency needs from growth or self-actualization needs. Rather than proposing stages through which children or adults mature, the humanists believe that individuals and those around them are responsible for any movement they make from one needs plateau to another; intrinsic forces do not move them along.

Ecological Theories of Development

Human ecology theory (Bronfenbrenner, 1979) emphasizes environmental influences more than most other developmental theories do. The key concepts of this perspective emphasize the interdependence of the settings (roles, interpersonal relations, and activities) that influence the developing child, both directly and indirectly. Children are viewed as dynamic entities who are increasingly able to restructure the settings in which they live. Environments also are seen as influencing children, leading to mutual accommodation and reciprocity. Children are influenced by the home and family, child care settings, schools, entertainment and recreational activities, their parents' work, and broad economic opportunities in society. The individual's perception of the environment influences behavior and development more than the objective reality does. Development is described as the growing capacity to discover, sustain, or alter the self or the environment. Finally, recognition is given to ecological transitions or changes in an individual's role or setting, such as the birth of a sibling or changes in family structure. The parent–child interaction also may be inhibited or enhanced by the parents' relationships. When the parent experiences positive mutual feelings, the parent–child relationship can be strengthened. Alternatively, when the parent experiences mutual antagonism or interference, the parent–child relationship may be impaired. These theories are especially useful to better understand the impact of domestic violence on a child's development and a child's future.

Temperament

Chess and Thomas (1995) have provided much of the understanding about the effect of temperament on a child's behavior. Their work seeks to explain the role that temperament plays in children's problem behavior. When a child is an infant, the practitioner can explain to parents the individual variations in temperament and help parents understand how temperament may impact the child's behavior (Carey, 1998). The intent is to alleviate guilt and frustration about the child's behavior and to assist parents in developing strategies that enhance rather than exaggerate difficult temperamental characteristics. Chess and Thomas (1995) also introduced the concept of goodness of fit to describe the degree to which the child's environment and parents' characteristics are congruous with the child's natural temperamental characteristics. Scales that can be used to assess an individual child's temperament are listed in the Chapter 6 Resource Box. Table 5-2 further defines characteristics of temperamental differences.

▩ PARENT DEVELOPMENT

Parental role development is described by many authors using the ecological model (Barnard, 1979; Bronfenbrenner, 1979; Sameroff & Chandler, 1975). These theories stress the fluid nature of early parent–child relationships and the importance of understanding the interactive

T A B L E 5-2
Characteristics of Temperament

TEMPERAMENT CHARACTERISTIC	DESCRIPTION
Activity	What is the child's activity level? Is the child moving all the time he or she is awake, some of the time, or rarely?
Rhythmicity	How predictable is the child's sleep/wake pattern, feeding schedule, and elimination pattern?
Approach/ withdrawal	What is the child's response when presented with something new such as a new toy, an experience, or new person? Does he or she immediately approach or turn away?
Adaptability	How quickly does the child get used to new things? Quickly or not at all?
Threshold of response	How much stimulation does the child require for calming? A quiet voice and touch or more intense, loud voice or firm grasp?
Intensity of reaction	Are the child's responses (crying or laughing) very subtle or extremely intense?
Quality of mood	Is the child's mood usually outgoing, happy, joyful, pleasant or unfriendly, withdrawn, or quiet?
Distractability	How easily is the child distracted from outside disturbance such as a phone ringing, TV, siblings?
Attention span and persistence	How long will the child continue to play with a particular toy or engage in a certain activity? Does this continue even when there are distractions?

and reciprocal influences between parent, infant, and environment. The significance of these models is emphasized in the evolving parental role that develops in concert with the development of the child. Barnard (1979) described two major parent–child nursing interventions to promote parental role development. One provides information to caregivers that assists them to facilitate the child's growth; the other provides support to parents so that their energy and motivation center on caring for their child.

The NP's responsibility for assisting parent role development through anticipatory guidance has often been more of a challenge than preventing serious illness through immunizations, early diagnosis, and treatment of disease. Anticipatory counseling is becoming even more difficult to do within the limits of the managed care environment. Creative strategies need to be developed and established as standards of care. NPs are far more likely to identify parent concerns by listening to the parents than by collecting data in a physical examination. One of the first questions that NPs must ask is how to address parenting issues or concerns. The answer to this question determines how prenatal visits, hospital discharge rounds, early discharge newborn follow-up, breastfeeding consultations, well-child visits, use of parent questionnaires, assessment of parent concerns, and parent consultation, education, and referrals are handled.

By organizing a parent support program in their practice settings, NPs can create a system that will help them listen, hear, and act on parent concerns. Without an organized plan that connects the child's developmental needs, parents' concerns and educational needs, providers' abilities and resources, and community resources, it is easy to overlook, delay, or deny important parenting issues.

The interview and counseling conducted during anticipatory guidance should be guided by a consistent framework. Programs such as Touch Points (Brazelton, 1992), Bright Futures (Green, 1994), and the Parenting Pyramid (Webster-Stratton, 1994) provide guidance to assist the NP. Trigger questions are suggested that can elicit responses from parents and guide the visit as well as provide anticipatory guidance and counseling. Sturner and Howard (1997a; 1997b) recommend the following questions for preschool children:

- How does your child communicate what he or she wants?
- What do you think your child understands?
- How does your child act around others?
- Does your child show an ability to understand the feelings of others?
- To what extent has your child developed independence in eating, dressing, and toileting?
- Tell me about your child's typical day.
- How does your child get from one place to another (e.g., running, walking)?

Stein (1998) emphasized the need of such an organized framework when approaching developmental and behavioral issues. He suggested focusing on four basic areas: developmental themes, temperament, family support, and resiliency or the ability to withstand stresses. He also stressed the use of the teachable moment and role modeling during the office visit. Other important aspects of facilitating parent development include eliciting parent questions, encouraging parent problem solving and decision making, engaging the parent during the visit, and reinforcing positive parent behaviors or actions. Providing parents with positive feedback builds parent confidence and establishes comfort for bringing forth more difficult concerns if such discussion is necessary.

Assessment tools are available when concerns require more in-depth assessment. Table 5-3 identifies parent "red flags" that should be assessed more fully. Tools for home and family assessment, parent-child interaction assessment, parent stress, and parental competency are most frequently used in research but may also be of value in the clinical setting. These tools can be used for more thorough assessment of the child within the family context and the parent–child interaction. The information provides the practitioner with greater opportunities to provide individualized interventions. These tools also can be used to evaluate nursing interventions related to parenting and educational programs.

CULTURAL FACTORS INFLUENCING DEVELOPMENT

Cultural and ethnic traditions are important considerations in the development of infants,

TABLE 5-3
Parenting Red Flags

MODERATE CONCERN	EXTREME CONCERN
Disinclination to separate from child, or prematurely hastening separation	Extreme depression and withdrawal; rejection of child
Signs of despondency, apathy, or hostility	Intense hostility; aggression toward child
Fearful, dependent, apprehensive	Uncontrollable fears, anxieties, guilt
Disinterested in or rejecting of infant or child	Complete inability to function in family role
Overly critical, mocking, and censuring of child; tendency to undermine child's confidence	Severe moralistic prohibition of child's independent strivings
Inconsistent in discipline or control; erratic in behavior	Domestic abuse or violence in the home
Very restrictive and overly moralistic environment	Self-destructive behaviors: alcohol or drug abuse

children, adolescents, parents, and families. Differences have been identified in achievement of childhood developmental milestones for some cultural groups. This information, however, is insufficient when providing individualized care for a particular child and family. More accurate assessments of families and children come from understanding the specific culture of a family and community. To gain this knowledge about a family, additional assessment is needed beyond the traditional health history and physical examination. The NP's ongoing relationship with a particular family and the families within a community may be most helpful in this regard. A nonjudgmental attitude must be used with families to gain insight into their beliefs and values.

Tools, such as the genogram, ecomap, and family functioning model (Minuchin, 1974), can be particularly helpful in identifying family structure, strengths, and resources. These tools also can be helpful in understanding individual

family health responses, beliefs, and practices (see Chapters 3 and 4). The interview process is valuable for clarifying families' unique qualities and resources and serving as an avenue for communicating interest in, and understanding of, individual families and their ethnic or cultural values, differences, and commonalities.

Nugent (1994) discusses three invaluable principles that can be achieved through cross-cultural studies of child development. First, these studies add an understanding of the diversity of parenting styles and belief systems, and, as such, they allow practitioners to move beyond their own world view. Second, cross-cultural research provides a better understanding of the dynamic aspects of child-environment relationships and development. Third, practitioners become sensitized to carefully examine conventional programs and assessment tools for their appropriateness with different populations.

METHODS OF DEVELOPMENTAL ASSESSMENT

Developmental Screening and Surveillance

One purpose of developmental screening is the identification of children with developmental delays. NPs should strongly consider doing developmental screening themselves, because completion of developmental screening and assessment provides opportunities to answer specific parent questions and address parenting issues. When developmental screening is omitted or delegated to medical assistants or volunteers, parenting issues and anticipatory guidance might not be addressed within the context of a child's development. NPs are skilled at integrating developmental screening with anticipatory guidance. One focus of developmental surveillance is to build parental competence and confidence, which, in turn, enhances the child's overall well-being. Learning about their own child's unique developmental strengths and skills allows parents to increase their knowledge of development and create their own parenting style. When parents feel success in their current parenting role, they do a better job meeting their child's future needs.

SCOPE OF DEVELOPMENTAL SURVEILLANCE

Developmental screening includes an evaluation of a child's physical, psychosocial, cognitive, language, fine motor, and gross motor progress and skills. Developmental surveillance requires an approach that evaluates how children's environments facilitate these skills and how children use these skills to interact within their environment.

Table 5-4 demonstrates the connection between children's developmental progress and needed anticipatory guidance. Knowledge of the connection allows the NP to individualize the anticipatory guidance for children and their parents. Trigger questions, such as the ones that follow, cover each area of development and, depending on the parent's responses, allow further questioning or the provision of anticipatory guidance:

- Tell me about your child's daily activities, such as sleep, play, and feeding.
- How does your child respond to you, family members, and others?
- What things does your child seem to enjoy learning about?
- How does your child communicate to you and understand you?
- What does your child try to do for himself or herself?
- How does your child move around or get from one place to another?

Anticipatory guidance provides parents with knowledge about what to expect during the child's current developmental phase and the next developmental phase. This counseling begins by assessing the parents' knowledge of child development and identifying actions they take to foster their child's development. Reinforcement of what a parent is doing well is critical in building a trusting relationship between parent and practitioner. Parental counseling that offers new information and clears up misconceptions can then be correlated with the individual child's development. This then provides the foundation for anticipatory guidance, which is intended to encourage parents to change their parenting styles and strategies in concert with their child's temperament and ever-changing growth and development.

SCREENING STRATEGIES AND TOOLS

Monitoring children's developmental progress brings the pleasure of watching their mastery of

TABLE 5-4
Developmental Screening and Anticipatory Guidance

DEVELOPMENTAL AREAS	DEFINITIONS	AREAS OF ANTICIPATORY GUIDANCE
1. Physical development	Physiological stability, physical growth, sexuality, and temperament	Rhythmicity, daily patterns, sexuality, disease prevention and treatment
2. Psychosocial development	Psychosocial skills, behavior, resiliency, and parent-child interaction	Emotional growth fostering
3. Cognitive development	Cognitive, adaptive, and intellectual skills	Cognitive and environmental stimulation
4. Language development	Receptive and expressive communication	Family communication
5. Fine motor development	Motor skills that facilitate feedings and self-care skills	Feeding and self-care
6. Gross motor development	Motor skills that facilitate locomotion	Health promotion and safety

expected developmental milestones. With time, many practitioners develop an intuitive sense about the ages at which particular milestones should occur. Experience also brings an appreciation of individual differences in infants, families, and ethnic groups. Despite the practitioner's intuitive knowledge of child development, using developmental screening tools can be helpful and, indeed, is necessary. The Resource Box in Chapter 6 lists a number of these tools.

It is often difficult for any practitioner to appreciate intuitively all the various developmental skills of a particular child. For example, a premature infant at or below the fifth percentile for height and weight may physically appear much younger. The discrepancy between size and age can result in an inaccurate estimate of the child's abilities. Specifically, consider an infant who is 15 months chronologically, 12 months adjusted age, but physically and developmentally at the 9-month level. If the NP evaluated this infant developmentally based on physical size, the development level might appear appropriate (size and development at 9 months). Consideration for age adjustment because of the infant's prematurity (adjustment to 12 months) still might not signal the need for intervention and referral. With the use of a screening tool, it is more readily apparent that, despite the history of prematurity, the infant requires referral and intervention services.

Screening is considered a first-level contact with an individual in which an attempt is made to identify specific problems. Developmental screening enables the practitioner to document developmental progress and developmental strengths objectively. It also serves as a tool for stimulating parent questions about development and facilitating parent education. Variation from the norm on a screening tool requires closer, more in-depth examination. Referrals are based on scores outside the defined normal limits of the tool.

NPs use a variety of developmental screening tools in their practices. Some of the more common screening tools include the Denver II and the Miller First Step. These tools require minimal training, have set standards for referral, and can be administered easily in a clinic setting.

ASSESSMENT STRATEGIES AND TOOLS

Assessment tools or diagnostic tests are significantly different from screening tools. They are considered to be at a second level of analysis, identifying more complicated problems. They tend to evaluate a narrower range of development or problem areas. Generally, these tests fulfill three functions (Teti & Gibbs, 1990):

1. Confirming a developmental problem
2. Describing an infant's level of functioning in one or more developmental domains
3. Identifying the type of problem

Because of the complexity of issues that might need evaluation, developmental assessment tools require more practice and skill to perform reliably. More knowledge and skill are required to interpret the findings and plan appropriate intervention strategies. These tools generally require special training or credentials to administer accurately. The NCAST Feeding Assessment to assess maternal-infant bonding is an example of a developmental assessment tool (Barnard, 1979).

WHEN THERE ARE CONCERNS ABOUT DELAYED DEVELOPMENT

Developmental Red Flags

There are red flags that should be kept in mind when seeing infants and children for well-child care or minor acute illnesses. Any child who fails to move ahead developmentally or, worse yet, begins to deteriorate developmentally requires immediate and in-depth evaluation. These red flags are highlighted in each of the following chapters in this unit. The etiologies for developmental delay may include the following:

- Central nervous system dysfunction
- Mental health problem
- Chronic disease affecting either functional abilities or activity tolerance (e.g., cardiovascular, visual, auditory)
- Child abuse and neglect
- Maternal or paternal stress

- Developmentally inappropriate animate or inanimate environment, or both
- Lack of parental knowledge of development
- Genetic syndromes
- Depression
- Attention-deficit hyperactivity disorder

Referral and intervention should be based on information from the history, physical examination, developmental testing, hearing and vision screening, and other tests as indicated. Understanding and managing the etiology are essential to planning appropriate developmental care, including parent counseling; educational programs; physical, occupational, and speech therapy; and social services. (See Chapter 28 for a discussion of the management of cerebral palsy, a condition that usually includes developmental delays.) One cannot assume that waiting will remedy the problem; even though developmental progress may occur, the rate and quality may be abnormal. Neither can one assume that all developmental problems can be fixed with home remedies (e.g., changing parenting or environmental factors). Sometimes, developmental problems are indicators of serious systemic, particularly neurological, dysfunctions.

Talking With Parents About Developmental Delays

Talking with parents about specific developmental problems is always a challenge. For this reason, it is particularly helpful to have an opportunity to complete developmental assessments on an ongoing basis. Each infant and child has areas in which development is progressing, even if the progress is not consistent with usual development. Discussing these areas first provides parents with a framework to understand their child's unique strengths along with any developmental challenges. Most often, parents notice differences in the child first and seek reassurance or confirmation of problems from their health care provider. It is always important to discuss the child's strengths and limitations as well as the parents' concerns.

Above all, it is important to be honest, positive, and realistic. Most often, the long-term prognosis for developmental delays is unknown

because of continuing brain development. Parents want to know what they can do and, specifically, how they can assist their child. They also need support and time to cope with their own feelings (Harnel & Feldman, 1998). Different families have different expectations for their children, so a child with mild delay may be more devastating to one family than a child with severe developmental delays may be to another.

Implementing Individualized Interventions

EARLY INTERVENTION PROGRAMS

Children with developmental delays should receive appropriate referral or more frequent visits, or both, particularly during the first year of life. Many later learning problems, difficulties with parent–child interaction, behavioral problems, and attachment problems can be managed effectively during the first year of life simply by offering parental counseling or referral to appropriate community services. The longer the problem lasts, the more difficult it is to resolve. Most communities have early infant education programs for infants and young children (birth to 3 years of age) under the federal 99-457 legislation. This federal legislation requires developmental screening and early intervention programs for infants and young children at risk for developmental delay. The individualized family service plan (IFSP) is a process that includes the family in planning services for children. These programs can be established through school systems, health departments, or developmental programs and vary significantly in quality and comprehensiveness from one community to another. NPs need to know the community resources and educate community leaders and legislators about the developmental and health needs of children and families. As primary care providers, NPs may be asked to participate in the meetings in which the IFSP is developed with the family.

Areas that require special attention to guide nursing interventions include assessment of feeding, sleep, elimination, activity, temperament, and behavior. Nursing interventions such as referrals to parent groups and recommendations regarding organization of the child's health records, are greatly appreciated by the family.

SCHOOL INTERVENTION RESOURCES

The federal 99-457 legislation also addresses the needs of children older than 3 years of age. Schools are mandated to provide developmental services to children with developmental delays, including opportunities for mainstreaming children with developmental delays or handicaps into regular classrooms. Special education services assist in this process through the development of an individualized education plan (IEP).

Planning sessions for IFSPs or IEPs determine the school services that will be provided during a designated period of time for a particular child. If a child's or family's needs are not identified, services are not made available. Often, health care services are omitted when the overall health history of the child is not addressed. As the primary care provider for children, the NP should be available to be an advocate for families and children. In this role, the NP can help clarify children's needs and ensure that parental concerns, health care services, and educational services are appropriately coordinated (Jackson & Vessey, 1996).

FAMILY-CENTERED CARE

One of the primary tenets of the federal 99-457 legislation is to emphasize family-centered care. This legislation also establishes a process in which families become active participants in determining the care of their children. The uniqueness of each family is to be respected, and families are considered to be active team participants. Nurses have stressed this focus with varying success. Educators are embracing the concept as well. The shift from child-centered to family-centered care is represented in Table 5-5.

CASE MANAGEMENT AND SERVICE COORDINATION

As a case manager, the NP's essential tasks are identification and development of community

TABLE 5-5

Family-Centered Care in Comparison to Child-Centered Care

CHILD-CENTERED CARE	FAMILY-CENTERED CARE
Goal: To take care of the child for the short term.	Goal: Parental empowerment and child advocacy for life of child.
• Child's needs are primary focus	• Family needs to assist the child are the focus
• Professionals decide on the plan of care	• Family and professionals decide on the plan of care
• Parents' opinions are not consistently requested	• Parents' ideas are requested and valued
• Families are considered part of a particular group	• Families are all considered to be unique
• Parents participate as observers	• Parents are considered to be equal members of the team at whatever level they are comfortable
• Parental differences are judged as not being in the best interest of the child	• Family culture, language, ethnicity, and structure are respected
• Test results of the child are the most important factor used to plan care	• Focus is on addressing parental concerns, issues, questions, and their need for assistance in problem solving
• One-way communication, professional to parent	• Communication is two-way with parents encouraged to have input into the child's care plan

resources and providing assistance to families so they can access these resources. It is important for the NP, however, to become "community wise" through professional networks, parent groups, and educational connections. These resources are invaluable in assisting families locally. However, it is not enough simply to give a family a name and phone number of a referring agency. All too often, parents' calls lead to busy signals, disconnected numbers, or the wrong agency for their needs. These deterrents can discourage even the most willing family from pursuing needed resources for their child. Parents can also hesitate to seek resources because of apprehension about the outcome of the referral, costs, time constraints, or lack of understanding about the need for timely follow-up. When the NP intervenes to guide families through the referral process and coordinate services, parents have greater confidence in the new health care or educational resource and are more likely to achieve appropriate follow-up for their child.

SUMMARY

Effective management strategies in primary care maximize the strengths of children, parents, and families and lead to optimal health outcomes. The role of NPs in this process is complex. Focusing on social and psychological needs of the child, NPs move beyond the standard well-child visit to comprehensive assessment of growth and development. NPs address parenting issues, examine the impact of environmental factors on health, facilitate access to community resources, and act to manage and coordinate interdisciplinary care. This holistic approach is essential to ensure that children have every opportunity to achieve healthful, responsible, and happy adulthoods.

REFERENCES

Ainsworth M, Bell S, Stayton D: Individual differences in strange-situation behavior of one year olds. *In* Schaffer HR (ed): The Origins of Human Social Relations. London, Academic Press, 1971.

Barnard K: NCAST Instructors' Manual. Seattle, NCAST Publications, 1979.

Bijou S, Baer D: Child Development II: Universal Stages of Infancy. New York: Appleton-Century-Crofts, 1965.

Bowlby J: Attachment and Loss: Vol 1. Attachment. New York, Basic Books, 1969.

Brazelton B: Touchpoints: Your Child's Emotional and Behavioral Development. New York, Addison-Wesley, 1992.

Bronfenbrenner U: The Ecology of Human Development: Experiments by Nature and Design. Cambridge, MA, Harvard University Press, 1979.

Buhler C, Allen M: Introduction to Humanistic Psychology. Monterey, CA, Brooks/Cole, 1972.

Carey WB: Let's give temperament its due. Contemp Pediatr 15(5):91–113, 1998.

Chess T, Thomas A: Temperament in Clinical Practice. New York, Guilford Press, 1995.

Colson ER, Dworkin PH: Toddler development. Pediatr Rev 18(8):255–259, 1997.

Dixon S, Stein M (eds): Encounters with Children: Pediatric Behavior and Development. St. Louis, Mosby–Year Book, 1992.

Dworkin PH: British and American recommendations for developmental monitoring: The role of surveillance. Pediatrics 83:619–622, 1989.

Emde R: Development terminable and interminable. I. Innate and motivational factors from infancy. Int J Psychoanalysis 69:23–42, 1988.

Emde R, Buchsbaum H: "Didn't you hear my mommy?": Autonomy with connectedness in moral self emergence. *In* Cicchetti D, Beeghly M (eds): The Self in Transition: Infancy to Childhood. Chicago, University of Chicago Press, 1990.

Erikson E: Insight and Responsibility. New York, Norton, 1964.

Flavell J: Cognitive Development. Englewood Cliffs, NJ, Prentice-Hall, 1977.

Fowler J: Stages of Faith: The Psychology of Human Development and the Quest for Meaning. New York, Harper & Row, 1981.

Freud A: The Writings of Anna Freud. Vol V. New York, International Universities Press, 1974.

Freud S: An Outline of Psychoanalysis. London, Hogarth, 1938.

Gesell A: The First Five Years of Life. New York, Harper, 1940.

Gilligan C: In a Different Voice: Psychological Theory and Women's Development. Cambridge, MA, Harvard University Press, 1982.

Green M (ed): Bright Futures: Guidelines for Health Supervision of Infants, Children, and Adolescents. Arlington, VA: National Center for Education in Maternal and Child Health, 1994.

Harnel SC, Feldman HM: Focus on families: Caring for children with special needs. Contemp Pediatr 15(4):141–155, 1998.

Havighurst R: Human Development and Education. New York, Longmans, Green, 1953.

Jackson PJ, Vessey J: Primary Care of the Child With a Chronic Condition, 2nd ed. St. Louis: Mosby–Year Book, 1996.

Klaus M, Kennel J: Maternal-Infant Bonding. St. Louis, CV Mosby, 1976.

Kohlberg L: Stage and sequence: The cognitive-development approach to socialization. *In* Gastin D (ed): Handbook of Socialization: Theory and Research. New York, Rand McNally, 1969.

Lewin K: Principles of Topological Psychology. New York, McGraw-Hill, 1936.

Mahler M, Pine F, Bergman A: The Psychological Birth of the Human Infant. New York, Basic Books, 1975.

Mahrer A: Experiencing: A Humanistic Theory of Psychology and Psychiatry. New York, Brunner/Mazel, 1978.

Maslow A: The Farther Reaches of Human Nature. New York, Viking, 1971.

Minuchin S: Families and Family Therapy. Cambridge, MA, Harvard University Press, 1974.

Mott S: Developmental theories: How the child grows. *In* Mott S, James SR, Sperhac A (eds): Nursing Care of Children and Families. New York, Addison-Wesley, 1990.

Nugent JK: Cross-cultural studies of child development: Implications for clinicians. Zero to Three 15(2):1–8, 1994.

Rogoff B: Apprenticeship in Thinking: Cognitive Development in Social Context. New York, Oxford University Press, 1990.

Sameroff A, Chandler M: Reproductive risks and the continuum of caretaking casualty. *In* Horowitz FD (ed): Review of Child Development Research. Chicago, University of Chicago Press, 1975.

Siegler R, Liebert D, Liebert R: Inhelder and Piaget's pendulum problem. Dev Psych 9:97–101, 1973.

Stein M: Preparing families for the toddler and preschool years. Contemp Pediatr 15(1):88–110, 1998.

Stern D: The Interpersonal World of the Infant: A View From Psychoanalysis and Developmental Psychology. New York, Basic Books, 1985.

Sturner RA, Howard BJ: Preschool development I: Communicative and motor aspects. Pediatr Rev 18(9):291–301, 1997a.

Sturner RA, Howard BJ: Preschool development II: Psychosocial/behavioral development. **Pediatr Rev** 18(10):327–336, 1997b.

Sullivan H: The Fusion of Psychiatry and Social Sciences. New York, Norton, 1964.

Teti D, Gibbs E: Interdisciplinary Assessment of Infants: A Guide for Early Intervention Professionals. Baltimore, Paul H. Brookes, 1990.

Thomas RM: Comparing Theories of Child Development. Belmont, CA, Wadsworth, 1985.

Webster-Stratton C: The Incredible Years: A Trouble Shooting Guide for Parents of Children Aged 3–8. Toronto, Ontario, Umbrella Press, 1994.

Wolraich ML, Felice ME, Drotar D (eds): Diagnostic and Statistical Manual for Primary Care (DSM-PC). Child and Adolescent Version. Elk Grove Village, IL, **American Academy of Pediatrics, 1996.**

CHAPTER 6

Developmental Management of Infants

Barbara Jones Deloian

INTRODUCTION

Statistics show that the 1996 birth rate in the United States was 14.8 births per 1000 population. In the same year, the infant mortality rate reached an all-time low of 7.2 deaths per 1000 births. Despite this decline, the United States continues to rank poorly in comparison to international infant mortality rates. Although there has been a decrease in the teen pregnancy rate, the percentage of low birth weight babies reached 7.4% in 1996, its highest level since 1975. Unintentional injury remains the leading cause of children's deaths in all age groups (Guyer et al., 1997). One in four infants and toddlers in the United States lives in poverty, 25% of children live in single-parent households, and 1 million children are affected by divorce (Barnard et al., 1993; Green, 1994). As a result, current studies of infant development have moved beyond studying the developmental milestones achieved during the first year of life to focus on infant mental health as well as the contextual and relational factors that have an impact on the infant's competent development. Management of infant's developmental health care emphasizes prevention and creation of programs to promote protective factors in children's lives (Barnard et al., 1993).

THEORIES OF INFANT DEVELOPMENT

Sameroff and Chandler (1975) emphasize a transactional model of development that includes active involvement of the individual with an active environment. In this model, developmental outcomes are a "result of the interplay between the child and context over time, in which the state of one affects the next state of the other in a continuous dynamic process" (Sameroff, 1993).

The influence of the family as a component of the infant's social context takes several forms. Mutual regulation between caregiver and infant is a predominant theme in current theories of infant development. From this perspective, external regulatory mechanisms, usually from the parent, are gradually internalized as self-regulation by the infant (Lyons-Ruth & Zeanah, 1993).

The work of Bronfenbrenner (1979), which examines family functioning as influenced by the social community's ability to support families and foster child development, particularly when family functioning is not optimal, is important.

Studies of temperament in infants and children have focused on dispositional differences accounted for by characteristics of the central nervous system. These differences affect how the infant approaches, interacts in, and experiences social relationships. Whether these differences are stable over time is, as yet, unknown.

Ainsworth and colleagues (1978) and Main and Solomon (1990) describe patterns of infant–parent attachment as secure, avoidant, ambivalent, or disorganized/disoriented. Parents of secure infants tend to be sensitive and responsive to the full range of their infants' behaviors and cues. Lyons-Ruth and Zeanah (1993) describe secure attachments as relationships that are "organized . . . by open emotional communication between partners."

Brazelton (1992) describes five touchpoints at which infants experience major developmental changes that require readjustments on the part of parents. Patterns of behavior that occur with regularity and smoothness are interrupted as the infant changes awareness of surroundings during cognitive and physiological growth spurts. During these phases, which occur at birth, 6 to 8 weeks, 4 months, 9 months, and 12 months, parents often experience frustration in knowing how to handle their infant's behavior consistently. Previous parenting behaviors no longer seem to be effective, and parents often begin to use inconsistent responses. A disruptive cycle of interactions can begin, which only increases the infant's behavior problems. When parents are prepared for these periods, they can provide more consistent caregiving and a dependable foundation for the infant. In this chapter, infant developmental progress and related anticipatory guidance suggestions are discussed within this framework.

DEVELOPMENTAL SCREENING AND ASSESSMENT OF INFANTS

Screening Strategies for Infants

THE PRENATAL VISIT

The opportunity to meet with parents prenatally provides a chance for the nurse practitioner (NP) to assess parental knowledge and receptiveness to anticipatory guidance. The prenatal visit should include a discussion of the partnership between the primary care provider and the parent. A variety of ways for pediatric providers to reach parents prenatally needs to be used, such as participation in Lamaze classes or parent preparation classes. Teenage mothers-to-be can be contacted through their local school programs. These meetings provide a foundation for later visits and establish the NP as a resource for the parents.

THE NEONATAL VISIT

The hospital visit may be the least opportune time to discuss infant care because of the short stay and the mother's physiological state, which reduces her ability to absorb new information. Ideally, a 48- to 72-hour postpartum home or office visit can be arranged to assess the infant's physiological and neurological status, especially as related to feeding and state regulation. Owing to the short length of hospital stay, a visit at 1 to 2 weeks after birth is also needed to monitor the infant's weight gain, elimination pattern, sleep and wake cycle, breastfeeding success, and parent–child interaction. The mutual regulatory patterns that are established during this period significantly influence later infant self-regulation and parental responses. Developmental screening tools are rarely sensitive enough to discern problems at this time. The NP's interviewing, observations, and clinical experience are the most useful factors for uncovering infant or parenting problems. Screening for metabolic conditions takes place at this visit as well.

THE 2 TO 12 MONTHS OF AGE VISITS

After the first month of life, more common screening tools, including the Denver Screening tools (Denver II or Denver PDQ Parent Questionnaire) and the Miller First Step, can be used. Many other tools are available that have been developed for use in clinical settings, such as the Well Child Check Sheet, the Revised Gesell, the Early Language Milestone (ELM), the Receptive-Expressive Emergent Language scale (REEL), and the KIDS chart. (See Resource Box 6–1 for more information about these tools.) Other tools developed by early education specialists and occupational therapists can be used in health care settings. These include the Battelle Development Inventory and the Chandler Movement Assessment of Infants screening tool.

It is recommended that a developmental screening test be completed and documented on all children during the first year of life. The visit at 8 months is an optimal time for this screening because of the significant developmental changes that have occurred by this time. This is also a time of change in parental control and the infant's developing autonomy.

Assessment Strategies for Infants

Developmental assessment tools include the Brazelton Neonatal Behavioral Assessment scale, the Assessment of Premature Infant Behavior (APIB), the HOME scale, the Bayley scales of infant development, and the Nursing Child Assessment Satellite Training (NCAST) scales (feeding scale, teaching scale, and sleep scale). These tools take longer to administer and are used for diagnostic assessments. Knowledge of developmental assessment tools offers the practitioner specialized skills that can ensure more appropriate referrals when necessary and help establish individualized intervention strategies for clients.

It is beyond the scope of this chapter to provide a complete review of the available screening and assessment tools in the areas of infant development, parent-child interaction, and family assessment. The Resource Box at the end of this chapter lists additional information about commonly used assessment tools.

ASSESSMENT AND ANTICIPATORY GUIDANCE DURING THE FIRST YEAR OF LIFE

Newborn to 1 Month of Age

DEVELOPMENTAL STATUS

The developmental assessment of the neonate must begin with a determination of gestational age using the Dubowitz or similar gestational age scale (see Chapter 39). It is important to be aware of significant prematurity, intrauterine growth retardation (IUGR), and size for gestational age (i.e., either too large [LGA] or too small [SGA]). The reported gestational age, birth weight and length, and head circumference data are compared for appropriateness with the infant's gestational age as assessed by observation. Primary reflexes, such as sucking, rooting, Moro, and grasp, should be assessed

for presence and symmetry. Arm and leg recoil provides information about the infant's active movements, particularly symmetry and coordination. Jerkiness and tremors need to be noted. Passive muscle tone is evaluated within gestational age scales through observation of shoulder (scarf sign) and knee flexibility (popliteal angle).

The stability of the infant's autonomic nervous system can be evaluated through heart rate, respiratory rate, temperature control, and color changes. The infant should demonstrate some degree of state regulation and ease of transitions from deep sleep through crying. Assessment for a normally pitched cry is important, because problems such as hypothyroidism and genetic disorders (e.g., cri du chat syndrome) involve alterations in voice.

With the use of a variety of techniques, the newborn can be aroused to an alert state for feedings. The newborn infant sleeps about 16 hours a day and breastfeeds every 2 to 3 hours. Nutritional needs to promote growth are about 110 kcal/kg per day. The infant initially loses up to 10% of birth weight but should regain the weight within 10 to 14 days after birth.

The newborn infant is able to give clear signals of distress, such as crying, arching, gagging, or hiccups. These help the caregiver respond to the infant's needs. The newborn also should be able to habituate to sound and light. Newborns use self-consoling or self-calming behaviors, such as sucking, moving hand to mouth, or grasping clothing, to keep organized or maintain their state.

Social skills are evident as the newborn quiets readily to the parent's voice and demonstrates a brief smile. Using a soft voice, touching, and picking up the baby are ways the caregiver can console the newborn. The sense of smell is most acute in newborns. Hearing is also fairly well developed. Vision is more limited, but the newborn does have the ability to focus briefly when an object is brought into visual range.

ANTICIPATORY GUIDANCE AND DEVELOPMENTAL INTERVENTIONS

On the basis of knowledge of newborn development, it is possible to provide parents with information about their infant that assists them in their transition to parenthood. By understanding the capabilities of the newborn, such as hearing, vision, states and state transition, and self-calming and self-consoling techniques, parents are better able to read infant cues and provide timely and appropriate care. In turn, the infant's responsive behaviors assist in building the parents' confidence and aid in their receptiveness to future anticipatory guidance. NPs can use the following interventions to help parents promote infant development during daily activities and routines.

Rhythmicity and Sleep/Wake Patterns

- Discuss the need for infants to develop day/night cycles, because infants' days and nights are often mixed up. Suggest that parents use consistent daily routines to help the infant establish a good sleep/wake cycle.
- Encourage parents to place the infant in a bassinet or crib during the day to allow an easier transition from the parent to bed at night.
- Describe the infant's need for variety of movement, voice, or touch to awaken or move up in sleep/wake states, and describe the infant's need for rhythmicity of voice, movement, or touch to calm or reduce state level.
- Explain that some infants benefit from external stimuli, such as music, voice, or movement to calm down and develop self-regulation.
- Explain the infant's startle or Moro reflex and encourage parents to use slow, easy movements in their caregiving activities.

Emotional Growth Fostering

- Describe the infant's ability to tolerate brief periods of social interaction by using visual orientation for state stability when in the alert state. It is helpful to demonstrate for parents how the infant achieves this alert state.
- Encourage parents to hold their infant and attend to the infant's crying. Many parents believe that holding spoils their child and do not understand the infant's need for emotional support.

- Discuss the role of sibling involvement with the new infant. Facilitating overall family development and emotional growth is important.

Cognitive and Environmental Stimulation

- Encourage opportunities for the infant to look at things in the environment, such as mobiles. Avoid having the same objects in the environment on the same side of the crib day after day. Variety encourages infants to move their heads from side to side. It is also helpful to place infants at different ends of the bed periodically.

Communication

- Discuss the communication skills of babies that are seen during state changes, periods of alertness, feeding, and sleep routines. Nonverbal infant communication (e.g., infant cues) must be used by parents to understand their infant's needs.
- Encourage timely parental response to infant crying. The contingency of the parental response to the infant's cries is an important aspect of the infant's developing sense of trust.
- Have parents reinforce their infant's comfort sounds through verbal responses.

Feeding and Self-Care

- Explain that the primary developmental activity of the newborn is organizing feeding responses. Bringing the infant slowly to an awake state for feeding must be the first step. Emphasize that if the infant becomes overstimulated or disorganized, it might be necessary to reduce external stimuli (e.g., lights and noise), increase the infant's flexion of arms and legs, or bundle the infant to assist with central nervous system control and improve feeding responses.
- Help parents understand the infant's need to set the suck–swallow pace for feeding. If milk flows through the breast or bottle too rapidly or too slowly, adjustments to help the baby manage the feeding pace are needed.
- Discuss how the face-to-face feeding position encourages eye contact, social smiles, and parent–child communication and interaction.

- Describe how the infant's reach for breast or bottle represents beginning exploratory learning and should be encouraged. Parents also can encourage the grasp reflex while the baby is feeding through finger play or finger holding.
- Parents often need information regarding volume expectations, urinary output, and burping. Discussion on how to avoid nipple confusion, stimulate milk production, and return to work while breastfeeding can be most productive (see Chapter 13). Helping parents feel successful promotes their development as parents. If parents have any concerns, they should be followed up closely with support, guidance, and reassurance. Early success with caregiving of the new infant is essential for parents to enjoy their new role.

Strength and Motor Coordination

- Infants' gradually increasing strength makes it possible for them to lift their heads. Parents sometimes worry about smothering when placing the infant on his or her stomach. With the current recommendation of the supine or side-lying position for infant sleeping, parents may hesitate to allow their infants to be positioned on their stomachs at all. Parents need to be encouraged to place their infants prone to play with toys or interact with the parent for periods of time, at least once or twice every day.

6 to 8 Weeks of Age

DEVELOPMENTAL STATUS

During the first 6 to 8 weeks of life, many changes occur physically and developmentally for the infant. By 6 to 8 weeks of age, the infant gains 0.5 to 1 ounce per day, feeding six to seven times daily. Length increases about 1 inch per month. The infant sleeps more regularly, about 15 to 16 hours per day, with defined sleep and wake patterns. Many infants begin to have fussy periods in the late evening.

The infant begins to become very social, imitating the parent's mouth movements and expressions and visually following the parent. Additionally, infants readily begin to take in more of their environment, vertically or horizontally following objects placed in front of them. They are more responsive to sounds in their environment, attending to sounds by quieting body movements or demonstrating visual responses. Infants also start to make cooing sounds, much to the delight of their parents.

Fine motor skills begin to emerge as primitive reflexes become integrated. Infants attempt to grasp rattles, fingers, and clothing. They also are able to demonstrate visible head control, lifting the head off the bed about 45 degrees and showing little head droop when held in suspension.

As infants become more active, alert, and responsive, parents can misinterpret this behavior and incorrectly assume that infants can handle more active and irregular stimulation than their true capacity. Regular feedings and appropriate stimulation are very important to the developing infant.

ANTICIPATORY GUIDANCE AND DEVELOPMENTAL INTERVENTIONS

Rhythmicity and Sleep/Wake Patterns

- Help parents understand that because of the infant's continued need for external routines to facilitate state organization, it is important to continue structuring the infant's day. Explore sleeping arrangements and begin discussion of the importance of establishing a nighttime ritual.
- Reemphasize the use of repetitive stimulation (e.g., rocking or a soothing voice) for quieting and stimulus variation (e.g., undressing, stroking or voice intonations) for awakening.
- Discuss the still immature nervous system, especially while the infant continues to show the Moro or tonic neck reflex.

Emotional Growth Fostering

- Advise parents of the increasing social needs of the infant and the infant's desire to play with the caregiver.
- Discuss the benefits of responding to infant cries as soon as possible. Consistent responses assist infants to trust that their needs will be met and decrease the chances of crying later on.

- Encourage social games and eye contact for longer periods of time but with sensitivity to the infant's level of tolerance.

Cognitive and Environmental Stimulation
- Explain that the infant's visual awareness is increasing and that the baby requires more visual diversity, such as changes in position and location and objects such as a mobile or mirror.
- Discuss the importance of equipment and toys that are semirigid, not painted but with varying textures. Toys that rattle and make sounds are appropriate. These encourage waving arms and kicking legs.

Communication
- Continue discussions of parents' observations and intuitions about their infant. Reinforce parental understanding and sensitivity to their infant's cues and sleep/wake states. Their confidence and competence grow with validation of their increasing skills. Recommendations associated with the parents' own observations are the most supportive.
- Discuss the emerging temperament of the infant and the parents' perceptions of the infant's behaviors (Carey, 1998).
- Support the parents' need to find time for their own relationship. Assist in identifying possible child-care resources and criteria for selection.
- Encourage parents to sing, to talk to, and to rock their infants.

Feeding and Self-Care
- Greater feeding control occurs at this time, and the infant begins to demonstrate a strong need for sucking.
- Discuss the purpose and use of a pacifier.
- Discuss the infant's need for non-nutritive sucking, such as sucking on fingers and toys as a way of learning about the environment.
- Discuss the importance of social and developmental, as well as nutritional, aspects of feeding.
- Give positive reinforcement for the parents' efforts to breastfeed. Offer problem-solving suggestions if the mother is returning to work.

- Remind parents to encourage infants to look at their hands and use their hands for self-consoling and hand-to-mouth exploration.

Strength and Motor Coordination
- Encourage parents to place the infant in different positions for playtime. Supine position stimulates movement of hands, feet, and legs; prone position strengthens upper torso, neck, and arms.

3 to 4 Months of Age

DEVELOPMENTAL STATUS

Infants 3 to 4 months of age usually begin to settle into regular patterns of eating, sleeping, and playing. Babies sleep 12 to 15 hours a day with five to six feedings a day. They begin to recognize their parents' responses to their needs, particularly preparation for feeding. Three- or 4-month-olds begin to demonstrate preferences for location and position of sleeping. Their growth, still quite rapid, should follow previous growth curves. Although the infant's primary source of nutrition comes from breast milk or formula, parents often want to begin feeding the infant cereal.

During this time, infants' social skills become more evident. Smiling spontaneously at parents and others while visually following the caregiver around the environment, moving the head a full 180 degrees, is usual behavior. Babies at this age should promptly look at an object when it is placed in front of them. They begin to look at their hands or a toy placed in their hands, particularly when they are lying on their back, and gradually are successful in placing their hands or a toy in their mouth.

Infants' social skills are increasing and verbal skills are becoming more evident. They begin babbling and cooing and laughing quietly. They begin to experiment with variations in tone, such as low-pitched chuckles and deeper laughs. Eventually, they begin to laugh out loud, much to the enjoyment of those around them. Their responses to sounds gradually become more localized, and they turn to the sound of a bell or rattle.

Fine motor skills are demonstrated as infants play with their hands and begin to scratch at clothing or other objects that are close. Eventually, they grasp toys and begin to grab at other objects, such as the parents' hair, earrings, or eyeglasses. They also start to place their hands on the breast or on the bottle in an attempt to hold or pat it.

Motor skills progress as the asymmetric tonic neck reflex is integrated, so there is no longer the obligation of arm extension with head turning. They begin to roll from front to back and then from back to front. Head control becomes stronger and more sustained as they learn to sit with the head held erect. When in the prone position, infants gradually begin to hold the head up at 45 degrees and then at 90 degrees for sustained periods of time. All their body movements should be symmetrical.

ANTICIPATORY GUIDANCE AND DEVELOPMENTAL INTERVENTIONS

The confidence of parents begins to strengthen as they resolve some of their earlier difficulties. They need reinforcement regarding the benefits of consistency in daily activities. Consistency helps infants to have internal control of their overall development. It is important to continue to discuss the benefits of the infant's sleep/ wake cycle and regularity of naps, feeding, and playtime. It is also important to help parents see the uniqueness of their infant and develop an individualized approach in their caregiving.

Rhythmicity and Sleep/Wake Patterns

- Discuss ways to help infants resume sleep independently when they awaken at night. This assists parents to prepare for future changes in the infant's sleep pattern.
- Discuss parents' perception of their infant's temperament. Note the parents' description of their infant as an easy, average, or challenging baby. Parents often compare their infant with other babies and need to understand the uniqueness of their infant, individualizing their activities to their baby's style of responsiveness.
- Discuss varied parenting approaches to infants of different temperaments, including patterns of eating and sleeping.

Emotional Growth Fostering

- Reassure parents that responding to their baby's cries promotes the infant's sense

of trust and will not cause the baby to be spoiled.
- Discuss the infant's continued need for non-nutritive sucking as a means of self-regulation. Sucking on fingers or toys requires different oral–motor movements from those needed to suck on a pacifier.

Cognitive and Environmental Stimulation

- Encourage parents to use a variety of types of stimulation, such as soft stuffed toys, rattles, a crib gym, or a busy box.
- Remind parents that at all ages, infants enjoy being talked to and played with affectionately.
- Explain that infants enjoy looking at themselves in a mirror. Putting a mirror by the changing table is a good diversion.
- Reinforce parents' efforts to provide new experiences for their infant, such as walks to the park, visiting neighbors, or trips to the grocery store.

Communication

- Reinforce parents' "back and forth talking" with their infant, especially using changes in voice inflection and intonation.
- Explore ongoing communication between parents about their roles and responsibilities. Fathers are often more comfortable handling their infant at this age, if not before, as the infant becomes responsive. Try to have both parents included in the well-child care developmental assessment visits in order to discuss parenting issues.
- Discuss mothers' feelings regarding their time to themselves, return to work, and particular life stresses. Mothers' feelings are often reflected in infants' behaviors.
- Discuss parents' thoughts about discipline and begin to open lines of communication for management of unwelcome infant behaviors.
- Discuss selection of good day care settings that are developmentally appropriate.

Feeding and Self-Care

- Counsel parents about salivary gland maturation, drooling, and the infant's developing ability to swallow excessive saliva.
- Advise parents that infants gradually become less dependent on external calming.

Encourage parents to note other methods of self-calming through play, vocalization, and visual stimuli that their babies use.

- Discuss the infant's individual cues for readiness to eat as well as satiation.
- Discuss the importance of allowing the infant to self-regulate the amount of feedings. Explain that the infant will be ready for solids as the gastrointestinal tract matures. Listen closely to parents' questions and beliefs and the influence of others on the introduction of solids (see Chapters 12 and 13).
- When solids are appropriate, discuss the importance of using a spoon instead of placing cereal in the bottle. This helps the development of new oral-motor skills, because skills needed to suck and swallow milk from a bottle or breast differ from those needed to take cereal from a spoon.
- Encourage parents to allow their infants to pat the breast or bottle and place their hands on the bottle in anticipation of self-feeding at a later date.

Strength and Motor Coordination

- Discuss the safety precautions needed when using jumpers and high chairs.
- Encourage parental holding and floor play.
- Discourage use of walkers.
- Discuss the need for childproofing (e.g., locks on cabinets and gates for stairs). Remind parents about the benefits of playpens as the child becomes more mobile.

5 to 6 Months of Age

DEVELOPMENTAL STATUS

By 5 to 6 months, infants have doubled their birth weight and are gaining 3 to 5 ounces per week. Their length increases about 0.5 inch per month. Their growth at this time begins to occur in spurts rather than evenly along the previously established growth curve. Weight gain can also be influenced by the amount of play activity and the sleep schedule.

Major developmental events that occur during this period include changes in the child's sleep cycle as the infant begins to have increased awake and play time, fewer feedings (four to six feedings per day), and fewer hours of sleep (14 to 15 hours per day). The infant demonstrates increased desire for play time with parents. Parents frequently interpret the infant's crying as hunger rather than a need for social interaction. Teething can begin at this time, and the first childhood illness might occur. Either of these events can disrupt the infant's previous sleep routine. Parents need counseling about helping their infant resume normal sleep/wake patterns.

Parents also become aware of their child's "temper" and are able to acknowledge their child's unique personality. Some parents are able to determine alternatives to responding to their infant's need for instant gratification through distraction, talking, and play. The infant's clear recognition of his or her parents is an important aspect of the attachment process that parents and infants greatly enjoy.

Vocalizations continue to show increasing variety in pitch, and imitation of speech sounds begins. Infants turn toward their parents' voices and other sounds, localizing directly.

At 5 to 6 months, the infant is making great strides in development of motor skills. Head control is well established, and there should be no head lag when the baby is pulled to sit. The Moro and asymmetrical tonic neck reflexes have become integrated by this time, and the Landau reflex emerges. The infant learns to sit, first in a tripod stance and then unassisted. Infants enjoy exploring their environment visually and gradually moving from place to place and rolling over. They are able to lift their legs and bring their feet to their mouth. They bear full weight when standing and enjoy bouncing up and down in their parent's lap.

Chewing and mouthing are other means of exploration that infants use to differentiate textures, tastes, and shapes. They actively reach for toys within their grasp and use both hands. They can follow a toy if it falls but remains within their visual field. They begin to rake at small objects and are able to hold a small cube momentarily, lifting it off the table. Gradually, they use fingers and thumb to pick up objects.

ANTICIPATORY GUIDANCE AND DEVELOPMENTAL INTERVENTIONS

This period of time can be one of enjoyment and pleasure for parents as they watch their infant accomplish new skills on a daily basis. At 5 to 6 months of age, infants are at a plateau before their next rapid growth and developmental spurt.

Rhythmicity and Sleep/Wake Patterns

- Discuss infants' needs for assistance to resume sleep/wake patterns after teething or illness. Encourage parents to be consistent. Have parents put infants to sleep in the crib while drowsy but not yet asleep. Then, if they awaken at night, they are more likely to resume sleep without comforting from the parent.
- Advise parents that crying still needs to be addressed in a consistent and timely manner. Demonstrate the use of gradually increasing caregiver facilitation (e.g., presence, face, voice, touch, holding) for quieting.
- Discuss the importance of starting nighttime rituals if this has not been done already.

Emotional Growth Fostering

- Discuss differences in parental expectations related to parenting (e.g., allowing or not allowing an infant to cry at bedtime) and processes used by the parents for resolution of these differences.
- Discuss the parents' ability to spend time together if this is not occurring. The parents' emotional well-being is a very important aspect of the infant's overall care.
- Discuss the parental role in discipline and teaching. Differentiate discipline and teaching from punishment. Help parents understand their role as the infant's first teachers. Offer examples of ways to handle infant behavior as the infant exerts his or her own personality.
- Recommend parenting classes that provide information on upcoming developmental milestones and changes.

Cognitive and Environmental Stimulation

- Discuss the infant's increasing activity and awake time. Counsel parents about their infant's increasing demands for adult attention and efforts to draw attention by smiling, making sounds, or crying.
- Reinforce the importance of parents en-

couraging play with toys of different sizes, weights, materials, and colors.
- Provide examples of home objects that infants see every day and how they can be used as "toys" for stacking, shaking, and rolling.

Communication

- Encourage parents to talk to their infant during caregiving activities. This holds the infant's attention, especially when fussy, and makes it easier to change diapers, dress the infant, prepare meals, and attend to the infant's needs in other ways.
- Discuss the benefit of looking at picture books and reading to infants even at this early age. The benefit of developing habits of quiet time together and reading as a nighttime ritual can be emphasized.

Feeding and Self-Care

- Encourage infant self-feeding. Encourage handling of utensils, holding the bottle, and taking solids from a spoon. Advise parents that using two spoons, giving one to the infant to hold, may make mealtimes more satisfying for all.
- Advise parents to offer finger foods when the pincer grasp appears or with the eruption of the first tooth. Caution parents about the need to engage infants socially, interacting with the child during feeding. Encourage making feeding a social and fun time, using utensils rather than toys for distraction.
- Encourage structured mealtimes, especially if there are feeding problems. Advise parents to use an infant seat or highchair and avoid opportunities for "grazing" (i.e., allowing small snacks).

Strength and Motor Coordination

- Encourage parents to allow space for their infant to move about under supervision. Explain that infants need opportunities to play on the floor and spend time on their abdomen.
- Review childproofing the home from the infant's eye level. Also encourage childproofing at relatives' homes and child care or day care settings; this is especially important when the infant does not visit these settings regularly.

7 to 8 Months of Age

DEVELOPMENTAL STATUS

Between 7 and 8 months, infant cognitive development demonstrates significant growth. This "touchpoint" is marked by the infant's increased awareness of surroundings and initiation of individual likes and dislikes. This is often a time when resistance to bedtime, feeding, and parental separation occurs. Feedings begin to follow a routine of breakfast, lunch, and dinner with midmorning, afternoon, and bedtime snacks.

Growth curves change as infants reduce their breast milk or formula intake and increase solids. Head circumference is still vital, owing to the rapid brain growth during this time, and measurements should be plotted on growth curves just as height and weight are. If concerns about a large head circumference exist, note each parent's "hat size" and continue to monitor the head circumference. Infants often get their first set of teeth during this time, and teething can interrupt previously established nighttime sleep patterns.

The infant's social development continues to show the effects of individual personality and temperament. Stranger anxiety varies among infants, based on the variety of caregivers they have experienced and their temperament. Infants use gestures, such as pointing, outstretched arms, and tugging, to get their parents' attention and communicate their needs.

Cognitive development allows the infant to see cause-and-effect relationships in activities, such as ringing a bell, pulling on a string to retrieve a ring, train, or phone, and dropping a toy from the crib or highchair. The infant's play and other activities become more spontaneous, whereas the parent begins to take a more passive role. Object permanence can be demonstrated as the child begins to play hide-and-seek or peek-a-boo, or looks for a toy placed under a cloth.

Although infants' expressive language skills are limited, their receptive language can clearly be seen as they listen and respond to their parents' instructions or requests. They initially stop or quiet when their parent uses "no" or a different tone of voice. They make single-consonant sounds such as "ah," "ba," "da," and "ga." Gradually they progress to making double-consonant sounds, "ah-ah," "da-da," and "ga-ga." They use "ma-ma" and "da-da" but not specifically for their parents. They also enjoy imitating oral sounds, such as raspberries and coughing.

Infants' increased ability to do things for themselves often puts them at odds with their parents. Their gradually increasing ability to feed themselves and their desire to partake of activities in their environment present many challenges. Even if parents have learned to understand their infant's cues and allow reciprocity between themselves and their infant, control issues begin to arise.

Babies become more adept at using their palm and all their fingers to pick up objects. They are now able to hold a toy in each hand at the same time and can transfer objects from one hand to the other. They also enjoy putting objects into containers and taking them out again.

Motor skills at this age need little encouragement for development. Infants sit erect for longer periods of time. They stand, fully supporting their weight, when their hands are held at shoulder height. They gradually stand by holding onto furniture and pull themselves up on the crib rails. They actively crawl on their hands and knees.

ANTICIPATORY GUIDANCE AND DEVELOPMENTAL INTERVENTIONS

This is one of the most challenging periods for parents. Often, previously successful parenting strategies and techniques are no longer effective. Recommendations from relatives and neighbors can undermine parents' confidence. Infants at this age demonstrate increasing developmental differences, with some beginning to walk while others are just beginning to crawl. Temperamental differences among 7- to 8-month-old infants are also striking. For these reasons, anticipatory guidance is particularly important to sustain parental confidence and increase parental knowledge about their infant's unique development.

Rhythmicity and Sleep/Wake Patterns
- Discuss the increased need to provide consistency and maintain a nighttime ritual

that transitions from play time (e.g., bath-time and bedtime story) to sleep time.

- Stress the importance of teaching infants to go to sleep in their own beds so that when they awaken at night they are able to return to sleep. Advise parents that night awakenings are best handled with the least amount of caregiver intrusion (e.g., use face, voice, touch, and then holding).
- Remind parents that infants are more able to wait for gratification. Parents can use tone of voice and talking to calm and reassure the infant.

Emotional Growth Fostering
- Discuss parents' feelings about the Infant's stranger anxiety and how parents handle this.
- Discuss parents' feelings regarding limit setting and consistency of care. Parental consensus in caregiving benefits the child.
- Discuss the infant's need for positive parental responsiveness and attention.

Cognitive and Environmental Stimulation
- Encourage toys that demonstrate cause and effect, stacking, and container play.
- Allow infants to initiate games and social activities on their own.
- Identify common favorite toys, such as wooden spoons, plastic bowls, pull toys, or telephone.
- Explore parents' expectations for later toilet training. Discuss the physiological and cognitive development that is necessary for learning this skill.

Communication
- Encourage parents to talk to their infant in their everyday activities, describing their caregiving and responding to their infant's vocalizations.
- Have the parents show the baby pictures in books, on the wall, or in magazines.
- Demonstrate naming body parts while examining the infant in order to show the parents the infant's responsiveness.

Feeding and Self-Care
- Discuss the continuing need for the infant to gain greater skill in self-feeding.
- Describe the benefits of offering finger foods, using a spoon, and drinking from a cup.
- Discuss parents' feelings about messiness of feeding, finding ways to minimize the mess (e.g., sheet on the floor, small-sized portions of food).
- Discuss eventual weaning from breast or bottle to cup at 12 to 15 months of age by encouraging cup feeding now.
- Discuss need to clean teeth and provide fluoride supplements if water supply is not fluoridated.

Strength and Motor Coordination
- Discuss opportunities for crawling and walking. Discourage use of walkers.
- Discuss safety needs related to the child's increasing mobility and poor understanding of dangers. Review aspects of child-proofing the home, such as checking gates on stairs, padding sharp corners, covering electrical outlets, and keeping the cord on an iron safely out of the way.

9 to 10 Months of Age

DEVELOPMENTAL STATUS

At 9 to 10 months, the infant's growth has begun to follow a growth curve possibly different from the one established early in infancy. Growth spurts become more apparent to parents as the infant outgrows clothes "overnight." At the same time, illnesses, decreased solid food intake caused by teething, and the infant's increased activity level can slow the rate of growth. It becomes important to estimate the infant's total caloric intake if there is a significant decrease in the infant's growth or if feeding problems are present. Early intervention in feeding problems at this time can result in a much easier resolution.

Infants begin to show regular patterns in bowel and bladder elimination. Some parents interpret their ability to predict their infant's bowel movements as toilet training. (See Chapter 14 for more information about toilet training.) Sleep problems, if managed with consistency, begin to resolve. Otherwise, there might still be struggles with bedtime.

Infants at this age demonstrate stranger wariness, and some demonstrate fear of new situations or experiences. However, once familiar with new people, particularly if introduced by their parents, babies enjoy initiating games and social interchanges. They assist in dressing by extending an arm or leg and are able to retrieve the bottle if it is dropped. They take great pride in mastering new skills or overcoming their fears. They look to others around them to take notice as well.

Their curiosity blossoms. Infants begin to explore not only visually and with mouthing and chewing, but also by grasping, poking, shaking, pushing, pulling, and stacking. They often develop their own games or explore different ways of playing with familiar toys or objects. Cognitive development increases.

Receptive language skills improve, and infants participate in games such as pat-a-cake and peek-a-boo. Words such as "da-da," "ma-ma," or "ba-ba" (for bottle) can be recognized. Babies at this age momentarily stop activity when they hear "no," but they do not truly understand what "no" means.

Fine motor development is exhibited through the ability to hold objects of different sizes and the ability to pick up small objects using the sides of the fingers and eventually a fine pincer grasp. They often begin to hold a cup with two hands but still have difficulty sealing their lips around the edge of the cup to take sips.

At 9 to 10 months, most infants sit for long periods and crawl on hands and knees. They begin to "cruise," walking around furniture holding on with both hands, and are able to pull themselves off the floor to a standing position. They may also begin to let themselves down from furniture with fairly good control.

ANTICIPATORY GUIDANCE AND DEVELOPMENTAL INTERVENTIONS

Depending on the transitions accomplished between 7 and 8 months, this period reflects some leveling out of previous changes or the actual beginning of new developmental changes requiring further parental adjustments. Because of frequent discrepancies between infant development and family readiness, it becomes increasingly important to individualize counseling to the infant and family at hand.

Rhythmicity and Sleep/Wake Patterns
- Discuss parental activities that provide consistent and contingent activities that facilitate the infant's sense of trust.
- Discuss the infant's need to rely on a favorite toy or blanket in new situations to maintain a sense of familiarity.

Emotional Growth Fostering
- Assess parents' coping with ever-increasing demands of busy infants.
- Provide positive reinforcement for parenting skills.
- Explore ideas about weaning, discipline, and how parental experiences are progressing.
- Discuss the infant's increasing need for control and initiative.
- Emphasize distraction and use of infant curiosity to deal with difficult situations.

Cognitive and Environmental Stimulation
- Discuss toys that demonstrate cause and effect. Advise parents that they might need to put some toys away and then bring them out at a later date to maintain curiosity and interest.
- Reinforce that the parents should allow the child to take the lead in play activities.
- Encourage books, music, blocks, stacking toys, container toys, pull toys, and toys that allow self-initiated activities.
- Encourage interactive games, such as peek-a-boo and pat-a-cake. Interaction with the caregiver is still the most important activity for the child.

Communication
- Discuss the continuing need to encourage the infant's verbalizations and to use a teaching style to help the infant learn about the environment.
- Encourage use of words in all interactions with the child (e.g., ear, nose, cup, shoe).
- If needed, demonstrate to parents how to encourage the infant's interest in picture books and willingness to pat and point to pictures on each page.

Feeding and Self-Care
- Encourage giving the infant meals in a highchair and having the infant eat or snack with the rest of the family.

• Discuss control issues that can arise as the infant increases self-feeding activities.

• Continue to encourage self-feeding and use of a cup vs. a bottle.

• Help keep the infant focused on meals by removing distracters, using verbal reinforcement, and talking about the meal.

• Reinforce the need to keep toys away from mealtime to differentiate from playtime. Some infants eat quickly and then want to socialize or play games. Assist parents to recognize satiation cues.

Strength and Motor Coordination

• Encourage the parents' natural tendency to "cheer" their children on as they refine old and achieve new motor skills. This parenting behavior can be used as an example of positive reinforcement for the child in other areas of development.

• Discuss the importance of childproofing the environment. Parents need help in anticipating their infant's next major developmental achievement and preparing for the child's natural curiosity. Babies at this age are often able to get into trouble but not get themselves out (e.g., falling into a bucket of water).

• Discuss the use of ipecac.

• Discuss the continuing need to check bath water temperature and avoid leaving the infant alone for even a few seconds in the tub. At this age, infants can sit well but are unable to right themselves if they fall over in a slippery tub.

11 to 12 Months of Age

DEVELOPMENTAL STATUS

Infant weight gain at this time is about 1 lb per month. Growth in length continues to occur in spurts. Eleven- to 12-month-olds are usually eating solids well, want to feed themselves, and are able to recognize their own hunger or satiation needs. They usually do not eat the same amount at each meal and demonstrate specific likes and dislikes.

Emotions such as affection, anger, jealousy, and anxiety become more evident at this age. Overall, 11- to 12-month-olds appear to be in love with the world, love to explore, and have little fear of those things that can cause them harm. Babies at 1 year enjoy playing interactive games and demonstrating their mastery of new skills. When in the mood, they are willing helpers in dressing and diaper changes. They also release an object if asked and love playing ball.

Cognitively, they are completing more complicated tasks, such as stacking and container play. They easily locate a toy placed out of sight or under a cloth. They hold a crayon or pencil with their whole hand and will make dots on a piece of paper imitating a drawn line.

Infants' expressive language has now expanded to a total of three or four words. They are able to name a picture in a book, visually look for an object when named, and follow simple one-step requests. They are still very focused on observing activities in their environment and, when given names of things, attend well to the new information.

Fine motor development usually allows infants to entertain themselves for extended times. They are able to stack blocks one on top of the other and can easily pick up an object with the tips of their fingers, most often transferring it directly to their mouth.

Gross motor skills improve as infants continue to walk around furniture with increasing confidence. They also take steps if someone holds two hands and then one hand. Eventually they take a few steps from one object or person to another. They may momentarily stand alone, and some infants walk independently.

ANTICIPATORY GUIDANCE AND DEVELOPMENTAL INTERVENTIONS

At this time, parents' needs vary considerably, depending on the needs of their particular infant. Parents continue to need to understand the developmental phases that their child faces, because each child's personality and temperament are unique. This can be done best by demonstrating the child's skills in each of the areas of development—physical growth, social-emotional growth, cognitive growth, feeding and self-care skills, communication, fine motor skills, and gross motor skills. Often, the parents and the child focus on those areas that come easiest for the child. The NP can support the parents' efforts in these areas while also guiding parents to assist their child's development in areas that are more challenging. Parents' efforts to develop positive child management strategies need to be reinforced.

Rhythmicity and Sleep/Wake Patterns

- Reinforce efforts to establish and maintain routine nighttime rituals, regular mealtimes, and consistency of caregivers. Discuss the child's need for predictability in the daily schedule in order to gain mastery over new situations.
- Discuss the child's temperament, which is becoming more evident in activity level, level of curiosity, and ease of adjusting to new situations. A child's temperament is not always consistent with that of other family members.

Emotional Growth Fostering

- Discuss the development of each child's will and desire for autonomy.
- Discuss the infant's ego growth and need to distinguish parent from self.
- Discuss the parent's "teaching role" and discipline vs. punishment.
- Introduce the teaching loop: attention, instruction, demonstration, practice, reinforcement (Table 6-1).
- Discuss the energy parents need to deal with busy toddlers and ways to cope when exhaustion occurs.
- Discuss negotiation of parental roles and responsibilities.

Cognitive and Environmental Stimulation

- Explore parental feelings when infants enjoy time away from the parent.
- Discuss infants' enjoyment of messy play (e.g., water, sand, and different textures).
- Encourage parents to play ball with the infant, rolling or throwing the ball back and forth interactively.

Communication

- Encourage "reading" stories for 1 to 5 minutes at a time, or as the child tolerates.
- Demonstrate teaching of body parts (e.g., eyes, nose, mouth).

Feeding and Self-Care

- Encourage weaning from the bottle or breast and counsel on dental hygiene and caries prevention (e.g., use a soft toothbrush or wrap a washcloth around the finger to cleanse teeth and gums).
- Encourage self-feeding and discuss letting the child practice using a spoon.

Strength and Motor Coordination

- Discuss the value of outings for both parents and child and the need to watch the child more closely, because the child is more mobile and apt to wander away from the parents.
- Continue to reinforce bath water temperature control and bath time supervision.
- Reinforce the need for placing medicine, cleaning agents, matches, and firearms in

T A B L E 6-1

The Teaching Loop

BEHAVIORS	DESCRIPTION OF BEHAVIOR
Alerting	The parent gets the infant's attention and makes sure that the child is paying attention. This may occur by calling the infant's name, making a noise, or directing the child to the toy.
Instruction	The parent gives a specific instruction to the infant or child about the toy or task and what is to be done. This instruction should be short and may be either verbal, or a demonstration, or both.
Performance	The parent then gives the infant or child time to explore the material, to attempt to practice the task or play with the toy as shown, or just to explore the toy depending on the child's age. Many parents have trouble allowing the child the time just to explore the task; others may offer excessive time without offering any assistance.
Feedback	The parent makes some comment that may be positive or negative, such as, "Good job," "Good try," or "No, that's not quite right; try it this way."

Data from Steward D, Steward M: The observation of Anglo-Mexican and Chinese-American mothers teaching their young sons. Child Dev 44:329–337, 1973.

locked cabinets, not just out of reach. These safety precautions are a must for mobile toddlers with increased fine motor skills and increasing curiosity.

COMMON DEVELOPMENTAL ISSUES OF INFANTS

Developmental Delays in Infants

Developmental delays that appear during infancy are usually connected to dysfunctions of major organs, physiological abnormalities, and physiological imbalances. Later presentations include feeding problems and poor interaction with caregivers or the environment and can indicate motor coordination problems or hearing and vision problems. Gross motor problems are most often identified after 9 months of age, although parents often report concerns earlier.

CLASSIFICATION OF DEVELOPMENTAL DISORDERS

Developmental disorders that need to be considered when evaluating an infant's developmental delay include disorders that manifest as motor problems, such as cerebral palsy, and disorders that manifest as cognitive problems, such as mental retardation, specific deficits in processing, and seizures. Processing disorders include peripheral problems such as deafness and blindness; central processing disorders reflected in motor, language, and perceptual dysfunction; and behavioral problems. Usually, the history best provides the clues to the diagnosis of developmental delay. Some problems, such as fetal alcohol syndrome, autism, or fragile X syndrome, may not have clear symptoms in infancy. It is important to determine whether the problems are the result of neurodegeneration as opposed to a static encephalopathy. Parental reports of developmental milestones are not always helpful because of incomplete parent recall (Shapiro, 1993).

RISK FACTORS FOR DEVELOPMENTAL DELAYS IN INFANTS

Factors associated with developmental problems in infancy include the following:

- Prenatal exposure to street drugs or alcohol
- Prematurity
- Low birth weight
- Anoxia or birth trauma
- Neonatal intensive care and long-term hospitalization
- Cardiovascular illnesses
- Endocrine and metabolic problems
- Genetic syndromes
- Failure to thrive
- Cerebral palsy
- Sensory problems
- Autism

DEVELOPMENTAL RED FLAGS

Table 6–2 identifies developmental findings that are indications for referral.

DEVELOPMENTAL SUPPORTIVE CARE

Developmentally supportive care is appropriate to the infant's age and abilities, is individualized to a particular infant, and is integrated throughout all aspects of caregiving. Parents and caregivers are responsible for providing an environment that is supportive of the child's development. For most parents, this means learning more about infant development and how to teach their infants. Many parents must also evaluate child care arrangements, finding those that will promote their infant's development.

Steward and Steward (1973) first introduced the concept of a teaching loop, in which teaching interactions between the parent and child consist of four specific teaching behaviors (see Table 6–1). These behaviors provide the infant with verbal instruction, modeling, and positive feedback. Parents are often observed using this technique at the age when infants begin to walk. By encouraging parents to use the same technique earlier and in other areas of development, the NP provides them with important skills that will assist their child's development.

PARENT EDUCATION AND ANTICIPATORY GUIDANCE

This same teaching loop can be used as a model for NPs to teach parents. NPs must be sensitive

T A B L E 6-2

Developmental Red Flags: Newborns and Infants

AGE	PHYSICAL DEVELOPMENT (AUTONOMIC STABILITY/ RHYTHMICITY/SLEEP/ TEMPERAMENT)	PSYCHOSOCIAL/ EMOTIONAL SKILLS	COGNITIVE AND VISUAL ABILITIES	LANGUAGE/ HEARING	FINE MOTOR (FEEDING/SELF-CARE)	GROSS MOTOR (STRENGTH/ COORDINATION)
Newborn/ 1 mo	Lack of return to birth weight by 2-wk examination Poor coordination of suck/swallow Tachypnea/bradycardia with feedings Poor habituation to external stimuli	Diffuse nonverbal cues Poor state transitions Irritable	Doll's eyes No red light reflex Poor alert state	No startle to sound or sudden noises No quieting to voice High-pitched cry	Hands held fisted Absent or asymmetrical palmar grasp	Asymmetrical movements Hypertonia or hypotonia Asymmetrical primitive reflexes
3 mo	Less than 1-lb weight gain in 1 mo Head circumference increasing greater than 2 percentile lines on growth curve or showing no increase in size Continuing problems with poor suck/swallow Difficulty with regulation of sleep/wake cycle	Lack of social smile Withdrawn or depressed Lack of consistent, safe child care	No visual tracking Not able to fix on face or object	Does not turn to voice, rattle, or bell No sounds, coos, squeals	Hands fisted with oppositional thumb No hand to mouth activity	Asymmetrical movements Hypertonia or hypotonia No attempt to raise head when on stomach
6 mo	Less than double birth weight Head circumference showing no increase Continuation of poor feeding or sleep regulation Difficulty with self-calming	No smiles No response to play Solemn appearance	Not visually alert Does not reach for objects Does not look at caregiver	No babbling Does not respond to voice, bell, rattle, or loud noises even with startle	Does not reach for objects, hold rattle, hold hands together Does not grasp at clothes	Persistent primitive reflexes Does not attempt to sit with support Head lag with pull to sit Scissoring
9 mo	Parent control issues with feeding or sleep	Intense stranger anxiety or absent stranger anxiety Does not seek comfort from caregiver when stressed	Lack of visual awareness Lack of reaching out for toys Lack of toy exploration visually or orally	Lack of single or double sounds Lack of response to name or voice Does not respond to any words	No self-feeding No highchair sitting No solids Does not pick up toys with one hand	Does not sit even in tripod position No lateral prop reflex Asymmetrical crawl, handedness, or other movements
12 mo	Less than triple birth weight Losing more than 2 percentile lines on growth curve for weight, length, or head circumference Poor sleep/wake cycle Extreme inability to separate from parent	No response to game playing No response to reading or interactive activities Withdrawn or solemn	Not visually following activities in the environment	Inability to localize to sound Not imitating speech sounds Not using 2–3 words Does not point	Persistent mouthing Not attempting to feed self or hold cup Not able to hold toy in each hand or transfer objects	Not pulling self to stand Not moving around the environment to explore

to parents' interest in and tolerance of the anticipatory guidance information presented. Information related to parental concerns will be the most openly received. Frequently, the time limitations in a clinic or office setting lead to use of a "laundry list" of topics for anticipatory guidance rather than individualized anticipatory guidance. Alternative approaches can be effectively used to provide parental education. For example, well-child care group visits and in-office evening parent education classes work well, especially because they bring parents together to problem-solve common issues.

The goal for parent education in the early years is to provide tools for parents that will be used in the many challenging years to come. It is also intended that parents become their child's advocates, capable and knowledgeable about their child's individual needs.

SUMMARY

Development is only one aspect of a child's overall health assessment. However, it is a very significant indicator of a child's physical, mental, and emotional progress. Surveillance of the child's developmental progress provides the NP with a window through which to observe and better understand the child's life. With this understanding and attention, the NP is able to advocate actively for the child and support the parents' continuing development of parenting skills.

RESOURCE BOX 6-1

SCREENING TOOLS

Ages and Stages Questionnaire (ASQ)
Diane Bricker and Jane Squires
(800) 638-3775

Battelle Developmental Inventory Screening Test (BDI)
(800) 323-9540

Bayley Infant Neurodevelopmental Screener
Glen Aylward
(800) 288-0752

Denver Screening Scales (Denver II, Denver Articulation Screening Scale [DASE], Denver Vision Screening)
(800) 419-4729

Gesell Developmental Screening Inventory (Revised)
Developmental Testing Materials, Inc.
(800) 724-5028

Hawaii Early Learning Profile: Activity Guide
Setsu Furuno, Katherine A. O'Reilly, Carol Hosaka, Takayo T. Inatsuka, Toney L. Allman, & Barbara Zeisloft
(650) 322-8282
e-mail: www.VORT.com

HOME Scale
Robert Bradley & Betty Caldwell
Order from Lorraine Coulson
(501) 565-7627
FAX: (501) 565-7627
e-mail: LRCOULSON@ualr.edu

Kent Infant Development Scale
(800) 648-8857

KIDS Chart
Grace Holmes & Ruth Hassanein
Published by Grace Holmes, M.D.
(913) 588-2749
FAX: (913) 588-2780
e-mail: gholmes@kumc.edu

Milani-Comparetti Motor Development Screening Test
Jack Trembath
(402) 559-7467
(800) 656-3937, X7467

Miller Assessment for Preschoolers (MAP) and **First Step: Screening Test for Evaluating Preschoolers**
Lucy J. Miller
(800) 228-0752

NCAST Parent Child Interaction Scales (Feeding and Teaching Scales)
[Training required to order NCAST] and
Community Life Scales [No training required to order]
Kathryn Barnard
(206) 543-8528
e-mail: NCAST@u.washington.edu

Neonatal Behavioral Assessment
T. Berry Brazelton
(800) 323-9540

Peabody Developmental Motor Scales
M. Rhonda Folio & Rebecca R. Fewell
(800) 323-9540

Revised Infant Temperament Questionnaire
William B. Carey & Sean McDevitt
(215) 836-2240

Continued on next page

RESOURCE BOX 6-1

SCREENING TOOLS Continued

Vineland Adaptive Behavior Scales
Sparrow, Balia, & Cicchetti
(800) 328-2560

REFERENCES

Ainsworth M, Blehar M, Waters E, et al: Patterns of Attachment. Hillsdale, NJ, Erlbaum, 1978.

Barnard K: NCAST Instructor's Manual. Seattle, NCAST Publications, 1979.

Barnard K, Morisset C, Spieker S: Preventive interventions: Enhancing parent-child relationships. *In* Zeanah C (ed): Handbook of Infant Mental Health. New York, Guilford Press, 1993.

Bradley R, Caldwell B: Using the home inventory to assess the family environment. Pediatr Nurs 14:97–102, 1988.

Brazelton B: Touchpoints: Your Child's Emotional and Behavioral Development. New York, Addison-Wesley, 1992.

Bronfenbrenner U: The Ecology of Human Development: Experiments by Nature and Design. Cambridge, MA, Harvard University Press, 1979.

Carey WB: Let's give temperament its due. Contemp Pediatr 15:91–113, 1998.

Dixon SD, Stein M (eds): Encounters With Children: Pediatric Behavior and Development. St. Louis, Mosby, 1992.

Green M (ed): Bright Futures: Guidelines for Health Supervision of Infants, Children, and Adolescents. Arlington, VA, National Center for Education in Maternal and Child Health, 1994.

Green M: Development in the first year of life. Contemp Pediatr 15:81–116. 1998.

Guyer B, Martin JA, MacDorman MF, et al: Annual summary of vital statistics—1996. Pediatrics 100:905–918, 1997.

Johnson CP, Blasco P: Infant growth and development. Pediatr Rev 18:224–242, 1997.

Lyons-Ruth K, Zeanah C: The family context of infant mental health: I. Affective development in the primary caregiving relationship. *In* Zeanah C (ed): Handbook of Infant Mental Health. New York, Guilford Press, 1993.

Main M, Solomon J: Procedures for identifying infants as disorganized/disoriented during the Ainsworth Strange Situation. *In* Greenberg M, Cicchetti D, Cummings EM (eds): Attachment in the Preschool Years: Theory, Research, and Intervention. Chicago, University of Chicago Press, 1990.

Sameroff A: Models of development and developmental risk. *In* Zeanah C (ed): Handbook of Infant Mental Health. New York, Guilford Press, 1993.

Sameroff A, Chandler M: Reproductive risks and the continuum of caretaking casualty. *In* Horowitz FD (ed): Review of Child Development Research. Chicago, University of Chicago Press, 1975.

Shapiro B: Detection and assessment of development disabilities. *In* Dershewitz R (ed): Ambulatory Pediatric Care. Philadelphia, JB Lippincott, 1993.

Steward D, Steward M: The observation of Anglo-Mexican and Chinese-American mothers teaching their young sons. Child Dev 44:329–337, 1973.

CHAPTER 7

Developmental Management of Toddlers and Preschoolers

Mary A. Murphy

▨ INTRODUCTION

Developmental changes in the second through fifth years of life are more subtle than those in the first year. The child refines abilities acquired in the first year, learning, for example, to walk smoothly with control and speed, to run and climb, and to combine words into phrases and sentences. A toddler is usually defined as a child aged 12 to 24 months, and a preschool child is aged 2 to 5 years. This chapter reviews some of the many changes that occur during these years.

▨ DEVELOPMENT OF TODDLERS AND PRESCHOOLERS

Theories of Toddler and Preschool Psychosocial Development

Toddlers show many of the characteristics described by various psychological theories. Freud thought that toddlers progress through an anal stage in which most of their gratification is sought through the anal opening. He argued that toddlers find pleasure in manipulation of the anal area and that they control their environment by manipulating the control of bowels and bladder. According to Freud, the preschool years represent a tremendously active stage, with the child's development evolving around the Oedipus complex, with love for the parent of the opposite sex and fear of the parent of the same sex.

Erikson believed that toddlers develop a sense of autonomy and move away from total dependence into more interdependence. During this process, toddlers discover themselves and explore their own bodies and their expanding world. With their increased mobility, they move away from their parents for short periods of time and look at the world outside their beds, houses, and yards. According to Erikson, preschoolers begin to develop a sense of initiative, learning new skills and exploring the larger outside world.

Kohlberg investigated moral development of children and described 12- to 18-month-old children as "amoral," with an ability to follow commands occasionally. He believed that 2-year-old children are in a preconventional stage, in which they follow commands more frequently. Preschool-age children are in a conventional stage of morality, able to follow commands consistently as they work to maintain approval of adults and to behave as "good" children are expected to do.

Temperament, another theoretical perspective important to child development, is discussed in Chapter 21. Resilience and vulnerability are two other characteristics under current discussion in the literature. Resilience (sometimes called *hardiness*) is a person's capacity to survive intact both psychologically and physically despite adversity. Vulnerability, in contrast, refers to a person's sensitivity and inclination to decompensate in the face of stressors in life. These characteristics are also found in children and they affect the outcomes in their lives as stressors come and go. Despite significant risks, some children manage to grow and prosper (Engle et al., 1996).

Physical Development

GENERAL

Physical and physiological changes in toddlers and preschoolers continue at a much slower pace than in the first year of life. The 2- to 3-year-old shows annual weight gains of 4.4 to 6.6 lb (2 to 3 kg). The average 2-year-old weighs 26 to 28 lb (12.5 to 13.5 kg), with boys being slightly heavier than girls. Height gains continue, with an average of 4.5 inches (12 cm) during the second year and 3 inches (6 to 8 cm) during the third year. An average 2-year-old is 34 to 35 inches (85 to 90 cm) tall. Head growth slows remarkably after the first year, with a yearly increase of 1 inch (2 cm). An average 2-year-old has a head circumference of 19 to 19.5 inches (48 to 50 cm). Most toddlers have no palpable fontanels by 12 months; for all, the anterior fontanel should be completely closed by 18 to 19 months. During the fourth and fifth years, skeletal growth continues as additional ossification centers appear in the wrist and ankle and additional epiphyses develop in some of the long bones. For the 4- to 5-year-old, the legs grow faster than the head, trunk, or upper extremities.

DENTAL

Dental growth is rapid for 2- and 3-year-olds. By the first birthday, the child usually has 6 to 8 primary teeth and, by 2 years of age, a complete set of 20 primary teeth. At this age, a few children are missing their second molars, which should erupt by the time they are 3 years old.

During the second year, calcification begins for the first and second permanent bicuspids and second molars. Visible dental growth is minimal for preschoolers, with most growth and calcification occurring for the permanent teeth within the gums. Around the fifth, sixth, or seventh year, the child loses the front primary incisors, which are replaced with adult permanent teeth.

ENDOCRINE

The toddler and preschool years are fairly quiescent times for sexual growth, with few physical or hormonal changes occurring.

NEUROLOGICAL

Neural growth continues during the preschool years, with additional myelinization and cortical development. Sensory function becomes more developed (e.g., visual acuity matures, from 20/70 in a 2-year-old to 20/30 in a 5- to 6-year-old). Neurological growth, combined with musculoskeletal development, allows the child to perform more complex physical tasks, and fine motor movements become more detailed and sustained. A 2-year-old can easily manipulate fingers to stack two blocks, whereas a 3-year-old can create a tower of eight or more blocks. A 4-year-old can easily build a 12-block step design, and a 5-year-old can use a pencil to copy simple geometrical designs accurately. Gross motor skills become smoother and more coordinated.

CARDIOVASCULAR

Little change occurs in the cardiovascular system in the second and third year, but by the fifth year the heart has quadrupled its size since birth. The heart rate continues to decrease and is usually around 70 to 110 beats per minute by age 5 years. Normal sinus arrhythmia may continue, and innocent murmurs are common. Components of the blood continue to mature, and the hematologic system should contain entirely adult hemoglobin. The hemoglobin level stabilizes at about 12 to 15 g/dl.

GASTROINTESTINAL

In the gastrointestinal system, salivary glands increase greatly in size and mature to adult size by 2 years of age. The stomach becomes more bowed and increases its capacity to 500 ml. During the second year, the liver matures, becoming more efficient in vitamin storage, glycogenesis, amino acid changes, and ketone body formation. The lower edge of the liver may still be palpable in some toddlers and preschoolers.

By 4 to 5 years of age, the gastrointestinal system is mature enough for the child to eat a full range of foods. Stomach capacity is still small enough that some children need a nutritional snack between meals to maintain blood glucose levels during growth periods. Owing to diet and maturation, stools are more like those of adults.

PULMONARY

Respiratory movements continue to be abdominal until the end of the fifth or sixth year. Because the chest wall is thin, respirations can be heard clearly and distinctly. The rate is slower and steadier than in infancy, around 20 to 30 per minute.

RENAL

The kidneys begin descending deeper into the pelvic area and grow in size. Ureters remain short and relatively straight. A normal 2-year-old may excrete as much as 500 to 600 ml of urine a day; a 4- to 5-year-old excretes between 600 and 750 ml.

DEVELOPMENTAL SCREENING AND ASSESSMENT OF TODDLERS AND PRESCHOOLERS

Screening Strategies for Toddlers and Preschoolers

Developmental surveillance is an essential part of each health maintenance visit and can include both screening and diagnostic testing.

The process begins by building rapport with the parents, encouraging them to share sensitive developmental concerns. The observation of the interactions between child and parents is part of data collection. Screening techniques provide a quick, inexpensive method of identifying potential problems. Screening is done for all children, assuming that some will be identified as outside normal limits. Screening techniques generally are viewed as appropriate for all children (although culture and experience affect outcomes and need to be taken into consideration). In contrast, assessments are done when a more individualized approach is required to decide whether a developmental problem exists and how to guide its management.

PHYSICAL DEVELOPMENT

Toddlers and preschool children should be screened for certain physical parameters with every well-child check. Specifically, 2-year-olds should have height, weight, and head circumference checked and graphed; blood tested for lead if screening identifies child at risk; plus hearing, vision, and dentition screened. Three- and four-year-olds need height and weight checked and graphed, blood pressure measured, and hearing and vision screened. Tuberculosis and cholesterol screening should be done for any toddler or preschooler who is at high risk (American Academy of Pediatrics, 1995).

DEVELOPMENTAL SCREENING

The child's development and progress should be reviewed periodically by the nurse practitioner (NP) in a variety of areas. For each area, ask questions directly of the parent, probing for the level of understanding. Observing the child during the history, looking for gross motor, fine motor, language, and social skills, may provide better information than that obtained through more formal testing. Chapter 6 lists a variety of screening tools to use. Broad developmental screening questions from *Bright Futures* (Green, 1994) include the following:

Screening Question	*Developmental Area Screened*
How does the child communicate needs and desires?	Language, psychosocial skills, self-control
What do you think the child understands?	Receptive language, cognitive level
How does the child act around others?	Receptive and expressive language, cognitive level, psychosocial skills
Does the child seem to understand the feelings of others?	Cognitive level, psychosocial skills
To what extent has the child developed independence in eating, dressing, and toileting?	Cognitive level, adaptability, fine motor control, psychosocial skills
Tell me about the child's typical play.	Receptive and expressive language, cognitive level, adaptability, fine and gross motor control, psychosocial skill
How does the child get from one place to another?	Gross motor control

Use of developmental screening tests such as the Denver Developmental Screening Test II (DDST II) and the Early Language Milestone (ELM) test is recommended annually. At every visit, the child's progress in gross motor and fine motor control, language, and personal social areas needs to be elicited and data compared with developmental norms. Stein (1998) has identified developmental themes that incorporate the developmental milestones, temperament, family support, and resilience of the child. The themes are introduced here because they can help to focus limited time for both developmental screening and parental anticipatory guidance and counseling. More in-depth discussions appear later in the chapter to help the clinician with assessments of various developmental areas.

The 12-Month Visit
- Independent walking helps the child develop a new perspective about the world
- Gross motor skills
- Individual style in motor skills
- Effect of walking on other skills and behaviors

The 18-Month and 2-Year Visits
- Autonomy vs. attachment
- Predictable regressions
- Discipline
- Self-determination
- Transitional object
- Behavior modifications

The 3- to 4-Year Visits
- Emergence of magical thinking
- Striving to gain a clearer sense of self

The 4- to 5-Year Visits
- Curiosity about people, objects, and events
- Rapid growth of language and motor skills
- Emergence of gender-specific behaviors
- Gender role identification with parental models
- Capacity for collaborative play
- Beginning mastery over aggressive impulses
- Social interactions with less adult supervision

Screening children from the age of 3 years on should include questions first to the child and then to the parent/caregiver. At the 4- and 5-year visits, the clinician should be sure to screen for articulation. Parents may not be fully sensitive to speech problems because they are accustomed to hearing the child's current speech.

Assessment Strategies for Toddlers and Preschoolers

Once a child has been identified through screening to have a possible problem, more definitive diagnostic testing needs to be done, or the child needs to be referred to an appropriate specialist. Diagnostic testing gives direction to treatment, management, and prediction of future needs. Tests can be invasive, costly, and time consuming and should be done only when necessary.

PHYSICAL DEVELOPMENT ASSESSMENT

Although it is assumed that physical problems are detected early in childhood, many children are not properly screened. Palfrey and colleagues (1987) studied 1726 children and found that only 4% of disabling conditions were identified at birth, 16.4% before age 3 years, 28.7% before age 5 years, 47.9% by early elementary school age, but more than 23% were not identified before age 8.

The following list is used to assess behavior related to physical development:

Questions Asked	*Purpose/Outcomes/ Goals of Questions*
Ask how the child usually feels	Invites discussion of somatic issues and complaints
Ask whether the child appears similar to other children of the same age	Assesses parent perceptions of physical development
Ask whether the child has been interested in his or her own body or those of others	Allows parents to discuss sexual curiosity and define this as normal behavior
Ask questions about bodily functions	Lays groundwork for later candid provider–patient relationship (especially helpful in children with a chronic illness)
Ask whether an illness has interfered with daily activities	Assesses chronic medical problem effects on development
Ask about toilet training, sleeping habits, and eating habits	Assesses parents' understanding of readiness, changing behaviors, and current status of child's habits

MOTOR DEVELOPMENT

Motor Development Concepts

Motor development is divided into two components—fine and gross. The former includes both hand and finger development as well as oromotor development, whereas the latter includes development and use of the large muscles. Table 7–1 identifies fine and gross motor milestones by age.

FINE MOTOR DEVELOPMENT. Five principles govern fine motor development (Dixon & Stein, 1992):

1. Primitive reflexes must disappear before voluntary behaviors appear (e.g., children do not walk until involuntary stepping disappears).

2. Development is proximal to distal (e.g., children reach before they grasp).
3. Development is ulnar to radial (e.g., children pick up objects with the little finger side of the hand before they use the thumb side of the hand).
4. The hand develops pronation before supination (e.g., children use the palm up to place objects in their mouth).
5. Grasp develops before release (e.g., a newborn reflexively grasps a rattle; a 12-month-old is able to grasp and voluntarily release the rattle).

Fine motor control in the hand moves from flexion and involuntary to voluntary pincer grasp and release movements. Use of the dominant hand may appear as early as 8 to 12 months but generally stabilizes between 2 and 4 years. The 4-year-old can thread small beads on a chain; grasp a pencil appropriately to copy some letters (v, h, t, o); draw a person with head and features, legs, trunk, and arms; use scissors to cut on a line; fasten buttons; and eat with a fork. By age 5 years, these movements expand to copying a square and additional letters (x, l, a, c, u, y), writing some letters spontaneously, producing identifiable pictures, counting fingers on one hand, and using all eating utensils appropriately.

GROSS MOTOR DEVELOPMENT. Gross motor development has four general principles:

1. Skills are built on neuromotor tone (e.g., a 1-year-old with poor muscle tone has difficulty standing, stepping, and walking).
2. Reflexive behavior progresses to volitional behavior (e.g., children move from a stepping reflex to a controlled walk).
3. More efficient behavior is easier and requires less energy (e.g., it is easier to walk than to crawl).
4. Speed and accuracy increase with practice (e.g., a wide-based waddle develops into a narrow-based, smooth walk).

Some behaviors expected of the average toddler include the following:

- Walking with control
- Stepping over a balance beam
- Climbing stairs while holding on

T A B L E 7-1

Fine Motor and Gross Motor Development Milestones for Infants and Preschoolers

AGE	FINE MOTOR MOVEMENT	ORAL MOVEMENT	GROSS MOTOR MOVEMENT
Birth	Flexion	Suckling tongue movements, extension-retraction of tongue, up and down jaw movements, low approximation of lips	Momentary head control when held sitting
1 mo	Extension, nondirected swipes	Rooting	Turns head when prone
4 mo	Directed swipes, corralling, reaching		Sits with support, rolls over, head steady in sitting
4–5 mo	Ulnar-palmar grasp		"Swims" in prone position, no head lag
6–7 mo	Radial-palmar grasp, raking	Sucking with negative oral cavity pressure, rhythmical jaw movements, firm approximation of lips	Sits independently, rocks on hands and knees, free headlift in supine
7–8 mo	Radial digital grasp	Phasic bite reflex, rhythmical bite and release pattern	Supports weight standing, bounces when held
7–9 mo	Scissors grasp	Munching, early chewing	Sits alone well, may crawl
9–10 mo	Voluntary release		Cruises, pivots while seated, pulls to stand
12 mo	Picks up pellet with pincer grasp	Chewing with spreading/rolling tongue movements, tongue lateralization, rotary jaw movements, controlled sustained bite	Walks with one hand held, stands alone momentarily
18 mo	Makes tower of four cubes, imitates scribbling, dumps pellet, puts blocks in large holes, drinks from cup with little spilling, can take off socks		Directed throwing, walks well independently, climbs into adult chair
24 mo	Makes tower of seven cubes, does circular scribbling, folds paper once imitatively, turns doorknobs, turns pages one at a time, unbuttons or unzips large fasteners, puts on coat with assistance		Throws overhand, runs well, kicks ball, up and down stairs 2 feet/step
30 mo	Makes tower of nine cubes, makes vertical and horizontal strokes, imitates circle, buttons large button, uses fork in fist, twists jar lids		Jumps off ground with both feet
36 mo	Makes tower of 10 cubes, imitates bridge of three cubes, copies circle, snips with scissors, can brush teeth but not well, puts shoes on feet		Broad jumps, walks up stairs alternating feet, may pedal tricycle, balance one foot 2–3 sec
48 mo	Copies bridge from model, copies cross and square, cuts curved line with scissors, dresses self, strings small beads		Pedals tricycle, runs smoothly, hops on one foot, catches large ball
60 mo	Some can print name, copies triangle, opens lock with key, bathes self, cuts out simple shapes, pours from small pitcher		Walks downstairs alternating feet, catches bounced ball, skips, stands on one foot 7–8 sec

Data from many developmental tests.

- Running around a corner
- Climbing to any height

The 4-year-old should be able to do the following:

- Walk up and down stairs using one foot to a stair tread
- Skillfully run around corners
- Climb ladders
- Ride a tricycle using the pedals
- Show improving skill in throwing, catching, bouncing, and kicking a ball

By age 5 years, the child should be able to do the following:

- Easily walk a narrow line
- Run lightly on the toes
- Skip with alternate feet
- Move rhythmically to music

Fine and Gross Motor Assessment Strategies

Toddlers and preschoolers continue to develop and refine their motor skills, driven by curiosity, desire for independence, and endless energy. Gross and fine motor skills are best assessed by standardized screening tests such as the Denver II.

Fine motor development is evaluated by assessing finger and hand movements and oral cavity movements. Gross motor development is evaluated by assessing the child's ability to crawl, sit, walk, run, hop, skip, and climb as well as the quality of the child's movements during these activities.

The following list is used to assess behavior related to motor development:

Questions Asked	*Purpose/Outcomes/Goals of Questions*
Ask how the child gets from place to place (walks, climbs, runs, rides tricycle)	Assesses gross motor development
Ask how the child feeds self (cup, spoon, fork)	Assesses fine motor skills
Ask about play activities	Assesses gross and fine motor skills

COGNITIVE DEVELOPMENT ASSESSMENT

Concepts

Cognitively, toddler thinking is quite concrete. According to Piaget, 1-year-olds, still in the sensory motor stage, demonstrate an increased ability to solve problems and will do trial-and-error experiments. They become more differentiated from the environment. They search for a hidden object where they last saw it, showing their increasingly thorough understanding of object permanence. From 18 to 24 months of age, children begin to use mental imagery and begin to infer a cause when they can see only the effect. By the end of the second year, children enter the preoperational stage with preconceptual and intuitive thinking. Primitive conceptualization processes begin with the development of symbolic thinking. A block becomes a car; words become symbols for ideas.

The 3-year-old continues to develop symbolic thinking, such as drawing and elaborate play scenarios. However, children at this age generally are unable to take another's perspective and view the world egocentrically from their own world view. Attending to one characteristic at a time is another feature of preschool thinking. For example, the child will try to fit a jigsaw puzzle piece using either color or shape but not both.

Parents have difficulty understanding the thoughts of preschool children. On the surface, preoperational thinking has many characteristics that resemble adult thinking, and parents are often deceived into believing that children are able to think as adults do. Preschool children, for example, are developing the use of language and the ability to symbolize concepts mentally. Some of their verbalizations appear quite precocious, as evidenced by the 3-year-old who stares out the window and then states "Look, Mommy, the trees are saying yes and no!" In fact, preschool children continue to be very concrete and egocentric in their thinking, and their logic is the source of many communication problems between parents and children. Table 7–2 identifies major characteristics of the thinking of preschool children and gives examples of each.

TABLE 7-2

Examples of Preschool Children's Thinking Using Piaget's Preoperational Stage

CHARACTERISTIC	EXAMPLE
Egocentricism	"It's snowing, so I can go play in it"
Unable to abstract to see other's viewpoint	If John is holding a doll with its face toward Ann, Ann thinks John can also see the doll's face
Mental symbolization of the environment	"The wind is crying," "The (flushing) toilet is an angry animal"
Incomplete understanding of sequence of time	Knows names of time components: today, tomorrow, yesterday, minutes, days, weeks, etc., but uses them inconsistently: "I'm not going to take a nap yesterday"
	Yesterday means any time before now; tomorrow means any time in the future
	Historical events are conceptualized in terms of the present: "Mommy, do you know George Washington?"
Developing sense of space: from experiencing space as a part of their activity to moving through it to understanding space in terms of detail and direction	Frequently used words: in, on, up, down, at, under
Evolving ability to categorize or order objects and phenomena	Early preschooler: no understanding of concept of class or groups; undisturbed to see new Santa Claus on every corner
	Cluster phenomena: when asked to sort a series of blocks, they may cluster a small, medium, and large block as a "baby," "mommy," and "daddy" block
	By 4–5 yr, child is able to consistently use one or two categories to arrange objects in some order (color, number, form, or size)
Developing ability to establish causality (realism, animism, artificialism)	Realism: child thinks self to be personally responsible for results; present in infancy
	Animism: 2- to 3-year-olds think objects possess innate person-like qualities that cause results: "The chair made me fall down"
	Artificialism: 3- to 4-year-olds think things are caused by some controlling force that controls the world
Transductive reasoning: from particular to particular	If the child does not like one particular vegetable, he or she will not like another particular fruit: "I can't eat my banana because my potatoes are burned"
Developing sense of conservation of quantity, weight, mass	Preschooler is usually unable to conceptualize that change in shape does not affect quantity, weight, or mass of an object
	Generally, 50% of 5-year-olds have mastered conservation of quantity and 50% of 6-year-olds of weight or mass

Language development through the toddler and preschool years remains one of the most sensitive indicators of cognitive development. Social development, too, is strongly affected by cognitive development. Differentiation of the self from others, with increasing sensitivity not only to the rules and norms for social interaction but also to the perception of the perspectives and feelings of others, requires ever-increasing cognitive capabilities. Finally, quality of play can be used as an indicator of cognitive development. Through play, children manipulate and learn to control their environment in safe yet stimulating ways.

Cognitive Development Assessment Strategies

Cognitive development is primarily expressed through motor activities in children younger than 2 years of age (Piaget's sensorimotor stage). After age 2 years, the child begins to use symbol systems as thinking moves into the preconceptual stage. The following list is used to assess behavior related to cognitive development:

Questions Asked	Purpose/Outcomes/ Goals of Questions
1- to 3-year-olds	
Ask about typical play	Assesses complexity of manipulation of objects, parallel and cooperative play, role playing
Ask name, age, gender	3-year-olds should know beginning facts
Ask about ability to follow simple instructions	Assesses ability to retain and process instructions and to respond to input
Ask about language development—both receptive and expressive	Assesses progress in decoding, encoding, and using a language system effectively
Ask about increasing social skills, relations with family, age mates, and others	Assesses understanding of social systems and norms
4- to 5-year olds	
Ask general information questions	Assesses general fund of information, e.g., colors, numbering objects
Ask what makes the sun come up	Illustrates child's beliefs about causality
Ask about concepts of time	Assesses a relatively sophisticated concept that becomes more differentiated over time
Ask about spontaneous puppet or doll play, imaginative use of clay, or other toys	Assesses imagination and magical thinking
Ask child to draw a man	Fifty percent of 4-year-olds can draw a person composed of three parts. Most 5-year-olds can draw a person composed of eight parts
Ask about preschool involvement and behavior	Assesses language, social, and play development in relation to peers in a setting in which expectations are different from those at home

PSYCHOSOCIAL AND EMOTIONAL ASSESSMENT

Concepts

Psychosocial changes in toddlers and preschoolers are remarkable. Emotions and cognition are interconnected so that assessment of any one area of development is somewhat arbitrary (Sturner & Howard, 1997b). Toddlers no longer spend most of their time sleeping; rather they are up, running around, verbalizing, and demanding to join in family activities. These are years of intense learning about and managing feelings, such as love, happiness, anger, frustration, aggression, and jealousy. A major developmental milestone for this age is the achievement of a sense of independence and autonomy.

SOCIAL INTERACTION. Learning how to interpret and manage feelings is a challenge for both toddlers and their parents, as is indicated by the birthday greeting some parents wrote in their local newspaper: "Roses are red, violets are blue. Watch out world, Charleen is two!!!" Toddlers need a great deal of love, warmth, and comfort, primarily from their parents. They also need to learn to give love and find satisfaction in pleasing their parents or caregivers. It is fun to give kisses and hugs and cuddle with mommy and daddy, especially when they respond with their own kisses, hugs, and cuddling. On the other hand, toddlers who make these early attempts at love giving and are rejected or ignored soon stop trying and begin to find pleasure elsewhere. They may find that the earlier comforts of thumb sucking, rhythmical body movements, and body manipulation are more pleasurable and reliable than person-to-person contacts. Maternal depression has a significantly negative effect on the development of normal infant engagement behaviors that can persist into the toddler and preschool years (Murray & Cooper, 1997). This can lead to serious social problems later. Even at this young age, problems of sibling jealousy and possessiveness emerge. These are based on the child's emerging sense of self-identity (Sturner & Howard, 1997b).

Preschoolers develop a broader understanding of the nature of social interactions. They discover that love is not all taking but comes with certain obligations and responsibilities. They also develop ideas about giving and sharing. The 4- to 5-year-old moves away from the very self-centered attitude of earlier toddlerhood. Parents are viewed as the epitome of wisdom, power, integrity, and goodness. If earlier stages of the love relationship have not been satisfied, preschoolers can show more fears, inhibitions, explosive behavior, and demands for attention.

Dependence vs. independence is a very important struggle for toddlers and preschoolers. The road from depending on mother for everything to doing some things for oneself is rocky and uneven. On some days, toddlers cling to mother's skirt, not letting her out of sight; on others, children play for short periods in the next room, trotting back every so often to see, touch, and hear the mother and be reassured by her presence. Gradually, the periods of separation lengthen, with children needing only to hear the mother's voice or to check occasionally for security. Separation anxiety is frequent during these years and can be very traumatic for both parents and children. Preschool children are much less dependent on their parents and frequently can tolerate physical separation for several hours. Peer dependence begins to be important.

Preschool-age children respond more verbally than toddlers and are able to perform many more self-care tasks. Children's increasing ability to care for themselves—feed themselves, blow their own nose, go to the bathroom unassisted, and verbally express needs and feelings—makes interactions easier and more enjoyable for parents.

Sturner and Howard (1997b, p. 328) write

Behavior around others is comprised of the quality of relationships, social skills and emotional development, temperament, family discipline, biologically determined behavioral dispositions, and contextual stresses and supports. Controlling emotional states, including delayed gratification, and tolerating frustration, separations, and fears without breaking down emotionally, are lifelong tasks that should be mastered during the preschool period.

SIBLING INTERACTION. Young children need to learn to share their lives in a family with siblings if there are other children. Opposite gender, temperament, insecure attachment, family discord, corporal punishment, and perceptions of unequal treatment affect interaction patterns. Many toddlers or preschoolers regress when a new baby comes into the family. On the other hand, older children also experience excitement, love, and enhanced self-esteem when the new baby arrives (Sturner & Howard,

1997a). Parents need to limit aggression promptly, provide love and attention, and talk about feelings. This may be the time to teach taking turns using lots of positive reinforcement for prosocial behaviors. When older children fight, parents need to describe the situation and provide even-handed control. Trying to lay blame, except in clear-cut instances, is usually unproductive: The first punch was probably not the start of the disagreement. Promoting support, loyalty, and friendship are important goals for sibling interactions.

MORALITY. Morality, or the ability to know right from wrong, is still controlled externally during the toddler years, stemming from the child's love of the parents and a desire to please them. Parent teaching generally focuses more on helping the child to make safe decisions than moral ones. Toddlers left alone cannot be trusted, because their internal sense of conscience is rudimentary. They cannot be expected to make correct choices if left alone in potentially dangerous situations. Any room with electrical sockets, knobs for technical equipment, open windows, or hot food represents a risk. As toddlers learn some language, they begin to echo the parent's firm "no," but they really do not understand the full meaning of the term. By 24 months, many toddlers show beginning internalization by saying "no" to themselves and stopping the act or going ahead with the act as they talk to themselves.

For the 4- to 5-year-old, morality becomes more internally controlled. Instead of basing all decisions on the knowledge of the consequences of the act (e.g., "If I take a cookie, I will be sent to my room"), older children show an elementary understanding of what is right and wrong, fair or unfair. They begin to think ahead and are able to plan and control their urges, thus avoiding punishment. Four-year-olds can internalize some demands from their parents, and feelings of guilt can be elicited after some transgressions.

PEER RELATIONSHIPS. Preschoolers learn to interact with peers as their social world grows. Play becomes interactive, with shared pretend play activities. These activities are culturally influenced. Farver and Shin (1997) videotaped the play of Korean American and Anglo American 4- and 5-year-old children, looking for frequency of pretend play, communicative strategies, and pretend play themes. Although there were no differences in the frequency of pretend play, the Korean American children included everyday activity and family role themes, whereas the Anglo American children enacted more environmental danger and fantasy themes. As they played together, the Anglo American children described their own actions, rejected their playmates' suggestions, and used directives. In contrast, the Korean American children described their partner's actions, used tag questions at the end of statements such as "right?" or "ok?", semantic ties which expanded on the statement just made by the other child, statements of agreement and polite requests. Thus, the culture of children colors their developing social skills and pretend play in significant ways.

BODY IMAGE. Toddlers are often very concerned about body image. As children realize that they are separate persons, they begin to take notice of their own bodies. They may become fascinated with the different parts of the body and how they work. Bodily injury becomes a concern, and cuts and bruises elicit much discussion. Toward the end of the second year, children may notice the inner feelings of their body (e.g., the urge and tension to move the bowels, the release and relaxation resulting from going to the bathroom, the discomfort of hunger, and the pleasure of eating). These are very abstract feelings that toddlers cannot put into words but that can be shown with actions. Toddlers quickly learn the pleasure of control in these situations and show it when they say, "Yes, I will go to the bathroom," or "No, I won't!" Toddlers discover the delights of control over others and themselves. This increases their sense of power but can also lead to misunderstandings and hurt feelings if their parents do not read their moods properly.

During the preschool years, the sense of separateness increases, and children are more aware that they are different from their surroundings, their families, and their friends. They begin to realize that other persons also have feelings, fears, and doubts. They reexamine themselves, and worries over a lost tooth or a skinned knee are common. Curiosity about their bodies and those of others generates a wealth of innocent questions. They learn that

genital manipulation brings pleasure; masturbation peaks around 3 to 4 years of age.

FEARS. As the 2- to 3-year-old's world expands and the ability to fantasize develops, fears can appear about things that might happen. Early fears include fear of separation and fear of strangers, water, loud noises, and crowds. Reassurance with words and presence usually helps the child work through the anxiety and tension of the fear. Preschool children may still express fear of the dark or of harm to their bodies, but if the fears do not decrease with time, the child and family need referral for counseling. By age 4 years, children can identify nightmares as "not real," although they may still be afraid. Aggression at this age can be a response to guilt associated with misbehavior. Aggression may also be used to avoid perceived aggression from others. Primary caregivers are essential to help children learn appropriate emotional reactions and responses to new situations (Sturner & Howard, 1997b).

PSYCHOSOCIAL AND EMOTIONAL DEVELOPMENT ASSESSMENT STRATEGIES

Assessment of psychosocial and emotional development addresses children's roles in the family, success in making friends and working with peers, self-esteem, and feelings of contentment and security. As previously suggested, social development is related to cognitive development with capacities to "read" situations, interpret the roles and behaviors of others in relation to self, and develop self-control and self-monitoring skills.

The following list is used to assess behavior related to psychosocial and emotional development:

Questions Asked	*Purpose/Outcomes/ Goals of Questions*
Ask about child's reaction to strangers (1-year-old) and reactions to new vs. familiar situations	Evaluates child's ability to deal with increasingly complex social situations
Ask how child acts around family members	Assesses child's development of roles and behaviors within the family system; attachments should be evident

Ask what child does for play	Indicates social and emotional well-being
Ask how child acts around other children	Considers social development with age-mates and development of appropriate play
Ask about tantrum behavior	Evaluates responses to stress, development of independence and social control. Tantrums are common in 2-year-olds but infrequent by age 5 years
Ask about responses to discipline and limit-setting	Assesses understanding of limits of appropriate behavior, social rules, and self-control
Ask how parent changes behaviors without always saying no	Evaluates adaptability, creativity, repertoire of parent's skills in response to child's behaviors
Ask what things cause fear for the child and how parent manages the child's fears	Considers parents' responses to child's emotional stresses and understanding of child's views and feelings
Ask about friends' names and shared activities	Indicates child's developing social circle and opportunities for development of social skills with peers
Ask about imaginary friends and fantasy play	Allows child to explore emotions and roles in a safe way

LANGUAGE DEVELOPMENT

Concepts

Language uses symbols for thoughts; thus, it emerges with Piaget's preoperational stage of development. Beginning around 2 years of age, toddlers use words to convey their thoughts and feelings. Once the process begins, it develops rapidly. Cognitive development is a basic requirement for language development because the child must decipher the rules of language independently, problem-solve to understand the communication of others, and create symbols understood by others, which reflect his or her ideas and emotions. Bilingual children should be equally competent in both languages by age 3 years.

The development of language requires mastery of the following:

- Oral-motor ability to articulate sounds
- Auditory perception in distinguishing words and sentences
- Cognitive ability to understand syntax, semantics, and pragmatics
- Psychosocial-cultural environment to motivate the child to engage in language use

Language milestones are evident in two general categories: receptive and expressive language. These are presented for children younger than 5 years of age in Table 7-3.

Oral-motor development is a prerequisite for speech. Oral development progresses from sucking and rooting to rhythmical biting and chewing. Between 6 and 24 months, the child learns to chew by moving the jaw up and down while flattening and spreading the tongue, and to control biting by using rotary jaw movements with lateralization of tongue placement. The motor skills for production of speech are the most complex movements that the young child must master.

ARTICULATION. Articulation, or the way that the structures of the nose and mouth mold the sounds emitted by the larynx, begins at birth with the infant's first cry. Infants proceed through making sounds of comfort, discomfort, vowels, and consonants to babbling and using *phonemes* (single-sound units that may be vowels or consonants or blends such as "ch" and "bl") at about 4 to 8 months of age. The child produces a few *morphemes* (one-syllable units of speech that may be a simple word) by about 4 to 8 months of age. Vowels are the predominant sounds made during the first year. Articulation skills are practiced daily and, by 24 months of age, speech sounds are 25% intelligible to a stranger. The intelligibility rate jumps to about 66% between 24 and 36 months of age, with 90% intelligibility by age 3 years. By 4 years of age, speech should be completely intelligible with the exception of particularly difficult consonants; by 5 years, the tongue-contact sounds of n, t, d, k, g, y, and ng are more intelligible. The f sound is added during the fifth year. Figure 7-1 identifies sounds articulated by children at certain ages.

During the second year, the child practices playful changes in pitch and loudness. Three- and 4-year-olds can show normal hesitance in speech or stuttering. These dysfluencies should

T A B L E 7-3

Speech and Language Milestones: Areas for Assessment

AGE	RECEPTIVE LANGUAGE	EXPRESSIVE LANGUAGE
0–3 mo	Attends to voice, turns head or eyes Startles to loud sounds Quiets in response to voice Smiles, coos, gurgles to voice	Undifferentiated but strong cry Coos and gurgles Single-syllable repetition /G/, /K/, /H/, and /NG/ appear
3–6 mo	Actively seeks sound source May look in response to name Responses may vary to angry or happy voice	Increased babbling, vocal play Laughs Increased repetitive babbling (gaga) Vocalizes to toys Spontaneous smile to verbal play Increased intensity and nasal tone Vocalizes to removal of toy Experiments with own voice
6–9 mo	May look at family member when named Inhibits to "no" Begins interest in pictures when named Individual words begin to take on meaning	Babbles tunefully Increased sound combinations Uses /M/, /N/, /B/, /D/, /T/ Initiates sounds such as click or kiss Uses nonspecific "mama" and "dada"
9–12 mo	Will give toy on request Understands simple commands Turns head to own name Understands "hot," "where's . . .?" Responds with gestures to "bye-bye"	Increased imitating efforts Has one word with specific reference Accompanies vocalizations with gestures Jargon increases Imitates animal sounds

12–18 mo	Follows simple one-step commands
	Understands new words weekly
	Increased interest in named pictures
	Differentiates environmental sounds
	Points to familiar objects and body parts
	   when named
	Understands simple questions
	Begins to distinguish "you" from "me"
		All vowels, many consonants present
		Increased use of true words
		Jargon is sentence-like
		Shows "no" behavior
		Names a few pictures
		10+ words
		Can imitate nonspeech sounds (cough,
		   tongue click)

18–24 mo	Follows two-step commands Vocabulary increases rapidly Enjoys simple stories Recognizes pronouns	Names some body parts Imitates two-word combinations Dramatic increase in vocabulary Speech combines jargon and words Names self Answers some questions Begins to combine words

24–30 mo	Understands prepositions in and on
	Seems to understand most of what is said
	Understands more reasoning ("when you are
	   done, then . . .")
	Identifies object when given function (wear
	   on feet, cook on)
		Jargon reduced
		Two- to three-word sentences
		Repeats two digits
		Increased use of pronouns
		Asks simple questions
		Joins in songs and nursery rhymes

30–36 mo	Listens to adult conversations Understands preposition under Can categorize items by function Begins to recognize colors Begins to take turns Understands "big/little," "boy/girl"	Can repeat simple phrases and sentences Answers questions (wear on feet, to bed) Repeats three digits Uses regular plurals Can help tell simple story

T A B L E 7-3

Speech and Language Milestones: Areas for Assessment *Continued*

AGE	RECEPTIVE LANGUAGE	EXPRESSIVE LANGUAGE
36–42 mo	Understands fast Understands prepositions behind and in front Responds to simple three-part commands Increasing understanding of adjectives and plurals Understands "just one"	Understands and answers (cold, tired, hungry) Mostly three- to four-word sentences Gives full name Begins rote counting Begins to relate events Lots of questions, some beginning prepositions (on, in)
42–48 mo	Recognizes coins Begins to understand future and past tenses Understands number concepts—more than one	Uses prepositions Tells stories Can give function of objects Repeats larger than six-word sentences Repeats four digits Gives age Good intelligibility
48–60 mo	Responds to three-action commands	Asks "how" questions Answers verbally to questions like "How are you?" Uses past and future tenses Can use conjunctions to string words and phrases together

Data from D. Anderson, Ph.D., Speech Pathologist, Portland, OR, using items from a variety of developmental tests.

pass if ignored and are no longer expected in 5-year-olds.

Children usually progress through a regular sequence of mispronunciation as they learn new articulation sounds. At first, they simply omit the new sound and then they try to substitute a more familiar sound for the new sound (e.g., the "w" for "r" substitution, as in "wabbit" for "rabbit"). Distortion is followed by "addition" as the child adds an extra sound ("gulad" for "glad"). Knowing each of these steps allows the examiner to reassure the parent that the child is developing normally.

LEXICON. Lexicon refers to vocabulary. Size of vocabulary is influenced by many factors, including environment, stimulation, intelligence, bilingualism, and personality. Children usually understand more words than they are able to express, and addition of words to their expressive vocabulary comes with continued practice. Girls usually say their first word between 8 and 11 months, boys at about 14 months. Most 2-year-olds have more than 200 words in their vocabulary, and most 4- to 5-year-olds add approximately 50 words a month to their vocabulary. Five-year-olds should be able to define words with other words.

SYNTAX. Syntax, or grammar, refers to the structure of words in sentences or phrases. The ability to construct sentences that convey meaning is a complex skill, proceeding through several stages in children: receptive, holophrastic, and telegraphic speech. Much of this skill is developed between 8 months and 3½ years. By 8 months of age, children are developing receptive language by which they understand others who use a new word or structure before they are able to use it themselves. When asked "Where is the ball?" an 8-month-old searches for the ball. Between 12 and 18 months, children begin to use holophrases or single words to express whole ideas. The child says "milk" to mean the whole sentence, "Give me a glass of milk." A complex idea is expressed in one succinct word. Holophrasic sentences are denominative (labeling) or imperative (commanding).

Age level

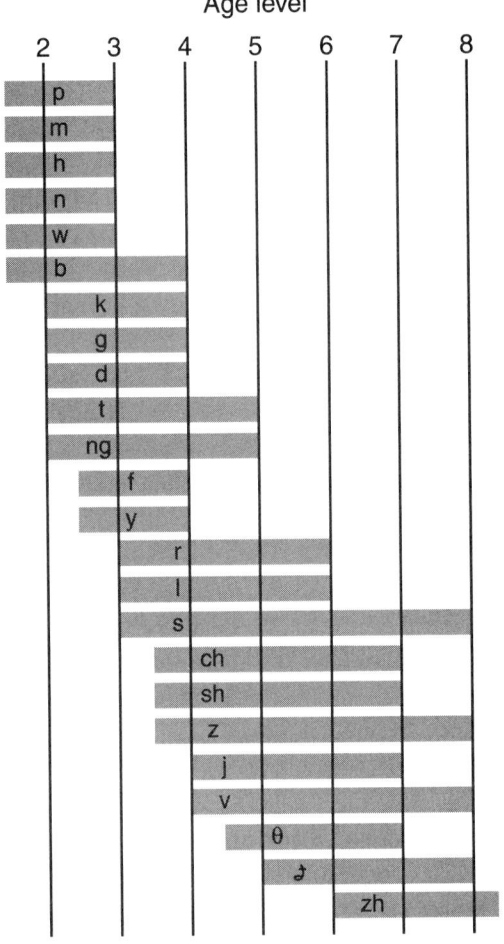

FIGURE 7-1
Norms for development of speech sounds. (From Van Riper C, Erickson RL: Speech Correction: An Introduction to Speech Pathology and Audiology, 9th ed, p 98. Needham Heights, MA, © 1996 by Allyn & Bacon. Reprinted by permission.)

Around 18 months of age, children begin using telegraphic speech, which is more complex and possesses two classes: pivot and open. The pivot class consists of a few frequently used words, and the open class contains newly learned words. Thus, the child may use the pivot word "daddy" with open-class words for "daddy eat," "daddy all gone," or "daddy sleep." From this stage, which lasts 2 to 3 months, the child further subdivides the pivot class into articles, demonstrative pronouns, and a second

pivot class. The second pivot class is subdivided into adjectives and possessives, and a third pivot class, and so on as the child developmentally progresses from simple to more complex language. Sentence structure also becomes more complex as children move from active sentences, questions, and passive and negative construction and add plurals (3 years of age) and past tenses (4 years of age) to their grammar. By 5 years of age, the child's syntax is close to adult style, including use of future tense and complete sentences of around 5 words' length.

SEMANTICS. Semantics, or the study of word meaning, is learned in stages from global to more specific. Words used in any language have both denotative (the specific, concrete referent of the word) and connotative (a broader range of feelings aroused by the word) meanings. Development of semantics is an ongoing process covering the years into young adulthood. Even though children may be quite adept at using words correctly, they may have only a vague, diffuse connotative understanding of these words (Ervin & Foster, 1960).

Bilingual Language Development

Bilingual preschoolers experience no delays in development of their vocabulary and are quite proficient in sorting one language from the other, although they may "code switch" to the other language for clarity as they talk. They switch languages depending upon whom they are speaking with and what the circumstances are. Some even translate for others, seeming to understand that not everyone speaks or understands both languages.

Simultaneous bilingualism occurs when children hear and learn two languages from infancy. Sequential bilingualism occurs when the child, usually 3 years of age or older, learns one language and then is immersed in another. Children learning sequentially may have more apparent differences in their skills from language to language until they have developed proficiency in both. Ultimately, whether learned simultaneously or sequentially, most children have one dominant language.

Parents may choose to raise their children bilingually or monolingually. Bilingualism may help preserve the family culture and heritage. Studies show that bilingual children have greater mental flexibility. They may also have enhanced employment and lifestyle opportunities. On the other hand, maintaining bilingualism requires time and effort as the child must learn to read and write and maintain fluency in both. For families anxious to integrate culturally in a place with a different language, emphasizing skill in the language of the new community may be viewed by the family as a first priority (Chiocca, 1998).

Language Development Assessment Strategies

Communication is a vital part of being a happy, functioning human being, and assessment of language is important during the early years of childhood. Assessment begins with screening of language, speech, and hearing and proceeds to diagnostic testing or referral as needed. It is important to remember that 80% of the essential information comes from a careful history, only 15% from a physical examination, and the remaining 5% from diagnostic testing.

Language screening is usually divided into expressive and receptive language skills. Because language and cognitive skills are intricately interwoven, most intelligence tests have language sections that can be useful in assessing the total child. Speech screening places emphasis on articulation and vocabulary. Both receptive and expressive areas must be included in assessing language (see Table 7-3).

The following list is used to assess behavior related to language development:

Questions Asked	Purpose/Outcomes/ Goals of Questions
Ask how child communicates wants	Assesses verbal and nonverbal strategies, vocabulary, expressive language
Ask what child understands	Evaluates cognitive level and receptive language
Ask whether child responds to simple commands	Evaluates receptive language
For 3-year-olds	
Ask about use of plurals, pronouns	Indicates increasing understanding of use of
Ask about sentence length	sounds and symbols in communication Three- to four-word sentences should be evident
Ask about intelligibility	Should be 75% intelligible to indicate speech maturation
For 4-year-olds	
Ask whether child follows two- or three-step commands	Evaluates short-term memory, auditory sequencing, and receptive language skills

▰▰▰ ANTICIPATORY GUIDANCE DURING THE TODDLER AND PRESCHOOL YEARS

1- to 3-Year-Olds

DEVELOPMENTAL STATUS

The toddler years are an exciting, albeit frequently frustrating, time for both children and parents. During the second year of life, children are growing more slowly, imitating adults more often, and becoming more skilled physically and socially. Their daily habits are governed by these developmental factors.

Nutrition and Feeding

Eating patterns reflect the toddler's needs and abilities. At approximately 12 months of age, there can be a drastic reduction in intake as growth slows, appetite declines, and the child becomes easily distracted and more interested in gross movement (walking and moving) than in sitting and eating. If the child has not been weaned from the breast or bottle, this will probably happen between 12 and 24 months of age, although there is wide variation. Most 18-month-old children eat the same foods as those around them, but finger foods are appealing and stimulating; they use utensils irregularly. Many 2-year-olds also have special preferences for foods and refuse or request the same foods day after day.

Elimination Behavior

Toilet training is a developmental task of the toddler and is discussed in Chapter 14. The toddler should be learning the concepts of toileting behavior long before actual training begins. If the principles of growth and development are applied, the child is generally ready for toilet training between 2½ and 3½ years of age, with a wide range of normal.

Rhythmicity and Sleep/Wake Behavior

Ritual activity in all areas of life seems to peak in the second year. Most toddlers have bedtime habits and rituals. There is a certain amount of washing, bathing, teeth brushing, hair combing, bedtime stories, and glasses of water required every night. Most children have a special place to sleep that may be referred to as "my bed" or "my room." Beds are often important to children because they are a personal territory and seem to give them the feeling of being safe and secure. Culturally, this may be one bed or the family bed. Children frequently need their special blanket or a toy in bed with them. They often have a favored sleep position and assume it on falling asleep. Most children sleep in the dark. By 12 months of age, many children sleep 8 to 15 hours per day, with 20 to 30% rapid eye movement (REM) sleep, and the majority of 2-year-olds sleep through the night. Toddlers are often resistant at bedtime. They also can experience nightmares, waking after 1 to 2 hours of sleep. Although very frightened, they can usually talk about the dream and can be easily calmed, reassured, and helped back to sleep. Bruxism (teeth grinding) occurs during non-REM sleep in approximately 15% of the population. If bruxism persists over a long period of time, the teeth have a blunt, sawed-off appearance. The child's dentist should be alerted and asked to check for temporomandibular tension. Bedwetting is common in toddlers who are out of diapers and should not be considered enuresis or treated with anything but time and patience.

Activities

Play is an important activity for toddlers. They are active, exploring individuals with rapidly changing interests. Play activities should provide toddlers an opportunity to practice their developing physical, social, and emotional skills. Parallel play is the norm.

Emotions

The emotional development of toddlers is an area in which parents may need a great deal of anticipatory guidance. The balance between dependence and independence is constantly in flux for toddlers and their parents, and conflict can develop as a result of inconsistent and extreme behavior. Children at this age vacillate between being a big boy or big girl and mommy's baby. They take great pride in doing as many things as possible for themselves, yet they need to feel totally secure in their parent's care. Toddlers like to have a choice in matters and quickly learn the power of the word no. They can become very negative, practicing the power of no every day for months. As toddlers practice making choices, they are clumsy, awkward, and frequently wrong. This can be very frustrating for them, and their outraged responses can be equally frustrating for their parents. With time, they become more skilled, make better choices, have more successes, and feel more powerful. They no longer have to work so hard to show others their power, and the negative stage passes.

"Having a toddler is a humbling experience" (Shelov, 1998). Discipline and limit setting are frequently discussed during the toddler years because parents find themselves changing limits as the child grows. Homan (1969) stated that discipline is necessary for survival in society, and if the child has "not learned life's requirements at an early stage, he will be taught them later, not by those whose love tempers the lesson with tenderness but by strangers who couldn't care less about the harm they may do to you." While children have to learn internal controls, the toddler years require more external control—as applied to a child by a parent.

The American Academy of Pediatrics (1998) recommends that effective discipline should include three essential components:

- A positive, supportive, loving relationship between parent and child
- Use of positive reinforcement strategies to increase desired behaviors

- Removing reinforcement or applying punishment to reduce or eliminate undesired behaviors

Discipline should be approached in the broadest sense of helping the child learn rules, regulations, and goals of living in a world with others, not just setting limits and punishing for wrongdoing. The learning process is easily seen in toddlers as they master the word no. First, they approach the forbidden object while watching their mother. The mother says no and removes the toddler. Then the toddler moves toward the object again, says "no," and leaves it alone. This process happens many times as toddlers learn to set limits for themselves. Early discipline is passive, gradually structuring the infant's life around the family routines. Later, families must begin setting some limitations on behavior, for safety reasons as much as anything else. As toddlers become preschoolers, they need to develop understanding about rules and socially acceptable behavior. Increasing responsibility for self-control is given to the child over the years.

Time-out is an effective approach to discipline, removing positive reinforcement for unacceptable behavior. It generally increases compliance from 25 to 80%. However, for success, it requires effort and practice by parents. At first, time-out increases negative behavior as the child tests new limits. Verbal or physical interaction with the child during time-out tends to negate its effects because attention is given to the child's disruptive behavior. Time-out needs to be short so that the child understands that good things lie ahead for better behavior. The child must also see that parents are, above all, good and not vindictive people. Verbal reprimands can be useful if used infrequently and targeted only toward specific undesirable behavior. Corporal punishment, generally spanking, increases the chances for physical injury in children less than 18 months of age. It also models aggressive behavior as a solution to conflict. Finally, it leads to altered parent–child relationships that make other forms of discipline more difficult, especially when the child becomes too old for spanking. Spanking is no more effective than other forms of discipline. Because spanking may provide the angry parent with some relief, it is likely to be a sustained

behavior (American Academy of Pediatrics, 1998). Discipline must be developmentally appropriate. Therefore, it should come up repeatedly as a developmental topic for discussion.

Coping and Tantrums

Negative feelings play a large part in the lives of children during the toddler years. Being a 2-year-old is frequently frustrating, often leading to anger and aggression. Temper tantrums can make their ugly appearance during this time. Tantrums usually consist of mounting frustration, crying, kicking, screaming, and turning red or blue in the face. About 5% of children hold their breath until they pass out (Sturner & Howard, 1997b). Basically, temper tantrums stem from the child's striving for power and control and the sudden loss of both. There are so many activities that toddlers want and struggle to do but are not developmentally ready to perform. There is no best way to deal with tantrums, and parents' responses usually depend on their comfort level. The goal is to restore the child's control and calm. This is not necessarily achieved by giving the child what he or she wanted in the first place. Some parents feel it is best to go to the children, hold them, comfort them, and offer some substitute. Others feel that children should be removed from the stimulation of the situation and placed alone in their rooms or on a chair until they can gain their own control. Still others feel that children need to be physically restrained in a bear hug until crying and thrashing-about behavior stops. In any case, parents need a plan to manage the tantrum while teaching the child that there are better ways to handle frustration. Expecting time-out quiet behavior for less than a minute's duration has been shown to be an effective strategy for many children.

Communication

Toddlers develop both verbal and nonverbal communication skills. Articulation, pitch, and loudness are practiced continually. Vocabulary builds and grammar becomes more complex. As with any learning situation, miscommunication can easily occur, and parents and children frequently spend time figuring out what each is trying to say and mean. While toddlers' speech increases daily, they also use gestures, touch, and postures to let the world know what they want. Touch continues to be important in forming early social attachments (Barnard & Brazelton, 1990) and should be encouraged between parents and children.

Developmentally, the second and third years are full of learning, growing, and excitement. The need for constant vigilance, supervision, and patience places special demands on parents (Gross & Tucker, 1994; Olson, 1994). Despite the demands, these are years of tremendous growth in language, movement, and thinking, and they set the stage for preschool development.

ANTICIPATORY GUIDANCE AND DEVELOPMENTAL INTERVENTIONS

Feeding and Self-Care
- Let child make food choices among healthy options.
- Anticipate slower weight gain with resulting decreased appetite.
- Offer finger foods that can be eaten on the run or in short periods of sitting to make mealtimes more pleasant for all.
- Share family meals whenever possible.
- Avoid making meals a power struggle.
- Food jags should be ignored or minimized.
- Encourage self-feeding to help child with mastery of environment and improving fine motor skills.
- Anticipate interest in genital differences, especially at around 3 years of age.
- Promote toilet training as readiness emerges.
- Promote hygienic habits, including hand washing and tooth brushing.
- Promote physical activities in safe places.
- Insist on use of a car seat.

Rhythmicity and Sleep/Wake Patterns
- Maintain nighttime rituals and bedtime.
- Provide opportunities for control at bedtime—choice of pajamas, story, toy to sleep with.

Strength and Motor Coordination and Safety
- Big muscles can be exercised with push-pull toys like a wagon.
- Balls can be fun and teach cooperative play.
- Sing and dance to music.
- Secure doors and windows.
- Remove toxic substances and dangerous objects.
- Supervise play constantly.
- Provide outdoor play opportunities in safe areas whenever weather allows.
- Provide opportunities for 2- and 3-year-olds to hold and manipulate pencils, crayons, utensils, and other small objects such as Legos and blocks.

Emotional Growth Fostering
- Teach child to manage anger and resolve conflicts and violence.
- Help child identify, name, and express feelings—both positive and negative.
- Show affection in family.
- Praise good behavior and accomplishments.
- Let child make choices wherever possible but do not offer choices when there are none.
- Avoid power struggles by sidestepping potential conflicts.
- Ignore tantrums but use time-out immediately for kicking or biting.
- Expect behavior within limits but know that the child is only just learning those limits; limits should be clearly set and consistent.
- Provide opportunities to play with other children.
- Provide transitional objects at around 2 years of age (e.g., blanket, toy).
- Consider providing a night light unless shadows increase fears.
- Provide reassurance if nightmares or fears occur.
- Avoid spanking, slapping, or yelling because these all do more harm than good in promoting desired behaviors.

Cognitive, Language, and Environmental Stimulation
- Read to child daily, but stories must be short, or simply describe and name pictures
- Limit television to between 1 and 2 hours per day or less; watch programs actively with child.

- Model appropriate language.
- Show interest in child's activities.
- Allow child to explore; guide child into new experiences that are fun.
- Point out events and things the child should attend to in the environment.
- Provide clear, simple explanations of what is happening around the child.
- Listen with care and respond actively to the child's verbalizations.

Preschool Children (4- and 5-Year-Olds)

DEVELOPMENTAL STATUS

During the preschool years, children have increasing verbal and social skills; they become less self-centered and more aware of the responsibilities of being a part of the family and group, sharing, contributing, and knowing right from wrong. This is often a time when conflict and worries decrease and family life is relatively calm.

Nutrition and Feeding

Daily habits reflect the child's growth and development. Eating patterns can be distinctive in preschoolers. Some children express specific likes and dislikes, engage in food fads and eat only one particular food, display erratic appetites and poor evening eating patterns, or dawdle over their food. Common dislikes are cooked vegetables, liver, and mixed dishes. Most preschool children are poor chewers and refuse some of the tougher meats. By the time children are 5 years old, their eating habits approximate those of their family.

Elimination

Independent toileting with few accidents is usually accomplished by 4 or 5 years of age, but children occasionally still wet the bed. Three-year-olds might resist using strange bathrooms, especially in large public areas, but by 4 years of age, children are more curious than frightened of new facilities. They continue to need some supervision of hygiene and hand washing.

Rhythmicity and Sleep/Wake Patterns

Sleep patterns are usually fixed by 4 to 5 years of age. Some 4-year-olds continue to need a short afternoon nap. Somnambulism (sleepwalking) may appear around 4 years of age and is usually seen more in boys than girls. Sleepwalking occurs during the non-REM stages of sleep, and the child can be at risk for injury. Night terrors may occur in the late preschool years. These issues are discussed in Chapter 16. Nocturnal erections occur in about 80% of boys during REM sleep.

Activities

Play for 4- to 5-year-olds is social, cooperative, and shared, with use of more symbolic language. Imaginary play leads to "let's pretend," role playing, and creation of imaginary friends. Fantasy and make-believe are very important during these years. Myths or fables can become important ways of teaching children abstract concepts of love, sharing, and giving. The Christmas holiday, for example, provides opportunities for the preschool child to learn about abstract feelings through concrete activities. Giving is a very abstract concept, but the child sees how a jolly man in a red suit gives gifts to children simply for being "good." Because children are still thinking transductively, from particular to particular, they do not connect one jolly man with another jolly man, nor do they have problems with the logistics of how he gets down the chimney or to all the homes of children around the world in one night. Parents can involve the child as they wrap and give gifts to others, discussing the pleasure they get from making others happy. By 5 to 6 years of age, thinking advances to more abstract terms and the child can be guided into the joy and love of giving.

Shared or cooperative play makes simple games of hide-and-seek and tag possible. Games with complicated rules can be frustrating to the preschooler, who prefers simple table games with the option of making up the rules as the game proceeds. Cheating in order to win is common, because the boundaries of acceptable play are not yet clear and the earliest stages of moral behavior are only beginning to emerge.

Emotions

Emotionally, preschool children continue to expand their sense of control over the world and become increasingly independent from parents. Security objects, such as a thumb, blanket, favorite toy, or even the parent's hand to hold may be helpful to the child. Social interaction with other children and adults, such as in day care and preschool centers, can stimulate and foster learning and allow children to form important attachments to persons outside the immediate family. Emotional development of preschool children can be fostered by parent's interactions. Children are learning to express simple concepts such as feelings of being happy, angry, hungry, tired, sad, and joyful. They learn the words that go with those feelings and, with guidance, the appropriate behaviors. Parents are the child's most important role models at this stage.

Cognitive

Cognitively, the 4- to 5-year-old continues to show concrete and magical thinking but with beginning threads of symbolic and more abstract patterns. Parents need to be ready to explain things over and over patiently, without expecting the child to understand the adult's interpretation clearly. "Why?" may be the most common question of 3- and 4-year-olds. Parents should avoid putting their own meaning on the child's behavior or statements. For example, the child's statement, "What if you just bought a new house, and I was allergic to something in the house? I guess you'd have to get rid of me," should not be interpreted to mean the parents have somehow failed to show the child how much they love him or her. Rather, the child can be exploring the concepts of place, ownership, belonging, size, or importance. In the child's mind, a house is much bigger than he or she is and may be more important. An appropriate response from the parent might be, "No, we'd probably have to get a new house or take out whatever you are allergic to. Even if we just bought it, you are more important than any house, and we wouldn't want to get rid of you!"

Communication

Children's language becomes more complex as they begin to use prepositions, understand past tense, and identify colors, letters, and numbers. Cognitively, children also begin to associate meaning with these concepts (e.g., letters can be used to make words, numbers can be put together, shapes and sizes can be labeled with names and numbers). This development allows for more sophisticated interaction between children and their parents. Children learn to sit to listen to a story, and parents can incorporate a story into the bedtime ritual. Learning letters of the alphabet and numbers and playing a game in which children go on, under, behind, between, or around are activities parents and children can share. These tasks show a readiness for the upcoming, more formalized learning within the school structure.

Whining can become a problem as the child learns to use words to express demands. The chronic whiner is the child who is physically well but engages the parent in a cycle of repeated requests ("Why can't I?", "There is nothing to do!", "Are we almost there?") that ends with both parent and child frustrated and angry. Parents can help to break the cycle with a friendly, firm manner, giving clear, explicit directions and follow-up (Spock & Parker, 1998).

ANTICIPATORY GUIDANCE AND DEVELOPMENTAL INTERVENTIONS

Feeding and Self-Care
- Promote hygienic habits.
- Do not worry about enuresis until after the child is 6 years of age.
- Encourage self-dressing and grooming by child.
- Maintain twice-daily, supervised teeth brushing.

Rhythmicity and Sleep/Wake Patterns
- Provide three meals and two nutritious snacks per day.
- Allow child to make choices among healthy food options.
- Maintain family mealtimes that are pleasant and interactive.
- Deal supportively with child's responses to dreams.
- Keep nighttimes regular; do not force nap times.

Strength and Motor Coordination

- Promote social and motor development through peer play and physical activities in safe places.
- Provide opportunities for drawing, painting, cutting, pasting, and other creative activities that develop fine motor skills.

Emotional Growth Fostering

- Encourage child to try new roles because fantasy play serves emotional development.
- Respond to fears that are common for toddlers and preschoolers.
- Discipline with limit-setting and clear rules for behavior.
- Recognize good behavior.
- Do not respond to aggressive behavior with aggression.
- Provide child with a feeling of safety to deal with fears.
- Support use of security objects as needed by child.
- Provide opportunities to play with other children.
- Help the child develop friendships.
- Explain about no one touching child's private parts without permission.
- Discuss sexual differences.

Cognitive, Language, and Environmental Stimulation

- Talk with child to help develop vocabulary and understanding of the world.
- Read to child to support language development.
- Limit television to 1 to 2 hours or less per day of appropriate programs.
- Discuss television programs to help child distinguish fantasy from reality.
- Provide toys that child can use creatively.
- Discuss differences among people openly and positively.
- Enlarge child's experiences through trips to many places of interest in the community.
- Encourage story telling and singing.

COMMON DEVELOPMENTAL ISSUES OF TODDLERS AND PRESCHOOLERS

Although a wide range of normal may be seen when assessing children, the NP needs to be alert to developmental red flags, signs of delayed or abnormal development. In addition to obvious abnormalities, minor problems that are left untreated can develop into major concerns; minor signs and symptoms that persist can indicate a more serious underlying problem; or a major problem can occur as a one-time event (e.g., child who sets a fire). Some children and families are at high risk and need careful monitoring and guidance to detect problems at an early stage or to prevent their occurrence (e.g., very early premature infants, families with history of potential violence, families with chronic medical or mental health problems, some single-parent families). The warning signs or red flags can be found in all of the developmental categories previously outlined (Table 7–4).

General Management of Developmental Issues

Anticipatory guidance provides parents with a direction for managing normal development. If the child has a developmental problem, more specialized care may be needed. Successful outcomes are clearly associated with early intervention.

Several key elements of appropriate, family-centered, early intervention have been identified by Donahue-Kolburg (1992). First, there must be parent and professional collaboration for assessment, management, and follow-up of any child and family. The family must be recognized as the pivotal constant in the child's life and the major source of care. Diversity in family strengths, values, and racial, ethnic, cultural, and socioeconomic characteristics must be respected and incorporated into care. Second, information and support should be shared with families continually and completely. Health care offered should be "flexible, culturally competent, and responsive to family-identified needs" (Donahue-Kolburg, 1992).

Prevention of developmental delays should be a primary effort of NPs working with families and children. Preventive programs include the following:

- Available, high-quality prenatal care
- Safe birthing options
- Immunization programs

TABLE 7-4

Red Flags of Development: Toddlers and Preschoolers

AGE	GROWTH/ RHYTHMICITY/ SLEEP/ TEMPERAMENT	PSYCHOSOCIAL/ EMOTIONAL SKILLS	COGNITIVE AND VISUAL ABILITIES	LANGUAGE AND HEARING	FINE MOTOR/ FEEDING/SELF-CARE	GROSS MOTOR/ STRENGTH/ COORDINATION
15 mo	No nighttime ritual Difficulty with transitions Parents express concern about temperament or control issues	Problems with attachment to caregiver	Lack of object permanence	Lack of consonant production Does not imitate words No gestures/pointing	No self-feeding	No attempts at walking
18 mo	Poor sleep schedule Problems with control/behavior	Doesn't pull person to show something	Primary play: mouthing of toys No finger exploration of objects Lack of imitation	Unable to follow simple directions (e.g., "no," "jump")	Does not try to scribble spontaneously Unable to use spoon	Not yet walking or frequently falls when walking
24 mo (2 yr)	Less than 4 times birth weight or falling off growth curve Poor sleep schedule Awakens at night; unable to put self back to sleep	Absent symbolic play No evidence of parallel play Displays destructive behaviors Always clings to mother	Unable to dump pellet from bottle	Use of noncommunicative speech (echolalia, rote phrases) Unable to identify five pictures Unable to name body parts No jargon History of >10 episodes of otitis media	Unable to stack four to five blocks Still eating pureed foods Unable to imitate scribbles on paper	Unable to walk downstairs holding a rail Persistent waddle walk Persistent toe-walking
30 mo	Resistance to regular bedtime Beginning behavior issues	Problems with biting, hitting playmates, parents	Doesn't try to get toy with stick	No two-word sentences Unable to name some body parts	Unable to feed self Unable to tower six blocks Unable to imitate circle shape Unable to imitate vertical stroke	Unable to jump in place Unable to kick ball on request

136

Age						
36 mo (3 yr)	Problems with toilet training Unable to calm self	Not able to dress self Doesn't understand taking turns		Unable to give full name Unable to match two colors Does not use plurals Does not know two to three prepositions Unable to tell a story Unclear consonants Unintelligible speech Unable to construct a sentence	Unable to build a tower of 10 blocks Holds crayon with fist Unable to draw circle	Unable to balance on one foot for 1 sec Toeing in causes tripping with running
48 mo (4 yr)	Lack of bedtime ritual Behavior concerns: withdrawn or acting out Stool holding Problems with toilet training	Unable to play games, follow rules Unable to follow limits/rules at home (e.g., put toys away) Cruelty to animals, friends Interest in fires, fire starting Persistent fears or severe shyness Inability to separate from mother	Unable to count three objects Unable to recall four numbers Unable to identify what to do in danger, fire, with a stranger Consistently poor judgment	Difficulty understanding language Problems understanding prepositions Limited vocabulary Unclear speech	Lack of self-care skills—dressing, feeding Unable to button clothes Unable to copy square	Unable to balance on one foot for 4 sec Unable to alternate steps when climbing stairs
60 mo (5 yr)	Continued sleep problems Concerns with night terrors Hair pulling—scalp or eyelashes	Difficulty making and keeping friends; no friends Difficulty understanding sharing, school rules, organization of daily activities Cruelty to animals, friends Interest in fires, fire starting Bullying or being bullied Prolonged fighting, hitting, hurting Withdrawal, sadness, extreme rituals	Unable to count to 10 Unable to identify colors Difficulty following three-step command	Speech pattern not 100% understandable Cannot identify a penny, nickel, or dime	Unable to copy triangle Unable to draw a person with a body	Difficulty hopping, jumping

- Family support programs
- Early intervention programs

Prevention is not always possible, and intervention focuses on attempts to arrest the problem or reduce the impact of the problem on the child's function.

Language and Speech Disorders

DESCRIPTION

The incidence of communication problems in toddlers and preschoolers is based on problems that are severe enough to require help. Those estimates range from 2 to 20%, depending on the study.

Language Disorders

Language delays or disorders are problems in learning systems of communication. Expressive and receptive language skills are the skills assessed. The inability to use the symbols of language may be characterized by the following:

- Improper use of words and their meanings
- Inappropriate grammatical patterns
- Improper use of speech sound

Language delays are caused by cognitive, familial, environmental, or cultural factors. Children with language delays have delays in receptive and expressive language. They can start saying words late, talk very little as toddlers, and have prolonged stages of normal stuttering, distortion, and substitution. Because language development is the best indicator of cognitive development, language delays can reflect serious issues needing developmental and educational help. Language delays or disorders also may occur if the child does not hear, speaks another language, is not immersed in a language-rich environment, or has a psychological disorder such as severe deprivation or autism. As a result, language evaluation must involve assessment of the total child—physically, cognitively, socially, emotionally, and perceptually.

Speech Disorders

Speech disorders involve difficulties producing correct speech sounds. Difficulties may be characterized by difficulty in

- Producing speech sounds (articulation)
- Maintaining speech rhythm (fluent speech)
- Controlling vocal production (voice)

Speech disorders are often associated with physical problems (cleft lip, cleft palate, cerebral palsy, hearing impairment), cognitive development (global developmental delays), or psychological disorders (severe deprivation, autism), or they can be idiopathic.

CLINICAL FINDINGS

History

A detailed history is essential, including

- Prenatal—especially use of ototoxic drugs and maternal illnesses
- Perinatal—toxemia, prematurity, premature membrane rupture, anoxia
- Neonatal—birth weight, jaundice, sepsis, anoxia or hypoxia, hypothyroidism, trauma
- Postnatal—accidents involving trauma to mouth, neck, head; recurrent otitis media; central nervous system infection; operations, hospitalizations; seizures; syndromes
- History of feeding difficulties—suck, swallow, chew
- Family history of other members with delays, cleft lip or palate, hearing loss, speech/language/reading problems
- Family structure and dynamics; family crises
- Language or languages spoken to child
- Description of child's language development, especially changes
- Developmental milestones—gross motor, fine motor, social, language

Physical Examination

Children with speech disorders may be seen with a range of clinical findings. Some children have no physical abnormalities; others have significant structural problems. Evaluation should include

- Ear, nose, throat—deformities of auricle, external ear canal, tympanic membrane, anomalies of first and second branchial structures of pharynx and neck

- Mouth—symmetry of structure, hard and soft palates, tongue size and control, lip and tongue movements while vocalizing, infant suck, chewing
- Dental—alignment
- General physical examination with focus on neurological, especially cranial nerve XII (tongue function)

Developmental Evaluation

Broad developmental assessment is important because problems with speech or language may be related to larger problems. Assessment includes the following:

- General developmental evaluation—Denver II or other
- Age profile of receptive and expressive language—Receptive and Expressive Emergent Language (REEL), ELM, Clinical Linguistic and Auditory Milestone test (CLAMS/CAT), Fluharty, or other language evaluation instrument (Table 7–5).

Ancillary Studies

Assessment of the child's hearing through audiometry may reveal hearing loss as the source of speech problems.

MANAGEMENT

Management of speech and language disorders depends on the identified cause, but management must be comprehensive, not focused solely on the speech or language problem, and must actively involve the family. Referral for specialty care may be necessary, including otolaryngology, speech pathology, audiology, neurology, or pediatric dentistry or orthodontistry.

Language Disorders

Discussing normal language development with parents and giving suggestions on how to encourage children to progress to the next stage of language may help mild delays. A referral is needed if:

- The child is not talking by age 2 years
- The child is not making sentences by age 3 years

- There is excessive, indiscriminate, irrelevant verbalizing after age 18 months
- Sentence structure is consistently faulty after age 5 years
- There are unusual confusions, reversals, or telescoping in connected speech
- There is a loss of previously acquired language skills

Speech Disorders

A referral is needed if

- Speech is largely unintelligible after age 3 years
- There are many omissions of initial consonants after age 3 years
- There is consistent and frequent omission of initial consonants, which are generally mastered very early
- There are many substitutions of easy sounds for difficult ones after age 5 years
- The child uses mostly vowel sounds in his or her speech at any age after 1 year
- Word endings are consistently dropped after age 5 years
- The child is distorting, omitting, or substituting sounds after age 7 years

STUTTERING. A referral is needed if:

- There is abnormal rate or rhythm of speech after age 4.5 years
- The child reacts to own speech by embarrassment or withdrawal at any age (see Box 7–1 for resources)

VOICING DISORDERS. A referral is needed if:

- The child's voice is monotone, extremely loud, largely inaudible, or of poor quality
- Pitch is not appropriate to the child's age and gender
- Hypernasality or lack of nasal resonance occurs

SUMMARY

Child development has been compared to a rose stem: an elegant spiral with smooth parts and thorns, the positive with the negative, the stressful with the placid. Monitoring children over time, both parents and providers learn that

T A B L E 7-5

Speech and Language Evaluation Tools

EVALUATION TOOL	TEST CHARACTERISTICS AND AGE ASSESSED	SOURCE
Clinical Linguistic and Auditory Milestone test (CLAMS/CAT)	0–36 mo Interview and some observation (Capute et al, 1986) Tests language and problem-solving skills to help clearly identify between the two	Arnold J. Capute Assoc. Professor of Pediatrics Johns Hopkins University School of Medicine JH Medical Institutions E Balt Kennedy-Krieger Institute Baltimore, MD 21203 (410) 502-9423 e-mail: capute@kennedykrieger.org
Denver Articulation Screening Examination (DASE)	3–6 yr Screens articulation only (not a complete assessment)	Denver Developmental Materials, Inc. P.O. Box 371075 Denver, CO 80237-5075 (800) 419-4729
Fluharty Preschool Speech and Language Screening Test	2–6 yr Direct testing Vocabulary, articulation, comprehension, repetition (expressive) (Fluharty, 1974)	Riverside Publishing Co. 8420 Bryn Mawr Ave. Chicago, IL 60631 (800) 323-9540
Early Language Milestone Scale (ELM)	0–36 mo Tests visual and auditory receptive, auditory expressive History, testing, observation 3–5 min (Coplan et al, 1982)	Pro-Ed 8700 Shoal Creek Blvd. Austin, TX 78757-6897 (800) 897-3202 (502) 451-3246 Website: www.proedinc.com
REEL—Receptive and Expressive Emergent Language	0–36 mo Interview or direct observation of expressive and receptive language	Riverside Publishing Co. 8420 Bryn Mawr Ave. Chicago, IL 60631 (800) 323-9540

children have ups and downs as they develop. The "terrible twos" are followed by the "terrific threes," the "fierce fours," and by the "fantastic fives." Normal growth and development changes happen with the parent's presence and guidance. Deviations, delays, and voids need to be assessed, monitored, and managed to foster optimal growth and achieve the goal of a functional, happy, productive adult. Participating in the process of their children's growth can be one of a parent's treasures. Having the support of an NP can make it easier.

BOX 7-1

RESOURCES FOR SPEECH AND LANGUAGE PROBLEMS

National Center for Stuttering
Website: www.stuttering.com
Informational materials (including Spanish), referrals to local resources, local chapters

Stuttering Foundation of America
(800) 992-9392
(901) 452-7343
Website: www.stutteringfa.org
Informational materials (including Spanish), referrals to local resources

REFERENCES

American Academy of Pediatrics, Committee on Practice and Ambulatory Medicine: Recommendations for preventive pediatric health care. Pediatrics 96:833, 1995.

American Academy of Pediatrics, Committee on Psychosocial Aspects of Child and Family Health: Guidance for effective discipline. Pediatrics 101:723-728, 1998.

Barnard K, Brazelton T (eds): Touch: The Foundation of Experience. Madison, CT, International Universities Press, 1990.

Capute A, Shipiro B, Wachtel R, et al: The clinical linguistic and auditory milestone scale (CLAMS). Am J Dis Child 140:694-698, 1986.

Chiocca E: Language development in bilingual children. Pediatr Nursing 24:43-47, 1998.

Colson E, Dworkin P: Toddler development. Pediatr Rev 18:255-259, 1997.

Coplan J, Gleason J, Ryan R, et al: Validation of an early language milestone scale in a high risk population. Pediatrics 70:677-683, 1982.

Dixon S, Stein M: Encounters With Children: Pediatric Behavior and Development. St. Louis, Mosby–Year Book, 1992.

Donahue-Kolburg G (ed): Family-Centered Early Intervention for Communication Disorders: Prevention and Treatment. Gaithersburg, MD, Aspen Publishers, 1992.

Eisenberg A, Murkoff H, Hathaway S: What to Expect in the Toddler Years. New York, Workman Publishing, 1996.

Engle P, Castle S, Menon P: Child development: Vulnerability and resilience. Soc Sci Med 43:621-635, 1996.

Ervin S, Foster G: The development of meaning in children's descriptive terms. J Abnorm Soc Psych 61:271-275, 1960.

Essa E: A Practical Guide to Solving Preschool Behavior Problems, 3rd ed. Boston, Delmar Publishers, 1995.

Farver J, Shin Y: Social pretend play in Korean- and Anglo-American preschoolers. Child Dev 68:544-556, 1997.

Fluharty N: The design and standardization of a speech and language screening test for use with preschool children. J Speech Hearing Dis 39:75-88, 1974.

Green M: Bright Futures: Guidelines for Health Supervision of Infants, Children, and Adolescents. Arlington, VA, National Center for Education in Maternal and Child Health, 1994.

Gross D, Tucker S: Parenting confidence during toddlerhood. Nurse Practitioner 19:25-34, 1994.

Homan W: Child Sense. New York, Basic Books, 1969.

Murray L, Cooper P: Postpartum depression and child development. Psychol Med 27:253-260, 1997.

Olson A: Depressive symptoms and work role satisfaction in mothers of toddlers. Pediatrics 94:363-368, 1994.

Palfrey J, Singer J, Walker D, et al: Early identification of children's special needs: A study of five metropolitan communities. J Pediatr 3:651-658, 1987.

Shelov S: Caring for Your Baby and Young Child. New York, Bantam, 1998.

Spock B, Parker S: Dr. Spock's Baby and Child Care. New York, Pocket Books, 1995.

Stein M: Preparing families for the toddler and preschool years. Contemp Pediatr 15:88-110, 1998.

Sturner R, Howard B: Preschool development I: Communicative and motor aspects. Pediatr Rev 18:327-336, 1997a.

Sturner R, Howard B: Preschool development II: Psychosocial/behavioral development. Pediatr Rev 18:291-301, 1997b.

Tschann J, Kaiser P, Chesney M, et al: Resilience and vulnerability among preschool children: Family functioning, temperament, and behavior problems. J Am Acad Child Adolesc Psychiatr 35:184-192, 1996.

Vaughn V: Child and Adolescent Development. Philadelphia, WB Saunders, 1990.

CHAPTER 8

Developmental Management of School-Age Children

Catherine Burns

▰▰▰ INTRODUCTION

Middle childhood is defined as ages 6 to 12 years. Developmentally, it begins with the ability of children to separate from home and family as they enter school and ends when they take on the tasks of adolescence. The transition to school both tests children's developmental achievements and provides the impetus for further development. Goals of school-age children's development include laying the groundwork for achievement, creating a sense of self-worth, developing the ability to contribute to the group, and, ultimately, gaining satisfaction with life.

Each child is unique and patterns of "normal" development have broad parameters. Nurse practitioners (NPs) must be familiar with the theoretical models of psychosocial development as well as the physical parameters of growth, because they are involved in diagnosing and managing psychosocial and developmental problems as well as healing physical problems. Parents often turn to their health care provider for understanding and guidance in issues related to their school-age child's psychosocial and physical development.

▰▰▰ DEVELOPMENT OF SCHOOL-AGE CHILDREN

Theories of School-Age Psychosocial Development

The school years have been described as a period of latency. Actually, the years from ages 6 to 12 are filled with immense developmental changes. Dworkin (1989) sees behavior maturing during these years in three domains: physical, cognitive, and affective, or psychosocial (Table 8–1).

COGNITIVE DEVELOPMENT

In Piaget's developmental theory, school-age children are in the concrete operations stage, capable of logical thought processes that are characterized by the following:

- Conservation—can understand that some aspects of things, such as weight, remain the same despite changes in appearance
- Reversibility—can mentally reverse a process or action (e.g., ice can melt to water and then refreeze)

T A B L E 8-1

Development of Behaviors in Middle Childhood

PHYSICAL	COGNITIVE	AFFECTIVE
Puberty changes can begin as early as 8 yr for girls and 9–10 yr for boys	Concrete operations stage emerges—ability to • Reason logically • See viewpoints of others • Focus on multiple aspects of problems at once • Solve problems mentally	Sense of competence and self-esteem
Gender identity solidifies		Importance of peers and social acceptance
Interest in body and functions increases		Influence of temperament on school performance, peer interactions, and family functioning
Body image concerns emerge	Mastery of language is followed by development of logical thought and relative morality	

- Decentration—can focus on more than one aspect of a situation at a time (e.g., keeping track of both color and shape when working on a jigsaw puzzle)
- Transitivity—can deduce new relationships from sets of earlier ones
- Seriation—can sequence in order (e.g., ordering triangle shapes from smallest to largest)
- Classification—can group objects on the basis of common features (e.g., separating out all the triangles from circles, squares, and stars)

Children's ability to mentally manipulate the world, relationships, and viewpoints of others is facilitated by the use of concrete materials. As children move from preoperational to concrete phases (Table 8-2), egocentricity ceases to dominate logical thinking. With the ability to understand the viewpoints of others, new social skills can emerge. Empathy, for instance, is a new school-age feeling.

PSYCHOSOCIAL AND EMOTIONAL DEVELOPMENT

The psychosocial models of development illustrate many critical tasks for children who are in the process of learning to interact with and master their environment. The stages are sequential and have been built upon since birth, with each being a prerequisite for the next

(see Table 8-2). In Freud's theory, school-age children (6 to 11 years old) are in the latency period. In this stage, sexual urges are submerged and energy can be put into acquiring cultural skills and forming friendships.

In Erikson's theory, school-age children (6 to 11 years old) are in the stage of industry vs. inferiority. Children in this stage are internally motivated (industry stage) to achieve, compete, and obtain recognition. They are eager to learn but feel inferior, develop a sense of failure, and lose interest in learning if their efforts to achieve are unsuccessful.

MORAL DEVELOPMENT

Kohlberg (1981) assessed the role of reasoning in the development of moral judgment, another aspect of psychosocial development. His theory of moral development uses a model divided into three levels of conscience, each with two stages. He did not correlate these stages to children's ages, but most experts agree that school-age children are at the first level, called the preconventional level (approximately ages 4 to 8 years of age). At this level, moral reasoning is determined by the consequences of behavior: punishment, reward, exchange of favors, and physical power of people in authority. Preconventional stage 1 behavior is primarily determined by efforts to avoid punishment or to seek the pleasure of rewards. Obedience to authority is automatic. By preconventional

T A B L E 8-2

Overview of Developmental Theories and Phases for the School-Age Child

FREUD	ERIKSON	PIAGET	KOHLBERG
LATENCY Sexual urges submerged Energy put into acquiring cultural skills and forming relationships Superego is internalized	**INDUSTRY VS. INFERIORITY** Internal motivation to achieve, compete, and obtain recognition Loss of interest in learning if not successful	**CONCRETE OPERATIONS** Conservation—some aspects of things remain the same despite changes in appearance Reversibility—can mentally reverse a process or action Decentration—can focus on more than one aspect of a situation at a time Transitivity—conceptualizes new relationships from sets of earlier ones Seriation—can sequence in order Classification—can group objects on the basis of common features	**PRECONVENTIONAL** Emphasis on avoiding punishment, getting rewards: *Stage 1*— Punishment-obedience *Stage 2*— Instrumental focus orientation (look out for self) **CONVENTIONAL** Emphasis on social roles: *Stage 3*—Approval from others important *Stage 4*—Dutiful citizen motivation **POSTCONVENTIONAL** Emphasis on moral principles: *Stage 5*—Social contract orientation *Stage 6*—Universal ethical principles motivation

stage 2, behavior is based on a desire to satisfy one's own needs and sometimes those of others. A child's view of reciprocity is concrete: "Do me a favor—I'll do you a favor." There is some consideration of the feelings of others but only of secondary conveyance. At the second level, the conventional level (ages 9 to 12 years), children act first to please others (conventional stage 3) and later to conform to authority. At the highest level, the postconventional level, people act morally from the perspective that individuals and society have a contract that benefits all. At the second stage of this highest level, individuals act from principles of conscience, even when those principles might differ from those of society as a whole. Kohlberg studied only men, which causes some to question the completeness and generalizability of his theory (see Table 8–2).

Loyalty and justice are not strong motivators for behavior among school-age children. Children discover that rules are not absolute but serve as mechanisms for maintaining and facilitating social order. This allows them to understand that rules may differ at home and school.

Physical Development

GENERAL

Generally, school-age children grow 2.5 inches per year and gain 5 to 7 pounds yearly. Head circumference increases slowly (typically from 20 to 21 inches), with the brain reaching adult size by age 12 years, marking near completion of growth of the central nervous system. School-age children have decreased fat, and organ development is complete. The spine usually becomes straighter, even though posture may be worse. Legs become straighter, often correcting knock-knee or flatfoot deformities. Although skeletal development is relatively minor, the facial bones are actively changing, particularly with growth of the nasal accessory sinuses. The lymphatic system is at its peak of development. Tonsils and adenoids are their largest at around 6 years of age and then later atrophy. Heart rate is normally 60 to 100 beats per minute, respirations 18 to 30 per minute, and blood pressure 90/60 to 108/60 mm Hg.

DENTAL

The first permanent teeth generally erupt after age 6 (6-year molars). When they arrive, the primary teeth begin to shed, usually in the same sequence in which they erupted. Approximately four teeth per year are replaced, one set in the lower jaw and one set in the upper.

ENDOCRINE

Puberty begins between ages 10 and 13 years in girls and between ages 11 and 14 years in boys but can be normal for either sex at any time after the age of 8. Before starting school, children typically establish their gender identity, but that identity is still under refinement. Children at 6 to 8 years of age are curious about their bodies and those of others. Sexually oriented behaviors emerge during this age, with 5- to 6-year olds often playing doctor and 8- to 9-year-olds of the same sex comparing their bodies. Masturbation or self-exploration is common at this age. There is an increasing sense of modesty.

DEVELOPMENTAL SCREENING AND ASSESSMENT OF SCHOOL-AGE CHILDREN

Screening and surveillance, as described in earlier chapters, requires periodic review of the child's progress. This review for school-age children involves discussion with the child and then the parent. Observations should continue to assess gross motor, fine motor, language, and social skills. Themes to pursue at various visits include the following:

The 6- to 8-year-old visit
- Adaptation to school
- After-school activities
- Development of peer relationships
- Family relationships
- Activities that support positive self-esteem
- Problem-solving away from home, without parents immediately available

The 9- to 10-year visit
- Progress at school
- After-school activities
- Peer relationships—friendships, bullying, or victimization
- Family relationships
- Sexual education
- Community safety; joining gangs
- Activities that support positive self-esteem
- Problem-solving away from home
- Handling emotions—sadness, anger, worries

The 11- to 12-year old visit
- Progress in school
- After-school activities
- Peer relationships
- Family relationships
- Community safety; membership in gangs
- Activities that support positive self-esteem
- Problem-solving away from home—avoiding drugs, alcohol, and smoking
- Handling emotions—sadness, anger, worries
- Completion of basic education in sexuality and reproductive health

Screening Strategies for School-Age Children

PHYSICAL DEVELOPMENT

Height, weight, and blood pressure should be measured and compared with age-appropriate norms at all visits. Hearing and vision should be screened annually. Tanner's staging should be a part of the physical examination because school-age children can begin pubertal changes as early as 8 years of age.

DEVELOPMENTAL SCREENING

Developmental screening is an essential part of each health maintenance visit. The process begins by building rapport with the parents, encouraging them to share sensitive developmental concerns. Directing questions first to the child and then to the parents expands on data collected, providing information not only about the child's abilities but also about the interactions between child and parents.

The child's development and progress should be reviewed periodically by the NP in a variety of areas: physical, cognitive, and social-emotional. For each area, the NP asks questions directly to the child, probing for the developmental level of understanding, language skills, and ability to interact socially with the examiner. It is also important to watch the interaction between parents and child during the examination.

Assessment Strategies for School-Age Children

Assessment involves more individualized analysis of a child's status than does screening that uses the same techniques for many children. It generally follows screening when possible problems are identified. Table 8–3 identifies red flags for development of school-age children.

PHYSICAL DEVELOPMENT ASSESSMENT

Concepts

Physical development by body system was discussed earlier. The child's increases in strength and coordination contribute to a sense of competence in physical abilities and set the stage for participation in sports, dance, gymnastics, and other activities. Social status among children is often based on physical competence; therefore, the child's feelings about physical development are as important as the growth parameters themselves.

Children with chronic illnesses or disabilities may have trouble adapting to their disorders during the school-age years and may need special help to foster independence and a sense of self-esteem (Green, 1994). Latchkey kids (those who spend the afternoon at home without supervision because their parents work) with chronic illnesses are especially vulnerable because they may need to make decisions about their health care without adult advice. For example, they may need to know whether they should have more medication or need to complete a treatment. Such children need to understand their illness, medications, where to go for emergency care, how to write down instructions or messages, and how to follow important

T A B L E 8-3
Developmental Red Flags: School-Age Child

AGE	PSYCHOSOCIAL/EMOTIONAL SKILL	COGNITIVE AND VISUAL ABILITIES	LANGUAGE/ HEARING	FINE MOTOR	GROSS MOTOR
6 yr	Problems with peer relationships Latchkey: stays home alone Unable to state special quality about self Flat affect, depression, withdrawn Cruelty to animals, friends Interest in fires/firesetting	School problems with grades, behavior, interest in grades Unable to sit still in class Unable to give age More than 2 hr per day watching television Unable to name interests	Language partially unintelligible	Unable to copy + Picture of self includes less than 8 parts	Unable to catch a ball
8 yr	Lack of hobbies Lack of best friend Cruelty to animals, friends Interest in fires/firesetting Flat affect, depression, withdrawn	Unable to state days of the week Unable to add and subtract Unable to identify right and left	Unable to read simple phrases Unable to relate simple story	Unable to copy a diamond and square Unable to print name Unable to tie shoes Picture of self includes less than 12–16 parts	Unable to walk a straight line Poor coordination/ endurance/ strength
10 yr	Lack of team sports or extracurricular activities at school Lacks understanding of rules Poor peer influence, interest in gangs Cruelty to animals, friends Interest in fires/firesetting Flat affect, depression, withdrawn	Lack of operational thinking: cause and effect, relationships of whole and parts, nonegocentric thinking	Problems with reading and math	Difficulty holding pencil with penmanship/ cursive writing	Problems throwing or catching
12 yr	Risk-taking behaviors: smoking, alcohol, sex Problems about sexuality Cruelty to animals, friends Interest in fires/firesetting Flat affect, depression, withdrawn	Difficulty with school work Lack of organizational skills for homework	Problems understanding/ following through with verbal instructions Problems with reading comprehension	Problems getting written homework done because of difficulties holding pencil or doing paper and pencil tasks	Unable to list strengths and physical things he/she likes to do

147

rules (Holaday et al., 1993). Children mature at different rates in their ability to manage their self-care throughout the school-age years.

Physical Development Assessment Strategies

Assessment of physical development in school-age children includes height, weight, and blood pressure measured at each health maintenance visit. Assessment of the trajectory using growth grids to identify growth norms is essential. If problems are suspected, additional testing can be performed (e.g., wrist radio-graphs can establish bone age). Tanner staging can help identify endocrine problems that may emerge in the school years. Further endocrine, nutrition, genetic, or other assessments may be necessary if the child does not meet the norms for size (Behrman et al., 1996).

Strength and coordination are harder to assess in the health visit, but inquiring about play and physical activities both during school and at home can provide information about the child's abilities and sense of confidence.

Capacity for self-care of chronic illnesses depends on the illness, its stability, and the child's age and cognitive skills.

ASSESSING BEHAVIOR RELATED TO PHYSICAL DEVELOPMENT

Questions Asked	*Purpose, Outcomes, and Goals of Questions*
Ask how child usually feels	Invites discussion of somatic complaints
	Obtains child's view of own health
Ask how child is feeling today	Communicates that you value child's information
Ask questions about body functions (especially helpful for children with chronic illnesses)	Lays groundwork for later candid adolescent provider–patient relationship
	Assesses compliance with treatment
Ask whether an illness has interfered with activities with friends and at school	Allows awareness of unnecessary restrictions of children with chronic medical problems
Ask about activities that the child engages in during school hours, and at home	Invites discussion about child's competence in relation to physical abilities

---

COGNITIVE DEVELOPMENT ASSESSMENT

Concepts

When children make the transition to concrete operational thinking, they are more likely to be ready for school. Concrete operational abilities allow children to read, write, and communicate thoughts effectively. Learning about the world, its people, and the views and values of others becomes possible.

The concepts of Piaget's cognitive development theory are useful for this assessment. Children should be able to classify or group material in relation to other information they have. Magical thinking and egocentric logic should fade, whereas concepts of conservation, transformation, reversibility, decentration, seriation, and classification emerge. Children should be able to view the world from another person's perspective.

The information processing model provides another useful conceptual framework for assessment of cognitive development in school-age children. For effective cognitive work, young people must recognize salient cues in the environment; organize their thoughts, consider relationships with other information; use short- and long-term memory retrieval and storage skills; make decisions based on the analysis of information; take action; and use feedback to further learning.

Cognitive Development Assessment Strategies

Assessment of cognitive development is difficult in school-age children. Generally, standardized paper and pencil tests are more accurate than clinical judgments. Knowledge about the child's performance compared with that of peers in the classroom, the child's grades, and information from conferences with teachers provide some data. Often a psychologist is asked to test children cognitively if more definitive information is needed.

ASSESSING BEHAVIOR RELATED TO COGNITIVE DEVELOPMENT

Questions Asked	*Purpose, Outcomes, and Goals of Questions*
5- to 8-year-olds:	
Ask about school, grade, likes and dislikes	A 6-year-old should be able to answer all questions
	May suggest problems at school
Ask child to give address and telephone number (7-year-olds)	Assesses basic information important to child's well-being
Ask child to copy square (5-year-olds), triangle (6-year-olds), diamond (7-year-olds)	Assesses visual and auditory memory skills
	Allows observation of handedness
	Assesses fine motor skills in using writing instrument
	Assesses visual-perceptual skills
Ask child to draw a person	Allows estimation of mental age using Goodenough's criteria
	Assesses cooperation
Ask what makes the sun come up	Assesses child's beliefs regarding cause
Ask how one can tell whether something is alive	Assesses magical and egocentric thinking: "The sun comes up so I can play," "Something is alive if I can talk to it"
Ask child how he or she gets from home to school	May suggest egocentric thinking, often leaving out important details
	Difficult to reverse thinking if asked
Ask about dreams. Are they real?	Assesses ability to distinguish reality vs. fantasy
9- to 12-year-olds:	
Ask general information questions (day, who is president, team names)	Assesses child's general fund of information
Ask how child gets from home to school	Assesses capacity for memory and ability to communicate; answer should be accurate
Ask how one can tell whether something is alive	Assesses knowledge of natural world
Ask child to point to examiner's right ear with the left hand	By age 10 years, children should be able to put themselves in another's place and respond correctly
Ask child's opinion of a current event	Assesses awareness of current events
All ages:	
Ask about the child's progress in school; invite parent to share after child answers	Child should be at grade level in all areas and should feel successful

SOCIAL AND EMOTIONAL ASSESSMENT

Social Development Concepts

FAMILY RELATIONSHIPS. The earliest school-age milestone in the psychosocial area occurs when children learn to separate easily from family, allowing them to go to school. As they move into the community, they need to develop their own sense of self. This sense of self includes their role and feelings of belonging to a family. Children in middle childhood need increasing opportunities for independence but with guidance and support from parents.

During the school-age years, children maintain their attachments with parents but also develop secondary attachments with other adults outside the home. Having good relationships with adults outside the home is especially important when the family is not wholly functional—not responsive and supportive—to the child (Schor, 1998).

PEER RELATIONSHIPS. A major task of school-age children is to develop competence in social relationships. "Friendships promote resilience, enhance self-image, fill emotional needs, and help compensate for stresses in other areas of life" (Coleman & Lindsay, 1998, p. 111). Relationship skills include initiating interactions, keeping them going, resolving conflicts, and terminating interactions positively. However, many other factors are necessary for children to be successful with their peers—reading social situations, being socially responsive, using the jargon of the group, making use of previous interactions to repeat successful behaviors, being appropriately assertive, and being empathetic, among others (Coleman & Lindsay, 1998).

Peer acceptance becomes a major factor with the development of social groups and pressure to conform. Children come to see themselves in the eyes of their friends. These early friendships are the basis for later relationships. Strong peer effects are seen in dressing, speaking, and eating as peers do. Family conflicts can arise when peer activities and expectations conflict with family rules and values.

Children's temperaments play a major role in the effect that interactions with peers, teachers, and family have on them as well as their responses to various situations. Emotional problems during these years often follow frustrations, losses, and situations in which the child's self-esteem is threatened. Temperament characteristics influence the responses children feel when faced with adversity.

MORALITY. School-age children tend to be rather rigid in their views of right and wrong. Their conscience is already developed but the ability to reason through difficult situations with a variety of factors operating is heavily dependent on cognitive development. The school environment, where rules and values differ from those of the immediate family, challenges children's moral thinking and must be confronted and negotiated daily. Social pressures may make it difficult to choose actions that the child believes are right. The pressures of gangs, drugs, and peers push many children to make decisions about their activities and behaviors before they are developmentally ready. Furthermore, the values of the family are challenged as the child learns that other families make decisions and have beliefs that are different from their own.

Discipline needs to be adjusted by parents of school-age children. Time-out may change to grounding. Natural consequences (losing out because the wrong decision was made) can become a more effective form of punishment. School-age children can understand the relationships between responsibility and privileges and that choices between right and wrong behaviors are in their control. They respond well to the use of reward systems to correct behaviors. These become contracts, ways of earning privileges or things of value by making choices that are honest and correct. Parents have the primary role as disciplinarians, although the school makes and enforces rules for that setting.

SELF-ESTEEM. Using Erikson's theory of psychosocial development, school-age children are in the stage of industry vs. inferiority. Thus, what they make and do directly impact their sense of self-esteem. Their activities, school performance, and social acceptance are key areas used to determine self-worth. Receiving positive feedback from family, peers, teachers, and others in the community allows them to gain in self-confidence and feelings of worth.

COPING. School-age children face a variety of stressors in society today. Violence is a constant problem for many, not only in neighborhoods where they live and play but also in schools where they go to learn. When parents work, many children must take responsibility for themselves after school. Latchkey kids remain alone, housebound and unsupervised, until adults return at the end of the day. Some are responsible for younger siblings during this time. Many schools lack resources to maintain small class sizes or offer special programs for children with learning difficulties. Children are simply passed on from grade to grade without remediation of their fundamental learning problems. Even for those children who live in relatively safe neighborhoods and attain success in their schoolwork, the pressures for achievement can be stressful.

School-age children are developing their ability to identify, label, and manage their feelings with increasing skill. However, they still need help labeling sadness, depression, worry, envy, anger, and other emotions. Furthermore, they need help in consciously managing those feelings in acceptable ways. Empathy, or the ability to share and understand another's feelings, emerges, and with it, the capacity for making deep friendships.

Psychosocial and Emotional Development Assessment Strategies

Assessment of social and emotional development includes children's roles in the family, success in making friends and working with peers, self-esteem, and feelings of contentment and security.

ASSESSING BEHAVIOR RELATED TO SOCIAL AND EMOTIONAL DEVELOPMENT*

Questions Asked	*Purpose/Outcomes/ Goals of Questions*
5- to 8-year-olds:	
Ask questions regarding sports team, favorite movie, television show, books read, favorite activities or games	Assesses knowledge of general information
Ask about friends	Assesses relationships with peers; should be able to name at least one friend
Ask what child does for play	Assesses solo vs. group activities
Ask who lives in the home and ask opinions about family members	Assesses child's perception of negative and positive family relationships Assesses sibling rivalry
Ask what the child does when feeling sad, angry, or hurt	Assesses sensitivity to emotions and coping strategies
Ask parent to comment on responses	
9- to 12-year-olds:	
Ask about best friends and what they do together	Assesses ability to form peer relationships
Ask child what he or she does to help at home	Assesses involvement with family in constructive activity
Ask child if he or she gets into trouble at home or school	Allows comment on child's conduct
Ask parent to comment—may discuss disciplinary techniques	
Ask child for three wishes, what they would be, and why	Allows child to express hopes and concerns

*Adapted from Dixon and Stein (1992).

Parent Development

Parents, too, must change when their children enter school. It is not always an easy transition. Parents must allow their children increased freedom and independence to meet the expectations of school entry. Their children are confronted with a new social system that in some ways evaluates the work that parents have done over the previous years. Are the children prepared for self-care throughout the day? Can they toilet; independently choose and eat a lunch; negotiate travel from home to school to classroom and home again; express needs to school personnel; participate appropriately in the classroom; make friends; and have enough self-control to resist peer pressures to act against family rules and expectations? Parents are expected to support the school's standards. The loss of the dependent child who relies on the family may be mourned by some parents, whereas others look forward to the new opportunities facing the child and the family. For most, school entry is a mixed blessing.

As school-age children move through the years from 6 to 12, parents must continue to extend freedoms along with adding new responsibilities. They need to provide opportunities that allow children to experience and master new challenges as well as adjust family patterns of nutrition, sleep, activities, health maintenance, safety, and communication to fit with the needs and emerging skills of the family's school-age child. Parents must reinforce and support the positive self-esteem and self-image of these vulnerable young people. Spending time with their children in positive, reinforcing ways is essential (Wolraich, 1997).

ANTICIPATORY GUIDANCE DURING THE SCHOOL-AGE YEARS

6- and 7-Year-Olds

DEVELOPMENTAL STATUS

Children at this age want to be independent but do not always have the decision-making strengths to allow them to do what they want. Making friends, starting school, and developing their new level of cognitive logical thinking are major areas for development.

Nutrition and Feeding

School-age children have good appetites. Diets can be deficient in iron or vitamin C and high-fat snack foods can become a habit, with resulting obesity. Choosing nutritious foods away from home and learning to eat new foods are areas for maturation. Because food is not readily available all day at school, eating well at breakfast and lunch becomes especially important.

Elimination

Elimination patterns are established for more than 90% of children, although encopresis or enuresis can be problematic for some children. For discussion, see Chapter 14 on elimination.

Rhythmicity and Sleep/Wake Patterns

Most school-age children sleep 8 to 12 hours per night without naps. Night terrors or sleepwalking may emerge.

Activities

Six-year-olds experience rapid cognitive, social, and emotional growth. Because of the maturity of the central nervous system and cognitive advances, children at 6 years of age generally can succeed in activities such as dancing, sports, and arts and crafts programs. Most enjoy playing hard to develop physical skills and coordination.

Children at this age need active exercise every day. Activities that are fun, involve family or peers, and require cognitive or social skills, including rules, strategies, and skills, are the most beneficial.

Emotions and Moral Development

By age 7 years, most children can name a site for their conscience (heart or brain). There is variability in moral development. Some children at this age act appropriately to get a direct reward, whereas others do their duty, viewing moral behavior as following the rules of higher authority (see Table 8–2). School-age children are learning to identify and control a wide variety of emotions and to behave in socially acceptable ways.

Coping

School-age children should be developing impulse control. Without control, random behavior occurs. Overcontrolled children appear hostile or noncreative, or both. By age 7 years,

children should have developed sufficiently to function in a variety of settings (home, school, playground) with increasing competence.

Seven-year-olds often use fantasy or identification with real or imagined characters to achieve their wishes. Fantasy becomes a healthy outlet for normal aggression and sexual feelings.

Cognition

Six-year-olds are entering the concrete operations cognitive development stage, beginning to understand relationships of mass and length. They are losing their magical thinking and are able to consider multiple variables relating to objects.

Communication

Six-year-olds have a well-developed vocabulary. They have simple syntactic abilities, not always understanding relative clauses (e.g., "the cat was chased by the dog"). There is often trouble with the concepts of "before" and "after." They may not be accustomed to attending to total auditory stimuli as in the classroom environment. Limited semantic and syntactic abilities make it difficult for them to follow complicated directions. With regard to expressive language, the ability to retrieve words quickly is developing at age 6 years. As school progresses, increased demand is made on recalling what is known within a specific time frame. Narrative skills can be poor. Thinking about language, such as what makes up a sentence, a skill needed for reading, can also be hard.

Seven-year-olds generally have language decoding mastered and are working on encoding information. In other words, these children can use previous knowledge, organize it, and verbally express or write it down. They are able to solve word problems.

Social Interactions

Learning to make friends is an important step for young school-age children. By age 7 years, some children are more concerned about a friend's opinion than about adults' opinions.

They develop "best friends" and dress and talk like their peers.

Children may need help in learning to initiate, sustain, and terminate relationships as well as in solving interaction problems. Parents and other adults should be available to help resolve problems with friends without having either party lose face or feel demeaned.

ANTICIPATORY GUIDANCE AND DEVELOPMENTAL INTERVENTIONS FOR 6- AND 7-YEAR-OLDS

Anticipatory guidance should be an individualized discussion with parents that helps them understand, respond to, and guide their child's behavior and development. Some discussion points are identified below. The lists are not intended to be used exhaustively at visits but to illustrate how parents can apply developmental concepts in everyday living. If problems emerge from discussions in these areas, the NP is referred to the appropriate chapter (generally, Chapters 12 to 22 are relevant) for ideas for assessment and management (e.g., sleep problems are discussed in Chapter 16).

Feeding and Self-Care

- Ensure that the child has three nutritious meals and two nutritious snacks daily.
- Provide a nutritious breakfast and lunch at school.
- As children enter middle childhood, help child to learn survival skills (e.g., name, telephone number, address, use of 911, asking adults for help, what to do if lost).
- For 6- and 7-year-olds, help the child learn how his or her body works as well as simple concepts for health maintenance— diet, hygiene, rest, and activities.
- Provide simple facts about pregnancy, intercourse, and human immunodeficiency virus (HIV) transmission (Wright, 1997).
- Help the child learn to think about safety in all activities.

Rhythmicity and Sleep/Wake Patterns

- Maintain regular bedtimes, especially during the school year.

Elimination

- Assist children who have not developed nighttime dryness to complete this step (see Enuresis Management in Chapter 14).

Activities

- Provide for physical activity every day.
- Limit television viewing and computer games to no more than 2 hours per day.
- Encourage sports that include other children, learning rules, and feelings of competence in the child.

Emotional Growth Fostering

- Enhance goal setting with charts, calendars, and tally sheets. Care should be taken not to overreward children, because this can decrease motivation.
- Play and work together as a family to enhance self-esteem and prepare children to work together with their class and to function as a team.
- Share family history and visits with relatives to help children be proud of their heritage.
- Help children feel that the home base is secure so they are confident in moving to other domains.
- Appreciate the products of the child's work at home and at school to promote self-esteem.
- Provide fantasy play opportunities to allow children to deal safely with their concerns and develop their creativity.
- Teach anger management skills.
- Help children identify and appropriately express their emotions.

Social and Moral Development

- Provide opportunities for children to make and develop friendships with a variety of children to develop their social skills and self-esteem.
- Include the child's friends in some activities and outings.
- Begin teaching conflict resolution skills that are nonviolent.

- Teach respect for authority and rules away from home.
- Help the child learn to communicate well with other adults.
- Discuss the reasons for family values and rules, and the differences that the child may face when away from home.
- Provide children with opportunities for appropriate behavior when values are challenged (e.g., "You can say, 'No, my Mom won't let me do that,' and then walk away").

Cognitive, Language, and Environmental Stimulation

- Stimulate thinking about comparisons (e.g., changes in shape, volume, directions to and from school) to facilitate concrete operations level cognition.
- Discuss variables in objects or situations as experienced, seen on television, or read about to help move the child's thinking away from the earlier egocentric style.
- Provide opportunities to gain knowledge through books, outings, classes, and family discussions.
- Establish a regular homework time and place to help the child maximize time for cognitive practice.
- Provide help early if children experience school problems to lessen secondary problems with emotions and conflict.
- Establish an environment that encourages children to focus and complete tasks with limits clearly defined.

8- to 10-Year-Olds

DEVELOPMENTAL STATUS

Between 8 and 10 years of age, children are mastering skills necessary for survival and productive living. These allow them to meet the demands of adult life at home and in society. They compete academically, socially, and in extracurricular activities. They are increasingly involved with clubs, sport teams, or music. During these years, children become separated more often from parents (e.g., at camp, sleepovers). They also develop a sense of hu-

mor, creativity, responsibility, leadership, and negotiation skills. The ability to get along with peers becomes even more important at this age.

Nutrition and Feeding

For school-age children, learning to take responsibility for health maintenance begins with simple goals and moves to more complex decision-making strategies. For example, children may begin by deciding to have a fruit or vegetable at each meal and then progress to helping plan some meals and participate in their preparation. Other areas in which children take increasing responsibility are dental health, hygiene and grooming, snacking, and exercise. Children at this age see health in positive terms and equate it with being able to participate in desired activities (Koster, 1983).

Elimination, Rhythmicity, and Sleep/Wake Patterns

Encopresis, enuresis, and sleep difficulties, if they have occurred, should be resolving.

Activities

As children immerse themselves in sports, clubs, music, and current fads, doing the "in thing" becomes critically important. All children should have at least one activity that they enjoy. Positive peer relations and social acceptance are central at this age.

Emotions

Family functioning seems to be the greatest protection for school-age children. Families can help children develop skills to deal with social and academic stress through parental modeling of coping skills, rules, and expectations. The expression of empathy becomes important at this time. Arguments with parents can increase, usually over homework or chores.

School expectations for performance increase (e.g., examinations, graded papers, and homework assignments determine school grades). Reading becomes a tool to master content in other subjects rather than being an end in itself. Thus, poor readers begin to experience broader academic failure. Social support helps children cope with stress. Interacting with healthy, interested, and caring adults is the strongest base children can have.

Cognitive

Children in the middle years of this stage should have well-developed concrete operational thinking. They should be able to focus on more than one aspect of a problem, use logical thinking, and do well in school.

Communication

Children at 8 to 9 years of age have had significant syntactic growth, allowing them to understand convoluted sentences. Second- or third-grade children have better use of pronouns. By age 8 years, children can follow complex directions. They can tell jokes because they understand different meanings of words. Expressively, children's ability to use words results in better narration and significantly improves storytelling and summarization skills needed for such activities as explaining a task to other children.

ANTICIPATORY GUIDANCE AND DEVELOPMENTAL INTERVENTIONS FOR 8- TO 10-YEARS-OLDS

Feeding and Self-Care

- Encourage application of life skills learned at school or other places to develop independence and appropriate decision-making.
- Teach safety skills.
- Encourage the successful completion of chores so that the child meets expectations and feels successful in tasks.
- Provide opportunities to participate in family and home activities to learn new skills and work with others to achieve goals.
- Have children begin to assume responsibility for health (e.g., diet, exercise, rest, hygiene) and encourage shared decision-making and self-care during illnesses and for chronic disease management.
- Teach about puberty changes.

Activities

- Encourage hobbies and activities, such as team sports, for fitness and self-esteem.
- Encourage participation in sports or other performance activities to learn about intense training, commitment, and physical risks.
- Limit television and computer game time to less than 2 hours per day.

Emotional Growth Fostering

- Provide guidance for how to express aggression and emerging sexual feelings appropriately.
- Support participation in activities that allow channeling feelings of aggressiveness plus giving a sense of group accomplishment.
- Recognize that fantasy play allows children to deal with feelings without loss of control.
- Recognize that children may identify with a person, such as a movie star, athlete, member of a military group, or member of a ball team.
- Encourage successful activities, because repeated failures at this age lead to a sense of inferiority.
- Provide positive expressions of love, concern, and pride to promote self-esteem, a sense of belonging to the family, and social support.

Social and Moral Development

- Provide social skills training and supervised social success experiences to promote social development.
- Teach children how to read social cues to promote their social acceptance.
- Recognize that parents are role models and that children internalize parental values as they begin to form a conscience.
- Teach conflict resolution without violence and help children with decision-making and accepting consequences of actions.

Cognitive, Language, and Environmental Stimulation

- Recognize academic achievement, because success motivates further work.

- Stay involved with school assignments and evaluate progress to support the child's work.
- Explore and explain the environment and community to the child to promote broader understanding of the world.
- Maintain a regular time and place for homework to help the child maximize cognitive work.
- Provide opportunities to plan and complete projects that use school skills (e.g., cooking and measuring ingredients, reading maps, calculating money, budgeting). Application of knowledge and skills promotes understanding and cognitive growth.

11- and 12-Year-Olds

DEVELOPMENTAL STATUS

At 11 and 12 years of age, children continue to master skills necessary for adulthood. They often become more aggressive in part as their interest in sexual matters increases. Their primary identity is with their social group, and they make an effort to develop culturally appropriate social behaviors. Independence is an increasing issue; as school-age children progress toward puberty, they should gradually assume more independent activities. By age 12 years, the conscience has become personified (e.g., children have the capacity to feel guilty). Values are explored and redefined during these years.

Self-Care

Ten- to 12-year-olds should be able to manage their own hygiene independently. Furthermore, they should have some home responsibilities and be learning to manage money. Their sexual education needs to be completed and discussions should occur regarding use of alcohol, drugs, and tobacco and the skills that will be required to avoid these substances when they spend time with their peers.

Activities

Children at this age may have selected particular activities at which they want to succeed at a high level of accomplishment. Family support is important to their achievement goals. At all times, regardless of stresses, it is important to maintain at least one positive area of activity. Parents need to share in their children's achievements while allowing the activity of interest to be the child's, not theirs.

Social Interactions

Friends are generally chosen because of shared skills, interests, personality, and loyalty. A special-friend phase should occur at around 10 years of age. This is a very intense attachment to a same-sex child. With that friend, the child expands the self, learns altruism, shares feelings, and learns how others manage problems. Talking on the telephone and sleepovers become more common. Social acceptance is especially important at this age. Even though they want to be like everyone else, children also want and need to have their own uniqueness recognized.

Cognitive

A sense of personal competence develops with a series of successful experiences.

Communication

By 10 years of age, children have better detail in verbal skills and understand inflections. Ten-year-olds should be able to discuss ideas. By age 12 years, children should be able to answer questions involving sophisticated concepts. Their sentences should be grammatically correct.

ANTICIPATORY GUIDANCE AND DEVELOPMENTAL INTERVENTIONS FOR 11- AND 12-YEAR-OLDS

Feeding and Self-Care

- Maintain family meals as much as possible to preserve family time.
- Maintain eating routines.
- Use snacking to complement planned meals.
- Help children learn safety skills and use of safety equipment for bicycles, in-line skates, and cars, for example.

- Encourage application of life skills learned at school or other places.
- Expect the successful completion of chores.
- Provide opportunities to participate in family and home activities.
- Have children take increasing responsibility for health (e.g., diet, exercise, rest, hygiene).
- Share decision-making and self-care during illnesses and in chronic disease management.
- Teach about menstruation, wet dreams, and sexual feelings and responses.
- Teach facts of pregnancy, contraception, adoption, and abortion (Wright, 1997).

Rhythmicity and Sleep/Wake Patterns

- Allow increased variation in sleep schedules on nonschool days but maintain a regular schedule during the school week to ensure adequate rest.

Activities

- Encourage extracurricular activities, because preteens are energetic and interested in doing many things.
- Avoid the stress of overactivity, which diminishes the pleasure of each experience.
- Encourage hobbies and activities, such as team sports and club activities.
- Encourage participation in sports or other performance activities to learn about intense training, commitment, and physical risks.
- Limit television viewing or playing computer games to a maximum of 2 hours per day.

Emotional Growth Fostering

- Recognize that having a strong sense of self-esteem helps "inoculate" children against some of the negative peer pressures they may experience.
- Help children learn delayed gratification and increase their frustration tolerance. However, parents need to remain sympathetic.

- Let children set goals while parents monitor activities and point out options.
- Help children learn appropriate expressions of aggression and emerging sexual feelings.
- Support participation in activities that allow feelings of aggressiveness plus giving a sense of group accomplishment.
- Encourage successful activities, because repeated failures at this age lead to a sense of inferiority.
- Provide positive expressions of love, concern, and pride.
- Discuss sexual values.

Social and Moral Development

- Provide social skills training and supervised social success experiences.
- Promote social acceptance of children, including assistance in reading social cues.
- Recognize that parents are role models and that children internalize parental values.
- Use natural consequences as the dominant form of discipline in this age group.

Cognitive, Language, and Environmental Stimulation

- Encourage problem-solving efforts.
- Recognize academic achievement.
- Stay involved with school assignments and evaluate progress.
- Explore and explain the environment and community to children.
- Maintain a regular time and place for homework.
- Provide more complex opportunities to plan and complete projects that use school skills, such as planning and cooking meals, planning family outings, and managing money and a budget.

COMMON DEVELOPMENTAL ISSUES FOR SCHOOL-AGE CHILDREN

First-Grade School Readiness

DESCRIPTION

School readiness assessment is an important first step in the successful achievement of school-age children. Because school entrance is based on chronological rather than developmental age, readiness problems occur for some children. School entry is stressful for all children, but immature children have increased stress because of unrealistic expectations for performance and poorly developed coping abilities. Children who lack necessary skills to meet school demands and expectations are unsuccessful, and early school failure has significant negative consequences.

School is stressful because it requires skills to perform self-care, interact with a variety of new people, act with a sense of responsibility, and emotionally separate from the family and home base. Children need to meet school standards, which may be different from those at home. There is a social expectation to become less egocentric and achieve awareness of "the group"—an ability to go along with the group while meeting some personal needs through the group's achievements.

INCIDENCE

Studies in the early 1990s indicated that teachers thought that 35% of children were not ready for school. Issues of concern, in decreasing order of importance, included language richness, emotional maturity, general knowledge, social confidence, moral awareness, and physical maturity (Boyer, 1993). Socially and economically disadvantaged children are at greatest risk (Byrd, 1998).

CLINICAL FINDINGS

History

- Experience away from home, practice in following directions, playing with other children, and interest in school are all important areas to assess.
- Assess the parents' feelings about their child's entering school. Reluctance on their part may be communicated to their child, a message that does not facilitate the child's positive regard for this anticipated event.

Physical Examination

The child should have a complete physical examination with special focus on the following:

- Neurological development
- Height, weight, blood pressure
- Immunization status
- Hearing
- Vision
- Urine
- Hematocrit
- Dental health

Developmental Evaluation

Developmental assessment is crucial to decisions about school entry and school placement. Normative skills are included in Table 8-4.

Ancillary Studies

A variety of tests are designed to look at educational readiness (Table 8-5). These tests have established norms and are generally reliable in predicting developmental outcomes. They should be used to consider all areas of readiness and to provide an explanation of readiness for parents. Test results should be evaluated in conjunction with history, observation, family situation, and previous experiences.

MANAGEMENT

Preventive strategies for high-risk children include enrollment in preschool, interactive reading with the child from an early age to promote language mastery, increased time for young children to play with peers and engage in creative play activities, and interaction with caring adults (Byrd, 1998).

Ensuring school readiness involves sharing data with school counselors and teachers, parents, and primary care providers, and offering anticipatory guidance in several areas.

- Encourage parents to visit the school, meet the teacher, and discuss their child's characteristics with the teacher.
- Before school starts, parents should rehearse school activities with their child.

T A B L E 8-4

Basic First Grade School Readiness Skills

Language skills	Counts 10 or more objects
	Uses complete sentences of at least five words
	Uses future tense
	Gives first and last name
	Recognizes four colors
	Defines five to seven words
	Communicates needs
	Recalls parts of a story
	Follows three-part commands
	Understands number concepts
Personal and social skills	Separates easily from parent
	Dresses without supervision
	Plays interactively with other children
	Has toilet skills
	Follows instructions
	Feels support from other adults
Fine motor and adaptive skills	Copies geometrical shapes (circle, square, triangle)
	Draws a person (six parts with distinct body)
	Prints some letters
	Classifies similar objects
Gross motor skills	Hops on one foot
	Catches bounced ball
	Walks backward heel/toe
	Balances on each foot 6 seconds

T A B L E 8-5

Screening Tests to Evaluate School Readiness

Denver Developmental Screening Test II	Denver Developmental Materials, Inc. P.O. Box 371075 Denver, CO 80237-5075 (800) 419-4729	Divided into four areas: Gross motor Language Fine motor Personal/social
VMI-4 (Beery, K. 1996)	Pro-Ed 8700 Shoal Creek Blvd. Austin, TX 78757-6897 (800) 897-3202 (502) 451-3246 Website: www.proedinc.com	Test of visual motor integration
Pediatric Examination of Educational Readiness (PEER) and Pediatric Examination of Educational Readiness at Middle Childhood (PEERAMID)	Educators Publishing Service, Inc. 31 Smith Place Cambridge, MA 02138-1007 (617) 547-6706 Fax: (617) 547-0412 Website: www.epsbooks.com	Combined neurodevelopmental, behavioral, and health assessment

Play that the child is getting to school, finding class, eating meals, going to the bathroom, asking for help, getting home, and following the rules.

- Help parents deal with their stress of separation. Review their expectations of the child and identify what will be new and different.
- Anticipate available community and school resources that parents may need to access to meet the developmental needs of their child.
- Encourage children to start school with their age-appropriate group. Children who are seen as not ready by parents often need extra support at school rather than spending another year at home.
- Be an advocate for parents and children with identified deficits to ensure that the school adequately assesses both strengths and weaknesses of children and develops a program of study that maximizes children's strengths.
- Counsel parents that deficits identified in a child's readiness are not always indicators of failure in parenting.
- Develop a care plan with parents to address deficits in a comprehensive way while preserving the child's self-esteem.
- Monitor the child's progress through the year, advocating as necessary.

Learning Problems

DESCRIPTION

Learning problems can be a hidden handicap that appears during the school-age years. Ability to manage school learning expectations requires growth in four areas: basic processing of information, memorization, increased attention span and recall of important events, and beginning problem-solving skills.

Knowledge (the sum of what children know) rapidly expands as a result of schoolwork, experiences at home, and activities with friends. The organization of knowledge improves as school-age children grow older and integrate knowledge into existing concepts. Self-awareness, reflected by children's ability to predict performance, develops slowly and in areas in which children have the most knowledge (Table 8-6).

Although children with learning problems generally have difficulties with basic thinking skills, they have specific problems in: linguistic skills, attention, and organizational skills; higher cognitive functions, such as memory, sensory; motor capacities; visual-spatial analysis and neuromotor function; and social awareness and behavior (Tanner, 1995).

CLINICAL FINDINGS

The history and physical examination should rule out the following:

- Neurological problems
- Hearing or vision deficits
- Developmental problems
- Social history to identify stressors in child's life at home or at school

Information needs to be obtained from the school system to evaluate the child's school performance and to review any educational testing that has been done. Testing must provide a picture of the child's strengths and weaknesses, revealing the cognitive styles that teachers and parents will be most successful in tapping. The Pediatric Examination of Educational Readiness at Middle Childhood (PEERAMID), a neurodevelopmental examination for 9- to 14-year-olds, may be administered (Levine et al., 1988).

DIFFERENTIAL DIAGNOSIS

The following diagnoses need to be considered in children with learning problems:

- Vision problems
- Hearing problems
- Mental retardation—genetic syndrome, neurological insult, or malformation
- Cognitive developmental delay
- Speech or language delay
- Depression
- Neurological problems
- Attention-deficit hyperactivity disorder
- Autism
- Toxin-related delay (e.g., lead, fetal alcohol syndrome)
- Medication-related delay (e.g., anticonvulsant, antihistamine)
- Substance abuse

T A B L E 8-6

Developmental Changes in Thinking Skills

COMPONENT	DEVELOPMENTAL CHANGES	EXAMPLES
Basic skills	Improvements in the speed and efficiency of memory, attention, language processing, motor implementation	Longer digit span Ability to work for longer stretches of time The use of adult-like logical principles The development of reading skills
Strategies	Use of active, complex strategies to improve basic skills	Greater spontaneous use of strategies Wider repertoire of strategies Greater likelihood of generalization to new areas
Knowledge	Expansion of what is known and greater organization of knowledge	Development of hobbies and special areas of interest More complex network of concepts
Metacognitive awareness	Development of explicit self-conscious knowledge about how to think	Ability to predict success or failure Ability to plan and to modify strategies

From Feldman H: Development of thinking skills in school-aged children. *Pediatr Ann 18*:358, 1989.

MANAGEMENT

NPs can encourage parents to obtain an early diagnosis and identify and access appropriate school programs. Some children qualify for special educational support. Parents need to review educational plans, provide an environment rich with experiences for children, and set realistic goals. They also need to act as advocates for their children during every school year, because classrooms and teachers change. Parents should work to minimize secondary problems such as poor self-esteem, hopelessness, or depression. Finally, parents need to be encouraged to avoid the use of the many unsubstantiated cures for learning disabilities. See Chapter 17 for further discussion of attention-deficit hyperactivity disorder and other cognitive-perceptual problems.

School Refusal (Phobia)

DESCRIPTION

School refusal or phobia is a form of anxiety. Children who refuse to attend school are generally suffering separation anxiety rather than a true phobia. Children request to stay home from school with a variety of physical complaints, including stomachaches, headaches,

dizziness, or fatigue, or a combination of these. The symptoms gradually improve as the day progresses and often disappear on weekends. Unexcused school absences peak in first grade and junior high school.

CLINICAL FINDINGS

The child's clinical examination, including the history, may point to school phobia and its cause:

- Frequent somatic complaints
- Sleep difficulties
- Parents' ambivalent feelings about children's attendance at school
- Difficult home situation; for example, children may try to stay at home, knowing that their mother drinks excessively when alone
- Recent loss

DIFFERENTIAL DIAGNOSIS

Somatic Illness

Physical examination and laboratory data need to rule out organic disease. Avoid overresponding with excessive diagnostic testing.

Depression

Isolation from peers, withdrawal from activities, sleep disturbances, erratic moods, poor self-esteem, and decreased activity level can indicate depression.

Attention-Deficit Hyperactivity Disorder and Conduct Disorder

The child who is unsuccessful in school, either academically or socially, may try to withdraw from the school environment.

Anxiety Disorder

This is the most common reason for school refusal, usually presenting as an inability to cope with anxiety, especially anxiety stemming from separation.

Sexual or Physical Abuse

Children who are being abused or who experience violence either at home or at school can feel intimidated to the point that they refuse to attend school.

MANAGEMENT

Intervention is generally successful when behavioral measures are combined with supportive counseling of parents. The physical complaints must be reasonably evaluated to rule out organic disease without excessive medical attention or diagnostic testing. Once the possibility of organic disease is set aside (or a plan is established to evaluate somatic problems), children must go to school. Generally, once they are at school, symptoms resolve.

- Support parents in getting children to school and insist on full attendance.
- Notify school personnel and encourage them to support and expect children's attendance and intervene to improve any situations related to children's anxiety.
- Referral for psychiatric care should be initiated immediately if no improvement occurs within 2 weeks (Van Buskirk, 1999).
- Assess home situation and identify issues that must be handled. Provide referrals as

needed for family and parent problems. These services may include counseling, social service, or other resources.

Recurrent Symptoms

DESCRIPTION

Complaints of recurrent symptoms such as headaches, abdominal pain, and limb pain are frequent in school-age children. There is no good medical explanation for these symptoms, but the frequency of complaints in school-age children suggests correlation with developmental factors. Children with recurrent symptoms often have parents with increased psychosocial problems and preoccupation with somatic complaints. Often, children get a great deal of attention for these symptoms.

CLINICAL FINDINGS

The clinical examination and history can include the following in children with recurrent symptoms:

- Vague and intermittent complaints of abdominal pain, headaches, nausea, or malaise but absence of significant findings on physical examination
- Normal function between episodes
- No objective findings such as vomiting, diarrhea, or constipation
- Family member with similar symptoms
- Stress in school or home environment (e.g., new social situation, school, teacher, examination, peer group conflict, moving, family illness or loss, parental pressure for achievement)

LABORATORY STUDIES

For discussion of abdominal symptoms, see Chapter 33.

DIFFERENTIAL DIAGNOSIS

The differential diagnosis includes insidious onset of a systemic problem. For chronic, recurrent abdominal pain, see Chapter 33. Consider irritable bowel syndrome, lactose intolerance, acid peptic disease, inflammatory bowel disease, sickle cell anemia, porphyria, hereditary angioedema, systemic lupus erythematosus, and dysmenorrhea in adolescent females. Consider the neurological conditions in the differential diagnosis of headaches. School refusal also needs to be considered.

MANAGEMENT

The following are keys to management of recurrent symptoms:

- Try not to "medicalize" the problem with a barrage of tests if the initial history and physical examination do not indicate systemic symptoms.
- Encourage child to keep a food or pain diary.
- Reassure child and expect normal participation in activities.
- Refer for mental health counseling if symptoms persist.
- Discuss coping strategies to deal with stressors.
- Discuss with family strategies that are supportive but that do not reinforce the illness behavior.

REFERENCES

Behrman R, Kliegman R, Arvin A: Nelson Textbook of Pediatrics, 15th ed. Philadelphia, WB Saunders, 1996.

Boyer E: Ready to learn: A mandate for the nation. Young Children 48:54–57, 1993.

Byrd R: School readiness: More than a summer's work. Contemp Pediatr 15:39–53, 1998.

Coleman W, Lindsay R: Making friends: Helping children develop interpersonal skills. Contemp Pediatr 15:111–129, 1998.

Dixon S, Stein M: Encounters With Children: Pediatric Behavior and Development. St. Louis, CV Mosby, 1992.

Dworkin P: Behavior during middle childhood: Developmental themes and clinical issues. Pediatr Ann 18:347–355, 1989.

Green M: Bright Futures: Guidelines for Health Supervision of Infants, Children, and Adolescents. Arlington, VA, National Center for Education in Maternal and Child Health, 1994.

Holaday B, Turner-Henson A. Harkins A, et al: Chronically ill children in self-care: Issues for pediatric nurses. Pediatr Health Care 7:256–263, 1993.

Kohlberg L: The Philosophy of Moral Development. San Francisco, Harper and Row, 1981.

Koster M: Self-care health behavior. Topics Clin Nursing April:29–40, 1983.

Levine M: Developmental and Behavioral Pediatrics. Philadelphia, WB Saunders, 1983.

Levine M, Rappaport L, Fenton T, et al: Neurodevelopmental readiness for adolescence: Studies of an assessment instrument for 9- to 14-year-old children. Dev Behavior Pediatr 9:181–188, 1988.

Schor E: Guiding the family of the school-aged child. Contemp Pediatr 15:75–93, 1998.

Tanner J: Neurodevelopmental variation in school-aged children. Contemp Therapy 21:499–506, 1995.

Van Buskirk D: School refusal. *In* Dershewitz R (ed): Ambulatory Pediatrics, 2nd ed. Philadelphia, JB Lippincott, 1999.

Wolraich M: Addressing behavior problems among school-aged children. Pediatr Rev 18:266–270, 1997.

Wright K: Anticipatory guidance: Developing a healthy sexuality. Pediatr Ann 26 (2 suppl):S142–S144, 1997.

Developmental Management of Adolescents

Linda Wildey and Judith Fisher

INTRODUCTION

Development from childhood to young adulthood is both a biological and a psychological process. *Puberty* is the term for the biological process that ultimately leads to fertility. *Adolescence* refers to the psychosocial and emotional transition from childhood to adulthood. This chapter focuses on the normal physical and psychosocial growth and development of adolescents. The common question on the mind of most adolescents is, "Am I normal?" Rapid change is the most characteristic trait of adolescents, and that change can create a tenuous sense of balance during this phase of development. Guidance and reassurance during well-child care are perhaps the most valuable services a health care provider can offer the adolescent.

DEVELOPMENTAL SURVEILLANCE PARAMETERS

The hormonal regulatory systems in the hypothalamus, pituitary, gonads, and adrenal glands undergo major changes between the prepubertal and adult states. Accompanying these changes are rapid growth in height and weight, development of secondary sex characteristics, and onset of fertility (Fig. 9-1; see Chapters 26 and 36). Limits of normal can be difficult to

define and are best understood as approximations rather than precise parameters. However, even though the timing (tempo) of adolescent development is variable, the sequence of events is orderly (Fig. 9-2).

The physical changes of puberty are accompanied by significant cognitive and psychosocial development that affects how adolescents view themselves and how the world views adolescents. Successful development in adolescence culminates in achievement of goals that can provide the basis for a healthy and productive adult life (see Table 9-1).

Physical Development

TANNER STAGES

Pubertal growth and maturation can be divided into five stages ranging from prepubertal (sexual maturity rating [SMR] of 1) to adult (SMR 5). These divisions are termed Tanner stages (Tanner, 1962) (Figs. 9-3 and 9-4). Pubertal changes occur on a continuum, with individual differences in sequence and tempo.

Female Stages

Females enter puberty earlier than males do and thus lose a year or so of the slow, but steady growth that males experience before the onset of puberty. Females also experience rapid

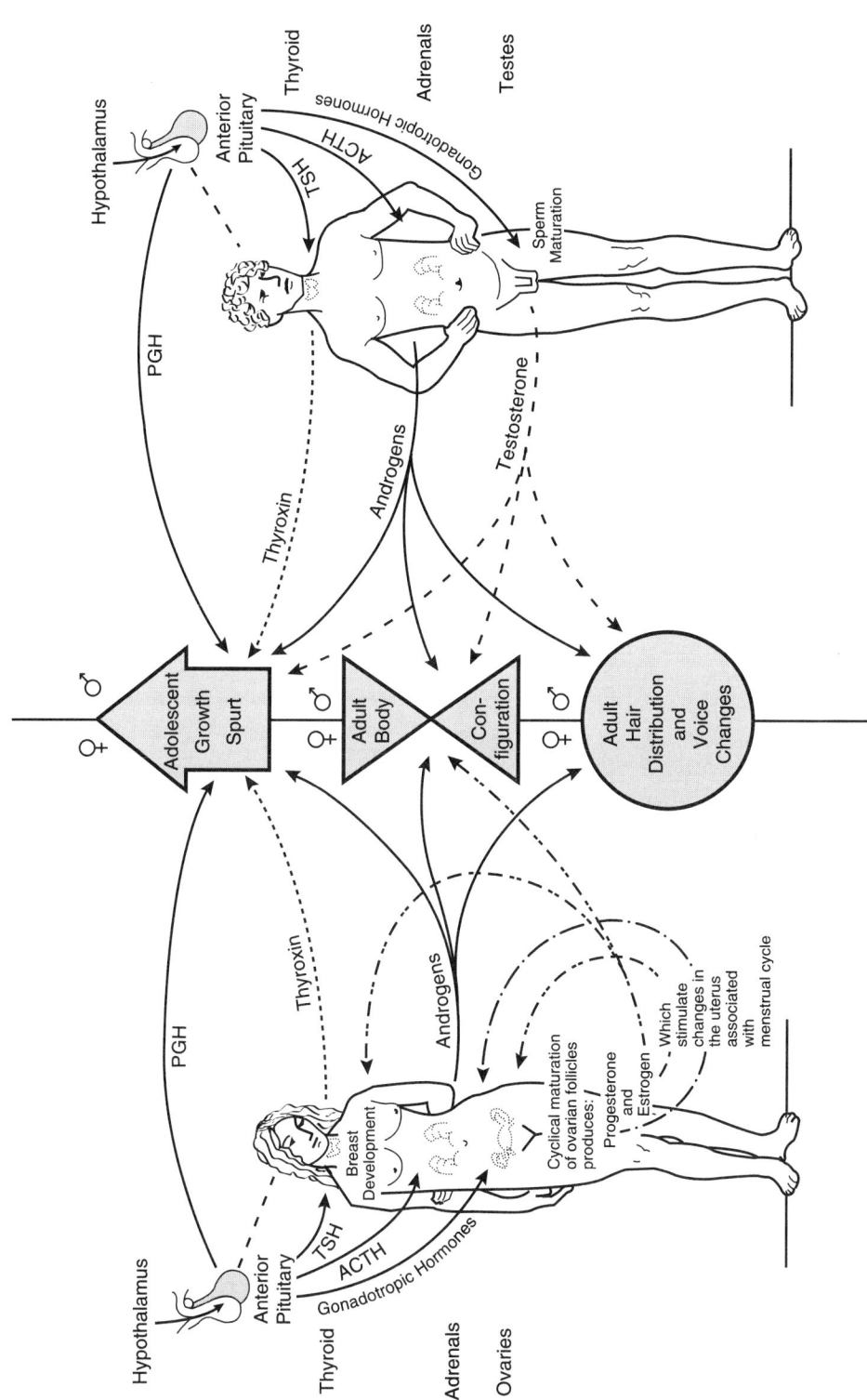

F I G U R E 9-1
The endocrine system at puberty. ACTH = adrenocorticotropic hormone; PGH = pituitary growth hormone; TSH = thyroid-stimulating hormone. (From Valadian I, Porter D: Physical Growth and Development From Conception to Maturity. Boston, Little, Brown, 1977.)

165

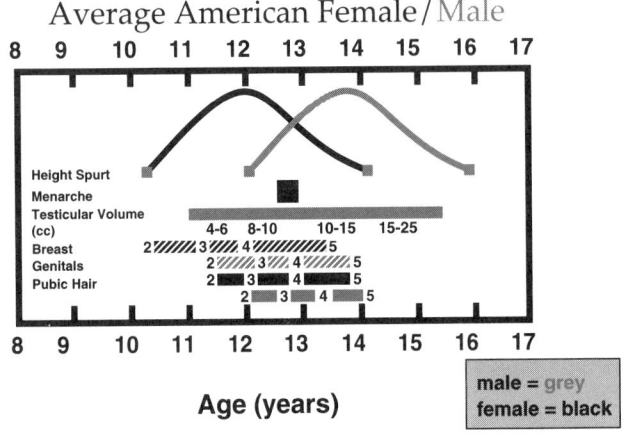

Average American Female / Male

Age (years)

male = grey
female = black

F I G U R E 9-2
Sequence of pubertal events. Breast, genital, and pubic hair development indicate Tanner stages 2 to 5. (From Division of Adolescent Medicine, Children's Hospital Medical Center, Cincinnati, OH, 1995.)

linear growth early in puberty and before menarche (SMR 2 to 3). The first pubertal change that occurs in females is internal, with the ovaries increasing in size. The first visible manifestation of puberty is usually breast budding (thelarche). Thelarche occurs, on average, at 11 years of age, with 95% of normal girls having initial breast development between 9 and 13 years of age.

Breast stage 1 is prepubertal; that is, no noticeable change is seen in the size of the breast. Stage 2 is the breast bud stage, in which a small mound is formed by elevation of the breast and papilla. The areolar diameter enlarges. Stage 3 is characterized by further enlargement of the breast and areola with no separation of their contours. Stage 4 involves a distinctive projection of the areola, with the papilla forming a secondary mound above the level of the breast. It is important to view the breast both anteriorly and laterally to appreciate this secondary mound. In stage 5, the breast is adult-like in appearance, the areola has recessed to the general contour of the breast, and the overall size of the breast is increased. Not all women complete SMR 5. The timing of onset of breast development in females has no relationship to breast size at the completion of puberty. Girls often have asymmetrical breasts and need assurance that breasts become more or less the same size within a few years after the onset of breast budding.

Most girls (85%) experience the develop-ment of breast buds approximately 6 months before the appearance of pubic hair (adrenarche or pubarche), which commences at about 11.5 years of age. However, some females have pubic hair before the development of breast buds. Pubic hair is included as a rating criterion but is less valid than other secondary sex characteristics in assessing sexual maturation because its appearance is related to adrenal rather than gonadal development and it is not related to thelarche.

In pubic hair stage 1, which is referred to as prepubertal or child-like in appearance, no pubic hair is present. Stage 2 is heralded by the first appearance of sexual hair. At this stage, pubic hair is sparse, long, slightly pigmented, downy, straight or only slightly curled, and primarily located along the labia. In stage 3 the hair is coarser, darker, and more curled. The hair spreads over the middle of the pubic bone. In stage 4 the hair is adult-like in appearance but not in distribution. The hair does not extend onto the thighs. Stage 5 hair is adult-like in appearance and extends onto the thighs. Some extension of growth of hair in the midline in the shape of a broad-based triangle is noted. Generally, females reach pubic hair stage 5 before reaching breast stage 5.

Changes in the body composition of females also occur during puberty. The female body shape changes (to the glee or chagrin of teenagers) as girls progress through puberty; broadening of the shoulders, hips, and thighs becomes

T A B L E 9-1

Adolescent Development and Related Anticipatory Guidance

AREA OF DEVELOPMENT	ANTICIPATORY GUIDANCE
PHYSICAL 1. Experience growth from prepubescence to sexual maturity 2. Reach adult parameters of height and physical growth by late adolescence 3. Become comfortable with one's body	1. Teach child about body functions (e.g., menstruation, nocturnal emissions) of both sexes 2. Provide prevention counseling regarding substance abuse, safety, and unintentional injuries (e.g., bicycle helmet use, seat belts, gun storage) 3. Offer reassurance that physical findings are normal. Explain what to expect; listen to adolescents' concerns. Encourage sports participation and body fitness
COGNITIVE 1. Move from concrete thinking to ability to reason abstractly 2. Develop personal value system and moral integrity	1. Emphasize value of successful completion of school 2. Engage adolescent in conversation, explain procedures, and answer questions 3. Encourage discussion of what the adolescent feels is important and what the adolescent finds of value 4. Help the adolescent develop skills in conflict resolution and avoidance 5. Discuss respect for rights, needs, and opinions of others
PSYCHOSOCIAL 1. Establish independence from parents 2. Develop sense of self-identity 3. Create new relationships with peers and other adults	1. Explain to parents an adolescent's need for privacy and that not joining in all family activities is not a sign of rejection 2. Discuss the notion that increased independence also requires increased responsibility 3. Encourage adolescents to take responsibility for their own health care 4. Encourage adolescent to take on new challenges. Discuss plans for the future (e.g., school, work, family) 5. Discuss importance of activities with peers. Identify healthy ways to be part of a group 6. Encourage the adolescent to participate in community activities 7. Provide information and opportunity to discuss questions regarding sexuality, how to differentiate between "love'" and "infatuation," how to be sexually responsible, and protect against pregnancy and sexually transmitted diseases

apparent. Girls experience a continuous increase in body fat during puberty. They enter puberty with approximately 80% lean body weight and 20% body fat. By the time puberty ends, lean body mass drops to 75%. Body fat is an important mediator for the onset of menstruation and regular ovulatory cycles.

The height spurt occurs relatively early in the female pubertal sequence. It usually begins shortly after the onset of breast budding and reaches its peak about a year later. Most girls experience peak height velocity (PHV) at about SMR 3. PHV is generally reached between ages 11 and 12 and is completed by age 13. Early developers may experience a height spurt between ages 9 and 10, whereas late developers may not experience a height spurt until between the ages of 13 and 14. Final height is determined by the amount of bone growth at the epiphyses of the long bones. Growth stops when hormonal factors shut down the epiphyseal plates.

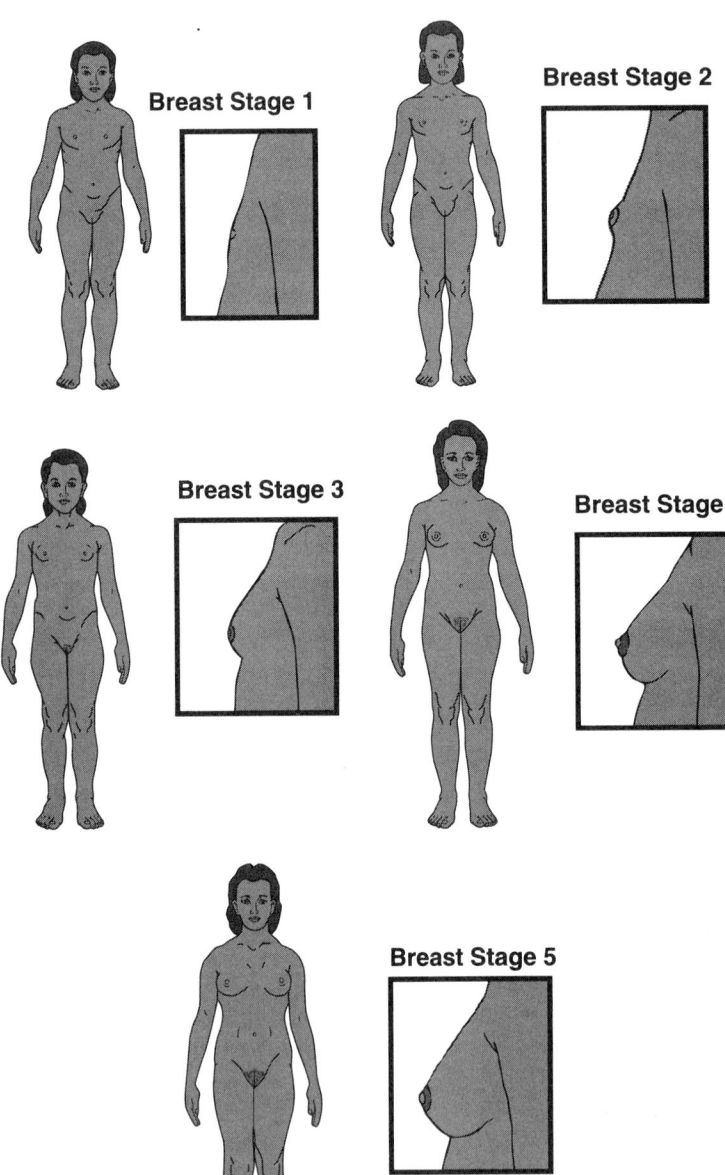

Breast Stage 1

Breast Stage 2

Breast Stage 3

Breast Stage 4

Breast Stage 5

F I G U R E 9-3
Tanner stages: Female. (From Division of Adolescent Medicine, Children's Hospital Medical Center, Cincinnati, OH, 1995.)

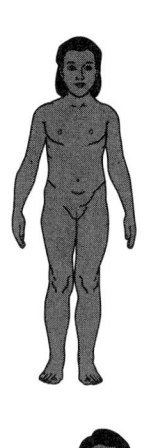
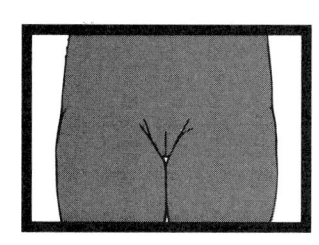

Pubic Hair Stage 1

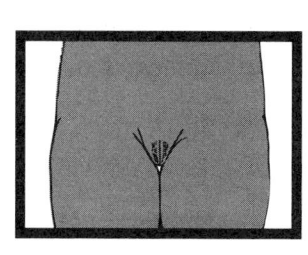

Pubic Hair Stage 2

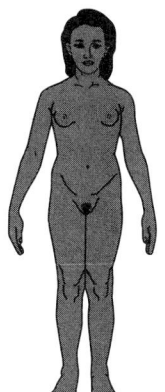
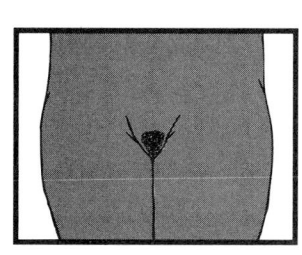

Pubic Hair Stage 3

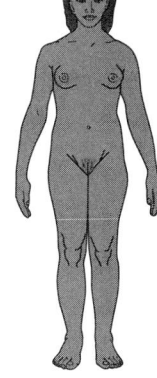
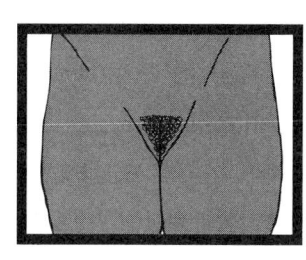
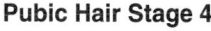

Pubic Hair Stage 4

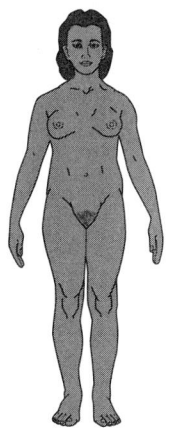
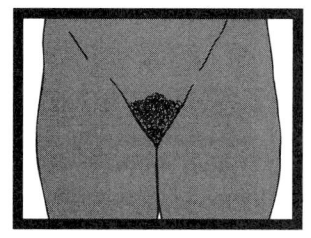

Pubic Hair Stage 5

FIGURE 9-3
Continued

169

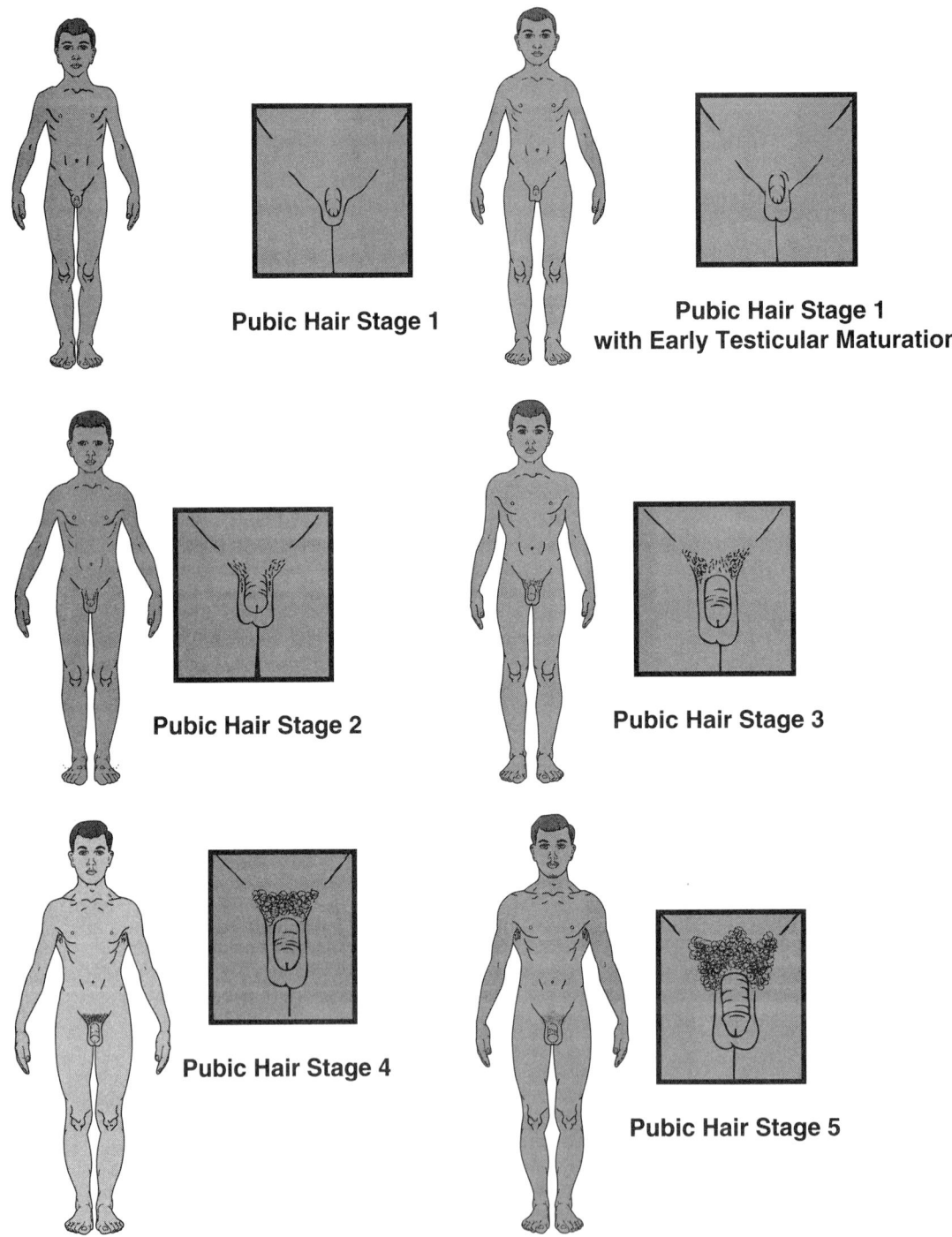

Pubic Hair Stage 1

**Pubic Hair Stage 1
with Early Testicular Maturation**

Pubic Hair Stage 2

Pubic Hair Stage 3

Pubic Hair Stage 4

Pubic Hair Stage 5

F I G U R E 9-4
Tanner stages: Male. (From Division of Adolescent Medicine, Children's Hospital Medical Center, Cincinnati, OH, 1995.)

One of the most significant events for adolescent females is their first period (menarche). The average age of menarche is 12.5 years, with more than 95% of girls experiencing menarche between 10.5 and 14.5 years of age. The mean age of menarche is highly dependent on ethnic, socioeconomic, nutritional, and to a lesser extent, the athletic activity of the female (Cameron, 1996). Menarche generally occurs 1.5 to 2.5 years after thelarche. An average of 17% of body fat is generally needed for menarche, and about 22% is needed to initiate and maintain regular ovulatory cycles. It may be 18 to 24 months after menarche before females establish regular ovulatory cycles.

Male Stages

The earliest pubertal body change in males is growth of the testes, followed by pubic hair development, elongation and widening of the penis, and finally rapid growth in height. Although the age for these changes may vary, testicular enlargement generally precedes these other events. If it does not, the nurse practitioner (NP) must consider whether the youngster is taking exogenous anabolic steroids.

Growth of the testes occurs approximately 6 months before the development of pubic hair in most males. Testicular growth can be directly assessed by palpation of the testes in the scrotum and comparison of their size with a standardized orchiometer. Self-assessment is generally reliable, and adolescent males can be asked to evaluate their own level of development if provided with standards against which to compare themselves. In stage 1, the penis, testes, and scrotum are child-like in size. A prepubertal testis is generally less than 4 ml in volume and less than 2.5 cm in greatest diameter. Stage 2 involves enlargement of the scrotum and testes, but the penis usually does not enlarge. The scrotal skin reddens. In stage 3, further growth of the testes and scrotum occurs, with enlargement of the penis, mostly in length. Stage 4 is characterized by further growth of the testes (10 to 15 ml) and scrotum. The penis increases in size, especially in width, because of growth of the corpora cavernosa in response to testosterone. In stage 5, genitals are adult-like in size. Growth of the penis is generally complete before full development of the testes or pubic hair.

Once puberty begins, the left testis generally hangs lower than the right. Varicocele, or enlarged veins palpable in the scrotum, may develop at sexual maturity and are not cause for alarm unless a discrepancy in testicular size is noted on examination. Spermarche is the first release of spermatozoa and generally occurs in midpuberty at a mean age of 13.5 to 14.5 years. However, it can occur at any stage of development from SMR 2 to 5.

Pubic hair development in males occurs in the same stages as in females. Pubic hair stage 1 is considered prepubertal, and no hair is visible. Stage 2 involves sparse growth of fine, downy hair along the base of the penis. In stage 3, the hair is darker, coarser, and curlier and extends over the middle of the pubic bone. In stage 4, the hair is adult-like in appearance but does not extend to the thighs. In stage 5, the hair is adult-like in appearance and distribution and may extend toward the umbilicus.

Along with changes in testicular size and pubic hair growth, development of axillary and facial hair occurs. The hair changes should not, however, be used as a parameter for assessing pubertal maturation related to changes in the endocrine system. Axillary hair generally does not appear before SMR 4 pubic hair. Facial hair appears only after SMR 4 pubic hair and does so in an ordered sequence. It starts at the outer corners of the upper lip and moves inward, then appears on the upper parts of the cheeks and middle of the lower lip, and finally grows along the sides and lower border of the chin. The extent of body hair is determined to a large extent by genetic factors. Body hair develops gradually after facial hair.

The PHV for males tends to occur late in middle puberty to early in late puberty. Boys generally lag about 2 years behind girls, but the height spurt can begin as early as 10.5 years or as late as 16 years. One fifth of normal adolescent males do not reach their PHV until SMR 5. Males can continue to grow, although minimally, well beyond their teenage years. The most outstanding feature of this stage of physical development is the male's increasing strength caused by an increase in muscle mass. Males develop the ability to endure prolonged periods of physical labor. Change in the male voice coincides with the PHV. In contrast to females, males experience progressive loss in the relative amount of body fat through puberty.

Some changes associated with puberty may be unwelcome. For males, approximately half the population experiences a transient enlargement of breast tissue called gynecomastia. Gynecomastia generally lasts 12 to 18 months and resolves completely in nearly all cases by late puberty. However, in a small percentage of males, some palpable breast tissue may persist. Acne starts in early puberty, and by midpuberty many males have moderate to severe acne, which becomes somewhat worse by the end of puberty. In cases of persistent gynecomastia or severe acne, the history should include questions to the patient regarding the use of alcohol, marijuana, and anabolic steroids, all of which can exacerbate these conditions.

HORMONAL EFFECTS ON EMOTIONS

Hormones present during puberty cause emotional as well as physical changes. As with physical growth and development, emotional changes appear differently in males than in females. Some males may experience an association between an increase in testosterone and sad and anxious affects, as well as acting out, aggressive behavior, and sexual activity.

Some emotional changes that occur in males are not directly associated with hormonal changes. Research has shown that boys with adult-like physiques are given more leadership roles, are more proficient in sports, are perceived as more attractive and smarter than their peers, and are more popular than others in their age group. In general, they also demonstrate high self-esteem in early adolescence. Late-maturing boys who are short and child-like in appearance until 15 or older tend to show more personal and social maladjustment over the entire course of adolescence. They tend to be insecure, suggestible, and vulnerable to peer pressure. Members of this group may be seen as weak, immature, and often less competent than average. Males, as they progress through puberty, typically develop a more positive self-

image and mood, whereas females feel a diminished sense of attractiveness as their bodies mature. Boys tend to be more satisfied with their body image and often want to gain weight, whereas girls are more likely to express dissatisfaction with changes in their body and want to lose weight. In one study, 40% of 9- to 10-year-old girls were trying to lose weight (Schreiber et al., 1996).

The emotional affect and behavior of pubescent females differ in other ways from those of boys. Early-maturing girls have more problems in adaptation than do girls who are late maturing (Ge et al., 1996). Often, these early bloomers get "bumped up" to an older group of peers and become the objects of sexual attention from older males. The developing body of early-maturing females may not match their chronological age or emotional maturity. For instance, a female fifth grader who is as tall as her teacher stands out from her peers. This difference can influence her behavior and place some females at risk for early sexual involvement, smoking, and drinking.

Psychosocial Development

PRINCIPLES OF ADOLESCENT PSYCHOSOCIAL DEVELOPMENT

Cognitive, emotional, and psychosocial developmental changes accompany the physical development of adolescence. Although each child develops in a unique fashion, all adolescents have specific psychosocial developmental milestones to achieve during the transition from childhood to adulthood. These milestones include

- Feeling a sense of belonging in a valued group
- Acquiring skills and mastering tasks that are important to the valued group
- Developing a sense of self-worth
- Developing at least one reliable relationship with another

A wide variety of normal behavior characterizes the process of psychosocial development. Three general principles may be used to understand the changes seen in adolescent development:

- Transition is continuous and generally smooth.
- Disruptive family conflict is not the norm.
- The quality of thinking changes from concrete to formal operational thinking.

TRANSITION IS SMOOTH. The first principle of adolescent psychosocial development is that the transition from adolescence to adulthood is continuous and generally smooth. A commonly held myth is that adolescence is a period of "storm and stress." This view was originally described by G. Stanley Hall in 1904 (Hall, 1904). Although his argument was not based on research, his ideas continue to be popular and influential today. It is important to remember that this period of development is only one of many transitional phases in life and may not be a difficult period for many.

FAMILY RELATIONSHIPS. The second principle of adolescent psychosocial development is that the biological, cognitive, and emotional changes experienced by adolescents prompt a reworking of family relationships. Some degree of adolescent-parent conflict is to be expected because of this reworking of relationships, but disruptive family conflict is not the norm. Despite societal changes, mundane, everyday issues such as what clothes to wear, hairstyles, household chores, curfew, and friends continue to be the usual sources of parent-adolescent conflict. It may also help to remind parents that verbal debate, or "arguing," is a normal behavior of teens that reflects their use of more abstract thinking skills. It is a way of engaging parents. However, the parent should not become too deeply engaged because the adolescent rarely is. The "storms" tend to blow over fairly quickly. The family should not be experiencing one crisis after another. If family crises are the norm, one should be concerned. When true turmoil exists, it usually represents psychopathology and will not be simply "outgrown." Careful assessment and treatment are required. Behavior that results in negative consequences is cause for concern (e.g., red hair dye grows out but being expelled from school has long-term consequences).

COGNITIVE CHANGES. The third principle of adolescent psychosocial development reflects change in cognitive processes. Adolescents develop what is referred to as formal operational thinking, which is characterized by the use of propositional thinking and abstract reasoning. The principal difference between concrete and formal operational stage thinking is the ability "to reason in terms of verbally stated hypotheses" rather than in terms of concrete objects and their manipulation. In early adolescence, thinking tends to be very concrete. The classic example is an adolescent who when asked, "Are you sexually active?" responds, "No, I just lie there." Or when asked, "What brings you here to see me today?" answers, "The bus."

Younger children think in concrete fashion. Around the age of 14 and throughout adolescence, most teenagers acquire increasing sophistication in abstract thought. They learn to conceptualize about past and future events and to relate actions to consequences. During this process, adolescents begin to

- Consider values. The ones they challenge most are those with which they are most familiar (e.g., in the past they always attended church on Sundays or always went to their grandmother's for Sunday dinner, but now they do not want to).
- Understand concepts of good and evil and understand human nature (e.g., not all authority figures are good people).
- Be aware of contradictions between what is said and what is done (e.g., parents may tell their children not to smoke or drink even though they do, or they may tell them to wear their seat belts although they do not).
- Understand the concept of time (past, present, future) and begin thinking about what they will be doing in the future (e.g., college, technical school, job, marriage, and family).

Although most teenagers become able to translate experiences into abstract ideas and think about the consequences of actions, approximately one third do not achieve more fully sophisticated thinking abilities even as adults.

EGOCENTRISM OF ADOLESCENTS

Changes in the quality of adolescent thinking coupled with physical and emotional changes give rise to a form of egocentrism. This change may result in a rather self-centered, but not necessarily selfish view of the world. Four major types of egocentrism that even adults exhibit at times are recognized:

- Imaginary audience: Everyone is thinking about them.
- Personal fable: They are special.
- Overthinking: They make things more complicated than they are.
- Apparent hypocrisy: Rules apply differently to them than to others.

IMAGINARY AUDIENCE. Abstract thinking allows teenagers to wonder what others are thinking about. At the same time, adolescents are obsessed by the physical changes brought about by puberty. These changes and their new thinking abilities create the notion that everyone is thinking about the same thing that they are (i.e., them). Teenagers may believe that one can read minds and know what others are thinking. For example, a boy who goes to the drugstore to purchase a condom may feel that he is "on stage," the object of everyone's scrutiny. An adolescent wearing orthopedic braces may think that everyone is staring at him. A young girl who has a pimple on her nose may feel that it is the first thing everyone sees when they look at her.

PERSONAL FABLE. The second type of egocentrism is the personal fable. If everyone is watching you and thinking about you (thanks to the imaginary audience), you must be someone special. The personal fable is the concept that the laws of nature do not apply to oneself and that one's thoughts and feelings are totally unique. Common examples include adolescents who believe that they will never grow old, cannot get pregnant (especially the first time), cannot get a sexually transmitted infection despite engaging in unprotected intercourse, or will not suffer long-term consequences from substance use.

OVERTHINKING. Overthinking involves making things more complicated than they need to be. An example might be an adolescent who attributes complicated motives to simple oversights (e.g., an adolescent boy who thinks that his parents would not have divorced if only he had helped more with the chores around the

house or an adolescent girl who breaks up with her boyfriend because she assumes that he does not like her because he did not compliment her on her new red dress).

APPARENT HYPOCRISY. Apparent hypocrisy is the notion that rules apply differently to adolescents than they do to others. For example, an adolescent girl may believe that she should have free access to her parent's clothes and electronic equipment (such as the stereo or home computer), whereas her parents entering her room to borrow a tape constitutes an invasion of privacy.

DEVELOPMENTAL SCREENING AND ASSESSMENT

Throughout infancy and the preschool and school years, the focus of the health-care visit is always clearly the parent or caregiver and the child as a unit. This dyad changes with adolescence. Teenagers must be evaluated independently of their parents, and discussions about developmental issues occur with the adolescents themselves. Nonetheless, parents remain concerned and should ideally be involved in their child's health care. Preserving confidentiality with the teenager while acknowledging the importance of parents to the child's development is essential. As at other developmental stages of childhood, parents are also changing in response to the adolescent's pressure on the family. Parents, too, need advice, support, and encouragement.

Physical Growth Assessment

Adolescents should have height, weight, and blood pressure measured at each health maintenance visit. Assessment of the growth trajectory with grids to identify growth norms is essential. Additionally, the Tanner stage for teenagers should be recorded at each visit to evaluate progression of the pubertal changes initiated by the endocrine system. Scoliosis may develop rapidly at this age. Gynecomastia in boys should be noted. The thyroid gland should be palpated because goiter may appear in this age group. Additionally, the teen should be questioned about attitudes regarding physical growth and development. Dissatisfaction with body appearance might warrant further probing to elicit unhealthy behavior (e.g., bingeing and purging, steroid use).

Cognitive Development

The cognitive development of young teenagers may not have reached the formal operational stage yet. Thus they do best in an interview situation in which they are asked direct questions rather than broad, open-ended questions such as, "Tell me how school is going for you." Discussions with adolescents in their later years follow a more adult pattern. Assessment should include questions about school attendance, school performance, and educational or career goals. Successful school performance is an important predictor for adolescent well-being. Children who are behind a grade have a 20 to 30% greater chance of dropping out of school. School failure could be viewed as "failure to thrive in adolescence" (Reiff, 1998). Chronic absenteeism, class skipping, and other types of school avoidance may indicate an underlying mental health problem and should be assessed in depth. Objective assessment of cognitive development, as with school-aged children, requires formal psychological testing, which is best done through schools.

Psychosocial Development

Key areas to assess in relation to psychosocial development include adolescents' emerging independence from family, relationships with peers, and goals for the future (an area that older teenagers should address more specifically than younger adolescents).

Adolescents should be interviewed about school, family, and peer relationships; exposure to violence or abuse in their home or community; mental health issues such as mood, anger problems, or suicidal ideation; concerns about sexuality; and involvement in risk behavior such as tobacco, alcohol, and prescription or street drug use and sexual activity (see Chapter 2). The American Medical Association has developed a thorough interview format for teens in their published *AMA Guidelines for Adolescent Preventive Services (GAPS)* program (Elster &

Kuznets, 1994). Questionnaires used to identify adolescent strengths have also been created by the Search Institute and have been used by communities to enhance adolescent self-concept (see Chapter 18).

Parent Assessment

GAPS (Elster & Kuznets, 1994) also offers recommendations for health guidance for parents. The parent interview should occur on three occasions during adolescence: early, middle, and late. The interview should consist of parents' concerns about adolescents relating to

• Health problems
• Physical development
• Psychosocial development
• Parenting issues
• Changing family structures

If problems exist in the parent's view or a discrepancy and potential conflict emerge in the interviews, the NP should bring the teen and parent together to clarify the concern and offer counseling.

INTERVENTION BY ADOLESCENT STAGE

One simple way to understand adolescence is to divide it into three psychosocial developmental phases: early, 11 to 14 years old or junior high school; middle, 15 to 17 years old or high school; and late, 18 to 21 years old or college, work, or vocational–technical school.

Each phase is characterized by certain behavior. Understanding such behavior can assist in identifying behavior of concern to the adolescent or family. Within each developmental phase, adolescents deal with issues of autonomy, body image, peer group involvement, and identity development.

Early Adolescence (11 to 14 Years)

PARAMETERS OF NORMAL DEVELOPMENT

Young adolescents may put away the objects of childhood, yet not be a part of an adolescent subculture. They may experience loneliness as they begin to renegotiate relationships with parents and other significant adults and develop more intimate contacts with their peers.

Wide mood swings—from euphoria to sadness—can occur within a matter of minutes. Normative fluctuations of mood are linked to adolescent developmental processes and are characterized by their transient nature, commonly measured in hours or days. These fluctuations can and should be distinguished from the unremitting, long-standing mood and behavior changes of serious depressive disorders. Teenagers may prefer to spend more time with friends than with family. At this stage they are antiadult and prefer that no one know that they have a parent! This behavior is a normal and healthy step toward maturity and a first step toward independence. One way of demonstrating independence is to challenge parental authority. The adolescent may become more argumentative and disobedient, refuse to do chores, and want to renegotiate rules (e.g., curfews, allowance, household responsibilities).

During this period, adolescents become extremely conscious of their bodies as they adjust to the physical changes they are experiencing. They begin to spend more time in front of the mirror ("increased mirror time") combing their hair, checking their skin, and putting on makeup. Clothes and appearance become more important for all teenagers in this group, including those with a developmental delay or chronic handicap.

The most important question for an early adolescent is, "Am I normal?" Health care providers for adolescents must never lose sight of this concern. Early adolescents often use their friends as the measure by which they determine standards of normal appearance. They become overly sensitive and critical of their own appearance, certain they are too tall, too short, too fat, too thin, too developed, or not developed enough. NPs can allay anxiety during an adolescent's examination by affirming normalcy rather than using a noncommittal "hmmm" or silence.

The onset of secondary sex characteristics increases anxieties about menstruation, wet dreams, masturbation, and size of the breasts or penis. This point is an opportune time to dispel myths, such as masturbation causes blindness and acne, and to provide anticipatory guidance (e.g., a premenarchal girl often has vaginal leukorrhea, which is generally a clear, mucoid discharge). Same-sex friendships occur, usually with one best friend. These strong friendships may lead to fleeting same-sex experimentation and the further development of a sexual identity. Contact with the opposite sex is usually in groups (e.g., middle school dances with boys on one side of the gym and girls on the opposite side). The peer group serves the purpose of aiding continued identity development.

The "imaginary audience" contributes to the adolescent's feeling of being on stage. As their thinking abilities develop, teenagers daydream frequently. Parents and teachers need to be reminded that daydreaming is cognitive work for adolescents and that they need time to participate in this activity.

Early adolescents set idealistic goals that change frequently. One day they want to be an engineer and the next day a pilot or a parent who stays home to raise children. Typically, these adolescents experience a drop in academic performance in junior high school, which is related to motivation rather than ability. Much of adolescents' time is used in the development of new friendships as a greater number of opportunities become possible.

Adolescents have a desire for greater privacy. They often spend more time in their room alone listening to music or talking on the phone. They magnify their problems and believe that no one could possibly understand what they are feeling.

Early adolescents begin to develop their own value system. They may try value systems other than the one that they have learned from their family, often leaving family members befuddled or even threatened. However, once adolescence is complete, young adults often have a modified value system very similar to the one with which they grew up.

Sexual feelings emerge, and behavior includes masturbating, telling dirty jokes, making lewd remarks to others, demonstrating interest in watching explicit sexual scenes in the media, or looking at magazines of nude individuals. The type of sexual experimentation may vary greatly, depending on the adolescent's subculture. For example, by this age some teenagers have already experienced sexual intercourse or pregnancy.

DEVELOPMENTAL ANTICIPATORY GUIDANCE

Anticipatory guidance should be an individualized discussion with teenagers that helps them understand, respond to, and take responsibility for their own behavior and development. Separate discussions need to be conducted with parents to help them understand and support their child's maturation and independence. Some discussion points are outlined here. These topics are not all-inclusive, nor are they intended to be covered exhaustively at each visit. They can be used by the NP to apply developmental concepts in everyday living. If problems emerge from discussions in these areas, the NP is referred to the appropriate chapter for ideas for assessment and management (e.g., sexuality problems are discussed in Chapter 20).

Physical and Sexual Development

- Rapid physical growth: Knowing what to expect and understanding the implications of growth (e.g., for injury) help adolescents become more comfortable with their bodies.
- Sexuality: Discussion should include
  - Menstruation and its management.
  - Masturbation and nocturnal emissions.
  - Pubertal development of the opposite sex.
  - Anticipated sexual changes.
  - Abstinence counseling.
  - Protection against sexually transmitted diseases and pregnancy.

Cognitive Growth

- Discuss with the adolescent how meeting academic responsibilities is a priority activity that needs to be integrated with other activities.

Psychosocial and Emotional Growth

- Family interaction: Not joining the family for all activities should not be interpreted by parents as rejection of the family.
- Feelings: Learning to identify feelings is the first step in understanding that "feelings" influence body processes.
- Peers: Peer interaction is important for all teenagers.
- Independence and responsibility: Developing increased independence as well as accepting responsibilities at home and school and in the community are essential to maturation.
- Privacy: Some privacy within the home should be expected.

Self-care

- Accident prevention: Correct and consistent use of helmets, seat belts, and proper sports equipment should be taught and encouraged.
- Weapons: Access to guns and other weapons should be restricted, with emphasis on safety and responsibility.
- Abusive behavior: Counseling should be provided on
  - Avoiding gang involvement.
  - Preventing the use of drugs, cigarettes, and alcohol.
  - Stopping substance use for those who are using.
  - Avoiding date rape or other abusive relationships.

Middle Adolescence (15 to 17 Years)

PARAMETERS OF NORMAL DEVELOPMENT

Parental conflict peaks as middle adolescents argue and renegotiate issues such as curfew, allowance, going to parties or movies, and dating. Physical development is nearing completion. Middle adolescents have less concern about body changes but increased interest in making themselves more attractive. As body attractiveness increases in importance, teenagers spend more time with hairstyles, clothes, and for some, activities to build muscle mass. Teenagers with apparent handicaps have no less concern about their body image and participate in the same activities to improve their appearance.

Middle adolescents defy the limits of their bodies, and many have periods of excessive physical activity followed by periods of lethargy. They cannot seem to find the energy to get out of bed on the weekends to help the family with chores, but if one of their friends asks them to wash cars to raise money for a local charity, they are out the door with lightning speed.

Middle adolescence is the essence of adolescence and its subculture. Picture in your mind's eye what typical adolescents look like and how they behave (e.g., jocks, nerds, punkers, druggies). What are they wearing? How do they act? What language are they using to communicate to adults and to one another? The picture that probably comes to mind is that of a middle adolescent. Middle adolescents stand out for their unique appearance. Peer group involvement is intense and includes the establishment of a dress code, communication style, and code of conduct. They tend to be more nonadult than antiadult, a characteristic of early adolescents. By this time, more than twice as much of adolescents' time is spent with peers as with adults. The need for peer contact is no less important for teenagers with developmental disabilities, chronic handicaps, or both. However, peer involvement may be more limited for this group for any number of reasons (e.g., ostracism by the peer group, parental overprotectiveness, lack of social skills).

Sexual drive emerges, and middle adolescents begin to explore their ability to attract a partner. Dating activity and sexual experimentation and intercourse are beginning at younger ages. Frequently, physical urges precede emotional maturity, and social pressure to experiment with sex is great. Without question, the adolescents of today are much more sexually tolerant than their predecessors. They are more sexually active than their parents were at the same age, and may be more sexually active than adolescents of any earlier time, including their older siblings. Ambivalence about desire for pregnancy is not uncommon, especially among adolescents lacking clear future goals.

Intellectual ability and creativity increase in middle adolescents. They demonstrate increased concern with neighborhood issues and certain societal issues, such as war or peace and the environment.

Because of the developing egocentrism and the concept of personal fable, with feelings of omnipotence, invulnerability, and immortality, risk taking and behavioral experimentation intensify. This stage may include smoking, use of alcohol, sexual activity, or drinking and driving.

DEVELOPMENTAL ANTICIPATORY GUIDANCE

Physical and Sexual Development

- Physical growth: Rapid growth and increasing skill allow adolescents to engage in a wider variety of activities.
  - Recommend fitness and sports activities; discuss the dangers of performance-enhancing drugs.
  - Recommend involvement in other activities (e.g., clubs, hobbies).
  - Discuss nutrition and the relationship between good nutrition and health and a positive body image.
- Sexuality: Provide discussion and counseling about
  - Implications of sexual intercourse.
  - Postponement of coitus or the choice of abstinence.
  - Prevention of sexually transmitted diseases.
  - Birth control.
  - Breast or testicular self-examination.

Cognitive Growth

- Discuss the importance of completing schooling and making plans for the future.
- Acknowledge and validate more abstract reasoning.

Psychosocial and Emotional Growth

- Family interactions:
  - Families should set reasonable limits for adolescents' behavior.

○ Families need to show interest in teenagers' work, interests, and activities.
- Peers: Adolescents should establish relationships with peers based on mutual respect, not promiscuous behavior.
- Independence and responsibility: Discuss how the adolescent is
  ○ Learning to constructively resolve conflicts and manage feelings of anger.
  ○ Learning to identify symptoms of stress.

Self-care

- Accident prevention: Encourage correct and consistent use of helmets, seat belts, and proper sports equipment.
- Weapons: Access to guns and other weapons should be restricted, with emphasis on safety and responsibility.
- Abusive behavior: Counseling should be provided on
  ○ Avoiding gang involvement.
  ○ Preventing the use of drugs, cigarettes, and alcohol.
  ○ Stopping substance use for those who are using.
  ○ Avoiding date rape and other abusive peer relationships.

Late Adolescence (18 to 21 Years)

PARAMETERS OF NORMAL DEVELOPMENT

Many late adolescents are preparing for high school graduation or entry to college. They are working, entering the military, marrying, or participating in a vocational or technical training program. These are all examples of normal behavioral autonomy. This period of late adolescence is a time when decisions are made about how to contribute to society as a responsible adult.

By now, adolescents usually relate to the family as adults. Relationships with parents and family are gradually renegotiated to a more adult-adult basis. The role of the parent during late adolescence should be one of support. By the end of late adolescence, this status has optimally progressed to autonomy for adolescents in the context of continuing strong affectional ties to the family.

Late adolescents have attained an adult level of reasoning skills. They are generally capable of understanding the consequences of their actions and behavior and can make very complex and sophisticated judgments about human relationships. They no longer base their judgments about people on overt behavior but have a good understanding of inner motivations, including multiple determinants of an action. Of course, this most mature level of cognition is not used by teenagers or adults all the time, and some never reach this level of cognitive maturity.

A substantial number of late adolescents have established their sexuality and entered into an intimate, committed partner relationship. Selection of a partner is based more on individual preferences and less on the peer group's values.

Much of the final shaping of identity centers on adolescents' perceptions of their future options as adults. Among contemporary late adolescents, roughly half attend college and the other half enter the adult world of work. In many significant ways, the years in college offer a "moratorium," a time to engage in further consolidation of identity. College life offers both maximal autonomy and a structured, supportive environment in which to complete developmental tasks in what could be considered a prolonged adolescence. Those adolescents who enter the work force immediately out of high school have quite different tasks and experiences. Their identity may be consolidated earlier because they do not have the added time and supportive structures of the college experience to delay facing the issues of earning a living, forming a family, and accepting other adult responsibilities. For adolescents who are unsuccessful in the educational system or the workplace (underemployed or unemployed), identity may be established by joining peers in gangs or by becoming socially isolated, both of which have negative implications for achieving healthy adult roles.

DEVELOPMENTAL ANTICIPATORY GUIDANCE

Physical and Sexual Development

- Physical growth: Exercise, nutrition, and rest are important to optimal physical growth.

- Sexuality: Discussion and counseling should be provided about
  - Implications of sexual activity. Sexual feelings for the same or opposite sex should be discussed with a trusted adult or health professional.
  - Postponement of coitus or the choice of abstinence.
  - Prevention of sexually transmitted diseases.
  - Birth control.
  - Breast or testicular self-examination.

Cognitive Growth

- Discuss the importance of completing academic work.
- Validate choices made to achieve positive future goals and plan for the future—college, vocational training, military, and job or career.

Psychosocial and Emotional Growth

- Family interactions:
  - Closer relationships with and an interest in the family should be re-emerging.
  - Families need to be supportive of independence efforts.
- Peers:
  - Intimate relationships are established.
  - Respect for the rights, needs, and views of others is a measure of maturity.
- Independence and responsibility: Adolescents should be encouraged to
  - Take on new challenges that increase self-confidence.
  - Identify talents and interests to be pursued.
  - Continue to clarify values and beliefs. Ethical and behavioral role modeling behavior is valued.
  - Develop skills in conflict avoidance; resolution reflects cognitive growth and maturity.
  - Learn to manage stress.
  - Find a balance between job and school or vocational training.

Self-care

- Accident prevention: Encourage correct and consistent use of helmets, seat belts, and proper sports equipment.
- Weapons: Access to guns and other weapons should be restricted, with an emphasis on safety and responsibility.
- Abusive behavior: Counseling should be provided on
  - Avoiding gang involvement.
  - Preventing the use and selling of drugs, cigarettes, and alcohol.
  - Stopping substance use for those who are using.
  - Avoiding date rape and other abusive relationships.
- Health care: Assist the adolescent to learn about health insurance, how to enter and use the health care system, and to take responsibility for self-care.

COMMON DEVELOPMENTAL ISSUES FOR ADOLESCENTS

Risk Behavior

DESCRIPTION

Risk behavior consists of actions that jeopardize adolescents' physical, psychological, or emotional health. It is a paradox of adolescence that developmental tasks (i.e., gaining independence, developing one's own values, becoming comfortable with one's body, and establishing meaningful relationships) may be achieved (albeit in negative ways) through risk-taking behavior (Alsaker, 1996). Adolescents needing peer affiliation and striving for increased autonomy are likely to explore, experiment, and otherwise push the limits of their personal experience—often in ways that put them at risk for health-compromising outcomes. However, many adolescents engage in risk behavior without apparent negative outcomes. Is an adolescent who is sexually active but uses condoms on a regular basis engaged in risk behavior? Is an adolescent who goes to a party on the weekend and has a beer or smokes marijuana at risk? On the other hand, some teenagers who seem situationally predisposed do not engage in risk behavior. What factors keep them from doing so?

ETIOLOGY

Although it is normal for behavioral experimentation to occur during this time, adolescents vary tremendously in their ability to think abstractly about the consequences of risky behavior. Their thinking is often characterized by the notion that "it can't happen to me" (personal fable). Even though adolescents have an increase in abstract cognitive skills, thinking related to emotionally charged topics (e.g., substance use, sex, school performance, peer pressure) is often less sophisticated. An adolescent who is drinking may be doing so in part to be accepted by friends or to feel a sense of independence and maturity. Because the behavior meets important developmental needs, it may be difficult for the adolescent to look at it objectively and relinquish it. Orr and Ingersoll (1995) found that "boys, whites, those of lower cognitive complexity, and those who began pubertal maturation earlier than peers" were most likely to engage in risk-taking behavior.

Environmental factors, both social and physical, can influence adolescents' decisions to take risks. Community support of positive adolescent behavior appears to minimize risk taking (see Chapter 18).

Examples of risk factors include but are not limited to

- Poverty
- Poor academic performance
- Attention-deficit hyperactivity disorder
- Role models for deviant behavior (e.g., parents who abuse drugs)
- Low self-esteem
- Sense of hopelessness/helplessness
- Child abuse
- Depression
- Illiteracy/lack of job skills
- Criminal behavior
- Early sexual activity

PROTECTIVE FACTORS

Protective forces may help counter the effects of risk factors and help adolescents make healthier lifestyle choices. Examples of possible protective factors are

- High self-esteem
- Sense of future
- Academic success
- Family involvement
- An interested adult
- Community involvement

Adolescents with multiple risk and few protective factors are more likely to engage in risk behavior, with potential health- and life-threatening results. These adolescents need prompt attention and assessment to determine the likelihood of negative outcomes. Conversely, resilient adolescents who are doing well, despite multiple risk factors, should be acknowledged and applauded.

ASSESSMENT

All adolescents should be assessed for their level of risk-taking behavior. The provider's approach to a discussion of sensitive issues should include ensuring confidentiality, providing privacy, using constructive body language and interviewing techniques, and establishing rapport (Ehrman & Matson, 1998).

The HEADSS technique for assessment is cited as a method of assessing risk behavior. Areas for assessment include **h**ome, **e**ducation/employment, **a**ctivities, **d**rugs, **s**exuality, and **s**uicide/depression (Ehrman & Matson, 1998; Goldenring & Cohen, 1988). NPs should also be alert for red flags at each developmental stage because delays in development may contribute to negative behavior (see Table 9–2).

CLINICAL FINDINGS

The following are considered examples of risk behavior:

- Substance use/abuse
- Poor academic performance
- Unprotected sexual intercourse
- Drinking and driving
- Delinquency or involvement with gangs
- Violence-related behavior such as carrying weapons

The consequences of such behavior can be

T A B L E 9-2

Developmental Red Flags: Adolescent

AGE	PHYSICAL AND SEXUAL DEVELOPMENT	PSYCHOSOCIAL DEVELOPMENT	COGNITIVE DEVELOPMENT

Early adolescence (11–14 yr)	Difficulty reading close or distant
	Female kyphosis/scoliosis
	Less than Tanner stage 2
	Female short stature or lack of height spurt
	Poor nutrition, poor oral health, caries, malocclusion
	Loss of appetite
	Chronic disease such as heart disease, diabetes, or a family member with a chronic or lifelong illness
	No physical activity; overweight
	Sleep disturbance
	Sexual experimentation
		Social habits:
		  Early experimentation with drugs or alcohol (including tobacco)
		Relationships:
		  Permissive or authoritarian parental style
		  No participation in home chores
		  History of family violence
		  School fights
		  No close or "best" friend
		  Friends or siblings in gangs
		  Cruelty to animals
		Sexuality:
		  Sexual orientation worries
		Mood:
		  Pervasive sad mood, feelings of hopelessness, suicidal thoughts or gestures, history of previous suicide attempt
		  Flattened affect without expressions of joy, sorrow, or excitement
		  Excessive worrying or rumination
		Self-concept:
		  Believes self to be "ugly" or "fat"; is dieting despite normal body size and shape
		  Negative feelings of self-worth
		  Does not fantasize or dream about adult career
			Low IQ
			Behind in grade or failing classes
			Chronic absenteeism or class skipping
			Attention problems
			Lack of organizational skills for homework
			Disruptive behavior
			Unable to identify feelings
			Unable to control own behavior (e.g., anger, impulsivity)

Middle adolescence (15–17 yr)	Difficulty reading close or distant
	Male kyphosis/scoliosis
	Less than Tanner stage 4
	Male short stature or lack of height spurt
	Male muscular growth without testicular maturation
	Male persistent gynecomastia and acne
	Female primary or secondary amenorrhea
		Social habits:
		  Recurrent experimentation or frequent use of drugs or alcohol; blackouts
		  Drinking and driving
		Relationships:
		  Excessively oppositional, defiant of all authority
		  Abusive dating relationships
		  School fights
		  No identified peer group
		  Gang association or involvement
		Sexuality:
		  Sexual orientation worries
			Low IQ
			Behind in grade or failing classes
			Chronic absenteeism or class skipping
			Attention problems
			Disruptive behavior
			Unable to differentiate emotional states from physical states
			Unable to control own behavior (e.g., anger, impulsivity)
			Poor judgment

T A B L E 9-2

Developmental Red Flags: Adolescent Continued

AGE	PHYSICAL AND SEXUAL DEVELOPMENT	PSYCHOSOCIAL DEVELOPMENT	COGNITIVE DEVELOPMENT
	Poor nutrition, poor oral health, caries, malocclusion Loss of appetite Chronic disease such as heart disease, diabetes, or a family member with a chronic or lifelong illness No physical activity; overweight Sleep disturbance Unprotected sexual intercourse Multiple sexual partners	Mood: Pervasive sad mood, feelings of hopelessness, suicidal thoughts or gestures, history of previous suicide attempt Flattened affect without expressions of joy, sorrow, or excitement Excessive worrying or rumination Self-concept: Believes self to be "ugly' or "fat"; is dieting despite normal body size and shape Negative feelings of self-worth No life goals	
Late adolescence (18–21 yr)	Difficulty reading close or distant Less than Tanner stage 5 Poor nutrition, poor oral health, caries, malocclusion Loss of appetite Chronic disease such as heart disease, diabetes, or a family member with a chronic or lifelong illness No physical activity; overweight Sleep disturbance Unprotected sexual intercourse Multiple sexual partners	Social habits: Substance abuse Drinking and driving Relationships: Lacks intimate relationships Abusive dating relationships Unable to separate from peer groups Unable to separate from parents Gang association or involvement Unable to keep a job Sexuality: Sexual orientation worries Mood: Pervasive sad mood, feelings of hopelessness, suicidal thoughts or gestures, history of previous suicide attempt Flattened affect without expressions of joy, sorrow, or excitement Excessive worrying or rumination Self-concept: Believes self to be "ugly" or "fat"; is dieting despite normal body size and shape Negative feelings of self-worth Does not fantasize or dream about adult career	Low IQ Behind in grade or failing classes Dropout Attention problems Disruptive behavior Persistent egocentrism Unable to control own behavior (e.g., anger, impulsivity) Unable to reason or plan based on future/ abstract concepts Poor judgment Chronic health care seeking for psychosomatic complaints

addiction, school failure, pregnancy and sexually transmitted diseases, accidents, death, convictions for driving under the influence, incarceration, or death. Engaging in chronic risk-taking behavior often arrests developmental progression toward adult emotional maturity.

MANAGEMENT

Interventions should be considered when the adolescent's behavior threatens the accomplishment of developmental tasks. As Alasker (1996) has noted, however, some adolescents strive to accomplish these tasks through risk-taking behaviors. In these cases, the NP has a responsibility to recognize and take action when the risk behavior begins to threaten the adolescent's safety and well-being.

Generally, when adolescents' behavior supports the achievement of developmental tasks, such behavior should be encouraged. Adolescents who pierce their noses, shave half their heads, and spend evenings with friends may be irritating to parents, but their behavior helps them establish their autonomy, identity, and ability to relate to others. It is important to understand the meaning of the behavior for the adolescent. Teenagers are more likely to engage in risk behavior if they are neglected, feel hopeless or powerless, and lack self-esteem.

Interventions specific to various risk-taking behaviors should be planned with consideration of the acuity of the problems at hand. For instance, an adolescent who is depressed and suicidal has an imminent risk of performing dangerous acts. Likewise, a young person with a serious drug problem needs immediate attention. Ideally, the NP identifies children at risk on the basis of the presence of risk factors and the absence of protective factors and intervenes before actual risk taking occurs. Unfortunately, the NP does not always see adolescents on a regular basis. Many adolescents have not established a consistent ongoing relationship with a primary care provider. Many, especially older adolescents, overuse emergency department services for conditions that could be managed in the primary care setting. Most adolescent visits to the emergency department are at night when access to supportive community re-sources for referral is limited. In addition, use of the emergency department compromises the continuity of care necessary to establish a trusting relationship with teenagers (Ziv et al., 1998). As a result, teenagers at risk may not receive the care they need.

The approach used when providing care to teenagers differs from that used with younger children. Earlier, parents were central to the success of interventions. Although parents are still critical to successful intervention, the NP must recognize that the teenager makes the decisions. The NP's role is to provide the adolescent with information and guidance to make the best decisions possible.

Confidentiality is an important issue, and the adolescent must be actively included in decisions about sharing information with others. Teenagers must be assured that information will be kept confidential unless (1) signs of them posing a risk to themselves or others are apparent, or (2) state laws mandate that information must be shared (e.g., some states require reporting teen sexual activity, even if consensual, if an age difference of 3 or more years exists between the couple). For many sensitive health issues, the NP will need to help the teenager weigh the risks and benefits of involving family members. NPs must also provide guidance and support on how to best inform the family, if that is the adolescent's choice. For example, a pregnant teen needs to know of the NP's concern that she inform her parent or another significant adult of her situation. This approach can help protect a teen from the parent who is abusive or unsafe. It also can reduce the problem of upset parents who are denied information about the child they love and for whom they feel responsible.

Generally, high-risk teenagers require numerous services. The NP needs to know how to access community resources and how to use other professionals collaboratively. The following list identifies basic services that at-risk teenagers may need:

- Food resources for teenage parents and their offspring
- Temporary shelters for teenagers
- Counseling and mental health services for teenagers and their families

- Foster care services for teenage parents and their offspring
- Local medical and social work services
- Local juvenile justice system and protective services
- Drug rehabilitation programs for teenagers
- Alternative school and vocational education programs
- Sports, fitness, and community activities for teenagers
- Support programs for teenagers such as Big Brothers/Big Sisters

Advocating for children and adolescents at risk, involving their families, communities, and schools, and helping the young person identify an individual who cares for them and trusts them are important actions an NP can take.

CONCLUSION

As adolescents struggle with issues of autonomy, body image, peer relationships, and ultimately, identity, parents and health care providers must be aware of and sensitive to the phase of development and the range of normal behavior. Both risk and protective factors must be assessed accurately. Intervention requires weighing the balance of risk vs. protective factors, the actual behavior, and the potential threat to health and well-being. At-risk situations cannot always be avoided; therefore, adolescents and their families need anticipatory guidance and strategies for managing risk. The desired outcome is for the teen to emerge into adulthood with a healthy mind, body, and identity.

REFERENCES

Alsaker FD: Annotation: The impact of puberty. J Child Psychol Psychiatry 37:249-258, 1996.

Cameron JL: Nutritional determinants of puberty. Nutr Rev 54(suppl):S17-22, 1996.

Ehrman WG, Matson SC: Approach to assessing adolescents on serious or sensitive issues. Pediatr Clin North Am 45:189-204, 1998.

Elster A, Kuznets N: AMA Guidelines for Adolescent Preventive Services (GAPS). Baltimore, Williams & Wilkins, 1994.

Ge X, Conger RD, Elder GH: Coming of age too early: Pubertal influences on girls' vulnerability to psychological distress. Child Dev 67:3386-3400, 1996.

Goldenring J, Cohen E: Getting into adolescent heads. Contemp Pediatr 7:75-90, 1988.

Hall G: Adolescence: Its Psychology and Its Relations to Physiology, Anthropology, Sociology, Sex, Crime, Religion and Education. Englewood Cliffs, NJ, Prentice-Hall, 1904.

Orr DP, Ingersoll GM: The contribution of level of cognitive complexity and pubertal timing to behavior risk in young adolescents. Pediatrics 95:528-533, 1995.

Reiff MI: Adolescent school failure: Failure to thrive in adolescence. Pediatr Rev 19:199-207, 1998.

Schreiber GB, Robins M, Streigel-Moore R, et al: Weight modification efforts reported by black and white preadolescent girls: National Heart, Lung, and Blood Institute Growth and Health Study. Pediatrics 98:63-70, 1996.

Tanner J: Growth at Adolescence. Oxford, Blackwell, 1962.

Valadian I, Porter D: Physical Growth and Development From Conception to Maturity. Boston, Little, Brown, 1977.

Ziv A, Boulet JR, Slap GB: Emergency department utilization by adolescents in the United States. Pediatrics 101:987-994, 1998.

Approaches to Health Management in Pediatric Primary Care

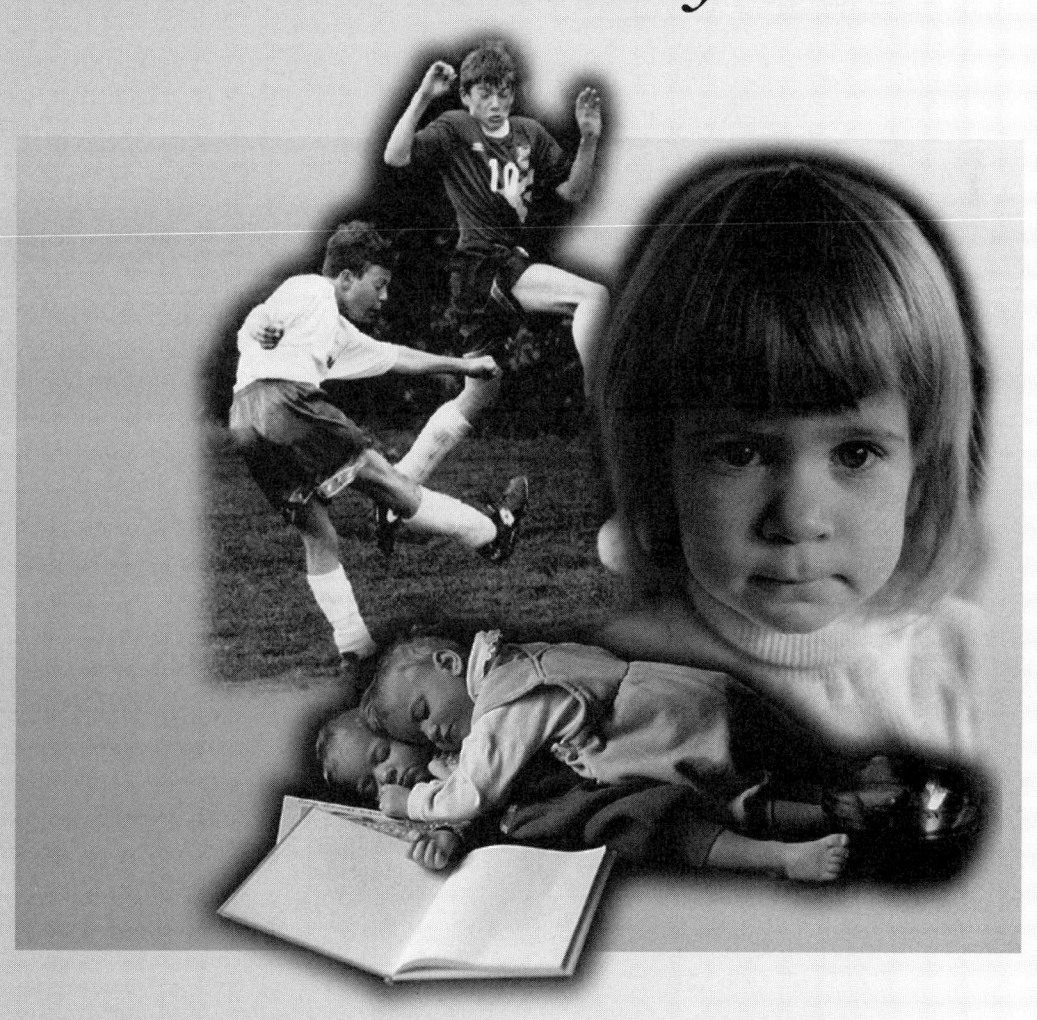

CHAPTER 10

Introduction to Health Promotion

Catherine E. Burns

INTRODUCTION

Health care is considered by many to be a birthright, and health is highly valued by all cultures in the world. Although valued, health is often compromised by behaviors of daily living. Lifestyle choices are the major causes of morbidity and mortality in infants, children, and adolescents. Thus, the majority of life-threatening and debilitating conditions of children are preventable. The goals of *Healthy People,* the health promotion and disease prevention objectives for the year 2000 and 2010 (United States [US] Department of Health and Human Services, 1990; US Department of Health and Human Services, 1998) focus on essential lifestyle and behavioral factors related to health. If these goals are to be met, proactive, comprehensive health promotion and disease prevention strategies directed at individuals, families, and communities are absolutely essential.

The nurse practitioner (NP) is in an excellent position to influence the health-care outcomes of the nation through work in the health promotion arena. Teaching and modeling healthy behaviors help children learn to promote their own health, and, because many health problems of children are carried into adulthood, working with children has long-term health effects on the whole population. The broad perspective used by NPs serves as a framework to encompass all the factors that have an impact on health. The use of functional health patterns, a construct unique to nursing, focuses one's practice directly on lifestyle and health behaviors. Consistent and vigorous attention to issues of nutrition, activity, coping and stress tolerance, accident prevention, and other factors of lifestyle has as much or more impact on achievement of national goals as time spent managing minor illnesses that occur in daily practice.

To provide maximal support for achievement of the nation's health goals, however, a much broader array of professionals and citizens must be involved. Nurses, teachers, health educators, city planners, legislators, the industrial community, volunteers, and others from all levels of society need to guide development of an infrastructure that supports health care for all. Although this section of the book focuses on management of individual children within families, a broader perspective on community intervention and support for health also needs to be maintained. When opportunities to work with communities on their primary health-care issues arise, the NP is strongly encouraged to become involved.

This chapter introduces the functional health patterns unit of the book. In this chapter, models that predict health behavior, factors that influence health-promotion behaviors, functional health patterns used to describe the lifestyle domains that health-promotion strategies must address, and specific management strategies for use with children and families are presented and discussed. Subsequent chapters in this unit examine each functional health pattern and its relationship to health.

MODELS TO PREDICT HEALTH BEHAVIOR

Four models are often used to predict health behaviors: the health belief model, the self-efficacy model, the health promotion model (Pender, 1987), and the transtheoretical (Stages of Change) model of behavior change (Prochaska et al., 1992; Prochaska, 1995; Prochaska et al., 1994). These models address issues of motivation, the first step toward action. They provide guidance for assessment of the motivation of the client as well as cues to plan efforts that will encourage the client to take positive action.

Health Belief Model

The health belief model was first described by Hochbaum (1958), Kegeles and colleagues (1965), and Rosenstock (1966). The model explains behavior that seeks to prevent disease better than behavior that attempts to promote health. According to this model, people engage in preventive behaviors if they have a reason or motive to do so and if they hold certain beliefs. They must meet the following criteria:

- Feel vulnerable or susceptible to the disease or health problem
- Believe that the disease will have negative consequences for them if they get it
- Be convinced that taking some action will reduce the risk
- Accept that the benefits of action outweigh the costs

Women are more likely than men to engage in preventive behaviors; social pressure appears to encourage or discourage preventive actions; and knowledge of, and prior experience with, the target disease influence the likelihood of acting preventively (Pender, 1987).

The health belief model can be illustrated by assessing the motivation for tooth-brushing behavior: the client must believe that caries are possible; that tooth loss, pain, or disfigurement would be unfortunate consequences of caries; that brushing teeth can prevent caries; and that the benefits of brushing outweigh the inconvenience, time, and costs of maintaining a supply of toothbrushes and toothpaste over time. This is a simple example. Getting a teenager to change the cholesterol content in his or her diet after considering the consequences of heart disease in later life is not so easy.

Self-Efficacy Model

Bandura's (1977) concept of self-efficacy augments the health belief model. Self-efficacy is the belief that the self is capable of acting effectively: "Expectations of personal efficacy determine whether coping behavior will be initiated, how much effort will be expended, and how long it will be sustained in the face of obstacles and aversive experiences." Bandura thought that two kinds of expectations were important. First, one estimates one's capacity to do what is required—expectancy that the behaviors used can achieve the goal. This expectation is based on performance accomplishments in the past, vicarious modeling experiences (watching the consequences of someone else's efforts), and verbal persuasion (someone saying, "You can do it"), with emotional arousal providing additional energy for action. Second, the outcome expectations (i.e., estimations that behavior will lead to intended outcomes) need to be considered. In other words, the person needs to believe that if he or she performs as well as expected, the outcome will be influenced favorably, being contingent on the actions taken rather than being independent of them.

Health-Promotion Model

Pender (1987) developed a comprehensive model with a focus on health promotion rather than on disease prevention. The model consists of two main domains—cognitive-perceptual factors and modifying factors—that explain participation in health-promotion behaviors (Fig. 10-1). The cognitive-perceptual factors include all the concepts in the health belief and self-effi-

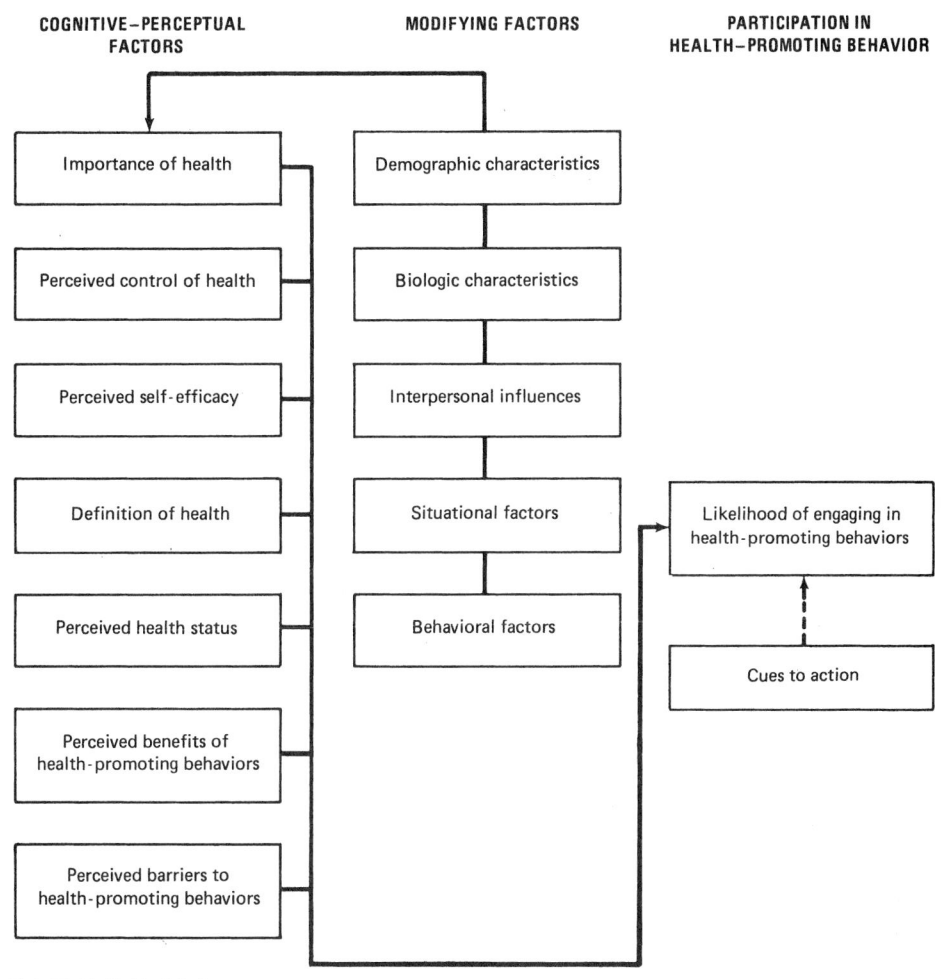

F I G U R E   10-1
Health-promotion model. (From Pender N: Health Promotion in Nursing Practice, 2nd ed. Norwalk, CT, Appleton & Lange, 1987.)

cacy models, locus of control notions, as well as individuals' definitions of health and their own health status estimates. Modifying factors in the model include demographic, biological, behavioral, and situational factors as well as interpersonal influences. Together, the two groups of factors are important in helping a person decide whether to engage in health-promotion behaviors.

The locus of control model also can be used to predict the likelihood that people will engage in particular health habits. Powerlessness and empowerment are more current concepts related to the ideas of locus of control. Persons with an external locus of control (feeling powerless) are less likely to engage in health-promotion behaviors.

Clark and colleagues (1988) found that the health belief model did not predict which children would engage in self-management activities to control asthma. The failure to predict behavior may be an issue of the child's developmental level or of measures that do not truly tap the health beliefs of the youngster. In any case, application of the models to child behaviors should not be assumed to be appropriate.

On the other hand, because pediatric primary care always has two clients, parent and child, it is worthwhile to assess the health beliefs and self-efficacy beliefs of both parties. Parents need to execute health-promotion activities for their children directly or take the initiative to guide older children in their own self-care.

Transtheoretical Model

The transtheoretical model is the newest of the four models. It incorporates elements from health belief and self-efficacy theories to develop a model that can be used to describe the stages of change that individuals go through as they initiate behaviors that promote health. The model describes 5 stages of change, 10 processes that facilitate movement from one stage to another, and 4 patterns that individuals use to progress through the various stages (Fig. 10–2) (Prochaska et al., 1992).

STAGES OF CHANGE

The stages include precontemplation, contemplation, preparation, action, and maintenance. Shifts in attitudes and behaviors occur at each stage. The time required in each stage depends on the individual and the task to be attempted.

- *Precontemplation.* At this stage, the individual does not acknowledge that a serious problem exists, although a wish to change may be expressed. Resistance to change is the hallmark of this stage and the reasons not to change are most clear to the individual.
- *Contemplation.* Awareness of the problem exists and the individual struggles with the costs and energy required for change. Many individuals remain stuck in this phase.
- *Preparation.* Planning begins in this stage. Small behavior changes may occur in preparation for commitment to the actual plan.
- *Action.* Behaviors to eliminate the problem occur in this stage. These may include initiating new behaviors, accessing resources, modifying the environment, and mitigating barriers.
- *Maintenance.* Plans occur here to prevent relapse, consolidate gains, and establish new behaviors as long-term changes. Maintenance occurs after at least 6 months in the action stage.

PATTERNS OF CHANGE

Most people are not able to proceed through all five stages in a linear way. Rather, there are *relapses* back to the precontemplation stage. Environmental barriers, external pressures to change beyond the individual's own desires, or problems with maintenance of steps not mastered at earlier stages can contribute to relapses. *Recycling* is defined as regression to the contemplation or preparation stages. The person actually spirals through small increments of change, recycling and moving forward again. Success with the change is increased with effort, action, and mastery of the tasks of each stage.

Many dieting, smoking cessation, and drug rehabilitation programs fail to sustain changes because assessment of readiness and readiness training to assist individuals to move through stages successively was not included in the initial plans. Drug and alcohol programs are frequently imposed externally on individuals (court-ordered drug treatment). As soon as the pressure is relieved from the source, the individual relapses because changes are not internally driven.

DECISIONAL BALANCE

Another component of the model is the cognitive exercise of weighing the pros and cons of change. The pros of change must predominate over the cons in the precontemplative stage for the individual to move to the contemplative stage. To sustain behavior in the action stage and move to the maintenance stage, the cons of returning to old ways must outweigh the pros of change. Because most people at risk for health problems are in a precontemplative stage, programs need to be designed to move them to the contemplative stage. Also, programs designed to maintain changes made are important.

Transtheoretical Model of Behavior Change

Stages of Change and Associated Processes of Change

STAGES:	Precontemplation	Contemplation	Preparation	Action	Maintenance

PROCESSES*:

Consciousness raising
Dramatic relief
Environmental reevaluation
                Self-reevaluation

Self-liberation
    Reinforcement management
    Helping relationships
    Counter-conditioning
    Stimulus control
Social liberation

PATTERNS:
  Relapse

  Recycling

DECISIONAL BALANCE:
    "cons" outweigh "pros"   "pros" outweigh "cons"

Explanations of Processes of Change	**Associated Interventions**
**Consciousness raising: gathering information about self & problem	Observation of others, Confrontations Classes, bibliotherapy, Interpretations
Dramatic relief: feeling and expressing feelings related to problem	Role play, psychodrama, grief work
Environmental reevaluation: Assessing one's behavior on environment	Documentary information, empathy training
Self-reevaluation: exploring one's feelings about self and the problem	Value clarification, Imagery Corrective emotional experience
***Self-liberation: choosing to act, changing belief in ability to change	Decision-making training Making resolutions, Commitment enhancing techniques
Social liberation: increasing alternatives and support for health behaviors	Empowerment & advocacy activities, policy interventions
Reinforcement management: establishing a reward system	Overt and covert reinforcement, contingency contracts
*Helping relationships: trusting and sharing problem with a caring person	Therapeutic alliance, buddy system, self help/support groups
Counter-conditioning: Substituting alternatives for problem behavior	Relaxation, desensitization, assertive skills, self-affirmations
Stimulus control: avoiding triggers of problem behavior	Restructuring environment, avoidance techniques, cue identification

*Most frequently used
**Second most frequently used
***Third most frequently used
*Used more frequently for psychologically distressing problems
***Used more frequently for weight control   Adapted from Prochaska, DiClemente, & Norcross, 1992.

F I G U R E 10-2

Transtheoretical (stages of change) model. (Adapted from Prochaska J, Diclemente C, Norcross J: In search of how people change: Applications to addictive behaviors. Am Psychol 47:1102–1114, 1992.)

▉▉▉ INFLUENCES ON CHILDREN'S HEALTH PROMOTION BEHAVIORS

Children's health-promotion behaviors are influenced by their own understanding of health and illness, the views and behaviors of their family, and community variables. The latter include direct effects of standards and practices in child care, school, and other community settings, as well as indirect effects, such as cultural and community values related to health.

Children's Concepts of Health and Illness

Children's concepts of health and illness must be considered within a developmental framework. Cognitive development is often used as a framework to analyze children's understandings of health and illness. Expectancy theory (from Bandura's work)—children's perceived vulnerability to health problems and the relationship of health problems to health behaviors—is also useful. Many studies offer evidence of children's views, but the knowledge base is relatively weak, with more research needed in the area. NPs need to understand the health beliefs of their young patients as well as their goals, hopes, priorities, health interests and concerns, perceptions about seriousness of problems, feelings of vulnerability to health problems, and perceptions of benefits and barriers to taking action (National Institute of Nursing Research, 1993).

One model for understanding children's cognitive processing of health information (used in the 1970s and 1980s) is Piaget's theory of cognitive development. Following this framework, preschoolers are in Piaget's preoperational stage of cognitive development. They have an egocentric view of health. Children at 3 to 5 years of age are just learning about the differences between being sick vs. well for themselves and their family members. They have little understanding of their internal bodies. Their lack of understanding of time and transformations means that the process of healing, for example, is not clearly understood.

School-age children are in the concrete operations cognitive development stage. They can list specific acts and rules used to maintain health and generally need overt signs of illness or health to recognize the health status of a person.

Adolescents, who are in the formal operations stage, are able to understand the difficulties of defining health (e.g., a person who looks well but has a cancerous tumor inside vs. a person whose mobility is limited but is actually very healthy). Teenagers understand the difference between the sick role and actual pathology, are sensitive to feeling states, and differentiate mental health from physical health.

Nevertheless, the provider should not consider adolescents ready for explanations at an adult level. Koff and Rierdan (1995) found that early adolescent girls had a very incomplete understanding of menstruation, with many misconceptions and gaps in their knowledge. They tended to focus on one particular element of the process rather than integrating elements. Cultural stereotypes and myths had been learned early.

Yoos (1994) offers an alternate view in which she argues that children's understanding may be better enhanced by use of a novice-expert model. Accordingly, with more experience and knowledge, children can incorporate more elaborate concepts into an understanding of how the body works, contagion, differences between physical and mental well-being, and the like. Similarly, adults may be cognitively sophisticated but demonstrate very elementary understanding of specific conditions based on lack of experience and knowledge rather than inability to process information. NPs should provide information based on the child's current base of knowledge and experience. If NPs assume, on the basis of a child's age, that he or she has a certain level of knowledge, experience, or cognitive abilities, they may fail to provide the most useful information to the child.

Other Determinants of Health Behavior of Children

A variety of studies have considered the determinants of health behavior of school-age children, not just their cognitive understanding of health or illness. A study of determinants of exercise behaviors in children (Stucky-Ropp & DiLorenzo, 1993) found that social and learning variables were major factors influencing physical activity for fifth and sixth graders. For boys, enjoyment of physical activity, support of friends and family for physical activity, mother's perceived barriers to exercise, and mother's perceived family support for exercise were most important. For girls, enjoyment of physical activity, number of exercise-related items at home, mother's perceived family support for physical activity, mother's perceived barriers to exercise, and direct parental modeling of physical activity were most important.

Olvera-Ezzell and associates (1994) demonstrated that among 4- to 8-year-old, low-income, Spanish-speaking Mexican American children, health knowledge about nutrition, hygiene, and safety varied and was significantly affected by age and gender. Older girls had better understanding of hygiene and safety health behaviors than did younger children and boys of the same age. Nutritional health was the least well understood area for all.

Farrand and Cox (1993) found gender differences, with girls reporting more health habits and more positive health self-concept and motivation from peers and others (extrinsic). Boys were more intrinsically motivated, with fewer family influences, such as family size and higher maternal education levels.

A significant health factor for adolescents is their risk-taking behavior. What is the adolescent's perception of risk? When do teenagers identify behaviors as risky but choose to engage in them anyway for the perceived social value? Busen (1991) developed an adolescent risk-taking instrument to help providers identify teenagers at risk. In a study using the instrument, Busen (1992) found that teenagers viewed aggressive, impulsive, and thrill-seeking acts as the most risky.

Sometimes, less knowledge leads to behaviors that are potentially unhealthful. One group of researchers (Massad et al., 1995) found that adolescent athletes with less knowledge about the effects of nutritional supplements were more likely to use them.

Among college students, Valois and colleagues (1993) found that early occurrence of any harmful behavior, poor performance in school, antisocial behavior, low resistance to peer influence, lack of parental bonding and supervision, and living in a subpoverty-level area or urban, high-density community were risk factors for violent behavior, a significant factor in adolescent and young adult morbidity and mortality.

FAMILY INVOLVEMENT WITH HEALTH OF CHILDREN

The family is the basic unit of health-care management. The family influences lifestyles and the health status of its members. The NP needs to understand family dynamics, especially the influence of the mother; decision-making patterns; and parenting styles, including autonomy and rewards for children and reasoning used to teach children. The psychological characteristics of the family, belief that members can make a difference, and the role of the family as a natural support system are all important in planning effective health-promotion strategies. Knowledge of the family's composition, health, lifestyles, nutrition, economic resources, and recent changes is helpful. Exercise, diet, hygiene, and rest patterns are family routines affecting the health of individual members.

A variety of studies provide some information about the health-promotion practices of families for their children. Chapter 11 identifies factors that facilitate families' choosing health-promotion behaviors.

The criteria mothers use to choose foods have been shown to influence the health behaviors of preschool Hispanic children (Contento et al., 1993). Mothers of 4- to 5-year-olds who believed food influenced health were more knowledgeable about foods and had children who ate healthier diets. Other mothers were more motivated by the taste of the food. Their children ate less healthy diets.

Competent parents take steps to protect the health and safety of their children. Hendricks and Reichert (1996) in a study of health and safety behaviors of parents of children enrolled in Head Start programs found that more than 90% reported using seat belts, taught handwashing and pedestrian safety, and kept medicines and alcohol out of children's reach. However, fewer than 60% kept guns and bullets stored separately and locked, kept a working fire extinguisher, or had the poison control telephone number at hand.

Skin cancer prevention is an area where fewer parents act on behalf of their children. In several studies (Rodrigue, 1996; Vail-Smith et al., 1997), many parents had relatively high levels of knowledge about sun exposure, used sunscreens themselves, and practiced adult skin cancer risk reduction, but they were less likely to provide sun protection to their children.

COMMUNITY INVOLVEMENT WITH HEALTH OF CHILDREN

The community influences health-promotion behaviors of families with children. The community provides options for health care, an economic base for family survival and prosperity, social norms, and regulation of the environment and behaviors of citizens. The community also provides many direct services, including schools, day care centers, social services, community organizations, and health-care centers, that support or impede family efforts to maintain the health of the members.

Use of community resources benefits families positively if recommendations for access and utilization are appropriate and timely. As is discussed in Chapter 11, appropriate use of community resources is an expected behavior in the maintenance and management of functional health patterns. Use of community standards and health values can effectively influence behaviors of individual families. According to Rogers' (1983) diffusion theory, innovators are the first to adopt new ideas in a community. They are followed by early adopters, then the early majority, the late majority, and finally late adopters. When between 10 and 25% of the population adopt an idea, it diffuses through the rest of the population. Thus, for example, when the use of bicycle helmets reaches a critical mass of 10 to 25%, use should become common enough so that the remaining families are persuaded to buy helmets and expect their children to use them.

In summary, many factors influence the health behaviors of children and their families. NPs helping families change lifestyle and behaviors to promote health need broad understand-ings of the health perspectives of their clients as well as an awareness of age, sex, education, and peer and community influences.

▬ FUNCTIONAL HEALTH PATTERNS—THE BEHAVIORS OF HEALTH

The functional health patterns that Gordon (1987) has used to describe the domain of nursing practice serve as the framework for the chapters in this unit. The patterns describe the health-related behaviors that people engage in that affect their health. These functional health patterns are universal, applying to all humans regardless of age, sex, culture, health status, or other factors. All people need to eat, sleep, and eliminate, for example. Each pattern is described as follows:

Health Perception–Health Management Pattern
- Describes client's perceptions of personal health and health care behaviors, and prevention as well as compliance with prescriptions for management of health and illness problems.

Nutrition-Metabolic Pattern
- Describes patterns of food and fluid intake. Includes choice of foods and food supplements, eating habits, and schedules.

Elimination Pattern
- Describes patterns of bowel and bladder excretion. Includes schedule and habit patterns, and use of laxatives or other methods to facilitate excretory functions.

Activity–Exercise Pattern
- Describes patterns of activity and exercise, including type of activity, schedule of participation, vigor, effect on leisure, physical state, and meaning of activity to the client.

Sleep–Rest Pattern
- Describes patterns of sleep and rest, including schedule, habits, aids to sleep, perceived feelings of renewal, fatigue, or exhaustion.

Cognitive-Perceptual Pattern

- Describes sensory-perceptual and cognitive patterns, including adaptations to hearing, vision, or other perceptual losses; includes the process of finding meaning from environmental stimuli and the effectiveness of efforts to compensate for deficits. Pain perception is a component.

Self-Perception–Self-Concept Pattern

- Describes pattern of perception and valuing of the self as well as evaluation of strengths and weaknesses, and sense of self-worth.

Role-Relationships Pattern

- Describes pattern of roles and responsibilities of the client and patterns of relationships with family and others.

Sexuality-Reproductive Pattern

- Describes patterns of satisfaction or dissatisfaction with sexuality and sexual relationships. Involves perception of and development of sexual identity as well as reproductive expectations, behaviors, and outcomes.

Coping–Stress Tolerance Pattern

- Describes patterns of coping with the range of stresses experienced. Includes strategies used, effectiveness, support systems, and perceived ability to control and manage difficult situations.

Values–Beliefs Pattern

- Describes patterns of values and beliefs that influence daily living activities, guide decision-making, and provide meaning to life. Involves religious and spiritual activities as well as personal values and beliefs.

Screening and Assessment of Functional Health Pattern Disorders

The same diagnostic reasoning methods are used by the NP to manage both health and illness issues. One must look at risk factors, comorbidities, etiology, differential diagnosis, and options for management that are acceptable to the client.

Screening for the presence of lifestyle and health behavior problems is a first step for NPs. In pediatric practice, the majority of screening is done in the clinical interview. Questions are asked about sleep, nutrition, elimination, play, discipline, utilization of primary care services, and others. Questionnaires can be used to ask about diet, smoking, exercise, use of seat belts, and feelings of satisfaction with self and health status. The clinical interview is more than taking a history of medical problems. It involves learning about concerns and worries as well as goals, lifestyle, family life, and cultural background. It produces information to put the child and family into a context necessary to plan for care. For instance, if a family has little money, decisions about care need to factor in the inability to pay for services, medications, or equipment.

If information generated by the clinical interview is appropriate, given the child's age and other factors, no further probing of the area is done. On the other hand, if an answer to a screening question is atypical, the NP begins the assessment mode to identify the nature, severity, duration, and effects of the problem to plan appropriate interventions. For example, if a mother notes that she has not been very happy lately, the Beck Depression Scale might be administered to assess whether she is depressed or not. Assessment might involve use of daily diaries of food intake, activity, or sleep-wake patterns. Screening methods are used for all children of a given age in the practice, whereas assessment is individualized and should yield information about the extent of the problem and comorbidities for a given client. The goal of assessment is development of a plan of care to manage the problem effectively and efficiently.

Health supervision using a clinical preventive services model involves regular visits timed to offer periodic screening opportunities. The visits need to be scheduled infrequently enough to be economical but frequently enough to identify changes in the patterns of growth and development or early physiological, psychological, or social changes that might be detrimental to the child's health. Health supervision includes the clinical interview, developmental and educational surveillance, observation of parent-child interaction, physical examination, and screening procedures such as measuring height, weight, head circumference, vision, hearing, blood pressure, and hemoglobin or hematocrit. The purpose of the health supervision visit is to assess strengths and weaknesses in health. The content of health supervision visits throughout infancy, childhood, and adolescence is addressed in Chapter 11. The details of screening, assessment, and management of functional health problems identified are found in the remaining chapters of this unit.

Nursing Diagnoses—A Way to Label Functional Health Pattern Problems

Nursing diagnoses developed by the North American Nursing Diagnosis Association (NANDA) provide a way to label, describe, and categorize the problems that nurses manage. One advantage to the use of nursing diagnoses lies in systematically identifying the health problems that nurses manage with labels that allow data retrieval for evaluation of practice outcomes and research purposes. Nursing diagnoses also provide a potential system for reimbursement of nursing care services. Using the labels in charting ensures that the range of services that NPs provide is explicit. Without labeling the problems of sleep, nutrition, coping, and so forth, no one knows what the NP does while in the room with the patient and family. The services provided become invisible, and the perception is left that NPs are slower in managing diseases than other primary care providers are. In order to be valued, the NPs' total work must be recognized. The use of nursing diagnosis labels can make the work in the health promotion domain of functional health patterns more visible.

Nevertheless, nursing diagnoses are not used systematically by all NPs. The first problem is that some NANDA diagnoses are not stated specifically enough for clinical application, although they identify an area of patient difficulty. For example, "sleep pattern disturbance" does not tell the NP whether the issue involves getting to sleep, staying asleep, or waking early. Each problem would be managed differently. Second, many senior NPs (those who are more likely to teach students) were educated as NPs

before the development of nursing diagnoses. Thus, students might not see role models using the system. Third, the nursing diagnosis taxonomy is not fully developed, so clinicians do not always find the diagnoses they need, and the terminology for some diagnoses has changed over the past several years. Fourth, there is a misconception on the part of some NPs that they should use nursing labels for medical diagnoses. This misconception has contributed to resistance to using nursing diagnoses and to NPs stating that nursing diagnoses are not appropriate for the patients they see. NPs should use medical diagnoses for the pathophysiological problems and nursing diagnoses for the problems of lifestyle and health behaviors not covered by medical diagnosis labels (Burns, 1991). The use of both sets of labels makes the scope of practice of the NP explicit. Therefore, "impetigo" is best for describing the skin infection but "alteration in parenting" alerts other professionals to look at parenting behaviors.

In the functional health patterns chapters (Chapters 11 to 22), nursing diagnoses that might be appropriate to label problems in a particular pattern are identified for those who wish to use them. However, the content of each chapter is organized conceptually around the nature of the pattern and not the nursing diagnosis framework.

▰▰▰ MANAGEMENT STRATEGIES FOR HEALTH PROMOTION

This section discusses some management strategies for promoting health and working with functional health-pattern problems. To provide excellent health-promotion care, the NP must

- Give consistent, credible health messages
- Merit trust and confidence
- Understand clinical preventive service recommendations and provide preventive services consistent with those recommendations
- Have working relationships with other health-care providers, social services, and educational professionals in the community

- Ensure that the clinic setting creates an environment consistent with good health and is developmentally appropriate
- Use motivational, patient education, and behavioral strategies effectively

In the Nursing Interventions Classification (NIC), McCloskey and Bulechek (1996) classified nursing interventions into six domains: (1) physiological: basic; (2) physiological: complex; (3) behavioral; (4) safety; (5) family; and (6) health system (Table 10-1). For the problems of functional health patterns and health maintenance and promotion, interventions in domains 1, 3, 4, 5, and 6 are most appropriate. The interventions of domain 2 (physiological: complex) are most appropriate for the disease/pathophysiological problems NPs manage. This text does not formally use the NIC. However, it is a useful tool when developing management strategies relevant to specific problems. For example, the interventions most specifically designed to result in behavioral changes desired for health promotion and disease prevention include those in NIC domain 3 (behavior therapy, cognitive therapy, communication enhancement, coping assistance, patient education, and psychological comfort).

Patient Education

Patient education is the most commonly used strategy for guiding patients to increase health promotion behaviors and manage lifestyle problems. Primary health education involves instructing clients about ways to avoid contracting preventable diseases, ways to change lifestyle to reduce risks, and methods to maintain a healthy environment. Secondary health education teaches people to recognize early illness and prevent disease progression, whereas tertiary health education relates to instruction of patients about their specific illnesses, treatments, and available health services and resources (Watts & Breindel, 1981).

Friere (1973) adds a sociopolitical dimension to learning that community health nurses find helpful. According to his model, education should be self-generated rather than simply receptive, with empowerment and liberation identified as outcomes for individuals who en-

TABLE 10-1

Nursing Interventions Classification: Domains and Classes of Interventions

1. *Physiological: basic:* Care that supports physical functioning
   A. Activity and exercise management
   B. Elimination management
   C. Immobility management
   D. Nutrition support
   E. Physical comfort promotion
   F. Self-care facilitation
2. *Physiological: complex:* Care that supports homeostatic regulation
   A. Electrolyte and acid-base management
   B. Drug management
   C. Neurologic management
   D. Perioperative care
   E. Respiratory management
   F. Skin/wound management
   G. Thermoregulation
   H. Tissue perfusion management
3. *Behavioral:* Care that supports psychological functioning and facilitates lifestyle changes
   A. Behavior therapy
   B. Cognitive therapy
   C. Communication enhancement
   D. Coping assistance
   E. Patient education
   F. Psychological comfort promotion
4. *Safety:* Care that supports protection against harm
   A. Crisis management
   B. Risk management
5. *Family:* Care that supports the family unit
   A. Childbearing care
   B. Family care
6. *Health system:* Care that supports effective use of the health-care delivery system
   A. Health system mediation
   B. Health system management
   C. Information management

From McCloskey J, Bulechek G (eds): Nursing Interventions Classification, 2nd ed. St. Louis, Mosby–Year Book, 1996.

gage in the educational process. Education occurs after the student and the teacher first come to a common understanding about the relationship between individual health problems and the social context of those problems. Part of the education focuses on addressing the social issues, such as barriers to care, that affect the management of the specific problem at hand.

PATIENT EDUCATION PROCESS

Patient education is the method used to provide patients and families with the knowledge they need to make decisions related to their health and to carry out self-care activities that will positively affect their health or allow them to manage their diseases.

The core methodology for patient education for individuals and groups is reviewed here and summarized in Table 10-2.

1. *Set the climate for learning.* Patients, families, or groups need to be in an environment that is comfortable and free of distractions and provides cues that learning activities will occur. Introductions and a mutually agreed-on time limit are helpful. For example, mothers who are worried about being home when the school bus drops off their children attend poorly to teaching, no matter how skilled the NP is.
2. *Establish a structure of mutual planning.*

T A B L E 10-2

The Patient Education Process

---

1. Set the climate for learning—make introductions, comfortable environment.
2. Establish a structure of mutual planning–identify learner and nurse practitioner goals.
3. Assess the learner—style of learning, level of knowledge and competency, readiness, physical and developmental capabilities, attitudes, and feelings.
4. Plan—provide knowledge, role modeling, practice, discussion. Various aids facilitate teaching–books, pamphlets, diagrams, videos, and models. The plan is formulated with objectives specifying the behaviors that the learner should exhibit to demonstrate learning.
5. Manage the learning intervention—use methods and resources for instruction with the patient and/or family to implement the plan.
6. Evaluate the outcomes—judge achievement of objectives and then reformulate the plan to move the learner to the next level.

Identify learner and NP goals. If learning is to be successful, the client must recognize a need for new knowledge. It becomes the NP's responsibility to identify the client (child, parent, class) need. Getting the client to express questions is the most direct way to identify client needs. The NP can also ask about the client's health goals. Sometimes it is necessary to provide information alerting clients to potential or emerging problems if lifestyle or behavior changes do not occur. In other words, the client does not always come to the NP with preestablished goals or needs; however, the client must agree with the NP that change is necessary in order for the mutual planning requirement of patient teaching to be met.

3. *Assess the learner.* Assessment includes readiness, attitudes and feelings, style of learning, level of knowledge and competency, and physical and developmental capabilities. Use of one of the health belief models identified earlier can provide the necessary information about the readiness and attitudes and feelings factors. Chow and colleagues (1984) suggest questions to evaluate the following areas:

Readiness
- Does the client ask questions?
- Does the client have multiple stresses in his or her life that would inhibit concentration on learning?
- Is the client coping with survival issues, such as chronic poverty, unemployment, or rehabilitation from substance abuse, that inhibit learning?
- When is the best time to meet with the client, given other daily expectations?

Attitudes and Feelings
- Have there been past attempts at learning with successful outcomes?
- Does the client have a sense of control over his or her future, as demonstrated by an ability to set and achieve goals, a positive feeling about life, and an ability to care for himself or herself adequately?
- Does the client have worries, depression, or a life situation that would decrease learning?
- Does the client feel vulnerable?

- Does the client feel that actions could make a difference?
- Does the client feel that the benefits of taking action outweigh perceived costs?
- Does the client feel capable of taking the necessary actions?

Style of Learning

- What are the preferred modalities of learning for the client? (e.g., "Do you learn best by reading or listening?" "Does watching a videotape help you learn?")
- What does the client already know about the subject?
- Judging from the developmental level of the client, how concrete or abstract can the teaching be?

4. *Plan.* The plan is formulated using objectives that specify the behaviors that will demonstrate learning. Objectives need to be realistic, achievable, and relevant to the goals of the client. Both short-term and long-term objectives are written if the goals are not achieved in one teaching session. The use of both types of objectives helps the client and NP set priorities and stage education in achievable steps. Generally in routine pediatric visits, objectives are stated, not written, but both client and NP should agree on what is to be achieved.

   Various aids facilitate learning—books, pamphlets, diagrams, videos, and models. Modalities for learning that are most appropriate for the client should be used. Methods for teaching include formal classes, role playing, demonstration and return demonstration, lecture and discussion, reading, viewing videos, or other activities. The plan should facilitate clear presentation of material to the client, provide for frequent reinforcement and feedback, and include some kind of active involvement of the client. Passive listening does not ensure learning.

5. *Manage the learning intervention.* During implementation of the teaching plan, the process is carefully orchestrated to actively engage the client in successful learning. Progress is constantly evaluated, new information added, success reinforced, the pace of feedback assessed, the pace adjusted, and outcomes and achievement of objectives evaluated.

6. *Evaluate the outcomes.* Judge achievement of objectives and then reformulate the plan to move the client to the next level. Learning is evaluated using a variety of methods, such as asking questions that require use of new knowledge to answer, watching for new behaviors, and looking for feelings of achievement and expressions of new understanding.

PATIENT EDUCATION WITH CHILDREN AND ADOLESCENTS

Teaching children includes all the aforementioned steps as well as careful assessment of the child's developmental level, because the concepts the child can learn vary with cognitive abilities. Children's attention spans are often short; therefore, information needs to be presented in smaller bites, with frequent reinforcement and opportunities for doing rather than just listening. Reading skills may not be developed, so verbal and demonstration strategies are more effective for younger children. Terminology might need to be adjusted to use simpler words and concepts. Verbal and nonverbal reinforcement and feedback need to be appropriate for the child. The use of star charts is a good way to reinforce behaviors visually and concretely. Such strategies are consistent with school-age children in Piaget's concrete operations cognitive stage.

For adolescents, assessment of developmental level is also important. The young adolescent (13 to 14 years of age) understands and engages in learning differently from the 18-year-old. Motivators for teenagers do not include knowledge of long-term effects. The use of several modalities, such as discussions with peers, reading, reviewing, and audiovisual media, is helpful. Advice needs to be practical. Teenagers do best when they are viewed as decision makers who need information to make good choices. Identification of strengths as well as weaknesses is always important. The use of peer groups is often effective.

After studying school-age children for 20 years, Lewis and Lewis (1990) concluded that children aged 9 to 12 years are capable of making decisions about self-care if given the opportunity. They are very likely to make their decisions after asking about risks and benefits of engaging or not engaging in health-related activities. The authors suggest that children are not allowed to participate in decisions involving their health because of control issues of parents and health-care providers. Elias and Kress (1994) reported on a project to teach social decision making for health promotion and prevention. Children in middle school are taught skills in self-control, social awareness, and social decision-making and problem-solving through discussions and practice. The skills learned have resulted in less cigarette, alcohol, and marijuana use, less aggression toward peers and parents, and less vandalism and other antisocial behaviors.

PATIENT EDUCATION WITH PARENTS

When working with parents, the provider must keep in mind that parents are experts for their child and home environment, whereas the health-care provider has more knowledge about children as an aggregate. Thus, collaboration between parents and providers produces the best outcomes for the child at hand. Adult education has some unique aspects. First, adults usually want knowledge to help them make decisions for change, not just to gain knowledge per se. Furthermore, they usually have expectations or goals and ideas about activities that will help them. Finally, adults may have to unlearn previous knowledge that is outdated or irrelevant to the situation at hand.

Roberts (1981) developed a model of levels of parent education that is useful to NPs (Table 10-3). The model identifies four levels of parental needs with related levels of responses by nurses. When parents have no obvious needs (level I), they may gain from anticipatory guidance. The nurse's role is one of providing prospective advice and information for future use. When parents feel uneasy about some aspect of child rearing (level II), the nurse begins to serve as a resource to help with the specific issue. At level III, problems overtly affect children in particular areas. The nurse, at this point, moves into a collaborative mode, taking more direct action to support the family rather than merely offering advice for the parents to

T A B L E   10-3

Levels of Parent Education

PARENT NEED LEVEL	NURSING INTERVENTION
I. No obvious needs.	"Prospective mode" —providing anticipatory guidance
II. Parents uneasy and/or engaging in some child care practices that may cause difficulties in the future.	"Resource mode" —responding to specific issues of parenting
III. Parents have obvious needs, because children display difficulties.	"Collaborative mode"—taking more direct actions to support family
IV. Parents' resources inadequate to meet the needs of their children.	"Protective mode"—protecting the children and sometimes the parents

Adapted from Roberts F: A model for parent education. Image 13:89, 1981.

use. For example, the nurse might begin to make telephone calls to arrange consultation appointments for the family or arrange transportation as needed. Finally, at level IV, the parents' resources are inadequate to meet the child's needs, so the nurse moves into a protective mode on behalf of the child.

Parent teaching is most effective at levels I and II. At level III, the parent generally needs more than teaching. And at level IV, the activities of the nurse are designed to support the child first.

Anticipatory Guidance

Anticipatory guidance is a particular form of patient teaching. It is used when the NP wants to be sure that the patient and family have information for decision-making about issues predicted to arise at some time in the future, usually between the current and the next scheduled visit. With the rapid growth and developmental changes occurring in childhood, anticipatory guidance is essential if competent child-rearing practices are to be maintained and developed. Skilled anticipatory guidance involves a process outlined in Table 10–4. The process involves a finely tuned cooperative discussion with the client about issues of client concern. It is *not* a rote recitation of information automatically provided at a specified visit. Skilled anticipatory guidance is individualized teaching, with outcomes mutually agreed on by provider and client. Part of the skill of the NP relates to making issues of anticipated change in the child relevant to the parent so that those issues can become topics for guidance (Pridham et al, 1977).

Providing Data

Often, providing data about a child's status to the parents or adolescent is a powerful yet easy patient education intervention. The height and weight grid and developmental screening or laboratory test scores with interpretation are often significant motivators or reinforcers for the work that parents have been doing. The key is interpretation of information so that the parents know how their child compares with the appropriate norms. Data provided should include both normal outcomes and areas of concern.

T A B L E 10-4
Anticipatory Guidance Steps

1. Scan. Discover the problem.
2. Formulate. Explore the issue, specify and name it.
3. Appraise. Patient decides whether the issue is worth working on—readiness and willingness.
4. Negotiate. Develop willingness on part of both parties.
5. Plan. Divide labor, plan action, and follow up.
6. Implement.
   Orient—develop or change feelings about the issue.
   Guide—identify actions to occur.
   Develop decision-making rules and problem-solving strategies.
   Practice.
7. Evaluate.

Role Modeling

Social learning theory suggests that modeling is an effective way for people to learn. Modeling appropriate parenting techniques can be most effective, especially when the parent then rehearses the desired behaviors with positive reinforcement. McCloskey and Bulechek (1996) classify interventions in this area as behavior therapy. The NP must be careful to create a situation in which parents are left feeling competent—that they are doing a fine job rather than that someone else could do it better. Parents need to feel new confidence as a result of working with the NP and trying out new behaviors. Parenting classes and support groups often provide more time for role modeling and practice of new behaviors than can occur during a primary care visit. Several visits are often needed to help parents learn new responses to children's behavior. Part of the developmental process requires that parents make decisions about when to use new responses they are learning.

Contracting

Establishing a contract with a client or family is an effective intervention that is interactive and collaborative in style. It requires shared responsibility and control on the part of patient and provider. Contracting can involve either contingencies (rewards) for completion of the client's actions to meet the contract or noncontingencies with the implied reward of better health consequences for progress made. It is important to make the contract with all the parties involved.

The contracting process involves three major phases. Phase one includes mutual identification of needs and problems, mutual agreement on goals, resources, and a plan of action. In phase two, the provider and client divide up the labor and responsibilities, establish a time frame, and then implement the plan. Mutual evaluation and renegotiation occur along the way. In phase three, the contract is terminated (Leavitt, 1982). A key factor is to keep the goals achievable.

Bibliotherapy

Promoting use of reading materials can be an excellent intervention in primary care. Books or pamphlets provide information that is well organized and presented in a manner that facilitates its retention. Furthermore, written materials allow patients or families to pace their learning at their own rate, and they serve as a familiar source of reference when needs arise at unexpected times. Redman (1993) refers to printed teaching material as a "frozen language that is selective in its description of reality (which is both a strength and a weakness). It encourages limited feedback but is constantly available." The good reader uses reading materials efficiently, scanning for important words, stopping to summarize the material learned, and using illustrations to enhance the meanings derived from the text. On the other hand, the unskilled reader either spends an inordinate amount of time trying to master the material at hand or sets aside the task, usually without letting the NP know of the difficulties encountered. Thus, the reading levels of the client and the materials must be considered.

Reading also provides vicarious role models for both children and parents, acts as a support by acknowledging the feelings and problems encountered by others with similar problems, and expands perspectives on various health-related issues.

Health System Interventions

McCloskey and Bulechek (1996) identify another domain of nursing interventions that address health system utilization problems. Families with children have many complex needs, which are often met by different organizations such as governmental agencies; health care resources, including clinics, screening programs, health promotion programs, and hospitals; and volunteer programs.

Referrals should be considered whenever there is need for expertise, a more accessible resource, more time for intervention than is available in the current setting, or special types of intervention such as a support group, class, or practice opportunities. Managed care settings, in some cases, seem to discourage use of referrals. However, solving problems efficiently and effectively, even if that means using another resource, is generally a cost-effective intervention.

Identifying and using various community resources requires knowledge and skills that some families do not have. Locating services and helping families learn to use them might be necessary. Transportation, financial resources, the process for entering the system, and the services that can be anticipated are all factors to be discussed with families.

CONCLUSION

Health-promotion management is as important to the health of children as is illness management. The process of diagnosis and treatment is the same for both domains of NP practice. Interventions for both health promotion and disease management include preventive and therapeutic strategies, with patient education essential to ambulatory management. The clients include children or their parents, or both. For adolescents, the client increasingly becomes the adolescent as the independent decision maker.

Because children change so rapidly, their functional health patterns are stable for only short periods of time. The patterns need continual reassessment in light of developmental progress. Parents also need continuing information and new skills to manage their children's evolving health-care needs adequately. In addition, a multitude of factors such as family practices and attitudes, peer influences, and community effects influence the health behaviors of children. Thus, in many ways, health-promotion care for children is more difficult than is management of their physical status. Developing skill as a manager of health promotion for clients is no easy task but it is worth the efforts. It is in the area of functional health pattern management that the unique contributions of NPs to the health care of their clients are confirmed.

REFERENCES

Bandura A: Self-efficacy: Toward a unifying theory of behavioral change. Psychol Rev 84:191–215, 1977.
Burns C: Development and content validity testing of a comprehensive classification of diagnoses for use by pediatric nurse practitioners. Nursing Diagnosis 2:93–104, 1991.

Busen N: Development of an adolescent risk-taking instrument. J Child Adolesc Psychiatr Mental Health Nursing 4:143–149, 1991.

Busen N: Counseling the high-risk adolescent. J Pediatr Health Care 6:194–199, 1992.

Chow M, Durand B, Feldman M, et al: Handbook of Pediatric Primary Care. New York, John Wiley & Sons, 1984.

Clark N, Rosenstock I, Hassan H, et al: Effect of health beliefs and feelings of self-efficacy on self management behavior of children with a chronic disease. Patient Educ Counseling 11:131–139, 1988.

Contento I, Basch C, Shea S, et al: Relationship of mother's food choice criteria to food intake of preschool children: Identification of family subgroups. Health Educ Q 20:243–259, 1993.

Elias M, Kress J: Social decision-making and life skills development: A critical thinking approach to health promotion in the middle school. J School Health 64:62–66, 1994.

Farrand L, Cox C: Determinants of positive health behavior in middle childhood. Nursing Res 42:208–213, 1993.

Friere P: Education for Critical Consciousness. New York, Seabury Press, 1973.

Gordon M: Nursing Diagnosis: Process and Application. New York, McGraw-Hill, 1987.

Hendricks C, Reichert A: Parents' self-reported behaviors related to health and safety of very young children. J School Health 66:247–251, 1996.

Hochbaum G: Public participation in medical screening programs: A socio-psychological study (U.S. Public Health Service Publication No. 572). Washington, DC, US Government Printing Office, 1958.

Kegeles S, Kirscht J, Haefner D, et al: Survey of beliefs about cancer detection and taking Papanicolaou tests. Public Health Rep 80:815–823, 1965.

Koff E, Rierdan J: Early adolescent girls' understanding of menstruation. Women's Health 22:1–19, 1995.

Leavitt, M: Families at Risk: Primary Prevention in Nursing Practice. Boston: Little, Brown, 1982.

Lewis C, Lewis M: Peer pressure and risk-taking behaviors in children. Am J Public Health 74:580–584, 1984.

Lewis C, Lewis M: Consequences of empowering children to care for themselves. Pediatrician 17:63–67, 1990.

Massad S, Shier N, Koceja D, et al: High school athletes and nutritional supplements: A study of knowledge and use. Int J Sports Nutr 5:232–245, 1995.

McCloskey J, Bulechek G (eds): Nursing Interventions Classification, 2nd ed. St. Louis, Mosby-Year Book, 1996.

National Institute of Nursing Research: Report of the Priority Expert Panel on Health Promotion for Older Children and Adolescents. Washington, DC, 1993.

Olvera-Ezzell N, Power T, Cousins J, et al: The development of health knowledge in low-income Mexican-American children. Child Dev 65:416–427, 1994.

Pender N: Health Promotion in Nursing Practice, 2nd ed. Norwalk, CT, Appleton & Lange, 1987.

Pridham K, Hanson M, Conrad H: Anticipatory care as problem-solving in family medicine and nursing. J Fam Practice 4:1077–1081, 1977.

Prochaska J: Disease management needs new paradigms. J Gen Intern Med 10:472–473, 1995.

Prochaska J, DiClemente C, Norcross J: In search of how people change: Applications to addictive behaviors. Am Psychol 47:1102–1114, 1992.

Prochaska J, Velicer W, Rossi J, et al: Stages of change and decisional balance for 12 problem behaviors. Health Psychol 13:39–46, 1994.

Redman B: Patient Education, 7th ed. St. Louis, Mosby-Year Book, 1993.

Richardson S: Child health promotion practices of parents. J Pediatr Health Care 2:73–78, 1988.

Roberts F: A model for parent education. Image 13:86–89, 1981.

Rodrigue J: Promoting healthier behaviors, attitudes, and beliefs toward sun exposure in parents of young children. J Consult Clin Psychol 6:1431–1436, 1996.

Rogers EM: Diffusion of Innovations. New York, Free Press, 1983.

Rosenstock I: Why people use health services. Milbank Memorial Fund Quarterly 44:94–127, 1966.

Stucky-Ropp R, DiLorenzo T: Determinants of exercise in children. Prev Med 22:880–889, 1993.

US Department of Health and Human Services: Healthy People 2000: National Health Promotion and Disease Prevention Objectives for the Year 2000. Washington, DC, US Government Printing Office, 1990.

US Department of Health and Human Services: Healthy people 2010: Draft. Washington, DC, US Government Printing Office, 1998.

Vail-Smith K, Watson C, Felts M, et al: Childhood sun exposure: Parental knowledge, attitudes, and behaviors. J Health Education 28:149–155, 1997.

Valois R, Vincent M, McKeown R, et al: Adolescent risk behaviors and the potential for violence: A look at what's coming to campus. J Am Coll Health 41:141–147, 1993.

Watts A, Breindel C: Health education: Structural vs. behavioral perspectives. Health Political Educ 2:47–57, 1981.

Yoos L: Children's illness concepts: Old and new paradigms. Pediatr Nursing 20:134–140, 1994.

Health Perception and Health Management Pattern

Ardys M. Dunn

INTRODUCTION

Maintenance of health in children depends on a multitude of factors, including appropriate rest, nutrition, stimulation, exercise, and emotional and social nurture. Effective health management is essential to the healthy growth and development of the child. This chapter discusses the ways in which nurse practitioners (NPs) can work with parents, children, and families to ensure that decisions made and actions taken regarding health management are best suited to growing children's needs. The chapter explores factors that influence the health behavior of children and their families and summarizes the health maintenance needs of infants, toddlers, preschoolers, school-age children, and adolescents.

Definition of Health Perception and Health Management Pattern

The health perception and health management functional health pattern provides an overview of children's health status and the behaviors that contribute to health. Relevant questions related to health perception and management include the following: How is health perceived? What characteristics of children contribute to their health status (e.g., is there an underlying chronic illness or genetic disorder)? What decisions have families made and what actions have

they taken to bring children to their current level of health? What resources to support good health are available to families? How can providers intervene to support healthy behaviors or to help change those that are unhealthy?

Significance for Nurse Practitioner Practice

Effective health management requires a commitment to good health, prevention of illness and injury, knowledge of ways to achieve optimum health, and access to and use of necessary health care resources. This functional health pattern is most concerned with the primary level of prevention—that is, actions taken to promote health or protect against specific factors that threaten health, or both.

Use of this functional health pattern gives NPs a better understanding of why certain decisions about health care are made. For example, in some communities, fewer than 50% of children younger than 2 years of age are fully immunized. Parents do not bring their children for regular well-child examinations or for scheduled immunizations. These behaviors could be attributed to the parents' belief that immunizations are unnecessary or even dangerous, or to a lack of knowledge about community health resources that provide immunizations. Transportation, child-care problems, and lack of financial resources can contribute to a parent's failure to bring children for regular well-child visits. By assessing factors that influence the decisions that families make, the NP can intervene effectively so that parents and children actively engage in positive health management.

Standards of Practice

Region X child health nursing standards for health perception and health management include the following outcomes (Region X Nursing Standards Board, 1998):

- Newborn and child receive health care and health screening on an accepted schedule based on health standards; care is appropriate for age.
- Newborn and child are evaluated and treated appropriately when ill or injured.
- Child or primary caregiver, or both know when and how to access health care.
- Child sees self as self-caregiver and self-care advocate.
- Newborn's and child's physical environment promotes health and safety and has been modified to keep hazards to a minimum.
- Newborn's and child's emotional environment is nurturing and fosters growth.
- For newborns and children with special health care needs or disabilities, services are available, appropriate, and coordinated.
- Adolescent is able to access health education, assessment, and treatment services for illness or accidents.
- Adolescent's health status is within normal range for age, development, and potential.
- Adolescent maintains a positive physical and social environment that limits hazards and high-risk behavior.
- Adolescent has adequate resources to meet basic needs.
- Adolescent demonstrates understanding of body changes and adjusts health practices accordingly.

Guidelines for Adolescent Preventive Services (GAPS) recommendations from the American Medical Association (1997) for the care of adolescents related to this functional health pattern include the following:

- Recommendations for delivery of health services:
  - From ages 11 to 21 years, annual age and developmentally appropriate preventive services visits should be available and should be sensitive to individual and sociocultural differences. Three complete physical examinations should be done during this period.
  - Physicians should establish (and communicate to adolescent and parent) office policies regarding confidential care of adolescents, including how parents will be involved.
- Recommendations for health guidance:
  - Parents or other adult caregivers should receive health guidance at least once during their child's early adolescence, once during middle adolescence, and, preferably, once during late adolescence.
  - Annual guidance should be provided to promote a better understanding of physical growth as well as psychosocial and psychosexual development, to promote the importance of becoming actively involved in health care decisions and to promote reduction of injuries.
  - Annual guidance should be given regarding dietary habits, healthy diets, and safe weight management; the benefits of physical activity and encouragement of physical activity; responsible sexual behaviors; and avoidance of tobacco, alcohol and other abusable substances, and anabolic steroids.
- Recommendations for screening:
  - Annual screening should be given for hypertension, risk for hyperlipidemia and adult coronary heart disease, eating disorders and obesity, tobacco use, alcohol and substance use, and use of over-the-counter or prescription drugs, including anabolic steroids, for nonmedical purposes.
  - Annual interviews should discuss involvement in sexual behaviors. In particular, sexually active adolescents should be screened for sexually transmitted diseases (STDs); adolescents at risk for human immunodeficiency virus (HIV) infection should be offered confidential

HIV screening, and sexually active female adolescents or those older than 18 should be screened for cervical cancer (Papanicolaou test).

  ○ Annual interviews should ask about behaviors or emotions indicating severe depression or risk of suicide; history of emotional, physical, and sexual abuse; and learning or school problems.

  ○ Annual tuberculin skin test should be given if the adolescent is at risk for tuberculosis.

  • Recommendations for immunizations:

  ○ All adolescents should receive prophylactic immunizations according to Advisory Committee on Immunization Practices (ACIP) guidelines.

The American Academy of Pediatrics (AAP) Committee on Practice and Ambulatory Medicine (1995) and the US Preventive Services Task Force (1996) have each developed recommendations and periodic schedules of preventive services for children (see Chapter 1, Figure 1–5, for a listing of recommended services).

NORMAL PATTERNS OF HEALTH PERCEPTION AND HEALTH MANAGEMENT

Health perceptions are the ways in which a person thinks about and defines health-related experiences, including the meanings given to illness (Aronowitz, 1998). Health management is based on health perceptions and reflects the judgments of individuals and families, the ways they solve problems, and the decisions or choices they make. Positive health management assumes that wise decisions are made. It also assumes that resources are available for families to implement these decisions. This section discusses normal patterns of behavior expected in this functional health pattern.

Components of Health Perception

By exploring a family's health perceptions, the NP can begin to see the logic of decision-making used by any particular family. Components of health perception include how individuals perceive and feel about their general state of health, past, present, and future, and the belief that there is a relationship between health status and health practices.

PERCEPTION OF HEALTH

How parents, caregivers, and children themselves perceive and feel about children's health status is shaped by several interrelated variables, including

  • Perception of one's susceptibility to the condition
  • Severity of the condition
  • Extent to which the condition has an impact on one's ability to function
  • Knowledge about the condition
  • Knowledge about how children's developmental stages affect their response to illness
  • Developmental stage of the child
  • Cultural or social cues about the condition

These perceptions are, in turn, reflected in health behaviors (Table 11–1).

BELIEF THAT HEALTH PRACTICES AFFECT HEALTH STATUS

The degree to which parents and children believe that they can influence their health status varies. In general, individuals and families with an internal locus of control believe that their behavior affects their health status. They are motivated to take action, seek information, and set goals, believing that such behaviors will make a difference in the outcome. Even when confronted with the stress and uncertainty of illness, they are active problem solvers, engaged in the process of decision-making. In contrast, many individuals and families with an external locus of control tend to believe that factors outside their control determine illness outcomes. These families are passive and dependent, lack motivation to engage in self-care, or fail to follow through with recommended treatments. Rather than actively seeking to change the condition, they let things happen to them. Outcomes for children tend to be poorer in families with external loci of control (Engstrom, 1991).

T A B L E 11-1

Relationship Between Health Perception and Health Behaviors

VARIABLE AFFECTING HEALTH PERCEPTION	RELATED HEALTH BEHAVIORS
Perception of susceptibility	• Increased sense of susceptibility contributes to taking precautions (e.g., immunizations) and seeking early treatment.
Severity of condition	• Severity of condition usually, but not always, results in health-seeking behaviors; if signs and symptoms are subtle or appear minor, care may be delayed. • Minor conditions with alarming signs (e.g., allergic hives) may be responded to aggressively.
Impact on ability to function	• Decreased function motivates health-seeking behaviors (e.g., child with minor illness may not be brought for care unless the condition disrupts sleep or eating patterns).
Knowledge about condition	• Increased understanding of condition usually increases family's ability to manage, either by seeking appropriate health care or providing self-care. • Increased education has not always contributed to health promotion activities. Foltz (1993) found that parents who were educated about dangers of sun exposure (skin cancer) did not consistently apply sunscreens to their children.
Knowledge regarding child development	• Knowledge of child development gives parents ability to anticipate behavior and recognize variations of normal. • Parents who lack knowledge of child development may interpret normal behavior as problematic, or may not perceive atypical behavior as a problem.
Developmental stage of child	• Children's conceptualization and response to illness vary by developmental stage (see Chapter 10).
Cultural or social cues	• Cultural beliefs shape health perceptions (see Chapter 4). • Messages or cues may be mixed (e.g., recent media emphasis on cigar smoking as the "in" thing to do) and can lead to positive and negative health behaviors.

A variety of factors appear to affect the extent of belief in one's ability to control health outcomes, and some research indicates that locus of control may change over time. Age and sex are two factors noted in children, with older children and girls having a more internal locus of control. Additionally, families who are usually self-directed can experience excessive stress related to their child's illness or other life circumstances and may temporarily feel inadequate to cope.

Components of Health Management

Health management is a process of seeking to maintain and promote health. It includes making decisions, taking action, and using resources within a particular environment.

DECISION-MAKING

When confronted with health issues, families are expected to take some action. The actions taken, however, do not always make sense to providers. For example, some parents choose to use harsh forms of discipline to manage their children's behavior, or they elect not to bring their children for regular well-child visits despite the need for immunizations or care of a chronic illness. The decisions behind these actions are a result of an active process tying together the subjective content of health perceptions with the objective reality of health behavior. Although the ways in which people make decisions vary greatly, forms of decisions may fall into categories in which the following occur:

- The decision maker examines and reexamines all options and selects one but may alter the choice if new information or variables arise.
- The person making the decision looks at options but is comfortable making a quick decision without excessive reflection.
- The person making the decision is overly concerned, shifts back and forth from one option to another, and never focuses on one as viable.
- The person elects not to make a decision, procrastinating or avoiding the situation entirely.

A family's decision-making is influenced by many factors, including the following:

- Social support structures
- Perception of health status
- Emotional competence of family members, which may be situational (e.g., the family is confronted with a condition that severely disrupts their emotional or psychological health, such as severe, unexpected trauma to a child)
- Past experience
- Education and knowledge level
- Cognitive abilities of family members
- Values and cultural perspectives
- Economic conditions
- Environment
- Information and advice from the health care provider

The decisions that a family makes lead directly to the health practices and behaviors in which they engage.

HEALTH BEHAVIORS

Several behaviors are expected by health care providers of families within this functional health pattern:

- Establishment of an ongoing relationship with a primary health care provider

- Use of health and community resources to promote health
- Demonstration of lifestyles that promote health and prevent illness and injury

Establishment of Primary Caregiver Relationship

It is expected that the family will establish an ongoing relationship with a primary health care provider, ensuring that the child receives regular physical and developmental evaluations; health maintenance care, such as immunizations; early intervention for minor acute health problems; and information and guidance related to growth and development issues of the child and the family. Having a regular provider also offers the family a stable contact and access to health care resources in case the child requires hospitalization, surgery, or long-term care.

Use of Health and Community Resources to Promote Health

A second behavior expected of a positive health management pattern is that families use health care services in the most effective and efficient manner possible, including appropriate interaction with the provider during the health visit. Effective health management depends on the family's ability to identify and gain access to appropriate social, community, family, and health related resources. For example, many communities have school nurses or school-based clinics, providing case management or primary care in the school setting. The NP can inform parents about these resources, explain their purpose, and encourage parents to communicate with school personnel about children's health needs. School-based health services are especially important for children with chronic illnesses.

Social supports offer a buffer against the stress of daily living, allowing the individual and family to respond more positively to both usual and unexpected events. Families isolated from a social network find it much more difficult to structure health maintenance into their lives or to cope with a child's illness. Connection to a network of community resources (e.g., schools, day care, recreational facilities) also provides structure to support families in daily living activities.

Families need both economic and experiential resources for optimal health management. The cost of health care services is often a barrier to access, contributing to delay or neglect in seeking essential treatment.

Past experience gives parents a base from which to evaluate and make decisions about how to care for their child's illness. Past experience reinforces beliefs about what causes illness, what is the most appropriate treatment, and how effectively parents can care for their children. For example, if parents of an ill child have once managed a fever successfully, they are more likely to feel confident coping with a fever in the child's current condition. If they believe that their child remains free of illness as a result of their care, they are more likely to continue health promotion activities. In contrast, if the child is healthy or ill, despite what the parents do, they can be more inclined to depend on the practitioner for advice or care or not to seek care at all.

There must also be a sufficient number of providers and health care services in the community. For many children, economic barriers prevent access to health care, but for others, adequate resources are simply not available.

Demonstration of Healthy Lifestyles

Finally, healthy families are expected to demonstrate lifestyles that enhance health and prevent illness and injury. Health, disease, illness, and injury are the results of multiple physical, psychological, and environmental factors, some of which are beyond the control of individuals. In many cases, however, health status is influenced by the lifestyle choices that individuals and families make. There are specific categories of individual and family behavior in which change has an impact on health status (Table 11-2). In addition, individuals can take actions that significantly change their external environment, thus influencing forces that affect their health and the health of family members.

ENVIRONMENT

Environmental conditions relate to health management on two levels: first, the nature of the

TABLE 11-2
Lifestyle Choices That Affect Health Status

Nutrition
Smoking
Alcohol use
Drug use
Exercise
Motor vehicle use
Sexual behavior
Social/interactional patterns (family and
  community relations)
Coping and stress management skills

environment affects health status and, second, as noted earlier, resources to support health may or may not be present in the physical environment. Environmental factors such as urban crowding, air pollution, streets with heavy traffic, inadequate housing, poor nutrition, lack of appropriate stimulation (e.g., no playgrounds or recreational facilities), violence, and physical and emotional stress are experienced by many children. In addition, families with limited economic resources have limited access to health care services, and frequent moves prevent families from establishing ongoing connections with a health care provider.

Rural environments often lack health related resources, with few providers, clinics, or hospital services easily available. Children living in rural settings are also at high risk of injury because they are exposed to farm machinery, pesticides, herbicides, unsafe transportation, and other physical hazards (Rivara, 1997; Daniels et al., 1997; Stueland et al., 1996).

CHILDREN WITH SPECIAL NEEDS

Health management of children with special needs is challenging. Chronically ill children receive expert illness care from a number of specialists, but their primary care needs are often neglected. Primary care NPs working with chronically ill children need to effectively coordinate health maintenance care with ongoing illness management. Communication and collaboration with the child's specialty physician are essential, as is clear communication with the parents about the role of each provider in the child's care.

NPs also need to adapt normal intervention techniques when providing primary care to chronically ill children. The regular immunization schedule may need to be adjusted, for example, or special techniques for obtaining height and weight or vital signs might be necessary. Parents and children should be assisted to develop ways to meet daily living needs consonant with the child's abilities. Children with spina bifida, for example, require special intervention to meet activity and exercise needs for growth and development.

■■■■ ASSESSMENT OF HEALTH PERCEPTION AND HEALTH MANAGEMENT PATTERN

Assessment of this functional health pattern focuses on health perception, health management, and decision-making.

History

COMPONENTS OF HEALTH PERCEPTION

Perception of Health

Health perception is assessed by examining the family's health belief structure and knowledge levels. During the initial intake history, a family's general perception of health is assessed. At subsequent visits, questions are focused on the particular presenting condition (e.g., "Tell me what this illness means to you"). General assessment questions include the following:

- How would you describe your child's health right now?
- Compared with other children, how healthy would you say your child is?
- What does it mean for you to say that your child is "healthy"?
- How do you describe good health in your family?
- Do you have any questions or concerns about your child's health, growth, or development?
- How important is it to you to have a regular health care provider?
- What makes you decide to call your health care provider or take your child in for an examination (e.g., as a way to stay well, for a serious problem such as a high fever, an accident, or a problem you've never seen before or one that won't go away)?
- What do you know about this current condition?
- Has your child had a problem like this before?
- How do you expect your child to respond when sick? To this particular sickness?
- What things can you do to help your child cope with being sick?

Belief That Health Practices Affect Health Status

General intake questions can give the NP important information about whether the family and child believe that their health practices affect outcomes. These include the following:

- Has your child ever had this type of problem before?
- What have you done for it in the past?
- What do you do or have you done that you believe makes a difference in how your child responds to illness?
- What kind of personality would you say your child has? How would you describe your child's temperament?
- When confronted with sudden changes in plans or a disruption of normal routine, feelings often change. What kinds of feelings do you have when this happens? How do you deal with those feelings?
- Describe the feelings you have when your child gets ill. How do you deal with those feelings?
- How do you think those feelings affect the way you handle your child's health and illness?

Locus of control can also be assessed using rating scales such as Rotter's (1966) internal-external scale, the health locus of control scale (Wallston et al., 1976), or the multidimensional health locus of control scale (Wallston et al., 1978).

COMPONENTS OF HEALTH MANAGEMENT

Decision-Making

Assessment of the family's decision-making examines how active the family is in making decisions about child's health care, the process used, and the factors that influence those decisions. Questions in this area include the following:

- What do you do when your child has health problems?
- Who makes decisions about health care in your family?
- How do you make those decisions? Do you talk things over? Do you get advice from others?
- Why do you think that you make decisions in that way?
- What are the most important things that you consider when making a decision about health care for your child?
- What is most difficult for you when you have to make decisions related to your child's health?

Health Behaviors and Use of Resources

The following questions refer to actions taken and resources used that promote health and contribute to healing:

- Do you have a regular health care provider for your child?
- What health care resources are available to you? Is there a primary care provider you can get to conveniently? Clinics? Pharmacies?
- When was the last time your child visited a regular health care provider or dentist?
- What makes it hard for you to follow the advice of your health care provider?
- What immunizations has your child received?
- What have you done to protect your child from injuries? What are your patterns of seatbelt use?

- Does your child have any special health problems? How do you manage them?
- There has been much focus on healthy lifestyles lately, such as eating right and exercising. What does your family do regularly to stay healthy?
- Does anyone in your family (adolescents, you yourself) smoke, drink, or use drugs? How often? What kind? Are there other things that your family does that you think are bad for your children's health?
- How does your family fit into your neighborhood? Do you feel like part of the community? Do you have relatives or neighbors on whom you can call if you need help or advice?
- Who cares for your child when you are not at home and the child is not in school?
- How are you managing household, work, school, and other child-care responsibilities during this illness? What is most difficult for you?
- Having sick children can create a financial strain on families. Is this a problem for your family? What is the most difficult part?
- How comfortable do you feel managing this illness? Have you had experience in the past that helps you manage?

Environment

Environmental conditions are difficult to assess during a clinic visit, even if the parent is open, cooperative, and willing to share information. If there is a question about the health of the child because of possible environmental problems, it may be appropriate to arrange for a community health nurse to visit the family at home to gain a thorough understanding of the family environment. Questions that can be asked in the clinic include the following:

- Do you use seatbelts or child restraints when riding in a car?
- Where does your child play? Do you believe it is safe? Why?
- Is your home childproof?
- How do you heat or cool your home? Is it comfortable?
- Is there any danger of falls? Does your child get enough to eat? Is he or she dressed

warmly for cold weather? Do you have a working smoke alarm?

- What would you do if your child had a health emergency? Do you have a car, or is there a friend, family member, or neighbor close by who could help you?
- What other conditions in your child's environment do you think could be a health risk?

Children With Special Needs

Assessment of the health perception and management pattern for children with special needs encompasses all the categories just discussed, with questions such as the following:

- What does it mean for you to say that your child is "healthy"?
- How did you feel when your child's problem was diagnosed? What did you do? What coping strategies do you currently use as you care for your child?
- How has managing a chronic illness changed your family functioning? How does your family function?
- Who is providing specialty care to your child? Do you believe this is adequate? What other special needs do you believe your child has that require care?
- How comfortable are you in providing home care? What would you need to be more comfortable?
- How are your child's regular health needs met—that is, those not directly related to the chronic illness, such as immunizations?
- What resources do you know about that can help you understand and manage your child's illness?
- What special physical arrangements have you made to accommodate your child's illness? At home? In the car? At school or day care?

▆▆▆ MANAGEMENT STRATEGIES FOR POSITIVE HEALTH PERCEPTION AND HEALTH MANAGEMENT

Parents and NPs work together to manage children's health. Each has a responsibility to en-

sure that children are receiving the best possible care. This section discusses areas of intervention relevant to health perception and health management.

Providing Health Maintenance for Children by Developmental Age

Health supervision visits for children are more than a simple physical checkup. Visits with the NP also allow assessment of home, family, and social life, teaching about growth and development, and problem-solving related to issues that affect children's health status. The visits can be used to enhance children's sense of independence and positive self-concept and to encourage children to make healthy lifestyle decisions. As children mature, they should be actively involved in the visit, with the NP asking them questions directly and providing appropriate feedback to their responses. In addition to screening interventions recommended by the American Academy of Pediatrics (1995) (see Fig. 1-5), the health supervision visit examines the child's daily living and functional health patterns as identified in Table 11-3.

Facilitating Communication Between Families and Nurse Practitioners

Effective communication between families and NPs requires sensitivity and skill. Families must be given the message that their values and beliefs are important, that NPs recognize they are making their best effort to do the right thing, and that those efforts are to be applauded. If families are listened to, they are more likely to participate in health care decision-making and be more invested in the process and outcome. Communication is facilitated by two strategies in particular, one focused on content and the other on process. These strategies relate to health promotion as well as illness management.

First, NPs, parents, and children must develop a mutual understanding of the perspectives that each brings to the encounter (Kleinman et al., 1978). To do this, family members must be encouraged to explain their understanding of the child's illness as well as their

Text continued on page 222

Health Supervision Visits: Assessment of Daily Living and Functional Health Patterns

	INFANT	TODDLER	PRESCHOOL CHILD	SCHOOL-AGE CHILD	ADOLESCENT
Parent–child interaction	Assess degree of mutual and reciprocal response between infant and parents Emotional status of parents Appropriateness of parental response to infant's cues	Assess parental confidence in role Emotional status of parents Appropriateness of parental response to toddler's cues Degree of affection demonstrated between toddler and parents Parental encouragement of independence, yet active involvement with child	Assess consistency in parents' behavior Emotional status of parents Appropriateness of parental response to child's cues Degree to which parents provide affection, praise, emotional support, and encourage child to express feelings Parental encouragement of independence, yet active engagement with child	Determine whether parents express clear, consistent but flexible expectations Appropriate limits set by parents Degree to which parents provide attention, affection, praise, approval, emotional support, and encourage child to express feelings Degree to which parents support independence, yet participate with child in activities Degree to which child demonstrates self-confidence, industriousness, cooperation, and consideration	Assess parental confidence and pleasure in role Open communication with mutual respect for privacy Parental encouragement of independence and activities with peers Reasonable and consistent limits Active parental interest in adolescent's activities, friends, school performance Parental pride and pleasure in adolescent's achievements
Developmental assessment to determine extent to which child has achieved milestones and received emotional nurturing	See Chapters 6 and 18	See Chapters 7 and 18	See Chapters 7 and 18; look for child who is friendly, secure, cooperative, proud and happy Conduct speech evaluation	See Chapters 8 and 18 Conduct speech evaluation	See Chapters 9 and 18

Table continued on following page

T A B L E 11-3

Health Supervision Visits: Assessment of Daily Living and Functional Health Patterns *Continued*

	INFANT	TODDLER	PRESCHOOL CHILD	SCHOOL-AGE CHILD	ADOLESCENT
Nutrition/metabolic	Discuss choice of feeding, breastfeeding versus bottle feeding (see Chapter 13); when to introduce solids; management of feeding problems or special nutritional needs (see Chapter 12) Fluoride beginning at 6 mo as indicated according to fluoride level in water source Skin care: Apply sun screen whenever child is exposed to sun	Discuss management of self-feeding, feeding problems, or special nutritional needs Explain pattern of dentition, need for good oral hygiene (see Chapters 12 and 34) Continue fluoride as indicated Skin care: Apply sun screen whenever child is exposed to sun	Discuss need for well-balanced diet Discuss parents' responsibility to provide nutritious foods, pleasant atmosphere for meals, and healthy role models for child; child's responsibility to select appropriate foods from those provided Explain pattern of dentition, need for dental assessment (see Chapters 12 and 34) Continue fluoride as indicated Skin care: Apply sun screen whenever child is exposed to sun	Discuss healthy food selections with child Encourage daily dental hygiene (see Chapters 12 and 34) Continue fluoride as indicated Skin care: Apply sun screen whenever child is exposed to sun	Discuss nutritional needs, dietary patterns Discuss body image and self-perception as they relate to eating habits Encourage good oral hygiene, regular dental care (see Chapters 12 and 34), orthodontia Fluoride until age 16, as indicated Skin care: Apply sun screen whenever child is exposed to sun Discuss acne management as appropriate
Sleep and rest: discuss sleep needs, patterns, and changes as child grows (see Chapter 16)	Discuss the importance of bedtime ritual, infant cues for sleep and wake states Instruct parents to position infant on back for sleep	Discuss the importance of bedtime ritual	Discuss typical night fears, night terrors	Discuss sleepwalking and night terrors	Discuss sleep needs during rapid growth of adolescence

Category					
Activity and exercise (see Chapter 15): discuss injury prevention (see Tables 11–7 through 11–10)	Discuss physical developmental needs and skills of infant	Discuss need to set limits and provide safe environment for expression of physical needs and developing skills	Discuss need to set limits and provide safe environment for expression of physical needs and skills Encourage child's active, pretend, and fantasy play; discourage passive activities such as watching television Discuss child's tendency to become overtired, often needing parent's help to calm down	Encourage regular physical activity Discuss bicycle, skateboard, swimming safety Discuss balance of nutrition with exercise to achieve appropriate weight gain Evaluate for scoliosis in child aged 10–12 years	Encourage regular physical activity, participation in fitness and organized sports activities Evaluate for scoliosis Evaluate for sports fitness
Elimination (see Chapter 14)	Discuss diapering, infant patterns of stooling and urination	Discuss toilet training	Discuss management of occasional "accidents" in toilet-trained child Teach good hygiene, handwashing	Discuss importance of good hygiene, handwashing Explain relationship between nutrition, exercise, and elimination	Discuss importance of good hygiene, handwashing Explain relationship between nutrition, exercise, and elimination

Table continued on following page

T A B L E 11-3
Health Supervision Visits: Assessment of Daily Living and Functional Health Patterns *Continued*

	INFANT	TODDLER	PRESCHOOL CHILD	SCHOOL-AGE CHILDREN	ADOLESCENT
Sexuality (see Chapter 20)	Discuss infant's sense of physical comfort and pleasure related to stimulation of genitalia Encourage parents to express their perceptions of sexuality in infant and child Assess testes and inguinal canal for abnormalities	Discuss toddler's sense of physical comfort and pleasure related to genital stimulation Encourage parents to express their perceptions of sexuality; discuss ways parents communicate with toddler about sexuality	Discuss child's natural curiosity related to sexuality Encourage parents to answer questions at age-appropriate level Discuss concept of "good" and "bad" touch; private body parts	Discuss children's natural curiosity and exploration related to sexuality Encourage parents to answer questions at age-appropriate level, set appropriate limits for sexual activity in child Assess sexual maturation in older school child	Discuss adolescent's developing sense of sexual identity, masturbation, degree of intimacy with others Counsel regarding sexual responsibility to self and others, including how to say "no" and how to deal with potential sexual abuse or "date rape" Discuss prevention of sexually transmitted diseases and pregnancy; discuss birth control options Assess sexual maturation stages, gynecomastia in boy

Role relationships (see Chapters 3 and 19)	Discuss infant's interaction with siblings and other family members; evaluate impact child has on family system, place of child in family	Discuss discipline strategies, interaction of toddler with siblings, other family members, impact child has on family system, place of child in family, day care needs and plans	Discuss discipline strategies, interaction of child with siblings, other family members, impact child has on family system, place of child in family, day-care needs and plans, school readiness for older preschool-age child	Discuss importance of increasing child's participation in family activities, taking more responsibility for tasks in household; discuss nature of child's interaction in school and with peer group; suggest that parents encourage and participate in hobbies, reading, other activities with child and peer group	Perform pelvic examination in sexually active girl, girl with menstrual problems, or those with history of mother taking diethylstilbestrol (DES) Teach breast and testicular self-examination Recommend folic acid 400 µg/day for girl Discuss importance of increasing independence in adolescents, taking responsibilities at home, school, or workplace; emphasize need to keep communication open among adolescent, peers, and parents

Table continued on following page

T A B L E 11-3
Health Supervision Visits: Assessment of Daily Living and Functional Health Patterns *Continued*

	INFANT	TODDLER	PRESCHOOL CHILD	SCHOOL-AGE CHILDERN	ADOLESCENT
Self-concept/self-perception (see Chapter 18)	Explain process of infant's developing an awareness of self as separate from parents and others	Explain importance of giving child positive feedback on achievements Encourage parents to relate to child in warm, loving manner; avoid harsh words and punitive parental behavior	Encourage parents to give children choices, allowing children to express selves and participate in family tasks Explain children's sense of absolutes at this age; discourage teasing and threats Encourage parents to participate in child's activities (e.g., school field trips)	Encourage parents to give child attention and positive reinforcement of choices, allowing child to express self and expecting participation in family tasks	Give adolescent opportunities to discuss changes in self and to openly ask questions about development Encourage parents to give adolescent positive attention, reinforcement for healthy choices and appropriate activities, allowing adolescent privacy, and expecting reasonable participation in family activities

Coping and stress tolerance	Identify family support network Assess knowledge of community resources Assess knowledge of child development Identify level of parenting skills Discuss how parents' health habits (e.g., smoking, exercise, diet) may affect child	Identify family support network Assess knowledge of community resources Assess parents' knowledge of child development Identify level of parenting skills Discuss discipline styles and options Encourage parent to guide and instruct child's positive social behavior (e.g., sharing, not hitting or biting)	Identify family support network Assess knowledge of community resources Assess parents' knowledge of child development Identify level of parenting skills Discuss discipline styles and options; need to set limits Encourage parents to help child name and identify feelings and discuss ways the child can manage feelings	Identify family support network Assess knowledge of community resources Assess parents' knowledge of child development Identify level of parenting skills Discuss discipline styles and options; need to set limits Encourage parents to praise child's efforts at self-control, management of feelings Assess for depression	Identify family support network Assess knowledge of community resources Assess parents' knowledge of child development Identify level of parenting skills Discuss discipline styles and options Encourage parents to provide appropriate limits while fostering independence Discuss adolescent's emotional states related to rapid growth and changes of puberty Assess for depression
Values and beliefs	Discuss parents' expectations of self and child as family grows	Encourage parents to identify their value and belief framework Discuss how they demonstrate their beliefs to their child	Encourage parents to provide opportunities for child to express ideas, feelings, and emotions Include child in family spiritual activities	Encourage parents to provide opportunity for child to explore understanding of emotions, values, and beliefs in more formal settings (e.g., religious institutions, spiritual activities)	Explain to parents that adolescent, as part of normal process of developing self-identity, may appear to reject family values Encourage adolescent to discuss values and beliefs

expectations for its outcome and the role each player has in working toward that outcome. NPs must explain their perspective, usually biomedical, focusing on similar areas of concern: cause, symptoms, pathophysiology, nature and course of the illness, and treatment.

Kleinman et al. (1978) outlined a set of questions to elicit information about a family's health beliefs. These questions can be adapted and used with parents when asking about their child's illness:

- What do you think caused your child's problem?
- Why do you think it started when it did?
- How has this illness affected your child?
- How severe is your child's sickness?
- Will it have a short or long course?
- What kind of treatment should your child receive?
- What are the most important results you hope to have happen from this treatment?
- What are the chief problems your child's sickness has caused?
- What do you fear most about your child's sickness?

With this information in hand, NPs, parents, and children can compare similarities and differences between their perspectives, develop a "clinical picture of the illness that is compatible with the [client's] experience" (Marshall, 1988), and create a mutually agreed upon plan of care.

A second strategy that strengthens communication and contributes to families having a greater sense of control in the situation relates to the process of the client–provider interaction. Marshall (1988) asserts that, in order to arrive at the appropriate interpretation of what the clinical situation means, clients and providers must engage in a process of interpretation at the conversational level. This "conversational cooperation" is enhanced when family members and the NP do the following:

- Use cooperative turn-taking in the conversation.
- Use similar patterns of conversation, such as open-ended questions or narrative discussion; communication is at risk, for example, if parents are using a narrative form

of discussion and the NP is using close-ended questions.
- Listen for the images clients use in speech patterns and try to respond in kind. Parents may use visual, auditory, or kinesthetic imagery when they talk, and may better understand providers who respond with similar imagery. For example, the parent may state, "I don't see any change..."; the provider responds, "You're looking for...". Or, the parent states, "I want to do something...," and the provider answers, "You'd like to take some action..." (Howard, 1998).
- Confirm assumptions.
- Develop a clear understanding of differences in perspectives or meaning of the illness.
- Remain open to alternative explanations and solutions, not limited to following an isolated path of clinical reasoning.
- Explain or provide the context of pronouns used; for example, if NPs say, "I'll check on that for you," they should be sure the parent understands what "that" means.

Helping Families Develop Sound Decision-Making Skills

A number of studies indicate that the health decisions people make are not necessarily shaped by the health education they receive (Rosenbaum, 1998; Marchand & Morrow, 1994). Nevertheless, health education, in which providers give information to clients, is still viewed as an essential component of intervention. The manner in which information is given, however, may be as important as the information itself. NPs who work with parents to establish effective communication, to generate mutual understanding of problems, and to listen actively to feelings, perceptions, fears, and anxieties are more likely to be heard by parents when they offer information or suggestions for care. Developing this level of rapport is important, because it is the information that NPs provide that allows parents to identify, evaluate, select, and implement options for care. NPs also serve an essential role in structuring the forum for parents to discuss feelings, clarify points of confusion, and receive validation for their choices in this decision-making process. The process of making health care decisions includes the following steps:

- Identify the problem being confronted. Review the facts and feelings one has about the problem.
- Generate alternative solutions to the problem.
- Evaluate the alternatives. Which are feasible? Which are cost effective? What are the consequences of each? Which best fits the family's belief system?
- Select a solution.
- Develop and implement a plan of action based on that solution.
- Review the outcomes of the decision and the action taken.

For this process to function well, families must be able, or be assisted, to communicate effectively, understand abstract concepts, and mobilize resources. Children should be encouraged to participate in the process consistent with their developmental abilities. Adolescents, especially, are at a stage at which they can make many decisions independently of their parents. NPs serve a vital role in helping families and children develop sound decision-making skills.

Helping Families Gain Access to Health Care Resources

Access to health care resources is influenced by a number of factors. Strategies to increase parents' ability to access resources occur on two levels: (1) giving parents the information to more easily and appropriately gain access and (2) removing barriers to access.

GIVING PARENTS INFORMATION TO GAIN ACCESS

Teaching Telephone Triage

An important parental skill involves effective use of the telephone to manage children's health. The nature of the telephone interaction between parent and NP can be a critical factor in accurately interpreting a child's condition, deciding on appropriate measures of care, and establishing confidence and trust. Chapter 23

presents a discussion of how pediatric care providers can use the telephone in the management of illnesses. The discussion here focuses on helping parents use the telephone as a resource for health care services (Brown, 1994; Schmitt, 1998). Tables 11–4 and 11–5 list criteria parents should use when deciding whether to call and how to manage telephone contacts (Brown, 1994).

An additional concern for parents is deciding when it is appropriate to call back about their child's condition. Parents should be instructed to contact the provider in the following circumstances:

- Symptoms persist
- Symptoms become worse
- There is a change in symptoms (i.e., symptoms become more severe or new symptoms appear) indicating deterioration of health status
- Parents feel a sense of increased anxiety

Identifying Resources

NPs serve as advocates by helping families locate local, regional, or national health care resources to serve their health needs. It is important that NPs develop and maintain a resource list relevant to their practice. Using a resource list facilitates making referrals and recommendations to parents; it gives the clear message that the family is not alone with their concern, that help is available, and that the NP is a knowledgeable ally in the family's effort to maintain good health.

Assisting in Contact of Support Networks

As an advocate, NPs make every effort to encourage independent action and decision-making by families, but if the family's coping abilities are compromised, it is not enough simply to give the name of a resource or contact to the family. In these situations, NPs need to contact the resource themselves or assist the family to make the contact. For some families in crisis, it is appropriate to refer them to a community or mental health nurse for assistance in establishing and maintaining contact with a supportive network.

T A B L E 11-4

General Rules When Calling the Nurse Practitioner or Physician: Guidelines for Parents

When calling for **nonurgent** matters, such as well-baby advice, prescription refills, or appointments, call during office hours whenever possible.

When calling for an **emergency**, tell the receptionist or answering service that your call is an emergency call.

Give the following **information on every call**: your child's name, age, sex, major problem, and telephone number where you can be reached.

Be ready to give **information related to your child's problem** as briefly and clearly as possible:

What are signs and symptoms?

How long has the problem been there?

What have you done for the problem?

How did your child respond to what was done?

How do you feel about your child's condition? What is your intuition? Is your child getting better, worse?

Be ready to give **information about your child's general health:**

Does your child have any chronic illnesses that need to be considered?

Is your child receiving medications for this problem, another problem, or has your child recently received immunizations?

Does your child have any allergies?

If you do not talk to your provider directly, **before hanging up**, ask when your call will most likely be returned.

If you do not receive a return call within a reasonable amount of time, **call back** to make sure your message was taken correctly.

If your provider decides not to examine your child, **before hanging up**, make sure you determine the following:

The most likely cause of your child's condition.

Which medicines or treatments should be given.

What signs or symptoms to watch for.

When you should call back for more advice or to report changes in your child's condition.

If you don't **understand the instructions** given, ask to have them repeated or call back for clarification.

If you are instructed to come to the office or go to an emergency department, make sure you **have clear directions on how to get there**. If you are too anxious to drive, ask a friend or neighbor to drive or call a taxi. If an ambulance is necessary, the provider may be able to call it for you.

Adapted from Brown JL: Pediatric Telephone Medicine: Principles, Triage, and Advice, 2nd ed. Philadelphia, JB Lippincott, 1994.

T A B L E 11-5

Deciding When to Call the Nurse Practitioner or Physician: Guidelines for Parents

WHEN TO CALL IMMEDIATELY FOR AN INFANT YOUNGER THAN 3 MO

If your baby manifests the following symptoms:

Is lethargic (very sleepy or difficult to arouse), has poor color, or appears limp and unresponsive

Has a rectal temperature of 100.4°F (38°C) or higher

Refuses to eat three or four times in a row

Has repeated bouts of diarrhea or vomiting

Has a labored, wheezing, or grunting breathing pattern that lasts longer than ½ hr

Has an illness associated with a rash that looks like bleeding under the skin

If your baby's eyes, hands, or feet have a yellow, jaundiced color or if the baby develops pumpkin-colored skin

If you feel very nervous about your baby's illness or general condition

WHEN TO CALL IMMEDIATELY FOR AN OLDER CHILD

If your child has the following symptoms:

Seems unresponsive, does not make eye contact with you, or has cold and clammy skin that is not associated with vomiting

Looks much sicker than usual with a routine illness

Has an illness associated with a rash that looks like bleeding under the skin

Has any symptom that you believe to be unusual or frightening; this includes labored breathing, severe headache, or very high fever

WHEN TO CALL IMMEDIATELY AFTER TRAUMA OR INJURY

If your child has struck his or her head and has lost consciousness, has nausea or vomiting, or complains of severe headache; also call if there is mental confusion, unbalanced walking, poor coordination, loss of memory, or a discharge coming from one or both ears

If there is a persistent swelling, tenderness, or deformity of the injured part

If your child refuses to use an injured extremity for more than ½ hr

If there is a deep puncture wound, a cut longer than ½ inch, or your child has not received a tetanus shot within the past 5–10 yr

If there is injury to an eye that causes redness, pain, or tearing for more than 15 min

If your child has been bitten by an animal and the bite has gone through the skin

If you need first aid instructions for uncontrolled bleeding or other problems

If you believe that your child may have swallowed a toxic or poisonous substance

WHEN TO CALL ABOUT SYMPTOMS

If you are concerned about your child's general appearance

If the symptoms seem to be getting progressively worse or last longer than expected

If fever of more than 101°F has persisted for longer than 24 hr

If cough, cold, sore throat, or runny nose has lasted longer than 48 hr

If vomiting has lasted longer than 8 hr or diarrhea longer than 24 hr, or when there is blood in the stool or vomit

If your child has severe stomach pains lasting longer than 4 hr

If the symptom seems more severe than it has in the past

If your child has a rash or other problem and you are not sure what is causing it

If you are not certain whether the child needs to be seen by the health care provider

Adapted from Brown JL: Pediatric Telephone Medicine: Principles, Triage, and Advice, 2nd ed. Philadelphia, JB Lippincott, 1994.

REMOVING BARRIERS TO ACCESS

Among the primary barriers to health care access are cost, geography, and lack of essential infrastructure services such as transportation and child care. NPs are aware of the relationship between the high cost of care and the failure of children to receive regular well-child care. Lack of primary care resources in rural and isolated areas also prevents families from obtaining regular care. Without adequate transportation or child-care services, the cost of seeking well-child care, or even treatment of minor acute problems that worsen without medical intervention, often outweighs the benefits perceived by the family.

NPs can work with parents and social workers to identify resources in the community that help overcome some of these barriers. For example, transportation may be available through some managed care plans or local volunteer organizations (e.g., churches), or a relative may have time to care for other children while the parent takes one child to the clinic. For other barriers, however, the solution lies in making changes in the way health care services are organized and financed. This task goes far beyond the primary care setting, but it is nonetheless the responsibility of NPs to be aware of and to participate in the process of restructuring and reorganizing the health care system within their community.

▇▇▇▇ ALTERED PATTERNS OF HEALTH PERCEPTION AND HEALTH MANAGEMENT

Ineffective Use of Health Care System

DESCRIPTION

Ineffective use of the health care system includes seeking care primarily when children are ill or when there is an external mandate (e.g., when immunizations are required to attend school), using emergency departments for routine care needs, using outpatient services for emergency care, not establishing an ongoing relationship with a primary care provider, underutilizing health care resources, or failing to comply or follow up with prescribed regimens. A key element of noncompliance is that the child or caregivers actively choose not to adhere to health recommendations despite knowledge of the benefits and risks.

ETIOLOGY

Ineffective use of the health care system can have many causes. Among these are long-standing patterns of misuse, knowledge deficit about how to gain access to and use the system, and knowledge deficit about health and illness, such as the seriousness of illness in children. Access to care can be limited by social, physical, or economic barriers. Health care in the United States is largely connected to employment, and the unemployed, or those with low incomes, may not be able to afford insurance. In addition, some employees receive no health insurance coverage benefits or, for others, insurance coverage is inadequate. The Medicaid program reimburses providers for primary health care services for families whose income is low enough to qualify for welfare.

Cultural perceptions of care and the perception that health care providers do not understand or value the family or their cultural beliefs can discourage use of health care services. Values, beliefs, and perceptions of risk and benefits contribute to the choices made. For example, a client may refuse chemotherapy for leukemia, believing that there is greater risk associated with the treatment than with the disease itself. Finally, a lack of health care resources can contribute to incomplete care. Health facilities in rural areas and poor urban areas are often absent or understaffed, leaving residents with no one to provide their care.

CLINICAL FINDINGS

The following are found with ineffective use of the health care system:

- No regular provider for child.
- History of fragmented care, lack of continuity of care.
- Lack of follow-up care for child seen in emergency department.
- Use of emergency department for nonemergent conditions.

- Failure to adhere to prescribed medical treatment or standards for well-child health supervision after having adequate information for decision-making.
- Child at risk for delayed or ineffective treatment or both.
- Poor health status of children as a result of untreated illness or other health problem.
- Underimmunization.
- Parents express dissatisfaction with health care providers.

DIFFERENTIAL DIAGNOSIS

- Dysfunctional family systems related to cognitive, emotional, or psychological variables

MANAGEMENT

Interventions vary depending on the reasons families ineffectively use the system.

Lack of an Identified Primary Care Provider

- Assist the family to establish a permanent relationship with a provider.
- Encourage and reinforce positive, ongoing communication with the primary care provider. As a primary care provider, the NP should establish a positive, accepting environment of trust and mutual respect, encouraging the family and child to take an active role in health care.
- Assist the child and family to develop an understanding of the importance of regular care.

Barriers to Access to Health Care Services

- Inform families of health care resources available in the community.
- Teach the family how to access and use health care services most effectively.
- Assist families to identify strengths and resources within their social and family network.
- Refer to social services or other resources to deal with financial concerns.

- Work with community, local, state, and federal leaders to change the way health care services are organized and financed.

Knowledge Deficit About Children

- Assess knowledge level of families related to development and health care needs of children.
- Educate parents about normal growth and development of children.
- Provide anticipatory guidance about variations of normal.

Knowledge Deficit Related to Illness

- Explain what can be expected during minor illnesses or with conditions that change the child's health status. For example: What signs and symptoms might be seen with an ear infection or following routine immunizations? What physiological changes can be expected in the child with an acute asthma attack? What factors might precipitate an asthma attack? Discuss what the caregiver can do to manage the condition in the home. For example: What can the parent do to control a fever if one should occur? How can the family manage the child's environment to minimize the possibility of an asthma attack?
- Establish a plan with the family about when and whom to call for help. Parents should be given clear instructions on when to use the telephone, when to bring the child back to the office, or when to use the emergency department (see Tables 11-4 and 11-5). The care of chronic or acute conditions is shared by family and provider. Although minor conditions can often be managed and more serious conditions prevented by actions taken in the home, many problems require professional intervention. Families should be encouraged to initiate contact with the NP when they have questions and doubts about their child's condition.
- Strengthen the family's ability to make appropriate decisions regarding care of ill children in the home. Support active participation in decision-making and provide

information needed to care for children in the home.

Noncompliance with Health Requirements

- Develop a partnership with the family around health care decision-making.
- Ensure that clients are active participants, invested in the decisions made.
- Assist the family to identify the bases of their decision-making.
- Identify differences between families' and NPs' approaches to health care.
- Clearly state when and why the NP disagrees with the client's decisions. In some cases, clients and NPs can "agree to disagree" on one issue, finding others on which they can work together. In other cases, NPs can feel so strongly about an issue that they need to refer clients to another provider.
- Provide positive reinforcement for healthy decisions.

Risk-Taking Behaviors

DESCRIPTION

Risk-taking behaviors include substance abuse, smoking, and other activities that threaten the health and well-being of the child or adolescent. This section focuses on smoking in adolescents. Smoking appears within a cluster of risk-taking behaviors and adolescent smokers tend to be poorer students, watch more television, have higher use of alcohol and marijuana, drive while drunk, use automobile seatbelts less frequently, and report more stress and depression than their nonsmoking peers (Coogan et al., 1998; Dappen et al., 1996).

ETIOLOGY AND INCIDENCE

It is estimated that in 1996, seventy-seven of every 1000 teenagers began smoking, a marked increase from 1988 when the incidence of new teen smokers was about 51 per 1000 (Centers for Disease Control and Prevention, 1998). The majority of teens begin smoking in early to middle adolescence (Dappen et al., 1996) and,

in one study of more than 30,000 students, the prevalence of smoking "increased precipitously between ages 14 and 15" (Coogan et al., 1998). Coogan's study found the highest rate of smoking among white female students. Having a close friend, sibling, or parent who smokes influences the adolescent's decision to begin smoking. Advertising by the tobacco industry has been shown to have a direct impact on encouraging teenagers to smoke (Centers for Disease Control and Prevention, 1998), and the tobacco industry is actively advertising to youth, especially from neighborhoods with large minority populations (Pucci et al., 1998).

CLINICAL FINDINGS

In the clinical setting, adolescents' smoking patterns are best assessed through direct questioning. Biochemical tests to measure tobacco by-products (e.g., carbon monoxide in serum or expired alveolar air, cotinine—a primary metabolite of nicotine, and thiocyanate—a detoxification product of hydrogen cyanide in tobacco smoke) are used primarily in the research setting. At every visit, children should be asked whether they or their friends smoke or use other forms of tobacco.

Increased incidence of respiratory disease in children, including asthma, is a clinical finding in smokers or in families in which parents smoke.

MANAGEMENT

Management of adolescent tobacco use takes place on two levels: (1) primary, with a goal of preventing the child from starting to use, and (2) secondary, with a goal of cessation (Table 11–6). Many adolescents experiment with tobacco use but stop after a short period of time before becoming addicted to nicotine. Addiction to nicotine appears to occur over about a 2-year period (Elster & Kuznets, 1994), giving providers an opportunity to intervene early for more effective cessation.

Many children are exposed to second-hand smoke of parents or other caregivers. Not only does this put them at risk for health and learning problems (Fried et al., 1997; Glantz & Parmley, 1995), but these children are also more

T A B L E 11-6

Primary and Secondary Prevention/Tobacco Use Cessation Strategies for Adolescents

PRIMARY PREVENTION	SECONDARY PREVENTION
Provide multimedia, multisite health information, not limited to schools	Ask at every visit whether adolescent or friends use tobacco
Emphasize skills to avoid peer pressure	Inform adolescent of health risks of tobacco use and process by which one becomes addicted to nicotine; emphasize that it is easier to stop early
Focus on adolescents' developmental need to belong to a social group	Develop mutual understanding of problem
	Determine realistic stop-use date
	Help adolescent identify barriers to stopping and ways to overcome those barriers
	Provide information about self-help and support groups; encourage adolescent to try to stop smoking with a friend
	Provide nicotine patches protocol if adolescent feels this will help
	Schedule follow-up visits to monitor progress; reinforce positive efforts

likely to become smokers themselves. Intervention with parents who smoke is appropriate for the pediatric primary care provider. One successful approach has been to provide parents with information about the hazards of passive smoking at delivery and at each subsequent well-child visit (Wall et al., 1995). Although pediatric NPs are not the parents' primary caregivers, they can encourage parents to make the decision to stop smoking, support any efforts they make toward decreasing smoking behaviors, and refer the parents for smoking cessation that involves the following:

- Asking about smoking at every medical visit
- Advising all smokers to stop
- Assisting patients with stop-smoking contracts, and self-help and motivating materials
- Setting a quit-smoking date and prescribing nicotine gum
- Arranging follow-up visits to reinforce the intervention (Elster & Kuznets, 1994)

In addition, medical practices could implement population-based interventions to help their clients stop tobacco use (McAfee et al.,

1998). These include tracking and monitoring smokers, providing insurance coverage for tobacco-cessation services, educating employees not to use tobacco, and lobbying for public antismoking campaigns and increased taxes on tobacco products.

Unintentional Injuries

DESCRIPTION

Unintentional injuries are traumatic events that are unanticipated and accidentally caused (see Chapter 40 for a more complete discussion of injuries in children).

ETIOLOGY AND INCIDENCE

Unintentional injury in children results from many factors, including the presence of hazards in the environment, unsafe or risky behaviors, and inadequate adult supervision. Injuries are one of the most serious health problems faced by the pediatric population, and morbidity secondary to injury is significantly more common than mortality. The nature and severity of childhood injuries vary by age, gender, race, and socioeconomic status (Behrman et al., 1996).

After 1 year of age, motor vehicle trauma is the major cause of pediatric mortality in the United States. Mortality and morbidity related to other injuries, such as falls, poisoning, drownings, near-drownings, fires and burns, and trauma secondary to weapons are significant in children. Male children are more likely to experience injury than female children. Native American children have the highest rate of injuries, followed in order by black, Hispanic, white, and Asian children. Children from lower socioeconomic groups experience more injuries than those from higher income groups.

CLINICAL FINDINGS

Clinical presentation of injuries varies, depending on the nature and extent of the trauma experienced.

A thorough history of the child with an injury is required to determine contributing factors. The following information should be gathered:

- Description of environment in which injury took place
- Condition of child before injury
- Actions of child and others immediately before injury
- Mechanism of injury
- Extent of supervision by adults
- First aid management at scene of injury

DIFFERENTIAL DIAGNOSES

The differential diagnoses for unintentional injuries include the following:

- Child abuse and neglect
- Suicide attempt
- Disease conditions that make the child more susceptible to injuries (e.g., osteogenesis imperfecta and hemophilia)

MANAGEMENT

A discussion of safety issues needs to be incorporated into the NP's anticipatory guidance at every well-child and adolescent visit, clarifying how the potential for injury as well as the type of injury varies by the child's age and developmental level. Effective management of unintentional injuries requires that parents understand how, at each age, developmental characteristics influence children's behavior and put them at risk for injury. Once aware of how children may be at risk, parents can more clearly see how they can intervene to prevent an injury from occurring. Tables 11-7 to 11-10 outline major injuries, developmental characteristics of children, the risks for injury these present, and strategies for intervention that parents can use to decrease the potential for injury.

Efforts to prevent injury include the following:

- Restructure the environment to make it safer.
  - Place devices in the environment (e.g., automobile restraint systems) to protect children.
  - Remove hazards from the environment (e.g., childproofing the home).
  - Adjust environmental conditions (e.g., lowering the water heater temperature).
- Implement school policies and procedures to ensure that playground equipment and activities are well maintained and suited for children's developmental abilities.
- Advocate for school curricula that teach safety at every grade level.
- Mandate behavior or use of devices that protect the child (e.g., wearing bicycle helmets).
- Teach importance of adult supervision of children's activities.
- Provide health education regarding safety and protection, including first aid and safety and cardiopulmonary resuscitation techniques for both children and adults.
- Encourage and instruct about proper training for sports in children and adolescents.
- Provide parents with syrup of ipecac and poison control center telephone numbers.
- Teach children age-appropriate safe behavior to decrease risks of motor vehicle accidents, burns, drowning, poisoning, weapons, and falls.

MANAGEMENT OF MOTOR VEHICLE TRAUMA

Although motor vehicle trauma is only one cause of pediatric injuries, it results in signifi-

---

NURSING DIAGNOSIS 11–1

NURSING DIAGNOSES FOR HEALTH PERCEPTION AND HEALTH MANAGEMENT FUNCTIONAL HEALTH PATTERN

Adjustment Impaired	Noncompliance
Decisional Conflict	Risk for Injury
Altered Health Maintenance	Self-Care Deficits
Health-Seeking Behaviors (Specify Area of Interest)	Ineffective Management of Therapeutic Regimen: Individuals
Home Maintenance Management Impaired	Ineffective Management of Therapeutic Regimen: Families
Knowledge Deficits (Specify Area)	

Source: North American Nursing Diagnosis Association: NANDA Nursing Diagnoses: Definitions and Classification 1997–1998. Philadelphia, 1996.

---

cant mortality and morbidity in all age groups, and a recent review of motor vehicle occupant death rates of children and adolescents by race, ethnicity, and sex found that black and Hispanic children and teenagers are at greater risk of death than their white counterparts (Baker et al., 1998). The data reviewed by Baker and her colleagues did not reveal a reason for this finding, but the researchers commented on the possible roles of safety belt and child-restraint use.

In many cases, motor vehicle injuries are preventable through the correct use of child restraint systems (CRSs) (Table 11–11). Still, despite clear evidence that CRSs are effective in preventing injury or death, despite the availability of CRSs, despite intense education programs directed at families, and despite legislation mandating use of CRSs, many children ride unrestrained. Failure to use CRSs increases the probability that an "injury" will become a "fatality."

In addition to not using restraints, a number of common errors have been found in the way adults use CRSs (Table 11–12). As many as 80% of children have been found to have their restraint improperly positioned or adjusted (National Highway Traffic Safety Administration, 1996a; Decina & Knoebel, 1997). Providers should assess the parents' use of CRSs by correcting errors. This may mean accompanying parents to the parking lot to observe how children are placed in the restraint. Use of CRSs

should be reviewed at each well-child visit, and children should be involved in the discussion from a very early age. Both parents and children should receive positive reinforcement for proper use of CRSs.

Airbags were developed to prevent serious injury in the event of a motor vehicle accident. Designed to protect a 165-pound, 5-foot, 9-inch-tall man who is not wearing a seatbelt in a 30-mph frontal crash, passenger-side airbags have caused fatalities in infants and children (Cooper et al., 1998; Giguere et al., 1998; Braver et al., 1998; Hollands et al., 1996) and can be equally hazardous for small adults. Based on the nature of these fatalities, children younger than 12 years of age should not ride in the front passenger seat if an airbag can be deployed. The optimal position for children is in the center back seat, with infants weighing less than 20 pounds placed in a rear-facing child seat (Braver et al., 1998; Graham et al., 1998).

Pedestrian injuries or injuries involving bicycles, skateboards, and automobiles are common in children. The NP should ask children about their pedestrian safety habits during the well-child visit, and educational efforts to instruct children on pedestrian safety and age-appropriate safe use of cycles or boards should be supported. In addition, children of all ages need adult supervision related to motor vehicles. Adult supervision is especially important for younger children who are unaware of the

Text continued on page 240

TABLE 11-7

Primary Injury Prevention Related to Developmental Characteristics of Infants

50% of injury-related deaths in infants occur before 4 mo of age
40% of all injury-related deaths in infants are due to asphyxiation
20% of all injury-related deaths in infants result from motor vehicle trauma
After 4 mo of age, falls account for a significant number of injuries

AGE AND DEVELOPMENTAL CHARACTERISTICS	POTENTIAL INJURIES	STRATEGIES FOR PREVENTION
BIRTH TO 6 MO		
Poor head control at younger ages	Injury to neck	Handle child with care when picking up or moving
		Support neck of young infant
		Supervise other children when they are playing with infant
		Never jiggle or shake infant
Reflex behavior; especially strong suck reflex in early months	Aspiration of foreign objects Suffocation	Keep occlusive materials, especially plastic, out of child's bed
		Check toys, mobiles for sharp, detachable parts, strings, or cords
Skin thin and sensitive	Friction burns	Handle child with care when picking up or moving
	Burns	Do not hold infant in lap when drinking hot beverage or smoking
		Set water heater thermostat at <120°F
	Sunburn	Use cover-up (e.g., hat) whenever child is exposed to sun; avoid exposure
Poor body temperature control	Hypothermia	Dress infant appropriately
	Hyperthermia	Never leave child alone in car
Rolls, turns, and scoots	Falls	Do not leave infant alone on bed, changing table, or other area from which infant may fall
		Use playpen as a safe area
	May slide between mattress and crib slats	Make sure mattress fits tightly against bed railings; railings are no more than 2⅜ inches apart
	Slips in bath	Place washcloth under infant in bath; stay with infant during bathing
	Motor vehicle trauma	Correctly use approved child safety restraint units in cars
	Fire	Install smoke detectors in home and check batteries routinely

T A B L E 11-7

Primary Injury Prevention Related to Developmental Characteristics of Infants *Continued*

AGE AND DEVELOPMENTAL CHARACTERISTICS	POTENTIAL INJURIES	STRATEGIES FOR PREVENTION
6 TO 12 MO Grasps and mouths objects	Aspiration of foreign objects Suffocation	Keep small, sharp objects off floor and play area, out of reach Check toys for detachable parts Keep balloons, plastic wrappers, and plastic bags out of reach
	Poisoning	Use childproof caps on medications Keep medications out of reach in locked cabinet Keep household, garden, and car products out of reach Supervise children's activity Keep syrup of ipecac in home Keep poison control numbers near telephone and alert older siblings and babysitters about them
Sits, rolls, scoots, crawls, may stand while holding support, cruises, may walk	Falls	Do not use walkers Supervise children's activities Survey home for all accident hazards, sharp objects, table edges, stairs, loose rugs; remove those possible, provide protection of infant for others; use gates
	Drowning	Keep pool or water ponds behind closed and locked gates Never leave children alone in bath Use playpen as a safe area
Pulls and reaches	May pull objects down onto self	Remove tablecloths, dangling cords, appliances that may be in infant's reach
	Burns	Do not drink hot beverages or smoke when holding infant
Developing fine pincer grasp	Electrocution	Insert plastic plugs in electrical outlets
	Swallowing, aspiration, or insertion of foreign body in body orifices	Keep small objects out of reach
	Motor vehicle trauma	Correctly use approved child safety restraint units in cars
	Fire	Install smoke detectors in home and check batteries routinely Install carbon monoxide detectors in home

T A B L E 11-8

Primary Injury Prevention Related to Developmental Characteristics of Toddlers and Preschoolers

44% of all deaths in children age 1 to 4 yr are injury related
Injuries cause more death and disability than all contagious diseases combined
Poisonings are the number one cause of injuries, followed by burns, drowning, and choking

DEVELOPMENTAL CHARACTERISTICS	POTENTIAL INJURIES	STRATEGIES FOR PREVENTION
Increased fine motor skills: Can open doors, gates, drawers, bottles, boxes Increased curiosity	Poisoning	Use childproof caps on medications; keep medicines locked in cabinet out of reach Keep household, garden, and car products locked or out of reach Keep bottle of syrup of ipecac in home Place Mr. YUK stickers on toxic materials Have telephone number of Poison Control Center readily available
Increased gross motor skills and control: Able to walk, run, climb, throw objects, ride tricycle Engages in more active play outdoors, with peers	Falls	Confine play to fenced area Supervise play, especially in areas where climbing occurs Use gates or screens to block off stair; lock windows and doors
	Sunburn	Use sunscreen whenever children are exposed to sun
	Motor vehicle trauma	Use approved child safety restraints Provide tricycle/bicycle helmet Teach children sidewalk, street, and highway safety Never let children cross street alone or play on sidewalks near streets unsupervised
	Contusions and bites	Supervise interactive play of children Teach children how to share, control tempers; use adult interaction or distraction to stop harmful behavior or tantrum trauma
Increased curiosity; reaches, stretches, and pulls	Burns, scalding	Turn handles of cooking utensils away from outer edge of stove Use caution in kitchen with children about Adjust hot water thermostat to 120°F Keep matches out of reach

Developmental Characteristics	Potential Injuries	Injury Prevention
Increased curiosity, desire to explore Easily distracted, lacks judgment, unaware of danger of heights, water, fire, toxic materials, electricity, weapons, animals, or strangers	Drowning Other injuries	Fence swimming pools Supervise use of swimming and wading pools Never leave children unattended in a car or alone at home Do not allow children to play near running machinery, mowers, cars, or tools Provide plastic covers for electrical outlets; teach children safety with electrical appliances and cords Do not allow children to use pointed objects in play Do not allow children to run or walk with sticks, lollipops, or other such objects Remove weapons from the house, or keep in locked cabinet, guns unloaded; store ammunition in separate, locked area Teach children to avoid strange animals, especially ones that are eating Teach stranger safety
Easily distracted, not always attentive	Abuse Choking, aspiration	Do not give foods that can be easily aspirated, such as nuts, gum, popcorn, hotdogs, grapes Supervise mealtimes and snacks

TABLE 11-9

Primary Injury Prevention Related to Developmental Characteristics of School-Age Children

51% of all deaths in children age 5 to 9 yr are injury related
58% of all deaths in children age 10 to 14 yr are injury related
Motor vehicle and pedestrian accidents, burns, drowning, and choking are the most common fatal injuries
1 in 10 injury fatalities is related to motor vehicle trauma or bicycle use

DEVELOPMENTAL CHARACTERISTICS	POTENTIAL INJURIES	STRATEGIES FOR PREVENTION
Motor skills improve: Becomes more physically agile and coordinated	Motor vehicle trauma as passenger, pedestrian, or cyclist	Use approved safety restraints in car Provide bicycle helmet and insist on its use Teach importance of seatbelt and helmet use Teach bicycle safety Do not allow children to ride tricycles or bicycles with training wheels in the street Prohibit use of all-terrain vehicles Teach pedestrian safety
Is adventurous and more independent, looks for new challenges; may accept dares	Falls	Use knee pads, elbow pads, wrist support, and helmets when skateboarding
	Drowning	Teach to swim; teach rules of water safety: swim in a supervised area with a buddy, check depth before diving, use life preservers in boats
Engages in sports and strenuous exercise Enjoys physical activity Works hard to improve skills Can strain self with excessive activity	Sprains and strains, fractures, and other bodily injuries	Encourage child to be active and stay conditioned; if engaged in organized sports, provide supervised strength training Ensure use of properly fitted equipment for each sport and safe playing area

Engages in group activities, subject to peer approval Is curious and exploring Easily distracted by environment Accepts explanations and is responsive to reasoning	Burns	Teach children dangers of flammable and toxic materials; how to handle them safely Supervise use of matches Develop a family plan for fires
	Poisoning Choking	Keep hazardous materials out of reach, in locked location; supervise their use Teach first aid, what to do in case of burns, choking, or poisoning Keep Poison Control Center telephone number readily available
	Sunburn	Use sunscreen whenever children will be exposed to sun
	Abuse	Teach child to memorize telephone number and address, use of 911 Warn child never to go with or accept things from strangers

237

T A B L E 11-10

Primary Injury Prevention Related to Developmental Characteristics of Adolescents

Nearly 80% of all fatal injuries are related to motor vehicles
1 in 50 teens is hospitalized for motor vehicle injury every year
Sports injuries are the most common nonfatal injury
Drownings, burns, and poisoning (drugs and alcohol) are the 2nd, 3rd, and 4th leading causes of injury, respectively

DEVELOPMENTAL CHARACTERISTICS	POTENTIAL INJURIES	STRATEGIES FOR PREVENTION
Able to legally drive motor vehicles	Motor vehicle trauma as passenger, pedestrian, or cyclist	Use approved safety restraints Take driver's education classes Use bicycle helmet Encourage to learn how to maintain bicycle Teach proper use of all-terrain vehicles Reinforce pedestrian safety Emphasize danger of driving, drinking, and drug use; support peer group efforts to control inappropriate behavior
Increased physical strength and ability	Falls	Use knee pads, elbow pads, wrist support, and helmet when skateboarding Use helmet when cycling
Perception of invulnerability; may take risks	Drowning	Teach to swim Reinforce rules of water safety: swim in a supervised area with a buddy, check depth before diving, use life preservers in boats and when water skiing
More participation in structured sports activities	Sprains, strains, fractures and other bodily injuries	Encourage adolescent to stay active and conditioned, engage in supervised strength training
Use of complex equipment, tools, weapons	Burns Bodily injury Choking	Teach first aid and cardiopulmonary resuscitation: what to do in the event of injuries, burns, choking, or poisonings Teach gun safety
Strong peer influence	Poisoning (drug and alcohol abuse)	Teach dangers of drug and alcohol use
Need for independence and peer approval Able to problem solve, reason, and think abstractly		Provide an opportunity to discuss values, perceptions, fears, and needs related to high-risk behaviors; discuss how adolescent deals with anger and violence, as well as how to prevent trauma related to violence; encourage healthy options

TABLE 11-11

Vehicle Child Restraint Systems: Recommendations for Use

AGE OF CHILD	WEIGHT OF CHILD	TYPE OF RESTRAINT
Infant <1 yr	Up to about 20 lb	Child restraint system (CRS) designed for infant; rear-facing; always in back seat, as automatic air bag for front passenger seat may strike child with injury-causing, even fatal, force; seated upright
Toddlers	20–40 lb	CRS designed for toddler; facing forward, although earlier research indicates serious or fatal neck injuries in children <18 mo riding in this position despite their weight (Fuchs et al., 1989), and a 13-yr study by Volvo demonstrated few injuries in children <5 yr riding in a rear-facing position (Carlsson et al., 1989); always in back seat
Preschool and early elementary school-age children	40–60 lb	Booster seat, without shield, used with seatbelt that has lap/shoulder belt Booster seat, with shield, used with seatbelt that has lap belt only
Older children	>60 lb	Adult lap/shoulder restraint that fits correctly: child sits with buttocks against the seat back, lap belt lies low and tight across the top of the thighs, shoulder strap crosses the shoulder and chest (not the neck or face) with no slack Lap belt alone if shoulder strap is unavailable
CHILDREN WITH SPECIAL NEEDS Very small infants	<7 lb	If in infant seat, have close-fitting harness and no shield Maximum distance from crotch strap to back of seat is 5.5 inches; height of harness straps should be <10 inches If too small for seat, use car bed with restraints that allow child to lie flat
Children with physical disabilities		The Spelcast child restraint, modified to hold a child weighing <40 lb in a hip spica cast; The modified E-Z-On Vest restrains a child who must lie flat

Adapted from Stewart (1993) and National Highway Traffic Safety Administration (1996b).

T A B L E 11-12

Common Errors in the Use of Child Restraint Systems

- Harness straps on the infant seat are too loose
- Harness straps on the infant seat are incorrectly threaded and positioned
- The infant is placed in a forward-facing position
- The child is either too small or too large for the child restraint system (CRS) or seatbelts
- Infant is wrapped in a cocoon of blankets before being strapped into CRS
- Seatbelts are incorrectly placed around CRS or booster seat
- Seatbelts are not adjusted tightly enough
- CRS has been found to be defective but continues to be used

dangers, and the NP should discuss this issue with parents at each well-child visit.

Adolescents, especially new drivers, are often involved in motor vehicle accidents because of their inexperience, immature judgment, or a tendency to take risks. Legislation has been passed in some states, Canada, and New Zealand to restrict adolescent driving. "Graduated licensing" legislation requires teenagers to complete driver education classes, restricts their driving to certain times of day, or prevents them from driving with other teenagers in the car. As adolescents gain experience and age, restrictions on driving decline. Successful implementation of the law depends on parents acting as advocates for safety and supporting their adolescents' compliance with the regulations. NPs also can reinforce the message to teenagers that driving is a privilege that requires skill and maturity.

REFERENCES

American Academy of Pediatrics Committee on Practice and Ambulatory Medicine: Recommendations for preventive pediatric health care. Pediatrics 96:373, 1995.

American Medical Association: Guidelines for Adolescent Preventive Services (GAPS): Recommendations Monograph. Chicago: American Medical Association, 1997.

Aronowitz RA: Making Sense of Illness: Science, Society, and Disease. Cambridge, UK: Cambridge University Press, 1998.

Baker SP, Braver ER, Chen L, et al: Motor vehicle occupant deaths among Hispanic and black children and teenagers. Archiv Pediat Adolesc Med 152:1209-1212, 1998.

Behrman RE, Kliegman RM, Arvin AM (eds): Nelson Textbook of Pediatrics, 15th ed. Philadelphia, WB Saunders, 1996.

Braver ER, Whitfield R, Ferguson SA: Seating positions and children's risk of dying in motor vehicle crashes. Injury Prev 4:181-187, 1998.

Brown JL: Pediatric Telephone Medicine: Principles, Triage, and Advice, 2nd ed. Philadelphia, JB Lippincott, 1994.

Carlsson G, Norin H, Yslander L: Rearward facing child seats: The safest care restraint for children? Proceedings of the 33rd Annual Association for the Advancement of Automotive Medicine, 1989.

Centers for Disease Control and Prevention: Tobacco use among high school students—United States, 1997. JAMA 279:1250-1251, 1998.

Coogan PF, Adams M, Geller AC, et al: Factors associated with smoking among children and adolescents in Connecticut. Am J Prev Med 15:17-24, 1998.

Cooper JT, Balding LE, Jordan FB: Airbag mediated death of a two-year-old child wearing a shoulder/lap belt. J Forensic Sci 43:1077-1081, 1998.

Daniels JL, Olshan AF, Savitz DA: Pesticides and childhood cancers. Environ Health Persp 105:1068-1077, 1997.

Dappen A, Schwartz RH, O'Donnell R: A survey of adolescent smoking patterns. J Am Board Fam Pract 9:7-13, 1996.

Decina LE, Knoebel KY: Child safety seat misuse patterns in four states. Accident Analysis Prev 29:125-132, 1997.

Elster A, Kuznets N: AMA Guidelines for Adolescent Preventive Services (GAPS): Baltimore, Williams & Wilkins, 1994.

Engstrom I: Family interaction and locus of control in children and adolescents with inflammatory bowel disease. J Am Acad Child Adolesc Psychiatry 30:913-920, 1991.

Foltz AT: Parental knowledge and practices of skin cancer prevention: A pilot study. J Pediatr Health Care 7:220-225, 1993.

Fried PA, Watkinson B, Siegel LS: Reading and language in 9- to 12-year olds prenatally exposed to cigarettes and marijuana. Neurotoxicol Teratol 19:171-183, 1997.

Fuchs S, Barthel MJ, Flannery AM, et al: Cervical spine fractures sustained by young children in forward-facing car seats. Pediatrics 84:348-354, 1989.

Giguere JF, St-Vil D, Turmel A, et al: Airbags and children: A spectrum of C-spine injuries. Pediatr Surg 33:811-816, 1998.

Glantz SA, Parmley WW: Passive smoking and heart disease: Mechanisms and risk. JAMA 273:1047-1053, 1995.

Graham JD, Goldie SJ, Segui-Gomez M, et al: Reducing risks to children in vehicles with passenger airbags. Pediatrics 102:e3, 1998.

Hollands CM, Winston FK, Stafford PW, et al: Lethal airbag injury in an infant. Pediatr Emerg Care 12:201-202, 1996.

Howard BJ: Working with difficult families. Paper presented at the 1998 Pediatric Update, Portland, OR, November, 1998.

Kleinman A, Eisenberg L, Good B: Culture, illness and care: Clinical lessons from anthropologic and cross-cultural research. Ann Intern Med 88:251-258, 1978.

Marchand L, Morrow MH: Infant feeding practices: Understanding the decision-making process. Fam Med 26:319–324, 1994.

Marshall RS: Interpretation in doctor-patient interviews: A sociolinguistic analysis. Culture Med Psychiatry 12:201–218, 1988.

McAfee T, Sofian NS, Wilson J, et al: The role of tobacco intervention in population-based health care: A case study. Am J Prev Med 14:46–52, 1998.

National Highway Traffic Safety Administration. Patterns of misuse of child safety seats. Final report. Washington, DC, U.S. Department of Transportation, 1996a.

National Highway Traffic Safety Administration. Size and weight guide for child safety seats. NHTSA Facts. Washington, DC, U.S. Department of Transportation, 1996b.

Pucci LG, Joseph HM, Siegel M: Outdoor tobacco advertising in six Boston neighborhoods: Evaluating youth exposure. Am J Prev Med 15:155–159, 1998.

Region X Nursing Standards Board: Prenatal and child health screening and assessment manual: Pregnancy and birth to adolescence. Seattle: Author, 1998.

Rivara FP: Fatal and non-fatal farm injuries to children and adolescents in the United States, 1990-3. Injury Prevention 4:79, 1997.

Rosenbaum M: "Just say know" to teenagers and marijuana. J Psychoactive Drugs 30:197–203, 1998.

Rotter JB: Generalized expectancies for internal versus external control of reinforcement. Psychol Monogr 80:1–25, 1966.

Schmid RE: Risks in children from air bags detailed. The Boston Globe, p. A3, Sept. 18, 1996.

Schmitt BD: Pediatric Telephone Protocols: The Quick Reference. Littleton, CO: Little, Decision Press, 1998.

Stewart DD: Child passenger safety: Current technical issues for advocates and professionals. Fam Community Health 15(4):12–27, 1993.

Stueland DT, Lee BC, Nordstrom DL, et al: A population based case-control study of agricultural injuries in children. Injury Prevention 2:192–196, 1996.

US Preventive Services Task Force: Guide to Clinical Preventive Services, 2nd ed. Baltimore, Williams & Wilkins, 1996.

Wall MA, Severson HH, Andrews JA, et al: Pediatric office-based smoking intervention: Impact on maternal smoking and relapse. Pediatrics 96:622–628, 1995.

Wallston BS, Wallston KA, Kaplan GD, et al: Development and validation of the health locus of control (HLC) scale. J Consult Clin Psych 44:580–585, 1976.

Wallston KA, Wallston BS, DeVellis R: Development of multidimensional health locus of control (MHLC) scales. Health Education Monogr 6:160–170, 1978.

CHAPTER 12

Nutrition

Ardys M. Dunn

INTRODUCTION

Definition of Nutrition Pattern

Nutrition is a complex science that includes the study of how food, nutrients, and other substances found in foods interact with the body to foster growth and health or contribute to disease. Nutrition examines the processes by which organisms ingest, digest, absorb, transport, utilize, and excrete food substances. In addition, knowledge of nutrition requires an understanding of social, economic, cultural, and psychological implications of food and eating. Adequate nutrition is essential for normal growth and development of children and plays a critical role in maintenance and restoration of good health. Nutrition impacts children's ability to interact with their environment. The effect of nourishment on children's behavior can be immediate and dramatic, as with the hungry, irritable infant who eagerly nurses and falls asleep; or nutrition can have long-range implications, as in the relationship between childhood cholesterol levels and adult coronary heart disease.

Significance for Nurse Practitioner Practice

The primary role of the nurse practitioner (NP) in relation to nutrition is to assess accurately the nutritional status of children, to determine parents' and children's knowledge related to nutrition, to identify ways in which food is managed and used, and to ensure that children are adequately nourished. The NP's interventions, aimed at helping children and families meet nutritional requirements and preventing problems related to poor nutrition, are based on certain assumptions, including the following:

- Children's nutritional needs vary as they grow.
- Children's nutritional needs are influenced by their state of health.
- A wide range of food choices and feeding behaviors are used to meet nutritional needs.
- Recommended dietary allowances are guidelines only.
- Parents and other caregivers are responsible for providing food choices that are nutritionally adequate and for establishing healthy eating patterns; they must be well informed in order to do so.
- The NP is a source of information regarding nutrition, feeding patterns, and health.
- The NP works with a network of specialists (e.g., registered dietitians) to manage children's nutrition.

Standards for Preventive Care

A number of recommendations and guidelines have been developed related to nutrition. The goals of the Region X child health nursing standards (Region X Nursing Network, 1998) are the following:

- The child receives nutrition that contributes to and promotes growth and wellness.
- The child develops nutrition patterns that contribute to physical growth, individual needs, and lifelong health.

The United States (US) Public Health Service (1997), in its Put Prevention into Practice (PPIP) initiative, presents the following nutritional recommendations:

- Encourage mothers to breastfeed for 6 to 12 months.
- Begin introducing single-ingredient foods when infants are developmentally ready, usually at 4 to 6 months of age.
- Counsel parents that children need a balanced diet that includes a wide variety of foods.
- Encourage use of iron-rich foods; advise children, especially adolescent girls, and their families to eat foods rich in calcium and iron.
- Do not use cow's milk for children younger than 1 year of age.
- Do not limit fat in children's diets during the first 2 years of life; do not use reduced-fat milk until the child is at least 2 years of age; help parents and children older than 2 years of age choose a diet that is low in total fat (30% or less of total calories), saturated fat (less than 10% of total calories), and cholesterol.
- Do not feed honey to infants during the first year of life; encourage moderate use of sugar and salt in the diet of all children.
- Vitamin supplements have not been proved necessary for healthy children with a well-balanced diet; vitamin D supplements may be necessary for dark-skinned children with little exposure to sunlight.
- Counsel parents and children about the importance of maintaining a healthy weight.
- Weight reduction through dieting or other means is not advisable for children and adolescents because they are still growing.

- Children 6 months of age and older who live in areas with low fluoride content in drinking water may need fluoride supplements.
- Adolescent girls should be counseled regarding folic acid intake.

The US Preventive Services Task Force (1996) recommends that practitioners counsel parents about the nutritional requirements of infancy and childhood, especially encouraging the following:

- Intake of breast milk to prevent infections
- A wide variety of foods in children's diets
- Iron-rich foods
- Attention to the intake of fats, particularly saturated fats and cholesterol
- Intake of calories and carbohydrates appropriate to metabolic needs and limiting sugar in those at risk for dental caries
- Extra calcium and iron in adolescent girls' diets
- Adequate fiber and sodium
- Adequate folic acid intake during childbearing years

The American Medical Association notes that "all adolescents should receive health guidance annually about dietary habits, including the benefits of a healthy diet and ways to achieve a healthy diet and safe weight management" (Elster & Kuznets, 1994).

▇▇▇ NORMAL PATTERNS OF NUTRITION

General Considerations

ENERGY

Energy intake, measured in kilocalories, should meet the basic needs of body metabolism and growth. In addition, activity, exercise, and other metabolic demands increase the level of calories needed to maintain good health. General energy requirements of children vary by age, body size, and composition, developmental stage, health, and activity level. *Resting energy expenditure,* a concept used interchangeably with *basal metabolic rate,* is the largest source of energy consumption in the body.

Exercise, the second major factor accounting for energy consumption, increases tissue demands for oxygen and nutrients, As exercise increases, caloric need increases. The body meets these demands by using stored energy sources or by consuming necessary nutrients and calories. Healthy individuals maintain a balance between the body's energy demands and caloric intake. Currently, many children have limited physical activity and are at risk for excess weight gain. These children should be encouraged to engage in regular physical exercise to balance energy use and caloric intake.

Table 12-1 presents recommended energy intake based on median height and weight. Before age 10 years, no distinction is made in energy requirements between boys and girls, but the demands of puberty and variations in activity levels in adolescence are reflected in higher caloric recommendations for teenage boys. Energy needs vary from one individual to another, however, and an athletic adolescent girl, for example, needs more calories than a teenage boy who has a sedentary lifestyle.

WATER AND ELECTROLYTES

Water

Water is the primary component of body tissue, and maintaining fluid balance is essential to good health. Because of the wide variation of healthful intake and output, there is no specific recommended daily requirement for water. Infants present special concerns. Factors such as their large skin surface per unit of body weight, the immaturity of their renal system to process solutes, their high daily water turnover (up to 15% of body weight), and their inability to express thirst make them uniquely susceptible to rapid variations in water balance.

Water loss is influenced also by illness, activity level, altitude, and temperature and dryness of ambient air. If a child has vomiting and diarrhea, water loss can be significant, leading to dehydration and other complications. A child who exercises strenuously, especially in a warm, dry environment, requires additional water intake. When more than 10% of body weight is lost without replacement, dehydration can become life threatening. Table 12-2 identifies fluid problems that require medical evaluation.

Sodium

Sodium functions primarily to regulate extracellular fluid volume. It also regulates osmolarity, acid-base balance, and the membrane potential of cells and is involved in the cell membrane transport pump, exchanging with potassium in intracellular fluid. Sodium loss occurs with vomiting, diarrhea, and perspiration.

Sodium requirements vary with the rate of extracellular fluid expansion, which is most rapid in infants and very young children. With the older child, it is not necessary to add sodium to the diet, even for children who exercise and perspire heavily. In fact, the typical North American diet far exceeds minimum requirements for sodium intake, with most sodium coming from salt added during processing and manufacturing of foods.

Potassium

Potassium serves to maintain intracellular homeostasis and contributes to muscle contractility and transmission of nerve impulses. Severe potassium deficit *(hypokalemia)* can lead to cardiac arrhythmias and death. Excessive potassium *(hyperkalemia)* can cause cardiac arrest. The urinary and gastrointestinal systems function to regulate potassium levels, and extreme imbalances are almost always due to disease processes or medication rather than to dietary factors. Potassium requirements are related to increases in lean body mass and are proportionally higher during the rapid growth of infancy and adolescence than during middle childhood. Fruits, vegetables, and fresh meat have high potassium content.

Chloride

Chloride functions in conjunction with sodium to maintain fluid and electrolyte balance. Loss of chloride occurs through the same routes as sodium loss: vomiting, diarrhea, and perspiration. The major source of chloride is salt (NaCl or KCl) added to foods during processing. There is no recommended daily allowance for chloride, but adequate amounts are ingested with a normal diet.

T A B L E 12-1
Recommended Daily Energy and Nutrient Intake by Age, Average Height, and Weight

Nutrient	INFANTS, TODDLERS, AND CHILDREN					BOYS AND MEN			GIRLS AND WOMEN			Pregnant
Age	0-6 mo	6-12 mo	1-3 yr	4-6 yr	7-10 yr	11-14 yr	15-18 yr	19-24 yr	11-14 yr	15-18 yr	19-24 yr	
Weight (kg)	6	9	13	20	28	45	66	72	46	55	58	
Height (cm)	60	71	90	112	132	157	176	177	157	163	164	
Energy (kcal/kg)	108	98	102	90	70	55	45	40	40	38	38	+300 kcal/d in second and third trimesters
Protein (g/kg)	2.2	1.6	1.2	1.1	1.0	1.0	0.9	0.8	0.8	0.8	0.8	
Vitamin A, µ RE	375	375	400	500	700	1000	1000	1000	800	800	800	800
Thiamin (B_1), mg	0.3	0.4	0.7	0.9	1	1.3	1.5	1.5	1.1	1.1	1.1	1.5
Riboflavin (B_2), mg	0.4	0.5	0.8	1.1	1.2	1.5	1.8	1.7	1.3	1.3	1.3	1.6
Niacin (mg NE)	5	6	9	12	13	17	20	19	15	15	15	17
Pyridoxine (B_6), mg	0.3	0.6	1	1.1	1.4	1.7	2	2	1.4	1.5	1.6	2.2
Folate, µg	25	35	50	75	100	150	200	200	150	180	180	400
Vitamin B_{12}, µg	0.3	0.5	0.7	1	1.4	2	2	2	2	2	2	2.2
Vitamin C, mg	30	35	40	45	45	50	60	60	50	60	60	70
Vitamin D, µg	7.5	10	10	10	10	10	10	10	10	10	10	10
Vitamin E, mg	3	4	6	7	7	10	10	10	8	8	8	10
Vitamin K, µg	5	10	15	20	30	45	65	70	45	55	60	65
Calcium, mg	400	600	800	800	800	1300	1300	1200	1300	1300	1200	1200-1500
Fluoride, mg*	0.1	0.2-0.5	0.5-1.5	1.0-2.5	1.5-2.5	1.5-2.5	1.5-2.5	1.5-4.0	1.5-2.5	1.5-2.5	1.5-4.0	1.5-2.5
Iron, mg	0 (if breast-fed); 6 (if not breast-fed)	10	10	10	10	12-15	12-15	12-15	15-30	15-30	15-30	30
Zinc, mg	5	5	10	10	10	15	15	15	12	12	12	15

*Fluoride supplement is not necessary if the water supply contains ≥3 ppm (parts per million) fluoridation.
RE, retinol equivalent. 1 retinol equivalent = 1 µg ß-carotene; NE, niacin equivalent. 1 niacin equivalent = 1 mg of niacin or 60 mg of dietary tryptophan.
Adapted from Recommended Dietary Allowances, 10th ed. Copyright 1989 by the National Academy of Sciences, Washington, DC; Dietary Reference Intakes for Calcium, Phosphorus, Magnesium, Vitamin D, and Fluoride, Copyright 1997 by the National Academy Press, Washington, DC; and US Public Health Service, 1992.

T A B L E 12-2

Fluid Problems Requiring Evaluation

- Diarrhea—watery bowel movements every 1–2 hr. Dehydration may be present and require fluid replacement therapy
- Chronic diarrhea (>2 wk) or acute diarrhea (<2 wk) that has not been evaluated
- Refusal to eat or drink, unexplained fever, unexplained vomiting
- Concentrated urine reported
- Increased thirst (ongoing), water craving, or excessive water intake

Adapted from Suskind RM, Lewinter-Suskind L: Textbook of Pediatric Nutrition. NY, Raven Press, 1992.

PROTEIN

Amino acids, essential for the synthesis of body protein and nitrogen-containing compounds, are constantly being resynthesized, allowing for muscle protein turnover and growth. The body requires sufficient caloric intake to use dietary protein for protein synthesis. Approximately 12 to 15% of daily calories should be supplied by proteins (see Table 12–1).

Protein and amino acid deficiencies rarely appear alone but follow other dietary deficits. Extreme stress and disease processes can deplete nitrogen, contributing to tissue wasting and creating an increased demand for protein. Growth needs of the premature infant require higher levels of protein intake than those of term infants. The demand for protein is not generally increased with normal activity except as needed to build additional muscle tissue during body conditioning or during some illnesses.

CARBOHYDRATES

Carbohydrates are the body's major dietary source of energy. It is recommended that more than half (55%) of the body's energy requirements be supplied by carbohydrates. In addition to providing energy, adequate carbohydrate intake is essential to facilitate protein synthesis. Because 1 g of carbohydrate provides 4 calories, the child who requires 2000 Kcal daily should ingest at least 250 g of carbohydrate. Carbohydrates are either simple sugars (the monosaccharides and disaccharides of sucrose,

fructose, and lactose found in fruits, vegetables, milk, and prepared sweets) or complex carbohydrates (starches found in cereal grains, potatoes, legumes, and other vegetables). Most dietary carbohydrates should be in the complex form. If dietary carbohydrates are extremely limited or absent (e.g., with a ketogenic diet used to manage intractable seizures of epilepsy; see Chapter 28), the body lipolyzes stored triglycerides, oxidizes fatty acids, and breaks down dietary and tissue protein. This process contributes to accumulation of ketone bodies.

FATS

Lipids, fats, and fatty acids are used by the body to provide energy, to facilitate absorption of the fat-soluble vitamins (A, D, E, and K), and to maintain integrity of cell membranes and myelin. Essential fatty acids, all of which are found in most vegetable oils, are not produced by the body and must be included in the diet.

The American Academy of Pediatrics Committee on Nutrition recommends that children older than 2 years of age gradually adopt a diet that by age 5 years includes daily intake of less than 10% saturated fats and a maximum of 30% and a minimum of 20% dietary fat to meet energy needs. Diets should include no more than 300 mg of cholesterol (AAP Committee on Nutrition, 1998). Before age 2 years, there should be no restrictions on dietary fat intake, although studies have shown that children receiving between 28 and 30% of their energy needs in fat have a healthy growth patterns (Kleinman et al., 1996). Canadian nutritional recommendations for dietary fat intake in children include no restrictions before age 2 years and a transition from age 2 until linear growth stops to a diet where 30% of energy needs are met by fat; 20% unsaturated and 10% or less saturated. During this time of transition, children should be encouraged to eat a variety of foods, including many complex carbohydrates, and to engage in vigorous physical activity (Zlotkin, 1996).

VITAMINS

A number of fat-soluble and water-soluble vitamins are essential for good health. Table 12–1 lists recommendations for daily vitamin intake. Table 12–3 identifies specific metabolic func-

T A B L E 12-3

Vitamins: Function, Dietary Sources, Interactions, Deficiency, and Excess

	FUNCTION	DIETARY SOURCES	INTERACTIONS AFFECTING ABSORPTION OR UTILIZATION	SIGNS OF DEFICIT	SIGNS OF EXCESS
Fat-soluble vitamins					
Vitamin A	Vision, cellular differentiaton and growth, reproductive and immune system function	Liver, fish liver oils, fortified milk, eggs, carrots, dark-green leafy vegetables	Absorption and utilization are facilitated by dietary fat, protein, and vitamin E. Absorption of vitamin A is hindered by lack of protein, iron, or zinc	Anorexia, dry skin, keratinization of epithelial cells of respiratory tract, night blindness, corneal lesions, increased susceptibility to infections	Headache, vomiting, double vision, hair loss, dry mucous membrane, peeling skin, liver damage. Toxic at 10 times the RDA. No toxicity with excessive intake of carotenoids (e.g., carrots)
Vitamin D	Bone growth and development; regulates intestinal absorption of calcium and phosphorus	Sunlight, artificial ultraviolet light, fortified food products, especially milk	Utilization compromised in patients with renal failure. Increased exposure to sunlight increases intake. Darker skin and aging skin inhibit synthesis	Inadequate bone mineralization, rickets or skeletal malformations, delayed dentition	Anorexia, nausea, vomiting, diarrhea, weakness, hypercalcemia, hypercalciuria, calcium deposits in soft tissue, permanent renal or cardiovascular damage
Vitamin E	Antioxidant, traps free radicals, prevents oxidation of polyunsaturated fats	Vegetable oils, margarine, nuts, wheat germ, green leafy vegetables	Low serum levels have been associated with prematurity and congenital defects of the hepatobiliary system (e.g., cystic fibrosis, biliary atresia)	Macrocytic anemia and dermatitis in infants; neurological defects in severe malabsorption	Unknown, if any
Vitamin K	Forms proteins that regulate blood clotting	Green leafy vegetables, milk, dairy products, liver	Inhibited by long-term antibiotic use, hyperalimentation, chronic biliary obstruction, or lipid malabsorption syndromes	Defective coagulation of blood, hemorrhages, liver injury	Vitamin K-responsive hemorrhagic condition, especially if patient is being treated with anticoagulants
Water-soluble vitamins					
Vitamin C	Essential for collagen formation and function; promotes growth and tissue repair; enhances iron absorption; improves wound healing	Vegetables and fruits, especially citrus fruits, broccoli, collard greens, spinach, tomatoes, potatoes, strawberries, peppers	Vitamin C is easily lost in food storage and preparation owing to exposure to heat, oxygen, and water. Exposure to cigarette smoke increases vitamin C requirement	Scurvy, cracked lips, bleeding gums, slow wound healing, easy bruising	Unknown; excessive vitamin is excreted in urine

Vitamin	Function	Sources	Comments	Deficiency	Toxicity
Thiamine (vitamin B₁)	Necessary for carbohydrate metabolism; promotes normal appetite and digestion	Whole grains, brewer's yeast, legumes, seeds and nuts, organ meats, lean cuts of pork	Availability inhibited by presence of thiaminase (found in raw fish); alcohol contributes to thiamine deficiency	Beriberi: muscle weakness, ataxia, confusion, anorexia, tachycardia, heart failure in infants	None by oral intake; excess excreted in urine
Riboflavin (vitamin B₂)	Necessary for oxidation-reduction reactions, essential for function of vitamin B₆ and niacin; helps maintain integrity of skin, tongue, and lips	Dairy products, meat, poultry, fish; enriched or fortified grains, cereals, and breads; green vegetables such as broccoli, spinach, asparagus, turnip greens	Positive nitrogen balance contributes to function of riboflavin	Oral-buccal cavity lesions, generalized seborrheic dermatitis, scrotal and vulval skin changes, normocytic anemia, dimness of vision	None known
Niacin	Essential for energy metabolism, glycolysis, fatty acids; maintains nervous system, integrity of skin, mouth, tongue	Meats, fortified grains, legumes Milk, eggs, and meats contain tryptophan	Requires riboflavin for absorption and utilization Grains treated with lime have more biologically available niacin Dietary tryptophan converts to niacin	Pellagra: dermatitis, diarrhea, inflammation of mucous membranes, indigestion	No known toxicity with dietary doses; heat rush flushing with excessive doses
Vitamin B₆ (pyridoxine)	Essential for metabolism of amino acids, lipids, nucleic acids, and glycogen	Chicken, fish, kidney, liver, pork, red meat, eggs, unrefined rice, soybeans, oats, whole wheat, peanuts, walnuts	Riboflavin enhances function Increased protein intake increases requirements for vitamin B₆ Processing of foods destroys vitamin B₆	Seen in combination with other B-complex vitamin deficiencies; dermatitis, anemia, convulsions, neurological symptoms, and abdominal distress in infants	Ataxia, sensory neuropathy when taken in gram quantities for months or years
Folate (folacin)	Essential for amino acid metabolism and nucleic acid synthesis; red blood cell formation	Liver, yeast, dark-green leafy vegetables, legumes, fruits, oranges, brewer's yeast, milk	Only about 25% of folate in foods is directly bioavailable for absorption in intestine; more efficiently absorbed if serum levels are low Boiling milk destroys about 50% of folate present	Poor growth, megaloblastic anemia in severe cases; macrocytic anemia, glossitis, gastrointestinal disturbances; increased risk of neural tube defects in infants of folate-deficient mothers	None known in dietary doses; excessive folic acid supplementation may inhibit uptake of phenytoin and contribute to seizures in epileptic cases controlled by phenytoin
Vitamin B₁₂	Essential for metabolism, adequate red blood cell formation	Animal products: meat, eggs, and milk; shellfish	Absorbed in ileum; intrinsic factor-mediated In strict vegetarians, the vitamin excreted in the bile is reabsorbed	Megaloblastic anemia, neurological symptoms, sore tongue, weakness	None known

tions, dietary sources, and signs of deficiency or excessive intake of these vitamins.

Fat-Soluble Vitamins

Several characteristics of the fat-soluble vitamins (A, D, E, and K) have implications for dietary assessment and management (Davis & Sherer, 1994):

- They can be stored for long periods of time in body tissues. As a result, temporary dietary deficiencies may not affect the body's growth and development. If stores are depleted and nutritional intake is inadequate, signs of vitamin deficiency appear. If intake is excessive, as can occur with supplementation, toxic effects can appear.
- These vitamins are absorbed in the intestines along with fats and lipids in foods. Low-fat diets, as well as increased intestinal motility or malabsorption syndromes, may put individuals at risk for vitamin deficiency.
- They are fairly stable to heat, as in cooking. Food preparation does not destroy fat-soluble vitamins as readily as water-soluble vitamins.
- They require bile for absorption. Conditions that compromise the hepatobiliary system put the individual at risk for decreased vitamin absorption.
- They do not contain nitrogen and do not act as coenzymes in cellular metabolism of nutrients.

Water-Soluble Vitamins

Unlike fat-soluble vitamins, water-soluble vitamins (C and B complexes) are stored in very small amounts in the body. If water-soluble vitamin intake is above that needed by the body, absorption (primarily in the jejunum) decreases and excess vitamins are excreted. As a result, daily intake of water-soluble vitamins is necessary and there is little risk of toxicity from large doses. The B vitamins also contain nitrogen and serve as essential coenzymes in the body's metabolism of nutrients.

MINERALS

Major minerals are defined as those present in the body in amounts larger than 5 g. Calcium, phosphorus, and magnesium are considered major minerals. Because of a lack of definitive data and research, only seven minerals have been given recommended dietary allowance (RDA) status: calcium, phosphorus, magnesium, iron, zinc, iodine, and selenium. Estimated safe and adequate dietary intakes have been identified for other trace elements known to be essential to humans. Table 12–1 identifies recommended allowances for calcium, iron, and zinc.

Peak bone density is directly related to calcium intake during the years of bone mineralization. Most mineralization takes place by the time an individual is 20 years old, but recent research indicates that calcification can continue for several years. To ensure maximum peak bone density, dietary calcium needs remain high until about 25 years of age. The National Institutes of Health Consensus Development Panel on Optimal Calcium Intake (1994) recommends a slightly higher calcium intake for older children than is listed in Table 12–1, with children aged 6 to 10 years receiving 800 to 1200 mg/d and adolescents and young adults (11 to 24 years) 1200 to 1500 mg/d. Breastfed infants or those who are fed an approved infant formula receive sufficient calcium and should not be given a supplement.

Minerals and essential trace elements, their functions, dietary sources, and signs of deficiency or excess are presented in Table 12–4. Foods rich in iron are listed in Table 12–5.

USE OF VITAMIN AND MINERAL SUPPLEMENTS

National surveys reveal that many U.S. children have suboptimal nutrient intakes. A national sample of more than 3000 children, aged 2 to 19 years, concluded that less than 1% meet all of the national standards for recommended dietary intake. Sixteen percent met none of the recommendations (Munoz et al., 1997).

Recommended daily requirements for most foods should be evaluated over a 3-day period (i.e., children do not need to eat an RDA diet every day in order to be healthy). Vitamin and mineral supplements are not necessary for children who consume a varied, healthy diet, but children at risk for nutritional deficit benefit by supplementation with multivitamins. Risk factors for vitamin and mineral deficiency may include economically deprived families, neglect or abuse, anorexia, poor and capricious appetites, fad diets, dietary restrictions to manage obesity, pregnancy, and vegetarian diets. Preterm or low birth weight babies and children with chronic illness also may need supplementation.

Age-Specific Considerations

NEWBORNS AND INFANTS

Energy

Rapid growth in infancy requires high caloric intake. From birth to 6 months of age, infants require 108 kcal/kg per day. This amount decreases to about 100 kcal/kg per day by 12 months of age and is 102 kcal/kg per day for children 1 to 3 years of age.

Fat

In order for proper myelinization to occur, infants must have adequate fat intake. Children younger than age 2 years require more than 30% dietary fat for neural development. The lipid content of breast milk and formulas meets infants' dietary requirements. During the second year of life, cow's milk can be included in children's diets. Because the majority of fat in the diet is derived from milk and milk products, skim milk is not recommended for infants. The AAP recommends whole milk for children between 12 and 24 months of age, although 2% milk, as part of a varied diet, can contribute to adequate fat intake.

Vitamins

Vitamin and mineral supplements, except iron, are usually not necessary for healthy term infants who are breastfed or formula fed and, after 4 to 6 months, receive mixed feedings of cereal, fruits, vegetables, and proteins. Breastfed infants whose mothers' diets are deficient in vitamin D, and infants who receive a formula not fortified with vitamin D (which is rare), need supplementation unless their exposure to sunlight provides adequate absorption of vitamin D. Infants also should have an adequate source of vitamin C, especially after 4 to 6 months of age. A multivitamin supplement is recommended for infants at nutritional risk as a result of lifestyle, economic status, or recurrent illness.

Iron

Iron deficiency is the leading cause of anemia in children, and iron supplementation is appropriate in some cases. Term infants who are breastfed usually have adequate iron supplies until 4 to 6 months of age. Premature or low birth weight infants, infants who are exclusively breastfed beyond 4 to 6 months of age, and infants who are fed cow's milk before age 12 months are at high risk for iron deficiency anemia. Iron-fortified cereals and iron-fortified formulas are excellent sources of dietary iron supplements for infants 6 to 12 months of age. Earlier supplementation may be necessary for breastfed premature infants.

Fluoride

The most recent guidelines from the American Dental Association recommend beginning fluoride treatment at 6 months of age. See Chapter 34 for recommended fluoride dosages.

Infant Formulas

Breast milk is the ideal food for newborns and infants and should be encouraged whenever possible. Most iron-fortified infant formulas provide adequate nutrition and, for some families, may be an appropriate alternative. Table 12–6 outlines the nutritional content of various commercial formulas and breast milk.

Occasionally, infants demonstrate an intolerance to formula, showing irritability, weight loss or slow gain, emesis, diarrhea, constipation, other gastrointestinal problems, or atopic dermatitis. The NP must work closely with parents to identify a formula tolerated by the in-

T A B L E 12-4

Minerals and Trace Elements: Function, Dietary Sources, Interactions, Deficiency, and Excess

	FUNCTION	DIETARY SOURCES	INTERACTIONS AFFECTING ABSORPTION OR UTILIZATION	SIGNS OF DEFICIT	SIGNS OF EXCESS*
Minerals					
Calcium	Development of bone tissue; vital role in nerve conduction, membrane permeability, blood clotting, and muscle contraction	Milk and milk products, green leafy vegetables, broccoli, kale, and collards, soft bones of fish, foods processed or fortified with calcium	Absorption enhanced in the presence of vitamin D, adequate protein intake, during periods of rapid growth, and if dietary intake of calcium is low	Decreased bone strength, increased risk for fractures	Constipation, increased risk for urinary stone formation; risk for decreased renal function
Phosphorus	Essential for bone integrity and general metabolism; provides essential energy during the metabolic process	Almost all foods, especially meat, poultry, fish, milk, cereal grains; food additives in processed foods	Aluminum hydroxide in antacids prevents absorption	Bone loss, weakness, malaise, anorexia, and pain	None known
Magnesium	Activates enzymes, facilitates cell metabolism, maintains electrical potential of cell membranes, enhances transmission of nerve impulses, assists to maintain adequate serum levels of calcium and potassium	Nuts, legumes, whole (unmilled) grains, green vegetables; bananas provide some magnesium	High-fiber diet may reduce absorption slightly	Nausea, muscle weakness, irritability	None in healthy individual; with impaired renal function, excess may contribute to nausea, vomiting, hypotension, bradycardia, central nervous system depression
Iron	Formation of the heme molecule; used in oxygen transport	Meat, eggs, vegetables, cereals, foods fortified with iron additives; Table 12–5 identifies a number of iron-rich foods	Absorption is enhanced if iron stores or daily intakes are low; presence of ascorbic acid increases absorption Heme iron in meats is more bioavailable than non-heme iron from grains, fruits, and vegetables Absorption inhibited if the iron-rich food is ingested with milk or caffeine or in presence of phytic acid, oxalic acid, and tannic acid	Anemia Children are particularly susceptible to iron deficiency during periods of rapid growth combined with low dietary iron intake: from about 6 mo to 4 yr of age and during early adolescence; adolescent girls are at risk owing to menstruation	Iron poisoning, can be fatal; for a 2-year-old, a fatal dose is approximately 3 g; for adolescents and adults, 200–250 mg/kg may be fatal

Mineral	Function	Sources	Interactions/Considerations	Deficiency	Toxicity
Zinc	Cellular metabolism, growth, and repair	Meats, animal products, seafood (especially oysters), eggs	Absorption may be decreased if taken with high-fiber diet	Anorexia, growth retardation, skin changes, immunological abnormalities	Gastrointestinal disturbances, vomiting, acute toxicity, impaired immune response
Iodine	Production of thyroid hormones	Water, seafood, airborne water from ocean mist, iodized salt, food processing related to milk and bread	None known	Thyroid dysfunction ranging from simple goiter to cretinism and mental retardation	Thyrotoxicosis; goiter, rare and not seen in children with intake up to 1 mg/d; toxic levels not known
Trace elements					
Selenium	Unknown	Seafood and organ meats; may be in grains grown in soil containing selenium	Intake linked to vitamin E intake; if vitamin E is adequate, selenium is likely to be also; may need to supplement in lactating women. Total parenteral nutrition (TPN) feedings contribute to deficiency	May be related to muscle weakness and pain, cardiomyopathy (Keshan's disease) in young children	Nausea, abdominal pain, diarrhea, fatigue, nail and hair changes or loss; toxic levels not known
Copper	Normal growth	Organ meats, seafood, nuts, seeds; infants store copper in liver during gestation	TPN feedings contribute to deficiency; high vitamin C, molybdenum, or zinc intake may reduce retention or bioavailability	Bone loss, anemia, neutropenia, growth impairment	Liver disease, gastrointestinal symptoms, diarrhea, vomiting
Manganese	Unknown, may be related to reproductive health, normal growth	Whole grains and cereals	Increased absorption during third trimester of pregnancy	Unknown, may be related to growth retardation	Unknown, may be related to learning disabilities, anemia
Fluoride	Prevents dental caries, enhances bone health	Fluoridated water, tea, meat and bones of marine fish, potatoes, wheat germ	Processing foods in fluoridated water or cooking with Teflon increases content; cooking foods in aluminum reduces fluoride	Dental caries, may be related to poor bone health	Mottling of teeth, kidney disease, bone disease, may affect muscle and nerve function
Chromium	Assists in glucose metabolism	Brewer's yeast, calves' liver, American cheese, wheat germ	TPN feedings can contribute to deficiency	May be related to impairment of glucose tolerance	Unknown, requires further study
Molybdenum	Enzyme function	Milk, beans, breads, cereals	TPN feedings can contribute to deficiency	Unknown	Related to loss of copper, may lead to gout-like symptoms

*Nearly all trace minerals are toxic in large quantities, because many are metals.

T A B L E 12-5
Iron-Rich Foods

	HIGH LEVELS (>5 mg/serving)	MODERATE LEVELS (2–4 mg/serving)	LOW LEVELS (<2 mg/serving)
Breads, grains, cereals, seeds	Almonds (1 cup, whole, oil roasted) Cashews (1 cup, dry roasted) Fortified cereals Mixed nuts (1 cup, dry roasted with peanuts) Brown glutinous rice (1 cup, cooked) Sunflower seeds (1 cup, dry roasted) Watermelon kernels (1 cup, dried) Wheat germ (1 cup, toasted)	Bagel (1, egg or plain) Bread, Indian fry (1 piece) Breadstick (10, plain, without salt) Filberts (1 cup, dried) Gingerbread (1 piece) Muffin (1 wheat) Peanuts (1 cup, dried) White rice (1 cup, enriched, regular, cooked) Waffles (2 each) Walnuts (1 cup, dried)	Biscuits (1 each) Bread (1 slice, whole wheat) Egg noodles (1 cup, cooked) English muffin (1 each) Pancakes (1 each) Peanut butter (2 tbsp)
Fruits	Apricot (1 cup, dried halves)	Avocado (1 whole) Currants (1 cup, dried Zante) Fig (10 each, dried) Pear (10 each, dried halves) Prune juice (1 cup) Raisins (1 cup)	Apple (1 medium, unpeeled) Apple juice (1 cup) Banana (1 medium) Dried mixed fruit (2 oz) Orange (1 medium) Orange juice (1 cup)
Vegetables	Kidney beans (1 cup, cooked, fresh) Lentils (1 cup, cooked) Soybeans (1 cup, cooked) White beans (1 cup, cooked) Spinach (1 cup, cooked)	Black beans (1 cup, cooked) Garbanzo beans (1 cup, cooked) Refried beans (1 cup, canned) Beet greens (1 cup, cooked) Potatoes (1 medium, with skin, baked) Snow peas with pods (1 cup, raw or cooked)	Kidney beans (1 cup, canned) Green beans (1 cup, raw or cooked) Broccoli (1 cup) Carrots (1 cup) Corn (1/2 cup) Lettuce (1 cup) Peas (1 cup, fresh, cooked) Potato chips (1 oz) Spinach (1 cup, raw) Sweet potatoes (1 cup, fresh, boiled, mashed) Tomatoes (1 cup fresh) Tomato juice (1 cup, canned) Turnip greens (1 cup, cooked)
Meats, poultry, fish, other protein sources	Beef heart meat (1/2 cup, cooked) Beef liver (3 oz, simmered) Clams (3.5 oz, 5 each, or 1 cup) Oysters (6 each, or 1 cup, Eastern) Veal liver (3 oz, simmered)	Ground beef (3.5 oz, cooked, lean) Catfish (1 piece, floured, fried) Tuna (1 cup, canned, water packed)	Roast beef (3 oz, lean) Chicken (1 cup, dark or light meat) Egg (one, whole) Halibut (1 piece, baked or broiled) Ham (1 cup, roasted) Bacon (3 pieces, cooked) Pork (3 oz, lean shoulder roast)

Adapted from Hands ES: Food Finder: Food Sources of Vitamins & Minerals, 3rd ed. Salem, OR, ESHA Research, 1995.

fant, being careful to allow sufficient time for the baby to respond to a new formula as it is introduced. This can be a time- and energy-consuming process in which parents need support, reassurance, and encouragement. Referral to a registered dietitian can be helpful. See the discussion on food intolerances (Altered Patterns of Nutrition) later in the chapter for management of the lactose- or protein-intolerant infant.

Introduction of Solids

A number of variables converge at about 6 months of age that make this an appropriate time to introduce solids into infants' diets. By 6 months, infants' sucking patterns have changed sufficiently to allow for chewing. Infants can sit with some support, and they are able to purposefully move their heads. Iron stores present at birth are being depleted, and growth demands require nutrients other than those provided in milk alone. Between 6 months and 1 year of age, infants master the ability to chew and control swallowing and to grasp, pick up, and bring objects to their mouths. New foods with their varied textures, smells, and tastes stimulate developmental needs of infants. As children grow, use of finger foods as well as utensils fosters motor, cognitive, and social skills. The period in which solid foods are first offered can be a creative, frustrating, learning-filled time for both children and caregivers.

The specific foods that parents provide for their children vary by cultural and family customs, and there are no set recommendations as to a sequence by which to introduce solids. Commercial baby foods provide adequate nutrition, but they should be examined to determine their content, especially looking at calories, fats, additives, salt, and sugar. Home-prepared foods, such as mashed bananas, applesauce, pureed squash, cooked peas, and blenderized meats can provide adequate nutrition if the diet is well-balanced. Table 12–7 lists some principles to keep in mind when beginning solids. NPs can offer suggestions and guidance to make feeding a positive experience.

TODDLERS AND PRESCHOOLERS

Energy and Protein

The growth rate of toddlers and preschoolers is slower than that of infants, resulting in decreased energy needs per unit of body weight. But because of increased size and activity, these children require an increased number of total calories. Addition of muscle mass also demands a high protein intake (see Table 12–1 for recommended protein intake).

Establishing Eating Habits in Early Childhood

Good nutrition for children is not simply a matter of meeting dietary requirements. When providing nutritional counseling, NPs must also consider the ways children and families eat. Lifelong patterns of eating are developed in the toddler and preschool years, and children learn how and what to eat by observing adults around them.

Establishing eating habits can be a positive growth experience for both children and parents. Among other things, children learn about textures, smells, and colors as well as taste. They learn physical skills of fine motor control, cognitive skills of relationships between action and consequence (the dog will eat whatever is dropped on the floor), and interactional skills of social exchange among family members. Parents are teachers in this process, both by instruction and by example. Often that teaching is done without conscious reflection or planning, but children learn nonetheless. NPs can help parents make the process more positive by having them examine their own values and patterns related to eating, identify and reinforce those they would like to foster in their children, and eliminate those they see as negative.

In the process of developing the child's eating habits, adults have the responsibility for what foods are presented to children and how those foods are presented; specifically, adults should provide a variety of nutritious foods that contribute to the child's optimal growth and development in a pleasant, supportive environment that enhances the child's desire to eat. Children have the responsibility to decide what

Text continued on page 262

T A B L E 12-6

Approximate Composition of Pediatric Formulas

	kcal/oz	PROTEIN SOURCE	(g/dl)	FAT SOURCE	(g/dl)	CARBOHYDRATE SOURCE	(g/dl)	Na (mEq/dl)	K (mEq/dl)	PHOSPHORUS (mg/dl)	CALCIUM (mg/dl)	OSMOLALITY (mOsm/kg WATER)
HUMAN MILK												
Mature human milk	20	Human milk	1.0	Human milk	4.4	Lactose	6.9	0.7	1.3	14	32	300
PREMATURE FORMULAS (HOSPITAL AND TRANSITIONAL)												
*Enfamil Human Milk Fortifier (3.8 g) added to 100 ml preterm milk (Mead Johnson)	24	Preterm human milk plus fortifier, whey, and caseinate	2.3	Preterm human milk fat	3.5	Preterm human milk, corn syrup solids, lactose	10.0	1.5	1.7	60	115	410–440
*Similac Natural Care Human Milk Fortifier (Ross)	24	Nonfat milk, whey	2.2	MCT 50%, soy, coconut oils	4.4	Lactose, polycose	8.5	1.5	2.7	85	159	280
*Enfamil Premature (Mead Johnson)	24	Whey, nonfat milk	2.4	MCT 40%, soy, coconut oils	4.1	Corn syrup solids, lactose	9.0	1.4	2.1	67	134	310
*Similac Special Care (Ross)	24	Nonfat milk, whey	2.2	MCT 50%, soy oil, coconut oils	4.4	Lactose, polycose	8.5	1.5	2.7	73	145	280
Similac NeoCare (Ross)	22	Nonfat milk, whey	1.9	Soy, coconut, MCT (25%), oils	4.1	Corn syrup solids, lactose	7.7	1.1	2.7	46	78	250
COW'S MILK-BASED FORMULAS												
Enfamil (Mead Johnson)	20	Whey, nonfat milk	1.4	Palm olein, soy, coconut, high-oleic sunflower oils	3.6	Lactose	7.3	0.8	1.9	36	53	300
Gerber (Gerber)	20	Nonfat milk	1.4	Palm olein, soy, coconut, high-oleic sunflower oils	3.6	Lactose	7.4	0.9	1.9	36	53	320
Lactofree (Mead Johnson)	20	Milk protein isolate	1.4	Palm olein, soy, coconut, high-oleic sunflower oils	3.6	Corn syrup solids	7.4	0.9	1.9	37	55	200

Product		Protein source		Fat source		Carbohydrate source						
Similac Improved (Ross)	20	Nonfat milk, whey	1.4	High-oleic safflower, coconut, soy oils	3.7	Lactose	7.3	0.7	1.8	28	53	300
Similac PM/60/40 (Ross)	20	Whey, sodium, caseinate	1.6	Soy, coconut oils	3.8	Lactose	6.9	0.7	1.5	19	38	280
PARTIALLY HYDROLYZED WHEY-BASED FORMULAS												
Good Start (Carnation)	20	Enzymatically hydrolyzed reduced mineral whey	1.6	Palm olein, soybean, coconut, high-oleic safflower oils	3.4	Lactose, maltodextrin	7.4	0.7	1.7	24	43	265
NUTRIENT-DENSE COW'S MILK-BASED FORMULAS												
*Enfamil (Mead Johnson)	24	Whey, nonfat milk	1.7	Palm olein, soy, coconut, high-oleic safflower oils	4.3	Lactose	8.8	1.0	2.3	43	63	360
*Similac (Ross)	24	Nonfat milk	2.2	Soy, coconut oils	4.3	Lactose	8.5	1.2	2.7	56	73	380
*Similac (Ross)	27	Nonfat milk	2.5	Soy, coconut oils	4.8	Lactose	9.5	1.3	3.1	64	82	410
SOY-BASED FORMULAS												
Alsoy (Carnation)	20	Soy protein isolate with L-methionine	1.9	Palm olein, soy, coconut, high-oleic safflower oils	3.3	Corn maltodextrin, sucrose	7.5	0.9	2.0	41	71	200
Gerber (Gerber)	20	Soy protein isolate with L-methionine	2.0	Palm olein, soy, coconut, high-oleic sunflower oils	3.6	Corn syrup solids, sucrose	6.8	1.0	2.1	56	71	230
Isomil (Ross)	20	Soy protein isolate with L-methionine	1.7	Soy, coconut oils	3.7	Corn syrup, sucrose	7.0	1.3	1.9	51	71	230
Isomil DF (Ross)	20	Soy protein isolate with L-methionine	1.8	Soy, coconut oils	3.7	Corn syrup, sucrose, soy fiber	6.8	1.3	1.9	51	71	240
Isomil SF (Ross)	20	Soy protein isolate with L-methionine	1.8	Soy, coconut oils	3.7	Polycose glucose polymers	6.8	1.3	1.9	51	71	180
ProSobee (Mead Johnson)	20	Soy protein isolate with L-methionine	2.0	Palm olein, soy, coconut, high-oleic sunflower oils	3.6	Corn syrup solids	6.8	1.0	2.1	56	71	200

Table continued on following page

T A B L E 12-6
Approximate Composition of Pediatric Formulas *Continued*

	kcal/oz	PROTEIN SOURCE	(g/dl)	FAT SOURCE	(g/dl)	CARBOHYDRATE SOURCE	(g/dl)	Na (mEq/dl)	K (mEq/dl)	PHOSPHORUS (mg/dl)	CALCIUM (mg/dl)	OSMOLALITY (mOsm/kg WATER)
CASEIN HYDROLYSATE (HYPOALLERGENIC) FORMULAS												
Alimentum (Ross)	20	Casein hydrolysate with added amino acids	1.9	MCT 50%, safflower, soy oils	3.7	Sucrose, modified tapioca starch	6.9	1.3	2.0	51	71	370
Nutramigen (Mead Johnson)	20	Casein hydrolysate with added amino acids	1.9	Palm olein, soy, coconut, high-oleic sunflower oils	3.4	Corn syrup solids, modified cornstarch	7.4	1.4	1.9	43	64	320
Pregestimil Powder (Mead Johnson)	20	Casein hydrolysate with added amino acids	1.9	MCT (55%), corn, soy, high-oleic safflower oils	3.8	Corn syrup solids, dextrose, modified cornstarch	6.9	1.1	1.9	43	64	320
Pregestimil Liquid (Mead Johnson)	20	Casein hydrolysate with added amino acids	1.9	MCT (55%), corn, soy, high-oleic safflower oils	3.8	Corn syrup solids, dextrose, modified cornstarch	6.9	1.4	1.9	51	78	280
AMINO ACID BASE (NONALLERGENIC) FORMULAS												
Neocate (SHS)	20	L-amino acids	1.9	Hybrid safflower, refined vegetable oils (coconut, soy)	2.8	Corn syrup solids	7.1	0.9	2.4	56	75	342
FOR SPECIAL FEEDING PROBLEMS												
Portagen (Mead Johnson)	20	Sodium caseinate	2.4	MCT (86%), corn oil	3.2	Corn syrup solids, sucrose	7.8	1.6	2.2	47	64	230
Product 3232A Monodisaccharide-free diet powder (Mead Johnson)	13 Using 81.0 g powder and water to make 1 quart	Casein hydrolysate with added amino acids	1.9	MCT (85%), corn oil	2.8	Modified tapioca starch May add: 59 g CHO/qt corn syrup solids, sucrose, glucose, fructose	2.8 9.1	1.3	1.9	43	64	Dependent upon additional CHO source; 250 without CHO source

Protein-Vitamin-Mineral Formula Component (Ross)	Add 30 g powder, CHO, and fat to 900 ml water	Casein	2.2	Coconut oils May add corn, soy, safflower, MCT oil	May add sucrose, polycose, dextrose, fructose	Tr	1.6	2.5	51	72	Dependent upon source and amount of CHO
RCF CHO-Free Formula Base (Ross)	12 Dilute 1:1 without added CHO	Soy protein isolate with L-methionine	2.0	Soy, coconut oils	May add sucrose, polycose, dextrose, fructose	—	1.3	1.9	50	70	Dependent upon source and amount of CHO

FOR ADVANCED FEEDING BEYOND 4 TO 6 MONTHS OF AGE WITH SOLIDS ADDED TO DIET

Follow-Up (Carnation)	20	Nonfat milk	1.8	Palm olein, soy, coconut, high-oleic safflower oils	Corn syrup, lactose	8.9	1.2	2.3	61	91	326
Follow-Up Soy (Carnation)	20	Soy protein isolate with L-methionine	2.1	Palm olein, soy, coconut, high-oleic safflower oils	Corn, maltodextrin, sucrose	8.1	1.2	2.0	61	91	200

FOR FEEDING BEYOND 1 YEAR OF AGE

Whole cow's milk Next Step (Mead Johnson)	20 20	Cow's milk Nonfat milk	3.3 1.8	Cow's milk Palm olein, soy, coconut, high-oleic sunflower oils	Lactose Lactose, corn syrup solids	4.7 7.5	2.1 1.2	3.9 2.3	93 57	119 81	288 270
Next Step Soy (Mead Johnson)	20	Soy protein isolate with L-methionine	2.2	Palm olein, soy, coconut, high-oleic sunflower oils	Corn syrup solids, sucrose	8.0	1.3	2.6	61	78	260

NUTRIENT DENSE

Compleat Pediatric Blenderized (Novartis)	30	Beef, sodium caseinate, calcium caseinate	3.8	High-oleic sunflower, soy, MCT (18%) oils beef fat, monoglycerides, diglycerides	Hydrolyzed cornstarch, apple juice, vegetables, fruits	12.6	3.0	3.8	100	100	380
Kindercal (Mead Johnson)	30	Calcium, sodium caseinates, milk protein concentrate	3.4	MCT (20%), canola, corn, high-oleic sunflower oils	Maltodextrin, sucrose, soy fiber	13.5	1.6	3.4	85	85	310

Table continued on following page

259

T A B L E 12-6

Approximate Composition of Pediatric Formulas Continued

	kcal/oz	PROTEIN SOURCE	(g/dl)	FAT SOURCE	(g/dl)	CARBOHYDRATE SOURCE	(g/dl)	Na (mEq/dl)	K (mEq/dl)	PHOSPHORUS (mg/dl)	CALCIUM (mg/dl)	OSMOLALITY (mOsm/kg WATER)
NUTRIENT DENSE *Continued*												
Nutren Junior (Nestle Clinical Nutrition)	30	Isolated casein and whey	3.0	Soy, MCT (25%), canola oils, soy, lecithin	4.2	Maltodextrin, sucrose	12.7	2.0	3.4	80	100	350
Nutren Junior with Fiber (Nestle Clinical Nutrition)	30	Isolated casein and whey	3.0	Soy, MCT (25%), canola oils, soy lecithin	4.2	Maltodextrin, sucrose	12.7	2.0	3.4	80	100	350
PediaSure (Ross)	30	Caseinate, whey proteins	3.0	High-oleic safflower, soy, MCT (20%) oils	5.0	Corn syrup solids, sucrose	11.0	1.7	3.4	80	97	365
PediaSure with Fiber (Ross)	30	Caseinate, whey proteins	3.0	High-oleic safflower, soy, MCT (20%) oils	5.0	Corn syrup solids, sucrose, soy fiber	11.0	1.7	3.4	80	97	365
Resource Just for Kids Vanilla (Novartis)	30	Sodium caseinate, calcium caseinate, whey protein concentrate	3.0	High-oleic sunflower, soy, MCT (20%) oils	5.0	Hydrolyzed cornstarch, sucrose	11.0	1.7	3.3	80	114	390
SPECIALIZED PEDIATRIC NUTRITION PRODUCTS—FREE AMINO ACID AND PEPTIDE-BASED FORMULAS												
L-Emental Pediatric (Nutrition Medical)	24	Free amino acids	2.4	MCT (68%), soy oils	2.4	Maltodextrin, modified starch	13.0	1.7	3.1	80	97	360
Neocate one + powder (SHS)	30	L-amino acids	2.5	Fractionated coconut, canola, hybrid safflower oils	3.5	Corn syrup solids	14.6	0.8	2.4	62	62	610
Neocate one + liquid (SHS)	30	L-amino acids	2.5	Fractionated coconut, canola, high-oleic safflower oils	3.5	Maltodextrin, sucrose	14.6	0.9	2.4	62	62	835
Peptamen Junior Plain (Nestle Clinical Nutrition)	30	Enzymatically hydrolyzed whey	3.0	MCT (60%), soybean, canola oils	3.8	Maltodextrin, corn starch	13.7	2.0	3.4	80	100	260

Pro-Peptide for Kids, Vanilla (Nutrition Medical)	30	Enzymatically hydrolyzed whey	3.0	Soy, canola, MCT (40%) oils	3.8	Maltodextrin, sucrose, cornstarch	13.7	2.0	3.4	80	100	360
Vivonex Pediatric (Novartis)	24	Free amino acids	2.4	MCT (68%), soy oils	2.4	Maltodextrin, modified starch	13.0	1.7	3.1	80	97	360
NITROGEN-FREE ENERGY SOURCE PRODUCTS												
Duocal (SHS)	4.9/g			Corn, coconut, MCT oils		Hydrolyzed cornstarch						
Product 80056 (Mead Johnson)	4.9/g			Corn oil		Corn syrup solids, modified tapioca starch						
Microlipid (Mead Johnson)	4.5/ml			Safflower oil		None						
MCT oil (Mead Johnson)	8.3/g			Fractionated coconut oil		None						
Safflower oil	8.8/g			Safflower		None						
Moducal (Mead Johnson)	3.8/g			None		Maltodextrin						
Polycose (Ross)	3.8/g 2.0/ml			None		Glucose polymers						
PROTEIN SUPPLEMENTS												
Casec (Mead Johnson)	3.8/g	Calcium caseinate	4.0 g/ Tbsp		tr							
Promod (Ross)	4.2/g	Whey protein	5.0 g/ scoop		tr							
ORAL ELECTROLYTE SOLUTIONS												
Beech-Nut Pediatric Electrolyte (Beech-Nut)	3.0					Glucose	2.5	5.0	2.0			280
CeraLyte (Cera)	4.9					Rice digest CHO	4.0	7.0	2.0			222
Infalyte (Mead Johnson)	3.7					Rice syrup, solids	3.2	5.0	2.5			200
Oral Rehydration Salts WHO (Jianas)	2					Dextrose	2.0	9.0	2.0			330
Pedialyte Unflavored (Ross)	3					Dextrose	2.5	4.5	2.0			250
Rehydralyte (Ross)	3					Dextrose	2.5	7.5	2.0			305

*Special order for hospital use only, not available commercially. Values are based on liquid formula unless otherwise indicated.
CHO = carbohydrate; MCT = medium chain triglyceride; WHO = World Health Organization.
Compiled 6/97 by J. Hattner, R.D., M.P.H., J. Kerner, M.D.
Stanford University Medical Center/Lucile Packard Children's Hospital Department of Nutrition and Food Services.

TABLE 12-7

Principles for the Introduction of Solids into the Infant's Diet

- Introduce one food at a time, waiting 3 to 5 d before offering another in order to assess for adverse reaction.
- Offer rice cereal, the least allergenic of cereal grains, as the first food.
- Introduce fruits, vegetables, and other cereals in any sequence desired.
- Feed only iron-fortified cereals.
- Avoid allergenic foods (e.g., wheat, nuts [especially peanuts], shellfish, egg whites, citrus) before 12 mo of age.
- Prepare food appropriate to child's developmental abilities (e.g., strained, mashed, or finger foods).
- Use commercially or home-prepared foods.
- Provide a variety of foods.
- Help child develop healthy patterns of eating:
  - Be alert and responsive to child's cues when eating.
  - Use a spoon to feed solids.
  - Offer about 1 tbsp per yr of age as a serving for infants; for older children, about one fourth to one half an adult serving.
  - Never force a child to eat.
  - Include the child in family meal times.

or even whether to eat. Negative patterns emerge when either party fails to perform its respective responsibility. Positive patterns are the result of healthy choices by both adults and children.

Appetite fluctuations are typical of toddlers and preschoolers, and parents should be aware that children often appear to eat less than the parent thinks is sufficient or too much of one particular food to the neglect of others. It is not unusual, for example, for 2-year-olds to refuse to eat. If parents punish a child for not eating or force a child to eat, they have taken away the child's responsibility to choose. Children, in response, may develop an aversion to certain foods or act out in other ways. Mealtimes can become contests of will between parents and children, creating feelings and patterns of interacting that extend far beyond the dinner table. If provided a nutritious variety of foods they like, children tend to select those necessary for their healthy growth, in terms of both amount of calories and other nutrients.

Use of Vitamin and Mineral Supplements

Evaluate a child's intake over the course of a week. If children persist with limited food choices or picky eating behavior, they might benefit from a complete type of children's multivitamin plus mineral supplement.

SCHOOL-AGE CHILDREN

Energy and Protein

Energy and protein needs of school-age children vary depending on body size, growth patterns, and activity and exercise levels. Younger children, aged 6 to 7 years, need about 90 calories/kg, those between 7 and 10 years need about 70 calories/kg, and children older than 10 years require a range of about 40 to 55 calories/kg, depending on age, size, and activity. Protein needs increase in older children as they acquire more muscle mass. Boys older than 10 years need between 2500 and 3000 calories a day, whereas girls require about 2200 calories daily.

Eating Habits

Food likes and dislikes carry over from the preschool years. There is great variation in appetite and intake as a result of uneven growth patterns and activity levels. School-age children have a tendency to skip meals and are more likely to snack as they become engrossed in activities. This tendency is exacerbated in families with hectic schedules, unstructured mealtimes, and reliance on fast foods.

School-age children are particularly at risk for excessive weight gain if caloric intake exceeds energy needs, and problems with obesity begin at this age. A discussion of obesity, including etiology and management, is found later in this chapter (Altered Patterns of Nutrition).

Use of Vitamin and Mineral Supplements

Poor eating habits place school-age children at risk for deficiencies in iron, thiamine, vitamin A, and calcium. Teaching children about specific nutrient sources and encouraging healthy eating habits can prevent many problems, but supplementation with a daily multivitamin may be necessary.

ADOLESCENTS

Energy and Protein

Requirements for adolescents vary greatly depending on body size, activity level, and growth patterns. The growth rate of adolescents is remarkable (Table 12–8), and the description by some parents that their children never seem to stop eating is apt. High levels of energy are needed to support adolescents' rapid growth, and if children participate in sports or other exercise programs, additional caloric intake can be needed. Adequate protein intake is essential to produce muscle mass. The average intake of protein in the US diet is significantly above the RDA, so additional supplementation is usually not necessary.

Eating Habits

Eating habits of adolescents are influenced by their increasing independence and social activity, perceptions of body image, and physical growth patterns. Adolescents often have erratic eating patterns, skip meals, eat high-fat, high-calorie, low-nutrient snack foods, and consume calories late in the day.

T A B L E 12-8

Average Weight and Height Gains in Infancy Through Adolescence

AGE	WEIGHT	HEIGHT
INFANT (mo)		
0–3	Average weekly gain 210 g (8 oz)	Average monthly gain 3.5 cm
3–6	Average weekly gain 140 g (5 oz); birth weight doubles by 4–6 mo	Average monthly gain 2.0 cm
6–12	Average weekly gain 85–140 g (3–5 oz); birth weight triples by 1 yr	Average monthly gain 1.2–1.5 cm
TODDLER (yr)		

1–3	Average yearly gain 2–3 kg (4.4–6.6 lb)	Average yearly gain:
		  1–2 years: 12 cm
		  2–3 years: 6–8 cm
		Height at 2 yr: approximately half of adult height

PRESCHOOL-AGE CHILD (yr)		
3–6	Average yearly gain 1.8–2.7 kg (4–6 lb)	Yearly gain 6–8 cm
SCHOOL-AGE CHILD (yr)		
6–12	Average yearly gain 1.8–2.7 kg (4–6 lb)	Average yearly gain 5 cm
PREADOLESCENT/ADOLESCENT (yr)		
Girl, 10–14	Average total gain 17.5 kg (38.5 lb)	Average yearly gain 6–8.3 cm 95% of adult height achieved by onset of menarche
Boy, 12–16	Average total gain 23.7 kg (52.1 lb)	Average yearly gain 6–9.5 cm 95% of adult height achieved by 15 yr

Adapted from Behrman RE, Kliegman RM, Arvin AM (eds): Nelson Textbook of Pediatrics, 15th ed. Philadelphia, WB Saunders, 1996.

Use of Vitamin and Mineral Supplements

Thiamine, riboflavin, niacin, folate, iron, zinc, and calcium needs increase during adolescence (see Table 12-1). Most adolescents who eat a well-balanced diet need no supplements, but their irregular eating habits put them at risk for many deficiencies.

Pregnancy in Adolescence

Pregnancy presents an added complication to the normal adolescent nutrient intake. Nutrition needs are high for the pregnant teenager, particularly those younger than 15 years old, in the midst of her pubertal growth spurt. During this period, teenagers' bodies are still growing and compete with their fetuses for nutrients. Infants born to teenage mothers are at higher risk for prematurity, low birth weight, chronic illness, disabilities, and death. Proper nutrition and early prenatal care can increase the chance of a successful pregnancy.

The nutrition needs of pregnant teenagers are the highest at a time when it is most difficult to meet them. Irregular eating patterns typical of adolescents contribute to poor nutrition status. Calcium, iron, zinc, vitamins A, D, and B_6, riboflavin, folic acid, and total calories—all of which are essential to fetal growth—are often found to be inadequate in the diets of female adolescents (Munoz et al., 1997).

When managing the pregnant teenager, the NP should carefully assess dietary intake and counsel the adolescent to eat a varied and healthful diet. A prenatal multivitamin and mineral supplement, including iron and folic acid, is advised, and, depending on dietary intake, calcium supplements can be indicated. The pregnant teenager should strive for a total of 1200 to 1500 mg of calcium through diet and supplements each day. Daily folic acid intake of 0.4 mg is recommended for 3 months before conception and through the first trimester (American Dietetic Association, 1994).

Weight gain in pregnant teens should be carefully monitored. Healthy teens should gain the amount they would normally gain in 9 months if they were not pregnant *plus* the upper limit of normal pregnancy weight gain. This amounts to an intake of about 38 to 50 kcal/kg per day and results in about 35 to 48 lb total weight gain. Adolescents who begin pregnancy when overweight should gain less (Gorrie et al., 1998). For those adolescents who meet income guidelines (185% of poverty level), a valuable resource is the federal supplemental food program for women, infants, and children (WIC). In addition to providing nutritious foods, the program offers nutrition education and counseling.

■ ASSESSMENT OF NUTRITIONAL STATUS

The goals of nutritional status assessment are to determine dietary adequacy and to identify deviation from normal growth and development. Data collected include a history of food and fluid intake, physical findings, and laboratory and diagnostic indicators.

History

The history of food and fluid intake includes the following:

- Nutritional status of mother during pregnancy.
- Type of feeding method used during infancy. Formula name and preparation. Any problems? When weaned? When solids started? Any allergies or intolerances noted?
- Current nutritional intake of child (if child is still an infant, ask more specifically about frequency and amounts of feedings in 24-hour period).
- Type of foods and fluids.
- Frequency of eating (nursings, meals, snacks).
- Amounts eaten (may use 24-hour recall, 3-day diet history, or length of time child is at breast).
- Additional intake (e.g., vitamin, fluoride, or iron supplements).
- Feeding patterns or behaviors for both child and family.
- Any reaction to particular foods (e.g., vomiting, diarrhea, rash).

- Food preferences or dislikes.
- Bottle feeding: Is bottle propped? Does child take bottle to bed at night or at naptime? Who feeds child?
- Breastfeeding: On demand or scheduled? How flexible is mother to demands of infant? Is mother working? Is breast milk frozen and fed by someone other than mother?
- Describe mealtimes: Does family sit down together? Are meals prepared at home? Does child eat at school? How often are "fast foods" eaten? What amount of time is spent eating? How long does it take to feed child?
- Who plans, purchases, and prepares food and meals for family?
- Does family eat out frequently?
- Economic and environmental factors that influence how food is managed. For example, are finances adequate to supply nutritious foods? Is there a refrigerator? Does family have a car to carry larger amounts of food from store? What is the socioeconomic status of family? Is food shopping budgeted? Are food stamps or other supplemental programs used?
- Cultural factors: What beliefs or attitudes does family have about how and what child should eat or how family should eat?
- What is child's attitude about foods and eating?
- Special considerations for children or family related to food. For example, does child have a chronic illness that requires a special diet? Are any medications being taken?
- Feeding abilities of child. For example, does child choke, gag, vomit, or refuse certain foods, perhaps due to texture or smell?
- Elimination patterns.
- Dental status and care of teeth.
- Patterns of wound healing.
- Any change in hair, nails, skin, or mucous membranes?
- Tolerance for hot or cold weather?
- Growth, activity, and exercise pattern. For example, has child been growing as parent expects? Has there been a history of unusual weight gain or loss? Does child have energy to play?

- Family history: hypertension, diabetes, hyperlipidemia, obesity, heart disease, allergies, eating disorders.

Physical Examination

The physical examination should include the following:

- Body temperature
- Height, weight, and head circumference for all children (see growth charts, Appendix B; also see Table 12-8 for average weight and height gains expected during childhood); arm circumference, and triceps and subscapular skinfold caliper measurements for children at risk for obesity or malnutrition
- Skin condition (clear, smooth, firm, with good turgor)
- Muscle tone, posture, skeletal development (body erect, tone good)
- Hair (smooth, full, shiny; no dryness, broken ends, bare patches, or discoloration)
- Mucous membranes, eyes (moist, shiny, no dark circles, conjunctiva pink)
- Teeth (erupted appropriate to age, gums healthy, no bleeding)
- Neck (thyroid, parotid glands of normal size)
- Abdomen (flat, soft)
- Cardiovascular (no murmur; normal heart size; skin warm, pink, less than 3-second capillary refill; peripheral pulses equal, strong)
- Neurological/behavior (alert, active, reflexes present, no complaints of headache, neuritis)

Laboratory and Diagnostic Tests

Laboratory and diagnostic tests are performed as indicated:

- Iron/ferritin levels (see Chapter 27)
- Serum levels for various elements: albumin, nitrogen balance, minerals
- Bone radiographs for suspected iodine, vitamins C and D, or copper deficiency, or to compare bone age with height age

MANAGEMENT STRATEGIES FOR OPTIMAL NUTRITION

NPs can work to ensure that dietary intake adequately supports optimal growth and development through nutritional education, counseling, and anticipatory guidance. Information and guidance are provided regarding children's nutritional requirements, eating behaviors, and strategies and foods used to provide adequate nutrition.

Children's Nutritional Requirements

Parents are not always aware of the nutritional needs of their children. NPs should explain the nutritional requirements of children and offer anticipatory guidance about how physical growth and development create demands for specific nutrients. Information about which foods are good sources of these nutrients can also be given. The relationship between disease and inadequate dietary intake should be discussed.

THE FOOD GUIDE PYRAMID

The food guide pyramid is a useful tool for educating families and children of all ages about a healthful diet. Designed to take the place of the four food groups model, the pyramid illustrates the proportions of a healthy diet and emphasizes a foundation of grains, fruits, and vegetables. The Oregon Dairy Council has adapted the pyramid to identify foods that are nutrient dense in each group. Called pyramid plus, this adaptation is presented in Figure 12-1.

Grains are rich in B vitamins, minerals, fiber, and complex carbohydrates and provide vital fuel for the body. Bread, cereal, rice, and pasta serve as the staples of a low-fat, nutrient-dense diet. The requirement for grains varies widely, depending on age, sex, and activity level. In general, the more active the child, the more carbohydrate is needed in the diet to fuel muscle work.

The second level of the pyramid features the fruit and vegetable groups. The groups are separated because of the different nutrients each provides. Most vegetables are virtually fat free and are rich in fiber, vitamins A and C, folic acid, iron, and magnesium. A minimum of three servings is recommended each day. Fruits and fruit juices provide important amounts of vitamin A, vitamin C, fiber, and potassium. A minimum of two servings daily is recommended, with emphasis placed on fiber-rich fresh fruit.

Protein and dairy foods remain important sources of essential nutrients, and two to three servings, the equivalent of 5 to 7 ounces of cooked lean meat, poultry, or fish per day, are recommended. While rich in B vitamins, iron, zinc, and protein, some foods in this group contribute high levels of fat and cholesterol to the diet. Moderation is the key to making wise choices from this group, and smaller amounts of lean protein foods contribute to better health.

Like the protein group, certain dairy products contribute significant fat, saturated fat, and cholesterol to the diet. However, there is a wide array of low-fat and nonfat dairy products available. Nonfat or 1% milk, nonfat yogurt, low-fat cheeses, and reduced-fat ice milk and frozen yogurt all offer the nutritional benefits of milk with less fat. The dairy group is a notable source of calcium, riboflavin, and protein. Three daily servings of dairy products are recommended for children.

The tip of the pyramid, which gives the caution "use sparingly," includes foods typically labeled "junk foods" or "sometimes foods." Pop, candy, cookies, butter, margarine, and jelly are all examples of "tip" foods. These foods provide taste and calories but little in the way of nutrition. Just as the tip of the pyramid is a small piece, "tip" foods should be a small piece of the diet. But overly restricting these foods, especially in children, can lead to unhealthy attitudes and eventual eating disorders. Moderate intake of sweets and fats can help to meet the caloric requirements of active youngsters.

Serving sizes change as children grow. A general principle to keep in mind is to serve 1 tablespoon of food per year of age. Thus, for children younger than 5 years of age, one serving is about one fourth to one third of an adult serving. Children's appetites vary, however, and parents should be alert to cues that the child wants more or less of any particular food.

Eating Behaviors

Children learn eating behaviors by observation and instruction. As noted in the previous discussion of age-specific considerations, children's eating patterns vary by age. The NP can inform parents about these age differences and offer suggestions for managing the eating experience so as to achieve a positive outcome. Parents should be encouraged to provide

- Positive examples of healthy intake
- An adequate supply of a wide variety of age-appropriate, nutritious foods
- Limits on consumption of non-nutritious sugars and "sometime" foods
- Food prepared in a form that stimulates children's appetites
- Regular, structured mealtimes
- A pleasant, relaxed environment for mealtimes
- Clear, developmentally appropriate expectations for children's behavior at mealtimes
- Developmentally appropriate access to and instruction in the use of utensils
- Appropriate supervision during mealtimes
- Healthy, age-appropriate snacks
- Developmentally appropriate opportunities to participate in preparation and serving of meals
- Adequate exercise, sleep, and rest to stimulate appetites

The introduction of new foods can create tension between parents and children, with children refusing to try or rejecting new tastes or textures. Parents should be informed that this is a normal reaction for many children. Strategies that can be used to increase the chances of children accepting a new food include the following:

- Offer the food when children are hungry.
- Allow children to taste a little of the food rather than eating a full portion.
- Expose children to the food by preparing and serving the food without expecting them to eat it.
- Never force food on children.

- Provide an example of parents eating and enjoying the food.
- Prepare the food the way children prefer: few spices, lukewarm, recognizable.
- Associate food with pleasant experiences.

Vegetarian Diets

An increasing number of individuals are adopting a meat-free lifestyle. Vegetarian diets are nearly as varied as the children who eat them and may be initiated based on religious, ecological or health beliefs, or economic necessity.

DESCRIPTION

Individuals who are vegetarians fall into one of the following categories:

- *Vegans,* or strict vegetarians, eat only foods of plant origin, including fruits, vegetables, grains, nuts, seeds, and legumes (e.g., beans, peas, lentils, tofu, and peanuts).
- *Lacto-vegetarians* include milk and dairy products in their diet as well as all plant-based foods.
- *Lacto-ovo-vegetarians* consume eggs, dairy products, and all plant-based foods in their diet.

For children who are lacto- or lacto-ovo-vegetarians, it is not difficult to achieve adequate amounts of protein, vitamins, and minerals needed for proper growth and development (ADA Reports, 1997). The diet of these children is often closer to the model of the food guide pyramid than that of their meat-eating peers. If they continue to follow a plant-based diet into adulthood, vegetarian children can expect to have a lowered incidence of obesity, high blood pressure, heart disease, and perhaps cancer.

On the other hand, the child who is a strict vegan faces greater difficulty meeting protein and nutrient needs. A high incidence of vitamin B_{12} deficiency and suboptimal zinc status has been noted in vegan children, and these children may be at risk for developmental retardation. Additionally, a vitamin B_{12} deficiency in pregnant women may retard myelination of nervous tissue in the fetus (Lovblad et al., 1997).

MILK & MILK PRODUCTS	MEAT & MEAT ALTERNATIVES	VEGETABLES	FRUITS	BREADS & CEREALS
Supplies: **Calcium,** riboflavin, protein	Supplies: **Iron, protein,** niacin, thiamine, zinc, B₁₂	Supplies: **Folic acid, vitamins A and C,** fiber	Supplies: **Folic acid, vitamins A and C,** fiber	Supplies: **Fiber, complex carbohydrate,** thiamine, iron, niacin
Amount recommended: 2–3 servings each day	Amount recommended: 2–3 servings each day	Amount recommended: 3–5 servings each day	Amount recommended: 2–4 servings each day	Amount recommended: 6–11 servings each day
★ ★ ★ ★	★ ★ ★ ★	★ ★ ★ ★	★ ★ ★ ★	★ ★ ★ ★
nonfat plain yogurt, nonfat milk, nonfat cream cheese, 1% milk, buttermilk, low-fat cheese, 2% milk	fish, shellfish, poultry (light meat, skinless), turkey, ham, beef (round and sirloin, well trimmed), pork (tenderloin, well trimmed), veal (leg and shoulder, well trimmed), lentils	red and green bell peppers, bok choy, spinach, leaf lettuce, broccoli, carrots, cauliflower	papaya, strawberries, kiwi, orange, grapefruit, orange juice, cantaloupe, mandarin oranges, mango	barley, bulgur, bran or whole grain cereals, popcorn (air-popped or lite microwave), whole grain breads, oatmeal, whole grain pasta, corn or whole wheat tortilla
★ ★ ★	★ ★ ★	★ ★ ★	★ ★ ★	★ ★ ★
part-skim ricotta cheese, whole milk, regular-fat cheese, low-fat chocolate milk, low-fat fruit yogurt, nonfat frozen yogurt	beef (rib, chuck, flank, and ground), ham (lean), tofu, veal and lamb (leg and loin), poultry (dark meat with skin), pork (loin and rib), Canadian bacon, poultry sausage, dried beans and peas, eggs	cabbage, chard, asparagus, kale, vegetable juice, brussels sprouts, iceberg lettuce, sweet potato, tomato, snow peas, zucchini, okra, winter squash, green beans	honeydew, raspberries, apricots, rhubarb, pineapple, watermelon, pineapple juice, blueberries	brown rice, bran muffin, whole grain crackers, soft pretzel or breadstick, English muffin, enriched pasta, popcorn (oil-popped)
★ ★	★ ★	★ ★	★ ★	★ ★
pudding, custard, low-fat frozen yogurt, ice milk	hot dogs, pork sausage, chicken nuggets, fish sticks, nuts and seeds	beets, cucumber, celery, jicama, artichoke, peas, mushrooms	peach, banana, plum, cherries, frozen fruit juice bar, canned fruit	flour tortilla, bagel, enriched breads, enriched rice, pancakes, waffles, graham crackers, saltines, sweetened cereal, dry pretzels or breadsticks
★	★	★	★	★
milkshake, cottage cheese, ice cream, nonfat sour cream	peanut butter, bologna	eggplant, corn, avocado, potato	pear, apple, dried fruit, grapes, raisins	cornbread, fruit or nut bread, biscuit, stuffing, croissant

Sometimes Foods: Alcoholic beverages, bacon, bouillon, butter, cakes, candy, coffee, cookies, condiments, snack crackers, cream, regular-fat cream cheese, doughnuts, french fries, fruit-flavored drinks, gelatin dessert, gravy, honey, jam, jelly, margarine, mayonnaise, nondairy creamer, olives, onion rings, pickles, pies, potato chips, salad dressings, sauces, seasonings, sherbet, soft drinks, sour cream, sugar, tea, tortilla chips, vegetable oils

F I G U R E 12-1
Pyramid Plus. Based on the United States Department of Agriculture Food Guide Pyramid, Pyramid Plus emphasizes foods from five major food groups. Each food group is important for the nutrients it provides, and no one food group is more important than another. For a healthy diet, you need foods from each group in the amounts recommended. The "Plus" in Pyramid Plus is nutrient density, a guide to the nutrient value of individual foods. Within each group, foods are listed according to the amount of key nutrients per calorie each provides. Key nutrients are listed in bold type. Four-star foods have the most nutrition per calorie. Generally, four-star foods are also lowest in fat. One-star foods should not be viewed as bad foods—they are merely less nutrient-dense. The most effective way to reduce fat, sugar, and calories without compromising nutrition is to cut back on sometimes foods, those foods that provide little or no nutrition. Young adults (11 to 24 years of age) and pregnant and breastfeeding women need four servings of milk and milk products each day. (Adapted from Nutrition Education Services/Oregon Dairy Council, 1994.)

How Many Servings Do You Need Each Day?

Use these ranges as your guide for how much food to eat each day. Choose the lower or higher number of servings based on your calorie needs. If you eat more or less than one serving, count as partial servings. For children under age 5, a serving is 1/4-1/2 of a standard serving. However to get enough calcium, all children need a total of at least 2 standard servings of milk or milk products each day.

SOMETIMES FOODS

Sometimes foods provide little or no nutrition and are often high in fat, sugar, salt, and calories. They should be eaten in moderation and not in place of servings from the five food groups.

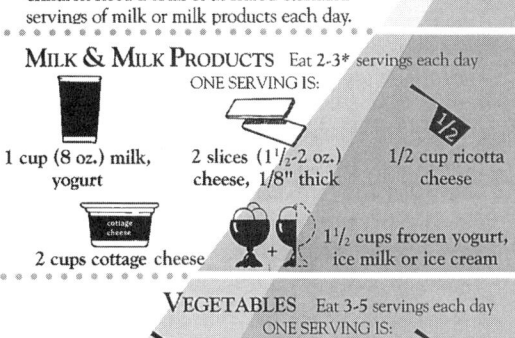

MILK & MILK PRODUCTS Eat 2-3* servings each day
ONE SERVING IS:

- 1 cup (8 oz.) milk, yogurt
- 2 slices (1½-2 oz.) cheese, 1/8" thick
- 1/2 cup ricotta cheese
- 2 cups cottage cheese
- 1½ cups frozen yogurt, ice milk or ice cream

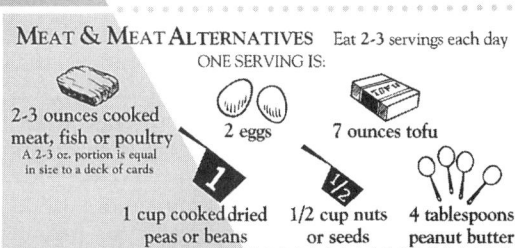

MEAT & MEAT ALTERNATIVES Eat 2-3 servings each day
ONE SERVING IS:

- 2-3 ounces cooked meat, fish or poultry *A 2-3 oz. portion is equal in size to a deck of cards*
- 2 eggs
- 7 ounces tofu
- 1 cup cooked dried peas or beans
- 1/2 cup nuts or seeds
- 4 tablespoons peanut butter

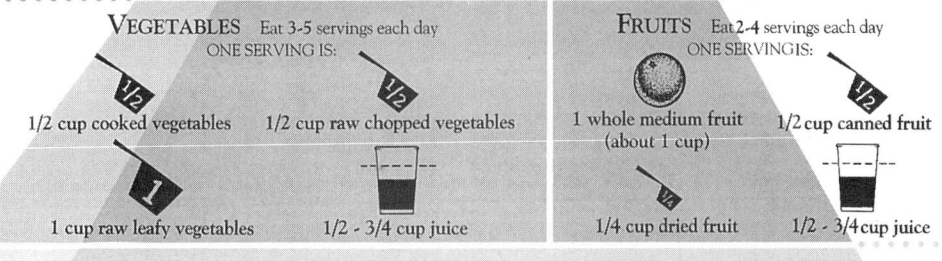

VEGETABLES Eat 3-5 servings each day
ONE SERVING IS:

- 1/2 cup cooked vegetables
- 1/2 cup raw chopped vegetables
- 1 cup raw leafy vegetables
- 1/2 - 3/4 cup juice

FRUITS Eat 2-4 servings each day
ONE SERVING IS:

- 1 whole medium fruit (about 1 cup)
- 1/2 cup canned fruit
- 1/4 cup dried fruit
- 1/2 - 3/4 cup juice

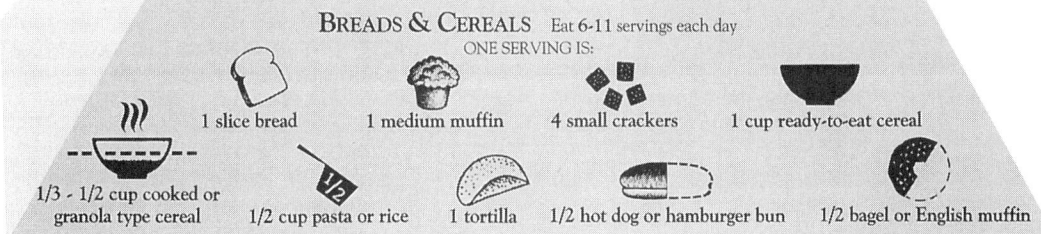

BREADS & CEREALS Eat 6-11 servings each day
ONE SERVING IS:

- 1 slice bread
- 1 medium muffin
- 4 small crackers
- 1 cup ready-to-eat cereal
- 1/3 - 1/2 cup cooked or granola type cereal
- 1/2 cup pasta or rice
- 1 tortilla
- 1/2 hot dog or hamburger bun
- 1/2 bagel or English muffin

*Young Adults (11-24 years), Pregnant and Breastfeeding Women need 4 servings   © 1994. Nutrition Education Services / Oregon Dairy Council.

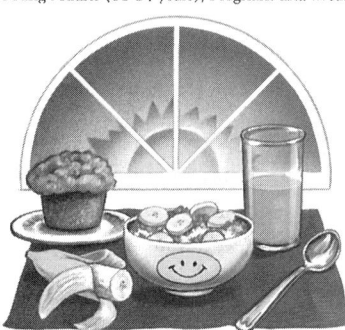

MILK = 1/2 SERVING
MEAT = 0 SERVINGS
VEGETABLES = 0 SERVINGS
FRUITS = 2 SERVINGS
BREADS & CEREALS = 2 SERVINGS

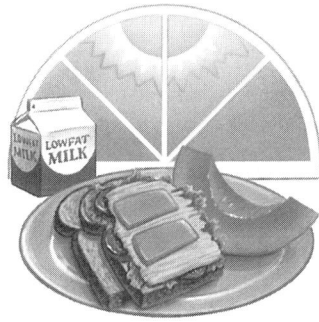

MILK = 2 SERVINGS
MEAT = 1 SERVING
VEGETABLES = 1/2 SERVING
FRUITS = 1 SERVING
BREADS & CEREALS = 2 SERVINGS

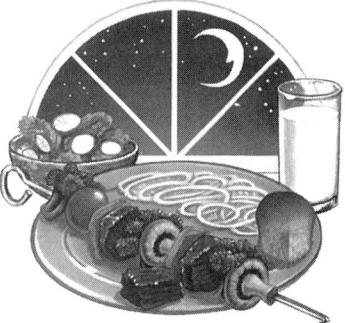

MILK = 1 SERVING
MEAT = 1 SERVING
VEGETABLES = 2 ½ SERVINGS
FRUITS = 0 SERVINGS
BREADS & CEREALS = 2 SERVINGS

F I G U R E 12-1 *Continued*

MANAGEMENT

Careful diet planning is needed if vegan children are to achieve optimal growth and development. Plant sources of protein are considered "incomplete" because they lack the full array of amino acids needed to synthesize new tissue. To ensure adequate intake of essential amino acids, vegans need to consume plant-based proteins that "complement" each other and that together provide a complete protein. The vegan's daily diet needs to include these complementary proteins but not necessarily in the same meal. Examples of foods that provide complete proteins include combinations of legumes and grains, nuts, or seeds (e.g., peanut butter/wheat bread, beans/rice, lentils/rice, lentils/sunflower seeds, peas/rye or wheat, or tofu/almonds).

Vitamin B_{12}, in the form of a supplement or in a supplemented food (such as fortified soy milk), is required for the vegan child, because bioavailable vitamin B_{12} is present only in animal-based foods. Use of algae as a source of vitamin B_{12} may be counterproductive, because vitamin B_{12} from algae does not appear to be bioavailable, and may, in excess, actually block vitamin B_{12} metabolism (Dagnelie et al., 1991). The vegan child can also require supplemental zinc, iron, calcium, and vitamin D (Table 12–9).

Because plant-based diets tend to be high in fiber and low in calories, the child may fill up before consuming sufficient calories and nutrients. Vegan children are advised to eat frequent meals and snacks, concentrating on foods that are nutrient dense in order to achieve adequate energy and nutrient intake.

TABLE 12-9

Vitamins and Minerals at Risk for Deficit in Strict Vegetarian (Vegan) Diets

VITAMIN AND MINERALS AT RISK FOR DEFICIT	USUAL SOURCES	ALTERNATIVE SOURCES IN VEGAN DIET
Vitamin D	Animal products: egg yolk, butter, liver, salmon, sardines, tuna; sunlight	Fortified cereals, milk, or margarine; sunlight (20–30 min/d, 2–3 times per wk)
Vitamin B_{12}	Animal products only: meat, fish, eggs, dairy products	Fortified soy milk, fortified soy-based meat substitutes, nutritional yeast, fortified cereals, vitamin supplements
Riboflavin	Milk and meat are best sources; also in eggs, dried yeast, grains, dark-green leafy vegetables, avocado, broccoli	Brewer's yeast, wheat germ, beans, almonds, soybeans, tofu, dark-green leafy vegetables, avocado, broccoli, orange juice
Calcium	Milk is best source; also in some fruits, nuts, dark-green leafy vegetables	Fortified soy milk, dried fruits, almonds, sunflower, filberts, whole sesame seeds, green leafy vegetables (avoid spinach, swiss chard, beet greens, whose oxalic acid hinders calcium absorption)
Iron	Iron in meat sources is more bioavailable than iron in plants; lentils, beans (cooked black, soy, garbanzo, lima) are good sources	All legumes, almonds, pecans, dates, prunes, raisins, fortified cereals, white or brown rice; absorption is enhanced by ascorbic acid–rich foods
Zinc	Meats, animal products, seafood (especially oysters), eggs; found in whole grains, brown rice, nuts, spinach; however, best plant sources also contain phytic acid, which inhibits zinc absorption	Whole grains, brown rice, almonds, wheat germ, tofu, pecans, spinach

Nutrition assessment of the vegan child should include regular growth measurements, diet recall and analysis, and laboratory assessment of vitamin B_{12}, zinc, and iron status.

It is important that the NP offer advice and counseling within the context of the child's and family's belief system. But in extreme cases, such as a highly restrictive macrobiotic diet resulting in growth failure, intervention on behalf of the child is necessary, with referral to appropriate health professionals and agencies as indicated.

ALTERED PATTERNS OF NUTRITION

Introduction

An estimated 10 to 20% of the general pediatric population is affected by chronic illness and handicapping conditions that affect nutrition status (American Dietetic Association, 1989a). Special health care needs affecting these children include chronic disorders, chronic illnesses, developmental disabilities, developmental special needs, and handicapping conditions.

Chronic conditions requiring specialized nutrition care are increasing, largely because of expanded screening programs, increased survival rates in children with certain chronic disorders, and improved prognosis for the very small (<1500 g), underdeveloped neonate. Increased rates of pediatric acquired immunodeficiency syndrome (AIDS) and prenatal exposure to drugs and alcohol also have enlarged the population of children with special health care needs.

Nearly two thirds of all children with special health care needs exhibit feeding problems (Ekvall et al., 1993). Nutrients often found to be inadequate in children with developmental disorders include iron, calcium, niacin, folic acid, vitamins A, C, and D, calories, and fluid.

The nutrition management of children with special health care needs requires input from an interdisciplinary team. Physical, occupational, and speech therapists, particularly speech pathologists, can assess head and trunk control, positioning, body mechanics, and oral-motor skills as they relate to feeding. For children who are socially or economically deprived, or both, social workers and psychologists are central to appropriate assessment, counseling, and referral to outside services and agencies. Depending on the child's presenting symptoms and diagnosis, gastroenterologists, allergists, endocrinologists, and other specialists may need to coordinate the child's care. The family should be included as an integral component of the team.

In addition to coordinating the medical management of children with special health care needs, the NP must be prepared to carefully assess the nutritional status of this population. Children who meet the criteria outlined in Table 12-10 should be referred to a registered dietitian for comprehensive nutrition assessment and treatment.

T A B L E   12-10
Suggested Criteria for Nutrition Referral

- Markedly overweight or underweight (height or length for weight below the 5th or above the 95th percentile)
- Mechanical feeding difficulties or neuromotor dysfunction
- Feeding skills below those anticipated for developmental level or mental age
- Unusual food habits (e.g., pica or food faddism)
- Inadequate or imbalanced dietary intake, according to dietary history or 24-hr recall
- Nutrition treatment central to medical management (e.g., inborn errors of metabolism, diabetes, malabsorption syndromes, allergy)
- Overt physical signs of nutritional deficiency (e.g., extremely underweight, anemia)
- Emotional disturbances and associated feeding and nutrition problems (e.g., anorexia nervosa, autism)
- At high risk for compromised nutrition status (e.g., takes stimulant or anticonvulsive drugs, family below poverty level, inadequate housing, pregnant adolescent)

Adapted from Ekvall SW, Ekvall VK, Frazier T: Dealing with nutrition problems of children with developmental disorders. Topics Clin Nutr 8(4):51–57, 1993. Copyright © 1993 Aspen Publishers, Inc.

Disorders Requiring Increased Caloric Intake

DESCRIPTION

A common nutrition problem in children with special health care needs is inadequate weight gain and delayed growth. Inadequate caloric intake should be suspected in any child with a weight-to-age ratio below the tenth percentile on standardized growth charts. For children who are genetically small or have a disabling condition that stunts growth, a weight-to-length ratio (if younger than 2 years old or unable to stand) or weight-to-height ratio below the tenth percentile indicates suboptimal nutrition.

INCIDENCE AND ETIOLOGY

The actual incidence of children requiring an increased caloric intake is not known, but it occurs commonly. An estimated 15 to 25% of children seen for developmental disabilities are underweight or growth retarded, or both (Ekvall, 1993).

Caloric needs of children are influenced by multiple factors, and a number of conditions put children at risk for insufficient caloric intake, including

- Conditions in which activity level is increased, either by purposeful or by involuntary muscle work, such as athetoid cerebral palsy, attention-deficit hyperactivity disorder, or chronic lung conditions
- A hypermetabolic state, sometimes complicated by secondary malabsorption, which may be present in the child who has AIDS, cancer, or frequent infections or is postsurgical
- Psychosocial factors such as inadequate resources, poor feeding relationship with caregiver, and improper dilution of formula, which can lead to delayed growth and require increased calories for the child's catch-up growth
- Oral-motor impairment or chronic conditions, such as congenital heart disease, which can contribute to fatigue and poor feeding
- Low birth weight or premature infants

CLINICAL ASSESSMENT AND FINDINGS

History

A thorough history should be taken, assessing for

- Type and amount of foods and liquids consumed (e.g., nutrient content and consistency)
- Amount of food lost from utensils, cups, or bottles during feeding
- Physical effort and time required for meals
- Any impaired oral functions (e.g., tongue thrust, drooling, difficulty chewing, choking, or aspiration)
- Family's pattern of feeding child (e.g., time, place, utensils used)
- Child's apparent food likes and dislikes

Physical Examination

Anthropometric measures are reliable indicators of a child's growth and development, especially if measured and compared over time. Appendix B provides standard growth charts as well as growth charts for premature infants. These charts can be used to determine whether the child is following a consistent growth curve. Growth charts specific to children with Down syndrome, myelomeningocele, Prader-Willi syndrome, sickle cell anemia, and Turner syndrome have also been developed (Ekvall, 1993; Hall et al., 1989). Anthropometric measures taken at each visit include

- Height
- Weight
- Weight-to-height ratio
- Head circumference
- Arm circumference
- Skinfold measurements

A feeding evaluation can be included in the physical examination, particularly for the child with oral-motor or behavioral problems associated with eating. Such an evaluation is usually conducted by a multidisciplinary team of primary health care provider, physician specialist such as a gastroenterologist, dietitian, speech pathologist, and physical or occupational therapist or both. In this type of assessment, parents or caregivers are asked to replicate the home experience, using the same types of foods, utensils, and positioning. If possible, the parents should videotape the child eating at home, and the video should be reviewed with them. By observing the interaction between the child and the caregiver during feeding, the health care team can more accurately assess feeding success and problems as well as emotional or psychological issues related to feeding.

Laboratory Studies

Laboratory studies are done as indicated:

- Hematocrit or hemoglobin
- Serum ferritin and transferrin levels
- Serum albumin

Clinical Findings

When a child is malnourished, regardless of etiology, the nutritional insult follows a predictable course. In the early stages, the child maintains or begins losing weight. If poor intake continues, the child's linear growth slows down or ceases. Finally, head circumference, indicating compromised brain development, levels off.

Other signs of inadequate nutrition include

- Anemia
- Pallor
- Fatigue
- Vulnerability to infections
- Delayed healing
- Behavior problems
- Inactivity
- Irritability
- Poor academic performance, poor vocabulary
- Perceptual difficulties

MANAGEMENT

The management of the child with delayed growth or poor weight gain varies with the underlying cause of the problem.

- A child with an increased activity level needs to receive calorically dense meals and snacks at 2- to 4-hour intervals.
- A child with a chronic disease that de-

creases the appetite (e.g., acquired immunodeficiency syndrome [AIDS], cancer) needs creative approaches that consider food preferences, optimal times of day for snacks and meals, and family dynamics that encourage eating.
- The child who is not receiving enough food because of neglect, inadequate financial resources, or other psychosocial factors requires referral to appropriate health care professionals and social services. The community health nurse can be an invaluable resource for these children.
- The child with a chronic condition that affects oral-motor control will benefit from a team approach. Special equipment, specific feeding techniques, proper positioning, and use of foods and liquids with appropriate consistency can all contribute to improved oral intake.

Although feeding by the oral route is preferable from a developmental perspective, tube feedings may be indicated when it becomes clear that a child's needs cannot be met orally. Frequently, a medical crisis precipitates the use of supplemental feedings. Although the NP can coordinate the plan of care for the child on supplemental feedings, a team approach to management is optimal.

Premature or low birth weight infants (particularly those with a poor suck) frequently require supplemental feedings. Breastfeeding is both possible and desirable for these infants (see Chapter 13). Human milk fortifiers or premature formulas that increase the caloric density from 20 kcal/ounce to 24 kcal/ounce are often fed to premature neonates. Regular infant formulas can be mixed to increase the kcal/ounce ratio from 20 kcal/ounce to 24 kcal or 27 kcal/ounce, and nutrient-dense formulas for older infants and children are available (see Table 12-6). Care must be taken that infants do not receive too much protein in concentrated infant formulas, because the breakdown and excretion of excess protein by the kidneys may place an excessive demand on the renal system.

Practical suggestions for increasing calories, protein, and nutrients needed for weight gain and growth are outlined in Table 12-11. Additionally, a "complete" multivitamin and mineral

T A B L E 12-11

Suggestions for Increasing Energy Intake

- Use readily available economical foods that are familiar to the child.
- Fortify milk by adding 1 c nonfat dry milk powder to 1 qt of whole milk. Drink or use to prepare cooked cereals, creamed soups, pancakes, pudding, milkshakes (do *not* use with children younger than 2 yr of age).
- Add additional margarine or cheese to potatoes, vegetables, casseroles, rice, pasta, cooked cereals, etc.
- Encourage high-calorie snacks such as fruit juice, dried fruits, nuts, bananas, cheese cubes, pudding or custard, cereal with whole milk, fruit yogurt (alone or as a dip for fruit), cheese or peanut butter on crackers, olives, sliced or mashed avocado (as a dip for vegetables or crackers).
- Add instant breakfast mixes to whole milk.
- Use commercially prepared formula with high caloric content (see Table 12-6).
- Use commercial liquid supplements such as Pediasure or Pediasure with fiber (Ross Laboratories) for children with lactose intolerance.
- Establish regular times for meals and snacks, 2 to 4 hr apart. Do not allow the child to nibble continually on small amounts of food.
- Keep mealtimes relaxed and pleasant. Avoid scolding, nagging, or force feeding.
- Allow the infant or child to provide cues regarding hunger and satiety.

supplement is recommended, because it contains the entire spectrum of these nutrients and can easily be chewed or crushed and mixed into soft foods.

Restoring calories, protein, and nutrients to age-specific norms is not adequate for children who are underweight or growth retarded. For catch-up growth to occur, children must receive an excess of calories and protein until growth is normalized. A method for calculating the calories and protein required for catch-up growth is presented in Table 12–12. (To determine recommended calories for weight age, use the kcal/kg values shown in Table 12–1.)

Frequent monitoring of the child with inadequate caloric intake is necessary. Infants should be weighed at least weekly and length and head circumference measured once a month. Children older than 2 years of age should be measured for height and weight at least once a month.

COMPLICATIONS

The child with inadequate caloric intake often displays a multitude of other nutrient deficiencies. A direct connection has been established between inadequate nutrition and mental and physical abilities. In the child with a chronic medical condition, compromised nutrition contributes to frequent illness, medical complications, and impaired development.

T A B L E 12-12

Estimating Catch-Up Growth Requirements*

$$\text{Catch-up growth requirement (kcal/kg/d)} = \frac{\text{Calories required for weight age (kcal/kg/d)} \times \text{Ideal weight for age (kg)}}{\text{Actual weight (kg)}}$$

1. Plot the child's height and weight on the NCHS growth charts.
2. Determine at what age the present weight would be at the 50th percentile (weight age).
3. Determine recommended calories for weight age (see Table 12–1).
4. Determine the ideal weight (50th percentile) for the child's present age.
5. Multiply the value obtained in (3) by the value obtained in (4).
6. Divide the value obtained in (5) by actual weight.

Estimated protein requirements during catch-up growth can be calculated similarly:

$$\text{Protein requirement (g/kg)} = \frac{\text{Protein required for weight age (g/kg)} \times \text{Ideal weight for age (kg)}}{\text{Actual weight (kg)}}$$

*Guidelines are used to estimate catch-up growth requirements: Precise individual needs vary and are mediated by medical status and diagnosis.

NCHS = National Center for Health Statistics.

From Rathbun JM, Peterson KE: Nutrition in failure to thrive. *In* Grand RJ, Sutphen JL, Dietz WH (eds): Pediatric Nutrition. Boston: Butterworth, 1987.

The etiology of growth retardation is multifactorial, including genetic disorders, in utero insults (e.g., maternal infection, fetal alcohol syndrome), neurological impairments, metabolic disorders, and environmental deprivation. In many of these physiological disorders, restoring nutrition status does not ultimately resolve growth deficits. In the case of environmental deprivation, the success of catch-up growth depends on the timing, length, and severity of the nutritional insult.

Complications of treatment must also be considered for children with caloric deficits. The NP must be alert to negative effects of a sudden change to a high-calorie, high-protein diet. As discussed previously, a dramatic increase in protein can increase renal solute load to the point where a child is at risk for dehydration. The child on a high-protein diet should be counseled to take in adequate fluids. Diarrhea can result from an abrupt increase in carbohydrates owing to their high osmolality. Gradually changing the child's diet can decrease these negative effects.

Disorders Requiring Decreased Caloric Intake

DESCRIPTION

Health conditions that contribute to decreased metabolic activity in children require changes in nutritional intake. If children's caloric intake exceeds their metabolic needs, excessive weight gain, even obesity, can occur, placing the child at risk for additional health problems. The assessment and management of obesity is discussed later as an eating disorder. This section looks specifically at medical conditions that contribute to excessive weight gain.

INCIDENCE AND ETIOLOGY

Any disorder or disability that reduces energy output places the child at risk for obesity. Obesity is common, for example, in children with Prader-Willi syndrome, myelomeningocele, or Down syndrome.

The child with Prader-Willi syndrome is hypotonic and may demonstrate dysphagia and failure to thrive as an infant. By 3 to 4 years of age, the child becomes hyperphagic, lacking the internal regulation responsible for satiety. In addition to abnormally high food intake, children with Prader-Willi syndrome are short in stature (Finberg, 1998).

Obesity occurs in 50% of children with spina bifida. Energy expenditure in nonambulatory children with myelodysplasia is estimated at only 25 to 50% of that of children who are walking (Ekvall, 1993).

Most children with Down syndrome have short stature, and obesity is common, but not inevitable (Finberg, 1998). Healthy eating and exercise habits begun in early childhood can help prevent obesity. Before age 3 years, children with Down syndrome may be light for their height, and the Down syndrome growth chart should be used to evaluate height and weight. As a result of a lower resting metabolic rate or hypothyroidism, the child with Down syndrome requires fewer calories than children without the syndrome.

CLINICAL ASSESSMENT AND FINDINGS

History

The history should assess for

- Level of physical activity in which child engages
- Diet recall (3 day)
- Mealtime patterns
- Concerns and attitudes of parents and child regarding weight gain
- Previous interventions or attempts to control weight

Physical Examination

Key components of the physical examination include:

- Weight for height or length ratio
- Triceps skinfold measurement
- Midarm circumference

- Body frame type
- Muscle mass
- Body mass index (BMI)

Laboratory Studies

Laboratory studies include those for thyroxine and circulating thyroid-stimulating hormone to rule out hypothyroidism. Because of sequelae associated with obesity, children should be monitored at least annually for

- Hypertension (blood pressure)
- Blood sugar
- Complete lipid profile
- Liver function

Clinical Findings

The following clinical findings indicate level of obesity:

- Weight for height ratio greater than 75% on growth chart may indicate mild obesity
- Weight for height ratio greater than 95% on growth chart may indicate significant obesity
- Triceps skinfold measurement greater than 85% of norm is diagnostic criterion for obesity in children
- BMI should fall within normal parameters over time

A child's growth pattern is evaluated over time. A child who is consistently in the 85% weight for height ratio may be genetically programmed to be big, whereas a child who suddenly zooms from the 60% to the 90% weight for height ratio can be developing a weight problem.

MANAGEMENT

Children with medical conditions that decrease caloric need often require special management. The goal of nutrition management is to ensure the child receives adequate nutrients without excessive caloric intake.

- Because of the reduced energy expenditure of children with impaired mobility, Prader-Willi syndrome, spina bifida, Down syndrome, or other such disorders, caloric intake needs to be restricted. A referral to a registered dietitian is recommended to establish an appropriate caloric level and eating plan individualized to each child's growth needs.
- A complete multivitamin with mineral supplement is recommended, because a restrictive diet can result in nutrient deficiencies.
- Whenever possible, children with a disorder that is associated with decreased caloric need should be encouraged to increase their energy expenditure through physical activity. The goal is to both increase calories used and increase the child's level of fitness. A team approach, involving a physical or recreational therapist, or both, is advised when developing exercise strategies for these children.
- In some cases, access to food needs to be rigidly enforced (e.g., in children with brain dysfunction affecting hypothalamic control or Prader-Willi syndrome). The family, school, and other care environments need to provide limited access to food, including locks on refrigerators, cupboards, and garbage cans.
- Frequent monitoring is necessary in order to assess compliance and devise alternate strategies as indicated; weekly weight and monthly height measurements are recommended.
- Support for families and children is essential. Despite the best efforts, many children gain excess weight. The NP needs to model and encourage a positive, accepting attitude toward the child, independent of weight gain or loss.

Disorders Requiring Restricted or Supplemental Diets

DESCRIPTION

The body's ability to absorb and metabolize nutrients is compromised when hormone, enzyme, or cofactor activity necessary for metabolism is either excessive or deficient or when physiological conditions limit absorption of nutrients. Under these conditions, nutritional intake must be adjusted to maximize the body's ability to use foods. Diet restrictions or supplemental nutrients, or both, can be essential for optimal growth and development.

Table 12–13 lists several metabolic conditions seen in the primary care setting that affect children's nutrition status. A number of defects of absorption or transport affect nutritional status in children; most are rare, but the NP may occasionally manage the care of a child with inflammatory bowel disease (Crohn's disease or ulcerative colitis), short bowel syndrome, or celiac disease.

INCIDENCE AND ETIOLOGY

Most metabolic disorders are rare, although diabetes mellitus type I affects about 1.9 in 1000 school-age children, and cystic fibrosis is seen in 1 in 2000 white infants. An estimated 1 in 70 individuals in the United States is a carrier of phenylketonuria (PKU); only about 1 in 10,000 persons has this autosomal recessive disease.

The etiology of metabolic disorders can differ from one individual to another. Some disorders are considered to be inborn errors of metabolism (e.g., PKU). Genetic conditions other than inborn errors of metabolism, autoimmune diseases, surgical intervention, drugs and medications, tumors, and infectious disease also contribute to metabolic dysfunction and problems of absorption or transport. For some individuals, a genetic predisposition to the disorder can be triggered by environmental factors, and the disorder appears later in life.

CLINICAL ASSESSMENT AND FINDINGS

Clinical findings related to specific disorders are discussed in Unit IV. If nutrition is inadequate in children with these chronic conditions, clinical signs and symptoms worsen, pathophysiological processes of the disorder accelerate, and growth is stunted.

MANAGEMENT

Disorders of absorption and metabolism are usually managed with specialized diagnostic tests and treatments and require the efforts of a coordinated health care team. Although not a cure for disease, nutrition is an essential component of treatment plans and can make a critical difference in the child's outcome. The goals of nutritional intervention include the following:

- Provide adequate nutrients for normal growth and development
- Maintain optimal level of health
- Prevent or delay development of complications associated with disease progression (e.g., diarrhea, fistulas)
- Prevent or delay need for more aggressive intervention (e.g., surgical bowel resection)

Nutritional intervention in chronic disorders can be extremely complex. Referral to a registered dietitian is necessary, and the NP should consult frequently with the dietitian when providing primary care to the child.

In some conditions, dietary restrictions are

TABLE 12-13

Metabolic Conditions Affecting Nutrition in Children

EXCESSIVE HORMONE/ ENZYME PRODUCTION	DEFICIENT HORMONE/ ENZYME PRODUCTION
PANCREAS	
Reactive hypoglycemia	Diabetes mellitus
Organic or fasting hypoglycemia	Cystic fibrosis
THYROID	
Hyperthyroidism	Hypothyroidism
Graves' disease	
PARATHYROID	
Hyperparathyroidism	Hypoparathyroidism
ADRENAL CORTEX	
Cushing's syndrome	Addison's disease
Corticosteroid therapy	
INBORN ERRORS OF METABOLISM	
	Phenylketonuria (deficiency of phenylalanine hydroxylase)
	Maple syrup urine disease
	Tyrosinemia
	Galactosemia

lifelong requirements; success of dietary intervention depends on the child's and family's willingness to adhere to the plan of care. Cooperation is enhanced if the child and family are actively included in decision making and if meal plans are developed that minimize disruption to the family's lifestyle while maximizing flexibility and normalcy for the child. Families and children must be given ample opportunity to express their concerns and frustrations regarding the child's condition. The NP's support, empathy, and encouragement can be vital elements in determining how well a family copes with the child's chronic condition.

Certain principles of nutrition related to dis-

orders of absorption and metabolism guide the dietitian, NP, and family as they create diet plans. Tables 12–14 through 12–17 outline these principles for several specific conditions.

COMPLICATIONS

See Unit IV for complications of specific disorders. Additionally, pregnant women with phenylalanine levels greater than 10 mg/dl are at great risk of injuring the fetus. When phenylalanines exceed 20 mg/dl, 90% of infants will have intrauterine growth retardation, microcephaly, and mental retardation (phenylketonuria [PKU]). Therefore, all pregnant women should

T A B L E 12-14
Principles for Dietary Management of Diabetes Mellitus

- Individualize diet. There are many types of meal planning systems for diabetics; identify one that works best for child and family.
- Space food intake to account for type of insulin used.
- Structure diet to include foods that everyone else eats; do not be overrestrictive; use insulin coverage to allow child to eat as typical a diet as possible.
- Vary specific nutrient intakes depending on child's age, size, and activity level.

General guidelines for nutrients include the following:

ENERGY
- Intake is essentially same as for child without diabetes; energy demands vary with growth spurts, exercise.
- Maintain plasma glucose as near normal physiological range as possible.

CARBOHYDRATES
- 55–60% of total calories from carbohydrates. Complex carbohydrates recommended; limit simple sugars, small amounts can be acceptable as part of a mixed meal.
- Emphasize consistent intake of carbohydrates from day to day.
- Include 25 to 40 g/1000 kcal/d of fiber; increase fiber as complex carbohydrates are increased.
- Increase carbohydrates 10 to 30 g/hr (depending on level of exertion) for intensive exercise; best effect if intake is several hours preceding exercise.

PROTEIN
- Same as for child without diabetes.

FAT
- Same as for child without diabetes.

VITAMINS AND MINERALS
- Same as for child without diabetes; if diabetes is poorly controlled, supplements are recommended.

SWEETENERS
- Noncaloric sweeteners such as aspartame and saccharine are acceptable but not encouraged; no long-term adverse effects of artificial sweeteners have been noted.
- Caloric sweeteners such as fructose, sucrose, glucose, sorbitol, and mannitol can be used (with caution) as substitute for carbohydrate calories.
- Excess sorbitol intake can contribute to diarrhea.

T A B L E 12-15

Principles for Dietary Management of Cystic Fibrosis

- Nutrients needed (high protein, high fat, high energy) may cause physical distress; work with family to help them understand the balance between comfort and adequate nutrition sought.
- Small, frequent meals, eaten slowly, are better tolerated.
- Consume nutrient-dense foods, avoid "empty calories."
- Increase fluid intake to prevent dehydration and help liquify secretions.
- Assess intake on a 3- to 5-day diet record rather than daily.

General guidelines for nutrients include the following:

ENERGY
- Energy needs are increased as a result of malabsorption of nutrients, extra effort needed for respirations and frequent pulmonary infections.
- Vary caloric intake for each child, depending on condition, activity, and growth.

CARBOHYDRATES
- 40–50% of total calories from carbohydrates. Simple sugars may be better tolerated than complex carbohydrates.
- Include extra fiber; increase fiber as complex carbohydrates are increased.

PROTEIN
- Higher need than for children without cystic fibrosis; 15–20% of caloric intake should be in proteins.
- Breastfed children may need supplements (e.g., casein hydrolysates).

FAT
- Increase to level of tolerance, as much as 40–50% of total caloric intake.
- Use medium-chain triglyceride oils to enhance absorption and decrease steatorrhea.
- Use corn or soy oil and include absorbable linoleic acid in diet to ensure essential fatty acid intake.

VITAMINS AND MINERALS
- Daily multivitamin supplement and water-soluble preparation of vitamins A, D, and E advised; 50–100 μg/d vitamin K recommended.
- Daily calcium supplements necessary.
- Normal diet is usually adequate to replace sodium lost through excessive sweat; can use salt tablets (intake is more easily monitored than adding salt to diet) if exercise or fever leads to profuse sweating.

SUPPLEMENTS
- Pancreatic enzymes are indicated.
- Other supplements include casein hydrolysates and powdered or liquid nutrient-dense preparations.

---

be questioned about a history of PKU or special diets during childhood. Also, approximately 1 in 30,000 women in the general population has a phenylalanine level high enough to damage her fetus or contribute to a spontaneous abortion, but not necessarily high enough to hurt her. Maternal PKU should be considered in any woman who has delivered a microcephalic offspring or experienced spontaneous abortion.

PREVENTION AND PATIENT EDUCATION, SUPPORT NETWORKS, AND GROUPS

A number of support groups are available for families of children with disorders of absorp-tion and metabolism. Many are national organizations, but some have local chapters as well (see Resource Box 12-1).

Disorders Requiring Physical Alterations in Diet Management

DESCRIPTION

Physical conditions such as cleft lip or palate, esophageal atresia, cerebral palsy, gastroesopha-geal reflux, and pyloric stenosis can create difficulty sucking, chewing, swallowing, or re-taining food and liquids in the gastrointestinal tract.

T A B L E   12-16

Principles for Dietary Management of Phenylketonuria

- Intervene promptly. Infants who begin treatment before 3 wk of age do not suffer mental retardation secondary to phenylketonuria (PKU).
- All children require phenylalanine in their diet.
- Recommended daily intake of phenylalanine decreases with age. Dietary restrictions continue for life.
- Most foods contain phenylalanine ($\approx$5% of all protein is phenylalanine).
- The goal of PKU dietary therapy is to prevent excess phenylalanine accumulation in the body.
- Involve older children in preparation of nutritional supplements.
- Supplements may be more palatable if served as frozen drinks or flavored with juices or fruits.

General guidelines for nutrients include the following:

ENERGY, CARBOHYDRATE, FAT, VITAMIN, AND MINERAL

- Requirements are same as for child without PKU. Restrictions on high-phenylalanine carbohydrates.
- Daily multivitamin recommended.
- Nutrient requirements not met by commercial formulas must be supplemented by a phenylalanine-deficient food.

PROTEIN

- Same protein requirements as for child without PKU.
- Phenylalanine intake restricted. Dietary intake to maintain serum phenylalanine levels between 2 and 10 mg/dl in children. Plasma phenylalanine levels >6 mg/dl should be controlled with dietary therapy.
- Low/minimal phenylalanine-deficient medical foods necessary in order to meet protein requirements.

INCIDENCE AND ETIOLOGY

Most of these conditions are congenital in nature, and a combination of environmental, hereditary, and behavioral factors appears to influence their development. Stenoses, atresias, or fistulas can also be secondary to environmental trauma such as a chemical burn. Incidence varies by condition, with approximately 1 in 600 children born with cleft lip and 1 in 1000 with cleft palate in the United States each year. Boys are more likely to have a cleft lip with or without a cleft palate (Behrman et al., 1996). Pyloric stenosis, occurring in about 1 in 200 births, is more common in boys and in children with Down syndrome. Esophageal atresia occurs in 1 in 3000 to 4500 live births and in more than 85% of cases is accompanied by a tracheoesophageal fistula (Behrman et al., 1996).

T A B L E   12-17

Principles for Dietary Management of Inflammatory Bowel Disease

- Restrict irritating and poorly absorbed foods.
- Decrease intake of foods that stimulate peristalsis (e.g., high-fiber foods) during inflammatory periods. High-fiber foods, especially those that retain water, can be introduced as clinical signs and symptoms decrease.
- Small, frequent meals are better tolerated.
- Vary specific nutrient intakes depending on child's age, size, activity level, and severity of disease. Mild disease can still require supplemental formulas; severe disease can require enteral elemental nutrition via tube feeding, or total parenteral nutrition.
- Condition can be complicated by lactose or gluten intolerance.

General guidelines for nutrients include the following:

ENERGY

- 40–50 kcal/kg of ideal body weight/d for teens; younger children need up to 120 kcal/kg ideal body weight/d.

PROTEIN

- >1.5 g/kg of ideal body weight/d.

FAT

- Low fat (40 g/d) intake necessary.
- Emulsified fats or medium-chain triglycerides (commercial preparation) are better tolerated.

VITAMINS AND MINERALS

- 100–150% daily multivitamin with minerals supplement.
- May need additional vitamin and mineral supplements (e.g., water-soluble vitamins, vitamin B_{12} intramuscularly), folic acid, iron, zinc, copper, calcium, potassium, and magnesium.

Gastroesophageal reflux (GER) is common in normal individuals following a meal and can be exacerbated by increased intra-abdominal pressure (as with crying, coughing, defecation, or external pressure from movement or position). GER in infants can occur during, immediately after, or several hours after a feeding. Premature infants, children with a weak lower esophageal sphincter, and neurologically impaired children are especially susceptible to GER. It is estimated that 1 in 300 to 1 in 1000 infants have significant reflux (Behrman et al., 1996).

Children with cerebral palsy or other neurodevelopmental problems can have difficulty chewing or maintaining coordinated suck-swallow skills. GER is also a common problem in children with cerebral palsy, and if the etiology for food refusal cannot be determined, GER may be a likely explanation.

CLINICAL ASSESSMENT AND FINDINGS

History

A thorough history of the infant's feeding patterns, incidence of gagging or vomiting, timing of emesis in relation to feeding, character and quantity of emesis, and associated symptoms is essential. Parents also should be asked about treatments they have tried and whether they have been successful.

Physical Examination

Clinical signs can be present at birth, and a diagnosis of the underlying condition, such as cleft lip or palate, made in the delivery room. Roentgenography or endoscopy, or both, are diagnostic techniques used to confirm atresias or fistulas. Some conditions, such as pyloric stenosis, present later in the neonatal period.

MANAGEMENT

The treatment goals related to conditions that require biomechanical or physical intervention include the following:

- Provide adequate nutrients for normal growth and development.

- Provide increased calories to add more weight if needed before surgical procedures.
- Strengthen infant's resistance to infection.
- Prepare infant to tolerate stress of surgical procedures.
- Facilitate healing processes postoperatively.
- Ensure correct development and use of oral-facial and oropharyngeal muscles and structures.
- Minimize disruption of family processes.
- Prevent development of feeding problems.

Some conditions require surgical correction of the underlying condition. In many cases (e.g., a simple cleft lip), initial surgical intervention is sufficient and the child progresses normally. In others, especially for the child with serious or multiple anomalies, long-term treatment is required. However, the treatment itself can lead to problems that require further management. For example, correction of esophageal atresia, tracheoesophageal fistulas, or presence of a tracheostomy can result in scarring and strictures, which, in turn, put the child at risk for impaired swallowing, choking, and aspiration. See Table 12–18 for strategies related to feeding in children with cleft lip or palate.

GER usually can be managed in the outpatient setting. Most babies "spit up," especially when burped or placed in certain positions directly after a feeding. A small regurgitation of undigested formula or breast milk is usually not of concern, but GER puts the infant at risk for esophagitis, pulmonary infection, and failure to thrive. See Table 12–19 for specific suggestions related to managing GER.

In addition to physical management, the NP must support parents emotionally and psychologically as they care for their children. Parents of a child with birth anomalies can suffer shock, loss, or disappointment and may find it difficult to accept their child; they can experience a wide range of feelings (e.g., guilt, rejection, anger). Difficult feeding or uncertainty about the child's long-term prognosis adds additional pressure to parents who are already facing an extremely stressful situation. Creating a positive feeding experience can facilitate a healthy par-

T A B L E 12-18

Strategies for Feeding in Children With Cleft Lip or Palate

AGE	PROBLEM PRESENTED	MANAGEMENT STRATEGY
Infants	Poor suction when nursing Nasal regurgitation	Individualize position used to feed infant; semiupright (60–90 degrees) position is often most effective. Breastfeed if possible; experiment with nipple position: position nipple toward side of mouth, do not put nipple into cleft. Use of longer, soft, or cross-cut nipples and squeezable bottles assists in infants with weak suck. Use of prosthetic device may be helpful. Wean child by 12 mo of age. Tube or gavage feedings may be necessary in severe cleft.
	Swallows air Fatigue	Burp frequently. Allow sufficient time for feeding; work toward providing adequate nutrients in 30 min.
Toddlers	Risk of aspiration Nasal regurgitation	Encourage use of cup, spoon, finger foods as developmentally appropriate. Avoid small, hard, sticky foods that can lodge in palate opening; supervise feeding.
School-age children and adolescents	Malocclusion Difficulty coordinating chewing, swallowing, and breathing Aspiration	Dental referral and treatment are essential. Teach child how to chew, swallow, and breathe, not to talk and chew at the same time. Cut food into small pieces; child can take sips of water while eating. Child will chew with mouth open.
	Anorexia secondary to decreased sense of taste/smell	Plan diets that stimulate appetite; provide child's favorite foods.

ent-infant bond. The NP can intervene in the following ways:

- Encourage parents to express their feelings.
- Listen nonjudgmentally, acknowledging those feelings.
- Demonstrate techniques that increase success in feeding.
- Explain the child's condition, treatments, and prognoses, both short and long term.
- Emphasize how the parent can be involved in the child's progress.
- Encourage parents to make decisions related to their child's care; provide suggestions and guidance as the child grows, as treatment is carried out, and as needs change.

COMPLICATIONS

Aspiration, failure to thrive, poor parent–child bond, esophagitis, and esophageal strictures are complications of difficulty in feeding.

PREVENTION AND PATIENT EDUCATION, SUPPORT NETWORKS, AND GROUPS

See Resource Box 12-1.

Eating Disorders

An eating disorder is defined as "a situation where the time spent (eating [or not eating] in response to an external stimulus) is greater than the time spent eating in response to internal hunger cues" (Hahn, 1998). Anorexia nervosa and bulimia are two common eating disorders seen in the pediatric population. Obesity can also be considered an eating disorder, especially because many people who are obese focus on food and its external cues rather than their body's messages about hunger and satiety.

ANOREXIA NERVOSA AND BULIMIA

Description

Individuals with anorexia nervosa claim to feel fat even when underweight or emaciated, have an intense fear of becoming obese (the fear does not decrease as weight loss progresses), and actively seek to reduce their weight further. A major clinical descriptor for *anorexia nervosa* is weight loss of 25% or more of ideal body weight for age with no known physical illness that would account for such loss.

Bulimia is defined as a pattern of binge

T A B L E 12-19

Strategies for Feeding in Children With Gastroesophageal Reflux

CONDITION	MANAGEMENT STRATEGIES
Mild	Keep child in very slightly upright position (10–15 degrees) after feeding; do not elevate head too much because it will cause scrunched over or slouched position that puts pressure on abdomen.
	Burp frequently during feeding.
	Thicken formula with rice cereal if bottle feeding.
Moderate to severe	Position infant on right side or supine after feeding; use folded and rolled blankets to keep child in position.
	Consult with pediatric gastroenterologist.
	Medical treatment can include cimetidine, metoclopramide, and cisapride (Behrman et al., 1996).
	Surgical referral may be necessary in cases that do not respond to medical management.

T A B L E 12-20

Characteristics of Individuals With Eating Disorders

- Poor self-esteem
- Perfectionism, unrealistically high expectations of self
- Feelings of powerlessness, lack of control
- Desire to be noticed, to be someone special
- Simplistic thinking
- Suppressed anger, hostility, rebellion, depression

eating, followed by attempts to lose weight through self-induced vomiting, severely restricted diets, fasting, and use of laxatives or diuretics.

Incidence and Etiology

Anorexia nervosa occurs most often in adolescent girls (about 1 in 100), although approximately 10% of anorexics are males; a bimodal distribution of the condition is present, with peaks at 14.5 and 18 years (Behrman et al., 1996). Bulimia peaks in later adolescence, at about age 18 to 19 years, with binge eating occurring approximately 2 years before purging begins (Stice et al., 1998).

A specific cause for these eating disorders is unknown, and factors that trigger these behaviors vary. A number of etiological theories are suggested, including psychodynamic, biological, behavioral, sociocultural, and family systems theories. Bulimia appears to have a significant element of learned behavior, acquired through modeling among peers (Stice et al., 1998). Characteristics of individuals with anorexia nervosa or bulimia and trigger factors related to the disorder (Tables 12–20 and 12–21) are similar and are helpful in understanding how to manage the disease.

Clinical Assessment and Findings

Diagnosing anorexia or bulimia can be difficult. Some clinical findings characteristic of these eating disorders are also seen in the healthy adolescent. For example, it is not uncommon for a 14-year-old girl who is neither

T A B L E 12-21

Trigger Factors Related to Eating Disorders

• Traumatic loss
• Sexual abuse
• Teasing about body shape, size
• Prolonged dieting
• Increased demands on performance
• Family problems
• Peer pressure

anorexic nor bulimic to express concern about her body appearance, stating that she is too fat or ugly. Additionally, adolescents with anorexia or bulimia, and their families, can work very hard to hide their condition, denying problems or presenting a very mature, self-sufficient, and successful facade. Early in the disease process, the family system may appear very coherent, making it difficult to collect accurate data about family relations and behavior patterns that contribute to eating disorders.

To draw accurate conclusions, assessment for anorexia and bulimia focuses on the number or combination of findings present and the patterns of behavior over time (see Table 12–22 for general assessment questions).

Clinical Assessment and Findings—Anorexia Nervosa

HISTORY. The history should assess for the following:

• Amenorrhea
• Dizziness, syncope
• Expressions of pleasure with weight loss
• Denial of hunger
• Statement of feeling fat, even though not overweight
• Preoccupation with food; often fixes elaborate meals but does not eat; has rituals associated with food
• Attempts to lose weight through diets, exercise, and/or self-induced vomiting
• Hides eating habits, lies about intake
• Displays social isolation and mood changes: irritable, sullen, hostile, intro-

verted, unhappy, intolerant of others, can have suicidal ideation
• Has fixed, highly structured schedule, inflexible to change

PHYSICAL EXAMINATION. The physical examination may reveal the following:

• Growth parameters: decreased height-to-weight ratio; weight 25% below ideal for age and height
• Abdomen: pain and distention, decreased bowel sounds
• Skin: dry, rough, cracked, yellowish or grayish color; mucous membranes dry, dull; edema
• Hair: thin, brittle, dull, can have alopecia, bristle hairs on scalp, lanugo on body
• Muscles: weak, decreased definition and mass
• Sensory: lack of concentration, drowsy, confused, irritable, apathetic
• Vital signs: decreased temperature, pulse, respirations, blood pressure

T A B L E 12-22

Quick Assessment Tool for Eating Disorders

	YES	NO
1. Do you spend most of your time thinking about food?	—	—
2. Do you panic if you gain a pound or two?	—	—
3. Do you ever eat uncontrollably?	—	—
4. Do you feel guilt and remorse after eating?	—	—
5. Do you ever fast or restrict your diet?	—	—
6. Do you vomit or use laxatives to control your weight?	—	—
7. Are your periods irregular, or have you stopped menstruating?	—	—
8. Do you have a strict exercise regimen?	—	—
9. Do you panic if you are unable to exercise as much as you'd like?	—	—

From Decker SD: Eating disorders: Anorexia and bulimia. *In* Johnson BS (ed): Psychiatric–Mental Health Nursing: Adaptation and Growth, 3rd ed. Philadelphia, JB Lippincott, 1993, p. 563.

LABORATORY. Laboratory studies are done as for bulimia.

Clinical Assessment and Findings—Bulimia

HISTORY. The history may include

- Excessive concern about weight
- Weight fluctuation
- Pattern of strict dieting followed by eating binges
- Plans for binge eating
- Frequent overeating, often used as a coping mechanism to manage stress
- Guilt expressed about eating
- Self-induced vomiting after binging; hematemesis
- Pattern of hiding binging and purging
- Complaints of frequent diarrhea or constipation
- Gregarious behavior but evidence of mood swings, especially depression
- Other destructive behaviors: shoplifting, substance abuse
- Family history of chaos, abuse, sexual abuse

PHYSICAL EXAMINATION. The physical examination may indicate

- Usually normal weight, can range from obese to severely underweight
- Tooth decay, lost enamel
- Enlarged parotid glands
- Skin: dry, rough, cracked, sores on mucous membranes of mouth and around fingernails, broken blood vessels in face; edema
- Weakness, fatigue
- Cardiac arrythmias

LABORATORY. Laboratory studies are done as indicated:

- Hematocrit, hemoglobin, transferrin (decreased amounts)
- Serum glucose, albumin, electrolytes (decreased); may have hypernatremia
- Liver enzymes (elevated liver function)
- Thyroid function (low thyroxine)
- Creatine phosphokinase (elevated)
- Electrocardiogram (ECG) (abnormalities)

DIFFERENTIAL DIAGNOSIS (ANOREXIA AND BULIMIA). The differential diagnoses for anorexia and bulimia include

- Diabetes
- Hyperthyroidism
- Inflammatory bowel disease
- Malignancy/central nervous system neoplasm
- AIDS
- Pregnancy
- Systemic lupus erythematosus
- Depression
- Substance abuse

Management

Management of adolescents with anorexia nervosa or bulimia is very difficult, in part because the adolescent, family, and even the health care provider often deny the significance of the problem. Diagnosis can be delayed and treatment inadequate. Because the issue is not food but, rather, sociopsychological dynamics of control in the adolescent's life, effective treatment is complex and long term. Treatment must include both psychological and physiological interventions, and referral to psychiatric therapists and medical specialists can be essential. Specific treatment modalities vary from one individual to another, depending on the severity of the condition and causal factors, and can include

- Hospitalization to stabilize fluids, electrolytes, and nutrient intake
- Medications and supplementation
  - Antidepressants
  - Metoclopramide
  - Estrogen
  - Progesterone
  - Minerals (potassium, calcium, phosphate, zinc, magnesium, iron)
  - Folate
- Individual psychotherapy
- Group psychotherapy
- Family therapy
- Nutritional counseling
- Assertiveness training
- Body work: relaxation, biofeedback, movement therapy

Complications

The complications of anorexia nervosa or bulimia include

- Death, usually secondary to cardiac arrhythmia, hypokalemia, or suicide
- Alcohol and drug addictions
- Osteoporosis
- Gastrointestinal disturbance: ulcers, motility disorders
- Fertility problems
- Gynecological problems related to prolonged amenorrhea
- Growth retardation
- Dehydration

Prevention and Patient Education, Support Networks, and Groups

See Resource Box 12-1.

OBESITY

Description

Excessive adipose tissue is the hallmark of obesity. A gain in adipose tissue can be related to an increase either in the size of fat cells (hypertrophy) or in the number of fat cells (hyperplasia). Childhood-onset obesity that is hyperplastic in nature is especially difficult to control, because fat cells can be reduced in size but not in number. Ideal body weight and body mass index (BMI) are used to define parameters of obesity. Ideal body weight is calculated based on the National Center for Health Statistics (NCHS) growth charts (Table 12-23). If weight is 20% above the ideal, the child is considered obese.

Normal BMI, in the adult, ranges from 20 to 26, and an individual is defined as obese if BMI is 27 or greater. For children older than 5 years of age, use of BMI for groups may be appropriate, but it must be used cautiously to assess individual children (Pietrobelli et al., 1998). Some children are genetically large-boned and have a body weight or BMI in excess of the norm for their age, gender, and height without having excess fat.

T A B L E 12-23

Calculation of Ideal Body Weight From National Center for Health Statistics Growth Charts*

% IDEAL BODY WEIGHT FOR HEALTHY CHILDREN	INTERPRETATION
>120%	Overweight
90–110%	Normal
80–90%	Mildly underweight
70–79%	Moderately underweight
<70%	Severely underweight

*% Ideal body weight = Current weight divided by weight at 50th percentile for current stature multiplied by 100.

Incidence and Etiology

Although studies indicate a decline in fat intake since 1990, rates of childhood obesity have increased dramatically. Studies have shown an incidence of obesity in more than 30% of children (Melnik et al., 1998; Hernandez et al., 1998). In the preschool age group, older children show a greater increase in being overweight than younger children (Mei et al., 1998; Ogden et al., 1997). Older children who are obese and obese children who have an obese parent are more likely to be obese as adults (Whitaker et al., 1997).

Obesity appears to result from a complex relationship between genetics, environment (e.g., exercise, caloric intake), and the body's response to environmental factors (e.g., neurohormonal regulation of the body's set point). Biological factors, particularly the role of the hormone leptin as a regulator of body weight and/or satiety, are currently being explored (Houseknecht et al., 1998; Sinha & Caro, 1998) and genetics may affect one's susceptibility to obesity. The contribution that genetics vs. environment makes in the obese child is not entirely clear, because, just as parents pass on genetic traits, they also influence lifestyle habits and set patterns associated with eating and activity.

Sedentary activity contributes to obesity (Maffeis et al., 1997). Although the average American child engages in 0.5 to 1.5 hours of moderate to vigorous activity per day, as many as 20 to 30% of children report being physically active less than one-half hour per day. A Centers for Disease Control and Prevention (CDC) survey indicated that 48% of girls and 26% of boys do not exercise vigorously on a regular basis (Centers for Disease Control, 1997). Children with chronic conditions that limit physical activity are especially susceptible to excessive weight gain.

Inactivity is fostered by the presence of television in the home. The average US child spends 25 hours a week in front of the television, and a positive relationship has been noted between the time spent watching television and levels of body weight and fat in children (Andersen et al., 1998). Besides replacing active play, the exposure to television advertising increases the likelihood that children will snack on low-nutrient-dense foods. Consumption of more than 12 ounces of fruit juice a day has been associated with obesity in preschool children (Dennison et al., 1997).

Psychosocial factors also contribute to the increased incidence of obesity, particularly in regard to family dysfunction. Children who suffer neglect or abuse or have an overcontrolling parent may turn to food for comfort and solace.

Clinical Assessment and Findings

HISTORY. The history looks at patterns of eating and exercise for both the child and the family system and includes the following:

- Dietary intake
  - Total caloric intake
  - Fat intake as percentage of total calories
  - Carbohydrate intake as percentage of total calories
  - Nutrient adequacy of diet
- Exercise pattern
- Parental obesity
- Time of onset of obesity
- Family history of diabetes
- Episodes of sleep apnea
- Social adjustment, peer group, friends
- Family readiness to participate in a weight management treatment program

PHYSICAL EXAMINATION. A complete physical examination to determine the child's level of

fitness is necessary, looking especially at the following:

- Blood pressure
- Vital signs
- Ideal body weight (see Table 12-23)
- Percent BMI (Table 12-24)
- Tricep skinfold
- Midarm circumference
- Height and weight

LABORATORY
- Lipid screen
- Glucose tolerance test may be indicated in children with a family history of diabetes

Differential Diagnosis

The differential diagnosis includes medical conditions such as hypothyroidism, Down syndrome, and Prader-Willi syndrome that contribute to obesity in children.

Management

The primary goal of weight management in children is to normalize weight, not reduce weight. Because most children are in a rapid growth and development phase, recommendations for treating obesity center on slowing the rate of weight gain, thereby allowing children to grow into their weight. Restricting fat and calories in infants is not recommended because of the rapid brain development occurring at this age. Young children's intake of fruit juice, however, should be limited to less than 12 ounces a day (Dennison et al., 1997).

Treatment goals include supporting the child and family as they change lifestyle patterns that

T A B L E 12-24

Calculation of Body Mass Index*

AGE	EXPECTED PARAMETERS
≤14 yr	19–20
15 yr	25
≥16 yr	28

*Body mass index (BMI) = Weight (in kg)/Height (in meters)^2

lead to excessive weight gain. Even though children must be monitored for height and weight on a regular basis, progress should be measured by other parameters as well. Improved dietary habits, increased physical activity, and enhanced self-esteem are significant endpoints that should be acknowledged and praised by the family and health care team alike.

For older children whose obesity is related to environmental conditions, the American Dietetic Association (1989b) recommends the following principles:

- Children should not be placed on restricted-calorie diets; rather, efforts should be made to encourage children to be physically active, to eat a well-balanced diet, and to return to internal control of eating.
- Intervention to treat obesity in children should not interfere with normal growth or promote the development of eating disorders.
- The feeding relationship between parent and child should be improved or normalized.
- Positive behavioral management techniques should be included and self-esteem, attitudes, and body image improved.
- Realistic goals should be set to achieve optimal weight through the growing years.

A Maternal Child Health committee of pediatric obesity experts (Barlow & Dietz, 1998) recommends:

- Use of either weight loss or weight maintenance, depending on child's age, baseline BMI percentile, and presence of medical complications
- Early treatment (in infancy if child is obese)
- Family-centered treatment, with emphasis on parenting skills
- Increased activity
- Decreased high-fat and high-calorie foods
- Stepwise interventions with a goal of long-term change
- Ongoing support for families

When counseling obese children and their parents, the NP is advised to emphasize a family-centered approach. When the entire family changes to a more healthy diet and engages in regular physical activity, the obese child has a much greater chance at weight normalization (Golan et al., 1998). This approach also tends to be positive rather than punitive and thereby helps to raise the child's self-esteem. Table 12–25 provides useful approaches and sugges-

---

T A B L E 12-25

Guidelines for Managing Childhood Obesity

- Do not put child on a diet. Instead, gradually modify the entire family's eating habits. For example, serve fruit as a substitute for dessert, switch to nonfat or 1% milk, experiment with low-fat recipes and methods of food preparation, and use reduced-fat margarine, salad dressings, and other low-fat condiments. Serve calorically dense foods that reflect the food guide pyramid, including whole grains, fruits, vegetables, lean protein foods, and low-fat dairy products.
- Do not force children to clean their plates. They should eat only until they are full.
- Schedule and enforce regular times for meals and snacks. Do not skip meals. Do not allow childen to nibble throughout the day.
- Have low-calorie, nutritious snacks readily available, such as air-popped popcorn, pretzels, low-fat yogurt, frozen fruit juice bars, skim milk, low-sugar cereals, fresh fruit, and raw vegetables.
- Do not have high-calorie snacks readily available (e.g., potato chips, cookies, cakes, pies, ice cream, candy, pop, and doughnuts).
- Promote physical activity. Make daily exercise a priority. Encourage family participation, individual exercise, and team sports and structured activities with peers.
- Limit television viewing. Children who watch 4 or more hours of television per day are twice as likely as other children to become obese. Children are more sedentary when they watch television, and frequent food advertising has been linked to increased snacking.
- Scale back television watching slowly, replacing time with activities, hobbies, or chores.
- Praise and reward children for the progress they make in reaching nutrition, activity, self-esteem, or weight goals. Emphasize the uniqueness of each child, pointing out special talents, abilities, and positive qualities.

tions to use when counseling obese children and their families.

The Shapedown program has been effective in treating obese children and teenagers. Using a variety of cognitive, behavioral, and affective techniques that make successive changes in diet, exercise, communication, and affect, the Shapedown program has produced significant long-term outcomes. The NP is an ideal provider of this program, which involves an interdisciplinary team approach.

Complications

Children who are obese are at much higher risk for related conditions, including hypertension, impaired glucose tolerance, sleep apnea, orthopedic problems (e.g., slipped capital epiphysis), social rejection, and lowered self-esteem. In the child with a physical disability, obesity can further impair mobility and reduce energy expenditure.

Prevention and Patient Education, Support Networks, and Groups

See Resource Box 12-1 for information on Shapedown program.

Adverse Food Reactions

DESCRIPTION

A distinction is made between *food allergy,* a hypersensitivity to a food or food additive with either an immediate or a delayed immune system response (e.g., anaphylactic reaction to ingestion of nuts), and *food intolerance,* a nonimmunological inability to process or tolerate the food product (e.g., PKU secondary to the body's inability to metabolize phenylalanine) (Fig. 12-2). Both are considered adverse reactions to food.

INCIDENCE AND ETIOLOGY

Many individuals believe they have a food allergy or intolerance. This perception, however, may not be accurate. Only about 1 to 2% of individuals meet the criteria of having "either a positive double-blind, placebo-controlled food challenge or an unequivocal report of a reaction with the typical features of an immunoglobulin E (IgE)-mediated severe allergic or anaphylactic reaction" (Hourihane, 1998). Eight foods, including cow's milk, hen's eggs, peanuts, soya, wheat, fish, crustacea, and tree nuts (including almonds and cashews), account for nearly 90% of actual IgE-mediated allergic reactions (Bock et al., 1988; Burks et al., 1998). *Any* food, however, can cause reactions in a specific individual. Factors contributing to adverse food reactions include the following:

- Heredity. A child with one parent with a food allergy has a 30 to 35% chance of developing the condition; if both parents have food allergies, the child's chances increase to 65%. Children born with a metabolic disorder (e.g., deficient lactase enzyme) can have adverse reactions to specific foods.
- Immature gastrointestinal tract. Before 7 months of age, the infant gastrointestinal tract is more permeable to large molecules, including most food proteins.
- Compromised gastrointestinal tract. As a result of injury or illness, the gastrointestinal system can be more permeable to allergens such as large proteins.
- Type of food. Some foods are more allergenic than others, and some individuals have greater sensitivity to certain foods.
- Allergic load or tolerance level. Conditions such as illness, stress, surgery, or trauma can place excessive metabolic demands on the body. An individual who is susceptible to food intolerance or allergy can have a reaction when these conditions are present. Additionally, frequent exposure or exposure to large quantities of the allergen can lead to a reaction.

CLINICAL ASSESSMENT AND FINDINGS

The goals of clinical assessment are to determine whether an adverse food reaction is present, distinguish between an allergy and a food intolerance, and identify the source or sources of the problem. This process is extremely challenging and can require referral to a registered

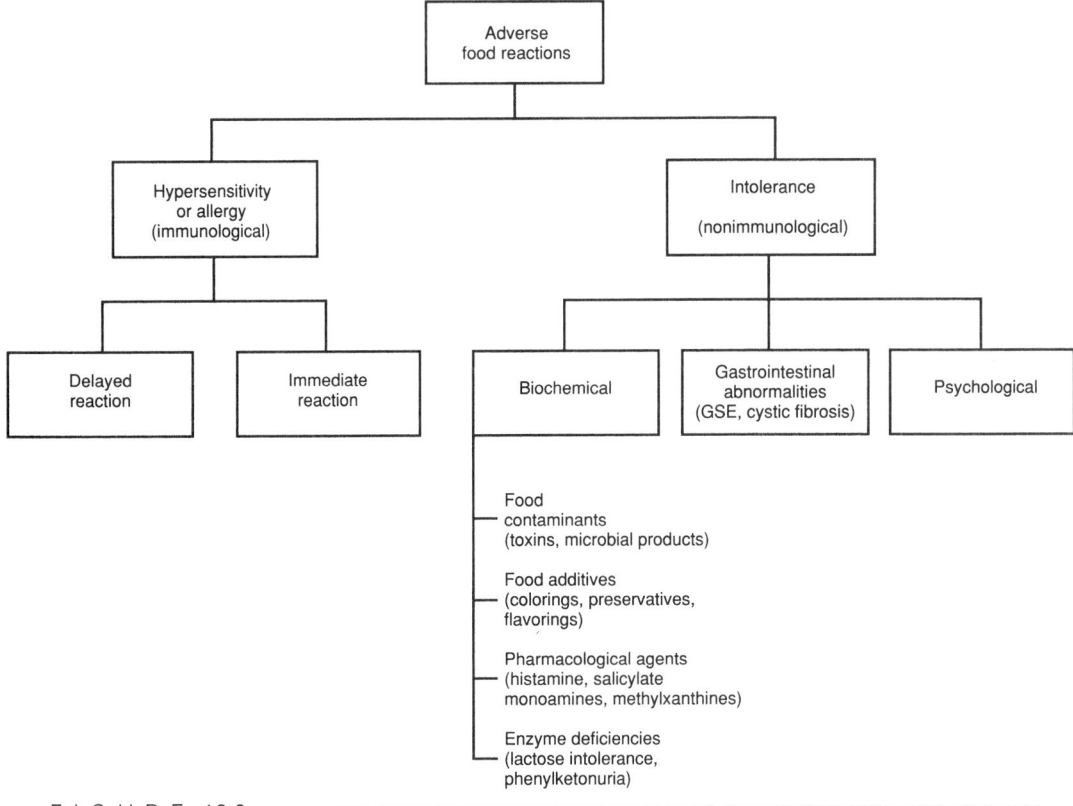

F I G U R E 12-2
Adverse food reactions. (From Davis J, Sherer K: Applied Nutrition and Diet Therapy for Nurses. Philadelphia, WB Saunders, 1994.)

dietitian or use of a team approach with NP, dietitian, and allergist for a more in-depth diagnostic workup. The basic examination includes the history, physical examination, laboratory studies, and food elimination and challenge.

History

The history should assess the following:

- Is there a family history of allergies, especially a history of reaction to certain foods?
- Does the child have a history of symptoms frequently seen in food allergies (e.g., eczema, urticaria, rashes, colic, vomiting, diarrhea), unaccompanied by other signs of illness, or history of exposure to infectious agents?
- Does the child have a history of symptoms following ingestion of food?
  - Description of symptoms
  - Time of onset of symptoms related to food intake
  - Type and quantity of food ingested
  - Description of other factors that are present and may contribute to or aggravate an allergic response (e.g., stress, environment, exercise)
- What is the child's diet history? When and what types of foods were introduced into the diet?
- Describe the child's usual intake. A food diary is an excellent mechanism for obtaining these data and includes
  - All foods and fluids ingested
  - How food is prepared (e.g., commercially, at home, fried, baked)
  - How food is stored and fed to the child
  - All medications

Physical Examination

Signs and symptoms of adverse food reactions vary by type and severity, from a mild local reaction to life-threatening anaphylaxis, making it difficult to diagnose the condition definitively. Table 12–26 lists possible clinical manifestations of food allergies or intolerances by body system.

Laboratory Studies

Laboratory studies assist in distinguishing between food allergies and intolerances. Tests include

- Serum IgE and eosinophil count (elevated serum IgE and eosinophilia >400/mm³ are related to allergies)
- Skin tests
- Radioallergosorbent tests
- Metabolic screening tests (e.g., PKU)

Food Elimination and Challenge

When a food has been identified as a potential source of the problem, the process of elimination and challenge is used to confirm the diagnosis. Referral to an allergist or immunologist for such a challenge is recommended. The suspected foods are completely eliminated from the child's diet for at least 2 weeks and reintroduced one at a time. An allergy or intolerance is confirmed if symptoms cease when the food is eliminated then reappear as it is reintroduced. If multiple foods are suspected or if the potential reaction to a food is severe, the process of elimination and challenge in the outpatient setting may not be feasible, and the child may need to be hospitalized for diagnostic evaluation.

Eliminating foods from children's diets can put them at risk for nutrient deficits. NPs should work with the allergist and a registered dietitian to ensure that children are receiving sufficient nutrients from other sources.

DIFFERENTIAL DIAGNOSIS

The differential diagnoses for food allergy and food intolerance include

TABLE 12-26

Possible Clinical Manifestations of Food Allergies or Intolerances by Body System

SYSTEM	SYMPTOMS
Respiratory system	Chronic rhinitis
	Asthma
	Croup
	Cough
	Serous otitis media
	Bronchitis
Gastrointestinal system	Swelling of lips, mouth, throat
	Nausea, vomiting
	Diarrhea
	Colic
	Protein-losing enteropathy
	Bloating, flatulence
	Constipation
	Gastrointestinal blood loss
	Malabsorption
Integumentary system	Eczema
	Pruritus
	Atopic dermatitis
	Rashes
	Urticaria
Central nervous system	Headaches (sinus, migraine)
	Fatigue
	Drowsiness, listlessness
	Irritability
	Depression
	Excessive sweating
Circulatory system	Hypotension
	Cardiac arrhythmias
	Anaphylaxis
	Pallor

From Davis J, Sherer K: Applied Nutrition and Diet Therapy for Nurses. Philadelphia, WB Saunders, 1994.

- Reactions related to other environmental allergens
- Psychological reactions to feeding
- Malabsorption syndromes
- Chronic diarrhea

MANAGEMENT

Care of children with adverse food reactions aims to maintain nutrition levels adequate for normal growth and development, prevent nutrient deficits, and avoid exposure to offending food or foods.

Balancing nutrient requirements with the need to restrict certain foods can be challenging. Not only must the restricted food be replaced with one of equivalent nutrient value, the physical signs of allergies (e.g., diarrhea, vomiting, eczema) can create a need for extra nutrients to maintain health and foster growth. The NP, family, and child should work with a dietitian to structure dietary care.

Once the offending food has been identified, elimination or rotation diets can be planned. Elimination diets seek to remove the food completely. Elimination of the food is required for highly allergenic foods. This can be difficult, especially when purchasing processed or prepared foods or eating in restaurants. Table 12-27 lists foods that are likely to contain more common allergens. With a rotation diet, items in "food families" are rotated every 4 to 5 days, reducing the potential food allergy load and allowing the child to tolerate a more diverse diet. Strict rotation diets appear to be most effective when the child has multiple, mild food allergies.

Because food allergies and intolerances are often outgrown, it may be appropriate to carefully challenge the child with most offending foods every year or two. There is some research to indicate that children may not outgrow their allergy, but its immediate effect is masked as the child grows. Obvious and immediate problems are gone, but long-term degeneration may occur (Hodson, 1992). Some foods appear to remain allergenic for longer periods (e.g., seafood). If the child's reaction has been serious or even life threatening, the parents may decide to continue to avoid the food. Children with allergies to nuts should *never* be challenged.

Management of food intolerances secondary to metabolic disorders was discussed earlier (see section on Disorders Requiring Restricted or Supplemental Diets).

COMPLICATIONS

Complications of adverse food reactions include the following:

- Anaphylaxis
- Convulsive coughing and sneezing, leading to aspiration or choking
- Malnutrition
- Gastrointestinal dysfunction
- Secondary skin infections
- Disruption of family processes

PREVENTION

The best treatment for food allergies and intolerances is prevention. Ideally, all infants should be breastfed for a minimum of 4 to 6 months and for 12 months if possible; infants who have been identified as high-risk for adverse reactions, especially allergies, should be exclusively breastfed until 6 months of age (Chandra, 1997). If formula is used, avoid soy-based or cow's milk–based formula for high-risk infants. Specially prepared formulas such as Nutramigen, Pregestimil, or Alimentum can be appropriate substitutes (see Table 12-6). The first foods introduced should be hypoallergenic (e.g., rice cereal, squash, bananas). At least 3 to 5 days are allowed between each new food introduced so that any adverse reaction has time to present. Cow's milk, wheat, corn, and citrus fruits should be avoided completely before 12 months of age.

Breastfeeding mothers of infants at high risk for allergies should avoid allergenic foods as well (e.g., cow's milk, nuts, fish), because the proteins from these foods may be passed to the infant via breast milk. Garlic, onions, cabbage, and broccoli also have been noted to cause reactions in infants.

Effect of Medications on Nutritional Status

DESCRIPTION

Medications are designed to alter the body's biochemistry in an effort to produce a healing effect. Biochemical processes inherent in drug therapy have implications for the individual's nutritional status. Some medications deplete essential nutrients from the body; others interfere with the body's ability to metabolize nutrients; still others have an adverse affect on the appe-

T A B L E 12-27

Common Foods Containing Allergens

FOODS LIKELY TO CONTAIN	MAY BE LISTED ON LABEL AS	SUBSTITUTES
MILK		
Milk	Milk	Soy milks
Buttermilk	Milk solids	Nut milks
Hot chocolate	Buttermilk solids	Milk-free shakes
Many nondairy products	Curds	Some nondairy creamers
Many baked goods	Whey solids	Baked goods without milk—most French
Many baking mixes	Whey	bread
Granola	Casein	Bagels, saltines
Cheese	Lactalbumin	Soy cheese
Prepared meats (hot dogs, luncheon meats)	Caseinate	Kosher-prepared meats
Macaroni and cheese	Cream	Products labeled parve or pareve
Canned spaghetti	Sodium caseinate	Foods prepared without milk or butter;
Potatoes mashed with milk or butter		e.g., potatoes, scrambled egg
Vegetables in cream, cheese, or butter sauces		casseroles
Many margarines		Milk-free margarines, salad dressings, sauces, and gravies
Many salad dressings		Milk-free sherbets, ices, and sorbets
Imitation sour cream		Frozen tofu desserts
Some gravies		Cornstarch puddings with fruit juice
Ice cream		Jello
Some sherbets		
Yogurt		
Puddings		
EGG		
Eggnog	Albumin	Egg-free baked goods and specialty items
Root beers	Egg white	Pasta, rice, potatoes, egg-free substitutes
Many baked goods	Egg white solids	Prepared meats and imitation seafood
Pancakes, waffles, French toast	Egg yolk	without egg products
Egg noodles	Yolks	Soups without egg products
Eggs		Imitation mayonnaise, sauces, and salad
Most egg substitutes		dressings prepared without egg
Many prepared meats (hot dogs, luncheon meats, imitation seafood)		products
Many batter-dipped foods		Cornstarch, tapioca puddings prepared without eggs
Noodle soups		Baked goods prepared without eggs
Mayonnaise		
Hollandaise sauce		
Many salad dressings		
Tartar sauce		
Custards		
Puddings		
Boiled frostings		
Meringues		
Macaroons		
Marshmallow products		
Fondants and other candies		
WHEAT		
Instant breakfast	Wheat	Breads and other wheat-free baked
Postum	Flour	goods
Many baked goods	Wheat bran	Wheat-free cereals, Rice Chex, cream of
Most baking mixes	Wheat germ	rice
Pancakes, waffles	Wheat starch	Rice cakes and crackers
Many cereals	Gluten	Rye crackers

Table continued on following page

T A B L E 12-27

Common Foods Containing Allergens *Continued*

FOODS LIKELY TO CONTAIN	MAY BE LISTED ON LABEL AS	SUBSTITUTES
WHEAT *Continued*		
Many crackers	Graham flour	Cornmeal coating
Breaded foods	Enriched flour	Corn tortillas
Wheat tortillas	Durum flour	Rice, corn pasta
Pasta, noodles	Vegetable gums	Meat products without wheat added
Prepared meat products, hot dogs, luncheon meats	Modified food starch	Gravies and sauces thickened with cornstarch, potato starch
Gravies and sauces thickened with flour	Vegetable starches	Homemade baked goods made without wheat
Cakes, cookies, pies	Malted cereal syrup	
Soy sauce	Hydrolyzed vegetable protein	Worcestershire sauce
Pretzels	Semolina	Salt
Beer, including nonalcoholic beer		Popcorn, corn chips
SOY		
Soy formula	Soy	Casein hydrolysate formula
Soy milks	Soy flour	Milk or nut milks
Nondairy creamers	Soy protein	Homemade breakfast shake
Instant breakfast	Soy protein isolate	Breads, cereals, and crackers made without soy
Many baked goods	Hydrolyzed vegetable protein	
Many baking mixes		
CORN		
Carbonated beverages	Corn	Flavored seltzer
Many sweetened fruit drinks	Cornstarch	Fruit juice
Instant breakfast	Corn syrup	Homemade breakfast shake
Many bread products	Corn oil†	Breads, crackers, and cereals made without corn products
Many cereals	Corn sweeteners	
Many crackers	Corn syrup solids	Wheat tortillas
Some baking and pancake mixes	High-fructose corn syrup	Processed meats made without corn products
Corn tortillas	Maltodextrin	
Some processed meats	Vegetable oil†	Peanut butter without added sweeteners
Imitation seafood		Foods without corn sweeteners or other corn products added
Imitation cheese		
Peanut butter with corn syrup added		Other oils
Canned spaghetti and sauces		Soy-free margarines or butter
Canned baked beans		Homemade dressings made without corn oil
Canned soups		
Au gratin potato mixes		Fresh fruit or packed in own juice
Vegetable starch		Sugar, pure maple syrup, or honey
Vegetable gums		Pure fruit spreads
Soybean oil*		Frozen desserts without added corn sweeteners
Vegetable shortening*		
Hydrogenated oils*		Featherweight baking powder
Corn oil†		Flour or potato starch
Corn oil margarine†		
Salad dressing†		
Pancake syrup		
Jellies and jams		
Popsicles and ice cream		
Most baking powders		
Catsup and barbecue sauce		

*Tolerated by most people with soy allergy. Caution is advised for those with a history of anaphylaxis.
†Tolerated by most people with corn allergy. Caution is advised for those with a history of anaphylaxis.
Adapted from Mahan LK, Arlin M: Krause's Food Nutrition and Diet Therapy, 8th ed. Philadelphia, WB Saunders, 1992.

tite or cause nausea. Although a medication can have an immediate effect on an individual, adverse changes in nutritional status are most often seen after prolonged therapy.

INCIDENCE AND ETIOLOGY

Drug-induced malnutrition results from drug-related alterations in the body's ability to absorb, distribute, metabolize, utilize, or excrete nutrients and their metabolites (Wynne et al., in press). Absorption is affected by characteristics of the molecule being absorbed (size, ionization, lipid solubility), gut motility (too rapid as with diarrhea or too slow as with Hirschsprung's disease), and environment of the gastrointestinal tract (e.g., gastric pH, lack of intrinsic factor). As medications change gastrointestinal motility or environment, they influence the absorption of nutrients.

Distribution of nutrients is affected by plasma protein-binding capabilities, total body water content, and relative fat content in the body. For example, if a drug that binds highly with plasma protein is taken for long periods of time, or if a child has low serum albumin, nutrients have to compete for protein-binding sites.

Metabolism occurs primarily in the liver, and drugs can either inhibit or stimulate hepatic enzyme activity, thus influencing the body's ability to metabolize nutrients for use at the cellular level.

The relationship of medications and nutrients in terms of excretion is less marked than with absorption, distribution, and metabolism, but drugs can have an effect on renal function, especially tubular reabsorption, which has an impact on nutritional status.

CLINICAL ASSESSMENT

Nutritional assessment of children on medication includes the general parameters discussed earlier, such as anthropometric measures, physical examination, and diet history. Specific attention should be paid to those nutrients for which drug therapy places the child at risk of deficiency.

MANAGEMENT

Management involves ongoing assessment and anticipatory intervention to prevent nutritional problems for children on drug therapy. Referral to a dietitian can be helpful. General interventions include the following:

- Alter dietary intake to include more foods containing nutrients affected.
- Supplement diet with required vitamins or minerals, or both.
- Administer medications in a manner that minimizes their impact on nutrition.
- Consider alternative medications and treatment modalities.

See Table 12-28 for dietary suggestions related to specific classes of medication. This list is limited, and a comprehensive pharmacology reference should be consulted for specific drugs.

COMPLICATIONS

Malnutrition, delayed healing, and drug toxicity are complications of the effects of medication on nutritional status.

Controversies in Pediatric Nutrition

COW'S MILK IN CHILDREN'S DIETS

During the first year of life, the use of unmodified cow's milk is contraindicated because of its high protein content, its inappropriate nutrient composition, and the risk of gastrointestinal bleeding and allergic reactions. Instead, infants should receive breast milk or an approved iron-fortified infant formula that closely matches the composition of breast milk. Although most pediatric providers agree on this recommendation, there is some debate about the use of cow's milk in the toddler's diet.

For some children, cow's milk has a detrimental effect, and parents may wonder whether the nutrition benefits of cow's milk are worth possible health risks. In most cases, children older than 1 year of age can safely drink cow's milk, and it can be recommended as a rich source of protein, calcium, riboflavin, and vita-

T A B L E 12-28

Nutritional Risk of Selected Drugs

DRUG CATEGORY OR NAME	NUTRITIONAL RISK	NUTRITIONAL INTERVENTION
Antibiotics/ chloramphenicol	Inhibits vitamin K–producing intestinal microflora Increases excretion of riboflavin Nausea, vomiting, diarrhea Decreases absorption of calcium, fat, and protein Decreases lactase activity Suppresses bone marrow (chloramphenicol) May cause aplastic anemia	Use acidophilus tablets, acidophilus milk, or yogurt to replace gastrointestinal organisms Supplement with vitamins C, B-complex, B_{12}, biotin, K, or well-balanced vitamin and mineral supplement Use lactose-reduced milk
Barbiturate/ phenobarbital	Breaks down vitamin D May cause calcium deficiency, rickets, or osteomalacia May decrease serum folate, vitamin B_{12}, pyridoxine, magnesium May cause nausea, vomiting, constipation	May need vitamin D and calcium supplements Give drug with meals Give high-fiber and fluid diet If folic acid supplementation is indicated, administer cautiously
Antihistamines/ cimetidine/ diphenhydramine	Decreases gastric acid secretion, increases pH Decreases absorption of iron, folate, vitamin B_{12} May lead to hyperglycemia May disrupt vitamin D metabolism	
Corticosteroids	Increases protein catabolism and gluconeogenesis; decreases protein synthesis, contributing to nitrogen wasting Stimulates appetite May cause hypokalemia, hyperglycemia, hypernatremia, hypocalcemia associated with osteoporosis May elevate serum lipids	If edema occurs, restrict sodium intake High doses require calcium and vitamin D supplements Supplement with vitamin B_6, vitamin C, and folic acid Increase dietary protein Monitor weight and restrict calories if there is excessive weight gain
Digoxin	May cause anorexia and nausea, weight loss May cause hypokalemia May increase urinary excretion of magnesium and calcium	Increase dietary potassium Evaluate need to increase dietary magnesium and calcium
Isoniazid	Interferes with enzyme pathway for creation of niacin Increases excretion of vitamin B_6 and folic acid May cause nausea and vomiting Decreases absorption of vitamin E Increases absorption of iron May cause hyperglycemia	Give pyridoxine supplement Increase foods high in folate, niacin, vitamin B_6, and magnesium Avoid foods with histamine and tyramine, such as tuna, mackerel, sardines, dry sausages and meats, imitation and hard cheeses, meat and protein extracts, and excessive amounts of caffeine (Davis & Sherer, 1994)

T A B L E 12-28

Nutritional Risk of Selected Drugs *Continued*

DRUG CATEGORY OR NAME	NUTRITIONAL RISK	NUTRITIONAL INTERVENTION
Methotrexate	Folate antagonist, contributes to folate deficiency May cause stomatitis, anorexia, diarrhea Decreases absorption of vitamins A, D, E, K, β-carotene	Give mineral oil Supplement with multivitamin given midway between times mineral oil is administered Give reduced folate
Oral contraceptives	Increases vitamin A and calcium absorption Causes low serum vitamin C; possibly contributes to low levels of vitamins B_1, B_{12}, B_6, B_2, folate, magnesium, zinc	Increase intake of vitamins C, B_1, B_{12}, B_6, B_2, folate, magnesium, zinc
Phenothiazides	Increases excretion of riboflavin	
Hydantoin, phenytoin	May cause nausea, vomiting, constipation May cause hyperglycemia Impairs metabolism and absorption of folate; may lead to megaloblastic anemia Inactivates vitamin D; can lead to osteomalacia Decreases serum vitamin K	Supplement with vitamins D, K, folate, but excessive folate levels can decrease action of anticonvulsants Administer drug with, or immediately after, a meal
Supplements	Reduces taste acuity Gingival hyperplasia Hyperglycemia	
Calcium	If taken with iron supplement, only calcium carbonate does not affect iron absorption; if taken with fluoride, absorption of both is decreased	
Zinc	>1500 mg/d: decreases copper absorption possibly leading to anemia-related fatigue	
Iron	Causes nausea, possibly anorexia	
Theophylline	May cause vitamin B_6 deficiency	Give pyridoxine supplements

min D. The calcium and vitamin D are present in highly absorbable forms, and the protein is highly bioavailable.

A small number of children, estimated at less than 5%, present with a true milk allergy, evidenced by skin rashes, digestive disturbances, or respiratory symptoms and confirmed by allergy testing. Most of these children eventually outgrow their milk allergy as they mature.

Another condition that can limit dairy product intake by children is lactose intolerance, a condition caused by a lack of the enzyme lactase, normally present in the small intestine. Lactose intolerance is rare in infants but common in older children and adults from Asian, Native-American, black, and Hispanic ethnic groups. The condition presents with symptoms of bloating, flatulence, abdominal cramps, and diarrhea between 15 minutes and 2 hours after the consumption of foods containing lactose.

Children with low lactase levels may be able to digest small amounts of milk and other dairy products. Yogurt, aged cheese, and fermented dairy products, much lower in lactose than milk, are usually better tolerated. Commercial preparations are also available (e.g., Lactaid) that break down the lactose in milk.

Findings from studies of Finnish children suggest that cow's milk antibodies may contribute to the development of insulin-dependent diabetes mellitus in children who are predisposed to the disease (Saukkonen et al., 1998; Virtanen et al., 1994). It is not recommended that children, diabetic or otherwise, give up milk on the basis of these findings.

THE EFFECTS OF SUGAR

Widely perceived as a causative agent of hyperactive behavior among children, controlled scientific studies have failed to demonstrate a link between sugar and behavior or cognitive performance (Wolraich et al., 1996; Krummel et al., 1996). Anecdotal reports from parents and teachers reinforce the misconception that sugar adversely affects behavior in children. In one Canadian study, 80% of primary school teachers stated that they believed sugar consumption contributed to increased activity of normal children and to behavioral problems in hyperactive children. Fifty-five percent of these teachers had counseled parents of children thought to be hyperactive to reduce sugar consumption (DiBattista & Shepherd, 1993). This misconception may stem from the association between sugar consumption and activities (e.g., birthday parties, Halloween) that often result in excitable behavior among children.

The role of the NP is to educate and reassure parents that moderate sugar consumption rarely results in adverse behavior. High sugar diets are to be avoided, however, because these foods tend to replace more nutrient-dense foods and contribute to dental caries if eaten frequently throughout the day. Current dietary recommendations are that 10% or less of calories should come from sugar. For the average child who consumes 2000 calories daily, this would amount to 50 g or about 10 teaspoons each day.

CHOCOLATE AND ACNE

Chocolate is often thought to initiate or worsen acne. Again, no controlled scientific studies have ever established a link between intake of chocolate and the incidence or severity of acne.

THE ROLE OF FAT IN CHILDREN'S DIETS

As the body of evidence pointing to diet as a major determinant of chronic disease continues to build, more emphasis has been placed on the importance of fat-restricted diets beginning in childhood. It is recommended that a diet low in fat (maximum of 30% of total calories), saturated fat (less than 10% total calories), and cholesterol (maximum intake of 300 mg daily) be phased in beginning at age 2 years. According to the AAP Committee on Nutrition (1998), this level of fat intake should be in place by age 5 years. A more restrictive diet may be indicated for children with established hyperlipidemia or a strong family history of coronary heart disease.

Dietary fat restrictions must be carefully managed because recommendations to decrease fat intake can be misunderstood. In some cases, excessively restricted fat and caloric intakes have contributed to loss of essential nutrients and resulted in growth failure (Lifshitz & Tarim, 1996). There is also a question as to what extent low-fat diets followed in childhood provide protection against disease or obesity in adulthood (Zlotkin, 1996; Seidell, 1998).

It appears that a moderate approach to fat restriction is in order. Lower fat diets (approximately 28% fat as a source of energy) in children aged 8 to 10 years (The Writing Group for the DISC Collaborative Research Group, 1995) and in children between 7 and 36 months who also had high vitamin and nutrient intake (Niinikoski et al., 1997) have been shown to reduce cholesterol levels safely without affecting normal growth and development. The NP should strive for balance when counseling parents about fat in their children's diets. A diet with about 30% of calories from fat easily provides for energy and growth needs; below 20% total fat, the child can be at nutritional risk.

NURSING DIAGNOSIS

NURSING DIAGNOSES FOR NUTRITION/METABOLIC FUNCTIONAL HEALTH PATTERN

Anorexia (not NANDA diagnosis)	**Altered Nutrition: Less than Body Requirements**
Bulimia (DSM-IV diagnosis)	**Altered Nutrition: Risk for More than Body**
Infant Feeding Pattern: Ineffective	**Requirements**
Altered Nutrition: More than Body Requirements	**Swallowing Impairment**

Sources: American Psychiatric Association: Diagnostic and Statistical Manual of Mental Disorders IV [DSM-IV]. Washington, DC, Author, 1994.

North American Nursing Diagnosis Association: NANDA Nursing Diagnoses: Definitions and Classification 1997–1998. Philadelphia, Author, 1996.

RESOURCE BOX 12-1

RESOURCE BOX FOR NUTRITION ISSUES

Allergies
Asthma and Allergy Foundation of America
(202) 466-7643
(800) 778-2232

The Food Allergy Network
(703) 691-3179
(800) 929-4040
www.foodallergy.org

Allergy Information and Referral Hotline
(800) 822-2762

American Allergy Association
(415) 322-1663
email: allergyaid@aol.com

Food Allergy Center
(800) 937-7354
www.nutramed.com/allergy/foodallergy.htm

Eating Disorders
American Anorexia Bulimia Association, Inc.
(212) 575-6200
www.aabainc.org

Anorexia Nervosa and Related Eating Disorders (ANRED)
(503) 344-1144
www.anred.com

National Association of Anorexia Nervosa and Associated Disorders
Hotline: (847) 831-3438
email: anad20@aol.com
www.members.aol.com/anad20

Shapedown
Child and Adolescent Obesity
University of California—San Francisco
Box 900
San Francisco, CA 94143

National Eating Disorders Centre (Canada)
(416) 340-4156
www.nedic.on.ca

SUSTAAN: Supporting the Struggle Against Anorexia Nervosa
(604) 734-0006
www.sustaan.direct.ca

Diabetes
American Diabetes Association
(800) 342-2383
www.diabetes.org
English and Spanish-speaking assistance

Juvenile Diabetes Foundation International Helpline
(800) 533-2873
(212) 785-9595
www.jdfcure.com

Gastrointestinal Diseases
American Celiac Society
58 Musano Court
West Orange, NJ 07052

Celiac Sprue Association/United States of America, Inc.
(402) 558-0600
www.csaceliacs.org

Box continued on following page

R E S O U R C E   B O X   12-1 *Continued*

RESOURCE BOX FOR NUTRITION ISSUES

Gastrointestinal Diseases *Continued*
Celiac Disease Foundation
(818) 990-2354
www.celiac.org

Canadian Celiac Association
(800) 363-7296
www.celiac.ca

Crohn's and Colitis Foundation of America
(212) 685-3440
(800) 932-2423
www.ccfa.org

Gluten Intolerance Group
(206) 325-6980
www.gig@accessone.com

Pulmonary Diseases
Cystic Fibrosis Foundation
6931 Arlington Rd.
Bethesda, MD 20814

Growth Charts for Children With Special Conditions
In Hall J, Frostr-Iskenius UG, Allanson JE: The Handbook of Normal Physical Measurements. Oxford, Oxford University Press, 1989.
  Achondroplasia height and head circumference, male and female
  Marfan syndrome height
  Noonan syndrome height
  Prader-Willi height
  Williams syndrome height
  Arthrogryposis-amyoplasia, height and distal heights, male and female
  Multiple ptergium height, male and female
  Diastrophic dysplasia height
  Pseudoachondroplasia height
  Spondyloepiphyseal dysplasia congenita height
  Turner syndrome

From Child Development and Rehabilitation Center, Genetics Clinic 503-494-8307:
  Myelomeningocele height and weight, male and female, ages 2–18 years
  Asian children, height and weight, male and female, ages 0–6 years

From Cystic Fibrosis Foundation, (800) FIGHT-CF:
  Cystic fibrosis growth chart

From Platt OS: Sickle cell anemia. N Engl J Med 311:7, 1984.
  Sickle cell anemia growth chart

Other
About Face USA
(800) 225-3223

American Cleft Palate Association
(800) 242-5338

Human Nutrition Information Service/USDA
Public Affairs Staff
(301) 436-8617

National Center for Nutrition and Dietetics (NCND)
The American Dietetic Association
(312) 899-0040
Consumer Nutrition Hotline: (800) 366-1655

American School Food Service Association
(703) 739-3900

National Association of School Nurses, Inc.
(207) 883-2117

REFERENCES

ADA Reports: Position of the American Dietetic Association: Vegetarian diets. J Am Diet Assoc 97:1317–1321, 1997.

American Academy of Pediatrics Committee on Nutrition: Cholesterol in children. Pediatrics 101:141–147, 1998.

American Dietetic Association: Position of the American Dietetic Association: Nutrition services for children with special health care needs. J Am Diet Assoc 89:1133–1137, 1989a.

American Dietetic Association: Position of the American Dietetic Association: Optimal weight as a health promotion strategy. J Am Diet Assoc 89:1814–1817, 1989b.

American Dietetic Association: Position of the American Dietetic Association: Nutrition care for pregnant adolescents. J Am Diet Assoc 94:449–450, 1994.

American Psychiatric Association: Diagnostic and Statistical Manual of Mental Disorders IV [DSM-IV]. Washington, DC, Author, 1994.

Andersen RE, Crespo CJ, Bartlett SJ, et al: Relationship of

physical activity and television watching with body weight and level of fatness among children: Results from the Third National Health and Nutrition Examination Survey. JAMA 279:938–942, 1998.

Barlow SE, Dietz WH: Obesity evaluation and treatment: Expert Committee recommendations. The Maternal and Child Health Bureau, Health Resources and Services Administration and the Department of Health and Human Services. Pediatrics 102:E29, 1998.

Behrman RE, Kliegman RM, Arvin AM (eds): Nelson Textbook of Pediatrics, 15th ed. Philadelphia, WB Saunders, 1996.

Bock SA, Sampson HA, Atkins FM: Double-blind, placebo-controlled food challenge (DBPCFC) as an office procedure: A manual. J Allergy and Clin Immunol 82:986–997, 1988.

Burks AW, James JM, Hiegel A: Atopic dermatitis and food hypersensitivity reactions. J Pediatr 132:132–136, 1998.

Centers for Disease Control: Guidelines for school and community health programs to promote lifelong physical activity among young people. Morbid Mortal Wkly Rep 46:RR-6, 1997.

Chandra RK: Five-year follow-up of high-risk infants with family history of allergy who were exclusively breast-fed or fed partial whey hydrosylate, soy, and conventional cow's milk formulas. J Pediatr Gastroenterol Nutr 24:380–388, 1997.

Dagnelie PC, Van Staveren WA, Van den Berg H: Vitamin B-12 from algae appears not to be bioavailable. Am J Clin Nutr 53:695–697, 1991.

Davis J, Sherer K: Applied Nutrition and Diet Therapy for Nurses, 2nd ed. Philadelphia, WB Saunders, 1994.

Decker SD: Eating disorders: Anorexia and bulimia. *In* Johnson BS (ed): Psychiatric-Mental Health Nursing: Adaptation and Growth, 3rd ed. Philadelphia, JB Lippincott, 1993.

Dennison BA, Rockwell HL, Baker SL: Excess fruit juice consumption by preschool-aged children is associated with short stature and obesity. Pediatrics 99:15–22, 1997.

DiBattista D, Shepherd ML: Primary school teacher's beliefs and advice to parents concerning sugar consumption and activity in children. Psychol Rep 72:47–55, 1993.

Ekvall SW (ed): Pediatric nutrition in chronic diseases and developmental disorders: Prevention, assessment, and treatment. New York, Oxford University Press, 1993.

Ekvall SW, Ekvall VK, Frazier T: Dealing with nutrition problems of children with developmental disorders. Topics Clin Nutr 8:51–57, 1993.

Elster AB, Kuznets NJ: AMA Guidelines for Adolescent Preventive Services (GAPS): Recommendations and Rationale. Baltimore, Williams & Wilkins, 1994.

Finberg L: Saunders Manual of Pediatric Practice. Philadelphia, WB Saunders, 1998.

Golan M, Weizman A, Apter A, et al: Parents as the exclusive agents of change in the treatment of childhood obesity. Am J Clin Nutr 67:1130–1135, 1998.

Gorrie T, McKinney E, Murray S: Foundations of Maternal-Newborn Nursing. Philadelphia, WB Saunders, 1998.

Hahn NI: When food becomes a cry for help: How dietitians can combat childhood eating disorders. Interview with Monika M. Woolsey. J Am Diet Assoc 98:395–398, 1998.

Hall J, Frostr-Iskenius UG, Allanson JE: The Handbook of Normal Physical Measurements. Oxford, Oxford University Press, 1989.

Hands ES: Food Finder: Food Sources of Vitamins and Minerals, 3rd ed. Salem, OR, ESHA Research, 1995.

Hattner J, Kerner J: Approximate Composition of Pediatric Formulas. Stanford, CA, Stanford University Medical Center/Lucile Packard Children's Hospital, 1997.

Hernandez B, Uphold CR, Graham MV, et al: Prevalence and correlates of obesity in preschool children. J Pediatr Nursing 13:68–76, 1998.

Hodson AH: Empirical use of exclusion diets in chronic disorders: Discussion paper. J R Soc Med 85:556–559, 1992.

Hourihane JO'B: Prevalence and severity of food allergy—Need for control. Allergy 53(suppl):84–88, 1998.

Houseknecht KL, Baile CA, Matteri RL, et al: The biology of leptin: A review. J Anim Sci 76:1405–1420, 1998.

Kleinman RE, Finberg LF, Klish WJ, et al: Dietary guidelines for children: U.S. recommendations. J Nutr 126(suppl):1028s–1030s, 1996.

Krummel DA, Seligson FH, Guthrie HA: Hyperactivity: Is candy causal? Crit Rev Food Sci Nutr 36:31–47, 1996.

Lifshitz F, Tarim O: Considerations about dietary fat restrictions for children. J Nutr 126(suppl):1031s–1041s, 1996.

Lovblad K, Ramelli G, Remonda L, et al: Retardation of myelination due to dietary vitamin B_{12} deficiency: Cranial MRI findings. Pediatr Radiol 27:155–158, 1997.

Maffeis C, Zaffanello M, Schutz Y: Relationship between physical inactivity and adiposity in prepubertal boys. J Pediatr 131:288–292, 1997.

Mahan LK, Arlin M: Krause's Food Nutrition and Diet Therapy, 8th ed. Philadelphia, WB Saunders, 1992.

Mei Z, Scanlon KS, Grummer-Strawn LM, et al: Increasing prevalence of overweight among US low-income preschool children: The Centers for Disease Control and Prevention Pediatric Nutrition Surveillance, 1983–1995. Pediatrics 101:E12, 1998.

Melnik TA, Rhoades SJ, Wales KR, et al: Overweight school children in New York City: Prevalence estimates and characteristics. Int J Obesity Rel Metabolic Dis 22:7–13, 1998.

Munoz KA, Krebs-Smith SM, Ballard-Barbash R, et al: Food intakes of US children and adolescents compared with recommendations. Pediatrics 100:323–329, 1997.

National Institutes of Health Consensus Development Panel on Optimal Calcium Intake: Optimal calcium intake. JAMA 272:1942–1948, 1994.

Niinikoski H, Lapinleimu H, Viikari J, et al: Growth until 3 years of age in a prospective, randomized trial of a diet with reduced saturated fat and cholesterol. Pediatrics 99:687–694, 1997.

North American Nursing Diagnosis Association: NANDA Nursing Diagnosis: Definitions and Classification 1997–1998. Philadelphia, Author, 1996.

Nutrition Education Services/Oregon Dairy Council: Pyramid Plus: A Star-Studded Guide to Food Choices for Better Health. Portland, OR, Author, 1994.

Ogden CL, Troiano RP, Briefel RR, et al: Prevalence of overweight among preschool children in the United States, 1971 through 1994. Pediatrics 99:E1, 1997.

Pietrobelli A, Faith MS, Allison DB, et al: Body mass index as a measure of adiposity among children and adolescents: A validation study. J Pediatr 132:204-210, 1998.

Platt OS: Sickle cell anemia. N Engl J Med 311:7, 1984.

Rathbun JM, Peterson KE: Nutrition in failure to thrive. *In* Grand RJ, Sutphen JL, Dietz WH (eds): Pediatric Nutrition. Boston: Butterworth, 1987.

Region X Nursing Network: Region X Nursing Network Standards for Prenatal and Child Health. Seattle, University of Washington, 1998.

Saukkonen T, Virtanen SM, Karppinen M, et al: Significance of cow's milk protein antibodies as risk factor for childhood IDDM: Interactions with dietary cow's milk intake and HLA-DQB1 genotype. Diabetologia 41:72-78, 1998.

Seidell JS: Dietary fat and obesity: An epidemiologic perspective. Am J Clin Nutr 67(suppl):545s-550s, 1998.

Sinha MK, Caro JF: Clinical aspects of leptin. Vitam Horm 54:1-30, 1998.

Stice E, Killen JD, Hayward C, et al: Age of onset for binge eating and purging during late adolescence: A 4-year survival analysis. J Abnorm Psych 107:671-675, 1998.

Suskind RM, Lewinter-Suskind L: Textbook of Pediatric Nutrition. NY, Raven Press, 1992.

The Writing Group for the DISC Collaborative Research Group: Efficacy and safety of lowering dietary intake of fat and cholesterol in children with elevated low-density lipoprotein cholesterol. JAMA 273:1429-1435, 1995.

U.S. Preventive Services Task Force: Guide to Clinical Preventive Services, 2nd ed. Baltimore, Williams & Wilkins, 1996.

U.S. Public Health Service: Put Prevention into Practice: The Clinician's Handbook of Preventive Services, 2nd ed. McLean, VA, International Medical Publishing, 1997.

Virtanen SM, Saukkonen T, Savilahti E, et al: Diet, cow's milk protein antibodies and the risk of IDDM in Finnish children. Diabetologia 37:381-387, 1994.

Whitaker RC, Wright JA, Pepe MS, et al: Predicting obesity in young adulthood from childhood and parental obesity. N Engl J Med 337:926-927, 1997.

Wolraich ML, Wilson DB, White JW: The effect of sugar on behavior or cognition in children. A meta-analysis. JAMA 274:756-757, 1996.

Wynne AL, Woo TM, Millard M: Pharmacotherapeutics for Nurse Practitioner Prescribers. Philadelphia, FA Davis (in press).

Zlotkin SH: A review of the Canadian "Nutrition recommendations update: Dietary fat and children." J Nutr 126(suppl):1022s-1027s, 1996.

CHAPTER 13

Breastfeeding

Pam Hellings

INTRODUCTION

Breast milk provides the ideal food for newborns and infants and supports infant nutrition essential for optimal growth and development. In addition, the parents and the infant receive psychological, physical, and emotional benefits that last a lifetime. A high priority should be placed on promoting and supporting breastfeeding whenever possible.

Breastfeeding is a learned skill for both the mother and the infant. Nurse practitioners (NPs) have an important role in assessing the mother's knowledge level and in providing information and support to increase the skills of the mother–infant dyad during the transition to a successful breastfeeding experience. More generally, NPs play an important part in the promotion, education, outreach, support, and management of breastfeeding. NPs can teach about the benefits of breast milk so that families can make educated choices about infant feeding. They can provide classes to increase knowledge in order to avoid common problems or assist in the decision to seek consultation for problems. Additionally, the NP's willingness to take the time required to determine the cause of a breastfeeding problem, to develop a plan to address the problem, and to support the family through difficulties may make the difference in continuation of breastfeeding. Among health-care professionals, the NP can play a ma-

jor role by contributing to hospital, clinic, and community committees, advisory boards, and task forces that develop policies to promote and support breastfeeding; advising and educating colleagues on breastfeeding issues; teaching breastfeeding content to students in the health professions; and serving as an expert contact for the media on issues related to breastfeeding. In all these activities, the NP serves an important leadership function in promoting and supporting breastfeeding.

Breastfeeding Recommendations

Major health professional organizations, including the National Association of Pediatric Nurse Associates and Practitioners (1993) and the American Academy of Pediatrics (1997), recommend breastfeeding for the first year of life. Despite these strong recommendations, much work remains to be done and NPs can make a major contribution to the success of breastfeeding efforts.

The Baby-Friendly Hospital Initiative

In 1991, a worldwide effort to recognize hospitals that provide optimal lactation support was developed by the World Health Organization (WHO) and the United Nations International Children's Emergency Fund (UNICEF) (UNICEF,

1992). This effort, known as the Baby Friendly Hospital Initiative, bases assessment of the quality of a lactation program on 10 steps for successful breastfeeding, delineated in a joint WHO/UNICEF statement (WHO/UNICEF, 1989). Every facility that provides maternity services and care for newborn infants should

- Have a written breastfeeding policy that is routinely communicated to all health-care staff.
- Train all health-care staff in skills necessary to implement this policy.
- Inform all pregnant women about the benefits and management of breastfeeding.
- Help mothers initiate breastfeeding within a half hour of birth.
- Show mothers how to breastfeed and how to maintain lactation even if they should be separated from their infants.
- Give newborn infants no food or drink other than breast milk, unless medically indicated.
- Practice rooming-in (i.e., allow mothers and infants to remain together) 24 hours a day.
- Encourage breastfeeding on demand.
- Give no artificial teats or pacifiers (also called dummies or soothers) to breastfeeding infants.
- Foster the establishment of breastfeeding support groups and refer mothers to them on discharge from the hospital or clinic.

CHARACTERISTICS OF HUMAN MILK

Benefits of Breastfeeding

With rare exception, breast milk is the ideal food for the human infant. Each mammalian species provides a unique milk for its offspring, and milk from the human breast is no exception. It is a living fluid rich in vitamins, minerals, fat, proteins (including immunoglobulins/antibodies), carbohydrates (especially lactose), enzymes, and cellular components, including macrophages and lymphocytes, as well as many other constituents that offer ideal support for growth and maturation of the human infant. Even as complementary foods are added after 5

to 6 months, breast milk continues to make an important nutritional contribution. Amazingly, as the infant grows and develops, the properties of the breast milk change. The sequence of colostrum, transitional milk, and mature milk meets the changing nutritional needs of the newborn and infant. In addition, some of the constituent properties in the milk are different from one time of the day to another and change with the passage of time over the months of the infant breastfeeding experience. Thus the milk of a mother of a 9-month-old has differences in concentrations of fat, protein, and carbohydrate, as well as differences in physical properties such as pH, when compared with the milk of the mother of a 1-month-old.

Breastfed babies have additional protection against bacterial, viral, and protozoan illnesses. Despite some methodological difficulties, various studies have documented decreases in the incidence and severity of allergies and gastrointestinal and respiratory diseases, including ear infections, diarrhea, and pneumonia (Cushing et al., 1998). Breast milk supports the growth of *Lactobacillus bifidus* in the intestine of the breastfed infant and creates an environment that discourages the growth of pathogens such as *Salmonella* and *Shigella*. Lactoferrin, an iron-binding protein, inhibits the growth of certain iron-dependent bacteria in the gastrointestinal tract.

Breastfeeding also provides an economic incentive as a free and plentiful source of excellent infant nutrition. The cost of formula and other necessary supplies can exceed $1000 each year.

Contraindications to Breastfeeding

In addition to all the beneficial nutrients that are provided to the infant during breastfeeding, certain infections and many drugs/medications can also be passed to the infant via breast milk. Although rare, contraindications to breastfeeding occur in some of these situations. In addition, a small number of infant conditions also preclude breastfeeding. Contraindications to breastfeeding include

- A human immunodeficiency virus (HIV)-positive mother (living in a developed nation)

- Maternal abuse of cocaine and intravenous drugs
- Maternal exposure to radioactive compounds
- Regular maternal use of drugs such as lithium, anticancer drugs, thiouracil, iodides or bromides, and ergot compounds
- Herpetic lesions on the mother's nipples, areolas, or breast
- Maternal diagnosis and treatment of cancer
- Infant with galactosemia

Special Situations

Additional circumstances require special consideration regarding the advisability or management of breastfeeding. These circumstances include:

- Significant maternal or infant illness affecting the ability to feed
- Maternal illness such as tuberculosis, chickenpox, or hepatitis B
- Invasive breast surgery, particularly breast reduction in which the areola was removed and reattached
- History of milk supply problems

Components of Human Milk

The uniqueness of human milk to support the growth and development of the human infant cannot be overestimated. Scientists continue to find new components and to clarify the purposes of known components. Over 200 constituents of milk have been identified (Lawrence & Lawrence 1999).

COLOSTRUM

Colostrum production begins at about 20 weeks of gestation. The pregnant woman may notice a small amount of yellow discharge on her nipple or clothing. After delivery of the baby, production of colostrum increases to 2 to 20 dl per feeding. This thick, rich, yellowish fluid has fewer calories than mature milk does (67 vs. 75 kcal/100 ml) and is lower in fat (2 vs. 3.8%). It is rich in immunoglobulins, especially IgA, and other antibodies. In addition, it is higher in sodium, chloride, protein, fat-soluble vitamins, and cholesterol than mature milk and facilitates the passage of meconium. Because of the outstanding contribution to the infant's immunological status, colostrum is often referred to as the infant's "first immunization." Colostrum provides everything that a normal term newborn needs for the first few days of life, and no routine supplementation is needed.

TRANSITIONAL MILK

Transitional milk appears several days after delivery. Significant variability is seen in the constituent properties of transitional milk between mothers and within samples from the same mother. However, as a general rule, transitional milk has more lactose, calories, and fat and less total protein than colostrum does.

MATURE MILK

Mature milk gradually replaces transitional milk by about the second week after delivery and provides, on average, 20 kcal/oz.

WATER. Approximately 90% of human milk is water. Breast milk can meet the fluid needs of the infant without any supplementation, even in tropical and desert climates.

FAT/LIPID CONTENT. The various fats/lipids make up the second greatest percentage of constituents of human milk. They are also the most variable component, with differences noted within a feeding, between feedings, in feedings over time, and between different mothers. On average, the fat content is approximately 3.8% and contributes 30 to 55% of the kilocalories in human milk. During feeding, the fluid content of the mammary gland becomes mixed with droplets of fat in increasing concentration. Thus the fat content is higher at the end of the feeding (hindmilk) than it is at the beginning (foremilk). The type and amount of fat in the maternal diet seem to affect the type of lipid but not the total amount of fat found in the mother's breast milk.

The cholesterol content varies little in human milk and is approximately 240 mg/100 g of fat. Changes in the maternal diet do not produce changes in these cholesterol values. Breastfed infants have higher plasma cholesterol levels than do formula-fed infants. In the animal world, it appears that rats given higher levels of cholesterol early in life had lower cholesterol values as they aged (Osborn, 1968), and a similar effect has been argued in the human world. Osborn (1968) also noted a lower incidence of coronary artery disease in individuals up to 20 years of age who were breastfed.

PROTEIN. Approximately 0.9% of the contents of human milk is protein. When milk is heated or exposed to enzymes as in digestion, a clot, or casein, is formed. The clear portion that remains is known as whey. In human milk, 60 to 70% of the protein is whey, which primarily consists of α-lactalbumin and lactoferrin, and 30 to 40% is casein. In contrast, cow's milk is 20% lactalbumin and 80% casein, with distinct chemical differences between the casein found in cow's milk and that found in human milk. The curds of human milk are more easily digested by the infant. Other proteins include immunoglobulins, nonimmunoglobulins, and lysozyme—a nonspecific antibacterial factor.

CARBOHYDRATES. The primary carbohydrate of human milk is lactose, which is synthesized by the mammary gland from glucose. Lactose is highly concentrated in human milk (6.8 vs. 4.9 g/100 ml in cow's milk) and appears to be essential for growth of the human infant. In addition, lactose enhances the absorption of calcium, a potentially important role because of the relatively low level of calcium in human milk.

VITAMINS AND MINERALS. Human milk has more than adequate amounts of vitamins A, E, K, C, B_1, B_2, and B_6. However, the level of vitamin D intake may not be adequate in breastfed infants who lack exposure to sunlight because of weather, living conditions, or being swaddled with the head covered. Thirty minutes per week of exposure to the sun while dressed in a diaper only or 2 hours per week clothed (as long as the head is not covered) provides adequate vitamin D for a breastfed infant (Specker et al., 1985). The NP needs to assess the situation for each infant individually to see whether supplementation is warranted because of the lack of any recommendation for universal vitamin D supplementation.

Iron is found in low levels in human milk. However, iron absorption from human milk is very efficient, with 49% of the available iron absorbed in contrast to 4% from formula. A full-term infant who is exclusively breastfed for 4 to 6 months is not at risk for iron deficiency anemia.

Zinc, another mineral identified as important to the human infant, is readily available in human milk and has an absorption rate of 41% vs. 31% from cow's milk protein formulas and 14% from soy formulas.

ANATOMY AND PHYSIOLOGY

Pregnancy brings about the final stage of mammogenesis—growth and differentiation of the mammary gland and development of the structures to support breast milk production. Estrogen, progesterone, placental lactogen, and prolactin all play a role in mammogenesis. By approximately 20 weeks, the breast is capable of milk production. The actual production of breast milk is triggered by the fall in progesterone concentration after birth of the baby. Placental retention inhibits milk production because of the influence of progesterone and other hormones.

Suckling by the infant plays an important role in the establishment and maintenance of lactation. The amount of milk produced is dependent on stimulation of the breast, removal of milk from the breast, and release of hormones. The concept of "supply and demand" is an important one for NPs and parents to understand. Suckling stimulates the hypothalamus to decrease prolactin-inhibiting factor, thus permitting release of prolactin by the anterior pituitary, leading to a rise in the level of prolactin. The hypothalamus also stimulates the synthesis and release of oxytocin by the posterior pituitary (Fig. 13-1).

Prolactin levels are directly proportional to the level of suckling by the infant. In addition, baseline levels vary greatly from one woman to another. Prolactin is more important to the initiation than to the maintenance of lactation.

Oxytocin reacts with receptors in the myoepithelial cells of the milk ducts to initiate a contracting action that results in forcing milk down the ducts. This action leads to an increase in milk pressure called the "let down reflex" or milk ejection reflex. Oxytocin also aids in maternal uterine involution.

Under the influence of the hormones mentioned previously, the mammary gland undergoes a dramatic change with an increase in size and rapid growth of the lobuloalveolar tissue. The alveoli are the site of milk production and combine in numbers of 10 to 100 to form lobuli. Twenty to 40 lobuli combine into lobes, and 15 to 25 lobes empty into a lactiferous duct. The ducts transport the milk to the nipple (Fig. 13–2).

The nipple and surrounding areola serve as a visual and tactile target to assist with latch-on. The size and shape of the woman's breast and areola vary greatly. Fortunately, the size of the breast is *not* a predictor of breast milk volume. Even women with very small breasts can successfully breastfeed. The NP should be alert, however, for the occasional presence of insufficient glandular tissue, which is characterized by the absence of breast changes associated with pregnancy, a unilaterally underdeveloped breast, or conical-shaped breasts (Neifert et al., 1985).

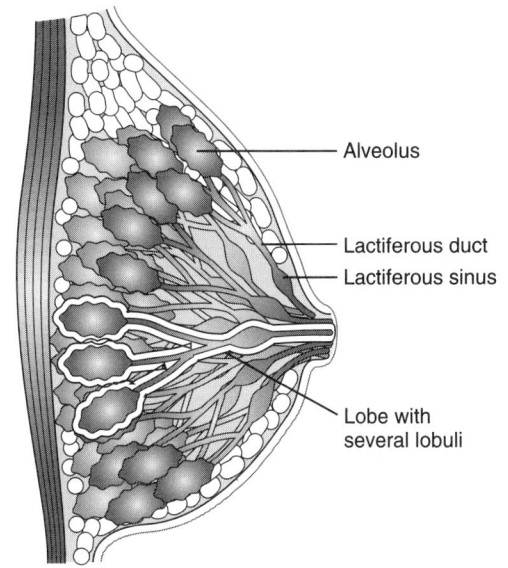

FIGURE 13-2
Anatomy of the breast.

The size, shape, and position of the nipple also vary among women. The nipple may be everted (protuberant from the breast), flat, or inverted. It is not always possible to detect an inverted nipple by observation only. The "pinch test" may be needed to identify nipples that invert with tactile stimulation to the areola. To accomplish the pinch test, the NP places the thumb and forefinger on opposite sides of the areola about 1 to 1½ inches back from the nipple-areolar junction. Gentle compression as though bringing the two fingers together will result in the nipple becoming more everted or inverted. This assessment should be conducted prenatally on every patient (Fig. 13–3). Management of inverted nipples is discussed later in the chapter.

Despite the complexity of the anatomical and physiological processes, the great news is that breastfeeding can proceed for the mother and the baby with little or no awareness on their part of these considerations!

ASSESSMENT OF THE BREASTFEEDING DYAD

Prenatal assessment focuses on maternal expectations for breastfeeding, knowledge about

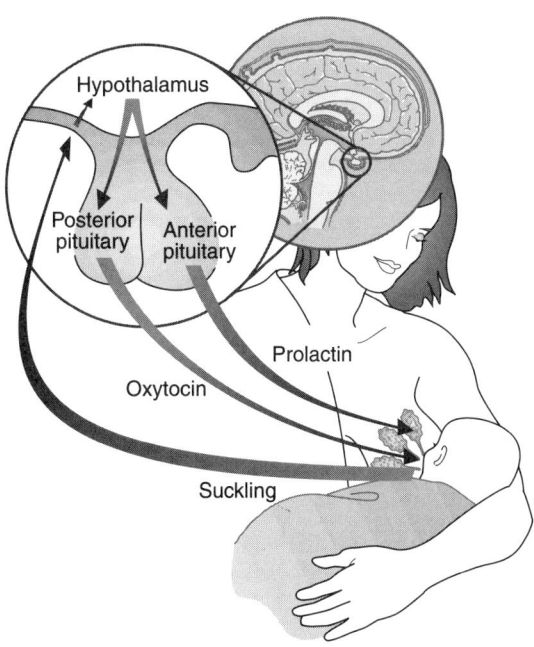

FIGURE 13-1
Neuroendocrine loop.

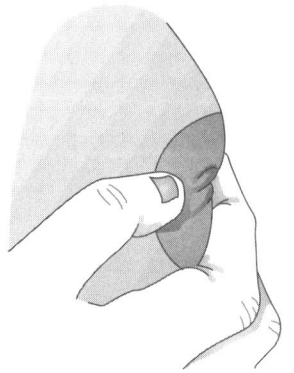

F I G U R E 13-3
Pinch test.

breastfeeding, especially techniques for getting off to a good start, and identification of any contraindications to breastfeeding. A nipple evaluation should be completed. All pregnant women should be assessed, not just primiparas. In the early postpartum period, assessment focuses on the transition to breastfeeding and should include observation of a feeding. In addition, signs of progress for successful breastfeeding should be reviewed, and contact persons for follow-up or questions should be identified by name and phone number.

Maternal History

In general, subjective data should be collected about the following areas:

- Overall health, including documentation of any chronic illnesses or allergies
- Previous breastfeeding experience
- Routine use of over-the-counter, prescribed, or recreational/street drugs, including tobacco
- Surgical interventions, especially to the breast or thoracic region
- Nutritional status
- Family and community support for breastfeeding
- Pregnancy history, especially any complications or need for medications
- Labor and delivery history, including medications, procedures, or complications

Infant History

Subjective data are gathered on the infant in the following areas:

- Overall health status
- Congenital conditions such as cardiac, respiratory, or orofacial conditions
- Trauma or complications during delivery
- Medications received during labor and delivery or in the early postpartum period
- Activities including circumcision, use of bilirubin lights, or use of bottle/cup/tube feeding
- Gestational age
- Early responses to feeding attempts

Maternal Examination

Examination of the mother should focus on an evaluation of the breast in the following areas:

- Type of nipples—everted, flat, or inverted
- Presence of surgical scars on the breast or thoracic area
- Any nipple bruising or bleeding

Infant Examination

Examination of the infant's oral–motor skills and structures serves as the basis for the examination. The infant should be able to suck smoothly and evenly as a finger is inserted into the infant's mouth. The examiner's finger should be inserted beyond the gum line nearly to the soft palate to assess the wave-like motion of the tongue as the infant draws the finger in for suckling. The hard and soft palate should be intact without palpable clefts or submucosal clefts. The infant should be able to extend the tongue over the lower gum with no evidence of a tight frenulum. In the process of the examination, the infant's state of alertness and readiness for feeding are also observed.

▬▬ POSITIONS FOR BREASTFEEDING

Getting off to a good start begins with positioning the baby at the breast in a way that is comfortable for both the mother and baby and that allows for good latch-on. The three most common positions include the cradle, side-lying, and football hold.

Principles of Correct Positioning

Several principles are common to all the various positions for breastfeeding. These principles include the following:

- Both the mother and the baby should be comfortable.
- The infant should be positioned "face-on" at nipple height so that no head turning or tilting is required. The nipple should be directed toward the center of the infant's mouth.
- The infant should be lying on the side, not the back.
- The infant's body should be in good alignment, with a straight line from the ear to the shoulder to the hips.
- The infant's top and bottom lips should be flanged out (Fig. 13–4).
- The infant's tongue should extend forward over the lower gum line and cup around the nipple and areola.
- Good latch-on results in quiet feedings. No "clicking" or "popping" sounds should be heard from the infant.
- After mother's milk is in, audible swallowing, like a "glug" or air blowing out the baby's nose, should be heard.

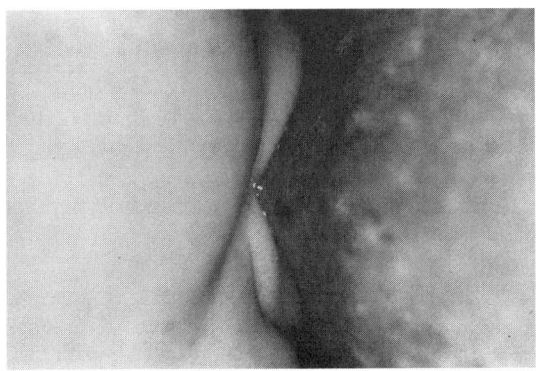

F I G U R E 13-4
Lip position. (Courtesy of UNICEF.)

Cradle Position

The cradle position (also called the Madonna or cuddle position) and its variation known as the cross-cradle position begin with the mother sitting upright or leaning slightly forward with her feet on the floor/stool or her legs crossed in front of her. The infant is held with the mouth at nipple height, and the mother and infant are in a tummy-to-tummy arrangement. The mother uses her free hand to support the breast, if needed, while keeping her fingers well back from the areola so that she does not interfere with latch-on. The "cigarette hold" or pinching of the breast tissue should not be used. In the regular cradle position, the baby's head is supported in the crook of the elbow on the same side as the breast being suckled (Fig. 13–5). In the cross-cradle position, the baby's head and shoulders are supported by the opposite hand. This position often works well for a premature infant because it provides extra support to the head and shoulders (Fig. 13–6).

After positioning the baby, the mother should touch the baby's lower lip with her nipple to stimulate mouth opening. As the mouth opens, the mother should bring the baby close so that the lips come up and over the nipple and back onto the areolar tissue and the nipple rests on top of the baby's tongue. Once the baby appears latched on, the mother can check the lips for a flanged, open placement. At this point the baby is very close to the breast, with the tip of the infant's nose touching it. Mothers often need to be shown that the baby is able to breathe without a need to press down on the breast tissue. If the baby appears to be pushed into the breast, the infant's buttocks should be brought closer into the tummy-to-tummy position. As the mother looks down at her baby, she should see a straight line from the baby's ear, to the shoulders, to the hips. Once the baby is suckling well, the mother can usually remove the hand that was supporting her breast and use it to cradle the baby in her arms. She can also relax back from the forward-leaning position that she used at the beginning.

Side-Lying Position

The side-lying or other lying-down variations are often helpful when the mother is uncomfortable sitting up or wishes to nap or sleep with her baby. In the early days of learning to achieve latch-on, the side-lying position is not easy to use because the mother cannot see her breast and nipple quite as well. In the hospital, a nurse should be available to help the mother and infant. At home and with practice, the mother and infant can achieve latch-on without assistance.

In the side-lying position, the mother lies on her side, cradles her infant in her elbow, and supports the infant's back and neck. The mother or the nurse should arrange one to two pillows under the mother's head and shoulders and a rolled towel or blanket along the infant's back to keep the infant in a side-lying position. As in the cradle position, the mother may sup-

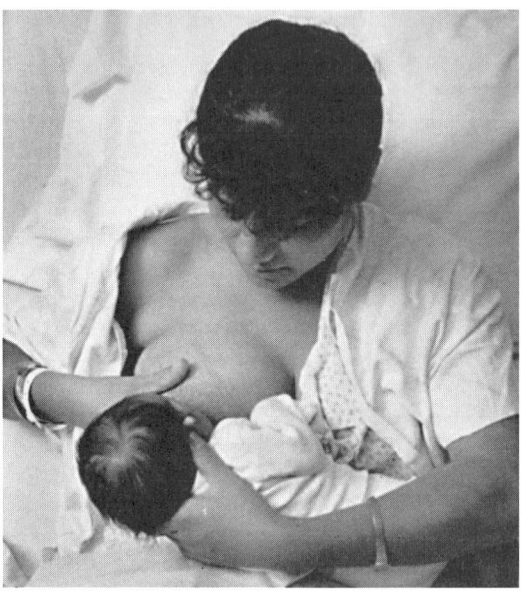

F I G U R E 13-6
Cross-cradle position. (From Gorrie TM, McKinney ES, Murray SS [eds]: Foundations of Maternal Newborn Nursing, 2nd ed. Philadelphia, WB Saunders, 1998.)

port her breast with her upper hand (Fig. 13-7).

Football Hold

In the football hold, the infant is supported off to the side of the mother. This position is often used by a mother who has had a cesarean delivery because it does not require that the infant be positioned along her abdomen. In addition, this position can be used by a mother of multiples when she would like to feed two babies at once. Finally, mothers with flat or inverted nipples are often able to achieve latch-on more easily with this position.

One or two firm pillows should be placed at the mother's side to help support the infant. The baby is in a side-lying position and flexed at the hips, with the buttocks back against the chair or couch. As in other positions, the mother may support her breast to assist with latch-on and remove her hand once the baby is suckling well (Fig. 13-8).

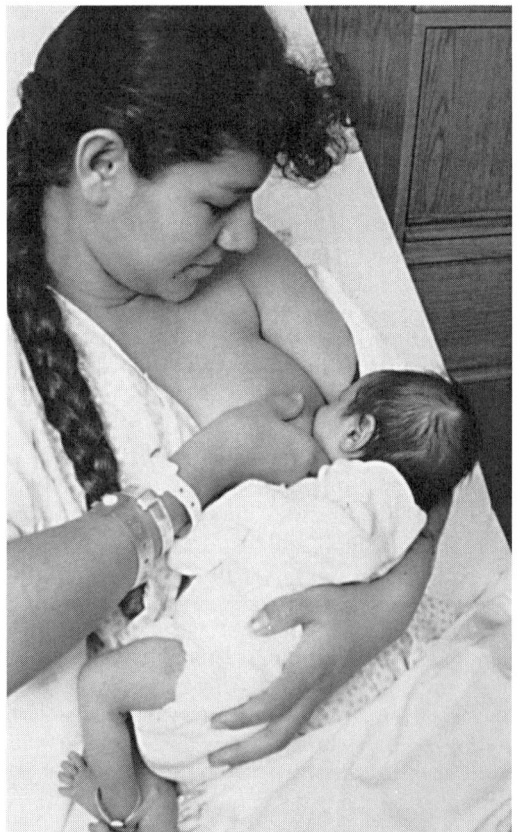

F I G U R E 13-5
Cradle position. (From Gorrie TM, McKinney ES, Murray SS [eds]: Foundations of Maternal Newborn Nursing, 2nd ed. Philadelphia, WB Saunders, 1998.)

DYNAMICS OF BREASTFEEDING

Early Feedings

The first breastfeeding should take place as soon after birth as possible. Full-term neonates often have an alert period for 30 to 60 minutes after delivery that is ideal for the first feeding practice. This first feeding can take place in the delivery area, if necessary, and should be encouraged by all in attendance. This early feeding will not delay, to any significant extent, any procedures required such as weighing and measuring the infant, instilling drops in the infant's eyes, and giving vitamin K injections. These procedures can be done one at a time in the delivery room or at the bedside after return to the room. The mother and infant should remain together as much as possible, with rooming-in preferable. The family needs to be encouraged and supported in making their wishes known to the staff about their desire to promote close contact and initiate breastfeeding. In addition, the NP should advocate changes in institutional policy to support the needs of breastfeeding families.

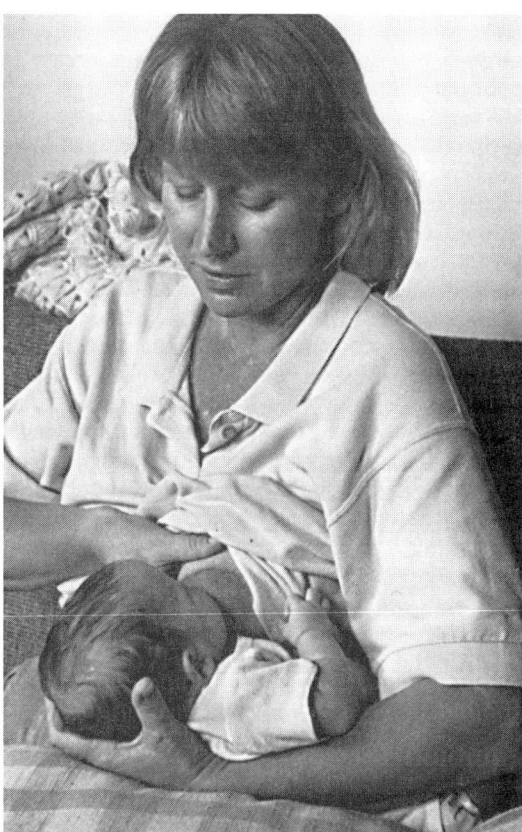

FIGURE 13-8
Football hold. (From Gorrie TM, McKinney ES, Murray SS [eds]: Foundations of Maternal Newborn Nursing, 2nd ed. Philadelphia, WB Saunders, 1998.)

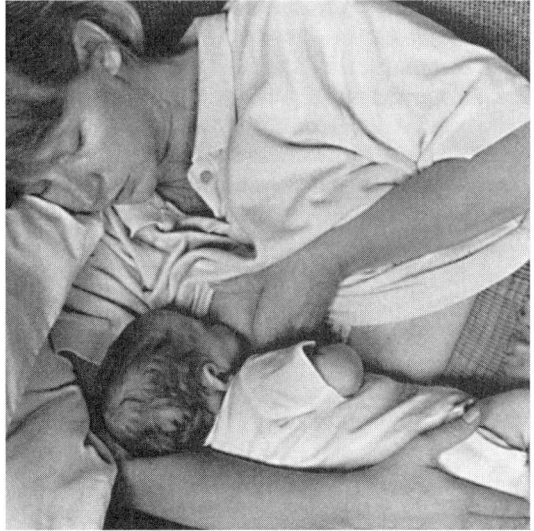

FIGURE 13-7
Side-lying position. (From Gorrie TM, McKinney ES, Murray SS [eds]: Foundations of Maternal Newborn Nursing, 2nd ed. Philadelphia, WB Saunders, 1998.)

The infant usually goes into a deep sleep after the initial alertness and is difficult to wake for feeding practice. Parents should be instructed to watch for any awakening behavior such as opening eyes or movement in the bed. Many newborns will not cry at this point, so parents need to be alert for these signs of feeding readiness. Full-term infants are born with stores of fluid and energy to carry them through this time of infrequent feeding and low volume of colostrum. During this period the infant is making the transition to the nonuterine environment. The stomach, liver, and kidneys are gearing up for the larger volumes of higher fat food that will come in a few days. It is not necessary to provide water, dextrose in water, or formula calories to a healthy, full-term neonate. In addition, the use of a rubber or silicone nipple that does not work like the breast in delivering milk may lead to nipple confusion.

During this transition time, assistance and support from an individual knowledgeable in breastfeeding can be helpful to the mother and infant as they practice latch-on and suckling. The infant should be encouraged to go to each breast for at least 10 to 15 minutes of active suckling, although some infants may spend even longer. The infant's behavior is much more important during this time than the clock. However, an infant who falls asleep in 5 minutes should be stimulated to continue active suckling. Attention to proper positioning and technique becomes important as the frequency and duration of the suckling behavior increase. A mother is unlikely to get sore or cracked nipples when her infant is latched on correctly. These early feedings are excellent "practice" sessions both for the mother, who gains confidence in her breastfeeding ability, and for the infant, who gets first colostrum and then milk for the efforts at suckling.

The goal of discharge planning is to maintain successful breastfeeding and includes the following:

- Review proper positioning.
- Review signs of good latch-on.
- Review signs of infant progress indicating adequate nutrition (Table 13–1).
- Arrange follow-up for 2 to 3 days after discharge.
- Provide a phone contact for questions and concerns.
- Encourage the mother to contact breastfeeding resources whenever she has questions.

These early efforts to provide contact and support during the transition to home can make all the difference in maintaining breastfeeding. Problems encountered during engorgement, sleep deprivation, and times of uncertainty or lack of confidence can be addressed quickly and directly rather than after a bottle has been introduced or the mother's nipples are cracked and bleeding.

Frequency and Duration of Feedings

After the first 24 hours, the infant should be going to the breast 8 to 12 times (or every 2 to 3 hours) in 24 hours for 20 to 45 minutes at each feeding. Frequent suckling stimulates milk production and establishes a regular routine early on. Exclusive breastfeeding for the first month should be encouraged to ensure the establishment of an adequate milk supply and avoid any nipple confusion. Parents need to be alert for an infant who sleeps for 4 to 5 hours at a time or who goes to sleep at the breast in 5 minutes. These infants must be actively wakened and stimulated for feeding.

If the mother and infant must be separated for one or more feedings or supplements are medically necessary, they may be given with a dropper, cup, or a 5-F feeding tube placed at the breast. Proper instructions, close supervision, and follow-up are needed for each of these methods, and they should not be used routinely.

Stool and Urine Output Guidelines

URINE

In the first 2 days of life as the volume of breast milk is increasing, the infant may urinate only one to three times in 24 hours. By day 3 the infant should have four or more wet diapers in 24 hours and then four to six wet diapers per 24 hours by day 4. Over time, the infant should have a minimum of six to eight wet diapers in a 24-hour period. The urine should be light yellow with no strong odor. If the parents are anxious or if they have a question about breastfeeding progress, a diary of wet diapers can be kept to aid in the accurate assessment of progress. Parents need to be alerted, however, to the difficulty of doing accurate diaper counts with disposable diapers and may elect to insert a tissue liner into the diaper or to use cloth diapers for the first few weeks. Ultra-absorbent diapers should be avoided when close monitoring of output is necessary.

STOOL

In the first 24 hours after delivery, the baby should have at least one meconium stool followed by another on day 2. By day 3, stools are beginning to make the transition to the characteristic loose, yellow, seedy stools of

T A B L E 13-1
Signs of Infant Progress: A Handout for Parents

	FIRST 8 H	8–24 H	DAY 2	DAY 3	DAY 4	DAY 5	DAY 6 ON
Milk supply	You may be able to express a few drops of milk		Milk should come in between the 2nd and 4th day			Milk should be in. Breasts may be firm or leak milk	Breasts should feel softer after nursing
Baby's activity	Baby is usually wide awake in first hr of life. Put to breast within ½ hr of birth	Wake your baby. Babies may not awaken on their own to feed	Baby should be more cooperative and less sleepy	Look for early feeding cues: rooting, lip smacking, hands to face. Note that baby swallows regularly while nursing			Baby should appear satisfied after feeding
Feeding routine	Baby may go into a deep sleep 2–4 hr after birth	Feed your baby every 1½–3 hr or as often as wanted	Feedings should be at least 8–10× each day			May go up to 5 hr between feedings (once in a 24-hr period)	
Breastfeeding	Baby will wake up and be alert and responsive for several more hours after the initial deep sleep	Nurse at both breasts as long as baby is actively suckling and mother is comfortable	Try to nurse on both sides at each feeding, aiming for 10–15 min each side Expect some nipple tenderness	Consider hand-expressing or pumping a few drops of milk to soften the nipple if the breast is too firm for the baby to latch on	Nurse at least 10–15 min each side every 2–3 hr for the first few months of life		Mother's nipple tenderness is improved or gone
Baby's urine output		Baby must have at least 1 wet diaper in first 24 hr	Baby should have at least 1 wet diaper every 8 hr	Wet diapers should increase to 4–6 in 24 hr	Baby's urine should be light yellow	Baby should have 6–8 wet diapers per day of colorless or light yellow urine	
Baby's stools	Baby should have a black-green stool (meconium stool)	Baby should have a black-green stool (meconium stool)	Baby may have a second very dark (meconium) stool	Baby's stools should be changing from black-green to yellow		Baby should have 3–4 yellow, seedy stools per day	The number of stools may slowly decrease after 4–6 wk

From Thilo EH, Townsend SF: Early newborn discharge: Have we gone too far? Contemp Pediatr 13:29–46, 1996.

breastfeeding, and the infant should begin having two to three stools in 24 hours. That number may continue to increase in the first few weeks of life. Some infants stool with every feeding. After the first month, the pattern may change again as some infants begin to stool less frequently and may go several days between stools. As long as the infant is healthy and gaining weight, there is no problem. However, infrequent stooling, especially in the first month, should stimulate a feeding history and possibly a weight check to make sure that the infant is getting enough breast milk.

Pumping

Routine pumping is unnecessary during early feedings. However, if the mother and infant must be separated for more than one or two feedings, pumping should be part of the plan to assist with milk production. If the mother and infant are separated right after birth, pumping should begin as soon as possible, within the first 24 hours. The mother should pump six to eight times in 24 hours for 15 minutes if she is using a double-pump setup or 10 minutes per breast if she is using a single-pump setup. She should be encouraged to save even the smallest amounts of colostrum to be given to her infant.

Hand expression and manual pumps work well for infrequent or short-duration pumping. However, a hospital-grade, piston-style pump that permits pumping both breasts at the same time is ideal for a mother who will have to pump for several weeks or months. No pump works as well as an infant in stimulating production, but frequent pumping goes a long way toward establishing a milk supply and provides the mother a concrete, healthful contribution to her sick or preterm infant. As the volume of milk goes up over the first few days, the mother can see the success of her efforts. She should be counseled about the increase in production in contrast to the small volume of colostrum produced in the first few days.

Collection and Storage of Breast Milk

A mother who is pumping should be reminded to wash her hands well before she begins pumping and to use clean containers for collection and storage. In addition, the pump parts should be thoroughly cleaned after each use. Many of the pump parts can go through a dishwasher, but the directions that come with the pump should be consulted for specific instructions on cleaning.

Milk collected from pumping should be stored in clean plastic bottles or disposable milk bags. It is preferable to store breast milk in small amounts so that only the amount that is needed is defrosted and used. Milk that has been defrosted and not used should be discarded. Pumped breast milk should be taken to the refrigerator as soon after pumping as possible and can be stored there for 24 to 48 hours. If it is not going to be used in that time, it should be immediately placed in the freezer. In a refrigerator freezer that maintains a steady temperature, breast milk can be stored for up to 3 months. Breast milk can be stored for more than 6 months in a freezer where 0°F is routinely maintained. The bottles or bags should be labeled with the date of collection so that the oldest milk can be used first. If the milk must be transported to the hospital or day care facility, it should be placed in ice or on a blue ice unit to minimize the amount of warming or thawing.

Infant Weight Gain

Normal newborn infants lose 5 to 10% of their birth weight in the first few days of life. It is helpful for parents to be aware of both the birth and discharge weights. Once the maternal milk volume increases, the infant begins to gain weight in the range of 1/2 to 1 oz/d or 4 to 7 oz/wk. Most breastfed infants have regained their birth weight by 2 weeks. One criterion for failure to thrive is lack of return to birth weight by 3 weeks. Breastfed infants usually double their birth weight by 5 to 6 months of age and triple it by 1 year.

An ongoing study of the growth patterns and nutrient intake of a cohort of breastfed and formula-fed infants (Dewey et al., 1992) has presented evidence that breastfed babies gain at a slower rate after the first 3 months. In fact, an infant who has followed the growth grid curves until 3 or 4 months may be growing at a normal rate for a breastfed infant. In addition, after combining these data with those of six other studies (Dewey et al., 1995), much supportive evidence has shown a need for new growth grids for breastfed infants. In the absence of appropriate growth grids for breastfed infants, an important consideration in the assessment of an apparently slowly gaining infant is developmental progress and other measures of growth. Characteristics of a *healthy*, but slowly growing, breastfed infant include the following:

- Active and alert state
- Developmentally appropriate progress
- Age-appropriate height and head circumference
- Good skin turgor and color
- Sufficient output of at least six wet diapers and several stools per day
- Content and satisfied behavior after feeding

Growth Spurts

Just when the parents begin to think that breastfeeding is going well, the first growth spurt occurs and can once again arouse their concern. The term "growth spurt" is often used to describe those recurring times during breastfeeding when the baby's growth exceeds the breast milk supply at that moment. For 2 to 4 days the infant feeds more frequently to increase milk production. However, an inexperienced parent may interpret this behavior as a sign of inadequate milk production and begin supplementation. This practice leads to inadequate breast milk volume, whereas allowing and even encouraging frequent breastfeeding results in an appropriate increase in milk production. Once the level of milk production has risen, the infant returns to the normal feeding pattern. Growth spurts tend to occur every 3 to 4 weeks, but parents seem to notice them less as time goes on. The behavior becomes an expected part of the breastfeeding experience.

Weaning

The decision about the time for weaning is an individual one. Certainly, breastfeeding should be encouraged for at least 1 year, but individual

circumstances may dictate a different choice for a family. Sometimes the weaning is led by the mother and other times by the infant. Typically, a natural weaning process occurs as other foods become a part of the infant's diet and the infant begins to participate in self-feeding. When a family inquires about the ideal time to begin weaning, the NP can counsel them to consider factors such as

- Beliefs and desires of individual family members
- Developmental readiness of the infant
- Nutritional replacements for breast milk
- Social and environmental issues affecting the decision

Whether weaning occurs as a planned or unplanned activity, it is best to implement it gradually. If necessary, the mother can use a breast pump to gradually decrease milk production and avoid breast engorgement, blocked ducts, and discomfort. A good approach is to pump when uncomfortable and pump only to comfort, not to empty. In situations where weaning was not an anticipated or planned event, the NP may help the mother deal not only with the act of weaning but also with her feelings about it. Some mothers grieve the early loss of the breastfeeding experience.

In an effort to avoid premature weaning, the NP should maintain close communication with families, especially those who are more likely to wean early. Early identification and support of these families may assist them to continue breastfeeding for a longer period. Factors associated with early weaning include:

- Younger, poorer mothers
- Lower maternal education
- Early return of the mother to work outside the home
- Lack of support from family or health professionals
- Previous breastfeeding failure

Maternal Nutritional Needs During Breastfeeding

Maternal nutritional needs increase during lactation. Characteristics of a good diet include:

- A minimum of 1800 calories
- An additional 500 calories over the prepregnant diet

- Generous intake of fruits and vegetables, whole grain breads and cereals, calcium-rich dairy products, and protein-rich meats, fish, and legumes
- Rich sources of calcium, zinc, folate, magnesium, and vitamin B_6
- Culturally appropriate foods
- Supplementation with calcium or prenatal vitamins or both only if the diet is poor (Institute of Medicine, 1991)

The mother should be encouraged to eat well for her own sake to keep herself healthy and to meet the energy demands of nursing. In addition, an adequate intake of fluid is necessary, but excessive use of fluids does not increase breast milk production. A good guideline for adequate fluid intake is maternal urine that is light yellow and has no strong odor. Eligible mothers and infants should be referred to the Women's, Infant's, and Children's (WIC) Special Supplemental Food Program for nutritional counseling, as well as for food supplements. Most WIC programs offer food supplements for the breastfeeding mother's diet because she does not need formula for the infant. Even with a diet that is adequate in nutrients and calories, a gradual maternal weight loss of 1 to 2 lb/mo usually occurs. In fact, breastfeeding is the ideal way for a mother to return to her pre-pregnancy weight.

No foods need to be routinely excluded from the maternal diet unless there is evidence that a particular food bothers the infant or the infant appears allergic to it. Sometimes the food does not need to be eliminated but merely decreased. Maternal intake of cow's milk products has been associated with colic, and some highly allergic babies are extremely sensitive to their mothers' intake of cow's milk protein (Jakobsson & Lindberg, 1983). When a mother has markedly decreased or eliminated cow's milk from her diet, another source of calcium must be identified. Certain foods such as onions and garlic may change the flavor and odor of the milk but do not negatively affect its quality. The nutrient characteristics of breast milk are fairly stable. One positive way to look at the variety of foods in the diets of mothers from all over the world is to acknowledge that infants are getting early exposure to the foods of their culture.

Increased alcohol intake does not improve lactational performance, and in fact, intake of an amount over 0.5 g/kg of maternal body weight (two cans of beer, 8 oz of wine, or 2 to 2.5 oz of liquor) can impair the milk ejection reflex (Institute of Medicine, 1991). The occasional use of small amounts of alcohol need not be avoided, but regular use should be discouraged.

Large amounts of caffeine from coffee, sodas, or chocolate should be discouraged because caffeine is associated with jitteriness in the infant and may have a negative effect on the iron content of the breast milk. However, the equivalent of one to two cups of coffee per day should pose no problem (Institute of Medicine, 1991).

Returning to Work

Women who return to work outside the home while breastfeeding should be encouraged to continue breastfeeding and supported in their decision with accurate information about how to manage both work and breastfeeding. The ideal work environment allows for breaks or lunch time or both in which the mother can pump or go to the infant; it has a private location for pumping with access to a refrigerator for storage, as well as supportive colleagues. NPs can support community initiatives that promote these conditions in employment settings, in addition to providing information regarding pumping, storing, and transporting breastmilk; introducing the bottle; and handling the challenges of multiple demands (Table 13-2). Even a minimal support program that provides access to an electric breast pump and help from the employee health department has been associated with a twofold increase in breastfeeding duration (Katcher & Lanese, 1986).

The world of work benefits from breastfeeding mothers. In one study (Cohen et al., 1995), a comparison of infant illnesses that resulted in 1 day of maternal absence from work demonstrated that 75% occurred in formula-fed babies. In addition, in the 28% of infants who experienced no illnesses, 86% were breastfed. Findings such as these may increase the likelihood that an employer will establish programs to support breastfeeding employees.

T A B L E 13-2

Breastfeeding and Returning to Work: Advice for Mothers

BEFORE RETURNING TO WORK
Practice pumping
Begin freezing milk
Introduce a bottle to your baby at 3 to 4 wk of age
Offer a bottle 1 or 2 times a week

STORAGE OF BREAST MILK
Refrigerate milk for only 24–48 hr
Freeze milk in refrigerator freezer for a maximum of 3 mo; deep-freeze for a maximum of 6 mo
Store milk in plastic baby bottles or disposable milk bags
Label with date and baby's name
Transport milk in cooler bag or container with ice/gel pak

HOW TO INCREASE MILK SUPPLY
Relax and avoid fatigue
Pump an extra time per day or add another feeding
Massage breasts before nursing
Have a picture of your baby at the pump
Play relaxing music or taped sounds of baby while pumping

RETURNING TO WORK
Pump 2–3 times a day, depending on the infant's age
Plan on 15–30 min per pumping session
Wear clothes to hide leaks and offer easy access to breasts

FEEDING BREAST MILK
Warm or thaw milk in warm water
Do not microwave because milk will heat unevenly and present a risk for burns
Refrigerate milk for no more than 24 hr after thawing
Can refeed milk once if the entire bottle is not finished
Refeed leftover milk at next feeding
Do not refeed leftover milk if baby has thrush
Do not add milk to a bottle that has already been used

GENERAL IMPORTANT REMINDERS
Wash hands before and after pumping
Clean pump parts with dish detergent after each use
Have care provider wash hands before and after feeding breast milk

Adapted from Humphrey N: Breastfeeding. Working moms can make it work. Adv Nurs Pract 2:22, 1994.

MEDICATIONS FOR BREASTFEEDING MOTHERS

Frequently, women question whether they can take certain medications while they are breastfeeding. Concerns relate primarily to two areas—the effect of the drug on maternal milk supply and the effect of the drug on the infant. General guidelines for maternal drug recommendations include the following:

- Give drugs that are normally safe for infants and/or have been tested in infants.
- Avoid long-acting forms of a drug.
- Schedule feeding at times when the drug level is lowest. Often, breastfeeding immediately after taking the drug is the safest time.
- Observe the infant for changes in feeding pattern, fussiness, vomiting/diarrhea, or rash.
- Consider all appropriate options and select the drug with the lowest level in breast milk.

- Avoid drugs that inhibit prolactin release such as estrogen, antihistamines, and ergot compounds.
- Be cautious about herbal preparations.

The American Academy of Pediatrics Committee on Drugs (1994) has developed eight categories of drugs grouped by their risk factors for breastfeeding. Four of these groups are summarized in Table 13-3, including drugs that

- Are contraindicated
- Require temporary cessation of breastfeeding

- Have an unknown effect on nursing but may be of concern
- Have been associated with significant effects on some infants and should be used with caution

A good drug reference should be available to the NP. Three excellent resources are shown in Table 13-4. Decisions about drug selection are difficult, especially when contraindicated drugs are being considered, but the consequences of weaning and loss of breast milk for the infant must be included in the deliberations.

T A B L E   13-3
Medications Affecting Breastfeeding

CONTRAINDICATED DRUGS	DRUGS REQUIRING TEMPORARY CESSATION OF BREASTFEEDING	DRUGS WHOSE EFFECT IS UNKNOWN	DRUGS ASSOCIATED WITH SIGNIFICANT EFFECTS
Bromocriptine	Radioactive compounds such as	Antidepressants	5-Aminosalicylic acid
Cocaine	^{64}Cu	Amitriptyline	Aspirin
Cyclophosphamide	^{67}Ga	Amoxapine	Clemastine
Cyclosporine	^{111}I, ^{123}I, ^{125}I, ^{131}I	Desipramine	Phenobarbital
Doxorubicin	Radioactive sodium	Dothiepin	Primidone
Ergotamine	^{99m}Tc	Doxepin	Sulfasalazine
Lithium	Need to stop	Fluoxetine	
Methotrexate	breastfeeding for a	Fluvoxamine	
Phencyclidine (PCP)	minimum of 5 half	Imipramine	
Phenytoin	lives of the drug	Trazodone	
		Antianxieties	
		Diazepam	
		Lorazepam	
		Midazolam	
		Prazepam	
		Quazepam	
		Temazepam	
		Antipsychotics	
		Chlorpromazine	
		Chlorprothixene	
		Haloperidol	
		Mesoridazine	
		Perphenazine	
		Others	
		Chloramphenicol	
		Metoclopramide	
		Metronidazole	
		Tinidazole	

T A B L E 13-4
Drug References

American Academy of Pediatrics Committee on Drugs: The transfer of drugs and other chemicals into human milk. Pediatrics 93:137–150, 1994.

Hale T: Medications and Mothers' Milk. Amarillo, TX, Pharmasoft Medical Publishing, 1998. Updated and reprinted annually. Order by mail from (800) 378-1317. Excellent, inexpensive reference.

Lawrence RM: Breastfeeding: A Guide for the Medical Profession, 5th ed. St Louis, CV Mosby, 1999.

COMMON BREASTFEEDING PROBLEMS

Flat or Inverted Nipples

Description

A nipple can look as though it is inverted, but a "pinch test" is necessary to determine what happens to the nipple during breastfeeding (see the previous description and Fig. 13-3 for the technique). If the nipple pulls in, it is considered to be inverted. If the nipple does not pull in or everts with compression, it is considered to be flat. In most cases the nipple everts when compressed.

Inverted nipples can make it more difficult for the infant to latch on in the early days because it is harder to pull the nipple into the mouth for suckling. As the baby continues to breastfeed, the nipple tissue elongates, and with time, the problem usually becomes less severe and successful breastfeeding is possible.

Flat nipples do not generally change over time, but the infant develops a style to more easily latch on successfully.

Etiology

Adhesions cause retraction or inversion of the nipples. Flat nipples are often found in women with larger breasts.

Differential Diagnosis

The differential diagnosis for flat or inverted nipples is dimpled, fissured, or unusually shaped nipples.

Management

PRENATAL. If the patient is not at risk for preterm labor, breast shells can be used during the third trimester for inverted nipples. The obstetrician or nurse midwife should be notified before their use. Shells are plastic, dome-shaped devices with small holes for ventilation. An opening in the portion that lies against the skin fits over the nipple, and gentle suction during use helps stretch the nipple tissue (Fig. 13-9). The bra cup holds the shell comfortably in place, and the use of shells during the last trimester generally helps stretch out adhesions in preparation for breastfeeding.

POSTPARTUM. The NP should stay with the mother during early feeding attempts; give extra praise, reassurance, and support; and emphasize the need for extra patience and persistence. Encourage use of the football hold position during feedings, and have the mother lean slightly forward as she latches the baby on.

The mother should

- Wear breast shells between feedings
- Manually pull or roll the nipple immediately before latch-on
- Use a breast pump for 1 or 2 minutes before latch-on
- Put a cold cloth or ice on the nipple for a few seconds
- Avoid pacifiers and bottle nipples until the infant is 4 to 6 weeks of age
- If supplementation is medically indicated, use a syringe, dropper, feeding tube, or

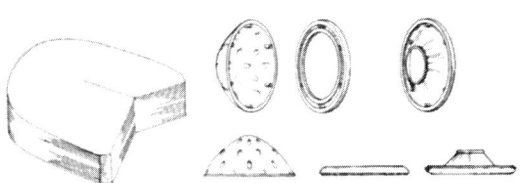

F I G U R E 13-9
Breast shells. (Courtesy of Medela, Inc.)

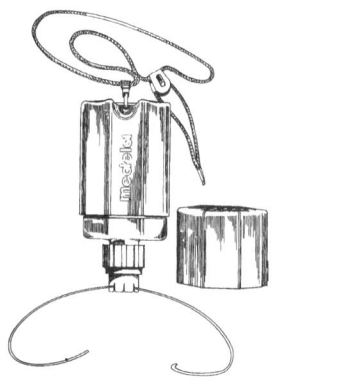

F I G U R E 13-10
Supplemental nursing system. (Courtesy of Medela, Inc.)

supplemental nutrition system (Fig. 13–10).

Complications

Complications of flat or inverted nipples include

- Frustration
- Loss of self-confidence
- Iadequate infant nutrition and its subsequent sequelae
- Severe maternal engorgement, plugged ducts, or mastitis

Sore Nipples

Description

Soreness of the nipples is pain caused by irritation or trauma to the nipples and areolae, often accompanied by a breakdown in skin integrity.

Etiology

Sore nipples have many causes, including

- Improper latch-on and positioning at the breast
- Prolonged negative pressure
- Inappropriate suction release from the breast
- Use of and/or sensitivity to nipple creams and oils
- Incorrect use of breastfeeding supplies (e.g., pumps, shells, shields)
- Thrush (candidiasis)
- Leaking nipples that are not properly air-dried

Clinical Findings

The nipples, areolae, and breasts are tender, bruised, raw, cracked, bleeding, blistered, discolored, swollen, or traumatized.

Differential Diagnosis

The differential diagnoses for sore nipples include the following:

- Mild tenderness, which is sometimes described by new mothers as they are getting used to the infant's suckling
- Breast or nipple trauma from another cause
- Thrush (candidiasis)
- Mastitis
- Abscess
- Milk plugs at the nipple pores

Management

The following measures can be taken to manage sore nipples:

- Assess breastfeeding at an early feeding. Prevent the problem by demonstrating and reinforcing the proper latch-on technique and positioning of the infant.
- Counsel mothers to seek help early for more than mild tenderness. Nipples can be damaged by constant high negative pressure and do not "toughen up" as breastfeeding progresses. Cracking and bleeding are not normal.
- Rub a few drops of colostrum or hindmilk onto the nipple and areola after every feeding and let it air-dry.
- Expose the nipples to air or sunlight for short periods several times a day.
- Use breast shells to prevent the bra or clothing from rubbing against the nipple.
- Nurse from the least sore side first.
- Use short, frequent feedings.
- Pump the affected breast if pain is too severe to allow nursing.

- Use mild analgesics as necessary.
- Refer to a lactation specialist as appropriate.

Severe Engorgement

Description

Severe engorgement is characterized by extremely full, sore, swollen breasts beyond the normal fullness experienced as the milk comes in.

Etiology

Engorgement is caused by milk stasis in the breast from inadequate emptying.

Clinical Findings

The following are seen in severe engorgement:

- Painful, hard, lumpy, swollen breasts
- Breasts usually warm to the touch
- Nipples flattened by the swelling
- Bruising or trauma to the nipples and areolae

Differential Diagnosis

The differential diagnosis for severe engorgement is bilateral mastitis.

Management

The following measures can be taken to manage engorgement:

- Take a hot shower or wrap the breasts with warm, wet compresses for 5 to 10 minutes before nursing. Disposable diapers can be wet with hot water and then wrapped around each breast and "tabbed" to hold them in place. The plastic liner holds the heat in longer than an ordinary washcloth or towel does.
- Gently massage the entire breast or use an electric pump with intermittent suction on the minimal setting for several minutes after using wet heat.
- Manually express milk before feeding to

soften the areola and make it easier for the infant to latch on properly.
- Nurse frequently and make certain that latch-on and position are correct and audible swallowing is heard.
- Avoid long stretches between feedings in the early weeks as the milk supply is being established. Pump the breasts if a feeding will be missed.

Mastitis

Description

Although rarely seen in the postpartum hospital setting, mastitis is an infection of the breast that can occur at any time during lactation. Occasionally, it has been identified during the third trimester of pregnancy.

Etiology

Staphylococcus aureus is most commonly associated with mastitis, but *Escherichia coli* and, more rarely, various streptococci are also found. Predisposing factors include:

- Stress, fatigue
- Cracked nipples, plugged ducts
- Constricting, improperly fitting bra
- Inadequate emptying of the breast
- Sudden weaning or a significant decrease in the number of feedings

Clinical Findings

The following are seen in mastitis:

- Malaise.
- Breast tenderness or pain.
- A reddened, warm lump in any quadrant, sometimes associated with red streaking.
- Flu-like symptoms, including fever, chills, and body aches. An old adage is that the "flu" in a breastfeeding woman is mastitis until proved otherwise.

Management

Recommendations for treatment of mastitis include

- Penicillinase-resistant penicillin or a cephalosporin that covers *S. aureus*. Currently, dicloxacillin is most commonly recommended to treat mastitis. Treatment should be maintained for 10 to 14 days.

- Rest (extremely important).
- Nurse frequently, or if pain is severe, pump milk carefully from the affected breast. Breast milk is not infected and is fine for the infant.
- Do not wean abruptly because of the possibility of mastitis progressing into an abscess.
- Take warm showers or use warm wet compresses.
- Increase fluids.
- Use analgesics as necessary.

Complications

Abscess and septicemia are complications of mastitis.

Nipple Confusion

Description

Nipple confusion is not commonly discussed in research literature but is seen anecdotally by experienced clinicians (Neifert et al., 1995). If babies accustomed to bottle feeding are offered the breast, they use the same sucking pattern as with a bottle: they thrust their tongues up against their mother's nipple, which makes it difficult to obtain adequate nourishment. They may cry, fuss, or push away with their arms during attempts to nurse. A similar phenomenon has been noted in breastfed infants who, when offered a bottle, may react by arching their back, crying, turning their head away from the nipple, and spitting out the formula (Egan, 1988).

Etiology

Different oral-motor skills are used in breastfeeding and bottle feeding, and infants who have been given a bottle or pacifier sometimes attempt to breastfeed as though they were bottle feeding. Nipple confusion cannot be predicted and can occur in some infants after a single bottle feeding (Newman, 1990).

Clinical Findings

The following are seen in nipple confusion:

- Ineffective suckling at the breast
- Breast refusal
- Sore, red, or bruised maternal nipples

Differential Diagnosis

The differential diagnoses for nipple confusion are other causes of fussiness and refusal to feed.

Management

The following are recommended to manage nipple confusion:

- Avoid all rubber bottle nipples and pacifiers for the first 4 to 6 weeks.
- Retrain the infant to suck correctly at the breast by correct positioning at the breast, proper latch-on technique, suck training to repattern tongue movements, and supplementation via alternative methods if required.
- Do not use nipple shields.
- Consult with a lactation specialist as indicated.
- If supplements are medically indicated, give with an eyedropper, spoon, syringe, or cup or through a 5-F feeding tube (attached to a 20- or 30-ml syringe) taped to the areola or breast. The end of the tubing protrudes slightly past the end of the nipple so that the tube, nipple, and areola are in the infant's mouth.

Complications

The following are complications of nipple confusion:

- Failure to thrive
- Hyperbilirubinemia
- Colic and crying
- Prolonged feedings
- Sore and cracked nipples
- Plugged ducts
- Mastitis
- Frustration

Breast Milk Jaundice

Description

Breast milk jaundice is an elevated serum indirect bilirubin concentration occurring on or after the fifth day of life in an infant drinking an adequate amount of breast milk with no other signs of liver pathology.

Etiology and Incidence

The exact cause of breast milk jaundice is unknown; however, an enzyme may be present in some mothers' milk that inhibits the action of glucuronyl transferase. Breast milk jaundice is more common in Asian and North American Indian infants. Siblings with the same mother are often affected. True breast milk jaundice is uncommon and occurs in only 1 to 2% of breastfed infants (Gartner & Auerbach, 1987).

Clinical Findings

PHYSICAL EXAMINATION. The following are seen with breast milk jaundice:

- Healthy and thriving infant
- Adequate stooling and voiding
- Appropriate weight gain
- Appearance of elevated bilirubin levels between the fifth and seventh day of life
- Bilirubin peaks around day 10 to 21
- Persistence into the third month of life

DIAGNOSTIC TESTS. The following tests are usually indicated:

- Serum bilirubin
- Urine and other cultures, which are sometimes necessary to rule out infection

Differential Diagnosis

The differential diagnosis for breast milk jaundice is pathological jaundice.

Management

In breast milk jaundice, breastfeeding should be continued unless clinical signs of pathological jaundice are observed. See Chapter 39 for a discussion of pathological jaundice. The family should be reassured that breast milk jaundice is not harmful.

Thrush

A discussion of thrush is found in Chapter 34. However, when oral candidiasis is diagnosed in the infant or found on the nipple/areolar areas of the nursing mother, both members of the dyad should be treated.

Poor Weight Gain

Description

Problems associated with poor weight gain occur at two different times and represent different challenges for management. During the newborn period, initiation of breastfeeding may not proceed normally and the infant may actually continue to lose weight or, at best, gain very slowly. After the newborn period, infants may gain weight more slowly than expected given normal parameters for their age (Stashwick, 1993).

Etiology

Poor weight gain has a number of contributing factors, including

- Infrequent or inadequate feeding because of poorly managed breastfeeding or environmental or social changes in the family system
- Inadequate milk production
- Genetic heritage
- Infection
- Organic disease
- Physical anomaly that prevents good suckling or swallowing

Clinical Findings

The following may be seen in poor weight gain:

INFANT FACTORS
- Continued weight loss after 5 to 7 days of age.

- Failure to regain birth weight by 2 to 3 weeks of age.
- Failure to maintain an ongoing weight gain of 1/2 to 1 oz/day.
- Weight below the third percentile for age. This finding can be a pattern over time or a sudden change.
- Lethargic, sleepy, inactive, unresponsive infant.
- Newborn or young infant sleeping longer than 4 hours between feedings.
- Dry mucous membranes.
- Poor skin turgor.

TECHNIQUE FACTORS
- Ineffective latch-on or sucking.
- Short time at the breast. The infant is removed before nursing is finished, thus reducing hindmilk consumption.
- Infant kept on a preset schedule despite cues for more feeding.
- Infant given water between feedings to "get through" to the next feeding.
- Infant encouraged or allowed to sleep through the night before 8 to 12 weeks of age.
- Fewer than eight feedings in 24 hours.
- Infant fed in a distracting environment.
- In older infants, breastfeeding offered after solids are given.
- Infant in a day care setting that does not facilitate breastfeeding.

MATERNAL FACTORS
- Does not initially respond to infant's cues for feeding or does not recognize that waking is needed to establish feeding.
- Uses nipple shields.
- Hectic schedule with limited time for breastfeeding.
- Recent illness or significant weight loss.
- Use of oral contraceptives or other hormones.

Differential Diagnosis

The differential diagnoses for poor weight gain are a pattern of slower but normal weight gain in healthy breastfed infants and failure to thrive.

Management

The following measures should be taken to manage poor weight gain:

- Complete a thorough history to elicit information regarding infant and maternal factors.
- Conduct a thorough assessment of breastfeeding techniques to accurately determine the extent to which mismanagement is a cause.
- Provide instruction, encouragement, and reinforcement for correct breastfeeding techniques.
- Refer for treatment of physical or organic causes.
- Be alert for any infant who has lost too much weight and is unable to feed with vigor at the breast; such infants require an immediate infusion of calories for energy.
- Use a supplemental system at the breast if supplementation is required (see Fig. 13–10).
- Encourage and reassure the parents.

Complications

Complications of poor weight gain include developmental delay, poor bonding, and severe dehydration. In situations of early failure to establish breastfeeding, some infants may appear to be in a septic state and require hospitalization for rehydration and further evaluation.

NURSING DIAGNOSIS 13-1

NURSING DIAGNOSES FOR BREASTFEEDING

Effective Breastfeeding

Interrupted Breastfeeding

Ineffective Breastfeeding

Source: North American Nursing Diagnosis Association: NANDA *Nursing Diagnoses: Definitions and Classification 1997–1998.* Philadelphia, North American Nursing Diagnosis Association, 1996.

RESOURCE BOX 13-2

RESOURCES FOR BREASTFEEDING

Ameda-Egnell
Tel: (800) 323-8750
Breast pumps and breastfeeding products

Best Start
Tel: (800) 277-4975
Videos and pamphlets for the economically disadvantaged. Also developed *Health Care Providers Breastfeeding Support Kit* funded by the US Departments of Health and Human Services and Agriculture. Every clinician should request a copy

Clearinghouse on Breastfeeding and Maternal Nutrition
American Public Health Association
Tel: (202) 789-5600

Florida Healthy Mothers/Healthy Babies
Tel: (904) 392-5667
Hospital breastfeeding protocols, in-service training package

Health Education Associates
Tel: (508) 888-8044
Website: www.aboutus.com/a100/hc2000
Continuing education programs, educational materials for families

Human Milk Banking Association of North America
Tel: (203) 232-8809
E-mail: milkbank@capecod.net
Guidelines and information on human milk banking; acts as clearinghouse for member milk banks. Currently lists eight regionally located human milk banks.

International Board of Lactation Consultant Examiners
Tel: (703) 560-7330
Website: www.iblce.org
International board certification program for lactation consultants

International Lactation Consultants Association (ILCA)
Tel: (919) 787-5181
Annual conference with continuing education programs, peer-reviewed professional journal *(Journal of Human Lactation)*

Center for Breastfeeding Information
La Leche League International
Tel: (800) LA-LECHE or (847) 519-7730
Website: www.lalecheleague.org
Educational materials for breastfeeding families, annual workshops for lactation consultants and primary care providers

Lactation Institute
(With Pacific Oaks College)
Tel: (818) 995-1913
Degree programs for lactation consultant preparation, educational materials for families and health-care providers, lactation educator program, specialized treatment center

Lactation Study Center
Department of Pediatrics
University of Rochester Medical Center
Tel: (716) 275-0088 or (716) 275-0036
Telephone hotline for health-care providers regarding unusual breastfeeding situations, specialized treatment center

Medela, Inc.
Tel: (800) 435-8316
Breast pumps and breastfeeding products, referral hotline for consumers, corporate lactation program

National Alliance for Breastfeeding Advocacy
Tel: (617) 893-3553
Continuing education programs, educational materials for families and health-care providers

National Capital Lactation Center & Community Human Milk Bank
Georgetown University Hospital
Tel: (202) 784-6455
Continuing education programs, lactation consultant preparation program

Rocky Mountain Drug Consultation Center
Tel: (800) 332-3073 or (303) 893-3784
Pharmaceutical and over-the-counter medication and drug information and consultation services

U.S. Committee for UNICEF
"Baby Friendly Hospital" Initiative
Tel: (202) 547-7946
Website: www.who.org

WELLSTART
Tel: (619) 295-5192 and (202) 298-7979
International educational programs, curricula, materials, speakers, conferences

World Health Organization
Publication Center
49 Sheridan Ave
Albany, NY 12210
Promotional materials (international in scope)

REFERENCES

American Academy of Pediatrics: Breastfeeding and the use of human milk. Pediatrics 100:1035-1039, 1997.

American Academy of Pediatrics Committee on Drugs: The transfer of drugs and other chemicals into human milk. Pediatrics 93:137-150, 1994.

Cohen R, Mrtek M, Mrtek R: Comparison of maternal absenteeism and infant illness rates among breastfeeding and formula feeding women in two corporations. Am J Health Promotion 10:148-153, 1995.

Cushing AH, Samet J, Lambert W, et al: Breastfeeding reduces the risk of respiratory illness in infants. J Epidemiol 147:863-870, 1998.

Dewey KG, Heinig MJ, Nommsen LA, et al: Growth of breast-fed and formula-fed infants from 0 to 18 months: The DARLING study. Pediatrics 89:1035-1041, 1992.

Dewey KG, Peerson JM, Brown KH, et al: Growth of breast-fed infants deviates from current reference data: A pooled analysis of US, Canadian and European data sets. Pediatrics 96:495-503, 1995.

Egan AM: Mothers' experiences with nipple confusion in their breast-fed infants who were introduced to bottles: A phenomenological study (unpublished doctoral dissertation). Texas Woman's University, Austin, 1988.

Gartner L, Auerbach KG: Breast milk and breastfeeding jaundice. Adv Pediatr 34:249-274, 1987.

Gorrie TM, McKinney ES, Murray SS (eds): Foundations of Maternal Newborn Nursing, 2nd ed. Philadelphia, WB Saunders, 1998.

Hale T: Medications and Mothers' Milk, 1998-99. Amarillo, TX, Pharmasoft Medical Publishing, 1998.

Humphrey N: Breastfeeding. Working moms can make it work. Adv Nurs Pract 2:21-23, 30, 1994.

Katcher A, Lanese M: Breastfeeding by employed mothers: A reasonable accommodation in the work place. Pediatrics 75:644-647, 1986.

Institute of Medicine Subcommittee on Lactation: Nutrition During Lactation. Washington, DC, National Academy Press, 1991.

Jakobsson I, Lindberg T: Cow's milk proteins cause infantile colic in breast-fed babies: A double blind crossover study. Pediatrics 71:268-274, 1983.

Lawrence RA, Lawrence RM: Breastfeeding. A Guide for the Medical Profession, 5th ed. St Louis, CV Mosby, 1999.

National Association of Pediatric Nurse Associates and Practitioners: NAPNAP position statement: Breast-feeding. J Pediatr Health Care 7:289, 1993.

Neifert M, Lawrence R, Seacat J: Nipple confusion: Toward a formal definition. J Pediatr 126 (suppl): S125-129, 1995.

Neifert M, Seacat J, Jobe W: Lactation failure due to insufficient glandular development of the breast. Pediatrics 76:823-828, 1985.

Newman J: Breastfeeding problems associated with the early introduction of bottles and pacifiers. J Hum Lactation 6(2):59-63, 1990.

Osborn GR: Relationship of hypotension and infant feeding to aetiology of coronary disease. Coll Int Cont Natl 169:93, 1968.

Specker B, Valanis V, Hertzberg N, et al: Sunshine exposure and serum 25-hydroxyvitamin D concentrations in exclusively breast-fed infants. J Pediatr 107:372-376, 1985.

Stashwick CA: When a breastfed infant isn't gaining weight. Contemp Pediatr 10:116-134, 1993.

Thilo EH, Townsend SF: Early newborn discharge: Have we gone too far? Contemp Pediatr 13:29-46, 1996.

UNICEF: Baby Friendly Hospital Initiative, Part II Hospital level implementation. *In* UNICEF Guidelines. Geneva, UNICEF, 1992.

WHO/UNICEF: Protecting, Promoting and Supporting Breastfeeding: The Special Role of Maternity Services: A Joint WHO/UNICEF Statement. Geneva, World Health Organization, 1989.

CHAPTER 14

Elimination Patterns

Ardys M. Dunn

▰▰▰ INTRODUCTION

Patterns of elimination involve normal developmental activities such as toilet training, as well as disease processes such as infections. This chapter discusses normal bowel and bladder function. Problems related more directly to pathophysiology are discussed in Chapters 33 and 35.

Developmental issues related to elimination can be troublesome and yet easily resolved for parents and nurse practitioners (NPs). Bowel and bladder habits and excretory function are indicators of how well the gastrointestinal, renal, and urinary systems are functioning. Assessment data related to elimination are vital pieces of information that must be complete and accurate. Collecting accurate data can be a challenge because cultural and social expectations about elimination can cause parents to become preoccupied with variations of "normal" and believe that their child has a problem when none exists. The words used by family members to describe bowel and bladder function and the understanding individuals have about the appropriateness of discussing elimination can distort information given to the NP.

Healthy children demonstrate an extremely wide range of "normal" elimination behavior, and NPs can help parents understand the parameters of those norms. NPs are also a valuable source of information about what parents can anticipate as their child develops and what parents can do to facilitate optimal bowel and bladder function.

▰▰▰ STANDARDS

The goals of the Region X child health nursing standards are that "the child's elimination pattern is normal for a healthy child" and that there be "adequate and regular functioning of bowel, bladder and skin" (Region X Nursing Network, 1998). The US Preventive Services Task Force (1996) states that "Routine screening for asymptomatic bacteriuria in . . . persons (other than pregnant women) is not recommended." The American Academy of Pediatrics recommends routine urinalysis at 5 years of age and a dipstick test for leukocytes in adolescence, preferably at age 15 (American Academy of Pediatrics, 1995).

▰▰▰ NORMAL PATTERNS OF ELIMINATION: BOWEL AND URINARY

Infants

BOWEL PATTERNS

Bowel patterns of infants are related to the frequency and amount of feeding and differ

327

between bottle-fed and breastfed babies. Breast-fed infants commonly have many small stools per day in the first weeks of life. As children grow, fewer stools are typical, with some older breastfed infants having a stool once a day or as infrequently as once every 10 to 14 days. The stools are usually soft, sticky or watery, and light yellow and have a "sour" but not unpleasant odor and a curd-like texture. Iron supplements can darken the stool.

Bottle-fed babies have two to four stools each day in the first month. As patterns become established, the number of stools decreases and older bottle-fed infants may have one to three stools each day. Stools of bottle-fed infants are firmer, darker, and smellier than those of breast-fed infants. They may be brown, greenish, or dark yellow, depending on the type of formula and whether iron supplements are given. They are soft and semiformed.

The stools of both breastfed and bottle-fed babies change in consistency and color as solid foods are introduced, at which point they become firmer and darker.

URINARY PATTERNS

Urination is associated with fluid intake and increases as infants take more fluids. Healthy, well-hydrated infants, whether breastfed or bottle fed, should urinate a minimum of 6 times a day and can void, in small amounts, 15 to 20 times a day. Fever in infants can quickly lead to dehydration, with less frequent urination.

Infants are not capable of voluntary bowel and bladder control because these functions are dependent on myelination of the pyramidal tracts in the spinal cord, a process probably completed between 12 and 18 months of age. Infants 9 to 12 months old generally have regular patterns in that they have a stool early in the morning or after feeding or stay dry for several hours and urinate immediately after waking from a nap.

Toddlers and Preschoolers

BOWEL PATTERNS

By the time children are 2 years of age, renal function is fully developed. Toddlers and pre-

schoolers usually have a regular pattern of elimination. Although they typically have one to three stools a day, it is not unusual for children in this age group to defecate every other day or every third or fourth day. It is a myth that healthy children must have a bowel movement every day. Stools are soft, formed, and various shades of brown, depending on the child's diet, and have an unpleasant odor.

URINARY PATTERNS

Fluid intake, environmental conditions, perspiration, fever, and diarrhea with significant fluid loss influence the urinary pattern of toddlers and preschoolers, who typically urinate 8 to 14 times a day. Cold weather, excitement, and stress lead to increased frequency.

School-Age Children

BOWEL PATTERNS

Elimination patterns in school-age children approximate those of adults. Depending on a child's intake, bowel movements occur from one to three times a day to once every 2 to 3 days. Stool is soft, formed, and brown and has an odor. School-age children should be completely toilet trained, although occasional soiling of underwear occurs as a result of poor hygiene or because children do not respond quickly to cues to defecate. It is important to remember children's increasing needs for independence and privacy during the school-age years and incorporate consideration of those needs into management of toileting.

URINARY PATTERNS

School-age children have essentially the same capacity as adults to produce urine—between 650 and 1500 ml in a 24-hour period—but the kidneys are still small and accommodate a smaller urine volume at any one time than those of adults. Children normally void 5 to 6 times a day. Girls appear to have slightly larger bladder capacity than boys. Dysfunctional voiding (too little, 1 to 3 times a day, or too much, 8 to 12 times a day), daytime incontinence, or nocturnal enuresis warrants further evaluation, especially because these conditions can be associated with infection, dehydration, or sexual abuse.

Adolescents

BOWEL AND BLADDER PATTERNS

Gastrointestinal and renal function is at adult levels in adolescents, and patterns of elimination are similar to those of adults. Abnormal variation can occur in teenagers who have eating disorders. Adolescents are also susceptible to the demands of schedules, stress, and irregular eating patterns. The need for privacy and personal space might inhibit normal elimination in public places such as school or dormitory restrooms. Sexual activity can contribute to changes in bowel or bladder function, including infections or constipation.

ASSESSMENT OF PATTERNS

Assessment of elimination patterns begins with a thorough health history, with questions being asked of the parent or the child, depending on the child's age and ability. As variations of normal behavior become evident, relevant follow-up questions should be asked to clarify and complete the health picture of the patient.

Health History

DESCRIPTION OF CURRENT STATUS

The patient's current health status can be assessed with the following questions:

- How often does your child urinate? How many wet diapers does your baby have in a 24-hour period?
- How often does your child have a bowel movement? Describe what the stools look and smell like. How does your child act when having a bowel movement?
- Describe your child's toileting habits. For example, at what time of day does your child have a bowel movement?
- Do you use any medications, including over-the-counter preparations or home remedies, to help your child with bowel movements?
- Tell me how you think the process of toilet training will happen? (Ask parents of a 12-month-old child.)
- Is your child toilet trained? When did training begin? Describe the process. How often do "accidents" happen? How do you (parent) feel toilet training is progressing?
- What names do you use in your family for stool and urine, for body parts, and for the process of using the toilet?

BIRTH HISTORY

It should be determined whether any problems with the child's urine or stool were present at birth. For example, did the baby pass a sticky, black (meconium) stool soon after birth? How soon after birth did the baby urinate?

REVIEW OF SYSTEMS

The review of systems should include the following questions:

- Has your child ever been constipated or had diarrhea? Was that condition related to anything in particular (e.g., a particular illness or a certain food or change in diet)? How does the parent define constipation and/or diarrhea?
- Has your child ever had a urinary tract infection? Describe.
- Has your child had any illness, injury, or operation related to the bowel or bladder? Describe.
- Does your child have a physical condition or chronic illness that affects voiding or bowel movements?
- What medications, including over-the-counter preparations, does your child take?

FAMILY HISTORY

The provider should determine whether any family members have had problems with urination or bowel movements and obtain a description of those problems.

ENVIRONMENTAL AND PSYCHOSOCIAL

Environmental and psychosocial issues should be assessed:

- How do you, as a parent, feel about the issue of toileting?
- How do you interact with your child around toileting issues?
- How do you deal with toileting "accidents"?
- What plans do you have for managing toilet training?
- Describe your child's typical diet.
- Tell me about the toileting facilities at your child's house/day care/school. How do you think they affect your child's toileting habits?

Physical Examination

The physical examination includes external examination of the perineum, anus, and urinary meatus and auscultation and palpation of the abdomen for bowel sounds, softness, masses, peristalsis, and tenderness.

Laboratory and Diagnostic Tests

A urinalysis is done as indicated, including once as a screening during the preschool years.

▬▬▬ MANAGEMENT STRATEGIES FOR NORMAL PATTERNS

Toilet Training

Toilet training occurs in the toddler and preschool years and is usually complete by age 4. Successful toilet training requires sensitivity, understanding of development, good communication, hope, humor, and patience. In addition to becoming self-sufficient in their toileting, children should also learn that elimination is a natural and necessary process. Both parents and children should experience pride and satisfaction in having worked together to accomplish an important developmental task.

Parents must have a clear sense of their own expectations for the child. The provider should introduce the topic of toilet training early in the second year, assess for parental expectations and plans, and provide ample opportunity for discussion of realistic toileting outcomes. Parents must be given correct information if their expectations are to be developmentally appropriate. Brazelton's (1962) classic study of 1170 children over a 10-year period describes behavior that might typically be expected of children during toilet training:

- Eighty percent of children were trained for bowel and bladder control at the same time.
- The average daytime training for both bowel and bladder control was completed at 28.5 months.
- The average day *and* nighttime training was completed at 33 months, 10 days.
- Girls were trained completely an average of 2½ months earlier than boys.
- Forty percent of children were still bedwetting at 4 years of age.
- Thirty percent of children were still bedwetting at 5 years of age.

Because true voluntary sphincter control is a function of psychological and social as well as physiological development, children are not usually ready for toilet training until 18 to 24 months of age or even older. Parents should be discouraged from attempting to toilet-train their children before this age because it is actually the parents who are being "trained" to toilet the children. Guidelines for assessing toilet-training readiness include physical, cognitive, interpersonal, and parental skills (Table 14–1).

When children and parents are ready to begin toilet training, several management techniques are helpful (Table 14–2).

If children resist training, the project should be put on hold for a few weeks before trying again. If toddlers seem to be toilet-trained for a brief period and suddenly regress to wetting and soiling consistently, they should be placed back in diapers and the process begun again within a few weeks.

Toilet training can be a source of extreme frustration for parents if their expectations do not match the abilities and performance of their

TABLE 14-1

Guidelines for Assessing Toilet-Training Readiness

Child's physical skills	Has voluntary sphincter control
	Stays dry for 2 hr, may wake from naps still dry
	Is able to sit, walk, and squat
	Assists in dressing self
Child's cognitive skills	Recognizes urge to urinate or defecate
	Understands meaning of words used by family in toileting
	Understands what toilet is for
	Understands connection between dry pants and toilet
	Is able to follow directions
	Is able to communicate needs
Child's interpersonal skills	Demonstrates desire to please parent
	Expresses curiosity about use of toilet
	Expresses desire to be dry and clean
Parental skills	Expresses desire to assist child with training
	Recognizes child's cues of readiness
	Has no compelling factor that will interfere with training (e.g., new job, move, family loss)

children, and the incidence of child abuse related to toilet training is high. Berkowitz (1996) notes that issues around toileting are the second most prevalent factor precipitating fatal child abuse. The NP can play a crucial role in preventing abuse by providing parents with information about child development, techniques for managing the process, and support and encouragement for their efforts.

▮▮▮ ALTERED PATTERNS OF ELIMINATION

The following discussion focuses on four relatively common conditions of childhood related to elimination: stool toileting refusal, encopresis, enuresis, and dysfunctional voiding. These conditions are considered here as developmental problems of normal urinary and bowel habits. If assessment reveals indicators of pathological problems, further investigation and different management are necessary.

TABLE 14-2

Management of Toilet Training

Keep child as clean and dry as possible:
    Change diapers frequently
    Introduce training pants when child stays dry for several hours. Use them during the day, and diaper at night
Talk to child about toilet training:
    Praise child for coming to you to have diaper changed
    Explain connection between being clean and dry and using toilet
    Encourage child to use toilet from time to time during the day, especially before going out to play, going on a trip, before naps, and at bedtime
Teach child how to use toilet:
    Allow child to observe while parents or older siblings use toilet
    Demonstrate how to sit on toilet, use toilet paper, flush, and wash one's hands
Provide practice time for child:
    Provide a potty chair or portable toilet seat for a regular toilet
    Allow child to sit on potty chair with clothes or diaper on
    Encourage child to use potty chair while parent uses regular toilet
    Have child sit on toilet without diapers for 5 to 10 minutes at a time
    Schedule practice sessions for times a child usually urinates or defecates
Provide a comfortable, safe-feeling environment:
    Seat child facing backward on a regular toilet or provide a footstool to rest the feet on
    Never flush the toilet when child is sitting on it
    Stay with child for safety reasons
Give consistent, positive feedback:
    Praise child for trying, as well as for success
    Never demand performance
    Never make child sit on toilet if child resists
    Be understanding of child's refusal to use toilet
    Ignore or minimize undesired behavior
    Never scold or punish a child for wetting or soiling

Stool Toileting Refusal

DESCRIPTION

Stool toileting refusal is present when a child demonstrates a pattern of successfully using the toilet to urinate but refusing to use the toilet for bowel movements. These children will usually defecate in a diaper, training pants, or "pull-ups." In some cases, these children will retain stool.

INCIDENCE AND ETIOLOGY

In a recent study (Taubman, 1997), 22% of healthy children between 18 and 30 months of age experienced at least 1 month of stool toileting refusal. The presence of younger siblings in the household and the parents' inability to set limits for the child appear to be related to refusal. Although children who displayed stool toileting refusal tended to have "a more difficult temperament" than did children who were toilet-trained (Blum et al., 1997), they did not have any more behavior problems. Constipation and painful bowel movements, a possible result of stool toileting refusal, may also be a cause of the problem.

CLINICAL FINDINGS

History

Parents or caregivers report that the child demonstrates the following:

- Bladder control but refusal to defecate on the toilet
- A regular pattern of stooling
- Signs that a bowel movement is imminent

Physical Examination

The physical examination will be unremarkable if the child has a pattern of regular bowel movements.

- Examine the anus for fissures or irritation that may cause a child to refuse to defecate.
- Check for signs of stool retention:
  - Abdominal distention
  - Abdominal tenderness on palpation
  - Palpation of a mass in the sigmoid colon

or at the midline in the suprapubic area (impaction)

DIFFERENTIAL DIAGNOSIS

The differential diagnosis includes stool withholding, constipation, and encopresis.

MANAGEMENT

Behavioral management is appropriate for younger children. Return them to diapers and reintroduce toileting training in about a month or when the child indicates interest. Some children prefer not to wear diapers all the time, but will ask to have one put on when they feel the urge to defecate. After stooling, they ask to be changed and return to wearing training pants. This pattern may continue for several weeks or months before the child is ready to use the toilet for stooling. Never flush the toilet while the child is sitting on it. Give positive feedback when the child successfully uses the toilet for stooling. If the child has constipation, fecal impaction, or both, initial bowel clean-out is necessary, in conjunction with increased fiber and fluid in the diet (Luxem et al., 1997). Mineral oil or suppositories may be useful (see Table 14-4 for management of a child with constipated encopresis).

COMPLICATIONS

Refusal to use the toilet for stooling may lead to stool withholding, constipation, and impaction, conditions that result in primary encopresis. Psychological complications include embarrassment, shame, conflict, and stress between children and parents, especially as the child becomes older. Child abuse is a significant complication (Berkowitz, 1996).

PATIENT EDUCATION AND PREVENTION

Prevention through appropriate toilet training is key (see Table 14-2). If a child refuses to defecate on the toilet, use of punishment or force may complicate the problem.

Encopresis and Constipation

DESCRIPTION

Encopresis is defined as stool incontinence after an age when children should be able to control stooling, usually 4 years of age. Primary, or continuous, encopresis is present in children who have never been toilet-trained. Secondary, or discontinuous, encopresis is seen in those who were previously trained but who begin to soil. Encopresis may or may not be associated with stool retention and constipation. In constipated encopresis, stool retention leads to distention of the colon, ineffective peristalsis, and decreased sensitivity to the defecation reflex. Stool becomes dry, hard, and difficult to evacuate (constipation), and bowel movements may be painful. Soft, semiformed or liquid stool from higher in the colon can leak around retained stool and pass through the rectum (soiling). Encopresis with constipation is involuntary, and the child is often unaware of the actual incontinence. Children with constipated encopresis may either refuse or be willing to use the toilet (Schmitt & Mauro, 1992). Children with nonconstipated encopresis have voluntary bowel movements, but in their clothing or other inappropriate places.

INCIDENCE AND ETIOLOGY

Encopresis is probably more common than believed because many families hesitate to inform their health care provider about it. It is estimated to be as much as six times more common in boys than in girls, and approximately 1% of school-aged children are believed to be affected (Behrman et al., 1996). The etiology of encopresis is unclear and appears to differ among children. Both physiological and psychosocial factors are involved. Abnormal pudendal nerve function is not a factor in the etiology of encopresis (Sentovich et al., 1998).

Physiological

Physiological factors related to encopresis and constipation include:

- Inadequate fluid intake
- Dehydration caused by illness and fever or during active play in hot weather
- A change in diet such as the introduction of solids or increased carbohydrates and decreased fiber
- Inappropriate use of laxatives, suppositories, or enemas by parents who do not understand normal bowel patterns in children and infants
- Stool retention and constipation secondary to
  - Painful bowel movements
  - Anal fissures
  - Paradoxical constriction of the external anal sphincter muscle during attempted defecation
  - Neurogenic conditions (e.g., aganglionic colon [Hirschsprung disease], cerebral palsy, myelomeningocele)
  - Endocrine and metabolic conditions (e.g., hypothyroidism)
  - Medications (e.g., medications with codeine)

Psychosocial

Psychosocial factors related to encopresis and constipation include:

- Major family or life adjustments such as loss of a parent, sibling, or other significant person
- Inappropriate toilet-training techniques. Children who are pushed might rebel in the only way they can, by refusing to cooperate
- Physical abuse and sexual abuse

CLINICAL FINDINGS

History

The history can include the following:

- Stained underwear
- Child suddenly becoming still during play
- Child running into a corner or attempting to hide
- Child crossing legs, grimacing, standing on tiptoe, or shifting from one foot to another in an attempt to retain stool
- Reports of a bloated sensation, abdominal pain, or both
- Odor of stool from leakage into underwear

Physical Examination

The physical examination should assess for the following:
- Overflow soiling
- Abdominal distention
- Abdominal tenderness on palpation
- Impactions felt on rectal examination
- Mass felt at the midline in the suprapubic area

Laboratory and Diagnostic Tests

An abdominal radiograph is obtained if structural anomalies are suspected. Results can indicate accumulation of stool in the sigmoid colon (see Chapter 33).

DIFFERENTIAL DIAGNOSIS

The differential diagnoses for encopresis and constipation are:

- Anorectal stenosis
- Spina bifida occulta
- Hirschsprung disease
- Mental retardation
- Hypothyroidism
- Hypercalcemia
- Cerebral palsy
- Normal red-faced grunting and straining of infants on defecation

MANAGEMENT

Treatment of children with encopresis differs depending on whether they have impactions, are constipated, or have normal but inappropriately placed bowel movements. In all cases, treatment should focus on establishing a regular bowel routine, and education should emphasize a "demystification" of the problem and removal of blame (Levine et al., 1999). Table 14-3 outlines approaches to managing a child with nonconstipated encopresis. Children who have constipated encopresis present a greater challenge and usually require medication. Table 14-4 provides guidelines to treating a child with encopresis and constipation, including appropriate medications (also see Fig. 14-1).

Management of encopresis is often multidisciplinary in that it combines medical and psy-

T A B L E 14-3

Management of Children With Mild Nonconstipated Encopresis

Avoid use of stool softeners or laxatives
Encourage child to take responsibility for own toilet habits
Use incentives or rewards to reinforce positive behavior
Establish a regular toileting routine

chological interventions (Stark et al., 1997). Psychological counseling of both the child and family may be necessary. In some cases, referral to a psychologist or behavioral pediatrician is appropriate. Biofeedback training does not appear to be an effective therapy (Loening-Baucke, 1996).

Because this problem often occurs in school-aged children, the NP may need to consult with the school nurse to ensure that the child receives appropriate medications, hygiene management, and essential psychological and emotional support.

COMPLICATIONS

Persistent encopresis is an unpleasant condition, and children with encopresis often experience ridicule and shame. Age group peers frequently treat children with scorn, hostility, and rejection. Teachers and other adults might be disgusted by children with encopresis, and parents, dealing with anger, guilt, embarrassment, and helplessness, find their children and the condition extremely difficult to manage. Social, interpersonal, and family relations are at grave risk.

PATIENT EDUCATION AND PREVENTION

The best treatment of encopresis is prevention. It is important for the pediatric provider to understand the relationship between constipation and encopresis, recognize conditions that may contribute to each, and provide parents with anticipatory guidance related to dietary and toileting management of their children to

T A B L E 14-4

Management of Children With Constipated Encopresis

TREATMENT PHASE	TREATMENT PROGRAM	COMMENTS

Catharsis	In the home: four 3-d cycles (12 d total):
	  Day 1: Fleet enema (adult size)
	  Day 2: Bisacodyl (Dulcolax) suppository
	  Day 3: Bisacodyl tablet
	  Day 13: Bisacodyl tablet
	Return to clinic
	Follow-up abdominal radiograph to confirm catharsis
		Catharsis may need to occur in the hospital if:
		  Retention is severe
		  Home compliance is poor
		  Parents prefer admission
		  Parents should not administer enemas for psychological reasons
		Goal of catharsis is to empty the bowel. The child may have soft stools for several days after catharsis; parents and patient should be informed that ongoing maintenance is essential for the bowel to return to fully normal functioning (see Fig. 14–1). Initial improvement can be falsely reassuring and may contribute to poor compliance to maintenance regimen

Maintenance	Stool softener (e.g., mineral oil), starting at 2 tbs bid. Titrate dose to facilitate soft stools without mineral oil leakage
	Daily multivitamin to counteract possible decreased absorption of fat-soluble vitamins
	Oral laxatives (e.g., milk of magnesia, senna concentrate [Senokot]) may be substituted for or used alternately with stool softener
	Toilet sitting at least twice a day for 10 min each time
	Increased activity, increased fluids (other than milk), increased fiber in diet
		Goals of maintenance:
		  No soiling
		  Regular, soft bowel movements (at least every other day)
		  Increased ability to sense the urge to defecate
		
		Toilet sitting should be scheduled at times the child is most likely to have a bowel movement (e.g., on wakening, after meals)

Follow-up	Regular visits (every 4–10 wk), depending on severity and need of family
	Telephone availability to discuss progress and adjust doses
	Counseling or referral as appropriate for psychosocial and developmental issues
	Continued education of normal bowel function (see Fig. 14–1)
		Goals of follow-up visits:
		  Monitor compliance
		  Provide encouragement and support
		  Detect and treat relapse early if it occurs

Adapted from Levine MD, Carey WB, Crocker AC: Developmental-Behavioral Pediatrics, 3rd ed. Philadelphia, WB Saunders, 1999.

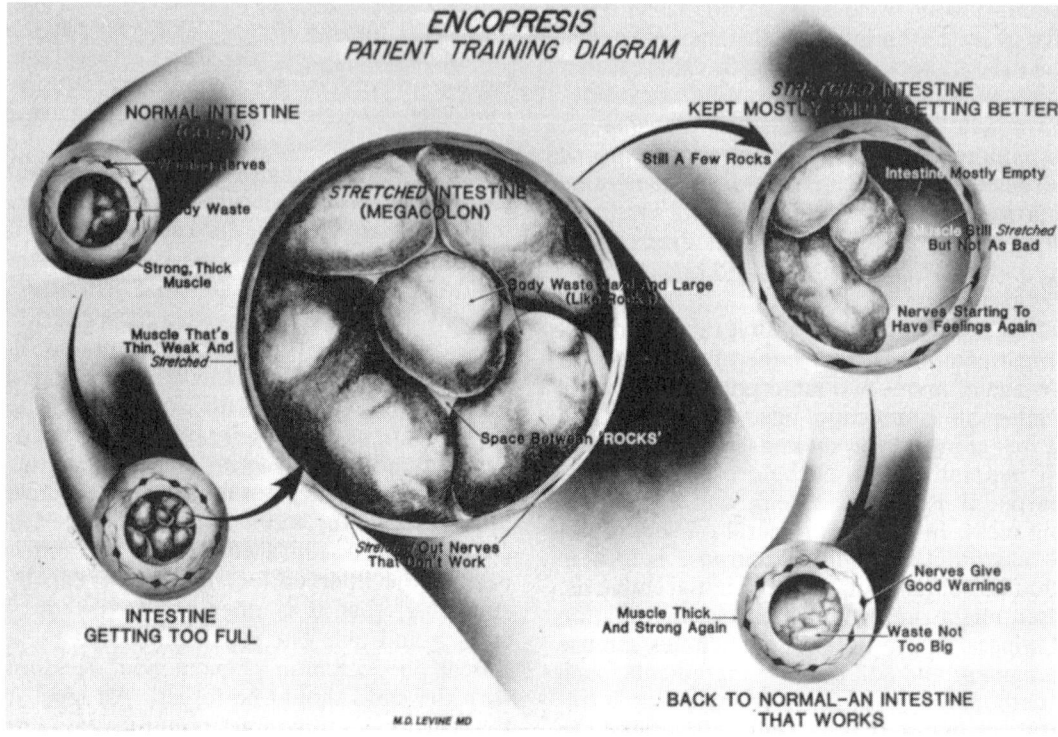

FIGURE 14-1
Encopresis: Patient training diagram. (From Levine MD, Carey WB, Crocker AC: Developmental-Behavioral Patterns, 3rd ed. Philadelphia, WB Saunders, 1999.)

prevent their occurrence. It is equally important to provide support during treatment. Although parents should be informed that treatment may be required for months or years, NPs should emphasize that by following a clear, consistent, aggressive treatment protocol, the condition can be managed. Finally, the NP, parents, and child must work together to prevent recurrence of symptoms after successful treatment.

Enuresis

DESCRIPTION

Enuresis is defined as involuntary urination at an age when voluntary control should be present. Children who have never established control have primary enuresis. Secondary enuresis is present when children have been dry for more than 6 to 12 months and begin wetting.

Nocturnal enuresis is incontinence during sleep. Diurnal enuresis occurs during waking hours.

INCIDENCE AND ETIOLOGY

Because a wide range of normal is seen in the age at which urinary continence is established, the incidence of enuresis is difficult to assess. Rates are estimated at 40% in 3-year-olds, 7 to 10% in 5-year-olds, and 2 to 3% in 10-year-olds. Boys are more likely to have nocturnal enuresis than girls, and black children have a greater incidence of enuresis than white children do. Generally, enuresis is not considered to be a problem before 6 years of age.

Approximately 95% of voiding problems are functional, whereas the remainder may represent an organic condition (Kelleher, 1997). Primary nocturnal enuresis has an organic etiology in only about 1% of cases (Behrman & Kliegman, 1998). Factors associated with enuresis include:

- Stress and family disruptions such as a divorce, move, or a new member.
- Inappropriate toilet training, especially when parents are overly demanding or punitive of the child.
- Familial disposition.
- Small bladder capacity. A bladder capacity of 300 to 350 ml is necessary for a child to sleep through the night without incontinence.
- Neurological developmental delay in which the child is unable to inhibit bladder contraction.
- Sleep arousal patterns. Children who "sleep deeply" are more prone to nocturnal bed wetting (Neveus et al., 1998).
- Hormonal regulation. Children with enuresis may require higher levels of antidiuretic hormone (ADH) to regulate the degree of plasma osmolality contributing to nocturnal polyuria (Eggert & Kuhn, 1995).
- Chronic constipation (Loening-Baucke, 1997).
- Stress incontinence.

CLINICAL FINDINGS

History

With daytime enuresis, parents often report that the child:

- Demonstrates an immediate urgency to void
- Becomes restless or jiggly, crosses the legs, or holds the penis or pubic area
- May smell of urine

Nocturnal enuresis is characterized by:

- Spot urination (the child wakes after beginning to urinate and is able to stop the stream)
- Bedwetting

Parents should be asked about the following:

- History of enuresis and treatment for child and other family members, including parents
- Frequency of wetting

- Time of wetting (daytime or nighttime)
- Volume of urine voided
- Type of urinary stream
- Any urgency, dysuria, polyuria, or dribbling
- History of toilet training
- Presence of other behavior problems
- Changes in the home, family, or school environment

Physical Examination

The physical examination includes the following:

- Assess the external genitalia for signs of irritation or infection.
- Assess for bladder capacity.
- Observe the size and velocity of the urine stream.
- Check for fecal impaction.
- Examine the abdomen for masses, especially at the suprapubic midline and in the left lower quadrant.

Laboratory and Diagnostic Tests

A urinalysis is recommended in all children with enuresis; urine culture is done if a urinary tract infection is suspected. Children with persistent enuresis should have a urine culture.

DIFFERENTIAL DIAGNOSIS

The differential diagnosis includes daytime or extraordinary urinary frequency syndrome, a benign condition seen in previously toilet-trained children. Daytime urinary frequency syndrome has no known cause but may be associated with viral cystitis/urethritis, stress, and hypercalciuria. It is usually self-limited (Robson & Leung, 1993).

Organic causes of enuresis must be identified; the most common is urinary tract infection, which occurs in 1 to 2% of cases. Urinary tract infections may be related to encopresis, and a child with enuresis should be examined for fecal impaction and a history of soiling.

Wetting can also be due to a primary detrusor instability in which the child has learned to inhibit sphincter relaxation and prevent complete emptying of the bladder. Detrusor instability in combination with delayed arousal from sleep and polyuria can be a factor in nocturnal enuresis (Chandra, 1998). Other organic causes to consider include:

- Diabetes mellitus
- Diabetes insipidus
- Sickle cell disease, in which treatment by means of forced fluids may lead to increased urine output
- Chronic renal failure, in which the kidneys are unable to concentrate urine
- Structural anomalies such as vesicoureteral reflux, ectopic ureter
- Neurological abnormalities, including neurogenic bladder
- Hypercalciuria
- Obstructive uropathy
- Vaginitis
- Sleep apnea

MANAGEMENT

Although most children maintain urinary continence after toilet training is established, wetting is a common phenomenon, and parents should be reassured that it rarely indicates disease. A thorough physical examination to distinguish between organic and nonorganic causes is the first step in treatment. Organic conditions are treated as appropriate; referral may be necessary.

Treatment of functional enuresis (i.e., from nonorganic causes) takes several forms. Use of an enuresis alarm appears to be the treatment of choice for families able to follow protocols (Gimpel et al., 1998). A combined treatment of enuresis alarm and desmopressin medication has been found effective in children with severe problems (wetting 6 or more nights per week) (Bradbury, 1997). Successful treatment has been correlated to family functioning and requires active involvement of both parents and children.

Because functional enuresis is self-limited, it is best to delay aggressive treatment until the child is 6 to 8 years of age. Strategies for use with a 6-year-old or older child include the following:

- *Enuresis alarm.* Behavioral modification involves the introduction of a stimulus that leads to a desired response from the subject. An electric alarm with a bell or buzzer

that wakes the child when the child begins to wet is the stimulus. Initially, the child learns to wake and use the toilet when stimulated by the buzzer; subsequently, the child learns to associate the beginning of urination with waking and toileting. Although this method has a significantly higher success rate than other methods do (Garber, 1996), some children object to continued use or relapse without the external stimulus.

- *Motivational therapy.* This strategy assumes that children will take responsibility for the problem and for learning how to resolve it. The family is expected to provide supportive reinforcement for positive behavior, such as use of a "star chart," rewards, and praise. Children are taught to be increasingly sensitive to their body's cues to urinate, encouraged to void in the toilet, and reinforced, either emotionally, materially, or both, for success. This therapy is emotionally time consuming and requires a high level of healthy communication between parents and children. Provider support of both parents and children is essential. Children should be seen by the provider every 2 weeks; 70 to 90% show improvement. Hypnosis and self-hypnosis have had more long-term efficacy than drug therapy (Banerjee et al., 1993), but they are not currently well established treatment strategies (Moffatt, 1997).

- *Bladder control training.* Because many children with enuresis have small bladder capacities, this technique is directed toward "training" the bladder to hold greater quantities of urine. Children are also taught to be more sensitive to cues of a full bladder and to control stopping and starting the urinary stream. Children are taught to postpone urinating until they "can't hold it any longer" and then start and stop the stream as they urinate. It is assumed that stretching the bladder leads to an increased threshold before the bladder is stimulated to empty. In a 6-year-old, a bladder capacity of 120 ml or less is small; 150 to 250 ml is normal. Techniques discussed earlier under toilet training can be helpful in bladder control training.

• *Drug therapy.* Drug therapy is sometimes used in conjunction with other strategies and often has high initial success rates. Unfortunately, extremely high relapse rates are seen when use of the drug is discontinued. Medications used include imipramine, desmopressin, and oxybutynin (Table 14-5 and Appendix A). Imipramine is a tricyclic antidepressant with an as yet unknown mechanism of action; its action in treating childhood enuresis appears to be separate from its antidepressant effect. The nasal spray desmopressin acetate (DDAVP) has been used for primary nocturnal enuresis and appears to be especially effective in children with a family history of enuresis (Hogg & Husmann, 1993). Oxybutynin chloride is an anticholinergic drug that relaxes the smooth muscle of the bladder, allows increased urine retention, reduces frequency, and has been useful in control of daytime incontinence. Children taking medications on a regular basis should have a drug "holiday" every 3 months to assess the need for continued pharmacotherapy. After 1 month without wetting, medications can be tapered over a 2- to 4-week period. Drug therapy is expensive and is associated with a high relapse rate. However, it can be extremely useful for overnight stays (e.g., camp), when staying dry is very important to the child.

COMPLICATIONS

Enuresis contributes to poor self-esteem and disrupted family interactions and threatens the child's ability to establish strong peer relationships. Although self-concept appears to improve with successful treatment, it has not been proved that failure of treatment causes an in-

T A B L E 14-5

Drug Therapy for Children With Enuresis

MEDICATION	DOSING	COMMENTS
Imipramine hydrochloride	Initially, 25 mg daily 1 hr before bedtime. After 1 wk can increase to 50 mg for children 6–12 yr, 75 mg for children older than 12 yr	Not recommended in children younger than 6 yr Has serious side effects and a high level of toxicity; has been fatal in some cases Administer with great care Use least amount effective
Desmopressin acetate (DDAVP)	*Oral:* 0.2 mg tablets once daily at bedtime; can be adjusted up to maximum of 0.6 mg/d *Nasal spray or solution:* 20 μg (2 sprays) or 0.2 ml solution intranasally at bedtime; can be adjusted up to 40 μg or down to 10 μg/d	Not recommended in children younger than 6 yr When switching from nasal spray to tablets, give first oral dose 24 hr after last intranasal dose When using nasal spray, administer one-half dose per nostril Changes in nasal mucosa (e.g., with upper respiratory infection) may compromise absorption; administer an antihistamine or decongestant 30–60 min before using or consider oral form Caution must be taken with patients who are hypertensive or have a potential for fluid-electrolyte imbalance (e.g., children with cystic fibrosis susceptible to hyponatremia) Manufacturer recommends that treatment beyond 7 d include electrolyte studies
Oxybutynin chloride	5 mg bid, maximum of 5 mg tid	Not recommended in children younger than 5 yr

crease in behavioral abnormalities in children with enuresis (Moffatt, 1989).

PATIENT EDUCATION AND PREVENTION

Supportive education of parents, positive reinforcement of children's efforts, and use of the toilet-training techniques described earlier can help prevent enuresis. For 3- to 5-year-old children, a nonjudgmental attitude of "benign neglect" in the face of accidents is the best approach.

Dysfunctional Voiding

DESCRIPTION

Dysfunctional voiding, or pediatric unstable bladder, is characterized by poor initiation of micturition, poor inhibition of voiding, or incomplete emptying of the bladder.

INCIDENCE AND ETIOLOGY

The cause of dysfunctional voiding is unknown but is believed to be related to voiding immaturity. It is more common in girls and is usually seen in children 4 to 8 years of age.

CLINICAL FINDINGS

History

Because of the various problems characteristic of dysfunctional voiding, children have a history of differing symptomatology. Reported symptoms include:

- Infrequent voiding
- Sudden daytime incontinence after having been dry
- Urgency
- Frequency
- Inability to stop the voiding stream
- Failure to void to completion
- Occasional nocturnal enuresis, but usually daytime wetting
- Constipation
- Urinary tract infection

Physical Examination

A complete physical examination should be done.

Laboratory and Diagnostic Tests

The following tests are indicated:

- Urinalysis
- Urine culture and sensitivity
- Renal and bladder ultrasound if structural abnormalities are suspected, with an abnormal ultrasound showing a normal upper renal system and a thick-walled bladder.

DIFFERENTIAL DIAGNOSIS

The differential diagnoses for dysfunctional voiding are:

- Urinary tract infection
- Structural abnormality, such as abnormal sphincters, ectopic ureter, duplicated urethra, or urethral valves
- Neurogenic bladder
- Vesicoureteral reflux
- Trauma or abuse
- Urethritis (may be caused by chemicals in soaps, bubble baths)

MANAGEMENT

The goal of management is to prevent or break the cycle of urinary dysfunction, infection, and irritable bladder. Intervention includes the following:

- Treat any urinary tract infection if present.
- Retrain the bladder. This process works well with 6- to 8-year-olds and requires a motivated child. Teach the child to void by the clock, every 2 hours, and not to wait for the urge to urinate (Kurtz et al., 1993) (see Table 14–6 for suggestions on bladder retraining).
- Treat constipation if present.
- Treat symptoms with anticholinergics such as oxybutynin chloride. This drug is not recommended for use in children younger than 5 years. The dose in children older

T A B L E 14-6

Bladder Retraining for Dysfunctional Voiding

Establish a schedule for voiding. Have child go to the bathroom every 2–4 hr, whether urgency is felt or not

Void with relaxation. Have child take a deep breath and relax sphincter when exhaling; use a straw to breathe through. Have child try grasping fingers together and pulling them apart

Void to completion. Teach child to use Credé maneuver or manual pressure over suprapubic area to complete voiding

Double void. After voiding completely, have child wait on toilet 2–3 min and attempt to void again

than 5 years is 2.5 to 5 mg every day or twice a day.

- Teach parents to perform intermittent catheterization if the effects of urinary retention progress to upper urinary tract infection (see Chapter 35 for a discussion of infections).

PATIENT EDUCATION AND PREVENTION

Effective toilet training can prevent urinary retention, especially if children learn to be sensitive and responsive to cues to urinate. Parents

NURSING DIAGNOSIS 14-1

NURSING DIAGNOSES FOR ELIMINATION FUNCTIONAL HEALTH PATTERN

Constipation

Encopresis (not a NANDA diagnosis)

Enuresis (not a NANDA diagnosis)

Source: North American Nursing Diagnosis Association. *NANDA Nursing Diagnoses: Definitions and Classifications 1997–1998.* Philadelphia, North American Nursing Diagnosis Association, 1996.

should be instructed to be alert to signs of dysuria. If urination is painful, children often struggle to retain urine or void incompletely. Early treatment for urinary tract infections is essential to prevent renal dysfunction.

RESOURCE BOX 14-1

NATIONAL RESOURCES FOR PROBLEMS WITH ENURESIS

National Enuresis Society
Tel: (900) NES-8080
Website: www.peds.umn.edu/centers/NES/

Enuresis Alarms

Nite train'r Alarm
Koregon Enterprises
Tel: (800) 544-4240
Cost: $69.00

Nytone Medical Products
Tel: (801) 973-4090
Cost: $48.50

Potty Pager
Ideas for Living, Inc.
Tel: (800) 497-6573
Cost: $49.95

Wet Stop Alarm
Palco Laboratories
Tel: (800) 346-4488
Cost: $55.00

REFERENCES

American Academy of Pediatrics: Recommendations for preventive pediatric health care. Committee on Practice and Ambulatory Medicine. Pediatrics 96:373–374, 1995.

Banerjee S, Srivastav A, Palan BM: Hypnosis and self-hypnosis in the management of nocturnal enuresis: A comparative study with imipramine therapy. Am J Clin Hypnosis 36:113–119, 1993.

Behrman RE, Kliegman RM (eds): Nelson Essentials of Pediatrics, 3rd ed. Philadelphia, WB Saunders, 1998.

Behrman RE, Kliegman RM, Arvin AM (eds): Nelson Textbook of Pediatrics, 15th ed. Philadelphia, WB Saunders, 1996.

Berkowitz CD: Pediatrics: A Primary Care Approach. Philadelphia, WB Saunders, 1996.

Blum NJ, Taubman B, Osborne ML: Behavioral characteristics of children with stool toileting refusal. Pediatrics 99:50–53, 1997.

Bradbury M: Combination therapy for nocturnal enuresis

with desmopressin and an alarm device. Scand J Urol Nephrol 183:61-63, 1997.

Brazelton TB: A child-oriented approach to toilet-training. Pediatrics 29:121-128, 1962.

Chandra M: Nocturnal enuresis in children. Curr Opin Pediatr 10:167-173, 1998.

Eggert P, Kuhn B: Antidiuretic hormone regulation in patients with primary nocturnal enuresis. Arch Dis Child 73:508-511, 1995.

Garber KM: Enuresis: An update on diagnosis and management. J Pediatr Health Care 10:202-208, 1996.

Gimpel GA, Warzak WJ, Kuhn BR, et al: Clinical perspectives in primary nocturnal enuresis. Clin Pediatr (Phila) 37:23-29, 1998.

Hogg RJ, Husmann D: The role of family history in predicting response to desmopressin in nocturnal enuresis. J Urol 150:444-445, 1993.

Kelleher RE: Daytime and nighttime wetting in children: A review of management. J Soc Pediatr Nurs 2:73-82, 1997.

Kurtz M, Murrey M, Salmonson K, et al: Daytime incontinence. J Pediatr Health Care 7:92, 99-100, 1993.

Levine MD, Carey WB, Crocker AC: Developmental-Behavioral Pediatrics, 3rd ed. Philadelphia, WB Saunders, 1999.

Loening-Baucke V: Incontinence and urinary tract infection and their resolution with treatment of chronic constipation of childhood. Pediatrics 100:228-232, 1997.

Loening-Baucke V: Biofeedback training in children with functional constipation: A critical review. Dig Dis Sci 41:65-71, 1996.

Luxem MC, Christophersen ER, Purvis PC, et al: Behavioral-medical treatment of pediatric toileting refusal. J Dev Behav Pediatr 18:34-41, 1997.

Moffatt ME: Nocturnal enuresis: A review of the efficacy of treatments and practical advice for clinicians. J Dev Behav Pediatr 18:49-56, 1997.

Moffat ME: Nocturnal enuresis: Psychologic implications of treatment and nontreatment. J Pediatr 114:697-704, 1989.

Neveus T, Lackgren G, Stenberg A, et al: Sleep and nighttime behaviour of enuretics and non-enuretics. Br J Urol 81(suppl 3):67-71, 1998.

North American Nursing Diagnosis Association: NANDA Nursing Diagnoses: Definitions and Classifications 1997-1998. Philadelphia, North American Nursing Diagnosis Association, 1996.

Region X Nursing Network: Region X Nursing Network Standards for Prenatal and Child Health. Seattle, University of Washington, 1998.

Robson WL, Leung AK: Extraordinary urinary frequency syndrome. Urology 42:321-324, 1993.

Schmitt BD, Mauro RD: 20 common errors in treating encopresis. Contemp Pediatr 9:47-52, 65, 1992.

Sentovich SM, Kaufman SS, Cali RL, et al: Pudendal nerve function in normal and encopretic children. J Pediatr Gastroenterol Nutr 26:70-72, 1998.

Stark LJ, Opipari LC, Donaldson DL, et al: Evaluation of a standard protocol for retentive encopresis: A replication. J Pediatr Psychol 22:619-633, 1997.

Taubman B: Toilet training and toileting refusal for stool only: A prospective study. Pediatrics 99:54-58, 1997.

US Preventive Services Task Force: Guide to Clinical Preventive Services, 2nd ed. Baltimore, Williams & Wilkins, 1996.

CHAPTER 15

Activities and Sports for Children and Adolescents

Catherine E. Burns

INTRODUCTION

Maintenance of activity is a basic health need of all people, including infants, children, and adolescents. Activity promotes motor and cognitive development, psychological well-being, and physical health. Activity also promotes psychological development through promotion of self-esteem as the child masters new skills and learns to interact with others in mutual activities. Activity is essential for optimal functioning of the body; body systems are influenced by the metabolic, physical, and neurological responses needed to execute and maintain a healthy level of activity. Further, activity patterns become long-term lifestyle habits that either promote or compromise health of the individual in the future. Youth in the United States (US) do not engage in sufficient exercise to develop and maintain cardiovascular endurance (Kuntzleman, 1993) and are less fit than youth in comparable countries (DiNubile, 1993). Only 25% of students in grades 9 through 12 were enrolled in daily school physical education in 1995 (US Department of Health and Human Services [DHHS], 1998). Thus, the nurse practitioner (NP) needs to assess and promote activities for health at all ages. The outcomes influence the health of children and their families in many ways.

CLINICAL PREVENTIVE SERVICES GUIDELINES AND STANDARDS FOR PHYSICAL ACTIVITY AND FITNESS IN CHILDREN

Healthy People 2010 Guidelines for Physical Activity and Fitness

Healthy People 2010: Objectives: Draft for Public Comment (US DHHS, 1998) includes objectives for physical activity and fitness in children that will likely be part of the final draft. These include:

1. Increase to at least 30% the proportion of people aged 6 years and older who engage regularly, preferably daily, in light to moderate physical activity for at least 30 minutes per day.
2. Increase to at least 20% the proportion of young people in grades 9 through 12 who engage in vigorous physical activity that promotes the development and maintenance of cardiorespiratory fitness 3 or more days per week for 20 or more minutes per occasion.
3. Increase to at least 50% the proportion of children in grades 9 through 12 who participate in daily physical education.

4. Increase to at least 50% the proportion of young people in grades 9 through 12 who spend at least 50% of school physical education class time being physically active, preferably engaged in lifetime physical activities at least 3 times per week.
5. Increase to at least 50% the proportion of primary and allied health-care providers who routinely assess and counsel their patients regarding their physical activity practices.

American Medical Association Guidelines for Adolescent Preventive Services (GAPS)

GAPS addresses the issue of physical activity for young people, including the following (Elster & Kuznets, 1994):

1. All adolescents should receive health guidance annually about the benefits of exercise and should be encouraged to engage in safe exercise on a regular basis.
2. All adolescents should receive health guidance annually to promote the reduction of injuries. This should include "counseling to promote appropriate physical conditioning before exercise."

The latter is based on information that athletic participation is a risk factor for injury. In fact, sports and recreational activities are the leading cause of nonfatal injuries among adolescents. Studies estimate that 20 million adolescents participate in recreational sports and another 5 to 7 million are involved in school sports. More than one study has shown that between 20 and 40% of athletes have injuries serious enough to cause them to miss a game or practice. Data from the Child Health Supplement of the 1988 National Health Interview Survey indicate that 2.9 million sports and recreational injuries occur annually in 5- to 17-year-olds in the United States, and almost a million of these are serious (Bijur et al., 1995). Football and wrestling are the most dangerous for male students, whereas gymnastics is most often associated with injuries in female students.

One of the goals of this chapter is to provide information to help young people engage in healthy sports and activities while minimizing

the risks of injury. Information about performing the preparticipation physical examination is important to identify those at most risk for injury. Preparticipation examinations are not required for many recreational activities of children and adolescents. The nurse practitioner also needs to evaluate the risks for youngsters participating in nonorganized recreational activities such as inline skating, skateboarding, cycling, swimming, and skiing.

Nursing Standards for Activity and Exercise Functional Health Pattern

The pediatric nursing standards for activity and exercise for children (Region X Nursing Network, 1998) are as follows:

ACTIVITY/EXERCISE PATTERN

Newborn, 1 month to 3 yrs: The child's play and activities are appropriate for his or her age.

School age: The child's exercise and activity levels are appropriate to maintain optimal health outcomes.

Adolescent: The adolescent's activity and exercise patterns promote physical and emotional health.

This chapter focuses on sports for older children and adolescents, recognizing that younger children also need daily activity and play to promote their growth and development. For younger children in elementary school, 30 to 60 minutes per day of age-appropriate physical activities most days of the week is recommended. Young children should engage in a variety of physical activities. Intermittent periods of 10 to 15 minutes of moderate to vigorous activity are recommended (Bykowski, 1998).

▓▓▓ ASSESSMENT

The Preparticipation Sports Examination

The preparticipation sports examination is one of the most common reasons for youths and adolescents to seek primary health care. Therefore, it offers an opportunity to identify children at risk for exacerbating preexisting medical conditions, to evaluate the general state of health, and to promote health. The examination is specifically used to identify conditions that are potentially life-threatening or disabling, identify medical or musculoskeletal conditions that put the child at risk for injury, assess general health and correct or take preventive measures to allow participation, suggest alternative sports if appropriate, and recommend treatment for any potentially serious condition (American Academy of Family Physicians [AAFP] et al., 1997). For the majority of youth, this examination is their only health assessment for the year (Bratton, 1997). The American Academy of Pediatrics (AAP, 1994) recommended sports examinations every 2 years. The examinations should be done at least 6 weeks before the season begins to allow time for follow-up of problems before engagement (Bratton, 1997; Overbaugh & Allen, 1994a; American Academy of Family Physicians et al., 1997). The American Heart Association also recommends preparticipation examinations including complete health history, physical examination, and brachial artery blood pressure (American Medical Association [AMA], 1997). A variety of studies report referral rates between 1.2 and 13.6%, most commonly for incompletely rehabilitated musculoskeletal injuries and heart murmurs (Harris & Runyan, 1991).

Ideally, the sports physical examination should be an individually scheduled appointment with the child's primary care provider. However, mass screenings are common in many school districts as an efficiency measure or because some youth may not be able to afford the examination or may have difficulty getting to such appointments. The mass screenings can be designed with stations for each part of the examination or organized with one-station visits for each child. One study has shown higher identification rates for problems when one examiner assesses hearts, another looks at backs, and so on (DuRant et al., 1985). However, there is a loss of continuity from history to physical examination and minimal opportunity to use the visit for health-promotion purposes. The NP needs to be clear about the goal of the examination: an opportunity to complete an annual health-promotion visit with special attention to sports, or solely a screening activity

TABLE 15-1
Psychosocial Implications of Sports Activities

POSITIVES	NEGATIVES
Fitness	Stress
Social skills	Meeting adult goals
Family activity and involvement	Potential for injuries
Self-esteem	Child may be made to feel inadequate;
Confidence	negative attributes
Coordination and physical skills	may be emphasized
Fun and recreation	

to identify children at risk for sports participation. Even if the latter choice is made, maximal health-promotion interventions need to be included in the project. For NPs working in school-based clinics, the sports physical can provide an opportunity to begin to introduce clinic services to the students and to encourage them to return for other health-related services. Communication with parents, coaches, and trainers is essential, whatever process for conducting the examinations is selected.

The psychosocial implications of sports participation need to be clearly identified both for practitioners and for the children and families with whom they work (Table 15–1).

RISK FACTORS

When assessing the young person for participation in sports, any history or physical findings in the following areas should be of special concern:

- Previous trauma, especially musculoskeletal or central nervous system injuries
- Cardiovascular disease, hypertension (>99th percentile) or exertional syncope
- Asthma or other allergic reactions
- Seizure disorder
- Infectious mononucleosis
- Skin infection
- Anatomical abnormalities or Down syndrome
- Obesity
- Conditions listed in Table 15–2

T A B L E 15-2

Medical Conditions and Sports Participation*

CONDITION	MAY PARTICIPATE?
Atlantoaxial instability (instability of the joint between cervical vertebrae 1 and 2) *Explanation:* Athlete needs evaluation to assess risk of spinal cord injury during sports participation.	Qualified yes
Bleeding disorder *Explanation:* Athlete needs evaluation.	Qualified yes
Cardiovascular diseases: Carditis (inflammation of the heart) *Explanation:* Carditis may result in sudden death with exertion.	No
Hypertension (high blood pressure) *Explanation:* Those with significant essential (unexplained) hypertension should avoid weightlifting and power lifting, body building, and strength training. Those with secondary hypertension (hypertension caused by a previously identified disease) or severe essential hypertension need evaluation.	Qualified yes
Congenital heart disease (structural heart defects present at birth) *Explanation:* Those with mild forms may participate fully; those with moderate or severe forms, or those who have undergone surgery, need evaluation.	Qualified yes
Dysrhythmia (irregular heart rhythm) *Explanation:* Athlete needs evaluation because some types of dysrhythmia require therapy or make certain sports dangerous, or both.	Qualified yes
Mitral valve prolapse (abnormal heart valve) *Explanation:* Those with symptoms (chest pain, symptoms of possible dysrhythmia) or evidence of mitral regurgitation (leaking) on physical examination need evaluation. All others may participate fully.	Qualified yes
Heart murmur *Explanation:* If the murmur is innocent (does not indicate heart disease), full participation is permitted. Otherwise, the athlete needs evaluation (see "Congenital heart disease" and "Mitral valve prolapse" listed earlier).	Qualified yes
Cerebral palsy *Explanation:* Athlete needs evaluation.	Qualified yes
Diabetes mellitus *Explanation:* All sports can be played with proper attention to diet, hydration, and insulin therapy. Particular attention is needed for activities that last 30 min or more.	Yes
Diarrhea *Explanation:* Unless disease is mild, no participation is permitted, because diarrhea may increase the risk of dehydration and heat illness (see "Fever" listed later).	Qualified no
Eating disorders: Anorexia nervosa, bulimia nervosa *Explanation:* These patients need both medical and psychiatric assessment before participation may be allowed.	Qualified yes
Eyes: Functionally one-eyed athlete, loss of an eye, detached retina, previous eye surgery, or serious eye injury *Explanation:* A functionally one-eyed athlete has a best corrected visual acuity of <20/40 in the worse eye. These athletes would suffer significant disability if the better eye was seriously injured as would those with loss of an eye. Some athletes who have previously undergone eye surgery or had a serious eye injury may have an increased risk of injury because of weakened eye tissue. Availability of eye guards approved by the American Society for Testing Materials (ASTM) and other protective equipment may allow participation in most sports, but this must be judged on an individual basis.	Qualified yes

T A B L E 15-2

Medical Conditions and Sports Participation* Continued*

CONDITION	MAY PARTICIPATE?
Fever *Explanation:* Fever can increase cardiopulmonary effort, reduce maximum exercise capacity, make heat illness more likely, and increase orthostatic hypotension during exercise. Fever may rarely accompany myocarditis or other infections that may make exercise dangerous.	No
Heat illness: History of *Explanation:* Because of the increased likelihood of recurrence, the athlete needs individual assessment to determine the presence of predisposing conditions and to arrange a prevention strategy.	Qualified yes
HIV infection *Explanation:* Because of the apparent minimal risk to others, all sports may be played that the state of health allows. In all athletes, skin lesions should be properly covered, and athletic personnel should use universal precautions when handling blood or body fluids with visible blood.	Yes
Kidney: Absence of one *Explanation:* Athlete needs individual assessment for contact, collision, and limited contact sports.	Qualified yes
Liver: Enlarged *Explanation:* If the liver is acutely enlarged, participation should be avoided because of risk of rupture. If the liver is chronically enlarged, individual assessment is needed before collision, contact, or limited contact sports are played.	Qualified yes
Malignancy *Explanation:* Athlete needs individual assessment.	Qualified yes
Musculoskeletal disorders *Explanation:* Athlete needs individual assessment.	Qualified yes
Neurological disorders: History of serious head or spine trauma, severe or repeated concussions, or craniotomy *Explanation:* Athlete needs individual assessment for collision, contact, or limited contact sports, and also for noncontact sports if there are deficits in judgment or cognition. Research supports a conservative approach to management of concussion.	Qualified yes
Convulsive disorder: Well controlled *Explanation:* Risk of convulsion during participation is minimal.	Yes
Convulsive disorders: Poorly controlled *Explanation:* Athlete needs individual assessment for collision, contact, or limited contact sports. Avoid the following noncontact sports: Archery, riflery, swimming, weightlifting, power lifting, strength training, or sports involving heights. In these sports, occurrence of a convulsion may be a risk to self or others.	Qualified yes
Obesity *Explanation:* Because of the risk of heat illness, obese persons need careful acclimatization and hydration.	Qualified yes
Organ transplant recipient *Explanation:* Athlete needs individual assessment.	Qualified yes
Ovary: absence of one *Explanation:* Risk of severe injury to the remaining ovary is minimal.	Yes
Respiratory: Pulmonary compromise, including cystic fibrosis *Explanation:* Athlete needs individual assessment, but generally all sports may be played if oxygenation remains satisfactory during a graded exercise test. Patients with cystic fibrosis need acclimatization and good hydration to reduce the risk of heat illness.	Qualified yes

Table continued on following page

T A B L E   15-2

Medical Conditions and Sports Participation* *Continued*

CONDITION	MAY PARTICIPATE?
Asthma	Yes
Explanation: With proper medication and education, only athletes with the most severe asthma have to modify their participation.	
Acute upper respiratory infection	Qualified yes
Explanation: Upper respiratory obstruction may affect pulmonary function. Athlete needs individual assessment for all but mild disease (see "Fever" listed earlier).	
Sickle cell disease	Qualified yes
Explanation: Athlete needs individual assessment. In general, if status of the illness permits, all but high-exertion, collision or contact sports may be played. Overheating, dehydration, and chilling must be avoided.	
Sickle cell trait	Yes
Explanation: It is unlikely that individuals with sickle cell trait (AS) have an increased risk of sudden death or other medical problems during athletic participation except under the most extreme conditions of heat, humidity, and, possibly, increased altitude. These individuals, like all athletes, should be carefully conditioned, acclimatized, and hydrated to reduce any possible risk.	
Skin: Boils, herpes simplex, impetigo, scabies, molluscum contagiosum	Qualified yes
Explanation: While the patient is contagious, participation in gymnastics with mats, martial arts, wrestling, or other collision, contact, or limited contact sports is not allowed. Herpes simplex virus probably is not transmitted via mats.	
Spleen: Enlarged	Qualified yes
Explanation: Patients with acutely enlarged spleens should avoid all sports because of risk of rupture. Those with chronically enlarged spleens need individual assessment before playing collision, contact, or limited contact sports.	
Testicle: Absent or undescended	Yes
Explanation: Certain sports may require a protective cup.	

*This table is designed to be understood by medical and nonmedical personnel. In the "Explanation" section, "needs evaluation" means that a physician with appropriate knowledge and experience should assess the safety of a given sport for an athlete with the listed medical condition. Unless otherwise noted, this is because of the variability of the severity of the disease or of the risk of injury among the specific sports listed in Table 15-2, or both.

Used with permission of the American Academy of Pediatrics. American Academy of Pediatrics Committee on Sports Medicine: Medical conditions affecting sports participation. Pediatrics 94:757–760, 1994. Copyright 1994 by the American Academy of Pediatrics.

Recommendations for participation given any of these conditions are discussed later in this chapter.

HISTORY

Coaches and others need to be aware of the athlete's health status in case problems arise during participation. Many medical history forms that are used to identify children with health conditions that might be adversely influenced by participation in a sport are available. A modification of the health history form rec- ommended by the AAFP and other organizations (1997) is found in Table 15-3. Many of the questions on the form relate to the risk factors listed earlier.

For a more holistic view, the NP should add questions about the following:

- The particular sports activity planned
- Extent of participation
- Level of competition
- Training schedule
- Use of protective devices, headgear, and new equipment

T A B L E 15-3

Preparticipation Physical Evaluation

HISTORY   **DATE OF EXAM** _____

Name _____ **Sex** _____ **Age** _____ **Date of birth** _____

Grade _____ **School** _____ **Sport(s)** _____

Address _____ **Phone** _____

Personal physician _____

In case of emergency, contact

Name _____ **Relationship** _____ **Phone (H)** _____ **(W)** _____

Explain "Yes" answers below. Circle questions you don't know the answers to.

	Yes	No
1. Have you had a medical illness or injury since your last check up or sports physical?	☐	☐
Do you have an ongoing or chronic illness?	☐	☐
2. Have you ever been hospitalized overnight?	☐	☐
3. Are you currently taking any prescription or nonprescription (over-the-counter) medications or pills or using an inhaler?	☐	☐
Have you ever taken any supplements or vitamins to help you gain or lose weight or improve your performance?	☐	☐
4. Do you have any allergies (for example, to pollen, medicine, food, or stinging insects)?	☐	☐
Have you ever had a rash or hives develop during or after exercise?	☐	☐
5. Have you ever passed out during or after exercise?	☐	☐
Have you ever been dizzy during or after exercise?	☐	☐
Have you ever had chest pain during or after exercise?	☐	☐
Do you get tired more quickly than your friends do during exercise?	☐	☐
Have you ever had racing of your heart or skipped heartbeats?	☐	☐
Have you had high blood pressure or high cholesterol?	☐	☐
Have you ever been told you have a heart murmur?	☐	☐
Has any family member or relative died of heart problems or of sudden death before age 50?	☐	☐
Have you had a severe viral infection (for example, myocarditis or mononucleosis) within the last month?	☐	☐
Has a physician ever denied or restricted your participation in sports for any heart problems?	☐	☐
6. Do you have any current skin problems (for example, itching, rashes, acne, warts, fungus, or blisters)?	☐	☐
7. Have you ever had a head injury or concussion?	☐	☐
Have you ever been knocked out, become unconscious, or lost your memory?	☐	☐
Have you ever had a seizure?	☐	☐
Do you have frequent or severe headaches?	☐	☐
Have you ever had numbness or tingling in your arms, hands, legs, or feet?	☐	☐
Have you ever had a stinger, burner, or pinched nerve?	☐	☐
8. Have you ever become ill from exercising in the heat?	☐	☐
9. Do you cough, wheeze, or have trouble breathing during or after activity?	☐	☐
Do you have asthma?	☐	☐
Do you have seasonal allergies that require medical treatment?	☐	☐

Table continued on following page

T A B L E 15-3

Preparticipation Physical Evaluation Continued

10. Do you use any special protective or corrective equipment or devices that aren't usually used for your sport or position (for example, knee brace, special neck roll, foot orthotics, retainer on your teeth, hearing aid)? □ □
11. Have you had any problems with your eyes or vision? □ □
    Do you wear glasses, contacts, or protective eyewear? □ □
12. Have you ever had a sprain, strain, or swelling after injury? □ □
    Have you broken or fractured any bones or dislocated any joints? □ □
    Have you had any other problems with pain or swelling in muscles, tendons, bones, or joints? □ □
    If yes, check appropriate box and explain below.

    □ Head   □ Elbow   □ Hip
    □ Neck   □ Forearm   □ Thigh
    □ Back   □ Wrist   □ Knee
    □ Chest   □ Hand   □ Skin/calf
    □ Shoulder   □ Finger   □ Ankle
    □ Upper arm   □ Foot

13. Do you want to weigh more or less than you do now? □ □
    Do you lose weight regularly to meet weight requirements for your sport? □ □
14. Do you feel stressed out? □ □
15. Record the dates of your most recent immunizations (shots) for:
    Tetanus _____ Measles _____
    Hepatitis B _____ Chickenpox _____

FEMALES ONLY

16. When was your first menstrual period? _____
    When was your most recent menstrual period? _____
    How many days do you usually have from the start of one period to the start of another? _____
    How many periods have you had in the last year? _____
    What was the longest time between periods in the last year? _____

Explain "Yes" answers here: _____
_____
_____
_____
_____

I hereby state that, to the best of my knowledge, my answers to the above questions are complete and correct.

Signature of athlete   Signature of parent/guardian   Date

T A B L E 15-3

Preparticipation Physical Evaluation Continued

PHYSICAL EXAMINATION

Name _____ **Date of birth** _____
Height _____ **Weight** _____ **% Body fat (optional)** _____ **Pulse** _____ **BP** __/__ (__/__, __/__)
Vision R 20/____ L 20/____   **Corrected: Y N**   **Pupils: Equal** _____ **Unequal** _____

	NORMAL	ABNORMAL FINDINGS	INITIALS*
MEDICAL			
Appearance			
Eyes/ears/nose/throat			
Lymph nodes			
Heart			
Pulses			
Lungs			
Abdomen			
Genitalia (males only)			
Skin			
MUSCULOSKELETAL			
Neck			
Back			
Shoulder/arm			
Elbow/forearm			
Wrist/hand			
Hip/thigh			
Knee			
Leg/ankle			
Foot			

*Station-based examination only

Table continued on following page

T A B L E 15-3

Preparticipation Physical Evaluation Continued

CLEARANCE

☐ **Cleared**
☐ **Cleared after completing evaluation/rehabilitation for:** _____
_____
_____
_____

☐ **Not cleared for:** _____
Reason: _____
Recommendations: _____
_____
_____

Name of health-care provider (print/type) _____
Date _____
Address _____ **Phone** _____
Signature of health-care provider _____

Modified from the American Academy of Family Physicians, American Academy of Pediatrics, American Medical Society for Sports Medicine, et al: Preparticipation physical evaluation. *In* American Academy of Family Physicians, American Academy of Pediatrics, American Medical Society for Sports Medicine, et al: The Physician and Sportsmedicine, 2nd ed. Minneapolis, MN, McGraw-Hill, 1997.

- Coaching and supervision
- Hazardous playing and field conditions
- Plans for the activity in the future
- Health promotion and preventive strategies planned
- Planned nutrition
- Preparticipation conditioning
- Risk behaviors such as increased alcohol consumption, driving while intoxicated, lack of seat-belt use, lack of helmet use while motorcycling, lack of contraception use, use of drugs or steroids, smoking, unprotected sexual activity, and numbers of sexual partners. (College athletes were found to have increased activity in these areas [Nattiv & Puffer, 1991])
- Family involvement and support
- Psychological issues as follow:
  ○ Stress management during the competitive season
  ○ Measures for success
  ○ Recent life changes
  ○ Strategies to maintain school work

PHYSICAL EXAMINATION

The physical examination should consist of two parts, the musculoskeletal examination and the general physical examination. The 2-minute orthopedic screening examination, which includes 12 simple steps, is recommended (Fig. 15-1). The examination focuses on musculoskeletal alignment, flexibility and proprioception, which are effective measures of abnormalities and injury sequelae. The additional musculoskeletal examination is done in conjunction with the regular physical examination, which focuses especially on the cardiovascular system, with blood pressure measurement, palpation of peripheral pulses, and auscultation.

LABORATORY EXAMINATION

Urinalysis and hematocrit or hemoglobin are not recommended by the AAP as part of the sports preparticipation examination. Although these can be useful for evaluation of a specific disease, there is no true indication from a health screening perspective. For adolescent girls, iron deficiency anemia is common enough that it may be appropriate to screen for the condition. Urine drug screening and human immunodeficiency virus (HIV) testing may be required by certain elite amateur or professional

EXAMINATION PARAMETERS
- Appropriate for interscholastic, intramural, and extramural sports activities.
- A screening evaluation created to direct attention to problems but *not* evaluate the problems.
- Identifies the following conditions that might be adversely affected by athletic participation:
  a. Congenital problems
  b. Acquired problems

HISTORY
Questions such as the following are to be answered by the athlete and signed by BOTH the athlete and parent:
- Have you ever had an illness, condition, or injury that required you to go to the hospital, either as a patient overnight or in the emergency room or for x-rays; required an operation; caused you to see a doctor; caused you to miss a game or practice?
- Are you now or have you been under the care of a physician for any reason?
- Do you currently have any medical problems or injuries?
- Have you ever had a broken bone, joint sprain or ligament tear, muscle pull, head injury, neck injury or nerve pinch, dislocated joint, back trouble or problems?

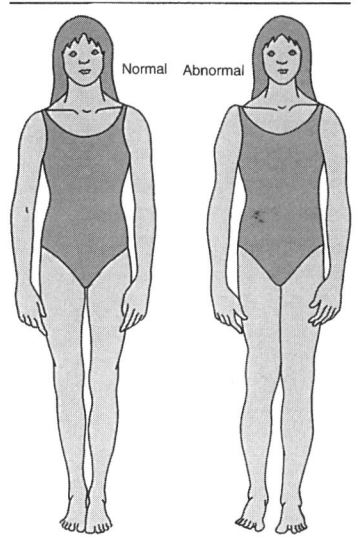

ACTIVITY 1

Normal   Abnormal

INSTRUCTIONS Stand straight with arms at sides.

OBSERVATIONS Symmetry of upper and lower extremities and trunk.
Common abnormalities:
1. Enlarged acromioclavicular joint
2. Enlarged sternoclavicular joint
3. Asymmetrical waist (leg length difference or scoliosis)
4. Swollen knee
5. Swollen ankle

ACTIVITY 2

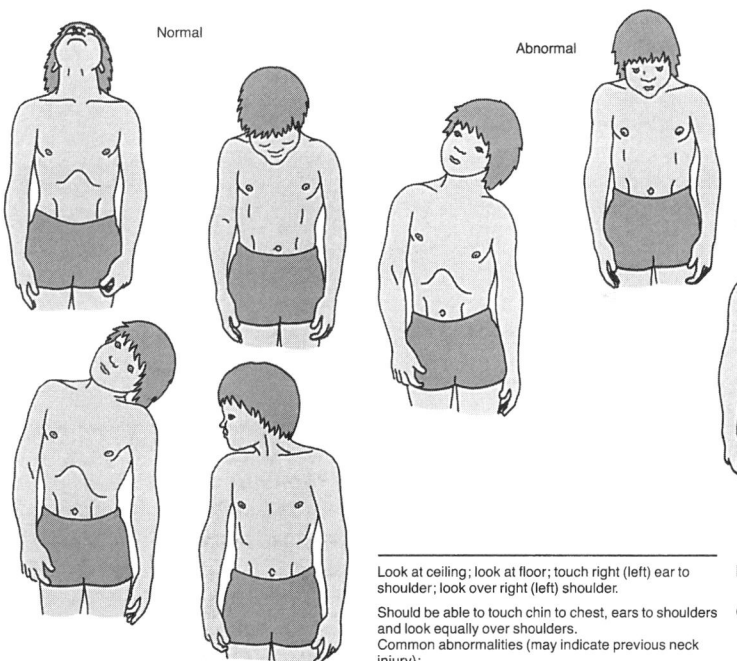

Normal   Abnormal

INSTRUCTIONS Look at ceiling; look at floor; touch right (left) ear to shoulder; look over right (left) shoulder.

OBSERVATIONS Should be able to touch chin to chest, ears to shoulders and look equally over shoulders.
Common abnormalities (may indicate previous neck injury):
1. Loss of flexion
2. Loss of lateral bending
3. Loss of rotation

F I G U R E 15-1
See legend on page 356.

Illustration continued on following page

ACTIVITY 3

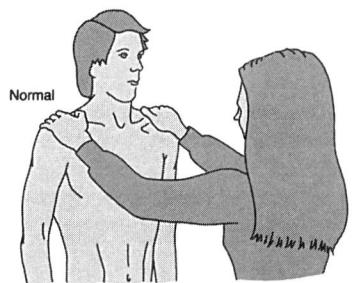

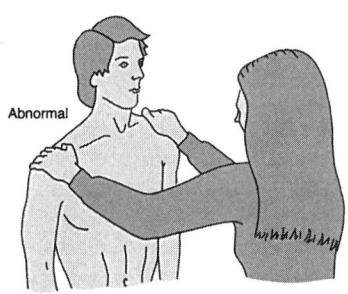

INSTRUCTIONS Shrug shoulders while examiner holds them down.

OBSERVATIONS Trapezius muscles appear equal; left and right sides equal strength.
Common abnormalities (may indicate neck or shoulder problem):
1. Loss of strength
2. Loss of muscle bulk

ACTIVITY 4

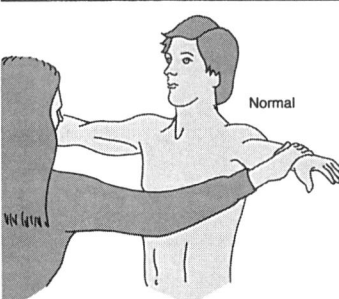

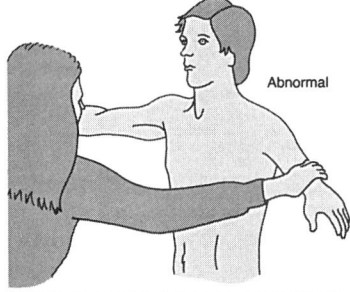

Hold arms out from sides horizontally and lift while examiner holds them down. **INSTRUCTIONS**

Strength should be equal and deltoid muscles should be equal in size. **OBSERVATIONS**
Common abnormalities:
1. Loss of strength
2. Wasting of deltoid muscle

ACTIVITY 5

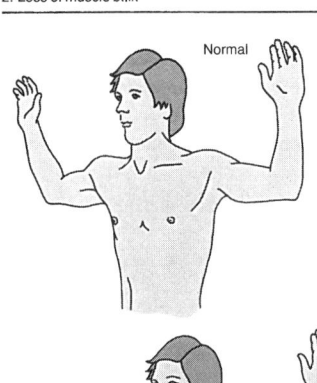

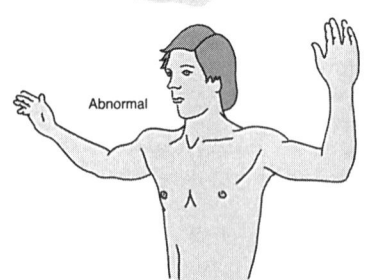

INSTRUCTIONS Hold arms out from sides with elbows bent (90°); raise hands back vertically as far as they will go.

OBSERVATIONS Hands go back equally and at least to upright vertical position.
Common abnormalities (may indicate shoulder problem or old dislocation):
1. Loss of external rotation

ACTIVITY 6

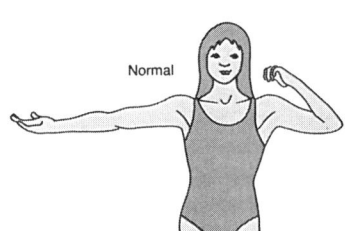

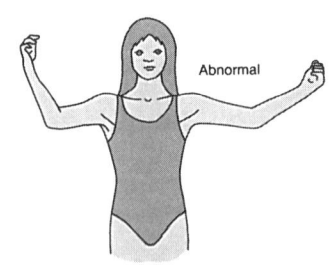

Hold arms out from sides, palms up; straighten elbows completely; bend completely. **INSTRUCTIONS**

Motion equal left and right. **OBSERVATIONS**
Common abnormalities (may indicate old elbow injury, old dislocation, fracture, etc.):
1. Loss of extension
2. Loss of flexion

FIGURE 15-1
Continued

ACTIVITY 7

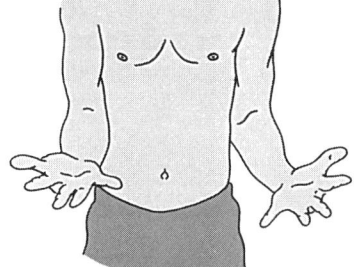

Normal   Abnormal

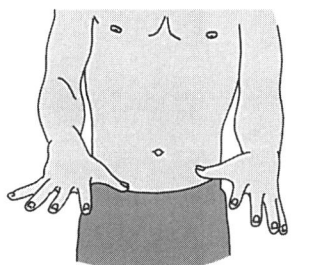

ACTIVITY 8

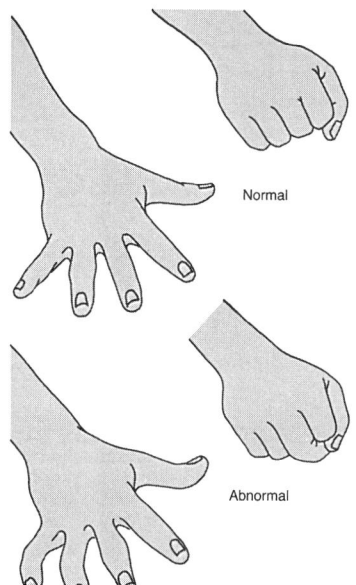

Normal

Abnormal

INSTRUCTIONS	Hold arms down at sides with elbows bent (90°); supinate palms ; pronate palms.
OBSERVATIONS	Palms should go from facing ceiling to facing floor. Common abnormalities (may indicate old forearm, wrist, or elbow injury):

1. Lack of full supination
2. Lack of full pronation

Make a fist; open hand and spread fingers.

Fist should be tight and fingers straight when spread. Common abnormalities (may indicate old finger fractures or sprains):
1. Protruding knuckle from fist
2. Swollen and/or crooked finger

INSTRUCTIONS

OBSERVATIONS

ACTIVITY 9

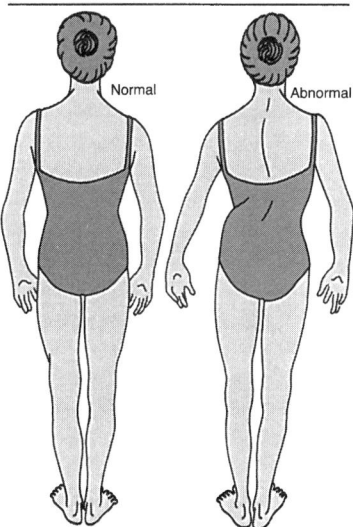

Normal   Abnormal

ACTIVITY 10

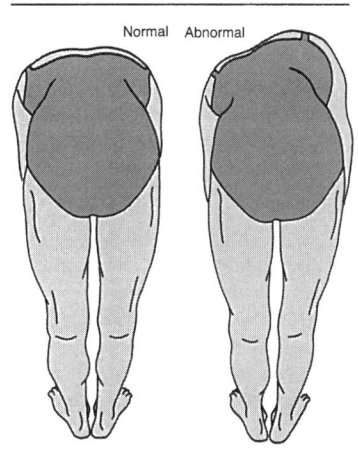

Normal   Abnormal

INSTRUCTIONS	With back to examiner stand up straight.
OBSERVATIONS	Symmetry of shoulders, waist, thighs, and calves. Common abnormalities:

1. High shoulder (scoliosis) or low shoulder (muscle loss)
2. Prominent rib cage (scoliosis)
3. High hip or asymmetrical waist (leg length difference or scoliosis)
4. Small calf or thigh (weakness from old injury)

Bend forward slowly as to touch toes.

Bends forward straightly and smoothly. Common abnormalities:
1. Twists to side (low back pain)
2. Back asymmetrical (scoliosis)

INSTRUCTIONS

OBSERVATIONS

F I G U R E 15-1
Continued

Illustration continued on following page

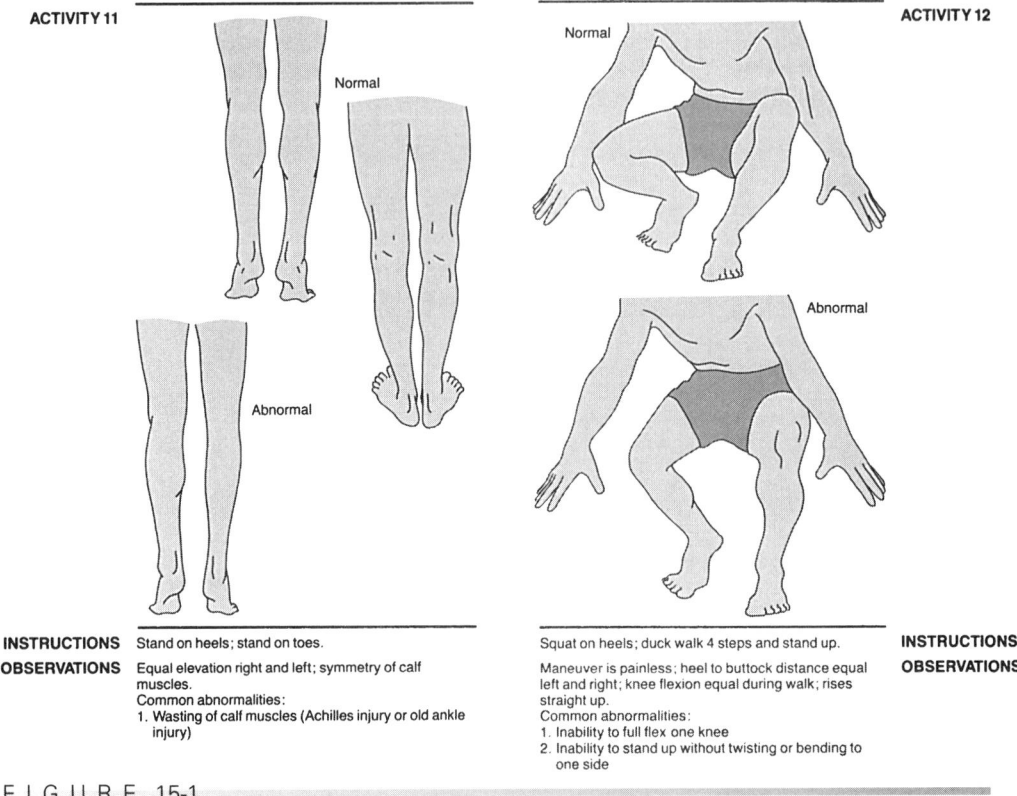

ACTIVITY 11

Normal

Abnormal

INSTRUCTIONS   Stand on heels; stand on toes.

OBSERVATIONS   Equal elevation right and left; symmetry of calf
muscles.
Common abnormalities:
1. Wasting of calf muscles (Achilles injury or old ankle
injury)

ACTIVITY 12

Normal

Abnormal

Squat on heels; duck walk 4 steps and stand up.

Maneuver is painless; heel to buttock distance equal
left and right; knee flexion equal during walk; rises
straight up.
Common abnormalities:
1. Inability to full flex one knee
2. Inability to stand up without twisting or bending to
one side

INSTRUCTIONS

OBSERVATIONS

F I G U R E 15-1
The orthopedic physical examination for sports participation. (Used with permission of Ross Products
Division, Abbott Laboratories, Columbus, OH 43216. From For the Practitioner: Orthopaedic Screening
Examination for Participation in Sports. © 1981 Ross Products Division, Abbott Laboratories.)

organizations. Voluntary testing should be encouraged if the athlete has any risk factors.

Classification of Sports for Risk

The AAP has classified the most common sports
activities into three types (Table 15-4). When
used with Table 15-2, Medical Conditions and
Sports Participation, the clinician can make specific recommendations as to which sports are
appropriate for young people with identified
health problems.

Recommendations for Participation in Sports for Children With High-Risk Conditions

Table 15-2 summarizes the AAP's recommendations for sports for youth with specific health

conditions. Tables 15-2 and 15-4 should be
available in the clinic setting. They lend credibility to sports participation recommendations
and should serve as guidelines for recommendations the NP makes to students and their families. Although families and schools will make
their own choices, the recommendations
should be recorded in both the student's permanent record and the form returned to the
school or sports facility. The goal is to find
safe, healthful activities for all children, not to
restrict their activities unnecessarily.

Several high-risk conditions are discussed in
the following section.

PREVIOUS TRAUMA

All musculoskeletal injuries require individual
assessment and decision-making. Referral to an

T A B L E 15-4

Classification of Sports by Contact

CONTACT/ COLLISION	LIMITED CONTACT	NONCONTACT
Basketball	Baseball	Archery
Boxing*	Bicycling	Badminton
Diving	Cheerleading	Body building
Field	Canoeing/kayaking	Canoeing/
hockey	(white water)	kayaking
Football	Fencing	(flat water)
flag	Field	Crew/rowing
tackle	high jump	Curling
Ice hockey	pole vault	Dancing
Lacrosse	Floor hockey	Field
Martial arts	Gymnastics	discus
Rodeo	Handball	javelin
Rugby	Horseback riding	shot put
Ski	Racquetball	Golf
jumping	Skating	Orienteering
Soccer	ice	Power lifting
Team	in-line	Race walking
handball	roller	Riflery
Water polo	Skiing	Rope jumping
Wrestling	cross-country	Running
	downhill	Sailing
	water	Scuba diving
	Softball	Strength
	Squash	training
	Ultimate frisbee	Swimming
	Volleyball	Table tennis
	Windsurfing/	Tennis
	surfing	Track
		Weightlifting

*Participation not recommended.
Used with permission of the American Academy of Pediatrics, American Academy of Pediatrics Committee on Sports Medicine. (1994). Medical conditions affecting sports participation. Pediatrics 94:757–760. Copyright 1994 by the American Academy of Pediatrics.

orthopedist may be required. In general, the athlete must be able to demonstrate, *without pain*, full range of motion, normal strength, endurance, and motor skills needed for participation before returning to the sport. Otherwise, repeated injury can be anticipated (Hergenroeder, 1998). Sprains, subluxations, dislocations, muscle contusions, and overuse injuries have the following characteristics:

- Effusion, swelling, or other signs of inflammation

- Decreased range of motion of the affected joint
- Strength less than 85% of the uninjured side or insufficient for the desired activity
- Ligamentous instability
- Loss of functional ability (AAFP et al., 1997)

For sports clearance, none of these characteristics should be found.

Use of supportive athletic devices such as knee or ankle braces can be accepted to achieve the tasks identified above (e.g., full range of motion, normal strength) (Nelson, 1992). Overuse injuries are caused by recurrent microtrauma resulting first in pain and inflammation and later in tissue failure and disability. Clearance criteria are similar to those for acute strains and sprains. Fractures need clearance by the treating physician (AAFP et al., 1997).

An estimated 300,000 sports-related traumatic brain injuries of mild to moderate severity occur annually in the United States (Centers for Disease Control [CDC], 1997). Central nervous system trauma is important to assess, because repeated concussions are often progressively more serious. Various concussion management protocols have evolved. The most recent and recommended is "Management of Concussion in Sports" (American Academy of Neurology, 1997) (Table 15–5). For the young person with a history of any serious head injury or intracranial surgery, consultation with a neurosurgeon should occur before participation. Athletes may suffer from a condition called second-impact syndrome in which a second brain injury occurring shortly after a mild concussion (generally within 2 weeks) causes massive brain swelling with significant mortality (Centers for Disease Control and Prevention, 1997). Because of this condition, properly identifying the concussion (Table 15–6) and accurately excluding the athlete from competition based on set criteria (Table 15–7) as well as preventing early reinjury are of utmost importance. Generally, athletes with a history of concussion who have been asymptomatic for a specified period of time and who have no neurological symptoms are allowed to participate in all sports (AAFP et al., 1997). A study by Guskiewicz and associates (1997) found that with mild head injury, it took

T A B L E 15-5

Recommendations for Management of Concussion in Sports*

GRADE 1 CONCUSSION

Definition: Transient confusion, no loss of consciousness, and a duration of mental status abnormalities of <15 min.

Management: The athlete should be removed from sports activity, examined immediately and at 5-min intervals, and allowed to return that day to the sports activity only if postconcussive symptoms resolve within 15 min.

Any athlete who incurs a second grade 1 concussion on the same day should be removed from sports activity until asymptomatic for 1 wk.

GRADE 2 CONCUSSION

Definition: Transient confusion, no loss of consciousness, and a duration of mental status abnormalities of ≥15 min.

Management: The athlete should be removed from sports activity and examined frequently to assess the evolution of symptoms, with more extensive diagnostic evaluation if the symptoms worsen or persist for >1 wk. The athlete should return to sports activity only after asymptomatic for 1 full wk. Any athlete who incurs a grade 2 concussion subsequent to a grade 1 concussion on the same day should be removed from sports activity until asymptomatic for 2 wk.

GRADE 3 CONCUSSION

Definition: Loss of consciousness, either brief (sec) or prolonged (min or longer).

Management: The athlete should be removed from sports activity for 1 full wk without symptoms if the loss of consciousness is brief or 2 full wk without symptoms if the loss of consciousness is prolonged. If still unconscious or if abnormal neurologic signs are present at the time of initial evaluation, the athlete should be transported by ambulance to the nearest hospital emergency department. An athlete who suffers a second grade 3 concussion should be removed from sports activity until asymptomatic for 1 mo. Any athlete with an abnormality on computed tomography or magnetic resonance imaging brain scan consistent with brain swelling, contusion, or other intracranial pathology should be removed from sports activities for the season and discouraged from future return to participation in contact sports.

*A concussion is defined as head-trauma-induced alteration in mental status that may or may not involve loss of consciousness. Concussions are graded in three categories. Definitions and treatment recommendations for each category are presented.

Data from Centers for Disease Control and Prevention: Sports-related recurrent brain injuries—United States. JAMA 277:1190–1191, 1997; American Academy of Neurology Quality Standards Subcommittee: Practice parameter: The management of concussion in sports (summary statement). Neurology 48:581–585, 1997.

athletes 3 days to resolve the neurological sequelae.

Burners, stingers, and transient quadriplegia must be asymptomatic before clearance for sports participation. Burners and stingers are nerve root or brachial plexus compression or traction injuries and generally cause unilateral symptoms. They may require cervical spine evaluation if recurrent or persistent. Transient quadriplegia is a much more significant problem that generally appears with bilateral symptoms. It is a contraindication for contact/colli-sion sports until fully evaluated or if any objective structural problems are found. Youths with burners, stingers, or transient quadriplegia symptoms need careful evaluation and must be free of symptoms before sports clearance (AAFP et al., 1997; Cantu, 1997).

CHRONIC MEDICAL CONDITIONS

Cardiac Disease

Most grade I–II/VI systolic murmurs without significant cardiovascular history do not need

T A B L E 15-6

Recognizing a Concussion in Athletes

SYMPTOMS	SIGNS FREQUENTLY OBSERVED (note early vs. late)

Early (min to hr)
  Headache
  Dizziness or vertigo
  Unawareness of surroundings
  Nausea or vomiting
Late (d to wk)
  Light-headedness
  Persistent mild headache
  Poor attention/concentration
  Memory dysfunction
  Fatigue
  Irritability/low frustration tolerance
  Sleep disturbance
	Vacant stare (befuddled facial expression)
	Delayed verbal and motor responses (slower to answer questions or follow instructions)
	Confusion/distractibility (easily distracted and unable to follow through with normal activities)
	Disorientation—time, place, date (walking in wrong direction; unaware of time, date, place)
	Slurred, incoherent speech (making disjointed or incomprehensible statements)
	Gross incoordination (stumbling, unable to walk tandem/straight line)
	Emotions out of proportion to situation (appearing distraught, crying for no apparent reason)
	Memory deficits (asking same question repeatedly, can't remember words, numbers for 5 min)
	Any period of loss of consciousness (paralytic coma, unresponsive to stimuli)

From American Academy of Neurology Quality Standards Subcommittee: Practice parameter: The management of concussion in sports (summary statement). Neurology 48:581–585, 1997.

further evaluation. However, louder or diastolic murmurs, unusual loudness, or wide splitting of S_2, and increased loudness with Valsalva maneuver or standing require further evaluation. A history of syncope with exertion, palpitations, or chest pain, or a family history of sudden unexpected death in the young or middle-aged should be evaluated for problems such as hypertrophic cardiomyopathy (formerly idiopathic hypertrophic subaortic stenosis) regardless of physical examination findings. Other cardiovascular causes of sudden death among teenagers engaged in athletic events include valvular aortic stenosis, mitral valve prolapse, ventricular arrhythmias, coronary arterial abnormalities, and coarctation of the aorta. Individuals with myocarditis, hypertrophic cardiomyopathy, severe aortic stenosis, or anomalous coronary artery disease should be excluded from all but nonstrenuous sports participation (Nelson, 1992). Asking about use of anabolic steroids and cocaine is important, because both have been linked to sudden cardiac death (AAFP et al, 1997). The *26th Bethesda Conference: Recommendations for Determining Eligibility for Competition in Athletes With Cardiovascular Abnormalities* may be a useful reference (Mitchell et al., 1994; AAFP et al., 1997). Specific exercise prescriptions can be developed under a cardiologist's direction for children with known cardiac disease.

Hypertension

Hypertension should be diagnosed only after elevated blood pressures have been demonstrated on three separate occasions with use of proper technique. Children with mild hypertension (95th-99th percentiles for normal blood pressure ranges for age) should not be restricted from any sports. Those with severe hypertension (>99th percentile for age) should

T A B L E 15-7

Sideline Evaluation for Assessment of Head and Neck Trauma

MENTAL STATUS TESTING

ORIENTATION	Time, place, person, activity, situation before and after the trauma
CONCENTRATION	Digits said backward: 3–1–7, 4–6–8–2, 5–3–0–7–4 Months of year said backward
MEMORY	Names of teams in prior contest Details of contest, such as plays or strategies used Recall of three words and three objects at 0 and 5 min Recent newsworthy events

EXERTIONAL PROVOCATIVE TESTS

EXERCISES*	40-yd sprint 5 push-ups, 5 sit ups, 5 knee bends

NEUROLOGICAL TESTS

PUPILS	Symmetry and reaction
COORDINATION	Finger-nose-finger Tandem walk
SENSATION	Finger-nose with eyes closed Romberg test

*Any associated symptoms are abnormal, including headache, dizziness, nausea, unsteadiness, photophobia, blurred or double vision, emotional lability, or mental status changes.

From American Academy of Neurology Quality Standards Subcommittee: Practice parameter: The management of concussion in sports (summary statement). Neurology 48:583, 1997.

not be cleared for participation until the condition is evaluated and treated (AAFP et al., 1997). The American Academy of Pediatrics recommendations are similar but also recommend counseling of hypertensive youth to adopt healthful lifestyle behaviors, including avoidance of anabolic steroids, growth hormone, alcohol, tobacco, and high sodium intake. For some athletic governing bodies, use of diuretics and β-blockers is prohibited.

Asthma

Children with asthma should be encouraged, not discouraged, from participation in sports. Properly managed asthma should not present such problems with exertion as were common in the past. The great majority of patients with asthma can engage in sports, even though most may experience exercise-induced asthma (EIA). Most commonly, exercise-induced bronchospasm occurs in 80 to 90% of children with asthma and in 40 to 50% of children with allergic rhinitis alone but no previous asthma. Progressive airway obstruction generally occurs *after physical activity ceases* with peak airway resistance occurring 5 to 10 minutes after activity stops and resolving within 60 minutes (Guill, 1996). There is a refractory period that lasts from 40 minutes to 3 hours after recovery from an initial EIA episode. Doing warmup drills before vigorous exercise can help athletes use this refractory period to their benefit. Breathing cold, dry air is more irritating than warm, humid air. Thus, swimmers are known to experience less EIA, whereas hockey players and figure skaters have high incidences of the condition. EIA is generally not life threatening.

Recommended management includes the use of inhaled albuterol or other β-adrenergic agonists (taken by aerosol 5 to 60 minutes before exercise) or cromolyn sodium (20 to 40 mg by Spinhaler or two puffs by metered-dose inhaler immediately before exercise) (Guill, 1996). Short-acting inhaled β-agonists can be repeated after 2 hours if exercise continues. Warmup drills for 10 minutes can prevent up to 50% of episodes. Athletic conditioning also helps to improve muscle and exercise efficiency. Warming down, or gradually decreasing exercise at the end of a session also seems to help decrease the magnitude of the attack. Covering the mouth and nose with a scarf when exercising in cold air can also help because exhaled air warms inhaled air. Teachers and coaches should be aware of exercise-induced asthma. Many children with well-controlled asthma experience some airway obstruction after exercise. (See Chapter 25 for further discussion of asthma and its management.) (Guill, 1996; Tan & Spector, 1998).

Seizures

Children and adolescents with seizure disorders can participate in most sports. They should be excluded only if having a seizure would put them or others at significant risk (e.g., swimming, high diving, rope or rock climbing, archery). Decisions about participation in specific sports should be made with information about the severity, frequency, etiology, and degree of control of the seizures.

Diabetes Mellitus

Children with diabetes, whether insulin dependent or not, should be the least restricted of all those with chronic diseases. Exercise is an essential component of their management. The child should be well controlled before entering a sports program and should have immediate access to a home blood glucose monitoring system. Assistance from a diabetic educator or the physician who plans the child's insulin therapy, nutrition, and exercise regimen is important. It is important to know that exercise can delay the hypoglycemic response from insulin.

ACUTE INFECTIONS

Infectious Mononucleosis

The risk of splenic rupture with mononucleosis needs to be considered. Ultrasonography may reveal splenomegaly that is not clinically palpable. Splenic rupture has not been reported longer than 4 weeks after resolution of clinical symptoms, so this can be a good guideline to follow for deciding when the young person can return to contact sports, assuming that splenomegaly is not present on examination.

Skin Infections

Skin infections are a special consideration for wrestlers. The incidence of contracting herpes gladiatorum from exposure to a person with a herpes simplex infection ranges from 20 to 50%. Lesions should be healed before wrestling is resumed. For other sports, bandaging may be sufficient to prevent transmission. Athletes with impetigo or other streptococcal or staphylococcal infections should be on antibiotics for at least 48 hours or until significant improvement is seen before participating in contact or collision sports. Scabies, lice, and molluscum contagiosum preclude participation in contact or collision sports, especially in sports in which mats are used and in sports such as baseball, in which equipment is shared. Tinea infections can also be passed from athlete to athlete.

PHYSICAL ANOMALIES

Hernia

Hernias should be repaired. However, the teen with a hernia need not be restricted from sports participation but should be aware of the symptoms of incarceration.

Absence of Paired Organs

Sports that involve objects, sticks, or racquets, or aggressive play, such as football or basketball, have greater risks for eye injuries. Baseball is the most dangerous eye sport. Face shields are now required for hockey, and the incidence of serious injuries in this sport has dramatically decreased. Eyewear is available for all sports except those such as boxing and full-contact martial arts.

The child with one eye or best-corrected vision in one eye worse than 20/40 should be required to wear molded polycarbonate sport frames with 3–mm-thick polycarbonate lenses for all sports involving rapidly moving objects, bats, or racquets. For collision sports involving headgear, such as football, hockey, or lacrosse, the same frames and lenses should be worn under the cage shield or mask. These children should not participate in sports in which the use of eye protection is not possible. A history of detached retina is significant, and participation should be limited to nonstrenuous sports until consultation with an ophthalmologist is complete.

The child with one kidney needs individual evaluation for participation in contact or collision and limited contact sports.

Young men with a single testicle can be adequately protected with the use of a hard-cup athletic supporter for contact and collision sports as well as those in which there are objects projected at high speed. Although somewhat uncomfortable to wear, most affected men comply if the risks of sterility are explained (AAFP et al., 1997). Girls with one ovary are not restricted because of the protected location of the organ.

Atlantoaxial Instability

Children with Down syndrome can have instability where the head joins the spinal column. Previously, radiographic screening for these children was recommended, and those with atlantoaxial separation greater than 4 mm were excluded. More recent review of the data has led to removal of this recommendation by the American Academy of Pediatrics in favor of individual evaluation (AAP Committee on Sports Medicine and Fitness, 1995). However, clearance for Special Olympics may still require radiographic screening. Any other youths with known problems in this area should not engage in contact or collision sports or limited contact or impact sports (see Table 15-4) or in such sports as diving. They may, however, engage in most of the noncontact sports listed in Table 15-4. The risk of spinal cord injury cannot be dismissed.

▓▓▓ MANAGEMENT STRATEGIES TO SUPPORT CHILDREN AND ADOLESCENT ACTIVITY PATTERNS

Injury Prevention

Few studies provide information about the numbers of youths injured in sports and recreational activities. The injury rate for youths participating in sports and recreational activities is 6.4% according to estimates from the Child Health Supplement of the 1988 National Health Interview Survey (Bijur et al., 1995). Injuries varied by age, with older youths having an adjusted rate of 13.5%, whereas 5- to 9-year-olds had an adjusted rate of only 5.8%. Male children

were four times more likely to experience injuries than were female children. In another study, the injury rate was 22% (McLain & Reynolds, 1989). Estimates of injury rates were 22% for girls and 39% for boys per season (Ostrum, 1993). In another study, injury rates increased with age, level of competition, and frequency of activity (Backx et al., 1989). Severity of injuries also increased with age (Landry, 1992). High school sports with the greatest injury rates included gymnastics, ice hockey, and football. For college participants, gymnastics, football, lacrosse, and basketball resulted in the most injuries (Ostrum, 1993). Strains and sprains were the most frequent injuries, followed by contusions and fractures (Overbaugh & Allen, 1994b). Overuse injuries exceed traumatic injuries (Ostrum, 1993).

A variety of strategies can be used to reduce the incidence and severity of injuries. Safety rules for games are designed to reduce injuries; protective equipment makes a significant difference; maintenance of playing fields, floors, and equipment is important; coaches need to teach good techniques and guide athletes through adequate warmup and stretching exercises before and after the game; and support personnel need to be qualified to manage acute trauma and cardiopulmonary resuscitation. Youngsters need to be matched for both skill and size. Maturational age is a better gauge than chronological age (Maffulli, 1990; Hergenroeder, 1998).

Injuries are of two main types—traumatic and overuse. Prevention strategies are different for the two types (Dyment, 1991a). Management of sports injuries is discussed in the Injuries chapter, and prevention strategies are summarized below.

TRAUMATIC INJURY PREVENTION

Strains and Sprains

- Do preseason stretching
- Tape site of previous injury
- Warm up body temperature before stretching
- Maintain playing surfaces
- Use proper footwear
- Limit practice time

Fractures

- Do strength-conditioning exercises
- Use proper techniques
- Take safety precautions
- Use protective gear that fits

Head and Neck Injuries

- Have appropriate supervision
- Adhere to safety rules of the games
- Strengthen neck muscles
- Use appropriate equipment—helmets, face and mouth gear

Eye

- Use headgear and protective glasses

OVERUSE INJURY PREVENTION

Stress Fractures

- Use soft running and playing surfaces
- Use proper footgear
- Do strengthening exercises
- Stop activity when pain occurs

Anterior Leg Pain Syndrome (Shin Splints)

- Stretch before and after activity
- Pronate and supinate feet while standing
- Use soft playing surface
- Use proper footwear—proper fit, impact-absorbing sole, support for hindfoot
- Avoid sudden increase in activity
- Limit forceful, extensive use of foot flexors

Plantar Fasciitis

- Use proper footwear (cushioned with fitted heel counters or lifts)
- Stretch calf and Achilles tendon
- Do ice massage after event
- Correct biomechanical errors
- Limit hills and speed work; increase soft-surface running

Blisters

- Wear socks
- Wear properly fitted shoes

- Use powder, petroleum jelly, or a product such as Second Skin on reddened or risk areas

Stress and Sports: Keeping Activities Fun

Children and adolescents need to enjoy sports and to find that they reduce rather than induce stress if they are going to include vigorous physical activity in their lifestyles. The athletic environment should foster psychological as well as physical well-being. It is part of the NP's role to assess the psychological dimensions of sports participation and intervene when problems appear.

ATHLETIC STRESS

The Problem

Athletic stress arises as a result of the interactions between situational factors, personality factors, and motivational factors. Situationally, athletes need to have sufficient resources to meet the demands of the event. Cognitively, athletes make an appraisal of the situation. They assess the demands and their resources, the consequences of success or failure, and their personal interpretation of the consequences. A person with low self-confidence might assess a particular event as more stressful than would a person with high self-confidence even if both have equal skills. Stress occurs when the assessment yields perceived negative outcomes. There is also a physiological component to stress. When the athlete becomes overexcited, performance decreases. Finally, stress is related to the coping and behavioral responses the athlete uses.

The consequences of excessive athletic stress can be withdrawal from sports, decreased enjoyment, decreased performance, and negative physical effects, including interference with eating and sleeping or possible increase in injuries.

Management of Athletic Stress

First, cognitive interventions can be taken to manage athletic stress. The following are key points that may be helpful to youngsters and their families (Smoll & Smith, 1990):

- Winning is not everything or the only thing.
- Failure is not the same thing as losing.
- Success is not winning but rather striving for victory (the effort).

Second, the organization and administration of sports programs can make a difference in the pleasure experienced by young athletes. Some strategies include the following:

- Establishing different skill and competition levels
- Organizing homogeneous groups by age and size
- Not scoring games, keeping season records, or calculating individual statistics
- Directly altering games to increase opportunities for success, such as playing T-ball instead of pitched softball, lowering the basket, decreasing the length of games, using a smaller playing field, and changing some rules, such as no press defense in basketball or no stealing in baseball

Third, coaching roles and relationships can be modified. A program called coach-effectiveness training has been shown to positively influence athletes' feelings of self-esteem, player attitudes, appreciation of the coach, and relationships among the players. Coaches should use positive control techniques, reframe winning into success for effort, work on team cohesion and development of positive desire. Coaches may also need to support the injured athlete's need for reduced training and rehabilitation. Coaches also should not overtrain athletes because this results in fatigue and a sense of being "stale." Again, reduced training may be needed (Hergenroeder, 1998).

Fourth, parents need to focus on supporting their children rather than identifying with them. Parental success and feelings of self-worth should not derive from having a child who wins at sports. Neither should the family build its identity around the young athlete to the extent that poor performance becomes a family catastrophe (Hergenroeder, 1998). At a minimum, parents should manifest the following behaviors:

- Remain seated in the spectator area during the activity
- Not yell instructions or criticisms to their child
- Not make derogatory comments to players, parents of the opposing team, officials, or league administrators
- Not interfere with the child's coach

Finally, stress management training can be recommended for the child who anticipates giving a significant amount of energy and commitment to a sport over several years (Smoll & Smith, 1990).

Health Teaching to Prevent Problems

NUTRITION

Adolescents are growing at a rate second only to that of infants. Thus, the nutritional intake of adolescent athletes must meet both growth and activity needs. Depending on the sport, calorie requirements for activity exceed baseline needs by 1500 to 3000 calories (Loosli & Benson, 1990). The recommended diet for the athlete is the same as for all people—high in carbohydrates (50 to 60% of calories), 25 to 30% of calories from fats, and 15 to 20% of calories from protein. Normal growth of children requires an intake of 60 kcal/kg of ideal body weight per day (Patient Care Nurse Practitioner, 1998). There are no changes in intake of nutrients such as vitamins and minerals. For females, eating red meat 2 to 3 times per week may prevent anemia. Teenage women, like all others, should consume 1200 mg of calcium daily.

Short-term, high-intensity activities, such as high jumping or diving, involve use of anaerobic fuel sources, whereas longer term activities, such as running or cross-country skiing, involve use of aerobic sources. Carbohydrates are used in both anaerobic and aerobic metabolic states, but fats and proteins are used only aerobically. "For athletes involved in moderate to heavy training on a daily basis, the diet needs to provide 5 to 10 g of carbohydrate per kg of body weight per day" (American Orthopaedic Society for Sports Medicine, 1992). Most of the carbohydrate intake should come from nutritional foods such as fruits and vegetables, grains, and milk sugars rather than refined sugars. Nutrition recommendations are summarized in Table 15-8.

In general, ingesting carbohydrate before activities has no effect on performance, although carbohydrate loading over several days can be of some benefit for those engaged in endurance events (Dyment, 1991b). Carbohydrate intake during physical activity lasting more than 1 hour improves performance. After competition, carbohydrate intake is again important to improve muscle glycogen resynthesis, which is most rapid in the first few hours after exercise. Consuming 100 g of carbohydrate in the first 30 minutes after performance is recommended. (American Orthopaedic Society for Sports Medicine, 1992). Weight gain of mostly muscle mass occurs primarily through eating extra carbohydrate calories and exercising. Adding 400 to 500 calories per day of carbohydrates plus the replacement for exercise energy expenditure should ensure building muscle (Kleiner, 1995).

Increasing protein intake can be of some benefit, but usually the active athlete meets protein requirements easily. No protein supplements are needed. In fact, hypercalciuria with calcium loss and dehydration can occur if protein intake is too high because the excess nitrogen, and hence water, is excreted. Protein requirements are easily met with normal diets of 0.4 g per pound of body weight. Strength training athletes probably need 0.6 to 0.8 g/lb per day, and endurance athletes 0.5 to 0.6 g/lb per day. Vitamins and minerals do not need to be supplemented except in women who have a diet low in both calcium and iron.

Weight loss by adolescent athletes can be a dangerous practice. Wrestlers may try to make weight, runners sometimes vomit to run lighter, and female gymnasts practice significant nutritional control to maintain size. Dancers, divers, figure skaters, and cheerleaders also control weight for appearance advantages. Body builders, rowers, distance runners, and swimmers also often try to control their weight. Starvation

T A B L E 15-8

Nutrition Recommendations for Athletes

NUTRIENT	RECOMMENDATIONS
CALORIES FROM CARBOHYDRATES/ FAT/PROTEIN	Maintain same as for all people—50–55% carbohydrate, 30% fat, 15–20% protein Do not decrease caloric intake during sports season May need added 500 to 3000 calories to meet activity requirements
VITAMINS AND MINERALS	Same as for all people Adolescent girls may need to bring calcium and iron intake up to recommended range Do not take salt tablets; they can increase dehydration
CARBOHYDRATES	5–10 gm/kg body weight is recommended intake Use nutritional foods such as fruits, vegetables, grains, and milk sugars Carbohydrate intake during prolonged activity may increase performance Carbohydrate intake of 100 g in first 30 min after performance is recommended to promote muscle glycogen resynthesis and rapid reloading
PROTEIN SUPPLEMENTS	None needed; hypercalciuria with calcium loss and dehydration can occur if protein intake is too high
FLUIDS	Plain water before, during, and after activity Athletic drinks containing electrolytes may be helpful for endurance athletes and those who sweat heavily (not preadolescents) 8 oz fluid every 15–20 min for events lasting more than 30 min Replace water loss after activity at 2 cups per lb of weight lost Avoid caffeine drinks because they can increase diuresis

can lead to suppressed growth hormones, can interfere with pubertal gonadal hormone changes, and may result in eating disorders. Nutritional counseling is essential, with a reminder that muscle weighs more than fat and that weight gain during adolescence with growth is normal (Overbaugh & Allen, 1994c). Weight loss by energy restriction (reduced calories) significantly reduces anaerobic performance by wrestlers. Further, wrestlers on high carbohydrate refeeding diets tend to recover their performance, whereas those on moderate carbohydrate diets do not (Rankin et al. 1996). Wrestlers, coaches, and parents may sign a contract requiring that the child eat three meals a day, that fluid be available at all times, and that no artificial means be employed to remove fluids from the body (e.g., sauna or sweatsuit, laxatives, diuretics, diet pills, licit or illicit drugs, nicotine, prolonged fasting, overexercising, or vomiting) (Ostrum, 1993; American Academy of Pediatrics, 1996).

The young person can avoid dehydration by drinking cool, plain water before, during, and after the activity. Athletic drinks containing electrolytes can help replace losses for endurance athletes performing under extreme conditions or for those who sweat profusely, but they are generally unnecessary. In fact, the principal effect of added sodium may be to make the athlete more thirsty so that he or she drinks more (Ryan-Krause, 1998). For the preadolescent who does not sweat well, use of electrolyte solutions is definitely not warranted. Exercise in the mature adolescent can cause fluid losses of more than a liter per hour. The athlete should drink 16 oz of water 2 hours before the activity. For events lasting more than 30 minutes, 8 ounces of water needs to be consumed every 15 or 20 minutes. Because the first sensations of thirst occur only after dehydration has already occurred, drinking needs to begin before the need is felt. Furthermore, performance is reduced by the amount of dehydration present; by the time the athlete feels thirsty, he or she already is at less than peak performance. A weight loss of more than 4% of body weight puts the athlete at risk for heat cramps, illness, stroke, and even death. After competition, rehydration is important. Generally, drinking 2 cups of water for each pound of weight lost is ade-

quate. Small amounts of sodium such as are found in sports drinks enhance rehydration, but additional sodium supplements are not recommended. Drinking fluids with caffeine should be avoided, because these beverages increase urine output, causing further dehydration (American Orthopaedic Society for Sports Medicine, 1992). Use of separate fluid containers for each child participating may help monitor the intake of each while decreasing the risk of disease spread. (See Table 15–8 for Nutrition Recommendations for Athletes). Scheduling fluid breaks and rotating players more frequently may also help avoid heat-related problems (Patient Care Nurse Practitioner, 1998).

HEAT AND HUMIDITY

Because children have a higher metabolic rate at a given submaximal walking or running speed, they produce more heat. This higher metabolic load, in addition to several other pediatric physiological factors, including poor sweating capacity, larger surface-to-mass ratio, and an immature cardiovascular system, results in a shorter tolerance for exercising in hot climates and greater susceptibility to heat stress for children. Hard exercise increases metabolic rate 8 to 10 times, with increases of core body temperature of 1 to 1.5°C in 20 minutes. With higher humidity and higher temperature, dissipation of body heat is reduced. In fact, at 98.6°F, there is no loss of body heat except by sweating and evaporation. Heavy uniforms or sweatsuits reduce evaporation further. Younger children dehydrate sooner and have higher core temperatures than adults do under the same conditions. Therefore, they are at greater risk of heat illness, heat exhaustion, and heat stroke. Acclimatization requires gradual heat stress over a period of at least 2 weeks (Conway & Zuckerman, 1997). The AAP recommends that activities lasting 30 minutes or more be reduced whenever the humidity or the temperature is high.

Heat Illnesses (Hyperthermia)

HEAT CRAMPS. Heat cramps are the mildest form of heat illness. Symptoms include painful muscle spasms of extremities and abdomen during or after strenuous exercise with profuse sweating. The subject is thirsty but well oriented and alert. Salted liquid (a sports drink or 0.5 to 1 teaspoon of salt to 1 quart of water) by mouth or normal saline given intravenously, rest in a cool area, and several days of avoidance of the activity causing the cramps is the treatment (Hay et al., 1997). Heat cramps occur most commonly when athletes are not adequately conditioned for participation at high temperature or humidity, or both. The condition is predominantly related to water and salt deficits (dehydration).

HEAT EXHAUSTION. Heat exhaustion symptoms include cramps as well as headache, fatigue, weakness, dizziness, and possibly nausea or diarrhea. Slow mentation, dry tongue and mouth, weight loss, and elevated body temperature may occur. The skin is ashen, cold, and clammy because of sodium depletion, or hot and dry from water depletion. Mild shock may be present, but there are no major central nervous system dysfunctions. Management includes rest; cooling measures, such as removing clothing and fanning to enhance evaporation, and spraying or sponging the skin with water; and oral or intravenous fluids. If the athlete is confused or refuses to drink, intravenous fluids are needed. A patient with the latter symptoms may need hospitalization (Hay et al., 1997).

HEAT STROKE. Heat stroke is a medical emergency. Rapid cooling is essential because the high body temperature damages tissues and alters heart, lung, brain, kidney, and other organ system functions. Symptoms include hyperthermia with rectal temperature over 40°C, headache, chills, nausea, vomiting, muscle cramps, ataxia, and incoherent speech. Sweating may or may not be present, depending on the degree of depletion of fluids that has occurred. Tachycardia and hypotension can occur. Loss of consciousness, circulatory failure, coagulopathy, and renal and hepatic failure occur as body systems decompensate. Rapid transport to an emergency department is essential for administration of intravenous fluids; rapid cooling with ice water immersion or lavages; and support of respiratory, cardiovascular, and renal functions (Hay et al., 1997). While waiting for transport, the patient should be placed in a cool environment, clothing should be removed, and ice

TABLE 15-9
Strategies to Prevent Heat Illnesses

Athletes should wear lightweight, dry, permeable clothing.

Athletes should be fully hydrated before activity begins.

Athletes should drink cool water at a rate of 100–150 ml every 15 min for activities lasting more than 30 min.

Athletes should have scheduled rest periods in the shade.

Athletes should be gradually acclimatized to heat over 7–10 d, if possible.

Athletes at greater risk should be observed carefully. Risk factors include cystic fibrosis; hyperthyroidism; obesity; previous heat stroke; general health problems; poor conditioning; diabetes; kidney disorders; and medications such as diuretics, antihistamines, antidepressants, and others.

Activities should be scheduled in early morning or evening to avoid direct sunlight and hottest time of day.

Activity should cease if any signs and symptoms of heat illness develop.

packs should be applied to the body with fanning to increase evaporation. Muscle massage can be helpful. Fluids should be given orally if the athlete is alert (Drake & Nettina, 1994).

PREVENTIVE MEASURES. Preventive measures for heat illnesses are found in Table 15-9. They include efforts to decrease metabolic effort, increase evaporation, and increase hydration.

Although not related to heat illnesses or their prevention, it is worth remembering that sunscreens are essential for sports activities played in direct sunlight. Products that do not sweat off easily are recommended.

ANABOLIC-ANDROGENIC STEROIDS AND THE ADOLESCENT

Endogenous anabolic-androgenic steroids start adolescent development in the prepubertal male. Exogenous anabolic-androgenic drugs used by teenage athletes are derivatives of testosterone. Androgenic refers to the effects on the male reproductive tract and the development of secondary male sexual characteristics.

Anabolic effects are changes that occur in non-reproductive tissues, such as closure of bony epiphyses, changes in the larynx, and increases in muscle bulk and strength. Aggressive male behavior is also thought to be related to androgenic effects.

In the late 1980s, several nationwide studies were reported in which anabolic steroid use was documented. Buckley and colleagues (1987) found that 6.6% of male high school seniors had used anabolic-androgenic steroids. A more recent review of prevalence studies indicates that 4 to 12% of boys and 0.5 to 2.9% of girls report having used anabolic steroids (Middleman & DuRant, 1996). Risk factors identified included the following:

- Strength training
- Injected drug use
- Use of multiple drugs such as amphetamines, heroin, tobacco, and alcohol

There are three types of agents that teenagers might use: testosterone, alkylated testosterones (oral), and other agents, such as testosterone esters (injected) and derivatives. Generally, these drugs are taken in cycles of use lasting 6 to 12 weeks each. Sometimes adolescents use more than one type at a time or alternate use to prevent developing tolerance (Hay et al., 1997). They increase the dose incrementally and then taper the dose at the end of a cycle.

Side effects include acne, seborrhea, and gynecomastia. With higher doses, some of the more serious side effects include priapism (sustained penile erection), edema, testicular atrophy, and liver dysfunction. Premature epiphyseal closure can leave the teenager shorter than expected. Hepatotoxicity is most related to the 17-alkylated derivatives. In adolescent females, irreversible effects include clitorimegaly, hirsutism, amenorrhea (may be partially reversible after termination of use), and deepening of the voice with larynx changes. Behavioral changes are not clearly documented in the literature, but some investigators report psychological dependence on the drugs—that is, preoccupation with drug use, inability to stop despite psychological effects, drug craving, mood swings with attempts to stop, violent behavior, heightened aggression, and depression possibly severe enough to be linked with suicide (Kashin &

Kleber, 1989; Middleman & DuRant, 1996; Hay et al., 1997).

Anticipatory guidance and education are essential in this area. Rapid weight gain, increased muscle bulk, increased acne, and behavioral changes with increased aggression and mood swings should raise suspicions in coaches, parents, and providers. Educational programs that offer alternatives to taking anabolic steroids can be helpful. Nutrition and strength-training techniques are important aspects of these programs (Rogul & Yesalis, 1992).

CREATINE SUPPLEMENTS

Creatine is an amino acid stored in muscle as phosphocreatine. During intense exercise, it is broken down to release energy for muscle contraction. Synthetic creatine is an over-the-counter supplement many athletes are using. The normal daily requirement is about 2 g for a 70-kg person. Some comes from animal protein and some is synthesized by the body. Supplementation increases muscle stores and results in greater muscle mass and weight gain. Athletes generally take 20 to 25 g per day for 5 to 7 days and then a maintenance dose of 2 to 5 g per day. It has been shown in studies to increase performance for high-intensity strength work and repeated sprints, as in football. Athletes for some other sports report poorer performance, perhaps because of excess weight gain. Weight gain is the only reported side effect (Schnirring, 1998). Unanswered questions in pediatrics include the following:

- Minimal dose for beneficial effect
- Effects and benefits in children
- Effects on endogenous synthesis
- Long-term health effects
- Ethics of societal rewards for performance enhanced by an exogenous substance

COUNSELING FAMILIES ABOUT SPORTS FOR THEIR CHILDREN

Physical activity needs to be encouraged from infancy. Playing outside and engaging in family physical activities serve important developmental needs. When children enter school, sports opportunities become organized, so children and their families need to make specific decisions and choices about the sports in which they want to participate. At this time, it is important to identify the parent who has sports goals for the child that may be meeting the parent's needs more than the child's. For the prepubertal child entering sports, the goals should be healthful activity, learning basic skills, and mastering the rules of the game. All children do not mature at the same rate. The skills of several children of the same age can be widely discrepant, and the performance of a 16- or 17-year-old is very different from that of the same child at age 12.

The following are some basic concepts to keep in mind for counseling:

- Noncontact team sports participation can begin at about age 6 years but should be guided by the child's development and individual interest. Contact sports such as basketball, soccer, and wrestling can be added at age 8 years. Collision sports such as tackle football and ice hockey should be delayed until 10 years (Patient Care Nurse Practitioner, 1998).
- The child who is an exceptional athlete may still have maturation difficulties in social and psychological areas. Finding a balance in supporting the development of an athletically gifted child can be difficult given the stress this child may face in the competitive arena.
- Children with handicaps can participate in sports. They should make the choice of which sport with advice about the health effects that can result as well as the conditioning that may be necessary.
- Children with academic problems should not be denied participation in sports. Sports can be the best arena for boosting self-esteem for the child who does not experience success in the classroom. Helping the child find a balance between academic work and sports participation is essential.
- Boys and girls can play together, especially in the prepubertal years. Differences in height and weight can make it unsafe for smaller girls to compete in contact sports with boys after puberty.
- Injuries occur in some sports more often

than in others. Football, hockey, gymnastics, and wrestling are especially high-risk activities. Good supervision and appropriate equipment can help minimize some of the risks. Trampolines are highly associated with head and spinal cord injuries. Although most US schools have heeded American Academy of Pediatrics' advice to ban trampolines from sports programs, many homes have trampolines (Smith, 1998).
- Parental coaching is difficult if the coach's child is on the team.

LEARNING SKILLS FOR RECREATIONAL ACTIVITY SAFETY

Swimming Lessons

All children should learn to swim. This is essential to their safety near water environments. Swimming is an excellent sports activity that can be engaged in throughout life.

Bike Safety Training

Bike riding can be an excellent aerobic activity. However, children need to wear helmets, learn to handle their bicycles with skill, and know the rules of the road for bicyclists.

In-Line Skating

In-line skating is a fun activity that can be risky if children do not wear helmets, knee pads, wrist guards, gloves, and elbow pads. Children need to learn to skate only in safe environments and to watch for traffic, irregular pavements, and other hazards. Since 37% of all in-line skating injuries involve the wrist and 67% of these are fractures, wrist guards are essential (American Academy of Pediatrics Committee on Injury and Poison Prevention and Committee on Sports Medicine and Fitness, 1998).

Skiing and Snowboarding

There are approximately 600,000 skiing injuries per year with beginners three to five times more likely to be hurt than advanced

---

NURSING DIAGNOSIS 15-1

NURSING DIAGNOSES FOR ACTIVITY AND EXERCISE FUNCTIONAL HEALTH PATTERN

Activity Intolerance

Diversional Activities Deficit

Physical Mobility Impairment

Source: North American Nursing Diagnosis Association. NANDA nursing diagnoses: Definitions and classification 1995–1996. Philadelphia, 1997.

---

skiers. Much of the decrease in injury rates over the past 20 years has been the result of improvements in equipment. Children should have well-fitting boots and poles with bindings

appropriately adjusted. Snowboarding results in fewer knee injuries than found in skiing, whereas ankle injuries are more frequent because soft-shell boots protect the ankle less well than ski boots do. Snowboarders have twice as many upper limb injuries than skiers. Fitness training can reduce fatigue injuries. Lessons can help both skiers and snowboarders learn proper techniques and principles of slope safety (Chissel et al., 1996).

Skateboarding

Skateboarding injuries are most often fractures (50%), with 33% of these occurring during the first week of skateboarding. Irregularity of the riding surface is often the etiological factor for the accident. As with in-line skating, recommended equipment includes helmet, knee and elbow pads, and wrist guards. The American

---

RESOURCE BOX 15-1

RESOURCES FOR PROFESSIONALS AND PARENTS

American Academy of Pediatrics
Website: www.aap.org
Pediatric health care focus with a committee on sports medicine that sets standards for children and sports.

American College of Sports Medicine
Website: www.acsm.org
Goal is diagnosis, treatment, and prevention of sports-related injuries and advancement of research related to exercise.

American College of Sports Dentistry
Dental Arts Building
Nine Linden St.
Worcester, MA 01609
Organization dedicated to the prevention of sports-related injuries to the head, face, mouth, and related oral structures.

American Orthopaedic Society for Sports Medicine
Tel: (847) 292-4900
Fax: (847) 292-4905
Provides a variety of pamphlets on nutrition for sports, heat, and athletic performance, flexibility, designing weight programs, preparticipation physical examination, and a resource directory for disabled athletes from their Committee on Athletes with Disability.

American Sport Education Program
Tel: (800) 747-5698
Provides information on sports and youth.

International Center for Sports Nutrition
502 S. 44th St., Suite 3012
Omaha, NE 68105
Association to stimulate research related to nutrition and human performance.

National SAFE KIDS Campaign
Tel: (202) 662-0600
Website: http://www.safekids.org

National Youth Sports Foundation, Inc. (NYSSF)
Tel: (617) 277-1171
Website: www.nyssf.org
An educational and research organization dedicated to promoting safety and well-being for children participating in sports. Fact sheets and bibliographies available.

Sports, Cardiovascular and Wellness Nutritionists
Tel: (303) 799-1950
Nutrition professionals with expertise in sports nutrition, health promotion, and fitness; associated with the American Dietetic Association.

Academy of Pediatics recommends education to learn the activity properly. Learning in a supervised environment with a smooth surface and no traffic can be helpful. Finally, the American Academy of Pediatrics recommends that children be 5 years of age or older to ride skateboards (Fountain & Meyers, 1996).

Trampolines

Although the American Academy of Pediatrics recommended that trampolines be banned from schools and competitive sports in 1977, trampolines are still popular for home recreational use by children. Injury rates increased 98% from 1990 to 1995 with an estimated 249,400 trampoline accidents treated in emergency departments during that period (Smith, 1998). The median age for injury was 10 years. Ninety-three percent of these accidents occurred at home. Injuries from trampoline use can be grouped as follows: injuries to extremities (70%), face injuries (11%), head and neck trauma (10%). Annually, about 1400 children require hospitalization for their injuries. Quadriplegia and death have been well described. The number of injuries seen in emergency rooms doubled between 1990 and 1995. Trampolines cannot be recommended for home use because there is no protective equipment that is helpful, and spotters cannot help when children collide or bounce out of reach (Smith, 1998).

REFERENCES

American Academy of Family Physicians, American Academy of Pediatrics, American Medical Society for Sports Medicine, et al: Preparticipation physical evaluation. In American Academy of Family Physicians, American Academy of Pediatrics, American Medical Society for Sports Medicine, et al: The Physician and Sportsmedicine, 2nd ed. Minneapolis, MN, McGraw-Hill, 1997.

American Academy of Neurology Quality Standards Subcommittee: Practice parameter: The management of concussion in sports (summary statement). Neurology 48:581-585, 1997.

American Academy of Pediatrics Committee on Injury and Poison Prevention and Committee on Sports Medicine and Fitness: In-line skating injuries in children and adolescents. Pediatrics 101:720-721, 1998.

American Academy of Pediatrics Committee on Sports Medicine: Medical conditions affecting sports participation. Pediatrics 94:757-760, 1994.

American Academy of Pediatrics Committee on Sports Med-

icine and Fitness: Athletic participation by children and adolescents who have systemic hypertension. Pediatrics 99: 637-638, 1997.

American Academy of Pediatrics Committee on Sports Medicine and Fitness: Atlantoaxial instability in Down syndrome: Subject review. Pediatrics 96: 151-154, 1995.

American Academy of Pediatrics, Committee on Sports Medicine and Fitness: Promotion of healthy weight control practices in young athletes. Pediatrics 97:752-753, 1996.

American Medical Association: Cardiovascular preparticipation screening of competitive athletes. Med Sci Sports Exerc 29: 1445-1452, 1997.

American Orthopaedic Society for Sports Medicine: Nutrition for Sports. Rosemont, IL, 1992.

Backx F, Erick W, Kemper A, et al: Sports injuries in school-aged children (ages 8-18): An epidemiological approach. Am J Sports Med 17:234-239, 1989.

Bijur P, Trumble A, Harel Y, et al: Sports and recreation injuries in US children and adolescents. Archiv Pediatr Adolesc Med 149:1009-1016, 1995.

Bratton R: Preparticipation screening of children for sports: Current recommendations. Sports Med 24:300-307, 1997.

Buckley W, Yesales C, Freidl K, et al: Estimated prevalence of anabolic steroid use among male high school seniors. JAMA 260:3441-3445, 1987.

Bykowski M: Guidelines make child's play of exercise recommendations. Pediatr News July:50, 1998.

Cantu R: Stingers, transient quadriplegia, and cervical spinal stenosis: Return to play criteria. Med Sci Sports Exerc 29, (suppl):S233-S235, 1997.

Centers for Disease Control and Prevention: Sports related recurrent brain injuries—US. JAMA 277:1190-1191, 1997.

Chissel H, Feagin J, Warme W, et al: Trends in ski and snowboard injuries. Sports Med 22:141-145, 1996.

Conway E, Zuckerman G: The long hot summer. Contemp Pediatr 14:127-136, 1997.

DiNubile N: Youth fitness—problems and solutions. Prev Med 22:589-594, 1993.

Drake D, Nettina S: Recognition and management of heat-related illness. Nurs Pract 19:43-47, 1994.

DuRant R, Escobido L, Heath G: Anabolic-steroid use, strength training, and multiple drug use among adolescents in the United States. Pediatrics 96:23-28, 1995.

DuRant R, Seymore C, Linder C, et al: The preparticipation examination of athletes: Comparison of single and multiple examiners. Am J Dis Child 139:657-661, 1985.

Dyment P: How to make the sports physical exciting. Contemp Pediatr 8:93-106, 1991a.

Dyment P: Sports Medicine: Health Care for Young Athletes. Elk Grove, IL, American Academy of Pediatrics, 1991b.

Elster A, Kuznets N: AMA Guidelines for Adolescent Preventive Services (GAPS): Recommendations and Rationale. Baltimore, Williams & Wilkins, 1994.

Fountain J, Meyers M: Skateboarding injuries. Sports Med 22:360-366, 1996.

Guill M: Exercise-induced bronchospasm in children: Effects and therapies. Pediatr Ann 25:146-153, 1996.

Guskiewicz K, Riemann B, Perrin D, et al: Alternative approaches to the assessment of mild head injury in athletes. Med Sci Sports Exerc 29: (suppl), S213–S221, 1997.

Harris S, Runyan D: The preparticipation examination. *In* Reider B (ed): Sports Medicine. The School-Age Athlete Philadelphia, WB Saunders, 1991, pp 88–101.

Hay W, Groothius J, Hayward A, et al: Current Pediatric Diagnosis & Treatment. Stamford, CT, Appleton & Lange, 1997.

Hergenroeder A: Prevention of sports injuries. Pediatrics 101:1057–1063, 1998.

Kashin K, Kleber H: Hooked on hormones? An anabolic steroid addiction hypothesis. JAMA 262:3166–3170, 1989.

Kleiner S: Healthy muscle gains. Physician Sports Med 23:27–28, 1995.

Kuntzleman C: Childhood fitness: What is happening? What needs to be done? Prev Med 22:520–532, 1993.

Landry G: Sports injuries in childhood. Pediatr Ann 21:165–168, 1992.

Loosli A, Benson J: Nutritional intake in adolescent athletes. Pediatr Clin North Am 37:1143–1153, 1990.

Maffulli N: Intensive training in young athletes: The orthopaedic surgeon's viewpoint. Sports Med 9:229–243, 1990.

McLain L, Reynolds S: Sports injuries in high school. Pediatrics 84:446–450, 1989.

Middleman A, DuRant R: Anabolic steroid use and associated health risk behaviors. Sports Med 21:251–255, 1996.

Mitchell J, Haskell W, Raven P: Classification of sports. 26th Bethesda Conference: Recommendations for Determining Eligibility for Competition in Athletes With Cardiovascular Abnormalities. Med Sci Sports Exerc 26 (suppl): S242–S245, 1994.

Nattiv A, Puffer J: Lifestyles and health, risks of collegiate athletes. J Fam Pract 33:585–589, 1991.

Nelson M: Medical exclusion from participation in sports. Pediatr Ann 21:149–155, 1992.

Ostrum G: Sports-related injuries in youths: Prevention is the key—and nurses can help! Pediatr Nurs 19:333–342, 1993.

Overbaugh K, Allen J: The adolescent athlete. Part I: Preseason preparation and examination. J Pediatr Health Care 8:146–151, 1994a.

Overbaugh K, Allen J: The adolescent athlete. Part II: Injury patterns and prevention. J Pediatr Health Care 8:203–211, 1994b.

Overbaugh K, Allen J: The adolescent athlete. Part III: Nutrition and hydration. J Pediatr Health Care 8:250–254, 1994c.

Patient Care Nurse Practitioner: Preventing sports injuries in kids. Patient Care Nurs Pract June:24–36, 1998.

Rankin J, Ocel J, Craft L: Effect of weight loss and refeeding diet composition on anaerobic performance in wrestlers. Med Sci Sports Exerc 28:1292–1299, 1996.

Region X Nursing Network: Region X Nursing Network Newborn, Child (Birth to Three), School Age, and Adolescent Manuals. Seattle, University of Washington, 1998.

Rogul A, Yesalis C: Anabolic-androgenic steroids and the adolescent. Pediatr Ann 21:175–188, 1992.

Ryan-Krause P: The score on high-tech sports nutrition for adolescents. J Pediatr Health Care 12: 164–166, 1998.

Schnirring L: Creatine supplements face scrutiny. Phys Sports Med 26:15–23, 1998.

Smith G: Injuries to children in the United States related to trampolines, 1990–1995: A national epidemic. Pediatrics 101:406–412, 1998.

Smoll F, Smith R: Psychology of the young athlete. Pediatr Clin North Am 37:1021–1044, 1990.

Tan R, Spector NS: Exercise-induced asthma. Sports Med 25:1–6, 1998.

United States (US) Department of Health and Human Services. Healthy People 2010 Objectives: Draft for Public Comment. Washington, DC, US Government Printing Office, 1998.

CHAPTER 16

Sleep and Rest

Catherine E. Burns

INTRODUCTION

Many of the common pediatric sleep disorders are related to sleep development issues. In their review of sleep studies, Rickert and Johnson (1988) note that 20 to 30% of 1- to 4-year-olds have frequent night awakenings, bedtime difficulties, or both. The highest incidence of disorders may occur in children 1 to 2 years of age (Zuckerman et al., 1987). They also found that 18% of 3-year-olds had trouble getting to sleep, whereas 22% had trouble with night waking. Perhaps of more importance, they found that 41% of children with sleep problems at 8 months of age still had problems at 3 years of age.

A number of psychological and physiological factors are related to sleep problems in infants and children. It is important to recognize that sleep problems of infants and children are interrelated with family problems. Pediatric sleep problems may produce sleep deprivation in the caregiver. Sleep problems can also be the result of family problems, stemming from maternal depression, social stresses, or problems such as child abuse, or a combination of these. Sleep problems may also result from a variety of other problems, including:

- Physical factors
  - Ear infections
  - Neurological disorders
  - Hypothyroidism
  - Colic or other pain
  - Perinatal complications
  - Pinworms
- Psychological factors
  - Developmental stage
  - Separation anxiety (Blum & Carey, 1996)
  - Depression or other psychiatric problems (Sheldon et al., 1992)
- Family factors
  - Parental mismanagement of sleep routines
  - Maternal depression
- Environmental and temperamental factors
  - Temperament characteristics, including low sensory threshold, negative mood, and decreased adaptability
  - Environmental factors, including sleeping arrangements, altered daily routines, and feeding practices
  - Toxins or substance abuse

As with all other primary care problems in pediatrics, the provider must be vigilant for a myriad of potential etiologies and recognize that the family disruption caused by a rebellious or noisy nonsleeper in a household may be significant. Attention to cultural definitions of normal sleep habits also is essential.

▰▰ NURSING STANDARDS

Nursing standards (Region X Nursing Network, 1998) recommend a goal for sleep and rest patterns for children as follows:

1. *GOAL*: Child's sleep, rest, and relaxation contribute to his or her health, growth, and development.
2. Outcomes:
   1. Child receives enough sleep, rest, and relaxation to meet his or her individual and developmental needs.
   2. Child's physical environment contributes to his or her sleep, rest, and relaxation.
   3. Child's social environment contributes to his or her sleep, rest, and relaxation.

It should be noted that the current nursing diagnosis term "sleep disturbance" is inadequate for clinical purposes. Several distinct clinical sleep problems require different interventions for children. These are discussed later in this chapter.

▰▰ NORMAL SLEEP STAGES AND CYCLES

Normal sleep can be divided into two distinct phases: rapid eye movement (REM) sleep and non-REM sleep. Non-REM sleep can be further divided into four distinct stages based on changes in electroencephalographic (EEG) patterns.

REM Sleep

REM sleep is considered to be the dreaming phase. Although nerve impulses to the spinal cord and muscles are blocked, leaving the body paralyzed except for minor twitching, the respiratory, eye, and middle ear muscles remain active. The child may smile in a transitory way or make short utterances. Breathing and heart rates become irregular and relatively rapid. Reflexes, kidney function, hormonal secretions, and auditory sensitivity are all altered. The rapid eye movements of this phase are of particular interest. People awakened during REM sleep may report dreams at the time. Children as young as 2 years of age have reported dreams

during REM sleep. The function of REM sleep is unclear. Newborns enter the sleep cycle with REM sleep. Some mothers are concerned about their infants' restless sleep when, indeed, it is only REM sleep that they are observing.

Non-REM Sleep

The four phases of non-REM sleep become distinguishable within 6 months of birth. After 3 months of age, it is the first type of sleep entered by the infant from the awake phase (Ferber, 1996).

STAGE 1

Stage 1 sleep is a state of drowsiness. There may be eye-rolling, decreased body movements, and perhaps opening and closing of the eyelids. Individuals may believe that they are awake, but they cannot report accurately events that occurred during this time. The electroencephalographic (EEG) pattern changes from the 8 to 12 waves per second waking rhythm to 5 to 7 waves per second. In mature individuals, stage 1 accounts for about 5% of sleep (Adair & Bauchner, 1993).

STAGE 2

Stage 2 sleep is somewhat deeper than that of stage 1, although the person can still be easily aroused. Eye movements slow as do breathing and heart rate. Muscles weaken. If aroused, the person may report thinking about things and may report dreams. EEG waves begin to show spindles and K complexes. Mature sleepers spend about 50% of their sleep in this stage, generally in the last half of the night (Adair & Bauchner, 1993).

STAGE 3

Stage 3 sleep is still deeper than that of stage 2. The body is deeply relaxed, breathing is shallow, and heart rate is slow. EEG waves slow to 1 to 2 per second, with very large delta waves occupying at least 20% of the EEG. Growth hormone appears to be secreted in larger amounts during stages 3 and 4 of sleep (Behrman et al., 1996). About 15 to 20% of sleep takes place in stages 3 and 4, occurring earlier in the night.

STAGE IV

When the delta waves occupy 50% of the EEG pattern, stage 4 sleep has begun. During both stage 3 and stage 4, the sleeper is hard to arouse. If awakened, the individual feels confused and disoriented. The transition from stage 4 to waking is related to the etiology of several common pediatric sleep disorders, such as night terrors and sleepwalking.

Sleep Cycles

Sleep onset is the time when the person enters stage 1 non-REM sleep. The *sleep period* begins with sleep onset and continues until full arousal occurs. The *sleep cycle* includes the repeated episodes of non-REM and REM sleep of the sleep period. *Waking* involves full alert and recall after the sleep period. *Semiwakefulness* or alerting to the immediate environment occurs easily in REM sleep or stages 1 or 2 in non-REM sleep. The child cycles between REM and non-REM phases throughout the night. Both total amount of sleep and proportion of REM sleep decrease with age (Fig. 16–1).

For newborns, REM sleep is the first phase of the sleep cycle, but by the age of 3 to 6 months, non-REM sleep initiates infant's sleep period. REM sleep usually precedes a brief period of semiwakefulness, after which the individual descends again through the non-REM stages to REM, followed by another brief awakening. Later in the evening, the REM phase becomes more pronounced. In older children and adults, the periods of semiwakefulness may last for a few seconds to a few minutes. It may be the time when one turns over, looks at the clock, or adjusts the covers. The infant sometimes has difficulty returning to the next sleep cycle from this normal waking episode. Young infants have more sleep cycles per night than older individuals do and each cycle has a brief waking that precedes the next sleep period. Therefore, more opportunities for sleep disturbance can arise with infants.

Adolescents also experience sleep problems; the most common is difficulty falling asleep. Middle adolescents seem to have more sleep disturbances than younger or older teenagers. (Yarcheski & Mahon, 1994).

Duration of Sleep

The typical neonate sleeps about 16 hours each day. Half of this is daytime sleep. The longest sleep period is 2.5 to 4 hours and can occur at

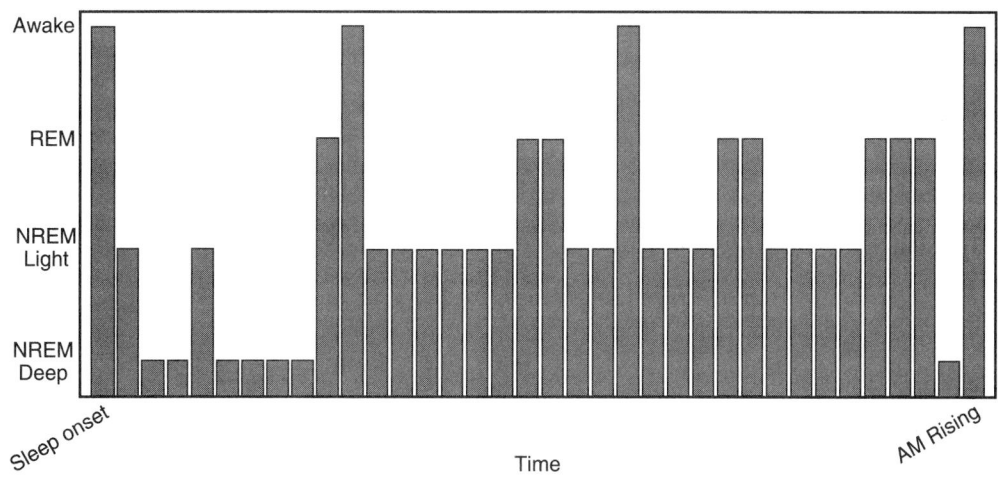

F I G U R E 16-1
Schema of typical night sleep pattern of sleep states and stages. REM = rapid eye movement; NREM = non-REM. (From Adair R, Bauchner H: Sleep problems in childhood. Curr Probl Pediatr April:150, 1993.)

any time during the 24-hour day. The neonate has only one or two sleep cycles during a sleep period. By 3 months of age, the baby sleeps almost 15 hours, but the sleep times are more clearly organized into daytime wakefulness and nighttime sleep. Most 6-month-old infants sleep through the night and have morning and afternoon naps. At 1 year of age, most children sleep about 13.5 hours. The morning nap is generally given up between 12 and 24 months, but the afternoon nap may persist to age 4 or 5 years. By age 2 years, the child is probably sleeping 11 to 12 hours at night with a 1- to 2-hour nap after lunch. Six-year-olds sleep 9.5 hours per night on average. Between 6 and 12 years of age, children spend less time asleep; the average sleep requirement for adolescents is believed to be about 8 to 9 hours per night (Adair & Bauchner, 1993; Blum & Carey, 1996).

Circadian Rhythms and Establishment of Normal Sleep Patterns

Many biological activities are set on a 24-hour cycle. These include sleep and wakefulness, body temperature regulation, hormonal activity, and respiratory, cardiac, renal, and intestinal functions. People use a variety of cues to set the cycle, including daylight, darkness, meals, and activities. Parents need to make these cues clear to infants and children to help them establish healthful bedtime and sleep patterns. Sleep hygiene is a term used to define healthful sleep behaviors.

FEEDING EFFECTS ON SLEEP

Breastfed infants need to eat more frequently than babies fed cow's milk. Probably this is due to the shorter emptying time for breast milk (Blum & Carey, 1996). Because of this, breastfed babies probably wake more frequently in the night. Bedsharing by mother and infant increases both the length and frequency of breastfeeding episodes in 3- to 4-month old infants (McKenna et al., 1997). By 6 months of age, most babies can go for a 6- to 12-hour period without being fed. This extended period coincides with the longest sleep period. Thus, after 6 months of age, feeding in the night

can be considered a learned behavior. Starting solids early to increase length of nighttime sleeping is a myth. Several studies have shown that solids do not help the baby sleep for longer periods.

CO-SLEEPING

Sleep habits are strongly influenced by culture. Co-sleeping is common in many cultures and has been the human norm for many thousands of years. Co-sleeping by family members is probably more common worldwide than is separate sleeping as advocated in the United States. Warmth, protection, and a sense of well-being are undoubtedly facilitated by having babies sleep with their mothers or siblings. It is most common in black and Hispanic families. Co-sleeping is also common with father absence (Madansky & Edelbrock, 1990; Lozoff et al., 1984). Infants between 11 and 15 weeks of age had more arousals from both stages 1 and 2 and 3 and 4 sleep when sharing the bed with their mothers than when sleeping alone. Researchers interpreted this as perhaps a protection against sudden infant death syndrome (SIDS) (Mosko et al., 1997). Sleep problems are found more often in children who frequently co-sleep all night with parents. Sharing the bedroom but not the bed is not associated with more sleep problems (Adair & Bauchner, 1993).

The American Academy of Pediatrics (AAP), in a 1997 statement, states that bedsharing should not be considered as a strategy to reduce SIDS risk. If a mother chooses to sleep with her infant, care should be taken to avoid using soft sleep surfaces—quilts, blankets, pillows, comforters, or other similar materials should not be placed under the infant. The bedsharer should not smoke or use substances that impair arousal. Finally, parents should understand that safety standards are in place for the design of infant cribs, but there are no standards for adult beds, so entrapment might be possible (AAP, 1997).

BEDTIME ROUTINES

Good sleep hygiene requires an environment that is dark, quiet, and slightly cool; a regular schedule for waking, nap lengths, and bedtime;

and sleep-conducive activities in the child's life that include non–fear-inducing stories, videos, or television; quiet activities before bedtime; and consistent parenting methods that are quieting before bedtime (Blum & Carey, 1996). Many authors believe that children from earliest infancy should be put into bed awake so that they learn to put themselves to sleep with self-soothing behaviors such as thumb-sucking (Ferber, 1996; Blum & Carey, 1996; Adair & Bauchner, 1993; Johnson et al., 1995). Bringing an inanimate transitional object to bed is helpful to many toddlers and preschoolers. Other sleep hygiene principles include avoiding hunger at bedtime but not taking in excessive fluids at bedtime or during the night, and avoiding stimulating drugs and foods such as caffeine, coffee, and chocolate in the evening (Sheldon et al., 1992).

Some sleep problems, such as trained night feeding and trained night crying, are learned. Sleep-onset problems can also be learned (Ferber, 1996; Blum & Carey, 1996). For instance, the child who is always rocked to sleep in mother's arms and then moved to the crib when asleep learns that the place to go to sleep is in mother's arms. During arousals in the night, the child then looks for those arms and not the sides of the crib to move into the next sleep cycle.

Sleep Positioning

Studies have provided strong evidence that positioning young infants on their backs significantly decreases the incidence of SIDS (Ponsonby et al., 1993; Spiers & Guntheroth, 1994; Willinger et al., 1994). The current recommendation of the AAP is to have all infants sleep side-lying or supine at naps and at bedtime during the first 6 months of life unless there is some specific medical contraindication to that position (AAP Task Force on Infant Positioning and SIDS, 1992). A 1997 study in Washington, DC, found that almost half of licensed daycare centers had caregivers who were unaware of the relationship between sleep position and SIDS (Gershon & Moon, 1997). Further education needs to be directed to this group to decrease this risk factor for young infants.

A 1997 study of 343 infants found that infants sleeping on their sides or supine were significantly less likely to be rolling over at their 4-month checkup visits (Jantz & Blosser, 1997). Whether this is a result of reluctance of parents to put their infants on their stomachs during the day or whether it stems from other developmental effects of back sleeping is unclear.

ASSESSMENT

Assessment of sleep patterns requires an understanding of the developmental progression of sleep patterns, a comprehensive history, and a physical examination. Assessment of sleep patterns should be included in all well-child visits. Before a decision is made that a sleep problem exists, the provider must be sure to determine whether the child's sleep pattern is problematic for the caregiver. Late bedtimes, early rising, night waking, co-sleeping, and so on, may be upsetting to some parents but not to others. Only sleep problems identified by the parent should be addressed, or cases in which there is evidence that the child's sleep patterns are disruptive to his or her health and well-being. Of course, preventive counseling is always in order.

History

The practitioner asks the parents, "Are you satisfied with your child's current sleep behaviors?" The normal sleep pattern, the general health history, the parents and family, and the sleep environment are assessed for factors that may affect sleep and rest.

NORMAL SLEEP PATTERN

1. Nighttime and daytime sleep hygiene patterns include the following:
   - Quality and quantity of sleep
   - Sleep hours, including naps
   - Awake time when parents are also awake
   - Longest night sleep interval
   - Number and frequency of feedings (for infants <3 mo old), day and night
   - Description of the state changes of the child, moving from wakefulness to sleep and then to waking again

- Cues given by the infant or child to indicate need for sleep or rest
- The routines used for getting the child to sleep and the child's behavior at these times

2. Sleep problem history includes the following:

   - Nighttime waking and the routine for managing these episodes
   - Nightmares and night terrors
   - Snoring and breathing problems during sleep
   - Jerks and twitches during sleep
   - Inappropriate sleep and awake times
   - Enuresis
   - Age when problem began and circumstances
   - Aggravating and relieving factors
   - Effects on daily living for child and family

3. The environment for sleeping, noise, light, temperature, safety, co-sleeping pattern.

GENERAL HEALTH HISTORY

1. Indicators of the health and well-being of the child: Energy and alertness for daily activities need evaluation. The child with chronic inadequate sleep may appear to the parents to be functioning quite well. However, with more sleep, the parents will notice a decrease in irritability and better performance in many arenas.

2. Past medical history and review of systems: Medical problems of the child are often associated with sleep difficulties. Ear infections, medications such as bronchodilators, some neurological problems, respiratory conditions, or anything that causes pain affects sleep. Developmental problems can affect the child's ability to learn appropriate sleep behaviors. Depression or other psychiatric problems may be significant in older children with sleep problems.

PARENTAL AND FAMILY ASSESSMENT

1. Indicators of the health and well-being and rest of the caregiver. Maternal depression

has been clearly associated with children's sleep disruptions (Zuckerman et al., 1987; Blum & Carey, 1996).
2. Parental knowledge and beliefs about infant and child sleeping patterns. Parental understanding of the relationships between illness, temperament, and sleep should be explored (Jimmerson, 1991; Blum & Carey, 1996).
3. Parental ability to modulate the child's sleep and rest state.
4. Family sleep routines and expectations.
5. Recent changes in family living arrangements.
6. Divorce, separation, or other family stresses.
7. Extent of disparity of problem with family's cultural expectations (Anders & Eiben, 1997).
8. Family history of sleep disorders (Anders & Eiben, 1997).

Physical Examination

It is important that a general physical examination be performed to detect signs of illness or pain. Signs of fatigue, irritability, or inattention may be associated with lack of adequate rest. Other clinical findings associated with sleep problems include upper respiratory infection, gastroenteritis, teething, pinworms, and injuries. Gastroesophageal reflux may affect sleep (Blum & Carey, 1996).

Diagnostic Studies

A 24-hour, 7-day chart for the parents to record the child's sleep patterns may be very useful for assessing the problem and establishing a baseline from which to evaluate improvement over time (Fig. 16–2). Sleep EEG studies are occasionally warranted. Temperament assessment is done by means of a tool such as the Carey infant temperament questionnaire (Carey & McDevitt, 1978).

STRATEGIES FOR PREVENTION AND MANAGEMENT OF SLEEP PROBLEMS

Usual management strategies include counseling parents, modifying diet, ignoring nocturnal

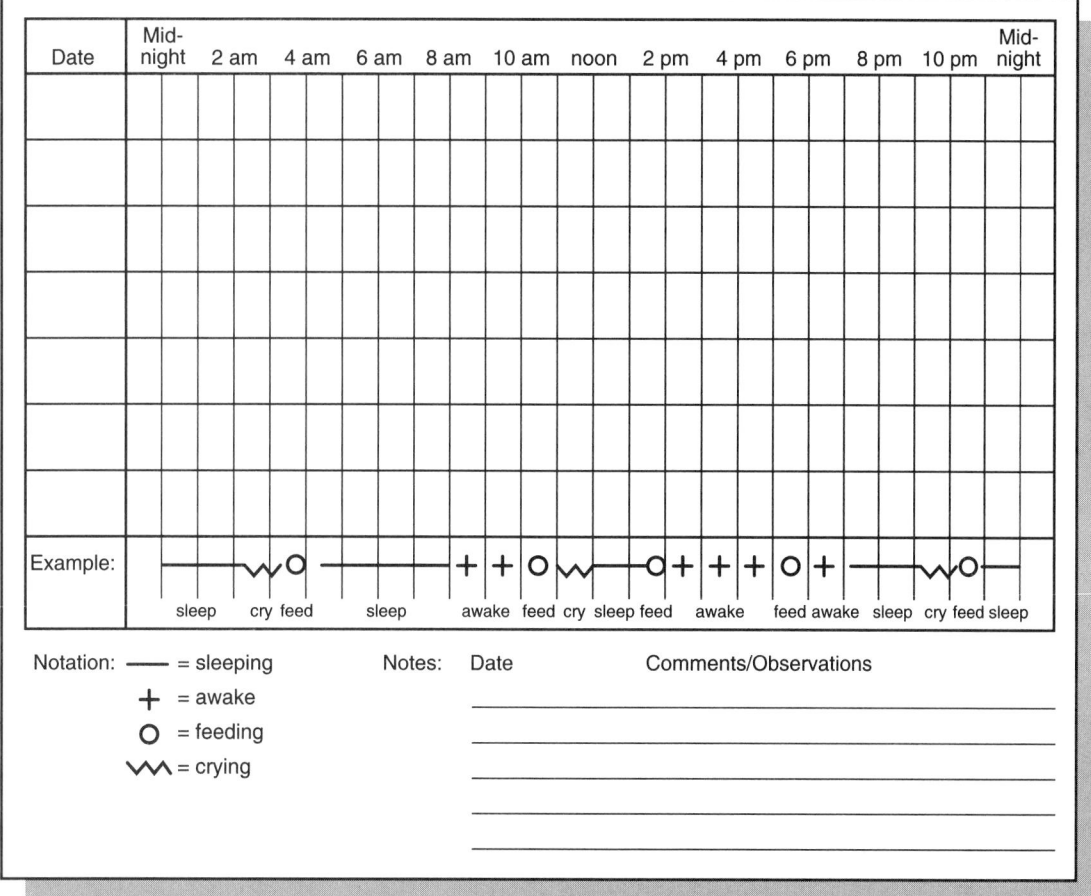

F I G U R E 16-2
Example of Sleep–Activity–Feeding Record.

crying, and scheduling awakenings. Sedation is sometimes helpful as a temporary measure. A study from New Zealand demonstrated that written instructions for parents about management of sleep problems were quite effective (Seymore et al., 1989). Deeper fears, depression, or family stresses may require counseling.

Parenting tips for managing the infant's state changes are helpful, and successful parenting strategies should be supported. A variety of parental behaviors help prevent sleep problems in children (Table 16-1).

For most infants and children, establishing a bedtime routine is probably the most important thing that parents can do. The routine should begin at a regular time with quieter activities

and then sleep-routine activities. Often this routine includes a bath; changing into pajamas; brushing teeth; and sharing a story, song, or prayer. Lights should be turned out, although a hall light or nightlight may be reassuring to the child. Toddlers often need to take a "transition object," such as a toy or blanket, to bed with them. Establishing consistent wake-up and nap-time routines and schedules are also useful strategies.

Helping parents to understand their child's temperament can be a useful intervention. For example, for the child who is less adaptable or who has tendencies to withdraw from new situations, changing the sleep routine in any way may be particularly difficult. For children

T A B L E 16-1

Prevention of Sleep Problems

NEWBORN

DURING THE DAY	Respond to crying; hold the baby when fussy Hold the baby frequently to avoid fussy episodes Schedule feedings with at least a 2-hour interval
DURING THE NIGHT	Put the baby to bed while drowsy but still awake Feed the baby at the parent's bedtime and then let the baby awaken for feedings and feed with little stimulation, dim lights, no play Avoid bringing the baby into the parents' bed unless co-sleeping is the family norm

2 TO 4 MONTHS OF AGE

DURING THE NIGHT	Move the baby to a separate bedroom unless this is not the cultural norm for the family Try to delay and then discontinue middle-of-the-night feedings No bottles in the crib Continue to keep middle-of-the-night feedings (if they are still occurring) as nonstimulating occasions

6 TO 12 MONTHS OF AGE

DURING THE NIGHT	Keep soft toy animal, doll, or blanket in the crib for snuggling Leave the bedroom door open and respond to any fears quickly and with reassurance

1 YEAR AND OLDER

DURING THE NIGHT	Keep bedtimes friendly and predictable occasions Always respond to nighttime fears with reassurance and comfort Allow the child to take increasing responsibility for self-management of body functions, including sleep Expect the child to remain in bed during the night

who are "difficult" (irregular, intense, with frequent negative moods), parents should be informed that sleep schedules and needs will be unpredictable, and reactions to parental interventions may be intensely resistant. Such behavior is certainly not reinforcing to the parents. Strategies parents have used with success in the past should be identified and similar parenting activities adapted for managing sleep difficulties. Children with low sensory thresholds also have more problems with night waking because they are more sensitive to light, sound, temperature, and tactile stimulation (Carey, 1974). All these stimuli must be considered by parents who are trying to promote sleep onset and maintenance behaviors in their children.

Family stressors need to be recognized and dealt with. Post-traumatic stress disorder, abuse, or other psychological problems in children may also be factors requiring family and individual counseling.

COMMON SLEEP PROBLEMS

The line between normal and problematic sleep may be somewhat fuzzy. The provider needs to identify that the child's sleep patterns are problematic for the caregivers and family or are resulting in problems for the child's health and well-being. There is an *International Classification of Sleep Disorders* (American Sleep Disorders Association, 1990). It is more complex than the system used in this chapter and refers to both adult and child sleep problems. It classifies sleep problems as dyssomnias, or problems of insufficient, excessive, or inefficient sleep; parasomnias, or problems that intrude upon the sleep state; and medical/psychiatric sleep disorders. This chapter identifies problems as found in Table 16–2.

Sleeplessness Problems

SLEEP-ONSET ASSOCIATION PROBLEMS (NIGHT WAKING)

Description

The child is unable to enter the sleep cycle easily unless a particular routine is carried out. For the infant, the problem results in frequent night waking and crying between midnight and 5 AM.

Etiology

This is learned behavior, often seen in infants who fall asleep while being rocked and who are then put in their beds.

Incidence

Sleep-onset association problems are very common. Studies identify incidence patterns ranging from 10% of 8-month-olds, 44% of 6- to 12-month olds, 20% of 9-month-olds, to 20 to 40% of 12- to 24-month olds (Adair & Bauchner, 1993).

Clinical Findings

The history reveals a baby or child who has frequent night awakenings. When the parent goes to the child and repeats a particular intervention, the child falls asleep promptly.

Differential Diagnoses

The differential diagnoses for sleep-onset association problems are pain or a medical condition affecting sleep, fear in the older child, and inappropriate expectations related to the amount of sleep the child needs.

Management

The infant or child must learn to go from the arousal phase into the next sleep cycle independently in the night. The parent must change the responses given during the night. Two strategies have been recommended in the literature:

1. Put the child down to sleep at night while he or she is awake. When the child awakens and cries in the night, the parent should go to him or her briefly to give comfort and reassurance but not to hold, rock, or feed. The parent's response must be supportive and comforting but should not reinforce a return to old patterns of infant behavior or parental response. Waiting for progressively longer intervals before going to the child over several nights may work if the parents can maintain compliance. Going "cold turkey" (not going to the child at all from the very beginning) is very hard for parents to do, although children learn to return to sleep alone within a few nights, crying for shorter periods each time (Blum & Carey, 1996).

2. Alternately, use a planned awakening approach. The first night, the parent should go to the child 30 minutes before night awakening is expected. The child is awakened, rocked for a few minutes, and then left again. When spontaneous awakenings stop, scheduled awakenings are gradually delayed 30 minutes more each night. The child learns to wait for the parents to come, knowing it will happen, and gradually learns to return to sleep. This pattern seems to be less stressful for parents and is as effective in teaching independent sleep onset within 6 weeks as is delayed comforting (Rickert & Johnson, 1988; Blum & Carey, 1996).

It may be easier to work on development of self-sleep during naps first, and then transfer this behavior to nighttime.

T A B L E 16-2

Summary of Common Pediatric Sleep Problems and Interventions

SLEEP PROBLEM	CLINICAL FINDINGS	DIFFERENTIAL	INTERVENTION
Dyssomnias			
Night waking	Needs help during the night to enter the next sleep cycle	Medical problem, pain, hunger, trained night feeder Depression	Always put the child to bed while still awake; keep day and nighttime cues very clear; do not reinforce calling out/crying behavior; try scheduled wakenings technique
Sleep refusals	Toddler/preschooler refuses to settle down to sleep when put to bed	Fears, separation anxiety, sleep needs less than parents' expectations Temperament irregular or low sensory threshold Emotional stress	Maintain consistent sleep routine and expectations; use transitional objects
Trained night feeder	Infant awakens predictably to be fed after age 4 mo	Night wakening, pain or medical problem, feeding needs	Move the child onto a 3–4 hr feeding schedule in the day; at first, feed the infant only once after the parents' bedtime; then, either eliminate that feeding or progressively decrease the volume of that feeding
Delayed sleep phase	Child goes to bed late and awakens late	Sleep refusal Depression	Have the child awaken progressively 15 min earlier until appropriate bedtimes and wakening times result
Advanced sleep phase	Child goes to bed early and awakens early		Progressively have the child stay up later; awakening will also occur later
Unpredictable schedule	Child goes to bed and awakens at random times	Family on erratic schedule; inconsistent parent expectations; excessive naps	Keep predictable eating, activity, and sleeping schedules for the family; maintain consistent expectation for bedtime and awakening but allow child to stay awake in bed if not disruptive to others

T A B L E 16-2

Summary of Common Pediatric Sleep Problems and Interventions *Continued*

SLEEP PROBLEM	CLINICAL FINDINGS	DIFFERENTIAL	INTERVENTION
Parasomnias			
Nightmares	Child awakens in fear/ crying; has memory of event; is interactive while upset; occurs in latter half of night; slow return to sleep	Night terrors; seizures; stress if nightmares recur frequently	Soothe and reassure the child; a nightlight or flashlight that the child can use may help if afraid of the dark
Night terrors and sleepwalking (variant)	Child awakens screaming/ crying but is not interactive with the parent at the time; has no memory of event; occurs in first third of night; rapid return to sleep; sleep walking is variant	Nightmares; seizures; physical exhaustion	Protect the child from injury if he or she is thrashing about or walking; help the child to lie down to return to sleep; protect child from stairways and other unsafe places sleepwalker might go
Medical/Psychiatric Problems			
Depression	Insomnia or hypersomnia with other symptoms of depression	Other psychiatric disorder, dyssomnia or parasomnia disorder	Manage the psychiatric condition first
Obstructive sleep apnea	Snoring with apneic periods against increased respiratory efforts, restless sleep, daytime sleepiness/ fatigue	Central apnea, benign snoring, seizure disorder	Refer for sleep studies and possible adenotonsillectomy

SLEEP REFUSAL

Description

In toddlers and preschoolers, the problem is one of difficulty with bedtime settling.

Incidence

A variety of studies report that approximately 20% of children between 15 and 48 months of age engage in bedtime resistance. One study found the problem peaked in 50% of 4-year-olds (Beltramini & Hertzig, 1983). It is very common in toddlers. Night wakers are also more likely to resist bedtime (Johnson, 1991; Richman, 1981).

Etiology

The child may experience an inability to make the transition from daytime activities to nighttime sleeping or may be making efforts to control another daily activity. Separation anxiety is a problem for some, as are nighttime fears.

Clinical Findings

The child makes repeated attempts to obtain parental attention (e.g., demanding snacks, asking for a drink, requesting another story, leaving bed to return to family activities, watching activities from afar).

Management

For the toddler or preschooler who exhibits sleep refusal try the following regimen:

- Maintain the bedtime routine and use transitional objects and a quiet environment for sleep.
- Set limits on the child's demands for attention. The parent should leave the room at the end of the bedtime routine, expecting good behavior. If the child arises, return the child to bed, saying, "It is time for bed," each time the child gets up (Blum & Carey, 1996).
- If the child has bedtime fears, leaving may increase the problem. In these cases, the parent may sit quietly in the room until the child falls asleep. When the child can fall asleep easily this way, then the parent should move to the bedroom door and eventually out of sight. The child needs to understand that the parent will only remain in the room if there are no tantrums and the child stays in bed (Blum & Carey, 1996).
- Use a sleep log to chart the child's pattern initially. It can then be used to mark progress toward the goal.
- Be sure that the child is not being expected to sleep earlier or for longer periods than expected for his or her age.
- For children older than 3 years of age, positive rewards, such as sticker charts, may help (Ferber, 1996).

TRAINED NIGHT FEEDER

Description

The child learns to nurse or feed at night with regularity. Ferber (1996) sees this as a problem of (1) feeding, which generates excessive fluid and increases wet diapers and associated discomfort, and (2) a disruption of circadian rhythms as a result of nutrient input into intestinal and hormonal systems, which are in a resting physiological state.

Etiology

Night feeding in volume, frequent daytime feedings (grazing), feeding until asleep, and leaving a bottle in the bed are all causes for this sleep disturbance.

Incidence

Trained night feeding is a common problem.

Clinical Findings

With this disturbance, middle-of-the-night feedings occur in a child older than 4 months of age.

Differential Diagnosis

The differential diagnosis is night waking not related to feeding.

Management

Four strategies are recommended:

1. Lengthen the time between daytime feedings.
2. Feed the child only once after the feeding given at the parent's bedtime.
3. Discontinue bottles in bed either cold turkey or, less stressfully, by gradually decreasing the volume of each feeding after the infant is on a 3-hour feeding schedule in the daytime.
4. The problem should resolve in 1 to 2 weeks (Ferber, 1996).

Complications

Night feedings should not be withheld from children who are not thriving for other reasons and who need the nutrition of another nighttime feeding.

Sleep-Cycle Problems

DELAYED SLEEP PHASE

Description

The sleep cycle begins at a late hour and is followed by a late awakening. This is commonly an adolescent problem.

Etiology

The child's internal clock for sleep and rest is not consistent with appropriate hours for sleep.

Management

Two approaches are suggested:

1. Keep the nighttime routine in place but awaken the child earlier each morning in 15-minute increments.
2. For the adolescent or older child who is off schedule by many hours (e.g., at the end of summer, when beginning the school year will require getting up earlier), it could take weeks to back up the cycle appropriately using 15-minute increments. In this case, it is better to go forward in time. In other words, have the child remain awake until the next evening and then go to bed at the desired hour, beginning the desired routine from that point.

Have the child or family keep a sleep log to document gradual change (Anders & Eiben, 1997).

ADVANCED SLEEP PHASE

Description

The sleep cycle begins too early with correlated early rising.

Management

Meals, naps, and bedtime should be delayed until the desired times. The early waking resolves itself.

INAPPROPRIATE OR UNPREDICTABLE SCHEDULES

Description

Some people have a poorly organized sleep-wake cycle. This is described by some as a temperament problem of rhythmicity.

Management

The routines of eating, activities, and sleeping should be kept as regular as possible. The older child may need to learn to play quietly in bed until others awaken or until a clock radio goes off. At night, the child may need to learn to read or listen to music in bed when bedtime comes.

The Parasomnias: Night Terrors, Nightmares, Sleepwalking

NIGHTMARES, MONSTERS, AND OTHER NIGHTTIME FEARS

Description

Nightmares occur as the child awakens from REM sleep, remembering dreams that are disturbing. Occasional nightmares are normal and benign. The child is awake, frightened, and able to describe the fears.

Differential Diagnosis

The differential diagnosis for nightmares is night terrors, in which the child is not fully conscious. The significance and severity of other nighttime fears need to be assessed. Separation anxiety in toddlers, parental fighting, or a scary event may make nighttime frightening.

Management

Parents should give comfort, reassurance, and a sense of security and not dismiss the fear as imaginary. The child may need to have the parent lie down with him or her for a period of time, or the child may even get into bed with the parent. However, this should not become habitual.

Monsters may be kept away by keeping on a nightlight, by using a flashlight to "sweep them away," or by keeping the bedroom door open.

Behavioral strategies or counseling may be required if nighttime fears are frequent or the degree of fear is exceptionally severe.

NIGHT TERRORS OR SLEEP TERRORS

Description

Night terrors are defined as a partial awakening from non-REM sleep in which the child is not fully conscious and aware of surroundings. Episodes occur 30 to 90 minutes after onset of sleep and may last from less than a minute to 5 minutes or more.

Etiology

These are related to the transition from the stage 4 non-REM sleep to the REM sleep cycle and are not psychological or developmental problems. Excessive fatigue or unusual daytime stresses may precipitate attacks in some children.

Incidence

Night terrors are most common in 3- to 8-year-olds, although they occur in children from 18 months to adolescence.

Clinical Findings

The child usually sits up screaming but cannot be reasoned with or consoled. Indeed, the child does not even seem to hear the caregiver. The child can have tachycardia and sweating (Anders & Eiben, 1997). The child is not awake or aware of the surroundings and does not remember the episode in the morning. It is the caregiver who is disturbed, not the child.

Differential Diagnosis

The differential diagnosis is seizures with stiffening, jerking, drooling, or nightmares.

Management

The child should be helped to lie down again and should be soothed back to sleep. The child is not disturbed by the incident in the morning and is unaware that anything has happened. The child should be protected from injury, and baby sitters should be prepared for these episodes.

SLEEPWALKING (SOMNAMBULISM)

Description

Sleepwalking is a variation of night terrors in which the manifestation is walking rather than sitting up and screaming.

Etiology

The cause is the same as that for night terrors.

Incidence

Sleepwalking is more common in boys and tends to be outgrown.

Clinical Findings

The child arises and walks about without being fully alert and responsive. The child may fall or bump into things.

Management

The child needs to be led back quietly to bed. A gate may need to be placed across the bedroom door if the sleepwalking becomes frequent. Doors may need to be secured to ensure that the child does not wander into unsafe areas. Stairways are particularly dangerous to the sleepwalking child.

Obstructive Sleep Apnea

Description

Obstructive sleep apnea is a serious problem for some infants and children because it is an indicator of severe airway obstruction. There is cessation of airflow at the nose and mouth associated with continuation of respiratory effort against the obstruction.

Associated clinical findings may include excessive daytime sleepiness, unusual daytime behavior, developmental delay or learning problems, growth disturbances (child is underweight), enuresis, morning headaches, cardiovascular findings of right ventricular hypertrophy and failure leading to cor pulmonale (Marcus, 1998).

Etiology

Collapse of the pharyngeal airway with increased airway resistance above the collapsing segment causes sleep apnea. The child makes repeated vigorous attempts to breathe. Snoring is associated with these efforts but will not be heard if obstruction is complete. Arousal may occur, and with it, upper airway muscle tone improves. The cycle may repeat many times during the night. The condition may also be partial, called obstructive hypoventilation. Other factors may include the following:

- Large adenoids or tonsils or both
- Nasal deformities
- Abnormally small oropharyngeal structures as in Pierre Robin syndrome
- Craniofacial structural problems such as midface hypoplasia
- Factors affecting neural control such as generalized hypotonia; central nervous system injury, and brain stem dysfunction, which includes cerebral palsy and muscular dystrophy. These conditions relate to incoordination of upper airway muscles.
- Idiopathic or genetic cause—Prader-Willi syndrome, sickle cell disease, mucopolysaccharidosis.
- Obesity (Marcus, 1998)

Incidence

Sleep apnea may occur in approximately 2% of 4- to 5-year-olds (Anders & Eiben, 1997).

Clinical Findings

HISTORY

The following should be assessed:

- Disrupted sleep patterns (timing, restlessness, positions, behavior while asleep)
- Snoring (pitch, periods of silence, intensity, onset, frequency, duration)
- Observed increased breathing effort (rib cage retraction, paradoxical chest wall movement)
- Alertness and functioning when awake
- Enuresis
- Associated conditions (e.g., craniofacial syndromes, tonsillar hypertrophy)
- Growth and development

PHYSICAL EXAMINATION

The physical examination should include the following:

- Vital signs, including blood pressure
- Height and weight if there is failure to thrive or obesity

- Complete ear, nose, and throat examination, including tonsils and adenoids, midfacial hypoplasia, retro- or micrognathia, patency of nasal passages, tongue size, signs of cleft palate
- Cardiac functioning for evidence of cor pulmonale
- Observation for digital clubbing, pectus excavatum
- Muscle tone

Laboratory Evaluation

Tape recording the apneic episodes may be helpful in assessing the problem. The child needs to be referred for a variety of sleep studies as well as electrocardiogram and echocardiogram if the problem is severe. Radiographs of the head and neck are usually not helpful.

Differential Diagnoses

The differential diagnoses are seizure disorder and central apnea, which are characterized by no airflow and no respiratory effort. Central apnea is a brainstem problem that is more commonly seen in premature or newborn infants (Anders & Eiben, 1997).

Management

The child should be referred for sleep studies and possible adenotonsillectomy. Nasal continuous positive airway pressure (CPAP) has also been used. Weight loss may help obese children. Drugs are ineffective.

Complications

Cardiac problems, including cor pulmonale resulting from hypoxic episodes, right ventricular hypertrophy, pulmonary hypertension, heart failure, systemic hypertension, and polycythemia can occur (Loughlin, 1992; Marcus, 1998). Neurological problems, including developmental delay, learning problems, hyperactivity, excessive daytime sleepiness, and morning headache, can occur. Finally, failure to thrive and enuresis have been associated with obstructive sleep apnea (Marcus, 1998; Marcus et al., 1994).

REFERENCES

Adair R, Bauchner H: Sleep problems in childhood. Curr Prob Pediatr 23:147-170, 1993.

American Academy of Pediatrics Task Force on Infant Positioning and SIDS; Positioning and SIDS. Pediatrics 89: 1120-1126, 1992.

American Academy of Pediatrics Task Force on Infant Positioning and SIDS: Does bed sharing affect the risk of SIDS? Pediatrics 100:272, 1997.

American Sleep Disorders Association: International Classification of Sleep Disorders: Diagnostic and Coding Manual. Lawrence, KS, Allen Press, 1990.

Anders T, Eiben L: Pediatric sleep disorders: A review of the past 10 years. J Acad Child Adolesc Psychiatr 36:9-20, 1997.

Behrman R, Kliegman R, Arvin A (eds): Nelson Textbook of Pediatrics, 15th ed. Philadelphia, WB Saunders, 1996.

Beltramini A, Hertzig M: Sleep and bedtime behavior in preschool-aged children. Pediatrics 71:153-158, 1983.

Blum N, Carey W: Sleep problems among infants and young children. Pediatr Rev 17:87-93, 1996.

Carey W: Nightwaking and temperament in infancy. J Pediatr 84:756-758, 1974.

Carey W, McDevitt S: Revision of the infant temperament questionnaire. Pediatrics 62:735-739, 1978.

Ferber R: Childhood sleep disorders. Neurol Clin 14:493-511, 1996.

Ferber; R: Solve Your Child's Sleep Problems. New York, Simon & Schuster, 1985.

Gershon N, Moon R: Infant sleep position in licensed child care centers. Pediatrics 100:75-78, 1997.

Jantz J, Blosser C: A motor milestone change noted with a change in sleep position. Archiv Pediatr Adolesc Med 151:565-568, 1997.

Jimmerson K: Maternal, environmental, and temperamental characteristics of toddlers with and toddlers without sleep problems. J Pediatr Health Care 5:71-77, 1991.

Johnson C: Infant and toddler sleep: A telephone survey of parents in one community. J Dev Behav Pediatr 12:108-114, 1991.

Johnson A, Wise M, Jimmerson K: The nurse practitioner's role in a pediatric sleep clinic. J Pediatr Health Care 9:162-166, 1995.

Loughlin J: Obstructive sleep apnea in children. Adv Pediatr 39:307-335, 1992.

Lozoff B, Wolf A, Davis N: Cosleeping in urban families with young children in the United States. Pediatrics 74:171-182, 1984.

Madansky D, Edelbrock C: Cosleeping in a community sample of 2- and 3-year-old children. Pediatrics 86:197-203, 1990.

Marcus C: Does your child snore? Contemp Pediatr 15:101-115, 1998.

Marcus C, Caroll J, Koerner C, et al: Determinants of growth in children with the obstructive sleep apnea syndrome. J Pediatr 125:556-562, 1994.

McKenna J, Mosko S, Richard C: Bedsharing promotes breastfeeding. Pediatrics 100:214-219, 1997.

Mosko S, Richard C, McKenna J: Infant arousals during mother-infant bedsharing: Implications for infant sleep and sudden infant death syndrome research. Pediatrics 100:841-849, 1997.

Ponsonby A-L, Dwyer T, Gibbons L, et al: Factors potentiating the risk of sudden infant death syndrome associated with the prone position. N Engl J Med 329:377-382, 1993.

Region X Nursing Network: Region X Nursing Network Newborn, Child (Birth to Three); School Age, and Adolescent Manuals. Seattle, University of Washington, 1998.

Richman N: A community survey of characteristics of one- and two-year-olds with sleep disruptions. J Am Acad Child Psychiatr 20:281-291, 1981.

Rickert V, Johnson M: Reducing nocturnal awakening and crying episodes in infants and young children: A comparison between scheduled awakenings and systematic ignoring. Pediatrics 81:203-212, 1988.

Seymore F, Brock P, During M, et al: Reducing sleep disruptions in young children: Evaluation of therapist-guided and written information approaches: A brief report. J Child Psychol Psychiatr 30:913-918, 1989.

Sheldon S, Spire J, Levy H: Pediatric Sleep Medicine. Philadelphia, WB Saunders, 1992.

Spiers P, Guntheroth W: Recommendations to avoid the prone sleeping position and recent statistics for sudden infant death syndrome in the United States. Archiv Pediatr Adolesc Med 148:141-146, 1994.

Willinger M, Hoffman H, Hartford R: Infant sleep position and risk of sudden infant death syndrome: Report of Meeting held January 13 and 14, 1994, National Institutes of Health, Bethesda, MD. Pediatrics 93:814-820, 1994.

Yarcheski A Mahon N: A study of sleep during adolescence. J Pediatr Nurs 9:357-367, 1994.

Zuckerman B, Stevenson J, Bailey V: Sleep problems in early childhood: Continuities, predictive factors, and behavioral correlates. Pediatrics 80:664-667, 1987.

CHAPTER **17**

Cognitive-Perceptual Patterns

Catherine E. Burns and Kathleen C. Shelton

INTRODUCTION

Cognition and perception are interrelated activities engaged in by all humans. Gordon (1987) describes the cognitive-perceptual functional health pattern to include "the adequacy of sensory modes, such as vision, hearing, taste, touch, or smell, and the compensation or prostheses utilized for disturbances. Also included are the cognitive functional abilities, such as language, memory, and decision-making." Gordon notes that "to hear, see, smell, taste, and touch are human functions taken for granted until deficits arise." Little has been written about children in terms of the cognitive-perceptual pattern per se. However, attention-deficit hyperactivity disorder (ADHD), deafness, blindness, and autism are all pediatric problems that involve use of sensory modes and are related to cognition, language, and the functional abilities of day-to-day life; that is, they represent problems within the cognitive-perceptual pattern.

Facilitating the developmental progress of children should be an overriding concern for families and health care providers. Cognition is an essential component of development. Assisting children and families to minimize the effects of perceptual problems on cognition and, thus, development as a whole, is an important role of the nurse practitioner (NP). In this chapter, selected cognitive-perceptual problems of children are addressed as they relate to functioning in daily life.

NURSING STANDARDS

The Region X Nursing Network (1998) goals related to childhood cognitive-perceptual functioning are as follows:

Goal for newborn, goal for 1 month to 3 years, and goal for school-age children: The child's cognitive-perceptual development is appropriate for age.
Goal for adolescent: The adolescent's cognitive-perceptual development is within normal limits.

The American Medical Association (AMA) Guidelines for Adolescent Preventive Services (GAPS)(Elster & Kuznets, 1994) recommend that "all adolescents should be asked annually about learning or school problems." Learning disability, ADHD, medical problems, and other factors are identified as areas for further assessment if the young person is not successful in school.

The draft of the 2010 Health Promotion and Disease Prevention Objectives (United States [US] Department of Health and Human Services, 1998) contains standards similar to those of *Healthy People 2000*. The *Healthy People 2000* standard reads: "Increase to at least

389

80 percent the proportion of providers of primary care for children who routinely refer or screen infants and children for impairments of vision, hearing, speech and language, and assess other developmental milestones as part of well-child care" (US Department of Health and Human Services, 1991).

▰▰ CONCEPTUAL BACKGROUND

Normal Cognitive-Perceptual Patterns

Cognition and general knowledge represent the accumulation and reorganization of experiences that result from participating in a rich learning setting with skilled and appropriate adult interventions. From these experiences, children construct knowledge of patterns and relations, cause and effect, and methods of solving problems of everyday life.

For children to develop, they must perceive and process information from varied stimuli. External stimuli include visual, auditory, proprioceptive, tactile, and other modalities, whereas internal stimuli include emotions, associations, fantasies, visceral-autonomic sources, and memory sources (Levine et al., 1980). When children experience problems perceiving their environment, both animate and inanimate, development is at risk. For example, the deaf child who fails to hear sounds or learn a communication system early in life can develop faulty language and experience decreased knowledge acquisition and storage skills, reading difficulties, and social difficulties.

Learning requires feedback related to behaviors exhibited. Feedback provides information to the child, positive reinforcement for correct responses to stimuli, and negative reinforcement for behaviors that are not appropriate. Parents, peers, and others provide important feedback to the child. For the child with perceptual problems, not only is the initial cue missed but also the feedback cues, which the child needs in order to know whether his or her response was appropriate. This feedback is an essential component of the learning process.

Information Processing Theories

Information processing is thinking or problem-solving. The collection of information-processing theories can serve as a useful framework for understanding learning from the perspective of cognitive and perceptual processes. The theories collectively focus on information presented, processes used to transform information, and memory limits that constrain the amount of information that can be represented and processed. Unlike Piaget's model, information-processing theories try to develop a complete theory of cognition, are relatively specific, and are testable. Information-processing theorists sometimes use computer models to develop and test their ideas.

Atkinson and Shiffrin (1968) have provided a broad theory of information processing. They proposed a system with structural and process components. Structural features include a sensory store with both visual and auditory registers, a short-term store, and a long-term store. There are also several processes or actions essential to the system. Rehearsal activity is used to keep information in the short-term store—the working memory. Automatic processing activities transform information outside the direct control of the individual to retain information not consciously remembered about the frequency of experiences. For example, children imitate same-sex models. They are affected by the numbers of times they see men vs. women engaged in certain activities and from those frequency data learn sex roles (Perry & Bussey, 1979). One should immediately see that blind or deaf children will have difficulty with the two registers, visual and auditory, with deficits in one as well as the necessity for greater skill in the other. Children with ADHD or autism can have serviceable visual and auditory registers but have difficulty screening input from the registers appropriately or have problems using the processes of rehearsal and automatic processing effectively and efficiently, or both.

The task environment or the context in which the child acts is also important. For example, a particular solution to a problem may create moral conflicts and thus alter the child's options. Encoding is also important. It involves identification of critical information in a situation and use of it to create internal representations (Newell & Simon, 1972). If children fail to identify or comprehend critical elements or do not know how to encode them efficiently, they do not learn from potentially useful experiences. A key role of parents and teachers is to help children learn to identify critical cues and encode and process the information so that it becomes useful knowledge.

Levine and associates (1980) applied information processing concepts to the clinical understanding and management of pediatric learning disorders. Their information processing model (Figure 17-1) asserted that selective attention is a gateway between the availability and perception of stimuli and the representational and storage processes the child mobilizes to use the information. A great deal of information in the form of various stimuli may be available to the child. Selective attention begins the processes of information management—taking in, manipulating, storing, and responding.

"Attention is a perpetual, self-reinforcing selection process. At any given instant, a display of internal and external stimuli compete for an individual's conscious focus. Such stimuli include immediate auditory or visual sensory data; information stored in long- or short-term memory; sensations originating in viscera, muscles, and joints; and fantasies, feelings, and associations. Through a process of conscious selection, one (or few) of these incoming stimuli can take priority or achieve conscious saliency, whereas the others are relegated, at least tentatively, to the status of background or noise (beyond immediate conscious awareness).

In childhood, as in adult life, the process of selective attention allows one to focus on those stimuli that will be beneficial. When attention is optimal, one can concentrate for appropriate lengths of time on data that will lead to productivity, acquisition of knowledge, and enhancement of skills. . . . Comprehension and problem-solving ability are optimized (Levine et al., 1980)."

Perception and attention are closely related phenomena. Perception is awareness of stimuli, whereas attention serves as a filtering process to focus on the most important perceptions at the moment. The primary-care provider needs to assess both perceptual and selective attention skills.

Cognitive-Perceptual Developmental Patterns

INFANTS

The infant uses perceptions in a very literal way to develop cognition as explained by Piaget's sensorimotor stage. The infant watches, listens, tastes, smells, and manipulates objects in the environment in order to learn. Eye-hand coordination is important; achieving object permanence as a concept is essential.

TODDLERS AND PRESCHOOLERS

Toddlers continue to develop cognitively in the sensorimotor stage, whereas preschoolers, sometime after age 2 years, move into the preoperational stage. In this egocentric phase, they continue mentally to construct models that explain how the world works. However, they are unable to do several critical operations, including considering several variables at once; recognizing that others have different perceptions, classifying proficiently; and understanding that some objects are inanimate, without intention and ability to act. Visual and auditory perceptions and selective attention are key factors in toddler learning. Language development assists them to encode and store information for retrieval and use.

SCHOOL-AGE CHILDREN

School-age children have increased perceptual skills. They have mastered the concept that others may have a different perception the world from theirs, an especially important step that helps them understand the world from psychosocial perspectives. Piaget described their thought processes as concrete operations. In other words, they reason best when actually manipulating variables so that the senses are directly stimulated rather than manipulating variables abstractly as they reason out problems. Reading becomes another type of coded language that allows further broadening of ex-

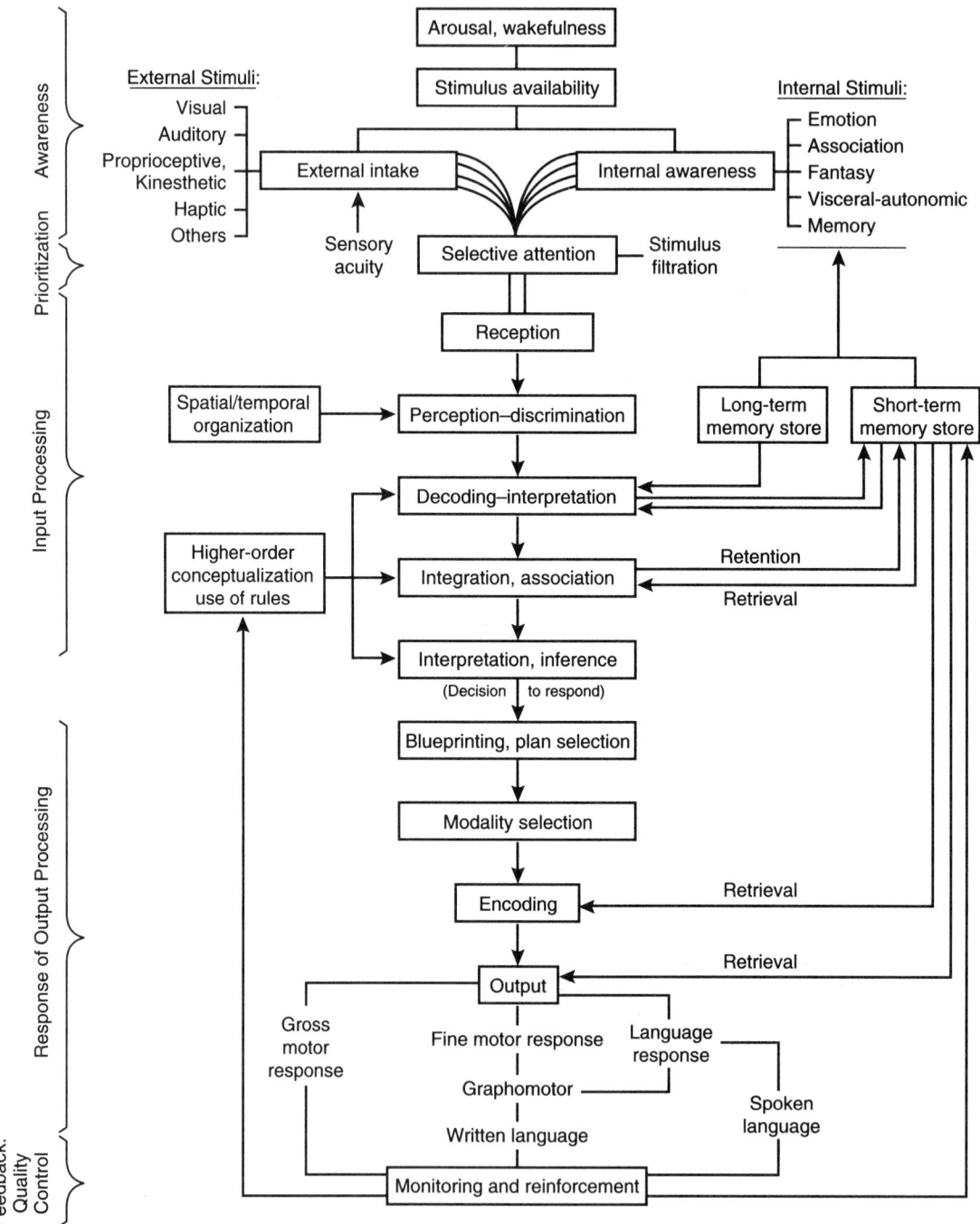

FIGURE 17-1
Information processing model. (From Levine M, Brooks R, Shonkoff J: A Pediatric Approach to Learning Disorders. New York, John Wiley & Sons, 1980, p 480)

perience beyond that which is directly observable.

ADOLESCENTS

Most adolescents can use formal operational thinking, including the capacity to reason from hypotheses and to identify various possible outcomes. Cognitive and perceptual skills are mature. (Of course, both adolescents and adults do not always use formal operational reasoning.)

The developmental milestones for children with cognitive-perceptual problems are altered from these normal patterns. A summary of some of the differences in blind and deaf children is found in Table 17-1.

Effects of Cognitive-Perceptual Pattern Problems on the Family

Family caregiving of children with impairments of all types is a related area that the NP must understand. Families adapt to achieve caregiving demands while trying to maintain family integrity. This adaptation is sometimes stressful. Because children with chronic conditions are rarely institutionalized, society relies on families to provide complex and time-consuming care.

TABLE 17-1

Developmental Milestones of Blind and Deaf Infants and Children

	BLIND	DEAF
Infants (0–1 yr)	Tend to lie quietly in crib. Attachment problems possible due to decreased social cues and visual following. Decreased use of hands and bringing hands to midline, decreased prone position, decreased facial expressions. Head control normal but delayed pull to sit; creep, stand, and walk delayed about 4 mo. Creeping delayed until reaching on sound cue is achieved. Increased separation anxiety may begin by 6 mo. Increased echolalia (Ryan, 1988). Sensorimotor delays common. Delayed object permanence.	Sensorimotor stage normal. Language development: deaf children exposed early to sign language develop language similarly to hearing children exposed to spoken language (Meadow-Orlans, 1990). Deaf children exposed to both spoken and sign language learn both and progress as hearing children (Meadow, 1980). Deaf children exposed only to spoken language have language delays (Gregory & Mogford, 1981). Language output decreased around 6–9 mo.
Toddlers (12 mo–2 yr)	Decreased aggression but increased tantrums and motor behavior when frustrated. Continued delayed object permanence. Walks at 17 mo on average. Blindisms appear—rocking, swaying, head turning (Phillips & Hartley, 1988).	Sensorimotor stage normal.
Preschoolers (3–5 yr)	Decreased social skills, decreased self-help skills. "I" sense of self delayed to 4 yr (Phillips & Hartley, 1988).	May have preoperational delays (Quigley & Kretschmer, 1982). Symbolic play may be delayed if language skills are decreased.
School-age children (6–12 yr)	Reading and mobility delays. Conservation delayed to 9 years (Tobin, 1972).	May have concrete operations delays (Quigley & Kretschmer, 1982). Decreased self-concept.
Adolescents (13–19 yr)	Delays may continue or adolescent may finally achieve developmental level with achievement in academic and social maturity areas.	Increased adjustment problems and decreased social maturity (Meadow, 1980), decreased self-concept. May have formal operations delays.

Families with blind children have been found to deal with the situation in four different ways. They may *realistically accept their child*, working to keep the child healthy despite the handicap. Other families are especially *devoted to the child*, often with a dominant parent. In the *perfect blind child* family, parents interpret the handicap as a challenge to be overcome. Their goal is for the blind child to become a perfect blind adult. Fathers dominate in these families, and achieving independence is essential for the child. Relationships among other family members, although appearing calm on the surface, are disturbed, often with parents or other family members seeking counseling. Finally, there is an *overwhelmed family* typology. The blindness diagnosis is accepted with sadness, anger, or despair. The goal for the child is survival, with independence discussed ambivalently. Parents have different agendas with little mutual support. Parents either focus on themselves or turn to relationships with other family members, often leaving the blind child alone or aligned with another family member. Relationships with outside agencies are ambivalent, with some complaints that too much is expected of them as parents (Kodadek & Haylor, 1990). Similar typologies probably exist for families with children with other cognitive-perceptual problems.

ASSESSMENT OF COGNITIVE-PERCEPTUAL PATTERNS

Normal Patterns

Assessment of normal cognitive-perceptual patterns have been discussed earlier in this chapter and elsewhere in this book. Developmental assessments appropriate to the age of the child and hearing and vision screening are the usual modes of assessment.

Assessment of Children with Cognitive-Perceptual Problems

No matter what the particular type of problem, an assessment should include three aspects:

1. Diagnosis or monitoring, or both, of the child's health from a primary care perspective

2. Evaluation of parent and family responses to the problem
3. Evaluation of the child's development

The details of these assessments vary with the condition. A variety of special assessment tools are available and are generally administered by experts. Mislabeling of children can occur when tools for sighted or hearing children, for instance, are adapted intuitively for children with visual or auditory disabilities.

MANAGEMENT STRATEGIES

Children and families with problems in this domain generally need support in four areas: social and adaptive skills, education, social support, and multidisciplinary health care team consultations.

Social and Adaptive Strategies

Social and adaptive care relates to helping children achieve maximal independence in living and learning to get along with family and others in a variety of social environments. Most of this care is delivered by the family, but some parents need help with knowing what social and adaptive developmental steps children should master at various ages. Sorting out what "normal" children do at given ages vs. what the handicapped child is doing requires thoughtful analysis. Particular strategies to help the impaired child learn new skills are often learned by trial and error or can be gleaned from parents of children with similar handicaps. Physical therapists, occupational therapists, and teachers with special education to help cognitively perceptually impaired children can be important resources. The NP can serve as case manager, help parents explore other ideas, or act as a conduit to help the parents find others who have solved similar problems.

Educational Strategies

Children with ADHD, deafness, blindness, and other problems are entitled to special education opportunities to maximize their learning potential. Infant stimulation programs are extremely important for blind and deaf children. Early-intervention preschool programs are essential. When children reach school age, decisions are made collaboratively between parents and school personnel about the best placement of the child, whether in a mainstream classroom, in a special classroom, or in a combination of settings. Blind and deaf children sometimes attend special schools designed to meet their needs in either residential or day programs. Children with ADHD or learning problems are usually managed in regular schools. Annual planning of the educational program is often a frustrating experience for parents. From the information processing model, the goals of educational programs are to help children perceive and utilize information for learning, using and developing all their skills to their maximum potential.

Social Support Strategies

Living with an unconventional child, whether the problem is blindness, deafness, hyperactivity, learning difficulties, or others, generally requires that the family develop a structure and organization to support the child without becoming overprotective or intrusive, and an environment that offers consistency for the child. For many families, maintenance of family organization and consistency is difficult.

Social support has been shown to provide significant benefits to families with children with health problems of all sorts. National organizations provide information and expert advice, and local groups can facilitate direct help. Connecting families to others with similar experiences is helpful. Further, the extended family, especially grandparents, can provide significant tangible support to families working to cope with the stresses (financial, temporal, energy, and emotional) of caring for a child with special needs. Siblings may also need support.

Multidisciplinary Team Strategies

The use of a variety of specialists can provide the best resources for children with special needs. Generally, these include medical special-

ists, physical and occupational therapists, social workers, and specially educated teachers. The NP helps families to identify appropriate teams, serves as a case manager among the parties, and ensures that primary health care needs are integrated with the special services provided.

▬▬ COGNITIVE-PERCEPTUAL PROBLEMS OF CHILDREN

Attention-Deficit Hyperactivity Disorder

DESCRIPTION

ADHD is the most commonly diagnosed behavioral problem in childhood. The cardinal features of this disorder are inattention, distractibility, impulsivity, and overactivity. These primary behaviors and their secondary manifestations have an impact on every aspect of life for affected children. The intensity and effect of ADHD behaviors vary widely among children. Behaviors can also change over time in response to normal maturational influences. ADHD is now regarded as a chronic condition that continues into adulthood (Biederman, 1998).

The nature and complexity of ADHD have been observed over time. While the actual behaviors associated with attentional difficulties still reflect the picture first described at the turn of this century, defining characteristics of the disorder have changed with time as scholars and clinicians have tried to tease out the essence of attentional problems and to differentiate the disorder from other diagnostic categories. This has led to confusion for practitioners who are trying to make accurate diagnoses (Barkley, 1990).

In an attempt to unify the understanding about ADHD, Barkley (1997) outlined a theoretical model of ADHD. Accordingly, the essential impairment is a deficit in behavioral inhibition, disrupting the developmental process of learning to self-regulate behaviors. Instead, external behaviors of inattention, distractibility, impulsivity, and hyperactivity, which may be age-appropriate in young children persist into school age and adolescence and result in the inability to regulate behavior internally as the child matures.

ATTENTION. Includes the ability to maintain concentration for an appropriate period of time and to resist attending to competing stimuli. Without these abilities, children and adolescents appear distracted at times when they are expected to concentrate on something else. Attention also implies skill at picking out salient vs. trivial information and choosing effective problem-solving strategies. Lacking this component of attention leads to missing the point in academic and social situations and doing things the hard way without careful thought about how to plan and solve a problem.

DISTRACTIBILITY. A byproduct of inattention that results when one pays attention to multiple stimuli at one time or in rapid succession. Difficulty maintaining enough mental effort to complete a task is related to distractibility. These characteristics lead to inconsistent performance in school and lost interest in activities and social plans.

IMPULSIVITY. Acting before thinking, is described in the Diagnostic Statistical Manual IV (DSM-IV) (American Psychiatric Association [APA], 1994) in part by the behaviors manifested: impatience; difficulty delaying responses, such as blurting out answers in class or interrupting conversations; and blundering without following directions.

HYPERACTIVITY. Describes the cluster of behaviors of overactivity, including fidgeting, an inability to remain seated when expected, and moving "as though driven." These behaviors interfere with attention. They are also regarded as disruptive to group activities and create negative social consequences for the ADHD child.

Longitudinal studies on ADHD, research using the newest imaging technology, and new conceptualizations about the nature of ADHD suggest that common ADHD behaviors occur when executive functions in the cortex of the brain fail to inhibit impulsive and hyperactive behaviors (Barkley et al., 1993: Faraone et al, 1996). This research also indicates that those with inattention without impulsivity and hyperactivity may have a disorder distinct from what is now called ADHD. Future revisions of the DSM will reflect this ongoing discussion among clinicians and researchers (Barkley, 1997; Schneider & Tan, 1997).

ETIOLOGY

ADHD has multiple etiologies, and many are controversial. Most findings are correlational rather than causal. A variety of antecedent factors seem to cause a disturbance in a final common pathway in the nervous system. Neurological and physiological factors associated with ADHD include perinatal hypoxic and anoxic insults, other injuries at birth, delayed brain maturation, imbalances in neurotransmitter functions, and differences in cerebral blood flow patterns. Elevated lead levels, cigarette smoking, and ingestion of alcohol or drug use during pregnancy are three environmental factors implicated with ADHD. A frequently found positive family history of ADHD implies a familial, if not genetic, predisposition (Hechtman, 1996). Extensive studies have failed to find connections between food additives or refined sugar and ADHD (Milich et al., 1986).

INCIDENCE

Psychiatric studies give the incidence of ADHD as 3 to 5% (APA, 1994). Most medical studies give the incidence as 3 to 10% (Barkley, 1990, 1997; Goldman et al., 1998). ADHD is more commonly diagnosed in boys than girls, with ratios ranging from 5:1 (epidemiological samples) to 9:1 (clinical samples). Confusion around diagnostic criteria and the unique manifestation of symptoms in each child contribute to wide discrepancies in reported incidence.

ADHD AND FAMILY FUNCTIONING

The effects of ADHD often produce stress in families, day care, and school environments. At home, disruption of family functioning and activities of daily living are most affected. Parents are often frustrated and exhausted. Frequently, there is increased physical fighting between the child with ADHD and his or her siblings or parents. Tolerance for this aggressive behavior results in the absence of successful family interventions. A cycle develops whereby families minimize the degree of aggression and violence as a coping strategy. Correlational studies indicate that increasing age and severity of ADHD symptoms are associated with more negative effects on family functioning (Lewis, 1992). Of course, some families accept the situation and cope better than others.

A family study has identified developmental trajectories for the child with ADHD, the parents, and other family members (Kendall, 1998) and indicates that early interventions are necessary to prevent the escalation of family violence, the deterioration of family functioning, and negative impacts on all family members.

ADHD CHILDREN AT SCHOOL

Children with ADHD may be unsuccessful in developing meaningful relationships with peers and other adults. Social interactions at school may involve aggressive behaviors, leading to exclusion from group activities or isolation and withdrawal on the part of the child with ADHD. Developmental tasks of adolescence frequently are negatively affected by ADHD.

The school experience comprises both educational and social aspects. Inattention, distractibility, and hyperactivity can interfere with learning directly by disrupting the child's ability to concentrate and complete work. Indirectly, the social consequences of the disruption produced by ADHD symptoms may alienate and frustrate the child, the teacher, and classmates, which reinforces the cycle of difficulty with learning, low self-esteem, and lack of satisfying friendships.

A cumulative effect can be seen when relationships at home, school, and in the community deteriorate, putting the child or adolescent with ADHD at risk for engaging in delinquent or socially unacceptable behaviors. High school dropout rates for adolescents with ADHD are significantly higher than those in the general population, as are rates for juvenile offenses, underemployment, and imprisonment in adulthood (Goldstein, 1997).

CLINICAL FINDINGS

DSM-IV criteria must be met and differential diagnoses ruled out to confirm the diagnosis and to plan treatment for this highly individualized problem. If problems have been identified by different observers and noted since early childhood, ADHD is more likely to be diagnosed. Children who display impulsive and hyperactive behaviors are more likely to be evaluated at a younger age than children who display inattentive and distractible behaviors.

History

The history must include assessment of the following:

- Family history: ADHD, neurological problems, learning difficulties, or psychological problems.
- Birth history: Prenatal history, maternal health, use of medications, recreational drugs, alcohol, and tobacco during pregnancy; birth anoxia, difficult delivery, postpartum complications, and postnatal history.
- General health history: Consider especially neurological status, vision, hearing, chronic diseases.

Questioning in a direct and nonjudgmental way often invites children and parents to share sensitive information.

DSM-IV criteria for ADHD signs and symptoms are found in Table 17–2.

A developmental, functional health pattern, and a family/social/environmental history is also taken. Suggestions for a complete history of the child who may have ADHD are found in Table 17–3.

Physical Examination

The physical examination should include the following:

- Complete health history and physical examination
- Neurological examination
- Minor congenital anomalies (e.g., fetal alcohol syndrome features)
- Auditory screening
- Visual screening
- Growth parameters
- Signs of anemia, chronic illness, allergy (Dulcan, 1997)

T A B L E 17-2

DSM-IV Criteria for Attention Deficit Hyperactivity Disorder

DOMAIN	CRITERIA
ESSENTIAL FEATURES	Symptoms occur in two or more settings (home, work, school, in public) *and* There is clear evidence of significant impairment in social, school, or work settings Symptoms have persisted for more than 6 mo Symptoms have been present before the age of 7 yr
INATTENTION TRAITS	At least *six* symptoms of inattention are present: Fails to tend to details, makes careless mistakes routinely in work and schoolwork Has difficulty sustaining attention on a task at work or at play Does not seem to listen when spoken to Fails to follow instructions or fails to complete tasks (not due to oppositional behavior or failure to understand instruction) Has difficulty organizing tasks and activities Often avoids or puts off tasks requiring sustained mental effort Often loses things necessary for performing tasks Is easily distracted by extraneous stimuli Is often forgetful in daily activities
HYPERACTIVITY/ IMPULSIVITY TRAITS	At least *six* of the following symptoms of hyperactivity/impulsivity are present: Often squirms in seat or fidgets with hands or feet Often leaves seat when remaining in seat is expected Often runs, climbs, or moves restlessly in situations when it is inappropriate Often has difficulty playing or enjoying quiet leisure activities Is often described as "on the go" or "driven" Often talks excessively Often answers before question is completed or blurts out answer Has difficulty taking turns Often interrupts or intrudes in others' activities

Other Studies

Additional studies may be needed, including the following:

- Neurodevelopmental examination with fine and gross motor skills test
- Brief mental status examination and screening for learning disabilities
- Laboratory work, including tests for anemia and lead, as well as a thyroid screen and levels of anticonvulsants if indicated by history and physical examination
- Behavior checklists completed by parents and teachers (Table 17–4)
- Psychoeducational tests to identify children with cognitive, language, visual-spatial-motor problems

DIAGNOSIS AND DIFFERENTIAL DIAGNOSIS

It is difficult to diagnose children with ADHD who are younger than 4 years of age when the characteristic features of ADHD may still be age-appropriate. Often, the diagnosis is only made in young children when behaviors are extreme (Adesman & Wender, 1991). Confusion about the diagnosis diminishes when careful consideration is given to the settings in which the behaviors in question arise (Schneider & Tan, 1997).

Other diagnoses to consider include normal variation; giftedness; language disorder; mental retardation; migraines; lead poisoning; hearing loss; thyroid dysfunction; visual disturbance; genetic disorders such as fragile-X syndrome; sei-

T A B L E 17-3

ADHD History

ASSESSMENT AREA	SUGGESTED TOPICS TO EXPLORE
CHIEF COMPLAINT/ HISTORY OF PRESENT PROBLEM	Major areas of concern First awareness of problem Beliefs about causation of problem Previous evaluations and results Medication history for behavioral, emotional, and/or learning problems
BIRTH HISTORY	Prenatal history, maternal health, use of medications, recreational drugs, alcohol and tobacco during pregnancy Birth anoxia, difficult delivery Postpartum complications, birth defects Neonatal behavior—feeding, sleep, temperament problems
GENERAL HEALTH	Neurological status, vision, hearing, chronic diseases Hospitalizations, prolonged illness Frequent injuries Poisoning or lead or environmental exposures Outbursts of uncontrollable sounds/words Tics, habit spasms, uncontrollable twitches Ongoing medications
ATTENTION/ HYPERACTIVITY SYMPTOMS HISTORY	Attention: paying attention, sustaining attention, listening, following through, organization, reluctant to engage in activities that need sustained attention, loses things, distracted, forgetful Activity: fidgets, leaves seat, runs/climbs when inappropriate, has difficulty with quiet games, talks excessively, has problems waiting turn, interrupts, "on the go"
DEVELOPMENTAL HISTORY	Milestones: motor, personal-social, language, cognitive Strengths (e.g., personality, activities, friendliness) Weaknesses
BEHAVIORAL HISTORY	Frequency that child complies when told to do something Methods used at home to improve behavior and effectiveness Parenting skills training Parental agreement about child management Counseling history for child and/or family
ACADEMIC HISTORY	Child's progress at each grade level Adjustment problems at school Difficulties with specific skills—reading, writing, spelling, math, concepts Performance problems—attention, grades, participation, excessive talking, disturbing others, fighting, abusive language, not completing work School assistance—tutoring, counseling, special help

Table continued on following page

T A B L E 17-3

ADHD History *Continued*

ASSESSMENT AREA	SUGGESTED TOPICS TO EXPLORE
Functional Health Patterns	
FEEDING	Not able to sit through a complete meal Messy and clumsy with utensils, dishes, and glasses Inadequate caloric intake can be result of symptoms and further exacerbated by medications used to treat ADHD Gastric distress may be a side effect of stimulant medication
SLEEPING	Difficulty falling asleep, night waking, needs less sleep than other family members Complains about fatigue interfering with completion of tasks
ACTIVITY	Difficulty maintaining routines for activities of daily living
COGNITIVE	Level of performance is below potential for achievement Tends to miss the point of conversations and activities Often does things the hard way in absence of established routines
SELF-CONCEPT	Struggles with low self-esteem, moodiness
ROLE RELATIONSHIPS	Inadequate social and relational skills Lies, steals, plays with fire, hurts animals, is aggressive with other children, talks back to adults
COPING/STRESS TOLERANCE	Low tolerance for frustration Outbursts of temper Moody, worried, sad, quiet, destructive, fearful/fearless, self-deprecating Somatic complaints
SOCIAL/ ENVIRONMENTAL HISTORY	Family stress and coping patterns Home, day care, and school environments Family social risk factors: recent moves, financial stress, parental job losses, births, deaths, divorces, remarriages, alcohol and drug use, involvement with law enforcement, weapons in the home
FAMILY HISTORY	ADHD, neurological problems, learning difficulties Mental health history of close family members, health or behavior problems in other family members
TEACHER HISTORY	Obtain information from school about child's problems, strengths, weaknesses, academic management of issues

zure disorder; Tourette syndrome; psychological disorders such as anxiety, oppositional defiant disorder, conduct disorder, post-traumatic stress disorder or depression; substance abuse; pervasive developmental disorder; environmental disorders (child abuse, family stress, domestic violence, parenting disruptions, parental psychopathology, inappropriate educational setting) and learning disabilities. Careful differentiation is needed to identify proper pharmacological and psychotherapeutic interventions (Spencer, et al., 1996).

Primary ADHD can exist simultaneously with family situations that predispose children to exhibit behaviors similar to those seen in children with ADHD. Since primary ADHD is the only form that is properly treated with medication, it is important to make an accurate diagnosis of ADHD to develop an appropriate management plan.

T A B L E 17-4

ADHD Behavior Rating Scales and Sources

ACTeRS: ADD-H II COMPREHENSIVE TEACHER'S RATING SCALE	MetriTech, Inc, 111 N. Market St., Champaign, IL 61820 Ages 5–12, grades K–8; 24 items rated on a 5-point scale to assess attention, hyperactivity, social skills, and oppositionality
ADDES: ATTENTION DEFICIT DISORDERS EVALUATION SCALE	Hawthorne Educational, 800 Gray Oak Dr., Columbus, MO 65201 Ages 4–18; items rated on 0–4 scale in Home and School versions to assess inattentiveness, impulsivity, and hyperactivity
ADHD-BEHAVIOR CODING SYSTEM (BCS)	Guilford Press, NY, or through ADD WareHouse Observational scale for use in a clinic or school setting to track behaviors: off task, fidgeting, vocalizing, out of seat, and playing with objects
ADHD RATING SCALE IV	George DuPaul, PhD, Education & Human Services, 111 Research Drive, Lehigh University, Bethlehem, PA 18015 Ages 5–18; items rated on a 0–4-point scale used for home and school; also a self-report version is available for use with older children
ANSER SYSTEM	Melvin D. Levine, MD, Educator's Publishing Service, Inc., 75 Moulton St., Cambridge, MA 02138 Ages 4–adolescents; questionnaires and task performance diagnostic tool yielding a descriptive, diagnostic statement of learning and behavioral problems
CHILD ATTENTION PROBLEMS (CAP)	Craig Edelbrock, PhD, University of Massachusetts Department of Psychiatry, 55 Lake Ave. N., Worcester, MA 01655
CHILD BEHAVIOR CHECKLIST	Thomas M. Achenbach, PhD, University of Vermont Center for Children, Youth, and Families, 1 S. Prospect St., Burlington, VT Ages 4–16; parent report and youth self-report forms rate items on a 3-point scale assessing social competence and behavior problems
CONNORS' RATING SCALES REVISED	Multi-Health Systems, Inc., 908 Niagara Falls Blvd., North Tonawanda, NY 14120 Ages 3–17; five versions varying in length and focus for parents and teachers using a 4-point rating scale to assess inattention, hyperactivity, and other behavioral problems; the Abbreviated Symptom Questionnaire assesses behavioral response to medication
SNAP-IV SCALE	J. Swanson, Child Development Center, University of California, Irvine, 4621 Tell, Suite 108, Newport Beach, CA 92660 Ages 3–14; parent and teacher versions use a 0–3-point scale to assess hyperactivity, undifferentiated ADHD, and oppositional defiant disorder

Primary Attentional or Behavioral Problems

These children have attentional problems that are chronic, permeate most areas of the child's life, and meet the DSM-IV diagnostic criteria (see Table 17-2). ADHD characteristics represent maladaptation and are often not consistent with age-specific developmental expectations. This type of inattention is also associated with concurrent difficulties with planning, self-monitoring, and completing tasks. Medica-

tion used to treat ADHD is targeted to this category of attentional problems and works well in about 70 to 80% of children in this group (Greenhill, 1992; Greenhill et al., 1996).

Situational Attentional or Behavioral Problems

These problems develop in specific situations and often reflect inappropriate environmental expectations. They do not permeate all settings (home, school, work, play). Problems with boredom, distractibility, and hyperactivity can be traced or related to family social problems (divorce, death, illness, moving); difficult temperament leading to a poor fit between child, parent, and school; parent-child relational problems; environmental overstimulation; and inappropriate reward systems. These children are still able to accomplish age-specific developmental tasks despite inattention and hyperactivity and do not meet the criteria for an ADHD diagnosis. Stimulant medication is not recommended when attentional or behavioral problems are situational.

Secondary Attentional or Behavioral Problems

These problems result from underlying deficits in cognitive abilities; specific learning disabilities; undetected vision and hearing problems; medical problems such as mild cerebral palsy, seizure disorders, allergies and asthma; and side effects to medications used for such conditions. The gifted child who is bored may also fit some of the behavioral patterns listed here but should be quickly identified as not having ADHD. Other significant and perhaps undiagnosed emotional problems, including unresolved anger, depression, anxiety, oppositional defiant disorder, conduct disorder, autism and abuse, may exist. These children do not meet the DSM-IV criteria for ADHD and should be diagnosed according to their other diagnostic features.

CO-MORBIDITY

A number of children with ADHD also have a concurrent diagnosis for learning disabilities (35%), or a psychiatric disorder such as anxiety (25%), depression (25%), oppositional defiant disorder, or conduct disorder (50%). The management of ADHD needs to include strategies for prioritizing needs and interventions in concert with these other conditions. If more than one health care provider is involved because of comorbid conditions, the NP may serve as case manager to keep family and other professionals informed and to coordinate treatment plans and services.

MANAGEMENT

Medication

Stimulant medication is often the most effective intervention. As many as 70 to 80% of children respond positively to stimulants, although response should not be used to confirm the diagnosis (Spencer et al., 1996). Medications should be used in conjunction with behavioral, family, cognitive-behavioral, and other interventions (see Table 17-5 for Medications).

Methylphenidate (Ritalin), dextroamphetamine (Dexedrine), and Adderal, a mixed salt preparation of amphetamines are the most commonly used drugs for treating children with ADHD (Greenhill et al., 1996). Stimulants have been shown to increase attention span, gross and fine motor coordination, and compliance while decreasing impulsiveness, hyperactivity, and aggression.

Both short- and long-acting medications are available. The short-acting forms provide greater flexibility to maximize positive behaviors at important times of the day. Usually, they are given at breakfast and again at lunch. The long-acting forms last 6 to 8 hours, getting a child through the school day. The potencies may differ between the two forms. Some families mix the forms, giving, for instance, the long-acting form for the day and then a short-acting dose to last until bedtime (Adesman & Wender, 1991).

Careful monitoring of children on medications for ADHD is necessary to minimize side effects. Antidepressants, stimulants, and allergy and asthma medications (especially over-the-counter preparations) should not be taken simultaneously without proper education; moreover, physicians should prescribe each medication with awareness of the other drugs the patient is taking. All medications for acute illnesses should be prescribed only with full knowledge of potential interactions with medications for ADHD and concurrent problems.

It is common for medication regimens to need periodic adjustment or complete change as the child grows. Increase in body weight or other medical conditions requiring medication may indicate the need to reassess the medication plan for ADHD. Social and emotional maturation may decrease or eliminate the need for

T A B L E 17-5

Medications Used to Manage ADHD Symptoms

MEDICATION	SIDE EFFECTS	MONITOR	COMMENTS
Stimulants			
Methylphenidate (Ritalin)	Anorexia, insomnia, stomachache, headache, irritability, "rebound" flattened affect, social withdrawal, crying, tics, weight loss, reduced growth rate	Height, weight, blood pressure, pulse	Do not chew or cut sustained-release tablets in half Avoid decongestants
Dextroamphetamine (Dexedrine, Dextrostat)	Anorexia, insomnia, stomachache, headache, irritability, "rebound," tics, stereopathy, weight loss, reduced growth rate	Height, weight, blood pressure, pulse	Avoid decongestants Risk of abuse
4 Mixed amphetamine salts (Adderall)	Same as dextroamphetamine		8–10 hour effect Tablet can be split Potential for abuse
Nonstimulants (not approved by FDA for ADHD use)			
Imipramine (Tofranil)	Constipation, fatigue, stomach upset, dry mouth, blurry vision, dizziness, tachycardia	Baseline ECG ECG and blood level with dose change Blood pressure, pulse	May affect cardiac conduction rate Increased levels with methylphenidate Use with ADHD + tics, enuresis, anxiety
Desipramine (Norpramin)	Tachycardia, dizziness, fatigue, stomach upset, dry mouth, blurry vision, constipation	Baseline ECG ECG and blood level with dose change Blood pressure, pulse	May affect cardiac conduction rate Increased levels with methylphenidate Use with ADHD + tics, enuresis, anxiety
Nortriptyline (Pamelor)	Dry mouth, constipation, weight gain	Baseline ECG ECG and blood level at steady state Blood pressure, pulse	Use with ADHD + tics, enuresis, anxiety
Bupropion (Wellbutrin)	Agitation, dry mouth, insomnia, headache, nausea, constipation, tremor		Lowers seizure threshold Contraindicated in patients with eating disorders or tics
Clonidine (Catapres)	Sedation, dizziness, nausea, orthostatic hypotension, clinical major depression, nightmares	Blood pressure at baseline, after dose adjustment and follow-up	Sedation decreases over time Rebound hypertension if stopped abruptly
Guanfacine (Tenex)	Sedation, dizziness, nausea, orthostatic hypotension, insomnia, agitation, headache, stomachache	Blood pressure at baseline, after dose adjustment and follow-up	

ADHD = attention deficit hyperactivity disorder; ECG = electrocardiogram; FDA = Food and Drug Administration.

medication in late childhood and adolescence. Changes in family or school schedules may necessitate a long-acting preparation or an adjustment in the timing of doses. For example, once a medication regimen has been established in early elementary grades, the plan may be successful for several years. As the child approaches middle school, the symptoms of greatest concern to the school and family may have changed or the child decides he or she no longer wants to take medication.

- Ask the parents and the child at regular intervals about how the medication is working and if they perceive a need to make adjustments.
- Assess the need to adjust medication at the beginning of each school year and at times when major changes are occurring in the family that affect the family system (births, deaths, divorces, remarriages, residential moves, death of pets, significant illness or injury)
- Include cognitive and behavioral strategies along with changes in medication to improve family functioning.

Nonstimulant medications may help children who respond poorly to an adequate trial of stimulants. This may be due to their comorbid conditions. These medications are used cautiously because they are not yet approved by the Food and Drug Administration (FDA) for these uses, but controlled studies and clinical data support their trial. Tricyclic antidepressants, including imipramine, desipramine, and nortriptyline are used. Bupropion is an antidepressant that has been used. Antihypertensives, such as clonidine and guanfacine, have been used also (Miller & Castellanos, 1998).

Family Education About Diagnosis

Families need to be well educated about the disorder because a large part of the treatment for ADHD involves parent-management techniques. The chronic nature of ADHD has a tremendous impact on family functioning. Parents often have to educate others about the special needs of their child. Because children with ADHD manifest a great variety of behaviors, parents become the experts who ultimately manage the problems and affect the outcome for their child.

Family education must be ongoing and reflect the developmental maturation of the child and unique expression of ADHD within each child and family. Educational needs at the time of diagnosis usually emphasize the broad scope of ADHD and address the parents' most pressing concerns. As parents and children adjust to the progression of this condition, their needs for education become more individualized to reflect the particular needs of the family. In addition, features of ADHD appear differently in early and middle childhood and adolescence. Parents and the children themselves need periodic assessment to ascertain which developmental tasks are being met and how education and support to accomplish those tasks should be focused.

- Designate at least one medication visit per year to assess developmental milestones, acknowledge gains in skills and abilities, and plan strategies with the family to address any developmental lags.

Another perplexing but predictable situation arises when behavioral modifications that have worked for a period of time seem to become ineffective. Education about how normal growth and development interacts with the symptoms of ADHD should be updated as children move through developmental stages.

- Routinely ask how the child's behavior is affecting the family. Plan with the family how to address the needs of the child with ADHD without eclipsing the needs of other family members.
- Routinely ask about significant changes within the family that may impact general family functioning. Individualize behavioral modifications for all family members to facilitate adjustment to changes within the family.

Family Support

Support is necessary initially to help parents understand the complexity of the diagnosis, to deal with feelings of shock or confusion, and to cope with guilt. The diagnosis of a child is often the first clue to the eventual diagnosis of an older sibling or a parent who is experiencing similar difficulties. National support groups with local affiliates can offer understanding and specific expertise in managing daily problems that come from living with the diagnosis. Support groups are often helpful around the time of the initial diagnosis. Many families use support services initially and then discontinue attending. Families need to know that they may return to such groups during times of increased stress as children move through developmental stages or other family stressors appear. Family therapy is sometimes useful and is frequently used for short terms with goals specific to the family's current situation.

- Periodically assess the need for family support.
- Ask families if there is aggressive behavior toward family members.
- Encourage family members to offer support to other families experiencing ADHD.
- Make referrals to professionals who are experienced with clients who have ADHD and their families.

Nutrition

Monthly height, weight, and blood pressure checks may be needed to monitor growth and potential weight loss as side effects of stimulant medications. When possible, give the morning dose before breakfast. Saltines offered with the morning dose of stimulant medication can decrease complaints of stomachaches. Suggestions of providing instant breakfast drinks to supplement calories when the child has low calorie intake because of difficulty sitting through meals may be helpful.

- Ask the child about his or her favorite foods and level of appetite. Diet therapy has not proven effective, and efforts to control the child's diet can put strains on the family. Guilt can result when inevitable indiscretions occur. If the whole family goes on the diet, some members may become resentful of the affected child. Further, once the child enters school, it is very difficult for the family to fully control the child's diet.

Sleep

Many children and adults with ADHD do not require as much sleep as other people. Sleep problems should be addressed in a comprehensive assessment and a parent training program. Ritualized bedtime routines are important to ADHD families; detailed instruction in massage, deep breathing, and relaxation techniques is sometimes helpful. It is necessary to ascertain the safety of children with ADHD who remain awake after other family members go to bed. Sleepwalking and night prowling sometimes cause safety concerns and should be addressed.

- Periodically ask if the child is sleeping well and staying in bed the entire night. Determine whether a safety plan is needed for night prowling.

Individual Educational Plan (IEP)

IEPs are usually necessary for ADHD children. Special accommodations at school are provided by the reauthorization of IDEA (Individuals with Disabilities Education Act). These plans should always include academic learning objectives as well as behavior modification objectives. NPs who are familiar with state and federal laws and local educational resources can guide parents as they work with the school to develop the child's plan. Frustration is common in ADHD students, their families, and school personnel. Inform parents that special assessments and evaluations can take 6 to 8 months of a school year, and children may be without special services during this entire time. IEP objectives are written in educational terms and may need to be restated in behavioral terms that children, parents, and classroom teachers can readily understand and implement. A helpful suggestion for parents is to ask that they be given a list of who is responsible for each aspect of the IEP. This spells out what is expected of the parents and individual teachers over the course of the year. Midterm or midyear monitoring of the IEP objectives is advised when children are not doing well in school.

- Ask parents what the IEP objectives are for the current school year and if they understand and support them. Help them to identify whom to contact for clarification.

Make sure that medication slips required by schools are completed and available at the time prescriptions are renewed. This simple office routine can provide significant help to parents and schools. Keep in mind that learning and language problems can coexist with ADHD. Therefore, psychoeducational testing is essential to develop an appropriate educational plan. (Table 17-6 provides suggestions for classroom adaptations.)

- Routinely ask if there are any problems when a child must take medication at school.

Psychological Interventions

Social skills training and cognitive-behavioral training are helpful when social skills deficits exist. However, recent reconceptualizations of ADHD suggest that this disorder is not caused by lack of knowing what behavior is appropriate, but by lack of ability to act on what is known (Barkley, 1997). In addition, counseling may help with problems related to anxiety, self-esteem, and depression.

Children with ADHD may be overwhelmed with the number of adults involved with managing their symptoms. When this situation occurs,

T A B L E 17-6

Suggestions for Classroom Adaptations for ADHD Children

MEMORY AND ATTENTION

Seat the child close to the teacher
Keep oral instructions brief with repetitions
Provide written directions
"Walk" the child through assignments to be sure they are understood
Break tasks and homework into small tasks
Use visual aids
Teach active reading with underlining and active listening with note taking
Provide remedial help in small sessions
Teach subvocalization to aid memorizing

IMPULSE CONTROL

Remind the child to slow down
Teach the child to monitor quality of work before turning it in

CLASSROOM ATMOSPHERE

Provide a structured classroom with clear expectations
Use moderate, consistent discipline
Rely on positive reinforcement for good behavior

ORGANIZATIONAL SKILLS

Establish a daily checklist of tasks
List homework assignments in a special notebook with the due date and needed resources
Follow up on homework not turned in

PRODUCTIVITY PROBLEMS

Divide work sheets into sections
Reduce the amount of homework and written classwork
Cut down on the number of math problems to be completed

WRITTEN EXPRESSION

Give extra time to complete written tests and assignments
Provide help with handwriting
Allow child to dictate reports and take tests orally
Reduce the quantity of written work required
Do not reduce grades for untidy work, spelling errors, poor handwriting

SELF-ESTEEM

Reward progress
Encourage performance in areas of child's strength
Avoid humiliation
Give hand signals only the child can see as private reminders of appropriate behavior

SOCIAL RELATIONSHIPS

Provide feedback about behavior involving other children
Make sure other children do not feel the child with ADHD is doing less or allowed unacceptable behavior. Change the rules for all children, if necessary.

Adapted from Baren M: Managing ADHD. Contemporary Pediatrics 11:33, 1994.

professionals should prioritize treatment recommendations in the following ways:

- Ask parents whether there is confusion or conflict about the management strategies of the professionals involved with their child to determine the best way to address these problems.
- Ask about daily and weekly schedules to determine whether the child has plenty of time for normal activities of childhood, including time to do nothing and daydream.
- Periodically assess the child and adolescent for anxiety or depression. Ask if other family members are in need of psychological assessment or support.

Advocacy

Families often need assistance in accessing educational services. Primary care providers are often in a position to exercise some influence in the local schools when services are not forthcoming. Some NPs specialize in the care and support of ADHD children and families. Those who monitor medications and provide family support should undertake these tasks only with adequate knowledge and experience and the availability of consultation with ADHD experts.

Case Management Issues

NPs may be in a unique position to offer case management services to ADHD families. Coordination of medical supervision, school programs, and family therapy or parent training programs is necessary for families to manage ADHD successfully.

- Ask whether the family thinks that the efforts to manage their child's ADHD are coordinated.

COMPLICATIONS

Children with ADHD can develop depression, problems with self-esteem, and failure to meet school educational expectations secondary to their attention and hyperactivity problems. Medication interactions and side effects are also potential complications for children with ADHD. Children with concurrent diagnoses of emotional disorders and chronic illness are at greatest risk for complications involving medication interactions. Often, medications are prescribed by different physicians; side effects can be missed because they mimic symptoms already present in a confusing and complicated disorder.

- At each visit, ask if anything new has arisen since the last visit or if the child's symptoms have changed in any way.

Deafness

DESCRIPTION

Deafness is classified as conductive or sensorineural. Conductive deafness is caused by a mechanical interruption of the sound waves from the external ear to the inner ear. It can sometimes be corrected through medical or surgical management. Hearing aids can be useful in assisting transmission of sound waves. Sensorineural deafness indicates inability of the inner ear or nerve to respond to sound waves. Sensorineural deafness can involve some frequencies more than others, resulting in a distortion of sound that is not helped by amplification. Central deafness is the least common hearing condition seen in children and is a problem between the brain stem and cortex in which sounds are heard but not understood. Mixed types also occur.

Profound deafness is deafness in which only sounds higher than 90 dB are perceived (41% of deaf children). Severe deafness is deafness to sounds 71 to 90 dB (19% of deaf children). Less than severe deafness is deafness to sounds less than 71 dB (33% of deaf children) (Center for Assessment and Demographic Studies, 1988).

ETIOLOGY AND INCIDENCE

The prevalence rate of newborns and infants with profound hearing loss is estimated to range between 1 and 3 per 1000 live births (American Academy of Pediatrics, 1999; Van Naarden et al., 1999). The incidence is about 15.3 per 1000 children younger than 18 years of age (Newacheck et al., 1993). Conductive deafness results from damage, inflammation, obstruction, or malformation of the outer or middle ear, or a combination of these. Sensorineural hearing loss is caused by damage or malformation of the inner ear or auditory nerve. It accounts for 90% of all cases of serious and profound hearing loss in children (Van Naarden et al., 1999). Heredity, encephalitis, intrauterine infections, exposure to loud noise, ototoxic drugs, and premature birth with anoxia, severe jaundice, or intraventricular hemorrhage are also causes. Syndromes involving renal, cardiac, musculoskeletal, dermatological, neurological, and ophthalmological systems can include deafness.

The American Academy of Pediatrics (1999) recommends universal hearing screening of all neonates. Methods may include evoked otoacoustic emissions (EOAE) and auditory brain stem response (ABR), either alone or in combination.

CLINICAL FINDINGS

History

The history must include assessment of the following risk factors:

- Pregnancy and birth history with intrauterine infections
- Premature birth weight less than 1500 g, birth trauma, hypoxia, mechanical ventilation lasting 5 days or longer
- Head and neck anomalies
- Bacterial meningitis
- Ototoxic drug exposure (e.g., aminoglycosides, furosemide, salicylates, naproxen, chemotherapeutics such as cisplatin [Kravitz & Selekman, 1992])
- Recurrent or chronic otitis media
- Trauma
- Tinnitus
- Hearing difficulties or difficulty discriminating speech sounds
- Exposure to loud noises
- Family history of childhood hearing loss

If loss is present:

- Onset, duration, progression, management, bilateral or unilateral, partial or complete, pain, tinnitus, vertigo, other medical conditions, viral infection history, immunization against mumps (Smeltzer, 1993)
- History of decreased verbal output beginning at 6 to 9 months of age

Physical Examination

The physical examination should include the following:

- Examination of the head, neck, and external ear
- Otoscopy
- Identification of relevant physical abnormalities
- Observation of responses to spoken and environmental sounds
- Voice volume
- Whisper test 18 inches from ear

Other Testing

The following tests may also be done (Bachmann & Arvedson, 1998):

- Behavioral testing for children younger than 5 years of age: responses to rattle, bell, whisper. Infant will open eyes, blink, startle, change sucking or breathing patterns in response to sounds. Children 4 to 7 months of age should look toward sound (Smeltzer, 1993). Visual reinforcement testing is used with children 6 months to 2 years of age.
- Tympanometry and acoustic reflex test.
- Audiology: For infants, brain–stem-evoked response (BSER) tests (also called the auditory brainstem response [ABR]) or otoacoustic emissions (OAE) tests are essential. An audiologist should provide definitive testing for deafness and its severity and type. Children older than 5 years of age can respond to a conventional hand-raising technique for specific threshold information
- Vision screening: This should be done because deaf persons need good sight. Also, Usher syndrome, which includes deafness and later retinitis pigmentosa, may need to be identified.
- Development needs to be monitored regu-

larly, especially in linguistic and cognitive areas.

DIFFERENTIAL DIAGNOSIS

Cerumen impaction, otitis media with effusion, and chronic suppurative otitis media with perforation of tympanic membrane are differential diagnoses. Consider tumor with sensorineural loss. For the child with significant hearing loss, comorbidities may exist, including developmental and communication problems, family disruptions, depression, and others.

MANAGEMENT

Multidisciplinary Team

The use of a multidisciplinary team working with the family provides the best support for the child with a hearing impairment. The team should include a primary care provider, physician, audiologist, speech and language pathologist, sign language specialist, teacher of the deaf, and others as needed. From an information-processing perspective, much of the management of the deaf child is directed at providing stimuli that the infant and child can use to understand and interact with the environment. Visual stimuli are used as the primary substitute for auditory deficits. Language serves not only as a communication device but also as a system for storing and using information.

Amplification Devices and Their Care

Different types of hearing aids have different purposes. The body box is used for children younger than 3 years of age and for those in need of more powerful or durable amplification. Postauricular devices are used for older children. Ear molds need a good fit (sometimes revised every 3 to 6 months with growth) and careful cleaning to avoid clogging. By ages 4 to 6 years, ear molds are changed yearly. Batteries last only about 100 to 150 hours and are toxic if ingested.

External otitis media can be avoided with use of petroleum jelly to decrease friction and adjustment of molds to reduce irritation. Ear molds should be washed with soap and water each night. If an infection occurs, it can usually be managed by using an antibiotic ointment and leaving the molds out for 1 to 2 days. For fungal infections, antifungal drops should be used and molds left out for 3 to 5 days.

Cochlear implants are used with some children who will not benefit from traditional hearing aids. They help children access some sounds in the environment.

Communication Needs

Communication needs can be supported by the use of text telephone devices, smoke alarms and doorbells with lights instead of alarms, a hearing ear dog, and other communication systems in the child's environment.

Family Support

Often there is stress for the family when the diagnosis is made. Siblings may need support as they cope in a family with a child identified as having a disabling condition. Parents often need counseling, support, and information related to their acceptance and parenting of the identified child. Grandparents and extended family can also need information and support (Burns & Madian, 1992).

Education

Children identified with hearing loss by 6 months of age who received early intervention services had better language development than children identified later (Yoshinaga-Itano et al., 1998). Deaf children need opportunities to learn by using their strongest modalities. Language and communication needs are paramount. There are several schools of thought related to education of the deaf. Oralists focus on amplification, speech reading, and speech training. They do not support exposure to sign language. Those who believe in the total communication approach counter that the use of sign language links the deaf to the deaf community and increases their acquisition of language and functioning in adulthood. Total communication methods include amplification, sign language, finger spelling, speech reading, and speech training. Parents are pressured to accept one approach over the other.

Parents also need education to communicate with their child effectively. One study indicates that two thirds of children learn sign language, but only one half of parents learn the same language (Center for Assessment and Demographic Studies, 1988). Lederberg and Everhart (1998) found that mothers of deaf 2-year-olds primarily communicated with their children by speech, even though the children did not visually attend. Thus, in some families, parents and children cannot fully communicate with one another. Early education for deaf children should begin in infancy. Educational services need to be family-centered and culturally sensitive. American Sign Language (ASL) is the language the deaf use with one another, and it provides the strongest link with the deaf community for the child.

Interpreter Services

If children sign, they should be provided with an interpreter during health care visits. Many deaf children have inadequate health care information and knowledge because of poor communication between provider and child (Badger & Jones, 1990; Jackson, 1990).

Genetic Counseling

Refer families for genetic counseling if the problem is inheritable.

Blindness

DESCRIPTION

Blindness varies from inability to distinguish light from darkness to partial vision, defined as visual acuity between 20/70 and 20/200 best corrected. Legal blindness is defined as distant visual acuity of 20/200 in the better eye or a visual field that includes an angle not greater than 20 degrees.

Children with visual impairments experience developmental delays. Table 17–1 shows a summary of milestones to be expected.

ETIOLOGY AND INCIDENCE

Blindness is caused by a variety of pathological conditions, including congenital cataracts, congenital glaucoma, high refractive errors, retinopathy of prematurity (ROP), detached retina, neurological conditions involving cranial nerve II, cortical blindness, and optic atrophy. ROP is the most common cause of severe visual impairment. Retinoblastoma, trauma, infection, hydrocephaly, and genetic conditions are also etiological factors.

About 1 in 500 children in the United States has partial vision, whereas about 35,000 children are legally blind (Behrman & Kliegman, 1998). Newacheck and associates (1993) report an incidence of blindness and vision loss of 12.7 per 1000 children less than 18 years. Up to 30% to 70% of visually handicapped children have additional handicaps, including mental retardation, deafness, seizures, and cerebral palsy (Teplin, 1990).

CLINICAL FINDINGS

Primary-care providers need to remember that the blind child needs special cues to understand the environment. Talk softly to the infant or child before touching and look for a variety of body cues rather than visual or facial signals. Be gentle in touching because the child has no warning that contact is coming. For older children, address the child by name, describe what you plan to do and how, warn the child of contacts or discomforts anticipated, and let the child touch or examine instruments when possible (Moller, 1993).

Signs and Symptoms of Blindness

Characteristics to assess include:

- History of failure of the infant to follow a moving object, or wandering eyes
- Poking the eyes or waving the hands in front of the face
- Nystagmus
- Failure to blink at a camera flash in front of the face
- Failure to fix and follow by 6 weeks
- Photophobia or chronic tearing

- History of prematurity with diagnosis of ROP
- Fixed strabismus or intermittent strabismus persisting longer than 6 months
- Lack of smiling in response to visual stimuli

The following should also be assessed:

- Family history of genetic visual impairments
- Family issues and environment
- General medical history
- Developmental history (attachment, midline play, reaching, gross motor skills, language skills)

Physical Examination

The physical examination should include a search for the following:

- Enlarged or cloudy cornea
- Abnormal or absent red reflex
- Lack of pupillary reflex
- Nystagmus
- Neurological disorder

Other Tests

An ophthalmological examination and developmental testing are also done.

DIFFERENTIAL DIAGNOSIS

See the etiological factors discussed earlier.

MANAGEMENT

Multidisciplinary Team

The primary care provider, ophthalmologist, special certification teacher, and orientation and mobility specialist are among the important team members for visually impaired children and their families. Genetics counselors, social workers, and other specialists can also be useful.

Family Support

As noted, families with blind children adapt in a variety of ways. Because visual cues are so important in language and social interactions, the family of the blind child may experience difficulties with attachment resulting from failure of eye contact and facial expressiveness. For instance, smiling is not recognized or imitated by the blind infant.

Parent support groups are valuable, and national organizations provide reading materials that are very helpful (see resource box). Sometimes families benefit from counseling.

Education

Public school educational programs for the visually impaired child include several distinct models. Infant early education and developmental preschool programs are essential. When children are ready to enter elementary school, full-time classes for blind children are sometimes available. These are taught by teachers with special certification to work with the blind. Some schools have resource-room programs where the child spends part of the day with a specially trained teacher, and the remainder of the day is spent in a regular classroom. Some school districts provide itinerant programs in which a specially trained teacher works with several teachers in regular classrooms, consulting with them about the learning needs of the visually handicapped children involved. Schools for the blind are generally reserved for children with multiple handicaps.

IEPs need to be developed annually, with input from both parents and school officials. When the child enters school, psychological assessments need to be done using tests designed for blind children to ensure correct educational placement and appropriate educational support systems.

Educational programs for visually handicapped children need to include some extra components. Blind children begin learning braille when sighted children learn to read. They learn to write braille in the early elementary grades by using a special typewriter. By fourth grade, blind children should also learn to use a regular typewriter. Developing additional listening skills and gaining proficiency in the use of computers with aids are also essential skills. The Optacon is a hand-held device that translates printed text into tactile displays. Children are ready to use this device at about 10 years of age. The ViewScan can be used by partially sighted individuals to enlarge type size for reading text on a screen.

Daily living skills include dressing, eating, hygiene, use of the telephone, and handling money. An orientation and mobility specialist teaches the visually handicapped child to travel with a sighted guide, use a cane, and use public transportation.

Physical education and fitness are as important to visually impaired children as to other children. Generally, individual sports, such as gymnastics and swimming, are more successful endeavors for a blind child than team sports, even if the child is partially sighted (Moller, 1993).

Developmental Interventions

Some strategies that parents can use to promote development in their visually impaired infant or child are found in Table 17-7.

Autism

DESCRIPTION

Autism is a type of pervasive developmental disorder. It is a lifelong disability that usually becomes apparent in the first 3 years of life. Communication and social interactions are impaired. Development is uneven, with occasional talent in a limited area such as music or mathematics coupled with severe deficits in other areas. Many autistic children have other impairments, such as mental retardation (70%) or seizures. Sleep disturbances are common.

Most children with autism have the following characteristics:

- Disturbances in development of physical, social, and language skills
- Abnormal responses to sensory stimuli, usually sound; abnormal sensory responses to pain, heat, and cold; tendency to taste and smell objects
- Speech, language, and nonverbal communication disturbances (the child may talk but have difficulty communicating; e.g., speech may be echolalic)

- Abnormal ways of relating to people, objects, and events

The disorder varies considerably in severity.

INCIDENCE AND ETIOLOGY

The incidence rate varies but ranges from around 0.7 to 4.5 in 10,000 children (Behrman & Kliegman, 1998). It is four times more likely to occur in male children. There is good evidence of a genetic link for some types of autism (10%). Other causes include prenatal infections, such as rubella or cytomegalovirus, as well as neonatal infections. The etiology is unknown for most cases.

CLINICAL FINDINGS

History

INFANTS. An autistic infant may be a passive, nonengaging, quiet, floppy infant or a difficult, colicky, stiff baby with poor eye contact. Attachment problems appear. There is failure to respond to name or gestures. Usually, autism is not identified in infancy.

TODDLERS. During the toddler stage, parents are convinced that something is wrong with their child. Language delays, lack of social relatedness, and severe behavior problems are common. Expressive language is delayed. Socially, the child exhibits detachment, decreased eye contact, a lack of fear, and poor creative play skills. Tantrums that persist; repetitive movements; a preference to line, stack, or spin toys; and insistence on routines are commonly observed behaviors. Use of echolalia is persistent.

PRESCHOOLERS. Language delays include lack of meaningful speech, decreased gestures, and gaze disturbances. Social interaction disturbances, such as lack of fear of strangers, invasion of the territory of others, preference to be alone, and lack of social awareness, are often seen. Persistent and insistent behaviors are common. Symbolic play is limited. The child may have precocious or average development of rote memory skills but often without comprehension of concepts.

SCHOOL-AGE CHILDREN. School-age children with autism often lack reciprocal friendships and continue with language, social, and behav-

T A B L E 17-7

Developmental Interventions for Visually Impaired Infants and Children

AGE	PSYCHOSOCIAL	COGNITIVE	MOTOR
Birth to 4 mo	Hold and talk to the infant to promote recognition through tactile and auditory modalities.	Stimulate the hands and mouth. Provide a cradle gym so that reaching and touching give feedback. Provide toys with feedback such as sound, interesting textures, or tastes.	Encourage the prone position at times while awake, a position that blind children do not generally like, since they have no reinforcement visually for lifting the head. Also encourage head turning. Bring the hands into midline. Exercise the legs and massage during baths and diaper changes. Put bells on booties.
5 to 8 mo	Stranger anxiety occurs early. Parents need to be available. Provide predictable routines.	Provide finger foods. Provide new temperatures, textures, toys with various sounds and sensations. Talk to the child. Call attention to music and other sounds in the environment.	Encourage play out of doors and on the floor. Dance and move the child actively.
9 to 12 mo	Provide routines that are predictable. Touch and voice are all-important. Cuddle.	Encourage reaching to find a sound source. Provide toys that respond to the actions of the child to develop cause-and-effect concepts. Name and describe the activities and items in the environment.	Encourage creeping about, which will occur after the child can reach for a sound. Help to stand and cruise. Touch and name body parts.
13 to 24 mo	Stranger anxiety continues. Reassure toddler of return. Fear and aggression are uncommon. Regression and tantrums are frustration responses. Guide behavior into more appropriate responses. Reduce frustrations when possible.	Continue to work on object permanence concept, which is delayed. Noncontingent sounds such as television or radio are not helpful.	Walking should begin. Crab walking is a common problem that needs to be eliminated. Walking with the child's feet on the adult's can help develop the reciprocal pattern. Blindisms may appear and can be altered with teaching. Walk together both indoors and outdoors.
2 to 5 yr	Interactions with peers and sighted children. Establish behavioral limits as with sighted children. Teach self-help skills—hygiene, feeding, dressing.	Teach games with directional concepts. Provide experiences in a variety of settings—park, grocery, etc.	Develop motor skills—walking, climbing, swimming.
6 to 10 yr	Continue to develop social skills and develop self-esteem through opportunities to be successful in activities. Provide opportunities to be with other children. Continue to develop self-help skills.	School with additional supports for the visually impaired. Braille and computer education.	Specific mobility training.

Data from Phillips S, Hartley J: Developmental differences and interventions for blind children. Pediatr Nurs 14:201–204, 1988; Teplin S: Visual handicaps. In Green M, Haggerty R (eds): Ambulatory Pediatrics. Philadelphia, WB Saunders, 1990, pp 319–322.

ioral problems. Transitions from place to place and activity to activity are difficult. Behaviors are ritualistic.

ADOLESCENTS. Adolescents usually continue with similar behaviors. Rote learning is possible, but comprehension lags (Church, 1995). It should be noted, however, that some high-functioning autistic children are mainstreamed and do very well in regular classrooms.

Family history may reveal other members with pervasive developmental disorder, autism, speech delay or language deficits, mood disorders, or mental retardation. Mildly affected persons may have social relationship problems.

The review of systems should investigate seizures, hearing loss, head injury, and meningitis.

Evaluation of the child for autism is best done at a specialty center. It is a diagnosis by exclusion.

Physical Examination

The child should be checked for general appearance of genetic syndromes and neurological findings of focal abnormalities.

Other Tests

A developmental test, a behavioral assessment, an electroencephalogram (EEG) for seizures, DNA testing for fragile-X syndrome or other syndromes, and a hearing test should be conducted.

Differential Diagnosis

Gifted child, elective mutism, obsessive-compulsive disorder, Tourette syndrome, schizophrenia of childhood, conduct disorder, mental retardation, Rett syndrome, hearing impairment, and fragile-X syndrome are all differential diagnoses for autism. Asperger syndrome includes characteristics of mild autism but without language or developmental delays. ADHD children may appear rigid, whereas autistic children may seem poorly focused.

MANAGEMENT

A focus on interactive patterns is the mainstay of management of autism. The use of a calm, firm voice, flexibility, few words, nonthreatening postures, and concrete communication is essential. Children need social skill training, early and intense developmental work, and assistance with learning.

Behavior

The most important aspect of management is behavioral training. The target behaviors vary according to age, developmental level, and disruptiveness of behaviors. Reasonable goals need to be set (Bauer, 1995).

Education

Cognitive testing with identification of strengths and weaknesses is essential to planning care. Social and behavioral functioning and language assessment are also important. School personnel need information and assistance to understand the clinical picture and management needs. Development of social and language skills is usually emphasized. "The long-term goal should be to permit the child to function as effectively and comfortably as possible in the least restrictive environment" (Bauer, 1995, p. 173).

NURSING DIAGNOSIS 17-1

COGNITIVE-PERCEPTUAL FUNCTIONAL HEALTH PATTERN

Disorganized Infant Behavior

Impaired Memory

Potential for Enhanced Organized Infant Behavior

Sensory or Perceptual Alteration

Thought Processes Alteration

Source: North American Nursing Diagnosis Association: NANDA Nursing Diagnoses: Definitions and Classification 1997–98. Philadelphia, North American Nursing Diagnosis Association, 1996.

RESOURCE BOX 17–2

RESOURCES FOR COGNITIVE-PERCEPTUAL PROBLEMS OF CHILDREN

Attention-Deficit Hyperactivity Disorder (ADHD)
Children & Adults with Attention Deficit Disorders
(CHADD)
Tel: (305) 587-3700
Website: chadd.org
600 local chapters, educational literature, newsletter
available with membership

Attention Deficit Information Network (Ad-In)
Tel: (617) 455-9895
Information on current research and regional meetings

ADD Warehouse Catalog
Tel: (800) 233-9273
Distributors for all ADHD literature published for chil-
dren, parents, professionals, and educators

National Attention Deficit Disorder Association
Tel: (440) 350-9595
Website: www.add.org

Texts for Professionals
Barkley RA: Attention-Deficit Hyperactivity Disorder:
A Handbook for Diagnosis and Treatment. New York,
Guilford Press, 1987.
Levine MD: Developmental Variation and Learning
Disorders. Cambridge, MA: Educators Publishing
Service, 1990.

Deafness
Alexander Graham Bell Association for the Deaf
(AGBAD)
Tel: (202) 337-5220
Website: www.agbell.org

**National Association of the Deaf (NAD) and
National Association of the Deaf-Blind**
Tel: (301) 587-1788
TDD/TTY: (301) 587-1789

National Information Center on Deafness
Gallaudet University
Tel: (202) 651-5051
TTY: (202) 651-5052
Website: www. gallaudet.edu/~nicd/

Blindness
American Council of the Blind (ACB)
Tel: (800) 424-8666
    (202) 467-5081
Website: www.acb.org

American Foundation for the Blind
Tel: (800) 232-5463
    (212) 502-7600

Blind Children's Fund (BCF)
Tel: (517) 333-1725

**National Association for Parents of the Visually
Impaired, Inc.**
Tel: (800) 562-6265
(617) 972-7441

National Federation of the Blind
Division for Parents of Blind Children
1800 Johnson St.
Baltimore, MD 21230

Autism
Autism Research Institute
Tel: (619) 281-7165

Autism Society of America
Tel: (301) 657-0881
Website: www.autism-society.org.

All Children With Disabilities
National Information Center for Children and
Youth with Disabilities
Tel: (800) 695-0285

Medications

None work well. Haloperidol is sometimes used, but it can have serious side effects, including dyskinesias. Usually, autistic children do not benefit from stimulant medications. Fluoxetine (Prozac) may be helpful for some if they are also depressed. Since 25% of autistic children also have seizures, they may be on anticonvulsants (Bauer, 1995).

Diet

No significant effects result from special diets.

Multidisciplinary Team

The team should include parents, teachers, primary care provider, physical therapist, and psychologist.

Family Counseling and Support

Families need a great deal of support and training to manage autistic children. They may benefit from assistance from members of the Autism Society of America (see resources box).

Since there are many unproved treatment programs touted for autistic children, parents need to be given information about programs that have proved useful and those that have not. Consideration of possible harm to child or family, scientific validation, individual assessment, and integration as a holistic part of the child's total program are factors for parents to consider before adopting a new treatment approach.

The family and siblings may need supportive counseling and referral because of the considerable stress found in families with autistic children.

Long-term care needs to be addressed because few autistic children become fully independent employed adults, although the prognosis for children with autism is highly variable and very difficult to predict. Those who are high-functioning as children will do best as adults.

REFERENCES

Adcock K, MacElroy D, Wolford E, et al: Pemoline therapy resulting in liver transplantation. Ann Pharmacother 32:422–425, 1998.

Adesman A, Wender E: Improving the outcome for children with ADHD. Contemp Pediatr 8:122–139, 1991.

American Academy of Pediatrics: Newborn and infant hearing loss: Detection and intervention. Pediatrics 103:527–530, 1999.

American Psychiatric Association. Diagnostic and Statistical Manual of Mental Disorders, 4th ed. Washington, DC, American Psychiatric Association, 1994.

Atkinson R, Shiffrin R: Human memory: A proposed system and its control processes. *In* Spence K, Spence J (eds): Advances in the Psychology of Learning and Motivation Research and Theory (Vol. 2). New York, Academic Press, 1968.

Bachmann K, Arvedson J: Early identification and intervention for children who are hearing impaired. Pediatr Rev 19:155–165, 1998.

Badger T, Jones E: Deaf and hearing children's conceptions of the body interior. Pediatr Nurs 16:201–205, 1990.

Baren M: Managing ADHD. Contemp Pediatr 11:29–38, 1994.

Barkley RA: Attention-Deficit Hyperactivity Disorder: A Handbook for Diagnosis and Treatment. New York, Guilford Press, 1990.

Barkley R: ADHD and the Nature of Self Control. New York, Guilford Press, 1997.

Barkley R, Fischer M, Edelbrock C, et al: The adolescent outcome of hyperactive children diagnosed by research criteria: I. An 8-year prospective follow-up study. J Acad Child Adolesc Psychiatr 29:546–557, 1990.

Bauer S: Autism and the pervasive developmental disorders: Part 2. Pediatr Rev 16:168–176, 1995.

Behrman R, Kliegman R: Nelson Essentials of Pediatrics, 3rd ed. Philadelphia, WB Saunders, 1998.

Biederman J: Attention-deficit hyperactivity disorder: A lifespan perspective. J Clin Psychiatr 59 (suppl):4–16, 1998.

Biederman J, Wozniak J, Kiely K, et al: CBCL clinical scales discriminate prepubertal children with structured interview-derived diagnosis of mania from those with ADHD. J Am Acad Child Adolesc Psychiatr 34:464–471, 1995.

Burns C, Madian N: Experiences with a support group for grandparents of children with disabilities. Pediatr Nurs 18:17–21, 1992.

Center for Assessment and Demographic Studies: Regional and National Survey. Washington, DC, Gallaudet University Press, 1988.

Church C: Lecture presented at the annual conference of the National Association of Pediatric Nurse Associates/Practitioners, Nashville, TN, 1995.

Dulcan M: Practice parameters for the assessment and treatment of children, adolescents, and adults with attention deficit/hyperactivity disorder. J Am Acad Child Adolesc Psychiatry 36 (suppl), 85S–121S, 1997.

Elster A, Kuznets N: AMA Guidelines for Adolescent Preventive Services (GAPS). Baltimore, Williams & Wilkins, 1994.

Faraone S, Biederman J, Mennin D, et al: A prospective

four-year follow-up study of children at risk for ADHD. Psychiatric, neuropsychological, and psychosocial outcome. J Am Acad Child Adolesc Psychiatr 35, 1449-1459, 1996.

Fischer M, Barkley R, Fletcher K et al: The adolescent outcome of hyperactive children: Predictors of psychiatric, academic, social, and emotional adjustment. J Am Acad Child Adolesc Psychiatr 32:324-332, 1993.

Goldman L, Genel M, Bezman R, et al: Diagnosis and treatment of attention-deficit/hyperactivity disorder in children and adolescents. J Am Med Assoc 279:1100-1107, 1998.

Goldstein S: Attention deficit/hyperactivity disorder: Implications for the criminal justice system. Law Enforcement Bull 6, 1997. http://www.fli.gov/library/leb/1997/june973.htm

Gordon M: Nursing Diagnosis: Process and Application. New York, McGraw-Hill, 1987.

Greenhill L: Pharmacologic treatment of attention deficit hyperactivity disorder. Psychiatr Clin North Am 15:1-26, 1992.

Greenhill L, Abikoff H, Arnold E, et al: Medication treatment strategies in the MTA study: Relevance to clinicians and researchers. J Am Acad Child Adolesc Psychiatr 34:1304-1313, 1996.

Gregory S, Mogford K: Early language development in deaf children. In Kyle WJ, Deuchar M: (eds): Perspectives on British Sign Language and Deafness London, Croom Helm, 1981, pp 218-237.

Hechtman L: Families of children with attention deficit hyperactivity disorder: A review. Can J Psychiatr 41:350-360, 1996.

Jackson C: Primary care for deaf children: Part II. J Pediatr Health Care 4:39-41, 1990.

Kendall J: Outlasting disruption: Process of reinvesting in families with ADHD children. Qual Health Res 8:839-857, 1998.

Kodadek S, Haylor M: Using interpretive methods to understand family caregiving when a child is blind. J Pediatr Nurs 5:42-49, 1990.

Kravitz L, Selekman J: Understanding hearing loss in children. Pediatr Nurs 18:591-594, 1992.

Lederberg A, Everhart V: Communication between deaf children and their hearing mothers: The role of language, gesture, and vocalizations. J Speech, Lang Hearing Res 41:887-899, 1998.

Lewis K: Family functioning as perceived by parents of boys with attention deficit disorder. Issues Mental Health Nurs 13:369-386, 1992.

Levine M, Brooks R, Shonkoff J: A Pediatric Approach to Learning Disorders. New York, John Wiley & Sons, 1980.

Marcotta P, Roberts E: Pemoline hepatoxicity in children. J Pediatr 132:894-897, 1998.

Meadow K: Deafness and child development. Berkeley, University of California Press, 1980.

Meadow-Orlans KP: Research on developmental aspects of deafness. In Moores DE, Meadow-Orlans KP (eds): Educational and Developmental Aspects of Deafness. Washington, DC, Gallaudet University Press, 1990, pp 283-298.

Milich R, Wolraich M, Lindgren S: Sugar and hyperactivity:

A critical review of empirical findings. Clin Psychol Rev 6, 493-513, 1986.

Miller K, Castellanos F: Attention deficit/hyperactivity disorders. Pediatr Rev 19:373-384, 1998.

Moller M: Working with visually impaired children and their families. Pediatr Clin North Am 40:881-890, 1993.

Musket C: Maintenance of personal hearing aids. In Roeser R, Downs M (eds.): Auditory disorders in school children. New York, Thieme Medical Publishers, 1988, pp 200-220.

Newacheck P, Stoddard P, McManus M: Ethnocultural variations in the prevalence and impact of childhood chronic conditions. Pediatrics 91:1031-1039, 1993.

Newell A, Simon H: Human Problem Solving. Englewood Cliffs, NJ, Prentice-Hall, 1972.

Perry D, Bussey K: The social learning theory of sex differences: Imitation is alive and well. J Personality Soc Psychol 37:1699-1712, 1979.

Phillips S, Hartley J: Developmental differences and interventions for blind children. Pediatr Nurs 14:201-204, 1988.

Quigley S, Kretschmer R: The Education of Deaf Children: Issues, Theory, and Practice. Baltimore, University Park Press, 1982.

Region X Nursing Network: Region 10 Nursing Network Newborn, Child (Birth to Three), School Age, and Adolescent Manuals. Seattle, University of Washington, 1998.

Ryan J: Hearing and speech assessment. In Ballard R (ed): Pediatric Care of the ICN Graduate. Philadelphia, WB Saunders, 1988.

Schneider S, Tan G: Attention deficit hyperactivity disorder. In pursuit of diagnostic accuracy. Postgrad Med 101:231-232, 235-240, 1997.

Smeltzer C: Primary care screening and evaluation of hearing loss. Nurs Pract 18:50-55, 1993.

Spencer T, Biederman J, Wilens T, et al: Pharmacotherapy of ADHD: A literature review. J Am Acad Child Adolesc Psychiatr 32:235-240, 1996.

Teplin S: Visual handicaps. In Green M, Haggerty R (eds): Ambulatory Pediatrics. Philadelphia, WB Saunders, 1990, pp 319-322.

Tobin M: Conservation of substance in the blind and partially blind. Br J Edu Psychol 142:192-197, 1972.

US Department of Health and Human Services: Healthy People 2000: Health Promotion and Disease Prevention Objectives for the Year 2000. Washington, DC, US Government Printing Office, 1991.

US Department of Health and Human Services: Healthy People 2010: Draft of Health Promotion and Disease Prevention Objectives for the Year 2010. Washington, DC: US Government Printing Office, 1998.

US Public Health Service: Clinician's Handbook of Preventive Services, 2nd ed, McLean, VA, International Medical Publishers, 1998.

Van Naarden K, Decouflé P, Caldwell K: Prevalence and characteristics of children with serious hearing impairment in metropolitan Atlanta, 1991-1993. Pediatrics 103:570-575, 1999.

Yoshinaga-Itano C, Sedey A, Coulter D, et al: Language of early-and later-identified children with hearing loss. Pediatrics 102:1161-1171, 1998.

CHAPTER 18

Self-Perception

Nancy Barber Starr

INTRODUCTION

All people—children and adults—have mental pictures of themselves that steer the course of their lives. This mental picture, or self-perception, begins to develop at birth, emerges in childhood, and is refined and crystallized in adolescence, but it continues to evolve throughout life. Significant relationships, temperament, heredity, and experiences in life all influence self-perception. Self-perception has to do with how individuals act, think, and feel about themselves, their abilities, and their bodies. It is also influenced by the response of others to them. This perception, in turn, influences the attitudes each person takes and the choices each person makes throughout life. A positive self-perception is a precious gift that provides the confidence and energy to take on the world, to withstand crises, and to focus outside one's self. It enhances the building of relationships and giving to others. People with a negative self-perception are handicapped, or "failure oriented" (Berne & Savary, 1992), focused on their own needs, trying to get and prove their self-worth. A negative self-perception drains energy, interferes with building relationships, and often leaves the person feeling like a victim.

Assessing self-perception is not a straightforward task but is interwoven with other data that the nurse practitioner (NP) collects. Routine anticipatory guidance, education, and counseling, individualized to the child and family, give the NP the opportunity to facilitate the development of positive self-perception and to assist in avoiding potential problems. Self-perception problems are often hidden within somatic complaints and require an awareness and sensitivity to the child or adolescent in order to identify and deal with them. If done successfully, the child's life can be significantly impacted.

STANDARDS OF CARE

The Region X Nursing Network (1998) self-concept/self-perception pattern goals are as follows:

- Newborn: The newborn's environment promotes development of self-respect.
- 1 month to 3 years: The child sees self in a positive way and knows he or she is competent.
- School age: The child sees self in a positive way and knows he or she is competent.
- Adolescent: The adolescent demonstrates a positive self-image as he or she moves through the stages of adolescence.

Goals in *Healthy Children 2000* (United States [US] Department of Health and Human Services, 1991), the upcoming *Healthy People 2010* (US Department of Health and Human

Services, 1999), the *Guide to Clinical Preventive Services* (US Preventive Services Task Force, 1996), the *AMA Guidelines for Adolescent Preventive Services (GAPS)* (Elster & Kuznets, 1994), and the *Put Prevention Into Practice (PPIP) Clinician's Handbook of Preventive Services* (US Public Health Service, 1998) all address screening for depression and potential suicide. These are potential complications of a negative self-esteem and should be considered by the NP working with children and adolescents (see Chapter 21 for an in-depth discussion of these topics).

Nursing diagnoses related to self-perception are listed in a box at the end of the chapter.

NORMAL PATTERNS OF SELF-PERCEPTION

Components of Self-Perception

The term "self-perception" is often used interchangeably with terms such as "self-concept," "self-esteem," and "self-image." "Body image" refers to one's picture of and feelings regarding the body.

Self-perception, being personal and subjective, includes both a *description* of the self and an *evaluation* of that description. The description a person draws and the evaluation a person makes come from thoughts and feelings, beliefs and convictions, observations, understanding, insight, and awareness received both from the self and from others. The three key components of self-perception are significance, worthiness, and competence (Table 18–1).

Significance refers to having a sense of belonging, feeling loved and lovable, secure, cared for and supported, accepted and understood unconditionally for who one is, not what one does. This is the most important component in

TABLE 18-1

Key Components of Self-Perception

- Significance: I am loved!
- Worthiness: I am OK! I like and respect myself!
- Competence: I can do it!

TABLE 18-2

External Measures Used to Build Self-Perception

- Physical appearance or attractiveness: How do I look?
- Intelligence: What do I know?
- Performance: How do I do?
- Importance: Who do I know?
- Financial status: What and how much do I have?
- Control: What and whom do I control?

developing and maintaining a healthy self-esteem.

Worthiness refers to being whole on the inside, feeling valuable and acceptable, meeting personal moral standards, respecting and feeling good about oneself.

Competence refers to feeling capable, confident, adequate, in control, and able to approach new tasks and to deal with life optimistically, hopefully, and with courage. Competence is measured in terms of cognitive, physical, or social skills.

Children who feel significant, worthy, and competent confidently initiate activities, explore the environment, take risks, and rebound from disappointments. Appreciating themselves, they are able to reach out to and interact with others, accepting and offering love, respect, and encouragement. Children who do not feel significant, worthy, and competent look increasingly to external measures such as those listed in Table 18–2 to try to create a positive self-perception.

External measures do play a role in self-perception. Physical attractiveness and intelligence are two measures frequently used in society to evaluate people. Financial status, state of physical health, temperamental coping style, and an overly protective environment are other measures that affect self-perception. However, undue or excessive emphasis on external measures causes children to compare themselves with others, adopting the description and evaluation others make of them. "Most of us are what we think others think we are" (Dobson, 1999), or, "self-attitudes develop in response to how children think others see them" (Hunsberger, 1994, p. 520). Children whose self-perception is based on a comparison of themselves with others, feel and describe themselves as insecure, inferior, and inadequate. Attempting to prove themselves, they often become both bossy and aggressive, or people pleasers and approval seekers.

Developmental Stages

The development of children's self-perception is closely tied to normal growth and development. Each stage of growth and development provides opportunities for learning about the self and interacting with and observing others and the environment. Transient periods of low self-esteem as a child masters new skills or sets new goals are a normal part of development. Self-perception can change as a result of relationships or experiences or can be maintained in spite of contrary evidence (e.g., the adolescent cheerleader who is loved—successful in school and relationships—yet is anorexic and feels she is never "good enough.")

One theoretical perspective that can be useful clinically is to view the development of self-perception as occurring in two stages (Table 18-3). The first stage, *emergence of the self,* occurs in infants, toddlers, and preschool-age children. Parents and caretakers play a key role during this stage. Infants are learning that they are separate individuals who affect others by their behavior. This is best accomplished in a supportive environment where the infants come to view the world (their parents and caretakers) as responsive to their needs, both physical and emotional. Toddlers, with their new motor, cognitive, and language skills, learn to explore their capabilities and limits and make others aware of their needs, desires, and concerns. They thrive with positive acceptance, praise, and guidelines that set limits while allowing them to make choices. Preschoolers begin to use "I" to describe their own activities. They become aware of discrepancies in abilities and discover their whole body, including the differences in sexes. The early feelings of competence begin to emerge, and preschoolers can be coached through early problem solving. Preschoolers internalize parents' demands and move away from seeing the self as the center

T A B L E 18-3

Developmental Stages of Self-Perception

EMERGENCE OF SELF (1ST STAGE)

- Infants—learn that they are separate individuals who affect others by their behavior, view the world as responsive or unresponsive to their needs.
- Toddlers—explore their capabilities and limits, and make others aware of their needs, desires, and concerns.
- Preschoolers—begin to use "I," become aware of discrepancies in abilities, discover their bodies, begin to do simple problem solving, move from seeing themselves as the center of the world.

REFINING THE SELF (2ND STAGE)

- School-age children—evaluate self on the basis of external evidence, compare themselves with others, criticize and ridicule deviations from normal.
- Early adolescents—finalize body image, focus on physical and emotional changes with peer acceptance determining self-evaluation.
- Late adolescents—refine and crystallize self-perception (physical, social, spiritual) with values, goals, and competencies guiding their future in place.

Data from Kump T: Self-esteem: Why little kids need BIG egos. Healthy Kids Oct/Nov: 53–58, 1998; Hunsberger M: Fostering self-esteem. *In* Betz CL, Hunsberger M, Wright S (eds): Family Centered Nursing Care of Children, 2nd ed. Philadelphia, WB Saunders, 1994, pp 513–526; Sieving RE, Zirbel-Donisch ST: Development and enhancement of self-esteem in children. J Pediatr Health Care 4:290–296, 1990.

of the world. Siblings and peers play an increasingly important role in the preschooler's life.

The second stage of self-development, *refining the self,* occurs in school-age children and adolescents. Friendships and peers, and the time spent in various activities, play an increasing larger role in shaping the child's character and personality, and thus self-perception. Cultural stereotypes such as those found in magazines, television, billboards, and the Internet all influence the child's perception of society's "ideal" self. School-age children are preoccupied with evaluating themselves on the basis of external evidence: cognitive and physical skills, achievements, physical appearance, social abilities and acceptance, and a sense of control. They are particularly prone to comparing themselves to others, making them more vulnerable to social pressure. Any deviation from normal is subject to criticism and ridicule.

Self-perception continues to be refined during early adolescence, solidifying in later adolescence. Early adolescents are still highly dependent on cultural stereotypes and peer acceptance, with physical and emotional changes being the main focus of self-evaluation. Body image formation, a crucial element in shaping identify, is finalized at this stage. Any defect, disability, or discrepancy between what is seen and what is visualized as ideal is magnified and significant in the adolescent's eyes. By late adolescence, a more established view of the self should be in place, with acceptance of that identity—physical, social, and spiritual. Teenagers with positive self-perception have values, goals, and competencies that guide them into adulthood. Areas to be evaluated in the adolescent include academic, physical, and social achievements, physical attributes, interpersonal acceptance, moral behaviors as compared with internal standards, sense of control over personal accomplishments, relationships, and participation in activities (Sieving & Zirbel-Donisch, 1990).

Developmental Assets

Developmental assets are basic life skills and attributes that are critical building blocks to help a child or adolescent grow into a caring, competent, contributing, and responsible adult. Developmental assets assist a young person to make wise decisions; they increase in value over time, provide a sense of security, are resources to draw on over and over; and they are cumulative. The more assets a young person has, the more likely he or she is to make wise decisions and choose positive lifestyles while avoiding risky behaviors or dangerous activities. Developmental assets have been identified and revised by the Search Institute based on nationwide surveys of more than 100,000 young people in 200 communities (Benson et al., 1998). There are two categories of assets: (1) *external assets*, things in the environment (home, school, community) that support, nurture and

empower, set boundaries and expectations, and make constructive use of time, and (2) *internal assets,* attitudes (commitment to learning and a positive identity), positive values, and social competencies that belong in the head and heart of every child (Benson et al., 1998). Forty developmental assets have been described (Table 18-4). Most children and adolescents have only 18. Girls tend to have more assets than boys do in a ratio of 19.5 to 16.5, and younger children have more assets than older ones do (Benson et al., 1998). The Search Institute believes that young people should have at least 31 assets.

Ten developmental deficits, or roadblocks to building assets have also been identified by the Search Institute (Benson et al., 1998). The more deficits a child has, the more likely he or she is to make negative choices and decisions. The deficits are as follows:

1. Spending 2 or more hours a day alone at home without an adult
2. Putting a lot of emphasis on selfish values
3. Watching more than 2 hours of television a day
4. Going to parties where friends drink alcohol
5. Feeling stress or pressure most or all of the time
6. Being physically abused
7. Being sexually abused
8. Having a parent with alcohol or drug problem
9. Feeling socially isolated from people who provide care, support, and understanding
10. Having numerous close friends who often get into trouble

Environmental Influences

Significant relationships in a child's life, temperament, traits endowed by heredity, and experiences in everyday life are all environmental factors that influence the development of self-perception.

Significant relationships include parents or parent figures, siblings and other family members, and ongoing caretakers. As children get older, peers and authority figures also have an influence. Constant unconditional acceptance and love, empathy, and an attitude of understanding, coupled with appropriate limits and

T A B L E 18-4

40 Developmental Assets

CATEGORY	ASSET NAME AND DEFINITION

EXTERNAL ASSETS

Support

1. *Family support*—Family life provides high levels of love and support.
2. *Positive family communication*—Young person and her or his parent(s) communicate positively, and young person is willing to seek advice and counsel from parent(s).
3. *Other adult relationships*—Young person receives support from three or more nonparent adults.
4. *Caring neighborhood*—Young person experiences caring neighbors.
5. *Caring school climate*—School provides a caring, encouraging environment.
6. *Parent involvement in schooling*—Parent(s) are actively involved in helping young person succeed in school.

Empowerment

7. *Community values youth*—Young person perceives that adults in the community value youth.
8. *Youth as resources*—Young people are given useful roles in the community.
9. *Service to others*—Young person serves in the community one hour or more per week.
10. *Safety*—Young person feels safe at home, at school, and in the neighborhood.

Boundaries and expectations

11. *Family boundaries*—Family has clear rules and consequences and monitors the young person's whereabouts.
12. *School boundaries*—School provides clear rules and consequences.
13. *Neighborhood boundaries*—Neighbors take responsibility for monitoring young people's behavior.
14. *Adult role models*—Parent(s) and other adults model positive, responsible behavior.
15. *Positive peer influence*—Young person's best friends model responsible behavior.
16. *High expectations*—Both parent(s) and teachers encourage the young person to do well.

Constructive use of time

17. *Creative activities*—Young person spends three or more hours per week in lessons or practice in music, theater, or other arts.
18. *Youth programs*—Young person spends three or more hours per week in sports, clubs, or organizations at school and/or in the community.
19. *Religious community*—Young person spends one or more hours per week in activities in a religious institution.
20. *Time at home*—Young person is out with friends "with nothing special to do" two or fewer nights per week.

INTERNAL ASSETS

Commitment to learning

21. *Achievement motivation*—Young person is motivated to do well in school.
22. *School engagement*—Young person is actively engaged in learning.
23. *Homework*—Young person reports doing at least one hour of homework every school day.
24. *Bonding to school*—Young person cares about her or his school.
25. *Reading for pleasure*—Young person reads for pleasure three or more hours per week.

Positive values

26. *Caring*—Young person places high value on helping other people.
27. *Equality and social justice*—Young person places high value on promoting equality and reducing hunger and poverty.
28. *Integrity*—Young person acts on convictions and stands up for her or his beliefs.
29. *Honesty*—Young person tells the truth even when it is not easy.
30. *Responsibility*—Young person accepts and takes personal responsibility.
31. *Restraint*—Young person believes it is important not to be sexually active or to use alcohol or other drugs.

T A B L E 18-4

40 Developmental Assets *Continued*

CATEGORY	ASSET NAME AND DEFINITION
INTERNAL ASSETS Continued	
Social competencies	32. *Planning and decision making*—Young person knows how to plan ahead and make choices.
	33. *Interpersonal competence*—Young person has empathy, sensitivity, and friendship skills.
	34. *Cultural competence*—Young person has knowledge of and comfort with people of different cultural/racial/ethnic backgrounds.
	35. *Resistance skills*—Young person can resist negative peer pressure and dangerous situations.
	36. *Peaceful conflict resolution*—Young person seeks to resolve conflict nonviolently.
Positive identity	37. *Personal power*—Young person feels he or she has control over "things that happen to me."
	38. *Self-esteem*—Young person reports having a high self-esteem.
	39. *Sense of purpose*—Young person reports that "my life has a purpose."
	40. *Positive view of personal future*—Young person is optimistic about her or his personal future.

Copyright © 1997 by Search Institute, Minneapolis, MN 55415; 800-888-7828; www.search-institute.org.

boundaries, are the most important interactions these significant others offer. Time spent with and encouragement given to the child, both in being together and in doing things, as well as in sharing life's happenings (listening, talking, and problem solving), are also essential ingredients (see the Parenting Pyramid discussed in Chapter 5). The sturdy base built by positive relationships is a key component in the child's developing positive self-esteem. By feeling, seeing, and hearing these continual reinforcements, children internalize or know that they are significant, worthy, and competent. Peers and authority figures serve to confirm or deny what is taught at home.

Temperament may also play a role in the child's development of self-perception. This is particularly the case when there is a mismatch of temperaments, especially between parent and child, or when a child has traits that are labeled difficult or challenging. If these traits are understood and managed correctly, the child's self-esteem can be positively affected. (See Kurcinka [1998] for an in-depth discussion.) However, if temperament is not understood, the child may carry negative perceptions and labels that adversely affect his or her self-perception (see Chapter 21 for a discussion of temperament).

The role of heredity in the development of self-perception is due to family traits over which the child has no control. Aspects such as appearance, intelligence, and family characteristics, including alcoholism, mental illness, and disfiguring disease are to be considered. Conditions in which the child exists, such as poverty and homelessness, also are important. Family traits and attributes either contribute to a positive self-perception or may become barriers to be overcome.

Children's social experiences provide an opportunity to observe the world, test skills and abilities, interact with others, and try various roles. Positive experiences such as success in solving problems, working out difficulties, and learning to carry on after setbacks contribute to significance, worth, and competence, encouraging further exploration and risk taking. Negative experiences cause children to retreat or attempt to compensate through other means.

ASSESSMENT OF SELF-PERCEPTION

The goal of assessing self-perception is to know how children describe and evaluate themselves and to identify the sources that provide them the input they use to develop their self-concept. These assessments then lay the groundwork for planning interventions for the child and family. Corresponding assessment of the parents' and caretaker's self-perception is important. Assessment of self-perception is not a simple task. It cannot be observed directly nor obtained from questioning alone, but must be inferred from observed behavior, self-statements or self-ratings, and other relevant information. Self-rating, observational scales, and draw-a-person tests are possible means of assessment. The draw-a-person test, used with younger children, asks the child to draw a picture of himself/herself, and also a picture of another child. A comparison of the two children often gives an idea of the child's self-perception. Somewhere between fourth and sixth grades, self-esteem inventories can be considered.

History

COMPONENTS OF SELF-PERCEPTION

Significance

- Does the child feel loved, lovable, cared for, secure, supported, accepted, understood?
- Is this conditional or unconditional? Is this based on who the child is or what the child does?

Worthiness

- Does the child feel valuable, acceptable?
- Are self-respect and self-liking evident?
- What beliefs or convictions does the child have? Do they match the child's lifestyle?

Competence

- Does the child feel capable, adequate, optimistic overall?
- Does the child approach new tasks with confidence?
- What are the child's cognitive, physical, and social strengths?

DEVELOPMENTAL STAGE

Infant

- Does the infant recognize self as separate from others?
- Does the infant realize his or her effect on others?

Toddler

- Does the toddler explore capabilities and limits?
- Does the toddler make others aware of needs, desires, and concerns?

Preschooler

- Does the child use "I"? Describe activities? Discover his or her body?
- Does the child internalize parental demands? Move away from self as center of world?
- Are siblings and peers increasingly important? How does the child think, feel, and act about self?

School-Age Child

- How does the child describe and evaluate self, including body image? Is the evaluation in comparison to peers?
- How does this view compare with the child's perceptions of peers' evaluation?
- What cognitive and physical skills and achievements are described?
- What friends, social abilities, and activities are described?
- Is there a sense of control over life? Confidence in self?

Early Adolescent

- How does the adolescent describe and evaluate himself or herself? What role do peers play?
- How are physical attributes described (body image)?
- What are academic, physical, social activities, and achievements?
- How do moral behaviors compare to internal standards?

- Is there a sense of control over personal activities, accomplishments, and relationships?

Late Adolescent

- How does the adolescent describe and evaluate self?
- What choices are being made? What values, goals, and plans are expressed? Is there a sense of optimism about that direction?

DEVELOPMENTAL ASSETS

In order to determine how many and what assets a child has, two checklists (Tables 18–5 and 18–6), one for children and adolescents and another for parents, have been developed (Benson et al., 1998). It is suggested that parents and children complete the lists separately, then sit down and share each other's responses. These checklists become helpful tools for parents and children to compare their perceptions and to identify strong and weak areas.

ENVIRONMENTAL INFLUENCES

Family Structure

- Who makes up the family? Significant others? Caretakers? What is the family like?
- What is the family's social and financial status?
- What is the physical living situation?
- Does anyone in the family have any physical disease? Any mental or social disease (e.g., mental illness or retardation, alcoholism)?

Parental Influences

- Who plays the parental role? How do parents describe themselves? Perceive their role?
- How does the parent describe the child? How valued is the child? How is that shown?
- What are parental expectations for the child? Is the child given age-appropriate guidance, responsibilities, freedoms?

Significant Others Outside Family

- Who are they? Peers? Authority figures? Social supports? Networks? Mentors?
- What are the relationships like?

Temperament Issues

- What temperament traits does the child have?
- How does the parent describe the child? React to the child? Interact with the child?

Environment

- What is the child's environment like? What experiences or opportunities are there? Within the family? In the neighborhood? More formally (e.g., play groups, extracurricular activities)?
- What opportunities are there to test skills and abilities? Interact with others? Try new roles? Is this encouraged?
- How protected is the child?

Discipline

- How is the child disciplined? What methods are used? Is guidance given?
- Are limits and consequences clear?
- Is the child allowed to try and not be rescued?

Communication

- What messages is the child receiving (e.g., "you are a helper," or "you are a bad boy")?
- Is he or she listened to? Are feelings acknowledged?
- What does the child say about himself or herself (e.g., describe self as "good" or "bad," "smart" or "dumb")?

Observations During the History and Examination

Direct questioning about all the areas previously listed gives the NP information about the child. However, equally important is observation of the child and interactions between

T A B L E   18-5

Developmental Assets: A Checklist for Kids and Teens

Check each statement that is true for you.
 1. I feel loved and supported in my family.
 2. I can go to my parents or guardians for advice and support. I have frequent in-depth conversations with them.
 3. I know three or more other adults (besides my parents or guardians) whom I can go to for advice and support.
 4. My neighbors encourage and support me.
 5. My school provides a caring, encouraging environment.
 6. My parents or guardians help me succeed in school.
 7. I feel valued by adults in my community.
 8. I am given useful roles in my community.
 9. I serve in my community 1 or more hours each week.
10. I feel safe at home, at school, and in my neighborhood.
11. My family has clear rules and consequences for my behavior, and they monitor my whereabouts.
12. My school has clear rules and consequences for behavior.
13. Neighbors take responsibility for monitoring my behavior.
14. My parents or guardians and other adults in my life model positive, responsible behavior.
15. My best friends model responsible behavior.
16. Both my parents or guardians and my teachers encourage me to do well.
17. I spend 3 or more hours each week in lessons or practice in music, theater, or other arts.
18. I spend 3 or more hours each week in school or community sports, clubs, or organizations.
19. I spend 1 or more hours each week in religious services or participating in spiritual activities.
20. I go out with friends with nothing special to do 2 or fewer nights each week.
21. I want to do well in school.
22. I like to learn new things.
23. I do an hour or more of homework each school day.
24. I care about my school.
25. I read for pleasure 3 or more hours each week.
26. I believe that it's really important to help other people.
27. I want to help promote equality and reduce world poverty and hunger.
28. I act on my convictions. I stand up for my beliefs.
29. I tell the truth—even when it's not easy.
30. I accept and take personal responsibility for my actions and decisions.
31. I believe that it's important not to be sexually active or to use alcohol or other drugs.
32. I'm good at planning ahead and making decisions.
33. I'm good at making and keeping friends.
34. I know and am comfortable with people of different cultural, racial, and/or ethnic backgrounds.
35. I resist negative peer pressure and avoid dangerous situations.
36. I try to resolve conflicts nonviolently.
37. I believe that I have control over many things that happen to me.
38. I feel good about myself.
39. I believe that my life has a purpose.
40. I'm optimistic about my future.

From Benson PL, Galbraith J, Espeland P: What Kids Need to Succeed. Minneapolis, MN, Free Spirit Publisher, 1998.

T A B L E 18-6

Developmental Assets: A Checklist for Parents

Check each statement that is true for you or your child.

1. I give my child a lot of love and support.
2. My child can come to me for advice and support. We have frequent in-depth conversations.
3. My child knows three or more other adults whom he or she can go to for advice and support.
4. Our neighbors encourage and support my child.
5. My child's school provides a caring, encouraging environment.
6. I'm actively involved in helping my child succeed in school.
7. My child feels valued by adults in our community.
8. My child is given useful roles in our community.
9. My child serves in our community one or more hours each week.
10. My child feels safe at home, at school, and in our neighborhood.
11. Our family has clear rules and consequences for behavior. We monitor each other's whereabouts.
12. My child's school has clear rules and consequences for behavior.
13. Our neighbors take responsibility for monitoring my child's behavior.
14. I model positive, responsible behavior, and so do other adults that my child knows.
15. My child's best friends model responsible behavior.
16. I encourage my child to do well, and so do my child's teachers.
17. My child spends three or more hours each week in lessons or practice in music, theater, or other arts.
18. My child spends three or more hours each week in school or community sports, clubs, or organizations.
19. My child spends one or more hours each week in religious services or participating in spiritual activities.
20. My child spends two or fewer nights each week out with friends "with nothing special to do."
21. My child wants to do well in school.
22. My child likes to learn new things.
23. My child does an hour or more of homework each school day.
24. My child cares about her or his school.
25. My child reads for pleasure three or more hours each week.
26. My child believes that it's really important to help other people.
27. My child wants to help promote equality and reduce world poverty and hunger.
28. My child acts on his or her convictions. My child stands up for his or her beliefs.
29. My child tells the truth—even when it's not easy.
30. My child accepts and takes personal responsibility for her or his actions and decisions.
31. My child believes that it's important not to be sexually active or to use alcohol or other drugs.
32. My child is good at planning ahead and making decisions.
33. My child is good at making and keeping friends.
34. My child knows and is comfortable with people of different cultural, racial, and/or ethnic backgrounds.
35. My child resists negative peer pressure and avoids dangerous situations.
36. My child tries to resolve conflicts nonviolently.
37. My child believes that he or she has control over many things that happen to him or her.
38. My child feels good about herself or himself.
39. My child believes that his or her life has a purpose.
40. My child is optimistic about her or his future.

From Benson PL, Galbraith J, Espeland P: What Kids Need to Succeed. Minneapolis, MN, Free Spirit Publisher, 1998.

the child and the accompanying person throughout the office visit.

- What is the relationship between the two?
- What actual words are said? With what tone of voice?
- What kind of nonverbal interaction occurs? What kind of physical interaction?
- Is the child encouraged to answer questions and perform tasks? Is rescuing occurring? Is guidance given?
- What expectations are voiced?
- How is discipline conducted within the examination setting? What limits are set?

Table 18–7 lists risk factors for low self-perception.

MANAGEMENT STRATEGIES FOR DEVELOPING POSITIVE SELF-PERCEPTION

Anticipatory guidance, education, and counseling are strategies the NP uses to guide and direct the family, child, and adolescent in developing healthy self-perception. If problems are significant, referral for more in-depth counseling is necessary. The strategies listed in Table 18–8 can be used by the NP to help the child, adolescent, and family set a foundation that builds a strong, positive self-perception.

T A B L E 18-7

Risk Factors for Low Self-Perception

1. *Physical alterations, including body image.* Chronic illness (visible or not), disfiguring disabilities, sensory disabilities, obesity, anorexia
2. *Mental/emotional alterations.* School problems such as slow learner, semi-illiterate, underachiever, culturally deprived, late bloomers, difficult temperament, emotional or mental illness or abuse
3. *Environmental/relational alterations.* Disrupted families and family relationships or inability to meet basic needs, unrealistic expectations or faulty thinking, temperament or personality misfits, social disorders, stress, past experiences of failure, rejection, criticism

T A B L E 18-8

Strategies to Help Build a Positive Self-Perception

- Facilitate good parenting
- Maintain appropriate expectations of the child
- Use discipline techniques that enhance self-esteem
- Communicate positively
- Provide helpful strategies for the child and adolescent
- Encourage asset building

While working with the child and family, specific strategies to improve self-esteem are chosen, keeping in mind that familial, generational, ethnic, or cultural practices influence the choice and use of strategies. Several books on developing children's self-esteem are listed in the references.

Facilitate Good Parenting

- Parental self-perception, either positive or negative, has a significant effect on the child's self-perception. Parents should be encouraged to understand and accept themselves, acknowledge their strengths and accept their uniqueness, take care of themselves, treat themselves with respect, and be aware of their own feelings.
- Parental roles include being available to the child both physically and emotionally, teaching the child, modeling behavior, and helping the child learn to relate to others. This is done by meeting basic needs (e.g., feeding, getting up at night, bathing) as well as spending time together, enjoying the child, having fun, touching, talking, and watching.
- Know your children (Dobson, 1999). See what they see, feel what they feel, hope what they hope. This provides needed empathy. Children have their own personality, temperament, dreams, and opinions and need to be known, loved, accepted, and respected for who they are.
- Value children. Appreciate and praise who they are rather than what they do. Show belief in their ability to learn, improve, and

grow. Look in their eyes when you talk to them. Recognize their unique means of self-expression. Delight in their discoveries. Contribute to their collections. Identify their strengths, focus on their efforts, structure situations for success, and offer thanks for what they do. Avoid shame, criticism, and humiliation.

- Be there. Presence endorses the child's involvement and reinforces the importance of their efforts. Do things with them, not just for them. Plan prescheduled times just to be together. Spend at least 20 minutes each day giving them undivided attention. Show up at their concerts, games, and events. Visit their schools.
- Know their friends. Encourage positive involvement with friends and activities. Help find the right niche (e.g., length of time, type of activity) that fits the child. Show an interest in friends (e.g., host a sleepover, take a group to the zoo). Steer them away from less constructive friends and activities.
- Avoid comparing children. Children are individuals who grow and develop in their own way and at their own rate. Celebrate their accomplishments. Tell them how terrific they are. Their individuality needs to be respected, and comparisons to siblings or peers avoided.
- Let go. Develop a gradual, planned granting of freedom and responsibility, beginning in infancy and ending in late adolescence. Letting go involves offering trust, providing opportunities, giving choices, instilling confidence, and refraining from rushing to aid a struggling child. As part of this process, each year the child should make more decisions and assume more routine responsibilities than during the prior 12 months (Dobson, 1999).

Maintain Appropriate Expectations of the Child

- Attempt to keep appropriate expectations. Expectations that are too high lead to a constant feeling of failure. Expectations that are too low diminish children's value and make them feel as if the parent has no faith in them. Expect their best, not perfection.
- Age-appropriate expectations involving tasks, toys, and roles are essential.
- Child-appropriate expectations are also important. Each child's individual personality, temperament, strengths, and weaknesses must be considered.
- Parent-driven vs. child-driven expectations need to be identified. Although this is a sensitive issue, knowing where expectations begin (with parent or child) and how they fit the child and family is important.
- Clearly stated expectations are essential for the child and parent alike to avoid frustration, distrust, and further problems.
- A positive response to failure, providing support and encouragement, putting the mistake in perspective, helping make repairs, as well providing feedback and evaluation, are critical in preparing children to approach future obstacles and disappointments.

Use Discipline Techniques That Enhance Self-Esteem

- Identify limits and consequences clearly and follow through. Knowing clearly what is expected provides security for the child.
- Help the child learn to choose acceptable behaviors and learn self-control. Establish house rules. Catch the child being good and offer praise. Be sincere.
- Foster problem-solving to build confidence. The steps (including stating the problem, expressing needs, considering alternatives, agreeing on a solution, and implementing and following through with the agreed upon solution) need to be used and taught. Part of the process is taking time and waiting to let the child work through the process.
- Avoid rescuing children. Allowing them to persevere, learn, and work through frustration empowers them for further success. Rescuing (providing unrequested assistance too soon) must be differentiated from guiding, encouraging, and being an ally to the child. Respect their choices.

- Provide guidance to understand the self and the surrounding world, to develop a conscience, and to steer clear of potential problems. This helps the child learn to do this independently.
- The manner and intent of providing discipline are as important as the techniques used.

Communicate Positively

- Listening to children includes taking them seriously, being interested, and letting them finish what they are saying. Show love by giving hugs and back rubs, by stroking hair, or by giving positive facial expressions. Say "I love you" often and in a variety of ways.
- Watching the words used as well as the tone of voice, the intent of the words, and body language are essential. Negative messages are sent in comparisons, putdowns ("you are such a baby"), humiliation ("you can't do anything right"), labeling ("you're such a slob"), and fault finding.
- Praise and encourage the child often, especially as they undertake new challenges or roles. Say "thanks" for their cooperation. Catch them doing well (e.g., "I like the way you..."). Acknowledge their help (e.g., "I appreciate..."). Love their person (e.g., "I love being with you...") (Hall, 1998).
- Help children identify, handle, and express their feelings by accepting and acknowledging those feelings. Avoid trying to change them or stop them by denial or reassurance. Listen. Parents should share their own feelings and failures. Intervention may take place at the thought and behavior level after feelings are brought forward.
- Reacting with "I" statements, not "you" judgments, separates performance from worth and validates children's behavior while still allowing behavior to be modified.
- Being aware of children's "self-talk" is worthwhile. What children say to themselves not only reflects what they believe but also further creates feelings about themselves. Positive statements enhance self-perception. "Stinkin' thinking" (Hart, 1990) or negative statements reflect low self-perception and require intervention.

Provide Helpful Strategies for the Child and Adolescent

- Support early and ongoing self-assertions as means of children expressing themselves (Kump, 1998). Allow your preschooler to wear the outlandish outfit chosen unless it's totally inappropriate (a bathing suit in November), or your school-age child to create the menu one night a week.
- Find the "island of competence" (Brooks, 1991; Kump, 1998). Every child has an interest, ability, or skill that can be developed and displayed to provide the child with a sense of success and a defense from failure. Identify what the child is interested in and good at, and encourage and praise those skills, talents, efforts, and achievements. Seven kinds of intelligence have been identified: linguistic, mathematical, spatial, musical, bodily, interpersonal, and intrapersonal (Dobson, 1999), and can be used to build and affirm the child's island of competence.
- Help your child compete (Dobson, 1999). A child needs encouragement to develop skills, opportunities to use the skills, and second chances when failure occurs. A child is empowered by having an ally in these endeavors.
- Encourage a healthy connectedness (Matiella, 1991; Meeks, 1990). Children need to belong to and feel that they are a part of both their family and groups outside their family through things as varied as social activities and links within their community, ethnic group, or geographical area.
- Promote a sense of ownership. Children who are given responsibility for themselves and their actions are also given a sense of control over their life.
- Keep a close eye on the classroom (Dobson, 1999). Problems in the classroom are often symptoms of other problems in a child's life. Temporary rough spots are normal and must be distinguished from more

pervasive problems that require intervention.

- Offer genuine encounter moments (GEMS) (Hall, 1998; Briggs, 1970). This refers to a mutually agreed upon time that is set apart for 100% attention and love, focused attention or direct involvement. The child takes the lead in how the time is spent.
- Defuse feelings of inferiority (Dobson, 1999). Throughout the school years and adolescence, comparisons are the norm, and feelings of inferiority often result. Children aware of this fact who have learned to compete and compensate are more likely to believe in themselves despite feelings of inferiority.
- Prepare for adolescence (Dobson, 1999). A special time set aside to talk with the preadolescent about the coming physical, social, and hormonal changes helps prepare them to handle the transitions with greater ease.

Encourage Asset Building

Fostering developmental assets can positively change a young person's life. Because all young people need assets, and building assets is an ongoing process, everyone (the child, parents, teachers, health care providers, and community members) can be involved in developing assets in the young people around them. Relationships are critical to building assets. *Consistent messages* about what is important in life and what is expected from the young person are essential. *Intentional redundancy,* hearing the same positive messages over and over again from many different people, is also important. One way for anyone to start developing assets in a young person is to use the checklists (see Table 18–5 and 18–6) to help identify an area in which to begin to build one or more assets. The Search Institute has many resources and programs to assist individuals and communities to build assets in young people. For information on how to contact the Search Institute, see Resource Box 18-1. Two particularly helpful items are *150 Ways to Show Your Kids You Care* and *What Kids Need To Succeed* (Benson et al., 1998), which define each asset and give

ideas for building that asset in the home, school, community, and congregational setting.

It is possible to overcome the deficits in a young person's life. Five areas identified by the Search Institute (Benson et al., 1998) that.are helpful in overcoming deficits are

1. Getting involved in structured adult-led activities
2. Setting boundaries and limits
3. Nurturing a strong commitment to education
4. Providing support and care in all areas of life, not just the family
5. Cultivating positive values and concern for others

SPECIFIC SELF-PERCEPTION PROBLEMS IN CHILDREN

Self-Esteem Problems

DESCRIPTION. When a child's sense of significance is disturbed, self-esteem problems arise. The child has a loss of confidence and feelings of insecurity are evidenced. This may, over time, emerge as aggressive behavior that eventually leads to violence.

ETIOLOGY. Self-esteem problems arise when children are unsure of belonging and of being loved, cared for, and accepted. Love is often conditional, with acceptance coming for what they do rather than who they are. Emotional maltreatment (abuse or deprivation) is an extreme example of this (see Chapter 19). Self-esteem problems may be situational or transient, or they may be chronic.

ASSESSMENT. The child with self-esteem problems seeks attention, importance, and security. Because of the desire for acceptance and love, these children are often people pleasers. Position and status are attempts to prove importance. Attention seeking may be extreme, causing aggression, leading to behavior problems. There may be a history of rejection or a dysfunctional family.

DIFFERENTIAL DIAGNOSIS. Differential diagnoses include personal identity problems, role performance problems, and body image problems.

MANAGEMENT. Unconditional love, acceptance, belonging, and security are needs that are not being met. Strategies for beginning to achieve these must be initiated. Refer to the management strategies discussed previously for specifics, especially "parental roles," "know your children," and "limits and consequences."

COMPLICATIONS. Anxiety, behavior problems, depression, and violence are complications of self-esteem problems.

Personal Identity Problems

DESCRIPTION. When children are uncertain of their worth, personal identity is shaky and feelings of inferiority are manifested. Children may feel confusion about who they are.

ETIOLOGY. Personal identity problems arise when children do not receive respect as individuals and are not valued for who they are. This results in questioning their worth and makes them wonder if they truly are OK. Potential parental factors that contribute to these feelings of inferiority include insensitivity to the child in words or attitude, fatigue and time pressure, guilt, and rivals for love.

ASSESSMENT. Children with personal identity problems do not feel good about themselves and often evidence lack of self-respect and self-liking, feeling as if they have not lived up to adult expectations. They may talk about themselves in degrading terms. There is a struggle to prove "I am OK." Coping may take the form of withdrawal, fighting, clowning, denying there is a problem, or striving for conformity (Dobson, 1999). There may be a history of the child being criticized, embarrassed, shamed or humiliated, or of familial mental illness or abuse.

DIFFERENTIAL DIAGNOSIS. Self-esteem problems, role performance problems, and body image problems are differential diagnoses for personal identity problems.

MANAGEMENT. Self-respect, self-value, and feeling good about the self are needs that are not being met. Time must be made to spend with the child in one on one interaction. Strategies for beginning to achieve these must be initiated. See the earlier discussion of management strategies for specifics, especially "value children," "maintain appropriate expectations of the child," and "defuse feelings of inferiority."

Helping the child learn to compensate can conquer low self-esteem. See section on "finding the island of competence."

COMPLICATIONS. Depression, guilt, anger, and hostility are complications of personal identity problems.

Role Performance Problems

DESCRIPTION. When children are unable to perform expected activities or behaviors because of physical, mental, or cognitive disability, or they feel incompetent, role performance problems emerge and feelings of inadequacy often result. A typical scenario involves a child with school problems.

ETIOLOGY. Role performance problems arise when children do not feel adequate, confident, and in control and can occur in cognitive, social, and physical performance arenas.

ASSESSMENT. Children with role performance problems may retreat and be hesitant to approach new opportunities and experiences. They may be perfectionists, always striving to prove competence: "I can do it." A history of "failure," or being a slow learner, semiliterate, an underachiever, a late bloomer, or culturally deprived, is not uncommon.

DIFFERENTIAL DIAGNOSIS. Self-esteem problems, personal identity problems, body image problems, and actual physical, mental, or cognitive problems are differential diagnoses for role performance problems.

MANAGEMENT. Competence, confidence, adequacy, and being in control are needs that are not being met. Strategies for beginning to achieve these must be initiated. See the previous discussion of management strategies for specifics, especially "letting go," "find the 'island of competence'" (a key), and "help your child compete." Working with the school to achieve these goals is helpful.

COMPLICATIONS. Complications of role performance problems include depression, withdrawal, and somatic complaints.

Body Image Problems

DESCRIPTION. Discrepancy between how children's bodies are and how they want them to be results in body image problems. The discrep-

NURSING DIAGNOSIS 18-1

NURSING DIAGNOSES FOR SELF-PERCEPTION AND SELF-CONCEPT FUNCTIONAL HEALTH PATTERN

Body Image Disturbance

Personal Identity Disturbance

Self-Esteem Disorder

Source: North American Nursing Diagnosis Association: NANDA Nursing Diagnoses: Definitions and Classification 1997–1998. Philadelphia, 1996.

DIFFERENTIAL DIAGNOSIS. Self-esteem, personal identity, or role performance problems are differential diagnoses for body image problems.

MANAGEMENT. The discrepancy between reality and the desired body as well as the cause of the discrepancy must be identified. Severity

ancy may be temporary or permanent, seen or unseen, occurring in terms of size, function, appearance, or potential. Attitudes, feelings, and fantasies all play a role in body image (Mayo, 1992).

ETIOLOGY. Disturbance in body image arises from sources as varied as physical illness or disability, chronic illness, emotional disturbances, abuse, or attitudes conveyed by others. Body image problems are most common in adolescence, when teenagers are most concerned about physical appearance in comparison to that of their peers. But they also occur in younger children. An example is immobilization resulting from a fracture; the child is no longer able to master his or her environment because of injury or illness and the subsequent treatment.

ASSESSMENT. Children with disturbed body image may have concerns related to body size, function, appearance, or potential, or these may be noted by questioning or techniques such as drawing a person. Possible behaviors include:

- Refusing to look at or touch the altered or missing part
- Preoccupation with the loss or change
- Feeling of shame and embarrassment
- Distorted perception of a normal body
- Fear of rejection or unwanted attention from others
- Overexposure or hiding of body part
- Actual or perceived change in structure and function of body or body part

RESOURCE BOX 18-1

RESOURCES FOR BUILDING SELF-PERCEPTION

Ms. Foundation for Women
Website: www.ms.foundation.org
From the creators and sponsors of Take Our Daughters to Work, an "empowering" GirlWorld site with information on organizations, publications, and websites for girls and their parents

NASE: National Association for Self-Esteem
Website: www.self-esteem-nase.org
Includes a book list, links to other sites, lots of information on self-esteem

Free Spirit Publishing, Inc.
Tel: (612) 338-2068
(800) 735-7323
Website: www.freespirit.com

Search Institute
Tel: (800) 888-7828.
E-mail: si@search-institute.org.
Website: http://www.search-institute.org
The researchers of developmental assets have multiple resources for individuals, schools, communities and congregations. Includes books, handouts, newsletter, and programs

Books That Teach Self-Esteem
Brave New Girls by Jeanette Gadeberg (Fairview Press, 1997) for ages 9 years and older
Corduroy by Don Freeman (Viking, 1968) for ages 3 to 8 years
I Like Being Me: Feeling Special, Appreciating Others and Getting Along by Judy Lalli (Free Spirit, 1997) for ages 4 to 8.
Leo the Late Bloomer by Robert Kraus (Harper Collins, 1971) for ages 4 to 8 years
On the Day You Were Born by Debra Frasier (Harcourt Brace, 1991) for ages 2 years and older
Those Can-Do Pigs by David McPhail (Dutton, 1996) for ages 5 to 9 years

and cause of the discrepancy guide the intervention:

- If the discrepancy is developmental and not severe, education and counseling should help.
- If the problem is significant, referral for psychiatric care is often necessary.

Some interventions that are helpful include:

- Identifying areas where assistance is needed
- Referral to counselors, dietary therapy, occupational or physical therapy
- Visits by the NP or other health team member to school or social arenas before child returns to that setting to educate and prepare the setting for the child
- Involvement with peer group of children with similar problems
- Ongoing support and encouragement from primary care provider with focus on positive aspects of body and functioning
- Verbalization of acceptance
- Use of play therapy to encourage verbalization
- Teaching new ways of handling situations to accommodate for loss or change
- Discussing ways to camouflage (e.g., wig or scarf for hair loss)
- Complimenting behaviors to indicate acceptance

REFERENCES

★Benson, PL, Galbraith J, Espeland P: What Kids Need to Succeed. Minneapolis, MN, Free Spirit Publisher, 1998.

★Berne PH, Savary LM: Building Self-Esteem in Children. New York, Continuum Publishing, 1992.

★Briggs D: Your Child's Self-Esteem. Garden City, NY, Doubleday, 1970.

★Brooks R: The Self-Esteem Teacher. Circle Pines, MN, American Guidance Services, 1991.

★Clark JI: Self-Esteem: A Family Affair. New York, Harper & Row, 1980.

★Clemes H, Bean R: Self Esteem: The Key to Your Child's Well Being. New York, Kensington Publication, 1981.

★Dobson J: The New Hide or Seek: Building Self-Esteem in Your Child. Grand Rapids, MI, FH Revell, 1999.

Elster AB, Kuznets, NJ: AMA Guidelines for Adolescent Preventive Services (GAPS). Baltimore, MD, Williams & Wilkins, 1994.

★Glenn, S. (1987). Raising Self-Reliant Children in a Self-Indulgent World. New York: St. Martin's Press.

Hall H: Ways to Enhance Your Child's Self-Esteem. Presentation at the NAPNAP National Conference. Chicago, IL, 1998.

★Hart L: The Winning Family: Increasing Self-Esteem in Your Children and Yourself. Oakland, CA, LifeSkills Press, 1990.

Hunsberger M: Fostering self-esteem. *In* Betz CL, Hunsberger M, Wright S (eds): Family-Centered Nursing Care of Children, 2nd edition. Philadelphia, PA, WB Saunders, 1994, pp. 513–526.

★Kump T: Self-esteem: Why little kids need BIG egos. Healthy Kids October/November:53–58, 1998.

★Kurcinka MS: (1998). Raising Your Spirited Child. New York, NY, HarperPerennial, 1998.

★Kvols KF: Redirecting Children's Misbehavior: Discipline That Builds Self-Esteem. Gainesville, FL, INCAF Publications, 1993.

Levine MD, Carey WB, Crocker AC: Developmental-Behavioral Pediatrics, 3rd ed. Philadelphia, WB Saunders, 1999.

★Matiella AC: Positively Different: Creating a Bias-Free Environment for Young Children. Santa Cruz, CA, Network Publications, 1991.

Mayo MA: Skin Deep: Understanding of the Powerful Link Between Body Image and Self-Esteem. Ann Arbor, MI, Servant Publications, 1992.

★McDowell J: Building Your Self Image. Wheaton, IL, Living Books, 1984.

★Meeks CA: Prescriptions for Parenting. New York, Warner Books, 1990.

Region X Nursing Standards Board: Nursing Standards for Prenatal and Child Health. Seattle, WA, University of Washington, 1998.

Sieving RE, Zirbel-Donisch ST: Development and enhancement of self-esteem in children. J Pediatr Health Care 4:290–296, 1990.

US Department of Health and Human Services: Healthy People 2010. http://web.health.gov/healthypeople, 1999.

US Department of Health and Human Services: Healthy Children 2000. Washington, DC, US Government Printing Office, 1991.

US Preventive Services Task Force. Guide to Clinical Preventive Services, 2nd ed. Baltimore, MD, Williams & Wilkins, 1996.

US Public Health Service: Put Prevention Into Practice (PIPP): Clinician's Handbook of Preventive Services, 2nd ed. McLean, VA, International Medical Publishers, 1998.

★Good reference for parents.

CHAPTER 19

Role Relationships

Margaret A. Brady

■ INTRODUCTION

Understanding family dynamics and role relationships is an important consideration in the delivery of primary care to children and adolescents. The nurse practitioner (NP) must be sensitive to the roles that parents or caregivers, siblings, extended family members, and peers have in shaping the developing child. Likewise, the community is an extension of the family and serves as a major component in the widening circle of influence that affects the child's or adolescent's life. This chapter discusses the family life cycle and family variations as well as the assessment and management of situations or events that the NP is likely to encounter in a primary care setting related to violence, family relationship problems, child maltreatment or neglect, and sibling rivalry. Preventive interventions for role relationship problems that are directed at the population as a whole (universal interventions) and specific individuals or groups at risk (selective interventions) also are identified. Because parents face many challenges in their parental role, a basic framework for positive parenting is presented. Advice about securing nurturing, safe, and developmentally appropriate child care is discussed to assist the NP in counseling parents about this important decision.

Family Life Cycle

Each family has its own unique pattern of growth and development. Just as a child goes through stages of development, so does the family unit. Family life with young infants and preschool children is vastly different from family life with school-age children, with early vs. late adolescents, or with young adults. Also, different types of family units—nuclear, single-parent, divorced, or blended—affect family life. However, common themes or denominators exist within all families. Family resources, stresses and changes, values, role structure, and coping strategies are five dimensions that influence and mold all family units regardless of how a family is classified or typed. These five dimensions have a significant impact on family functioning (Table 19-1), which, in turn, affects feelings of satisfaction as a family unit. The levels of family cohesiveness, adaptability, and family communication patterns are key to how well a family functions at different stages in the family life cycle (Friedman, 1992).

Family cohesion addresses the emotional bonding between family members and affects how the family functions. Family cohesion can range from the extremes of very low (disengaged) to very high (enmeshed) bonding, with moderate to high (connected) bonding representing the middle ground.

The concept of family adaptability represents the ability of a family system to change its power structure, role relationships, and relationship rules in response to situational and developmental stress. The range of adaptability varies from very rigid (very low) to chaotic

T A B L E 19-1

Five Key Factors That Shape the Family Unit

FACTORS	EXAMPLES
Family resources	Social support network, financial assets, spiritual beliefs
Family stresses and changes	Financial adversity, illness, marital strain, family transitions
Family values	The importance of productivity, individual achievement, the family unit, materialism
Role structure	Sharing of power or caregiving, marital, parental and kinship roles
Family coping strategies	Ability to adapt to adversity, family group reliance, seeking social support

(very high), with a midground between structured and flexible. A key element in adaptability is the ability to change when appropriate. Communication patterns range from positive communication skills that reflect such messages as empathy, reflective listening, and supportive comments to negative communication skills that reflect double messages, double binds, or criticism and minimize opportunities to share feelings. Communication is one of the most crucial elements within an interpersonal relationship. Family cohesion and adaptability are threatened and thwarted with negative communication patterns.

Family Resources, Stresses, and Coping Styles

To assist parents and children across the family life cycle and during times of stress, the NP must carefully assess three elements that both mold families and predict their level of family functioning or dysfunction. These dimensions are family resources, stresses, and coping styles. Family resources include (1) a social support network that includes extended family members, friends, and community; (2) financial assets; and (3) spiritual beliefs and values, which support a family in its everyday life and in times of challenge. Families with limited re-

sources or social support networks are more vulnerable to stressful life events than are families with resources and support systems in place.

Potential family stresses and changes are numerous and include financial strains, illness, marital strain, family transitions, losses, and lack of effective coping strategies. Life brings transitions that necessitate change. Many transitions are normal, some are anticipated, and others are unexpected. Family life and family members change over time as children grow and develop. The way in which transitions are handled and resolved depends on family adaptability. Coping is a lifelong process that occurs both at the individual and at the family unit level. Positive or effective coping is characterized as a creative response to a change or stressor that results in a new behavior or attitude. *Coping styles* reflect habitual patterns of action. In contrast, *coping efforts* refer to specific actions taken as a direct result of a specific situation.

The Interactive Family Life Cycle

Family resources, stresses, and coping styles affect family cohesion, adaptability, and communication patterns, which, in turn, influence the quality of and satisfaction with marital and family life. The degree of satisfaction as a married couple and as parents is an important outcome measure of how well the family is functioning as a family unit. Single-parent households face many challenges that can have a negative impact on the family unit. However, family-life satisfaction in a single-parent household is enhanced if there are nurturing relationships in both the parent's and the child's life.

The family life cycle is interactive. Each family member influences all others in the family and is likewise affected by them. Maladaptive patterns of interaction among family members can place a child and family at risk for negative outcomes. For example, if the family unit does not provide a protective, supportive, and loving environment to nurture the child or fails in its responsibility to help the child learn self-discipline and the ability to socialize with others, the child often develops maladaptive behaviors.

In addition, children are at risk for developing mental health problems as a result of environmental factors such as living in poverty, living in a community with a high crime rate, living in a home marked by marital conflict or domestic violence, living in a home in which they or their siblings are the victims of child maltreatment or neglect, or having a parent who abuses alcohol or other substances or has mental illness. In contrast to at-risk factors, there are factors that are protective and foster child resiliency. Certain temperaments, a caring relationship, and effective parenting can counter the negative effects of adverse risk factors and contribute to a child's positive mental health.

ASSESSMENT OF FAMILY RELATIONSHIPS AND DYNAMICS

In an assessment of family dynamics, the health provider must investigate the relationship between child, parent or caretaker, and social and environmental factors. Each factor must be analyzed separately, with its various component parts identified. The interactive effect of these factors must then be explored. The goal of assessment is to determine whether there are factors that have a negative impact on the child's ability to achieve his or her optimum level of physical, social, cognitive, or emotional growth and development. After problem areas and strengths are identified, appropriate interventions can be planned to avoid negative outcomes.

Significant points to identify as part of the child factor are the following:

- Chronological age and developmental level
- Present or past history of physical, emotional, or cognitive problems
- Personality traits and characteristics as well as temperament
- Prior maltreatment or significant negative life events
- Special care needs
- School performance for the older child

Significant points to identify as part of the parent or caregiver factor are these:

- Physical, intellectual, or emotional abilities or limitations
- Level of involvement in child care and life events of child
- Awareness, responsiveness, and availability to the child
- Level of parenting skills and pattern of communication
- Structure of family—two-parent or single-parent household
- History of maltreatment as a child
- A victim or perpetrator of domestic violence
- Previous parental history of child neglect or maltreatment
- Current drug use in the home or previous history of substance abuse (drugs or alcohol, or both)
- Financial resources
- Child-rearing practices experienced as a child
- Beliefs about discipline and corporal punishment

Significant points to identify as part of social and environmental factors are the following:

- Type and strength of family social support network or social isolation of a family
- If older child, peer group relationships
- Sibling assessment
- Cultural belief system

- Environmental condition of home
- Community characteristics—both needs and assets
- Availability and accessibility of community support systems and partnerships
- Stresses, crises, or conflicts in the home environment
- Stresses in neighborhood environment

The preceding outline of significant child, parent or caregiver, and social and environmental factors does not contain a complete listing of all relevant areas that must be addressed for each child–parent dyad. Rather, key elements are identified in each of these areas to alert the NP to areas that need investigation.

Preventive Interventions

Parent- or child-initiated concerns, situations and events related to violence, family relationship problems, and child maltreatment or neglect are significant problems that NPs are likely to encounter. Families and children who are either experiencing or who are at risk for these stressful situations must be identified. In addition, family strengths and attributes that sustain and help families effectively deal with stress are important factors to evaluate in the assessment process. NPs also can expect to be involved in some aspect of intervention strategies to ameliorate emotional or behavioral problems associated with role relationships.

The NP is typically involved in *universal* interventions and, depending on background and education, can be involved in *selective* and *indicated* preventive interventions. Universal preventive interventions are directed at enhancing the parent–child relationship and are an essential part of routine pediatric health care supervision. Universal preventive interventions are directed to the population as a whole and are focused on wellness promotion, improving communication, and relationship enhancement. Selective preventions are directed at individuals or groups at risk for the development of mental health or relationship problems, or both. Indicated preventive interventions are for high-risk individuals who are experiencing symptoms or who have biological markers for mental illness. Selective and indicated preventions often em-

ploy a multidisciplinary approach, with community resources and other professionals from various social fields joining together. NPs must always remember to focus their efforts on the need for preventive services for children and their parents and families.

HEALTH PROMOTION AND DISEASE PREVENTION OBJECTIVES AND GOALS

Healthy People 2000: National Health Promotion and Disease Prevention Objectives for the Year 2000 (United States [US] Department of Health and Human Services, 1991) addressed the issues of violence and abusive behavior and their negative effect on children, families, and society. The updating of the national health promotion and disease prevention objectives will continue to highlight these important issues as unintentional injuries continue to be a major threat to the health of children and a leading cause of death in childhood. Important strides have been made in reducing injury-related deaths resulting from motor vehicle crashes. In contrast, the number of child homicides have not declined. Violence toward children and youths continues to be a significant health concern, as evidenced by the increasing rate of reported cases of child deaths caused by violence. Homicide and suicide in the adolescent population are escalating problems.

Health organizations and health professionals recognize that national attention must continue to focus on homicides and assault injuries resulting from interpersonal and intrafamilial violence. National, state, and local efforts must be dedicated to the reduction of preventable death and disability and to the enhancement of the quality of life for all children. Health professionals in their individual practice settings and as a collective group must commit their time and talents to improving the quality of life by incorporating health promotion and disease prevention as integral components of health care for children and their families.

NPs who work with families and children experiencing role relationship problems often need to assist parents and their children to establish mutually agreed-on goals that are both child and parent focused. After management goals are established, outcome measures are identified. The work done by the Region X Nursing Network (1998) is used here as an example of goal setting with outcome measures to evaluate progress within families who are faced with role relationship issues or problems.

Goal: Child's behavior shows he or she has developed roles and relationships within the family and other social environments appropriate for age.

Child Outcomes

1. Child's attachment to primary caregiver and family is appropriate for his or her development.
2. Child behaves positively when interacting with others.
3. Child understands his or her role in the family and his or her social environment. Child understands his or her social environment offers opportunities for success and independence.

Parent Outcomes

4. Parent promotes his or her child's health, cognitive and physical growth, and overall development.

Primary care providers are frequently approached by parents with concerns about developmental or role relationship issues that do not require intervention by mental health therapists. The NP is in a strategic position to empower parents and children by acting as a supportive professional who provides education, resources, and opportunities for counseling. However, the NP must develop a plan of action with goals and outcome measures and specific criteria that indicate when there is need for referral to a mental health professional.

ROLE RELATIONSHIP PROBLEMS

Violence

Violence has surfaced as a major social and health problem. It has become a way of life for many of today's youth, who are either perpetrators, victims, or witnesses of violent acts (see Chapter 21 for additional discussion). Violence is the outcome of aggressive behavior that becomes destructive and results in physical injury to people or damage to property. Violent behavior has certain antecedents: emotional factors and situational crises or events. Feelings of anger, shame, low self-esteem, a sense of powerlessness, and hostility lead to aggressive behavior. In addition, a sequence of events precedes violent acts and results in a predictable pattern of violent behavior unless there are interventions to interrupt, minimize, or prevent violence (Brady, 1994; Ginsburg, 1997).

Violence is characterized by certain key features:

- Continuity
- Reciprocity
- Sameness
- Addiction
- Limitations of options or alternative actions
- Escalation

Once violence is used as a coping mechanism, it becomes a habit that is difficult to break; violence then becomes a continuous behavior. Violence generates violent behavior in others; violence is reciprocal. Violent behavior becomes an acceptable behavior for oneself and one's opponents, and one form of violence is just as acceptable as another. Violent behavior is never viewed by the perpetrators as unjustified; violence is characterized by sameness in that it becomes a way of life that permeates one's existence. Violence is addictive in that it gives a temporary sense of power. Violence destroys the ability to problem-solve, to reason, or to develop alternative solutions to problems. Finally, violent acts increase in intensity and potential for serious sequelae.

Impact of Violence on the Lives of Children and Their Families

The five main categories of violence that can have an impact on children and their families are

1. Domestic violence, including child abuse, corporal punishment, sibling violence, and spousal abuse
2. Predatory violence (e.g., a crime or assault)

3. Peer violence, such as fighting and gang violence
4. Sexual assault and rape
5. Dating violence

NPs are likely to become involved with young people who are involved as either witnesses, victims, or perpetrators of crime related to one or more of these five categories.

Homicide and injury to another are typically the end-results of violence. Firearm homicides are increasing in rate faster than any other cause of death in youths. In 1995, firearm-related death rates, including homicides, suicides, and accidents for children aged 5 to 14 and 15 to 19 years old, were 1.9 and 27.1 per 100,000 population, respectively (Centers for Disease Control and Prevention [CDC], 1997). From 1987 through 1994, there was a 155% increase in firearm homicides for youths ages 15 to 19 years (CDC, 1996). Although there are major differences in rates of violence-related injuries and death by ethnic groups, poverty is the most significant factor that predicts violence. The majority of homicides involve people who know each other and are of the same race. The typical scenario is played out: An argument occurs, alcohol has been consumed, a weapon is available, and a homicide is the end-result.

Youths are often the innocent victims of a crime or assault and at the same time perpetrators of crime. In 1994, almost 20% of all violent crime arrests involved a juvenile younger than the age of 18 years (Snyder et al., 1996). The youth (15 to 24 years) homicide rate in this same year was an average of 22 youth victims per day (CDC, 1996). Between 1987 and 1994, there was a 41% increase in arrests of youths 14 to 17 years of age for homicide (Fox, 1996).

Risk Factors and Predictors of Violence

The following factors are associated with youth violence:

1. Gender
   - Males predominate as perpetrators of violence.
   - Males predominate as victims of violence except for sexual assault.
   - Female gang membership is increasing.
2. Age
   - Risk increases with age and escalates rapidly around age 15 years.
3. Socioeconomic status
   - Poverty, discrimination, and the lack of opportunities for education and employment are significant risk factors.
4. Possible biological triggers
   - Brain injury is associated with aggressive behavior.
   - Genetics—it is unclear whether there is an association with sociopathic mental illness in families or as a result of poor nurture.
   - Low intelligence and attention-deficit hyperactivity disorder.
   - Lead poisoning.
5. Psychological profile
   - Temperament—child who is easily frustrated and has difficulty with transitions.
   - No sense of the future.
6. Family situation
   - Inappropriate parenting, lack of parental supervision, authoritarian child rearing.
   - Use of corporal punishment.
7. School/peers
   - Dropout from school or poor school achievement.
   - Antisocial and/or bullying behavior.
   - Peer rejection.
8. Substance abuse
   - Alcohol use.
9. Weapon use
   - Possession of firearms, handguns, knives, and baseball bats.
10. Exposure to violence
    - Past victim of violence.
    - Witness to a violent event in the home or community.

Assessment

The assessment of youths who are victims or perpetrators of violent crime should focus on certain key pieces of historical information and the presence of risk factors to help determine the potential for future violence. If possible, the youth and parent should be interviewed separately.

1. History of the episode
   - What seemed to cause the incident?

- Did the child or family know who was involved, or was this a random event?
- Were alcohol or drugs involved?
- Did either the victim or the perpetrator have or threaten to use a weapon? If yes, what type of weapon?
- Is the youth attending school? If yes, have there been any academic or behavioral problems?

2. Past history
   - Have there been prior incidents of violence or assault?
   - What is the usual pattern of drug or alcohol use?
   - Does the child have a history of mental health problems, or was the youth a victim of child abuse?
   - Does the youth have a criminal or police history?
   - Is there gang involvement or membership, or do friends carry weapons?
   - Does the youth have access to or carry a weapon or weapons?

3. Family and social history
   - How is the youth supervised by his or her parent?
   - Is there a family history of child abuse, substance abuse, domestic violence, mental illness, or a criminal record?
   - Are there handguns or rifles in the home?
   - Does the youth have a job? How is free time spent? Are the youth's friends in gangs or in trouble with the law?
   - Are siblings involved in gangs? Do they have a criminal history? Have any family members ever been victims, witnesses, or perpetrators of crime?

Management

The NP is likely to become involved with (1) the health-care management of minor trauma resulting from assault, (2) counseling after an incident of violence or threat of violence, and (3) the prevention of youth violence. In brief, the following are the key points in the management of minor assaults:

- Treatment of minor trauma or referral
- Alcohol and drug screening
- Reporting the incident to law enforcement
- Referral to social worker or mental health professional

Prevention of Youth Violence

1. Key strategies in the prevention of youth violence include the following:
   - Supervision of youths and their activities by parents or guardians
   - Educating youths about violence at an early age
   - Assessment for violence risk factors at all health supervision and illness visits
   - Limiting access to and carrying of lethal weapons (handguns and knives)
   - Having after-school programs for youths and community commitment to youth programs
   - Legislating control of handguns
   - Teaching self-defense strategies such as teaching youths martial arts and the use of mace
   - Teaching anger management and strategies for avoiding a fight (role playing)
   - Providing parents with skills for effective parenting
   - Regulating alcohol sales and use
   - Addressing the issue of media violence and of condoning violence as a way of life
   - Making neighborhoods and schools safe places for youth
   - Involving the community in a commitment to preventing violence

2. Practical hints for talking with teens on how to keep out of trouble include discussing the following issues (Ginsburg, 1997):
   - Do not carry a weapon, rather "fight clean" (i.e., discuss the issue in conflict). Carrying weapons only makes one less safe; pulling out a weapon begins a cycle of retaliation.
   - Do not go into harm's way. Avoid being around fights because the cycle of escalation and retaliation often involves innocent people.
   - If one becomes involved in a fight, try to end the incident on equal ground; that way, anger is more likely to be diffused. The person who wins often takes on the aggressor role; the loser then becomes the

scapegoat. Thus, violence continues and becomes cyclical.

- Avoid being caught alone; stay with friends.
- Do not be provoked into fighting. Words are said and names are called, not because the names are true, but rather to provoke anger and a fight.
- Suggest discussions with friends about ways to handle potential situations in which a gun or knife might be brandished.
- Do not join gangs or associate with individuals who turn to violence as a way of settling differences.

3. Talking with teens about the prevention of date or gang rape should stress the following points:
- Both males and females can be victimized.
- Alcohol intoxication or the use of drugs is a major factor in date rape. Prevention includes not placing oneself in harm's way by using such substances.
- Manipulative verbal threats and physically trapping the victim are common tactics used by perpetrators.
- Reluctance to report gang or date rape is common. However, keeping the rape a secret only leads to self-doubt and delays healing. The teen should report the rape immediately and seek professional counseling.

Child Maltreatment

In 1997, child protective services agencies investigated more than 3 million reports of child abuse and neglect and determined that almost 1 million of these reports about children were substantiated or indicated abuse and neglect. Sadly, the national rate of victimization for child abuse and neglect in 1997 was 15 victims per 1000 children (Wang & Daro, 1998; US Department of Health and Human Services, 1998). Child maltreatment or child abuse includes physical abuse, physical neglect, sexual abuse, and emotional maltreatment. The acts of inflicting injury (commission) and allowing injury to occur (omission) are the key determinants for intervention on behalf of the child. All categories of child abuse endanger the child's physical or emotional health and development. The

severity of injury is always an important consideration in treatment and disposition of the child but does not determine, per se, whether intervention should occur. The burden to report minor injury or emotional maltreatment is just as great as the burden to report significant trauma resulting in grave bodily injury.

NPs delivering primary care to children are in a unique position to identify children who are maltreated and to institute strategies for primary prevention aimed at high-risk families. Each state has its own laws related to the various categories of child maltreatment. Nurses are mandated reporters in all states and must report known or suspected child abuse. Both civil and criminal immunity is ensured to mandated reporters who are acting within their professional role in making a required or authorized report. In most instances, if the history or physical examination is suspicious for child abuse and the child is not in acute danger, the NP only need notify the child abuse registry. If the child requires protection and is in imminent danger, both the police and the child abuse registry must be called. Most states have a system of cross-reporting cases with their social service agency, usually referred to as child protective services, responsible for child abuse investigations and law enforcement. NPs should contact the department of social services or the office of the attorney general in their state for written guidelines about individual state reporting laws and procedural policies related to child abuse. The telephone number for reporting suspicion of child abuse should be readily available in each practice setting. In addition, consultation with experts in the field of child maltreatment is appropriate for those situations that are problematical or questionable for the NP.

Physical Abuse

DESCRIPTION

Any act that results in nonaccidental physical injury to a child is physical abuse. Physical abuse often occurs when the parent or caregiver is frustrated or angry. In these instances, the injury is frequently due to shaking, striking, or throwing the child and can involve unreasonably severe corporal punishment or unjustifiable punishment. Physical injury also can represent intentional, deliberate assault such as burning, biting, cutting, poking, twisting limbs, or torturing.

INCIDENCE

See Table 19-2 for relevant incidence statistics.

ASSESSMENT

Suspicion of physical abuse can involve a disclosure of inflicted injury or discrepancies in the history of the injury (type and severity of injury together with age and developmental capabilities of child) as well as behavioral or physical findings, or both. Behaviors are not definitive signs of physical abuse but are important areas to investigate for additional information. Specific physical findings are often the key to a diagnosis of nonaccidental injury resulting from physical abuse.

History

The history should assess the following:

- Child states that injury was caused by abuse.
- Injury is unusual for a specific age group.
- Parent or caregiver delays seeking care for child or seeks inappropriate care.
- Child or parent or caregiver, or both, hides

injury (e.g., child wears excessive layers of clothing), or child is kept out of school.
- There is presence of triggering behaviors such as inconsolable, colicky crying in an infant, toilet training accidents, or sleeping or discipline problems that may have led to a violent response by a caregiver.
- There is a report of a crisis or stressful time for the family (e.g., financial difficulties) or domestic violence.
- There is a problem with substance abuse in the family, currently thought to be a primary contributor to child maltreatment (Wang & Daro, 1998).
- Injuries are unexplained or implausible (e.g., parent or caregiver cannot explain injury, is vague about how the injury occurred, gives discrepant accounts of what happened or blames someone else; explanation does not match the type or mechanism of injury; or child is not developmentally capable of reported injurious behavior).

Behavioral Signs

See Table 19-3 for behavioral signs that should be investigated in a child suspected of having been abused.

Physical Findings

The location of the physical injury as well as the type of injury are two key indicators of physical abuse. See Tables 19-4 and 19-5.

TABLE 19-2

Statistics for 1997 Child Abuse and Neglect Cases Reported to Child Protective Services in the United States

GENERAL FACTS	
Number of reports	3,195,000
Increase over 1996 reports	1.7%
Number of reports confirmed	1,054,000
TYPE OF CONFIRMED CHILD MALTREATMENT (%)	
Physical abuse	22
Sexual abuse	8
Neglect	54
Emotional maltreatment	4
Other forms	12

Data from Wang CT, Daro D: Current Trends in Child Abuse Reporting and Fatalities: The Results of the 1997 Annual Fifty State Survey. Denver, CO: American Humane Association, 1998.

T A B L E 19-3

Behavioral Signs Associated With Child Maltreatment

Overly compliant or exhibits exaggerated fearfulness
Clingy and indiscriminate attachment
Extremes in behavior (aggressive/passive)
Apprehensive when other children cry
Wary of physical contact with adults
Frightened of parents or of going home, or both
Exhibits drastic behavioral changes in and out of parental or caregiver presence
Depressed, hypervigilant, withdrawn, apathetic, antisocial, exhibits destructive behavior
Suicidal (suicide attempts and/or plans) and/or engages in self-mutilation
Overprotective of parents or caregivers
Displays sleep or eating disorders

I. General considerations
   A. Location
      1. The location of injury typically associated with most physical abuse is the back surface of the body from the neck to the knees. However, injury to other parts of the body can be intentionally inflicted.
      2. Injuries to shins, elbows, or knees are typically associated with accidental, unintentional injuries that commonly occur during childhood activities.
      3. Typical sites for nonaccidental, intentional injuries by common type of injury are found in Table 19-4.
   B. Types of injuries associated with physical abuse include damage to the skin and surface tissue, brain, other internal organs, or skeleton, as well as poisonings.
II. Characteristics by type of physical injury
   A. Damage to skin and surface tissue
      1. Bruises or soft tissue injuries
         a. The location of bruising is a key indicator: bruises found on multiple surfaces, especially the buttocks, trunk, back, genitals, ears, and face.
         b. Characteristic pattern, shape, or

outline of bruising (e.g., outline of a paddle, coat hanger, or jewelry; pinch marks; strap or loop marks; hand or finger imprints).
      c. Colorations of bruising from red, red-blue, to pale green or yellow reflect various stages of healing and vary by intensity of injury and location. See Table 19-6 for general dating of contusion injuries by color change; however, color changes are subject to many factors, including the depth and severity of the injury.
      d. Multiple bruises of different colors reflect a series of injuries over varying time periods.
   2. Burns
      a. The location of a burn and its characteristics (i.e., shape, depth, and

T A B L E 19-4

Physical Abuse of Children: General Considerations Related to the Location of the Injury

Typical sites of accidental injuries
  Shins, elbows, knees
Common site of intentional injuries
  Back surface of the body—neck to knees
Common type of intentional injury by location
  Head area
    Eyes—bilateral black eyes
    Earlobe—pinch and pull marks
    Cheek—slap marks, squeeze marks
    Upper lip and frenulum—lacerations or bruises
    Scalp—bare and broken hair, bruises
  Neck—choke marks
  Trunk
    Chest—bite marks, fingertip encirclement marks
    Buttocks and lower back—paddling and strap marks
  Genitals—pinch marks, penile wrapping with constrictive materials
  Extremities
    Upper arms—grab marks
    Ankles or wrists—tethering, friction burn marks
    Feet—pin or razor tattoo marks

T A B L E 19-5

Common Characteristics of Physical Abuse by Type of Injury

TYPE OF INJURY	KEY CONSIDERATIONS
Bruises—surface and soft tissue	Pattern, shape, outline Location Stages of coloring
Burns	Location Patterns, such as sharply demarcated or circumferential (e.g., sock, glove, zebra, branding, bite, mark, doughnut or cigarette shaped)
Bites	Pattern such as doughnut or double-horseshoe shape; adult >3 cm between canine teeth
Abrasions and lacerations	Location "C" or "U" shape typical of belt buckle mark
Central nervous system	Radiographic findings (e.g., subdural hematomas, subarachnoid hemorrhages, skull fractures), retinal hemorrhages
Shaken infant syndrome	Retinal hemorrhage, subdural hematoma, posterior rib and metaphyseal fractures
Internal organs	Liver, bowel, spleen, pancreas, kidney consistent with blunt-force trauma
Skeletal	Spiral fractures of long bones, avulsion of metaphyseal tips, multiple rib fractures in different stages of healing, subperiosteal proliferation reaction
Poisoning/ingestion of medication	Deliberate poisoning or exposure to substance abuse
Munchausen-by-proxy syndrome	Creates a fictitious illness or induces illness in child

margins) are important in the differential diagnosis of accidental vs. nonaccidental injury. Children tend to accidentally burn themselves on a hand, arm, or leg. Burns on both palms, both soles, flexor surfaces of the thighs, or perineum are pathognomonic for child abuse (Krugman et al., 1998).

  b. Splash marks—caused as child at-

T A B L E 19-6

General Dating of Contusion Injury

BRUISE CHARACTERISTIC	AGE OF BRUISE
Swollen, tender	0–2 d
Red/purple/blue	0–5 d
Green	5–7 d
Yellow	7–10 d
Brown	10–14 d
Clear	2–4 wk

tempts to escape or withdraws from the source of burn injury—are common in accidental injuries from hot liquids.

  c. Scalding by hot liquid is the most common intentionally inflicted burn injury; infants or young children are typically immersed, and older children have hot liquid thrown or poured on them.

  d. Sharply demarcated or circumferential burns ("sock" or "glove" burn) occur when children are held in hot water.

  e. A "doughnut-shaped" burn on the buttock occurs in a child who is forcibly held down in a tub of hot water and the center part of the buttock is spared from burning.

  f. "Zebra" burns are a typical pattern that results when the child is held by the hands and legs under a faucet of hot water; the creases in the abdomen and upper legs fold up and are spared from burning, resulting in a zebra-stripes effect.

g. Branding burns reflect the outline of an object (e.g., iron, electric heater, grill).

h. Cigarette burns are often multiple and are usually found on the palms or soles.

i. Rope burn marks typically appear around the wrists and ankles.

3. Bite marks

a. Bite marks can be found on any part of the body.

b. A doughnut shape or double-horse-shoe shape is the typical pattern.

c. Adult bite marks are diagnostic if the space between the canine teeth marks is greater than 3 cm.

4. Abrasions and lacerations

a. Number and location of abrasions or lacerations, or both, are important.

b. Belt buckles typically cause lacerations resembling a "C" or "U" shape or loop or linear marks; other instruments of injury can leave distinctive shapes.

B. Damage to the brain

1. Head injuries

a. Radiographic findings are often distinctive.

b. Typical types of inflicted head injuries include subgaleal hematomas and cephalhematomas—violent and sudden hair pulling or blunt impact trauma; scalp bruise and soft tissue swelling—direct blows by objects; subdural hematomas, subarachnoid hemorrhages, and retinal hemorrhages (see shaken baby/infant syndrome); and skull fractures and suture spread—indicative of blunt force trauma.

c. Head injuries are the most common cause of child abuse–related deaths and an important cause of chronic neurological disability.

d. Most research of nonabusive falls less than 4 feet onto hard surfaces

shows less than a 1% incidence of skull fractures (Brodeur & Monteleone, 1994).

2. Shaken baby/infant syndrome—intentional shaking

a. Retinal hemorrhages are classic signs of shaken baby syndrome and can be associated with subdural hematoma, posterior rib fractures, and metaphyseal fractures of the long bones.

b. Many children with subdural hematomas caused by child abuse have no visible scalp injuries or associated skull fracture.

c. Central nervous system symptoms can have an acute or subtle presentation (see Chapter 28).

C. Damage to other internal organs

1. Blunt force trauma to the abdomen is typically from forceful blows such as punching, kicking, or being stepped on and can cause injury to the liver, bowel, spleen, pancreas, kidneys, or other internal organs.

2. Injury might not leave visible marks or bruises on the abdomen.

3. Child can have symptoms of shock; internal injury is the second leading cause of death in child abuse cases.

D. Damage to the skeleton

1. Unexplained fracture in an infant or toddler is cause for investigation.

2. Spiral fractures of long bones in a child who is not yet walking are almost always caused by physical abuse.

3. Suspicious fractures include the following:

a. Avulsion of the metaphyseal tips—"chip" fractures at the end of long bones

b. Multiple rib fractures, especially back rib fractures

c. Sternal fractures and scapular fractures

d. Healing or healed fractures that are without explanation and are revealed by radiographs

e. Multiple fractures in different stages of healing

4. Subperiosteal proliferation reaction is suspicious.
5. Fractures from birth injury are healed by 4 months of age.
6. Documentation of approximate date of fracture is important (recent vs. old).

E. Other
1. Deliberate poisoning or ingestion of medication.
2. Substance abuse exposure in infants and children from breast milk, passive inhalation of marijuana smoke, or accidental contamination of formula feeding equipment or cocaine used as topical anesthetic on sore nipples.
3. Munchausen syndrome by proxy—parent or caretaker reports a fictitious illness in the child or induces illness in the child to obtain medical attention. The acute signs and symptoms cease when the suspect no longer has contact with or unsupervised access to the child.

Diagnostic Studies

These should include (1) blood coagulation studies (platelet count, bleeding time, prothrombin time, and partial thromboplastin time) on any child who is severely bruised or has a history of "easy bruising" and suspicious bruises and (2) radiographic studies. A child with limited range of motion or bony tenderness on examination should have a local radiological evaluation. A radiological skeletal survey should be ordered for any child with soft tissue findings who is nonverbal or unable to give a clear history (usually younger than 4 to 5 years) or for infants suspected of failure to thrive (FTT). The minimum radiological survey is a skull series, long bones, and ribs. Bone scan, computed tomography scan, and magnetic resonance imaging study should be ordered on the basis of physical findings on examination or symptoms. Serum calcium, phosphorus, and alkaline phosphatase levels are useful measurements if bone disease is suspected. Ultrasonography is useful if visceral injury is suspected. Other studies are ordered depending on physi-

cal findings (Behrman & Kliegman, 1998; Krugman et al., 1998; Reece, 1994).

DIFFERENTIAL DIAGNOSIS

Differential diagnoses are identified by type of intentional physical injury:

1. Soft tissue injuries
   • Normal bruising from accidental injuries that typically involve the knees, anterior tibia, and forehead
   • Mongolian spots and allergic shiners
   • Bleeding disorders
   • Cultural practices such as "coining," sometimes practiced by Southeast Asian groups
2. Burns
   • Impetigo, bullous impetigo, or toxic epidermal necrolysis (scalded skin syndrome)
3. Fractures
   • Osteogenesis imperfecta and rare bone diseases such as scurvy, congenital syphilis, and neoplasms

MANAGEMENT

Medical treatment of specific types of injuries is discussed in Unit 4 of this text under the appropriate illness-related heading. If physical abuse is suspected, certain general management strategies should be followed. The NP must

1. Report suspicions of child maltreatment to child protective services or law enforcement agencies, or both.
2. Carefully document findings and any statements made by parent or caregiver or child, or both.
3. Secure photographic documentation of soft tissue injury or burn injury; this can be done by law enforcement personnel or health care provider as appropriate.
4. Refer for appropriate medical treatment of injuries depending on type and severity of injury.

The child should be referred for psychological counseling; this is generally handled by child protective services. The need for long-term or intermittent therapy often depends on the individual child, the severity of the physical injury, and other life events.

PATIENT EDUCATION AND PREVENTION

Prevention of physical abuse involves the following steps:

1. Screening for parental history of abuse during childhood, history of domestic violence, and absence of a social support network in the family. Pursue positive screens.
2. Identification of at-risk families and children with early referral to social service agencies. At-risk families include those with any of the following characteristics:
   - A prior history of child maltreatment, drug abuse, violent behavior, or serious mental illness
   - Evidence that the mother is not showing attachment to her infant, makes negative remarks about the child, or lacks basic parenting knowledge, skill, and motivation
   - Evidence of spanking of young infants
   - Isolated parent who lacks social support network
   - A history of infant or child death resulting from child maltreatment (categorized as extremely high risk)
3. Referral for supportive service, including social service referrals, parenting classes, self-help groups (Parents or Alcoholics Anonymous plus battered women's services), respite care, public health nurse visits, or a combination of these.
4. Close primary care supervision and ill child follow-up visits of at-risk families and children.
5. Management of at-risk or high-risk families by a team approach (ideally, a multidisciplinary team). A team approach gives objectivity to a situation.
6. Early and prompt reporting to child protective services.
7. Support of community child abuse prevention programs.

Neglect

DESCRIPTION

Physical neglect refers to the negligent treatment or maltreatment of a child that can harm or threaten harm to a child's health or welfare.

Neglect by the parent or caregiver can be divided into categories of severe or general neglect. Severe neglect includes instances in which the parent or caregiver fails to protect the child from such dangers as severe malnutrition or medically diagnosed nonorganic FTT. Another example of severe neglect involves the willful placing of a child in a situation in which the child's health is endangered (i.e., physical injury occurred) because of intentional failure to provide adequate food, clothing, shelter, education, or medical care. General neglect refers to failure to provide basic needs such as adequate food, clothing, shelter, medical care, or supervision where no physical injury to the child occurred as a result of the negligent actions by the caregiver. A key factor in neglect is the extreme or persistent presence of these conditions in the child's home.

INCIDENCE

See Table 19-2 for relevant incidence statistics.

ASSESSMENT

The general indicators of possible neglect and specific criteria for psychosocial FTT are addressed separately. The general indicators of neglect are divided into child, home, and supervision factors (Table 19-7).

Child factors include the child's appearance and general status as well as having access to needed dental and health care. Home factors focus on a safe and sanitary environment. To determine lack of proper adult supervision, child protective workers investigate such factors as the child's age and level of functioning, the length of time the parent was away, where the parent went, whether the parent left a plan of supervision (e.g., relative or adult living next door or nearby who was readily available to the child), and how often the minor was left alone. The key issue is whether the child's safety and welfare were threatened. Most child protective services hold parents to the standard of a "reasonable or prudent" parent.

DIFFERENTIAL DIAGNOSIS

Differentiating willful neglect from neglect resulting from poverty or mental retardation or

T A B L E   19-7

General Indicators of Neglect: Child, Home, Supervision Factors

CHILD

Dirty, malnourished, poor hygiene, inadequately dressed for weather

Inadequate medical and dental care (has multiple caries)

Always sleepy (chronic fatigue) or hungry

HOME

Fire hazards or other unsafe conditions

No heating or plumbing

Nutritional quality of the food inadequate

Meals not prepared; food spoiled in refrigerator or cupboards

SUPERVISION

Child has history of repeated physical injuries or ingestion of harmful substances with evidence of poor supervision by adult caregiver

Child cared for by another child

Child left alone in the home, car, or anywhere without supervision (typically defined as a child younger than 12 years of age who is left unsupervised during the daytime, or child aged 16 to 18 years, left unsupervised by an adult at night)

mental illness is necessary. Educational neglect differs from truancy (child is sent to school but never arrives) in that the parent makes no provisions for the child to attend school.

MANAGEMENT

Referral to child protective services is needed in cases of neglect.

Psychosocial Failure to Thrive

DESCRIPTION

Infancy is the major period of time when FTT due to nonorganic reasons is diagnosed. Children older than 2 years of age can get their own food. However, purposeful starvation in older children by their caregiver does happen. FTT is defined as an underweight condition or malnourishment in a child because the child is not fed enough. The term FTT is used to de-

scribe children younger than age 5 years whose growth persistently and significantly deviates below the norms for their age and sex. The infant with psychosocial FTT is generally below the fifth or third percentile in weight with signs of malnourishment (Behrman & Kliegman, 1998; Frank, 1995).

ETIOLOGY

Depending upon the population studied, between 50 and 90% of children seen for FTT were not growing adequately because of inadequate food intake due to educational, economic, or psychological inadequacy (Barness, 1997).

ASSESSMENT

The assessment includes the history, physical examination, and diagnostic studies.

History

The history can include the following:

- Feeding and dietary history—can be helpful in distinguishing accidental feeding or formula-preparation error from neglect and organic or psychological causes; dietary history should be obtained but might not be truthful.
- Past history—might be suggestive of neglect (e.g., little or no health care supervision, immunizations not up to date, earlier removal of a sibling for neglect).
- Interview with mother—might reveal mother's negative feelings toward infant, a state of feeling overwhelmed or depressed, plus feelings of being deprived or unloved; mother may be cognitively delayed.
- Observations of mother–infant interaction —might indicate a lack of attachment or presence of anger.
- Inquire about financial hardships related to inability to provide for basic food needs.

Physical Findings

The physical findings in FTT include

- Depressed weight-for-height ratio; short stature with a proportional weight can reflect chronic malnutrition or a genetic or endocrine-based problem.

- Failure to maintain previously established growth trajectory.
- Signs of general neglect: poor hygiene such as filthy fingernails, clothes, body, rampant diaper rash, or untreated impetigo.
- Flattened occiput from lying in one position.
- Ravenous appetite; should observe the caregiver feed the infant.
- Avoidance of eye contact: does not like to be cuddled or has an expressionless face.
- Associated developmental delays resulting from little psychosocial stimulation.

Diagnostic Studies

Dietary management should be undertaken for 1 week to determine whether there is significant weight gain before laboratory studies are ordered to rule out organic causes of FTT (see Chapter 33).

DIFFERENTIAL DIAGNOSIS

The differential diagnoses for FTT include accidental feeding or formula errors and organic causes of FTT, including endocrine, metabolic, gastrointestinal, cardiovascular, genetic, neurological, infectious, and renal conditions.

MANAGEMENT

Depending on the severity of malnourishment, the child is placed in either a hospital setting or a foster home. Demonstration of adequate weight gain while out of the home is diagnostic. Dietary management should include an appropriate diet for age that provides 120 Kcal/24 hour times median weight (kg) for measured length. Most children younger than 6 months of age with caloric-deprivation FTT gain weight by 2 to 3 days; children 6 to 24 months gain weight by 2 to 17 days (Behrman & Kliegman, 1998). Close and long-term health care supervision and follow-up plus psychosocial intervention and local case management by child protective services are needed.

PATIENT EDUCATION AND PREVENTION

Prevention of physical neglect and psychosocial FTT generally involves the same prevention strategies as identified under physical abuse. The importance of frequent health visits to monitor weight gain for infants who are falling behind is essential to prevent significant growth problems.

Sexual Abuse

DESCRIPTION

Sexual abuse or maltreatment is defined to include acts of sexual assault or sexual exploitation of minors, or both. These acts can occur over an extended period of time or involve a one-time incident; they may or may not involve force; they can involve threats of physical harm to a child or others in their family, or involve emotional entrapment of the child; and they can often involve a secret between the victim and the perpetrator. The perpetrator is usually known to the child and is often a "trusted" adult (Leventhal, 1997; Heger & Emans, 1992). A growing group of perpetrators are adolescents who commit sexually aggressive acts on young children.

Sexual assault of children includes a range of acts including rape, rape in concert, incest, sodomy, lewd or lascivious acts on a child younger than 14 years of age (e.g., fondling or touching of genital areas and breasts or inappropriate kissing), oral copulation, and penetration of genital or anal openings by a foreign object. Sexual exploitation includes activities such as pornography depicting minors and promoting prostitution by minors.

INCIDENCE

Multigenerational abuse is not uncommon in cases of child sexual abuse. Reported abuse among girls is more prevalent than among boys, with estimates of lifetime prevalence being from 7 to 62% for females and 3 to 19% for males (Leventhal, 1997; Heger & Emans, 1992). In 1997, a total of 84,320 cases of reported child sexual abuse (see Table 19-2) were accepted by social service agencies in the United

States, which represents 8% of the total number of child abuse and neglect cases (Wang & Daro, 1998). Proving sexual abuse in young children is difficult.

ASSESSMENT

Chapter 36 discusses the examination of the genitalia in girls. The child or adolescent who has been sexually assaulted by a stranger usually discloses the abuse and comes in for an immediate evaluation. This type of assessment is straightforward and involves the usual taking of a history and performing the medical examination with collection of possible evidence. If the incident occurred within 72 hours, evidence (e.g., semen, nail scraping, and pubic hair) is collected, and testing for sexually transmitted diseases should be done. These children are often seen in the emergency department of a local hospital or at a special center that treats victims of child sexual abuse.

The NP in a primary care setting is likely to become involved in a child sexual abuse case in any of the following circumstances: There is a spontaneous disclosure by the child; a parent voices concerns about the possibility of abuse or reports a disclosure by their child; there are suspicious physical or historical findings, or both; or laboratory tests indicative of sexually transmitted diseases (STDs) are positive. In many instances, sexual abuse occurs over several years before the child discloses.

If possible, the assessment of the child should be done by a health care provider who is an expert in the field of sexual abuse of children. The assessment of a child who has been molested in the past but whose molestation has only recently been disclosed, or who is suspected of being sexually abused should focus on three areas: behavioral findings, medical findings, and the interview of the child. Each of these three areas is addressed separately.

Behavioral Indicators

- Loss of bowel and bladder control
- Regressive behaviors such as newly manifested clinging and irritability in young children, thumb sucking, renewed need for a security object
- Night terrors, inability to sleep alone, bed wetting after having been dry at night
- Overeating or lack of appetite; compulsive behaviors or unusual fears and phobias
- Change in school performance; loss of concentration or easy distractibility
- Sexualized behavior or play inappropriate for developmental level
- Depression or inactivity, poor peer relationships, poor self-esteem, acting out, excessive anger
- Runaway, suicide attempts, prostitution or promiscuity, substance abuse, teen pregnancy, psychosomatic gynecological and gastrointestinal complaints

Behavioral indicators in and of themselves are not diagnostic of sexual molestation but indicate a need for a thorough investigation (Krugman et al., 1998; Heger & Emans, 1992).

Medical Indicators—Nonspecific

- Pain on urination; vaginal or penile discharge; vaginal, rectal, or penile bleeding; enuresis and encopresis
- Urethral or lymph gland inflammation; genital or perianal rashes; labial adhesions
- Pain in anal, gastrointestinal, pelvic, and urinary areas
- Genital injuries or signs such as bruising, scratches, bites, grasp marks, swelling of the genitalia that are unexplained or inconsistent with history

Medical Indicators—Specific

- Blunt force trauma (lacerations, bruising, abrasions, tears) to the genital or rectal areas, or both, that is inconsistent with the history, or these same findings with a history of sexual contact or penetration
- Commonly encountered STDs (by probability of sexual abuse in prepubertal infants and children from certain to uncertain)*:

*The verification of STDs that are categorized as certain, probable, and possible should be reported (American Academy of Pediatrics, 1991). Common warts on the hands of parents or caregiver can infect a child when touching the genitals during nonsexual activity such as bathing or helping with toileting or with activities involving sexual abuse (Cohen, 1999).

- ◦ Certain—gonorrhea (by culture) and syphilis if not perinatally acquired
- ◦ Probable—chlamydia (culture is only reliable diagnostic method), condyloma acuminatum (if not perinatally acquired), *Trichomonas vaginalis*, herpes type 2
- ◦ Possible—herpes type 1 (in the genital area)
- ◦ Uncertain—bacterial vaginosis
- • Pregnancy and semen are certain indicators of sexual abuse in young children

Lack of Significant Physical Findings

- • Most child victims of sexual abuse do not have any significant physical findings.
- • Lack of findings is often the result of delayed disclosure and the nature of the abuse.
- • Most sexual abuse of young children does not involve penetrating trauma.

Interview of the Child

- • If the child gives a spontaneous or clear disclosure of sexual abuse during a primary care visit, report the case. Children rarely lie about such matters. Always think, How would a child that age know about such sexual details?
- • When talking with a child who is disclosing sexual abuse, or whom you suspect was or is being sexually abused, be nonjudgmental, use language that the child understands, identify the words the child uses for the genital and rectal areas, have the child tell you what happened in his or her own words, and ask open-ended questions. Try not to ask leading questions.
- • Consider separate questioning of the child and parent or caregiver if the child is 4 years or older.
- • The purpose of the health provider interview is to collect adequate information to decide whether to report the case. A social worker, psychologist, or law-enforcement person with experience in evaluating sexually abused children will conduct a detailed interview after the case is reported.
- • Recanting a disclosure of sexual abuse is

not uncommon because of fear of what disclosure can bring to the family or child.

Diagnostic Studies

Any sexual abuse of children that involves oral, genital, rectal, or penile contact or penetration within the previous 72 hours requires that appropriate forensic specimens be collected. In addition, the rectal, throat, urethral, and/or endocervical areas should be cultured for *Neisseria gonorrhoeae* and *Chlamydia trachomatis*. Blood to test for syphilis should be obtained. In selected cases, additional diagnostic tests for human immunodeficiency virus (HIV), hepatitis B, herpes simplex, bacterial vaginosis, human papillomavirus, and *T. vaginalis* can be performed if indicated.

Testing for STDs in children who were molested in the past (more than 72 hours previously) is a judgment call. Recency of exposure and the possibility of penile contact are key indicators for whether specimens need to be collected for possible STDs. Testing for *N. gonorrhoeae*, *C. trachomatis*, and syphilis should be considered in all children with a history of sexual abuse. A colposcopic examination of the genital and rectal areas by an expert in the field is often requested by law enforcement agencies to determine whether there is evidence of acute traumatic or past healed injury to the genital or rectal areas.

DIFFERENTIAL DIAGNOSIS

Differential diagnoses include straddle injury to the genitalia or rectal area, which produces labial ecchymosis, abrasions, or tears; penetrating vaginal trauma from accidental injury such as jumping from dresser onto bedpost (needs careful investigation); perinatally acquired STDs or STDs acquired through close contact but not sexual abuse; lichen sclerosus, poor hygiene, and pinworm infestation, resulting in vulvar skin irritation; and foreign body (frequently toilet paper) and other nonsexually transmitted bacteria causing vaginal discharge.

MANAGEMENT

An immediate forensic examination for a chain of evidence is required if the child gives a history that sexual abuse including ejaculation occurred within 72 hours. Specimen collection for semen, STDs, pregnancy, and other evidence is done according to the local law enforcement protocol for child or adolescent rape. If possible, the child should be referred to health providers who are skilled in performing this special examination on children and adolescents. An expert in the medical examination of children suspected of being sexually abused should evaluate the child if the incident or incidents occurred more than 72 hours before the disclosure. A psychosocial interview with an expert in the field of child sexual abuse is often part of the evaluation.

If the NP is the first health care provider to see the child, he or she is likely to become involved in the following management issues:

* Careful documentation of the history and physical examination findings for medicolegal purposes
* Reporting of the case to law enforcement and social service agencies as required by law
* Referral for medical and psychosocial evaluation by experts in the field of child sexual abuse
* Referrals for crisis counseling of the child and other family members as needed
* Prescribing medication for treatment of STDs; follow-up STD cultures or blood work as indicated
* Referrals for therapy as well as support and encouragement for the child and family

PATIENT EDUCATION AND PREVENTION

Prevention of sexual abuse involves the following steps (Daro, 1994; Leventhal, 1997):

1. Primary prevention includes instructing parents and caregivers about the need for early and consistent education of their children about good, bad, and questionable touching of private parts; how to say no or the use of self-defense techniques (e.g., yelling, kicking, or fighting back) if someone inappropriately touches them; to tell a responsible adult; and not to keep secrets. In addition, instructing parents about not leaving their child in high-risk situations is important.

2. Referrals for individual and family counseling are essential if sexual abuse is confirmed or suspected. Daughters and Sons United is a self-help group for older children and teenagers (see Resource Box 19-1). Prevention of later psychological problems related to child sexual abuse and revictimization are key issues.

3. Multigenerational abuse is common. Many women who have been abused themselves as children by a family member keep this a secret but unwittingly allow their child access to the perpetrator. These women blame themselves for what happened and often erroneously believe that the perpetrator will not sexually abuse their child. Counseling that children are never safe around a pedophile is an important topic to address.

4. The need for parents to periodically discuss the topic of good and bad touching and sexual molestation should be emphasized. Parents should again bring up this subject as their child progresses through the various developmental stages. Young children who have been molested by a trusted adult often do not disclose for many years because they were threatened not to tell anyone or they interpreted the sexual activity (if it is not painful) as a sign of affection from the trusted adult and not as molestation. Later, feelings of guilt, fear, and/or betrayal emerge when children realize they were molested.

5. Efforts to target high-risk groups for intervention to avoid the continued spread of child abuse should be supported (e.g., adolescents who have exhibited sexual curiosity beyond the bounds of normal or have experimented with but not yet victimized younger children).

6. Handouts and educational reading materials about the topic of sexual abuse of children should be available for families. Teaching should be tailored to the child's cognitive and learning abilities.

7. Early and prompt reporting to child protective services is essential if one is at all suspicious.

8. Support of public education efforts and com-

munity child sexual abuse prevention programs is needed.

9. Educate parents about the need to talk to their children about their daily activities, especially what their children did during the time they were not with the parents.

Emotional Maltreatment

DESCRIPTION

There are two forms of emotional maltreatment: emotional abuse and emotional deprivation. Emotional abuse is characterized by excessive and distorted parental attitudes and actions that lead to emotional and behavioral problems in children. Parents or caregivers can emotionally abuse their children in any number of ways by subjecting them to unpredictable responses, continual negative moods, constant family discord, double messages, and verbal insults such as belittling, screaming, threats, terrorizing, blaming, or sarcasm. Witnessing acts of domestic violence is another example of emotional abuse of children. The communication pattern between the parent or caregiver and the child is one of negative messages that hinder the child's positive emotional development. The issue of consistency or recurrence of negative parental behaviors, as well as willful cruelty or unjustifiable emotional punishment, is a key indicator.

Emotional deprivation is another form of emotional maltreatment of children. Parents or caregivers can ignore or reject their child for any number of reasons, including drug use, psychiatric disturbances, personal problems, or other preoccupying situations. Parents or caregivers who do not provide the normal experiences necessary for a child to feel loved, wanted, secure, or worthy are depriving their child of the emotional security that is critical for positive self-esteem. The issue of consistency in these types of negative behaviors or the serious consequences to the child as a result of these behaviors, or both, are key in proving emotional deprivation.

INCIDENCE

Emotional maltreatment is often difficult to prove from a legal standpoint. Accumulative documentation is generally needed (see Table 19-2).

ASSESSMENT

Behavioral indicators often lead to suspicions of emotional maltreatment but can also be due to other causes; therefore, a careful history is important. Interviewing both parent or caregiver plus any child older than 3 years of age is essential. A range of behavioral indicators can be exhibited by children who are emotionally deprived or abused (Table 19-8).

Diagnostic Studies

Diagnostic evaluation by a mental health professional is needed to determine whether the behaviors or psychopathology, or both, in the child are due to parental emotional abuse or deprivation.

DIFFERENTIAL DIAGNOSIS

Psychopathology in the child resulting from other causes is the differential diagnosis.

MANAGEMENT

Because emotional maltreatment is generally difficult to prove, the NP must carefully document what was said in the interview or what behavioral indicators were found. Referral to a mental health professional for evaluation should be considered if the NP has concerns. Reporting concerns to the appropriate child protective services agency is essential, as is close supervision of these families.

PATIENT EDUCATION AND PREVENTION

Prevention of emotional abuse involves the same strategies as identified under physical abuse. Early recognition and intervention are the key to prevention of subsequent mental health problems.

TABLE 19-8

Behavioral Findings Associated With Emotional Maltreatment

BEHAVIORAL FINDINGS SUGGESTIVE OF EMOTIONAL ABUSE

1. Behavioral indicators seen in children
   Withdrawn, depressed, apathetic
   Act out or have behavioral problems
   Overly rigid in conforming to instructions or attention to details as if fearful of doing something wrong
   Somatic signs of emotional distress (e.g., repetitive rhythmical movements, enuresis, encopresis)
   Talk about or report negative comments made by parent about themselves
2. Behavioral indicators seen in parents or caregivers
   Unrealistic demands or impossible expectations placed on child in terms of child's developmental capacity
   Child used to satisfy parents' ego needs or as a battleground for marital conflicts
   Child referred to as "it" or treated as an object

BEHAVIORAL FINDINGS SUGGESTIVE OF EMOTIONAL DEPRIVATION

On presentation, these children can have the following characteristics:
   Be developmentally delayed for age with no organic reason
   Appear frail or refuse to eat adequate amounts of food (see Psychosocial Failure to Thrive)
   Display any of the following behaviors: antisocial behavior, delinquency, unresponsiveness, sadness, and/or withdrawal
   Exhibit exaggerated fears
   Crave attention and affection from other adults, such as teachers or neighbors

VARIATIONS IN FAMILY PATTERNS

Separation and Divorce

DESCRIPTION

The increasing rate of divorce is troublesome because of its profound effect on family life. Divorce results in a major disruption and dis-equilibrium in the lives of most children. The US Census Bureau (1997) reported a divorce rate of 52% compared with a 43% rate in 1988. Custodial and visitation arrangements for children are variable. Joint custody is an option that allows both parents the opportunity to participate in mutual decision-making about their child's life and welfare. There are instances in which single custody is in the best interest of the child; however, the noncustodial parent may have sporadic contact with the child and limited involvement in the child's life in these circumstances. Various living arrangements and visitation rights are possible with joint custody.

Research studies investigating the psychological consequences of divorce on children have reported varying data on its negative effect. Wallerstein (1992) reported that children in families in which the parents were separated or divorced tended to have significantly more psychological problems than their counterparts in intact families. Problems with aggression and conduct disorders, especially among boys, is reported in the literature as a consistent finding in studies focusing on children of divorce. There also are data to support that children can adapt to and successfully cope with marital separation and divorce with no long-term negative effect (Melnyk & Alpert-Gillis, 1997). Many researchers hold the opinion that the difference in psychological functioning between children from married and divorced families more likely is the result of conflict or poor parenting that began before the divorce than as a direct result per se of the divorce experience (Emery, 1997). Parental conflict is the most significant predictor of long-term adjustment of children after divorce.

INCIDENCE

Almost 50% of all children experience the divorce of their parents. Divorce occurs in marriages with children of all age groups. However, the number of young couples divorcing has increased dramatically, and the children in divorcing families tend to be younger.

ASSESSMENT

The NP must remember several important points in assisting families in which the parents are separated or divorced (Foster & Pascoe, 1995; Wallerstein, 1992). They include the developmental stage of the children, the common psychosocial issues that these children experience, the psychosocial impact of the divorce on the parents, and the economic consequences of divorce on the family unit (Tables 19-9 and 19-10).

MANAGEMENT

Parents who are in the process of separating and divorcing need assistance and counseling

---

T A B L E 19-9

Child-Related Assessment Factors in Divorce

DEVELOPMENTAL STAGE OF CHILDREN
Age and developmental stage of children greatly affect their response to separation and divorce of parents
Common reactions of children to divorce by age group:
2–5 yr: Regression, irritability, sleep disturbances, aggression
6–8 yr: Open grieving and feelings of rejection or being replaced; whiny, immature behavior, sadness, fearfulness
9–12 yrs: Fear and intense anger at one or both parents
≥13 years: Worried about own future, depressed, and/or acting-out behaviors (e.g., truancy, sexual activity, alcohol or drug use, suicide attempts)

COMMON ISSUES FOR CHILDREN OF DIVORCING PARENTS
Continued tension, conflict, and fighting between parents
Litigation disputes over custody and visitation arrangements
Abandonment by one parent or sporadic visitation (decreased availability) vs. denial of visitation
Diminished parenting resulting from such factors as availability issues or emotional inaccessibility, distress, or instability
Limited social support system outside nuclear family
Feelings of loneliness or emotional abandonment, or both

T A B L E 19-10

Parental and Family Unit Assessment Factors in Divorce

IMPACT OF DIVORCE ON PARENT
Psychological functioning of parent and availability to child are often negatively impacted
Feelings of bitterness and acrimony toward divorcing spouse are common
Feelings of helplessness and depression can overwhelm parent, who may no longer be able to maintain household standards or standards of behavior for child

ECONOMIC CONSEQUENCE OF DIVORCE
Often devastating economic hardships and decline in living standard are problems that families (especially women) face as a result of divorce
Nonpayment or delinquency in payment of child support is a widespread problem

---

about certain key issues of anticipatory guidance and the need to seek health care for symptoms or behaviors brought on by this crisis.

Anticipatory guidance given to parents should cover four main topics: the need to prepare the child for the impending separation if possible; the need to give ongoing explanations about the divorce and custody issues, plus assurances that the child will be taken care of and is loved; suggestions about self-help measures; and indications when referral for mental health counseling is needed (Table 19-11).

PATIENT EDUCATION AND PREVENTION

Promoting a healthy adjustment to divorce should be the goal as the child experiences an acute crisis in family structure and family life that is usually followed by an extended period of disequilibrium and reorganization. In working with children of divorce and their parents, the NP must stress those factors that have been shown to significantly affect whether the child will experience a healthful adjustment to the divorce (Table 19-12).

In an early research study, Wallerstein (1983) identified six psychological tasks that children

TABLE 19-11

Key Anticipatory Guidance Issues for Families Experiencing Divorce

Advise parents to prepare the child for the impending breakup.
- If possible, prepare the child for the impending breakup of the family and departure of a parent from the home. Children who are told of the impending divorce before the departure of a parent handle the situation in a calmer manner than those who are given no preparation and wake up to find the parent gone.
- Discussions about the impending divorce should be an ongoing supportive process for the child.

Explain the need for parents to discuss with their children the following key issues about the separation and decision to divorce.
- Assure children that they will continue to see the departing parent if this is true.
- Explain what divorce means in language that the child can understand, what the family structure will be like afterward, and what imminent changes will occur in the living arrangements and daily routines.
- Reassure children that they will be cared for and are not being abandoned by either parent unless a parent has disappeared or indicates noninvolvement.
- Explain the visitation arrangements as soon as established.
- Offer an explanation of the reasons for the divorce appropriate to age and level of understanding of the child. Young children can simply be told that their parents are unhappy and that the purpose of the divorce is to end the unhappiness and conflict between their parents.

- Reassure children that they did not cause the divorce, they can do nothing to correct their parents' unhappiness in the marriage, and the divorce is the parents' decision.
- Tell children that they are not expected to take sides against one parent or the other. They should love both parents, and feelings of sadness, anger, and disappointment are normal.

Suggest self-help measures.
- Attendance at divorce recovery workshops or classes about families in transition as well as participation in support groups for children can be helpful.
- Working with school counselors, religious groups, or community and government agencies is another option that can be explored.

Discuss indications for referrals for mental health counseling.
- Professional counseling can be an essential component of the recovery process. The type of referral depends on the nature of the problem, the severity of symptoms, and the continuance of symptoms or problems without signs of improvement.
- Referrals can include individual or family counseling with mental health practitioners.

of divorce must master beginning from the time of parental separation and culminating in young adulthood. These tasks continue to be relevant for children whose parents are divorced. If these psychological tasks are not achieved, the child's mastery of normal developmental tasks associated with growing up is negatively impacted. Therefore, the goal of education is to prevent future psychological trauma and to help children restore a sense of wholeness and integrity in their lives. Long-range and preventive interventions need to focus on helping the child to achieve these six tasks or goals:

1. Acknowledging the reality of the marital breakup
2. Disengaging from parental conflict and distress and resuming customary pursuits
3. Resolving loss of familiar daily routine, traditions, and symbols, and the physical presence of two parents
4. Resolving anger and self-blame
5. Accepting the permanence of the divorce
6. Achieving realistic hope regarding relationships—the capacity to love and be loved

The NP should offer support and may schedule additional visits or telephone contacts with

TABLE 19-12

Factors Affecting a Child's Ability to Achieve Healthy Adjustment to Divorce in Their Families

The opportunity for continued participation of the noncustodial or visiting parent in the child's life on a regular basis

The ability of the custodial parent to handle and successfully parent the child

The ability of parents to separate their own feelings of anger and conflict and resolve their own hostility toward the other parent so that the child's need for a relationship with both parents is met

The child does not become involved in parental conflict and does not feel rejected

The availability of a social support network

The ability of parents to meet the child's developmental needs and to help the child master the developmental tasks before him or her

The child's overall personality and personal assets as well as deficits

the family to monitor their adjustment. Be careful not to use terminology that is offensive such as "broken home," "intact family," and "child of divorce." In addition, look at each family as a unique situation and avoid negative stereotyping (e.g., "deadbeat dad" or "angry mom"). In addition, help the family cope by focusing on their positive strengths and ability to be resilient.

Single-Parent Families

DESCRIPTION

Numerous circumstances lead to a single-parent household, including divorce, births to unmarried mothers, abandonment of the family by a parent, incarceration of a parent, or death of a parent. Being a single parent is often a difficult, challenging role. Approximately 40% of American families are headed by a single parent (Emery, 1997). The majority of single-parent households are headed by women. However, fathers raising children in single-parent households are a growing population.

INCIDENCE

The traditional two-parent family has gradually faded over the past few decades. The escalating divorce rate and the birth rate to unmarried mothers (a rate of 4 in 10 reported by the US Census Bureau in 1997) are two key factors. Incidence varies by racial and ethnic demographics; black and Hispanic children are more likely than white children to be members of single-parent households. Children living in single-parent households generally experience significantly lower standards of living and family income than children in two-parent households.

ASSESSMENT

Several key areas are important to assess when working with single parents and their children. They can be divided into parent- and child-related factors. Parent-related factors include

- The availability of emotional support from a social network such as extended family members, friends, or church and community groups
- The presence of financial difficulties and economic hardships, which are often major concerns
- Living situation and insurance coverage
- The availability and quality of child care for parents who must work
- Opportunities for the single parent to have a social life and relationships or personal time
- The emotional and physical well-being of the parent: the capacity to parent when exhausted or overwhelmed is problematic
- The ability of the parent to maintain consistency in discipline as well as a positive outlook and commitment to parenting (e.g., Does the parent have the energy and temperament to parent in a consistent fashion?)
- The availability of financial and emotional support from a noncustodial parent

Child-related factors to assess include

- The availability of emotional support from a social network such as extended family members and friends
- The role of the child in the family related

to his or her responsibilities to care for siblings and opportunities to participate in activities outside of home

- Relationships with custodial parent (e.g., Is the child the single parent's primary source of emotional support or contact?)
- Location of and relationship with the non-custodial parent
- The availability of opportunities to accomplish age-appropriate developmental tasks (e.g., child is doing well in school, has friends, and/or is participating in sports or club activities)
- Signs of problem behavior at school, home, or with social activities, or the presence of children in the home with special needs (e.g., developmental disability, cognitive delay, or chronic illness)

MANAGEMENT

Signs of exhaustion, depression, or being overwhelmed, burdened, or socially isolated in the parent signal the need for mental health intervention. Similar signs in children plus deviant behaviors, emotional adjustment problems, or school disciplinary, academic, or behavioral problems are indicators for mental health intervention. The type of referral depends on the nature of the problem, the severity of symptoms, and the continuance of symptoms or problems without signs of improvement. Referrals can include individual or family counseling with mental health practitioners. (See Management section under Divorce.) Social organizations such as Big Brothers and Big Sisters offer a supportive role model for children in single-parent families. Parents Without Partners is a national organization that offers social activities and support for single parents.

PATIENT EDUCATION AND PREVENTION

Several critical factors promote successful child rearing in single-parent homes (Tanner, 1995). They involve the availability of a social support network and positive communication patterns (Table 19-13). The NP should encourage the development of a social support network and

---

T A B L E   19-13

Significant Determinants for Successful Child Rearing in a Single-Parent Home

The presence of support persons in the child's life who can collaborate effectively with the single parent, who are able to develop quality relationships, and who are used by the parent as available support figures for the child

The capacity of a parent to communicate with his or her child in an open, direct, and understanding manner

The ability of the parent to recognize the child's need for and to provide social opportunities for enjoyment and accomplishment outside the home

The presence of a supportive person or relative for the parent

Economic well-being that is perceived as adequate to meet the family needs

Supportive adults who are concerned about the child, including school officials, teachers, and health-care providers

---

suggest community resources or give referrals to assist in parenting.

Remarriage: The Blended Family

DESCRIPTION

The blended family is a term used to describe family reorganization or reconstitution associated with divorce and remarriage. Because of past negative connotations of the term "stepfamily," blended family is the term that is currently used to describe these families.

INCIDENCE

The majority of women and men who divorce remarry. Children whose parents are divorced spend an average of 5 years in single-parent households. With remarriage, children become members of blended families. Blended families can present unique parenting challenges in family adaptation, cohesiveness, coping, and role relationships.

ASSESSMENT

The introduction of a stepparent and possibly stepsiblings can be beneficial for a child or can be a time of difficult adjustment. The majority of children within blended families gradually adjust well to their new family situations. However, role relationship problems do arise related to the special needs of reconstituted families. The NP must remember several important points when assisting blended families during times of transition or problems. They include the developmental stage of the children, the common psychosocial issues that these children experience, and characteristics of problem behaviors in blended families (Table 19–14).

MANAGEMENT

The goal of primary care interventions is to focus on fostering of positive parenting behaviors and protecting the development of the stepchild. A careful assessment of the behavioral concern should be done. Whether the family is given guidance and followed closely by the primary care provider or given a referral to mental health services depends on the presence of significant behavioral problems or pathology. NPs should investigate community services that assist blended families, such as a self-help group for stepparents or a parenting group. Written information about and telephone numbers of community resources should be maintained in a handbook or resource guide kept in the practice setting.

PATIENT EDUCATION AND PREVENTION

Premarriage counseling and guidance about coping with transition in a blended family should be explored with parents. Relationships develop and are created over time. Many children go on to develop strong and meaningful

T A B L E 19-14
Assessment of Children in Blended Families

DEVELOPMENTAL STAGE OF CHILD
Age and developmental stage of child greatly affect child's response to the remarriage and ability of child to cope with change and new family relationships
Early adolescence is often a time of greatest difficulty in adjustment to remarriage
A mother's subsequent pregnancy is often a time of increased frequency and intensity of problems with young children

COMMON ISSUES FOR CHILDREN IN BLENDED FAMILIES
Complex relationship with new family members
Altered relationships with own family members and possible feelings of betraying other biological parent or being torn between parents
Possible relocation and separation from family members and friends
Continued or new tensions between parents and tensions between stepparents; rivalries between parents and stepparents
Jealousy among stepsiblings
Establishing new family traditions and values
Continuing to respect earlier family history, traditions, and loyalties that may be in conflict with new family ties
Unrealistic expectations by child of stepparent
Unrealistic expectations of child by stepparent for instant love, respect, and obedience
Tensions within blended family household creating anxiety and fear of another family breakup

CHARACTERISTICS OF PROBLEM BEHAVIORS IN BLENDED FAMILIES
Problems can occur both at home and at school
Children in divorced and blended families experience more behavioral, social, emotional, and educational problems than do children from nondivorced families
Parental conflict more than family structure is the critical factor that influences both marital and family adjustment

attachments to their stepparents if the relationship is cultivated over time with careful sensitivity to the needs of the child.

Adoption

DESCRIPTION

Adoption is the legal process that gives a child permanent family membership. Birth parents terminate their rights, and the adoptive parents are awarded legal custody. The adoption process has changed greatly in the past two decades from that of the traditionally married couple adopting a newborn. Single-parent adoption; subsidized adoption of children with special needs; independent, identified, and international adoptions; surrogacy arrangements; and open adoptions are examples of the changing pattern of adoption. Public and private agencies, independent adoption through attorneys, and foreign adoption services are potential avenues to assist in the placement of children.

INCIDENCE

Since 1975, there have been no federal agencies or nonprofit organizations that collect data on the annual number of total adoptions in the United States. Statistics are kept on the adoption of foster children. It is known that adoption rates have declined markedly over the past 20 years as more unwed women elect to keep their babies and not place them for adoption. Adoption of children from minority backgrounds continues to be a problem because of the limited availability of adoptive parents of the same race or ethnic group.

ASSESSMENT

Important information that the NP should attempt to ascertain when assisting adoptive families includes the following:

Legal Arrangements and Circumstances Surrounding Adoption Process

- What, if any, contact will the birth parent or parents have with the child?

- When will the adoption be finalized? How long is the waiting period?
- Are there support services available for the adoptive family if an agency is arranging the adoption?

Knowledge of Medical and Psychosocial History of Birth Parents and Child

- Was the presence of any inherited diseases or mental illnesses reported about the birth parents? Does the child have any known or suspected medical problems?
- Is information about the pregnancy, delivery, and neonatal period or subsequent medical problems available?
- Children adopted from foreign countries can be at risk for medical problems. Routine recommended screening tests are outlined in Table 19–15.

Availability of Social Supports for Adoptive Parents and Older Child

The presence of a social support network is important. Adoptive parents face the same parenting challenges as biological parents do when their child passes through the various developmental stages of childhood. In addition,

---

T A B L E   19-15

Recommended Screening Tests for Children Adopted From Foreign Countries

Complete blood count and differential, platelet count, and indices
Hemoglobin electrophoresis and G6PD screening
Hepatitis B panel, HIV, and RPR
Urinalysis, tuberculosis skin test, lead level, and stool for ova and parasites
If a young infant, standard newborn screening
Thyroid function test (if not done as part of newborn screen)
Developmental, dental, hearing, and vision screening (Barnett & Miller, 1996)

G6PD = glucose-6-phosphate deficiency; HIV = human immunodeficiency virus; RPR = rapid plasma reagin.

adoption is a special circumstance and can present special challenges to parents.

MANAGEMENT

Close monitoring and support by the NP during the initial adoption period are important. Scheduling of additional or more frequent health supervision visits is appropriate if high-risk situations or conditions are identified. If problems arise, prompt referral to mental health or social service agencies is imperative. Children with known special needs who are adopted are often eligible for federal and state financial support and services. Excellent books about adoption for adults and children are available in local bookstores. The NP should select and recommend those books that best fit the needs of the parents and children in the practice.

PATIENT EDUCATION AND PREVENTION

In considering adoption, the parent or parents often benefit from a preadoption visit to the health-care provider who will take care of their child. Parents often have many questions to ask about the initial adoption period and the establishment of a family relationship. Adoption is a lifetime commitment. Issues that the NP should address with parents include the following:

- There should be a gradual disclosure of the adoption to the child.
- Discussions of the adoption should be open, keeping in mind the child's developmental stage, cognitive abilities, and emotional needs.
- Discussions with the parents should address any myths, concerns, or fears that the parents might have about adoption and their adopted child.

Other issues that often arise in the family include the following:

- Parents need to understand that their child's wish to know about or seek out the biological parents is not a rejection of them.

- The adolescent years can be difficult for adoptive children as they seek their own identity and deal with the fact that they are adopted.
- If teenagers wish to seek out their biological parents, they should be encouraged to wait until they are older.

Teenage Parents

DESCRIPTION

Teens who become pregnant and give birth face the challenge of raising an infant at a period in their lives when they are seeking to learn who they are and what they are about. The phrase often used to describe teen mothers is "children having children." Adolescent pregnancy is linked with poor educational and vocational outcomes for the mother, which, in turn, is associated with socioeconomic disadvantage. Yet, there are teens who can successfully parent their infant if given support. Maternal age is an important predictor of successful parenting; however, pre-existing family and individual factors that lead a teenager to become a mother before completing the educational and developmental tasks necessary for adult life are the more relevant predictors of successful parenting. Cultural and racial variables also play a role in teen motherhood (Stevens-Simon & McAnarney, 1997; Kohlenberg, 1995).

INCIDENCE

In 1996, the birth rate for teenagers was 54.7 live births per 1000 women aged 15 to 19 years. The teen birth rate recently has been declining (National Vital Statistics System, 1998).

ASSESSMENT

Key issues to address in assessment of at-risk status vary depending on the stage of the teen: prepregnancy, pregnancy, birth and postpartum period, infancy, and later years. Assessment issues related to each of these stages are separately addressed.

Prepregnancy Issues

Adolescent sexuality is an issue that should be discussed as a routine part of every health care encounter (see Chapter 20). Early identification and targeting of at-risk teens (both female and male) for intervention is an important role of the NP. Predictors of teen motherhood include the following:

- Sexual molestation as a child
- Abuse or neglect in childhood
- Being a child of an addicted parent or family history of mental illness
- Lack of family involvement; an intolerable home situation
- Poor academic achievement or school dropout
- Loss of a parent by death, separation, divorce, or foster placement
- Living in an impoverished social environment where adolescent pregnancy is commonplace and accepted

Pregnancy

- Disclosure of pregnancy to family, the baby's father, peers, or other significant people. Who has the teen told about the pregnancy and are they supportive? Many teens and their families are in turmoil during the pregnancy.
- Access to prenatal care and compliance with pregnancy health supervision. Does the teen need to access federal- and state-sponsored programs for medical financial coverage and general assistance?
- Adjustment to the emotional and physical changes of pregnancy.
- Preparation and plans for the delivery and after the baby is born: current living arrangements; plans for future living and child-care arrangements, returning to school or work, and financial support.

Birth and Postpartum

- Preparation for childbirth and postpartum care.
- Identify who is available to give emotional support and physical help at this critical time.

Infancy

- Time of major transition: A teen mother may lack confidence to take care of an infant or be more interested in reestablishing her adolescent lifestyle. Monitor to determine whether the teen develops a growing sense of competence and pride in her ability to care for her baby.
- Adolescent mother–infant attachment: Is there evidence of emotional, general, or physical neglect?
- Living arrangements: With whom and where are the teen mother and baby living?
- Plans for birth control.
- Degree of involvement of the social support network in the mother's and infant's life: Is the baby's father invested in the child? Is the teen mother's or father's family supportive, overprotective, or not involved?
- Return to school or the work force: What are the child-care arrangements? How has this affected the teen mother and baby?
- Conflicts between the teen's needs and those of her infant.

Later Years

Toddler years are challenging, particularly for teens who themselves are survivors of abuse or neglectful parenting. Typically, the teen mother and young child, if living with family, move out on their own or with the mother's partner.

The NP needs to assess

- Mother's ability to cope with the normal inquisitive and provocative behaviors of her toddler
- How well the family unit is functioning
- Progress made by the mother toward reaching her life goals

As the child gets older, the teen mother is thought of as a young mother. Studies have shown that the children of these mothers, especially those who are poor and living in urban settings, are more likely than their peers to have behavioral problems. When their own children are adolescents, they find this a difficult period, and often they become young grandmothers as the teen pregnancy circle is perpetuated (Kohlenberg, 1995).

MANAGEMENT

Key points in management include the following:

1. Maintain regular and frequent contact with the teen mother during her pregnancy and during the child's infancy and early childhood.
2. Remember that both the teen mother and the infant or child have their own separate needs for health supervision and guidance.
3. Provide a supportive environment for the teen mother. Have a plan for follow-up so that teen mothers do not get lost in the system.
4. Provide referrals for resources and community agencies that can assist teen mothers (e.g., parenting classes or literature; support groups; special clinic programs that see both infants and teen mothers; Women, Infants, and Children [WIC] Program).
5. Involve other family members (e.g., grandparents, the father) in discussions about child-rearing issues depending upon the teen's wishes.
6. Emphasize the strengths of the teen mother and praise her positive efforts.
7. Intervene early when warning signs of potential neglect or abuse are evident.

Other Variations in the Family Unit

Other variations in the family unit that reflect changes in American family life and the diversity in experiences of parental structures include households in which children live with grandparents or extended family members, foster parents, homosexual parents, or two parental figures who are not married. Each of these situations is unique and requires a thorough assessment. Key issues to consider when working with these families follow.

CHILDREN LIVING WITH GRANDPARENTS OR EXTENDED FAMILY MEMBERS

- Often, children have lived with one or two biological parents before either voluntary

or court-ordered placement with relatives. Such children frequently bring with them a history of significant stress, hardship, and emotional turmoil.
- Children can be involved in continuing conflict with their biological parent or parents and may experience emotional reaction to separation from or abandonment by the parent or parents.
- Children can experience the loss of friends, schoolmates, and familiar surroundings.
- Caring for children can be an overwhelming responsibility, especially for older relatives or grandparents; the parenting experience can be physically, emotionally, and financially draining on relatives. In 1997, the number of children living with grandparents was 3.9 million, or 5.5% of children (US Bureau of the Census, 1998).
- Children need a supportive environment and consistency in discipline.
- Such families need significant support from social service agencies, the educational system, and health-care providers.

CHILDREN LIVING IN FOSTER OR GROUP HOMES

- Children are generally placed in protective custody because of concerns of neglect, physical abuse, sexual abuse, or other forms of child maltreatment or because of their parents' inability to care for them.
- Children frequently have a history of significant stress, hardship, and emotional turmoil in their family life.
- Children can experience multiple placements and separation from siblings.
- Children in foster homes are rapidly increasing in numbers, and meeting their psychosocial needs is an escalating problem in the United States. More than 382,000 children were reported to be in foster care placement in 1997 (US Bureau of the Census, 1998).
- Foster children are often involved in family reunification programs and are placed back with their parents under the supervision of the child protective services, with home-based family preservation services available

to monitor the situation, assist the parents, and safeguard the children.

- Foster children are placed under legal mandates in foster homes that mirror the children's ethnic, racial, and cultural identities as much as feasible.
- Foster children often receive erratic health care before and after their placement; a medical passport should be used as a means to keep track of medical problems, treatments, and special needs.
- Foster children have special needs, should be followed closely, and should receive preventive health services.
- Children are emancipated from the foster care system at age 18 years and need to be prepared for this major life change.

CHILDREN LIVING WITH HOMOSEXUAL PARENTS

- Children living with homosexual parents can be the "biological products" of former heterosexual relationships, or they may have been adopted, or conceived by artificial technology. Perrin (1998) reports that between 6 and 10 million children are currently living with one parent who is lesbian or gay. These families reflect every ethnic, racial, and socioeconomic group in the United States.
- Children can experience problems because of teasing or social isolation and stigmatization by peers, secrecy of parents, or negative reaction of the noncustodial biological parents (Gershon, 1995).
- Children do well if parents are committed to their children, are sensitive to the children's needs, and are patient.
- Children do well if the homosexual stepparent is supportive of the other parent and the child or children. Some states allow adoption by the nonbiological parent; this is called co-parent adoption.
- Children find it easier to deal with questions posed about their parents if they learn about their parents' sexual orientation during childhood rather than during adolescence.
- Children are not at risk to develop a homo-

sexual identity based on their living situation.
- Children of homosexual parents show no significant differences in their emotional and social adaptation, self-esteem, gender identity, sexual behavior, or sexual orientation than their counterparts raised with heterosexual parents (Perrin, 1998).

CHILDREN LIVING WITH TWO PARENTAL FIGURES WHO ARE UNMARRIED

- Children can be the biological children of two adults who decide not to marry but live together, the biological children of one of the adults but not the other, or children who live with their guardian and the guardian's unmarried partner.
- Such children face significant developmental risks if they sense a lack of permanence or uncertainty in the relationship between the two adults or if there is major conflict in the relationship between these adults.
- Children can be torn emotionally if other significant adults in the children's lives (other biological parents, grandparents, or other extended family members) express distress about the relationship between the unmarried adults.
- Children can experience turmoil in their lives if their family life is characterized by conflict, inconsistency in who lives in the home, frequent breakups, new adult relationships, or frequent changes in living arrangements.

In each of these family situations, consistency in discipline, a continued commitment to the child, and the development of a quality parent–child relationship are the hallmarks of successful parenting and child rearing. The NP is in a unique role to identify and support the development of healthy parenting strategies.

HOMELESS CHILDREN AND THEIR FAMILIES

The homeless family and homeless children are an increasing special-need population. A survey conducted in 29 US cities in 1997 found that 25% of the homeless population were children. In 1997, there were approximately 400,000 homeless families in the United States (National Coalition for the Homeless, 1998). Characteristics of these children include:

- A significant minority representation, with the majority of these children being younger than 5 years of age
- A teen population composed of runaway and "throwaway" adolescents who are often victims of physical and sexual abuse and neglect, or teens alienated from their parents for multiple reasons (e.g., homosexual youth)
- Living in poverty because of parental job layoff, substance abuse, domestic violence, mental illness, or unexpected family or economic crisis
- Living in a variety of environments, such as a car, motel, makeshift shelters of cardboard or tents, or homeless shelters
- Three times more likely to be placed in remedial classes in school and to become school dropouts (National Coalition for the Homeless, 1998)

Health care problems for which these children are at high risk include the following:

- Early initiation of and sustained substance abuse
- Diseases linked to poverty, including tuberculosis, multiple caries, impetigo
- STDs for runaway teens who prostitute themselves

Homeless children face many emotional health problems. Those who attend school may be ostracized by other children because of their unkempt appearance, poor hygiene, or substandard living conditions. Many experience social isolation because they are not in places (such as schools) where they can interact with peers.

PARENTING STRATEGIES

Regardless of the type of family unit, the role of a parent or caregiver is often challenging. Positive parenting strategies can help promote a relationship between the child or adolescent and parent that is based on mutual support, love, trust, and respect. To build a positive relationship, parents should:

- Encourage positive behaviors by paying attention to and praising good behavior. Be observant for times when their child or teen shows good behavior or acts responsibly and praise this behavior.
- Try to understand why their child or teen acts in a certain way, such as feeling hurt, disappointed, sad, angry, fearful, or needing attention.
- Act the way they want their child or teen to act by responding in a loving and helpful manner.
- Discuss feelings with their child or teen—their own and their child's or teen's feelings—especially when upset or angry.
- Set clear rules for safety—rules vary depending on the child's developmental stage.
- Establish routines for family life (e.g., for sleeping and eating; curfews, watching television, doing homework).
- Make sure that the child or teen knows which behaviors are acceptable and which are not; set clear standards of behaviors.
- Establish fair rules (e.g., do not discipline a child for something that he or she cannot help, such as vomiting, or for normal behaviors, such as thumbsucking).
- Be consistent in following rules and family routines.
- Respond every time the child or teen does something wrong by explaining what rules were broken and why the rules are important.
- Have as few rules as possible, make sure that the rules are simple, repeat the rules as often as necessary, and have reasonable consequences or sanctions.
- Set boundaries and define acceptable behavior.
- Encourage good behavior by giving hugs, kisses, smiles, and verbal feedback; provide a warm, responsive, cohesive family environment.
- Listen to, talk with, and spend special time with the child or teen.
- Give children reasonable choices and responsibilities within the home setting.

- Have realistic expectations for the child or teen and their role as a parent; being the super parent or a super child or teen is an unrealistic expectation.
- Work on being a positive thinker and enjoying life.
- Laugh at themselves and at situations, and promote the child or teen's sense of humor.
- Have brainstorming discussions with children or teens and discuss healthy lifestyle choices.
- Help children or teens to identify ways to express anger in a healthy way.

OTHER CHALLENGES IN THE FAMILY UNIT

Sibling rivalry and multiple births are two challenges to the family unit that can cause a period of disequilibrium. Sibling rivalry is a familiar problem, with tales of sibling rivalry recorded in early historical writings. With advances in reproductive technology and the use of fertility drugs, multiple births of two or more infants are much more common, particularly to women older than 30 years of age.

Sibling Rivalry at the Birth of a New Sibling and Between Other Children

The birth of a younger sibling is often an occasion marked by some degree of unrest and distress for an older sibling. Sibling jealousy or rivalry is dreaded by parents who frequently voice concern about the possibility of transient behavioral regressions occurring after the new infant is brought home from the hospital. The developmental stage of the older sibling at the time of the new sibling's birth is an important consideration in helping parents prepare their older sibling for the new arrival and in dealing with rivalry behaviors afterward. For example, the 2-year-old who is working on developing autonomy often feels very vulnerable with the appearance of a new sibling. However, many school-age children also experience feelings of sibling rivalry with the birth of an infant, and

this sibling rivalry may continue in varying degrees as the children grow and develop.

Parents often seek guidance about dealing with regressive behaviors and jealous feelings exhibited by older siblings after the birth of a new child. Anticipatory guidance about this common challenge is critical. The NP needs to prepare parents before the birth of the new sibling for the possibility of sibling rivalry and to guide them in managing this situation.

Birth of a New Infant

ASSESSMENT

The following key issues to discuss with parents about sibling rivalry after the birth of a new infant are whether the older child has:

- Manifested regressive behaviors since the birth (e.g., bed wetting, return to the bottle, temper tantrums); and, if so, what they are
- Made negative comments about the new sibling or become more demanding of the parent
- Voiced psychosomatic complaints

In addition, the NP should ask the parent to describe how he or she has reacted to the older sibling's behaviors or verbal comments and if and how they have disciplined the child.

Sibling Rivalry Between Older Children

ASSESSMENT

To assess sibling rivalry, ask parents to do the following:

- Describe sibling behaviors that concern them—fighting, verbal abuse, bickering.
- Identify any precipitating events or situations that seem to elicit negative behaviors between the siblings.
- Identify how rivalry behaviors between siblings were handled in the past.

MANAGEMENT

Management strategies include the following:

1. Explain to parents that sibling rivalry is a common, probably universal response of

older siblings at the time of the birth of a younger sibling and does continue throughout childhood.

2. Help parents plan ways to spend special time with the older sibling; suggest ways that parents can support their older child so that he or she feels appreciated and valued. Plan to do simple activities around the house or amusing outdoor activities (e.g., going to the park).

3. Explain the need for tolerance when a child younger than 4 years exhibits regressive behaviors such as toileting accidents, wanting the bottle or pacifier again, willful destruction of toys, books, or valuables, or temper tantrums.

4. Reassure the parents that regressive behavior associated with the birth of a new sibling is not a reflection of poor parenting.

5. Educate parents about teaching children to distinguish between acceptable and unacceptable behaviors (see Parenting Strategies).

6. Emphasize the need to see the individuality of each child and his or her uniqueness.

7. See Table 19–16 for additional suggestions for parents.

Multiple Births

There are several important points to cover in anticipatory guidance for parents who experience multiple births. Characteristically, these children:

- Often develop a special sibling relationship marked by loyalty and cooperative play
- Have periods in which they get along well or quarrel with each other just as other siblings do
- Work out relationships among themselves and function more independently, needing less parental attention
- May develop their own language among themselves as young children
- Display sibling rivalry, especially if they are fraternal rather than identical twins

Advise parents who have multiple births to do the following:

- Organize the home for daily activities and plan ahead to have sufficient supplies such as bottles, diapers, and car seats

---

T A B L E 19-16

Clues for Parents for Coping With Rivalry Between Siblings

DO

Allow children to vent negative feelings
Encourage children to develop solutions
Anticipate problem situations
Foster individuality in each child
Spend time with children individually
Compliment children when they are playing together
Tell children about the conflict you had with your siblings when you were children
Define acceptable and unacceptable behaviors

DON'T

Take sides
Serve as a referee
Foster rivalry by comparing siblings or their accomplishments
Use derogatory names
Permit physical or verbal abuse between siblings

From Berkowitz CD: Sibling rivalry. *In* Berkowitz CD (ed): Pediatrics: A Primary Care Approach. Philadelphia, WB Saunders, 1996, p 98.

- Schedule daily activities to accomplish all that needs to be done—this is crucial.
- Breastfeed if possible. Twins can be breastfed at the same time or one right after the other. Develop a plan to rotate breastfeeding if the mother has more than two infants.
- Take time out for themselves and as a couple.
- Keep a sense of humor.
- Promote individuation of each child (e.g., discipline and praise as individuals, build a one-to-one relationship with each child).
- Seek out support people to help (e.g., enlist the aid of extended family members) during early infancy when the tasks of physically caring for multiple infants can be overwhelming.
- Contact support groups such as The National Organization of Mothers of Twins Clubs, Inc. (See Resource Box.)
- If an older sibling or siblings are in the family, be cognizant of their needs and feelings during this time of major family

T A B L E 19-17

Guidelines for Selecting a Child-Care Provider: A Four-Step Approach

STEP 1: INTERVIEW POTENTIAL CHILD-CARE PROVIDERS AND OBSERVE THE PROGRAM OR SETTING
Ask questions about
1. Cost—cost calculation per hour, daily, weekly, monthly; any late fees; policy about fee structure and rules (e.g., if the child is absent)
2. Enrollment—number of children enrolled in the program, the maximum daily capacity of setting
3. Child factors—age of the children served in the setting/program
4. Daily activities or program plan—structured vs. unstructured activities
5. Accreditation and licensing regulations related to the provider or setting; review copy of any license or certificate
6. Caretaker issues—credentials and/or experience (e.g., academic degrees, course, cardiopulmonary resuscitation certification)
7. Policies—open visiting, illness in the child, emergency care, nutrition and feeding policies
8. Preventable illness prevention—immunization requirements for child and staff

Carefully observe the environment
1. Look at provider–child interactions—check for evidence of nurturing, responsive, comforting interactions
2. Look at safety issues of the physical environment—the play areas, toileting and diaper changing areas, outdoor environment, napping and eating areas
3. Assess the quality of the learning materials and/or toys (from an educational and safety perspective)

STEP 2: CHECK REFERENCES
1. Talk to parents with children enrolled in the program or being cared for by the provider; ask about their experience relative to how the providers handled the care (discipline) and whether they were nurturing and responsive to parents as well as the child; ask about reliability and consistency of the providers.
2. Talk to local child-care resource and referral program or licensing office; Child Care Aware (800) 424-2246 provides information about the nearest child-care resource and referral programs

STEP 3: MAKE A DECISION BASED ON SPECIFIC CRITERIA
1. The child will be happy with this care provider and have a safe, nurturing, and developmentally appropriate environment
2. If the child has special needs, these will be met
3. The values of the provider and parents are compatible
4. The child care is affordable

STEP 4: BE AN INVOLVED PARENT
1. Regularly talk to the provider about how the child is doing
2. Talk to the child daily about activities and experiences at the facility
3. If possible, visit the setting unannounced and observe at various times of the day
4. Communicate with other parents and become involved in child-care events as much as possible

From US Department of Health and Human Services Administration for Children and Families. March 1999. (http://www.acf.dhhs.gov/programs/ccb/faq/4steps.htm)

RESOURCE BOX 19-1

NATIONAL RESOURCES FOR ROLE RELATIONSHIP PROBLEMS

General Information
Check local telephone book for the following organizations:
  Big Brothers and Sisters
  Daughters and Sons United
  Parents Anonymous
  Parents Without Partners

American Professional Society on the Abuse of Children
Tel: (312) 554–0166
Website: www.apsac.org

Center to Prevent Handgun Violence
Tel: (202) 289–7310
Website: www.handguncontrol.org

Child Care Aware
Tel: (202) 393–5501 x111
(800) 424–2246
Website: www.childcarerr.org

Kempe Children's Foundation
Tel: (303) 864–5300 x5250

National Adoption Center
1500 Walnut St., Suite 701
Philadelphia, PA 19106

National Clearinghouse of Child Abuse and Neglect Information
Dept. Health and Human Services (DHHS)
Tel: (800) 394–3366
Website: www.calib.com/nccanch/

National Committee for Prevention of Child Abuse
Tel: (312) 663–3520
Website: www.childabuse.org

National Organization of Mothers of Twins Club, Inc.
Tel: (616) 595–0936
(877) 540–2200
Website: www.nomotc.org

National Organization of Single Mothers, Inc.
Midland, NC 28107

National Resource Center on Child Sexual Abuse
Tel: (205) 534–6868
(800) 543–7006

National Resource Center for Health and Safety in Child Care
Tel: (800) 598–KIDS
Website: http://nrc.uchsc.edu

North American Council on Adoptable Children (NACAC)
Tel: (651) 644-3036
Fax: (651) 644-9848
E-mail: NACAC@aol.com

Stepfamily Association of America, Inc.
Tel: (402) 477–7837
(800) 735–0329

NURSING DIAGNOSIS 19-1

NURSING DIAGNOSES FOR ROLE RELATIONSHIPS FUNCTIONAL HEALTH PATTERN

Abuse (not a NANDA diagnosis)

Altered Role Performance

Altered Family Process: Alcoholism

Caregiver Role Strain

Impaired Verbal Communication

Ineffective Family Coping: Compromised

Ineffective Family Coping: Disabling

Family Coping: Potential for Growth

Family Process Alteration

Parenting Alteration

Risk for Altered Parent/Infant/Child Attachment

Parental Role Conflict

Impaired Social Interaction

Social Isolation

Risk for Loneliness

Source: North American Nursing Diagnosis Association: NANDA nursing diagnoses: Definitions and classification 1997–1998. Philadelphia, North American Nursing Diagnosis Association, 1996.

---

transition. Suggestions for strategies to handle this are discussed under the birth of a new sibling.

CHILD CARE

Selecting a child-care provider and a setting that offers safe, nurturing, and developmentally appropriate child care are challenges for many parents. The individual needs of the child together with parental needs for work coverage and flexibility must be matched with the philosophy and constraints of the child-care setting. The NP is often called upon to advise parents about how to select a suitable provider. The Administration for Children and Families, US Department of Health and Human Services provides information to assist parents in this task (1999). The four-step approach outlined in Table 19-17 is recommended for parents to follow.

REFERENCES

American Academy of Pediatrics: Guidelines for the evaluation of sexual abuse of children. Pediatrics 87:254–260, 1991.

Barness LA: Failure to thrive. *In* Hoekelman RA, Friedman SB, Nelson NM, et al (eds): Primary Pediatric Care, 3rd ed. St. Louis, CV Mosby, 1997, pp 949–952.

Barnett ED, Miller LC: International adoption: The pediatrician's role. Contemp Pediatr 13(8):29–46, 1996.

Behrman RE, Kliegman RM: Nelson Essentials of Pediatrics, 3rd ed. Philadelphia, WB Saunders, 1998.

Berkowitz CD: Sibling rivalry. *In* Berkowitz CD (ed): A Primary Care Approach. Philadelphia, WB Saunders Company, 1996.

Brady MA: Educating youths and their parents about the prevention of handgun injuries. J Pediatr Health Care 8:127–129, 1994.

Brodeur AE, Monteleone JA: Child Maltreatment: A Clinical Guide and Reference. St. Louis, Mosby–Year Book, 1994.

Centers for Disease Control and Prevention: National Summary of Injury Mortality Data 1987–1994. Atlanta, GA, National Center for Injury Prevention and Control, 1996.

Centers for Disease Control and Prevention: Deaths and Death Rates for the 10 Leading Causes of Death in Specified Age Groups: United States, Preliminary 1997. Atlanta, GA, National Center for Health Statistics, 1997.

Cohen BA: Pediatric dermatology: What's your DX? Contemp Pediatr 16:35-36, 1999.

Daro DA: Prevention of child sexual abuse. The Future of Children: Sexual Abuse of Children. 4(2):198-223, 1994.

Emery RE: Children of divorce. *In* Hoekelman RA, Friedman SB, Nelson NM, et al (eds): Primary Pediatric Care, 3rd ed. St. Louis, CV Mosby, 1997, pp 629-631.

Foster SW, Pascoe JM: *In* Parker S, Zuckerman B (eds): Behavioral and Developmental Pediatrics: A Handbook of Primary Care. Boston, Little, Brown, 1995, pp 359-362.

Fox JA: Trends in Juvenile Violence: A Report to the United States Attorney General on Current and Future Rates of Juvenile Offending. Washington, DC, US Department of Justice, Bureau of Justice Statistics, 1996.

Frank D: Failure to thrive. *In* Parker S, Zuckerman B (eds): Behavioral and Developmental Pediatrics: A Handbook of Primary Care. Boston, Little, Brown, 1995, pp 134-139.

Friedman MM: Family Nursing: Theory and Practice, 3rd ed. Norwalk, CT, Appleton & Lange, 1992.

Gershon T: Lesbian and gay parents. *In* Parker S, Zuckerman B (eds): Behavioral and Developmental Pediatrics: A Handbook of Primary Care. Boston: Little, Brown, 1995, pp 371-373.

Ginsburg KR: Guiding adolescents away from violence. Contemp Pediatr 14(1):101-111, 1997.

Heger A, Emans SJ: Evaluation of the Sexually Abused Child: A Medical Textbook and Photographic Atlas. New York, Oxford University Press, 1992.

Kohlenberg TM: Teen mothers. *In* Parker S, Zuckerman B (eds): Behavioral and Developmental Pediatrics: A Handbook of Primary Care. Boston, Little, Brown, 1995, pp 396-401.

Krugman SD, Wissow LS, Krugman RD: Facing facts: Child abuse and pediatric practice. Contemp Pediatr 15(8):131-144, 1998.

Leventhal JM: Sexual abuse of children. *In* Hoekelman RA, Friedman SB, Nelson NM, et al (eds): Primary Pediatric Care, 3rd ed. St. Louis, CV Mosby, 1997, pp 651-656.

Melnyk BM, Alpert-Gillis LJ: Coping with marital separation: Smoothing the transition for parents and children. J Pediatr Health Care 11:165-174, 1997.

National Coalition for the Homeless: Fact Sheet: Homeless Families With Children. NHC Fact Sheet #7, May 1998.

National Vital Statistics System: Teenage Births in the United States: National and State Trends. 1990-1996. Public Health Service 98-1120, 4/30/98.

Perrin EC: Children whose parents are lesbian or gay. Contemp Pediatr 15(10):113-130, 1998.

Reece RM: Child Abuse: Medical Diagnosis and Management. Philadelphia, Lea & Febiger, 1994.

Region X Nursing Network: Region X Nursing Network Prenatal and Child Health Screening and Assessment Manual: Pregnancy and Birth to 36 Months. Seattle, University of Washington, 1998.

Snyder HN, Sickmund M, Poe-Yamagata E: Juvenile Offenders and Victims: 1996 Update on Violence. Washington, DC, US Department of Justice, Bureau of Justice Statistics, 1996.

Stevens-Simon C, McAnarney ER: Adolescent pregnancy and parenthood. *In* Hoekelman RA, Friedman SB, Nelson NM, et al (eds): Primary Pediatric Care, 3rd ed. St. Louis, CV Mosby, 1997, pp 834-839.

Tanner JL: Single parents. *In* Parker S, Zuckerman B (eds): Behavioral and Developmental Pediatrics: A Handbook of Primary Care. Boston, Little, Brown, 1995, pp 387-390.

US Bureau of the Census. Co-resident grandparents and their grandchildren: Grandparent maintained families. Washington, DC: Population Division Working paper No. 26, March, 1998.

US Census Bureau: Marital status and living arrangements. Current Population Survey Updates. Washington, DC, US Government Printing Office, 1997.

US Department of Health and Human Services. Healthy People 2000: National Health Promotion and Disease Prevention Objectives for the Year 2000. Washington, DC, US Government Printing Office, 1991.

US Department of Health and Human Services. Child Maltreatment 1996 Reports from the States to the National Child Abuse and Neglect Data System. Washington, DC, US Government Printing Office, 1998.

US Department of Health and Human Services, Administration for Children and Families. March, 1999. (http://www.acf.dhhs.gov/programs/ccb/faq/4steps.htm)

Wallerstein JS: Children of divorce: The psychological tasks of the child. Am J Orthopsychiatry 53:230-243, 1983.

Wallerstein JS: Separation, divorce and remarriage. *In* Levine MD, Carey WB, Crocker AC (eds): Developmental-Behavioral Pediatrics, 2nd ed. Philadelphia, WB Saunders, 1992, pp 136-146.

Wang CT, Daro D: Current Trends in Child Abuse Reporting and Fatalities: The Results of the 1997 Annual Fifty State Survey. Denver, CO: American Humane Association, 1998.

CHAPTER 20

Sexuality

Ardys M. Dunn and Jeanette M. Broering

INTRODUCTION

Sexuality is an integral part of the human experience for people of all ages and lifestyles. The sexual health of patients, therefore, must be a consideration for the primary care provider. In order to provide comprehensive primary health care, nurse practitioners (NPs) must understand how variations in health status relate to an individual's sexuality, assess an individual's sexual functioning and concerns as a part of health status, and make appropriate decisions for anticipatory guidance, intervention, or referral to resources. Much of the literature on sexuality deals with problems. This chapter focuses on health promotion, emphasizing that sexual development is a necessary and healthy part of human growth.

STANDARDS

The Region X Nursing Network's (1998) goal related to childhood sexuality is that "the child develops age-appropriate sexuality." For the infant and child, outcomes involved in meeting this goal are the following:

- There will be supports in the environment to promote positive feelings and healthy development of sexuality and reproductive health.

- The child is knowledgeable and has access to information about human sexuality and reproduction as expected for age or cognitive development.
- The child has positive feelings about his or her own gender and that of others.

For adolescents, outcomes are that the individual:

- Has developed positive feelings and experiences satisfaction regarding his or her sexual identity
- Demonstrates responsible decision-making regarding sexual behavior and disease prevention
- Feels positive about sexual orientation of self and others

The *AMA Guidelines for Adolescent Preventive Services (GAPS)* recommends a comprehensive primary and secondary prevention strategy for promoting healthy adolescent psychosexual development and preventing the negative consequences of sexual behaviors (American Medical Association, 1997). This strategy includes the following:

- Health guidance to promote a better understanding of psychosexual development
- Health guidance regarding responsible sexual behaviors, including abstinence

- Latex condoms to prevent sexually transmitted diseases (STDs), including infection with human immunodeficiency virus (HIV), and appropriate methods of birth control with instructions on how to use them effectively
- Annual interviews about involvement in sexual behaviors that may result in unintended pregnancy and STDs, including HIV infection
- Screening sexually active adolescents for STDs
- Confidential HIV screening of adolescents at risk for HIV infections
- Annual screening of sexually active females or females older than 18 years for cervical cancer by use of a Papanicolaou (Pap) test
- Annual interviews about a history of emotional, physical, and sexual abuse
- Universal vaccination of adolescents for hepatitis B
  - Vaccinating all 11- to 12-year-olds for hepatitis B
  - Vaccinating older, unimmunized adolescents with identified risk factors for hepatitis B infection
  - Widespread use of hepatitis B vaccination because risk factors are not always easily identifiable among adolescents

NORMAL PATTERNS OF SEXUALITY

Definition of Sexuality, Sexual Health, and Sexual Identity

Parents, children, and adolescents have a right to information, education, and health care services that promote, maintain, and restore optimal sexual health. There is little consensus, however, regarding the scope of issues involved in the areas of sexuality and sexual learning. This lack of consensus is exacerbated by the lack of clarity in terminology. The definitions presented herein form the basis for the following discussion of sexuality in children.

SEXUALITY

The term sexuality is imprecise, referring variously to the process of development, a dimension of personality, and an expression of behavior (Roberts, 1980). Sexuality has been defined by the Sex Information and Education Council in the United States (SIECUS) as encompassing "the sexual knowledge, beliefs, attitudes, values, and behaviors of individuals. It deals with anatomy, physiology, and biochemistry of the sexual response system; with roles, identity, and personality; with individual thoughts, feelings, behaviors, and relationships. It addresses ethical, spiritual, and moral concerns, and group and cultural variations" (Haffner, 1990).

SEXUAL HEALTH

Sexual health has been defined in a holistic perspective by the World Health Organization (1975) as the positive integration of somatic, emotional, intellectual, and social aspects of sexual being in ways that are positively enriching and that enhance personality, communication, and love. Sexual function, sexual self-concept, and sexual relationships are dimensions of sexual health.

Sexual function incorporates the biological component of the human sexual response cycle and refers to the ability to give and receive sexual pleasure. Sexual self-concept is the psychological component of sexuality, the image one has of oneself as a man or a woman, and the evaluation of one's adequacy in masculine and feminine roles. Sexual relationships refer to the social domain of sexuality and include the interpersonal relationships in which one's sexuality is shared with others.

SEXUAL IDENTITY

Sexual identity as a component of sexuality evolves over the life span of an individual and encompasses four elements: biosexual identity, gender identity, sex role identity, and sexual orientation:

1. Biosexual identity ("What sex am I?") is determined from conception and is based on chromosomes. Morphologically, by 12 weeks' gestation, the anatomy of the fetus' gender can be observed. Gender assignment occurs during ultrasonography or at birth with the pronouncement of "It's a girl!" or

"It's a boy!" From then, the process of gender role scripting begins.

2. Gender identity, or one's sexual self-concept, is the internal belief or sense of being male or female and is achieved in the toddler and preschool years.

3. Sex role identity ("How do I appear?") is characterized by the emergence of behaviors, attitudes, and feelings that are labeled as male, female, or neutral. This process begins at preschool age and continues into adulthood.

4. Sexual orientation ("Whom do I love?") refers to an individual's feelings of sexual attraction and erotic potential. Sexual orientation emerges over the life span, although it has been suggested that sexual attraction to one sex or the other is identified in late infancy and prepubertal childhood (Money, 1988).

Developmental Patterns of Sexuality

A full discussion of normal child development is found in Chapters 5 to 9. This section briefly emphasizes those components of development related to sexuality, especially those that are used in assessment of the child's health status (Table 20-1) (Smith, 1993).

INFANT

Newborn infants are reflexive beings, responding to their physical environment without hesitation or cognition. Sexual reflexes are present prenatally and are easily stimulated in the infant. It is not uncommon to observe a penile or clitoral erection in the nursing child, for example, and infants clearly enjoy the sensual feelings of warm water or air on their naked bodies. As infants mature, self-stimulation is a natural part of exploring their environment and most frequently begins between 6 and 12 months of age. The sexual meaning attributed to such spontaneous or reflexive behavior is absent for the infant.

Healthy parent–infant bonding requires physical contact as well as social interaction. Parents must hold, cuddle, stroke, talk to, look at, and respond to children if the children are to develop a sense of trust, upon which intimacy will be based in later years.

TODDLER AND PRESCHOOL CHILD

Toddlers are able to recognize and pronounce themselves as "I'm a girl" or "I'm a boy," but they can easily confuse gender in others and, sometimes, in themselves. Changing one's style of clothes, for example, can be perceived as a change in gender. Children cannot integrate gender identity into their self-concept until they understand that gender is a permanent condition, usually by age 3 or 4 years.

Children in this age group are extremely curious about their environment (including their own and other people's bodies); they love to explore and experiment. They have a cognitive awareness of the pleasure self-stimulation gives them and frequently masturbate, but, as with infants, they attribute no erotic or sexual meaning to their actions. The combination of curiosity and lack of self-consciousness characteristic of toddlers can contribute to embarrassing social incidents for their parents.

The ways in which parents communicate about sexuality are important for the toddler and preschooler. Because children at this age interpret statements so literally and have "magical" thinking, their understandings of the physical self can be distorted and lengthy explanations about body functions can be misunderstood. Parents should give children the message that they and their bodies—including its sexual parts— are valuable and important. Defining limits of appropriate and inappropriate behavior is also a parent's responsibility (e.g., it is not acceptable for a 3-year-old girl to discuss with a stranger on the bus the fact that she and her mother have "ginas" but her father and brother have penises). Clearly articulated limits help the child to better understand the social meanings given to sexuality.

SCHOOL-AGE CHILD

School-age children continue to have a high level of curiosity about sexuality, their bodies, and their environment and, aware of the pleasure stimulation gives, may actively seek sexual arousal. Masturbation and sex games are typical

T A B L E 20-1

Sexual Function, Self-Concept, and Relationships During Childhood Through Young Adulthood

	SEXUAL FUNCTION	SEXUAL SELF-CONCEPT	SEXUAL ROLE/RELATIONSHIP
Infancy	Orgasmic potential present Erectile function present	Gender identity reinforced Association of sexuality and good/bad Distinction between self and others	
Toddler	Genital pleasuring and exploration Sensual activity (e.g., hugging, stroking)	Core gender identity solidified by age 3 years	Sex role differences learned Discrimination between male and female role models Sexual vocabulary learned
Preschool	Sex play—exploration of own body and those of playmates Self-pleasuring (masturbation)		Sex roles learned Parental attachment and identification
School age		Curiosity about sex Sexual fears and fantasies Interest in aspects of sexual development Self-awareness as sexual being	Same-sex friends Off-color humor related to sexuality
Adolescence, prepubertal	Menarche (female) Seminal emissions (male)	Concerns about body image	Same-sex friends Sexual experiences as part of friendship
Adolescence, early	Awkwardness in first sexual encounter Masturbation, petting May or may not be sexually active	Anxiety over inadequacy, lack of partner, virginity	Appropriate sex friendships Dating
Adolescence, late	May or may not be sexually active	Responsibility for sexual activity	Intimacy in relationships learned
Young adult	Experimentation with sexual positions, expressions Exploration of techniques	Responsibility for sexual health, e.g., contraception, sexually transmitted disease prevention Development of adult sexual value system, tolerance for others	Giving and receiving pleasure learned Long-term commitment to relationship developed

(e.g., playing "house" or "hospital"), and both homosexual and heterosexual encounters are commonly seen. Older school-age children are less sexual in their behavior than younger children (Friedrich et al., 1991). Younger school-age children tend to be modest about body exposure and may react negatively to nudity in the home; older children can demonstrate a certain "sexual prudery" that may, it is suggested, be a mechanism used to deal with negative messages received about sexuality (Money, 1988).

By the time children reach school age, or about 8 years of age, they begin to understand the significance of sexuality. They have often learned that "good" children do not demonstrate sexual behavior, that questions about sex are "dirty." In response, their sexual activity can become secretive or silly, and, unless parents actively communicate with their children, sexual lessons will be learned from peers, the media, jokes, and movies. Parents and teachers are in key positions to teach children that their sexual curiosity and feelings are normal and to help both boys and girls better understand how sexual development is an integral part of growing up.

ADOLESCENT

Adolescence is a period of rapid physical, psychological, and social change that presents a developmental challenge to both children and parents. In terms of sexuality, adolescents fit their sense of sexual being into their evolving self-image and personal identity; they learn about their bodies' sensual and sexual responses to stimulation (sometimes quite unexpected and embarrassing), and they develop a sense of the moral significance of sexuality.

Privacy is essential for the adolescent to explore this emerging self, and activities such as group social functions, dating, participation in sports, and interactions at work and school provide opportunities to learn social and interpersonal skills of intimacy.

Learning how to communicate about sex, how to set limits, how to avoid misunderstandings, how to say yes or no, are important skills for adolescents. Equally important is the process of developing a set of sexual values. Whether the adolescent practices abstinence, has a double standard for men's and women's sexual behavior, or is exploitative or nurturing in close personal relationships is a reflection of the adolescent's sexual values.

ASSESSMENT OF NORMAL PATTERNS

Sexuality is an integral component of a child's development. Although for the majority of children the onset of the first sexual intercourse, or sexual debut, occurs in adolescence, sexual development, questions, and concerns are present throughout childhood.

Assessment of sexuality and sexual maturation should be integrated into the health history and physical examination at all health maintenance visits. Recent data suggest that adolescents are quite honest when responding to a self-report sexual questionnaire (Siegel, 1998).

History

FUNCTIONS OF THE SEXUAL HISTORY

The sexual history is designed to achieve several purposes. First, it is used to collect information. Second, by including it within the health history, permission is given to the child, adolescent, or parent to ask questions and receive reliable information regarding issues of sexual concern. Third, it allows the NP to incorporate sexuality-specific education as a normal component of anticipatory guidance (Laube, 1982).

TYPES OF SEXUAL HISTORIES

The sexual history can be either comprehensive or problem oriented. The comprehensive sexual history is detailed, encompassing all aspects of sexual information about individuals, their family of origin, siblings, and peer relationships. It includes information about each phase of sexual development, body image, masturbation, learned attitudes, feelings about sexuality, sexual debut, sexual orientation, and a range of sexual behaviors. A comprehensive history is lengthy and may not be accomplished at the first visit or in a single interview, because it can be anxiety-producing to have the client disclose such a level of detail during early visits, and clients can become fatigued by one lengthy interview.

In contrast, the problem-oriented sexual history usually focuses on the current complaint or assessment of specific behaviors such as the risk of exposure to pregnancy or the acquisition of STDs. Problem-oriented sexual histories are shorter, more direct, and specific to the issue at hand.

APPROACH TO TAKING A SEXUAL HISTORY

Sexual history-taking should be integrated as one part of the health history. In taking a sexual history, the interviewer should:

- Convey an aura of comfort with the client and respond to the client without embarrassment.
- Give appropriate, factual information.
- Create a nonjudgmental environment.
- Use language that validates the client's understanding of terms and concepts. For example, when talking with adolescents, the question "Are you sexually active?" can denote a meaning of current activity on a planned and regular basis. The adolescent who has concrete cognitive abilities may respond negatively. However, the question "Have you ever had sex or are you currently having sex?" allows for a more inclusive description of sexual activity.
- Use open-ended questions. For example, use of phrases such as "explain how that happened," "what happened next," or "tell me about a typical date" elicit more complete information than do close-ended questions. Questions that contain "why" can require a level of analysis beyond the capabilities of children operating at a concrete level of cognition.
- In the questioning process, move from the least to most sensitive information.

CONTENT OF A SEXUAL HISTORY

The content of a comprehensive adolescent sexual and reproductive history is contained in Table 20–2. Table 20–3 lists questions for a problem-oriented sexual history. Questions for parents about their children follow (Region X Nursing Network, 1998; Finan, 1997). As the child grows, questions can be reworded and asked directly of the child or adolescent. Questions and the answers to them should be age appropriate (e.g., an 8- to 10-year-old should have some awareness of sexually transmitted disease, but a 4-year-old would not; it would not be necessary to ask the parent of a 2-year-old if the child has a healthy awareness of alternate sexual preferences).

- Does your child have meaningful interactions with men and women who have positive self-images?
- Do you have positive feelings about your child's gender?
- Is your child aware of physical sexual differences between men and women?
- What does your child know about his or her body parts? Does he or she know the correct terminology for body parts?
- What does your child know about sexuality? About gender differences?
- What does your child know about how babies are born and cared for (e.g., pregnancy, childbirth, breastfeeding)?
- What does your child know about STDs and acquired immunodeficiency syndrome (AIDS)?
- Does your child (older than 8 years of age) have a healthy awareness of alternate sexual preferences?
- How do members of your family demonstrate affection?
- Does your child seek and receive positive touching from others?
- Does your child experience a variety of sensory stimuli?
- Does your child have friends (same or opposite sex)? In what types of interactions do they engage? Is exploration (e.g., masturbation, playing "doctor") occurring? How is it handled?
- How does your child express sexuality? In play? By touching? Verbally?
- What sorts of questions does your child ask about sex?
- How do you respond to your child's sexual behavior and questions?
- What do you know about human sexuality? What are your feelings and attitudes about it?
- Does the child's school provide appropriate information about sexuality and reproduction?
- Is your child at risk for sexual abuse?

Physical Examination

The physical examination serves to identify normal (and variations of normal) sexual anatomy, stage of sexual development (Tanner stages),

The Comprehensive Adolescent Sexual and Reproductive History

BACKGROUND DATA
Adolescent
  Age (birth date)
  Sex
  History of risky behaviors (e.g., drug history: onset,
    duration, and frequency of use of cigarettes,
    alcohol, other illicit drugs)
Parents
  Ages
  Religions
  Educational levels
  Occupations
  Marital status
  Affectional relationship (parent to parent)
  Child's feelings toward parent(s)

CHILDHOOD SEXUALITY
  What were your parents' attitudes about sexuality
    when you were a child?
  How did your parents handle nudity?
  When do you first recall seeing a nude person of the
    same sex? Opposite sex?
  Who taught you about sex, sex play, pregnancy,
    intercourse, masturbation, homosexuality, venereal
    disease, birth?
  How often did you play doctor–nurse or other sex
    play with another child?
  Tell me about any other sexual activity or experience
    that had a strong effect on you.

ADOLESCENT SEXUALITY
Girls
  Onset of breast development?
  When did pubic hair appear?
  Onset of menstruation (age, regularity of periods;
    initially, now)?
  When was your last normal menstrual period
    (LNMP)?
  What hygienic methods are used (pads, tampons)?
  How were you prepared for menstruation? By whom?
  What were feelings about early periods? Later
    periods?
  Have you had unusual bleeding or pains?
Boys
  How were you prepared for adolescence? By whom?
  Age of first orgasm (ejaculation)?
  What were "wet dreams" like? How did they make
    you feel?
  When did pubic hair appear?
Body image
  How do you feel about your body?
  What about your breasts, genitals?
  How much time do you spend nude in front of a
    mirror?
Masturbation
  How old were you when you began?
  What are others' reactions to your masturbation?
  What methods do you use?
  What are your feelings about it?

ADOLESCENT SEXUALITY Continued
Necking and petting
  How old were you when you began? How often?
  How many partners do you currently have?
Intercourse
  How often have you had intercourse?
  How many partners?
  How often do you initiate sex?
  How often do you currently have sex?
  How often have you had oral sex?
Contraceptive use
  What kinds of contraceptives have you used?
  What are you using now?
  Do you have any problems with contraceptives?
  Do you use condoms with a new partner?
  How do you communicate about contraception with
    your partner?
Homosexuality
  What does it mean to be a homosexual?
  How many homosexuals have you known?
  How often have you had homosexual feelings?
  How often have you been approached?
  How often have you had homosexual experiences?
    What kinds of experiences? What were the
    circumstances?
Seduction and rape
  When have you seduced someone sexually?
  When has someone seduced you?
  Have you been raped?
  Have you raped someone? How often have you
    forced someone to have sex?
Incest and abuse
  What kinds of touching did you receive in your home?
  From your mother? Father? Brother(s)? Sister(s)?
    Other relatives? Others?
Prostitution
  What feelings do you have about prostitution?
  Have you ever accepted money for sex?
  Have you ever had sex with a prostitute?
Sexually transmitted diseases (STDs)
  How old were you when you learned about STDs?
  Have you ever had an STD? Gonorrhea? Syphilis?
Pregnancy
  Have you ever been pregnant? At what age?
  How resolved—miscarriage, abortion, adoption,
    marriage, single parenthood?
  Have you caused a pregnancy?
Abortion
  What are your feelings about abortion?
  Have you (or a partner) had an abortion? If yes, at
    what age? What were your feelings?
  What about your feelings now? What about your
    feelings immediately afterward? What about your
    feelings after 1 year?

Adapted from Laube HH: The use of a sexual history with adolescents. *In* Blum RW (ed): Adolescent Health Care: Clinical Issues: New York, Academic Press, 1982.

T A B L E 20-3
Adolescent Sexual Problem History

Describe the sexual concern, problem, issue, or difficulty that you have.

How do you feel about discussing this problem?

How long have you had it? When did this problem begin?

What do you think caused you to have this problem?

What might be contributing to this problem?

What kinds of things have you done to treat or solve this problem?

What health professionals have you seen?

What, if any, medication have you taken or are you taking?

Have you talked to a friend or relative?

Have you read any books to solve this problem? What books?

Adapted from Laube HH: The use of a sexual history with adolescents. *In* Blum RW (ed): Adolescent Health Care: Clinical Issues. New York, Academic Press, 1982.

and pathology. The physical examination should include examination of the breasts, female genitalia and pelvis (in sexually active adolescents or when a pathology is suspected), male genitalia, and rectum, as indicated. Laboratory studies, including a Pap test, cultures or blood work for STDs, and genetic studies to determine gender are performed as indicated. Recent analysis of smears and cultures in more than 10,000 patients between 10 and 19 years of age found an unusually high level of infectious processes, leading researchers to stress the importance of "early cervical Pap smear screening in the sexually active pediatric and adolescent population" (Mount & Papillo, 1999). NPs are frequently asked to determine whether a child has been sexually abused. Knowing variations of normal genital anatomy is important in making this assessment (see Reece, 1994, for specific variations; also see Chapter 19 for discussion of sexual abuse in children).

The physical examination should be performed with care and sensitivity to the child's or adolescent's feelings. A girl's first gynecological examination can influence her attitude toward future gynecological care, and subsequent examinations can reinforce positive or negative feelings toward her body. Very young children and toddlers make no distinction between examination of external genitalia and other body parts; school-age children can be extremely modest, act embarrassed, and resist taking off their clothes for the examination. Older school-age children and adolescents can misinterpret the examination procedures and may feel violated or abused. By providing clear explanations of procedures, using straightforward techniques, and involving the child in the examination (e.g., asking if the child wishes to have the parent or another adult present), the NP can better achieve the fine balance necessary to perform a thorough, respectful examination (Kahn & Emans, 1999).

MANAGEMENT STRATEGIES OF NORMAL PATTERNS

The NP has two primary goals related to management of sexual development in children: to help children achieve healthy sexual identity and function and to provide support for parents to enable them to guide their children through the process of sexual development. By counseling parents about children's sexual development, both goals can be achieved. In particular, the NP must

- Assess the parent's level of understanding regarding normal physical and psychosocial sexual development in children.
- Provide or clarify information as needed.
- Provide strategies and support for teaching children about sexuality.
- Assist the parent to connect to community-based resources.

Setting the Stage

When working with children, the NP focuses on establishing and maintaining a positive relationship, based on mutual trust and respect, in which the child is validated and feels comfortable revealing concerns and asking questions. In addition to using a constructive approach to taking a sexual history (see earlier text), a positive relationship can be achieved by:

- Asking questions to give the message that the child is expected to be changing and is aware of and curious about those changes (e.g., "How are you feeling?" "How's your body?" "Do you notice that you're getting taller?").
- Asking questions to give the message that sexual changes are to be expected and are as normal as other body changes (e.g., "Have you noticed your breasts getting any bigger?" "Boys' penises begin to get longer and wider as they become teenagers. Have you noticed any changes in yours?").
- Asking questions to give the message that you care about the child's feelings (e.g., "How does that make you feel?" "Do you wonder sometimes about what's happening to your body?").
- Listening thoughtfully and carefully to the child's input.
- Responding positively by answering the child's questions as fully as possible and being nonjudgmental, calm, friendly, open, and having a sense of humor, yet taking the child seriously.
- Using growth charts to give the message that this child is special (e.g., explain the child's personal development, discuss what the numbers of height and weight mean).
- Utilizing appropriate teachable moments during the health visit. For example, when examining a 3-year-old for inguinal hernia, the NP can discuss appropriate and inappropriate touching with the child and his or her parent.
- Providing accurate information and referral resources as appropriate.
- Respecting the child's need for privacy (e.g., knocking before entering the examination room, providing appropriate gowns, examining the child semiclothed).
- Maintaining confidentiality as appropriate, especially with an adolescent; however, children of any age may give information that need not be shared with the parent.

Sex Education

For the child, developing healthy sexuality means gaining knowledge about physical changes, shaping a positive gender identity, clarifying one's sexual identity as a boy or a girl, establishing close, intimate relationships with others, and demonstrating the ability to make healthy judgments about sexuality and sexual activity. It is the parents' responsibility to facilitate this learning. Human sexuality, however, is an emotionally charged issue for many parents, and they can find it difficult to be comfortable with their child's normal, innocent curiosity about sex, gender, and body parts and functions. The questions a child asks and the behaviors displayed can embarrass some parents, who may respond in a manner that frightens, shames, or confuses the child. Each parental response helps shape the child's perception of sexuality:

> *Although we may not like it, children are born as sexual beings, and parents, whether or not they are aware of it, are constantly providing lessons in sex education. The way parents respond to a child's innate sexuality and allow it to unfold is the core of a child's sex education. This response does more to mold that child's mature sexual behavior than all the information or misinformation parents may provide*
> —*Ehrenberg & Ehrenberg, 1988.*

Parents should be encouraged to take advantage of teaching opportunities in normal childhood sexual play and to answer questions simply and directly, at the child's level of understanding (Table 20-4).

The content of sex education is controversial, but a comprehensive approach includes emphasis on human development, relationships, personal skill, sexual behavior, sexual health, and society and culture (SIECUS National Guidelines Taskforce, 1991) (Table 20-5).

In most states, schools have a responsibility to provide sex education to children. Curricula that address the content outlined in Table 20-5 have been shown to have a positive impact on adolescent sexual behavior. Use of the theory-based, sexuality education curriculum, Reducing the Risk, for example, appeared to contribute to a delay in initiating sexual intercourse, an increased use of protection against STDs and pregnancy by those who were sexually active, and an increase in parent–child communication on sexuality issues (Hubbard et al., 1998). The

T A B L E 20-4

Approaches to Teaching Your Child About Sex

Discuss sex in a matter-of-fact way.

Avoid lecturing about sex. Keep the topic short and to the point, remembering the child's attention span.

Include values, emotions, feelings, and decision-making in your discussion. Don't focus just on biological facts.

Don't worry about telling children too much about sex. They tune out what they don't understand.

When your child uses "four-letter words," calmly explain what they mean and why it is not appropriate to use them. Do not laugh or joke about your child's four-letter words because this can serve as encouragement.

Use correct terminology when talking about body parts.

Discuss anticipated changes of puberty before they occur. Don't wait until your child is a teenager.

Discuss menstruation with boys as well as with girls.

Be direct in bringing up topics of sexually transmitted diseases, including acquired immunodeficiency syndrome (AIDS).

Encourage questions. Never embarrass children or tell them they are too young to understand or that they will learn that when they grow up.

If you don't know the answer to your child's question, say so, and then look it up. Ask your nurse practitioner or other pediatric primary care provider.

Check with your child to be sure your answer is understood. Make sure you answer the question that is asked, and give your child a chance to ask more.

Adapted from Masters WH, Johnson VE, Kolodny RC: Human Sexuality, 5th ed. New York, HarperCollins College Publishers, 1995.

sex education curricula in most states, however, are not as comprehensive as the SIECUS guidelines and children may not be taught what they need to learn (SIECUS 1993; Klein et al., 1994; Haignere et al., 1999).

Contraception

CONTRACEPTIVE COUNSELING

For NPs to provide reproductive health and contraceptive services to adolescents requires significant and specific knowledge. An in-depth discussion is beyond the scope of this text; however, several excellent management references are available (Hatcher et al., 1998; Dickey, 1998). NPs who provide contraceptive counseling to adolescents should understand that the successful use of a contraceptive device requires a complex process of knowledge, decision-making skills, and public behaviors. To use contraceptives successfully, an individual must master the following:

Knowledge

The person must acquire, process, and retain accurate information regarding the specific methods of birth control under consideration. For most adolescents, this means mastery of a barrier method such as condoms, spermicides, or diaphragm to prevent an STD, as well as a variety of hormonal methods for contraceptive purposes.

Ability to Plan for the Future

Planning for the future requires self-admission that the adolescent will have sex in the future, as well as the ability to take the steps necessary to use a method consistently and correctly. Adolescents must be willing to use the chosen method of contraception consistently, not just when it is convenient to do so.

Willingness to Acquire Needed Contraceptives Publicly

The adolescent must be willing and able to be public with requests for contraceptives; for example, to purchase condoms at a local pharmacy or to seek services at the local clinic, school-based health facility, or private practice.

Communication Skills

Adolescents must have the ability to communicate with another person such as their partner, health care provider, or salesperson about birth control needs. Communication also involves adolescents' willingness and ability to articulate how they feel about sexual activity, how it affects them, and the thinking behind their decision to be sexually active. Successful

T A B L E 20-5

Comprehensive Sexuality Education

CONTENT AREA	EXAMPLES
• Human development	• Differences in anatomy between the sexes • Puberty, menstruation • Pregnancy and where babies come from
• Relationships	• Family values about sexuality • Dating • Respect for others and self • Respect for privacy
• Personal skill	• Communication • How to say no • How to be affectionate • Importance of responsible behavior • Judgment and decision-making • How to talk with parents about sexual questions
• Sexual behavior	• Appropriate limits on behavior • Abstinence • Masturbation • Sexual intercourse
• Sexual health	• Sexually transmitted diseases (STDs) • Mechanisms for contraception and prevention of STDs
• Society and culture	• Gender roles • Sexuality in the law and religion • Sexual diversity

Based on Sex Information and Education Council of the United States (SIECUS) National Guidelines Task Force: Guidelines for Comprehensive Sexuality Education: Kindergarten–12th Grade. New York, SIECUS, 1991.

communication with partners appears to contribute to safer sex practices (Cobb, 1997).

INITIAL SCREENING TO ASSESS FOR APPROPRIATE CONTRACEPTION

History

- Examine developmental maturity and cognitive status, chronological age, and the coexistence of other risk-taking behaviors.
- Obtain thorough personal and family medical history with attention to absolute and relative contraindications for oral contraceptives.

Physical Examination

- Height and weight
- Blood pressure
- Thyroid examination
- Breast examination, including Tanner staging
- Auscultation of heart and lungs
- Abdominal examination
- Pelvic examination

Laboratory Studies

- Pap smear.
- Cultures for gonorrhea and chlamydia.
- KOH and saline preparation when indicated by presence of abnormal vaginal discharge.
- Complete blood count or hemoglobin and hematocrit and rubella titer as indicated.
- Venereal Disease Research Laboratories (VDRL) test or rapid plasma reagin (RPR) with known STD, particularly condylomas or genital ulcers.
- Hyperlipidemia screen measuring serum cholesterol and triglycerides initially (fast-

ing or nonfasting) and lipid profile if initial screen is elevated. Screen if first-degree relative, especially a female relative, had a myocardial infarction before age 50 years or if client is a smoker, or is hypertensive, with a history of first-degree relative with a myocardial infarction before age 65 years.

• HIV

HORMONAL METHODS OF CONTRACEPTION (ORAL CONTRACEPTIVE PILL)

Protocol for Initial Use of Oral Contraceptives

The initial use of an oral contraceptive pill (OCP) requires special attention to dosing, preparation, timing, patient education, and follow-up.

DOSING. Initial dosing for an OCP should be at 35 μg or less estrogen, with low progestin potency per tablet. The selection of an OCP can also be individualized based on menstrual characteristics or patient sensitivity. For example, a client with a history of cystic acne can be tried on a low androgenic pill, such as Ortho Tri-Cyclen, the only contraceptive with Food and Drug Administration (FDA) approval for use in acne. For clients with hirsutism, a low androgenic potency pill is used. Adolescents who demonstrate estrogen sensitivity can be tried on a more androgenic pill such as Lo/Ovral, Nordette, Triphasil, or Loestrin. For short-term therapeutic considerations, such as treatment of dysfunctional uterine bleeding, a 50-μg preparation with increased progestational activity (e.g., Ovral, Ortho-Novum 1/50, or Norinyl 1 + 50), is used. Otherwise, it is important to use the lowest dose estrogen possible.

PREPARATION. Since 1994, there have been 10 new oral contraceptive formulations released. Given the vast selection of products available to the NP, Hatcher and associates (1998) developed a flow chart to assist clinicians in choosing a combined oral contraceptive with low-dosage estrogen. The selection process contains four steps:

1. Does the adolescent have a contraindication to estrogen use?

2. If yes, consider the use of a progestin-only pill.
3. If the client can use estrogen, the NP can select between numerous products. Considerations are
   • The number of micrograms of estrogen in the preparation
   • Availability of the pill
   • Ease of understanding the packaging of the pill
   • Price of the pill to the adolescent and possibly the clinic
   • Previous adverse event or experience the adolescent may have experienced in reaction to a specific preparation
4. Consider other clinical factors such as acne, nausea or vomiting, or both, spotting or breakthrough bleeding, and absence of withdrawal bleeding.

TIMING. Ideally, oral contraceptives should not be started until 1 year after the initiation of menses, but high-risk teens can be put on OCPs even before menarche (Hatcher et al., 1998). If an adolescent has had two periods and is sexually active, consider prescribing an OCP.

PATIENT EDUCATION. Emphasize correct and consistent use of the OCP. Remember that adolescents may not perceive the daily ingestion of an OCP as a medication.

FOLLOW-UP MANAGEMENT. Provide an emergency follow-up number, and instruct the client on indications for calling. Schedule a return appointment. The return visit gives the NP an opportunity to assess the physiological effects of the OCP as well as the adolescent's acceptance and use of this particular contraceptive method.

Adolescents tend to be acutely aware of and sensitive to body changes and processes. As a result, they may incorrectly interpret physical signs, exaggerate the effects of oral contraceptives on their bodies, and discontinue the OCP use without consulting their health care provider. At the follow-up visit, the NP should reemphasize the benefits of the OCP, discuss the lower risks of OCPs compared with those of pregnancy, and review and clarify side effects.

The use of the acronym ACHES can help guide assessment questions but should be used carefully to help the teenager understand more clearly the advantages and risks of OCPs without unduly concerning her:

- Have you experienced *A*bdominal pain (severe)?
- Have you noticed *C*hest pain (severe), cough, or shortness of breath?
- Do you have *H*eadaches (severe), dizziness, weakness, or numbness?
- Have you had a change in vision (loss or blurring) or other *E*ye problems or speech problems?
- Have you had any *S*evere leg pain, especially in the calf or thigh?

Also, interview the client for STD exposure, drug compliance, satisfaction with medication, and perceived side effects. Physical examination parameters during the return visit include weight, blood pressure, and laboratory follow-up.

Estrogen/Progesterone Preparations

TYPES OF PREPARATIONS. Two basic preparations are available: a combination formulation that contains estrogen ($< 50 \ \mu g$) and progestin in a low dose, and a progestin-only minipill. Most women in the United States use the combination formulation, either monophasic or triphasic. Progestin-only pills are prescribed for women for whom estrogens are contraindicated (e.g., lactating women). (See Table 20–6 for summary of available formulations.)

MECHANISMS OF ACTION
- Prevention of ovulation through hypothalamic and pituitary secretion secondary to estrogenic and progestational activity
- Alteration of cervical mucus, creating hostile environment for sperm
- Alteration of endometrial lining

THEORETICAL AND USE EFFECTIVENESS
- Lowest expected failure rate is 0.1%.
- Typical first-year failure rate in all women is 2%.
- Typical first-year failure rate in women younger than age 20 years is 4.7%.

BENEFITS
- High rate of effectiveness
- Simple method to use
- Ease of discontinuing use

- Rapid reversal of effects after discontinuing medication
- Beneficial effects on the menstrual cycle

MEDICAL BENEFITS
- For women younger than age 20 years, the estimated death rate while on an OCP is 1.3 per 100,000 users, as compared with that of childbirth, for which the estimated maternal death rate is 11.1 per 100,000 live births.
- Reduction of premenstrual symptoms (e.g., dysmenorrhea).
- Reduction of anemia.
- Decreased incidence of pelvic inflammatory disease (PID), which results in less morbidity in the areas of chronic pelvic pain, decreased incidence of ectopic pregnancies, and less infertility.
- Suppression of ovarian cysts.
- Reduction of endometriosis.
- Reduction of ovarian and endometrial cancer.
- Ortho Tri-Cyclen is approved by FDA for treatment of acne.
- Decreased effect on high-density lipoproteins (with use of triphasics).
- Decreased effect on blood pressure (with use of triphasics).
- Decreased effect on carbohydrate metabolism (with use of triphasics).

DISADVANTAGES OF TRIPHASIC OCP
- Confusion about color of package.
- Increased incidence of breakthrough bleeding as compared with straight preparations.
- No studies reliably document long-term effect on lipids.
- Less flexibility of use by the prescribing person (e.g., difficult to use for periods greater than 21 days or for management of ovarian cysts, endometrial bleeding, or dysfunctional uterine bleeding).
- Some adolescents find the triphasic preparation confusing, especially if they forget to take a pill.

DISADVANTAGES OF PROGESTIN-ONLY OCP
- Irregular bleeding.
- Effectiveness of these pills decreases dramatically if only one pill is missed. The

T A B L E 20-6
Composition of Oral Contraceptive Preparations

TYPE	NAME	ESTROGEN	μg	PROGESTIN	mg
LOW ANDROGENIC ACTIVITY OF PROGESTIN COMPONENT					
Monophasic	Modicon	EE	35	norethindrone	0.5
	Brevicon				
	Nelova 0.5/35E				
	N.E.E. 0.5/35				
	Ovcon-35	EE	35	norethindrone	0.4
	Ortho-Cyclen	EE	35	norgestimate	0.25
	Ortho-Cept	EE	30	desogestrel	0.15
	Desogen				
Triphasic	Ortho Tri-Cyclen	EE	35/35/35	norgestimate	0.18/0.215/0.25
MEDIUM ANDROGENIC ACTIVITY OF PROGESTIN COMPONENT					
Monophasic	Norlestrin 1/50	EE	50	norethindrone acetate	1.0
	Ovcon-50	EE	50	norethindrone	1.0
	Genora 1/50				
	Norethin 1/50M				
	Ortho-Novum 1/50	mestranol	50	norethindrone	1.0
	Norinyl 1 + 50				
	Demulen 1/50	EE	50	ethynodiol diacetate	1.0
	Demulen 1/35	EE	35	ethynodiol diacetate	1.0
	Ortho-Novum 1/35	EE	35	norethindrone	1.0
	Norinyl 1 + 35				
	Genora 1/35				
	Norethin 1/35E				
	Norcept-E 1/35				
	Nelova 1/35				
	N.E.E 1/35				
	Loestrin 1/20	EE	20	norethindrone acetate	1.0

Type	Product	Estrogen	Estrogen dose (µg)	Progestin	Progestin dose (mg)
Biphasic	Ortho-Novum 10/11	EE	35/35	norethindrone	0.5/1.0
	N.E.E. 10/11				
	Jenest-28				
Triphasic	Ortho-Novum 7/7/7	EE	35/35/35	norethindrone	0.5/0.75/1.0
	Tri-Norinyl	EE	35/35/35	norethindrone	0.5/1.0/0.5
	Triphasil	EE	30/40/30	levonorgestrel	0.05/0.075/0.125
	Tri-Levlen				

HIGH ANDROGENIC ACTIVITY OF PROGESTIN COMPONENT

Type	Product	Estrogen	Estrogen dose (µg)	Progestin	Progestin dose (mg)
Monophasic	Ovral	EE	50	norgestrel	0.5
	Norlestrin 2.5/50	EE	50	norethindrone acetate	2.5
	Loestrin 1.5/30	EE	30	norethindrone acetate	1.5
	Lo-Ovral	EE	30	norgestrel	0.3
	Nordette	EE	30	levonorgestrel	0.15
	Levlen	EE	30	levonorgestrel	0.15

COMPOSITION OF PROGESTIN-ONLY OCs

Type	Product	Estrogen	Estrogen dose	Progestin	Progestin dose (mg)
Monophasic	Micronor	None	N/A	norethindrone	0.35
	Nor-Q.D.	None	N/A	norethindrone	0.35
	Ovrette	None	N/A	norgestrel	0.075

From Health Learning Systems, Inc.: Dialogues in Contraception. Vol. 5, no. 4. (Fall 1997). Copyright 1997, Health Learning Systems, Inc., Wayne, NJ. Composition of Combination OCs: Low Androgenic; Medium Androgenic; High Androgenic. Composition of Progestin-Only OCs.
EE = ethinyl estradiol.

manufacturer recommends that progestin-only pills be taken at the same time every day and that a backup method of control be used if even one pill is missed or late.

FAILURE/LACK OF EFFICACY. Reasons for failure of OCPs include the following:

- Method failure or method ineffectiveness.
- Patient failure/user effectiveness—50 to 70% of women still use OCPs 1 year after initiation, with most discontinuing for non-medical reasons.
- Concurrent drug interaction such as with anticonvulsants or antibiotics. With pheno-barbital, prescribe any OCP with 50 µg of estrogen or greater; with antibiotics such as rifampin, use a backup method (if the antibiotic is a short course); otherwise, consider an alternative method to an OCP.

Medroxyprogesterone Acetate (Depo-Provera)

PROTOCOL FOR INITIAL USE. Always evaluate for pregnancy before giving initial dose. A single 150-mg injection inhibits ovulation for 13 weeks. Dosage adjustment for body weight is not necessary. It is preferable to deliver the initial injection before day 5 of the menstrual cycle to minimize pregnancy potential. Injections are usually given at 12-week intervals. If more than 13 weeks have transpired between injections, evaluate for pregnancy before giving the injection.

MECHANISM OF ACTION
- Inhibits ovulation by inhibiting luteinizing hormone surge
- Creates shallow, atrophic endometrium, unsuitable for implantation
- Increases thickening of cervical mucus, decreasing sperm penetration

THEORETICAL AND USE EFFECTIVENESS. The lowest expected pregnancy rate is 0.3 per 100 women years.

BENEFITS
- Failure rate less than 1%
- One-time dosing every 3 months
- Good method for adolescents who want

to keep their contraception private from family and friends
- Inhibits intravascular sickling; increases hemoglobin and red blood cell survival rate
- Beneficial effect on duration and quality of lactation in lactating females
- Gynecological benefits (e.g., decreases in pelvic inflammatory diseases [PID], ectopic pregnancy, and endometriosis)

DISADVANTAGES
- Menstrual irregularities
- Amenorrhea or decreased menstrual flow
- Weight gain
- Headache
- Breast tenderness
- Acne
- Hirsutism
- Psychological effects such as moodiness, depression, change in libido
- Increased risk for low birth weight in infants exposed in utero
- Evidence of bone density loss in adolescents; osteoporosis
- Intramuscular injection

PATIENTS APPROPRIATE FOR DEPO-PROVERA
Depo-Provera is a contraceptive method of choice for patients with the following characteristics:

- Seeking a long-term, reversible, highly reliable, private method of contraception
- Those for whom use of estrogen is contraindicated (e.g., patients with a previous thromboembolic episode, lupus, sickle cell anemia)
- Those with poor compliance using other contraceptive methods
- Those with menstrual hygiene issues, such as individuals who are mentally retarded, because Depo-Provera often causes amenorrhea after two injections

Postcoital Hormonal Contraception or Emergency Contraception

PREPARATION. Preven is the only FDA-approved emergency contraceptive marketed in the United States. It is packaged as four tablets of a high-dose combination of 50 µg ethinyl estradiol and 0.25 mg levonorgestrel, a pregnancy test, and a patient education booklet (Contraception Report, 1999). Regular OCPs may be used at recommended dosage (see Clinical Management).

CLINICAL MANAGEMENT
- Assess for pregnancy using rapid high-sensitivity urine pregnancy test. If last normal menstrual period has been within 1 month, a pregnancy test is not necessary.
- Have patient sign consent and follow-up agreement.
- Administer 100 μg of ethinyl estradiol and 0.5 mg of progestin (two tablets of Preven) as soon as possible but no later than 72 hours from time of unprotected coitus, then 100 μg of ethinyl estradiol and 0.5 mg progestin (2 tablets Preven) 12 hours after first dose (can also use "Yuzpe" regimen: 100 to 130 μg of ethinyl estradiol and 0.5 to 1.2 mg of progestin. This dosage is found in two tablets of Ovral or four tablets of Lo/Ovral, Nordette, Levlen, or four of the yellow Triphasil or Trilevlen tablets. Administer the first dose within 72 hours followed by second dose 12 hours later [Kahn et al., 1999]).
- Instruct patient to keep menstrual calendar.
- Instruct patient to abstain from intercourse until the start of her next cycle.
- Schedule return visit in 2 to 3 weeks.

MECHANISM OF ACTION. Same as for oral contraceptives.

EFFECTIVENESS. Controversy exists within the medical literature as to the effectiveness of postcoital hormonal contraception in preventing unintentional pregnancy—it may have an average effectiveness rate of about 76%. Risk of pregnancy overall is 0 to 26% if the event occurs during a menstrual cycle. At midcycle, the average likelihood of conception from 3 days prior to ovulation to the day of ovulation is 15 to 26%.

BARRIER METHODS OF CONTRACEPTION: CONDOMS

Condoms are the most common barrier method of contraception. Used effectively, they can prevent pregnancy and STD. The most recent data available indicate that teenagers are more likely to use condoms than young adults. Fifty-seven percent of men and 37% of women aged 15 to 19 years old claim to use condoms, whereas 39% of men and 26% of women between 20 and 24 years of age do so (Sonenstein et al., 1989; Tanfer et al., 1993; Piccinino & Mosher, 1998). This finding may be related to an increased availability of condoms to high school students, a relatively high sense of self-efficacy (i.e., that one can successfully complete the behavior required to produce a desired outcome) among older adolescents (Hanna, 1999), or the use of coitus-independent methods of contraception (e.g., oral contraceptives) (Roye, 1998). Among all teens, the rate of condom use increased from 46 to 54% between 1991 and 1995 (Warren et al., 1998) and it appears that those who have had an STD are more likely to use them (Roye, 1998).

Protocol for Use

- *Use every time!*
- Apply correctly, allowing for ½-inch tip at end and removing any trapped air.
- Remove correctly after intercourse. Hold onto the condom while withdrawing the penis from the vagina to avoid the condom coming off in the vagina.
- Avoid use of petroleum-based lubricants such as petroleum jelly, shortening, oil-based vaginal therapeutics such as Monistat or Femstat, and some sexual lubricants.
- Check expiration date on the package and make sure package is intact.

Mechanism of Action

- Prevent sperm from entering vagina.
- Spermicidal condoms inactivate motile sperm ejaculated into the condom. It is unknown whether a spermicidal condom is more effective in actual use than a non-spermicidal condom.

Theoretical and Use Effectiveness

- First-year failure rate among typical users is 12%.

- First-year failure rate among perfect users is 2%.
- Concomitant, perfect use of condoms with a spermicide has an estimated probability of contraceptive failure of 0.1%. This is equivalent to perfect-use failure rate with an OCP.

Benefits

- Encourages male participation
- Is inexpensive and accessible
- Use of lubricated condoms reduces mechanical friction and vaginal or penile irritation
- Decreases the risk of transmitting STDs
- Prevents development or enhances regression of cervical intraepithelial neoplasia
- Eliminates postcoital vaginal discharge
- Helps maintain erection for some men
- Has few contraindications

Disadvantages

- Condom breakage or slippage. Approximately 2 to 6% of condoms fail as a result of breakage or slippage.
- Natural-skin condoms are contraindicated if there is a risk of infection by sexually transmitted viruses (e.g., hepatitis B virus, human papillomavirus, herpes simplex virus, and HIV).
- Either partner may be allergic to latex.
- Male partner may fail to accept responsibility for use.
- Some men cannot maintain an erection when condom is used.

OTHER BARRIER METHODS

Diaphragm

Available for 100 years, there are currently four types of diaphragms in sizes from 50 to 105 mm, available by prescription only. For most adolescents, the 65- to 75-mm sizes are commonly prescribed. These are:

- Flat spring (Ortho-White)
- Arching spring (Koroflex, Allflex, Ramses Bendex)
- Coil-spring rim (Koromex, Ortho, Ramses)
- Wide-seal rim (Milex)

The diaphragm can be placed in the vagina up to 1 hour before intercourse and can be left in place for 24 hours, but it must be left a minimum of 6 to 8 hours. Reapplication of spermicide is required with subsequent intercourse.

Cervical Cap

Manufactured in England, there are three types of cervical caps: Prentif, Dumas, and Vimule. In 1988, the FDA approved Prentif for use in the United States. Sizes range from 50 to 75 mm. The cap can be left in place for 48 hours, and subsequent intercourse is possible without reapplication of spermicide. The use of the cervical cap among adolescents has not been well researched. It should probably be reserved for those adolescents who are older and more motivated to comply with contraception.

Female Condom

The female condom is a device with an inner ring or dome that fits next to the cervix. An outer ring fits around the external opening to the vagina. The single-use condom acts as a barrier to prevent sperm from entering the vagina.

Protocols for Use

These vary depending on the barrier method.

Theoretical and Use Effectiveness

Effectiveness of any of these methods is influenced by the patient's ability to use the method consistently and correctly, along with her own personal fertility characteristics. Patients who are younger than 30 years of age and have intercourse four or more times a week experience higher failure rates.

- Diaphragm failure rate is 14.3 to 18.6% in typical users.

- Cervical cap failure rate averages 17.4%, ranging from 8 to 27%.
- Female condom pregnancy rates are reported to be 24 to 26%.

Benefits

- Diaphragms help prevent transmission of STDs and decrease risk of PID, bacterial and viral infection, and cervical neoplasia.
- Female condoms are accessible over the counter.

Disadvantages

- Barrier methods are contraindicated if there is a history of toxic shock syndrome.
- Caps are contraindicated if there has been a full-term delivery within the last 6 weeks, recent spontaneous or induced abortion, or there is vaginal bleeding from any cause, including menstrual flow.
- Allergic reaction may occur in those sensitive to spermicide, rubber, latex, or polyurethane.
- Abnormalities in vaginal anatomy can interfere with satisfactory fit or placement of any of the devices.
- Diaphragm can cause recurrent urinary tract infections that do not resolve after diaphragm has been refitted.
- For diaphragms and caps, trained personnel may not be available to fit device or they may lack time to instruct patient adequately on use of method.
- Patient may be unable to learn correct insertion technique.
- Patient may not feel comfortable touching self, or may find procedure messy and unpleasant.

Controversy

Association of Pap smear abnormalities with the use of the cervical cap is unresolved. FDA protocol recommends obtaining a Pap smear at the time of fitting, then 3 months after onset of use and annually thereafter.

SPERMICIDES

Protocol for Use

- *Use every time!*
- Keep adequate supply and store properly.
- Be alert to timing of product placement before intercourse. Place in vagina at appropriate time.
- Insert new application of product before every episode of repeated intercourse.

Mechanism of Action

Spermicides are a combination of an inert base or carrier (foam, cream, jelly, suppository, or tablet) with active spermicidal agent nonoxynol-9 or octoxynol, which kills sperm by permeating the cell membrane. Spermicides are marketed in various formats:

- Foams, creams, or jellies that can be used alone or in combination with a condom or diaphragm.
- Spermicidal suppositories that are intended for use alone or with a condom. These require a 10- to 15-minute wait time before intercourse in order to allow the product to effervesce.
- Vaginal contraceptive film that can be used alone or with a condom or diaphragm. The film contains 72 mg of nonoxynol-9 in a thin sheet that is placed next to the cervix 5 minutes before intercourse.

Theoretical and Use Effectiveness

- Estimate among perfect first-year users is 6% failure rate.
- Among typical users, failure is about 21%.

Benefits

- Medically safe, with same efficacy as barrier methods or condoms
- Available over the counter without a prescription; no need to access medical system
- No need for partner involvement with decision-making or implementation
- Used at midcycle to augment effectiveness of intrauterine device (IUD) or condom

- Used as backup option while waiting to start OCPs, for missed OCPs, or between relationships
- Emergency use when condom breaks (insert immediately)
- Effective against bacteria such as gonorrhea and chlamydia

Disadvantages

- Can cause allergic reaction in those sensitive to spermicidal agent or base
- Can be difficult or impossible for some people to learn correct insertion technique
- Abnormalities in vaginal anatomy can prevent correct placement or product retention (e.g., septum, prolapse, double cervix)

MANAGEMENT OF ALTERED PATTERNS

Sexual development is an integral part of children's whole development. Children's sense of self, personality, relationship to others and to the physical world, cognitive, emotional, and spiritual abilities, perceptions, and expressions are all influenced by and, in turn, influence their sexual development. If children experience problems with sexuality, all other aspects of development are affected. Issues of major concern include child sexual abuse (see Chapter 19) and adolescent pregnancy. Homosexuality, although an alternate rather than an altered pattern, is discussed later in this chapter, because the establishment of sexual orientation and intimacy often occurs during adolescence.

Adolescent Pregnancy

DESCRIPTION

Adolescent pregnancy occurs in girls or young women between ages 13 and 19 years, although pregnancy is possible for any girl who has begun ovulation. Pregnancy has been seen in girls before their first menstrual cycle and in those as young as 10 or 11 years of age.

INCIDENCE

Following a sharp increase from 1985 to 1990, the rate of teen pregnancy has declined steadily in the past decade. Between 1991 and 1995, the rate decreased by 13% to 83.6 per 1000, and there was an overall decrease of 15% between 1991 and 1997. Teen abortions also decreased significantly (21% from 1991 to 1995). Birth rates declined more for girls age 15 to 17 years than for older teenagers (18 to 19 years), and more for black teenagers than other racial groups. Second pregnancies, or repeat childbearing during adolescence mirrored this trend, decreasing 21% between 1991 and 1996. Despite these declines, pregnancy rates continue to be higher among adolescents than in the mid-1980s, and a growing number of pregnancies and births are attributed to unmarried teenagers (Kaufmann et al., 1998; Ventura & Curtin, 1999).

ETIOLOGY

The decline in teen pregnancy is due to a variety of factors, among which may be the use of condoms, especially at first intercourse. Although there are some conflicting data, school-based programs that make condoms available and provide education about sexuality and sexual responsibility appear to decrease pregnancy rates effectively without increasing sexual activity (Polaneczky, 1998). Not all studies indicate a positive relationship between condom availability and use, however. Surveys of students in 10 Seattle high schools in 1993 and 1995 revealed that, although condoms were readily accessible and students took them, there was no corresponding increase in condom use. On a positive note, neither was there a corresponding increase in sexual activity (Kirby et al., 1999).

Research on adolescent pregnancy has established risk factors that may be helpful in identifying youth at risk for adolescent pregnancy. Periods of vulnerability to unwanted pregnancy in the sexual career of women have been described by using a developmental approach for known risk (Adler, 1984) (Table 20-7).

A number of factors have been identified as predictors of failure or success with contraception. These include the following:

T A B L E 20-7

Developmental Risk Factors for Sexual Activity

DEVELOPMENTAL PHASE OF RELATIONSHIP	ASSOCIATED RISK FACTORS
Early adolescence	No self-concept of being fertile (fecundity)
Initiation of a relationship	No self-concept of being fertile (fecundity)
	Feels conflict or guilt over planning to be sexually active
Developing relationship	Change from using coitus-dependent methods of contraception (condoms or spermicides), which have lower use effectiveness rates, to using coitus-independent (hormonal) methods, which have a reported higher use effectiveness rate; change involves learning new technique
Change in relationship	Shift in established communication skills from a known to an unknown partner
	Persons with immature interpersonal communication skills may be unprepared to negotiate the use of a contraceptive device with a new partner
Geographical mobility	Lack knowledge needed to access local systems of care that dispense contraceptive devices
Following each pregnancy	Lack understanding of reproductive physiology
	Unaware that ovulation may return within 2 wk after the termination of a pregnancy
	Perceive self to be at reduced risk of pregnancy

Adapted from Adler NE: Contraception and unwanted pregnancy. Behav Med Update 5:28–34, 1984.

- Age: Adolescents 15 years of age and younger are at highest risk for pregnancy, because 46% report using no method of contraception at their first episode of intercourse. In comparison, only 17% of females age 19 years or older report using no method.
- Noncompliance with the first method chosen (previous method failure).
- Not acquiring a method of contraception at the first reproductive health visit.
- Frequency of family planning visits in the preceding 12 months: Increased compliance with clinic attendance appears to correlate with effective contraceptive use by client.
- Coital frequency: Adolescent females who have sexual intercourse more than six times per month are at greater risk of becoming pregnant.
- Length of time between first coitus and initiation of birth control use: The longer adolescents delay seeking services for contraception, the less likely they are to use a highly reliable method consistently and correctly.

Antecedent risk factors to unintentional pregnancy include the following:

- Early onset of sexual activity, especially before age 15 years
- Early onset of substance use, including cigarettes, alcohol, and illicit drugs
- Low educational expectation
- Low perception of life options
- Poor grades and academic achievement
- Behavior problems, including truancy and delinquency
- Negative peer influence
- Poor contraceptive compliance or failure with a contraceptive device
- Nonintact families (those without both biological mother and father present)
- Depression

CLINICAL FINDINGS

History

The history should include the following:

- Menstrual history: last normal menstrual period, any oligomenorrhea or amenor-

rhea, hypomenorrhea or irregular period, intermenstrual spotting
- Sexual history (see Table 20-2)
- Associated symptoms: breast sensitivity, nipple tenderness (1 to 2 weeks after conception); fatigue, nausea, urinary frequency (2 weeks after conception)
- Presenting complaints: patients often present with vague unassociated complaints (e.g., headache, abdominal discomfort, dizziness)

Physical Examination

There are three classic signs of pregnancy, each of which can be observed during the pelvic examination:

1. Hegar sign. Softening of the isthmus of the uterus (the area between the cervix and the uterine body). This may be observed before there is uterine enlargement.
2. Chadwick sign. Dark-bluish or purplish discoloration of the vaginal and cervical epithelium, the result of increased blood supply to the pelvis. This is usually observed before uterine growth.
3. Uterine enlargement. Occurs at 5 to 6 weeks and initially is due to changes in the uterine muscle rather than growing gestation. Uterine sizing is traditionally done by bimanual examination and recorded in weeks of estimated gestation.

Laboratory Studies

The following laboratory studies are done in cases of suspected pregnancy:

- Pregnancy testing: Quantitative serum human chorionic gonadotropin (HCG) is the most specific, accurate by 6 to 10 days after conception, and expensive. Quantitative serum HCG testing is indicated for serial measurements to evaluate ectopic pregnancy or molar pregnancy or to rule out gestational trophoblastic neoplasia (GTN). Urine testing is the chosen test for the ambulatory setting, because results can be obtained in 5 minutes and the test is very accurate. Reliability allows for accurate results 6 to 8 days after ovulation or

from 2 days after the last missed menstrual period.
- If pregnancy test is positive, laboratory diagnostics include
  ○ Cervical cultures for *Neisseria gonorrhoeae* and *Chlamydia trachomatis*
  ○ Cervical cytology if indicated
  ○ Vaginal pH with saline and KOH wet mounts
  ○ If the pregnancy is to be continued, additional serum testing, including syphilis serology, complete blood count, blood type and Rh status, screening for hepatitis B serology, and, potentially, screening for HIV infection
  ○ Urinalysis and urine culture
  ○ Possibly, pelvic ultrasonography to determine gestation accurately

DIFFERENTIAL DIAGNOSIS

The differential diagnoses for pregnancy are as follows:

- Nonviable intrauterine pregnancy with partial spontaneous abortion
- Ectopic pregnancy
- Molar pregnancy to exclude GTN

MANAGEMENT

Prompt diagnosis assists with pregnancy planning, early onset of prenatal precautions (e.g., avoidance of medications, alcohol, and smoking), and medical care. Early care also allows women considering an abortion ample time for counseling, decision-making, and obtaining an abortion in the first trimester, when the procedure is safest.

The NP should schedule a health visit to include pregnancy test, physical examination, and health counseling. If the pregnancy test is negative, counsel the adolescent regarding risk of potential pregnancy and reliable methods of contraception. If the pregnancy test is positive, schedule for a health visit to include the following:

- Pelvic examination to determine gestational age
- Counseling for pregnancy options, including continuing pregnancy and retaining

custody of child, continuing pregnancy and placing child for adoption, or terminating pregnancy
- Assessment of need for involvement of social support system, including family, male partner, and any significant others; NP may need to serve as mediator for teenager in informing others
- Initiation of referrals as appropriate for the decision made:
  - If the choice is continuing pregnancy, refer to adolescent pregnancy program to initiate comprehensive medical, nutritional, psychosocial, and educational services.
  - If adoption is the option of choice, refer to appropriate legal or social service agency, or both.
  - If the choice is terminating pregnancy, refer to appropriate source for abortion.
- Make additional referrals as indicated (e.g., Women, Infants and Children [WIC] program or insurance coverage). Public health–based research indicates there is a significant positive effect on pregnancy, parenting, and child rearing outcomes if home visits are made by public health nurses (Olds et al., 1997). Refer all pregnant teens to a public health nursing service.

COMPLICATIONS

Young age in a pregnant woman is an inherent risk factor, even with good prenatal care. Adverse outcomes are common in pregnant teenagers (Fraser et al., 1995; DuPlessis et al., 1997).

Maternal

- Anemia
- Pregnancy-induced hypertension
- Excessive weight gain
- STDs
- Cephalopelvic disproportion (CPD)
- Puerperal complications
- Potential social consequences (e.g., educational, economic, and occupational delay)

Fetal/Neonatal

- Low birth weight
- Intrauterine growth retardation
- Prematurity
- Sudden infant death syndrome (SIDS)
- Minor acute infections
- Perinatal death
- Potential medical, social, behavioral, and educational sequelae

Prevention and Resources

Prevention goals include the following:

- Maintain sexual health
- Promote sexual responsibility
- Assist adolescents to make informed choices, recognizing educational, social, and economic impact of choices
- Delay onset of intercourse
- Provide contraceptive counseling and selection of a contraceptive device for any adolescent who has recently experienced a spontaneous abortion, as part of third-trimester health teaching before delivery, or at the time of an elective termination of pregnancy

These goals can be achieved by supporting a positive or protective environment, connecting the adolescent to an intervention program, and providing appropriate health care services. Common components of successful intervention programs have been described by Dryfoos (1990) as including the following:

- Intensive individualized attention
- Community-wide multiagency collaborative approaches
- Early identification of at-risk children
- Early intervention to prevent high-risk behavior
- Adequate staff training
- Social skills training for children
- Engagement of peers in interventions
- Parental involvement
- Link to the world of work

An environment that protects against pregnancy has been described (Jaskiewicz & McAnarney, 1994; Fehring et al., 1998) as:

- Consistent and predictable
- Emphasizing educational achievement
- Having high parental education levels
- Having religious values

Appropriate health-care services include the following:

- Confidential services with minimal or no financial barriers
- Easy availability (e.g., timed for easy access, onsite at school, or easy transportation to site)
- Full range of contraceptive services for male and female adolescents (see section on Contraception for specific methods)

Homosexuality

DESCRIPTION

Sexual orientation refers to a person's sexual responsiveness to partners of the same or opposite gender. The concept of sexual orientation includes at least three distinctive components: sexual imagery (fantasies or attraction), actual sexual behavior, and the person's self-identification as heterosexual, bisexual, or homosexual. Homosexuality is sexual orientation toward individuals of the same gender. It is not a mental disorder nor is it a choice that individuals voluntarily make.

INCIDENCE

Sexual orientation received considerable attention after the release of data from the Kinsey studies of comprehensive sexual histories (Kinsey et al., 1949). Kinsey concluded that 4% of men in the cohort born between 1920 and 1930 were exclusively homosexual throughout their lives and 10% were more or less exclusively homosexual for at least 3 years. The estimates of the prevalence of homosexuality for American women were half those of corresponding male rates (Kinsey et al., 1953). Criticism has been raised as to whether Kinsey's data can be generalized, because the small convenience samples of students and tradesmen in the studies may have skewed findings. Adolescent-specific data on sexual orientation are sparse. Remafedi and associates (1992) surveyed a representative sample of 34,706 Minnesota junior and senior high school youths and reported that 10.7% were unsure of their sexual orientation, 88.2% described themselves as exclusively heterosexual, and 1.1% described

themselves as bisexual or predominantly homosexual. Random-probability nationally based survey data on adolescent sexual orientation are absent.

ETIOLOGY

The etiology of sexual orientation, either homosexual or heterosexual, is unknown. Sexual orientation appears to develop in phases, from the prenatal period through latency. Although the dynamics of its evolution are unknown, sexual orientation tends to be fixed by the end of the child's prepubertal years.

Because there is no scientific evidence to explain the development of sexual orientation, controversy continues as to "causes" of homosexuality. Some clinicians believe that it is a purely biological phenomenon, largely determined in utero. The work of Bell and colleagues (1981) served to rule out many psychosocial components when the researchers concluded that homosexuality does not result from a cold, distant father, poor peer relationships, sexual abuse, or sexual experimentation in childhood.

CLINICAL FINDINGS

People with a homosexual orientation are diverse individuals and their behavior cannot be stereotyped. The daily lifestyles of those with a homosexual orientation and their ability to function in occupational, educational, and family structures are as varied as those of heterosexual individuals. The development of a homosexual orientation, however, involves a process of acknowledging and integrating one's sexual identity.

A proposed model of homosexual identity formation includes sensitization, identity confusion, identity assumption, and commitment (Troiden, 1988).

- *Sensitization* occurs during childhood when individuals identify themselves as feeling different from others of the same gender. Girls describe themselves as "unfeminine," whereas boys often report feelings of disinterest in sports and a proclivity for artistic endeavors. Boys state that they are often called "sissies."

- *Identity confusion* usually occurs during adolescence when individuals begin to question whether they may be homosexual. On average, this occurs for males at age 17 years and for females at age 18 years. Feelings of inadequacy, insecurity, self-deprecation, poor self-esteem, and depression can result from unresolved identity confusion.
- *Identity assumption* is the stage at which the child assumes a homosexual identity that is shared with others. The age at which this occurs varies by gender, with males reporting an average age of 19 to 21 years and females 21 to 23 years. Exploration of the homosexual role can lead to multiple sexual experiences with accompanying risks of acquiring STDs, including AIDS. In contrast, close, long-term relationships can develop. The late adolescent–young adult homosexual, sexually active male is at risk for having the same problems as his heterosexual counterpart.
- *Commitment* is an internalized pledge to live as a homosexual and enter into a same-sex relationship. This process can be referred to as "coming out." External disclosure to others who are not homosexual may vary, depending on what is perceived to be safe to the individual. A stigma management strategy of blending or acting gender appropriate may be adopted in an attempt to be safe in environments that are not tolerant or accepting of homosexuality.

DIFFERENTIAL DIAGNOSIS

The differential diagnoses for homosexuality are gender identity disorders and transvestism.

MANAGEMENT

A number of professional articles describe management issues for the primary care provider (Bidwell, 1988; Remafedi et al., 1992; Sturdevant & Remafedi, 1992; Kreiss & Patterson, 1997). It is important that the provider support and validate the adolescent throughout the process of developing his or her awareness of and commitment to a homosexual orientation. Specific interventions include the following:

- Providing a safe environment in which to access health care
- Providing appropriate counseling, nonjudgmental listening, assistance in problem-solving, and communication between adolescent and others
- Educating about the high risk for STDs

Counseling varies from one adolescent to another and can require referral to a psychologist. Several principles have been identified to guide counseling of homosexual adolescents (Schneider & Tremble, 1986):

- Homosexuality is not a barrier to developing and maturing into a happy, productive adult.
- Homosexual adolescents must not be allowed to use their sexual orientation as an excuse to ignore the responsibilities of growing up and maturing.
- Issues and concerns of homosexual youth are often the same as those of heterosexual youth.

COMPLICATIONS

A high incidence of mental health problems such as suicide ideation, suicide attempts, substance abuse, runaway behavior, school truancy, and other emotional trauma can be present among homosexual adolescents, especially if the normal process of developing one's homosexual identity has been conflictive and is not progressing toward resolution. The NP should assess for conflicts regarding sexual orientation as an etiological factor if an adolescent has these clinical issues.

NURSING DIAGNOSIS 20-1

NURSING DIAGNOSES FOR SEXUALITY FUNCTIONAL HEALTH PATTERN

Sexual Dysfunction

Sexual Pattern Alteration

Source: North American Nursing Diagnosis Association: *NANDA Nursing Diagnoses: Definitions and Classifications 1997–1998.* Philadelphia; NANDA, 1996.

RESOURCE BOX 20-1

RESOURCES FOR SEXUALITY, PREGNANCY, AND HOMOSEXUALITY ISSUES

For Young Children and Parents

Mayle P: *Where Did I Come From?* Secaucus, NJ, Lyle Stuart, 1973.

Mayle P: *What's Happening to Me?* Secaucus, NJ, Lyle Stuart, 1976.

Leight L: *Raising Sexually Healthy Children.* New York, Avon Books, 1990.

Adolescents

American Medical Association
Website: http://www.ama-assn.org/adolhlth/adolhlth.htm

Gans-Epner J: *Policy Compendium on Reproductive Health Issues Affecting Adolescents.* Chicago, American Medical Association, 1996.

Pregnancy

Planned Parenthood Federation of America
Tel: (212) 541-7800 Check local sources for the Planned Parenthood group in your community.

Homosexuality

Federation of Parents and Friends of Lesbians and Gays, Inc. (PFLAG)
Tel: (202) 638-4200
Website: www.pflag.org
The national organization can provide referrals to local chapters.

Gay and Lesbian Parents Coalition International
Tel: (202) 583-8029
Resource on support groups throughout the United States.

Sexual Assessment and History Taking

American Medical Association (1999). Talking to patients about sex: Training program for physicians.
Website: http://www.ama-assn.org/sexhist

Davis CM, Yarber, WL, Bauserman, R, et al: *Handbook of Sexuality-Related Measures.* Thousand Oaks, CA, SAGE Publications, 1998. Includes a wide range of standardized measurement tools and questionnaires with discussion of their use, reliability, and validity.

Sexuality and Prevention and Treatment of Sexually Transmitted Infections

American Social Health Association
Tel: (919) 361-8400
Fax: (919) 361-8425
Tel: (800) 783-9877
Website: http://www.ashastd.org

General Health Education

ETR Associates
Tel: (800) 321-4407
Fax: (800) 435-8433
Website: http://www.etr.org
Reducing the Risk
Sex education program for high school students.

REFERENCES

Adler NE: Contraception and unwanted pregnancy. Behav. Med Update 5:28–34, 1984.

American Medical Association (AMA): Guidelines for Adolescent Preventive Services (GAPS): Recommendations Monograph. Chicago, AMA, 1997.

Bell AP, Weinberg MS, Hammersmith SK: Sexual Preference. Bloomington, Indiana University Press, 1981.

Bidwell RJ: The gay and lesbian teen: A case of denied adolescence. J Pediatr Health Care 2:3–8, 1988.

Cobb BK: Communication types and sexual protective practices of college women. Public Health Nurs 14:293–301, 1997.

Contraception Report: Specially-packaged emergency contraception comes to U.S. Contraception Report 9:11–12, 1999.

Dickey RP: Managing Contraceptive Pill Patients, 9th ed. Durant, OK: EMIS, 1998.

Dryfoos JG: Adolescents at Risk: Prevalence and Prevention. New York, Oxford University Press, 1990.

DuPlessis HM, Bell R, Richards T: Adolescent pregnancy: Understanding the impact of age and race on outcomes. J Adolesc Health 20:187–197, 1997.

Ehrenberg M, Ehrenberg O: The Intimate Circle: The Sexual Dynamics of Family Life. New York, Simon & Schuster, 1988.

Fehring RJ, Cheever KH, German K, et al: Religiosity and sexual activity among older adolescents. J Religion Health 37:229–247, 1998.

Finan SL: Promoting healthy sexuality: Guidelines for the school-age child and adolescent. Nurse Pract 22:62, 65–67, 71–72, 1997.

Fraser AM, Brockert JE, Ward RH: Association of young

maternal age with adverse reproductive outcomes. N Engl J Med 332:1113-1117, 1995.

Friedrich WN, Grambsch P, Broughton D, et al: Normative sexual behavior in children. Pediatrics 88:456-464, 1991.

Haffner DW: Sex Education 2000: A Call to Action. New York, Sex Information and Education Council in the U.S. (SIECUS), 1990.

Haignere CS, Gold R, McDanel HJ: Adolescent abstinence and condom use: Are we sure we are really teaching what is safe? Health Educ Behav 26:43-54, 1999.

Hanna KM: An adolescent and young adult condom self-efficacy scale. J Pediatr Nurs 14:59-66, 1999.

Hatcher RA, Trussell J, Stewart F, et al: Contraceptive Technology, 17th ed. New York, Ardent Media, 1998.

Hubbard BM, Giese ML, Rainey J: A replication study of Reducing the Risk, a theory-based sexuality curriculum for adolescents. J School Health 68:243-247, 1998.

Jaskiewicz JA, McAnarney ER: Pregnancy during adolescence. Pediatr Rev 15:32-38, 1994.

Kahn JA, Emans SJ: Gynecologic examination of the prepubertal girl. Contemp Pediatr 16:148-159, 1999.

Kahn JA, Mansfield J, Emans SJ, et al: Special problems in the adolescent: Adolescent gynecology. *In* Burg FD, Ingelfinger JR, Wald ER et al (eds): Gellis & Kagan's Current Pediatric Therapy, 16th ed. Philadelphia, WB Saunders, 1999, pp 1181-1195.

Kaufmann RB, Spitz AM, Strauss LT, et al: The decline in US teen pregnancy rates, 1990-1995. Pediatrics 102:1141-1147, 1998.

Kinsey AC, Pomeroy WB, Martin CE: Sexual Behavior in the Human Male. Philadelphia, WB Saunders, 1949.

Kinsey AC, Pomeroy WB, Martin CE: Sexual Behavior in the Human Female. Philadelphia, WB Saunders, 1953.

Kirby D, Brener ND, Brown NL, et al: The impact of condom distribution in Seattle schools on sexual behavior and condom use. Am J Public Health 89:182-187, 1999.

Klein NA, Goodson P, Serrins DS, et al: Evaluation of sex education curricula: Measuring up to the SIECUS guidelines. J School Health 64:328-333, 1994.

Kreiss JL, Patterson DL: Psychosocial issues in primary care of lesbian, gay, bisexual, and transgender youth. J Pediatr Health Care 11:266-274, 1997.

Laube HH: The use of a sexual history with adolescents. *In* Blum RW (ed): Adolescent Health Care: Clinical Issues. New York, Academic Press, 1982.

Money J: Gay, Straight, and In-Between. New York, Oxford University Press, 1988.

Mount SL, Papillo JL: A study of 10,296 pediatric and adolescent Papanicolaou smear diagnoses in Northern New England. Pediatrics 103:539-545, 1999.

Olds D, Eckenrode J, Henderson C, et al: Long-term effects of home visitation on maternal life course and child abuse and neglect. JAMA 278:637-643, 1997.

Piccinino L, Mosher W: Trends in contraceptive use in the United States: 1982-1995. Fam Plan Perspect 30:4-10, 46, 1998.

Polaneczky M: Adolescent contraception. Curr Opin Obstet Gynecol 10:213-219, 1998.

Reece RM: Child Abuse: Medical Diagnosis and Management. Philadelphia, Lea & Febiger, 1994.

Region X Nursing Network: Region X Nursing Network Standards For Prenatal and Child Health. Seattle, University of Washington, 1998.

Remafedi G, Resnick M, Blum R, et al: Demography of sexual orientation. Pediatrics 89:714-721, 1992.

Roberts EJ: Childhood Sexual Learning: The Unwritten Curriculum. Cambridge, MA, Bollinger Publishing, 1980.

Roye CF: Condom use by Hispanic and African-American adolescent girls who use hormonal contraception. J Adolesc Health 23:205-211, 1998.

Schneider MS, Tremble B: Training service providers to work with gay or lesbian adolescents: A workshop. J Counsel Dev 65:98-99, 1986.

Sex Information and Education Council of the United States (SIECUS): Unfinished Business: A SIECUS Assessment of State Sexuality Education Programs. New York, SIECUS, 1993.

Sex Information and Education Council of the United States National Guidelines (SIECUS) Task Force: Guidelines for Comprehensive Sexuality Education: Kindergarten-12th Grade. New York, SIECUS Task Forces 1991.

Siegel DM: Self-reported honesty among middle and high school students responding to a sexual behavior questionnaire. J Adolesc Health 23:2-28, 1998.

Smith M: Pediatric sexuality: Promoting normal sexual development in children. Nurse Pract 18:37-44, 1993.

Sonenstein F, Pleck R, Ku L: Sexual activity, condom use and AIDS awareness among adolescent males. Fam Plan Perspect 21:152-158, 1989.

Sturdevant MS, Remafedi G: Special health needs of homosexual youth. Adolesc Med 3:359-371, 1992.

Tanfer K, Grady W, Klepinger D, et al: Condom use among U.S. men 1991. Fam Plann Perspect 25:61-66, 1993.

Troiden RR: Homosexual identity development. J Adolesc Health Care 9:105-113, 1988.

Ventura SJ, Curtin SC: Recent trends in teen births in the United States. Statistical Bulletin/Metropolitan Insurance Companies 80:2-12, 1999.

Warren CW, Santelli JS, Everett SA, et al: Sexual behavior among U.S. high school students, 1990-1995. Fam Plan Perspect 30:170-172, 1998.

World Health Organization: Education and Treatment in Human Sexuality: The Training of Health Professionals (Technical Report Series No. 372). Geneva, Author, 1975.

Coping and Stress Tolerance

Gail M. Houck

INTRODUCTION

Coping with a variety of challenges, potential threats, and adverse experiences is a central feature of human development. Influenced by temperamental and developmental differences, coping with stressful events and circumstances is crucial to children's immediate adjustment. The ways children cope can alter the course of their development and influence their responses to subsequent life events.

Most young children have experienced at least one major negative event by early adolescence. There are consistent relationships between stressful events and children's adjustment. Typically, higher levels of stress, whether caused by undesirable life events or daily circumstances, are associated with higher levels of behavioral symptoms. Problem behaviors, which are viewed as a manifestation of children's responses to stress and as a reflection of their coping efforts, affect 10 to 30% of families with youngsters.

The nurse practitioner (NP) must assess children's adverse life experiences as well as potential or actual behavioral problems that accompany them. Because preschool behavior problems tend to continue through the school-age (Egeland et al., 1990; Fagot & Leve, 1998; Prior et al., 1992) and adolescent years (Tubman et al., 1993), and because they are linked to adult psychopathology, early identification and intervention in childhood behavior problems is crucial. Improvement in children with early behavior problems is related to reduction in occurrence of adverse life experiences or enhancement of children's environmental circumstances. If NPs take a proactive stance toward early intervention in children's stressful experiences and toward the development of their coping efforts and behavioral manifestations, children's subsequent development can be influenced in a positive direction.

NURSING STANDARDS

The Region X Nursing Network (1998) identified the following goal and outcomes for the Coping/Stress Tolerance Pattern for children:

Newborn	The newborn copes and tolerates stress in a way that promotes health, growth, and development
1 month to 3 years	The child copes and tolerates stress in a way that promotes health, growth, and development
School age	The child's coping patterns promote health, growth, and development

| Adolescent | The adolescent develops and demonstrates patterns of coping and stress reduction that promote optimal physical and emotional health |

At the minimum, according to the *AMA Guidelines for Adolescent Preventive Services (GAPS),* all adolescents should be asked annually about behaviors or emotions that indicate recurrent or severe depression or risk of suicide (Elster & Kuznets, 1994).

DEVELOPMENTAL CONTEXT

Psychopathology can be considered a distortion in the normal developmental process when children lack integration of the cognitive, social, and emotional competencies crucial to adaptation at a given developmental period. Failure to achieve competencies at one developmental period makes adaptation more difficult at the subsequent period and affects adaptation throughout the life span. In short, early deviations or disturbances in functioning contribute to the emergence of later disturbed patterns (Cicchetti, 1987).

Poor behavioral adaptation requires early intervention with a view toward prevention of later maladaptation. Two features of child development provide some optimism and direction for early intervention. First, children possess a self-righting and self-organizing tendency that encourages normal development in the face of pressure for deviation. A single instance of stress or negative forces at one traumatic point in time do not usually interfere with the child's development and adaptation. Rather, maladaptive outcomes result from continuous malfunction in the caretaking environment, such as poor parenting (Sameroff & Chandler, 1975). Second, many factors—family changes, day care, foster care, reduced stress—mediate between early and later maladaptation to permit more positive outcomes (Cicchetti, 1987). Changes in children's experiences allow the achievement of adaptive competencies and the successful negotiation of subsequent developmental tasks. Efforts that target children's cop-

ing problems and their behavioral manifestations by intervening with parenting and family environments at the earliest opportunity allow children to "self-right." The parent–child relationship and family functioning are critical to children's effective coping with inevitable stress.

STRESS DURING CHILDHOOD

The stresses that children face can be organized into three categories of life events that represent *sets of events* formulated by Rutter (1981):

1. Those that tend to occur as part of a broader network of chronic problems or circumstances
2. Those that require lasting or permanent life changes
3. Those that stem from the person's own behavior

In addition, the child's perception of those events must be considered.

Although change itself has been viewed as intrinsically stressful, more recent research shows that negative outcomes are largely confined to unpleasant or adverse experiences, especially those that continue over time (Egeland et al., 1990; Goodyer, 1990; Rutter, 1989).

Perceptions of events and reactions to them are filtered through children's developing cognitive, emotional, and social capacities. The relevance of life events and the child's vulnerability to their impact depend on the given developmental period. The salient tasks and issues that constitute each developmental period are listed in Table 21–1.

Developmental differences account, in part, for how some life events may be "nonshared" between siblings. An experience that is salient and perceived negatively by one child may be irrelevant to or perceived positively by another sibling. Experiences of short duration with immediate impact and no long-term consequences are relatively benign. In contrast, acute events with long-term impact or consequences carry psychosocial risk, and negative chronic experiences carry a long-term threat because they present ongoing or enduring factors that make

T A B L E 21-1

Developmental Tasks and Issues by Age Group

0 to 1 yr	Biological regulation; formation of attachment
1 to 3 yr	Exploration of physical and social environment (with caregiver as secure base); development of self: separation, individuation, and autonomy; responding to external control of impulses
3 to 5 yr	Flexible self-regulation; self-reliance and initiative; gender concept; empathy; development of peer relationships
6 to 12 yr	Gender constancy; school adjustment; same-gender friendships; social understanding; sense of competence
13+ yr	Perspective taking; loyal friendships; beginning heterosexual relationships; identity; emancipation

From Stroufe LA, Rutter M: The domain of developmental psychopathology. Child Dev 55:17–29, 1984.

the child vulnerable (Sandberg et al., 1993). On the whole, the most difficult life events are those that persistently alter personal relationships or foster negative self-evaluation, for example, divorce, family discord, and harsh or neglectful parenting styles.

CHILDHOOD COPING

Definition

Coping refers to the responses to stressful events or experiences and is differentiated in three ways (Compas, 1987):

1. Coping is distinguished from instinctive responses and includes all purposeful reactions to stress regardless of their effectiveness.
2. Coping responses are generally of two types, those intended to act on the stressor and those intended to regulate emotional states. Also known as *problem-focused coping* (Folkman & Lazarus, 1980), efforts to act on the stressor include problem-solving or altering the situation. Examples of efforts to regulate the emotional state include avoidance, cognitive reframing, and selective attention to positive aspects of the situation.
3. Coping mechanisms differ depending on resources, styles, and situation. Resources are the personal and environmental characteristics that facilitate effective adaptation to stress. Personal characteristics that help shape children's coping responses include

temperament, cognitive development, and social development. The nature of the social environment and the availability of environmental coping resources (e.g., a supportive network) also influence the development of coping strategies.

Coping styles flow from personal and environmental resources and develop in response to particular types of stressful episodes.

Role of Temperament in Coping

Temperament serves as a foundation for coping and has generally come to be accepted as inborn. Temperament involves an individual's characteristic style of emotional and behavioral response across situations, especially those involving change or stress (McClowry, 1992). Although biological in origin, temperament is influenced by environmental characteristics and is patterned in significant ways by the social environment. This view of temperament is clinically important because both short- and long-term psychosocial adjustment are shaped by the goodness of fit between the individual's temperament and the social environment. Goodness of fit refers to the consonance of a given child's temperament with the expectations, demands, and opportunities of the social environment (Chess & Thomas, 1984). This includes those of parents, family, day care setting, and school setting.

Infants' first coping efforts are determined by temperament and are expressed by a range of responsiveness to stress (Compas, 1987). A variety of dimensions of temperament have been proposed (Table 21-2). Overall, there appears to be consensus that three factors are inherent in temperament: sociability, activity, and emotionality (Coffman et al., 1992; Prior, 1992).

TEMPERAMENT TYPES

Three types of temperament have clinical utility and can be generalized cross-culturally: difficult, easy, and slow to warm up. Children with *difficult temperaments* tend to be characterized by an intense and negative mood, slow adaptability, withdrawal from new situations, and irregularity in biological functions (McClowry, 1992). Children with *easy temperaments* typically exhibit a prevailing positive mood, low intensity, ready adaptability, and regularity and predictability of biological and behavioral patterns. In other words, these children are easygoing. Children with *slow to warm up temperaments* are characterized by initial quiet alertness and subdued emotionality. This reserve in the face of new situations and stimuli gives way to features of an easy or difficult temperament. There is no absolute standard for any of these classifications, and all features of temperament must

be considered in the context of the parents' evaluations.

TEMPERAMENT AS A RISK FACTOR

Temperament predicts behavioral disturbance in preschool (Mehregany, 1991; Prior et al., 1992), elementary school (McClowry, 1995; Prior et al., 1992), and adolescence and young adulthood (Goodyer et al., 1993; Tubman et al., 1993). Difficult temperaments seem to be most consistently related to behavior disorders (see Prior et al., 1992, for review). Temperament alone is not a risk factor for maladjustment. Rather, temperament exerts an influence on children's psychosocial adjustment by way of its effect on caretaker–child interactions (Egeland et al., 1990; Prior et al., 1992). Difficult temperamental features tend to engender parental criticism and irritability as well as conflicted and coercive interactions. Critical mediators of the role of temperament in the development of behavioral disorder include parental psychological functioning, marital adjustment, child-rearing attitudes and practices, and social support factors. Although temperament is unrelated to intelligence quotient (IQ), it impacts academic outcomes and some children

T A B L E 21-2
Temperament Dimensions

BUSS & PLOMIN (1984)	THOMAS & CHESS (1977)	ROTHBART (1989)	BATES (1989)	STRALAY (1983)
Activity	Activity level	Activity level	Attention regulation	Activity
Emotionality	Persistence	Attention span	Emotionality	Reactivity
Sociability	Rhythmicity (regulation)	Self-regulative functions	Adaptability	
	Mood (prevailing positive/negative)	Smiling and laughing	Reactivity	
	Intensity of response	Fear		
	Distractability or ease of soothing	Reaction to frustration		
	Approach vs. withdrawal to new stimuli	Soothability		
	Adaptability to new experiences	Reactivity		
	Threshold of responsiveness			

Data from Prior M: Childhood temperament. J Child Psychol Psychiatry 33:249–279, 1992.

are clearly disadvantaged by their more difficult temperaments in the majority of school environments (McClowry, 1995).

TEMPERAMENT MANAGEMENT

The goal for the NP is to help parents achieve goodness of fit for their children. Specific strategies for intervening with temperament issues have been developed for parents of infants (Medoff-Cooper, 1995), toddlers (Gross & Conrad, 1995), preschoolers (Melvin, 1995), and school-age children (McClowry, 1995). These can be readily integrated into well-child care:

- Assist parents, other caregivers, and teachers to recognize the child's innate behavioral qualities as expressions of temperament. Perceptions of the child can be obtained through an interview about typical situations (e.g., changes in activities, new situations, changes in routines, new people, task completion) or by completing a standard temperament questionnaire.
- Assist parents and others to understand how temperament is related to behavior and is not amenable to change. This means allowing the parents, for example, to express their feelings about their child or their child's behavior, and assisting them in reframing their assessment more positively. Members of the extended family who often advise parents may need to be included to help alleviate feelings of failure.
- Assist parents, caregivers, and teachers to develop temperament-based management strategies. Such strategies can be applied to new situations, such as those that occur in infancy (Medoff-Cooper, 1995), or during routine situations, such as mealtime and bedtime for preschoolers (Melvin, 1995), or during school-related activities, such as doing homework (McClowry, 1995).

Role of Development in Coping

Strategies that children use to cope vary according to their cognitive, motor, and affective capacities, social abilities, and feelings about themselves. Although little research has been conducted on the relationship between development and coping strategies, some general points can be made.

From birth to age 2 years, children are highly dependent on the primary caretaker, typically the mother, to cope effectively with the world. Dominant coping strategies include those behaviors and strategies that serve to meet the child's needs. The behaviors and strategies become more complex as autonomy and increasing sociability begin to emerge at about 1 year of age. Also at around 12 months of age, goal-directed behavior and a sense of causality reflect children's developing reasoning capacities. At about 15 to 18 months, capacities for fantasy and problem-solving emerge, and language development facilitates shared communication.

From 2 to 6 years of age, several capacities emerge that help children learn about coping from parents: maintaining self-generated goals, modeling adult activities, naming and describing feelings, referring to the self as an objective entity, using language to share words and ideas, engaging socially with others, and reflecting on the self (self-awareness). Memory for events develops, with salient features retained and perhaps distorted. During this period, children can reason in familiar contexts about experiences but have difficulty reasoning with novel experiences. A search for causal explanations often results in magical thinking. Children's strategies for coping at this age include asserting themselves, engaging in limited problem-solving, and using adults as resources. Symbolic play is a dominant medium for effective coping.

During middle childhood (6 to 12 years), a more integrated self emerges. As cognitive and perspective-taking skills mature, school-age children can make logical inferences based on what is known. Dominant coping strategies include a focus on the self, problem-solving, and overt and direct action toward adapting to challenges. Children who are less adept at generating and using problem-focused coping strategies have more behavior problems (Compas et al., 1988). Older school-age children and young adolescents use emotion-management strategies and intrapsychic coping. These strategies reflect increasing cognitive capacities but are not as effective as problem-focused strategies (Compas et al., 1988; Wertlieb et al., 1987).

Stress and Ineffective Coping: General Behavior Problems

There are two broad categories of problem behaviors for preschool and school-age children: "internalizing" and "externalizing." Internalizing behavior is constituted by social withdrawal, depressive symptoms, sleep problems, and somatic problems. Internalizing disorders are conditions whose central feature is disordered mood or emotion (Kovacs & Devlin, 1998). Externalizing behavior consists of aggressive and destructive behavior. Externalizing disorders are ones whose central feature is dysregulated behavior. Both behavior types demonstrate consistency from preschool through school age, with stability for the externalizing behavior remarkable for its link to adult pathology and antisocial outcomes.

From 12 to 20% of young children are believed to exhibit behavior problems at some time during their early years in the home or school setting, or both. Even when stringently defined by clinical severity, behavioral maladjustment is a significant concern for 10% of families (Prior et al., 1992). Transitory behavior symptoms might be argued as "normative," particularly in response to transient stresses, such as birth of a sibling, beginning school, or reaching developmental periods such as toddlerhood and adolescence. Whereas transitory behavior difficulties might be no cause for alarm, behavior problems in early childhood are good predictors for adverse long-term outcomes.

BEHAVIOR PROBLEMS AS RISK FACTORS

Children with behavior problems in preschool do not outgrow their problems as many clinicians and some researchers believe. The majority of preschoolers with behavior problems continue to have them in early grade school (Egeland et al., 1990; Fagot & Leve, 1998), especially those with externalizing behavior problems. These children are subsequently less competent and have greater pathology in adolescence and adulthood.

A 20% prevalence estimate for a psychiatric disorder rooted in behavioral problems was consistently identified in earlier epidemiological studies of the general population of children. A more recent epidemiological study reported that one third of 9- to 20-year-olds received a diagnosis for at least a mild disorder (Cohen et al., 1993a). Furthermore, substantial persistence of the diagnoses was found for all but one disorder (major depression) over a 2½-year period. These prevalence estimates are much larger than service data that estimate that 2 to 3% of children receive treatment for emotional or behavioral problems (Cohen et al., 1993b). Pediatric behavior problems are common but usually remain undiagnosed or untreated (Herman-Staab, 1994).

Higher levels of stress, whether assessed in terms of negative life events or negative circumstances ("daily hassles"), consistently predict higher levels of behavior problems (Egeland et al., 1990; Goodyer, 1990). The level of family stress is related to the quality of the caretaking style (degree of nurturing and aversiveness) and the quality of the home environment, especially the degree of predictability and organization (Fagot & Leve, 1998). When children with behavior problems improve (e.g., between preschool age and school age), a reduction in stressful life events and more optimal parenting and home environments have been found. These relationships between life events and psychosocial dysfunction do not appear to be influenced by gender or age (Egeland et al., 1990; Fagot & Leve, 1998).

ASSESSMENT

Self-report, which is central to adult diagnosis, does not occur in children. The diagnosis of behavior problems usually depends on complaints by parents or teachers when the child's behavior is inconvenient, embarrassing, or imposes on others. Assessment must, therefore, explore possible negative life events and circumstances as well as behavioral symptoms in the event that problems have yet to meet the nuisance criteria. The goal is not simply to relieve symptoms but to facilitate and strengthen long-term behavioral adaptation and progress in cognitive, social, and emotional development.

History

RECENT LIFE EVENTS

Assess recent events: "What important events or changes have occurred in your family in the past year?"

1. Objectively defined events:
   - Moves
   - Changes in household composition (births, departures)
   - Separations from family
   - Illnesses and hospital contacts
   - Changes in parents' work
   - Changes in family relationships
   - Changes in school
   - Major traumatic incidents
   - Changes in routines
2. Developmental context of events and whether most age mates would find the incident threatening, upsetting, or unsettling
3. Contextual threat—short-term and long-term consequences:
   - Loss or risk of loss of attachment figure
   - Physical jeopardy
   - Witness to trauma
   - New role or responsibilities (psychological challenge)
4. Enduring change in life circumstances, for better or worse
5. Consequent changes in the child's perception of self, family, or relationship security
6. Extent to which events stem from the child's behavior (resulting in self-blame) or stem from the actions of other family members, especially parents (creating a sense of betrayal)

CHRONIC EXPERIENCES

Determine chronic events: "What sorts of difficulties or hassles in parenting or family life do you have on a daily basis?"

1. Chronic conditions or circumstances, such as:
   - Parental overprotection
   - Lack of effective parental supervision
   - Ineffective control strategies
   - Ineffective conflict resolution
   - Parental failure to protect child in risky situations

   - Control struggles
   - Mental health problems of parents, especially maternal depression
   - Child's chronic illness or handicap
2. Major life happenings that have lasting influence:
   - Loss of parent by death or separation
   - Loss of sibling by death or separation
   - Chronic illness or handicap of any family member
   - Any hospitalization
   - Any separations (e.g., in home of relatives or foster care)
   - Victim of sexual or physical abuse
   - Witness of trauma
   - Major psychiatric illness in a parent
3. Duration of experiences or circumstances

BEHAVIORAL MANIFESTATIONS

Seek information about how the child's behavior problems manifest.

- Parental description of undesirable and desired behaviors
- Parental perceptions about the nature of the child's problems, including cause and severity as measured by frequency and duration
- Situational context that elicits or maintains problem behavior (setting, timing, who is present, triggers)
- Situational context in which the problem behavior does not occur
- Responses to and consequences of problem behavior

PARENT AND FAMILY ASSESSMENT

The parent and family assessment includes the following:

- Parental knowledge and beliefs about child behavior problems
- As thorough a child and family history of behavior problems as is possible, especially given the role genetically driven biological processes play in internalizing disorders (Kovaks & Devlin, 1998)
- Any indicators of parental psychopathology, particularly maternal depression (Egeland et al., 1990; Sandberg et al., 1993)

- The parents' perception of the child, especially temperament
- The parents' knowledge and beliefs about harsh discipline or coercive parent–child interactions (Sandberg et al., 1993; Weiss et al., 1992)
- The parents' knowledge and beliefs about the development of autonomy and self-esteem should be assessed, especially in relation to parenting strategies (e.g., praise and affection) and conflict resolution
- Parental understanding of the relationship between life events and behavior
- Parental strategies to facilitate their child's coping given the child's developmental level and temperament

GENERAL HEALTH HISTORY

The general health history should include the following:

- Prenatal history, including mother's use of substances
- Birth history, including complications or medical conditions
- Childhood illnesses
- Neurological injuries or soft neurological signs
- Developmental progress and achievement of milestones to reveal any existing vulnerability or risk status

Physical Examination

A complete physical examination and developmental screening should be included in the assessment. If warranted by suspicious or ambiguous findings, the child should be referred for a more thorough developmental evaluation.

Diagnostic Studies

LABORATORY

Pertinent laboratory tests (hemoglobin or hematocrit, blood lead level, urinalysis) rule out physical health problems with behavioral manifestations (Herman-Staab, 1994).

STRUCTURED PARENTAL REPORTS

An assessment of temperament is useful for infants, toddlers, preschoolers, and school-age children (see Resource Box 21-1 for a list of assessment tools). A behavioral diary or log kept by parents, by the school-age child, and by the teacher informs the practitioner and family about the situational context for and severity of the behavior problem or problems. Often, this monitoring process itself serves as an effective intervention. Behavior rating scales or checklists are valuable screening tools, especially because they usually have established reliability and validity and provide norms as a basis for comparison. The Child Behavior Checklist provides separate checklists for age groups (2 to 3 years and 4 to 16 years), with norms provided by age and gender, and with separate report forms for parents and teachers. Other checklists with clinical utility include the Eyberg Child Behavior Inventory (ECBI) (Eyberg & Ross, 1978) for 2- to 16-year-olds and the Pediatric Symptom Checklist (PSCL) (Jellineck & Murphy, 1997) for 6- to 12-year-olds (see Resource Box 21-2). Even if children's scores do not reach a clinical level by normative standards, attention must be paid to notably high scores, stable problem behavior, and attending circumstances.

BEHAVIORAL OBSERVATION

Behavioral observation of parent–child interactions and family dynamics can be made in the course of the assessment. Features to observe include the tone and quality of verbal communication, the emotional tone or warmth of the parent–child relationship, patterns of control and submissiveness, degree of involvement (enmeshed vs. distant), acceptance and rejection, and affection. If necessary, children and their parents can be referred for further assessment, with concerns and observations documented.

▓▓▓ STRATEGIES FOR MANAGEMENT

Pediatric primary care providers can manage some coping and stress problems whereas others should be referred. Generally speaking, if the cause of the problem is a life event with acute, short-term consequences, such as the death of a pet or the loss of a friend, it is probably manageable in primary care settings. More enduring problems, such as loss of a parent, should be referred. The strategies that primary care providers can use effectively include primary prevention of behavior problems and secondary prevention.

Primary Prevention

Primary prevention of behavior problems occurs through positive, nurturing parent–child relationships. It is crucial for children to experience a secure attachment relationship, with a sense of worth and lovableness, as a foundation for effective coping. Healthy parenting strategies are positive in tone and regard for the child, responsive to the child's autonomy and individuality, neutral in response to unwanted behavior, and attentive to the child's needs (Herman-Staab, 1994) (Table 21-3).

NPs can also assist parents to anticipate predictable life events that are likely to influence children, such as changes in day care or care providers, moves, or changes in schools. Chil-

dren's developmental and temperamental needs must be assessed and strategies identified for facilitating the transition in a way that meets those needs. Parents can be educated to facilitate the uses of developmentally appropriate coping strategies available to children. Encouraging symbolic play or expression through developmentally appropriate media contributes to adaptive coping.

Secondary Prevention

Secondary prevention or early intervention is required for unanticipated life events. Such events occur, and behavior problems can emerge, even with positive parenting approaches. At the level of secondary prevention, appropriate parental management strategies must often be employed to deal effectively with the problem behavior (see Chapters 5 to 9). Harsh discipline or physical punishment is consistently linked to negative outcomes for children in terms of behavioral maladaptation, low self-esteem, and poor social competence. A va-

---

T A B L E 21-3
Positive Parenting Strategies

ATTENDING TO THE CHILD INDIVIDUALLY
Allow the child to make reasonable choices
Respond to child's bids for attention with eye contact, smiles, and/or physical contact
Comment on child's appropriate/desirable behavior frequently and positively throughout the day
Provide guaranteed special time daily: no interruptions, no directions, no interrogations
Avoid secondary gains for the child's minor transgressions by having no discussion, physical contact,
   perhaps even eye contact; be neutral and simply state the preferred behavior

LISTEN ACTIVELY
Paraphrase or describe what child is saying
Reflect the child's feelings
Share the child's affect by matching the child's body posture and tone of voice
Avoid giving commands, judging, or editorializing
Follow the child's lead in the interaction

CONVEY POSITIVE REGARD
Communicate positive feelings (e.g., love) directly
Give directions positively, firmly, specifically
Provide notice before requiring child to change activities
Label the behavior, not the child
Praise competency and compliance; say thank you
Apologize when appropriate
Avoid shaming or belittling the child
Strive for consistency

riety of strategies, excluding coercive control efforts, must be explored, with emphasis placed on positive parenting strategies that are highly important in primary prevention.

Tertiary Prevention

Tertiary prevention and intervention are required for major losses and traumas, especially that of victimization through sexual or physical abuse, as well as marital problems, divorce, substance abuse, and parental psychopathology. Even in the absence of behavioral manifestations, a referral to a mental health specialist for further assessment and intervention is fruitful given the difficulties that can result and affect behavioral adaptation at a later point.

Referrals in these situations must be firmly presented with a direct appraisal of the circumstances that necessitate it. It is most helpful to frame the behavior problem as a "normal response to an unusual or stressful situation." The goal can be clarified as one that maximizes the child's development and growth. A release of information allows direct contact with the consultant to ensure follow-through. Ongoing follow-up is essential with children, families, and other professional providers.

Table 21-4 presents information about common psychotropic medications that may be prescribed by mental health specialists for children and adolescents.

▇▇▇ COMMON BEHAVIOR PROBLEMS

Fears, Phobias, and Anxieties

FEARS AND PHOBIAS

Description

Fear is the occurrence of various avoidance responses to particular stimuli; it is a state of apprehension or response to a threatening situation. A phobia is a persistent, extreme, and irrational fear. The onset of fears occurs during the transition to toddlerhood.

Etiology and Incidence

Fears actually have a developmental function, and the nature of predominant fears varies

with age. Childhood fears are a part of normal development. In a classic study by MacFarlane and colleagues (1954, as cited by Barrios & Hartmann, 1988), 90% of 2- to 14-year-olds were found to have at least one specific fear. Children from 3 to 11 years of age average 9 to 13 fears (Ollendick, 1983); adolescents (15 to 17 years) average 2 to 3 intense fears. A significant minority of children, however, have fears that interfere with their functioning: specific phobias occur in about 5% of the population and in 15% of children referred for anxiety-related problems (King & Ollendick, 1997). Phobias are determined by multiple factors, with genetic influences, temperament, parental mental health problems, and individual conditioning histories converging in specific phobias (King & Ollendick, 1997).

Clinical Findings

Infants typically react defensively to loss of support, height, and unexpected stimuli. Toddlers experience separation anxiety and fear physical injury and strangers. Preschoolers fear imaginary creatures, animals, darkness, and being alone, and they also demonstrate some persistent separation anxiety. Fear of animals and darkness extends into school age, but safety, natural events, and school- and health-related fears dominate. In preadolescence and adolescence, fears of bodily injury, economic and political catastrophes, and social fears are central. Fear and phobic reactions typically involve symptoms of autonomic arousal. In phobias, the symptoms of autonomic arousal may evolve into panic attacks in addition to phobic avoidant reactions.

Differential Diagnosis

Distinction must be made between abnormal fears and normal developmental fears that encourage the acquisition of boundaries, caution, and safety. Clinical phobias are defined on the basis of persistence, magnitude, and maladaptiveness (Barrios & Hartmann, 1988).

Management

Most fears are short lived, are not serious, and do not predict adult mental health prob-

T A B L E 21-4

*Understanding Common Pediatric Psychotropic Medications**

PRESCRIBING GOALS

Lowest effective dose

Minimal side effects: ½ daily dose the first wk; if no problems, advance to full dose

Simple dosing regimens to facilitate child acceptance and minimize parent stressors

Avoid need for ongoing laboratory and electrocardiographic (EKG) monitoring when possible

DRUG	PHARMACOLOGY (PREDOMINANT NEUROTRANSMITTER EFFECTS)	INDICATIONS	CONCERNS
DRUGS FOR DEPRESSION			
Selective serotonin reuptake inhibitors (SSRIs) Fluoxetine (Prozac) Sertraline (Zoloft) Paroxetine (Paxil) Fluvoxamine (Luvox)	Complex series of changes in reuptake at multiple serotonin (5HT) receptors and autoreceptors may be responsible for the delay in therapeutic response Allow 4 wk to experience benefits before increasing dose Poor response to one SSRI does not indicate similar response to others Low toxicity Once-daily dosing	Depression Anxiety Obsessive-compulsive disorder (OCD) Panic disorder Social phobia	Low side effect profile, but may experience GI upset, headache with initial doses If increase in anxiety, diminish dose as benefits are experienced Infrequent—increased menstrual flow, dizziness with missed doses or discontinuation, paresthesias
Norepinephrine and dopamine reuptake blockers Bupropion (Wellbutrin)	A unicyclic antidepressant whose action is primarily due to its active metabolite, hydroxybupropion, which reaches higher concentrations in the brain Benefits seen within the first 2 wk; may be less likely to trigger mania ADHD application: Bupropion inhibits reuptake of norepinephrine and dopamine, whereas stimulants (methylphenidate, dexedrine, pemoline) cause release *and* inhibit reuptake of norepinephrine and dopamine Available in SR form: b.i.d. dosing for >200 mg, smoother response than the immediate-release form	Depression Anger ADHD when stimulants not appropriate	At daily doses of 450 mg or less of SR form, seizure incidence approximates that of other nontricyclic antidepressants; earlier guidelines for immediate-release form recommended doses of 5 mg/kg Ensure that child can swallow SR tablets whole Generally well tolerated, initial transient effects May increase anxiety/arousal that (unlike SSRIs) does not diminish over time
Dual reuptake (serotonin-norepinephrine) inhibitors Venlafaxine (Effexor)	Primarily inhibits reuptake of serotonin and norepinephrine; some dopamine reuptake inhibition at high doses Simulates beneficial actions of classic tricyclic antidepressants without the muscarinic/alpha-1 anticholinergic and antihistamine side effects Once-daily dosing of XR form Low toxicity	Depression, may be more effective in severe forms	Generally see benefits sooner than with SSRIs Generally well tolerated, possible initial transient GI side effects, headache Complaint of bad taste to immediate-release form not seen with XR form
Tricyclic antidepressants (TCAs) Tertiary amines Imipramine (Tofranil) Amitriptyline (Elavil) Clomipramine (Anafranil) Secondary amines Desipramine (Norpramin) Nortriptyline (Pamelor)	Blocks serotonin and norepinephrine reuptake Muscarinic anticholinergic side effects include dry mouth, constipation, urinary retention, blurred vision Alpha-1 anticholinergic side effects include orthostatic hypotension, dizziness Antihistamine side effects include sedation, weight gain	Depression Enuresis Insomnia ADHD	No longer first choice because available alternatives with fewer side effects and lower toxicity Require baseline and ongoing EKGs in children Lethal in overdose

Table continued on following page

T A B L E 21-4

Understanding Common Pediatric Psychotropic Medications* Continued

DRUG	PHARMACOLOGY (PREDOMINANT NEUROTRANSMITTER EFFECTS)	INDICATIONS	CONCERNS
Serotonin-2 antagonist/ reuptake inhibitors Trazodone (Desyrel)	Blocks serotonin-2 receptors and weakly inhibits serotonin reuptake Blocks alpha-1 adrenergic receptors (dizziness, orthostatic hypotension) Blocks histamine receptors (sedation, weight gain)	An antidepressant that is primarily used in children to improve sleep	Well tolerated at the low doses effective for insomnia Priapism is a rare side effect (1:15,000) Explain priapism to male clients/ parents, requesting they notify prescriber if erectile changes occur
DRUGS FOR ANXIETY			
Serotonin-1A partial agonists Buspirone (Buspar)	Acts directly to desensitize (downregulate) 5HT-1A receptors Delayed response, as with SSRIs	Anxiety	Alternative to benzodiazepines—nonsedating, no tolerance/withdrawal More effective when benzodiazepines have not been used previously May be used to augment SSRIs Not as effective as benzodiazepines for severe anxiety
Benzodiazepines Clonazepam (Klonopin)	The benzodiazepine receptor is part of a complex of receptors modulating gamma aminobutyric acid's fast inhibitory effects on chloride ion channels in the brain There are multiple subtypes of benzodiazepine receptors, which accounts for the variety of benefits and side effects of benzodiazepines	Anxiety	Chronic administration results in dependence and withdrawal
Alpha-2 adrenergic agonists Clonidine (Catapres) Guanfacine (Tenex)	Acts like norepinephrine at alpha-2 receptors, reducing release of more norepinephrine	Anxiety Tourette's ADHD (Primary use is in adults for hypertension)	Reduces physiological arousal (i.e., hypertension, tachycardia, dilated pupils), but not as effective at blocking emotional aspects of anxiety Useful in conjunction with Wellbutrin for ADHD impulsivity/ hyperarousal Requires baseline cardiac evaluation, gradual taper up, and monitoring for blood pressure changes Inform client/parent of orthostatic hypotension symptoms and prevention (e.g., adequate fluids)—usually transient side effect Avoid sudden withdrawal of medication (rebound hypertension)

ADHD = attention deficit–hyperactivity disorder; GI = gastrointestinal; SR = sustained release; XR = extended release.

*This table is intended to provide clinical guidelines for understanding the uses and effects of commonly used medications for children and adolescents with mental health issues. Children who need these drugs should be under the care of a mental health specialist. For prescribing recommendations, refer to standard references.

Table contributed by Mary Beth Kaufman, MS, PMHNP.

References:

Bezchlibnyk-Butler K, Jeffries J, Martin B (eds): Clinical Handbook of Psychotropic Drugs, 4th ed. Toronto, Hogrefe & Huber Publishers, 1994.

Kaplan H, Sadock B: Pocket Handbook of Psychiatric Drug Treatment, 2nd ed. Baltimore, Williams & Wilkins, 1996.

Stahl S: Essential Psychopharmacology: Neuroscientific Basis and Practical Applications. Cambridge, Cambridge University Press, 1996.

lems. Parents absolutely must be cautioned against using fears as a form of behavioral control (e.g., threats of abandonment with toddlers) or as a strategy for discipline (e.g., leaving a preschooler alone in a dark room). The key to whether to refer for treatment is the impact of the fear on the child's functioning, developmental progress, learning experiences, and level of comfort. Various management strategies are available for treatment of phobias: systematic desensitization, contingency management, cognitive-behavioral procedures, and family interventions (King & Ollendick, 1997).

ANXIETY

Anxiety is distinguished from fear on the basis of its diffuse apprehension in response to less specific stimuli. Anxiety that persists at high levels and is reflected in maladaptive behavior warrants diagnosis and treatment. Children diagnosed with anxiety disorders tend to have multiple problems, are impaired in important areas of social functioning, and live with parents who experience symptoms of anxiety or mood disorders (Kovacs & Devlin, 1998). Anxiety disorders typically appear earlier than behavior disorders which, in turn, appear earlier than mood disorders (Kovacs & Devlin, 1998).

A temperamental disposition for affective sensitivity or negative emotionality may be a predisposing factor. Youngsters with anxiety disorders are at high risk for subsequent anxiety disorders, for comorbid anxiety or mood disorders, and for adolescent substance use disorder. Anxiety disorders show distinct clustering in families (Kovacs & Devlin, 1998).

Separation Anxiety Disorder

DESCRIPTION. The essential feature of separation anxiety disorder is excessive anxiety on separation from major attachment figures, home, or familiar surroundings. Separation anxiety is a normal developmental phenomenon from about age 7 months through the preschool years (Bernstein & Borchardt, 1991; Dashiff, 1995). Separation anxiety disorder manifests at from 5 to 16 years of age; the mean age for clinical presentation is 9 years.

ETIOLOGY AND INCIDENCE. Separation anxiety

is thought to evolve from a poor attachment relationship or the interaction between physiological, cognitive, and overt behavioral factors in response to life events that threaten safety or primary relationships, or both. Separation anxiety is probably the most common anxiety disorder in school-age children (Bernstein & Borchardt, 1991) and the most common reason for referral (Last et al., 1992). The rate decreases with age, being present in 13% of girls and 11% of boys at 10 to 13 years of age, 5% of girls and 1% of boys aged 14 to 16 years, and 2% of girls and 3% of boys aged 17 to 20 years (Cohen et al., 1993a).

CLINICAL FINDINGS. The following are found in separation anxiety disorder:

- Developmentally inappropriate or excessive anxiety about separations (American Psychiatric Association, 1994)
- Unrealistic worry about harm to self or attachment figures or about abandonment during periods of separation
- Reluctance to sleep alone or sleep away from home
- Persistent avoidance of being alone
- Nightmares about separation
- Physical complaints and signs of distress in anticipation of separation
- Social withdrawal during separations

Environmental stress and maternal depression are risk factors for separation anxiety disorder, especially with panic disorder or agoraphobia (Dashiff, 1995).

DIFFERENTIAL DIAGNOSIS. Anxiety can be a response to trauma or a manifestation of posttraumatic stress disorder. It is essential to attend to cues that a traumatic experience or situation (e.g., sexual or physical abuse) underlies the symptoms of anxiety. Anxiety disorder not associated with separation is also a differential diagnosis. Common comorbidities with separation anxiety include social phobia and overanxious disorder, followed by major depression and behavior disorder (Kovacs & Devlin, 1998). In adolescence, comorbid substance use disorder increases in prevalence (Kovacs & Devlin, 1998).

MANAGEMENT. This is a family system or relationship-based problem that is preferably treated as such (Dashiff, 1995). The symptoms must be treated and then the sources of the problem pursued. The role of attachment figures must be noted. This diagnosis can be a precursor for agoraphobia or panic disorder in adolescence or adulthood. Refer the patient to a child therapist for early intervention; cognitive-behavioral approaches have been effective, with added benefits obtained from family intervention (Barrett et al., 1996; Ginsburg et al., 1995). Small, diverse studies point to antidepressants and benzodiazepines as having benefit (Bernstein & Borchardt, 1991); refer the patient to a child psychiatrist or mental health NP for a medication evaluation.

Generalized Anxiety Disorder

DESCRIPTION. Generalized anxiety disorder, or overanxious disorder, is cognitive and obsessive in nature. There are excessive anxiety, worry, and apprehensive expectations that are not focused on a specific object or situation, nor are they the result of a recent stressor. It is generalized anxiety about a number of events or activities. These children are characterized as "worriers." The exact onset is not known, but older children and adolescents (9 to 18 years) tend to be represented (Cohen et al., 1993b).

ETIOLOGY AND INCIDENCE. There is a familial association for anxiety that suggests a genetic vulnerability to anxiety as a consequence of social learning; twin studies suggest that shared environment is far less important than genetic factors (Kovacs & Devlin, 1998). The prevalence is relatively stable for girls from 10 to 20 years of age at 14 to 15%; a declining rate is found for boys, with 13% from 10 to 13 years of age and 5% thereafter (Cohen et al., 1993b).

CLINICAL FINDINGS. Major symptoms of generalized anxiety disorder are

- Worry about future events
- Preoccupation with past behavior
- Overconcern about competence
- Marked self-consciousness
- Somatic complaints without physical basis
- Need for reassurance

Additional symptoms include restlessness, fatigue, difficulty concentrating, irritability, tension, and disturbed sleep (American Psychiatric Association, 1994). Comorbidity with other anxiety disorders or mood disorder is common.

DIFFERENTIAL DIAGNOSIS. It is important to attend to cues that might point to traumatic experiences or conditions as the source of anxiety symptoms. Differential diagnoses are separation anxiety, adjustment disorder associated with a specific stressor, and attention deficit disorder. The last does not involve worry about the future.

MANAGEMENT. Refer the patient to a child therapist for treatment of the manifest symptoms through relaxation techniques or cognitive-behavioral therapy. The source of anxiety must be pursued through individual or family counseling. Treatment outcomes are more positive when parents are involved in interventions that target familial contextual processes (Ginsburg et al., 1995). Younger children especially seem to benefit from a combination of cognitive-behavioral strategies and family intervention (Barrett et al., 1996). Pharmacological intervention may be warranted, especially if there is comorbid social phobia or separation anxiety disorder.

Obsessive-Compulsive Disorder

DESCRIPTION. Obsessions are recurrent thoughts or images that are disturbing to the child and difficult to dislodge. They often involve a sense of risk or fear of harm to the child or family members; concerns for contamination are common. Compulsions are repetitive behaviors or mental acts that the child feels driven to perform to prevent harm or remove contaminants, such as washing (e.g., hands, objects, body), counting, or arranging objects (Scahill, 1996). Recurrent worries, rituals, and superstitious games are common in children at various stages of development. These behaviors are attended by mild anxiety but do not cause distress. Abnormal compulsive behavior is distinguished by a sense of urgency or a profound discomfort until the ritual is completed. Children often deny the fear and lack recognition of the "senselessness" of the ritual (Scahill, 1996). Obsessional thoughts are intrusive, recurrent, and disturbing and, unlike anxious worries, are generally unrelated to events or situations.

ETIOLOGY AND INCIDENCE. Obsessive-compulsive disorder (OCD) is more common than previously thought. Neurobiological underpinnings include a role for serotonin and involve abnormalities in the basal ganglia and functionally related cortical structures. Although OCD appears to affect primarily preadolescents and adolescents, OCD is increasingly diagnosed in younger children, some as young as 2 years of age (Rapoport et al., 1993). The rate seems to be about 2.5% of the population (Valleni-Basile et al., 1994). Familial transmission is evident (Kovacs & Devlin, 1998; Scahill, 1996). Studies of OCD show that this condition is chronic, with high rates of comorbidity, typically with some other anxiety disorder, major depression, or substance use disorder (Kovacs & Devlin, 1998).

CLINICAL FINDINGS. OCD is characterized by obsessions and compulsions, as previously defined. Children do not recognize that the obsessions or compulsions are excessive or unreasonable. No pleasure is derived from ritualistic activity. The obsessions and compulsions are time consuming and can significantly interfere with the child's or adolescent's normal routine, academic performance, and social functioning. Washing, checking, and ordering rituals are more common in children (American Psychiatric Association, 1994).

DIFFERENTIAL DIAGNOSIS. If the obsessions or compulsions are a direct physiological consequence of a specific medical condition, the diagnosis is anxiety disorder caused by a general medical condition. If a substance is etiologically related to the obsessions or compulsions, a substance-induced anxiety disorder is assigned. A diagnosis of OCD is warranted if the content of the obsessions and compulsions is unrelated to another disorder (e.g., social phobia, trichotillomania, body dysmorphic disorder). A major depressive episode is diagnosed if the obsessions are mood congruent (e.g., guilt), and generalized anxiety disorder is diagnosed if the obsessions are experienced as excessive worry about real-life circumstances (American Psychiatric Association, 1994.)

MANAGEMENT. Clinical and emerging empirical evidence suggests that cognitive-behavioral psychotherapy, alone or in combination with pharmacotherapy, is an effective treatment for OCD in children and adolescents (March,

1995). Anxiety management training and OCD-specific family interventions play an adjunctive role, especially in preventing the avoidant behavior that is a complication of OCD (Rapoport & Inoff-Germain, 1997). Most OCD patients respond to antidepressant agents that have prominent blocking properties of serotonin uptake. Clomipramine's usefulness is limited by side effects (Rapoport & Inoff-Germain, 1997). See Scahill (1996) for a thorough review of pharmacotherapeutic treatment of children and adolescents with OCD.

Responses to Trauma
DESCRIPTION

Childhood trauma is the result of one sudden traumatic event or exposure to repeated trauma over time, such as physical and sexual abuse (Bernstein & Borchardt, 1991). Childhood trauma begins with events generated outside the child. Studies have identified four characteristic responses to childhood trauma regardless of the child's age or where in the course of the problem the child is assessed (Terr, 1991):

- Strongly visualized or otherwise repeatedly perceived memories
- Repetitive behaviors
- Trauma-specific fears
- Changed attitudes about people, aspects of life, and the future

There are two categories of childhood responses to trauma:

- Acute stress disorder, with symptoms experienced within 2 days of the event for a duration of no more than a month
- Post-traumatic stress disorder (PTSD), with a delayed onset of trauma responses or a duration of symptoms over 4 weeks, or both

For children, it is helpful to consider the nature of the traumatic event as well as whether the responses are acute and of relatively short duration or chronic and long term. Symptoms caused by a one-time traumatic event and those caused by repeated trauma, usually physical and sexual abuse, are discussed separately.

RESPONSES TO A SINGLE TRAUMA

Etiology and Incidence

A single trauma is an unanticipated solitary event directed at the child or witnessed by the child, such as an act of violence that involves threat, injury, or death. It includes learning about unexpected or violent death, harm, or threat experienced by a family member or close friend (American Psychiatric Association, 1994). Proximity to the event influences the severity of the response. Retrospective reports of adults with mental health problems indicate that stress disorder is more common than previously believed. However, actual incidence rates for children have not been reported.

Clinical Findings

In general, children older than 28 to 36 months of age do not become amnestic for the event; they retain full, detailed memories. Younger children (18 to 28 months of age) retain fragments of memories to the extent that they have the verbal capacity to articulate them. Responses to exposure to a single traumatic event tend to be characterized by anxiety (Famularo et al., 1990). With a single traumatic event, children often do not experience psychic numbing, sudden intrusive visual flashbacks, or prolonged effects on school performance, such as adults do. Depending on proximity, the more commonly experienced responses include the following (Bernstein & Borchardt, 1991; Famularo et al., 1990):

- Agitated and disorganized behavior
- Hypervigilance
- Avoidance of reminders of the trauma
- Intrusive memories
- Emotional constriction
- Diminished concentration
- Distorted sense of time
- Sleep disturbances
- Nightmares without recognizable content

Post-traumatic play that expresses themes or aspects of the trauma and reenactment behavior are typical coping strategies.

Differential Diagnosis

The most typical differential diagnosis is an anxiety disorder not precipitated by a traumatic event.

Management

Crisis intervention is often necessary for child and parents. Parents should be educated by the NP about trauma and PTSD. Referral for mental health assessment and counseling is essential.

RESPONSES TO REPEATED TRAUMA

Etiology and Incidence

Repeated trauma is long standing or repeated exposure to a painful event, usually maltreatment (e.g., physical or sexual abuse, or both). Ongoing trauma is typically accompanied by other family dysfunctions, including emotional abuse, neglect, and substance abuse. Estimates for at least one childhood sexual victimization experience range from 19 to 38% for girls and 3 to 15% for boys (Dubowitz et al., 1993). The rate of PTSD is high among those who have been physically and sexually abused, with estimates ranging from 25 to 75% of sexual abuse victims, depending on the perpetrator. The closer the perpetrator is in relation to the victim, the greater the trauma; for example, PTSD is more likely when the perpetrator is a member of the immediate family as opposed to an extended family member, family friend, or stranger.

Clinical Findings

The profile for responses to repeated exposure to trauma is similar to that of depression, detachment, or both (Famularo et al., 1990). However, a high level of anxiety is also prominent. Responses characteristic of PTSD include the following:

- Insomnia
- Poor concentration
- Restricted range of affect
- Sadness
- Thoughts that life is too hard

- Detachment or estrangement from others
- Depersonalization and dissociative episodes

Characteristic coping strategies (Dubowitz et al., 1993) include the following:

- Denial and psychic numbing (not present with single trauma)
- Self-hypnosis and dissociation
- Rage directed against self or others
- Avoidance of reminders of the trauma
- Internalizing or externalizing behavior problems

The trauma can be persistently re-experienced through repetitive play with themes of the trauma, frightening dreams, or behavioral reenactment, or a combination of these. Sexualized (i.e., seductive) behavior is a hallmark sign of sexual abuse. Preschoolers display behavioral or physical symptoms that prompt the caregiver's or other adults' suspicions of sexual abuse. Disclosures by school-age children tend to be purposeful and unrelated to a precipitating event. However, repression and dissociation often preclude disclosure until adulthood.

Differential Diagnosis

With depression or externalizing disorders, such as conduct disorder unrelated to trauma, memory is intact and psychic numbing and dissociation are not present.

Management

During assessment, do not use prompting or leading questions. Instead, ask questions about whether someone has invaded the child's privacy, how it may have happened, and how the injuries came to be. With young children, the use of dolls or drawings provides a basis for disclosure. Crisis intervention is necessary for the child or family in the event that maltreatment is disclosed. Reporting to appropriate authorities is essential for children younger than 18 years of age. Referral to a child mental health specialist is crucial when symptoms are evident, even in the absence of a disclosure. Behavioral problems and psychological sequelae persist, so consistent follow-up assessment is important.

Mood Disorders

DEPRESSION

Description

There are three categories of depression that may be assigned regardless of age: major depressive disorder, dysthymic disorder, and adjustment disorder with depressed mood (American Psychiatric Association, 1994). A *major depressive disorder* is defined as a depressed or irritable mood and/or a markedly diminished interest and pleasure in almost all of the usual activities for a period of at least 2 weeks. A *dysthymic disorder* is characterized by a depressed or irritable mood, more often than not extending over a year-long period of time with symptom relief for no more than 2 months. *Adjustment disorder with depressed mood* typically occurs within 3 months after a major life stressor and is relatively mild and brief.

Etiology and Incidence

Like that of other disorders, the rate of depression increases with age (Kovacs & Devlin, 1998). Depression is estimated to affect between 1 and 9% of school-age children; the rate increases to between 4 and 7% of adolescents (Laraia, 1996). Depression accounts for more than half of the admissions of children and adolescents to psychiatric inpatient units (Laraia, 1996). Kovacs and Devlin (1998) concluded from their review of the empirical literature that gender differences in rates of depressive disorders are neither compelling nor consistent among children or young adolescents, whereas Brent (1993) found depression to be four times higher among adolescent girls. Genetic factors underlie the risk for major depression, especially for childhood onset. The offspring of depressed parents are 3 times as likely to be diagnosed with depression, with a peak incidence at 15 to 20 years of age (Weissman et al., 1997).

Three biological theories of depression are used to understand the psychopharmacology of depression: impaired neurotransmission, endocrine dysfunction, and biological rhythm dysfunction (see Laraia, 1996, for review). Given this biological predisposition, certain life events may trigger the onset of depression. These include loss of a parent or significant other, losses that attend a disability or injury, family dysfunction, and physical or sexual abuse. There is a high risk of recurrent depression in depressed children and adolescents that appears to persist into young adulthood. An important feature of early-onset depressive illness is a switch from unipolar depression to bipolar depression (Kovacs, 1996). The most common comorbidity with depression is an anxiety disorder, which co-occurs two to three times more often than conduct disorder (Kovacs & Devlin, 1998).

Clinical Findings

Any disturbance in mood that is attended by functional impairment should be assessed (Brent, 1993). Talking directly with the child or adolescent is essential because it is thought that half of depression cases are missed when parents alone are interviewed. The following depressive symptoms may exist:

- Depressed mood: sad, "blue," down, angry, bored
- Loss of interest and pleasure in usual activities
- Change in appetite/weight (loss or increase)
- Insomnia or hypersomnia
- Low energy and fatigue
- Difficulty concentrating; indecision
- Feelings of worthlessness or inappropriate or excessive guilt
- Recurrent thoughts of death or suicidal ideation

Tearfulness and depressed affect, observable psychomotor agitation or retardation, and somatic complaints are common. A diagnosis of major depressive disorder is made if there have been at least 2 weeks of depressed mood or loss of interest and at least four additional symptoms of depression. The symptoms cause considerable distress and impairment in social and academic functioning. Therefore, it is important to assess the following:

- Recent life events and losses
- Family history of depression or other psychiatric disorders
- Family dysfunction

- Changes in school performance
- Risk-taking behavior, including sexual activity and substance use
- Deteriorating relationships with family
- Changes in peer relations, especially social withdrawal

Possible warning signs for suicide are listed in Table 21–5.

Dysthymic disorder is diagnosed if the child or adolescent has had depressed mood for the majority of days in the past year and has other symptoms but not to the extent of a major depressive episode. *Adjustment disorder with depressed mood* involves less severe symptoms and functioning is less impaired.

In infants and preschoolers, depressive symptoms may include anorexia with lack of expected weight gain, weight loss, or failure to thrive; sleep problems; apathy and social withdrawal; and developmental delays. School-age children may manifest externalizing behavior, such as hyperactivity or difficulty handling aggression. School phobia or school problems are common. On the other hand, school-age children may have internalizing symptoms such as anxiety, irritability, social withdrawal, somatic complaints (gastrointestinal, headaches, chest pain), eating or sleeping disturbances, and enuresis or encopresis. Depressive symptoms in adolescents additionally include impulsivity, fatigue, and hopelessness. Substance abuse is a problem for about 20%.

Depression Scales

Both patient self-report and clinician-completed rating scales are available. The following are used in pediatrics:

- Child Behavior Checklist (4 to 18 years)
- Children's Depression Inventory (6 to 12 years)
- Pediatric Symptom Checklist (6 to 12 years)
- Zung Self-Rating Depression Scale (adolescents)
- Beck Depression Inventory (adolescents)

Differential Diagnosis

Some medications (steroids, phenobarbital, antihypertensives) and certain chronic illnesses

T A B L E 21-5

Warning Signs for Suicide

AREA OF FUNCTIONING	SIGNS*
Change in behavior	Accident prone
	Drug and alcohol abuse
	Physical violence toward self, others, or animals
	Loss of appetite
	Sudden alienation from family, friends, coworkers
	Worsening performance at work/school
	Putting personal affairs in order
	Loss of interest in personal appearance
	Disposal of possessions
	Writing letters, notes, or poems with suicidal content
	Taking unnecessary risks
	Buying a gun
Changes in mood	Expressions of hopelessness or impending doom
	Explosive rage
	Dramatic swings in affect
	Crying spells
	Sleep disorders
	Talk about suicide
Changes in thinking	Preoccupation with death
	Difficulty concentrating
	Irrational speech
	Hearing voices, seeing visions
	Sudden interest (or loss of interest) in religion
Major life changes	Death of a family member or friend (especially by suicide)
	Separation or divorce
	Public humiliation or failure
	Serious illness or trauma
	Loss of financial security

*These signs must be interpreted in context. Many of them are common outside the realm of presuicidal behavior. From Oregon Health Division: Suicidal thoughts, suicidal deaths. CD Summary 46:24, 2, 1997.

(hypothyroidism, multiple sclerosis, inflammatory bowel disease, and type 1 diabetes) predispose for mood disorder. If a substance (e.g., medication, toxin, or drug of abuse) is related to the mood disturbance, a substance-induced mood disorder is diagnosed. A depressive episode with irritable mood can be difficult to distinguish from a manic episode with irritable mood; careful evaluation of the presence of manic symptoms (e.g., excessive activity, inflated self-esteem, little need for sleep, talkativeness) is required. Mood disturbance that reflects irritability rather than sadness or loss of interest must be differentiated; mood disorder can be overdiagnosed in youths with attention deficit–hyperactivity disorder (ADHD) (American Psychiatric Association, 1994).

Management

The first goal of management is determination of suicidal risk. In a recent follow-up study, approximately 37% of those with childhood-onset depression reported suicide attempts in the 12 years after they were diagnosed (Wolk & Weissman, 1996). *Acute suicidal intent,* which includes a plan, requires immediate psychiatric evaluation. *Cumulative suicidal risks*—prior suicidal behavior or attempts, depression, and alcohol or drug use—require psychiatric intervention as well, but attention must also be paid to the establishment of a safe environment (removal of firearms and lethal medications), provision of community resources such as hotlines, and commitment to a no-suicide agreement by which the adolescent agrees to refrain from harming himself or herself and promises to notify the caretaker or care provider if suicidal ideation returns.

A major depressive episode requires intervention by a mental health specialist (NP or psychiatrist). Therapies typically include cognitive-behavioral strategies in a group or individual psychotherapy format. Often, family therapy or psychoeducation is indicated. A central issue in psychopharmacological approaches is that children and adolescents are not usually included in clinical drug trial research; safety and efficacy data from the literature about adults are often extrapolated. In general, the use of tricyclic antidepressants (imipramine is approved for children age 12 years and older) is declining as the newer agents prove safer and more tolerable (Laraia, 1996). The use of selective serotonin reuptake inhibitors (SSRIs) in clinical practice is increasing, although there is little research documenting their safety and efficacy in depressed children. There is no compelling evidence for the use of monoamine oxidase inhibitors (MAOIs) in children (Laraia, 1996). See Table 21-4.

BIPOLAR DISORDER

Description

Bipolar disorder is determined from a clinical course characterized by one or more manic episodes and, typically, one or more episodes of major depression. There is evidence that depression precedes mania early in the course of bipolar disorder in children and adolescents (Bowden & Rhodes, 1996). It is a recurrent disorder in which nearly all of those (90%) who have a single manic episode will have future episodes. A characteristic pattern usually evolves for a particular person, with manic episodes preceding or following major depressive episodes. Most individuals with bipolar disorder return to a full level of functioning between episodes; 20 to 30% experience persistent

mood lability and interpersonal difficulties (American Psychiatric Association, 1994). Sometimes psychotic symptoms develop after several days or weeks; such features tend to predict that the individual with subsequent manic episodes will again experience psychotic symptoms. There is growing evidence that bipolar disorder is comorbid with panic disorder, bulimia, conduct disorder, and ADHD (Bowden & Rhodes, 1996).

Etiology and Incidence

There is evidence of a genetic influence for bipolar disorder from twin studies and adoption studies; bipolar disorder tends to cluster in families. Although the lifetime prevalence of bipolar disorder varies from 0.4 to 1.6% (American Psychiatric Association, 1994), there is concern that the prevalence of childhood onset (prepubertal) may be increasing (Geller, 1997). There is no differential incidence based on race, ethnicity, or gender. Children with ADHD seem to be vulnerable to bipolar illness (Lombardo, 1997). If children are also bipolar, treatment of ADHD with psychostimulants or antidepressants may precipitate a manic episode. Tricyclic antidepressants in depressed children (6 to 12 years of age) may also precipitate mania and the onset of bipolar illness (Lombardo, 1997).

Clinical Findings

The hallmark feature of a bipolar disorder is a manic episode and usually at least one major depressive episode (previously described). A manic episode is a defined period (at least 1 week) during which there is a persistent, abnormally elevated, expansive, or irritable mood. This disturbance of mood is accompanied by three or more of the following symptoms: inflated self-esteem or grandiosity, decreased need for sleep (e.g., 3 hours), talkativeness or compulsion to talk, racing thoughts, distractibility, and psychomotor agitation or increase in goal-directed activity (socially or at school). The mood may shift rapidly to anger or depression; behavioral aggression may be manifested. In adolescents, manic episodes are more likely to include psychotic features and may be associated with school truancy, school failure, substance use, or antisocial behavior. No laboratory findings diagnostic of a manic episode have been identified, so a careful history and assessment is crucial.

Differential Diagnosis

A manic episode must be distinguished from a mood disorder caused by a medical condition (e.g., brain tumor) and a substance-induced mood disorder (e.g., cocaine, amitriptyline). A manic episode must also be distinguished from a hypomanic episode; a hypomanic disturbance is not sufficiently severe to cause marked impairment in functioning but may precede a full manic episode. ADHD is also characterized by excessive activity, poor impulse control and judgment, and denial of problems that are found with a manic episode. ADHD is distinguished from a manic episode by its lack of clear onsets or episodes, absence of mood disturbances, and lack of psychotic features. However, recent evidence that children with ADHD are vulnerable to bipolar disorder and that pharmacological treatments may precipitate manic episodes points to the need for very careful evaluation and referral to the provider (usually a psychiatrist) who is treating the ADHD.

Management

Referral to a child psychiatrist or child mental health NP is critical. Options in the pharmacological treatment of mania include valproate, divalproex, and carbamazepine, as well as lithium (Bowden & Rhodes, 1996). The use of lithium in children is gradually increasing (Laraia, 1996), especially in combination with methylphenidate, anticonvulsive agents, calcium channel blockers, thyroid medications, and electroconvulsive therapy (ECT) (Botteron & Geller, 1995). Psychotherapy and psychoeducation for the family are recommended to facilitate the management of this episodic disorder.

The Aggressive Child

SOCIAL AGGRESSION

Description

Social aggression is a pattern of social behavior based primarily on aversive control of situations and others. Onset occurs in toddlerhood.

Etiology and Incidence

Acute, stressful life events or transitions can precipitate a brief period of social aggression. A range of antecedents has been found, including a history of maltreatment (physical or sexual abuse, or both); inconsistent or harsh discipline, or both; separations from parents, shifts in parent figures, or parental rejection; and other stressful life events or enduring circumstances. Social aggression can be a precursor to conduct disorder or oppositional disorder. The incidence rate is thought to be higher than that for clinical diagnoses because most cases are untreated.

Clinical Findings

Excessively high levels of aggressive behavior involve the following (Hops & Greenwood, 1988):

- Destruction of property
- Name calling
- Physical pestering
- Threatening
- Hitting, biting, kicking
- Frequent engagement in disagreements with peers
- Temper tantrums
- High activity level
- Carrying expectations of others' hostility
- Misinterpreting social cues and responding aggressively
- Limited problem-solving in social situations

When social aggression becomes a pattern of behavior rather than an isolated response to stress, peer rejection is common. In fact, negative behavior in preschool play groups is predictive of externalizing behavior problems in the classroom when children are in kindergarten (Fagot & Leve, 1998).

Differential Diagnosis

Oppositional disorder is directed primarily toward parents and teachers and is more defiant than aggressive. Conduct disorder is a clear pattern of behavior established over a 6-month period and typically diagnosed at school age.

Management

It is important to ascertain whether a difficult temperament underlies the behavioral difficulty, especially in conjunction with a lack of fit with parental temperament. A difficult temperament may account for a child's being harder to discipline, having social behavior problems in school (e.g., poor fit with the teacher), or having poor academic achievement (Carey, 1998). In these situations, the use of positive parenting strategies does not have to change, but supportive counseling for the parents should be provided regarding temperament, its manifestations, and strategies for managing transitions and other difficult times or behaviors. A conference with the teacher may be valuable to provide similar information and to explore strategies to facilitate the child's learning and positive behavior (Carey, 1998).

When social aggression is a response to acute stress, the problem usually resolves if parents employ positive parenting strategies and facilitate developmentally appropriate coping efforts. If peer relationship development is hampered, close monitoring of and intervention with peer interactions by day care or preschool personnel, especially with the parents present for observations, enhance appropriate social behavior and competence. Changing schools in an effort to ameliorate problems is not advised, because children have been found to carry their social difficulties with them and assume the same roles in new groups. The teacher needs to be supportive and facilitative.

When social aggression becomes a pattern of social behavior, referral for intervention is critical. Aggressive behavior is highly stable and accurately predictive of academic problems and later behavior problems, especially antisocial and criminal behavior. Early intervention is a must.

CONDUCT DISORDER

Description

Conduct disorder is a repetitive and persistent pattern of behavior in which either the basic rights of others or major age-appropriate societal norms and rules are violated. The onset of aggressive behavior is observed in toddlerhood. Early-onset conduct problems are diagnosed from 4 to 6 years of age; a formal diagnosis is typically made when the child is about 7 years of age or older.

Etiology and Incidence

The etiology of the disorder rests in chronic negative circumstances, as described for social aggression. Most common referrals for clinical treatment are for aggressive behavior patterns. Conduct disorder is about twice as prevalent in boys as in girls: 16% of boys and 4% of girls aged 10 to 13 years; 16% of boys and 9% of girls aged 14 to 16 years; 9.5% of young men and 7% of young women aged 17 to 20 years (Cohen et al., 1993a). Gender differences in behavioral symptoms tend to reflect the gender of the person reporting the behavior (Webster-Stratton, 1996). Comorbidity with major depression is common (Kovacs & Devlin, 1998). The expression of behavioral disregulation tends to become notable during the transition from early to middle childhood and is mediated by changes in the structure and demands of the social environment—peers and school settings (Kovacs & Devlin, 1998).

Clinical Findings

Physical aggression toward others is common, including the following:

- Hitting, kicking, fighting
- Physical cruelty to animals or people
- Physical destruction (including fire setting)
- Frequent engagement in temper tantrums and a high activity level
- Engagement in a high rate of annoying behavior, such as yelling, whining, threatening
- Disobedience to adult authorities
- Lying
- Cheating
- Covert stealing
- Truancy
- Running away from home

Social role functioning tends to be impaired, with poor academic performance, poor family and peer relationships, and poor self-management (Riley et al., 1998). For adolescent girls, a conduct disorder is predictive of medical problems and substance abuse in early adulthood (Bardone et al., 1998).

Differential Diagnosis

Oppositional disorder is more disobedience than aggressiveness and is evidenced in preschool or early school age. Attention deficit disorder, with which there is considerable overlap, is characterized by inattention, impulsiveness, and hyperactivity. Conduct disorder is distinguished from isolated acts of aggressive behavior by the repetitive and persistent pattern over at least 6 months (American Psychiatric Association, 1994).

Management

If aggressive behavior is identified before a conduct disorder develops, parent education and support for positive parenting strategies and healthy, consistent approaches to discipline may be fruitful. Such early intervention efforts are more successful if the etiological sources are addressed. Once a conduct disorder is evident, referral for child and family intervention is crucial.

Promising treatments include parent management training, problem-solving skills training, functional family therapy, and multisystemic therapy (Kazdin, 1997). Videotaped parent training programs, such as those developed by Webster-Stratton in the Parenting Clinic at the University of Washington School of Nursing, have been found very effective in the treatment of conduct disorder (Webster-Stratton, 1994). In a comparison of interventions, combined child training groups and parent training were found to produce the most significant improvements in child behavior 1 year later (Webster-Stratton & Hammond, 1997). For adolescents, the results are generally supportive of family therapy for conduct disorder, although there were some negative findings (Chamberlain & Rosicky, 1995). Collaboration between the family and the school is of critical importance, and the NP can assist with strategies in this regard (Webster-Stratton, 1993). Psychopharmacological intervention tends to be reserved for explosive aggression.

OPPOSITIONAL DISORDER

Description

Oppositional disorder is a pattern of negative, hostile, and defiant behavior that exceeds that seen in other children of the same age. Precursors appear in early childhood, from 3 to 7 years of age. The disorder typically begins by 8 years of age.

Etiology and Incidence

Etiological factors include many of the parenting and family dysfunctions identified for social aggression. The disorder is fairly common in early childhood, especially the precursors of social aggression, defiance and negativism. More common in boys before puberty, the gender distribution is fairly equal thereafter. Estimates for 10- to 13-year-olds include 10% of girls and 14% of boys, 15% of all 14- to 16-year-olds, and 12% of 17- to 20-year-olds.

Clinical Findings

Behavior is typically directed at family members, teachers, or peers whom the child knows well. The child manifests the following behaviors:

- Actively defies or refuses adult requests or rules
- Is argumentative, angry, resentful, touchy, or easily annoyed
- Easily loses temper
- Blames others for own mistakes or difficulties
- Deliberately does things to annoy others

Children often see their own behavior as justifiable, not oppositional or defiant (American Psychiatric Association, 1994).

Differential Diagnosis

Conduct disorder involves more serious violations of the rights of others.

Management

Attend to the early signs of defiant and oppositional behavior or aggression, or both, by educating parents about positive parenting strategies and by exercising consistent, healthy discipline, as with the management of conduct disorders. Because these children typically do not perceive themselves as having a problem and the etiology rests with the family system, referral for intervention is indicated. As described for conduct disorder, videotaped parent training programs, such as Webster-Stratton's (1994), are successful. Child training groups provide added benefit and the most successful outcomes if combined with parent training groups. Again, collaboration with the school is important. These multiple approaches, conducted simultaneously, are most effective.

▄▄▄ THE SHY CHILD

Shyness

DESCRIPTION

Shyness is a pattern of social inhibition with unfamiliar people, with novel objects, or in unfamiliar situations. Inhibition is evident in infancy as an inborn bias to respond to unfamiliar events with anxiety, distress, or disorganization (Rubin et al., 1997). Shyness appears as a social behavior pattern in toddlerhood with stability by early school age. Extremely inhibited toddlers may be at risk for becoming socially withdrawn in later childhood (Rubin et al., 1997).

ETIOLOGY AND INCIDENCE

Shyness is caused by a rather stable temperamental disposition toward withdrawal that is linked to family factors. Shyness is common. Behavioral inhibition in social situations may be adaptive if handled effectively by the mother and can be indicative of optimal self-regulation and development of conscience.

CLINICAL FINDINGS

Retreat and withdrawal from social stimulation are noted in infancy. In toddlerhood, general inhibition persists, evidenced by irritability, withdrawal, and clinging to the mother in new situations. Shy children are slower to approach peers or initiate play with an unfamiliar child and often spend more time observing the situation and other children in play before engaging. School-age shy children continue to make fewer social approaches. They usually "warm up slowly" or tend to engage in solitary but appropriate play. Viewed by their peers as likable but shy, these children may be neglected by their peers (Harrist et al., 1997). One or both parents also usually identify themselves as shy.

DIFFERENTIAL DIAGNOSIS

Children with social withdrawal rather than shyness have a lower rate of social interaction overall and do not warm up to social situations.

MANAGEMENT

Parenting strategies that provide warmth, sensitivity, and responsiveness to the child's inhibition and shyness foster security in attachment relationships and facilitate social competence. In preschool and school-age children, insensitivity and a lack of responsiveness foster a sense of insecurity and predict social withdrawal, with associated internalizing disorders, including depression. It is helpful to have parents prepare shy children for new situations with visits to the new settings, by identifying a sensitive adult to whom they may turn with requests or concerns, and by negotiating for them to be allowed to watch and observe before engaging in play or other activities.

Social Withdrawal

DESCRIPTION

Social withdrawal is a pattern of social behavior characterized by a low rate of social interaction with peers. Onset occurs in school-age children. Some withdrawn children avoid peers because of their own fearfulness, some simply prefer to play alone, and some are socially unskilled and are rejected by their peers (not allowed to play) (Harrist et al., 1997).

ETIOLOGY AND INCIDENCE

A rather stable inhibited temperament is usually antecedent and linked to a lack of family sensitivity and warmth with consequent insecurity, or to a highly stressful experience or an exacerbation of stressful life events (Rubin et al., 1997). Social withdrawal is less common than shyness.

CLINICAL FINDINGS

Low interaction entails few social approaches and limited or compliant (or both) responsiveness to initiations by peers. These children tend to be isolated in solitary play. In group play, they are less communicative, deferential, submissive, and immature. Preschoolers are described as anxious and fearful. In early school age, similar patterns persist with attendant social failures. By middle childhood, social anxiety and low self-esteem are more prominent and depressive symptoms become evident. Peer rejection is concomitant, and social problem-solving is poorly developed.

DIFFERENTIAL DIAGNOSIS

A differential diagnosis is depression, which is usually not diagnosed until the child is 10 years of age.

MANAGEMENT

The key is to intervene as early as possible to prevent negative consequences of poor social development. Addressing any acute or chronic life events alleviates the source of the problem. In addition, parent education and positive parenting strategies support efforts to restore social behavior. Confidence-boosting social experiences can be developed, such as opportunities to interact with or help younger playmates. Such situations provide opportunities for self-assertion and successful play. Similarly, assigning responsibilities in the social setting can serve to enhance the withdrawn child's social behavior (e.g., introducing and orienting a new child). Finally, structured intervention, such as assertiveness training and social skills training, might be necessary.

▓▓▓▓ BEREAVEMENT

Description

Bereavement is the sad or lonely state resulting from loss or death. Grief is the effect of bereavement and typically involves distress, sorrow, and painful regret. Mourning is the psychological process set in motion by loss of a loved one. For children and adolescents, parental and sibling deaths are the most profoundly disturbing.

Etiology and Incidence

The clinical picture of bereavement and grief depends, to some extent, on the concept of death. Children younger than 6 years of age perceive death as a continuation of life under different circumstances. From 6 to 9 years of age, children begin to personalize death. After 9 years of age, death is conceived as a finality and is akin to the adult concept. At any given developmental stage, a child can resolve the impact of the death only at that developmental level. Thus, bereavement resurfaces and the significance of the loss needs to be reworked at each subsequent developmental stage (Sekaer, 1987). It is expected that most children and adolescents experience at least one significant loss before they reach adulthood. Two thirds of school-age children and adolescents have experienced a loss (Finke et al., 1994). It is estimated that 5% of children lose one or both parents to death before the age of 15 years.

Clinical Findings

Depressive symptoms are a normal reaction to loss: sadness, feeling depressed, poor appetite, weight loss, insomnia, crying, anxiety, guilt, and idealization are common behaviors (Finke et al., 1994). Rage is a common reaction to the death of a parent; the parent who died is often idealized, and the rage is typically directed at the surviving parent and others in the immediate family (Mishne, 1992). Angry behavior may be directed at peers as well, compounding a sense of inferiority and alienation. Fears of dying, disease, and growing old are often stimulated (Mishne, 1992). Identification with the deceased is common and needs to be assessed for whether this furthers or inhibits development. Similarly, a fantasy tie to a dead parent can develop and may be helpful (Sekaer, 1987). Guilt and responsibility are typical issues for children but are less problematic for adolescents (Kuntz, 1991). Adolescents often manifest a sudden "maturity" along with numbness, regrets, disorganization, and despair before closure and reorganization are achieved (Kuntz, 1991).

Differential Diagnosis

Children at high risk for pathological bereavement or depression generally have a previous history of individual and family problems. Symptoms of pathological bereavement (American Psychiatric Association, 1994) include the following:

- Guilt about things other than circumstances surrounding the death
- Thoughts of death other than feeling as if death might be better or that the child should have died instead of the deceased person
- Morbid preoccupation with worthlessness
- Notable psychomotor retardation
- Prolonged and marked functional impairment
- Hallucinations other than the transitory experience of hearing the voice of, or seeing the image of, the deceased

Management

Parent education can facilitate effective management of bereavement in children and adolescents. Children need parental help to understand the facts of death and to correct misunderstandings as they develop; children cannot understand, however, beyond their cognitive level. Children need to be allowed to participate in the rituals around death as much as they choose (Mishne, 1992; Sekaer, 1987). Sensitivity to the child's reactions of grief and restlessness is important, as is support for the child's assimilation and mastery of the loss and emotional experience. Children need to express and work through feelings and fantasies related to the loss; open communication is a must (Finke et al., 1994). It is critical for children to have an attachment to an adult who can be an effective source of support and involvement as well as a focus for reactions to

loss (Sekaer, 1987). The child must be sensitively prepared for any consequent changes, with the family advised to minimize these as much as possible. Any parental loss before the age of 5 years probably warrants treatment (Mishne, 1992). Because bereavement resurfaces at subsequent developmental phases, early parental loss should be determined and current symptoms assessed as a possible manifestation of recurring bereavement issues.

SUBSTANCE ABUSE

Description

Substance use is a precursor to abuse or dependence, and regular use clearly increases the risk for developing a substance use disorder (SUD). However, the American Academy of Child and Adolescent Psychiatry (AACAP) (1997) clarified in its practice parameters that the use of substances per se is not sufficient for a substance use disorder diagnosis. *Substance abuse* is a maladaptive pattern of the use of alcohol or drugs manifested in significant impairment or distress. The criteria for *substance dependence* in adults include tolerance, withdrawal, and compulsive drug use. For children and adolescents, tolerance and loss of control are not good indicators for a diagnosis. Instead, alcohol-related blackouts, craving, and impulsive sexual or risk-taking behavior tend to be more important criteria (AACAP, 1997). Onset is often in early adolescence, about 12 years of age. However, nearly half of problem drinkers are thought to have tried alcohol by the age of 10 and two thirds by the age of 13 (Finke & Bowman, 1997; Heyman & Adger, 1997).

Two factors emphasize the need for pediatric primary care providers to be responsible for discussion about substance use at an early age and for screening for substance use. First, a recent research report concluded that addiction treatment providers and purchasers with limited resources should concentrate on improving the services for "visible" users already in contact with the health-care system rather than attempting to uncover "invisible" users (those who use substances but who are not identified or concerned) (Robson & Bruce, 1997). Second, young people are making the choice to experiment with substances at earlier ages (Heyman & Adger, 1997). Pediatric primary care providers are crucial in prevention and early intervention.

Etiology and Incidence

The etiology of a substance use disorder is multifaceted (AACAP, 1997; Heyman & Adger, 1997; Tweed, 1998). Many contributing factors are included in the following:

- Genetic vulnerability (family history)
- Parental substance use
- Dysfunctional family relationships, such as rigidity, distant relationships, neglect or lack of supervision, history of abuse
- Negative life events
- Psychiatric conditions (e.g., conduct disorder, ADHD, depression)
- Ineffective coping (poor emotional regulation)
- Peer network that uses substances

Precipitating life events tend to center around loss of relationships (e.g., parental separation, divorce, or death; death of a close friend) and chronic negative circumstances (e.g., parental substance abuse, maltreatment).

By the end of high school, 90% of students have tried alcohol and more than 40% have tried an illicit substance (AACAP, 1997; Tweed, 1998). Boys tend to be more involved in both alcohol and drugs of all kinds than girls are at the same age (Finke & Bowman, 1997; Tweed, 1998). Generally, estimates reveal that, for both boys and girls, abuse of alcohol and other drugs is negligible from 10 to 13 years but doubles between mid-adolescence (12 to 16 years) and late adolescence (17 to 20 years) (Cohen et al., 1993a). Recent surveys revealed that 25% of eighth grade students and 39 to 42% of 10th grade students reported alcohol use during the preceding month (AACAP, 1997; Tweed, 1998); 12% of eighth graders, 20% of 10th graders, and 23.8% of 12th graders reported illicit drug use other than alcohol during that time (AACAP, 1997). Trends in adolescent use indicate that substance use and abuse are increasing (Tweed, 1998).

Clinical Findings

Identifying an adolescent's problem with substance abuse requires a careful assessment, conducted with an accepting, nonjudgmental, nonthreatening, matter-of-fact attitude (Tweed, 1998). The covert nature of substance abuse and the dynamic of denial make it crucial to avoid a critical tone.

HISTORY

Meeting with the adolescent and parents is helpful to explore changes they have observed. Interviewing the adolescent with the parents is a key strategy for obtaining information about etiological factors and behavioral, cognitive, emotional, and physical changes in the adolescent. However, it is essential that the adolescent be interviewed alone at every visit (Heyman & Adger, 1997) in order to assess mental health and family issues.

When talking about substance use with an adolescent, it is important to begin with general questions that are not overly personal (Tweed, 1998). Begin by asking the adolescent about acquaintances who smoke, drink, or use drugs; whether anyone in the family has had problems with these; whether friends smoke, or use alcohol or drugs; what the adolescent does with friends when they get together. It is helpful to ask about experimentation, under what circumstances it occurred, and the adolescent's feelings about it. To obtain a chronological history of tobacco, alcohol, or drug use, it may be helpful to approach the subject by inquiring about prescription drugs and moving to illicit substances. The key is to remain nonjudgmental in order to elicit information that will indicate whether the adolescent is experimenting, a regular user, or dependent on substances. A helpful question asks about the adolescent's source of drugs or alcohol; the adolescent who uses substances provided by a friend or acquaintance is less advanced than one who purchases them directly.

A two-item conjoint screening test (TICS)

for alcohol and other drug problems has been developed for adults, including 18- to 20-year-olds (Brown et al., 1997). The TICS asks "In the last year, have you ever drunk or used drugs more than you meant to?" and "Have you felt you wanted or needed to cut down on your drinking or drug use in the last year?" Respondents in a primary care setting who replied to both items with "no" had a 7.4% chance of having a current substance use disorder, those with one positive response had a 45.5% chance, and those with positive responses to both items had a 75% chance of having a current substance use disorder. This may also be helpful for screening adolescents. Significant behavioral changes include the following:

- Disinhibition, lethargy, hyperactivity or agitation, hypervigilance
- Deviant or risk-taking behavior
- Repeated absences from school; suspensions from school
- Decline in academic performance
- Loss of interest in activities previously enjoyed
- Change in friends to those involved in drugs and alcohol
- Withdrawal from family and usual friends
- Angry or violent outbursts
- Early sexual activity

Parents may also be able to report on changes in personal habits, such as the following:

- Use of eye drops
- Altered sleep pattern (lack of or excessive sleep)
- Loss of appetite
- Less attention to hygiene

Cognitive changes may include the following:

- Impaired concentration
- Changes in attention span
- Perceptual and overt changes in thinking (e.g., paranoia, delusions)

Mood changes include swings from depression to euphoria, nervousness, unreasonable anger, and frequent expressions of hopelessness or failure. Low self-esteem typically characterizes those who abuse substances.

PHYSICAL EXAMINATION

Physical signs that indicate a substance use problem include the following:

- Weight loss
- Red eyes
- Nasal irritation
- Frequent "colds" or "allergies"
- Hoarseness, chronic cough, wheezing
- Accidents, trauma, injuries
- Intoxication

LABORATORY STUDIES

Urine toxicology can be helpful to verify adolescent truthfulness, although a positive drug screen does not indicate substance abuse or dependence but only indicates substance use; a negative drug screen does not rule out a substance use disorder (AACAP, 1997). The approximate duration that drugs can be detected in the urine (AACAP, 1997) is as follows:

- Stimulants—1 to 2 days
- Cocaine and its major metabolite—1 to 3 days
- Sedative-hypnotics—1 day to 1 week
- Barbiturates—2 to 4 weeks
- Quaaludes—2 to 3 weeks
- Opiates—1 to 2 days
- Marijuana—Up to 1 month

Duration of detection from last substance use varies according to the laboratory and type of testing used. The AACAP recommends that, to obtain a valid result, a positive result on immunoassay should be followed by confirmation with a more sensitive method, such as gas chromatography or mass spectrometry.

Differential Diagnosis

Substance abuse is distinguished from social drinking or nonpathological substance use by the presence of compulsive use, craving, or substance-related problems (AACAP, 1997).

Management

The exposure to tobacco and alcohol—even illicit substances—begins in early childhood. Heyman and Adger (1997) recommend that the pediatric primary care provider begin to discuss parental modeling of the use of alcohol, tobacco products, and other substances in early childhood during routine well-child visits. It becomes more important to provide education to school-age children and their parents about substance use and its consequences. For adolescents, a direct assessment and an interview about substance use become essential.

Substance abuse must be treated, and referral to a substance abuse program is crucial. However, the initial goal may be best defined as helping adolescents take positive steps toward changing their substance use and abuse behaviors (Tweed, 1998). If the adolescent denies any problem, efforts can be directed to helping the adolescent acknowledge problems. Clarifying reported negative consequences, creating doubts about substance use, and raising awareness of the risks related to current use are strategies that may be helpful. It is important to remain empathic and yet leave responsibility with the adolescent. If the adolescent has not reached a level of chronic use, harm reduction is the thrust of the intervention. Guide the adolescent to examine his or her substance use or abuse responsibly and identify ways to avoid harmful consequences. If the adolescent has progressed to chronic substance use, a range of options exist. Outpatient or day treatment programs are effective for those who can live and be managed at home. For adolescents with serious addiction, comorbid psychiatric conditions, or suicidal ideation, residential treatment or hospitalization may be necessary. Given the prominence of family dysfunction and family life events in the etiology of the problem, family-based treatment programs are essential. Follow-up assessments should include not only substance use issues but also life events (a risk factor) and the presence of positive support within or outside of the family (a protective factor). Self-help or 12-step groups are thought to be an essential element in the recovery process.

NURSING DIAGNOSIS 21–1

NURSING DIAGNOSES FOR COPING AND STRESS TOLERANCE FUNCTIONAL HEALTH PATTERN

Anxiety
Defensive coping
Depressive episode (DSM-IV diagnosis)
Ineffective denial
Ineffective individual coping
Fear
Post-trauma response
Rape trauma syndrome
Dysfunctional grieving
Anticipatory grieving
Hopelessness
Powerlessness
Risk for self-mutilation
Risk for violence: self-directed or directed at others
Substance misuse (not a NANDA diagnosis)
Risk for violence: dIrected at others
Risk for violence: self-directed

Source: North American Nursing Diagnosis Association (NANDA) (1996); American Psychiatric Association (1994).

RESOURCE BOX 21–1

RESOURCES FOR ASSESSMENT

Temperament
Revised Infant Temperament Questionnaire
Carey WB, McDevitt SC: Revision of the infant temperament questionnaire. Pediatrics 61:735–739, 1978.

Toddler Temperament Questionnaire
McDevitt SC, Carey WB: The measurement of temperament in 3-7 year old children. J Child Psychol Psychiatry 19:245–253, 1978.

Middle Childhood Temperament Questionnaire
Hegrik RI, McDevitt SC, Carey WB: The Middle Childhood Temperament Questionnaire. J Dev Behav Pediatr 3:197–200, 1982.

EAS (Emotionality, Activity, Social Ability) Scale
Buss AH, Plomin R: The EAS approach to temperament. *In* Plomin R, Dunn J (eds): The Study of Temperament: Changes, Continuities, and Challenges. Hillsdale, NJ, Erlbaum, 1986.

(Continues on next page)

RESOURCE BOX 21–1 *Continued*

RESOURCES FOR ASSESSMENT

Dimensions of Temperament Survey
Lerner R, Palermo J, Spiro A, et al: Assessing the dimensions of temperamental individuality across the life span: The Dimensions of Temperament Survey (DOTS). Child Dev 53:149–159, 1982.

Infant Characteristics Questionnaire
Bates J, Freeland C, Lounsbury M: Measurement of infant difficultness. Child Dev 50:794–803, 1979.

Temperament Inventory
Strelau J: Temperament, Personality, Activity. New York, Academic Press, 1983.

Behavior Problems
Anxiety Disorders Website
National Institute of Mental Health (NIMH)
www.nimh.nih.gov/anxiety
1-88-88-ANXIETY

Child Behavior Checklist for ages 2 to 3 years
Child Behavior Checklist for ages 4 to 18 years
Youth Self-Report for ages 11 to 18 years
Teacher's Report Form for ages 5 to 18 years
Ordering information:
Child Behavior Checklist
(802) 656-8313

Behavior Screening Questionnaire
Richman N, Graham PJ: A behavioral screening questionnaire for use with three-year-old children: Preliminary findings. J Child Psychol Psychiatry 12:5–33, 1971.

Preschool Behavior Questionnaire
Behar L, Stringfield SA: Behavior rating scale for the preschool child. Dev Psychol 10:601–610, 1974.

Conners Parent Rating Scale
Sattler JM: Assessment of Children. San Diego, Jerome M. Sattler, 1986.

Eyberg Child Behavior Inventory
Eyberg SM, Ross AW: Assessment of child behavior problems: The validation of a new inventory. J Clin Child Psychol 7:113–116, 1978.

Pediatric Symptom Checklist
Jellineck MS, Murphy JM: The recognition of psychosocial disorders in pediatric practice: The current status of the Pediatric Symptom Checklist. J Dev Behav Pediatr 11:273–278, 1990.

REFERENCES

American Academy of Child and Adolescent Psychiatry: Practice parameters for the assessment and treatment of children and adolescents with substance use disorders. J Am Acad Child Adolesc Psychiatry 36(suppl):140S–156S, 1997.

American Psychiatric Association: Diagnostic and Statistical Manual of Mental Disorders, 4th ed. Washington, DC, 1994.

Bardone AM, Moffitt TE, Caspi A, et al: Adult physical health outcomes of adolescent girls with conduct disorder, depression, and anxiety. J Am Acad Child Adolesc Psychiatry 37:594–601, 1998.

Barrett PM, Dadds MR, Rapee RM: Family treatment of childhood anxiety: A controlled trial. J Consult Clin Psychol 64:333–342, 1996.

Barrios BA, Hartmann CP: Fears and anxieties. In Mash EJ, Terdal LG (eds): Behavioral Assessment of Childhood Disorders, 2nd ed. New York, Guilford, 1988, pp 196-262.

Bernstein GA, Borchardt CM: Anxiety disorders of childhood and adolescence: A critical review. J Am Acad Child Adolesc Psychiatry 30:519–532, 1991.

Botteron KN, Geller B: Pharmacologic treatment of childhood and adolescent mania. Child Adolesc Psychiatric Clin North Am 4:283–304, 1995.

Bowden CL, Rhodes LJ: Mania in children and adolescents: Recognition and treatment. Psychiatric Ann 26 (suppl):430–434, 1996.

Brent DA: Depression and suicide in children and adolescents. Pediatr Rev 14:380–388, 1993.

Brown RL, Leonard T, Saunders LA, et al: A two-item screening test for alcohol and other drug problems. J Fam Pract 44:151–160, 1997.

Carey WB: Let's give temperament its due. Contemp Pediatr 15:91–113, 1998.

Chamberlain P, Rosicky JG: The effectiveness of family therapy in the treatment of adolescents with conduct disorders and delinquency. J Marital Fam Ther 21:441–459, 1995.

Chess S, Thomas A: Origins and Evolutions of Behavior Disorders. New York, The Guilford Press, 1984.

Cicchetti D: Developmental psychopathology in infancy: Illustration from study of maltreated youngsters. J Consult Clin Psychol 55:837–845, 1987.

Coffman S, Levitt MJ, Guacci N, et al: Temperament and interactive effects: Mothers and infants in a teaching situation. Issues Compr Pediatr Nurs 15:169–182, 1992.

Cohen P, Cohen J, Kasen S, et al: An epidemiological study of disorders in late childhood and adolescence—I. Age- and gender-specific prevalence. J Child Psychol Psychiatry 34:851–867, 1993a.

Cohen P, Cohen J, Brook J: An epidemiological study of disorders in late childhood and adolescence—II. Persistence of disorders. J Child Psychol Psychiatry 34:869-877, 1993b.

Compas BE: Coping with stress during childhood and adolescence. Psycholog Bull 101:393–403, 1987.

Compas BE, Malcarne VL, Fondacaro KM: Coping with stressful events in older children and young adolescents. J Consult Clin Psychol 56:405–411, 1988.

Dashiff CJ: Understanding separation anxiety disorder. J Child Adolesc Psychiatric Nurs 8:27-38, 1995.

Dubowitz H, Black M, Harrington D, et al: A follow-up study of behavior problems associated with child sexual abuse. Child Abuse Neglect 17:743-754, 1993.

Egeland B, Kalkoske M, Gottesman N, et al: Preschool behavior problems: Stability and factors accounting for change. J Child Psychol Psychiatry 31:891-909, 1990.

Elster A, Kuznets N: AMA Guidelines for Adolescent Preventive Services (GAPS). Chicago, American Medical Association, 1994.

Eyberg SM, Ross AW: Assessment of child behavior problems: The validation of a new inventory. J Clin Child Psychol 7:113-116, 1978.

Fagot B, Leve LD: Teacher ratings of externalizing behavior at school entry for boys and girls: Similar early predictors and different correlates. J Child Psychol Psychiatry 39:555-566, 1998.

Famularo R, Kinscherff R, Fenton T: Symptom differences in acute and chronic presentation of childhood post-traumatic stress disorder. Child Abuse Neglect 14:439-444, 1990.

Finke LM, Birenbaum LK, Chand N: Two weeks post-death report by parents of siblings' grieving experience. J Child Adolesc Psychiatric Nurs 7:17-25, 1980.

Finke LM, Bowman CA: Factors in childhood drug and alcohol use: A review of the literature. J Child Adolesc Psychiatric Nurs 10:29-34, 1997.

Folkman S, Lazarus RS: An analysis of coping in a middle-aged sample. J Health Social Behav 21:219-239, 1980.

Geller G: "BPD and ADHD": Commentary. J Am Acad Child Adolesc Psychiatry 36:720, 1997.

Ginsburg GS, Silverman WK, Kurtines WK: Family involvement in treating children with phobic and anxiety disorders: A look ahead. Clin Psychol Rev 15:457-473, 1995.

Goodyer IM: Family relationships, life events, and childhood psychopathology. J Child Psychol Psychiatry 31:161-192, 1990.

Goodyer IM, Ashby L, Altham PME, et al: Temperament and major depression in 11 to 16 year olds. J Child Psychol Psychiatry 34:1409-1423, 1993.

Gross D, Conrad B: Temperament in toddlerhood. J Pediatr Nurs 10:146-151, 1995.

Harrist AW, Zaia AE, Bates JE, et al: Subtypes of social withdrawal in early childhood: Sociometric status and social-cognitive differences across four years. Child Dev 68:278-294, 1997.

Herman-Staab B: Screening, management, and appropriate referral for pediatric behavior problems. Nurse Pract 19:40-49, 1994.

Heyman RB, Adger H: Office approach to drug abuse prevention. Pediatr Clin North Am 44:1447-1455, 1997.

Hops H, Greenwood CR: Social skills deficits. *In* Mash EJ, Terdal LG (eds): Behavioral Assessment of Childhood Disorders, 2nd ed. New York, Guilford, 1988, pp 263-314.

Jellineck MS, Murphy JM: Screening for psychosocial disorders in pediatric practice. Am J Dis Child 142:1153-1157, 1997.

Kazdin AE: Practitioner review: Psychosocial treatments for conduct disorder in children. J Child Psychol Psychiatry 38:161-178, 1997.

King NJ, Ollendick TH: Treatment of childhood phobias. J Child Psychol Psychiatry Allied Disciplines 38:389-400, 1997.

Kovacs M: Presentation and course of major depressive disorder during childhood and later years of the life span. J Am Acad Child Adolesc Psychiatry 35:705-715, 1996.

Kovacs M, Devlin B: Internalizing disorders in childhood. J Child Psychol Psychiatry Allied Disciplines 39:47-63, 1998.

Kuntz B: Exploring the grief of adolescents after the death of a parent. J Child Adolesc Psychiatric Mental Health Nurs 4:105-109, 1991.

Laraia MT: Current approaches to the psychopharmacologic treatment of depression in children and adolescents. J Child Adolesc Psychiatric Nurs 9:15-26, 1996.

Last C, Perrin S, Hersen M, et al: DSM-III-R anxiety disorders in children: Sociodemographic and clinical characteristics. J Am Acad Child Adolesc Psychiatry 31:1070-1076, 1992.

Lombardo GT: BPD and ADHD. J Am Acad Child Adolesc Psychiatry 36:719-720, 1997.

March JS: Cognitive-behavioral psychotherapy for children and adolescents with OCD: A review and recommendations for treatment. J Am Acad Child Adolesc Psychiatry 34:7-18, 1995.

McClowry SG: Temperament theory and research. IMAGE: J Nurs Scholarship 24:319-325, 1992.

McClowry SG: The influence of temperament on development during middle childhood. J Pediatr Nurs 10:160-165, 1995.

Medoff-Cooper B: Infant temperament: Implications for parenting from birth through 1 year. J Pediatr Nurs 10:141-145, 1995.

Mehregany DV: The relation of temperament and behavior disorders in a preschool clinical sample. Child Psychiatry Hum Dev 22:129-136, 1991.

Melvin N: Children's temperament: Intervention for parents. J Pediatr Nurs 24:152-159, 1995.

Mishne J: The grieving child: Manifest and hidden losses in childhood and adolescence. Child Adolesc Social Work J 9:471-490, 1992.

North American Nursing Diagnosis Association: NANDA Nursing Diagnoses: Definitions and Classification 1997-1998. Philadelphia, Author, 1996.

Ollendick TH: Reliability and validity of the Revised Fear Survey Schedule for Children. Behav Res Ther 21:685-692, 1983.

Prior M: Childhood temperament. J Child Psychol Psychiatry 33:249-279, 1992.

Prior M, Smart D, Sanson A, et al: Transient versus stable behavior problems in a normative sample: Infancy to school age. J Pediatr Psychol 17:423-443, 1992.

Rapoport JL, Inoff-Germain G: Tourette syndrome. Medical and surgical treatment of obsessive-compulsive disorder. Neurol Clin 15:421-428, 1997.

Rapoport JL, Leonard HL, Swedo SE, et al: Obsessive compulsive disorder in children and adolescents: Issues in management. J Clin Psychiatry 54:27-29, 1993.

Region X Nursing Network: Region 10 Nursing Network Newborn, Child (Birth to Three), School Age, and Adolescent Manuals. Seattle, University of Washington, 1998.

Riley AW, Ensminger ME, Green B, et al: Social role functioning by adolescents with psychiatric disorders. J Am Acad Child Adolesc Psychiatry 37:620-628, 1998.

Robson P, Bruce M: A comparison of "visible" and "invisible" users of amphetamine, cocaine and heroin: Two distinct populations? Addiction 92:1729-1736, 1997.

Rubin KH, Hastings PD, Stewart SL, et al: The consistency and concomitants of inhibition: Some of the children, all of the time. Child Dev 68:467-483, 1997.

Rutter M: Stress, coping and development: Some issues and some questions. J Child Psychol Psychiatry 22:323-356, 1981.

Rutter M: Pathways from childhood to adult life. J Child Psychol Psychiatry 30:23-51, 1989.

Sameroff AJ, Chandler MJ: Reproductive risk and the continuum of caretaking casualty. In Horowitz F, Hetherington M, Scarr-Sclapatek S, et al (eds): Review of Child Development Research, Vol IV. Chicago, University of Chicago Press, 1975, pp 187-244.

Sandberg S, Rutter M, Giles S, et al: Assessment of psychosocial experiences in childhood: Methodological issues and some illustrative findings. J Child Psychol Psychiatry 34:879-897, 1993.

Scahill L: Contemporary approaches to pharmacotherapy in Tourette's syndrome and obsessive-compulsive disorder. J Child Adolesc Psychiatry Nurs 9:27-43, 1996.

Sekaer C: Toward a definition of "childhood mourning." Am J Psychother 41:201-219, 1987.

Terr LC: Childhood traumas: An outline and overview. Am J Psychiatry 148:10-20, 1991.

Tubman JG, Lerner RM, Lerner JV, et al: Temperament and adjustment in young adulthood: A 15-year longitudinal analysis. Am J Orthopsychiatry 62:564-574, 1993.

Tweed SH: Intervening in adolescent substance abuse. Nurs Clin North Am 33:29-45, 1998.

Valleni-Basile LA, Garrison CZ, Jackson KL, et al: Frequency of obsessive-compulsive disorder in a community sample of young adolescents. J Am Acad Child Adolesc Psychiatry 33:782-791, 1994.

Webster-Stratton C: Strategies for helping early school-aged children with oppositional-defiant and conduct disorders: The importance of home-school partnerships. School Psychol Rev 22:437-457, 1993.

Webster-Stratton C: Advancing videotape parent training: A comparison study. J Consult Clin Psychol 62:583-593, 1994.

Webster-Stratton C: Early onset conduct problems: Does gender make a difference? J Consult Clin Psychol 64:540-551, 1996.

Webster-Stratton C, Hammond M: Treating children with early-onset conduct problems: A comparison of child and parent training interventions. J Consult Clin Psychol 64:93-109, 1997.

Weiss B, Dodge KA, Bates JE, et al: Some consequences of early harsh discipline: Child aggression and a maladaptive social information processing style. Child Dev 63:1321-1335, 1992.

Weissman MM, Warner V, Wickramaratne P, et al: Offspring of depressed parents. Arch Gen Psychiatry 54:932-940, 1997.

Wertlieb D, Weigel C, Feldstein M: Measuring children's coping. Am J Orthopsychiatry 57:548-560, 1987.

Wolk SI, Weissman MM: Suicidal behavior in depressed children grown up: Preliminary results of a longitudinal study. Psychiatric Ann 26:331-335, 1996.

CHAPTER 22

Values and Beliefs

Ardys M. Dunn

INTRODUCTION

This functional health pattern examines values and beliefs and their impact on health. The nurse practitioner's (NP's) role in this pattern is to assess the nature of social, cultural, and spiritual dimensions of children's and family's values and beliefs, determine their impact on health care decisions, and identify means to support values, beliefs, and subsequent actions that are health promotive.

STANDARDS OF PRACTICE

The Region X Nursing Network's (1998) goal is that children will develop health promotive values that are a source of strength and hope. To achieve this goal, children's environments should contribute to a sense of security, belonging, autonomy, hope, initiative, and confidence. The environment should promote the development of a value and belief system, helping children as they become aware of right and wrong and of how other people view their behavior. For adolescents, outcomes include being able to express their belief system, incorporating values and beliefs into decision-making and future goals, tolerating diversity, and accepting others.

The American Medical Association (AMA) Guidelines for Adolescent Preventive Services (GAPS) (Elster & Kuznets, 1994) include the following points related to values and beliefs:

1. Preventive services should be appropriate for age and development and sensitive to individual and sociocultural differences.
2. All adolescents should receive health guidance annually to promote a better understanding of their physical growth, psychosocial and psychosexual development, and the importance of being actively involved in decisions regarding their health care.
3. All adolescents should be asked annually about behaviors or emotions that indicate recurrent or severe depression or risk of suicide.

Although the United States (US) Preventive Services Task Force (1996) does not set specific standards for values and beliefs, emphasis is placed on the importance of being alert to behavioral disorders, parent and family dysfunction, signs of child abuse or neglect, abnormal bereavement, and, among adolescents, depressive symptoms and suicide risk factors. Problems in these areas may reflect dysfunction or inappropriate development of values and beliefs.

NORMAL PATTERNS OF BEHAVIOR

Values and Beliefs: Definitions and Relationship to Behavior

Values have been defined as perceptions held about the worth or importance of a certain thing, person, or idea. Beliefs are attitudes representing a "personal confidence in the validity of some idea, person, or object" (Steele & Harmon, 1979).

Values and beliefs influence actions, both consciously and unconsciously. They are guides that individuals use as they make decisions. Values and beliefs are learned phenomena, and recognition and acceptance of shared values and beliefs are fundamental to the integrity of the individual, the family, and the social group. Although perceptions, attitudes, values, and beliefs are transmitted from one generation to another, they remain open to change and are responsive to social contexts and situations. Values clarification is the process by which one examines behavior in light of values and changing circumstances and asks why a certain action is taken or whether that action is consistent with the values one claims to have. Change in values and behavior can result from the process of values clarification.

Expected Patterns of Behavior Related to Values and Beliefs

The creation of values and beliefs in children is related to their developmental stage, and those values and beliefs are reflected in behaviors expressed by children of different ages. In general, healthy behaviors are expressions of positive values. In particular, the development of moral integrity, or conscience and spirituality, or faith, is expected of the healthy child.

Children's responses to illness are also related to their values and beliefs. In her review of attribution theory, Pehler (1997) notes that "children, like adults, need to find meaning in illness." Children are more likely than adults to attribute the cause of illness to internal factors (e.g., believing that an illness is a punishment for being bad) and these beliefs may be related to their level of spiritual understanding. If this is the case, the child may experience spiritual distress and require spiritual interventions.

As they develop moral and spiritual values, healthy children achieve a positive sense of self, internalize the cultural values and beliefs related to their social group, learn to value themselves and their contribution to the family and larger social system, and feel a sense of understanding and belonging to their community. Chapter 18 discusses stages and factors influencing the development of healthy self-perception in children. See Chapter 4 for a discussion of the cultural dynamics that occur as children grow within the context of family, cultural group, and society. This chapter focuses on definition, assessment, and management of moral and spiritual development.

Development of Moral Integrity or Conscience

Moral integrity involves demonstrating an understanding of right and wrong; engaging in reflection on ethical issues of justice and fairness; and expressing a sense of responsibility to oneself, others, and the environment. The development of moral integrity is enhanced if children believe that they and their contributions to the family and community are valued; if they are rewarded emotionally, psychologically, and intellectually for their participation in the community; and if their peer groups support positive behavior. Simply stated, children must believe that they make a difference and have a future.

Moral judgment is also dependent on the developmental stage of children. Developmental theorists have presented several perspectives on moral development in children: Freud asserted that children develop a conscience through identification with a significant caregiver and the processes of guilt and shame; Piaget claimed that children's moral development parallels their intellectual development and ability to reason; Kohlberg theorized that moral development proceeds sequentially through three levels related to intellectual development and social interactions. Social learning theory states that positive role modeling teaches moral behavior. Developmental theories suggest that younger children have little sense of right and wrong and are often concrete in their thinking, whereas older children and adolescents are more likely to be reflective as they examine moral dilemmas, and they are able to articulate and understand motivation or conditions that influence behavior.

Other theorists have suggested that gender plays a significant role in the way children interpret situations and make choices based on moral judgment (Gilligan, 1990). Research also indicates that children as young as 36 months "are able to articulate coherent stories about rules, reciprocity, empathy, and internalized prohibitions" and to generate alternatives to resolve moral dilemmas (Buchsbaum & Emde, 1990).

Development of Spirituality

Spirituality has been defined as a unifying force that gives meaning to life. It is the acceptance of a nonmaterial higher power that encompasses all of life's affairs and is mediated through the individual's relationships to others, to the community, and to the environment. Although related to religion, spirituality should not be confused with religious activities, rituals, and behaviors. Characteristics of spirituality are listed in Table 22-1 (Howden, 1993).

The development of spirituality in children has been conceived as paralleling cognitive and moral development. Table 22-2 presents that relationship and outlines age-specific interventions to enhance healthy growth (Aden, 1976; Fowler, 1980; Westerhoff, 1976; Stilwell et al., 1998). As children develop a spiritual sense, they engage in the process of finding meaning in life (Kegan, 1982). In the infant and toddler, this takes the form of establishing autonomy or separateness of self from the parent, and becoming a part of a bigger culture (i.e., the family). Preschool and early school-age children gain an understanding of the meaning of life through fantasy play, active engagement with their environment, strong attachments to their parents, and growing relationships with their peers. Although they have finished the task of defining themselves as separate individuals, their thinking and behavior in relation to faith issues is still an expression of the family's faith and practice. School-age children and adolescents define life's meaning within the context of their "self-sufficiency, competence, and role differentiation," and in their relationship to both

T A B L E 22-1
Characteristics of Spirituality

COMPONENTS OF SPIRITUALITY	CHARACTERISTICS
INNER RESOURCES AND IDENTITY	Those who possess inner resources have a sense of wholeness, competence, and direction. They are capable of responding to crises or turmoil and draw on inner strengths to maintain a sense of stability and control
INTERCONNECTEDNESS	Interconnectedness is the sense of being an integral part of the world, attached to others, to one's environment, and to a universal or supreme being
PURPOSE OR MEANING OF LIFE	A sense of direction and meaning and a reason for existence are developed in the relationships individuals have with others and their world
TRANSCENDENCE	The ability to go beyond, or transcend, the experiences of daily life is evident in the expression of hope, meaning, and direction when an individual is faced with fear, inability to effect change, uncertainty, and ambiguity

From Howden J: Development and Psychometric Characteristics of the Spirituality Assessment Scale. In Dissertation Abstracts International 54, 1993, p 166.

Developmental Outcomes and Appropriate Interventions Related to Values and Beliefs

	INFANT (0–12 mo)	TODDLER AND PRESCHOOLER (1–5 yr)	SCHOOL-AGE CHILD (6–12 yr)	ADOLESCENT
Area of Development				
Moral integrity and conscience (right and wrong; sense of responsibility to oneself, others, and the environment)	Develops sense of trust in caregivers (Erikson, 1963); learns to adjust to family routine (e.g., sleeping, eating)	Believes rules are absolute; behaves well for fear of punishment or to receive rewards (Kohlberg, 1969); develops sense of autonomy, initiative, and purpose; differentiates self from others (Erikson, 1963)	Believes rules exist to keep order and protect people and that everyone benefits from them; behaves well to please others, to avoid guilt and, to maintain status of "good" child (Kohlberg, 1969); develops sense of industry, faith in self-competence; explores, creates, collects; understands cause and effect (Erikson, 1963)	Rules are based on ethical judgment; believes individual answers to personal conscience, has moral obligation to a social contract; behaves to maintain respect of self, peers, and larger community (Kohlberg, 1969); integrates personality and develops sense of identity, loyalty to group and significant others (Erikson, 1963)
Faith development	Primal or undifferentiated faith (Fowler, 1980); faith is trust (Aden, 1976); primary caregivers represent superordinate beings; infant develops object permanence, sense of trust, attachment, and sense of being nurtured	Intuitive-projective faith based on images, feelings, and symbols (Fowler, 1980); faith as courage and obedience—younger child learns to let go and take hold in order to affirm self, and older child develops more realistic perspective of self in relation to others, learns to balance self desires with demands of others; egocentric thinking may contribute to misconceptions; child begins to participate in family's religious practices and rituals	Mythic-literal faith, with concrete beliefs, rigid system of order and activities (Fowler, 1980); faith as assent, as child learns to master environment and become competent (Aden, 1976); child begins to explore ultimate issues, develop understanding of the meaning of life, develop and express moral decision-making	Synthetic convention stage—ideas about spirituality are synthesized from peers, parents and other significant adults, and life experiences (Fowler, 1980); faith as identity (Aden, 1976) as child seeks identity, understanding of self in the world; child demonstrates self-reflection, insight, sense of inner spiritual process and presence in the world, and continues to more fully develop understanding of ultimate questions, life's meaning

Experienced faith (infancy through early adolescence)

Affiliative faith (late adolescence)

Children experience faith through relationships with others and others' faith traditions (Westerhoff, 1976)

Adolescent actively participates in a faith community, feels a sense of belonging, awe and wonder; acknowledges authority of faith community (Westerhoff, 1976)

Parental Interventions to Foster Healthy Development

Respond to infant's physiological and emotional needs promptly and adequately; demonstrate loving, gentle approach in communication and interaction

Treat child with respect and acceptance; set realistic limits on behavior; remove temptation from environment; provide positive role model; provide guided opportunities to interact with adults and other children as well as active play alone; be patient; involve child in family religious practices; begin to establish regular tasks for child in family activities

Treat child with respect and acceptance; set realistic limits on behavior; provide opportunities for active play alone and with other children; encourage group activity; allow children to make decisions as appropriate, helping them to explore meanings of feelings, events, and interactions; choose stories related to children's experience of moral dilemmas to explore right and wrong (Vitz, 1990); regular tasks for child as member of family are established

Treat adolescent with respect and acceptance; set realistic limits on behavior; enforce family's moral standards; encourage involvement in family activities; allow children to make more of own choices regarding values and beliefs; allow experimentation in dress, hair, makeup as child develops sense of self; don't overreact to adolescent "crises," provide opportunities to discuss values, ethics, and moral behavior; provide support and encouragement for successes and failures in school, social, athletic, and work activities peers and adults. Children at this age need to explore their understanding of the ultimate questions in life (Harding & Snyder, 1991). They are interested in issues such as life, death, war, evil, good, and creation, but, because of their cognitive limitations, they need help to think about these important matters.

ASSESSMENT

The goals of assessing values and beliefs include the following:

- Determine the nature of the child's and family's belief system.
- Identify ways that the family interacts to support their beliefs.

Because children are in the process of developing values and beliefs and because much of their development depends on their interaction with the parent or caregiver, assessment questions are often directed to or focused on the parent or caregiver.

Measures of spirituality are necessarily subjective, and assessment of spirituality is often part of the psychosocial assessment; questions should elicit information about the individual's subjective perceptions as well as objective religious practices.

History

MORAL INTEGRITY OR CONSCIENCE

The following points can be used in the assessment:

- How does the child define right and wrong? How does the child's behavior reflect his or her moral understanding?
- What are family attitudes about right and wrong?
- How are parents teaching the child about right and wrong?
- What other influences affect the child's concept of right and wrong (e.g., day care, teachers and counselors, peer group)?
- How do parents set limits on the child's behavior?
- How does the child respond to discipline and limits?

- What messages do parents give about the value and importance of the child's contribution to the family and the community?
- What opportunities do parents give the child to make independent, age-appropriate decisions?
- What traditions and activities does the family have? How is the child included in these activities?

SPIRITUALITY

The following information should be identified in relation to spirituality:

General

Tell me about your religious beliefs related to the following issues:

- Family relations, gender roles, and children's and parents' responsibilities
- Sexuality issues (e.g., homosexuality, premarital sex)
- Dietary restrictions
- Rituals (e.g., at mealtime or bedtime)
- Use of drugs, alcohol, or tobacco
- Medical treatment

Inner Resources and Identity

- What are your child's goals in life? Your family's goals?
- What are your child's strong points? Your family's strong points?
- What do you like about yourself? Your child? Your family?
- How important is faith in your child's life? In your life?
- What brings you, your child, and your family joy and peace?

Interconnectedness

- How do you feel about your child? About yourself? About your family?
- What do you do as a family to show love for each other?
- Who are significant people in your child's and your family's life?
- Whom do you ask for support when your family needs help?

- How do members of your family share feelings with others?
- Do you feel that you and your family are part of a community? Of a larger world or universe?
- Does the family belong to a religious or spiritual group?

Purpose or Meaning of Life

- What are your family's religious and cultural beliefs? What ethics or values are important in your family's life? What gives life meaning? What is the most important thing in life?
- How does your family express religious and cultural beliefs? How is your child involved?
- What religious rituals or practices contribute to a sense of spiritual fulfillment or peace?
- How do you teach your child about values and beliefs? How else does your child learn about values and beliefs?
- Are you comfortable talking about your beliefs with your child?

Transcendence

How do members of your family deal with spiritual distress during a crisis?

Physical Examination

Observe the child's behavior, especially noting interaction with parents, other adults, and peers. The child exhibits the following behavior:

- Appears at ease, although behavior may vary (e.g., shy, quiet, active, talkative, engaging) depending on developmental level and temperament
- Responds to parent or caregiver cues; follows directions and conforms to limits set without demonstrating guilt or fear of punishment
- Shares toys
- Respects people and property
- Is not physically aggressive
- Is able to articulate moral reasoning (older child)

- Is able to articulate a faith statement, depending on spiritual, religious, and cultural background (older child)

MANAGEMENT OF NORMAL PATTERNS

Parents should function in the following ways:

- Be a loving, responsive, and accepting presence in their children's lives.
- Set realistic standards or limits for right and wrong behavior.
- State what is acceptable behavior and what is unacceptable behavior.
- Provide a rationale for limits set; the explanation varies depending on the cognitive and developmental level of the child.
- Articulate personal values, beliefs, and faith statements for the child. Give clear, age-appropriate explanations of God and spiritual lessons.
- Be a role model for constructive and positive behavior.
- Give reinforcements for positive behavior and for attempts at positive behavior.
- Hold children accountable for negative behavior.
- Teach children strategies to avoid misbehavior; teach constructive coping skills.
- Use creative parenting strategies (e.g., distraction, diversional activities) to help children avoid misbehavior.
- Provide a developmentally appropriate environment to minimize children's misbehavior. It is usually easier to remove a breakable object from a table than to keep saying no or to discipline a child for breaking it.
- Provide opportunities for children to make age-appropriate decisions independently.
- Praise children in front of others.
- Do not give false praise.
- Articulate and reinforce messages that children belong and are valued for themselves, not just for their behaviors.
- Establish family traditions and projects that actively involve children (e.g., family outings, family value sessions, during which family members share a meal with directed conversation). Don't expect perfection.

- Involve children in the family's religious and cultural practices.
- Provide opportunities for the child to explore moral and ethical dilemmas and to develop possible solutions.
- Discuss moral and spiritual implications of events in the child's life (e.g., death of a grandparent, birth of a sibling, sharing, stealing, violence portrayed in media).

Nurse practitioners should do the following:

- Be aware of their own values and beliefs.
- Distinguish between moral and medical advice. Be willing to offer both.
- Recognize and appreciate differences between own and client's values.
- Provide an opportunity for parents to express values and beliefs and to discuss their child's moral and spiritual development.
- Provide information about parenting strategies, discipline, and effective communication between child and parents.
- Assist parents and child in values clarification as appropriate.
- Provide a role model of positive behavior.
- Refer the family for religious or spiritual counseling as indicated or requested.

ALTERED PATTERNS

Lack of Moral Integrity

DESCRIPTION

Children who lack moral integrity demonstrate little regard for people and the rights and property of others and are unable to judge behavior as right or wrong.

ETIOLOGY

The complexity of moral judgment makes it likely that a multitude of factors contribute to poor moral reasoning and antisocial behaviors. Research indicates that moral reasoning is clearly related to children's real-life situations (Elbedour et al., 1997) and that children develop morals through a process of shifting from external to internal regulation, much of which occurs during the toddler period (Grusic & Goodnow, 1994). Moral development, based on

a protective spirituality, is enhanced when children have positive adult–child interactions, characterized by respect, acceptance, value, and active participation of the children (Haight, 1998; Sutherland, et al., 1997). Failure to treat children in this manner can contribute to lack of moral reasoning. Research also indicates that "maternal power-assertive discipline is detrimental to conscience development" (Grusic & Goodnow, 1994).

CLINICAL FINDINGS

Many behaviors seen are typical of normal children, depending on developmental and cognitive levels (e.g., lying, hitting, refusing to share), but the child expresses little or no remorse for negative behavior and demonstrates no internalization of a sense of justice, fairness, or right or wrong.

DIFFERENTIAL DIAGNOSIS

Attention deficit hyperactivity disorder, conduct disorder, oppositional defiant disorder, and depression are differential diagnoses.

MANAGEMENT

In addition to strategies listed here, see the earlier discussion of management strategies for normal moral development. In extreme cases, referral for psychiatric management may be necessary.

- Assist child in values clarification process.
- Use storytelling to explore moral and ethical issues.
  - Watch films and discuss books with adolescents.
  - Tell stories to younger children.
- Encourage interaction with older children who demonstrate higher levels of moral reasoning (McCown, 1984).

COMPLICATIONS

Antisocial behavior and delinquency are behavioral disorders in which lack of moral integrity is a key component.

Spiritual Distress

DESCRIPTION

Spiritual distress is "a disruption in the life principle that pervades a person's entire being and that integrates and transcends one's biological and psychosocial nature" (North American Nursing Diagnosis Association [NANDA], 1996). For children, issues of death and dying and serious illness are major reasons for seeking spiritual counsel. The question of "why" is often asked by parents and the child. These conditions relate to two factors that contribute to spiritual distress: "intense suffering" and a challenge to the child and parents' belief and value system (Pehler, 1997).

ETIOLOGY

Because of the complex nature of spirituality, spiritual distress can result from a number of factors. These factors challenge the child's or family's belief system or contribute to separation from spiritual ties and can include the following:

- Trauma or violence
- Loss of significant other, especially parent or sibling
- Debilitating disease
- Chronic disease
- Separation of child from his or her family
- Recommended medical therapies in conflict with child's or family's religious or spiritual beliefs (e.g., Christian Science)
- Barriers in health care setting to practicing spiritual rituals
- Beliefs of health care providers, family members, or peers that conflict with those of child or parent

CLINICAL FINDINGS

The following may be seen in spiritual distress:

- Depressive behavior (may be suicidal)
- Withdrawal
- No participation in usual religious practices
- Disparaging family's spiritual beliefs and values

- Questioning one's own value, meaning, and purpose of life
- Expressions of anger, resentment, fear of God, suffering, death
- Expressions of inner conflict and doubts about beliefs
- Expressions of sense of spiritual emptiness
- Sleep disturbance
- Behavior changes with mood swings
- Request for spiritual assistance

DIFFERENTIAL DIAGNOSIS

Depression, poor coping mechanisms, conduct disorders, and antisocial behavior are differential diagnoses for spiritual distress.

MANAGEMENT

The nurse practitioner should take the following management steps:

- Identify situational factors that contribute to distress.
- Consult with parents as appropriate to identify family values and belief system.
- Assist parents to help their child process experiences contributing to distress (Garbarino et al., 1991). Referral may be necessary in cases in which child is experiencing significant psychological trauma. An integrated team composed of psychologist, clergy, and parish nurse can be appropriate.
- Encourage child to participate in spiritual practices as desired.
- Encourage child to express feelings about spiritual distress.
- Encourage child to talk about beliefs and understandings of stressors such as death and illness.
- Answer questions honestly, according to the child's age and developmental level.
- Advocate for the child and parent when they express beliefs in conflict with those of other health care providers or other family members.
- If parents refuse treatment for their child:
  - Consider use of alternative methods of care.
  - Provide opportunity for parents to dis-

cuss implications of decision and possible court order for temporary guardian who will give consent to treat the child.

○ Provide opportunity for parents to express negative feelings.

COMPLICATIONS

Depression, suicide, and conduct disorders are complications of spiritual distress.

NURSING DIAGNOSIS 22-1

NURSING DIAGNOSES FOR VALUES AND BELIEFS FUNCTIONAL HEALTH PATTERN

Potential for Enhanced Spiritual Well-Being
Spiritual Distress

Source: North American Nursing Diagnosis Association: NANDA Nursing Diagnoses: Definitions and Classification 1997–1998. Philadelphia, 1996.

REFERENCES

Aden L: Faith and the developmental cycle. Pastoral Psychology, 24:215-230, 1976.

Buchsbaum HK, Emde RN: Play narratives in 36-month-old children: Early moral development and family relationships. Psychoanalytic Study of the Child 45:129-155, 1990.

Elbedour S, Baker AM, Charlesworth WR: The impact of political violence on moral reasoning in children. Child Abuse & Neglect 21:1053-1066, 1997.

Elster AB, Kuznets, NJ: AMA Guidelines for Adolescent Preventive Services (GAPS): Recommendations and Rationale. Baltimore, Williams & Wilkins, 1994.

Erikson EH: Childhood and Society, 2nd ed. New York, Norton, 1963.

Fowler J: Moral stages and the development of faith. *In* Munsey B (ed): Moral Development, Moral Education, and Kohlberg. Birmingham, AL, Religious Education Press, 1980, pp. 130-160.

Garbarino J, Kostelny K, Dubrow N: What children can tell us about living in danger. Am Psychol 46:376-383, 1991.

Gilligan C: Mapping the Moral Domain. Cambridge, MA, Harvard University Press, 1990.

Grusic JE, Goodnow JJ: Impact of parental discipline methods on the child's internalization of values: A reconceptualization of current points of view. Dev Psychol 30:4-19, 1994.

Haight WL: "Gathering the spirit" at First Baptist Church: Spirituality as a protective factor in the lives of African American children. Soc Work J Nat Assoc Soc Workers 43:213-221, 1998.

Harding CG, Snyder K: Tom, Huck, and Oliver Stone as advocates in Kohlberg's just community: Theory-based strategies for moral development. Adolescence 26:319-329, 1991.

Howden J: Development and Psychometric Characteristics of the Spirituality Assessment Scale. *In* Dissertation Abstracts International 54, 1993, p 166.

Kegan R: The Evolving Self. Cambridge, MA, Harvard University Press, 1982.

Kohlberg L: Stage and sequence: The cognitive-development approach to socialization. *In* Gastin D (ed): Handbook of Socialization: Theory and Research. NY, Rand McNally, 1969.

McCown DE: Moral development in children. Pediatr Nurs 10:42-44, 1984.

North American Nursing Diagnosis Association: NANDA Nursing Diagnoses: Definitions and Classification 1997-1998. Philadelphia, 1996.

Pehler S-R: Children's spiritual response: Validation of the nursing diagnosis spiritual distress. Nurs Diagn 8:55-66, 1997.

Region X Nursing Network: Region X Nursing Network Standards for Prenatal and Child Health. Seattle, University of Washington, 1998.

Steele SM, Harmon VM: Value Clarification in Nursing. New York, Appleton, 1979.

Stilwell BM, Galvin MR, Kopta SM, et al: Moral volition: The fifth and final domain leading to an integrated theory of conscience understanding. J Am Acad Child Adolesc Psychiatr 37:202-210, 1998.

Sutherland MS, Hale CD, Harris GJ, et al: Strengthening rural youth resiliency through the church. J Health Edu 28:205-218, 1997.

US Preventive Services Task Force: Guide to Clinical Preventive Services, 2nd ed. Baltimore, Williams & Wilkins, 1996.

Vitz PC: The use of stories in moral development: New psychological reasons for an old education method. Am Psychol 45:709-720, 1990.

Westerhoff J: Will Our Children Have Faith? New York, Seabury Press, 1976.

Approaches to Disease Management

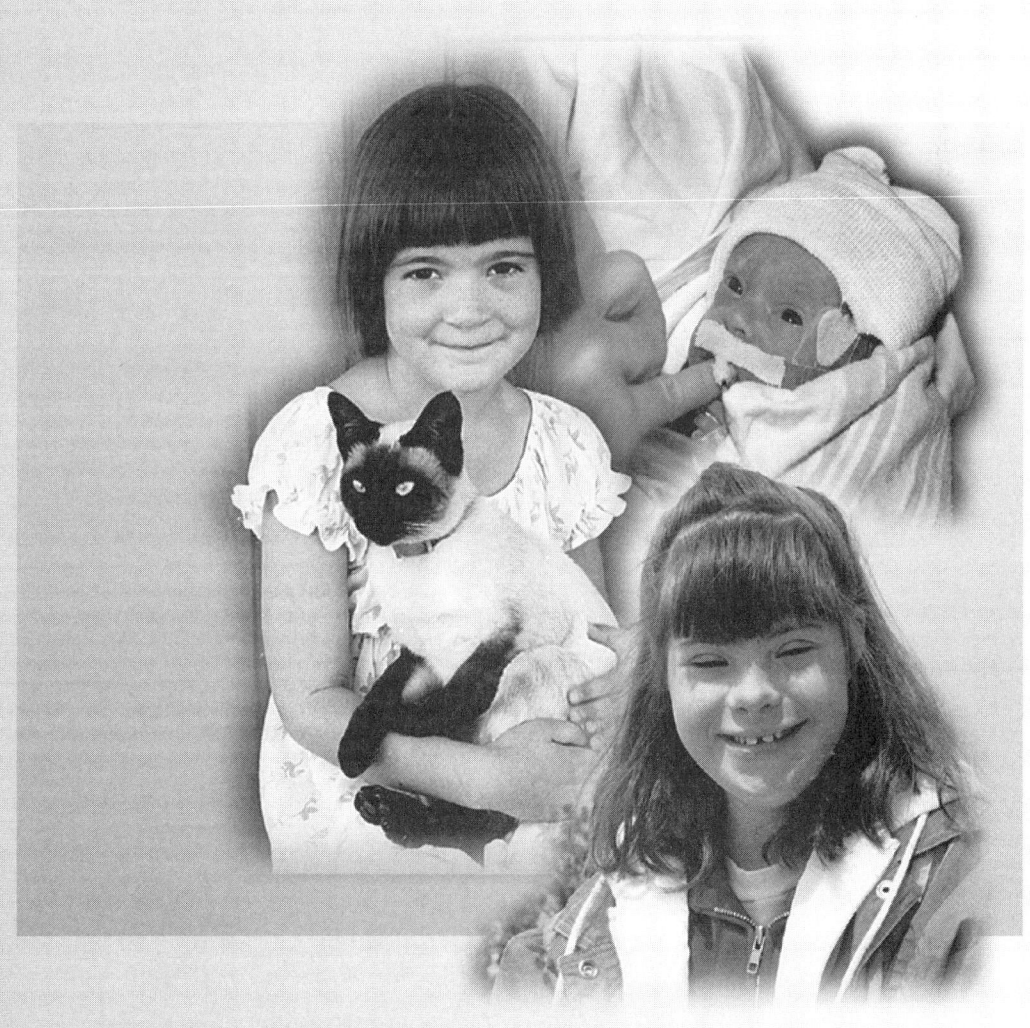

CHAPTER 23

Introduction to Disease and Pain Management

Margaret A. Brady

APPROACHES TO ACUTE DISEASE IN CHILDREN

A major role of a primary care provider in pediatrics is to arrive at a diagnosis and to treat common illnesses of childhood with a management plan that is consistent with the community standard of practice. This process begins with a thorough assessment of the child and the presenting complaint. In caring for children with acute illnesses, the nurse practitioner (NP) must always remember that an accurate assessment of the ill child is contingent on the following five points:

1. Careful observation of the child
2. Attention to pertinent positive and negative historical and physical findings
3. Knowledge of physiological functions and developmental considerations that vary by age
4. Consideration of the trajectory of the problem over time
5. Inclusion of the parents or caretakers and, if appropriate, the child as participants in the evaluation process

When satisfied that these five parameters have been given adequate attention, the NP forms an action or management plan that can include ordering basic laboratory and radiological studies and other special testing, if needed,

to arrive at a final diagnosis. Extensive laboratory and radiographic testing are often not in the best interest of children, especially for those who would be best served by being referred to a pediatrician or pediatric specialist for diagnosis or treatment of their disease.

NPs are responsible for the assessment and management of children with common pediatric illnesses or conditions. The effectiveness of NPs in primary care is due in large part to their ability to educate patients and their families about the prevention of disease and the management of common illnesses. The patient–parent educational component of the management plan must be individualized but should always include the following essential points:

- Information about the length of time it can take before the child improves and symptoms wane; description of what the course of the disease or illness is likely to be
- Identification of specific signs and symptoms that indicate the need for immediate medical attention or for a return visit sooner than planned
- Instructions about when to return for a follow-up visit or telephone conference if needed
- Written instructions about any special treatment or therapy that is required
- Careful instructions about medication,

545

both prescription and over-the-counter (OTC) drugs (see Use of Medication)

- Specific information about any dietary needs or changes, special hydration needs such as electrolyte solutions or increase in fluid intake, plus any changes in eating patterns that can be expected
- Information about the etiology, transmission, and communicability of an infectious disease
- Information about the etiology and recurrence risks of noninfectious illnesses or medical conditions
- Information about prevention and recurrence
- Determination of impediments that prevent the parent or the child from complying with the management plan (e.g., limited financial resources, inability to read, dysfunctional family, transportation problems) and discussion about steps to correct these difficulties
- Recognition and discussion of cultural practices and beliefs about illnesses, including the potential benefit or harm from specific folk medicine or complementary practices if used either alone or concurrently with prescribed or OTC medications
- Information for the working parent about resources for sick care in the community, if available in the area and affordable for the parent

It is important to allow time for the natural defense system of the body to fight disease. Premature and excessive pharmacological therapy can result in needless iatrogenic disease and often serves to confuse the clinical picture. The drug of first choice—the one that is least harmful—should be given time to work. Prematurely changing to a new drug, adding additional drugs, or using more toxic drugs are dangerous practices.

For the most part, parents are alert to subtle changes in their children, so the NP should listen attentively when parents voice concerns about their children. Any sick child who is at high risk because of physical or social problems merits closer observation and follow-up than does the average thriving child who becomes ill. Finally, if the child returns and is not signifi-cantly improved or is more symptomatic, the NP should reassess the situation by carefully analyzing the symptoms, investigating problems related to compliance issues, and repeating the physical examination. The NP should rethink the original diagnosis and review likely differential diagnoses before deciding on another management plan.

Management of an ill child also can include a short stay in an outpatient clinic or private office for intravenous hydration, pulmonary therapy, medication, and close observation to determine whether the child's condition stabilizes. Hospitalization might not be needed if the child's condition stabilizes, the parent is reliable, the child can be monitored closely at home, the home has a telephone, and the parent has transportation available to return for follow-up or an emergency visit. However, before discharging an ill infant or child to home rather than admitting the child to the hospital, the NP must carefully assess the parent's ability to cope with a significantly ill child and to identify signs or symptoms of increasing illness.

The number of infants and young children in group day care is expanding as the number of women in the work force increases. The disease pattern in this cohort of children is often related to group exposure to illnesses. The issue of multiple caregivers can complicate history taking. In these situations, obtaining accurate information about the manifestation or pattern of an illness can be difficult. Often, parents express feelings of guilt about being a poor parent because their child has been exposed at day care and they must work. Addressing these issues during the health encounter is often helpful for parents.

▓▓▓ APPROACHES TO CHRONIC DISEASE IN CHILDREN

It is estimated that between 5 and 10% of American children experience a prolonged period of illness or disability, the severity of which varies, as does its interference with the child's usual daily activities (Bechtold & Barkley, 1999). Some chronic conditions are not permanent, serious, or obvious, whereas other conditions are nonreversible, serious, and readily apparent.

There also can be great variability in both the presentation and the course of illness among children. Children with chronic medical or psychiatric conditions have special health needs. They and their families often face a range of problems that are as diverse as the conditions that cause these difficulties. A variety of genetic, congenital, and acquired conditions can lead to permanent or persistent problems that have a significant impact on the child's lifestyle and family functioning. The NP must be cognizant of several key points when working with these children and their families:

- Prevention of special health problems is a primary goal of care and includes
  ◦ Early prenatal care for all pregnant women
  ◦ Genetic counseling as indicated
  ◦ Elimination of environmental triggers or toxins
- Early identification of the condition or disease is of paramount importance.
- Amelioration of any functional problem that is treatable is as essential as prevention of secondary complications.
- Early intervention whenever possible to prevent secondary psychosocial difficulties is crucial; the developmental aspects of long-term illness must be addressed.
- Counseling is needed for the child and family to handle psychosocial and behavioral problems
- The child, the family, and school personnel must be consulted to ensure that the child is able to attain realistic developmental milestones.
- Appropriate educational support in school is a right. Public law 94–142, the Education for All Handicapped Children Act of 1975, mandates an appropriate education for all school-age children with developmental disabilities in the least restrictive environment.
- Public law 99–457 (1986) provides states with the opportunity to extend benefits of public law 94–142 to children from birth to 2 years of age.
- Early intervention from birth is optimal and encouraged.
- NPs should be prepared to participate in the child's individual education plan, if warranted, to ensure that school officials understand the often complex health care needs of the child.
- Prevention of discrimination is a right and is mandated under legislation related to individuals with disabilities. The Americans With Disabilities Act (1990) is a law that provides federal protection in the areas of employment, transportation, public accommodations, and communications for individuals with disabilities. The scope of protection covers both private and public sectors.
- Advocacy for children with chronic conditions and their families includes assisting them to secure coordinated and comprehensive health care and community-based services as needed.
- Provision of primary care services—regular health maintenance supervision and anticipatory guidance—must not be overlooked.
- Social service support is essential to assist parents who need special services for their child and to help determine financial eligibility for SSI (Supplemental Security Income) or state program benefits for individuals with handicaps or specific chronic diseases.

Medically fragile and technology-dependent children are living longer than in the past and are reaching adulthood mainly as a result of improved technology and major advances in medical and surgical care. These children require a multidisciplinary team approach to their care.

Although chronic illnesses are diverse in their severity and effect on the child, certain issues are often common concerns for children with chronic conditions and their families. They include the following:

- The high cost of treatment
- Lack of, or difficulties and barriers in, acquiring health-care insurance coverage
- Family lifestyle alterations that may be required of parents or siblings, or both, in caring for the child
- The need for supervised care by multiple health-care providers and the frequent lack

of coordination of services in providing continuity of care

- Unpredictability of the condition and the potential for complications, frequent medical visits, hospitalizations, and death
- The developmental impact that chronic disease can have on a child, especially during adolescence and early adulthood
- Longevity concerns—ability to live and function independently as an adult, including the need for career and vocational counseling
- The level of knowledge parents need about the pharmacological management of pain and the disease process or other therapeutic treatments, including nutritional support for the at-home care of the child
- The impact of stress on emotional and psychological well-being of the child and family members
- Acceptance by peers
- Dealing with feelings (e.g., anger, sorrow) while attempting to cope with chronic illness
- Developing advocacy skills for these children to access services through schools, state and community agencies, or special federally sponsored programs
- Securing special illness-related equipment (e.g., movement and mobility aids such as walkers, wheelchairs, or braces) or acquiring communication aids such as hearing aids or special computers with voices
- Finding respite care
- Legal conservatory issues and the concern about who will care for the child as an adult when parents are no longer capable of providing physical care or are deceased

A multidisciplinary team approach is best for children with complex chronic diseases. These teams offer the expertise of many individuals in a united approach. Involvement of a clinical social worker, a community health nurse, or a nurse case manager is important to secure essential community resources for child and family. Family support groups are often beneficial; they offer a chance to interact with others who have experienced many of the same challenges, difficulties, sorrows, and triumphs. Sibling issues and feelings such as anger, embarrassment, a sense of being overwhelmed with added responsibilities, or believing they need to be the protector for their brother or sister also must be addressed.

ASSESSMENT

History and Physical Examination

Chapter 2 discusses the complete history and physical examination of children from infancy through adolescence. In addition, each of the pediatric disease management chapters in this unit focuses on key questions to ask in history taking and highlights significant findings to be alert to if found on physical examination. Careful attention must be given when analyzing the signs and symptoms of the illness, including the presentation of clinical findings, the course of the disease process, and its associated manifestations. The NP should listen to what parents say about their child. The physical examination is often a challenge when a young child is ill and uncooperative. Patience is important when examining children who are sick. The sick child should be carefully assessed so that significant physical findings are not missed during a hurried or cursory examination.

Chapter 24 discusses an overall assessment and management plan for sick, febrile children. It also identifies specific infectious diseases and assessment criteria for illnesses or problems commonly seen in childhood. In general, with infectious diseases, the NP must remember that the age of a child is a significant factor to consider in any management plan. The immune response in infants aged 0 to 90 days is particularly poor. Infants and young children are at increased risk for overwhelming bacteremia with any infection. Similarly, in other noninfectious diseases and conditions, age often continues to remain a key factor in the assessment of the child. To assess the severity of illness in infants and young children, careful attention must be given to the following four key indicators during both the history and the physical examination:

1. Level of consciousness
2. Hydration

3. Respiratory status
4. Activity level

Diagnostic Studies

When deciding whether to order diagnostic tests, the NP should keep the following goals in mind. Order only those tests that give the most information for the least money, and order a test only if it is a crucial factor in the establishment of a concrete diagnosis or if it is a critical element in the treatment plan. If radiographic or imaging tests are necessary, order the test that is the least invasive. There are several useful points to remember about common imaging tests:

1. Conventional radiographs are
   - Useful diagnostic tools
   - The least expensive of the imaging tests
   - Readily available
2. Computed tomography (CT) imaging
   - Provides excellent bone and soft tissue detail
   - Can be used with contrast material for special evaluations
   - Shows relationships well; images can be presented in the frontal, transverse, and/or sagittal planes or obtained in three-dimensional imaging
   - Requires sedation of infants and young children
   - Has greater radiation exposure
   - Is costly
3. Magnetic resonance imaging (MRI)
   - Provides excellent images of soft tissue without exposure to ionizing radiation; bone imaging is poor
   - Is expensive
   - Often requires sedation or anesthesia in infants and young children, because immobilization is necessary
4. Ultrasonography
   - Gives two-dimensional images and measurements of internal organ systems; however, air-filled lungs and gas-filled bowel loops are impenetrable to ultrasound
   - In the form of Doppler ultrasound, blood flow direction and velocity can be measured; a still picture of the image can be recorded as a permanent record, or sonog-

raphy can be viewed as the image is being projected on a video screen
   - Is highly dependent on operator skill and experience
   - Does not require sedation
   - Involves no radiation exposure

Chapter 27 contains a detailed discussion of the complete blood count (CBC) and provides insight as to the information that can be gained from a CBC as well as indications for ordering this basic laboratory study. Chapter 27 also discusses frequently ordered coagulation studies. Chapter 24 discusses the laboratory workup for young children with a fever of undetermined origin. All disease entities or conditions addressed in this text include information about diagnostic studies and laboratory tests. Diagnostic studies and tests are valuable but are only one part of the entire database. Tests should be ordered only when the results are necessary to guide clinical decision-making.

▨ USE OF MEDICATION

Several key principles should guide the NP in the use of prescription drugs and OTC medications.

Safe Prescription-Writing Practices

Prescriptions should be written in a manner that conveys accurate information to the pharmacist and the patient or parent. The following suggestions are made to ensure safe prescription writing for children (Taketomo et al., 1998):

1. Never place a decimal and a zero after a whole number, because the decimal point might not be read correctly (e.g., 3.0 ml can be mistaken for 30 ml).
2. Place a zero before fractions less than one. For example, write 0.3 ml rather than .3 ml, which can be confused with 3 ml if the decimal point is inadvertently missed.
3. Never use the abbreviations q.d. (every day) or U or u (unit), which may be misinterpreted for q.i.d. or zero, respectively. Write out in full the words "every day" or "unit."

The abbreviation O.D. means right eye; never use O.D. as an abbreviation for once daily.

4. Use the metric system only.
5. Write legibly.
6. Issue a complete prescription that contains
   • Patient's full name, age, and weight (for infants and young children)
   • Name of the drug, dosage, and strength
   • Instructions if a brand name drug is to be used rather than the generic drug option
   • Total amount to be dispensed
   • Route of administration (e.g., take by mouth, instill in both ears, insert in rectum, instill in right eye)
   • General instructions to the patient or parent about indications for or the purpose of taking the medication and for how long (e.g., take until completed, take for wheezing)
   • Special instructions to the patient or parent about the drug or other instructions (e.g., translate to the primary language of the parent if English is not spoken or read)
   • Number of refills

Prescribing Pharmacological Agents

When prescribing pharmacological agents or recommending OTC drugs, the NP must be knowledgeable of the pharmacokinetics of the drug, the usual dosage, its side effects, and the indications and contraindications for its use in children. The NP must have a clear purpose in mind for using a particular drug and should not prescribe or recommend agents because of pressure from a parent or any other individual. Keep the following points in mind when prescribing drugs or OTC medications:

1. Lack of compliance in taking medications can be a major problem. Factors that affect compliance include the following:
   • The more often a drug must be given per day the greater the chance that a dose or doses will be missed.
   • Drugs that have a bitter or repulsive taste are difficult and sometimes impossible to get a child to take.

   • The greater the number of drugs that a child is given, the greater the potential for a drug dose to be missed or the wrong drug taken.
   • Waking a child to take a medication is difficult for parents; prescribe round-the-clock dosing only when it is essential to maintain tight therapeutic drug levels.
2. Poorly given or inadequate instructions increase the risk that the prescribing agent will be misused.

Educating Parents and Children About Pharmacological Agents

The success of any pediatric health care encounter depends on the ability of the health provider to educate parents or children, or both. The NP is in a unique position to educate parents and children about preventive care and common childhood illnesses. Before patients and their parents leave the health care setting, they should have a basic understanding about the pharmacological effect of any medication or OTC drug that is prescribed or recommended. Points of information that the NP should emphasize include:

• The purpose of the drug, how much should be given, and the frequency of administration
• Instructions about the indications for using a drug that is given on an "as necessary" basis or under specific circumstances (e.g., a rescue plan for the child with asthma whose symptoms are worsening)
• Signs or symptoms that indicate that a drug is either effective or not producing the desired effect or effects
• Possible drug interactions, precautions, or adverse reactions that can occur
• If applicable, any monitoring parameters that are required for safe administration of the drug or to maintain effective therapeutic blood levels
• Pregnancy risk factor of a drug and the need to screen for pregnancy when giving specific drugs to female teenagers.

Return demonstration can be a useful adjunct to evaluate the ability of the parent or child to administer a drug or drugs in the desired fashion. Return demonstration is a desired teaching tool in many situations. Examples of such circumstances include the following:

- Administering oral suspensions to infants and young children
- Measuring small or exact dosages (e.g., when a syringe is needed to measure amounts)
- Giving injectable, intravenous, gastrostomy, or nasogastric tube medications
- Instilling ophthalmic drops or ointments or nasal sprays or drops
- Using a metered dose inhaler (MDI), spacers, or inhalation equipment
- Ensuring that parents of limited cognitive abilities can safely administer medication to their children

Prescriptive Authority for Nurse Practitioners

NPs must be knowledgeable about the individual state regulations that govern their prescription-writing privileges in primary care. Some states do not use the term "prescribe" to identify what NPs do when writing medication prescriptions for patients. For example, in California, the term "furnish" is used to describe this activity. The individual State Board of Registered Nursing identifies the terminology to be used for this activity and regulates (either as a single state regulatory entity or jointly with medicine or pharmacology state boards) the activities and procedures related to this particular function. Regulations about prescriptive activity vary from state to state. NPs are governed by individual state guidelines and are legally obliged to follow all state regulations and mandates related to any prescriptive authority granted to them.

▨▨▨ EDUCATIONAL STRATEGIES

When educating parents and children about a particular illness or disease entity, the NP must use terms easily understood by the parent or child, or both. The health professional must include information as appropriate to the individual situation about the following topics:

- Etiology of the disease if known
- Epidemiology and communicability issues as well as prevention guidelines if applicable
- The management strategy
- Use of pharmacological agents
- Nutritional counseling
- Need for special treatments, adaptive devices, or in-home monitoring tests; how to do the testing or monitoring; and how to use adaptive devices
- Need for laboratory or radiographic tests and the meaning of results
- Specific information on the signs and symptoms that indicate either a worsening or an improvement in the child's condition or illness
- Availability of telephone follow-up contact with the health care provider
- Issues related to administration of medications at school—appropriate forms completed and school personnel instructed on key issues related to pharmacological therapy
- Specific directions about when to schedule follow-up appointments

The severity of the illness or disease and the child's age, maturity, and cognitive level are key factors that determine the child's degree of involvement in self-care activities related to acute illness and chronic disease management. Children should be taught basic health promotion and disease prevention behaviors from early childhood. Likewise, they should be involved in the management of their illness to the fullest extent possible considering their developmental capabilities; health professionals frequently ignore or forget to include the school-age child or adolescent as a partner in the management plan. Children should be consulted regarding their responsibilities for self-care. The NP also might be called on to be a liaison with school personnel to optimize the child's educational and social experience at school.

Written instructions and easy-to-read handouts are useful for parents and children, whether the instructions deal with common illness management, complex treatment needs, or information about developmental milestones and anticipatory guidance issues. *Instructions for Pediatric Patients* (Schmitt, 1999) and *Guide to Your Child's Symptoms* (Schiff & Shelov, 1997) are excellent resources to suggest to parents for guidance about common infections of childhood, preventive pediatrics, common behavioral problems, and other frequently encountered pediatric concerns.

PREVENTION OF ILLNESS

Prevention of illness and communicable diseases is a significant responsibility for NPs providing primary health care services for children or managing the care of children with chronic diseases or conditions. Education of children and their parents or caretakers is a key component of all prevention programs or activities. NPs must be vigilant in their practice settings to prevent or reduce the possibility of exposure to communicable diseases and to control the spread of infectious diseases that are a threat to infants, children, and youth. Therefore, NPs must strive to ensure the following:

- All children are appropriately immunized against vaccine-preventable diseases according to the recommendations of the Advisory Committee on Immunization Practices (ACIP), the American Academy of Pediatrics (AAP), and the American Academy of Family Physicians (AAFP).
- Communicable diseases are identified and treated appropriately and are reported in a timely fashion to public health departments as required by law.
- Health practices to prevent or control the spread of infectious disease are carried out in home, out-of-home child care programs, schools and health care settings, and hospitals. Key practices are included in the following list:
  - Effective personal hygiene—hand washing to prevent fecal-oral and person-to-person skin contact spread of disease
  - Appropriate environmental sanitation—disposing of waste (e.g., blood, urine,

feces, vomit, saliva) together with proper cleaning and disinfection of equipment; toys, toilets, eating areas, and diaper changing surfaces
  - Reducing respiratory spread of disease—covering mouth when sneezing or coughing and disposal of tissue after wiping nose; eliminating passive smoke and providing adequate ventilation
  - Sanitary food handling and preparation
  - Reducing exposure to communicable disease by separating sick children from well children
- Education about the prevention of sexually transmitted diseases is provided to youth.
- Young children and teenagers are educated about not sharing food, liquids, personal hygiene products, cosmetics, hair coverings, grooming products, or towels with others.
- Preventive health guidance is given about avoidance of second-hand smoke, especially in cars or confined areas.

The American Public Health Association and the American Academy of Pediatrics (1992) participated in a joint project that resulted in the publication of *Caring for Our Children. National Health and Safety Standards: Guidelines for Out-of-Home Child Care Programs.* This book outlines preventive health practices that promote a safe environment for infants and children and addresses the issues of disease prevention and management in child care programs. Preventing and controlling the spread of illness in these group settings are important issues in maintaining health.

PAIN IN CHILDREN

NPs must be familiar with the assessment and effective management of pain in the pediatric and adolescent population. Unrelieved pain has both negative physiological and psychological consequences. Pain can result from injury or disease process, or as a side effect of procedures or surgery. Assessment and management of minor pain in the primary care setting is the focus of this section. The NP should seek other references for the treatment of chronic pain in pediatric patients.

Key factors that can influence effective pain management in children include the following:

- Established pain is difficult to control; therefore, prevention of pain is an important goal of pain management.
- Pediatric and adolescent patients and their families should be involved in pain assessment and management as much as possible.
- Culture and family learning patterns must be considered (e.g., beliefs about pain, folk remedies, how pain is expressed verbally, and language barriers).
- Genetic stressors (those physiological and psychological differences between individuals, memories, and possibly prenatal and perinatal stressors can influence a child's perception of pain (Zeltzer et al., 1997).
- Developmental issues (e.g., cognitive, emotional, and physical), age, and temperament significantly impact how pain is interpreted, expressed, and controlled
- Cognitive issues that influence pain perception include the child's memory and level of understanding, ability to control what will happen, attachment of a meaning to the situation with regard to pain, and expectations of the intensity of the pain.
- Emotional issues that impact a child's pain perception include anxiety, fear, frustration, anger, and depression.
- Social issues, such as how others react (their behaviors) to the child in pain, can influence the treatment plan.
- Pain perception involves complex neural interactions that send out impulses generated by tissue damage.
- Pediatric or adolescent patients and their parents must be educated about the assessment and management of pain.
- For a variety of reasons (e.g., fear of getting a shot), some children do not report pain to health-care providers.

Pain Assessment

A systematic assessment of pain in children and adolescents begins by obtaining a pain history from the child or the parent. When talking with younger children, ask the parent what words the child uses for pain (e.g., "owie," "boo-boo," "ouchie") and use these words with the child. Behavioral observations and physiological findings provide additional information to complete a comprehensive pain assessment.

Clinical Findings

HISTORY

In assessing pain, the following information should be obtained:

1. Pain history (symptom analysis):
   - Intensity (mild, moderate, severe, overwhelming)
   - Location (areas of pain and without pain)
   - Quality—how pain is described by child or parent (e.g., stinging, burning, "big ouchie") and any pain behaviors noted
   - Duration (how long has the pain been present)
   - Temporal features or chronology (when and how did the pain start, precipitating factors, any variations in intensity and quality)
   - Previous treatments
   - What makes the pain worse or better
   - Other associated symptoms, such as anxiety
2. Past experience with pain including child's memory of the painful experience and how the pain was treated
3. Cultural beliefs about pain and its treatment
4. Self-reports of pain in the verbal child (if possible, obtain pain history as noted), if needed, identify a tool that is reliable, valid, sensitive and simple for the child to understand and use the tool consistently. The use of self-report tools and other objective pain measures helps to objectively quantify pain pretreatment and serves to evaluate the outcome of treatment. (See Fig. 23-1 for information about child pain scales and tools and Table 23-1 for a listing of interview tools and pediatric pain questionnaires.)

BEHAVIORAL INDICATORS

Behavioral observations include vocalizations (e.g., crying, whimpering, whining), social

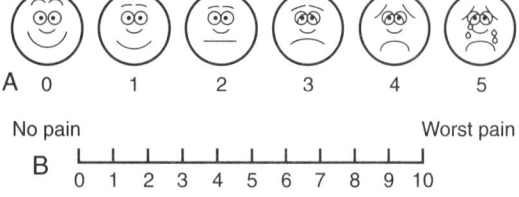

A   0   1   2   3   4   5

No pain   Worst pain

B | 0 1 2 3 4 5 6 7 8 9 10 |

F I G U R E 23-1
Common pain rating scales used to measure pain in pediatric and adolescent patients: Important considerations. Age factors (basic principles): Most children older than 4 years of age are developmentally able to provide accurate self-report information. Around the age of 7 to 8 years, children who understand the concept of ordering and numbering can use numerical rating scales or a horizontal word-graphic rating scale. Specific Tools (basic instructions and principles): *A*, Five faces showing expressions of pain with a sixth face representing no pain or hurt are shown to the child, who is asked to select the face that best describes his or her own pain. The number under the face is used to quantify the level of pain. A similar tool is the Oucher scale developed by Beyer in 1989. It uses six photographs of a child's face to represent levels of pain from "no hurt" to the "biggest hurt you could ever have." A vertical scale using numbers from 0–100 also can be used. Again, the end points represent "no pain" to the "most or worst pain." Points in between are given ranges with a qualifying statement. For example, 1 to 2 represents "just a little pain," and the child who has just a little pain selects a number within this range to rate his or her own pain. (From Wong D, Baker C: Pain in children: Comparison of assessment scales. Pediatr Nurs 14:9–14, 1988.) *B*, Numeric Scale: A straight line is used with divisions of 10 units, with 0 signifying "no pain" and 10 signifying "the worst pain imaginable." The numbers 1 to 9 represent "little pain to a lot of pain." The child is asked to select one number to best describe his or her own pain. Older children can be asked to rate their pain on a scale of 0 to 10 without showing them a visual line. The instructions are the same regarding 0 representing "no pain" and 10 the "worst possible pain." (From Wong DC, Wilson D: Waley and Wong's Nursery Care of Infants and Children, 5th ed. St. Louis, Mosby, 1995.)

withdrawal, changes in sleep patterns (more or less), verbalizations, facial expressions of guarding, grimacing, vigilance or anger, motor responses, body posture, and activity such as rubbing or touching the painful site, avoiding or guarding the affected area (e.g., not letting anyone touch the abdomen). These may be the only cues of pain in preverbal or nonverbal children.

PHYSIOLOGICAL INDICATORS

Physiological parameters (e.g., heart rate and blood pressure) are neither sensitive nor specific indicators of pain, particularly in children who experience chronic pain. Other physical indicators include such findings as diaphoresis and pallor.

Management

If there is a known etiology or underlying disease causing the pain, treat its causes. Other measures also may be needed to control for pain symptoms. Principles of effective pain management include the use of a combination of pharmacological and nonpharmacological measures.

Common nonpharmacological measures include

- Sensorimotor techniques for infants such as pacifiers, swaddling, holding, and rocking
- Cognitive/behavioral strategies such as relaxation procedures, music and play therapy, and preparatory information before painful procedures
- Physical strategies such as application of heat (if muscle spasm) or cold (if swelling, bleeding, or pain), massage, acupuncture, exercise, rest, or immobilization
- Distraction techniques such as having the

T A B L E 23-1

Structured Interviews, Pain Questionnaires, and Other Tools for Assessing Pain in Pediatric Patients: Used With Children Experiencing Long-Term, More Complex, or Intense Pain

TOOL	AUTHOR
Adolescent Pediatric Pain Tool (APPT)	Savedra et al., 1989
Patient pain diary or journal	
Varni/Thompson Pediatric Pain Questionnaire	Varni et al., 1987

child watch a video, look out the window, or play with a toy, praising the child, giving the child a party blower and asking the child to blow the pain away, providing stickers or stamps, gently stroking the child, or giving multiple injections (e.g., immunizations) at the same time.

Pharmacological measures used in primary care settings for acute pain include

- Analgesic for mild to moderate pain: acetaminophen—10 to 15 mg/kg every 4 hours; use of an anti-inflammatory agent is more effective if inflammation is a key factor causing pain.
- Oral nonsteroidal anti-inflammatory drugs (NSAIDs): The usual pediatric dosage for children weighing less than 50 kg is listed (U.S. Department of Health and Human Services, 1993). See Appendix A for additional information about drugs:
  - Aspirin—10 to 15 mg/kg every 4 hours contraindicated in children because of its association with Reye's syndrome. Use only in the management of selected pediatric conditions (e.g., juvenile rheumatoid arthritis and Kawasaki disease).
  - Ibuprofen—10 mg/kg every 6 to 8 hours for children 6 months of age or older.
  - Mefenamic acid (Ponstel)—250 mg every 6 hours; use in adolescent patients.
  - Naproxen (Naprosyn)—5 mg/kg every 12 hours for children older than 2 years.
- Opioid agonists for moderate or severe pain:
  - Codeine—oral, 1 mg/kg every 3 to 4 hours.
  - Hydromorphone (Dilaudid)—oral, 0.06 mg/kg every 3 to 4 hours for children 6 to 12 years.
  - Hydrocodone (in Lorcet, Lortab, Vicodin)—child dose not established; adolescent, 1 to 2 tablets or capsules every 4 to 6 hours.
  - Oxycodone (in Percocet, Percodan, Tylox)—oral, 0.05 to 0.15 mg/kg every 4 to 6 hours.
  - Morphine—oral, 0.3 mg/kg every 3 to 4 hours; parenteral, 0.1 mg/kg every 3 to 4 hours. This drug is not used commonly in primary care settings for the management of acute pain.
- Topical analgesic creams such as EMLA and ionophoresis delivery of drugs—used with procedures involving skin punctures.

Pharmacological measures used in primary care settings for chronic pain management include (Shapiro, 1995)

- The primary treatments used to treat chronic pain unrelated to disease or trauma are the NSAIDs, acetaminophen, and tricyclic antidepressants (TCAs). Assess for the efficacy of the drug as follows:
  - Have the child or parent use a pain intensity rating scale and keep a diary of the child's activities and pain.
  - On follow-up visits, question whether symptoms have improved.
- Selective serotonin reuptake inhibitors, opioids, certain anticonvulsants, and other selected medications may be needed. Children requiring these agents for the management of their chronic pain are best handled by referral.

FEVER IN CHILDREN

Fever is a common phenomenon seen in children and involves neurologic, endocrine, and metabolic functions. Viral infections are responsible for most fevers in children. Bacterial infection, malignancy, reaction to immunizations, and connective tissue disease are other known etiologic factors. Associated symptoms of headache, malaise, anorexia, and irritability are uncomfortable for the child and always worrisome to parents. Those parents who have fever phobia need reassurance because they believe that temperatures greater than 40 to 40.1°C cause brain damage or, if not treated, will go higher. Most health care providers treat fevers to provide comfort to the child and use pharmacological agents when a temperature exceeds 102°F or 38.9°C and the child is uncomfortable or if the child has a persistent temperature above 101°F. Some clinicians use temperatures greater than 101.5°F as their guide to treatment (Berlin, 1996).

Management strategies for fever control include the following:

- Nonpharmacological measures
  - Providing adequate hydration
  - Providing appropriate clothing—not bundled in additional clothing or coverings
  - Providing ambient environment temperatures of around 72°F (22°C)
  - Sponging with tepid water for temperatures above 104°F (40°C). Sponging should be stopped if the child starts to shiver. Ice water baths and alcohol sponging should *not* be done.
- Pharmacological measures—antipyretic agents (Taketomo et al., 1998)
  - Acetaminophen 10 to 15 mg/kg/dose every 4 to 6 hours, not to exceed five doses in 24 hours; temperature generally is reduced by 1 to 2°C within 2 hours.
  - Ibuprofen in children 6 months to 12 years: for temperature less than 102.5°F (39°C), 5 mg/kg/dose; for temperature greater than or equal to 102.5°F (39°C), 10 mg/kg/dose every 6 to 8 hours with a maximum daily dose of 40 mg/kg/day.

TELEPHONE MANAGEMENT OF ILLNESSES

Several excellent resources address telephone management of illnesses in children (Brown, 1994; Schmitt, 1998a, 1998b, 1998c). Many daytime telephone calls represent routine questions or common pediatric problems and can be effectively managed by office nurses with special training. NPs with their specialty education and background in primary care are frequently called on to give advice to parents over the telephone or are assigned to take telephone calls either during the daytime or after regular office hours. All NPs should ensure that their practice settings have developed a safe system for managing sick child calls and follow-up calls on patients seen by the NP or physician.

Nonemergency calls to a practice about a sick child during the day are usually routed through a telephone receptionist who can make an appointment if appropriate, transfer the call over to a triage nurse or the NP who can determine the urgency of the need to see the child, give home care advice, or refer to the physician. If home care advice is given, the triage person should use standards of care or telephone advice protocols addressing a particular set of symptoms, complaints, or a diagnosis that is agreed upon for use in that particular setting.

Triage Categories

Schmitt's (1998b; 1998c) triage categories for sick calls are

- Life threatening situation—call 911.
- Emergent—see patient immediately.
- Urgent—see patient within 4 hours.
- Urgent or uncomfortable patient—see the patient that day.
- Nonurgent—see the patient that day or the next day.
- Recurrent or persistent—see the patient within 2 weeks.
- Mildly ill—give home care advice.

The development of telephone protocols is a key factor to ensure an effective telephone management system for a busy practice setting. Schmitt developed a quick reference for pediatric telephone protocols that can be reviewed for ideas about how protocols can be developed. Whatever protocols are used or developed in an individual practice setting, any management-by-telephone protocol should accomplish the following objectives:

- Allow the telephone triage person to manage sick child calls safely.
- Provide a standard of care.
- Prevent omissions resulting from forgetfulness or fatigue.
- Prevent harmful triage or recommendations.
- Improve quality of care.

The NP who is doing telephone triage must be a perceptive, conscientious, and calm individual who carefully listens to the caller, asks selected questions, processes the information, determines the correct management protocol to use for a particular situation, gives the necessary instructions to parents, and writes notes in a log book. In addition, all these activities must be performed in a relatively short period of time. The sequence of steps that one must go through in using telephone protocols includes the ability to

- Identify the problem or main symptom.
- Select the correct protocol.
- Collect data about the symptoms through open-ended and direct questioning.
- Determine a diagnosis or working assessment.
- Decide on a triage category for the patient.
- Educate the parent about the plan of care.

Documentation

Documentation of the telephone call and disposition is an important element in a successful system for managing telephone calls for sick children. A documentation system, whether it consists of a log sheet or note pad, should be simple and brief. Written documentation serves several purposes, including

- A medicolegal defense
- A method to review charts for quality improvement and assurance purposes
- An avenue to assist in complaint resolution if parents are upset about the advice given to them
- A tool to use when making follow-up calls to the family

Important items to include in any telephone log are

1. Date and time
2. Patient data—name, age, sex, telephone number—and history of chronic disease or condition
3. The chief complaint and a brief list of symptoms and signs, including their duration and frequency
4. Diagnosis or working assessment
5. Triage category
6. Instructions given about follow-up
7. List of medications and their dosage if prescribed by the NP
8. An "other" section for any additional comments that are deemed important information

When using telephone protocols in a practice setting, training of all individuals who are doing telephone triage is essential and is the best method to ensure consistency in the use of the system. Staff sessions set up to review the written documentation are also useful teaching tools and should be encouraged. Perhaps the most important point to emphasize in training and about the use of any telephone management system is the need to assess the comfort of the parent with the advice given. Parents should be asked at the end of the telephone contact whether they are comfortable with the advice and plan. If the parent is not satisfied or is uneasy about the plan, physician or NP consultation should be an option. Finally, parents should be told to call back if their child's condition worsens or the problem persists too long.

Relating to Parents Via the Telephone

Brown (1994) emphasizes several points about telephone management of common pediatric illnesses, conditions, or concerns. These include method of interaction, screening questions to ask, and points at which intervention is necessary. The individual should be receptive to the parent's call, using language and taking the necessary time to give the message that the call is as important to the provider as it is to the parent. Parents can be anxious and find it difficult to calmly state the problem. The individual also must be calm, direct, and comforting in order to help parents manage their child's illness.

Screening questions that should be asked of parents include

- Duration: How long has the problem been present?
- Description: Tell me about the problem. What signs and symptoms are present?
- Clinical changes: How has the child's behavior changed (e.g., eating, sleeping, interaction with peers and family members)?
- Environmental problems: Has there been any recent exposure, change, or stress in the child's environment?
- Cause: What does the parent believe is contributing to or causing this condition?

- Management: What has the parent done for the condition, and with what effect?
- Feelings: Does the parent feel anxious about how the child is behaving?

Questions should be asked in an effort to narrow the problem clinically and to assist the parent to be clear and focused. Questions should be clustered by area of concern, should move from most to least serious, and should follow a logical algorithm based on initial data obtained.

Call centers are another avenue that pediatric practices use for handling sick calls after office hours. These centers employ nurses and NPs who use telephone protocols to guide parents in the management their child's illness until their regular health provider is available. These call centers alleviate the burden of night call and are set up to use telephone protocols and a software program for documentation (Schuman, 1998).

Educating Parents About Telephone Management of Illness

Practice settings should have a telephone call policy about sick calls and should acquaint parents with this policy. The policy should cover basic information about the office protocol for handling calls about sick children during office hours, well-child questions, prescription refills, nighttime (after-hours) calls, and weekend and holiday calls. Who screens calls, when calls are returned (e.g., during the noon hour or from 4 to 5 PM), and after-hours coverage are points to cover in the policy.

Parents should be encouraged to handle minor illnesses at home without unnecessary calling in for advice. Home instruction sheets for managing fevers (including dosage charts) and common childhood illnesses or books on common pediatric illnesses designed for parents are excellent resources to provide to parents. Pamphlets can be given to parents at anticipatory guidance visits. During illness visits, parents should be told what to expect when their child is ill, preparing them for the increasing temperature, vomiting or diarrhea, as well as what to do if they occur.

Parents need to know what type of situations

require a call for emergency medical services or the poison control center. If sick care is necessary after scheduled office hours, parents will need to give the following information about their child:

- The main symptoms
- Any chronic disease or health problem
- Temperature (and route it was taken)
- Approximate weight
- Names and dosages of current medications
- Type of insurance coverage

In addition, the parent should have the name and telephone number of the pharmacy available to give the provider (Schmitt, 1998c).

REFERRALS AND CONSULTATIVE SERVICES

Referrals and Use of Consultants

On many occasions, NPs identify clinical or behavioral problems that they are uncomfortable managing for any number of reasons, such as being out of the scope of their practice parameters or a problem that requires the expertise of a provider in a subspecialty practice. In these instances, patients should be referred to other providers for management of that problem. In other situations, the NP may wish to continue to manage the patient's care but seeks consultation with other experts in the field. The NP uses this individual as a case consultant. Whether the NP refers the patient and family out to or consults with another health care expert, certain information must be shared with the referral or consultant provider in an organized, logical fashion. Guidelines for presenting this information are as follows:

- Give the patient's name, age, and actual or tentative diagnosis or chief clinical findings.
- Briefly discuss, in a sentence or two, why the patient or family is being referred to another provider or the reason that a consultation is being requested.
- Give a synopsis of the patient's history, clinical findings, prior management plan, and outcome of treatment if applicable.

- Identify any pertinent past medical history such as chronic illnesses or conditions.
- Provide pertinent family, educational, or social information, including insurance coverage if this is problematic.

If the NP is referring the patient out for problem-focused care, this should be made clear to the referral provider. In addition, guidelines should be established for when the patient should be seen again by the NP for primary care supervision and how information about the child's progress will be shared with the NP. If the child is to be seen by the NP for primary care services and at the same time by the referral provider for speciality care, coordination of responsibilities between the two providers relative to the need for follow-up testing, monitoring, treatments, or therapy should be identified.

The NP should maintain a listing of specialty providers in the local area who take referrals from the NP's work setting. If the NP is employed in a large health maintenance organization, then the NP should maintain a list of pediatric specialty providers in the organization. Important information to include about these individuals includes their specialty or subspecialty practice area, evaluation of their effectiveness (can be an informal notation such as "great resource person") and, if applicable, their fees for service (e.g., full fee or sliding scale) or which insurance plans will reimburse for their services.

Whether consulting formally or informally with another provider about the care of a particular patient, the NP should present information about the patient, as listed, and discuss potential management options. At the end of the consultation, the NP should summarize the key areas that were discussed and the recommendations that were agreed upon. A notation about the consultation, the main discussion points, and the recommendations should be made in the patient's chart.

Often overlooked sources of free consultation are state and local public health departments or agencies and health-related professional organizations, as well as some major medical centers that provide telephone consultation about patients for providers in their service area. Again, a notation should be placed in the child's file if the case is discussed with a consultant in such an agency. Connecting with colleagues on the Internet is another option. Real-time chat sessions and e-mail exchanges are possible sources of consultation; however, information secured from unknown sources should be verified for accuracy.

When a patient is referred to another provider, the NP must explain the reason for the referral to the child and parent, how the transfer of care will be managed, and when the patient is to return to see the NP. The information should be presented in such a manner as to dispel fears of abandonment or giving up. The bond between the child, the parent, and the primary care provider is a strong relationship that individuals rely on. If the NP plans to seek a consultation, the child and parent should be informed by explaining the need for a second opinion or the desire to collaborate with others to ensure that nothing has been missed. After the consultation, parents should be informed about what was decided. Finally, the parent may seek consultation with another health-care provider. If so, treat this as the parent's need to collaborate in the child's care and listen to the recommendation by this consultant. Be sure that the consultant's reports are filed in the child's chart.

NATIONAL AND LOCAL ORGANIZATIONS AND RESOURCES

Parents and their children with specific disease entities or health conditions can benefit from the educational materials, resources, and support that national health organizations provide. Learning to live with a chronic disease or handicapping condition presents a special challenge to families. Most national organizations provide written materials that parents and children can easily understand about the etiology, management, and treatment of the particular disease in question. These materials also help parents explain their child's condition to teachers and others. Many of these national organizations can guide parents and children to support groups with other families and children who are similarly challenged and to health professionals and other related groups who specialize in the treatment of a particular disease entity. Likewise, these organizations can assist parents in accessing unique services to benefit their children; for example, enrolling in special camps and sports activities, learning about the various legal rights of children with disabilities or handicapping conditions, and acquiring special adaptive equipment.

Many national and local health organizations and foundations provide educational materials and valuable information designed for health professionals about a variety of subjects related to their target population of children. Often these organizations can provide up-to-date information about new treatment modalities or management strategies. These groups are a source of valuable information and assistance to health professionals and their patients. NPs should take advantage of the services that national health organizations and local chapters offer and inform parents about national organizations and local chapters that can assist them in meeting their child's special needs. In addition, every clinical or practice setting should have a listing of local community resources. One can make up a personal local resource guide and keep this information along with a listing of national organizations. Many such resources are listed at the end of each chapter in this textbook.

REFERENCES

American Public Health Association and the American Academy of Pediatrics: Caring for our children. National Health and Safety Standards: Guidelines for Out-of-Home Child Care Programs. Ann Arbor, MI, Edwards Brothers, 1992.

Bechtold DW, Clark RB: Psychosocial aspects of pediatrics and child and adolescent psychiatric disorders. *In* Hay WW, Hayward AR, Levin MJ, et al (eds): Current Pediatric Diagnosis and Treatment. Stamford, CT, Appleton & Lange, 1999, pp 161–194.

Berlin CM: Fever in children: A practical approach to management. Contemp Pediatr Educational Supplement: 1–8, 1996.

Beyer JE: The Oucher: A User's Manual and Technical Report. Denver, CO, University of Colorado, 1989.

Brown JL: Pediatric Telephone Medicine: Principles, Triage and Advice, 2nd ed. Philadelphia: JB Lippincott, 1994.

Hester NO: Comforting the child in pain. *In* Funk SG, et al (eds): Key Aspects of Comfort. New York, Springer, 1989.

Savedra MC, Tesler MD, Holzemer WL, et al: Adolescent Pediatric Pain Tool (APPT) Preliminary User's Manual. San Francisco, University of California, 1989.

Schiff D, and Shelov S: Guide to Your Child's Symptoms. Elk Grove, IL, American Academy of Pediatrics, 1997.

Schmitt BD: Instructions for Pediatric Patients, 2nd ed. Philadelphia, WB Saunders, 1999.

Schmitt BD: Calls about sick children: A triage system for the office. Contemp Pediatr 15(7):138–152, 1998a.

Schmitt BD: Calls about sick children: Launching your own triage system. Comtemp Pediatr 15(8):49–71, 1998b.

Schmitt BD: Pediatric Telephone Protocols: The Quick Reference, 2nd ed. Littleton, CO, Decision Press, 1998c.

Schuman AJ: Is there a pediatric call center in your future? Contemp Pediatr 15(8):75–94, 1998.

Shapiro BS: Treatment of chronic pain in children and adolescents. Pediatric Annals, 24, 148–156, 1995.

Taketomo CK, Hodding JH, and Kraus DM: Pediatric Dosage Handbook, 5th ed. Hudson, OH: Lexi-Comp Inc, 1998.

U.S. Department of Health and Human Services: Acute Pain Management in Infants, Children, and Adolescents: Operative and Medical Procedures. AHCPR Pub. No. 92-0020. Rockville, MD, 1993.

Varni JW, Thompson KL, and Hanson V: The Varni-Thompson pediatric pain questionnaire. I. Chronic musculoskeletal pain in juvenile rheumatoid arthritis. Pain 28:27–38, 1987.

Wong D, and Baker C: Pain in children: Comparison of assessment scales. Pediatric Nursing 14:9–14, 1988.

Zeltzer L, Bursch B, and Walco G: Pain responsiveness and chronic pain: A psychobiological perspective. Dev Behav Pediatr 18:413–422, 1997.

CHAPTER 24

Infectious Diseases

Mark H. Goodman and Margaret A. Brady

INTRODUCTION

Infections are a way of life for all children at one time or another. Viruses are the leading cause of most pediatric infections. Bacterial infections, particularly of the respiratory and gastrointestinal tracts, whether primary or secondary to viral illnesses, are also common problems seen in pediatric practice (Hay et al., 1999). Most childhood illnesses resolve completely. The skilled nurse practitioner (NP) quickly needs to differentiate the insignificant illness from the more serious condition. In addition, parental anxiety and frustration in dealing with a sick child require the NP to communicate with, educate, and support the family during those trying times.

PATHOGENESIS OF INFECTIOUS DISEASES

Humans are host to a variety of microbes, most of which are harmless and, in fact, beneficial to the host. Microbial colonization occurs soon after birth. Normal host flora are protective in that they limit colonization of pathogenic organisms.

An infectious process starts when a microorganism attaches to and invades host cells. For example, viruses attach and bind to the host cell surface structures by glycoproteins that are recognized by cell surface structures. Many microbes express factors that allow them to invade cells. In addition, there are other microbe–host cell interactions that permit colonization.

Illnesses occurring after colonization of viruses and bacteria result not only from cell lysis but also from cellular dysfunction or tissue destruction. For example, infection can cause an inflammatory response that is meant to defend the host against invasion by microbes but also results in destruction of both infected and adjacent tissue. This inflammatory response can occur at the local site of infection or can lead to systemic effects. With tissue infection, polymorphonuclear neutrophils (PMNs) and macrophages migrate to the site as part of the host immune response. Certain infections also have been associated with malignant changes. Chronic hepatitis B infection and Epstein-Barr viral infections are associated with hepatocellular carcinoma and Burkitt's lymphoma, respectively.

CLINICAL·FINDINGS

The diagnosis of a common infectious disease in pediatric patients often is based solely on clinical findings. The history and physical examination constitute the cornerstones. The history must be comprehensive.

History

Important historical items for the NP to investigate include the following:

- Evolution of the symptoms—the order and timing of their presentation
- Epidemiology—looking for family, day care, school, or neighborhood contacts
- History of all recent and previous travel
- Recent medical intervention or instrumentation—dental, gastrointestinal, genitourinary, vaccinations, transfusions
- Unusual occurrences, including loss of consciousness or trauma
- Possible drug use
- Contact with animals or animal byproducts such as hides, waste, or blood
- Unusual dietary practices—ingestion of raw milk or meat
- Preexisting illness that may compromise the child
- Congenital anomalies that increase the likelihood of illness
- History of pica
- Medication history—previous and current medications used, including all over-the-counter and prescription medications
- Genetic background of family
- Hereditary diseases
- Cultural practices of family or community

Physical Examination

A complete physical examination must be undertaken. The specific examination procedures mentioned in other chapters concerning the various organ systems should be employed. Special attention should be given to the skin and mucous membranes for exanthemas and enanthemas.

Nonspecific signs of infection can include the following:

- Fever (temperature instability with severe infections in young children)
- Respiratory distress
- Vomiting or diarrhea or both
- Skin rashes, including petechiae
- Tachycardia
- Apnea and bradycardia (in infants)
- Irritability, high-pitched cry, bulging fontanel, convulsions
- Lethargy
- Weak suck or poor appetite

DIAGNOSTIC AIDS

Laboratory Studies

The laboratory is only an adjunct to help confirm clinical suspicions. One can easily succumb to the lure of the laboratory and order all the tests necessary to rule out every illness in the differential diagnosis. This practice is ineffective and costly, and it can create confusion. Common tests used to diagnose infectious diseases include the following.

COMPLETE BLOOD COUNT (CBC)

Bacterial and viral infections cause changes to the white blood cell count. Generally, bacterial infections cause leukocytosis with a differential left shift (e.g., increased polymorphonuclear leukocytes [polys] and bands). Viral infections usually cause leukopenia. There are some specific exceptions to this rule, (e.g., pertussis causes an elevated white blood cell count with lymphocytosis). The clinical state of the patient is important in interpreting the CBC. Overwhelming sepsis, immunosuppressive drugs, and corticosteroids can alter the CBC and confuse the clinical picture.

ERYTHROCYTE SEDIMENTATION RATE (ESR)

An elevated ESR, either zeta or Westergren method, suggests inflammation. While not specific for infectious disease, it may suggest the need for further workup. It also is useful to evaluate treatment and resolution of many types of infections, such as osteomyelitis.

CULTURES

Depending on the clinical presentation, one can obtain specimens for culture from all natural body orifices and, if necessary, create some additional ones (e.g., blood, cerebrospinal fluid [CSF], pleura, joints, and abscesses). Different types of bacteria and viruses require different media. This can result in handling problems. One should notify the laboratory of clinical suspicions to ensure proper handling. Gram stains also can be performed on all body fluids and can help in the choice of proper antibiotics before the culture and sensitivity tests are available.

SKIN TESTS

These include purified protein derivative (PPD) and Schick tests.

FLUORESCENT STAINING TECHNIQUES

Specific antisera are combined with fluorescein dye. If a sensitive organism is present, antibodies concentrate around it, and the resultant mixture illuminates.

SEROLOGICAL TESTS

Specific antisera can cause an agglutination reaction. The tests are measured by dilutional factors. A fourfold rise is considered positive and suggests the diagnosis. There are false-positive and false-negative reactions owing to cross-reactivity of antisera.

ANTIBODY DETECTION TECHNIQUES

Besides fluorescent staining techniques and serological tests, other techniques of antibody detection include complement fixation, hemagglutination inhibition, and ELISA (enzyme-linked immunosorbent assay) testing.

ANTIBIOTIC SENSITIVITY TESTING

Standard zone diameters indicate sensitivity or resistance of a microbe to a specific antibiotic.

OTHER TESTS

DNA probes are DNA-segment specific, radioactively labeled reagents used to identify various bacteria. Rapid antigen detection tests are useful in helping to make a quick diagnosis (e.g.,

rotavirus and respiratory syncytial virus). Polymerase chain reaction (PCR) is a process that increases the amount of DNA sequences to be analyzed by multiplying copies of the original DNA segment.

IMAGING TECHNIQUES

Radiographs can be useful in the diagnosis of infections. Chest radiographs, sinus series, and mastoid studies assist the NP in the evaluation of children with unusual or minimal findings. Radioactive scans are advantageous in the detection of osteomyelitis or abscesses. Computed tomography (CT) scans and magnetic resonance imaging (MRI) can detect abscesses or other purulent material collections.

GENERAL MANAGEMENT STRATEGIES

Principles for Preventing the Spread of Infections

Education of parents and children in the prevention of the spread of infectious diseases should be routinely done. Potential areas to cover include the following:

1. The spread of respiratory disease may be decreased by hand washing, covering one's mouth when coughing, properly disposing of saliva-infected tissues, not sharing foods or liquids that someone else has eaten, and limiting exposure to ill contacts.
2. Skin infections can be reduced, again, by careful hand washing and limiting contact with fluid from skin lesions (e.g., covering lesions if appropriate; use of separate towels for personal hygiene; keeping nails trimmed).
3. Enteric infections are transmitted by the fecal-oral route; meticulous hand washing after toileting or changing diapers is critical. Attention to proper food handling and preparation to prevent growth of, or contamination with, bacteria, viruses, fungi, and parasites also is an area to discuss. Proper disposal of pet waste and washing of hands after contact with pets should be stressed.
4. Parents of infants and young children in day

care should be familiar with the day care setting's policies related to cleaning of toys and sleep equipment, toileting practices, diaper-changing procedures, routine hand washing procedures for both staff and children, sick child procedures, and environmental sanitation procedures.

Principles Guiding the Judicious Use of Antimicrobial Agents in Pediatrics

The increasing emergence of bacterial strains that are resistant to antimicrobial agents is worrisome. Vancomycin-resistant enterococci, multidrug-resistant tuberculosis, and antimicrobial-resistant respiratory pathogens are now major threats to children who become infected with these organisms. Scientific data have shown that the key factor responsible for the emergence and spread of resistant organisms is the widespread use of antimicrobials, whether inappropriately or appropriately prescribed. Parental pressure to prescribe unnecessary antimicrobials for the common cold, bronchitis, and viral pharyngitis is no longer an acceptable reason to prescribe an antibiotic. Parental education about the course and treatment of viral illnesses and the link of antimicrobial resistance to the overuse of antibiotics is a key point that NPs must address with parents. In addition, when antimicrobials are prescribed, completion of the prescribed course of therapy should be stressed.

Practice guidelines have been developed by the American Academy of Pediatrics (AAP) for the judicious use of antimicrobial agents for pediatric upper respiratory tract infections in hope of curtailing this dangerous trend (Dowell et al., 1998b). Principles developed for the treatment of otitis media, pharyngitis, acute sinusitis, cough illness or bronchitis, and the common cold follow.

Principles of Treatment

OTITIS MEDIA

(Dowell et al., 1998a)

1. Otitis media should be classified as acute otitis media (AOM) or otitis media with effu-

sion (OME). AOM is diagnosed when there is fluid present in the middle ear with signs of acute local or systemic illness such as otalgia, otorrhea, or fever. With OME, fluid is present in the middle ear but without signs or symptoms of acute infection.

2. Antimicrobials are indicated to treat AOM if there *is documented middle ear effusion and signs or symptoms of acute local or systemic illness.* Pneumatic otoscopy can be used to assess the tympanic membrane for color, position, translucency, and mobility. Tympanometry and acoustic reflectometry also can be used to validate effusion. Fever without other findings, such as ear pain or a red or bulging tympanic membrane, may be unrelated to middle ear effusion.

3. A short course of antimicrobials (i.e., a 5- to 7-day course) is acceptable for treating uncomplicated AOM in certain patients. Data support short-course therapy in older children (>2 years of age) with mild AOM.

4. Antimicrobial agents are not indicated for the initial treatment of OME. Antibiotic therapy or bilateral myringotomy with insertion of tympanotomy tubes is recommended in children with documented bilateral effusion that persists for 3 months and significant bilateral hearing loss (see Chapter 30).

5. Persistent middle ear effusion after treatment of AOM does not require antimicrobial therapy.

6. The use of antimicrobial prophylaxis is appropriate treatment for the use of recurrent AOM with the following criteria: three or more distinct and well-documented episodes of AOM in a 6-month time frame or four or more episodes in 12 months.

PHARYNGITIS

(Schwartz et al., 1998)

1. The diagnosis of group A streptococcal pharyngitis must be based on results of a throat swab culture or antigen-detection test with a culture backup (if this test is negative) in association with clinical and epidemiologic findings.

2. A child with signs and symptoms of pharyngitis should not be given antimicrobial ther-

apy in the absence of diagnosed group A streptococcal or other bacterial infection. Viral pharyngitis is common. Thus, starting children on antimicrobial agents pending culture results is not advised.

3. The drug of choice for the treatment of group A streptococcal infection continues to be penicillin (see Chapter 32).

SINUSITIS

(O'Brien et al., 1998a)

1. Bacterial sinusitis is diagnosed clinically using the following criteria: prolonged nonspecific upper respiratory signs and symptoms (i.e., rhinosinusitis and cough for >10 to 14 days), or more severe upper respiratory tract signs and symptoms (i.e., fever >39°C, facial swelling, and facial pain).

2. Radiographic evidence of sinus involvement can be seen with the common cold; therefore, sinus x-rays should be interpreted and ordered cautiously. Indications for the use of radiographs to diagnose sinusitis are as follows: recurrent episodes of sinusitis; complications of sinusitis are present or suspected; or the diagnosis is unclear (see Chapter 32).

3. The most narrow-spectrum antimicrobial agent that is active against the suspected organism should be the initial drug of choice.

COUGH ILLNESS OR BRONCHITIS—PRINCIPLES OF TREATMENT

(O'Brien et al., 1998b)

1. Antimicrobial therapy is rarely indicated in children with nonspecific illness or bronchitis regardless of duration of symptoms. Fever with symptoms and signs of bronchitis is not by itself an indication to prescribe antibiotics (see Chapter 32).

2. Antimicrobial agents may occasionally be indicated in the treatment of prolonged cough (>10 days). Pertussis or *Mycoplasma pneumoniae* is associated with prolonged cough (>10 days) and requires antibiotics. Children with chronic pulmonary disease (ex-

cluding asthma) may benefit from antimicrobial therapy with acute exacerbations of pulmonary disease marked by coughing.

THE COMMON COLD

(Rosenstein et al., 1998)

1. Antimicrobial agents are not beneficial and should not be prescribed for the common upper respiratory infection.

2. Thick, opaque, or discolored nasal discharge (mucopurulent rhinitis) is a frequent manifestation of the common cold and part of the natural course of viral rhinosinusitis. It is not an indication for antimicrobial therapy unless it persists for more than 10 to 14 days (see Chapter 32).

▬ PREVENTION OF INFECTION THROUGH THE USE OF VACCINES

Prevention is always better than treatment. Vaccination is the single best technique for the prevention of infectious disease. Vaccines now exist to combat many childhood diseases (e.g., *Haemophilus influenzae* type B, meningococcus, diphtheria, pertussis, tetanus, polio, measles, mumps, rubella, hepatitis, and varicella), but NPs still see some of these illnesses. Practitioners must continue to educate patients about the need to keep current with necessary immunizations. Failure to do so results in unnecessary epidemics.

Informed consent is critical when discussing the benefits and risks of vaccination. The National Childhood Vaccine Injury Act (public law 99-660, amended by Public Law 101-239) became effective in 1988. This act has provisions that call for standardized consent forms. All practitioners are required to use these forms to fulfill their duty to warn the public. The act also requires that the vaccine lot number, site of inoculation, name of the person administering the vaccine, and parental signature are included in the medical record.

The National Childhood Vaccine Injury Act also requires health care providers to report selected adverse events that occur after immunization. These are discussed in detail later. The events are to be reported to the Vaccine Adverse Event Reporting System (VAERS), established by the United States (US) Department of Health and Human Services. A standard confidential form for reporting suspected vaccine-related problems has been in existence since 1990. A VAERS staff member contacts the provider at 60 days and 1 year after the report to follow up on the patient's condition. The VAERS telephone number is 800-822-7967.

ACTIVE IMMUNITY

Inoculating a child with modified parts of a microorganism evokes an immune response. Whole organisms (live, attenuated, or killed), modified proteins, and sugars are used to prepare certain vaccines. The response to vaccination is often as protective as the natural infection. Anti-invasive, antitoxin, or neutralizing antibodies can be found soon after the vaccination is given. Some types of vaccines give life-long immunity. Others require periodic boosters. The active and inert vaccine ingredients differ among manufacturers. One must be aware of these components because of a patient's possible hypersensitivity to the ingredients used. Thimerosal, a preservative containing ethyl mercury, is contained in various vaccines to reduce bacterial growth. Manufacturers have been urged to eliminate or reduce the mercury content of thimerosal-containing vaccines.

Live or attenuated vaccines usually confer broader and longer lived immunity than killed types. Killed and inactivated vaccines can provide systemic protection (immunoglobulin G [IgG] antibodies) but may fail to provide local mucosal antibody (IgA). Thus, although protected from systemic illness, a recipient of a killed vaccine can have local colonization or infection that can be a problem during an epidemic.

The AAP, American Academy of Family Physicians (AAFP), and the Advisory Committee on Immunization Practices (ACIP) of the Centers for Disease Control and Prevention (CDC) approved a new unified recommended childhood immunization schedule (Table 24-1).

Maternal antibodies neutralize vaccines; therefore, infants vaccinated in the first year of life require more inoculations than older children. Children who are not immunized in the first year of life should be vaccinated according to the schedule listed in Table 24-2. Missed vaccinations should be given when possible. One does not need to repeat the entire series again; just continue normally from that point. Proper storage of vaccines and correct immunization technique are critical for optimum results. The manufacturer's package inserts provide this information.

Diphtheria and Tetanus Toxoids With Pertussis Vaccines (DTP/DTaP)

DTP comes in two distinct forms. DTP is a trivalent vaccine and is composed of the diphtheria and tetanus toxoids and killed whole-cell pertussis vaccine. DTaP is also composed of diphtheria and tetanus toxoids but has an acellular pertussis vaccine and is the preferred vaccine for the prevention of childhood diphtheria. DTP is an acceptable alternative to DTaP, but because of its higher likelihood of vaccine-associated reactions, it is quickly falling out of favor. Scheduling for these vaccines is given in Table 24-1 and Table 24-2. Universal immunization with DTaP (or DTP) is the only effective control measure for these illnesses. Diphtheria and tetanus toxoids are very effective vaccines as proved by the rarity of these diseases in the United States. The usual dosage is 0.5 ml intramuscularly (IM). There are currently four licensed DTaP vaccines in the United States: Tripedia, Infantrix, Acel-Imune, and Certiva. They are equally effective but differ slightly in their ingredients.

Interchangeability of these vaccines has not been studied. When possible, one should continue the same vaccine for the primary series. Any licensed product is acceptable for the 4th and 5th dose if any of the previous doses were DTP. Tripedia and Infantrix are not licensed for the 4th or 5th dose if all the previous doses were DTaP. Certiva currently is not licensed for the 5th dose. Children younger than 7 years of age must be vaccinated with DT if they cannot receive pertussis vaccine. Td vaccine contains

T A B L E 24-1

Recommended Childhood Immunization Schedule, United States

							Age					
VACCINE*	**Birth**	**1 mo**	**2 mo**	**4 mo**	**6 mo**	**12 mo**	**15 mo**	**18 mo**	**4–6 yr**	**11–12 yr**	**14–16 yr**
Hepatitis B[2]	Hep B										
		Hep B			Hep B					Hep B	
Diphtheria, tetanus, pertussis[3]			DTaP	DTaP	DTaP		DTaP[3]		DTaP	Td	
H. influenzae type b[4]			Hib	Hib	Hib	Hib					
Polio[5]			IPV	IPV	IPV				IPV[5]		
Measles, mumps, rubella[6]						MMR			MMR[7]	MMR[6]	
Varicella[7]						Var				Var[7]	

*Vaccines[1] are listed under routinely recommended ages. | Bars | indicate range of recommended ages for immunization. Any dose not given at the recommended age should be given as a "catch-up" immunization at any subsequent visit when indicated and feasible. (Ovals) indicate vaccines to be given if previously recommended doses were missed or given earlier than the recommended minimum age.

Approved by the Advisory Committee on Immunization Practices (ACIP), the American Academy of Pediatrics (AAP), and the American Academy of Family Physicians (AAFP).

[1]This schedule indicates the recommended ages for routine administration of currently licensed childhood vaccines. Combination vaccines may be used whenever any components of the combination are indicated and its other components are not contraindicated. Providers should consult the manufacturers' package inserts for detailed recommendations.

[2]*Infants born to HBsAg-negative mothers* should receive the 2nd dose of hepatitis B vaccine at least 1 month after the 1st dose. The 3rd dose should be administered at least 4 months after the 1st dose and at least 2 months after the 2nd dose, but not before 6 months of age for infants.

Infants born to HBsAg-positive mothers should receive hepatitis B vaccine and 0.5 mL hepatitis B immune globulin (HBIG) within 12 hours of birth at separate sites. The 2nd dose is recommended at 1–2 months of age and the 3rd dose at 6 months of age.

Infants born to mothers whose HBsAg status is unknown should receive hepatitis B vaccine within 12 hours of birth. Maternal blood should be drawn at the time of delivery to determine the mother's HBsAg status; if the HBsAg test is positive, the infant should receive HBIG as soon as possible (no later than 1 week of age).

All children and adolescents (through 18 years of age) who have not been immunized against hepatitis B may begin the series during any visit. Special efforts should be made to immunize children who were born in or whose parents were born in areas of the world with moderate or high endemicity of HBV infection.

[3]DTaP (diphtheria and tetanus toxoids and acellular pertussis vaccine) is the preferred vaccine for all doses in the immunization series, including completion of the series in children who have received 1 or more doses of whole-cell DTP vaccine. Whole-cell DTP is an acceptable alternative to DTaP. The 4th dose (DTP or DTaP) may be administered as early as 12 months of age, provided 6 months have elapsed since the 3rd dose and if the child is unlikely to return at age 15–18 months. Td (tetanus and diphtheria toxoids) is recommended at 11–12 years of age if at least 5 years have elapsed since the last dose of DTP, DTaP, or DT. Subsequent routine Td boosters are recommended every 10 years.

[4]Three *H. influenzae* type b (Hib) conjugate vaccines are licensed for infant use. If PRP-OMP (PedvaxHIB and COMVAX [Merck]) is administered at 2 and 4 months of age, a dose at 6 months is not required. Because clinical studies in infants have demonstrated that using some combination products may induce a lower immune response to the Hib vaccine component, DTaP/Hib combination products should not be used for primary immunization in infants at 2, 4, or 6 months of age, unless FDA-approved for these ages.

[5]IPV: The ACIP recommends the use of an all-IPV schedule (effective January 1, 2000). Give 4 doses, at 2, 4, 6–18 months, and 4–6 years of age.

[6]The second dose of measles, mumps, and rubella vaccine (MMR) is recommended routinely at 4–6 years of age but may be administered during any visit, provided at least 4 weeks have elapsed since receipt of the first dose and that both doses are administered beginning at or after 12 months of age. Those who have not previously received the second dose should complete the schedule by the 11- to 12-year-old visit.

[7]Varicella vaccine is recommended at any visit on or after the first birthday for susceptible children, i.e., those who lack a reliable history of chickenpox (as judged by a health care provider) and who have not been immunized. Susceptible persons 13 years of age or older should receive 2 doses, given at least 4 weeks apart.

Adapted from Centers for Disease Control and Prevention. Recommended childhood immunization schedule—United States, MMWR Morb Mortal Wkly Rep, 48:8–16, 1999.

TABLE 24-2

Recommended Schedule for Children Not Vaccinated in the First Year of Life

TIME	IMMUNIZATION
CHILDREN <7 YEARS OLD	
First visit	HepB, DTaP, IPV, MMR (if >12 mo of age), Hib (15–59 mo of age), Mantoux
1 mo later	HepB, DTaP, varicella (if >12 mo)
2 mo later	DTaP, IPV, Hib (if first dose was given at <15 mo of age)
8 mo or later	DTaP, HepB, IPV
4–6 yr	DTaP, IPV, MMR
11–12 yr	MMR (if not given at entry to kindergarten), Td can be given if 5 yr since previous dose (then repeat Td every 10 yr)
CHILDREN >7 YEARS OLD	
First visit	HepB, Td, IPV, MMR
2 mo later	HepB, Td, IPV, varicella
8–14 mo later	HepB, IPV, Td
5 yr later	Td (then repeat Td every 10 yr)
11–12 yr	MMR

a smaller amount of diphtheria toxoid and is given to patients older than 7 years of age. Older children and adults require less stimulation for antibody production. If tetanus toxoid is required for contaminated wound management, consider using either DTaP (or DTP), DT, or Td, as indicated, to provide adequate diphtheria immunity as illustrated in Table 24-3.

There are a few relative contraindications to vaccinating a child with DTP or DTaP. The first is an immediate anaphylactic reaction and the second is encephalopathy within 7 days. If DTP or DTaP is given and any of the following events occurs, they are listed as precautions to further administration of DTP or DTaP: convulsion, with or without fever, within 3 days of immunization; persistent inconsolable screaming (≥3 hours) within 48 hours; collapse or shock-like state within 48 hours; and unexplained temperature higher than 104.9°C within 48 hours. DTaP, as previously noted, has a significantly lower probability of vaccine-associated reac-

tions, such as moderate or high fever and local reactions.

Mild to moderate fever is not uncommon after a DTP vaccination. Vaccinating a febrile child can confuse the clinical picture (i.e., Was the fever caused by the illness or the vaccination?). Minor respiratory illnesses, however, are not a contraindication to vaccination.

Children who have progressive developmental delay or a changing neurological picture should not be vaccinated with DTP because of its association with encephalopathies. No studies exist either proving that DTP causes brain damage or fully exonerating the vaccine. As with fever, confusion regarding the cause of the neurological disorder can occur. For this reason, immunization should be deferred until the problem is stabilized. Defer DTP or DTaP vaccination in any child with a personal history of seizures until a progressive neurological disease is ruled out or the child's diagnosis is established and the seizures controlled. Infants and children who have or are suspected to have neurological disorders or degenerative diseases that could induce convulsions must be reassessed at each visit. The decision to vaccinate should be based on the risk–benefit ratio. If one withholds pertussis, DT should be withheld as well for the first year, as it too may confuse the picture and be associated with adverse events. Subsequent doses of DTP or DTaP should be

TABLE 24-3

Tetanus Prophylaxis in Wound Management

PREVIOUS TETANUS IMMUNIZATION	CLEAN MINOR WOUND	DIRTY WOUND
Uncertain or <3 doses	Td only*	Td* and TIG within 3 d
3 doses	Td (fourth dose)*	Td (fourth dose)*
>3 doses	Td* if last dose >10 yr ago	Td* if last dose >5 yr ago

*In children older than 7 years, use Td for vaccination. In children younger than 7 years of age, use DTaP (or DTP) or DT if pertussis is contraindicated.

held until the neurological disorder is either stabilized, corrected, or resolved, and a reevaluation should be made after 1 year. In the United States, there is a remote risk of children younger than 1 year of age acquiring diphtheria or tetanus. Children who develop neurological disorders after their first year usually have already received DTP vaccine. If the neurological condition is stabilized, controlled, or resolved and pertussis vaccination is contraindicated, DT vaccination can be given. Children with culture-proved pertussis do not need to receive further pertussis vaccinations.

DTP reactions in children can be mild or severe, life-threatening events. *Mild* reactions include local swelling, pain, and discomfort at the injection site as well as irritability and low to moderate fever. *Serious* reactions encompass fever of 104.9°F or higher, drowsiness or somnolence, anorexia, vomiting, persistent high-pitched crying for more than 3 hours, and a shock-like state that may last for many hours. Depending on the clinical picture, these reactions usually warrant consultation with a physician or pediatric neurologist about further DTP or DTaP immunizations. Serious reactions do not leave sequelae. *Severe* neurological reaction in children, such as seizures (1 of 1750 DTP doses) or encephalopathy (1:140,000 DTP doses) after vaccination, are specific contraindications to further use of the vaccine (AAP, 1997). The reactivity of the pertussis component of the vaccine is not dosage dependent. Decreasing the dose of DTP has not been shown to significantly alter the incidence of adverse effects and is not recommended (AAP, 1997). If the child has a severe reaction to DTP, the series should be continued with DT vaccine.

DTP and *H. influenzae* type B (HIB) vaccine have been combined into DTP-HIB. DTP-HIB can be given when both DTP and HIB are scheduled simultaneously. It carries the same likelihood of causing adverse events as plain DTP. For children scheduled to receive DTP and PRP-T (a conjugated HIB vaccine) at the same visit, PRP-T can be reconstituted with DTP manufactured by Connaught Laboratories. Other conjugated HIB vaccines cannot be mixed in the same syringe with DTP. Reportable vaccine-associated events related to the various diphtheria, tetanus, and pertussis combination vaccines are found in Table 24-4.

Bacille Calmette-Guérin (BCG) Vaccine

BCG vaccine was developed in the early part of this century to prevent the spread of tuberculosis (TB). Studies of vaccine efficacy demonstrate inconsistent findings, but the vaccine is still recommended as a public health measure in developing countries with a high prevalence of TB. Two strains are currently licensed in the United States. The last field trials were done in 1955. The efficacy of the current vaccines is unknown.

In the United States, BCG is indicated only for uninfected children who are at unavoidable exposure and who cannot be protected by any other method of prevention, including prophylatic isoniazid (INH). They include children and infants living with persons who are untreated, ineffectually treated, or who have drug-resistant forms of TB, and children living in areas where TB is excessive and a source of health care is not readily available. Health-care workers in high-risk settings also may be candidates for BCG (AAP, 1997).

BCG is given to infants from birth until 2 months of age without prior tuberculin testing as long as the child is not further exposed to tuberculosis. Older children must have a negative tuberculin test before the vaccine is given. The vaccine is given intradermally; the usual dose is 0.05 ml for a neonate and 0.1 ml for an older child. If given properly, a small papule forms at the site of injection. The papule enlarges, crusts, and lasts approximately 2 to 3 months. PPD testing should be repeated 2 months later. If the second PPD is not reactive, repeat the vaccination.

One percent to 10% of those vaccinated with BCG experience side effects. These include localized ulceration, lymphadenopathy, and lupus vulgaris. Osteomyelitis and death are rare reactions (AAP, 1997). BCG is contraindicated in patients with immunological disorders. Children who are receiving corticosteroids or other immunosuppressive agents should not be vaccinated. Although no fetal problems have been

T A B L E 24-4

Vaccine Associated Events Reportable to Vaccine Adverse Events Reporting System*

VACCINE	ILLNESS, DISABILITY, INJURY, OR CONDITIONS COVERED	TIME PERIOD FOR THE FIRST SYMPTOM OR MANIFESTATION OF ONSET OF SIGNIFICANT AGGRAVATION AFTER VACCINE ADMINISTRATION
DTaP, DTP, DTP/HIB, DT, TT	Anaphylaxis or anaphylactic shock	4 hr
	Encephalopathy (or encephalitis)	3 d
	Brachial neuritis	2–28 d
	Any acute complication or sequela (including death) of an illness, disability, injury, or condition referred to above, which illness, disability, injury, or condition arose within the period prescribed	Not applicable
ORAL POLIO	Paralytic polio in	
	• A nonimmunodeficient individual	30 d
	• An immunodeficient individual	6 mo
	• A vaccine-associated community case	Not applicable
	Vaccine-strain polio viral infection in	
	• A nonimmunodeficient individual	30 d
	• An immunodeficient individual	6 mo
	• A vaccine-associated community	Not applicable
	Any acute complication or sequela (including death)	Not applicable
INACTIVATED POLIO	Anaphylaxis or anaphylactic shock	4 hr
	Any acute complication or sequela (including death) of an illness, disability, injury, or condition referred to above, which illness, disability, injury, or condition arose within the period prescribed	Not applicable
HIB (UNCONJUGATED, PRP)	Early onset HIB disease	Any time after immunization
	Any acute complication or sequela (including death) of an illness, disability, injury, or condition referred to above, which illness, disability, injury, or condition arose within the period prescribed	Not applicable
HIB (CONJUGATED VACCINES)	No condition specified	
MMR OR ANY MEASLES, MUMPS, OR RUBELLA-CONTAINING VACCINES	Anaphylaxis or anaphylactic shock	4 hr
	Encephalopathy (or encephalitis)	5–15 d
	Chronic arthritis	42 d
	Thrombocytopenia purpura	7–30 d
	Any acute complication or sequela (including death) of an illness, disability, injury, or condition referred to above, which illness, disability, injury, or condition arose within the period prescribed	Not applicable
HEPATITIS B	Anaphylaxis or anaphylactic shock	4 hr
	Any acute complication or sequela (including death) or an illness, disability, injury, or condition referred to above, which illness, disability, injury, or condition arose within the period prescribed	Not applicable

*Section 2114.(a) of the National Childhood Vaccine Injury Act effective March 24, 1997.

reported, pregnant women should not be inoculated with BCG.

Children with symptomatic human immunodeficiency virus (HIV) infection should not receive BCG (US Public Health Service, 1998). Asymptomatic HIV-infected children living in areas where the incidence of TB is low (e.g., the United States) should not be vaccinated. However, asymptomatic or suspected HIV-infected children living in areas where the incidence of TB is high should receive BCG as close to birth as possible according to World Health Organization guidelines. BCG vaccine can produce a mild to severe hypersensitivity reaction to tuberculin. It also can cause a false-positive reaction in children who receive tuberculin skin testing.

Polio Vaccine

Before January 2000, two forms of polio vaccine were licensed in the United States: live oral trivalent polio vaccine (OPV) and inactivated trivalent polio vaccine (IPV). The difference between OPV and IPV is that IPV does not protect against intestinal infection with wild virus, as does OPV.

Cases of vaccine-associated paralytic polio (VAPP) have occurred in vaccinees and close contacts. In children, the risk is 1 in 1.5 million doses of vaccine given. In contacts, it is 1 in 2.2 million doses. The risk of paralysis is higher with administration of the first dose of vaccine and when immunocompromised persons are exposed to live polio vaccine (AAP, 1997). When polio was epidemic, these vaccine-induced cases were acceptable. IPV was less potent than the vaccine now. The current strain of IPV is stronger (IPV-e, injectable poliovirus vaccine of enhanced potency).

The ACIP, AAP, and AAFP currently recommend an all-IPV schedule for routine childhood polio immunization. All children should receive 4 doses of IPV at 2 months, 4 months, 6 to 18 months, and 4 to 6 years (see Table 24-1). The dose of IPV is 0.5 ml IM. The need for booster dosages of enhanced IPV has not been determined.

OPV should be used only in the following special circumstances:

- If mass vaccination is needed to control outbreaks of paralytic polio
- If an unvaccinated child is traveling in less than 4 weeks to an area where polio is endemic
- If a parent does not accept the recommended number of vaccine injections despite counseling

These children should receive OPV for only doses 3 and 4.

For reportable vaccine-associated events related to the various polio vaccines, see Table 24-4.

Haemophilus Influenzae Type B (HIB) Vaccine

The HIB vaccines consist of purified bacterial protein joined to a poly- or oligosaccharide that is linked to a protein to enhance immunogenicity. PRP-D (ProHIBiT), HbOC (HibTITER), PRP-T (ActHIB or OmniHIB), PRP-OMP (PedvaxHIB), and combination HIB/Hepatitis B (Comvax) are currently licensed HIB vaccines. HbOC, PRP-T, and PRP-OMP are given to infants beginning at 2 months of age. HIB vaccine must not be given to children younger than 6 weeks of age, as there is a possibility that they may not respond to subsequent doses (Humiston & Atkinson, 1998). Therefore, *ComVax vaccine cannot be used at birth*. PRP-D is licensed only for children 15 months of age and older. Any child younger than 2 years of age who had had invasive *H. influenzae* disease should be vaccinated with any of the conjugated HIB vaccines according to the schedule recommended for their age. This is because of the decreased natural immunity in this age group. Unlike DTaP (or DTP) or polio vaccine, the number of doses of HIB vaccine changes depending on when immunization for this illness is begun. The older the child is, the fewer doses the child receives. For all vaccines the dosage is 0.5 ml IM. Table 24-5 lists the HIB immunization schedule. The same vaccine should be used for the primary series, but studies have not shown a decline in antibody production if regimens involving different vaccine products are used. Any licensed single HIB vaccine may be used for the booster when the child is 12 or 15 months old.

T A B L E 24-5

Haemophilus Influenzae *Type B Dosing Schedule*

VACCINE	AGE (MO) FIRST DOSE GIVEN	NUMBER OF DOSES	SCHEDULE
HbOC/PRP-T	2–6	4	Three at 2-mo intervals Fourth at 12–15 mo
	7–11	3	Two at 2-mo intervals Third at 12–18 mo, given at least 2 mo after dose 2
	12–14	2	Two at 2-mo intervals
	15–59	1	One dose only
PRP-OMP	2	3	If given at 2 & 4 mo, 3rd dose not needed Otherwise, two at 2-mo intervals Third at 12–15 mo
	7–11	3	Two at 2-mo intervals Third at 12–18 mo, given at least 2 mo after dose 2
	12–14	2	Two at 2-mo intervals
	15–59	1	None
PRP-D*	15–59	1	None
ComVax	2–6	3	Two at 2-mo intervals Third at 12–15 mo
HbOC-DTP	2–6	4	Three at 2-mo intervals Fourth at 12–15 mo, given at least 2 mo after dose 3

*PRP-D can be used for the booster dose after completion of the primary series.

The HIB vaccines are safe. PRP-T (ActHIB, OmniHIB), PRP-D (ProHIBit), and HbOC (Hib-TITER) use carrier proteins related to those components in the DTP vaccines. These formulations should not be used in children with suspected DTP reactions. PRP-OMP (Pedvax-HIB) is the recommended vaccine. No severe side effects have been reported, but low-grade fever and local pain have been observed. There are no major contraindications to giving the vaccine. Children who are receiving chemotherapy or immunosuppressive agents should receive HIB vaccine 2 weeks before or 3 months after therapy. The caveat concerning use of vaccine during a febrile illness should be observed.

Children with immunological disorders or certain chronic illnesses are at increased risk for invasive HIB. They also may have decreased ability to make HIB antibodies. Children with HIV infection, sickle cell disease, functional or anatomical asplenia, or those who are receiving chemotherapy or immunosuppressive therapy may require additional doses of HIB vaccine:

- *Asplenia*: If the child has received a complete primary series and booster, no additional vaccinations are needed. A child undergoing elective splenectomy for a medical condition may benefit from an additional dose of vaccine one week before the procedure.
- *HIV infection, chemotherapy, immunosuppressive therapy, or IgG2 deficiency*: There is not enough information at this time to determine whether additional doses of vaccine will be helpful. If these children have an incomplete course, they should be vaccinated to finish the series. Unvaccinated children older than 59 months of age should receive two doses of vaccine at least 1 to 2 months apart.

For reportable vaccine-associated events related to the various HIB vaccines or combination vaccine, see Table 24-4.

Measles–Mumps–Rubella (MMR) Vaccine

MMR is a trivalent vaccine. It is still possible, but often difficult, to obtain each component individually. The dosage is 0.5 ml subcutaneously (SC) for either MMR or its singular components.

MEASLES

The Moraten strain is the only licensed measles vaccine available in the United States. It is a live attenuated chick–embryo-prepared virus. Ninety-five percent of vaccinees develop antibodies to measles. The immunity is lifelong in most persons, but a second dose at entry to kindergarten is recommended. Children who do not receive the second dose at kindergarten should be revaccinated at the earliest possible time. The Year 2000 goal for protection against measles is that all school-age children will have received two doses of MMR (AAP, 1997). Persons vaccinated with killed vaccine or live vaccine/IgG and those vaccinated before 12 months of age should be revaccinated.

The measles component is responsible for almost all the adverse reactions to the MMR vaccine. A fever of 103°F beginning approximately 1 week after vaccination occurs in up to 15% of vaccine recipients. Transient rashes are common. Encephalopathy and encephalitis are rare complications of the vaccine. They occur at a much lower rate than they do after the natural disease. Febrile convulsion is an infrequent occurrence in children after they receive the vaccine. In children with a history of seizure disorders, vaccinations are still recommended. The benefits outweigh the risks. Subacute sclerosing panencephalitis has been reported in vaccinees without a history of clinical measles. These persons possibly had unrecognized disease. Allergic reactions to one of the components and thrombocytopenia have been reported, but they are very rare occurrences.

Contraindications to measles vaccine include the following:

- *Pregnancy:* Women vaccinated with measles vaccine should not become pregnant for 3 months after MMR vaccination. If measles monovalent vaccine is given, the woman has to wait only 30 days before conceiving.
- *Immunodeficiency or therapeutic immunosuppression:* Patients with compromised immune systems should not receive any live vaccine. These include children receiving cancer therapy and children with other immunosuppressive disorders. The vaccine can be given to medically suppressed children at least 3 months after the therapy is stopped. Measles vaccine as part of MMR is *recommended* for both symptomatic and asymptomatic HIV-infected children who are not severely immunocompromised. Symptomatic HIV-infected children should be given IgG at the time of exposure to measles (unless they have received intravenous gamma globulin [IGIV] within 3 weeks) because they may not be able to manufacture antibodies.
- *TB:* Measles vaccine can cause anergy to tuberculin skin tests. Skin testing can be done on the day of measles vaccination or postponed for 4 to 6 weeks.
- *Allergy:* Persons with anaphylactic reaction to either egg or neomycin should not be vaccinated without previous referral to an allergist. Vaccination should be done with extreme caution.
- *Febrile illness:* This is a relative contraindication. If fever suggests a serious illness, the child should not be vaccinated.
- *Corticosteroids:* Immunocompetent children on high-dose, long-term steroid therapy (>14 d) should wait at least 1 month after discontinuing steroids before being vaccinated.

Immune globulin (IG) affects the body's ability to react to measles vaccine. Children who receive IG must be vaccinated according to the following schedule:

- Children who receive a relatively low dose of IG for tetanus or hepatitis (A or B) prophylaxis may be vaccinated with MMR 3 months after receiving IG.
- Children who receive rabies IG should wait 4 months before receiving MMR vaccination.
- Children (especially those who are immunocompromised) who receive large doses

of IG in the range of 0.25 to 0.5 ml/kg for the prophylaxis of either varicella or measles should wait 5 to 6 months before being vaccinated with MMR.

- Children who are receiving replacement therapy or therapeutic IG in doses of 300 to 400 mg/kg per month, should wait for approximately 8 months after the last dose of IG before receiving MMR vaccine.
- Children who receive adenine-saline red blood cells (RBCs), unwashed packed RBCs, whole blood cell transfusions, plasma, or platelets must wait 3, 5, 6, and 7 months, respectively, before being vaccinated with MMR.
- Children who are being treated for immune thrombocytopenic purpura or other disorders with a single dose of IG of 400 to 1000 mg/kg should be deferred from MMR vaccination for 8 to 10 months. With doses of IG of 1000 to 2000 mg/kg, MMR should be held for 10 to 11 months.
- If exposure to measles is imminent, vaccination may be given after a shorter interval and a second dose of the vaccine may be given after the recommended time period.

MUMPS

Live mumps virus vaccine is effective, with a 95% seroconversion rate. Immunity is usually lifelong. Reactions to mumps vaccine are very rare. Febrile seizures, rash, pruritus, nerve deafness, encephalitis, purpura, and orchitis have been reported. Encephalopathy and encephalitis are rare complications of the vaccine. They occur at a much lower rate than they do after the natural disease. Contraindications are the same as for measles.

RUBELLA

RA 27/3 is the current vaccine licensed in the United States. Seroconversion is 98%. Reactions to the vaccine include fever, lymphadenopathy, rash, arthritis, arthralgia, paresthesia, pain in the extremities (usually occurring at night), and morning knee pain with decreased range of motion. Contraindications are the same as for the measles vaccine. Rubella vaccine can be given postpartum with RhoGAM. The vaccine

should not be given to pregnant women. The fetus is at maximum theoretical risk of 1.4% to develop congenital rubella.

Adverse reactions to the vaccine include:

- Rash, fever, and lymphadenopathy occur 5 to 12 days after vaccination.
- Arthritis as is similarly seen with natural disease occurs in 0.5% of children and 1 to 3% of adolescent girls. It is more frequent in previously unvaccinated postpubertal women. Onset of arthralgia is usually 7 to 21 days after vaccination.
- Neuritis occurs rarely.

For reportable vaccine-associated events related to the various measles, mumps, and rubella vaccines, see Table 24-4.

Hepatitis A (HA) Vaccine

Havrix and Vaqta are the two inactivated Hepatitis A vaccines licensed by the FDA for use in persons 2 years of age or older who are at risk for contracting hepatitis A virus (HAV). These vaccines have seroconversion rates of 100%. Hepatitis A vaccine can be administered simultaneously with other childhood vaccines but should be given at a separate injection site (intramuscular injection in the deltoid). The vaccines are currently recommended for those children and adults who are at risk of exposure (Harris & Edwards, 1998):

- Children 2 years of age or older who live in communities with high case rates—Native Alaskans and Native Americans and children in day care centers with high rates of HAV
- Homosexual and bisexual men
- Severe illness (e.g., chronic liver disease)
- Illicit or intravenous (IV) drug users
- Healthy persons who are older than 2 years of age at the health care provider's discretion:
  ○ Child care staff and attendees
  ○ Custodial care workers
  ○ Hospital care workers
  ○ Food handlers
  ○ Hemophiliacs

Hepatitis A vaccine is required in Oklahoma for children entering school or day care. Rou-

T A B L E 24-6

Hepatitis A Vaccination Schedule (AAP, 1997)

AGE	VACCINE	ANTIGEN	DOSAGE	#DOSE	SCHEDULE
2–18 yr	Havrix	360 EL.U	0.5 ml	3	Initial, 1 mo, and 6–12 mo later
	Havrix	720 EL.U	0.5 ml	2	Initial and 6–12 mo later
	Vaqta	25 U	0.5 ml	2	Initial and 6–18 mo later
19 yr	Havrix	1440 EL.U	1.0 ml	2	Initial and 6–12 mo later
	Vaqta	50 U	1.0 ml	2	Initial and 6–18 mo later

tine vaccination with hepatitis A vaccine is recommended in other states that experience two to three times the national average incidence of this illness. Table 24-6 lists the recommended hepatitis A vaccination schedule.

Hepatitis B (HB) Vaccine

Two recombinant HB vaccines are currently licensed in the United States: Engerix-B and Recombivax HB. They are produced from common baker's yeast and differ in antigen concentration. They are equally immunogenic when used as directed according to manufacturer's guidelines. Seroconversion is 95%. Side effects are rare, but pain and soreness at the immunization site are common complaints. Between 2 and 5% of children who receive the vaccine develop fever to 102°F and irritability (Behrman et al., 1996; Greenberger, 1993). Ta-

ble 24-7 lists recommended dosage and scheduling.

Although current recommendations call for universal immunization of all infants with HB vaccine and immunization for young children and adolescents not previously vaccinated, there are specific individuals who should also receive hepatitis B immunization (AAP, 1997):

- Hemophiliac patients and other recipients of certain blood products
- IV drug users
- Heterosexual persons with a history of multiple sex partners in the previous 6 months and recent STDs
- Sexually active homosexual or bisexual males
- Household and sexual contacts with chronic carriers of hepatitis B virus (HBV)
- Household members of adoptees from

T A B L E 24-7

Dosage and Scheduling for Immunization Against Hepatitis B Virus

	VACCINE DOSE		
	Recombivax HB	Engerix-B	SCHEDULE*
Infants of HBsAg-negative mothers	5 μg	10 μg	0–2 mo, 1–4 mo, and 6–18 mo
Children 0–19 yr (not vaccinated)	5 μg	10 μg	1–2 mo, 4 mo, and 6–18 mo
Infants of HBsAg-positive mothers†‡	5 μg	10 μg	Day 0, 1–2 mo, and 6 mo
Infants of HBsAG status unknown mothers§	5 μg	10 μg	Day 0, 1–2 mo, and 6 mo

*If a thimersol-free vaccine is not available, consult 1999 AAP interim alterations for hepatitis B vaccine schedule.
†Give HBIG and HepB vaccine within 12 hours of birth.
‡0.5 ml HBIG should also be given at birth.
§Give HepB vaccine within 12 hours of birth, and give HBIG within first 7 days of life if mother found to be HBsAG positive.

HBV-endemic, high-risk countries who are hepatitis B surface antigen (HBsAG) positive.

- Specific infants, children, and other household contacts in populations of high HBV endemicity
- Staff and residents of institutions for the developmentally disabled
- Staff of nonresidential day care and school programs for the developmentally delayed if attended by a known HBV carrier; other attendants in certain circumstances
- Hemodialysis patients
- Health-care workers and others with occupational risk
- International travelers who live for more than 6 months in areas of high HBV endemicity and who otherwise may be at risk
- Inmates of long-term correctional facilities

Engerix-B and Recombivax HB are not interchangeable vaccines, but either can be given with IG to ensure even better protection rates in postexposure vaccination. For reportable vaccine-associated events related to HB vaccination, see Table 24–4.

Influenza Vaccine

Influenza virus vaccine is a multivalent embryonic egg vaccine. Two preparations are currently available: whole and split cell. Only the split cell can be given to children younger than 13 years old. The vaccine is formulated yearly based on epidemiological forecasts. Major changes in viral antigens occur at 10-year intervals. This process is called antigenic shift. Minor variations that occur are called antigenic drift. These changes within the virus can prevent the body's immune system from recognizing the altered strain and mounting an immunological response. Because other common childhood viral agents can lead to diseases that look like influenza, the impact of the vaccine is less likely to be evident in children. The efficacy rate for either preparation is 70 to 80% (range, 50 to 95%). The vaccine should be given at the beginning of October through mid-November (it can be started in September if vaccine is available), before the onset of the yearly influenza season that begins in December. Influenza immunization is not recommended for normal healthy

children and adolescents. Efficacy in infants younger than 6 months of age has not been assessed.

Two doses of vaccine, given 1 month apart, are required for children younger than 9 years of age who are first-time vaccine recipients. Only one dose is needed in subsequent years and for children aged 9 years or older. Children 6 to 35 months of age receive 0.25 ml IM. Children older than 3 years require 0.5 ml IM.

Specific individuals who should receive influenza vaccination include:

- High-risk children: Children with chronic pulmonary disease (mild to severe asthma, bronchopulmonary dysplasia, cystic fibrosis) or hemodynamically significant heart disease, immunosuppressed children (should be off chemotherapy 3 to 4 weeks if possible), children with hemoglobinopathies such as sickle cell anemia. Children with other conditions, such as diabetes mellitus, chronic renal disease, severe metabolic illness, symptomatic HIV, rheumatoid arthritis, and Kawasaki disease, and children who are household contacts of high-risk patients, should be vaccinated.
- Children who are on long-term aspirin therapy and who are at risk for developing Reye syndrome.
- Residents of nursing homes and those in other chronic care facilities housing patients of any age with chronic medical conditions.
- Persons 65 years of age or older
- Health care workers or others attending or living with high-risk persons.

Young children, 6 to 24 months old, occasionally have fever in the first 6 to 24 hours after vaccination. The vaccine can also exacerbate underlying disease. The vaccine can be given simultaneously with DTP and IPV but at a different site and with a different syringe. DTaP is the recommended vaccine to be given because it is less likely to produce a febrile reaction. With the exception of the 1976 swine flu vaccine, there has been no increased risk of Guillain-Barré syndrome. Other side effects include tenderness, redness, and pain at the site of injection. Fever, malaise, myalgia, headache, and other flulike symptoms are also reported after immunization. A nasal spray vaccine to prevent influenza has shown promising results in children during clinical trials. It is currently licensed for use in adults only.

There are a few contraindications to the influenza vaccine. Children with severe anaphylactic reaction to egg rarely experience a similar type of reaction to killed influenza vaccine. If there is concern about this, an immediate-reacting IgE skin test using a dilution of influenza vaccine can be used to judge the potential risk of vaccination. If the skin test confirms hypersensitivity, the vaccine should not be given. Children with a neurological disorder characterized by progressive developmental delay or a changing neurological picture should not receive influenza vaccine until the neurological problem is stabilized. The occurrence of any neurological symptom or sign after administration of influenza vaccine is a contraindication to further use.

The vaccine should not be given to a patient with a febrile illness. The use of influenza vaccine in pregnant women (>14 weeks) is considered safe. Children who receive prolonged high-dose corticosteroid therapy (more than 2 mg/kg per dose or 20 mg of prednisone/d) may have impaired antibody response to the vaccine. Immunization should be deferred until the steroid dose is lowered. However, if it is not possible to lower the steroid dose before the influenza season starts, the influenza vaccine should be administered and no longer deferred.

Varicella Vaccine

The Oka/Merck vaccine has been tested for more than 20 years. The vaccine is reported to be well tolerated, immunogenic, and effective in healthy and high-risk children (AAP, 1997). However, vaccinated children can develop modified clinical disease after exposure to wild virus. The infection is usually very mild, with little or no systemic illness and few lesions. A small percentage of vaccinees develop a mild zoster-like rash a week or so after vaccination. Vaccine virus has been isolated from these lesions. Normal immunocompetent children who have not yet acquired varicella immunity have less than a 1% risk of infection from recently

vaccinated individuals. Immunosuppressed individuals have a higher risk of infection when exposed to the modified varicella vaccine and should avoid direct contact with children who have been vaccinated until all lesions are dry.

Current AAP (1997) recommendations for the varicella vaccine are:

- A one-time dose of vaccine for healthy children 12 to 18 months old who have not had chickenpox can be given at the same time as MMR.
- A one-time dose of vaccine for children 18 months to 13 years old who have not had chickenpox nor been previously immunized.
- Two doses of vaccine for children older than age 13 years who have never been immunized and have no known history of chickenpox. Give two doses 4 to 8 weeks apart.

The vaccine is not recommended for children with immune system deficiencies, including HIV, those being treated for leukemia and lymphoma, and those taking high doses of steroid, nor for pregnant teenagers.

Pneumococcal and Meningococcal Vaccines

These two vaccines are indicated for routine use in selected children. The 23-valent pneumococcal vaccine is composed of purified, capsular polysaccharide antigens. It is given subcutaneously or IM at a dose of 0.5 ml. Children who should routinely receive pneumococcal vaccine include those with sickle cell disease; functional or anatomical asplenia; nephrotic syndrome or chronic renal failure; conditions associated with immunosuppression (e.g., organ transplantation or HIV infections); CSF leaks; and chronic pulmonary, cardiac, and liver disease. Likewise, children living in environments with high risk of invasive pneumococcal disease (e.g., Alaskan Natives and certain American Indian groups) should be vaccinated. Pneumococcal vaccine is generally given to children 2 years and older as a single dose. The practitioner should consult the AAP Red Book for specific recommendations about when to revaccinate with pneumococcal vaccine and about which children should receive it.

Clinical studies are in progress investigating a new conjugate heptavalent pneumococcal vaccine for use in children younger than 2 years of age. This vaccine has worked well in clinical trials related to the prevention of otitis media, pneumococcal bacteremia, and meningitis and is predicted to be on the market soon.

The meningococcal vaccine is a quadrivalent vaccine composed of groups A, C, Y, and W-135 *Neisseria meningitidis.* It contains bacterial capsular polysaccharides of the respective groups and is given to children older than 2 years of age unless there is an epidemic. This vaccine is administered SC, at a dose of 0.5 ml, and is generally given as a single dose. Children who should routinely receive meningococcal vaccine include those with functional or anatomical asplenia and terminal complement component deficiencies. It may be used as an adjunct to chemoprophylaxis. Children who are first immunized when they are younger than 4 years of age may be revaccinated after 2 to 3 years. The vaccine can be used for general vaccination during an epidemic. The American College Health Association recommends that college students consider meningococcal vaccine to reduce their risk of this disease. It also is given routinely to all military recruits in the United States. Travelers to areas where the disease is either epidemic or hyperendemic may benefit from vaccination.

Rotavirus Vaccine

Rotaviral gastroenteritis affects almost all children between the ages of 3 and 5 years and accounts for a significant number of healthcare visits and hospitalizations of infants and toddlers. It is a widespread and highly contagious disease. RotaShield, the live oral tetravalent rotavirus vaccine, did well in clinical trials. However, a significant number of cases of intussusception were reported, within the first year of its use, and the vaccine was removed from the market in late summer 1999.

PASSIVE IMMUNITY

Passive immunization entails immunizing an individual with a solution of preexisting antibod-

ies to prevent or amend an infectious disease. These antibodies are derived from pooled human IG, illness-specific human IG, or IG formulated from animals. Passive immunization is reserved for patients who suffer from immunodeficiencies, in whom a live or attenuated vaccine could be dangerous, or who have a problem making antibodies. The procedure is also indicated for nonimmunized or underimmunized patients who have been exposed to an infectious disease whose incubation period is not long enough to allow complete active immunization. Patients at high risk for developing severe complications from an infectious disease should receive passive immunization when exposed. Some patients who suffer from disease-produced toxins benefit from antitoxin passive immunization. A poisonous snake bite, tetanus, diphtheria, and botulism are examples of this. Some of the more routine passive immunizations given to pediatric patients include those in the following lists.

Hepatitis A

Hepatitis A prophylaxis is recommended for the following individuals:

- Household contacts and sexual partners of known cases
- Persons accidentally inoculated with a contaminated needle
- Newborn infants of infected, jaundiced mothers
- Persons with open lesions directly exposed to body secretions of known cases
- Children in schools where more than one case is reported
- All children and employees of day care centers where a case is reported
- Custodial care residents and staff in close contact with an active case
- Persons traveling to developing countries for less than 3 months

The dose of IG is 0.02 ml/kg IM. It should be given within 2 weeks of exposure. It is approximately 80 to 90% effective in preventing infection. The dosage for those with continuous exposure to HAV is 0.06 ml/kg every 5 months.

Hepatitis B

Hepatitis B prophylaxis is recommended for the following unvaccinated people:

- Newborns whose mothers are hepatitis B surface antigen (HBsAG) positive
- Household contacts younger than 12 months of age and all contacts if index case becomes a carrier
- Sexual partners of known cases
- Persons accidentally inoculated with a contaminated needle
- Individuals with percutaneous or permucosal exposure to body secretions of known cases

Newborns exposed to hepatitis B virus should receive 0.5 ml hepatitis B immune globulin (HBIG) within 12 hours after birth. They should also begin hepatitis B (HepB) vaccine at the same time. Infants born to mothers not tested during their pregnancy should also receive HepB vaccine, and HBIG must be given within 7 days after birth if the mother tests positive to HBsAG. Sexual partners of known cases should receive 0.06 ml/kg HBIG (maximum dose, 5 ml) along with HB vaccine up to 14 days after the last exposure. Repeat the dose 1 and 6 months later (AAP, 1997). Household contacts younger than 12 months should receive HBIG and three doses of vaccine. For children older than 12 months of age and other household contacts, follow the index case's antibody statement. If carrier status is determined, vaccinate all household members. For patients with percutaneous or permucosal exposure, give 0.06 ml/kg HBIG within 24 hours if possible. Follow up with HB vaccine within 7 days. Revaccinate at 1 and 6 months.

Measles

Unvaccinated children exposed to measles can be immunized with live attenuated vaccine if given within 72 hours of exposure. The vaccine provides protection in most cases. IG can be given within 6 days of exposure. The dosage of IG is 0.25 ml/kg (15 ml maximum dose). In immunocompromised children, 0.5 ml/kg (15 ml maximum dose) is recommended. For patients who receive immune globulin intrave-nous (IGIV), use the same dosage as for IG given IM. Children with symptomatic HIV infection should receive 0.05 ml/kg IG regardless of vaccination status unless they were given IGIV within the previous 3 weeks. Asymptomatic children with HIV infection should be dosed at 0.25 ml/kg (15 ml maximum dose) when exposed to wild measles.

Mumps

Mumps vaccine is not effective in preventing infection after exposure. Mumps IG is ineffective and is no longer manufactured.

Polio

Pooled human globulin may be used in sudden virulent nursery outbreaks. The dosage is 0.2 ml/kg IM (Behrman et al., 1996).

Respiratory Syncytial Virus (RSV) Prophylaxis

Palivizumab (Synagis) is an RSV-specific monoclonal antibody produced by biotechnology and approved for use in infants at high risk for adverse outcomes after RSV infection. At-risk candidates include premature infants (less than 35 weeks' gestation) and those with bronchopulmonary dysplasia. Synagis has been shown to be safe and effective in reducing RSV hospitalizations in high-risk infants. In clinical trials, there were no statistically significant differences in adverse side effects in infants treated with palivizumab vs. placebo group.

Palivizumab is given in monthly IM injections during RSV season in dosages of 15 mg/kg and is generally well tolerated. It does not interfere with routine immunizations (AAP, 1998).

Rubella

In exposed persons (nonpregnant adult women, adult men, adolescents, and children), rubella is considered a benign disease. The routine use of IG after exposure in early pregnancy is not advised. The available evidence suggests that the use of IG modifies or suppresses the clinical manifestations of the disease without preventing the viremic stage. Live RA 27/3 vaccine given after exposure does not prevent illness. If a pregnant woman is exposed to rubella, either wild or as a result of being accidentally vaccinated within 3 months of conception, a blood specimen should be obtained as soon as possible. The presence of serum antibodies suggests that the fetus is not at risk (1.4 to 2% theoretical risk factor). If no antibody is detected, a second sample should be obtained 2 weeks later. A positive test indicates infection. A negative test calls for a third sample 2 weeks later. A positive test again indicates maternal infection. A negative test at 6 weeks after exposure indicates that maternal rubella infection has not occurred. IG is recommended only if termination of the pregnancy is not an option. IG may prevent or modify rubella infection; the dose is 0.55 ml/kg. The administration of IG and the absence of clinical manifestation of rubella infection in the mother do not guarantee that the child will be born without congenital rubella syndrome.

Tetanus

Undervaccinated patients or those with unknown vaccination status should receive tetanus immune globulin (TIG), 250 to 500 units IM, for prophylaxis. Immunodeficient patients, including HIV-infected patients, should be considered undervaccinated regardless of actual status. If TIG is not available, tetanus antitoxin (TAT) is used. TAT is either equine or bovine antibodies and should not be used without hypersensitivity testing before the first dose. The dosage for TAT is 3000 to 5000 units IM. The type of wound and the state of immunization are critical to the management and use of prophylaxis. (See Table 24–3 for tetanus prophylaxis information.)

Varicella Vaccine

Varicella zoster immune globulin (VZIG) is indicated for use in persons exposed to varicella who are in the following categories:

- High-risk children: Immunocompromised children younger than 15 years of age, including HIV-infected children
- Normal adults and adolescents who are nonimmune

- Pregnant women, particularly in the first and second trimester: Subclinical infection is linked to fetal involvement; a "healthy" mother does not rule out congenital disease
- Newborns whose mothers experience the onset of infection within 5 days before or 2 days after delivery
- Premature infants less than 28 weeks' gestation or less than 1000 g who have been exposed to varicella
- Premature infants older than 28 weeks' gestation (with a nonimmune mother) who have been exposed to varicella

The dosage of VZIG is 125 units for each 10 kg, with 125 units as the minimum and 625 units as the maximum dose, given as soon as possible after exposure for up to 96 hours.

SPECIFIC INFECTIOUS DISEASES

Viral Diseases

COXSACKIE VIRUS

Etiology

This virus is in the Enterovirus family. It is related to both polio and echo viruses. These RNA viruses are divided into groups: A (23 subtype) and B (6 subtype).

Epidemiology

Enteroviruses are spread by fecal-oral contamination, especially in diapered infants. They are also transmitted during parturition. Coxsackie virus has a worldwide distribution, with increased prevalence during the warm months of the year. Epidemics transpire from May to October. Infection is most commonly reported in children from 1 to 4 years of age.

Incubation Period

The incubation period is 3 to 6 days. The virus is shed for several weeks after the infection begins.

Clinical Findings

TYPE A INFECTION

1. *Acute respiratory infection:* A mild upper respiratory infection (URI) is very common. Cases of pneumonia have been described.
2. *Nonspecific febrile illness:* In young children, there is an undifferentiated febrile illness associated with myalgias and malaise.
3. *Herpangina:* There is a sudden onset of high fever lasting 1 to 4 days. Loss of appetite, sore throat, and dysphagia are common, with vomiting and abdominal pain in 25% of cases. Minute vesicles or ulcers appear on the anterior pillars of the fauces, tonsils, uvula, pharynx, and the edge of the soft palate. The vesicles are gray-white with red areolas. They are usually 1 to 2 mm in diameter. The lesions enlarge and evolve into 5-mm gray-yellow ulcers. The entire course usually lasts 4 to 6 days with complete recovery.
4. *Acute lymphonodular pharyngitis:* This manifests as an acute sore throat lasting approximately 1 week.
5. *Hand-foot-mouth disease:* This is a clinical entity evidenced by fever, vesicular eruption of the buccal mucosa of the mouth, and a maculopapular rash involving the hands and feet. The rash evolves to vesicles, especially on the dorsa of the hands and the soles of the feet, and lasts 1 to 2 weeks.
6. *Aseptic meningitis:* There are the usual signs of fever, stiff neck, and headache. Altered sensorium and seizures are common. Most patients recover completely.
7. *Paralytic disease:* A Guillain–Barré-type syndrome has been described.

TYPE B INFECTION

Type B infections are similar to type A infections, but type B herpangina does not exist. Other type B infections include the following:

1. *Congenital or neonatal infection:* Transplacental infection occurs and serious disseminated disease affects the fetal liver, heart, meninges, and adrenal cortex. The neonatal infection often presents as a sudden onset of vomiting, coughing, fits, cyanosis, and dyspnea. It is often mistaken for pneumonia. There is pallor and tachycardia that progresses to congestive heart failure. No murmur is heard. Infants often go into cardiac collapse and die. For those who survive, the recovery can be quite rapid.
2. *Pleurodynia (devil's grip):* This condition is most often caused by type B disease, but type A virus has been implicated. There is sudden severe chest pain, pleuritic in nature and aggravated by deep breathing, coughing, or sudden movements. The pain is described by patients as feeling like being stabbed with a knife, or being squeezed in a vise. It can be mistaken for coronary artery disease. There may be a prodrome 1 to 10 days before the onset of chest pain ushered in by headache, malaise, anorexia, and myalgia. Fifty percent of patients have abdominal pain. Low to high fever occurs, and a pleural friction rub often is heard. The disease lasts from 1 to 10 days (mean 3.5 d).
3. *Orchitis:* This type B infection is clinically similar to mumps.
4. *Myocarditis or pericarditis:* Type B infection can cause mild to severe acute and chronic heart disease. Fatalities have been reported (Zaoutis & Klein, 1998).

Differential Diagnosis

Includes other causes of the above conditions (e.g., viral bacterial, connective tissue diseases).

Diagnostic Tests

Viral cultures obtained from throat, stool, and rectum. The best specimens for results should be sent to the laboratory frozen at 4°C. Polymerase chain reaction (PCR) is a very sensitive test but has limited availability. Serologic specific titers 2 to 4 weeks apart can also confirm the diagnosis.

Management

There is no therapy available for treatment. IgG may be helpful in immunocompromised patients.

Prevention

Enteric precautions and good hand washing are the only efficient control measures.

ERYTHEMA INFECTIOSUM

Etiology

Erythema infectiosum, or fifth disease, is caused by parvovirus B19. The virus is a member of the Parvoviridae family. It is called fifth disease because it was the fifth eruptive rash described. These rashes are the following:

1. Scarlet fever
2. Measles
3. Rubella
4. Dukes' disease (erythema subitum)
5. Erythema infectiosum
6. Roseola

Epidemiology

The first recorded outbreak occurred in Germany in 1889. Humans are the only reservoir. Upper respiratory secretions and blood during the viremic stage are considered infectious. Distribution is worldwide. Erythema infectiosum is a disease of childhood, usually attacking 2- to 15-year olds, but infants and adults are not immune. Secondary spread to household contacts is approximately 50%. The disease occurs most commonly in late winter and early spring.

Incubation Period

The incubation period is approximately 4 to 14 days. The rash erupts between 2 and 3 weeks after exposure. The period of communicability lasts until the rash appears. In patients with aplastic crisis (sickle cell) or chronic anemia, the period of communicability is extended 1 week.

Clinical Findings

The following two phases are seen in erythema infectiosum:

1. *Prodrome:* Occurs in 15 to 30% of cases. It is usually mild with low-grade fever and malaise.
2. *Rash:* Appears in three stages: It first appears on the face and is "slapped cheek" in nature. There is an intense red eruption on the cheeks with circumoral pallor that lasts 1 to 4 days. Next, a lacy maculopapular eruption appears on the arms, face, thighs, and buttocks, moving caudally. Palms and soles are occasionally involved. This phase can last a month. Finally, the rash subsides. There may be periodic recurrences precipitated by trauma, heat, sunlight, or cold, or both (see Color Fig. 1).

Differential Diagnosis

This is not a difficult disease to diagnose. The differential diagnoses include rubella, enterovirus disease, lupus, atypical measles, and drug rashes.

Diagnostic Tests

Serological tests for parvovirus are limited in availability. Serum B19-specific immunoglobulin M (IgM) confirms the presence of infection. Serum B19-specific immunoglobulin G (IgG) confirms past infection and immunity. There are ELISA and radioimmunoassay tests for B19. The virus is difficult to grow.

Complications

These are few and typically not significant. All previously healthy patients usually recover without sequelae. The most frequently reported complications are

- Arthritis: Symptoms begin 2 to 3 weeks after the onset of initial symptoms. Joint manifestations are transient and self-limited. Adults are more prone to develop arthritis and arthralgia than are children.
- Hemolytic anemia: Most common in patients with immunodeficiency.
- Aplastic crisis: Most common in patients with chronic hemolytic anemias, especially sickle cell anemia.
- Proved maternal infection during pregnancy has a less than 10% probability of fetal death. Fetal hydrops is reported; there are no reports of congenital anomalies.
- Pneumonia.

Management

There is no specific treatment.

Prevention

Women who are exposed to children with the disease either at home or at work are at increased risk for infection with parvovirus B19. Because B19 has a low risk for fetal infection and there is widespread inapparent infection in children and adults, all women are at some risk of exposure. Because avoidance can reduce but not eliminate the risk of exposure, routine exclusion of pregnant women from the workplace where B19 infection is present is not recommended. When IgG-specific testing becomes more available, the serological status of women can help assess exposure risks.

Pregnant health-care workers should not care for aplastic B19 patients because they are highly contagious (AAP, 1997). Pregnant women who are exposed to B19 can have fetal ultrasonography and alpha-fetoprotein testing to help assess if there is any fetal damage.

Children in the rash stage can attend school.

Whether IG is effective in preventing infection in exposed persons is unknown.

HUMAN IMMUNODEFICIENCY VIRUS

Etiology

HIV is an RNA cytopathic human retrovirus with at least two serotypes: HIV-1 and HIV-2. They are in the lentivirus subgroup. Both serotypes cause clinically indistinguishable disease. There are some reports that HIV-2 could, in fact, be a milder form of infection, but deaths are reported. Mixed infections are also documented. Retroviruses integrate into the target cell's genome as proviruses, and the viral genome is copied during cell replication. HIV persists in infected individuals for life, and its protein envelope mutates frequently. This antigenic drift creates havoc with the body's immune system. The body's defense system recognizes only previously encountered immunogenic forms. At least 100 variants of HIV virus have been identified. Its mutation rate is believed to be 100 to 1000 times greater than the influenza virus (AAP, 1997; Legal Economic Guidelines, 1993). Any information about HIV is subject to immediate change, and the NP is cautioned to check with the CDC regarding any new changes in HIV or autoimmune deficiency syndrome (AIDS) diagnosis or treatment.

Epidemiology

Although there are AIDS syndromes in other primates and felines, infection cannot be obtained from pets, animals, or insects. Humans are the only source of HIV. The mode of transmission is intimate sexual contact, sharing of contaminated needles for injection, transfusion of contaminated blood or blood products, and perinatal exposure, similar to the transmission of HBV. Before December 1993, transmission through casual contact in families or households, day care centers, schools, or with routine care in hospitals or clinics was never documented. Subsequently, a child in a foster home contracted HIV from an HIV-infected toddler. There was no documented exposure to the infected child's blood. However, there might have been unrecognized exposure (Fitzgibbon et al., 1993). There was another report of a household transmission of HIV from an infected hemophiliac to his younger adolescent brother through the use of a contaminated razor (Brownstein & Fricke, 1993). One HIV-infected sister with open, bleeding oral lesions reportedly bit and infected her sister. The case was not documented but only suspected (Rogers et al., 1990).

HIV has been isolated from blood (lymphocytes, macrophages, and plasma), CSF, pleural fluid, cervical secretions, human milk, tears, saliva, and urine. However, only blood, semen, cervical secretions, and human milk are implicated in transmission. Infectivity is low. The risk of sexual transmission from just one episode of intercourse with an infected person is low (1.0%) but possible (AAP, 1997). Male-to-male and male-to-female transmission is more common than female-to-male transmission (Legal Economic Guidelines, 1993). Two undocumented incidences of lesbian transmittal were reported (Chu et al., 1990). Accidental needle sticks rarely account for seroconversion and have a low infectivity rate. Less than 0.3% of the documented cases occurred this way (AAP,

1997). Plasma levels of HIV-positive individuals are only 10 to 50 infectious particles/ml, as compared with the levels of those with HBV, which are 100 million to 1 billion particles/ml (Legal Economic Guidelines, 1993).

The incidence of AIDS in children and adolescents younger than 19 years old is approximately 2% of the total number of reported cases. Ninety percent of these children are affected perinatally. Five percent of cases have no identifiable risk factor on first glance, but with further investigation most do fall into an identifiable risk category. One percent were infected from contaminated blood products. Three percent of the adolescents obtained HIV in the adult manner (AAP, 1997). In 1996, the CDC reported the first-ever decline in AIDS diagnoses (National Institute of Health Press Release, 9/17/97).

Transplacental infection is well documented. Most babies born to HIV-infected mothers are initially HIV positive owing to the placental transfer of maternal antibodies. If the mother has been infected with HIV during late pregnancy and has not had time to develop antibodies, both mother and child will be antibody negative. Risk of an untreated HIV-infected woman giving birth to an infected infant is 13% to 39%. In vaginal twin deliveries, the first born twin has a greater risk of developing HIV than the second. The question of whether cesarean delivery prevents fetal infection is unknown (AAP, 1997).

Infection through human milk transmission is documented. Most of these mothers had postpartum blood transfusions and nursed their children. The donors later developed clinical AIDS. Mothers and their infants on subsequent testing were seropositive. These were unique situations in that there was viremia and no time to develop circulating antibodies. The viral load of the breast milk seems to be a factor in possible infection. The actual risk of HIV transmission through human milk of mothers infected before pregnancy or early in gestation is unclear (AAP, 1997). The AAP guidelines (1997) for HIV-infected mothers follows:

- Women and their health-care providers need to be aware of the potential risk of transmission of HIV infection to infants during pregnancy and in the postpartum period as well as through human milk.

- Documented, routine HIV education and routine testing with consent of all women seeking prenatal care are strongly recommended in order that each woman knows her HIV status and the methods available to prevent the acquisition and transmission of HIV and to document whether breastfeeding is appropriate.

- At the time of delivery, provision of education about HIV and testing with consent of all women whose HIV status is unknown are strongly recommended. Knowledge of the woman's HIV status assists in counseling on breastfeeding and helps each woman understand the benefits to herself and her infant of knowing her serostatus and the behaviors that decrease the likelihood of acquisition and transmission.

- In general, women who are known to be HIV-seronegative should be encouraged to breastfeed. However, women who are HIV-seronegative but at particular high risk of seroconversion, (e.g., injection drug users) should be educated about HIV with an individualized recommendation concerning the appropriateness of breastfeeding. In addition, during the perinatal period, information should be provided on the potential risk of transmitting HIV through human milk and about methods to reduce the risk of acquiring HIV infection.

- Each woman whose HIV status is unknown should be informed of the potential for HIV-infected women to transmit HIV during the peripartum period and through human milk and the potential benefits to her and her infant of knowing her HIV status and how HIV is acquired and transmitted. The health-care provider needs to make an individualized recommendation to assist the woman in deciding whether to breastfeed.

- Neonatal intensive care units should develop policies that are consistent with these recommendations for the use of expressed human milk for neonates. Current standards of the Occupational Safety and Health Administration (OSHA) do not require gloves for the routine handling of expressed human milk. However, gloves should be worn by health care workers in situations where exposure to breast milk might be frequent or prolonged, such as in milk banking.

- Human milk banks should follow the guidelines developed by the United States Public Health Service, which includes screening all donors for HIV and assessing risk factors that predispose to infection as well as pasteurization of all milk specimens (AAP, 1997).

Incubation Period

The incubation period is variable. Perinatal infection usually results in clinical disease during the first year of life, usually by 6 months of age. The mean onset of age of first symptoms is 3 years. The infection can have a long latency period. Seroconversion usually occurs between 6 and 12 weeks after exposure, and 95% of HIV-infected persons seroconvert within 6 months. In transfusion-associated infection, the time between exposure and clinical disease is months to years, with a mean of 3.5 years.

Clinical Findings

The CDC revised the diagnosis and clinical categories for children with HIV infection in 1994 (CDC, 1994b). Table 24–8 and Table 24–9 list the diagnostic guidelines and outline the signs, symptoms, and conditions associated with the four clinical categories for children with HIV infection.

Children with AIDS manifest symptoms similar to those of adults, with interstitial pneumonia, weight loss, failure to thrive, hepatomegaly, splenomegaly, generalized lymphadenopathy, chronic diarrhea, and candidiasis of the esophagus, trachea, bronchi, or lungs. *Pneumocystis carinii* pneumonia (PCP) is the most common finding later in the disease and the most common cause of death. Other opportunistic diseases are *Mycobacterium avium* infection, severe cytomegalovirus (CMV) (after 6 months of age), disseminated herpes, and disseminated histoplasmosis. Malignancies are uncommon in pediatric AIDS but do occur. Children can pre-

sent with Kaposi sarcoma, lymphoma, and non-Hodgkin B-cell lymphoma (Burkitt type).

Pediatric AIDS patients often have recurrent serious bacterial infections. *Streptococcus pneumoniae, H. influenzae* type b, *Staphylococcus aureus,* and *Salmonella* organisms are common infections in pediatric AIDS patients. Lymphoid interstitial pneumonitis occurs in 30 to 40% of children with AIDS.

Differential Diagnosis

The differential diagnosis includes other causes of immunological deficiency, such as recent therapy with an immunosuppressive agent, lymphoproliferative disease, congenital immunological states, severe malnutrition, graft-vs.-host reaction, congenital CMV, or toxoplasmosis.

Diagnostic Tests

Laboratory tests are nonspecific in that a number of immunodeficiency states can give similar findings. The diagnosis of infection is usually made serologically by ELISA testing, which is generally highly sensitive and specific. The test is repeated, and, if positive, confirmation is made by Western blot, immunofluorescent antibody testing, or radioimmunoprecipitation assay (RIPA).

Infants born to HIV-infected, seropositive mothers also are seropositive at birth owing to passive transfer of maternal antibodies. Maternal HIV IgG can persist for as long as 15 to 18 months. HIV proviral DNA testing (polymerase chain reaction [PCR]) will identify HIV-infected newborns very early in the neonatal period. Serial HIV testing can be performed to assess the origins of the antibodies present. Positive cultures of the virus from blood or body fluid, increased HIV antibody, clinical disease, or the development of a new antibody to a specific viral protein indicates infant infection.

Viral culture is not widely available. Serum antibodies are present in all infected persons. Some AIDS patients become seronegative late in the disease because the weakened immune system cannot manufacture antibodies. Tables 24–8 and 24–9 list the diagnostic criteria.

As the disease progresses, lymphopenia oc-

TABLE 24-8

*Diagnosis of Human Immunodeficiency Virus (HIV) Infection in Children**

DIAGNOSIS: HIV INFECTED

1. A child <18 mo of age who is known to be HIV seropositive or born to an HIV-infected mother *and*:
   • Has positive results on two separate determinations (excluding cord blood) from one or more of the following HIV detection tests:
     —HIV culture
     —HIV polymerase chain reaction
     —HIV antigen
       or
   • Meets criteria for acquired immunodeficiency syndrome (AIDS) diagnosis based on the 1987 AIDS surveillance case definition
2. A child ≥18 mo of age born to an HIV-infected mother or any child infected by blood, blood products, or other known modes of transmission (e.g., sexual contact) who:
   • Is HIV-antibody positive by repeatedly reactive enzyme immunoassay (EIA) and confirmatory test (e.g., Western blot or immunofluorescence assay [IFA]);
       or
   • Meets any of the criteria in 1. above.

DIAGNOSIS: PERINATALLY EXPOSED (PREFIX E)

A child who does not meet the criteria above who:
   • Is HIV seropositive by EIA and confirmatory test (e.g., Western blot or IFA) and is <18 mo of age at the time of test
       or
   • Has unknown antibody status but was born to a mother known to be infected with HIV.

DIAGNOSIS: SEROREVERTER (SR)

A child who is born to an HIV-infected mother and who:
   • Has been documented as HIV-antibody negative (i.e., two or more negative EIA tests performed at 6–18 mo of age or one negative EIA test after 18 mo of age)
       and
   • Has had no other laboratory evidence of infection (has not had two positive viral detection tests, if performed)
       and
   • Has not had an AIDS-defining condition.

*This definition of HIV infection replaces the definition published in the 1987 AIDS surveillance case definition. From Centers for Disease Control and Prevention (1994b). 1994 revised classification system for human immunodeficiency virus infection in children less than 13 years of age. MMWR: Recommendations Rep 43:1–10, 1994b.

curs. There are decreased circulating CD4+ cells (T-suppressor, T-helper cells), and the helper-suppressor ratio is less than 1.

Complications

HIV becomes a multisystemic illness with multiorgan complications. Management becomes complicated. The mortality rate is extremely high.

Management

Treatment with antiretroviral agents such as zidovudine (formerly known as azidothymidine, or AZT) with IVIG, didanosine (ddI), or zalcitabine (ddC), stavudine (d4T), lamivudine (3TC), saquinavir (SQV), indinavir (IDV), or ritonavir (RTV) is based on the immunologic, virologic, and HIV-associated conditions. Treatment of associated conditions with appropriate medical therapy is indicated. The Red Book (AAP, 1997) lists specific recommendations but because this material is constantly being reevaluated, the CDC should be contacted for the latest information regarding treatment.

RECOMMENDATIONS FOR CHILDHOOD VACCINATIONS AND THE REDUCTION OF PERINATAL TRANSMISSION OF HIV

Specific immunization recommendations are as follows:

- Children with symptomatic HIV infection: As with other immunizations for children suffering from immunological deficiencies, live viral vaccines (with the exception of MMR, unless severely immunocompromised) and BCG should not be given. DTP, DTaP, IPV, HIB, and HB vaccines are administered according to the usual schedule. Pneumococcal vaccine should be given to children at 2 years of age. Yearly influenza vaccine should be given when children are 6 months of age. Passive immunization must be given when symptomatic HIV-infected children are exposed to wild disease regardless of immunization status. Children with asymptomatic HIV infection should follow the same schedule.
- Children who live with a symptomatic HIV-infected person: The use of live vaccines is contraindicated with the exception of MMR. The immunosuppressed patient is at risk from the normal child. MMR can be given because these viruses do not shed. Yearly influenza vaccines should be given to household members who live with infected persons.
- Passive immunization of children with HIV infection has been discussed previously.
- The use of zidovudine to reduce perinatal transmission of HIV is recommended: Research has demonstrated that zidovudine administered to a selected group of HIV-infected pregnant women and their infants significantly reduced the risk of perinatally acquired HIV transmission. The CDC (1994a) has specific guidelines for the use of this drug during pregnancy and for infants born to HIV-infected women.

Because this material is constantly being reevaluated, the CDC should be contacted for the latest information regarding treatment.

Prevention

There is no preventive vaccine as yet. Patient education remains the only method to reduce the risk of acquisition and transmission.

Control Measures

The following control measures should be taken:

- Work-related exposure: Health-care workers with parenteral or mucosal membrane exposure to HIV should confirm that the exposure indeed came from an HIV-infected person. Serial HIV testing should be obtained after exposure. AIDS counseling should be provided. Use of antiretroviral chemoprophylaxis for postexposure prophylaxis (PEP) must balance the risk of transmission against the toxicity of the medications (Table 24–10).
- Adolescent education: Adolescents must be counseled about the risk of HIV transmission (e.g., sexual transmission, sharing of needles or syringes) and the use of condoms.
- School attendance: Children with AIDS or HIV infection should go to school if they are healthy enough to do so. Factors that must be taken into account include the risk to the immunosuppressed child of "normal germs" from "healthy kids and school personnel." The benefit from attendance far outweighs the risks. As casual transmission is unknown, there is no real risk to other children as long as the infected child can control body secretions. Children who display biting behavior or have oozing wounds should be cared for in a setting that minimizes risk to others. The child's primary care provider is the only person with an absolute need to know the child's primary diagnosis. If the

T A B L E 24-9

Clinical Categories for Children Younger Than 13 Years of Age With Human Immunodeficiency Virus (HIV) Infection

| | IMMUNOLOGICAL CATEGORIES | | | | AGE-SPECIFIC CD4+ T LYMPHOCYTE COUNT AND % OF TOTAL LYMPHOCYTES | | | | | |
| | | | | | <12 mo µl | % | 1–5 yrs µl | % | 6–12 yr µl | % |
	No	**Mild**	**Moderate**	**Severe**						
Immunologic definitions	S&S	S&S	S&S	S&S						
No evidence of suppression	N1	A1	B1	C1	≥1500	≥25	≥1000	≥25	≥500	≥25
Evidence of suppression	N2	A2	B2	C2	750–1499	15–24	500–999	15–24	200–499	15–24
Severe suppression	N3	A3	B3	C3	<750	<15	<500	<15	<200	<15

CATEGORY N: NOT SYMPTOMATIC

Children who have no signs or symptoms that are considered to be the result of HIV infection or who have only one of the conditions listed in Category A

CATEGORY A: MILDLY SYMPTOMATIC

Children with two or more of the conditions in the following list but none of the conditions listed in Categories B and C
- Lymphadenopathy (≥0.5 cm at more than two sites; bilateral = one site)
- Hepatomegaly
- Splenomegaly
- Dermatitis
- Parotitis
- Recurrent or persistent upper respiratory infection, sinusitis, or otitis media

CATEGORY B: MODERATELY SYMPTOMATIC

Children who have symptomatic conditions other than those listed for Category A or C that are attributed to HIV infection; examples of conditions in clinical Category B include, but are not limited to, the following:
- Anemia (<8 gm/dl), neutropenia (<1000/mm^3), or thrombocytopenia (<100,000/mm^3) persisting ≥30 days
- Bacterial meningitis, pneumonia, or sepsis (single episode)
- Candidiasis, oropharyngeal (thrush), persisting (>2 mo) in children >6 mo of age
- Cytomegalovirus infection (CMV), with onset before 1 mo of age
- Diarrhea, recurrent or chronic
- Herpes simplex virus (HSV) stomatitis, recurrent (more than two episodes within 1 yr)
- HSV bronchitis, pneumonitis, or esophagitis with onset before 1 mo of age
- Herpes zoster (shingles) involving at least two distinct episodes or more than one dermatome
- Lymphoid interstitial pneumonia (LIP) or pulmonary lymphoid hyperplasia complex
- Persistent fever (lasting >1 mo)
- Toxoplasmosis, onset before 1 mo of age

T A B L E 24-9

Clinical Categories for Children Younger Than 13 Years of Age With Human Immunodeficiency Virus (HIV) Infection *Continued*

CATEGORY C: SEVERELY SYMPTOMATIC

Examples of conditions included in clinical Category C for children infected with HIV:

- Serious bacterial infections, multiple or recurrent (i.e., any combination of at least two culture-confirmed infections within a 2-yr period), of the following types: septicemia, pneumonia, meningitis, bone or joint infection, or abscess of an internal organ or body cavity (excluding otitis media, superficial skin or mucosal abscesses, and indwelling catheter-related infections)
- Candidiasis, esophageal or pulmonary (bronchi, trachea, lungs)
- Coccidioidomycosis, disseminated (at site other than, or in addition to, lungs or cervical or hilar lymph nodes)
- Cryptosporidiosis or isosporiasis with diarrhea persisting >1 mo
- CMV disease with onset of symptoms at age >1 mo (at a site other than liver, spleen, or lymph nodes)
- Encephalopathy (at least one of the following progressive findings present for at least 2 mo in the absence of a concurrent illness other than HIV infection that could explain the findings):
  a) Failure to attain or loss of developmental milestones or loss of intellectual ability, verified by standard developmental scale or neuropsychological tests
  b) Impaired brain growth or acquired microcephaly demonstrated by head circumference measurements or brain atrophy demonstrated by CT or MRI (serial imaging is required for children <2 yr of age)
  c) Acquired symmetrical motor deficit manifested by two or more of the following: paresis, pathological reflexes, ataxia, or gait disturbance
- Herpes simplex virus infection causing a mucocutaneous ulcer that persists for >1 mo; or bronchitis, pneumonitis, or esophagitis for any duration affecting a child >1 mo of age
- Kaposi sarcoma
- Lymphoma, primary, in brain
- Lymphoma, small, noncleaved cell (Burkitt), or immunoblastic or large cell lymphoma of B-cell or unknown immunological phenotype
- *Mycobacterium tuberculosis*, disseminated or extrapulmonary
- *Mycobacterium*, other species or unidentified species, disseminated (at a site other than or in addition to lungs, skin, or cervical or hilar lymph nodes)
- *Pneumocystis carinii* pneumonia
- Wasting syndrome in the absence of a concurrent illness other than HIV infection that could explain these findings

*See the 1987 AIDS surveillance case definition for diagnosis criteria.
Adapted from Centers for Disease Control and Prevention: 1994 revised classification system for human immunodeficiency virus infection in children less than 13 years of age. MMWR: Recommendations Rep 43:1–10, 1994b.
S&S = signs and symptoms.

T A B L E 24-10

Human Immunodeficiency Virus (HIV) Postexposure Prophylaxis (PEP)

EXPOSURE	SOURCE	MATERIAL	PEP	ANTIRETROVIRAL REGIMEN
Percutaneous	Blood	Highest risk*	Recommended[1]	ZVD, 3TC, + IDV
		Increased risk†	Recommended[2]	ZVD, 3TC, ± IDV
		No increased risk‡	Offered[2]	ZVD, + 3TC
		Fluids containing visible blood, other potentially infectious fluid, or tissue[5]	Offered	ZVD ± 3TC
		Other body fluids	Not offered[3]	
Mucous membranes		Fluids containing visible blood, other potentially infectious fluid, or tissue	Offered	ZVD ± 3TC
		Other body fluids (e.g., urine)	Not offered	
Skin, increased risk[5]		Blood	Offered	ZVD, 3TC, ± IDV
		Fluids containing visible blood, other potentially infectious fluid, or tissue	Offered	ZVD ± 3TC
		Other body fluids (e.g., urine)	Not offered	

IDV = indinavir; 3TC = lamivudine; ZVD = zidovudine.

[1]Recommended: PEP should be recommended to the exposed person with counseling.

[2]Offered: PEP should be offered to the exposed person with counseling.

[3]Not offered: PEP should not be offered to the exposed person because it is not considered a potential occupational exposure to HIV.

[4]Includes semen, vaginal secretions, and cerebrospinal, synovial, pleural, pericardial, and amniotic fluids.

[5]High HIV titer, prolonged contact, extensive area, or an area in which skin integrity is visibly compromised. For skin exposure without increased risk, the risk for drug toxicity outweighs the benefit of PEP.

*Highest risk: Exposure that involves either a larger volume of blood (deep injury with a large-diameter hollow needle) or blood containing a high titer of HIV.

†Increased risk: Exposure that involves either a larger volume of blood (deep injury with a large-diameter hollow needle) or blood containing a high titer of HIV.

No increased risk: Exposure that involves neither a larger volume of blood (deep injury with a large-diameter hollow needle) nor blood containing a high titer of HIV.

From Centers for Disease Control: Update: Provisional Public Health Service recommendations for chemoprophylaxis after exposure to HIV. MMWR 45:468–472, 1996.

family decides to inform the school, those informed should maintain confidentiality.

- Routine screening of school-age children for HIV antibodies is not recommended (AAP, 1997).

HEPATITIS A

Etiology

Hepatitis A virus (HAV) is a picornavirus and causes a primary infection in the liver.

Epidemiology

HAV is a highly contagious infection spread through person-to-person contact and fecal-oral contamination of food and water. It is rarely transmitted by contaminated blood transfusion. Human infection from nonhuman primates is also reported. Transmission occurs readily in households and day care centers. Eighty percent of cases in infants younger than 2 years of age and 50% of infected children between 3 and 4 years of age have nonsymptomatic (anicteric hepatitis) or nonspecific illness. Adults tend to have more severe disease. The high anicteric disease incidence allows considerable spread of disease before the index case is identified. Infants are protected by maternal antibodies during the first few months of life. The infection is more common in lower socioeconomic groups. Young adults are affected more than children. There is increasing incidence of HAV in intravenous drug users. There is no seasonal variance.

Incubation Period

The period of contagion is as long as the patient sheds virus and usually lasts 1 to 3 weeks. The patient is most contagious from 2 weeks before the onset of illness until 1 week after the onset of jaundice. The incubation period is 15 to 50 days.

Clinical Findings

The following two phases may be seen:

1. *Preicteric phase:* Presents as an acute febrile illness. Malaise, nausea, anorexia, vomiting, digestive complaints, and occasional abdominal complaints occur. This phase goes unnoticed in many children. There can be dull right upper quadrant pain during exercise.
2. *Jaundiced phase:* Jaundice appears shortly after the onset of symptoms. Urine darkens and stools become clay colored. Often these are the only apparent signs of the illness. Diarrhea is common in infants, whereas constipation is more common in older children and adults. Patients feel sick. Infants have poor weight gain during the icteric phase. Fulminant disease is rare. There is no chronic disease. The icteric phase lasts from a few days to almost a month.

Differential Diagnosis

Any cause of jaundice is in the differential diagnosis of HAV.

- Infancy: Physiological jaundice, hemolytic disease, galactosemia, hypothyroidism, biliary metabolic disorders, biliary atresia, alpha$_1$-antitrypsin deficiency, and choledochal cysts. Hypervitaminosis A causes a yellow pigmentation of the skin often mistaken for jaundice in children. Infections such as toxoplasmosis, rubella, CMV, and herpes (TORCH) also cause hepatitis.
- Older infants, children, and adolescents: Hemolytic-uremic syndrome, Reye syndrome, malaria, leptospirosis, brucellosis, chronic hemolytic diseases with gallstone development, Wilson disease, cystic fibrosis, Banti syndrome, collagen-vascular disease, infectious mononucleosis, CMV, coxsackievirus, toxoplasmosis, Weil disease, yellow fever, acute cholangitis, amebiasis, and hepatitis B, C, and D. Drugs and poisons such as pyrazinamide, isoniazid, zoxazolamine, gold, cinchophen, phenothiazines, and methyltestosterone are among others that also cause hepatitis.

Diagnostic Tests

Serological testing is widely available. IgM-specific antibodies indicate recent infection. These are replaced by IgG-specific antibodies 2 to 4 months later. These indicate past infection. Changes in liver enzymes indicate the degree of injury. There is elevation of serum transaminases (SGOT, AST, SGPT, ALT). Prothrombin time can be elevated.

Management

Therapy is supportive in nature. The use of gamma globulin was discussed earlier in this chapter.

Complications

Although patients can become very ill, most cases of HAV heal completely. Fulminant hepatitis with liver failure is rare.

HEPATITIS B

Etiology

Hepatitis B virus (HBV) is a hepadnavirus. It is highly contagious and causes severe liver disease.

Epidemiology

The most common method of transmission is percutaneous or mucous membrane exposure to contaminated blood or sexual secretions, or both. Saliva has not been shown to be infectious. Fecal-oral transmission cannot be demonstrated experimentally. HBV survives in a dried state for almost 1 month. Prolonged percutaneous contact with contaminated fomites can be a source of infection. Surface and core antigens are useful markers for epidemiological studies. Patients are infectious when they are hepatitis B surface antigen (HBsAg) positive or if they are chronic carriers of HBV. Hepatitis B e-antigen (HBeAg) correlates with viral replication and indicates chronic carriage. Antibodies to core and surface antigen lessen infectivity.

The major reservoir for HBV is healthy chronic carriers and patients with acute disease. Eskimos, Southeast Asians, Pacific Islanders, Africans, and other populations living in high endemic areas have a high infection and carriage state. Perinatal transmission from female carriers (HBsAg positive or HBeAg positive, or both) to their newborn children has a 70 to 90% infant infection rate unless intervention is undertaken. Adolescents and adults who abuse intravenous drugs or who engage in sexual activity with multiple partners, or both, have the greatest risk of acquiring HBV. There is also a higher incidence of infection in the gay community. Health care workers who are exposed to blood and blood products or who care for the developmentally disabled are also at a high risk, as are chronic renal dialysis patients. Tattooing with contaminated instruments is another route of infection.

Incubation Period

The incubation period is 45 to 160 days.

Clinical Findings

HBV has a range of illness from asymptomatic seroconversion to fulminating disease and death. HBV usually has a gradual onset. Arthralgia and skin problems such as urticaria or other rashes can be the first apparent signs. Papular acrodermatitis has been described in infants. Acute hepatitis B infection is somewhat similar to the icteric phase of HAV, but it is usually more severe. Skin, mucous membranes, and sclerae are icteric. The liver is enlarged and tender. Ten percent of patients develop chronic disease.

Differential Diagnosis

Any cause of jaundice is in the differential diagnosis of HBV. See listing under HAV differential diagnosis.

Diagnostic Tests

Changes in liver enzymes indicate the degree of injury. There is elevation of serum transaminases (SGOT, AST, SGPT, ALT). Prothrombin time can be elevated, especially in fulminating disease. Serological tests are available to detect HBsAg, HBcAg (core), HBeAg, and antibodies to these antigens (Table 24-11).

Laboratory markers can be useful in determining the stage of infection (Table 24-12).

Complications

There are hepatic and extrahepatic complications.

CHRONIC PERSISTENT HEPATITIS. Most patients with this diagnosis are asymptomatic. Some have minimal nonspecific constitutional complaints such as fever, nausea, and minimal hepatomegaly. The condition is benign in childhood, although there is inflammatory liver disease.

T A B L E 24-11

Serologic Tests to Detect Hepatitis B

ANTIGEN OR ANTIBODY	USE
HBsAg	Identifies acute illness and carriage state
Anti-HBs	Identifies past infection and vaccine-induced immunity
HBeAg	Identifies carriers at high risk of infectiousness
Anti-HBe	Identifies carriers at low risk of infectiousness
Anti-HBc	Identifies past infection with HBV
IgM Anti-HBc	Identifies acute or recent infection

T A B L E 24-12

Laboratory Markers for Infection With Hepatitis B Virus: The Stages of Infection and When They Are Generally Present

TEST	PREICTERIC	ICTERIC	CONVALESCENT	CARRIAGE
HBsAg	+ + + +	+ +	+	+ +
Anti-HBs		+ or −	+ +	−
IgM anti-HBc		+ +	+ + +	
Anti-HBc		+ or −	+ + +	+
Anti-HBe		+ + +	+ +	+ or −
Bilirubin	+ + + +	+ +		+ or −
Transaminase	+ + +	+ or −	+ +	+ or −

+ indicates laboratory values will be present; on a scale of 1 to 4, 4+ indicates very high levels; − indicates this laboratory marker is not present.

Adapted from Behrman RE, Kliegman R, Nelson WE (eds): Nelson Textbook of Pediatrics, 14th ed. Philadelphia, WB Saunders, 1992.

Chronic persistent hepatitis can progress to cirrhosis, liver failure, or liver cancer in adults. Chronic persistent hepatitis is usually diagnosed by liver biopsy. Often the disease follows a mild anicteric hepatitis.

CHRONIC ACTIVE HEPATITIS. This condition has increased likelihood of progressing to cirrhosis and liver failure. There is recurrent episodic jaundice, elevated liver enzymes, and increased prothrombin time. Evolution of portal hypertension and ascites can begin. Often the disease follows a mild anicteric hepatitis.

FULMINATING HEPATITIS. This is a progressive course that is distinguished by liver failure and can occur a few days to a month after acute hepatitis. Elevated bilirubin (>20 mg/dl), elevated ammonia levels, marked elevated transaminases, encephalopathy, bleeding, coma, ascites, and abnormal EEG occur. There is a 30% mortality rate.

HEPATOMA. Primary hepatocellular carcinoma is associated with HBV.

EXTRAHEPATIC MANIFESTATIONS. Polyarteritis nodosa, glomerulonephritis, mixed cryoglobinemia, a serum sickness–like prodrome, and polymyalgia rheumatica are associated with HBV.

Management

Therapy is supportive in nature. The use of active and passive vaccination was discussed previously.

HEPATITIS C

Etiology

Hepatitis C virus (HCV), a single-stranded RNA virus with seven genotypes in the flavivirus family, causes the chronic form of non-A, non-B hepatitis.

Epidemiology

The risk factors associated with HCV are illicit IV drug use (40%), occupational or sexual exposure (10%), and transfusions (10%). Hence children with hemophilia or those on chronic hemodialysis are at greatest risk for this type of hepatitis. Transmission from HIV positive mothers to their infants is documented. Transmission from breastfeeding is thought to be rare.

Incubation Period

HCV has an incubation period of 1 to 5 months.

Clinical Findings

Onset of symptoms is often insidious and most children are symptomatic. Flu-like prodromal symptoms followed by jaundice occur in fewer than 25% of cases. Chronic hepatitis with cirrhosis is associated with hepatosplenomegaly, ascites, clubbing, palmar erythema, or spider angiomas.

Diagnostic Studies

Mild to moderate fluctuations in aminotransferase elevations can occur. Confirmation of anti-HCV by ELISA or radioimmunoblot assay or HCV RNA by PCR is diagnostic. A newborn can be anti-HCV positive from maternal transfer for up to 12 months. Liver biopsy may be performed.

Differential Diagnosis

Hepatitis A and B and other causes of chronic hepatitis.

Management

Treatment of acute hepatitis is supportive. Chronic HCV infections respond to therapy with interferon-α in 40 to 50% of cases.

Prognosis

Chronic hepatitis and cirrhosis are known problems. Liver transplantation is an option, although reinfection is common and gradually progressive. The outcome of chronic HCV disease in children is less known. Hepatocellular carcinoma is seen with adults who are HCV infected (Sokol & Narkewicz, 1999).

HERPESVIRUS

Etiology

Herpes simplex virus (HSV) is among the most widely disseminated infectious agent in humans. HSV has two antigenic types. HSV-1 is associated chiefly with nongenital infections of the mouth, lips, eyes, and central nervous system. HSV-2 is most commonly associated with genital and neonatal infection. Type 1 strains can be found in the genital tract (autoinoculation or oral-genital contact). Type 2 lesions found in the mouth or pharynx usually result from oral sexual activity.

Epidemiology

Primary infection with type 1 virus usually occurs in infants and children between 1 and 4 years of age. Distribution is worldwide, but the infection is more frequent in crowded environments. It is spread by intimate, direct contact. The virus has been recovered from stool, urine, skin lesions, saliva, and respiratory secretions. The primary site of clinical infection is gingivostomatitis (12.1%), usually occurring in the second year of life. There is no seasonal variation, and adults are the chief source of infection. Type 2 infections usually occur as a result of sexual activity. Sexual molestation must always be ruled out when the infection is found in non-neonates.

Neonatal HSV infection is usually acquired from the mother during the birthing process. Direct exposure occurs as the fetus passes through the vaginal vault. Viral migration from the vault to the fetus is the most common method of infection. Occasionally, a scalp monitor probe becomes contaminated and is the source of infection. Although the majority of neonatal infections are caused by HSV-2, approximately 15 to 20% are HSV-1. Risk of infection for an infant born to a mother with a primary genital infection is 40 to 50%. The risk for infants born to mothers with recurrent HSV genital infection is only 3 to 5%. This is an incidence of 1 in 3000 to 1 in 20,000 live births (AAP, 1997). Most infants with congenital HSV infection are born to women without a history or clinical findings of active infection during pregnancy. Postnatal transmission is described but is less common. Mothers can inoculate their babies from oral, breast, or skin lesions. Fathers also can inoculate infants with nongenital lesions. There can be lateral transmission from an infected baby in the nursery. Postnatal transmission from nursery personnel with fever blisters is extremely rare.

Incubation Period

Period of communicability for types 1 and 2 is unknown, probably less than 1 week. Some cases of congenital infection occur more than 6 weeks after birth. Infection can be transmitted during either primary or recurrent infections, whether children are clinically ill or asymptomatic.

Clinical Findings

Manifestations are determined by the port of entry of the host, age, state of health, and immune competence. Eczema alone or in combination with other manifestations is also a complicating factor.

GINGIVOSTOMATITIS. This is the most common primary infection. One- to 4-year-olds are most commonly involved. In upper socioeconomic groups, onset begins in older children. The illness begins with abrupt fever, 103° to 105°F, irritability, and a sore mouth. Lesions appear on the mucous membranes and oropharynx. Gums become swollen, reddened, and friable and bleed easily. Shallow plaque-like ulcers with red areolas appear in the buccal mucosa, tongue, plate, and fauces. They are white in color and approximately 2 to 3 mm in diameter. Anterior cervical nodes enlarge and are tender. Satellite lesions can spread around the mouth. Lesions on the hands of children who suck their fingers are not uncommon. The disease can last up to 2 weeks and varies in clinical severity from mild discomfort to a raging viral illness with extensive bleeding lesions coupled with severe dehydration (see Chapter 34).

NEONATAL HERPETIC INFECTION. This infection of premature and full-term infants is usually caused by HSV-2. Transplacental maternal antibodies are not protective. The infant presents with signs of sepsis, fever or hypothermia, jaundice, poor feedings, gastrointestinal symptoms, lethargy, and respiratory problems. If untreated, these cases are fatal. Even with treatment, the overall mortality rate is 70%, with 75% of survivors having severe morbidity. Early diagnosis and treatment can lower the mortality rate to 50% (see Chapter 39).

KAPOSI VARICELLIFORM ERUPTION. This herpetic reaction occurs in children with atopic eczema or chronic dermatitis. It occurs most often during primary infection and starts abruptly with high fever to 105°F, irritability, and restlessness. Crops of vesicles occur mostly on the eczematous skin. Some of the vesicles rupture and crust over like varicella. The infection can be mild to fatal. There are extensive areas of weeping, oozing skin that may be associated with severe fluid loss and bacterial superinfection.

TRAUMATIC HERPETIC INFECTION. This is a localized infection that occurs in a susceptible child because an abrasion, laceration, or burn is inoculated with herpesvirus by an orally infected parent who kisses the "booboo." Vesicles appear at the site of the lesion. There may be fever, constitutional symptoms, and regional lymph node involvement.

ACUTE HERPES VULVOVAGINITIS. The vulvovaginal area becomes swollen and erythematous with multiple painful shallow white ulcers 2 to 4 mm in diameter. Many of the ulcers coalesce and create large ulcers. Swollen, painful inguinal lymph nodes, fever, and constitutional symptoms last 5 to 7 days. Typing the virus in prepubescent children is important because of the possibility of sexual molestation (see Chapter 36).

ACUTE HERPETIC KERATOCONJUNCTIVITIS. This is a rare primary herpes infection of the eye. Fever and other constitutional symptoms of primary herpes occur. Preauricular lymphadenopathy occurs. Eye involvement is usually unilateral. The cornea appears hazy with purulent membranous exudate. Vesicles are often seen on the eyelid, and the patient has trouble closing the eye. If the infection is confined to the conjunctiva, the infection clears in approximately 14 days. Sight impairment can occur if there is corneal involvement (see Chapter 29).

ACUTE HERPETIC MENINGOENCEPHALITIS. Primary central nervous system involvement is an unusual manifestation outside the neonatal period. HSV-1 causes a rapidly progressing infection with a 70% fatality rate. Encephalitis can be focal, mimicking a mass lesion. Diagnosis is made by brain biopsy. In contrast, HSV meningitis is usually a relatively benign disease most often caused by HSV-2.

RECURRENT INFECTIONS. As with varicella, the body does not truly eradicate the virus, and recurrent infections are common. The usual manifestation of recurrent infections is herpes labialis, the common fever blister, and involvement of skin adjacent to the lips. However, acute herpes encephalitis is more common with recurrent infections. Constitutional symptoms are rare except in immunocompromised patients.

Differential Diagnosis

The diagnosis is usually not a problem if vesicles are present. Coxsackievirus can cause a vesicular stomatitis.

Diagnostic Tests

Viral culture, cytology-Papanicolaou smears, Tzanck stains, HSV serial antibody testing 2 weeks apart, ELISA testing, TORCH-IgM specific antibody, or brain biopsy, or a combination of these, can be ordered if the HSV diagnosis needs confirmation or is questionable, for medicolegal purposes, or for treatment considerations.

Complications

Usually the infection is mild. Major problems have been discussed. Bacterial superinfection is always a problem. There is an increased incidence of cervical cancer in women with HSV-2 infections.

Management

Treatment is supportive in nature except in life-threatening illness (neonatal infection or immunocompromised patients). Herpetic eye infection must be treated immediately by an ophthalmologist. The medications for ocular infections include multiple DNA inhibitors. These include 1 to 2% trifluridine, 1% iododoxyuridine, and 3% vidarabine. Corticosteroids are contraindicated in herpetic ocular infections (see Chapter 29).

Pharmacotherapy

Acyclovir and *vidarabine* are used in adults and children. Acyclovir for 14 to 21 days is the preferred drug in treating neonates.

The dosage of acyclovir is as follows:

SERIOUS INFECTION. Newborn: 30 to 60 mg/kg per day divided every 8 hours IV for 14 to 21 days; children (<12 yr): 250 mg/m² per dose every 8 hours IV for 14 to 21 days.

HERPES ENCEPHALITIS. Children (<12 yr): 500 mg/m² per dose every 8 hours IV for 14 to 21 days.

PRIMARY GENITAL AND MUCOCUTANEOUS INFECTION. Oral acyclovir diminishes the duration of illness and viral shedding in primary genital and mucocutaneous infection if used within 6 days of onset of signs and symptoms. The dose for children older than 2 years is 200 mg every 4 hours (5 doses/24 h) for 10 days. The topical preparation (5%) is used every 3 hours (6 doses/24 h) for 7 days for mild genital and mucocutaneous infection.

RECURRENT GENITAL INFECTION. If there are more than six recurrent infections in 1 year, oral acyclovir daily for 12 months is the treatment of choice. It is not recommended for use during pregnancy (see Chapter 36).

Prevention

The prevention of neonatal infection is directly tied to the monitoring of women during pregnancy and labor. All pregnant women must be asked about HSV infection in themselves and all sexual partners. Signs and symptoms of HSV should be carefully monitored throughout pregnancy. Again, during labor, all women must be requestioned about HSV. The mother must be carefully examined for signs and symptoms of infection. Cesarean delivery is indicated in women with apparent infection unless membranes are ruptured for more than 4 to 6 hours. Scalp monitoring should be avoided.

After birth, the infant must be carefully examined for vesicular lesions. Any lesions found should be cultured. The child should be started on acyclovir while awaiting culture results if HSV is strongly suspected. Infants born to mothers with a history of HSV but no signs of active disease follow the same protocol. Intrapartum cultures from mother and child should be obtained on the day of delivery (see Chapter 39).

Children with "fever blisters" may attend school as long as they have control over their saliva. Covering lesions with a bandage is appropriate for children with active nonmucosal involvement.

INFECTIOUS MONONUCLEOSIS

Etiology

Infectious mononucleosis is part of the Epstein–Barr family of herpesvirus.

Epidemiology

Infectious mononucleosis is worldwide in distribution. By 3 to 6 years of age, 80 to 100%

of children in poor urban settings or developing countries are seropositive for Epstein–Barr virus. In these children, primary infection tends to produce only mild symptoms or is subclinical. In more affluent social economic groups, this viral infection tends to occur between the ages of 10 and 30 years and is associated with clinical symptoms (Peter & Ray, 1998). The mode of transmission is close personal contact (e.g., kissing). Pharyngeal secretions are the main source of transmission; fomite contamination can be a problem. About 15 to 20% of healthy immune individuals secrete virus at any one time. Up to 50% of patients on immunosuppressive therapy, including those on steroids, shed virus.

Incubation Period

Because infectious mononucleosis virus is found in the saliva and blood of both clinically ill and asymptomatic infected persons for many months, the period of communicability is difficult to assess. The period of incubation is thought to be from 2 to 8 weeks.

Clinical Findings

IM is the great impostor and can mimic any disease imaginable. It is a disease of the primary lymphoid tissue and peripheral blood. There is enlargement of lymphoid tissue: regional lymph nodes, tonsils, spleen, and liver. Atypical lymphocytes are seen in the peripheral blood. Almost all body organs are involved, including but not limited to the lungs, heart, kidneys, adrenals, central nervous system, and skin. Clinical presentation can include the following:

- Fever: Moderate to high fever lasting 1 to 3 days is very common.
- Sore throat: Usually begins a few days after the fever. The throat is very painful. There is marked tonsillar enlargement, ulceration, and pseudomembrane formation. Petechiae are found on the palate.
- Lymphadenopathy: Usually the anterior and posterior cervical nodes are involved, but any lymphoid tissue can be affected. Nodes are firm, tender, and discrete in nature.

- Splenomegaly: Occurs in 50 to 75% of cases. Rupture is rare.
- Hepatomegaly: Is common. Almost all patients have abnormal liver function tests; 5 to 25% have clinical hepatitis.
- Skin rash: Occurs in 5 to 15% of cases. Can be maculopapular, urticarial, scarlatiniform, hemorrhagic, or nodular. The rash occurs more frequently in patients taking ampicillin and probably represents a form of arteritis or vasculitis.
- Bilateral periorbital edema: Reported in 30% of cases.
- Other systemic manifestations reported as primary disease and not complications include myalgia, arthralgia, chest pain, ocular pain, photophobia, conjunctivitis, gingivitis, abdominal pain, diarrhea, cough, pneumonia, rhinitis, epistaxis, bradycardia, aseptic meningitis, Guillain-Barré syndrome, Bell palsy, Reye syndrome, and acute cerebellar ataxia.

Differential Diagnosis

Infectious mononucleosis is in the differential diagnosis of almost every infectious disease. Conditions and infections typically associated with a mononucleosis-like syndrome are malignancies, adenoviruses, toxoplasma, rubella, HIV, hepatitis A, and diphtheria (Peter & Ray, 1998).

Diagnostic Test

The CBC has a classic picture of more than 10% atypical lymphocytes. There are a number of serological tests. Monospot and the serum heterophile test are positive in 90% of infected patients. Children older than 4 years of age usually must be ill for approximately 2 weeks before seroconverting. Viral culture and Epstein–Barr specific core and capsule antibody testing are usually used for diagnosis if the primary screening tests are negative and there is continued suspicion of IM. Test for CMV in patients who are negative on primary testing. CMV can appear exactly like infectious mononucleosis, and it is often impossible to differentiate the two clinically.

Complications

Usually most clinically healthy patients experience few sequelae. Rare complications include the following:

- Splenic rupture
- Thrombocytopenia
- Agranulocytosis
- Hemolytic anemia
- Orchitis
- Myocarditis
- Fatal disseminated disease or B-cell lymphoma: Occurs in patients with congenital or acquired cellular immunity deficiencies
- Chronic infectious mononucleosis
- Burkitt B-cell lymphoma and nasopharyngeal carcinoma: Also caused by Epstein–Barr virus; these conditions are more commonly found in Central Africa and Southeast Asia.

Management

Treatment is supportive. Corticosteroids can be used for tonsillar swelling and other lymphadenopathy but are not recommended for routine disease. Antiviral drugs such as acyclovir have little effect.

Prevention

Persons with a recent history of infectious mononucleosis or an infectious mononucleosis–like disease should not donate blood.

INFLUENZA

Etiology

This is the only remaining pandemic disease with no effective control. Influenza virus is an orthomyxovirus of three antigenic types, A, B, and C. Types A and B are still responsible for epidemic disease. Type A is further classified into numerous subtypes, depending on the antigenic strain, hemagglutinin (H), and neuraminidase (N). H_1, H_2, H_3, N_1, and N_2 are known to cause disease in humans. These proteins are identified by the hemagglutination inhibition tests. Specific antibodies to the virus are important in immunity. Influenza has major changes in these antigens at 10-year intervals. This process is called antigenic shift. Minor variations in cell protein occur in both influenza A and B. This is noted as antigenic drift. Animals may be reservoirs and account for the constant genetic reassortment of the viral antigenic code (AAP, 1997).

After the emergence of a newly shifted strain, the highest incidence of the illness occurs in infants and children 5 to 14 years old, with an attack rate of almost 50%. One percent are hospitalized. Subsequent outbreaks, with variants (drifts) of the same subtype, approach attack rates of only 15% in children of the same age. The attack rate of type B is higher in children than in adults.

Epidemiology

Influenza is a very contagious disease and is spread person to person by direct contact, droplet contamination, and fomites recently contaminated with infected nasopharyngeal secretions. Viremia is a rare occurrence. In temperate climates, epidemics always occur in the winter months, last approximately 4 to 8 weeks, and peak 2 weeks after the index case. In recent years, some epidemics have lasted 3 months.

Incubation Period

The incubation period is 1 to 3 days. Patients become infectious 24 hours before the onset of symptoms. Viral shedding usually ceases 7 days after the onset of illness.

Clinical Findings

Influenza patients are sick! There is a sudden onset of high fever, 102°F to 106°F, headache, vertigo, dry sore throat, pain in the back and extremities, and hacking cough that can resemble pertussis. Vomiting, diarrhea, and croup occur in young children. Infants can appear septic. Conjunctival injection, epistaxis, and myocarditis (evident by weak heart sounds and rapid, weak pulse) are common. In severe infection, there can be involvement of the lower respiratory tract with pneumonia and anoxia. Severe myocardial involvement can cause distention of the right side of the heart and congestive heart failure.

Differential Diagnosis

The differential diagnosis includes other viral respiratory infections (common cold, parainfluenza, respiratory syncytial virus), allergic croup, epiglottitis, and bacterial upper respiratory infections.

Diagnostic Tests

With the exception of the direct fluorescent antibody tests, diagnostic tests are of little help. Direct fluorescent antibody tests are hampered by false-positive and false-negative reactions. There are numerous serological tests: viral agglutination, complement fixation, immunofluorescence testing, and ELISA. Results from the ELISA or immunofluorescence techniques are available within several hours. Cultures taken within 72 hours of the onset of illness can isolate the virus in 2 to 6 days to confirm the diagnosis.

Complications

These include respiratory infections followed by a bacterial superinfection, usually *H. influenzae*. Reye syndrome is associated with type B infections and A subtype (H_1N_1). *Do not give aspirin to influenza sufferers!*

Management

Treatment is supportive in nature. Amantadine (5 mg/kg per day or 150 mg/d in 1 dose or 2 divided doses for children aged 1-9 years who weigh less than 40 kg; for children older than 10 years of age or who weigh 40 kg or more, a dose of 200 mg/d) diminishes the severity of type A illness but has no effect on type B. Antiviral therapy should be reserved for high-risk patients (AAP, 1997). It should be started as soon as possible and continued for 2 to 5 days until the patient is asymptomatic for 48 hours. Newer medications (oral and inhaled) for the treatment of influenza are on the market but are not yet approved for use in pediatric patients. Zanamivir has been effective in preventing familial spread of influenza A and may

be active against influenza B. Bed rest helps reduce cardiopulmonary problems (AAP, 1997).

Prevention

As previously discussed, influenza vaccine should be used. Both amantadine and rimantadine are approved for use in children and adults for prophylaxis against influenza A infections. The prophylactic doses are the same as listed under treatment. An alternative dosage for children who weigh more than 20 kg is 100 mg/d in 1 or 2 divided doses (AAP, 1997).

MEASLES

Etiology

Measles (rubeola) is a morbillivirus in the Paramyxoviridae family and is similar to mumps and influenza. There is only one antigenic type. Measles involves a rash indicating viremia. It is a serious illness in children! The disease is associated with high mortality and morbidity worldwide.

Epidemiology

Humans are the only reservoir of infection. The source of the infection is respiratory secretions, blood, and urine of infected persons. Virus is transmitted through droplet contact, fomites, and, less likely, aerosol transmission. Peak incidence of infection in susceptible persons occurs during the winter and spring months.

Successful vaccination programs during the 1960s and 1970s decreased the number of cases reported. However, in the 1980s there were major outbreaks among nonvaccinated preschool children (<5 years), primarily in urban settings. Older children and young adults, most of whom were vaccinated, also became ill with measles. These outbreaks led to a reevaluation of the vaccination schedule.

Incubation Period

The incubation period is 10 to 12 days. The person becomes infective around the ninth day and is contagious for approximately 1 week. The attack rate is 90% in susceptible households and 25% from school, bus, or hospital exposure. There is no carrier state; disease or vaccination usually carries lifelong immunity.

Clinical Findings

The clinical manifestations are divided into three stages:

1. *Incubation period*: There are no specific symptoms.
2. *Prodromal period*: This is the first sign of the illness and lasts 4 to 5 days. This stage consists of upper respiratory infection symptoms, low to moderate fever, cough, coryza, and conjunctivitis (the three "Cs" of measles). An enanthem can be found on the oral mucosa opposite the lower molars. These Koplik spots last 12 to 15 hours. They are small, irregular bluish-white granules on an erythematous background and are pathognomonic of measles infection.
3. *Rash stage*: The rash of unmodified measles usually appears on the third or fourth day of the illness. As the rash appears, temperature rises, often to 105°F. The rash first appears behind the ears and on the forehead. It is maculopapular in nature. Papules enlarge, coalesce, and move progressively downward, engulfing the face, neck, and arms over the next 24 hours. By the end of the second 24 hours, the rash has spread to the back, abdomen, and thighs. As the legs become more involved, the face begins to clear. The entire process takes approximately 3 days. Respiratory symptoms are most severe on day three of the rash. The more severe the rash, the more severe the illness. It can become hemorrhagic. This type of measles can be fatal because of disseminated intravascular coagulation (DIC). After the fourth day of the rash stage, the rash begins to fade. The disease peaks and defervesces. After the rash clears, a residual light pigmentation occurs, lasting approximately 1 week. This desquamates finely. Maternal antibody level and improperly given vaccine can alter the presentation and clinical course of measles.

Atypical Measles (Fulginiti Syndrome)

A severe illness can occur in children 2 to 4 years of age after they receive inactivated measles vaccine. The illness manifests with fever, pneumonitis, pneumonia with consolidation and pleural effusion, an unusual rash, and an extraordinarily high measles titer (>1:25,000 to 200,000) early in the disease. The vaccine that caused this problem was withdrawn in 1967. Consequently, atypical measles is an illness of young adults.

Modified Measles

This most commonly appears in children who have been passively immunized with IG after exposure to the disease. It can occur in infants with partial maternal immunity. The incubation period can persist as long as 20 days. The illness is an abbreviated version of typical disease. The prodrome period can be as early as 1 to 2 days with normal to low grade fever. Upper respiratory infection symptoms are minimal to absent. Koplik spots usually do not appear. The rash is so mild that it is often missed. There are usually no complications.

Differential Diagnosis

Any viral rash (e.g., roseola, echovirus, coxsackievirus, adenovirus, and Epstein–Barr virus), toxoplasmosis, scarlet fever, meningococcemia, Rocky Mountain spotted fever, drug rashes, and serum sickness are included in the differential diagnosis.

Diagnostic Tests

These include viral isolation in tissue culture and serial antibody titers drawn 3 weeks apart. A single measles IgM level is useful if drawn after the rash appears but not later than 30 to 60 days after the onset of the rash.

Complications

Measles is a severe disease. The measles virus is responsible for a significant inflammatory reaction that extends from the nasopharynx to the bronchi. One must carefully document complications before specific treatment is undertaken.

BACTERIAL SUPERINFECTION AND VIRAL COMPLICATIONS. These usually manifest as upper respiratory infections, obstructive laryngitis, otitis, mastoiditis, cervical adenitis, bronchitis, and pneumonia. The causative organism is usually the measles virus or group A β-hemolytic streptococci, pneumococci, *H. influenzae,* or an exacerbation of TB. Bacterial and viral infections can sometimes be differentiated by leukocytosis seen on the CBC.

MYOCARDITIS. This is a rare but reported complication. Transient EKG changes are common.

PURPURA FULMINANS (BLACK MEASLES). This is a severe complication with multiorgan bleeding.

DISSEMINATED INTRAVASCULAR COAGULATION. Activation of the coagulation system leads to intravascular fibrin deposit and platelet destruction.

NEUROLOGICAL COMPLICATIONS. EEG changes are common, especially during the rash stage, but are usually not significant. However, 1 in 1000 to 2000 cases suffers from an acute measles encephalitis that occurs between the second and sixth day of the illness. The child seems to be either doing well or recovering from the disease. Then there can be a sudden onset of fever, headache, vomiting, drowsiness, convulsions, and possibly coma. Frequently, there are signs of meningeal irritation. The CSF demonstrates increased protein and lymphocytic pleocytosis. An acute demyelinating encephalomyelitis can develop. Depending on the study, 15 to 33% of patients with measles encephalitis die, and 25 to 50% demonstrate significant neurological sequelae. A possible etiological role of measles virus in multiple sclerosis is suggested but not proven (Behrman et al., 1996).

SUBACUTE SCLEROSING PANENCEPHALITIS. This is a rare condition that is considered a late complication of measles. It usually occurs 5 or more years after infection and is considered a "slow virus." The incidence is 1 in 100,000 cases. The infection is slow, progressive, and invariably fatal, frequently within 6 months. It is diagnosed by EEG changes, marked elevation of CSF globulin (especially IgG), exceptionally high serum measles antibody titer, and measles antibodies in the CSF.

Management

Treatment is supportive in nature. Bacterial superinfections are treated with appropriate antibiotics.

VITAMIN A THERAPY. Children with severe measles have low vitamin A levels. Although the data are incomplete, vitamin A supplementation is recommended in the following circumstances (AAP, 1997):

* All children diagnosed with measles in areas where vitamin A deficiency is a recognized problem.
* Children between the ages of 6 months and 2 years of age who are hospitalized with severe measles, manifested by pneumonia, croup, or diarrhea, or both.
* Infants who are younger than 6 months of age diagnosed with measles with the following risk criteria: immunodeficiency, ophthalmologic evidence of vitamin A deficiency or xerophthalmia, impaired intestinal absorption (e.g., cystic fibrosis, short bowel syndrome), moderate to severe malnutrition, and recent travel from an area where measles has a high mortality rate.

The dosage of vitamin A is a one-time dose of 100,000 units for children between 6 months and 1 year of age and 200,000 units for children who are older than 1 year of age. Vitamin A is repeated the next day and 1 month later if there is ophthalmologic evidence of vitamin A deficiency.

Care of Exposed Persons

This is done with active and passive immunization, as discussed previously.

MUMPS

Etiology

Mumps is an acute generalized viral disease with painful enlargement of the salivary glands as the apparent sign. Mumps is a paramyxovirus. Only one serotype is known. Humans are the only natural reservoir.

Epidemiology

The source of infection is the saliva of infected persons. The virus is spread by direct contact, aerosol transmission, fomites, and, possibly, urine from infected persons. Viremia exists, and the virus is found in blood, urine, CSF, saliva, and upper respiratory secretions. Mumps is a disease of childhood; 85% of infections occur in children younger than 15 years of age. Death from this virus is rare, but half the fatalities occur in patients older than 19 years. Infection occurs during all seasons but is most common during late winter and spring. Mumps virus crosses the placenta, and infection during the first trimester increases the abortion rate to as much as 27% (AAP, 1997).

Incubation Period

The incubation period is 14 to 21 days, with a mean of 18 days. The period of communicability is 1 to 7 days. The virus has been isolated 6 days before to 9 days after the onset of parotid swelling. One third of patients are asymptomatic but infectious. One attack usually confers lifelong immunity. The recurrence rate is only 4%; most cases probably reflect an error in diagnosis. Transplacental antibodies to mumps are protective for 6 to 8 months. Neonatal infection reflects maternal disease just before delivery.

Clinical Findings

There are two clinical stages:

1. *Prodromal stage:* Rare in children but presents with fever, headache, anorexia, neck pain, and malaise.
2. *Swelling stage:* Approximately 24 hours after the prodromal stage, one (in 25% of patients) or both of the parotid glands begin to swell in a characteristic manner. The gland fills the space between the posterior border of the mandible and mastoid, pushing downward and forward to the zygoma. The ear is pushed forward and upward. This

can take a few hours to a few days. The area becomes swollen and painful. The enlarged glands decrease in size and return to normal in 3 to 7 days. Occasionally, an urticarial, maculopapular rash is seen on the trunk (Behrman et al., 1996). Pain on the affected side can be elicited by having the patient eat something sour. This is known as the "pickle sign." Stensen's duct is red and swollen. Twenty percent of patients are afebrile during this time. Fever is usually moderate and rarely high, with 10 to 15% of cases involving only submandibular gland swelling. Little pain is associated with the submandibular infection. However, the redness subsides more slowly. Wharton's duct is frequently swollen. Sublingual salivary glands are not commonly involved. When they are involved, there is bilateral swelling in the submental region in the floor of the mouth. Edema caused by lymphatic obstruction of the manubrium and upper chest is reported.

Differential Diagnosis

Cervical or preauricular lymphadenitis, suppurative parotitis by either bacterial or viral (coxsackievirus, parainfluenza 3) infection, idiopathic recurrent parotitis, ductal stones, Mikulicz syndrome, uveoparotid fever, and cancer (especially lymphosarcoma) are included in the differential diagnosis.

Diagnostic Tests

These include viral isolation and culture, serological tests (complement fixation, ELISA, hemagglutination inhibition, specific mumps antibody), and elevated serum amylase (70% of cases).

Complications

The following complications can occur:

MENINGOENCEPHALITIS. This is a frequent occurrence in 65% of all cases having CSF changes (pleocytosis). It is usually benign and follows the course of aseptic meningitis with no permanent sequelae. However, 2% of cases are fatal. Males are affected three to five times more often than females. Facial neuritis, myelitis, and a measles-like postinfectious encephalitis are rare complications.

NEPHRITIS. Viruria is a common complication, reported in 75% of patients studied. Fatal nephritis is reported. Abnormal renal functions occur in all patients at some time during the illness.

ORCHITIS/EPIDIDYMITIS. Rare in the prepubescent male, this is the second most common complication in the adult. It is ushered in by fever, chills, headache, nausea, and lower abdominal pain. The testes become swollen (up to four times normal size), tender, edematous, and red. Thirteen percent of affected males have fertility problems; sterility is rare.

OOPHORITIS. Manifested by fever, nausea, vomiting, and lower quadrant pain, this occurs in 7% of affected postpubertal women. There is no evidence of infertility problems.

PANCREATITIS. A rare complication with severe onset of sudden epigastric pain, tenderness, fever, chills, extreme weakness, prostration, nausea, and vomiting. Symptoms can last approximately 7 days and recovery is complete.

THYROIDITIS. This can occur along with the development of antithyroid antibodies.

MYOCARDITIS. Seen in 13 to 15% of adults, serious complications of myocarditis are rare.

MASTITIS. Mastitis is common.

DEAFNESS. Deafness occurs in 1 in 15,000 cases. Although this is a rare complication, mumps is the leading cause of unilateral nerve deafness. It can be transient or permanent.

OCULAR COMPLICATIONS. These include dacryoadenitis, neuritis, uveokeratitis, exophthalmos, and central vein thrombosis.

ARTHRITIS. Arthritis is manifested by arthralgia, swelling, and redness of the joints. The larger joints are usually affected, and involvement is migratory in nature. Recovery is usually complete.

THROMBOCYTOPENIA AND HEMOLYTIC ANEMIA. These can be severe but are usually self-limited.

Management

Treatment is supportive.

Prevention

School and day care students should be kept home until 9 days after the onset of parotid swelling. Active and passive immunization as discussed previously.

PARAINFLUENZA VIRUS

Etiology

Parainfluenza virus, a paramyxovirus, is similar to the influenza virus. Parainfluenza is the major cause of croup. It also is an important cause of bronchitis, bronchiolitis, and pneumonia. There are four antigenic types. These are classified as 1, 2, 3, and 4. Type 4 has two subtypes, A and B. Types 1, 2, and 3 are associated with croup.

Epidemiology

The disease is spread by direct contact through infected nasal-pharyngeal secretions. Transmission occurs by person to person contact as well as fomite contamination. Infection occurs throughout the year depending upon the type. Type 3 is a major cause of lower respiratory tract disease in children during the first year of life. Types 1 and 2 usually strike children 2 to 6 years of age, and reinfections occur at any age. Type 4 infections usually are mild.

Incubation

The incubation period is 2 to 6 days. Normal children usually shed type 1 virus for 4 to 7 days with a range of up to 14 days. Type 3 virus generally sheds 8 to 9 days with a range of up to 3 weeks.

Clinical Findings

Eighty percent of parainfluenza infections affect the upper airways. This virus accounts for 50% of those admitted for bronchitis, bronchiolitis, and pneumonia. Sore throat is a common complaint in older children. Fever is found in only 20% of cases and is inversely proportional to the age of the child. Discrete maculopapular rashes of short duration can be found if the patient is carefully examined. Types 1 and 3 also have been associated with acute parotitis, causing an illness clinically indistinguishable from mumps virus. A type 3 strain was found in the CSF of an adolescent with Guillain-Barré syndrome. Reye syndrome has occurred in association with parainfluenza viral infection. Parainfluenza viruses have been recovered from the spinal fluid of victims of sudden infant death syndrom (SIDS).

Differential Diagnosis

The differential diagnosis includes other viral URIs (e.g., common cold, influenza, RSV), allergic croup, and bacterial URIs. The most important clinical differential diagnostic consideration is laryngotracheitis and other acute upper airway obstructive diseases, such as acute angioneurotic edema, epiglottitis, and foreign body aspiration.

Diagnostic Tests

These do not need to be done routinely. Direct fluorescent antibody tests are hampered by false-positive and false-negative reactions. There are numerous serological tests: viral agglutination, complement fixation, immunofluorescent testing, and ELISA. Parainfluenza virus infection may not always cause a rise in antibody titers. Cultures can isolate the virus in 4 to 7 days. Serologic results can be confusing because of cross-reaction among paramyxovirus.

Complications

These are infrequent. Secondary bacterial infections, including otitis media and pneumonia, may occur. Immunocompromised hosts can have significant secondary infections such as bacterial tracheitis, bronchitis, and pneumonia.

Management

The treatment is supportive. Ribovirin is active against parainfluenza. It is currently being investigated for use in children. Antibiotics in cases of severe upper airway infection are reasonable until definitive test results are available. Cefuroxime covers most of the usual opportunistic bacterial organisms. No vaccine is available.

POLIOMYELITIS VIRUS

Etiology

The agent for poliomyelitis (polio) is a picornavirus. The disease ranges from an asymptomatic illness to lower motor neuron paralysis.

Epidemiology

Humans are the only documented source of infection. Transmission is through fecal-oral and infected upper respiratory secretions. The last North American epidemic occurred in 1979 in a group of individuals who declined immunization (AAP, 1997). Since 1980, almost all cases were associated with vaccine as discussed earlier.

Asymptomatic disease occurs in 90 to 95% of those infected. Communicability is greatest 1 week before the onset of clinical illness due to respiratory secretions and high fecal excretion. Contagion exists as long as the organism is secreted, which can take months. The incubation period is 3 to 6 days for abortive polio and 7 to 21 days for the paralytic form.

Clinical Findings

There are three clinical forms:

1. *Nonspecific febrile illness (abortive polio):* A mild and brief illness. There is an acute onset of fever to 103°F. Malaise, pharyngitis, headache, nausea, vomiting, abdominal pain, constipation, and anorexia are common findings. The entire illness lasts a few hours to a couple of days.
2. *Nonparalytic polio:* Presents as aseptic meningitis. The patient manifests abortive symptoms and becomes sicker. Pain and stiffness of the neck, trunk, back, and legs are common. Headache is severe. Hyperesthesia and paresthesia occur. There may be a fleeting bladder paralysis. Usually there is a 1- to 2-week symptom-free period between the abortive and the nonparalytic stages.
3. *Paralytic disease:* Produces aseptic findings plus weakness of one or more muscle groups. The incubation period for paralytic polio is from 4 to 21 days. This most likely coincides with the replication of the virus

in the oropharyngeal and gastrointestinal tracts. There is asymmetrical distribution of weakness. Cranial or skeletal muscle can be involved, with lower extremities more commonly affected. Bladder paralysis occurs, and up to 20% of the cases have bowel paralysis. The muscle paralysis is a flaccid type, with subsequent atrophy due to denervation and disuse.

Differential Diagnosis

Polio is rare. Differential diagnoses include other conditions causing muscular weakness: Guillain-Barré syndrome, peripheral neuritis, encephalitis, rabies, tetanus, botulism, demyelinating encephalomyelitis, tick-bite paralysis, spinal cord tumors, familial periodic paralysis, myasthenia gravis, and hysterical paralysis. Conditions that cause decreased limb movement or pseudoweakness are also differential diagnoses and include unrecognized trauma, toxic synovitis, acute osteomyelitis, acute rheumatic fever, scurvy, and congenital syphilitic osteomyelitis.

Diagnostic Tests

Viral culture of two stool samples within the first 2 weeks after the beginning of symptoms is the diagnostic test of choice.

Complications

The following may be seen:

- Gastrointestinal problems, including bleeding and acute gastric dilatation
- Cardiopulmonary problems, consisting of mild hypertension and myocarditis
- Acute pulmonary edema
- Pulmonary embolism
- Metabolic problems (hypercalciuria and renal stones)

Management

There is no specific treatment. Patients with paralytic disease should be hospitalized.

Prevention

Prevention is active and passive vaccination, as discussed previously.

ROSEOLA INFANTUM

Etiology

Roseola infantum is also known as exanthem subitum. The causative agent is human herpesvirus 6.

Epidemiology

Humans are the only natural reservoir. The method of transmission is still unknown. The disease is most common in children between 6 and 24 months of age. It is rare in children younger than 3 months or older than 3 years of age. Most children are seropositive by 4 years of age. This would indicate that there is asymptomatic illness or roseola without rash. Secondary cases are rare, and occasional outbreaks are reported. Cases occur all year long but tend to cluster in the spring and early summer.

Incubation Period

Incubation is still unknown but is probably 7 to 17 days. The period of communicability is probably greatest during the fever phase before the rash erupts.

Clinical Findings

There is a sudden onset of high fever to 105°F for 3 to 5 days, but the child does not seem particularly ill. There may be signs of an upper respiratory infection and, occasionally, a febrile convulsion. As the fever breaks, a diffuse, discrete, pinkish, maculopapular rash, 2 to 3 mm in diameter, appears. It fades on pressure and rarely coalesces. The roseola exanthema is quite similar to the rash of rubella. The rash lasts 1 to 2 days, begins on the trunk, and spreads centrifugally.

Differential Diagnosis

Most viral rashes are included in the differential diagnosis. However, the clinical course usually makes this illness easy to diagnose. A roseola-like illness is associated with parvovirus B19, echovirus 16, other enteroviruses, and adenoviruses. Until the rash develops, fever of unknown origin and bacterial sepsis are in the differential diagnosis. Continued high fever without a ready source usually leads to a septic workup for some of these children. If a febrile seizure occurs, meningitis is usually added to the differential diagnosis.

Diagnostic Tests

No specific tests are available. There may be initial leukocytosis with white counts as high as 20,000/mm^3 during the first 24 to 26 hours. Then classic viral leukopenia occurs.

Complications

Rare complications include febrile convulsions and encephalitis.

Management

There is no specific treatment.

RUBELLA

Etiology

Rubella is an acute disease of childhood that occurs in two forms, postnatal and congenital. Rubella is an RNA virus in the Togaviridae family.

Epidemiology

Humans are the only reservoir. Infection is spread through nasopharyngeal secretions of either apparent or silent infections and is worldwide in distribution. The virus has been isolated in blood, stool, and urine of infected individuals. It also has been isolated on fomites for as long as 24 hours. With the arrival of immunization, the numbers of epidemics declined. Most cases occur in unvaccinated children, teenagers, and young adults. In closed populations (boarding schools and the military), the attack rate is close to 100%. Males and females are equally affected. The ratio of subclinical to clinical infection is 2 to 1. There is transplacental immunity for approximately 5 to 6 months if the mother is immune. There is probable lifelong immunity for naturally occurring disease. Verified second attacks are rare.

Incubation Period

The incubation period is 14 to 21 days. The period of maximum communicability is approximately 7 days before to 5 to 7 days after the onset of rash.

Clinical Findings

Postnatal disease is marked by three stages:

1. *Prodrome:* There are mild catarrhal symptoms. This stage is occasionally missed.
2. *Lymphadenopathy:* Can begin as early as 7 days before the rash appears and can last for 2 weeks. The postauricular, posterior cervical, and posterior occipital are the primary lymph nodes involved. There is generalized lymph node involvement and at times splenomegaly is noted.
3. *Rash:* An enanthem can appear just before the general rash. These Forschheimer spots, which consist of small rose-colored to reddish spots located on the soft palate, were first noted in 1898. They are not considered pathognomonic for rubella and are noted in scarlet fever and other upper respiratory infections. The rubella rash can be the first obvious sign of illness. It begins on the face and can fade before it spreads to the chest during the next 24 hours. The rash is composed of discrete maculopapules that occasionally coalesce. It spreads caudally, lasting a mean of 3 days. There can be a fine branlike desquamation. Rubella without rash is also possible. A low-grade fever can occur during the eruption. There is no photophobia.

Differential Diagnosis

The disease can be difficult to diagnose unless there is an epidemic. The rash can be confused with scarlet fever, mononucleosis, echovirus, roseola, and drug eruptions.

Diagnostic Tests

Viral cultures and serological testing of acute and convalescent titers at least 2 weeks apart are done. Hemagglutination inhibition studies are the most widely used method but are being supplanted by ELISA and fluorescence immuno-assay, among others. Rubella-specific IgM is an important test in the newborn.

Complications

Complications in postnatal rubella are rare. They include the following:

ARTHRITIS. This is the most common complication. It usually develops as the rash fades but can be delayed for up to 2 months. The pain and occasional swelling last 5 to 10 days, affecting the hands, wrists, feet, and ankles. Adolescents and adults are affected more often than children. Women are affected more commonly than men.

NEURITIS. Neuritis occurs in two forms. In the "night reaction," the child awakens at night complaining of pain and paresthesia of the arms, wrists, and hands. These pains cease during the day and resume nightly over a few days. Nerve conduction and velocity tests demonstrate marked slowing. The second form is the "catcher's crouch." These children complain of popliteal pain and have trouble getting out of bed. When they walk, they assume a squatting gait. Onset of rubella neuritis can be delayed 1 to 2 months after the clinical infection and occasionally occurs after the vaccination.

ENCEPHALITIS. Encephalitis occurs in 1 of 6000 cases and is most common during the eruptive stage. Its presentation is similar to most postinfectious encephalitis. While there is usually complete recovery, fatalities have been reported (Levin, 1999).

IDIOPATHIC THROMBOCYTOPENIC PURPURA. This is a rare but serious complication of rubella. Cutaneous hemorrhage, epistaxis, bleeding gums, hematuria, and rare cerebral hemorrhages are reported.

Management

There is no specific therapy.

Prevention

Children with postnatal rubella should be kept home from school or day care for approximately 1 week after the rash erupts. Active and passive immunization was discussed previously.

Reinfection

There are conflicting studies. Because illness without rash exists, the actual numbers of reinfections are unknown. Rubella virus has many antigenic sites, causing the production of numerous antibodies. Their duration is unknown. In serologically immune persons, reinfection from wild virus is 3 to 10%. Reinfection rate in those immunized is approximately 14 to 18%. Many of these reinfections are subclinical. Infection was demonstrated in pregnant women who were reinfected as well as in pregnant women who were accidentally immunized, creating a question about the risk of congenital malformations for infants of women who are serologically immune (Behrman et al., 1996). There is no evidence that rubella vaccine inadvertently given to pregnant women causes congenital rubella syndrome.

CONGENITAL RUBELLA

Etiology

Congenital rubella was first described approximately 100 years after the disease was initially reported. Approximately 15% of women of childbearing age have no detectable antibodies, and maternal infection is acquired in the usual manner. After nasopharyngeal replication, viremia occurs. Timing of the viremia is critical in determining whether fetal infection will develop. If exposure occurs during the first trimester, there is a 50 to 80% chance of fetal infection. Maternal infection during the second trimester has a fetal infection rate of 10 to 20%. Third trimester infection rarely results in fetal infection (Behrman et al., 1996). The earlier the infection occurs in pregnancy, the more severe the fetal involvement. Regardless of the severity of fetal infection, the infant is chronically ill, shedding virus from nasopharyngeal secretions, stool, urine, and tears for at least 1 year. Children with congenital rubella are considered contagious for the first year of life unless they possess negative urine and nasopharyngeal cultures for the virus.

Clinical Findings

These range from subclinical to very serious. Infants are usually born with low birth weight.

There are eye defects such as cataracts, glaucoma, retinopathy, and microphthalmia. Cardiac defects include patent ductus arteriosus, ventricular septal defect, pulmonary stenosis, and myocardial necrosis. Central nervous system anomalies encompass psychomotor retardation, microcephaly, spastic quadriplegia, mental retardation, and progressive panencephalitis. Autism and deafness are common. Other problems noted are hepatitis, thrombocytopenia (blueberry muffin babies), splenomegaly, bony lesions, pneumonia, diabetes mellitus, thyroid disorders, and precocious puberty.

VARICELLA

Etiology

Varicella is a common, highly contagious virus. It is a herpesvirus with only one antigenic strain, *Herpesvirus varicellae*. Chickenpox is the primary illness. Shingles (herpes zoster) is the reactivation infection (see Chapter 37).

Epidemiology

Humans are the only reservoir of infection, and illness is spread by direct contact, droplets, and airborne transmission. Victims of shingles are also infectious. Immunity is usually lifelong. Symptomatic reinfection is rare, but asymptomatic reinfection occurs. Secondary attacks are usually mild. Asymptomatic primary infection is rare. Immunocompromised patients are at risk of developing generalized zoster. Ninety percent of varicella patients are younger than 10 years of age, and all but a few individuals contract the disease. There seems to be a shift in the epidemiology as adolescents and young adults contract the disease. Chickenpox is worldwide in distribution and endemic in most large cities. Epidemics occur but at irregular intervals. The incidence is greater in late autumn, winter, and spring.

Incubation Period

The incubation period is 10 to 21 days, with a mean of 14 days. The period of communicability is 1 to 2 days before the rash erupts until all lesions are dry. This can be prolonged to 28 days in VZIG recipients (AAP, 1997).

Clinical Findings

The following two phases are seen in varicella:

1. *Prodrome:* Not always present. It is composed of low-grade fever, listlessness, headache, backache, abdominal pain, and occasionally upper respiratory infection symptoms.
2. *Rash:* Classic appearance. It is centripetal, beginning on the trunk. Crops of lesions progress from spots to "teardrop vesicles" to scabs in 6 to 10 hours. After a few days, all morphological forms can be seen simultaneously. Scabs last from 5 to 20 days, depending on the depth of the lesions. There can be high fever, to 105°F. The more severe the rash, the higher the fever. Lesions can develop on all mucosal tissue, mouth, pharynx, larynx, trachea, vagina, and anus.

Differential Diagnosis

The rash is classic; therefore, the diagnosis is usually not a problem. Occasionally, impetigo, cigarette burns, and insect bites can cause some confusion in children with a mild rash.

Diagnostic Tests

These are of little importance except in the case of exposure of pregnant women. The virus can be cultured. Tzanck smears of lesions demonstrate multinucleated giant cells containing intranuclear inclusion bodies that are diagnostic of herpesviruses. ELISA or FAMA (fluorescent antibody against membrane antigen) tests are the most sensitive for assessing immune status.

Complications

The following complications can occur:

PYODERMAS. These occur as a result of the patient's scratching the lesions. Usual organisms are group A β-hemolytic streptococci and staphylococci.

BLEEDING MANIFESTATIONS. Idiopathic thrombocytopenic purpura is not uncommon in severe infections.

PNEUMONIA. Pneumonia is preceded by a sudden onset of cough 1 to 6 days after the rash begins, with possible cyanosis and hemoptysis. It is most often caused by a bacterial superinfection. Pneumonia is rare in children; 10 to 20% of adolescents and adults develop it.

CENTRAL NERVOUS SYSTEM PROBLEMS. Encephalitis occurs in 1 of 1000 cases. Cerebellar ataxia is common; if this is the only complaint, the clinical course is usually mild with few residua. Cerebral involvement is manifested by seizures, changes in the sensorium, paralysis, or coma. The morbidity rate is 15 to 45%. One percent of cases are fatal and include children receiving corticosteroids or antimetabolites. Guillain-Barré syndrome is a rare complication.

REYE SYNDROME. Chickenpox victims who take aspirin are at increased risk of developing Reye syndrome. *Aspirin is contraindicated in chickenpox patients!*

OTHER PROBLEMS. Other, less common problems include glomerulonephritis, orchitis, myositis, myocarditis, arthritis, and appendicitis (especially with intestinal lesions).

Management

Chickenpox is usually a benign infection in normal children. Treatment is supportive in nature. Intravenous acyclovir and vidarabine are effective in treating varicella in immunocompromised patients. VZIG can prevent or modify the course of the infection if given shortly after exposure. It is not effective after the disease has progressed. Oral acyclovir (20 mg/kg [800 mg maximum dose] q.i.d. for 5 d) given to otherwise healthy children within 24 hours after eruption of the rash usually results in a decrease in the symptoms and duration of the illness. The drug is expensive and is not routinely recommended for most children. Indications for the use of acyclovir include children older than 12 years with chronic pulmonary disorders, receiving chronic salicylate therapy, or receiving intermittent or short courses of oral or aerosolized corticosteroids.

Prevention

The following are recommended:

- Children exposed to chickenpox can attend school for about 1 week. If they begin to show signs of illness, they must be kept home for 1 week. If they do not break out in a rash, they can return to school. Children with active disease are to be kept home until all lesions are dry.
- Exposed patients: Use of VZIG has already been previously discussed. VZIG is associated with asymptomatic infection. Varicella titers should be obtained 2 months after VZIG is given to assess immune status.
- Chickenpox vaccine.

CONGENITAL VARICELLA

Neonatal involvement is directly tied to the timing of the maternal infection. Infection early in pregnancy can result in significant anomalies and scarring. Prenatal maternal infection less than 5 days from the estimated date of delivery to 2 days after delivery has a poor prognosis for infants. There is no time for maternal antibodies to develop and cross the placenta. Seventeen percent of infants whose mothers become infected develop the disease, with a 30% mortality rate; therefore, these infants should be given VZIG as soon as possible.

Bacterial Infections

CAT SCRATCH DISEASE (CSD)

Etiology

Bartonella henselae is the organism thought to be responsible for CSD. CSD is the most common cause of chronic persistent lymphadenopathy (Behrman et al., 1996). It is a slow-growing, gram-negative bacillus.

Epidemiology

CSD is believed to be a very common infection (9.3 cases: 100,000 population/year) with 80% of the contacts under 20 years of age. Infection occurs after direct contact with an infected animal. In 95% of the cases, a cat is involved. Four percent of the cases occur after dog contact (Behrman et al., 1996). Monkeys and fomites have also been associated in the transmission of this disease (AAP, 1997). Most of these animals are healthy and are CSD skin test negative. Association with mucous membrane lesions, canker sores, and regional lymphadenopathy has been postulated, but person-to-person contact has not been reported (Behrman et al., 1996). The CSD agent may be the cause of bacillary angiomatosis and peliosis hepatis. These infections have been reported in HIV-infected patients.

Incubation Period

The incubation period between injury and primary skin lesion is 3 to 10 days. The lymphadenopathy may take 5 to 50 days to develop but averages 12 days.

Clinical Findings

In approximately one third of cases, patients manifest systemic illness; the rest are not very sick. The illness appears in two stages:

1. *Skin lesion:* A cutaneous lesion arises approximately 1 week after inoculation and can persist for months. This nonpruritic lesion initially begins as a vesicle or pustule and evolves into a papule. It may be misdiagnosed as impetigo secondary to an insect bite. The cutaneous lesion heals completely without scarring. Up to 10% of the patients may have the inoculation lesion present as nonsuppurative conjunctivitis or ocular granuloma. Mucous membrane ulcers have been found at the onset of the lymphadenopathy stage. Two weeks after the inoculation, the preauricular, submandibular, cervical, supraclavicular, axillary, epitrochlear, or inguinal nodes closest to the lesion begin to swell. There can be single or multiple nodes involved. Multiple node-site involvement usually indicates several different inoculation sites. The node may swell up to 5 cm. The area around the infected node is usually warm, tender, indurated, and erythematous during the first few weeks. Cellulitis is uncommon, but large nodes may suppurate. The lymphadenopathy usually lasts approximately 2 to 4 months. In up to 2% of the cases, the lymphadenopathy can last for as long as 3 years.

2. *Systemic cat scratch disease (SCSD):* In one third of cases, patients manifest systemic illness. This can be associated with fever up to 106°F (41.2°C), malaise, fatigue, anorexia, emesis, headache, splenomegaly, sore throat, exanthema, blindness, arthralgia, seizures, coma, and conjunctivitis. Enlarged mediastinal or pancreatic nodes can cause pleurisy, obstructive phenomena, and splenic and hepatic abscesses. Significant weight loss is reported.

Differential Diagnosis

The differential diagnosis includes any cause of lymphadenopathy. The most common of these are bacterial and viral infections (e.g., streptococci [especially group A β-hemolytic], staphylococci, anaerobic bacteria, mycobacteria [both typical and atypical], tularemia, brucellosis, CMV, HIV, Epstein–Barr virus, systemic fungal infections, toxoplasmosis). Neck masses from other sources (e.g., cystic hygromas, bronchogenic cysts, tumors) are in the differential.

Diagnostic Tests

A diagnostic test is available from the CDC. It is an indirect immunoassay antibody test. The skin test antigen (0.1 ml) is applied to the volar forearm. The test is read in 72 to 96 hours. Five millimeters of induration is considered positive. A negative test should be reread 7 to 10 days later. Again, a 5-mm area of induration is considered positive. PCR for cat scratch antigen is also available. Computed tomography (CT) and MRI scans may be useful in identifying hepatic or splenic abscesses and granulomas. The CBC may show leukocytosis and increased eosinophils. The erythrocyte sedimentation rate (ESR) may be elevated early in the disease process. Lymph node biopsy stained with Warthin-Starry silver stain also is diagnostic.

Complications

ATYPICAL CSD. This may appear in up to 10% of cases. Complications include Parinaud oculoglandular syndrome, encephalopathy, severe chronic systemic disease, erythema nodosa, neuroretinitis, thrombocytopenia purpura, hepatosplenomegaly, primary atypical pneumonia, breast tumor, angiomatoid papules, and osteo-myelitis. Almost all of these problems resolve completely. No fatal cases or severe sequelae have been reported (Behrman et al., 1996).

Management

Symptomatic treatment is usually sufficient in most cases. Antipyretics can be used if there is moderate fever. Painful nodes can be treated with moist wraps. Incision and drainage of suppurative lesions should be avoided because of the high risk of sinus tract formation. Needle aspiration can yield material for diagnostic testing. Biopsy may be required if neoplasm is in the differential. Systemic antibiotics may be used for SCSD. Biaxin, ceftriaxone, cefotaxime, cefoxitin, amikacin, gentamicin, tobramycin, ciprofloxacin and imipenem/cilastin are effective IV medications for severely ill children. Trimethoprim/sulfamethoxazole (Bactrim), rifampin, and ciprofloxacin (Cipro) have been used orally with some success.

LYME DISEASE

Etiology

Borrelia burgdorferi, a spirochete, is the causative agent.

Epidemiology

Lyme disease is the most commonly reported vector-borne infection in the United States. It has been diagnosed in 49 states and over 50 countries. In the United States, three clusters (the Northeast [Maryland to Massachusetts], the Midwest [Wisconsin and Minnesota], and the West [California and Oregon]) have reported the most cases. In the East, the natural host to *B. burgdorferi* is the white-footed mouse. The eastern deer tick (*Ixodes scapularis*) becomes infected by feeding on the mouse and transmits the organism to humans. The western deer tick (*Ixodes pacificus*) feeds mostly on lizards, and they are not effective hosts for *B. burgdorferi.* Lyme disease has been reported in habitats that are inhospitable to the tick. The vector in these cases has not been identified. The risk of infection after a tick bite is directly related to

how long the tick has fed. It takes hours for the tick to fully implant its mouth into the host's skin and days to become fully engorged. Nymphal ticks must feed for 36 to 48 hours, and adult ticks for 48 to 72 hours before the risk of transmission of *B. burgdorferi* is significant (Behrman et al., 1996).

Incubation Period

The incubation period from the bite to the rash stage is approximately 1 to 2 weeks (range 3 to 31 days). Late manifestation of the disease may appear more than 1 year later.

Clinical Findings

Lyme disease is divided into 3 stages:

1. *Stage 1 (Early Localized Disease):* Within 1 to 2 weeks after the bite, a typical rash appears at the inoculation site. Erythema migrans begins as a red macule or papule and progresses into large annular erythematous lesions 5 to 15 cm in diameter. Erythema migrans can vary in morphology. The center of the lesion may be clear, vesicular, or necrotic. The lesion may be pruritic or painful. Organisms are present in the lesions. They may be cultured or seen in biopsy material. The rash remains for a few weeks and will fade even if untreated. The patient may experience fever, malaise, headache, arthralgia, and stiff neck during this phase. Without treatment these symptoms, including the rash, may become intermittent, lasting for weeks to months.

2. *Stage 2 (Early Disseminated Disease):* Through spirochetemia, the organism disseminates through the skin causing multiple skin lesions. These are morphologically similar to, but smaller than, the local lesion. They develop several days to several weeks after the primary lesions. The other systemic manifestations noted in the local disease may return. Infections of eye, bone, heart, synovium, muscle, liver, spleen, and central nervous system (CNS) occur due to the hematogenous and lymphatic spread of the organism. The patient may experience retinitis, uveitis, conjunctivitis, osteomyelitis, peri-

carditis and myocarditis (manifested by varying degrees of heart block), mild arthritis, hepatitis, lymphadenitis, aseptic meningitis, and cranial neuropathies (especially 7th nerve palsy in children). State 2 can last from weeks to 2 years without treatment. Most of the symptoms wax and wane during this time.

3. *Stage 3 (Late Disease):* Stage three usually begins with pauciarticular arthritis. The knees are most commonly affected. They are red, hot, and swollen but not as painful as with other types of bacterial arthritis. Untreated, the arthritis initially resolves in a few weeks but becomes recurrent and chronic. Lyme arthritis has been described in patients without initial skin lesions. Adults suffer late CNS sequela (progressive encephalopathy) much more frequently than children.

Differential Diagnosis

The rash is characteristic but may not be present in all cases. Lyme disease should be included in the differential of osteomyelitis, septic arthritis, infectious hepatitis, nonresponsive lymphadenopathy, meningitis, multiple sclerosis, amyotropic lateral sclerosis, Alzheimer disease, and juvenile arthritis.

Diagnostic Tests

Cultures from leading-edge biopsy are possible. The organism is slow growing and may take up to 4 weeks to isolate. The organism, if found, can be stained with Warthin-Starry silver or immunohistochemical (with mono- or polyclonal antibodies). Since *B. burgdorferi* occurs in such low concentrations, it is often either missed or confused with normal skin structures. In patients without rash, manifesting late stage signs and symptoms, the diagnosis of Lyme disease should be based upon clinical findings, with serologic testing as an adjunct (AAP, 1997).

IgM-specific antibodies appear 3 to 4 weeks after the infection begins. The antibodies persist 6 to 8 weeks and then decline. IgG-specific antibodies appear 6 to 8 weeks after inoculation and peak at 4 to 6 months. They can remain elevated indefinitely. Due to the timing of anti-body formation, serologic testing is useful in stage 2 or 3 disease only. Note that early antimicrobial intervention may prevent the production of Lyme antibodies. ELISA and Western blot test have been developed for Lyme disease. These tests are very hard to interpret and should be performed in reference laboratories. There are many false-positive cross-reactions with other spirochetes, lupus, and varicella organisms.

Complications

These have been mentioned previously.

Management

Clinical judgment is crucial in determining whether to treat a patient for Lyme disease. False-positive and false-negative test results are frequently reported. There are many clinically asymptomatic but serologically positive cases, and Lyme disease may not be the cause of a patient's multisystemic illness.

EARLY LOCALIZED DISEASE (STAGE 1)

1. Amoxicillin (patients younger than 8 years of age), 50 mg/kg per day PO divided into three doses a day (maximum dose 500 mg) for 21 days
2. Doxycycline (patients aged 8 years or older), 100 mg, PO twice daily for 21 days. For patients unable to take either amoxicillin or doxycycline use erythromycin, 30 to 50 mg/kg per day PO (maximum 250 mg), divided four times daily for 21 days.

EARLY DISSEMINATED DISEASE WITHOUT FOCAL FINDINGS

Same as early focal disease.

EARLY DISSEMINATED DISEASE WITH FOCAL FINDINGS

1. *Isolated facial palsy:* Same as stage 1 but for 28 to 30 days. Do not use corticosteroids.
2. *Arthritis:* Same as stage 1 but for 28 to 30 days. If symptoms fail to resolve after 8 weeks or there is recurrence, repeat treatment either PO or use ceftriaxone, 20 to 100 mg/kg per day (maximum 2000 mg) every day IV or IM or penicillin, 200,000 to 400,000 u/kg/day (maximum 20 million

units/d) IV divided every 4 hours for 14 to 21 days.

3. *Carditis*: Ceftriaxone, 50-100 mg/kg/day (maximum 2000 mg/d) once a day IV or IM or penicillin 200,000 to 400,000 u/kg/day (maximum 20 million units/d) IV divided every 4 hours for 14 to 21 days. Do not use corticosteroids.

4. *CNS disease:* Ceftriaxone, 50-100 mg/kg per day (maximum 2000 mg/d) once a day IV or IM or penicillin 200,000 to 400,000 u/kg per day (maximum 20 million units/d) IV divided every 4 hours for 14 to 21 days.

Prevention Measures

1. Avoid tick-infested areas. Use tick skin repellent with diethyltoluamide (DEET). Inspect skin carefully every day during the tick season.
2. Infection risk is low. Chemoprophylaxis is not necessary.
3. A three-dose vaccine (LYMErix) is licensed by the Food and Drug Administration (FDA) for persons 15 to 70 years of age.

MENINGOCOCCAL DISEASE

Etiology

Neisseria meningitidis is a gram-negative diplococcus. It is a common commensal organism in the human upper respiratory tract. It was first described in 1805. It has no animal or environmental reservoirs. There are 13 serotypes identified, and groups A, B, C, L, W, X, Y, and Z are known to cause invasive disease. Groups B and C are the most common in the United States.

Epidemiology

The organism is spread from person to person via respiratory tract secretions and in most cases causes asymptomatic colonization. This can persist for weeks to months. Carriage rates range from 2 to 30% in nonepidemic periods depending upon the study (Behrman et al., 1996). Carriage rate is higher in areas of crowding especially in day care centers. During epidemics, the carriage rate can rise to 100%. Dis-

ease occurs most often in children who are younger than 5 years of age during winter and early spring. The peak attack rate occurs in children 3 to 5 months of age. Epidemics occur in semi-closed communities (e.g., day care centers, schools, colleges, and military bases). Patients with functional or anatomic asplenia, complement 5-9 deficiency, and properdin deficiency are at increased risk of invasive or recurred meningococcal disease (AAP, 1997).

Incubation Period

The incubation period is 1 to 10 days. Patients are contagious until 24 hours after treatment.

Clinical Findings

Colonization can lead to invasive disease. Bacteremia and sepsis result and, depending upon hematogenous spread, multiple patterns of illness can result, including bacteremia without sepsis, meningococcemia without meningitis, meningitis with or without meningococcemia, meningoencephalitis, and specific organ infection (Behrman et al., 1996).

1. *Occult bacteremia:* This appears in a febrile child with URI or gastrointestinal-like symptoms. There may be a maculopapular rash. Often these children are treated as having a viral illness. Some have recovered without antimicrobial intervention, whereas others have developed meningococcal meningitis.
2. *Acute meningococcemia:* Abrupt fever, chills, pharyngitis, headache, myalgias, weakness, malaise, prostration, and a maculopapular rash may quickly progress into septic shock manifested by hypertension, DIC, acidosis, adrenal hemorrhage, renal failure, myocardial failure, and coma. Bacteremia can result in endophthalmitis, meningitis, pericarditis, pneumonia, or septic arthritis. Seventy-one percent manifest petechiae or purpura or both (Behrman et al., 1996).
3. *Chronic meningococcemia:* This is rare. A nontoxic appearing child has fever, headache, and rash. The rash consists of painful, discrete pinkish-red macules up to 20 mm

in diameter that progress into lesions on an erythematous base. The rash usually spares the face and scalp but is concentrated on the extremities. The symptoms are recurrent, lasting 6 to 8 weeks. Bacteremia can occur, and without treatment, acute infection can result.

Differential Diagnosis

The list of differential diagnoses is long and includes septicemia caused by other invasive bacteria (e.g., pneumococcus or *H. influenzae,* viral meningitis, leptospirosis, syphilis). Collagen vascular diseases, primary hematology/oncology disease, erythema nodosa, erythema multiforme, Rocky Mountain spotted fever, mycoplasma, coxsackievirus, echovirus, rubella infections, and Kawasaki disease are also in the differential.

Diagnostic Tests

The diagnosis is confirmed with a positive culture from blood, CSF, or synovial fluid. Latex agglutination testing exists, but the sensitivity is less than 50%. It may be of some value in cases where oral antibiotics were given and organism growth has been suppressed. PCR testing exists but is used only in research labs.

Complications

These are caused by inflammation, vasculitis, and shock. Abscesses and infarcts cause necrosis of tissue and gangrene. Skeletal deformities and limb amputations are not infrequent. Meningitis can lead to ataxia, seizures, deafness, blindness, palsies, paralysis, developmental delays, and hydrocephalus. Immune-complex reactions are responsible for arthritis symptoms.

Management

Penicillin G (250,00–300,000 u/kg per d IV divided every 4 h for 7 d) is the drug of choice. The patient is kept in respiratory isolation until 24 hours after the induction of treatment. Four percent of isolates studied by the CDC are resistant to penicillin. In these cases, or if the patient is allergic to penicillin, cefotaxime, ceftriaxone, or chloramphenicol may be substituted.

Control Measures

Exposed contacts must be carefully monitored. Household, school, or child contacts who develop a febrile illness must be evaluated for invasive disease promptly. If the child is suspected of having meningococcemia, IV antibiotics should be started pending culture results.

1. *Chemoprophylaxis:* Close contacts of the index case are at increased risk of invasive disease. Medical personnel are usually not considered at high risk unless they performed mouth-to-mouth resuscitation, intubation, or suctioning before antibiotic therapy was instituted (AAP, 1997). Rifampin, 10 mg/kg per dose (maximum dose 600 mg) PO twice daily for a total of 4 doses, is the prophylactic treatment of choice. Infants younger than 1 month of age should be given 5 mg/kg per dose PO twice daily for a total of 4 doses. Ceftriaxone, 125 mg IM, in one dose is also useful and can be given to pregnant women. Ciprofloxacin, 500 mg PO, in a single dose can be given to nonpregnant adults. IV antibiotic therapy does not eradicate carriage; therefore, chemoprophylaxis is recommended for the index case before hospital discharge unless the child was treated with ceftriaxone or cefotaxime.
2. *Vaccine:* This has been discussed previously.

STREPTOCOCCAL DISEASE

Etiology

Streptococci are gram-positive spherical cocci that are classified based on their ability to hemolyze red blood cells. Complete hemolysis is known as β-hemolytic. Partial hemolysis is α-hemolytic. Nonhemolysis is γ-hemolytic. Cell wall carbohydrate differences further subdivide the streptococci. These differences are identified as Lancefield antigen subgroups A–H and K–V. Subgroups A–H and K–O are associated with human disease.

GROUP A β-HEMOLYTIC STREPTOCOCCI (GABHS)

Epidemiology

There are more than 80 M-protein types of GABHS. Transmission is through infected upper respiratory tract secretions. Fomites, especially unwashed hands, are a common source of indirect contact. Foodborne epidemics, especially via water, milk, ice cream, and eggs, are reported. The two most common infections are pharyngitis and impetigo. Both are associated with crowding and lower socioeconomic status. Pharyngitis is rare in infancy, but the incidence rises with age until adolescence. It is not common in adults unless there is an epidemic. Upper respiratory infections occur year round but are most common in the winter. Temperate climates have greater incidences of infection than tropical climates. Carriage state is high, and 15 to 50% of asymptomatic children have GABHS cultured from their throats. By contrast, impetigo is more common in toddlers and preschool-age children and occurs more often during summer and early fall in tropical areas.

Incubation Period

The incubation period is 2 to 5 days for pharyngitis and 7 to 10 days for skin acquisition to lesions of impetigo. The period of communicability is from the onset of symptoms up to a few months in untreated persons.

Clinical Findings

The following may be seen in GABHS:

RESPIRATORY TRACT INFECTION. Pharyngitis and pneumonia are described in Chapter 32.

SCARLET FEVER. This is caused by erythrogenic toxin. The incubation period is 2 to 4 days (range, 1 to 7 days). There is abrupt illness with sore throat, vomiting, headache, chills, and malaise. Fever can reach 103°F. Tonsils are erythematous, swollen, and usually covered in exudate. The pharynx also is inflamed and can be covered with exudate. The palate and uvula are erythematous and reddened, and petechiae are present. The tongue is usually coated red. Desquamation of the coating leaves prominent papillae (strawberry tongue).

The rash appears 12 to 24 hours later. The exanthema is red and finely papular and makes the skin feel coarse, akin to sandpaper. The rash begins in the axilla, groin, and neck, spreads centripetally, is generalized within 24 hours, and blanches on pressure (Schultz-Charlton sign). The face is usually spared. There is circumoral pallor, and the cheeks are flushed. There is increased rash density on the neck, axilla, and groin. Pastia's lines, transverse linear hyperpigmented areas with tiny petechiae, are seen in the folds of the joints. In severe disease, small vesicles (miliary sudamina) can be found on the hands, feet, and abdomen. Rash, sore throat, and constitutional symptoms resolve in approximately 7 days. The rash begins to desquamate shortly thereafter. Fine branlike flakes begin on the face and slowly spread to the trunk and extremities. This process takes up to 3 weeks.

Scarlet fever can occur after wound infection (surgical scarlet fever) or burns. The disease is similar to regular scarlet fever, but there is no pharyngeal or tonsillar involvement.

SKIN INFECTIONS. The characteristic lesion for streptococcal impetigo is a honey-colored scab on an erythematous base (Color Fig. 14). Localized lymphadenopathy is common. A small, transient, vesicular lesion may precede the scab lesion. Deep soft tissue infection may develop after impetigo. Streptococcal soft tissue abscesses result from puncture wounds contaminated with GABHS. Infants having weepy eczema can have secondary GABHS skin infection. The eczema area develops the typical impetiginous lesions. Erysipelas is an acute cellulitis and acute lymphadenitis. The skin becomes red and indurated. It begins as a small lesion and spreads marginally for 4 to 6 days. The lesion's borders are firm, raised, and tender. Fever, chills, vomiting, irritability, and other constitutional symptoms are present. These subside when the rash stops spreading. Bacteremia, abscesses, metastatic foci, and death are reported (see Chapter 37).

BACTEREMIA. This can occur after pharyngitis, tonsillitis, and localized skin infection. Some children have no obvious source of infection. Meningitis, osteomyelitis, septic arthritis, pyelonephritis, and bacterial endocarditis are associated with GABHS bacteremia.

VAGINITIS. GABHS causes severe vaginitis in

prepubertal females. Vulvar erythema, serous discharge, and pain are common findings. Although the infection is usually the result of autoinoculation, it can be a symptom of sexual molestation if infected saliva is used as a sexual lubricant.

PERIANAL STREPTOCOCCAL CELLULITIS. This is uncommon and occurs in either sex. Manifestations include local itching, pain, blood-streaked stools, erythema, and proctitis. While infection is usually the result of autoinoculation, it can be a symptom of sexual molestation if infected saliva is used as a sexual lubricant.

NECROTIZING FASCIITIS. This occurs in children and often is associated with varicella.

STREPTOCOCCAL TOXIC SHOCK SYNDROME. Toxic shock syndrome caused by GABHS appears as an acute multiorgan disease. There is hypotension, renal damage, DIC, adult respiratory distress syndrome, rash, and tissue necrosis. The mortality rate can be 70%. Hypotension is the key to making the diagnosis of GABHS toxic shock (Table 24-13).

Differential Diagnosis

A differential diagnosis is acute pharyngitis caused by viruses, especially infectious mononucleosis. Other bacterial upper respiratory diseases, such as diphtheria, tularemia, toxoplasmosis, tonsillar tuberculosis, salmonellosis, and brucellosis, are in the differential. Staphylococcal impetigo must be differentiated from GABHS pyoderma. Septicemia, meningitis, osteomyelitis, septic arthritis, pyelonephritis, and bacterial endocarditis can result from other bacteria causing similar infections. Culture differentiates the offending organism.

Diagnostic Tests

Culture of the organism is the most useful method of establishing the diagnosis. A positive throat culture confirms the diagnosis; however, a positive culture may identify a carrier state. Many rapid streptococcal identification tests are not as sensitive as a culture in picking up GABHS; therefore, a negative rapid test must be followed up by a culture unless the rapid streptococcal identification test is highly sensi-

T A B L E 24-13

CDC Case Definition of Streptococcal Toxic Shock Syndrome

1. **ISOLATION OF GROUP A STREPTOCOCCI**
   A. From a normally sterile site (e.g., blood, CSF, peritoneal fluid, tissue biopsy, surgical wound)
   B. From a nonsterile site (e.g., throat, superficial skin lesion, etc.)

2. **CLINICAL SIGNS OF SEVERITY**
   A. Hypotension: systolic blood pressure ≤90 mm Hg in adults or <5th percentile for age in children

   and

   B. Two or more of the following signs:
   • Renal impairment: creatinine ≥2 mg/dl for adults or ≥2× the upper limit of normal for age
   • Coagulopathy: platelets ≤100,000/mm³ or DIC
   • Liver involvement: elevated SGPT, SGOT, or bilirubin concentration greater than or equal to twice the upper limits of normal
   • Adult respiratory distress syndrome
   • A generalized erythematous macular rash that may desquamate
   • Soft-tissue necrosis, including necrotizing fasciitis, myositis, or gangrene

An illness fulfilling criteria 1A and 2A and B can be defined as a definite case. An illness fulfilling criteria 1B and 2A and B can be defined as a probable case if no other etiology can be found.

Modified from Centers for Disease Control, the Working Group on Severe Streptococcal Infection: Defining the group A streptococcal toxic shock syndrome: Rationale and consensus definition. JAMA 269:390–391, 1993; American Academy of Pediatrics (AAP): 1997 Red Book: Report of the Committee on Infectious Diseases, 24th ed. Elk Grove Village, IL, 1997, p 484.

tive. The specificity of most rapid tests is good (95%); therefore, if the rapid test is positive, the diagnosis of GABHS is confirmed. The Strep A Optical Immuno Assay (OIA) is reportedly a highly sensitive and specific test that has proved reliability and accuracy. Documentation of past GABHS infection is done by drawing a titer for antibodies to various streptococcal enzymes, such as antistreptolysin O (ASO).

Complications

These are usually caused by spread of the disease from the localized infection and have already been discussed.

Management

Antimicrobial therapy is the treatment of choice (AAP, 1997):

1. Benzathine penicillin G IM (600,000 units if child is <60 pounds, or 1.2 million units for larger children and adults).
2. Potassium penicillin V PO (250 mg t.i.d. for 10 d). If compliance is good, penicillin PO (500 mg/d in two divided doses for 10 d) can be given.
3. Erythromycin ethyl succinate (20 to 30 mg/kg per day in two to four divided doses for 10 d), if allergic to penicillin. Lincomycin, clindamycin, and oral cephalosporins (cephalexin, cephradine, cefadroxil, cefaclor, cefixime, cefuroxime) can also be used but are much more expensive.
4. Topical antibiotics may be used with simple uncomplicated impetigo (one to two single lesions). Mupirocin, bacitracin, and neosporin are effective.

SUPPORTIVE CARE. This includes antipyretics, fluids, and rest. If clinical relapse occurs, another culture should be done. If positive, a second course of penicillin is indicated, preferably benzathine penicillin IM. If recurrent infection is a problem, simultaneous culturing of the family for chronic carrier state is advised. Children can return to school as soon as they are afebrile and on antibiotics for at least 24 hours. Asymptomatic carriers generally do not need treatment.

GROUP B β-HEMOLYTIC STREPTOCOCCI (GBBHS)

GBBHS is a leading cause of perinatal bacterial infection. There are nine serotypes (Ia, Ib, Ia/c, II, III, IV, V, VI, and VII) associated with human infection. Type III is the most frequent cause of neonatal meningitis. GBBHS colonizes the gastrointestinal tract and vagina, with rates in pregnant women and newborns that range from 5 to 35% (AAP, 1997). Infection occurs in approximately 1 to 5 per 1000 live births, and the incidence of early-onset disease is 1 in 100 to 200 colonized women. Transmission occurs by direct contact, mother to child during parturition, and after birth by contact with colonized persons, usually through hand contamination. Early-onset disease is more common in high-risk deliveries or premature infants, small-for-gestational-age infants, infants born after prolonged rupture of membranes, and in mothers with genital tract infections. It can cause disease in older persons with diabetes mellitus or immunological disorders. Chapter 39 discusses this problem and the management of the disease in infants.

NON-GROUP A OR B STREPTOCOCCI

These organisms are associated with invasive disease. They are frequent causes of urinary tract infections (UTIs), endocarditis, respiratory disease, and meningitis. The incubation period and communicability times are unknown. Culture is the best method of establishing the diagnosis.

Management

Groups C, D, and G are less susceptible to penicillin and cephalosporins. Ampicillin or vancomycin with an aminoglycoside is the combination of choice. The other groups are usually susceptible to penicillin.

TUBERCULOSIS

Etiology

TB is caused by *Mycobacterium tuberculosis*, an aerobic, nonmotile, nonsporulating, pleomorphic rod. *M. tuberculosis* does not stain with the usual tests and is a very slow-growing organism, averaging approximately 21 days to culture. This organism is spread primarily by droplet contamination; fomite transmission is uncommon.

Incubation Period

The incubation period is 2 to 10 weeks. Risk of disease is highest in the first 2 years after infection. Infection is defined as converting from a negative to a positive tuberculin skin test.

Clinical Findings

PRIMARY PULMONARY TB. Most children aged 3 to 15 years are asymptomatic when first noted to have a positive TB skin test. Eighty percent of infected children who are older than 4 years of age and prepubertal do not progress to disease. Chest radiographs are usually negative for signs of pulmonary disease. There may be a nonspecific low-grade fever, malaise, decreased appetite, weight loss, erythema nodosum, and (or) phlyctenular keratoconjunctivitis (a hypersensitivity reaction marked by elevated clear nodules with surrounding hyperemia near the limbus). Enlarging lymph nodes can encroach on mediastinal structures, causing compression, obstruction, or erosion. Compression on the esophagus causes dysphagia or aspiration. Major arteries and veins can also be compressed by enlarging nodes with resulting edema. Superior vena cava syndrome can occur.

Fistulas can occur between the lymph node and the bronchial lumen and cause fibrosis, bronchiectasis, and pneumonia. Recurrent cough, stridor, and wheezing are signs of increasing pulmonary infection. Most children do not suffer significant pulmonary infection, and most reinfections resolve even without chemotherapy. However, progressive primary TB does occur in immunosuppressed children. Instead of resolving, the lesions continue to evolve, often involving an entire lobe. Older children and adolescents suffer from upper lobe infiltrates and cavitation. Calcification and lymphadenitis may be minimal.

MILIARY TB. Infants and children younger than 3 years of age frequently develop miliary TB. During early stages of the disease, bacilli reach the blood stream directly from the initial focus or by way of the regional lymph nodes. Necrosis and caseation of multiple organs can occur. Lesions are the size of millet seeds; hence the name "miliary" TB. It is also common in very old and immunosuppressed patients, especially those with AIDS. The disease has a precipitous onset. Moderate to high fever is common. Malaise, decreased appetite, weight loss, and fatigue are constitutional symptoms at the outset. Lymphadenopathy, hepatomegaly, splenomegaly, tachypnea, dyspnea, rales, wheezes, and stridor are often found on physical examination. Other signs and symptoms are present, depending on which organs are involved.

Differential Diagnosis

This includes mycotic infections, staphylococcal pneumonia, sarcoidosis, chronic pneumonia, and Hodgkin lymphoma.

Diagnostic Tests

Chest radiographs showing hilar adenopathy suggest TB, but culture of the organism is essential to establish the diagnosis. *M. tuberculosis* is a slow-growing organism. It often takes 2 to 10 weeks to isolate it in the bacteriology laboratory. Acid-fast bacilli stains can be helpful. DNA probes are useful but have limited availability. Histological examination for acid-fast bacilli is helpful.

Tuberculin skin testing is based on the delayed hypersensitivity to *M. tuberculosis* antigens. The test usually becomes positive 2 to 10 weeks after infection with the bacilli. The preparation currently available for skin testing is PPD. The Mantoux test uses 0.1 ml of 5 TU PPD. It is injected intradermally into the volar surface of the forearm, producing a 6- to 10-mm wheal.

Tuberculin skin tests (Mantoux) are read 48 to 72 hours later by experienced health care professionals. The induration is measured, not the erythema. Pediatric patients are considered at high risk for TB if they meet any of the following medical risk criteria:

- Contacts with adults who have active TB
- Born in or have parents from TB-prevalent parts of the world
- Have clinical signs suggestive of TB on chest radiograph or other clinical evidence
- HIV positive or have an immunosuppressive disorder
- Have other risk factors, including Hodgkin disease, lymphoma, diabetes mellitus, chronic renal failure, or malnutrition

- Incarcerated adolescents
- Exposed to high-risk adults (AAP, 1997)
- Residents of homeless shelters or some medically underserved, low-income populations (US Public Health Service, 1998)

A Mantoux skin test is defined as positive with reactions of

- Induration (≥15 mm) in children 4 years of age or older without any risk factors
- Induration (≥10 mm) in children younger than 4 years of age or with medical risk factors as listed above
- Induration (≥5 mm) in children who are household contacts of active or previously active TB cases suspected to have TB because of either a chest radiograph consistent with active or previously active TB or clinical findings of TB diagnosed with immunosuppressive disorders or HIV infection (AAP, 1997).

Of children with culture-proven infection, especially those with miliary TB, 5 to 10% can have a negative skin test. Skin testing is not always valid in immunocompromised patients, infants younger than 6 months of age, BCG recipients, and those with early TB infection. Patients sensitized to nontuberculous mycobacteria can cross-react and have a less than 10 mm sized reaction to TB skin testing. BCG cross-reaction was discussed previously. High-risk groups and patients living in areas where TB is endemic or on the rise should be skin tested yearly. Low-risk groups should be tested periodically, at 1, 4 to 6, and 11 to 16 years of age.

Complications

The following complications can occur:
CHRONIC PULMONARY TUBERCULOSIS. This complication is a progression of the primary disease, usually occurring 1 to 2 years after the infection, in less than 5% of children younger than 15 years of age. It is most common in adolescents.

PLEURAL EFFUSION. This occurs in approximately 8% of children with primary disease. It is caused by an extension of the bacillus into the pleural space by subpleural foci or hematogenous spread, or both. It usually occurs within 6 months of the primary infection.

TUBERCULOUS MENINGITIS. This is the most serious complication of TB. It generally follows primary pulmonary disease in infants and young children, usually developing within 6 months. Meningeal infection is also common in miliary TB. Caseous lesions can enlarge, encapsulate, and form a tuberculoma that can act just like any other CNS mass lesion.

SKIN TB. This variant is rare in the United States. It occurs in two forms: the TB chancre, and multiple skin lesions resulting from hematogenous spread. Ingestion of contaminated raw milk is the usual cause of this infection.

TUBERCULOSIS OF THE EYE. Ocular structures such as the cornea, choroid, retina, iris, sclera, and conjunctiva are most commonly involved. Bacilli usually reach the eye by hematogenous spread. Infected upper respiratory secretions can spread to the cornea, sclera, and conjunctiva by sneezing or by contaminated fingers. Yellow-gray nodules appear at the posterior pole or palpebral conjunctiva. Coalescence of the nodules can form small ulcers. Phlyctenular conjunctivitis, small jelly-like gray nodules seen on the conjunctiva, is the result of a hypersensitivity reaction.

HEMATOGENOUS SPREAD OF TUBERCULOSIS TO OTHER ORGANS OR BODY SYSTEMS. Spread can be to endocrine and exocrine glands, urogenital tract, heart and pericardium, skeleton, abdomen, tonsils, adenoids, larynx, middle ear, and mastoids.

Management

The AAP (1997) recommends the use of the following drugs and treatment regimen based on disease state:

Drug	Daily Dose
Isoniazid (I)	10 mg/kg prevention (maximum, 300 mg);
	10 to 15 mg/kg treatment (maximum, 300 mg)
Rifampin (R)	10 to 20 mg/kg (maximum, 600 mg)
Pyrazinamide (Z)	20 to 40 mg/kg (maximum, 2000 mg)
Streptomycin (S)	20 to 40 mg/kg (maximum 1000 mg)
Ethambutol (E)	15 to 25 mg/kg (maximum, 2500 mg)

Drug	Twice-weekly dose
I	20 to 30 mg/kg/dose (maximum, 900 mg)
R	10 to 20 mg/kg/dose (maximum, 600 mg)
Z	50 mg/kg/dose (maximum, 2000 mg)
S	20 to 40 mg/kg/dose (maximum, 1000 mg)

Disease State	Regimen
Prophylactic treatment (asymptomatic infection with positive skin test only)	6-9 months of isoniazid (I) daily (I susceptible). 9 months I and R; if resistant, consult TB specialist
Pulmonary disease	6-month regimen (standard): 2 months of I, R, and Z daily followed by 4 months of I and R daily or 2 months of I, R, and Z daily followed by 4 months of I and R twice weekly. 9-month regimen (for hilar adenopathy only): 9 months of I and R daily or 1 month of I and R daily followed by 8 months of I and R twice weekly
Meningitis, miliary, bone, and infection	2 months of I, R, Z, and S daily followed by 10 months of I and R daily (12 months total) or 2 months of I, R, Z, and S daily followed by 10 months of I and R twice weekly (12 months total)
Extrapulmonary other than meningitis, miliary, bone, or joint	Same as pulmonary disease

In situations in which compliance with daily therapy cannot be ensured, twice-weekly administration of medication can be considered after 2 months of daily therapy (1 mo prevention). Patients with HIV infection should be treated for at least 3 months initially and continued for a minimum of 9 months thereafter. They should be treated for at least 6 months after documented cure with three negative cultures.

TEMPERATURE AND FEVER

Fever is defined as an abnormally elevated body temperature with a temperature of 38°C (100.4°F) or higher or 38.2°C (100.8°F) or higher considered a fever by most practitioners.

Fever results from a resetting of the hypothalamic heat regulatory center or when heat production exceeds heat loss. Peripheral warm and cold neurons and the temperature of blood circulating in the hypothalamus act on the heat regulatory center to keep the human body at a preset core temperature of 37°C (98.6°F). Axillary temperature may be 1°F lower. Body temperature is lower in the morning and peaks in the late afternoon. The human body generates heat by metabolic processes (increased cellular metabolism, muscle activity, and involuntary shivering). Heat conservation is maintained by vasoconstriction and heat preference behaviors. Heat loss occurs by sweating, evaporation, conduction, radiation, convection, vasodilatation, and cold preference behaviors. These factor inputs are integrated by the heat regulatory mechanism to keep the human body at 98.6°F ± 3.18°F (Behrman et al., 1996). The normal hypothalamic setpoint is altered by many different agents. Fever is caused by bacterial and viral infections, vaccines, biological agents, tissue damage, malignancy, drugs, collagen-vascular disorders, endocrine disorders, inflammatory disorders, and other disease states.

Fever-causing agents produce endogenous pyrogens that reset the hypothalamic center. This process takes approximately 90 minutes. Clinically, this means that blood cultures should be obtained before the fever spikes, as there would be a greater bacterial or fungal yield.

A temperature of 107°F or higher is considered a harmful fever and has the potential complication of death or brain damage if not treated (Berlin, 1996). The increased metabolic processes can exacerbate problems in children with chronic illness.

Fever is the most common presenting complaint in pediatric practice. There are two situations that are particularly worrisome for any NP: fever without source in infants and young children and fever of unknown origin. Each of these situations is discussed separately, and guidelines for their management are given.

Fever Without Source in Infants and Young Children

Managing fever without source in infants and young children is a challenge. The assessment of the child who has an acute fever often involves a careful investigation for a source of infection. Potential differential diagnoses include the following:

- Upper respiratory tract disease such as viral URI, otitis media, and sinusitis
- Lower respiratory tract disease such as bronchiolitis and pneumonia
- Gastrointestinal disease, primarily bacterial, or gastroenteritis
- Musculoskeletal infections such as cellulitis, septic arthritis, and osteomyelitis
- Urinary tract infection
- Bacteremia
- Meningitis

Research studies and analysis of data have established practice guidelines for the outpatient management of infants and children from 0 to 36 months of age (Prober, 1999; Baker et al., 1993; Baraff et al., 1993). The practice guidelines of Baraff and colleagues for the management of infants and children 0 to 36 months of age with fever without source include the following definitions:

1. Fever is defined as a temperature of 38.0°C or greater
2. Fever without source is defined as "an acute febrile illness in which the etiology of the fever is not apparent after careful history and physical examination"
3. An infant or young child is considered *low risk* if the following clinical and laboratory low-risk criteria are met:

   - Clinical—previous good health (no chronic illnesses, prematurity, previous hospitalizations); no focal bacterial infection on examination (except otitis media); negative laboratory screening; nontoxic clinical appearance; and reliable parents who can manage the child as an outpatient;
   - Laboratory—WBC count 5 to 15,000 mm^3, fewer than 1500 bands/mm^3; normal urinalysis (fewer than 5 WBCs/hpf); and, when diarrhea is present, <5 WBCs/hpf in stool

The practice guidelines of Baraff and colleagues recommend the following management strategy:

1. Hospitalization of all toxic-appearing 0- to 36-month-old infants and children for parenteral antibiotic therapy after prompt laboratory workup.
2. Febrile infants younger than 28 days of age, regardless of whether they meet the low-risk criteria identified above, should have a sepsis evaluation (culture of CSF, blood, and catheterized or suprapubic urine specimen; a CBC and differential and complete analysis of the CSF) and hospitalization for parenteral antibiotics.
3. Infants 28 to 90 days old who are nontoxic-appearing and meet the low-risk criteria listed above can be managed as outpatients with use of either an option 1 or an option 2 strategy, discussed later. Febrile infants 28 to 90 days old who do not meet the laboratory low-risk criteria should be hospitalized.

OPTION 1

- Blood and urine cultures
- Lumbar puncture
- Ceftriaxone at 50 mg/kg IM (maximum 1 g) after laboratory tests are drawn
- Return visit within 24 hours or sooner if worse; a second injection of ceftriaxone can be given in 18 to 24 hours if cultures are pending; and if otitis media is present, give oral amoxicillin at 40 mg/kg per day for 10 days

OPTION 2

- Urine culture
- Careful observation

4. Hospitalize all toxic-appearing children 91 days to 36 months of age for sepsis workup and parenteral antibiotics.
5. Children 91 days to 36 months of age can be managed as outpatients using the low-risk criteria as follows:

FEVER LOWER THAN 39.0°C

- No laboratory test or antibiotics if the fever without source of infection is less than 39.0°C
- Prescribe acetaminophen 15 mg/kg per dose every 4 hours for fever
- Return if fever persists longer than 48 hours or child is worse

FEVER HIGHER THAN 39.0°C

- Urine culture: boys younger than 6 months of age; girls younger than 2 years of age
- Stool culture if diarrhea (positive if blood and mucus in stool or ≥5 WBCs/hpf)
- WBC count
- Blood culture: option 1, do on all children if fever ≥39.0°C; option 2, do only if fever ≥39.0°C and WBC count ≥15,000
- Chest radiograph if respiratory symptoms
- Antibiotic therapy with ceftriaxone pending cultures: option 1, all children if temperature ≥39.0°C; option 2, if temperature ≥39.0°C and WBC count ≥15,000
- Acetaminophen 15 mg/kg per dose every 4 hours if temperature ≥39.0°C
- Follow up in 24 to 48 hours

An important point to remember in treatment is that bacteremia can be an occult infection in young infants and children. A useful axiom to remember is that the higher the WBC and the greater the absolute number of neutrophils or bands, the greater the risk of bacteremia in a febrile child. Remember that all toxic-appearing infants need immediate hospitalization. Also the younger the infant, the greater the uncertainty about the possibility of a serious bacterial infection and the need to rule out this possibility. Parents of infants who are managed as outpatients need detailed instructions on signs and symptoms that indicate a worsening of their infants' illness. Instruct parents to bring their infant in immediately if any of these signs and symptoms appear: change in or new rash; duskiness, cyanosis, or mottling; coolness of extremities, poor feeding or vomiting; irritability; difficulty in comforting or arousing; seizure activity (eye rolling or jerking of extremities); or bulging anterior fontanel. Careful follow-up of such infants must be assured (Prober, 1999).

Fever of Unknown Origin (FUO)

The definition of FUO is variable; however, when a child has a prolonged fever (>38.5°C) for more than 2 weeks without an apparent cause or a noninfectious etiology, this is considered an FUO. The approach to infectious disease outlined in this chapter is the best approach to finally establishing the diagnosis. A child with an FUO requires that the health caregivers frequently rethink and reevaluate historical, clinical, and laboratory data. Many FUOs are atypical presentations of common disorders. Few are exotic. Infectious diseases, collagen-vascular disease, malignancies, and Münchausen syndrome by proxy are included in the differential diagnosis of an FUO.

The approach to evaluating a child with an FUO should include a detailed history, thorough physical examination, and screening laboratory studies.

HISTORY

- Careful analysis of any appearance of symptom or sign, a meticulous review of systems, and history of the fever pattern
- Past medical history of recurrent infections, surgery, transfusions, travel, and contact with ill individuals
- Medication use and family medical history, including autoimmune disease or inflammatory bowel disorder

PHYSICAL EXAMINATION

- Skin findings (e.g., rashes, lesions)
- Local or generalized lymphadenopathy or hepatosplenomegaly
- Joint examination and palpation of bones
- Palpation of sinus and mastoid areas
- Eye examination looking for conjunctivitis, and ophthalmologic examination if juvenile arthritis suspected
- Pelvic examination in adolescent females
- Rectal examination and guaiac test

SCREENING LABORATORY STUDIES

- CBC with differential
- Urinalysis plus blood and urine cultures
- PPD with controls
- Chest and sinus radiographs
- Liver chemistries
- Serum protein analysis
- Heterophil antibody and antinuclear antibody titer in older children

MONITORING OR HOSPITALIZATION

If the child is systemically ill, failing to thrive, or very young, hospitalization is appropriate. Otherwise, the child should be followed up with frequent visits, documented fever pattern, and other specialized tests if screening tests indicate the need or if other physical findings develop (Nizet et al., 1994).

REFERENCES

American Academy of Pediatrics (AAP): 1997 Red Book: Report of the Committee on Infectious Diseases, 24th ed. Elk Grove Village, IL, 1997.

American Academy of Pediatrics: Palivizumab, a humanized respiratory syncytial virus monoclonal antibody, reduces hospitalization from respiratory syncytial virus infection in high-risk infants. Pediatrics 102: 531-537, 1998

Baker MD, Bell LM, Avner JR: Outpatient management without antibiotics of fever in selected infants. N Engl J Med 329: 1437-1441, 1993.

Baraff LJ, Bass JW, Fleisher GR, et al: Practice guidelines for the management of infants and children 0 to 36 months of age with fever without source. Pediatrics 92: 1-12, 1993.

Behrman RE, Nelson WE (eds). Nelson Textbook of Pediatrics, 14th ed. Philadelphia, WB Saunders, 1992.

Behrman RE, Kliegman R, Arvin AM, et al: Nelson Textbook of Pediatrics, 15th ed. Philadelphia: WB Saunders; 1996.

Berlin CM: Fever in children: A practical approach to management. Contemp Pediatr (suppl): 1-8, 1996.

Brownstein A, Fricke W: HIV transmission between adolescent brothers with hemophilia. MMWR Morb Mortal Wkly Rep 42: 948-951, 1993.

Centers for Disease Control and Prevention: 1993 revised classification system for HIV infection and expanded case surveillance for AIDS among adolescents and adults. MMWR Morb Mortal Wkly Rep 41:1-19, 1992.

Centers for Disease Control and Prevention: Recommendations of the US Public Health Service Task Force on the use of zidovudine to reduce perinatal transmission of human immunodeficiency virus. MMWR Morb Mortal Wkly Rep: Recommendations Rep, 43:1-20, 1994a.

Centers for Disease Control and Prevention: 1994 Revised classification system for human immunodeficiency virus infection in children less than 13 years of age. MMWR Morb Mortal Wkly Rep: Recommendations Rep 43:1-10, 1994b.

Centers for Disease Control and Prevention: Recommended childhood immunization schedule—United States, January-December 1999. MMWR Morb Mortal Wkly Rep 48:8-16, 1999.

Chu SY, Buehler JW, Fleming PL, et al: Epidemiology of reported cases of AIDS in lesbians, United States 1980-1989. Am J Public Health 80:1380-1381, 1990.

Coffin SE, Offit PA: At last: A vaccine for rotavirus. Contemp Pediatr 16:105-116, 1999.

Dowell SR, Marcy SM, Philips WR, et al: Otitis media—principles of judicious use of antimicrobial agents. Pediatrics 101:165-171, 1998a.

Dowell SR, Marcy SM, Philips WR, et al: Principles of judicious use of antimicrobial agents for pediatric upper respiratory tract infection. Pediatrics 101: 163-165, 1998b.

Fitzgibbon JE, Guar S, Frenkel LD, et al: Transmission from one child to another of human immunodeficiency virus type 1 with zidovudine-resistance mutation. N Engl J Med 329:1835-1841, 1993.

Greenberger NJ: Issues in Hepatitis. National Hepatitis Detection, Treatment and Prevention Program, Special Bulletin, Fall 1993.

Harris N, Edwards K: A progress report on hepatitis A vaccination. Contemp Pediatr 15:64-69, 1998.

Hay WW, Groothuis JR, Hayward AR, et al (eds): Current Pediatric Diagnosis and Treatment, 14th ed. Norwalk, CT: Appleton & Lange, 1999.

Humiston S, Atkinson W: 1998 Immunization schedule changes and clarifications. Pediatric Ann 26:6, 1998.

Legal Economic Guidelines: Bloodborne Pathogens: Exposure and Risk Reduction Based Upon OSHA Bloodborne Pathogen Standard. North Miami; FL, Physician's Update ENSA Continuing Education, March 1993.

Levin MJ: Infections: Viral and rickettsial. In Hay WW, Hayward AR, Levin MJ, et al (eds): Current Pediatric Diagnosis and Treatment, 14th ed: Stamford, CT: Appleton & Lange, 1999, pp 960-994.

National Institute of Health Press Release: CDC reports first-ever decline in AIDS diagnosis. US Department of Health and Human Services Press Release. September 18, 1997. Website: http://www.HIVpositive.com/f.drugadvisories/nih-nov97/hhs-pr.htm

Nizet V, Vinci RJ, Lovejoy, FH: Fever in children. Pediatr Rev 15:127-135, 1994.

O'Brien KL, Dowell SR, Schwartz B, et al: Acute sinusitis—principles of judicious use of antimicrobial agents. Pediatrics 101:174-177, 1998a.

O'Brien KL, Dowell SR, Schwartz B, et al: Cough illness/bronchitis—principles of judicious use of antimicrobial agents. Pediatrics 101:178-181, 1998b.

Peter J, Ray CG: Infectious mononucleosis. Pediatr Rev 19:276-279, 1998.

Prober CG: Managing the febrile infant: No rules are golden. Contemp Pediatr 16:48-55, 1999.

Rogers MF, White CR, Sanders R, et al: Lack of transmission of human immunodeficiency virus from infected children to their household contacts. Pediatrics 85:210-214, 1990.

Rosenstein N, Philips WR, Gerber MA, et al: The common cold—principles of judicious use of antimicrobial agents. Pediatrics 101:182-183, 1998.

Schwartz B, Marcy DM, Philips WR, et al: Pharyngitis—principles of judicious use of antimicrobial agents. Pediatrics 101:171-174, 1998.

Sokol RJ, Narkewicz MR: Liver and pancreas. *In* Hay WW, Hayward AR, Levin MJ, et al: Current Pediatric Diagnosis & Treatment, 14th ed. Stamford, CT: Appleton & Lange, 1999, pp 559-598.

US Department of Health and Human Services: Put Prevention Into Practice: Clinician's Handbook of Preventive Services, 2nd ed. Bethesda, MD: International Medical Publishing Inc., 1990.

Zaoutis T, Klein JD: Enterovirus infections. Pediatr Rev 19: 183-191, 1998.

CHAPTER 25

Atopic Disorders and Rheumatic Diseases

Margaret A. Brady

▩ INTRODUCTION

Atopic disorders and rheumatic diseases of children share certain characteristics that lend to their combined discussion in this chapter. Inflammation, chronicity, and genetic predisposition are common to both groups of disorders. The triad of atopic disorders that may or may not coexist includes atopic dermatitis, allergic rhinitis, and asthma.

The two most common childhood rheumatic diseases are juvenile arthritis (JA) and systemic lupus erythematosus (SLE). Both are collagen-vascular disorders that nurse practitioners (NPs) are likely to encounter in their practice. Fibromyalgia is a rheumatic disease that is gaining attention in the literature. Brief discussions of this disease as well as chronic fatigue syndrome are presented. Finally, although the incidence of rheumatic fever has diminished significantly in the United States, it is still a disease that merits attention by NPs; therefore, review of its clinical presentation and treatment also is included.

▩ ANATOMY AND PHYSIOLOGY

Information related to the anatomy and physiology of the organ systems involved in atopic disorders and rheumatic diseases is contained in Chapters 31, 32, 37, and 38.

▩ PATHOPHYSIOLOGY AND DEFENSE MECHANISMS

Atopic or Allergic Disorders

Allergy results as part of a specific acquired alteration in the body that has an immunological basis. The union of antigen and antibody creates a cascade of events that culminates in biochemical reactions. There are four types of allergic reactions: I (anaphylactic reactions), II (cytotoxic reactions), III (Arthus-type reactions), and IV (delayed-type hypersensitivity). All four types of allergic reactions are mediated by circulating or cellular antibodies and generally can occur in any individual. In contrast, atopic disorders are forms of allergic reactivity that occur only in certain susceptible individuals with some unknown and probably genetic predisposition. Certain antigens (e.g., cat dander, ragweed) are problematic for atopic individuals but not for others. These atopic individuals become sensitized to the offending allergen, and an atopic disorder is the end result.

The development of an atopic disorder or allergic response involves a susceptible individual who is both exposed to an offending antigen and has a predisposition to selective synthesis of immunoglobulin E (IgE) when in contact with common environmental antigens. If these conditions are in place and contact with an offending antigen occurs, the following biochemical chain of cascading events unfolds:

- CD4 cells, that is, lymphocytes (TH_2-like cells), respond to an antigen-presenting cell by producing cytokines: interleukin (IL)-4, IL-5, and IL-13.
- Cytokines are involved in IgE synthesis and activation of eosinophils.
- IgE binds to receptors on mast cells, basophils, and Langerhans cells.
- Chemical mediators that cause biochemical reactions and allergic-related injury to target organs (skin and respiratory tract) are released. Examples of chemical mediators include
  - Histamine
  - Prostaglandins
  - Leukotrienes
  - Eosinophil chemotactic factor of anaphylaxis
  - High-molecular-weight neutrophil chemotactic factor
  - Platelet-activating factor
  - Arachidonic acid—cyclooxygenase and lipoxygenase products

The end result of this biochemical process is tissue injury of a target organ. Examples of tissue injury include inflammation and hyperresponsiveness, resulting in such symptoms as obstruction, increased mucus discharge, and pruritus.

Immediate allergic reactions can involve sneezing, hives, wheezing, vomiting, or anaphylaxis. Acute reactions can be followed by a late-phase response resulting from the release of toxic mediators by activated eosinophils and mononuclear cells recruited to the site of the acute allergic reaction (Boguniewicz & Leung, 1999).

The pathogenesis of atopic diseases involves a complex interrelationship of genetic, environmental, and immunological factors. The main defense mechanism to protect against atopic disorders is the elimination of the offending substance to prevent IgE development and antigen–antibody interaction. For example, if there is a family history of atopic disorders, breastfeeding offers the protection of limited exposure to cow's milk protein and the benefit of maternal IgA and IgG antibodies. Once chemical mediators are released, the body's protective responses reduce inflammation and repair tissue damage. Pharmacological therapy cannot cure atopic disorders but reduces symptoms and checks the allergic process. For example, drugs may be used to control inflammation (corticosteroids), compete with histamine for receptor sites on target tissues (antihistamines), and prevent mast cell degranulation and mediator release (cromolyn sodium).

Rheumatic Diseases

Juvenile arthritis is the term currently used in the United States to describe a group of conditions involving chronic inflammation of synovial joints in children younger than 16 years of age. The British use the term *chronic juvenile arthritis* (CJA) to describe these same conditions. Both JA and SLE are connective tissue disorders marked by inflammatory changes in connective tissues throughout various parts of the body. The exact cause of these collagen diseases is unknown; however, an autoimmune basis is postulated as a key factor in rheumatic disease.

There is no natural defense mechanism identified to prevent either of these diseases; however, periods of remission do occur in some children with SLE for unknown reasons, and many children with JA achieve complete remission with puberty. Because inflammation is a significant factor in these two rheumatic diseases of childhood, administration of corticosteroid preparations is a key therapy to control inflammation responsible for tissue injury.

Considerations in the Pathogenesis of Juvenile Arthritis

The exact etiology of most forms of JA is unknown; however, there are two theories about its causation. Genetics is believed to be a predisposing factor to most forms of this disorder. JA associated with clinical findings of iritis and the production of antinuclear antibodies is found in children with histocompatibility complex antigens—human leukocyte antigen (HLA)-

DR5. Children with seropositive, polyarticular disease are found to have HLA-DR4. Infectious agents also have been implicated in JA, including *Yersinia enterocolitica* and related enteric pathogens and *Klebsiella.*

The pathophysiology of JA is marked by proliferation of macrophage-like and fibroblastoid synoviocytes with subsequent infiltration of neutrophils and lymphocytes, evidence of autoimmunity, and cytokine production. The end-result is nonsuppurative inflammation of the synovium that can lead to articular cartilage and joint structure erosion. Children with JA have no demonstrable immunodeficiency (Hollister, 1999; O'Neil, 1998a).

Considerations in the Pathogenesis of Systemic Lupus Erythematosus

Various immune phenomena are associated with SLE, including altered immunological reactions in the T- and B-lymphocyte function. There is a strong link between a faulty immune mechanism and SLE. The disease is sometimes familial. Approximately 20% of children with SLE have a first-degree relative with the disease, and more than 50% of monozygotic twins are concordant for SLE. This familial pattern suggests altered cellular immunity in genetically predisposed individuals as a key factor in the pathogenesis of SLE.

There is an HLA and complement deficiency association with SLE. Other factors such as hormones (in patients older than 10 years, SLE is ninefold more common in females than males and is often precipitated by menarche, oral contraceptive use, or pregnancy), infectious agents (viral agents mostly), temperate climates, exposure to ultraviolet light, and certain drugs (e.g., hydralazine and procainamide) seem to play a role in its pathogenesis. Characteristic pathological findings include the production of numerous autoantibodies and impairment in the normal suppression of autoreactive B-cell clones. Immune complexes are abundant and their clearance may be impaired. In addition, the deposition of immune complexes causes inflammation of the endothelium of blood vessels leading to vasculitis in many organs that results in ischemic damage (O'Neil, 1998b).

ASSESSMENT

History

Additional key factors to consider in the history of a child who has an atopic disorder include the following:

- A family history or personal history of allergies, asthma, atopic dermatitis (eczema), hay fever, or allergic rhinitis is frequently found.
- Pruritus is a significant finding in atopic dermatitis and allergic rhinitis.
- The rash of atopic dermatitis is characteristically found in certain locations of the body.
- Nighttime coughing and wheezing are characteristic of asthma.
- Signs and symptoms of allergic rhinitis and asthma may be associated with certain allergens or key triggering agents and may be seasonal.
- Coughing or shortness of breath with exercise or exertion is characteristic of asthma.

Additional key factors to consider in the history of a child who has a rheumatic disease include the following:

- History of a characteristic rash or joint involvement, or both, is common.
- The child can have other systemic manifestations of disease.

Physical Examination

The physical examination sections in Chapters 31, 32, 37, and 38 should be reviewed.

Diagnostic Studies

Various diagnostic studies or procedures can be used in the outpatient evaluation and management of children with either atopic disorders or rheumatic diseases.

ATOPIC DISORDERS. Chest radiographs can be useful in selected cases of asthma or suspected asthma: in a child with atypical signs or symptoms; if a secondary infection does not clear with standard therapy; or if there are signs and symptoms of significant pulmonary involvement. Routine chest radiographs are not indicated in most children with asthma.

Pulmonary function tests, such as peak expiratory flow (PEF) rate and pulse oximetry, can provide additional information useful to the diagnosis and management of asthma.

Eosinophil count, determination of serum IgE concentration, and radioallergosorbent test (RAST) or prick test are not needed to confirm the diagnosis nor to monitor treatment of the majority of children with an atopic disorder.

RHEUMATIC DISEASES. Laboratory blood studies, including antinuclear antibodies (ANA), anti-DNA antibody, and determination of serum complement levels, are common tests ordered in children with SLE. Other related blood and serological laboratory studies are indicated, depending on organ involvement (e.g., renal involvement is a frequent complication). A positive rheumatoid factor by latex fixation, ANA, or erythrocyte sedimentation rate (ESR) may be useful markers in JA.

Imaging studies are done to assess and manage joint pathology.

MANAGEMENT STRATEGIES

The atopic disorders and rheumatoid diseases tend to be chronic conditions with exacerbation and remission of symptoms. Individual management strategies are based on the specific disease process and are discussed in each of their respective sections. However, certain key concepts apply to these conditions.

General Measures

The following general measures should be taken in the management of atopic disorders and rheumatic diseases:

- Encourage self-care and learning about one's disease
- Address issues of living with a chronic disease, such as
  ○ School, peer, and family dynamics
  ○ Body image
  ○ Adolescent adjustment
  ○ Patient–parent role in management of a long-term illness or chronic condition

Medications

The control of inflammation associated with atopic disorders and rheumatoid diseases is a key principle in the management of these illnesses. Corticosteroids, whether used topically on the skin, inhaled via the nostrils or throat, taken orally for systemic effect, or taken intramuscularly or intravenously for rapid systemic absorption, are a mainstay of treatment. Other pharmacological agents commonly used are as follows:

- For atopic conditions:
  ○ Antipruritic agents—to control itching
  ○ Antihistamines—to control symptoms associated with the release of chemical mediators
  ○ Anticholinergics—to reduce vagal tone in the airways (may also decrease mucous gland secretion)
  ○ Bronchodilators—to control bronchospasm
  ○ Cromolyn sodium and nedocromil—to inhibit mast cell release of histamine
  ○ Leukotriene modifiers—to disrupt the synthesis or function of leukotrienes
  ○ Antibiotics—to treat secondary infections
- For rheumatic diseases:
  ○ Analgesics (salicylates or nonsteroidal agents)—to relieve arthritis or joint pain; to relieve pain in general
  ○ Other therapeutic agents—to relieve signs and symptoms specific to the disease process and organ system involvement

Parent and Patient Education

Both patients and parents need to be instructed about the following:

- Signs and symptoms necessitating the immediate reevaluation of the child
- Medications—clear instructions are needed on how much to give, when to give, side effects to watch for, how to administer, and how long medication should be taken.
- Correct administration of inhaled medications (e.g., when two puffs or sprays are ordered, the child should activate one puff or spray then inhale followed by a second puff or spray and second inhalation. A parent or child may think incorrectly that be-

ing told to take two puffs or two sprays means to activate two puffs or sprays and then inhale.)

- Any other measures relevant to the treatment plan (e.g., bathing instructions, monitoring peak flow rate, avoidance of allergens, and environmental control).
- Parent support groups and professional organizations and resource groups.

SPECIFIC IMMUNOLOGICAL PROBLEMS OF CHILDREN: COMMON ATOPIC DISORDERS

Asthma

DESCRIPTION

Asthma is a chronic respiratory disease and is characterized by the following features (National Heart, Lung, and Blood Institute [NHLBI], 1997; Boguniewicz & Leung, 1999):

- Immunohistopathological responses produce
  - Shedding of airway epithelium and collagen deposition beneath the basement membrane
  - Edema
  - Mast cell activation
  - Inflammatory infiltration by eosinophils, lymphocytes (TH$_2$-like cells), and neutrophils (especially in fatal asthma)
- Airway inflammation contributes to airflow limitations including
  - Acute bronchoconstriction
  - Airway edema
  - Mucus plug formation
- Persistent inflammation can result in airway wall remodeling and irreversible changes. Airflow obstruction is often reversible, either spontaneously or with treatment.
- Airway inflammation also triggers hyperresponsiveness (to any of a variety of stimuli, such as physical, chemical, or pharmacological agents, allergens, exercise, cold air) and is a factor in disease chronicity

Asthma in children is classified as mild intermittent, mild persistent, moderate persistent, or severe persistent depending on symptoms, recurrences, need for specific medications, and pulmonary function measurements (Table 25–1). Children classified at any level of asthma can have episodes involving mild, moderate or severe exacerbations. Exacerbations involve progressive worsening of shortness of breath, cough, wheezing, chest tightness, or any combination of these symptoms. The degree of airway hyperresponsiveness is usually related to the severity of asthma. Children younger than 5 years of age experience greater airway hyperresponsiveness than do older children.

Many children experience early- and late-phase responses to their asthma episode. The early asthmatic response (EAR) phase is characterized by activation of mast cells and their mediators, with bronchospasm being the key feature. EAR starts within 20 to 30 minutes of mast cell activation and resolves within approximately 1 hour if the individual is removed from the offending allergen. The late-phase asthmatic response is a prolonged inflammatory state that usually follows the EAR within a few hours, is often associated with respiratory symptoms more severe than the EAR presentation, and can last from hours to days (May, 1998).

Exercise-induced bronchospasm describes the phenomenon of airway narrowing during or minutes after the onset of vigorous activity. Most asthmatics exhibit airway hyperirritability after rigorous activity and display exercise-induced bronchospasm. However, for some children, exercise is the only stimulus that triggers their asthma. Although asthma is not always associated with an allergic disorder in children, many pediatric patients with chronic asthma have an allergic component. For this reason, asthma is discussed in this chapter.

ETIOLOGY AND INCIDENCE

It is not known for certain whether hyperresponsiveness of the airways is present at birth in genetically predisposed children or acquired. However, the genetic predisposition for the development of an IgE-mediated response to common aeroallergens, known as atopy, remains the strongest identifiable predisposing risk factor for asthma.

The morbidity and mortality statistics of asthma in childhood demonstrate an alarming

T A B L E 25-1

Classification of Asthma Severity in Children: Clinical Features Before Treatment

CLASSIFICATION & STEP	SYMPTOMS*	NIGHTTIME SYMPTOMS	LUNG FUNCTION
Step 1: Mild intermittent	Symptoms ≤2 times per wk Asymptomatic and normal PEF between exacerbations Exacerbations brief (few hr or d); varying intensity	≤2 times per mo	FEV_1 or PEF ≥80% predicted PEF variability <20%
Step 2: Mild persistent	Symptoms >2 times per wk but <1 time per d Exacerbations may affect activity	>2 times per mo	FEV_1 or PEF ≥80% predicted PEF variability 20–30%
Step 3: Moderate persistent	Daily symptoms Daily use of inhaled short-acting β₂-agonist Exacerbations affect activity, ≥2 times per week; may last days	>1 time per wk	FEV_1 or PEF >60%; ≤80% predicted PEF variability >30%
Step 4: Severe persistent	Continual symptoms Limited physical activity Frequent exacerbations	Frequent	FEV_1 or PEF ≤60% predicted PEF variability >30%

*Having at least one symptom in a particular step places the child in that particular classification.
FEV_1 = forced expiratory volume in 1 second; PEF = peak expiratory flow.
Adapted from Highlights of the Expert Panel Report 2: Guidelines for the Diagnosis and Management of Asthma (National Heart, Lung, and Blood Institute [NHLBI] Publication No. 97-4051). Bethesda, MD, National Institutes of Health, 1997.

increase in the prevalence of asthma and its complications. Asthma has become a leading reason for pediatric hospital admissions and accounts for more than 2 million visits annually to pediatric settings (Nimmagadda & Evans, 1999). Occupational or environmental exposure can cause airway inflammation associated with asthma. Factors known to precipitate or aggravate asthma in children include the following:

- Atopic individual response to allergens—inhaled, topical, ingested
- Viral infections
- Exposure to known irritants (paint fumes, smoke) and occupational chemicals
- Gastroesophageal reflux
- Exposure to tobacco smoke (for infants, especially smoking by mother)
- Environmental changes—rapid changes in barometric pressure, weather, especially cold air
- Exercise

- Psychological factors (e.g., anxiety attack or panic disorder)
- Allergic rhinitis and sinusitis
- Emotional stress (both positive and negative emotions)
- Drugs (e.g., aspirin, β-blockers)
- Food additives (sulfites)
- Endocrine factors

Allergen-induced asthma results in hyperresponsive airways. The majority of children with asthma show evidence of sensitization to any of the following inhalant allergens:

- House dust mites, cockroaches, indoor molds
- Saliva and dander of cats and dogs
- Outdoor seasonal molds
- Airborne pollens—trees, grasses, and weeds

Food allergens (cow's milk protein) can cause asthma but are generally problematic only in infants. The mechanism by which allergens cause asthma is explained in the earlier section on pathophysiology and defense mechanisms (Boguniewicz & Leung, 1999).

CLINICAL FINDINGS

History

The history of a patient being seen for asthma can include the following:

- Family history of asthma or other related allergic disorders (e.g., eczema, hay fever, or allergic rhinitis)
- Conditions associated with asthma (e.g., chronic sinusitis, nasal polyposis, and chronic otitis media)
- Complaints of chest tightness
- Cough, particularly at night and in the early morning
- Cough or shortness of breath with exercise or exertion
- Seasonal, continuous, or episodic pattern of symptoms
- Episodes of recurrent "bronchitis" or pneumonia
- Precipitation of symptoms by known aggravating factors

Physical Examination

The following may be seen on physical examination:

- Wheezing (may be absent if severe obstruction), dyspnea, coughing
- Prolonged expiratory phase, high-pitched rhonchi
- Diminished breath sounds
- Signs of respiratory distress, including retractions, nasal flaring, use of accessory muscles, increasing restlessness, apprehension, agitation, drowsiness to coma
- Tachycardia, hypertension or hypotension, pulsus paradoxus
- Cyanosis of lips and nail beds if underlying hypoxemia
- Other possible associated findings include sinusitis, flexural eczema, and rhinitis

Diagnostic Studies

Use of various laboratory and radiographic tests should be individualized to the child and based on symptoms, severity or chronology of the disease, response to therapy, and age. Tests to consider include the following:

- A complete blood count (CBC) if secondary infection or anemia is suspected (also check for elevated numbers of eosinophils)
- Chest radiograph *only* if secondary respiratory infection or other pulmonary disorders are suspected
- Sinus radiograph if sinusitis is suspected
- Allergic workup, including skin testing, immunoglobulins, or RAST
- Sweat test if cystic fibrosis is a possibility
- Pulmonary function tests
  - Start with PEF rate assessment in children 4 to 5 years of age or older: used to assess the severity of airflow obstruction and to monitor the effectiveness of β-agonist treatment (measurements before and after treatments)
  - Consider the use of more sophisticated pulmonary studies for the child with severe asthma

Pulmonary monitoring and typical findings include the following:

- Can use PEF rate in some children as young as 4 to 5 years. Use child's personal best value as a guideline to help detect possible changes in airway obstruction; can use predicted range for height and age if personal best rate is not available (Table 25-2 and Fig. 25-1).
- Interpretation of PEF rate reading (see Table 25-3 for use of peak flow meter and interpretation of results)—if PEF rate is in the
  - Green zone: 80 to 100% of personal best signals good control
  - Yellow zone: 50 to 80% of personal best signals caution
  - Red zone: below 50% of personal best signals major airflow obstruction
- Oxygen saturation by pulse oximetry to assess severity of acute exacerbation: pulse oximetry measures the oxygen saturation (Sao_2) of hemoglobin—the percent of total

TABLE 25-2

Predicted Average Peak Expiratory Flow for Normal Children and Adolescents

HEIGHT (in)	MALES AND FEMALES (L/min)
43	147
44	160
45	173
46	187
47	200
48	214
49	227
50	240
51	254
52	267
53	280
54	293
55	307
56	320
57	334
58	347
59	360
60	373
61	387
62	400
63	413
64	427
65	440
66	454
67	467

Note: It is recommended that peak expiratory flow rate (PEFR) objectives for therapy be based on each individual's "personal best," which is established after a period of PEF rate monitoring while the individual is under effective treatment.

From National Heart, Lung, and Blood Institute: Executive Summary: Guidelines for the Diagnosis and Management of Asthma [Publication No. 94-3042A]. Bethesda MD, National Institutes of Health, 1994. Adapted from Polger G, Promedhar V: Pulmonary Function Testing in Children: Techniques and Standards. Philadelphia, WB Saunders, 1971.

hemoglobin that is oxygenated—as follows:
- ○ Greater than 95%, mild
- ○ 90% to 95%, moderate
- ○ Less than 90%, severe lack of oxygen
- • Chest radiograph findings: hyperinflation of the lungs with flattening of the diaphragm on radiograph with or without patchy infiltrate or atelectasis (Boguniewicz & Leung, 1999; May, 1998)

DIFFERENTIAL DIAGNOSIS

Numerous conditions can cause airway obstruction and be incorrectly confused with asthma, especially in young children and infants. Examples include the following:

- • Acute bronchiolitis, laryngotracheobronchitis, bronchopneumonia
- • Bronchial foreign body aspiration
- • Congenital malformations of the respiratory, cardiovascular, or gastrointestinal systems
- • Cystic fibrosis
- • Tracheal or foreign body compression (e.g., aortic ring, tumors)
- • Chronic lower respiratory tract infections caused by immunodeficiency disorders
- • Recurrent aspirations

TABLE 25-3

Use of the Peak Flow Meter and Its Interpretation

STEPS TO FOLLOW IN USING A PEAK FLOW METER
1. Have child stand up.
2. Make sure that indicator is at the base of the numbered scale.
3. Ask child to take a deep breath.
4. Have the child place the peak flow meter in the mouth with the lips sealing the mouthpiece.
5. Tell the child to blow out as hard and fast as possible.
6. Record the rate.
7. Repeat steps 2 through 6 two more times.
8. Record the highest of the three values.

PEAK EXPIRATORY FLOW RATE (PEFR)
The maximum flow rate that is produced during forced expiration with fully inflated lungs.

PERSONAL BEST VALUE
The highest value that an individual achieves in measuring PEFR is known as one's "personal best" value or rate. Using the personal best value is the most accurate gauge to use to interpret changes in peak flow measurements, as the child's own scores are used as the standard for comparison.

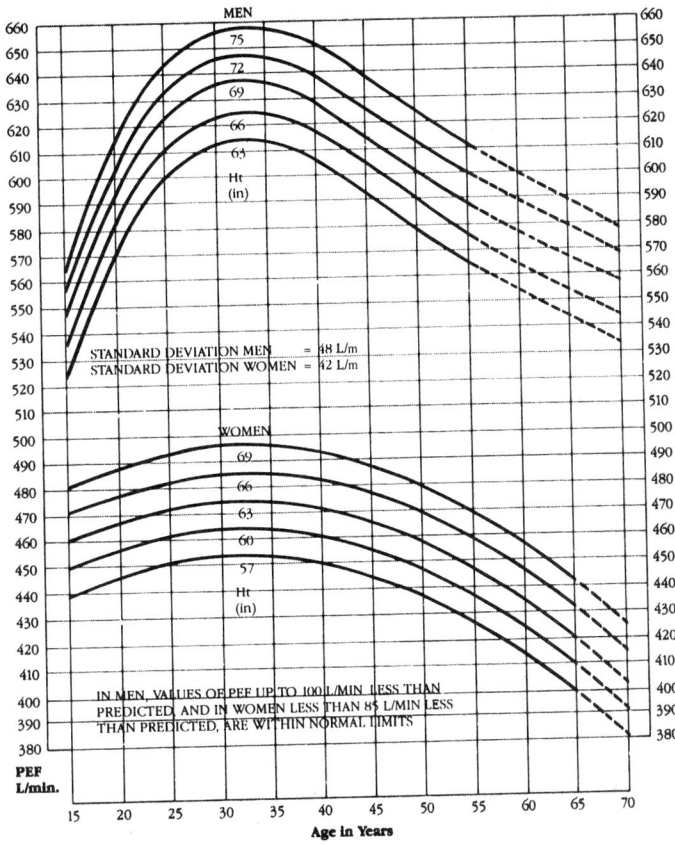

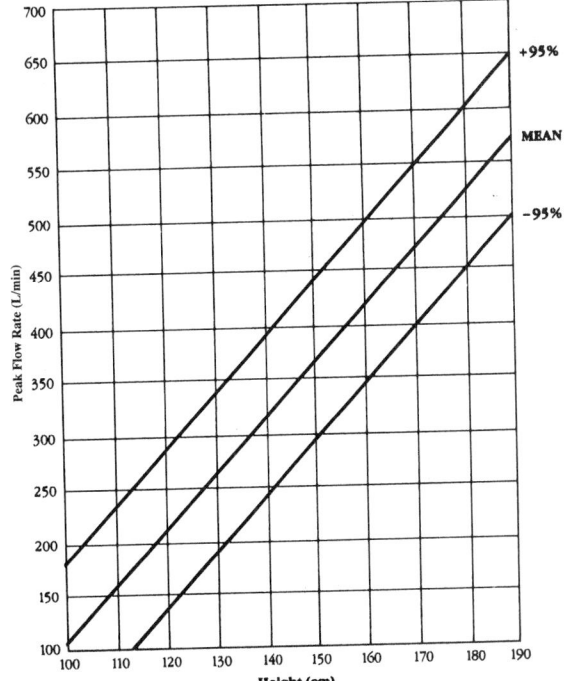

FIGURE 25-1

Sample peak expiratory flow rate nomogram. (From National Heart, Lung, and Blood Institute. Executive Summary: Guidelines for the Diagnosis and Management of Asthma [Publication No. 94-3042A]. Bethesda, MD, National Institutes of Health. *Top,* Adapted from Nunn AJ, Gregg I: New regression equations for predicting peak expiratory flow in adults. BMJ 298: 1068–1070, 1989. *Bottom,* Adapted from Godfrey S, Kamburoff PL, Nairn JR: Spirometry, lung volumes and airway resistance in normal children aged 5 to 18 years. Br J Dis Chest 64:15–24, 1970.)

MANAGEMENT

The *Highlights of the Expert Panel Report 2: Guidelines for the Diagnosis and Management of Asthma* (NHLBI, 1997) are the most recent standards for the treatment of asthma in children. Management strategies are based on whether the child has mild intermittent, mild persistent, moderate persistent, or severe persistent asthma. A stepwise approach is recommended. If control of symptoms is not maintained at a particular step of classification and management, the health-care provider first should reevaluate for compliance and administration factors. If these factors do not appear to be responsible for the lack of symptom control, then the health-care provider should go to the next higher step. Likewise, gradual stepdowns in treatment may be considered every 1 to 6 months.

In this chapter, the outpatient management of mild intermittent, mild persistent, moderate persistent, and severe asthma is discussed as is the outpatient management of acute exacerbations. The practitioner should refer to other textbooks for management of severe asthma requiring hospitalization.

Chronic Asthma

Treatment of chronic asthma in children is based on general control measures and pharmacotherapy.

General control measures include the following:

- Avoid exposure to known allergens or irritants.
- Administer yearly influenza vaccine.
- Control environment to eliminate or reduce offending allergen.
- Provide allergen immunotherapy.
- Treat rhinitis, sinusitis, or gastroesophageal reflux.
- See Patient Education section for other measures.

The pharmacological management of asthma in children is based on the classification of the severity of asthma and the child's age. A child's classification can change over time. Also, within any classification, a child may experience mild,

moderate, or severe exacerbations. Table 25–1 lists the four classifications of asthma based on severity of clinical manifestations. A stepwise approach to treatment is based on severity of symptoms and the use of pharmacotherapy to control chronic symptoms, maintain normal activity, prevent recurrent exacerbations, minimize adverse side effects, and maintain nearly "normal" pulmonary function. Tables 25–4 and 25–5 show the management plan for children younger than 5 years of age and for children older than 5 years of age, respectively.

Important considerations to note in the pharmacological treatment of asthma include the following:

- Control of asthma should be gained as quickly as possible by starting at the classification step most appropriate to the initial severity of the child's symptoms or at a higher level (e.g., a course of systemic corticosteroids or higher dose of inhaled corticosteroid). After control of symptoms, decrease treatment to the least amount of medication needed to maintain control.
- Systemic corticosteroids may be needed as a rescue medication at any time and step if there is a major flare-up of symptoms.
- Children with intermittent asthma may have long periods in which they are symptom-free; they can also have life-threatening exacerbations, often provoked by respiratory infection. In these situations, a short course of systemic corticosteroids should be used (NHLBI, 1997).
- Variations in asthma necessitate individualized treatment plans.
- The β-agonist can be given by nebulization with a compressor (e.g., Pulmo-Aide). Nebulization can be a more effective route than metered-dose inhaler (MDI) therapy for young infants (2 years of age or younger) or children who progress to moderate or severe airway obstruction.
- A spacer or holding chamber enhances the delivery of MDI medications to the lower airways of a child and is strongly recommended.
- Dry powder inhalers (DPI) such as Serevent Diskus, Pulmicort Turbuhaler, and Flovent Rotadisk do not need spacers or shak-

Stepwise Approach* for Managing Asthma in Infants and Children 5 Years of Age and Younger for Long-Term Control and Quick Relief

LONG-TERM CONTROL	QUICK RELIEF

STEP 1: MILD INTERMITTENT ASTHMA
No daily medications
	• For symptoms <2 times per wk, use bronchodilators; frequency of medications depends on severity of exacerbation
	  Use one of the following:
	    Inhaled short-acting β_2-agonist by way of nebulizer or face mask and spacer/holding chamber
	        or
	    Oral β_2-agonist for symptoms
	• With viral respiratory infections use bronchodilator q 4–6 hr up to 24 hr (longer use, consult with asthma specialist); repeat no more than every 6 wk without further review
	• Consider systemic corticosteroids if severe exacerbation or previous history of severe exacerbations
	• Use of short-acting bronchodilators >3 or 4 times in 1 d or daily use indicates need for additional therapy

STEP 2: MILD PERSISTENT ASTHMA*
Daily anti-inflammatory medications
Use either of the following:
  Cromolyn (nebulizer preferred or MDI) or nedocromil (MDI) 3 or 4 times per d. Usually try these drugs first in infants and young children
        or
  Low-dose inhaled corticosteroid via spacer/holding chamber and face mask
	Bronchodilators as needed for control of symptoms (see step 1 recommendations)

STEP 3: MODERATE PERSISTENT ASTHMA*
Daily anti-inflammatory medications
Use either of the following:
  Medium-dose inhaled corticosteroid by way of spacer/holding chamber and face mask
        or
  Once symptoms controlled
  Medium-dose inhaled corticosteroid and nedocromil
        or
  Medium-dose inhaled corticosteroid by way of spacer/holding chamber and face mask
	Bronchodilator as needed for symptoms up to 3 times a day (see Step 1 recommendations)

STEP 4: SEVERE PERSISTENT ASTHMA[a]
Daily anti-inflammatory medications
Use either of the following:
  High-dose inhaled corticosteroid via spacer/holding chamber and face mask
  If needed, add systemic corticosteroids at 2 mg/kg per day, reducing to lowest daily or alternate-day-dose that will stabilize symptoms
	Bronchodilator as needed for symptoms up to 3 times a day (see Step 1 recommendations)

*NHLBI Guidelines recommend consultation with an asthma specialist for infants and young children (≤5 years old) in step 3 and 4 classifications; a step 2 classification merits consideration of a consultation.

MDI = metered dose inhaler.

Adapted from Highlights of the Expert Panel Report 2: Guidelines for the Diagnosis and Management of Asthma. (National Heart, Lung, and Blood Institute [NHLBI] Publication No. 97-4051A). Bethesda, MD, National Institutes of Health, 1997.

Stepwise Approach for Managing Asthma in Children Older Than 5 Years of Age for Long-Term Control and Quick Relief

LONG-TERM CONTROL	QUICK RELIEF

STEP 1: MILD INTERMITTENT ASTHMA
No daily medications
	Short-acting bronchodilator for symptom control
	  Inhaled short-acting β-agonist is preferred
	  Intensity of treatment depends on severity of exacerbation
	  Use of short-acting inhaled β-agonists >2 times per week indicates need to consider long-term control therapy

STEP 2: MILD PERSISTENT ASTHMA
Daily medication:
Anti-inflammatory medications
  Low-dose inhaled corticosteroid or cromolyn or nedocromil is the *preferred treatment*. Usually begin with trial of cromolyn or nedocromil in children
  Sustained-release theophylline is an alternate but not preferred therapy in pediatrics. Used only with older children. Zafirlukast or Zileuton may be considered for children 12 years of age or older.
	Short-acting bronchodilators:
	  Prefer inhaled β-agonist for relief of symptoms
	  Intensity of therapy depends on severity of exacerbation
	  Daily or increasing use of a short-acting bronchodilator indicates need for additional long-term control therapy

STEP 3: MODERATE PERSISTENT ASTHMA
Daily medication
Either
  Anti-inflammatory: inhaled medium-dose corticosteroid is the *preferred treatment*
       or
  Inhaled low-medium dose corticosteroid and add a long-acting bronchodilator, especially for nighttime symptoms: either a long-acting inhaled β-agonist (for children 12 years or older), which *is preferred*, or sustained-release theophylline, or long-acting β-agonist tablets
If needed:
  Anti-inflammatory: inhaled corticosteroid (medium-high dose)
       and
  Long-acting bronchodilator, especially for nighttime symptoms: either a long-acting inhaled β-agonist (for children 12 years of age or older), which *is preferred*, or sustained-release theophylline, or long-acting β-agonist tablets
	Short-acting bronchodilators:
	  Prefer inhaled β-agonist for relief of symptoms
	  Intensity of therapy depends on severity of exacerbation
	  Daily or increasing use of short-acting bronchodilator indicates need for additional long-term therapy

STEP 4: SEVERE PERSISTENT ASTHMA
Daily medications
  Anti-inflammatory: Inhaled high-dose corticosteroid *is preferred*
       and
  Long-acting bronchodilator: either a long-acting inhaled β-agonist for children 12 years of age or older, sustained-release theophylline, or long-acting β-agonist tablets
       and
  Corticosteroid tablets or syrup long term (2 mg/kg per d, generally not to exceed 60 mg per d) reducing to lowest daily dose or alternate day dose that stabilizes symptoms
	Short-acting inhaled bronchodilator as needed for symptoms
	  Intensity of treatment depends on severity of exacerbation
	  Daily or increasing use of short-acting bronchodilator indicates need for additional long-term control therapy

T A B L E 25-6

Daily Doses of Inhaled Corticosteroids (Long-Term Control Medications) for Children: Comparison of Agents and Frequency of Delivery

DRUG	LOW DOSE	MEDIUM DOSE	HIGH DOSE	FREQUENCY
Beclomethasone dipropionate 42 μg/puff	84–336 μg 2–8 puffs	336–672 μg 8–16 puffs	>672 μg >16 puffs	Divided doses 2 or 3–4 times per d
84 μg/puff (double strength)	1–4 puffs	4–8 puffs	>8 puffs	Divided doses twice a day
Budesonide Turbuhaler 200 μg/dose	100–200 μg	200–400 μg 1–2 inhalations	>400 μg >2 inhalations	Once or twice daily (divided doses)
Flunisolide 250 μg/puff	500–750 μg 2–3 puffs	1000–1250 μg 4–5 puffs	>1250 μg >5 puffs	Divided doses twice daily
Fluticasone MDI: 44 μg/puff 110 μg/puff 220 μg/puff	88–176 μg 2–4 puffs	176–440 μg 4–10 puffs 2–4 puffs	>440 μg >4 puffs >2 puffs	Divided doses twice daily
Triamcinolone acetonide 100 μg/puff	400–800 μg 4–8 puffs	800–1200 μg 8–12 puffs	>1200 μg >12 puffs	Divided doses 3–4 times daily

From Highlights of the Expert Panel Report 2: Guidelines for the Diagnosis and Management of Asthma (National Heart, Lung, and Blood Institute [NHLBI] Publication No. 97-4051A). Bethesda, MD, National Institutes of Health, 1997, and from information in Taketomo CK, Hodding JH, Kraus DM: Pediatric Dosage Handbook, 5th ed. Hudson, OH: Lexi-Comp, 1998.

ing before use. Dry powder systems should not be used in children younger than 5 years.

- AeroChamber and InspirEase work well in young children.
- Spacers eliminate the need to synchronize inhalation with activation of MDI.
- Different inhaled corticosteroids are not equal in potency to each other on a per puff or microgram basis. Table 25-6 compares the daily low, medium, and high doses of the various inhaled corticosteroids used for children.
- For treatment of exercise-induced bronchospasm:
  - Use either an inhaled short-acting β_2-agonist or a mast cell stabilizer (cromolyn or nedocromil) or both. Combination of both types of drugs is the more effective therapy. A long-acting β_2-agonist can be used in older children.
  - Use two puffs of a β_2-agonist, cromolyn,

or nedocromil 20 minutes before exercise.
  - An extended warming-up period may promote a refractory state and eliminate the need for repeat medications (Boguniewicz & Leung; 1999, May, 1998).

Table 25-7 identifies the usual dosages for long-term control medications (exclusive of inhaled corticosteroids) used to treat asthma in children. Quick-relief medications are listed in Table 25-8.

Practice parameters are guides and should not replace individualized treatment based on clinical judgment and unique differences in patients.

Acute Exacerbations of Asthma

The treatment of acute episodes of asthma is based on classification of the severity of the episode. Acute episodes are classified as mild, moderate, and severe (Table 25-9). Early

Text continued on page 644

T A B L E   25-7

Long-Term Control Medications for the Treatment of Asthma

MEDICATION	DOSAGE FORM	ADULT DOSE	CHILD DOSE	COMMENTS
SYSTEMIC CORTICOSTEROIDS				
Methyl-prednisolone	2, 4, 8, 16, 32 mg tablets	7.5–60 mg daily in a single dose or every other day as needed for control	0.25–2 mg/kg daily in single dose or every other day as needed for control	For long-term treatment of severe persistent asthma, administer single dose in morning either daily or on alternate days (alternate-day therapy may produce less adrenal suppression). If daily doses are required, one study suggests improved efficacy and no increase in adrenal suppression when administered at 3:00 PM.
Prednisolone	5 mg tabs, 5 mg/ 5 ml, 15 mg/5 ml	Short-course "burst": 40–60 mg/d as single or 2 divided doses for 3–10 d	Short course "burst": 1–2 mg/kg/day, maximum 60 mg/d for 3–10 d	Short courses or "bursts" are effective for establishing control when initiating therapy or during a period of gradual deterioration.
Prednisone	1, 2.5, 5, 10, 20, 25 mg tablets: 5 mg/ml, 5 mg/5 ml			The bursts should be continued until patient achieves 80% PEF personal best or symptoms resolve. This usually requires 3–10 days but may require longer. There is no evidence that tapering the dose following improvement prevents relapse.
CROMOLYN AND NEDOCROMIL				
Cromolyn	MDI 1 mg/puff Nebulizer solution 20 mg/ampule	2–4 puffs tid–qid 1 ampule tid–qid	1–2 puffs tid–qid 1 ampule tid–qid	One dose before exercise or allergen exposure provides effective prophylaxis for 1–2 hr.
Nedocromil	MDI 1.75 mg/puff	2–4 puffs bid–qid	1–2 puffs bid–qid	See cromolyn above.

	Dosage Forms	Dose		Comments
LONG-ACTING β₂-AGONISTS				
Salmeterol	**Inhaled** MDI 21 μg/puff, 60 or 120 puffs DPI 50 μg/blister	2 puffs q12h 1 blister q12h	1–2 puffs q12h 1 blister q12h	May use one dose nightly for symptoms. Do not use as a rescue inhaler for symptom relief or for exacerbations.
Sustained-release albuterol	**Tablet** 4-mg tablet	4 mg q12h	0.3–0.6 mg/kg/day, not to exceed 8 mg/day	
METHYLXANTHINES				
Theophylline (numerous manufacturers)	Liquids Sustained-release tablets and capsules	Starting dose 10 mg/kg per d up to 300 mg maximum; usual maximum 800 mg/d	Starting dose 10 mg/kg per d: usual maximum: ≥1 yr of age: 16 mg/kg per d <1 yr: 0.2 (age in wk) + 5 = mg/kg per d	Routine serum theophylline level monitoring is required; not commonly used with pediatric patients.
LEUKOTRIENE MODIFIERS				
Montelukast	5 mg chewable tablet 10 mg tablet	10 mg tablet daily in evening (≥15 years of age or older)	5 mg chewable tablet daily in evening (6–14 years of age)	Approved for use in children 6 years of age or older
Zafirlukast	20 mg tablet	40 mg daily (1 tablet bid)		Take zafirlukast at least 1 hr before or 2 hr after meals
Zileuton	300 mg tablet 600 mg tablet	2400 mg daily (two 300 mg tablets or one 600 mg tablet qid)		Monitor hepatic enzymes (ALT)

T A B L E 25-8

Quick-Relief Medications for the Treatment of Asthma

MEDICATION	DOSAGE FORM	ADULT DOSE	CHILD DOSE	COMMENTS
SHORT-ACTING INHALED BETA$_2$-AGONISTS				
	MDIs			
Albuterol	90 µg/puff, 200 puffs	2 puffs 5 min before exercise	1–2 puffs 5 min prior to exercise	An increasing use or lack of expected effect indicates diminished control of asthma.
Albuterol HFA	90 µg/puff, 200 puffs	2 puffs tid–qid	2 puffs tid–qid	Not generally recommended for long-term treatment. Regular use on a daily basis indicates the need for additional long-term control therapy.
Bitolterol	370 µg/puff, 300 puffs			Differences in potency exist so that all products are essentially equipotent on a per puff basis.
Pirbuterol Terbutaline	200 µg/puff, 400 puffs 200 µg/puff, 300 puffs			May double usual dose for mild exacerbations. Nonselective agents (i.e., epinephrine, isoproterenol, metaproterenol) are not recommended because of their potential for excessive cardiac stimulation, especially at high doses.
	DPIs			
Albuterol Rotahaler	200 µg/capsule	1–2 capsules q4–6h as needed and before exercise	1 capsule q4–6h as needed and before exercise	
	Nebulizer solution			
Albuterol	5 mg/ml (0.5%)	1.25–5 mg (0.25–1 ml) in 2–3 ml of saline q4–8h	0.05 mg/kg (min 1.25 mg, max 2.5 mg) in 2–3 ml of saline q4–6h	May mix with cromolyn or ipratropium nebulizer solutions; may double dose for mild exacerbations
Bitolterol	2 mg/ml (0.2%)	0.5–3.5 mg (0.25–1 ml) in 2–3 cc of saline q4–8h	Not established	May not mix with other nebulizer solutions

ANTICHOLINERGICS				
Ipratropium	**MDIs** 18 μg/puff, 200 puffs	2–3 puffs q6h	1–2 puffs q6h	Evidence is lacking for producing added benefit to β_2-agonists in long-term asthma therapy
	Nebulizer solution 0.25 mg/ml (0.025%)	0.25–0.5 mg q6h	0.25 mg q6h	
SYSTEMIC CORTICOSTEROIDS				
Methylprednisolone	2, 4, 8, 16, 32 mg tablets	Short course "burst": 40–60 mg per d as single or 2 divided doses for 3–10 d	Short course "burst": 1–2 mg/kg/d, maximum 60 mg/d, for 3–10 d	Short courses or "bursts" are effective for establishing control when initiating therapy or during a period of gradual deterioration.
Prednisolone	5 mg tabs, 5 mg/5 ml, 15 mg/5 ml			The burst should be continued until patient achieves 80% PEF personal best or symptoms resolve; this usually requires 3–10 d but may require longer; there is no evidence that tapering the dose following improvement prevents relapse
Prednisone	1, 2.5, 5, 10, 20, 25 mg tablets: 5 mg/ml, 5 mg/5 ml			

From the Highlights of the Expert Panel Report 2: Guidelines for the Diagnosis and Management of Asthma. NHLBI Publication No. 97-4051A, 1997.

T A B L E 25-9
Classifying Severity of Asthma Exacerbations*

	MILD	MODERATE	SEVERE	RESPIRATORY ARREST IMMINENT
SYMPTOMS				
Breathless	While walking Can lie down	While talking (infant—softer, shorter cry; difficulty feeding) Prefers sitting	While at rest (infant—stops feeding) Sits upright	
Talks in	Sentences	Phrases	Words	
Alertness	May be agitated	Usually agitated	Usually agitated	Drowsy or confused
SIGNS				
Respiratory rate	Increased	Increased	Often >30/min	

Guide to rates of breathing in awake children:

Age	Normal rate
<2 mo	<60/min
2–12 mo	<50/min
1–5 yr	<40/min
6–8 yr	<30/min

	MILD	MODERATE	SEVERE	RESPIRATORY ARREST IMMINENT
Use of accessory muscles; suprasternal retractions	Usually not	Commonly	Usually	Paradoxical thoracoabdominal movement
Wheeze	Moderate, often only end expiratory	Loud; throughout exhalation	Usually loud; throughout inhalation and exhalation	Absence of wheeze
Pulse/min	<100	100–120	>120	Bradycardia

Guide to normal pulse rates in children:

Age	Normal rate
2–12 mo	<160/min
1–2 yr	<120/min
2–8 yr	<110/min

	MILD	MODERATE	SEVERE	RESPIRATORY ARREST IMMINENT
Pulsus paradoxus	Absent <10 mm Hg	May be present 10–25 mm Hg	Often present >25 mm Hg (adult) 20–40 mm Hg (child)	Absence suggests respiratory muscle fatigue

FUNCTIONAL ASSESSMENT

PEF % predicted or % personal best	80%	Approx. 50–80%	<50% predicted or personal best, or response lasts <2 hr
Pao_2 (on room air) *and/or*	Normal (test not usually necessary)	>60 mm Hg (test not usually necessary)	<60 mm Hg: possible cyanosis
Pco_2	<42 mm Hg (test not usually necessary)	<42 mm Hg (test not usually necessary)	≥42 mm Hg: possible respiratory failure
Sao_2 % (on room air) at sea level	>95% (test not usually necessary)	91–95%	<91%
Hypercapnia (hypoventilation) develops more readily in young children than in adults and adolescents			

*The presence of several parameters, but not necessarily all, indicates the general classification of the exacerbation. Many of these parameters have not been systematically studied, so they serve only as general guides.

Pao_2 = partial pressure of oxygen in arterial blood; Pco_2 = partial pressure of carbon dioxide; PEF = peak expiratory flow rate; Sao_2 = oxygen saturation in arterial blood.

From the Highlights of the Expert Panel Report 2, Guidelines for the Diagnosis and Management of Asthma. NHLBI Publication No. 97-4051A, 1997.

recognition of warning signs and treatment should be stressed in patient or parent education, or both.

Characteristics of a *mild acute episode* are

- Cough and audible wheezing
- No signs of respiratory distress, cyanosis, increased respiratory rate, or activity restriction
- PEF or forced expiratory volume (FEV) greater than 75% of expected value
- Ability to speak in normal sentences between breaths (Warner et al., 1998)

Children with a *moderate acute episode* of asthma manifest the following:

- Audible wheeze
- Use of accessory muscles
- Slight increase in respiratory rate
- Unable to walk or utter more than three to five words between breaths

Manifestations of a *severe acute episode* of asthma in children include the following signs of severe respiratory distress:

- Cyanosis
- Use of accessory muscles plus lower rib and suprasternal retractions
- Agitation and the ability to say only words between breaths
- Loud wheezing both on inhalation and expiration (Warner et al., 1998)

The *initial pharmacological treatment* for acute asthma exacerbations is inhaled short-acting β_2-agonists two to four puffs every 20 minutes for three treatments by way of MDI with or without a spacer or a single nebulizer treatment (0.05 mg/kg; minimum 1.25 mg, maximum 2.5 mg of 0.5% solution of albuterol in 2 to 3 ml of normal saline).

If the initial treatment results in a good response (PEF rate >80% of patient's best), the inhaled short-acting β_2-agonists can be continued every 3 to 4 hours for 24 to 48 hours. If a child has been on corticosteroids, the dose should be doubled for 7 to 10 days.

An incomplete response (PEF rate between 50 and 80% of personal best or symptoms recur within 4 hours of therapy) is treated by continuing β_2-agonists and adding an oral corticosteroid. The β_2-agonist can be given by nebulizer.

Parents should contact their child's health care provider for additional instructions. If there is marked distress (severe acute symptoms) or a poor response (PEF rate <50%) to treatment, the child should have the β_2-agonist repeated immediately and should be taken to the emergency department. Emergency medical rescue (911) transportation should be used if the distress is severe and nonresponsive.

Children who experience acute asthma exacerbations more than once every 4 to 6 weeks should be reevaluated as to their treatment plan (Boguniewicz & Leung, 1999; NHLBI, 1997).

Complications

Complications from asthma can range from mild secondary respiratory infections to respiratory arrest. Unresponsiveness to pharmacological agents can lead to status asthmaticus and ultimately to death. Chronic high-dose steroid use leads to growth retardation and other related side effects.

Patient and Parent Education and Prevention

The practitioner needs to remember that day-to-day management of asthma is the responsibility of the child or parent. Education should be tailored to meet the patient's individual and family needs. Therefore, the NP should provide instruction on the following:

- Factors responsible for asthma symptoms (i.e., inflammation, airway hyperresponsiveness, and obstruction).
- Environmental control of allergens or triggers such as smoking and dust.
- Medication use (when to take, how often to take, side effects).
- Home PEF rate monitoring.
- How to use inhalers, spacer devices, or aerosol equipment (Table 25–10).
- Proper cleaning of aerosol equipment.
- What to do if symptoms worsen (what medications to add or increase; how frequently to use inhaled medication; specific indications about when to seek additional medical treatment for worsening of symptoms). Develop a written action plan with the child or parent to cover these issues.

T A B L E 25-10

How To Use a Metered-Dose Inhaler

CHILDREN <5 YEARS

1. The use of a mask chamber, such as the InspirEase, with an MDI allows the delivery of inhaled medications even in an uncooperative child.
2. The child should be placed in the parent's lap and the mask placed around the child's mouth.
3. Press down on the MDI while firmly holding the mask around the child's mouth. The child will eventually take a deep breath and inhale the medication.

CHILDREN ≥5 YEARS

1. Remove the cap and hold the MDI upright.
2. Shake the MDI.
3. Tilt head back slightly and breathe out.
4. Position the inhaler in one of the following ways:
   a. If a spacer is used, put the spacer in the mouth and seal with the lips.
   b. If a spacer is not used, the most effective method of delivery is to open the mouth and hold the inhaler 1 to 2 inches away.
   c. If a spacer is not used and the child cannot coordinate the method outlined in b, have the child put the inhaler in his or her mouth and seal with the lips.
   d. If a breath-activated β_2-agonist MDI is used, place inhaler in mouth.
5. Press down on the MDI to release the medication while slowly taking a deep breath (3 to 5 seconds) through mouth.
6. Hold breath for 10 seconds.
7. Wait for at least 1 minute between inhalations.

- Need to have an adequate supply of all medications (including oral corticosteroids) at home and medications readily accessible to the child at school or other settings where the child frequents.
- Management of the child at school, camp, or other places away from home.

The NP should stress that asthma is a chronic disease that can be controlled—the goal of therapy is to maintain normal activity. The child should wear a medical alert bracelet. Patients and parents should be acquainted with local asthma education programs and activities such as asthma camp. Also, written instructions and handouts should be provided for parents, child, and other significant individuals (e.g., school personnel).

PROGNOSIS

Asthma is a chronic disease that, for most children, can be successfully managed with proper pharmacological therapy, allergen and environmental control, and patient education. Mild asthma is more likely to disappear with increasing age than is moderate or severe asthma.

Allergic Rhinitis

DESCRIPTION

Allergic rhinitis (AR) is a disorder that results in nasal edema and other related local manifestations owing to the release of chemical mediators from the antigen–antibody reaction. Manifestations can be seasonal or perennial depending on exposure and subsequent sensitization to the offending allergen.

ETIOLOGY AND INCIDENCE

AR is second only to asthma as the most common atopic disorder. There is an increased incidence in families with an atopic history. A combination of genetic (the presence of an abnormal sensitivity that is associated with IgE production) and environmental factors are linked to its etiology. Many of the allergens that cause asthma produce allergic rhinitis in the same child. Food allergens can occasionally cause rhinitis.

The nasal mucosa is particularly vulnerable to inhaled allergens. The nasal mucosa of a susceptible individual comes in contact with an allergen that binds to a specific IgE antibody. Superficial mucosal mast cells and basophils then degranulate and release chemical mediators. This causes an early-phase reaction of edema, cellular recruitment, and increased vascular permeability with hyperemia and increased serous and mucoid secretions. A late-phase response can occur that results in additional release of chemical mediators and nasal obstruction (Nimmagadda & Evans, 1999).

AR tends to be seasonal, perennial, or episodic. Seasonal allergic rhinitis, hay fever, or seasonal pollenosis is rarely observed in children younger than 4 or 5 years of age but can occur anytime after 2 years of age. Seasonal AR results from sensitization to windborne allergens such as pollens of:

- Trees
- Grasses
- Weeds (ragweed and other weeds)
- Outdoor molds

There can be geographic variations in seasonal AR depending on climate and when the allergens are released into the environment.

Perennial allergic rhinitis has year-round signs and symptoms that may be more severe in the winter. Onset of manifestations can occur before the second year of life and offending substances tend to be indoor allergens, including:

- Dust mites
- Cockroaches
- Feathers
- Allergens or danders of household pets
- Indoor mold spores

CLINICAL FINDINGS

Common nasal symptoms and findings on physical examination include the following:

- Reduced patency from chronic or recurrent bilateral nasal obstruction
- Mouth breathing, snoring, nasal speech
- Mucosal hyperemia to purplish pallor and edema (bogginess) of nasal mucous membranes
- Clear, watery to seromucoid rhinorrhea
- Horizontal crease across the lower third of nose
- Itching and rubbing of nose or "allergic salute"
- Nasal stuffiness, postnasal drip, sneezing, congested cough
- Nasal turbinates pale blue and swollen

Associated manifestations include the following:

- Itching of palate, pharynx, or eyes
- Redness of the conjunctiva, tearing, lid and periorbital edema, infraorbital cyanosis or allergic shiners
- Enlarged tonsillar and adenoid tissue
- "Cobblestone" appearance of the pharynx due to increased lymphoid tissue
- Malocclusion if problem is chronic

Diagnostic Studies

Characteristic symptoms and clinical findings are the key to diagnosis. A history of atopy in the child or family member is helpful in making the diagnosis of AR. The presence of eosinophils on nasal smear can help substantiate the diagnosis but is a nonspecific, nonuniversal finding. Referrals for skin or serological testing for IgE antibody to specific allergens should be reserved for the child with significant symptoms who does not respond to traditional management. The RAST, an in vitro test, can be done for suspected allergens (Boguniewicz & Leung, 1999).

DIFFERENTIAL DIAGNOSIS

Conditions to include as differential diagnoses are the common cold, purulent rhinitis, sinusitis, adenoidal hypertrophy, foreign body obstruction, nasal polyposis of cystic fibrosis, nasopharyngeal tumors, choanal atresia or stenosis, and vasomotor rhinitis. Overuse of topical nasal decongestants can cause drug-induced rhinitis.

MANAGEMENT

There are three strategies for the management of AR: avoidance, pharmacology, and immunotherapy.

Avoidance Strategies

Avoiding exposure to the offending allergen as much as possible is essential. Allergens causing seasonal rhinitis are more difficult to avoid than are the indoor allergens such as molds because pollens are smaller and lighter and, thus, remain in the air.

Key avoidance measures for indoor allergens include the following:

- Control house dust, paying special attention to the child's bedroom.
- Eliminate smoking from the child's environment; if household members still smoke despite education, stress that they should smoke outside the house.
- Keep pets outdoors; consider not having pets.
- Reduce mold; avoid damp basements.
- Use dehumidifiers, air conditioners with efficient filters, and air-cleaning devices with an electronic precipitator or with a high-efficiency particulate air (HEPA) filter.
- Eliminate milk, egg, or wheat for infants with perennial allergic rhinitis, if these prove to be offending substances

Pharmacological Therapy

Oral antihistamines, nasal cromolyn, nasal antihistamine, and nasal corticosteroids are part of the therapy for AR. Pharmacological agents should be started 1 to 2 weeks before pollen season for children with seasonal AR. For perennial AR, start with maximum recommended doses and then taper to minimal dose needed to control symptoms. Some practitioners still occasionally use decongestants or combination decongestant and antihistamine preparations. Antibiotics need to be prescribed for secondary infections. Consult Appendix A for drugs and their administration.

ORAL ANTIHISTAMINES

- Oral antihistamines are especially helpful in seasonal allergic rhinitis.
- Oral antihistamines relieve symptoms of itching, sneezing, and rhinorrhea, but do little to relieve nasal obstruction.
- Oral antihistamines are divided into different classes (Table 25-11).
- Dosage of drug may need to be increased until relief of symptoms is obtained or side effects are experienced (see Appendix A).
- Patient can develop a tolerance to a particular antihistamine and may need to rotate drugs if tolerance develops.
- If side effects with one antihistamine are experienced, switch to another antihistamine in a different class or one in the same class but with different actions.
- Sedating antihistamines may interfere with daytime activities and negatively impact school performance.

NASAL ANTIHISTAMINE

- Azelastine is a nasal antihistamine spray approved for use in seasonal AR in children 12 years of age and older.
- Azelastine acts by competing with histamine for H_1-receptor sites.

DECONGESTANTS

- Decongestants may help relieve nasal congestion.
- Decongestants may be used alone or in combination with an antihistamine.
- Topical decongestants can cause rebound rhinorrhea if used for more than 3 to 5 days; errors in administration can cause systemic absorption and side effects.

NASAL CROMOLYN

- Nasal cromolyn can be used for both seasonal and perennial AR.
- Prophylaxis prevents the mast cell release of histamine and other chemical mediators.
- Best results occur when therapy is initiated before seasonal exposure.
- One to two sprays are administered in each nostril four times a day with tapering if symptoms are controlled (Boguniewicz & Leung, 1999).

INTRANASAL CORTICOSTEROIDS

- Corticosteroids are effective agents to reduce inflammation and subsequent nasal

T A B L E 25-11

Antihistamine Classes

CLASS	NAME	COMMENTS
Ethanolamines	Diphenhydramine (Benadryl) Clemastine (Tavist) Carbinoxamine (Clistin, Rondec)	Combination antihistamine and decongestant
Ethylenediamines	Pyrilamine (in Rynatan, Atrohist) Tripelennamine	
Alkylamines	Chlorpheniramine (Chlor-Trimeton) Brompheniramine (in Dimetane, Bromfed)	
Piperazines	Hydroxyzines (Atarax, Vistaril)	
Piperidines	Cyproheptadine (Periactin)	
Nonsedating antihistamine	Loratadine (Claritin)	Approved for children ≥6 yr old
	Cetirizine (Zyrtec)	Approved for children ≥2 yr old
	Fexofenadine (Allegra)	Approved for children ≥12 yr old

obstruction. Have child clear nasal passages of mucus before their use.

- Use when symptoms are not relieved with antihistamine therapy or if child has severe symptoms.
- Corticosteroids can be effective alone or together with antihistamines.
- Corticosteroids can take 1 week or more before clinical benefit is observed.
- Side effects can include local burning, irritation, soreness, or epistaxis.
- Table 25–12 lists usual dosages per nostril for intranasal corticosteroid preparations (Taketomo et al., 1998).

ANTIBIOTICS
- Treat secondary infections (e.g., sinusitis and otitis media) with appropriate antibiotic coverage.

Immunotherapy

Allergen immunotherapy is indicated when symptoms are severe and have not improved with avoidance measures and pharmacological therapy or when complications of chronic or recurrent sinusitis or otitis media and hearing loss are problematic. It should only be performed in a facility that has both the necessary

equipment and health-care professionals who are prepared to treat anaphylaxis.

COMPLICATIONS

Sinusitis may complicate allergic rhinitis owing to associated swelling of the mucosal lining of the sinuses with secondary infection. Likewise, eustachian tube dysfunction and its sequela, serous otitis media, are common complications. Malocclusion, the development of a high-arched palate, and the typical allergic facies can result from long-standing allergic rhinitis.

PATIENT AND PARENT EDUCATION AND PREVENTION

Because allergic rhinitis is often a chronic problem, parents and children need to have specific information about control of this disorder.

- Instruct on environmental control. Handouts and a review of ways to individualize this information are essential.
- Review pharmacological therapy, including
  - Indications for and changes in medications
  - Frequency of use
  - Common side effects and contraindications

T A B L E 25-12
Intranasal Corticosteroid Preparations Used for Allergic Rhinitis: Usual Doses

DRUG	DOSE	No. INHALATIONS OR SPRAYS & DAILY FREQUENCY	AGE
Beclomethasone (Vancenase, Beconase inhaler)	42 μg/inhalation	1 tid 1 bid–qid or 2 bid	6–12 yr ≥12 yr
Beclomethasone—aqueous inhalation (Vancenase AQ, Beconase AQ)	42 μg/inhalation	1–2 b.i.d.	≥6 yr
(Vancenase AQ 84 μg)	84 μg/spray	1–2 once daily	≥6 yr
Budesonide* (Rhinocort)	32 μg/spray	2 sprays bid or 4 sprays daily (in morning)	≥6 yr
Dexamethasone (Dexacort Turbinaire, Decadron Turbinaire)	84 μg/spray	1–2 sprays bid 2 sprays bid–tid	6–12 yr ≥12 yr
Flunisolide (Nasalide, Nasarel)	25 μg/spray	1 spray tid or 2 sprays twice daily; maintenance dose is 1 spray daily 2 sprays bid	6–14 yr ≥14 yr
Fluticasone (Flonase)	50 μg/spray	1 spray daily; 2 sprays daily if severe or poor response	≥4 yr
Triamcinolone (Nasacort)	55 μg/spray	2 sprays daily 2 sprays daily; after 4–7 days may increase to 4 sprays daily or 2 sprays bid or 1 spray qid	6–11 yr ≥12 yr
Triamcinolone AQ (Nasacort AQ)	55 μg/spray	2 sprays daily; maintenance dose 1 spray daily	>12 yr

*Reduce slowly every 2–4 wk to smallest effective dose.
Adapted from Taketomo CK, Hodding JH, Kraus DM: Pediatric Dosage Handbook, 5th ed. Hudson, OH, Lexi-Comp, 1998.

○ How to use intranasal sprays or inhalers if prescribed

PROGNOSIS

Perennial allergic rhinitis can be a chronic problem unless offending allergens are identified and eliminated from the environment. If this is not possible, pharmacological therapy is usually helpful in reducing symptoms. As the child grows and the nasal passages increase in size, symptoms may also lessen. Symptoms from seasonal allergic rhinitis resulting from hay fever allergy often worsen from the adolescent years to mid-adulthood. Moving to a new environment often results in a short respite (1 to 3 years) from symptoms. However, the child frequently becomes sensitized to new airborne pollens, and symptoms of seasonal AR return.

Atopic Dermatitis

DESCRIPTION

Atopic dermatitis (AD) is a common skin disorder of childhood that is characterized by acute and chronic skin eruptions. The term eczema is sometimes used interchangeably with atopic dermatitis. Eczema means flaring up, which describes the acute symptom complex (erythema, scaling, vesicles, and crusts) seen with atopic dermatitis but does not adequately describe the chronic skin changes that can result from this disorder. Atopic dermatitis manifests a typical morphology and distribution of flexural lichenification or linearity in adults and facial and extensor involvement in infants and children. AD is frequently referred to as the "itch that rashes." With AD, the skin's ability to act as a protective barrier is impaired, resulting in dryness, cracking, and susceptibility to skin infection (Color Fig. 13).

ETIOLOGY AND INCIDENCE

AD affects approximately 1 to 3% of the general population in the United States with higher incidence in other countries; AD develops in 80% of cases by the first year of life and in another 10% by their second birthday. Asthma also develops in approximately 20 to 60% of those with AD, and AR develops in 30 to 45% of those with AD.

The exact etiology is unknown and may vary from individual to individual. Although many children have high IgE levels, an exact immune mechanism for this disorder is not evident. Abnormalities in histamine production (increased in the skin), chemotaxis, monocytes, and cytokines are associated with AD. The strongest predictor of AD is a positive family history of AD; a family history of asthma is also a predictor but less so than AD. Sweating increases itching in the atopic skin. A predisposition to development of pruritus is believed to be a key factor (Nimmagadda & Evans, 1999; Krafchik, 1998).

CLINICAL FINDINGS

The following are seen in atopic dermatitis:

- More than one third of cases begin before age 3 months. Dry skin is the only presenting sign. These infants are generally not brought in for health care until pruritus and the itch-scratch-itch cycle develops, generally around 2 to 3 months of age.

- Acute manifestation (more common in infants):
  ○ Intense itching
  ○ Redness
  ○ Papules, vesicles, and edema
  ○ Serous discharge, and crusts
  ○ Generalized dry skin (xerosis) with dry hair and scalp; diaper area usually spared

- Chronic manifestation (more common in children and adolescents)
  ○ Thickened, leathery, hyperpigmented skin
  ○ Scratch marks
- Characteristics of infantile phase
  ○ Begins at age 2 to 3 months; resolves around 2 to 3 years of age, with approximately one third of cases continuing into the childhood phase
  ○ Cheeks, forehead, scalp, extending to trunk as oval patches or to the extremities; lateral extensor surface of arms and legs
  ○ Tends to be acute
- Characteristics of childhood phase
  ○ Beginning around age 18 months to 24 months and lasting to adolescence; again, approximately one third of cases progress to adolescent AD
  ○ Wrists (hands), neck, ankles (feet), popliteal and antecubital fossae, buttock–thigh crease, flexural areas
  ○ Eyebrows can be thin and broken off
  ○ Tends to be chronic; possible lichenification
  ○ Involvement only of the feet in some children
- Characteristics of adolescent phase
  ○ Often manifested by hand dermatitis only; can involve the popliteal and antecubital fossae, face, neck, upper arms and back, dorsa of hands, fingers, feet, and toes
  ○ May be new occurrence or recurrence of a chronic condition
  ○ Dry skin and lichenification prominent findings
  ○ Erythema and scaling with less exudate
  ○ Postinflammatory hypopigmentation or hyperpigmentation that disappears
  ○ Continuing disease as adults in approximately 30% of children with AD
- Other key features of AD
  ○ Tendency toward dry skin and a lowered threshold for itching (itch-scratch-itch cycle)
  ○ Tendency to worsen during dry winter months or with heat in the summer
  ○ Chronic AD often secondarily infected

with *Staphylococcus aureus* or *Strepto-coccus pyogenes*

- Possible associated features
  - Atopic pleats—extra groove in lower eyelid called Dennie-Morgan fold or pleat, nasal crease across top of nose
  - Accentuated palmar creases
  - Allergic shiners, mild facial pallor, or dry hair
  - Keratosis pilaris, nummular eczema, dyshidrotic eczema, juvenile plantar dermatitis, or ichthyosis vulgaris
  - White dermatographism—red line, flare and wheal reaction following stroking of the skin (Morelli & Weston, 1999; Krafchik, 1998)

Diagnostic Studies

Diagnosis of atopic dermatitis is based on characteristic historical and physical findings. A chronic or recurring rash that is pruritic and has a characteristic distribution and appearance, together with a family or personal history of atopy is key in leading to the diagnosis of atopic dermatitis. Histological examination of the skin is rarely needed and is reserved only for cases that are difficult to diagnose. Serum IgE concentration is elevated in many children with this problem; for the vast majority of children, immunological testing (e.g., IgE, RAST, or prick test) is not needed to confirm the diagnosis or to monitor treatment. Skin testing and hyposensitization are not recommended for children with atopic dermatitis only.

DIFFERENTIAL DIAGNOSIS

Other types of dermatitis, including seborrheic dermatitis, contact dermatitis, allergic contact dermatitis, nummular dermatitis, psoriasis, and scabies, are included in the differential diagnosis. A few genetic conditions are associated with similar skin eruptions (e.g., phenylketonuria, Wiskott-Aldrich syndrome, histiocytosis X, and acrodermatitis enteropathica). Pityriasis alba can also be a differential diagnosis.

MANAGEMENT

Treatment strategy is based on key concepts:

1. The itch-scratch-itch cycle must be interrupted.
2. Dryness of the skin must be corrected.
3. If there are known offending agents, they must be eliminated.
4. Secondary bacterial or viral infections must be treated.

Acute vs. chronic care management is also a consideration. The following therapies are key factors in the control of atopic dermatitis:

1. Antipruritic/sedative agents are essential to control pruritus (Taketomo et al., 1998). These agents are essential to help control active exacerbations of AD and also are helpful as maintenance therapy.
   - Hydroxyzine (Atarax, Vistaril) has excellent antihistaminic and antipruritic qualities but can cause drowsiness and behavioral changes. If an antihistamine is needed throughout the day, the usual oral dose of Atarax in children is 2 mg/kg per day divided every 6 to 8 hours (Takemoto et al., 1998). This dose may need to be increased. If itching is mainly problematic at nighttime, a dose of Atarax at 0.5 mg to 1 mg/kg at bedtime will keep the child comfortable (Eichenfield & Friedlander, 1998).
   - Diphenhydramine hydrochloride (Benadryl) is also a useful antihistamine, especially if sedation is also needed. Usual oral dose in children: diphenhydramine hydrochloride (5 mg/kg per day in divided doses every 6 to 8 hours, not to exceed 300 mg/day).
   - Nonsedating antihistamines may be considered in older children and adolescents (see Table 25–11 and Appendix A). Cetirizine has been shown to be beneficial for AD (Eichenfield & Friedlander, 1998).
2. Use wet compresses if there are weeping, oozing lesions and signs of acute skin inflammation. They also help to rehydrate the skin.
   - Aluminum acetate (Burow solution in a 1:20 or 1:40 preparation). Solution should be tepid, lukewarm, or body temperature.
   - Use a soft cloth that is moderately wet; remoisten as needed. Corticosteroid topical preparations can be applied either before or after application of compresses.

- Can use up to 5 days; effective during the acute stage of atopic dermatitis.
- Aveeno or oatmeal baths help to soothe acute episodes of pruritus, followed by application of a heavy cream emollient.

3. Limit daily bath or shower to 5 to 10 minutes to reduce skin dryness. Excessive soaking in the bathtub depletes the skin of natural moisturizers. Use warm, not hot, water. Some recommend two baths daily, each less than 5 minutes, immediately followed by lubricating oils or ointments as a way to restore water to the skin. Avoid bubble baths.

4. Immediately after bath or shower, gently pat dry and within 2 minutes emolliate with a heavy cream. Lubricants maintain the skin's hydration, and emollients are the treatment of choice for dry skin.
   - An emollient (e.g., petrolatum [Vaseline] or Aquaphor [Beiersdorf]) can be applied just before getting out of the bath water or just after getting out of the bath while still damp. This is also a good time to apply topical corticosteroid preparations, because absorption of the agent is more effective if the skin is hydrated.
   - Use mild soap such as Dove or Neutrogena for the axilla and groin. Do not use drying or deodorant soaps and no oils in bath water.
   - Cetaphil is a nondrying soap-free cleansing agent and can be substituted for bathing. Instruct parents to leave Cetaphil on the skin; it should not be wiped off after applying.

5. Topical corticosteroid preparations are a mainstay of therapy. Do not apply topical steroids containing propylene glycol.
   - When applied over large areas of dermatitis or if occlusion (covering with plastic wrap) is used, the possibility of significant systemic absorption is greatly increased, especially in infants and young children.
   - Apply a thin layer of 1% hydrocortisone cream (acute stage) or ointment (chronic stage) to affected areas three or four times a day.
   - Mix corticosteroid preparation with Eucerin cream or Aquaphor and apply to-

gether to enhance the effect. The combination of emollient and steroid cream has a steroid-sparing effect (Eichenfield & Friedlander, 1998).
   - Use of fluorinated, topical corticosteroid preparations in children should only be done in consultation with a physician. Never use fluorinated, topical corticosteroid preparations on the face; instead, use 1% hydrocortisone ointment sparingly 2 to 3 times a day until symptoms improve and then withdraw. Do not use for an extended period of time because corticosteroids cause thinning of the skin. (See Appendix A for a listing of topical corticosteroids by potency rating.)

6. Emollients can be applied two or three times a day as needed, such as fragrance-free Eucerin cream, Crisco (plain, not butter flavored), or petroleum jelly. If a child is sensitive to fragrances, scented creams such as Nivea should be avoided.

7. Systemic antibiotic agents are essential if secondary skin infection with *S. aureus* or *S. pyogenes* is suspected.
   - Oral erythromycin and cloxacillin should be prescribed for 10 to 14 days depending on resistance of staphylococcus to a particular antibiotic.
   - If bacterial skin infections are recurrent or frequent, a 3-week course of oral antibiotics is recommended.
   - Topical antibiotic preparations are contraindicated although the use of mupirocin has been demonstrated to reduce colony counts of *S. aureus*.
   - Topical antibacterial scrubs are contraindicated because they dry out the skin and cause irritation.

8. Tar preparations may be added to help manage chronic and lichenified forms of dermatitis.
   - These are topical agents that have limited use.
   - Patients should be cautioned about photosensitivity.

9. Systemic corticosteroid agents are rarely needed.

10. Eliminate known or suspected offending agents.

- Avoid nonbreathable fabrics—nylon, or wool; wool is irritating whereas soft cotton clothing is not.
- Avoid chlorine, turpentine, harsh soaps, fragrances, and bleach.
- Known atopic agents should be avoided (e.g., feather pillows, fuzzy toys, stuffed animals, pets).
- Dietary restrictions may include the elimination of cow's milk from infants predisposed to atopy. Eggs, fish, chocolate, nuts, and citrus fruits are generally not allowed until 12 months of age.
- Control of house dust to reduce mite exposure is encouraged. Careful attention to the child's bedroom is important.
- Commercial powders (e.g., benzyl benzoate [Acarosan, Capture]) may help to control dust mites in carpets.

11. Manipulate the environment. A decrease in environmental humidity and an increase in antigen presentation are key causative factors. Therefore, increase environmental humidity and decrease exposure to antigens. Cool temperatures (air conditioning) help.
12. Refer to a dermatologist if child is unresponsive to traditional therapy or has an unusual manifestation (Morelli & Weston, 1999; Krafchik, 1998).

COMPLICATIONS

Secondary skin infections are a frequent complication of AD. *S. aureus* is the most frequent bacterial organism associated with skin infection. Treatment of secondary skin infection is imperative in the management of atopic dermatitis. Kaposi varicelliform eruption (eczema herpeticum) is a significant complication that can result in severe illness in children. Lichenification, a secondary skin change marked by thickening of the skin, is associated with chronic itching. Keratoconus is occasionally seen and is associated with chronic rubbing of the eyelids. Individuals with AD may be prone to molluscum contagiosum, tinea, and warts.

PATIENT AND PARENT EDUCATION AND PREVENTION

Practitioners should provide patients and parents instruction on the following:

- Environmental control of allergens or triggers
- Medication use (when, how much, and how often to use; side effects; and proper application of topical preparations)
- What to do if symptoms worsen or signs of secondary skin infection appear and when to seek additional medical treatment for worsening of symptoms
- Precipitating factors:
  - Extreme temperatures/humidity
  - Excess sweat
  - Emotional stress
- New clothes—wash with mild detergent (with no dyes or perfumes) before wearing them to remove formaldehyde and other chemicals
- Harsh washing detergents—add second rinse cycle when washing clothes
- Coarse clothes
- Excess soap and water
- Allergies
- Cutaneous or systemic infection
- Keeping fingernails trimmed

The practitioner should stress that AD is often a recurrent disease that can be controlled. The goal of therapy is to prevent the itch-scratch-itch cycle and hydrate the skin. Specific written instructions and handouts should be provided to parents regarding bathing, skin care, and use of soaps and other skin cream or lotions.

PROGNOSIS

With appropriate treatment, AD can generally be controlled. In most children, the symptoms of AD become quiescent by age 5 years; however, there is an adolescent and adult stage of the disease. Approximately 25% of children with atopic dermatitis go on to have persistence of symptoms throughout adulthood. Self-image problems may result if atopic dermatitis is severe.

DISEASES WITH AN AUTOIMMUNE BASIS

Juvenile Arthritis

DESCRIPTION

JA is a disease with an autoimmune basis and represents a group of conditions with onset of symptoms in children younger than 16 years of age that causes chronic inflammation of synovial joints for 6 weeks or more. There are various subtypes of JA disease in children that are categorized based on differences in their disease onset, severity, duration, and pattern of complications. The subtypes are systemic arthritis, polyarthritis–rheumatoid factor (RF) negative, polyarthritis–RF positive, oligoarthritis (inflammation of one to four joints), extended oligoarthritis, enthesitis-related arthritis (characterized by joint inflammation at the sites of insertion of fascia or tendons [enthesitis] and spine arthritis), and psoriatic arthritis (O'Neil, 1998a).

ETIOLOGY AND INCIDENCE

The exact etiology of JA is unknown. Genetics is believed to be a factor in most forms of JA. Certain histocompatibility complex antigens are more prevalent in the JA population. Infectious agents such as rubella, parvovirus, *Klebsiella, S. pyogenes*, and *Y. enterocolitica* also have been implicated in the etiology of JA. Cytokine production, proliferation of macrophage-like synoviocytes, infiltration with neutrophils and lymphocytes, and autoimmunity are thought to be the major pathological processes causing chronic joint inflammation.

Prevalence estimates of JA in children are 1.1 in 1000 to 1 in 1500. The rate of JA in girls is significantly higher than in boys except for two subtypes: systemic arthritis and enthesitis-related arthritis. Oligoarthritis comprises approximately 50 to 60% of the cases of JA, and its peak age is early childhood. Systemic arthritis (representing 10 to 15% of JA cases) and polyarthritis–RF negative (representing 15 to 20% of JA cases) occur throughout childhood. Polyarthritis (RF positive) and enthesitis-related arthritis have a peak age of 8 years of age and older (O'Neil, 1998a).

CLINICAL FINDINGS

History

The major complaints of the child with JA are:

- Pain—generally a mild to moderate aching
- Joint stiffness—worse in the morning and after rest

Physical Examination

Typical manifestations of JA are:

- Nonmigratory monoarticular or polyarticular involvement of large or proximal interphalangeal joints for more than 3 months.
- Systemic manifestations—fever, erythematous rashes, leukocytosis, and nodules. Less commonly seen are ocular disease (e.g., iridocyclitis, iritis, or uveitis), pleuritis, pericarditis, anemia, fatigue, and growth failure.

Key physical findings are:

- Swelling with effusion or thickening of synovial membrane, or both
- Heat over inflamed joint and tenderness along joint line
- Loss of joint range of motion and function; child typically holds the affected joints in slight flexion and may walk with limp

There are three major patterns of presentation:

1. *Acute febrile pattern* with an evanescent pale or salmon pink macular rash, arthritis, hepatosplenomegaly, leukocytosis and polyserositis; this group does not develop iridocyclitis.
2. *Polyarticular (five or more synovial joints) pattern* of chronic pain and symmetrical joint swelling; low-grade fever, fatigue, nodules, and anemia may be present but are not prominent as in acute form; iridocyclitis is a common feature in this group.
3. *Pauciarticular pattern* with involvement of few joints, typically the weightbearing joints; synovitis may be mild and painless, joint involvement is asymmetrical, and approximately 30% of these children have asymptomatic iridocyclitis.

Each of the seven subtypes of JA has a typical pattern of presentation. For more information on their specific presentation, the NP should consult other texts on this subject. In addition to joint involvement, in some children with JA, iridocyclitis, pleuritis, pericarditis, anemia, and fatigue may develop (O'Neil, 1998a; Hollister, 1999).

Diagnostic Studies

Diagnosis is based on physical findings and history; there is no diagnostic laboratory test for RA. A positive RF by latex fixation may be present, and ANA may be present in pauciarticular disease with iridocyclitis. Other laboratory findings that may be useful include ESR, leukocytosis, anemia, hyperglobulinemia, and hypoalbuminemia. Imaging studies (magnetic resonance imaging [MRI]) can help in managing joint pathology. Analysis of synovial fluid is not helpful in diagnosis of JA.

DIFFERENTIAL DIAGNOSIS

The various causes of monoarticular arthritis are differential diagnoses and include tumors, leukemia, cancer, bacterial infections, toxic synovitis, rheumatic fever, SLE, Lyme disease, inflammatory bowel disease, septic arthritis, toxic synovitis, and chondromalacia patellae.

MANAGEMENT

Children with severe involvement should be followed up by a specialist in pediatric rheumatology. Other pediatric subspecialists, such as orthopedists, ophthalmologists, and cardiologists, may be consulted as needed. Therapy depends on the degree of local or systemic involvement.

Pharmacological agents include the following (Hollister, 1999; O'Neil, 1998a):

- Nonsteroidal anti-inflammatory drugs (NSAIDs): Children with oligoarthritis generally respond well to NSAIDs.
  - Aspirin: 80 to 100 mg/kg/day (qid)
  - Ibuprofen: 30 to 40 mg/kg/day (tid to qid)
  - Tolmetin: 20 to 30 mg/kg/day (tid)
  - Naproxen: 10 to 20 mg/kg/day (bid)
- Oral or parenteral corticosteroids, sulfasalazine, Enbrel (a newly approved drug that soaks up tumor necrosis factor, an immune-system protein), or methotrexate is indicated in severe forms of JA.
- Intra-articular corticosteroid injections are used if there is severe joint involvement.
- Pharmacological therapy for iridocyclitis is given as indicated by an ophthalmologist.

Physical therapy—range of motion muscle-strengthening exercises and heat treatments—is used for joint involvement, and occupational therapy is beneficial. Rest and splinting are used if indicated.

COMPLICATIONS

Systemic involvement can include iridocyclitis, pleuritis, pericarditis, and hepatitis. Residual joint damage due to granulation of tissue in the joint space can be a problem. Children most likely to develop permanent crippling disability are those with hip involvement, unremitting synovitis, or positive RF tests.

PATIENT AND PARENT EDUCATION AND PREVENTION

The following education and preventive measures are taken:

- For children on aspirin therapy
  - Educate parents about the risk of Reye syndrome and its signs and symptoms.
  - Recommend influenza vaccine.
- Offer chronic disease counseling as indicated in Chapter 23.
- Educate about side effects of medications.
- Instruct about need to follow up with an ophthalmologist. Frequency of follow-up for uveitis screening is based on subtype of JA. Those with systemic arthritis, polyarthritis (both RF-negative and RF-positive subtypes), and enthesitis-related arthritis should be seen every 6 months. Those classified as oligoarthritis, extended arthritis, and psoriatic arthritis are seen every 3 months if ANA positive or every 4 months if ANA negative.

PROGNOSIS

The course of the disease is variable, and there is no curative treatment. After an initial episode, the child may never have another episode, or the disease may go into remission and recur months or years later. The disease process of JA wanes with age and subsides in 95% of children by puberty. Onset of JA in the teenage years is related to progression to adult rheumatoid disease.

Systemic Lupus Erythematosus

DESCRIPTION

SLE is a chronic systemic disease that can involve many organ systems. Autoantibody formation resulting from activation of B lymphocytes is a key characteristic of this immune complex disease. It is more acute and severe in children than in adults.

ETIOLOGY AND INCIDENCE

The exact cause is unknown, but SLE is believed to be a disease of altered immune regulation. In SLE, immune complexes are deposited in various tissues of the body and their clearance is impaired. Deposits of immune complexes trigger a generalized inflammatory response that can lead to tissue damage such as vasculitis and numerous organ system abnormalities.

The presence of lymphocytes, neutrophils, and complement results in antigen–antibody complex formation and causes tissue damage in various organs. The mechanism triggering immune complex formation is unknown. Females are predominantly affected, frequently between the ages of 9 and 15 years. SLE is often precipitated by menarche, pregnancy, or use of oral contraceptives. Onset before age 3 years is rare; adult onset tends to occur at around 30 to 40 years of age. Altered cellular immunity in genetically predisposed individuals is postulated as a key factor in this disease. Approximately 20% of children with SLE have a first-degree relative with SLE (O'Neil, 1998b).

CLINICAL FINDINGS

These depend on organ involvement.

History

The history may include the following:

- Joint involvement—the most common presenting finding
- Nondeforming arthritis—often symmetrical joint involvement
- Arthralgia
- Systemic manifestations

- Fever—intermittent or sustained
- Fatigue
- Anorexia and loss of weight
- Malaise

Physical Examination

The following may be seen on physical examination (Hollister, 1999; O'Neil, 1998b):

- Malar or "butterfly" rash—bluish or scaly erythematous maculopapular rash covering malar areas extending over the bridge of the nose and cheeks; may spread down the face to the chest and extremities; "butterfly" rash and other lesions can be photosensitive
- Discoid rash with plugging of the follicles, hypopigmentation and hyperpigmentation, and scarring
- Lesions may also include small ulcerations in the skin and mucous membrane, indurations, purpura, and erythema nodosum and multiforme
- Alopecia
- Mucous membrane manifestations
- Gingivitis, mucosal hemorrhage, erosions, ulcerations
- Silvery whitening of the vermilion border of the lips or thickening, redness, ulceration, or crusting of the lips
- Raynaud's phenomenon is present in some children
- Polyserositis—pleurisy, pericarditis, and peritonitis
- Hepatosplenomegaly and lymphadenopathy
- Signs and symptoms of central nervous system and renal involvement

Diagnostic Studies

The ANA test is positive in 95% of children who have active, untreated SLE. A negative ANA excludes SLE from the diagnosis except for the rare false-negative test. A positive ANA test should be followed up with testing for disease-specific types of ANA. Elevated titers of anti-DNA antibody and depressed levels of serum complement are found in active disease involving the skin and central nervous and renal systems. Leukopenia, anemia, elevated sedimentation rate, and hypergammaglobulinemia are frequent laboratory findings. Other laboratory and radiographic studies depend on organ involvement (e.g., histopathological studies and serological testing).

DIFFERENTIAL DIAGNOSIS

Diseases that resemble SLE include rheumatic fever, RA, and viral infections. A temporary, drug-induced SLE can be caused by several pharmacological agents, including hydantoin compounds, hydralazine, isoniazid (INH), procainamide, and sulfonamides.

MANAGEMENT

Children with SLE need to be followed up by a specialist in collagen-vascular disorders. Other pediatric subspecialists may be consulted. Therapy depends on the degree of local or systemic involvement. General measures include avoiding sun exposure and daylight fluorescent light as well as applying sunscreen for ultraviolet A (UVA) and ultraviolet B (UVB) protection. In addition

- NSAIDs are used for relief of arthritis, serositis, or pain (if nephritis is present, use with caution).
- Oral steroids are prescribed if renal, cardiac, or central nervous system involvement is present. The dose is adjusted depending on clinical and laboratory findings.
- Antimalarial drugs may be used to treat cutaneous manifestations.
- Immunosuppressant agents may be added if the response to steroids is inadequate.
- Use of other pharmacological agents or therapies depends on the type and level of organ system involvement.

COMPLICATIONS

Currently, SLE is considered, for the most part, a controllable disease in children. The severity of the illness is variable. A diagnosis of SLE in childhood does not always mean a poor prognosis, especially if renal involvement is not pres-

ent. Renal failure, central nervous system lupus, myocardial infarction, cardiac failure, and infection are the leading causes of death in children. Exposure to ultraviolet light may bring out or worsen skin lesions and can also result in exacerbation of systemic problems that can cause death. Side effects resulting from chronic use of high-dose corticosteroids can be a problem.

PATIENT AND PARENT EDUCATION

The practitioner should educate patients and parents as follows:

- About the effect of sun exposure and the need for sunscreen protection
- About the need to rest between activities, because fatigue is a frequent problem for children with SLE
- That SLE is a chronic disease that can have periods of remissions followed by exacerbations

PROGNOSIS

SLE is a chronic disease with periods of exacerbations with waxing and waning of symptoms; however, complete remission can occur. Children with mild disease do well; patients with severe major organ involvement have a poor prognosis.

Fibromyalgia

DESCRIPTION

Fibromyalgia is a benign, intermittent, noninflammatory musculoskeletal pain syndrome. It is a complex syndrome that involves fatigue and generalized pain involving muscles, ligaments, and tendons. Symptoms are often vague and variable, with no major organ system abnormalities found. Its presentation can range from a generalized increased sensitivity to pain to a more classic pattern of specific symptoms. Fibromyalgia can occur as a primary condition or in conjunction with other rheumatologic disorders (secondary fibromyalgia). Fibromyalgia was first described in children in 1985.

ETIOLOGY AND INCIDENCE

The cause of fibromyalgia is unknown. There are data associating hypermobility and fibromyalgia and possible neuroendocrine involvement. Females are affected more often than males in a 5 to 1 ratio (Olson, 1998; Ballinger & Bowyer, 1997).

CLINICAL FINDINGS

History

The history may include the following symptoms (Hollister, 1999; Ballinger & Bowyer, 1997):

- Headache
- Blurry vision
- Dizziness
- Fatigue
- Chest pain or shortness of breath
- Bowel problems: constipation or diarrhea
- Myalgias and arthralgias with morning stiffness that lasts only minutes
- Tingling in limbs
- Insomnia or prolonged night awakenings (universal complaint)
- Widespread musculoskeletal pain
- Complaints of swelling of hands and feet without objective findings

Physical Examination

Local areas of tenderness or trigger points in muscles (usually at areas of tendon insertion) with pressure are characteristic physical findings. Pressure causes pain at the site and also in a circumferential or linear pattern surrounding the site.

Diagnostic Criteria

The criteria for the diagnosis of fibromyalgia established by the American College of Rheumatology are as follows:

- History of widespread pain that involves both sides of the body, is above and below the waist, and includes axial skeletal pain.
- Pain in 11 of 18 bilateral point sites on digital palpation using approximately 4 kg of pressure. Sites to evaluate are occiput, trapezius, supraspinatus, gluteal, greater trochanter, low cervical, second rib, lateral epicondyle, and knee (Ballinger & Bowyer, 1997).

Diagnostic Studies

Laboratory studies are of little benefit. Blood count, liver functions, and muscle enzymes are normal. If secondary fibromyalgia, order appropriate tests to diagnose rheumatoid disorder.

DIFFERENTIAL DIAGNOSIS

In chronic fatigue syndrome, tiredness rather than pain is the major complaint. Fibromyalgia initially may be mistaken for other rheumatoid diseases but does not have the associated rashes, weight loss, fever (over 101°F) or joint swelling.

MANAGEMENT

Children and their parents need reassurance that they do not have a life-threatening disease but have a chronic condition that can be a lifelong problem. Treatment focuses on relieving symptoms and can include the following:

- Physical therapy for range of motion exercises, mild low-impact aerobic exercises (e.g., swimming, bicycling, and walking), and muscle strengthening.
- Amitriptyline (10 to 25 mg) taken before bedtime has been helpful in stabilizing abnormal sleep patterns and in reducing pain *or* cyclobenzaprine (10 mg at bedtime) also has helped to stabilize sleep patterns but should be used for no longer than 2 to 3 weeks at a time.
- Psychotherapy to help cope with this condition and deal with stress.

Analgesics and NSAIDs do not help relieve the pain and should not be prescribed.

PATIENT AND PARENT EDUCATION

The practitioner should educate patients and parents as follows:

- About fibromyalgia and that it is not a psychosomatic disorder
- About the possibility that this could be a chronic problem and they can have periods of remissions followed by exacerbations

PROGNOSIS

The outcome of fibromyalgia in children appears to be better than that in adults. However, the prognosis for young patients is not clear (Hollister, 1999; Ballinger & Bowyer, 1997).

Chronic Fatigue Syndrome

The existence of or cause of chronic fatigue syndrome continues to be a debated topic. Criteria to assist in the classification of this syndrome have been developed by the National Institutes of Health. The presentation of chronic fatigue syndrome in children and adolescents is similar to that seen with adults. The key patient complaint is fatigue that must have a defined day of onset, is unexplained, and is persistent or relapsing. This fatigue is not relieved by rest or sleep and results in reduced activity. Other significant clinical findings include impaired memory or concentration, low-grade fever, sore throat, painful cervical or axillary lymph nodes, muscle pain, and neuropsychiatric problems. These clinical findings must have been present for 6 months or longer.

Epstein-Barr virus (EBV) infection has been implicated in the etiology of chronic fatigue syndrome. However, EBV does not explain all the symptoms. No single immunological abnormality has been consistently identified as the causative factor. The etiology of chronic fatigue syndrome remains undetermined and treatment is based on symptoms. Care must be taken in diagnosing this disorder in children, and other conditions (e.g., hypothyroidism, sleep apnea, hepatitis B or C, SLE, cancer, major depressive and other psychiatric disorders) must first be ruled out (Hollister, 1999; National Institute of Allergy and Infectious Diseases, 1997).

Acute Rheumatic Fever

DESCRIPTION

Acute rheumatic fever (ARF) is a nonsuppurative complication of a group A β-hemolytic streptococcus (GABHS) pharyngeal infection that results in an inflammatory process involving the joints, heart, central nervous system, and subcutaneous tissue. ARF is diagnosed based on a set of criteria called the Jones criteria that were updated in 1992. Recurrent ARF can follow subsequent GABHS pharyngeal infections.

ETIOLOGY AND INCIDENCE

The exact pathological mechanism that is responsible for the inflammatory changes in various organs and tissues is unknown. Abnormalities in the host immune response to streptococcal cell wall proteins are believed to be involved. Serotypes 1, 3, 5, 6, 18, and 24 are associated with ARF. There appears to be a genetic influence on susceptibility to GABHS infection. The risk of an initial attack of ARF following a GABHS pharyngeal infection is 1 to 3%; the risk for recurrent ARF following subsequent episodes of GABHS pharyngitis (symptomatic or asymptomatic infection) is 75%. The most commonly affected group are children between 5 and 15 years of age (Billigmeir & Loeffler, 1999; Kaplan, 1998).

CLINICAL FINDINGS

The diagnosis of an initial attack of ARF is based on the following:

- Evidence of documented (culture, rapid streptococcal antigen test, or ASO titer) GABHS pharyngeal infection
- Findings of two major manifestations or one major and two minor manifestations of ARF (Olson, 1998):

  Major Manifestations
  Carditis (pancarditis)
  Polyarthritis (migratory and painful)
  Sydenham chorea
  Erythema marginatum
  Subcutaneous nodules
  Minor Manifestations
  Clinical:
    Fever, polyarthralgia, prior history of ARF
  Laboratory:
    Elevated acute phase reactants (ESR, WBC, C-reactive protein), prolonged PR interval on electrocardiogram.

Children may be diagnosed with ARF without evidence of a preceding streptococcal infection in the following two situations: a child with Sydenham chorea or with acquired heart disease (commonly mitral valve regurgitation without a congenitally abnormal or prolapsed valve) that can only be linked to ARF.

DIFFERENTIAL DIAGNOSIS

No single diagnostic test exists for ARF, and many diseases are included in the differential diagnosis (e.g., JA, connective tissue diseases, infective endocarditis, and Lyme disease).

MANAGEMENT

The treatment of ARF includes the following:

1. Antibiotic therapy to eradicate GABHS infection. Benzathine penicillin G is the drug of choice (see Appendix A) unless there is an allergic history; erythromycin is then the drug of choice. A patient with a history of ARF who has an upper respiratory infection should be treated for GABHS whether or not GABHS is recovered.
2. Anti-inflammatory therapy. Aspirin can be used for arthritis at 30 to 60 mg/kg per day in four divided doses for 2 to 6 weeks with a reduction in dosage as symptoms are relieved. Corticosteroids are indicated only with severe carditis and manifestations of heart failure (Wolfe et al., 1999).
3. Referral for treatment of congestive heart failure if needed. Medical management and/or valve replacement may be necessary.
4. Bed rest is generally indicated only for children with congestive heart failure. Children with Sydenham chorea may need to be kept in bed to protect them until their choreiform movements are controlled (Wolfe et al., 1999; Kaplan, 1998).
5. Children with severe chorea may benefit with a trial of haloperidol (0.01 to 0.03

RESOURCE BOX 25-1

NATIONAL ORGANIZATIONS AND RESOURCES FOR ASTHMA AND ATOPIC DERMATITIS

Allergy and Asthma Network–Mothers of Asthmatics, Inc.
Tel: (800) 878-4403
Tel: (703) 641-9595
Website: www.aanma.org
An excellent resource for parents.

American Academy of Allergy and Immunology
Tel: (800) 822-2762
Tel: (414) 272-6071

American College of Allergy, Asthma, and Immunology
Tel: (800) 822-2762
Website: www.ACAAI.org

American Lung Association
Tel: (800) 586-4872
Website: www.lungusa.org

Asthma and Allergy Foundation of America
Tel: (800) 727-8462

Asthma and Allergy Information Center and Hotline
Tel: (800) 727-5400

National Asthma Education Program Information Center
Tel: (301) 951-3260
Provides an excellent resource packet titled "Managing Asthma: A Guide for Schools and an Asthma Management Kit for Clinicians."

National Eczema Association for Science and Education
Tel: (800) 818-7546
Fax: (503) 224-3363
Website: www.eczema-assn.org
E-mail: nease@teleport.com

National Heart, Lung, and Blood Institute
National Asthma Education and Prevention Program
NHLBI Information Center
Tel: (301) 251-1222
Website: www.nhlbi.nih.gov

National Jewish Center for Immunology and Respiratory Medicine
Tel: (800) 222-5864
Website: www.njc.org

Some organizations have local branches listed in local telephone directories.

mg/kg per day in two divided doses (Billigmeir & Loeffler, 1999).

The prevention of ARF includes the following:

1. Treat GABHS pharyngeal infections with the appropriate antibiotics. Antibacterial prophylaxis for those with a prior history of ARF is required because of their greatly increased risk of recurrent ARF with subsequent inadequately treated GABHS infections. Intramuscular penicillin G every 21 to 28 days is more effective than daily penicillin V.
2. Antibacterial prophylaxis is continued for 3 to 5 years of therapy or discontinued at adolescence for children with transient cardiac involvement. For those with persistent myocardial or valvular disease, treatment is lifelong (Wolfe et al., 1999).
3. Children with a history of ARF need bacterial endocarditis prophylaxis treatment for dental or surgical procedures in addition to their regular antibiotic prophylaxis (See Tables 31-11 to 31-15).

COMPLICATIONS

Chronic congestive heart failure (CHF) can occur after an initial episode of ARF or follow recurrent episodes of ARF. Residual valvular damage is responsible for CHF.

REFERENCES

Ballinger SH, Bowyer SL: Fibromyalgia: The latest "great imitator." Contemp Pediatr 14(4):140-154, 1997.

Billigmeir SL, Loeffler AM: Acute rheumatic fever. *In* Burg FD, Ingelfinger JR, Wald ER, et al (eds): Gellis & Kagan's Current Pediatric Therapy, 16th ed. Philadelphia, WB Saunders, 1999, pp 594-595.

Boguniewicz M, Leung YM: Allergic disorders. *In* Hay WW, Hayward AR, Levin MJ, et al (eds): Current Pediatric Diagnosis and Treatment, 14th ed. East Norwalk, CT, Appleton & Lange, 1999, pp 917-942.

Eichenfield LF, Friedlander SF: Coping with chronic dermatitis. Contemp Pediatr 15(10):53-68, 1998.

Hollister JR: Rheumatic diseases. *In* Hay WW, Hayward AR, Levin MJ, et al (eds): Current Pediatric Diagnosis and Treatment, 14th ed. East Norwalk, CT, Appleton & Lange, 1999, pp 715-722.

Kaplan EL: Rheumatic fever. *In* Finberg L (ed): Saunders Manual of Pediatric Practice. Philadelphia, WB Saunders, 1998, pp 596-599.

Krafchik BR: Atopic dermatitis. *In* Finberg L (ed): Saunders Manual of Pediatric Practice. Philadelphia, WB Saunders, 1998, pp 905-911.

May JN: Asthma. *In* Finberg L (ed): Saunders Manual of Pediatric Practice. Philadelphia, WB Saunders, 1998, pp 244-248.

Morelli JG, Weston WL: Skin. *In* Hay WW, Hayward AR, Levin MJ, et al (eds): Current Pediatric Diagnosis and Treatment, 14th ed. East Norwalk, CT, Appleton & Lange, 1999, pp 341-359.

National Heart, Lung, and Blood Institute: Executive Summary: Guidelines for the Diagnosis and Management of Asthma (NIH Publication No. 94-3042A). Bethesda, MD, National Institutes of Health, 1994.

National Heart, Lung, and Blood Institute. Highlights of the Expert Panel Report 2: Guidelines for the Diagnosis and Management of Asthma (NIH Publication No. 97-4051A). Bethesda, MD, National Institutes of Health, 1997.

National Institute of Allergy and Infectious Diseases. Chronic Fatigue Syndrome: Information for Physicians (NIH Pub. No. 97-484). Bethesda, MD, Author, 1997.

Nimmagadda SR, Evans R: Allergy: Etiology and epidemiology. Contemp Pediatr 20:111-115, 1999.

Olson JC: Rheumatic diseases of childhood. *In* Behrman RE, Kliegman RM (eds): Nelson Essentials of Pediatrics, 3rd ed. Philadelphia, WB Saunders, 1998, pp 299-314.

O'Neil KM: Juvenile arthritis. *In* Finberg L (ed): Saunders Manual of Pediatric Practice. Philadelphia, WB Saunders, 1998a, pp 265-272.

O'Neil KM: Systemic lupus erythematosus. *In* Finberg L (ed): Saunders Manual of Pediatric Practice. Philadelphia, WB Saunders, 1998b, pp 272-277.

Taketomo CK, Hodding JH, Kraus DM: Pediatric Dosage Handbook, 5th ed. Hudson, OH, Lexi-Comp, 1998.

Warner JO, Naspitz CK, Cropp GJ: Third international pediatric consensus statement on the management of childhood asthma. Pediatr Pulmonol 1-17, 1998.

Wolfe RR, Boucek MM, Schaffer MS, et al. *In* Hay WW, Hayward AR, Levin MJ, et al (eds): Current Pediatric Diagnosis and Treatment, 14th ed. East Norwalk, CT, Appleton & Lange, 1999, pp 465-527.

CHAPTER 26

Endocrine and Metabolic Diseases

Jean Betschart

INTRODUCTION

The endocrine system is a secretory feedback system in which glands secrete circulating hormones that affect multiple organs and tissues. Primary care nurse practitioners (NPs) are in a position to assess whether physical findings related to growth or sexual development are normal variants or indicators of a disease process. When growth and sexual development are involved, there is always the possibility of an abnormal secretion of a particular hormone or combination of hormones. Normal variations commonly occur in the timing and pattern of growth and sexual development and can present a diagnostic challenge for the practitioner. In contrast, other symptoms and physical findings that the primary care practitioner might note are clearly associated with specific endocrine disorders marked by either hyposecretion or hypersecretion of hormones. The primary care NP has a responsibility to identify children with these disorders and refer them to an endocrinologist for additional diagnostic studies and treatment.

Diabetes mellitus is an endocrine disorder but is discussed under metabolic disorders, because the pathogenesis involves alterations in glucose metabolism. In diabetes mellitus, the hormone insulin is diminished, absent, or ineffective, and glucose metabolism is adversely affected at the cellular level. Type 1 diabetes is the most common endocrine-metabolic disorder of childhood and adolescence.

Metabolic disorders generally affect multiple organs and tissues by altering metabolic processes to produce deleterious end products or cause the presence of abnormal substances. Early identification of metabolic disorders is imperative, because metabolic diseases can cause significant, irreversible changes in multiple organ systems. Metabolic diseases can cause significant problems, some of which are life threatening, such as galactosemia. Newborn screening programs can identify a variety of inborn errors of metabolism and congenital hypothyroidism that are treatable endocrine disorders. Early intervention can alter the outcomes for children born with these problems and prevent mental retardation and other consequences associated with untreated metabolic and endocrine disorders.

STANDARDS FOR SCREENING

Screening for congenital hypothyroidism is recommended for all neonates during the first week of life. Routine screening for thyroid disorders is otherwise not warranted in asymptomatic adults or children. Persons with a history of upper-body irradiation may benefit from regular physical examination of the thyroid.

Screening for phenylketonuria (PKU) is recommended for all newborns before discharge from the nursery. Infants who are tested before 24 hours of age should undergo a repeat screening test before the third week of life (US Preventive Services Task Force, 1998). Routine prenatal screening for maternal PKU is not recommended. Table 26–1 lists available newborn screenings for common metabolic disorders.

ANATOMY AND PHYSIOLOGY

The endocrine system is a looped regulatory system that involves the hypothalamus, the pituitary gland, and other endocrine glands outside the central nervous system. The pituitary gland secretes various protein hormones that stimulate other endocrine glands or body cells. These in turn respond by secreting specific hormones that affect hormone production in the pituitary gland (Fig. 26–1). The following is an outline of the endocrine loop system:

1. The hypothalamus secretes hormones that regulate specific anterior pituitary cells:
   - Growth hormone-releasing hormone (GHRH) and somatostatin-regulated growth hormone (GH)
   - Prolactin-releasing factor (PRF)
   - Thyroid-stimulating hormone (TSH)-releasing hormone (thyrotropin-releasing hormone [TRH])
   - Corticotropin-releasing hormone (CRH)
   - Luteinizing hormone-releasing hormone (LHRH)
2. The anterior pituitary responds to the above hormones by releasing the following corresponding hormones:
   - GH
   - Prolactin
   - Thyrotropin (TSH)
   - Corticotropin (adrenocorticotropic hormone [ACTH])
   - Gonadotropic hormones: follicle-stimulating hormone (FSH) and luteinizing hormone (LH)
3. These anterior pituitary hormones affect the following target organs or endocrine glands:
   - Growth plate of bones

- Breast tissue to maintain lactation
- Thyroid gland
- Adrenal glands
- Gonads
4. The following endocrine glands secrete the identified hormone, which then influences hypothalamic hormone production:
   - Thyroid: T_3 (triiodothyronine) and T_4 (thyroxine)
   - Adrenals: corticosteroids
   - Gonads: LH stimulates synthesis of progesterone and androgens; FSH stimulates estradiol
5. The posterior pituitary is an extension of the ventral hypothalamus and secretes arginine vasopressin, the antidiuretic hormone, and oxytocin, a hormone significant in parturition and breastfeeding.

The metabolism of essential amino acids, carbohydrates, and lipids involves complex biochemical functions that transform these substances so that they can be used at the cellular level. When metabolic pathways are altered, fundamental biochemical processes are adversely affected in multiple ways and with varying degrees of severity.

PATHOPHYSIOLOGY

Endocrine pathology occurs when there is an alteration in regulation of the normal feedback system that results in hypo- or hypersecretion of one or more hormones. Multiple factors cause alterations in hormone production. They include tumors, trauma, infection, systemic disease, genetic disorders, congenital malformation or agenesis of an endocrine gland, idiopathic causes, and iatrogenic causes (medications). The defect or problem can originate at the pituitary-hypothalamic level, in end-organ abnormalities, or for unknown reasons that lead to unresponsiveness to endogenous hormone. Hypothyroidism and hyperthyroidism are examples of disease entities in which the interrelationships of the hypothalamic-pituitary-thyroid axis are altered at any one of several possible sites (Fig. 26–2).

Many metabolic diseases are caused by inborn errors of metabolism. Alteration in genetic

T A B L E 26-1

Newborn Screenings for Metabolic Disorders

SCREEN	DESCRIPTION	STATES MANDATING SCREENING	SEVERITY	TEST	COMMENTS
Biotinidase deficiency	Autosomal recessive, multiple carboxylase deficiency	19 states, District of Columbia, United States (US) Virgin Islands	Neurological signs including hearing loss and optic atrophy	Colorimetric assay for biotinidase using dried blood spot	Zero mortality with screening and treatment
Branched-chain ketoaciduria: maple syrup urine disease	Autosomal recessive, branched-chain ketoacid decarboxylation and high body fluid ketoacids	23 states, District of Columbia, and US Virgin Islands	Lethal if unrecognized and untreated; irreversible retardation	Bacterial inhibition assay (BIA) for leucine using dried blood spot	Infants often have irreversible damage by the time they are identified
Congenital adrenal hyperplasia	Family of disorders; defects in enzymes required for biosynthesis of adrenal corticosteroids	11 states	Life-threatening adrenal crisis	Enzyme/radioimmuno-assay for 17α-hydroxy-progesterone (17OHP) in 21-hydroxylase deficiency on dried blood spot	
Congenital hypothyroidism	Insufficient thyroid hormone	50 states, District of Columbia, Puerto Rico, and US Virgin Islands	Mental retardation, poor growth	Radioimmunoassay for T4, thyroid-stimulating hormone (TSH), or both	Mortality not expected but may be underestimated as a result of failure to diagnose
Galactosemia	Inherited disorder of galactose metabolism	44 states, District of Columbia, and US Virgin Islands	Failure to thrive, vomiting, liver disease, mental retardation; lethal in most cases	Elevated blood galactose content	
Homocystinuria	Autosomal recessive defect in catabolism of sulfur-containing amino acids	20 states, District of Columbia, and US Virgin Islands	50% mortality by 25 yr of age; developmental delay; marfanoid habitus	BIA for elevated levels of blood methione	
Phenylketonuria	Autosomal recessive disorder of phenylalanine hydroxylation	50 states, District of Columbia, Puerto Rico, and US Virgin Islands	Developmental delay, severe mental retardation, seizures	Measurement of blood phenylalanine level by BIA using dried blood spot; automated fluorometric assay	Registries of affected females are being developed to track those at risk

Data from American Academy of Pediatrics Policy Statement: Newborn Screening Fact Sheet (RE9632). Pediatrics 98:467–472, 1996.

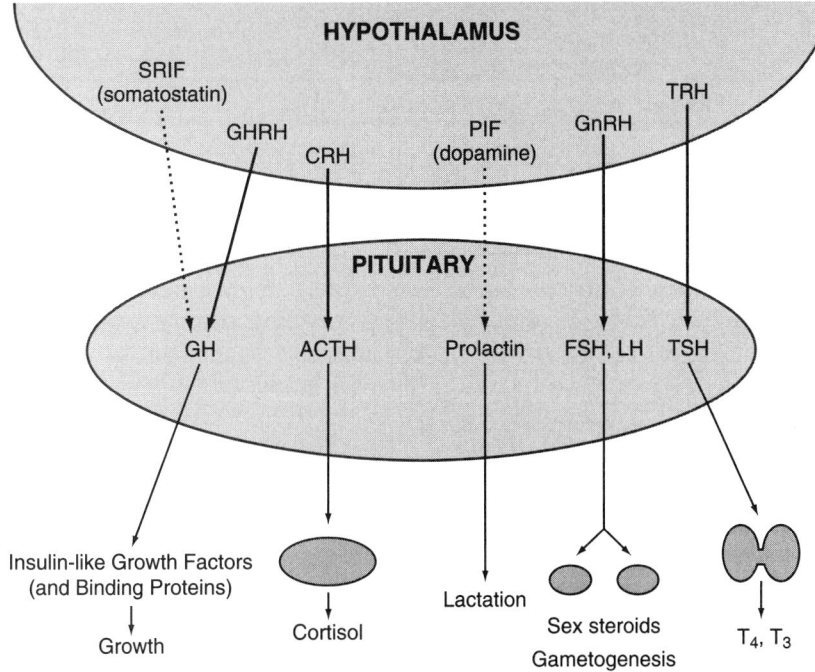

F I G U R E 26-1

Hormonal influences of the hypothalamus and pituitary gland. Solid line represents stimulatory influence; dotted line represents inhibitory influence. SRIF = somatotropin release–inhibiting factor; GHRH = growth hormone–releasing hormone; CRH = corticotropin-releasing hormone; PIF = prolactin inhibitory factor; GnRH = gonadotropin-releasing hormone; TRH = thyrotropin-releasing hormone; GH = growth hormone; ACTH = adrenocorticotropin; FSH = follicle-stimulating hormone; LH = luteinizing hormone; TSH = thyroid-stimulating hormone; T_4 = thyroxine; T_3 = triiodothyronine. (From Behrman RE, Kliegman RM, et al: Nelson Essentials of Pediatrics, 3rd ed. Philadelphia, WB Saunders, 1998, p 649.)

constitution results in disrupted biochemical functioning. In children with PKU, a deficiency of the enzyme phenylalanine hydroxylase, or of its cofactor tetrahydrobiopterin, results in an excessive accumulation of phenylalanine, an essential amino acid. In galactosemia, the defect involves deficiency of galactose-1-phosphate uridyltransferase and the resulting inability to metabolize galactose. Type 1 diabetes is an example of an acquired immune-mediated metabolic disease. In diabetes mellitus, a reduction in insulin production or deficiency of its action results in abnormal metabolism of carbohydrate, protein, and fat.

ASSESSMENT

Endocrine and metabolic disorders can be manifested in various organs throughout the body and can alter numerous body functions. Assessment of endocrine pathology most commonly seen in children in ambulatory care settings is best approached by dividing these problems into five classifications:

1. Disturbance of growth and sexual development
2. Posterior pituitary gland dysfunction
3. Thyroid problems
4. Adrenal disorders
5. Primary and secondary gonad dysfunction

History

Endocrine disorders and metabolic diseases are either congenital or acquired, with symptoms differing based on age of the patient at the time of manifestation. Key factors to consider in the

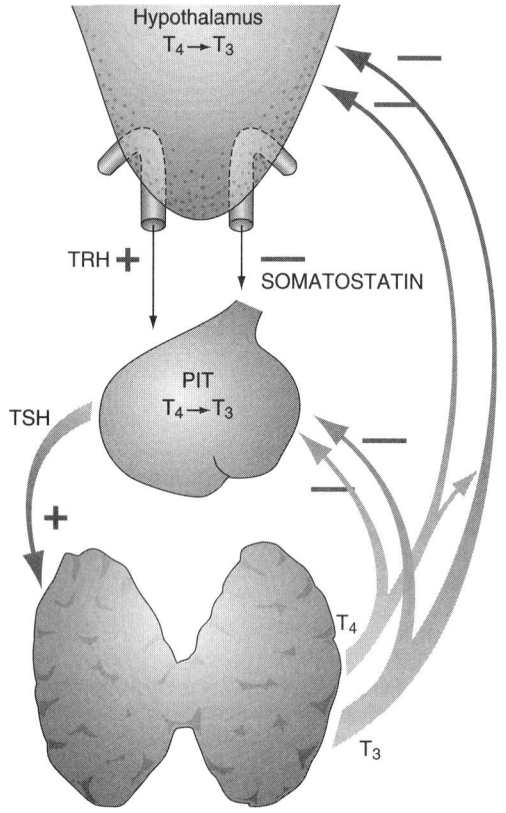

F I G U R E 26-2
Interrelationships of the hypothalamic-pituitary-thyroid (HPT) axis. (From Wilson JD, Foster DW [eds]: Williams Textbook of Endocrinology, 8th ed. Philadelphia, WB Saunders, 1992, p 169.)

history of a child who is suspected of having an endocrine or metabolic disorder are identified using the classification previously described under Assessment.

1. Disturbance in growth and sexual development
   - Is the child growing less or more than 2 inches per year? Is the child still wearing last year's clothes?
   - What are the heights of mother, father, and other family members?
   - Is the child showing signs of sexual development (pubic hair, breast development, axillary or beard/facial hair or both, menses, scrotal and testicular growth)? If yes, at what age did these occur?

- Is the child taking any medications that affect growth (e.g., steroids)?
- Are past measurements of stature available for review? Have the plots on standard growth curves crossed percentile lines?

2. Posterior pituitary gland dysfunction
   - Are there symptoms of hypofunction, including polydipsia and polyuria?

3. Thyroid problems
   - Are there symptoms of hypo- or hyperfunction of this gland (as identified later under each of these problems)?
   - Does the child have another condition associated with secondary thyroid problems, such as trisomy 21, Turner syndrome, exposure to radiation, or type 1 diabetes mellitus?
   - Was there maternal exposure to radioiodine, goitrogens (e.g., thiourea or thiouracil), or iodine medication during pregnancy?

4. Adrenal disorders
   - Are there symptoms of adrenal hypofunction that manifest as either acute adrenal crisis with vomiting, dehydration, and collapse or as a chronic form of disease with weakness, fatigue, and pallor?
   - Are there symptoms of adrenal hyperfunction in the newborn that manifest as alterations in sexual development or present as significant electrolyte and water disturbances?
   - Are there symptoms of acquired hyperfunction (Cushing syndrome) that present with classic symptoms such as moon face, truncal adiposity, muscle wasting and weakness, lethargy, and hypertension?

5. Primary and secondary gonad dysfunction
   - When did the child show signs of sexual development (pubic hair, breast development, axillary or beard/facial hair, menses, scrotal and testicular growth)? This is a key question in premature pubertal development.
   - How has the child been growing? Has growth accelerated? If delayed sexual development is suspected, questions regarding growth rate are important.
   - What are the child's diet and exercise history? Diet and exercise history are im-

portant if secondary amenorrhea resulting from anorexia or bulimia is suspected.

6. Metabolic diseases
   - Are there classic signs and symptoms of diabetes mellitus, PKU, or galactosemia present as identified in this chapter under the specific disease entity?
   - Is there a positive family history of diabetes mellitus, PKU, or galactosemia? Type I diabetes mellitus is associated with certain markers found on chromosome 6 in specific human leukocyte antigen (HLA) regions; PKU and galactosemia are autosomal recessive diseases.

Physical Examination

Endocrine and metabolic disorders can affect numerous body systems. When performing a physical examination on a child with a suspected disorder, the NP should be careful to do the following:

- Measure stature. Supine length is the preferred position for measuring children younger than 2 years of age. Use a stadiometer in children older than 2 or 3 years of age. Height and weight are plotted on a standardized growth chart. Serial measurements of growth to determine growth rate or velocity are essential facts needed to assess growth problems.
- Check for proportionate appearance. Measure sitting and standing heights for upper to lower segment ratio, and check for height age.
- Inspect the child's genitalia carefully. Look for signs of either normal or ambiguous genitalia.
- Identify the stage of sexual development using Tanner staging criteria.
- Note facial, axillary, and body hair as to their presence, distribution, and any unusual texture.
- Examine the skin for striae, acanthosis nigricans of the neck, axilla, or breast.
- Palpate the neck carefully for enlargement of the thyroid gland.
- Perform a detailed physical examination of the newborn, and record any dysmorphic features; some endocrine problems may be manifested at birth.

Acquired endocrine disorders can be manifested by systemic crises caused by either hypo- or hypersecretion of a specific hormone or combination of hormones. Signs of dehydration, exophthalmos, and tachycardia are examples of physical findings associated with endocrine pathology. Newborns with PKU and galactosemia have normal newborn examinations but physical findings develop as the deleterious effects of metabolic alterations become apparent.

Other characteristic physical findings are identified later under the specific disease entity.

Diagnostic Studies

Laboratory studies measuring hormone levels are key indicators of endocrine disorders. Many of these studies are expensive. Accurate interpretation of data requires strict adherence to laboratory protocol for timing the collection of blood specimens.

Specific blood and urine studies that identify end products of abnormal metabolism or elevated or diminished levels of various substances, such as glucose, galactose, amino acids, calcium, or sodium, are important in the diagnosis of metabolic disorders.

Radiographic and imaging studies (e.g., bone age, skull radiographs, ultrasonography, radioactive isotopes, computed tomography [CT], and magnetic resonance imaging [MRI]) are also important diagnostic tools in evaluating certain endocrine disorders.

MANAGEMENT STRATEGIES

General Measures

Chronic disease issues and the effects of these diseases on lifestyle must be addressed:

- Family, school, peer, and emotional adjustment
- Body image, self-esteem, and social competence
- Disease understanding, acceptance, and self-care

Receiving encouragement in self-care and learning about one's disease and the patient–

parent role in management of a long-term illness or chronic condition are essential for successful outcomes.

Genetic Counseling

There are significant implications for the family of a child with endocrine and metabolic disorders that are genetically linked. Genetic counseling is necessary (see Chapter 41).

Medications

Hormone replacement, whether temporary or lifelong, and therapy with other pharmacological agents are often essential components of management of these disorders. Clear instructions about medications are important: how much to give, when to give, side effects to watch for, how to administer, and when to make adjustments in medication.

Dietary Considerations

Many metabolic diseases require rigid adherence to dietary plans and restrictions. Parents and patients must be knowledgeable about dietary needs and restrictions and the effect of diet on the disease process.

Patient and Parent Education

Close supervision and frequent follow-up are necessary for children with metabolic and endocrine disorders. Therefore, it is best that children and teens with such conditions be evaluated initially and periodically by a multidisciplinary health-care team of providers with expertise in pediatric endocrinology. Parents and children will need to learn about the nature of the disorder, the treatment, possible complications, and the plan for long-term follow-up. The team of specialists should keep the primary care provider informed about the plan of care so that the NP can support and reinforce that care. Primary health care needs and anticipatory guidance must not be overlooked in these children.

▓▓▓ SPECIFIC ENDOCRINE AND METABOLIC DISORDERS OF CHILDREN

Common Disorders Detected in the Newborn Period

AMBIGUOUS GENITALIA

Description

The diagnosis of ambiguous genitalia is made when a child is born with varied degrees of both male and female external genitalia. The term *true hermaphrodite* refers to a child who has both male and female gonadal structures. This is rare. It is more common to see either female pseudohermaphroditism, a female with ambiguous external genitalia and female gonads, or male pseudohermaphroditism, a male with ambiguous external genitalia and male gonads. Children born with ambiguous genitalia should be treated as a medical emergency in order to ensure the correct assignment of sex as quickly as possible. There are many causes leading to abnormal sexual differentiation. A referral to a pediatric endocrinologist is necessary to determine the exact etiology as quickly as possible and to institute a treatment plan.

CONGENITAL ADRENAL HYPERPLASIA

Description

The most common cause of ambiguous genitalia is congenital adrenal hyperplasia (CAH), an autosomal recessive disorder. CAH is caused by a deficiency of one of the several enzymes necessary for the adrenal cortex to produce cortisol and aldosterone. The most frequent enzyme deficiency is 21-hydroxylase (95%). The most common form of CAH is caused by overproduction of ACTH, leading to hyperplasia of the adrenal gland and excessive adrenal androgen secretion. When aldosterone and cortisol pathways are blocked or inhibited, excessive sodium is lost through the kidneys, resulting in an inability to maintain serum electrolyte balance. The androgen pathway is overstimulated, and virilization ensues. Patients with CAH fall into two categories: those who are salt losers and those who are not.

Clinical Findings

HISTORY. In CAH, unexplained death in previous infants and other siblings with the same disorder.

PHYSICAL EXAMINATION. Patients with CAH who are not salt losers display varied features. There may be enlargement of the clitoris or penis, development of pubic hair, acne, and acceleration of growth. In affected females, diagnosis is usually made at birth because of ambiguous genitalia. In females, there are normal internal genitalia with varying degrees of virilization of the external genitalia ranging from enlarged clitoris to complete fusion of the labial-scrotal folds, forming a penile urethra. Males often appear normal at birth. Signs of precocious sexual growth may appear in the child by 6 months of age or develop more gradually over the next 4 to 5 years.

Infants who are salt losers begin to have symptoms shortly after birth. Females are more easily identified because of the virilization of their external genitalia (although a female case may be missed because mild virilization is missed). Males have normal genitalia and appear normal. These males are often diagnosed at 7 to 14 days in adrenal crisis. Precocious sexual growth may appear by 6 months of age.

In the salt-losing variety of CAH, symptoms begin shortly after birth and present as

- Failure to regain birth weight
- Progressive weight loss
- Vomiting
- Lack of appetite
- Dehydration
- Symptoms of acute adrenal insufficiency if untreated:
  - Hyponatremia
  - Hypochloremia
  - Hyperkalemia
- Vascular collapse
- If untreated, other symptoms include the following:
  - Rapid somatic growth
  - Advanced epiphyseal maturation leading to short stature as adults
  - Progressive penile or clitoral enlargement
  - Early appearance of facial, axillary, and pubic hair
  - Acne

About 75% of newborns with CAH detected with newborn screening are salt losers (DiGeorge & Levine, 1996).

DIAGNOSTIC TESTS. Laboratory findings include high plasma renin activity, low serum and urinary aldosterone levels, and elevated 17α-hydroxyprogesterone.

Management

The diagnosis and treatment of infants with suspected salt-losing CAH constitute a medical emergency and require an immediate endocrine evaluation and treatment. The NP may follow up with the child between endocrinology visits for well-child care and sick visits and should be familiar with the medical therapy involved. Surgical repair is required for those children with ambiguous genitalia.

Children with salt-losing CAH are given the following:

1. Hydrocortisone (Cortef). This replaces deficient cortisol and suppresses ACTH overproduction, thus inhibiting excessive production of androgen and further virilization. The administration of glucocorticoids suppresses ACTH secretion and produces atrophy of the adrenal cortex. The pituitary–adrenal axis may take 1 to 18 months to return to normal.

   Adjustments in the dosages of the glucocorticoids are based on periodic evaluation of plasma renin activity, 17α-hydroxyprogesterone, and serum androgens and on clinical assessment of growth and pubertal development. The initial dosage for congenital adrenal hyperplasia is 30 to 36 mg/m² with one third of the dose every morning and two thirds every evening or one fourth every morning and midday and one half every evening; maintenance is 20 to 25 mg/m²/day in divided doses (Taketomo et al., 1998).

2. Fludrocortisone (Florinef). This mineralocorticoid is administered to salt-losing patients to replace aldosterone at a dose of 0.05 to 0.15 mg orally daily given as a single dose or in two divided doses.

3. Sodium chloride. Salt is administered to patients with salt-losing forms of CAH at 3 to 5 mEq/kg/day in two to four divided doses.

Assessment of the child's feelings about body changes and differences can be important. Play therapy can be a useful strategy to help children play out and cope with their differences. In addition, a home health referral can be helpful for follow-up, support, and reinforcement to ensure that medications are taken properly and the child and family are adjusting.

Complications

Children with ambiguous genitalia or precocious virilization are at risk for developing disturbances in self-concept and self-esteem. Precocious development can enhance feelings of being different. In addition, there can be other problems such as inability to fight infection, hypoglycemia, and hyponatremia, which can lead to vascular collapse and death.

Patient and Parent Education

The NP's role is to listen to parent and patient concerns and provide anticipatory guidance, referrals, and reinforce the following:

1. Children with CAH should wear medical identification bracelets. Patients or parents also need to carry medical information about the child's condition in case medical therapy is needed from an unfamiliar provider.
2. Families must learn the need for lifelong medication therapy and medical follow-up.
3. Caretakers must know the symptoms of acute adrenal insufficiency (vomiting, lethargy, dehydration) that require immediate medical attention.
4. Education must also include when and whom to call for help in times of unusual stress. At these times there may be a need to triple the dose of hydrocortisone (e.g., illness with fever, pain, or vomiting). The parents should be prepared to give their child an intramuscular injection of hydrocortisone sodium succinate before transport to an emergency department if there are signs of acute adrenal insufficiency.

PHENYLKETONURIA

Description

PKU is a disorder of amino acid metabolism in which phenylalanine cannot be converted to tyrosine because of a deficiency of the enzyme phenylalanine hydroxylase. As a result, toxic levels of phenylalanine accumulate in the blood (hyperphenylalaninemia). If undetected and untreated, PKU causes progressive neurological dysfunction with psychomotor retardation. At present, in all 50 states, routine screening tests are performed on all infants in the first few days of life after the initiation of feeding. Hyperphenylalaninemias can be classified as follows:

Disorder	Plasma Phenylalanine Level (mg/dl)	Mental Retardation (if not treated)
Classic PKU	>20	Severe, profound
Atypical (variant) PKU	6-20	Mild to moderate
Benign persistent hyperphenylalaninemia	2-6	None (no treatment necessary)
Biopterin defects	4-40	None to severe

Etiology and Incidence

PKU most often occurs in whites, with an incidence of 1 in 10,000 to 15,000 live births (US Preventive Services Task Force, 1998). It is inherited as an autosomal recessive trait.

Clinical Findings

The neonate with PKU appears normal at birth, but if the PKU is untreated, signs and symptoms such as vomiting, irritability, and a musty odor in the urine develop.

On physical examination, the child with more advanced disease has a light complexion, eczematoid rash, hypertonicity with hyperactive deep tendon reflexes, seizures, and mental retardation.

DIAGNOSTIC TESTS. Routine screening is done by the collection of blood on filter paper from the heel of an infant. Patients with classic PKU who are on normal diets have serum concentrations of phenylalanine greater than 30 g/dl and a low concentration of tyrosine.

Management

Successful prevention of mental retardation caused by PKU is possible by limiting dietary phenylalanine intake to amounts that permit normal growth and development. The use of a low-phenylalanine, tyrosine-enriched diet with a low-phenylalanine milk substitute such as Lofenalac constitutes treatment. It is generally recommended that the phenylalanine restriction be followed strictly until the child is 6 years of age, when it can be relaxed. However, adolescent females with PKU should be aware that strict dietary adherence must resume if they become pregnant.

Management of a child with PKU should be done at a facility where blood levels of phenylalanine can be followed up and dietary adjustments made. Consultation with or referral to a dietitian is essential.

GALACTOSEMIA

Description

Galactosemia is a disorder of galactose metabolism in which there is a deficiency of galactose-1-phosphate uridyltransferase. Galactose is broken down from the disaccharide lactose, which is primarily found in milk. Without galactose-1-phosphate uridyltransferase, galactose metabolites accumulate in the tissues, leading to the clinical manifestations.

Etiology and Incidence

The incidence of galactosemia is about 1 in 60,000 to 80,000 live births; it is an autosomal recessive trait (US Preventive Services Task Force, 1998).

Clinical Findings

The neonate born with galactosemia appears normal, with clinical manifestations beginning after milk feeding.

HISTORY. In galactosemia, there may be a history of vomiting, weight loss, diarrhea, and lethargy.

PHYSICAL EXAMINATION. If therapy is delayed or therapy is not yet effective, the following may be seen: jaundice, hepatomegaly, hypoto-

nia, severe neonatal *Escherichia coli* infections, cataracts, and death.

DIAGNOSTIC TESTS. Urine testing for glucose with a glucose oxidase method for reducing substance can be done for the initial workup. Confirmation of the diagnosis depends on assay of transferase activity in erythrocytes.

Management

A galactose-restricted diet is the mainstay of therapy for a child with galactosemia. Foods that contain galactose (milk and milk products) are restricted. Milk substitutes such as soybean and casein hydrolysate are used instead of milk. Clinical manifestations subside after galactose intake is restricted. Galactose tolerance generally increases with age; however, pregnant teenagers should be advised to continue the restricted diet throughout the pregnancy.

Growth Hormone Disorders

Assessment of growth is an important component in the routine health care of children. Growth is an indicator of a child's mental and physical health and the quality of the environment. Differentiation of abnormal growth patterns from normal variants is integral to the practice of the NP. Recognition and referral of those children whose abnormal growth pattern is indicative of a pathological process are extremely important. Children with poor growth should be carefully monitored to assess genetic, prenatal, endocrine, nutritional, metabolic, psychological, or systemic chronic illness. GH deficiency (GHD) and GH excess are two endocrine disorders that require referral to a pediatric endocrinologist for appropriate treatment.

GROWTH HORMONE DEFICIENCY

Description

GH is released in response to sleep, exercise, and hypoglycemia. It is responsible for the stimulation of growth in children, whose long bones are not fused. A deficiency is suspected with low levels of human growth hormone (hGH) in the serum or if the level fails to increase in response to sleep, exercise, and hypoglycemia.

Etiology and Incidence

The incidence of GHD is approximately 1 in 4000 (Gotlin et al., 1999). GHD in children can be either congenital or acquired. The majority of the cases of GHD are idiopathic. It is suspected that there is a deficiency or impairment in the secretion of hGH-releasing hormone, or it can be associated with a minor organic hypothalamic lesion. Other causes of GHD include pituitary or hypothalamic disease, trauma, infection, embryological defects, tumors, and irradiation.

Clinical Findings

HISTORY. A history of GHD can include the following:

- Poor growth rate (<4 cm/year) with history of normal birth weight
- Prolonged labor or breech delivery
- Headache, visual field disturbances, polyuria, polydipsia if a tumor is present
- Normal intelligence

PHYSICAL EXAMINATION. The following may be noted on physical examination:

- Proportional short stature
- Increased subcutaneous adiposity
- Hypoglycemia
- Microphallus in males
- Delayed bone age
- Childlike face with large, prominent forehead
- High-pitched voice

DIAGNOSTIC TESTS. Diagnostic evaluation of a child with a suspected growth disorder is highly individualized and should be conducted in conjunction with a pediatric endocrinologist. Constitutional growth delay can be differentiated from genetic short stature by the level of skeletal maturation, which in the latter is consistent with chronological age. In addition to a complete history, the diagnostic evaluation includes

- Growth measurements and evaluation of growth charts

- Complete blood count
- Sedimentation rate
- Urinalysis
- Stool for occult blood and ova and parasites
- Chemistry panel
- Thyroid function tests
- Bone age
- Karyotype (short girls)

A diagnosis of GHD is made when serum hGH is low and hGH levels fail to increase after specific stimulation tests.

Management

The patient should be referred to a pediatric endocrinologist for treatment. The NP should be aware of the type of therapy being used, including expected response and possible adverse reactions. The treatment of GHD has expanded owing to the increased availability of synthetic GH. The range of doses is 0.025 mg/kg per day (a low recommendation) for the younger child to a higher dose of 0.05 mg/kg per day in the older child when there is a need to maximize growth before epiphyseal fusion occurs (Rosenfeld, 1999). However, children with chronic renal failure may receive 0.05 mg/kg per day given subcutaneously. The initial starting dose and dosing schedule are still under consideration. The younger the child is when GH therapy is initiated, the greater the effects. Before age 10 years, doubling of the growth rate is often seen. Side effects include hyperglycemia and increased incidence of slipped capital epiphysis and infection at the administration site.

The average annual cost of GHT is approximately $15,000, which may place a burden on the family. Some states offer assistance through programs for children with special health care needs. The manufacturers also offer a program for financial assistance.

EXCESSIVE GROWTH SYNDROME: PITUITARY GIGANTISM

Description

Pituitary gigantism is a result of hypersecretion of GH, usually caused by a pituitary adenoma. The adenoma also can interfere with the functioning of other pituitary hormones. Hyposecretion of gonadal hormones can lead to pubertal delay or menstrual disturbances.

Clinical Findings

HISTORY. If the tumor occurs before the fusion of the epiphyses, the child is extremely tall with a history of sudden growth. If the tumor occurs after closure of the epiphyses, the child shows signs of acromegaly. Complaints of impaired vision from compression of the optic nerve and symptoms of increased intracranial pressure occur.

PHYSICAL EXAMINATION. Signs of acromegaly that occur after fusion of the epiphyses include coarse facial features, protruding jaw, rapid increase in height, large hands and feet, and thickened skin.

DIAGNOSTIC TESTS. The definitive test for the diagnosis of acromegaly is failure of serum GH level to decrease to less than 2 μg/L after ingestion of glucose (Wilson & Foster, 1992). In normal children, an increase in blood glucose suppresses GH secretion. The presence of a tumor is confirmed with skull films and CT or MRI.

Differential Diagnosis

Other conditions associated with excessive growth include

- Precocious puberty
- Hyperthyroidism
- Constitutional tall stature
- Klinefelter syndrome
- Syndromes of XYY, XXYY
- Marfan syndrome
- Soto syndrome

Management

The patient should be referred to a pediatric endocrinologist. The goal of therapy is to eliminate excessive GH secretion. In those with a pituitary lesion, the treatment regimen includes surgery, radiation, or pharmacological therapy.

CONSTITUTIONAL SHORT STATURE

Description

The most common cause of short stature is constitutionally delayed growth. In most cases, children with constitutional short stature do not have GH abnormalities or any other detectable alteration. Constitutional delay in growth is a variation of normal growth and is not a disease. By adulthood, the child's final height is within the normal adult range. This entity needs to be differentiated from those of a pathological nature.

Clinical Findings

HISTORY. The history may include the following:

- Normal growth velocity with impaired growth during the first several years of life (i.e., the child does increase in height but does so at a below-average rate)
- Delayed pubertal development
- Family history of delayed growth and pubertal development

PHYSICAL EXAMINATION. The following may be seen on physical examination:

- Delayed bone age
- Final height in lower part of the range predicted for family height

DIAGNOSTIC TESTS. The same screening tests are indicated as listed for GHD to rule out pathological processes.

Management

Because it is difficult at times to differentiate constitutional short stature from that due to GHD, an endocrine referral is necessary. Before pharmacological intervention, reassurance and support should be provided to the child regarding ultimate height and development. If the decision is made to treat, males can be started on testosterone at 14 years of age (50 to 100 mg intramuscularly per month for 3 to 6 months). Testosterone provides immediate temporary increased growth velocity, increased virilization, and increased self-esteem. Females can be started on low-dose estradiol. This hormone promotes some growth in addition to breast development.

Secondary to an abundance of recombinant DNA-derived human growth hormone (hGH), GH therapy is being considered for the treatment of non–GH-deficient children; however, current studies suggest that the short-term, long-term, and psychological benefits of GH therapy are minimal (Allen et al., 1994).

DIABETES MELLITUS

Description

Diabetes mellitus is a group of metabolic diseases causing hypoglycemia. It results from defects in insulin secretion, insulin action, or both. Type 1 diabetes is immune-mediated, and there is beta cell destruction in the pancreas, which leads to absolute insulin deficiency. Type 1 diabetes occurs most frequently in children and adolescents but can occur at any age. Type 2 diabetes includes disorders that range from predominantly insulin resistance with relative insulin deficiency to predominantly an insulin secretory defect with insulin resistance. Type 2 diabetes is most commonly associated with the obese, sedentary, and those with strong genetic predisposition. There are also other specific types of diabetes, including gestational diabetes (American Diabetes Association, 1998a).

Etiology and Incidence

Type 1 diabetes occurs in children and adolescents at a rate of 13.8 to 16.9 per 100,000 for white American children and from 3.3 to 11.8 per 100,000 for African-American children. (Tull & Roseman, 1995). Approximately 100,000 children and adolescents younger than 19 years have diabetes (US Department of Health and Human Services, 1995).

Type 1 diabetes previously had been called juvenile-onset or insulin-dependent diabetes mellitus. It is most common in childhood and adolescence but can occur at any age. This form of diabetes results from a cell-mediated autoimmune destruction of the beta cells of the pancreas. Markers of the immune destruction include islet cell antibodies (ICAs), insulin auto-

antibodies (IAAs), autoantibodies to glutamic acid decarboxylase (GAD65) and autoantibodies to the tyrosine phosphates. Also, this disease has strong histocompatibility antigen (HLA) associations (American Diabetes Association, 1998a).

Some forms of type 1 diabetes have no known etiology. People with these forms of the disease may have insufficient insulin and be prone to ketoacidosis, but have no evidence of autoimmunity. Most often these individuals are of African or Asian origin.

Type 2 diabetes has been called adult, maturity-onset, or non–insulin-dependent diabetes. Affected individuals have insulin resistance and relative insufficiency. This type of diabetes is strongly associated with a strong genetic predisposition. Type 2 diabetes can occur in children and youth and has been called maturity-onset diabetes in youth (MODY).

Clinical Findings

HISTORY. The history of patients with diabetes may include

- Polydipsia
- Polyphagia
- Polyuria
- Nocturia
- Blurred vision
- Weight loss
- Fatigue

Onset is usually acute for type 1 diabetes, slower and less acute for type 2; ketonuria and ketonemia occur in type 1 diabetes.

PHYSICAL EXAMINATION. The following signs of ketoacidosis may be found on physical examination:

- Dehydration
- Slow, labored breathing, or air column
- Flushed cheeks and face
- Mental confusion
- Lethargy
- Fruity odor (acetone) on breath

DIAGNOSTIC TESTS

1. Symptoms of diabetes plus a random plasma glucose concentration greater than or equal to 200 mg/dl (11.1 mmol/L).

2. Fasting plasma glucose ≥126 mg/dl (7.0 mmol/L).

3. A 2-hour after-meal plasma glucose greater than or equal to 200 mg/dl (11.1 mmol/L) during an oral glucose tolerance test (OGTT) (American Diabetes Association, 1998c).

It is most likely that children, adolescents and young adults will have type 1 diabetes. Onset of illness is acute, ketones are present in blood and urine, and blood glucose levels can be very high. However, in children with a strong family history of type 2 diabetes and obesity, non–type 1 diabetes is possible. Verification through use of autoantibodies substantiates type 1 diabetes but is not universally recommended at this time because of cost-effectiveness issues. Glycohemoglobin HbA1c measurements are not currently recommended for the diagnosis of diabetes (American Diabetes Association, 1998a).

Management

Traditional multidisciplinary team approaches are one way to manage a newly diagnosed case in a child, especially when the child is ill at the time of diagnosis. However, when the child is not ill, many centers are successfully managing their patients and providing education on an outpatient basis. The goals are to educate the child and family about diabetes management and to stabilize blood glucose levels.

The management team includes the child, parents, primary care provider, pediatric endocrinologist, nurse educator, dietitian, and social worker. All members are essential for the physical and psychological well-being of the child. Diabetes management must integrate education and support for daily insulin, medical nutrition therapy, and exercise into daily life.

The general goals of therapy for children include achieving normal growth and development, optimal glycemic control, minimal acute or chronic complications, and a positive psychosocial adjustment to diabetes. There has been no consensus for adapting glycemic goals for pediatric use (American Association of Diabetes Educators, 1998). Goals must be individualized for each child based on age, ability to recognize hypoglycemia, and self-care skills. Target ranges for blood glucose levels of children and teens vary depending on the judgment of the provider and individual goals set with the child and his or her parents. Guidelines for target levels can range from 80 to 120 mg/dl at fasting and from 80 to 180 mg/dl at other times of the day. Younger children (younger than 6 years) may have goals of 90 to 130 mg/dl fasting and from 90 to 200 mg/dl at other times (Porter et al., 1997). A major study has shown that those who keep blood glucose levels as close to normal as possible had a 60% reduction in the risk, the development, and progression of eye, kidney, and nervous system complications (American Diabetes Association, 1998b). However, the study was done only on older children and cannot be generalized, although most practitioners feel strongly that the effects of hyperglycemia are common to all people with diabetes.

Diabetes control is determined based on HbA1c levels, a daily log of metered glucose values, and clinical symptoms. HbA1c levels determine an approximate level of glycemic control over the past 60 days. Acceptable control for children younger than 7 years is a value around 8 to 8.5% or less, and for older children and teens, levels less than 8.0% are desirable. However, this value must be used in consideration of metered serum glucose values. If the HbA1c level is acceptable but daily values have wide excursions (e.g., moving between 40 and 400 mg/dl), diabetes is not well controlled. Clinical symptoms would include the frequency and severity of hypoglycemia, ketonuria, or weight loss.

Hypoglycemia is the most immediate reason for making adjustments in insulin doses; however, the presence of ketonuria is also an indication for immediate action. Table 26-2 identifies key points to consider for insulin adjustment.

In general, it is wise to decrease insulin doses if there is any unexplained or severe hypoglycemic event. However, in raising insulin doses, it is most acceptable to look for patterns of control over a 3- to 4-day period before increasing insulin doses. Children who are treated with pork NPH insulin generally require approximately ⅔ of their dose in the morning and ⅓ in the evening, whereas those on Hu-

T A B L E 26–2

Considerations for Insulin Adjustments

HYPOGLYCEMIA

Is there a known reason for the hypoglycemia?
  Insufficient food; delayed meal?
  Exercise?
  Extra insulin taken?
Was hypoglycemia severe? Easily treated by
  mouth?
Is there a long period of time between meals and
  snacks?
Which insulin is most likely to be peaking at the
  time of hypoglycemia?

HYPERGLYCEMIA

Is there a known reason for hyperglycemia?
  Too much food; sweets?
  Meals/snacks too close together?
  Insufficient exercise?
  Less insulin given; insulin leaked out of
    pump if used?
Are ketones present in the urine?
Which insulin is most likely to be peaking at the
  time of hyperglycemia?
Does the high blood glucose follow
  hypoglycemia?

mulin NPH most often require a ½ to ½ split. In addition, for those who require 2 or 3 injections daily, there is approximately ⅔ to ⅓ ratio distribution between the NPH (or Lente) and Regular insulin (or Humalog).

The usual diabetes regimen includes medical nutritional therapy and insulin injections 2 to 4 times daily with blood glucose monitored before meals and bedtime. After initial management, frequent follow-up visits at a minimum of 3-month intervals are essential. At first, the family may be in contact with the health care provider on a daily basis until blood glucose levels are stabilized. At each visit, the management plan is reviewed with the child and family and modified based on the physical and pyschosocial needs of the patient and family. Follow-up visits may focus on obtaining information regarding hypoglycemic episodes or ketonuria, results of blood glucose self-monitoring, insulin dose adjustments, and social or emotional issues.

The physical examination visit should include assessment of the following:

- Adequate physical growth and sexual development (children in poor control may not grow normally)
- Blood pressure
- Fundus and vision

Laboratory examination should include

- Glycosylated hemoglobin every 3 months
- Total urinary protein excretion measured once yearly in children who have had diabetes for more than 5 years or after puberty (American Diabetes Association, 1998b)
- Lipid profile done on children older than 2 years of age at time of diagnosis and when glucose control is established (American Diabetes Association, 1998b)
- Thyroid screen yearly

INSULIN THERAPY. Most children are started on an injection regimen 2 to 4 times a day of human or purified pork NPH or Lente insulin along with Regular and/or Humalog. Commercially prepared premixed insulins generally do not allow for the flexibility of daily dosage adjustment based on blood glucose values and exercise levels. Total insulin dosage is 1 unit/kg per day unless the child is in remission. A range of 0.5 to 1.5 units/kg per day is acceptable and allows for individual differences such as age, activity, eating habits, and metabolic requirements. The type and schedule of insulin delivery is highly variable and depends on a number of factors such as the child's routine schedule and the need for flexibility in daily routine. A multiple daily insulin regimen (four injections per day) or an insulin pump can provide the ability to be more flexible in the daily regimen. (See Table 26–3 for a description of the commercially available insulins.) Many children use a "pen," an insulin delivery device that looks like a pen and that can provide insulin easily when they are on the go. Generally, adjustments of the insulin dose are based on the patterns of the blood glucose over several days. However, most often, parents are given a scale or algorithm of Regular or Humalog insulin doses based on before-meal blood glucose. Parents and teens are taught to make adjustments in insulin based on patterns of control. They are helped to adjust insulin to avoid hypoglyce-

TABLE 26-3

Commercially Available Insulin

PRODUCT	MANUFACTURER	ONSET (HR)	PEAK (HR)	DURATION	ORIGIN
RAPID ACTING					
Humalog	Lilly	0.25	1–2	3–4	Human analog
Humulin R	Lilly	0.75	2	6	Human
Novolin R	Novo Nordisk	0.5	2–5	8	Human
Velosulin BR (buffered regular for insulin pump therapy)	Novo Nordisk	0.5	1–3	8	Human
Iletin II Regular	Lilly	0.5–1	2–4	6–8	Pork
Purified Pork R	Novo Nordisk	0.5	2–5	8	Pork
INTERMEDIATE ACTING					
Humulin N	Lilly	3	6–7	13	Human
Novolin N	Novo Nordisk	1.5	4–12	24	Human
Iletin II (NPH)	Lilly	1–3	6–12	18–24	Pork
Purified Pork R	Novo Nordisk	1.5	4–12	24	Pork
Humulin L	Lilly	1–3	6–12	12–28	Human
Novolin L	Novo Nordisk	2.5	7–15	12	Human
Iletin II (Lente)	Lilly	1–3	6–12	12–28	Pork
Purified Pork L	Novo Nordisk	2.5	7–15	22	Pork
LONG ACTING					
Humulin U	Lilly	4–6	14–24	36	Human
MIXTURES					
Humulin 50/50	Lilly	0.5–1	6–12	24	Human
Humulin 70/30	Lilly	0.5–1	6–12	24	Human
Novolin 70/30	Novo Nordisk	1.5	4–12	24	Human

mia and hyperglycemia. Usually, a 10% adjustment in insulin can be safely made by parents. However, in young children, dose adjustments must be made in increments of one-half units.

The usual sites for insulin injection are the legs, arms, and upper outer quadrant of the buttocks. School-age children and adolescents can be encouraged to use their abdomen as a regular injection site; however, young children with minimal subcutaneous abdominal fat have difficulty with this site. Rotation of injection sites is necessary to avoid lipohypertrophy and prevent poor absorption of insulin. It is not clear whether findings from adult studies about insulin absorption are applicable to children (McNabb et al., 1994).

MEDICAL NUTRITIONAL THERAPY. The principles of medical nutritional therapy (MNT) for children and adolescents differ from those for adults primarily because children and teens have unique caloric requirements and do not usually require weight reduction. However, children do need sufficient calories and protein for growth and development.

Nutrition recommendations for children and teens are based on a nutrition assessment. The distribution of calories from fat and carbohydrate can vary and can be individualized based on the nutrition assessment and treatment program (i.e., insulin regimen).

The goals of MNT for children are to maintain normal growth, weight, and sexual development; to prevent obesity, excessive glycemic excursions, hypoglycemia, and hyperlipidemia; to control blood pressure; and prevent future complications of diabetes (American Association of Diabetes Educators, 1998). Generally, calories are split between three meals and two to three snacks daily. Caloric intake is based on body size and surface area and can be calculated from a standard RDA table with the division of calories at approximately 55% carbohydrate, 30% fat, and 15% protein (Sperling, 1996). There are various approaches to nutrition therapy currently being used for children and teens. The American Diabetes Association's traditional exchange diet provides guidelines for a food plan for meals and snacks. Increasingly, carbohydrate counting is an approach being used that allows for a total number of grams of carbohydrate for meals and snacks. Frequently a modified approach of both methods can be successful. MNT for children and adolescents includes the following:

1. Taking in recommended nutrients and vitamins
2. Maintaining a consistent day-to-day intake of food
3. Eating meals and snacks within 1 hour of the usual time
4. Using a protein or fat snack in the evening to prevent hypoglycemia
5. Carefully monitoring carbohydrate intake
6. Avoiding overtreatment of hypoglycemia
7. Decreasing cholesterol, total fat, and saturated fat intake
8. Maintaining ideal body weight
9. Avoiding excessive protein intake (Chase, 1995)

Reevaluation of the nutritional program should occur at least annually in consideration of the growth and development of the infant, child, and adolescent. Consultation with a dietitian should be sought whenever nutritional questions arise that the NP cannot answer.

EXERCISE. Exercise may not result in improved glycemic control in children with type 1 diabetes but is encouraged to promote cardiovascular fitness and long-term weight control and to enhance social interaction and self-esteem through team play (American Diabetes Association, 1998c). Exercise improves glucose utilization, leading to an increased uptake of glucose and, thereby, lowering blood glucose levels. Therefore, additional carbohydrates with protein or fat can be eaten before exercise. Because there is commonly a prolonged hypoglycemic effect from exercise, there can be a possibility of nocturnal hypoglycemia on active days. To replenish glycogen stores depleted during high-intensity exercise, a child or teen with diabetes may require additional food at bedtime and may need to test his or her blood glucose at 3 to 4 AM (American Diabetes Association, 1998a).

Complications

The acute complications of diabetes include ketoacidosis, severe or prolonged hypoglycemia, vaginal yeast infections or thrush, and cellulitis resulting from infection or injury. Chronic complications include microvascular disease such as retinopathy, nephropathy, neuropathy, eating disorders, depression, and cognitive defects as well as macrovascular disease such as arterial obstruction with gangrene of extremities and ischemic heart disease.

Patient and Parent Education

The cornerstone of treatment has and continues to be education regarding diabetes issues and management for the child and family. Diabetes is a relentless illness in that it impacts every facet of daily life. Therefore, it is crucial for parents to have a sound understanding in order to fit diabetes tasks into the activities of daily living. Education of the child, family, and care givers should include insulin therapy, self-monitoring of glucose, nutrition and meal planning, exercise, managing sick days, school issues, coping skills, and prevention of complications. Those with diabetes should always wear a form of medical identification. School personnel must be informed of the plan of care and must implement an individualized care plan for the child. The American Association of Diabetes Educators provides excellent resources (see Resource Box 26–1).

Thyroid Disorders

Thyroid disorders result from inadequate or excessive production of thyroid hormone resulting from congenital anomaly or biosynthetic alteration. The thyroid gland, located below the larynx in the anterior middle portion of the neck, is necessary for growth and development in children, including mental development, sexual maturity, and metabolism.

CONGENITAL HYPOTHROIDISM

Hypothyroidism is a deficiency in thyroid hormone that can be either congenital or acquired (juvenile hypothyroidism).

Description

Congenital hypothyroidism (CH) results from an inadequate production of thyroid hormone, which may be due to a number of causes. CH is the most common cause of preventable mental retardation. Untreated hypothyroidism leads to irreversible brain damage and variable degrees of growth failure, deafness, and neurological abnormalities.

Etiology and Incidence

CH has an overall incidence of 1 in 3600 to 5000 births (US Preventive Services Task Force, 1998). More female than male infants are affected (2:1). The majority of cases of CH are due to partial or complete failure of the thyroid gland to develop, most likely resulting from an autosomal recessive genetic condition. Enzymatic deficiencies are known to cause CH; however, these defects are rare.

Clinical Findings

Often the signs and symptoms of CH are difficult to assess, because most newborns with CH look normal at birth. Normal newborn thyroid test results may decrease vigilance for clinically symptomatic patients. The most common neonatal signs are prolonged jaundice, constipation, and umbilical hernia.

HISTORY. The patient's history may include the following:

- Family history of CH
- Prolonged gestation
- Increased birth weight
- Lag in first stooling
- Feeding or sucking difficulties
- Constipation
- Lethargy

PHYSICAL EXAMINATION. The following may be seen on physical examination:

- Respiratory distress
- Large posterior fontanel, delayed closure
- Abdominal distention with umbilical hernia
- Hypotonia, hypoactivity
- Macroglossia
- Poor peripheral circulation
- Peripheral cyanosis
- Hypothermia
- Jaundice (prolonged)
- Dry, cool, scaly skin
- Delayed mental responsiveness
- Delayed osseous development

DIAGNOSTIC TESTS. Symptoms of hypothyroidism can be clinically unrecognizable during the first month of life. Newborn screening is performed in all 50 states, the District of Columbia, Puerto Rico, and the US Virgin Islands. Screening tests use T_4 measurements of blood collected on filter paper before hospital discharge of the newborn. If the T_4 result is low, a TSH level is obtained on this blood. If this TSH level is elevated, the newborn screen is reported as abnormal. The practitioner may repeat the thyroid screen to determine whether laboratory values are still abnormal before referral. When the TSH level is greater than 15 to 20 mU/L, a pediatric endocrinology workup is necessary (Loechner & Levitsky, 1999). Hypothyroidism can develop in neonates with normal T_4 and TSH levels on newborn screening during the first weeks of life. Infants with the symptoms of hypothyroidism should always be retested. Children with Down syndrome should also be retested at 3 months of age, because they are at increased risk of development of late-onset hypothyroidism. It is recommended that they be tested annually (Bellisario et al., 1987; Roizen, 1999).

Management

The American Thyroid Association Committee on Neonatal Screening recommends a starting dose of levothyroxine sodium (Synthroid) of 10 to 15 µg/kg per day to maintain serum T_4 levels within a 10- to 15- µg/dl range (American Academy of Pediatrics, American Thyroid Association, 1987; DiGeorge & LaFranchi, 1996). Improvement is usually noted within 7 to 21 days. Linear growth and skeletal maturation respond dramatically. Intellectual capacity improves with early treatment. Two key points need to be followed throughout the treatment:

1. Thyroid tests (T_4, free T_4, and TSH levels) need to be done every month for the first 6 months; every other month between 6 and 12 months; and every 3 months thereafter.
2. Bone age needs to be determined at the start of therapy and at 1 year of age.

Differential Diagnosis

Thyroid failure secondary to hypothalamic or pituitary insufficiency must be differentiated from primary hypothyroidism resulting from a defect in the thyroid gland.

Prevention

Neonatal screening programs are the mainstay of prevention.

ACQUIRED HYPOTHYROIDISM

Etiology

The majority of the cases of juvenile hypothyroidism are due to autoimmune chronic lymphocytic thyroiditis, or Hashimoto thyroiditis. Other causes include thyroidectomy, ingestion of a goitrogenic substance (propylthiouracil), iodine deficiency, and irradiation of the thyroid tissue.

Clinical Findings

Manifestations of juvenile hypothyroidism are even more subtle than manifestations of CH.
HISTORY. A child's chief complaint may be only delayed growth. The following are other symptoms:

- Decreased appetite
- Lethargy
- Poor school performance
- Cold intolerance
- Delayed puberty

PHYSICAL EXAMINATION. The following may be noted on physical examination:

- Goiter
- Tenderness of the anterior neck
- Weakness
- Delayed dentition
- Cool, dry, carotenemic skin
- Reflexes diminished or absent

DIAGNOSTIC TESTS. If acquired hypothyroidism is suspected, a referral to a pediatric endocrinologist is suggested to determine the cause of the disease. Initial laboratory tests that may be ordered before referral include:

- T_4, free T_4, and TSH assays
- Serum thyroid antibody measurement

Management

The drug of choice in children and adolescents with acquired hypothyroidism is levothyroxine sodium. Dosage must be individualized based on age and ranges from 8 to 10 μg/kg per day for newborns to 100 to 200 μg/kg per day for adults. In follow-up, serum TSH should be monitored 2 to 3 months after a change in dosage and with symptoms of hypothyroidism or hyperthyroidism (McGhee et al., 1997).

HYPERTHYROIDISM

Description

Hyperthyroidism is present when there are excessive levels of circulating thyroid hormone.

Etiology and Incidence

Hyperthyroidism in children and adolescents is uncommon but is usually due to Graves disease. Graves disease occurs 5 to 7 times more often in girls than in boys. There is an increased frequency of occurrence during the adolescent years (Fisher, 1986; Loechner & Levitsky, 1999). The precise etiology is still unclear; however, an autoimmune component is postulated. Chronic thyroiditis, tumors of the thyroid, and exogenous thyroid hormone excess also can cause hyperthyroidism.

Clinical Findings

Symptoms most often occur in children between 10 and 14 years of age and usually develop over several months.

HISTORY. The history may include the following:

- Emotional instability
- Increased sweating
- Weight loss
- Insomnia
- Tremors
- Behavioral problems or deterioration in school performance

PHYSICAL EXAMINATION. The following may be noted on physical examination:

- Goiter
- Eyelid lag
- Tachycardia
- Systolic hypertension
- Thyroid bruit

DIAGNOSTIC TESTS. The following tests may be ordered before referral:

- Serum T_4 assay
- T_3 resin uptake measurement
- Measurement of antithyroid antibodies

Differential Diagnosis

Diseases that are associated with hypermetabolism, such as leukemia, severe anemia, and chronic infections, need to be ruled out by the appropriate diagnostic tests.

Management

The patient should be referred to an endocrinologist. In mild cases, therapy may not be necessary. Treatment includes the use of propylthiouracil, which blocks the formation of T_4 and T_3. Propranolol may be added to control nervousness and tachycardia. Alternative therapy includes radiation and surgical removal.

Pubertal Disorders

PRECOCIOUS PUBERTY

Description

Precocious puberty is diagnosed when pubertal development occurs before age 8 years in girls and 9 years in boys. True precocious puberty refers to a premature maturation of the hypothalamic–pituitary axis, which initiates sexual development, as opposed to pseudoprecocious puberty, which refers to autonomous secretion of sex steroids as a result of an adrenal or gonadal tumor or exogenous hormones. Girls are more apt to have precocious puberty with no underlying pathology. On the other hand, boys with symptoms of true precocious puberty are found to have central nervous system pathology such as hamartomas, astrocytomas, or gliomas.

Etiology

Causes of precocious puberty are numerous. Common etiologies include idiopathic causes, central nervous system disorders such as trauma, postinflammation and postsurgical damage, hypothalamic hamartomas, tumors and space-occupying lesions, CAH, gonadal tumors, and variants of normal development such as premature thelarche and premature adrenarche (Gotlin et al., 1999; Lee, 1990).

Clinical Findings

Clinical manifestations often associated with precocious puberty may be seen on the history and physical examination.

HISTORY. The history may include the following:

- Breast development
- Pubic hair growth
- Menstruation
- Behavioral changes

PHYSICAL EXAMINATION. Findings on physical examination include the following:

- Accelerated linear growth
- Advanced bone age
- Genital maturation
- Acne

DIAGNOSTIC TESTS. Referral to a pediatric endocrinologist is necessary because of the large number of possible causes and treatments. Laboratory tests that may be ordered before referral include the following:

Blood

- Testosterone (boys)
- Estradiol (girls)
- Thyroid function test
- Serum LH
- Serum FSH
- Dehydroepiandrosterone sulfate (DHEAS) or 24-hour urine 17-ketosteroids

Radiological

- Pelvic ultrasonography (girls)
- Testicular ultrasonography (boys)
- Skeletal age determination
- MRI
- CT

Differential Diagnosis

Benign conditions such as premature thelarche and premature adrenarche must be ruled out.

Management

Treatment of precocious puberty is aimed at eliminating the cause. In the case of central nervous system tumors, radiation, surgery, or chemotherapy is indicated. When a definitive diagnosis is not found, as is usually the case in girls, the treatment of choice is administration of a long-acting gonadotropin-releasing hormone agonist to decrease the circulating gonadotropin and return the sex steroids to the prepubertal levels. It is important to treat precocious puberty in order to increase final adult height.

DELAYED PUBERTY

Description

Puberty is considered delayed if the initial changes of puberty have not occurred by age 13 in girls and age 14 in boys, or if 5 years have elapsed since the first signs of puberty and menarche in girls or the completion of genital growth in boys (Allen et al., 1994; Lee, 1990).

Etiology

There are multiple causes that can delay the onset or progression of puberty. Some causes include the following:

- Chromosomal abnormalities such as Klinefelter and Turner syndromes
- Acquired disease, infection
- Chemotherapy
- Trauma
- Testicular torsion
- Temporary conditions such as chronic illness, stress, malnutrition, or anorexia nervosa
- Permanent deficiencies such as hypothalamic or pituitary gonadotropin deficiency or tumors

Clinical Findings

HISTORY. The history may include cryptorchidism or amenorrhea.

PHYSICAL EXAMINATION. Underdeveloped genitalia, short stature, and immature body proportions may be seen on physical examination.

DIAGNOSTIC TESTS. Initially, plasma LH and FSH level assays should be ordered in addition to bone age determination. Additional tests might include the following:

- GH secretion
- Thyroid function tests
- Blood and urinary pH
- Urine specific gravity
- Sedimentation rate
- Karyotype
- Radiological examinations—MRI, CT, lateral skull films

Management

Because there are various causes of delayed puberty, a pediatric endocrinology referral is necessary. Once the underlying cause is identified, hormonal replacement or hormonal stimulation therapy is the treatment of choice for hypogonadism or low gonadotropin levels.

HYPERCHOLESTEROLEMIA AND HYPERLIPIDEMIA

Description

Cholesterol levels should be less than 170 mg/dl (low-density lipoprotein [LDL] <110 mg/dl). Borderline acceptable results are 170 to 190 mg/dl (LDL 110 to 129 mg/dl). High results are greater than 200 mg/dl (LDL ≥130 mg/dl). For a number of years, attention has been focused on the control and prevention of coronary artery disease (CAD). Because of the relationship between dietary factors (fat and cholesterol) and atherosclerotic disease, it is important to identify children at risk in early childhood. However, the prediction of adult cholesterol levels based on multiple childhood screenings of serum cholesterol levels does not provide an accurate classification of all individuals (Schieken, 1999).

Etiology and Incidence

Atherosclerosis begins in childhood and is related to elevated levels of cholesterol in children as young as 10 years old. Approximately 5 to 25% of children and teenagers have cholesterol levels in excess of 200 mg/dl. Children with elevated serum cholesterol, particularly LDL cholesterol levels, frequently have a family history of CAD, often as a result of blood cholesterol elevation tendency, which leads to early CAD and premature death. Aortic fatty streaks are seen in children as young as 10 years. Genetic disorders for familial hypercholesterolemia, familial combined hyperlipidemia, and familial hypertriglyceridemia are found in 0.5 to 1% of the population. Familial hypercholesterolemia, the best understood of this group of disorders, is an autosomal dominant disease resulting from defective LDL cholesterol receptors with a resultant disorder of lipoprotein metabolism and transport (Schieken, 1999)

The risk factors that indicate the need to screen children for hypercholesterolemia are as follows:

- Family history of heart disease—if parent or grandparent at age 55 years or younger underwent coronary angiography for coronary atherosclerosis, balloon angioplasty, or coronary bypass surgery; had a documented myocardial infarction, angina pectoris, peripheral vascular disease, cerebrovascular accident, or sudden cardiac death
- Either parent has a known total cholesterol level of 240 mg/dl or higher (Schieken, 1999)

Children with incomplete or unknown family histories or with other risk factors should be screened at the discretion of the NP (Tershakovec et al., 1996). The National Institutes of Health (NIH) has published a childhood risk assessment and a screening algorithm that includes the classification, education, and follow-up of patients based on LDL cholesterol levels (Figs. 26-3 and 26-4).

Clinical Findings

HISTORY. Risk factors for hyperlipidemia and hypercholesterolemia are:

- Family history of heart disease as identified earlier
- High-cholesterol, high-fat diet
- Obesity
- Lack of exercise, physical inactivity
- Smoking
- Hypertension
- Diabetes mellitus

DIAGNOSTIC STUDIES. See Figure 26-4. The lipoprotein analysis should be repeated and the two averaged to obtain an average LDL cholesterol level.

Differential Diagnosis

Differential diagnoses include:

1. Secondary hyperlipidemia
   - Exogenous factors such as drugs (e.g., corticosteroids, isotretinoin, thiazides, anticonvulsants, anabolic steroids, certain oral contraceptives), alcohol, obesity
   - Endocrine and metabolic disorders (e.g., hypothyroidism, diabetes mellitus, lipodystrophy, pregnancy)
   - Storage diseases (e.g., glycogen storage disease)
   - Obstructive liver disease (e.g., biliary atresia, cirrhosis)
   - Other causes such as anorexia nervosa, collagen disease, or Klinefelter syndrome
2. Homozygous familial hypercholesterolemia (rare)
   - Plasma cholesterol levels of 600 mg/dl or higher
   - Cutaneous xanthomas develop during the first 6 years of life
   - Atherosclerosis onset before 10 years of age

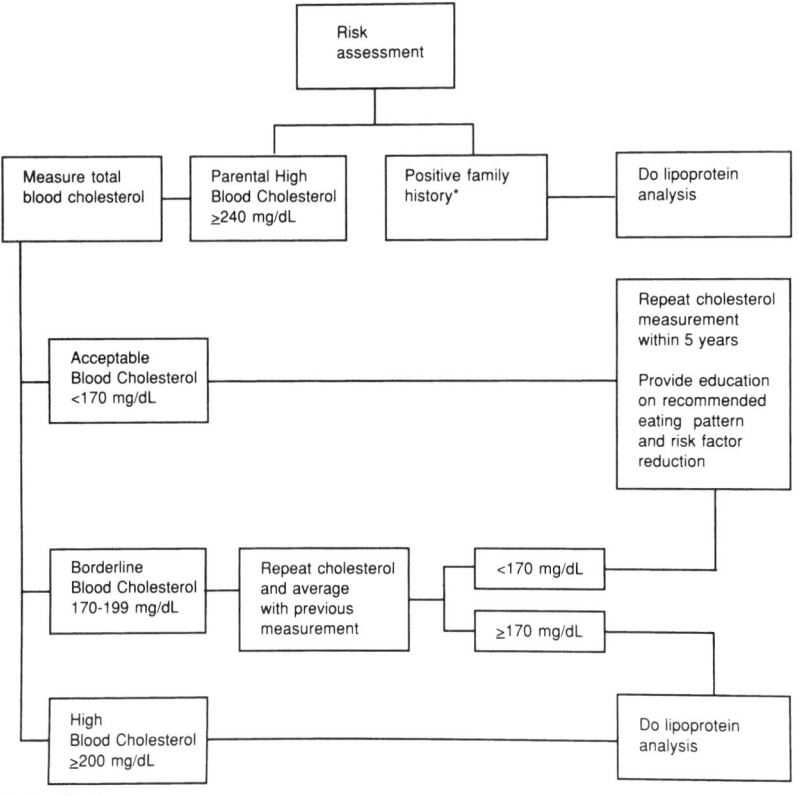

F I G U R E 26-3
Risk assessment of children based on high parental blood cholesterol or a positive family history of premature atherosclerotic disease. (Reprinted from NIH Publication No. 91–2732. September 1991, p 46.)

• Most affected persons die of complications of myocardial infarction before age 30 years (Tershakovec et al., 1996)
3. Heterozygous familial hypercholesterolemia (1 in 500 in the general population)
    • Affected children's total cholesterol levels of greater than 250 mg/dl with LDL cholesterol greater than 200 mg/dl
    • Tendon xanthomas seen in teenagers
    • Xanthomas seen in adults (Tershakovec et al., 1996)

Management

The following plan of action should be taken:

1. Rule out secondary causes of hypercholesterolemia before a treatment regimen is begun (Schieken, 1999).

2. Perform hyperlipidemia screening if family risk factors are identified or if history cannot be ascertained.

3. Manage other risk factors including a history of smoking, low HDL cholesterol concentration (<35 mg/dl), hypertension, severe obesity, or diabetes mellitus. These risk factors may contribute to earlier onset of coronary heart disease. Counsel about their link to cardiovascular disease in adults and the need for lifestyle changes beginning in childhood or adolescence to promote and prevent future cardiovascular disease.

4. Manage blood cholesterol (see Fig. 26-3).

5. Manage blood LDL-cholesterol (see Fig. 26-4).

6. Provide nutritional management: See Table 26-4 for Step-One and Step-Two diets and see Table 26-5 for dietary interventions based on total and LDL cholesterol levels.

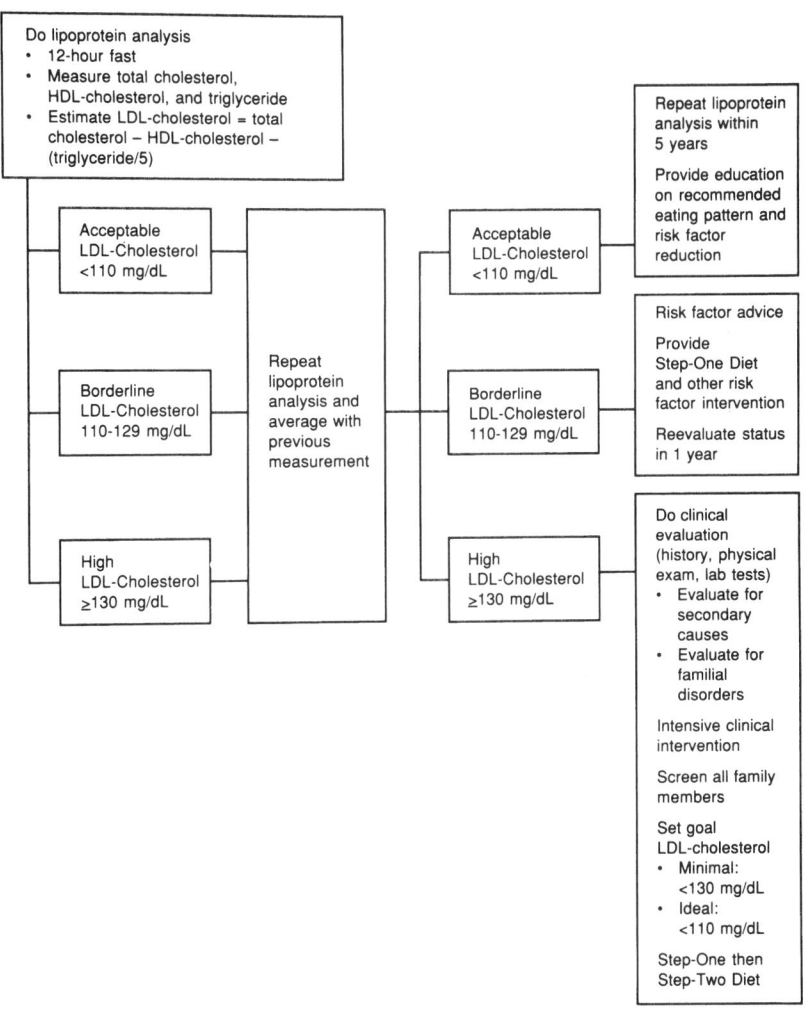

F I G U R E 26-4
Classification, education, and follow-up of patients based on low-density lipoprotein (LDL) cholesterol level. (Reprinted from NIH Publication No. 91–2732. September 1991, p 47.)

7. Drug therapy is recommended for children age 10 years or older under the following conditions: if, after a trial of dietary intervention for 6 months, LDL cholesterol is greater than or equal to 190 mg/dl, cholesterol is greater than 160 mg/dl in a child with a positive family history of premature cardiovascular disease, or two or more other risk factors (see 3) are still present after concerted efforts to control them.

8. Recommended drugs include bile acid sequestrants (such as cholestyramine and col- estipol); however, compliance is frequently problematic. Nicotinic acid and other cholesterol-lowering drugs must be used with caution in children, and referral to a specialist in this area is best (Schieken, 1999).

Prevention

Although the genetic component is fixed in disorders of lipoprotein metabolism and transport, the environmental components that are

T A B L E 26-4

Characteristics of Step-One and Step-Two Diets for Lowering Blood Cholesterol

NUTRIENT	RECOMMENDED INTAKE	
	Step-One Diet	Step-Two Diet
Total fat	Average of no more than 30% of total calories	Same
Saturated fatty acids	Less than 10% of total calories	Less than 7% of total calories
Polyunsaturated fatty acids	Up to 10% of total calories	Same
Monounsaturated fatty acids	Remaining total fat calories	Same
Cholesterol	Less than 300 mg/d	Less than 200 mg/d
Carbohydrates	About 55% of total calories	Same
Protein	About 15–20% of total calories	Same
Calories	To promote normal growth and development and to reach or maintain desirable body weight	Same

From National Cholesterol Education Program: Report of the Expert Panel on Blood Cholesterol Levels in Children and Adolescents. National Heart, Lung, and Blood Institute, US Department of Health and Human Services, Public Health Service. NIH Publication No. 91–2732. Washington, DC: Government Printing Office, 1991.

associated with adult CAD are subject to intervention. Promotion of a healthy lifestyle should begin in childhood.

1. Risk reduction is essential. Health education that emphasizes exercise, weight control, prudent diet (including breastfeeding, late introduction of appropriate solids, control of salt intake, and reduced saturated fat intake), and stress management is the best preventive approach.
2. Early and sustained management of hypertension and diabetes is essential.
3. Smokers (patient or family members) should be counseled and referred to effective intervention programs. The effect on children's personal health and the negative impact of passive smoking should be emphasized.

T A B L E 26-5

Cutoff Points of Total and LDL Cholesterol for Dietary Intervention in Children and Adolescents With a Family History of Hypercholesterolemia or Premature Cardiovascular Disease

CATEGORY	TOTAL CHOLESTEROL (mg/dl)	LDL CHOLESTEROL (mg/dl)	DIETARY INTERVENTION
Acceptable	<170	<110	Recommended population eating pattern: normal diet with reduced cholesterol intake
Borderline	170–199	110–129	Step-One diet prescribed, other risk-factor intervention
High	≥200	≥130	Step-One diet prescribed, then step-Two diet if necessary

From National Cholesterol Education Program: Report of the Expert Panel on Blood Cholesterol Levels in Children and Adolescents. National Heart, Lung, and Blood Institute, US Department of Health and Human Services, Public Health Service. NIH Publication No. 91–2732. Washington, DC: Government Printing Office, 1991.

R E S O U R C E   B O X   26-1

NATIONAL ORGANIZATIONS AND RESOURCES FOR PROBLEMS OF ENDOCRINE AND METABOLIC DISEASE

Ambiguous Genitalia Support Network
Tel: (209) 727-0313

American Association of Diabetes Educators (AADE)
Tel: (312) 424-2426
Website: http://www.aadenet.org

American Diabetes Association
Tel: (800) DIABETES
Website: http://www.diabetes.org

American Dietetic Association
Website: http://www.eatright.org

Barbara Davis Center for Childhood Diabetes
Tel: (303) 315-8796
The book *Understanding Insulin Dependent Diabetes,* by Peter Chase, M.D., can be ordered from this organization.

Children's Diabetes Foundation at Denver
700 Delaware St.
Denver, CO 80204

Human Growth Foundation (HGF)
Tel: (800) 451-6434

Juvenile Diabetes Foundation (JDF)
Tel: (800) JDF-CURE
Website: http://www. jdfcure.com

Magic Foundation for Children's Growth
1327 N. Harlem Ave.
Oak Park, IL 60302

Medic Alert Foundation
Tel: (800) 432-5378

Pediatric Endocrinology Nursing Society (PENS)
PO Box 2933
Gaithersburg, MD 20886

Pituitary Tumor Network Association
Tel: (805) 499-9973

Short Stature Foundation
Tel: (800) 243-9273

Thyroid Foundation of America
Tel: (800) 832-8321
Tel: (617) 726-8500
Website: www.tfaweb.org/pub/tfa

REFERENCES

Allen D, Brook C, Bridges N, et al: Therapeutic controversies: Growth hormone treatment in non-growth hormone deficient subjects. J Clin Endocrinol Metabol 79: 1239–1247, 1994.

American Academy of Pediatrics, American Thyroid Association: Newborn screening for congenital hypothroidism: Recommended guideline. Pediatrics 80: 745–749, 1987.

American Association of Diabetes Educators: *In* Funnell MM (ed): A Core Curriculum for Diabetes Education, 3rd ed. Chicago, IL, Author, 1998, p 544.

American Diabetes Association: Clinical Practice Recommendations 1998: Report of the Expert Committee on the Diagnosis and Classification of Diabetes Mellitus. Diabetes Care 21(suppl 1): S5–S17, 1998a.

American Diabetes Association: Standards of medical care for patients with diabetes mellitus. Diabetes Care 21(suppl 1): 1998b.

American Diabetes Association: Nutrition recommendations and principles for people with diabetes mellitus. Diabetes Care 21(suppl 1):32–35, 1998c.

Barkan AL, Kelch, RP, Hopwood NJ, et al: Treatment of acromegaly with a long acting somatostatin analog SMS 201-995. J Clin Endocrinol Metabol 66:16–23, 1988.

Bellisario R, Brown D, Beblowski D, et al: Newborn screening for hypothyroidism in New York State. *In* Therrel BL Jr (ed): Advances in Neonatal Screening. Amsterdam, Excerpta Medica, 1987, pp 35–39.

Chase PH: Understanding Insulin-Dependent Diabetes, 8th ed. Denver, Hirschfeld Press, 1995.

DiGeorge AM, LaFranchi S: Disorders of the thyroid gland. *In* Behrman RE, Kliegman RM, Arvin A (eds): Nelson Textbook of Pediatrics, 15th ed. Philadephia, WB Saunders, 1996, pp 1587–1605.

DiGeorge AM, Levine LS: Adrenogenital syndrome. *In* Behrman RE, Kliegman RM, Arvin A (eds): Nelson Textbook of Pediatrics, 15th ed. Philadephia, WB Saunders, 1996, pp 1617–1623.

Fisher DA: Thyroid physiology in the perinatal period and during childhood. *In* Ingbar SH, Braverman LE (eds): The Thyroid. Philadelphia, JB Lippincott, 1986, pp 1387–1395.

Gotlin R, Kappy MS, Slover RH, et al: Endocrine disorder. *In* Hathaway W, Groothuis J, Hay W, et al (eds): Current Pediatric Diagnosis and Treatment, 14th ed. Stamford, CT, Appleton & Lange, 1999, pp 812–850.

Lee PA: Disorders of puberty. *In* Lifshitz F (ed): Pediatric Endocrinology: A Clinical Guide, 2nd ed. New York, Marcel Dekker, 1990, pp 217–248.

Loechner KJ, Levitsky LL: Thyroid disorders. *In* Burg FD, Ingelfinger JR, Wald ER, et al (eds): Gellis & Kagan's Current Pediatric Therapy, 16th ed. Philadelphia, WB Saunders, 1999.

McGhee B, Howrie D, Kraisinger M, et al: Pediatric Drug Therapy Handbook & Formulary 1998-1999. Department of Pharmacy, Children's Hospital of Pittsburgh. Cleveland, Lexi-Comp, 1997.

McNabb W, Quinn M, Murphy D, Thorp F, et al: Increasing children's responsibility for diabetes self-care: The In Control study. Diabetes Educator 20:121-124, 1994.

Porter PA, Keating B, Byrne G, et al: Incidence and predictive criteria of nocturnal hypoglycemia in young children with insulin dependent diabetes mellitus. J Pediatr 130:366-372, 1997.

Roizen NJ: Down syndrome. *In* Burg FD, Ingelfinger JR, Wald ER, et al (eds): Gellis & Kagan's Current Pediatric Therapy, 16th ed. Philadelphia, WB Saunders, 1999, pp 422-429.

Rosenfeld RG: Hypopituitarism and growth hormone therapy. *In* Burg FD, Ingelfinger JR, Wald ER, et al (eds): Gellis & Kagan's Current Pediatric Therapy, 16th ed. Philadelphia, WB Saunders, 1999, pp 731-733.

Schieken RM: The child at risk for coronary heart disease as an adult. *In* Burg FD, Ingelfinger JR, Wald ER, et al (eds): Gellis & Kagan's Current Pediatric Therapy, 16th ed. Philadelphia, WB Saunders, 1999, pp 578-582.

Sperling MA: Diabetes mellitus. *In* Behrman RE, Kliegman RM, Arvin A (eds): Nelson Textbook of Pediatrics, 15th ed. Philadephia, WB Saunders, 1996, pp 1646-1666.

Taketomo CK, Hodding JH, Kraus DM: Pediatric Dosage Handbook. Cleveland, Lexi-Comp, 1998.

Tershakovec AM, Coates PM, Cortner JA: *In* Behrman RE, Kliegman RM, Arvin A (eds): Nelson Textbook of Pediatrics, 15th ed. Philadephia, WB Saunders, 1996, pp 377-384.

Tull ES, Roseman JM: Diabetes in African-Americans. *In* Diabetes in America, 2nd ed. Bethesda, MD, National Institute of Diabetes and Digestive and Kidney Diseases, 1995, pp 613-625.

US Department of Health and Human Services: Diabetes Statistics (NIH Publication #96-3926). Bethesda, MD, 1995.

US Preventive Services Task Force: Guide to Clinical Preventive Services: An Assessment of 169 Interventions. Baltimore, Williams & Wilkins, 1998.

Wilson JD, Foster DW (eds): Williams Textbook of Endocrinology, 8th ed. Philadelphia, WB Saunders, 1992, pp 221-259.

CHAPTER 27

Hematological Diseases

Martha K. Swartz

INTRODUCTION

Blood is a major homeostatic force of the body. Essential body functions carried out by blood include the transfer of respiratory gases, hemostasis, phagocytosis, and the provision of cellular and humoral agents to fight infection. Abnormalities of blood cells are seen in various disease states and alterations in nutrition. Therefore, diagnostic hematological studies are an essential part of pediatric practice. For the pediatric provider, the types of hematological diseases encountered in the clinical setting range from common nutritional deficiencies in which treatment is straightforward to those rare disorders with a genetic or chronic component that necessitate extensive referral and a multidisciplinary approach. In pediatrics, particularly, early diagnosis of blood disorders is important to ensure the best possible prognosis.

ANATOMY AND PHYSIOLOGY

Blood is made up of a cellular component with specialized functions and a fluid component or plasma. The cellular component consists of red blood cells (RBCs), or erythrocytes; white blood cells (WBCs), or leukocytes; and platelets, or thrombocytes. Leukocytes are further differentiated into granulocytes, monocytes, and lymphocytes. Plasma is a clear yellow fluid in which proteins (primarily albumins, globulins, and fibrinogen) are the major solutes. These plasma proteins maintain intravascular volume, contribute to the coagulation of blood, and are important in acid–base balance.

Blood formation in the human embryo initially takes place in the yolk sac during the first several weeks of gestation. In the second trimester, blood is formed primarily in the liver, spleen, and lymph nodes. During the last half of gestation, hematopoiesis shifts from the fetal liver and spleen to the bone marrow, where by birth, most blood formation takes place. Bone marrow produces erythrocytes, granulocytes, monocytes, and platelets and provides lymphocytes and lymphocytic precursors to the spleen, lymph nodes, and other lymphatic tissues.

Erythrocytes

Production of RBCs is regulated by the specific hormone erythropoietin, produced primarily by renal glomerular epithelial cells. In response to a decrease in the number of circulating RBCs or a decrease in the PaO_2 of arterial blood, erythropoietin stimulates the bone marrow to convert certain stem cells to proerythroblasts. Substances essential for RBC formation include iron, vitamin B_{12}, folic acid, amino acids, and other nutrients. The RBC matures through the following stages: proerythroblast, erythroblast, normoblast, reticulocyte, and erythrocyte.

As cellular differentiation occurs, the nucleus present in the early forms of the cell is extruded and replaced by hemoglobin (Hb). The RBC assumes its characteristic non-nucleated biconcave disk shape, which is easily distorted, thereby enabling it to pass through small capillaries and sinuses without being destroyed. The large surface-to-volume ratio also facilitates rapid gas exchange.

The youngest red cells are the reticulocytes; after release from the bone marrow, they stay in circulation about 1 day before becoming mature RBCs. The reticulocyte count is about 4 to 6% for the first 3 days of life, which reflects the relatively greater amount of erythropoiesis that occurs in the fetus. This increased reticulocyte count is followed by a sudden drop to the normal range of 0.5 to 1.5% (see Appendix C). A mature RBC lasts about 120 days before it is destroyed through phagocytosis in the spleen, liver, or bone marrow.

Hemoglobin

Hemoglobin is the oxygen-carrying protein molecule in the RBC. Each hemoglobin molecule is made up of two pairs of polypeptide chains (the globin portion) attached to heme groups, which are large disks containing iron and porphyrin, a nitrogen-containing organic compound. Various forms of hemoglobin are found in the embryo, fetus, and adult, depending on changes in globin chain synthesis. At birth, approximately 70% of hemoglobin is made up of fetal hemoglobin (Hb F). By 12 months of age, 95% of hemoglobin consists of the normal adult hemoglobin molecules (Hb A), which are composed of two α- and two β-polypeptide chains attached to four heme groups. Hb F remains present at levels of less than 2%. Hb A_2, another type of normal hemoglobin composed of two α- and two δ-globin chains, makes up about 2.5% of the total hemoglobin.

Each of the four iron atoms in the hemoglobin molecule combines reversibly with an atom of oxygen to form oxyhemoglobin. This reaction occurs when the oxygen concentration is relatively high, as in the lungs, where oxygen crosses the alveolocapillary membrane and saturates about 96% of the hemoglobin. This percentage is the arterial oxygen saturation (Sao_2), and it is measured through pulse oximetry or arterial blood gas determination. When the oxygen concentration is lower, as in the tissues, oxygen is released to meet cellular needs.

The level of hemoglobin in a newborn ranges from 15 to 22 g/dl and then drops to its lowest point at 3 to 6 months, which is a physiological anemia caused by the shortened survival of fetal RBCs and the rapid expansion of blood volume during this period. A decrease in hemoglobin can also develop secondary to a decrease in RBC production, blood loss, or increased RBC destruction. Because of these processes, transport of oxygen to the tissues is adversely affected, and the individual can become clinically anemic.

Antigenic Properties of Red Blood Cells

Red cells are classified into different types according to the presence of antigens on the cell membrane. The most common antigens are A, B, and Rh. A person inherits either A or B antigen (type A or B blood), both antigens (type AB blood, which is the universal recipient), or neither antigen (type O blood, which is the universal donor). Of the six types of Rh factors, the most common is D, which accounts for the Rh+ designation. In the United States, 85% of whites and 95% of blacks are Rh+ (Guyton & Hall, 1996). Clinically, these distinctions become important when blood transfusions are necessary or in assessment for maternal–fetal blood incompatibilities.

Leukocytes

Leukocytes, or WBCs, are larger and fewer in number than erythrocytes. Normally, about 5000 to 10,000 leukocytes are contained in a microliter of blood. The primary function of WBCs is protection of the body from invasion by foreign organisms and distribution of antibodies and other factors of the immune response.

Five distinct types of WBCs can be grouped into two broad classifications: *granulocytes* (also known as polymorphonuclear leukocytes

[PMNs], or "polys") and *agranulocytes* (Table 27-1). Granulocytes contain large granules and horseshoe-shaped nuclei that become segmented and are connected by thin strands (Fig. 27-1). With Wright's stain, the cytoplasm stains blue or pink. Granulocytes are further divided into *neutrophils; eosinophils,* which absorb the acid dye eosin; and *basophils,* which absorb a basic dye. The agranulocytes include *lymphocytes* (also known as *immunocytes*) and *monocytes.*

Granular Leukocytes

In children, granulocytes make up 30 to 60% of all WBCs. They mature in the bone marrow through the following stages: stem cells, myeloblasts, promyelocytes, myelocytes, metamyelocytes, band forms, and mature segmented neutrophils. This maturational process takes approximately 6 to 11 days. Once a neutrophil is released into the bloodstream, it circulates about 6 to 9 hours before entering the tissues, where the major function of PMNs is phagocytosis of harmful particles and cells, particularly bacterial organisms.

A frequency distribution of the types of WBCs is obtained by the *differential count,* and quantitative alterations within the categories are important diagnostically (see Table 27-1). A relative increase in the number of band (or other immature) cells is often called a "shift to the left," a term derived from how the differential count used to be tabulated on written forms. This phenomenon is indicative of the body's immunological response to an infectious process.

Basophils and eosinophils are also important in the body's inflammatory and allergic responses. Basophils, which account for less than 1% of circulating leukocytes, release heparin and histamine into the bloodstream during systemic allergic reactions. They contain receptor sites for immunoglobulin E (IgE), levels of which are elevated in people with allergies; they also prevent clot formation in the microcirculation. Eosinophils are found in the mucosa of the gastrointestinal tract and in the lungs. They are weakly phagocytic. Eosinophilia is also associated with allergic reactions, as well as parasitic infections and drug reactions.

Monocytes

Monocytes, which contain a large lobulated nucleus, are relatively immature cells that circulate for about 8 hours before migrating to tissues, where they assume their mature form as macrophages. Like granulocytes, which are the first line of defense against microbe invasion, their primary function is phagocytosis of bacteria and cellular debris. Fixed and mobile macro-

TABLE 27-1

Normal Leukocyte Differential Count

	GRANULOCYTES				AGRANULOCYTES	
AGE	Segmented Neutrophils (%)	Band Neutrophils (%)	Eosinophils (%)	Basophils (%)	Lymphocytes (%)	Monocytes (%)
Birth	47 ± 15	14.1 ± 4	2.2	0.6	31 ± 5	5.8
6 mo	23	8.8	2.5	0.4	61	4.8
12 mo	23	8.1	2.6	0.4	61	4.8
2 y	25	8.0	2.6	0.5	59	5.0
4 y	34 ± 11	8.0 ± 3	2.8	0.6	50 ± 15	5.0
6 y	43	8.0	2.7	0.6	42	4.7
8 y	45	8.0	2.4	0.6	39	4.2
10 y	46 ± 15	8.0 ± 3	2.4	0.5	38 ± 10	4.3
12 y	47	8.0	2.5	0.5	38	4.4

Data from Wallach J: Interpretation of Diagnostic Tests, 6th ed. Boston, Little, Brown, 1996.

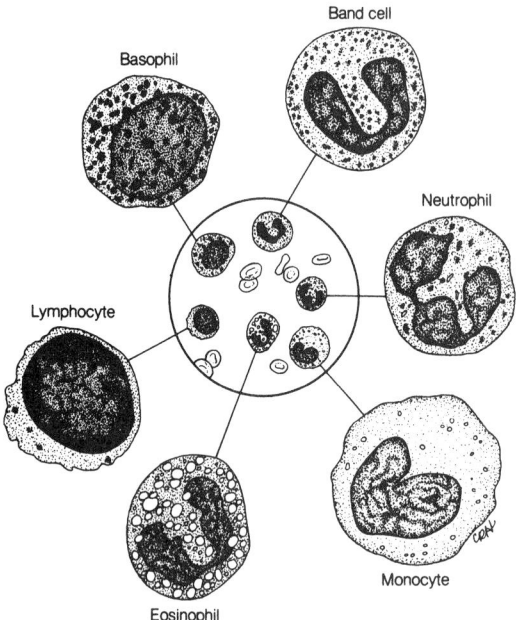

F I G U R E 27-1
Types of white blood cells (leukocytes) in comparison with red blood cells (the smaller cells) in the *circle*. (From Jackson DB, Saunders RB: Child Health Nursing. Philadelphia, JB Lippincott, 1993.)

phages are located primarily in the liver, spleen, lymph nodes, and gastrointestinal tract and make up the monocyte–macrophage system, also known as the reticuloendothelial system (Guyton & Hall, 1996).

Lymphocytes

Lymphocytes (or immunocytes), although not phagocytic, protect the body against specific antigens. They originate in the bone marrow but differentiate in lymphoid tissues such as the spleen, liver, thymus, lymph nodes, and intestines. Thymus-dependent lymphocytes, or *T cells,* are part of the cell-mediated immune response in which cytotoxic agents and macrophages are synthesized. *B-cell* lymphocytes are precursors of the humoral immune response whereby the cells are transformed into plasma cells that release immunoglobulins or antibodies into the bloodstream.

Platelet Cells and Coagulation Factors

The smallest cellular components in blood are the platelets, or thrombocytes, which are essential to hemostasis and clot formation. Circulating platelets are fragments of megakaryocytes, which are precursor cells that form in the bone marrow. The normal platelet count ranges from 150,000 to 300,000 cells/mm^3.

When a blood vessel is injured (or in the presence of intrinsic damage to the blood), platelets adhere to the inner surface of the vessel and form a hemostatic plug. As the platelets are degraded, a series of at least 13 clotting factors or proteolytic enzymes are released that bring about the clotting process in a cascading sequence of successive reactions (Fig. 27-2).

T A B L E 27-2

Blood Coagulation Factors

FACTOR (INTERNATIONAL NOMENCLATURE)	COMMON SYNONYMS
I	Fibrinogen
II	Prothrombin
III	Tissue thromboplastin, thrombokinase
IV	Calcium
V	Proaccelerin, labile factor, accelerator globulin
(VI)	Obsolete term
VII	Proconvertin, stable factor
VIII	Antihemophilic globulin (AHG), antihemophilic factor (AHF), antihemophilic factor A
IX	Plasma thromboplastin component (PTC), Christmas factor, antihemophilic factor B
X	Stuart-Prower factor, Stuart factor
XI	Plasma thromboplastin antecedent (PTA), antihemophilic factor C
XII	Hageman factor, contact factor, antihemophilic factor
XIII	Fibrin-stabilizing factor (FSF), plasma transglutaminase

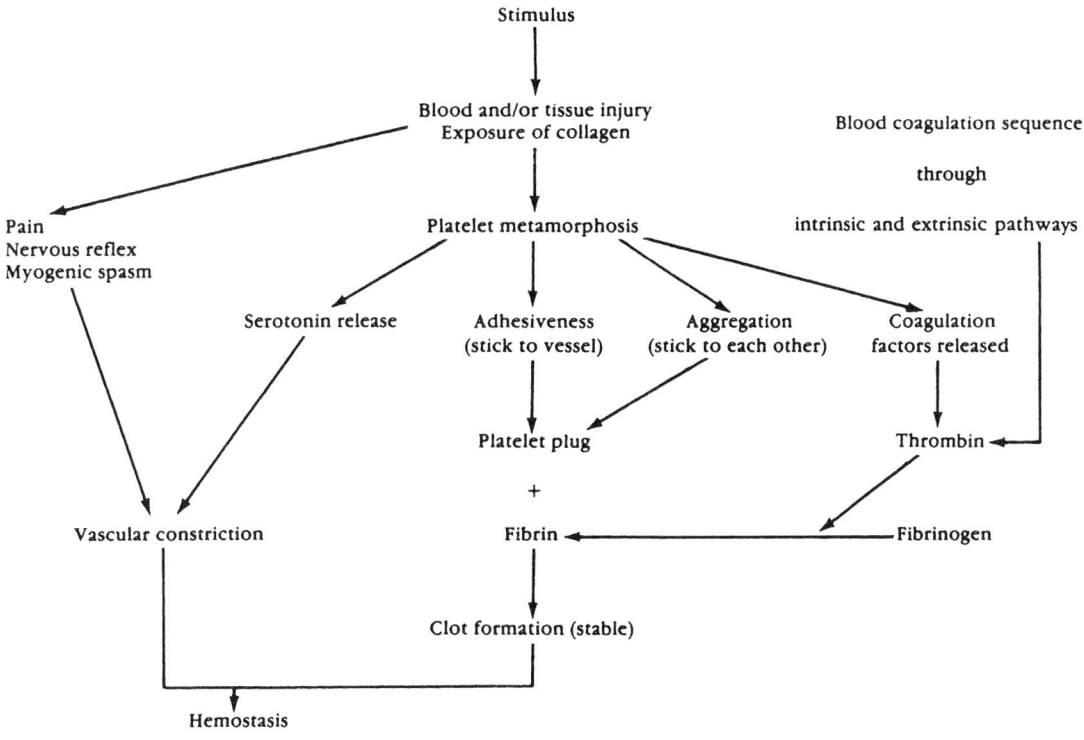

F I G U R E 27-2
Hemostatic mechanisms. (From Bullock B, Rosendahl P: Pathophysiology: Adaptations and Alterations in Function. Philadelphia, JB Lippincott, 1995.)

The basic reactions that occur in the sequential process of blood coagulation are as follows: As factor X is activated, prothrombin (factor II) is converted to thrombin, which then catalyzes the conversion of fibrinogen (factor I) to fibrin (Table 27-2). Fibrin provides the matrix in which blood cells aggregate to form a clot. A deficiency of any of the proteins in the pathway leads to a clotting disorder. In particular, if factor VIII is deficient (as in classic hemophilia) or the number of platelets is inadequate (thrombocytopenia), activation of factor X is impaired.

PATHOPHYSIOLOGY

Hematological problems are generally classified as disorders of RBC function, WBC function, and platelet and coagulation function. These three broad categories are further divided into disorders of blood cell production, maturation,

or destruction. Knowledge of these pathophysiological classifications gives the provider a rationale for routine screening and useful algorithms to guide further clinical investigation.

Classification of the Anemias

Anemia is generally defined as a reduction in blood hemoglobin concentration or a decrease in red cell mass below the normal range. The reduction in the amount of circulating hemoglobin also causes a decrease in the oxygen-carrying potential of the RBC. Morphologically (according to RBC size, shape, and color), anemias are described as hypochromic, microcytic; as macrocytic; or as normochromic, normocytic. This approach is a useful method for ruling out particular causes of anemia when trying to determine the underlying etiology (Table 27-3). In toddlers and young children, approximately 90% of cases of anemia are accounted for by

T A B L E 27-3
Acute Anemia in Childhood and Adolescence

CLASSIFICATION	HISTORY	PHYSICAL FINDINGS	SCREENING TESTS	DIAGNOSTIC TESTS	TREATMENT
I. Microcytic Iron-deficiency anemia	Infant and toddler Excessive cow's milk ingestion Poor solid food intake	Waxy, sallow appearance of skin	Hb: <7 g/dl MCV: <60 fl Retic: ↓ to sl ↑	Serum Fe: ↓ TIBC: ↑ % Saturation: ↓	Ferrous sulfate, 6 mg/kg/d of elemental iron Discontinue cow's milk Limit formula to <24 oz/d and encourage solid food
Homozygous thalassemia (Cooley anemia)	Infant and toddler Growth failure Ethnic background consistent	Hepatosplenomegaly Frontal bossing	Hb: var ↓ MCV: 50–60 fl		
II. Macrocytic Diamond-Blackfan anemia		*See III. Normocytic*			
Megaloblastic anemia	Variable, depending on etiology	Variable, depending on etiology	Hb: var ↓ MCV: ↑ Retic: ↓ Platelets and WBC: ↓ Hypersegmented polys	Bone marrow: megaloblastic Vitamin B$_{12}$ Folate Others	Variable, depending on etiology
III. Normocytic A. Productive defect Diamond-Blackfan anemia	Age: 65% <6 mo; 90% <1 y Insidious onset	25% with physical abnormalities	Hb: 2–3 g/dl MCV: ↑ in 30% (100% after treatment) Retic: <1%	Bone marrow: erythroid hypoplasia and lymphocytosis Hb F: ↑ RBCi antigen: ↑	Prednisone: 2 mg/kg/d in 3–4 doses until Hb >10 g/dl
Transient erythroblastopenia of childhood	1 to 3 y of age Viral illness in preceding 3 mo	None	Hb: 3–9 g/dl MCV: normal Retic: <1%	Bone marrow: erythroid hypoplasia	Supportive
Aplastic crisis of hemolytic anemia	Underlying hemolytic anemia Viral syndrome in preceding 1 to 3 wk Sudden exacerbation of pallor	Splenomegaly	Hb: <7 g/dl Retic: <1% Smear: abnormalities of chronic anemia	Bone marrow: erythroid hypoplasia	Supportive

Marrow infiltration	Variable, depending on etiology Bleeding Infection	Petechiae, purpura Infection Hepatosplenomegaly	Hb: var ↓ Retic: ↓ to nl Platelets: ↓ WBC: ↓ or ↑ Smear: variable	Bone marrow: infiltration by nonhematopoietic cells	Variable, depending on etiology (e.g., leukemia, neuroblastoma)
Aplastic anemia	Bleeding Infection Multiple anomalies possible with Fanconi anemia	Petechiae, purpura Infection	Hb: var ↓ MCV: ↑ in Fanconi anemia Retic: ↓ Platelets and WBC: ↓	Bone marrow: hypoplasia of all hematopoietic elements	Variable
B. Hemolytic Autoimmune hemolytic anemia	Jaundice Gastrointestinal symptoms Dark/red urine	Icterus Hepatosplenomegaly	Hb: var ↓ Retic: ↑ (occ ↓) Smear: microspherocytes	Direct Coombs test: positive	Corticosteroids: prednisone or intravenous equivalent: 2–6 mg/kg/d Transfusion indicated
Hemolytic-uremic syndrome	Infant and toddler Viral prodrome Gastrointestinal bleeding in 20% Sudden pallor, purpura ± Central nervous system symptoms	Purpura Hypotension ± Central nervous system abnormalities	Hb: 7–8 g/dl Retic: ↑ Platelets: ↓ Smear: microangiopathy	None Renal failure—supportive	Supportive: early dialysis ? Plasma infusion/exchange ? Antiplatelet drugs
C. Blood loss Splenic sequestration crisis of sickle cell (SS) disease (internal blood loss)	SS disease: 5 mo to 2 y of age Hb SC or S-thalassemia: all ages Sudden weakness, dyspnea, abdominal distention Shock	Hypotension Massive splenomegaly	Hb: <4 g/dl Retic: ↑ Smear: sickle cells	None	Plasma expanders: whole or reconstituted blood

Fe = iron; Hb = hemoglobin; MCV = mean corpuscular volume; nl = normal; OCC = occasionally; polys = polymorphonuclear leukocytes; RBCi = red blood cell i antigen; Retic = reticulocytes; sl = slightly; TIBC = total iron-binding capacity; var = variably; WBC = white blood cell count.
Adapted from Green M, Haggerty R: *Ambulatory Pediatrics IV.* Philadelphia, WB Saunders, 1990, pp 378–379.

iron deficiency, lead poisoning, infections, and hemoglobinopathy.

Anemias that are caused by *inadequate production* include acquired and constitutional aplastic anemia, red cell aplasia, and transient erythroblastosis of childhood (TEC). Maturational anemias are caused by nutritional disturbances such as iron deficiency, lead poisoning, and deficiencies in folic acid and vitamin B_{12}. Anemias are also a common occurrence in chronic illnesses in which either red cell survival time is decreased or the bone marrow response or transport of iron is impaired. Such conditions include chronic inflammatory illnesses, chronic infections, renal and liver disease, endocrine disorders, and malignant neoplastic diseases.

Anemias that are the result of *increased cell destruction* are hemolytic anemias and are caused by defects in the red cell membrane, hereditary hemoglobinopathies (as in sickle cell anemia), and congenital enzyme defects. These syndromes also include hereditary spherocytosis (HS) and glucose-6-phosphate dehydrogenase (G6PD) deficiency.

White Blood Cell Dysfunction

The WBC count and differential are useful diagnostic guides in the management of a variety of childhood illnesses. The normal range of granulocyte and lymphocyte counts varies throughout childhood (see Table 27-1). Neutrophilic leukocytosis (absolute neutrophil count [ANC], >7500/µl) occurs in pathological conditions such as acute infections, cancer, hemorrhage, hemolysis, tissue necrosis, or toxic exposure. A relative increase in the number of circulating immature band neutrophils (i.e., a shift to the left) is also indicative of an inflammatory process or acute bacterial infection.

Alterations of Granulocytes

Neutropenia (ANC, <2500 cells/mm³) results from decreased cellular production (as in various hematological diseases, infections, drug-induced states, and nutritional deficiencies), increased peripheral destruction (as in autoimmune disorders), or peripheral pooling (as in bacterial infections, hemodialysis, and cardio-

pulmonary bypass). Most cases of neutropenia are discovered during evaluation of the WBC count in a child with an acute febrile illness. In an otherwise healthy child who is not taking any medication, the neutropenia should be monitored at least twice weekly. If it does not resolve over a 6-week period, the child should be managed in consultation with a hematologist and immunologist (Platt, 1999). In rare cases when the ANC is less than 500 cells/mm³, the child should be hospitalized for extensive culturing and coverage with broad-spectrum antibiotics.

Qualitative abnormalities of granulocytes are usually related to defects in the function of phagocytosis. These defects occur with collagen-vascular disorders and bacterial infections. The ingestion of certain drugs such as aspirin or corticosteroids leads to dysfunction of the phagocyte (Bullock, 1996). *Granulomatous diseases* are relatively rare disorders of granulocytes, particularly neutrophils, in which the enzymes necessary for bactericidal activity are lacking. Such diseases result in severe, recurrent infections of the skin, lymph nodes, lungs, liver, and bone.

Lymphocytic Disorders

Lymphocytosis is produced by viral illnesses, including mumps, measles, rubella, rubeola, varicella, and hepatitis. Pertussis and chronic lymphocytic leukemia also elevate the lymphocyte count. An increase in the number of atypical lymphocytes is evident in infectious mononucleosis, cytomegalic inclusion disease, and toxoplasmosis.

Malignant White Blood Cell Disorders

Leukemia refers to a group of malignant diseases with qualitative and quantitative changes in circulating leukocytes. Leukemia is characterized by diffuse, abnormal growth of leukocytic precursors in the bone marrow. Such an uncontrolled increase in immature WBCs leads to anemia and thrombocytopenia. Life-threatening infections occur because of a decrease in the function of circulating WBCs. Leukemias are further classified according to the course of the illness and the types of cells and tissues involved.

Malignant lymphomas, as in Hodgkin disease, are solid neoplasms that are lymphocytic in origin. They are associated with lymphadenopathy and tumor development in the liver, spleen, thymus, bone marrow, and submucosa of the gastrointestinal and respiratory tracts. Lymphomas are classified according to the type of cell involved (B cells, T cells, or monocytes). As the cell becomes more undifferentiated, the tumor becomes more aggressive (Bullock, 1996). As in leukemia, immune deficiencies develop and are followed by infection.

Platelet and Coagulation Disorders

In pediatrics, the most common cause of thrombocytopenia (platelet count, $<100,000/mm^3$) is idiopathic thrombocytopenic purpura (ITP). It is associated with destruction of circulating platelets brought about by an immune-mediated process.

When thrombocytopenia occurs, it is critical to rule out acute lymphocytic leukemia (ALL). If the child is febrile, meningococcemia should be considered (Platt, 1999). Secondary thrombocytopenia results from drug hypersensitivity, viral infections, and autoimmune conditions. Thrombocytosis, or an elevation in the platelet count, is associated with certain malignancies or with polycythemia vera.

Disorders of coagulation can be brought about by deficiencies of any of the clotting factors. Single–coagulation factor deficiencies are usually hereditary. The most common are deficiencies in factor VIII (classic hemophilia), factor IX (hemophilia B or Christmas disease), and factor XI (hemophilia C or Rosenthal syndrome).

▰▰▰ ASSESSMENT

History

A comprehensive, focused history and physical assessment are important aspects of the evaluation of a child with anemia or other suspected hematological disorder. Many hematological processes are inherited. Therefore, the family history, nationality, and geographical origins are aids to diagnosis. For example, thalassemia occurs most often among patients of Mediterranean or Asian descent; G6PD deficiency is found in these ethnic groups and is also common among blacks. Information should also be obtained about family members with a history of the following:

- Anemia
- Jaundice
- Splenomegaly
- Gallbladder disease
- Sickle cell or thalassemia disease or trait
- Bleeding tendencies
- Drug and toxin exposure
- Bone marrow failure
- Chronic illnesses
- Lead exposure

The child's medical history and a review of systems are important, with particular attention paid to the following:

- Episodes of jaundice (including in the newborn period)
- Extremity pain
- Abdominal pain
- Blood loss (particularly from mucous membranes)
- Weight loss
- Recent infections
- Drug exposure
- Travel
- Behavioral changes
- Pallor
- Petechiae, ecchymoses
- Adenopathy
- Gastrointestinal and genitourinary disorders
- Changes in stool characteristics indicating gastrointestinal bleeding (i.e., black, tarry stools)

The nutritional history of the child (and of the breastfeeding mother) should include the following:

- Dietary intake of iron sources, vitamins, milk, and meat
- A 24-hour dietary recall
- Any history of pica (particularly when iron deficiency or plumbism is suspected)

Physical Examination

The physical examination of the child should be comprehensive, and vital signs and growth parameters should be documented. The following positive signs are particularly important to identify:

- Pallor (especially of the conjunctivae and palmar creases)
- Jaundice
- Petechiae
- Fundal hemorrhages
- Excessive bruising
- Bleeding from mucous membranes
- Lymphadenopathy
- Frontal bossing
- Joint or extremity pain
- Heart murmurs and signs of congestive heart failure
- Hepatomegaly or splenomegaly
- Congenital anomalies

Screening

In many states, routine screening is done on the cord blood of newborns to detect sickle cell disease, sickle cell trait, and other hemoglobinopathies. Routine hemoglobin screening should be done (American Academy of Pediatrics, 1997):

- At 9 to 12 months of age, when fetal stores are depleted
- In menstruating adolescents

Lead screening should also be an integral part of pediatric primary care (see Chapter 42):

- At 6 months of age, the potential risk for high-dose environmental lead exposure should be assessed (Centers for Disease Control, 1991). If the child is considered to be at high risk, a blood lead level should be obtained at that time.
- A child considered to be at low risk for exposure should have blood drawn to determine the level of lead at 9 to 12 months of age. Universal screening of children is recommended (American Academy of Pediatrics, 1997).
- If the result is less than 10 μg/dl, the test should be repeated at 24 months because blood lead levels peak at that time.

- If the initial blood lead level is 10 μg/dl or greater, the child should be retested more frequently and may need individual case management. Two test results with levels less than 10 μg/dl are necessary before follow-up is discontinued.

WORKUP OF ANEMIA

Anemia may be suspected on the basis of clinical judgment and the established norms of hematocrit (i.e., the percentage of blood volume occupied by RBCs) and hemoglobin values. The initial laboratory approach is to obtain:

- A complete blood count (CBC)
- Reticulocyte count
- Peripheral smear to examine the morphological characteristics and staining properties of the RBC

In the description of the smear, *anisocytosis* refers to cells of unequal size, *poikilocytosis* denotes cells of abnormal shape, and *hypochromic* describes cells that are paler than usual.

The results of the RBC indices obtained in the CBC are useful in classification of the anemia, first according to the size of the RBC and then based on the pathophysiology (see Table 27-3):

- Mean corpuscular volume (MCV) is a measure of the average volume or size of the RBC and is calculated by dividing the hematocrit by the total number of RBCs. A decrease in the MCV is seen in iron deficiency or thalassemia when the RBC is microcytic or smaller than usual. The MCV is increased in the megaloblastic anemias (such as folic acid anemia or juvenile pernicious anemia) when the RBC is abnormally large.
- Mean corpuscular hemoglobin (MCH) represents the average amount of hemoglobin in an RBC and is computed by dividing the hemoglobin concentration by the number of RBCs.
- The mean corpuscular hemoglobin concentration (MCHC) is the average percentage of hemoglobin in an RBC and is obtained by dividing the hemoglobin by the hematocrit.

In addition to the aforementioned screening tests, further diagnostic studies may be indicated to identify the type of acute anemia seen in childhood (Fig. 27–3). These measures include the following:

- Free erythrocyte protoporphyrin (FEP), which is a measure of the porphyrin precursors that have not been converted into heme.
- Serum iron (SI or Fe), which indicates iron concentration levels in plasma.
- Total iron-binding capacity (TIBC), which denotes the number of binding sites available for iron (the ratio SI/TIBC expresses the saturation).
- Serum ferritin (SF) concentration, which indicates the level of iron stores in the liver, spleen, and bone marrow.
- Red cell distribution width (RDW), which is the coefficient of variation of the MCV (or the standard deviation of the measured MCVs divided by their mean MCV $\times$ 100). A larger RDW indicates greater diversity in cell size. The most common use of RDW is to differentiate thalassemia minor (in which the RDW is elevated) from iron deficiency.
- Hemoglobin electrophoresis, which identifies the percentages of different types of hemoglobin and is useful in the diagnosis of sickle cell anemia, thalassemia, and other hemoglobinopathies.
- Bone marrow aspiration, which examines for the presence of precursors of all the hematological lines: erythroid elements, myeloid elements, and platelets/megakaryocytes. This procedure is necessary for the diagnosis of aplastic anemia (complete bone marrow failure), leukemia, and other malignancies.

White Blood Cell Count

The WBC count and differential are obtained on a smear of blood one cell layer thick, usually with a Wright stain procedure that contains both basic and acidic dyes.

The ANC is calculated from the results of the differential: if WBCs = 3600, segmental neutrophils = 20, band neutrophils = 5, lymphocytes = 60, monocytes = 10, and eosinophils = 5, then

$$\begin{aligned} ANC &= WBC \times (\% \text{ Seg} + \text{Band}) \\ &= 3600 \times 0.25 \\ &= 900 \end{aligned}$$

Tests for Coagulation Disorders

- Platelet count (normal range, 150,000 to 300,000/mm^3).
- Prothrombin time (PT) (normal range, 11.5 to 14 seconds).
- Partial thromboplastin time (PTT) (normal range, 25 to 40 seconds) (Corrigan, 1996).
- Specific coagulation factor assays determine which clotting factors are absent.

The PT and PTT measure all of the clotting factors except factor XIII. If the PT and PTT are elevated in association with thrombocytopenia, the probable diagnosis is disseminated intravascular coagulation. If the platelet count is normal, the PTT or PT is prolonged, or both, a coagulation factor deficiency is possible (Platt, 1999).

Bone Marrow Aspiration

Bone marrow aspiration or biopsy may be necessary to evaluate the specific types of cells present, including any foreign or malignant cells and maturation of the blood cell lines. In infants, the usual sites of aspiration are the proximal end of the tibia and posterior aspect of the iliac crest. In older children, the posterior part of the iliac crest or sternum can be used.

▨ MANAGEMENT STRATEGIES

The types of management strategies used to treat children with hematological problems are as varied as the disorders themselves. Most commonly, the plan of care focuses on provision of adequate nutrition and iron supplementation. Changes may be needed in the child's environment because of lead exposure. For some problems, management centers on teach-

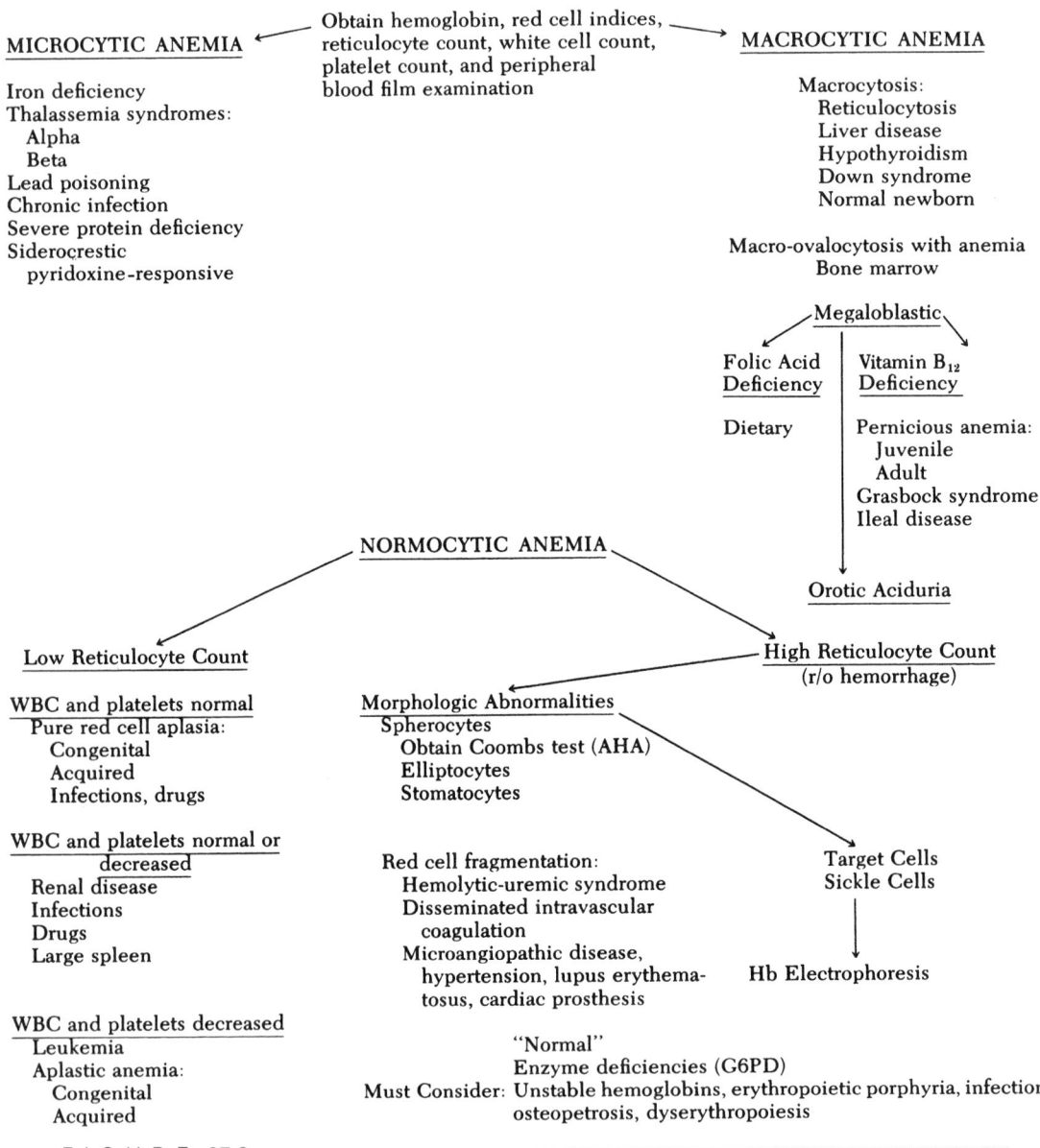

A diagnostic approach to anemia. AHA = antihuman globulin antibody; G6PD = glucose-6-phosphate dehydrogenase; Hb = hemoglobin; WBC = white blood cell count. (From Nathan D, Oski FA: Hematology of Infancy and Childhood, 4th ed. Philadelphia, WB Saunders, 1993, p 352.)

ing the family ways to prevent symptom exacerbation. For other, rarer disorders, the focus is on helping the child and family cope with a chronic or potentially fatal condition and on collaborating with pediatric hematologists and oncologists in the delivery of care. Effective patterns of communication and referral among all the interdisciplinary providers, including laboratory personnel, are crucial.

Improvements in technology have brought about positive changes in the clinical management of children with hematological disorders. The recognition of blood group antigens and infectious agents makes red cell transfusion a relatively safe procedure. Advances in pediatric hematology have led to an understanding of coagulation proteins and have dramatically improved the clinical course of children with coagulopathies. Unparalleled progress in the treatment of malignant hematological diseases is likely to continue, and future breakthroughs will be possible as a result of gene replacement therapy.

▪▪▪ SPECIFIC HEMATOLOGICAL PROBLEMS

Anemias

Anemias are classified on the basis of two overall functional disturbances: anemias caused by nutritional deficiencies or inadequate production of RBCs and anemias brought about by increased destruction (hemolysis) of RBCs. Anemias occurring in the neonatal period are generally secondary to blood loss, isoimmunization, or congenital hemolytic anemias.

Anemias Caused by Inadequate Production of Red Blood Cells

IRON-DEFICIENCY ANEMIA

Description

Mild to moderate iron deficiency (hemoglobin, 7 to 10 g/dl) is the most common cause of childhood anemia (Martin & Pearson, 1994).

Etiology and Incidence

Iron-deficiency anemia is seen in approximately 3% of white children and 15% of black children, usually between the ages of 9 and 24 months and earlier in preterm infants (Poncz, 1997). Two factors that account for this relatively high rate of anemia are the rapid increase in body size and blood volume during the first 2 years of life and insufficient iron in the diet. Typically, the young child has a history of a diet low in iron-containing foods and high intake of milk (>1 qt/d). Milk impairs iron absorption and can cause gastrointestinal irritation leading to occult blood loss, which compounds the problem. Iron deficiency is also common among girls in the adolescent years after menarche, when iron intake is often inadequate.

Clinical Findings

HISTORY. Two features are noted.

- Irritability and restlessness are often noticed only in retrospect, after treatment.
- Pica may be present in unusual circumstances.

PHYSICAL EXAMINATION. The child appears normal, or pallor may be present. Rarely, in anemias that develop slowly, the physical examination may reveal tachycardia, systolic murmurs, and signs of congestive heart failure.

DIAGNOSTIC TESTS. The following may be seen:

- A microcytic, hypochromic anemia on CBC
- Low reticulocyte count
- Elevated FEP (40 to 160 μg/dl) (Poncz, 1997)

Differential Diagnosis

If resistant to treatment, iron deficiency should be differentiated from other microcytic, hypochromic anemias such as lead poisoning, thalassemia minor, anemia of chronic disease, and hereditary sideroblastic anemia (see Fig. 27–3). In lead poisoning, the FEP may be above 200 μg/dl, and basophilic stippling may be seen on the RBCs in the peripheral smear. β-Thalassemia is indicated by elevations in Hb A_2.

Management

Responses to treatment with iron supplementation are important diagnostically as well as therapeutically. In a child whose laboratory data reveal a microcytic, hypochromic anemia and an elevated FEP panel and whose history and physical examination are consistent with iron deficiency, a trial of iron is started (4 to 6 mg/kg per day of elemental iron in three divided doses) (Martin & Pearson, 1994). Peripheral reticulocytosis may be seen after the first 4 days of treatment, and hemoglobin should return to a normal level within 4 to 6 weeks. At the least, the hemoglobin should be rechecked 1 month after treatment. If a therapeutic response is observed, iron supplementation should continue for 2 months to ensure adequate stores (Poncz, 1997). Otherwise, alternative diagnoses should be explored.

Complications

The lack of a therapeutic response may be due to poor compliance, inadequate dosage, the presence of unrecognized blood loss, or an alternative diagnosis. A more extensive determination of the child's iron status is obtained by measuring serum iron, iron-binding capacity, and the venous lead level.

Children with extremely low hemoglobin (<7 g/dl), hypotension, or signs of congestive heart failure should be referred and may need to be hospitalized. Laboratory results that also indicate referral are neutropenia, thrombocytopenia, nucleated RBCs, or immature myeloid elements (Platt, 1999)

Education and Prevention

Parents or caretakers should be counseled about the adequacy of the child's diet. Whole cow's milk should be avoided in infants younger than 12 months. For full-term infants, dietary iron supplementation (as in iron-enriched infant cereal) should begin at 4 to 6 months of age. For preterm infants, supplementation with oral iron drops should begin as early as 2 months. If the child is treated therapeutically with oral iron supplements, parents should be advised that they should avoid giving the iron with meals, that juice enhances absorption, and that the child's stools will probably turn black. Parents should also be cautioned to keep the medi-

cation safely out of reach to avoid accidental ingestion.

MEGALOBLASTIC ANEMIAS

Description

Megaloblastic anemias are characterized by oval macrocytes and hypersegmented PMNs in the peripheral blood and megaloblasts in the bone marrow.

Etiology

The relatively rare megaloblastic anemias are due primarily to a lack of folic acid, vitamin B_{12} or both. These two substances function as coenzymes in the synthesis of nuclear protein. Megaloblastic anemias may develop if the diet lacks these two substances or if the gastric intrinsic factor necessary for the absorption of vitamin B_{12} is absent.

Clinical Findings

HISTORY. Patients with megaloblastic anemia may include:

- Young infants who are being fed powdered milk products or goat's milk, which are deficient in folic acid and vitamin B_{12}.
- Older children who are exclusively vegetarian or who have severe nutritional deficiencies, absorption problems, or tapeworm infestations

PHYSICAL EXAMINATION. The following may be seen:

- Weakness, pallor
- Beefy-red, smooth, sore tongue

DIAGNOSTIC TESTS. The following results may be seen:

- Elevated MCV (>95 fl) and MCHC
- Blood smear showing macro-ovalocytes with anisocytosis and poikilocytosis
- Normal white cell count and platelet count, but possibly decreased in more severe cases
- Large and hypersegmented neutrophils

Management

In general, management of folic acid deficiency and juvenile pernicious anemia (caused by a lack of vitamin B_{12}) is best done in consultation with a pediatric hematologist. Treatment is through dietary supplementation and correction of the underlying disorder (e.g., infection) if possible.

In folic acid deficiency confirmed by measurement of the RBC folate level,

- Folic acid may be administered in a dose of 1 to 5 mg/24 hr and continued for 3 to 4 weeks. Prolonged use of folic acid should be avoided (Schwartz, 1996).

In vitamin B_{12} deficiency, a prompt hematological response is usually seen after parenteral administration of vitamin B_{12}. If neurological involvement is present, 1 mg should be given intramuscularly daily for at least 2 weeks. A maintenance dose of a 1-mg intramuscular injection of vitamin B_{12} is administered monthly throughout the patient's life (Schwartz, 1996).

TRANSIENT ERYTHROBLASTOPENIA OF CHILDHOOD

Description

Idiopathic erythroblastopenia of childhood, or TEC, is a benign disorder of unknown cause that occurs in children during the first few years of life. It is characterized by anemia, reticulocytopenia, and erythroid hypoplasia of the bone marrow. The cause of this acquired decrease in red cell production is not clear, although it frequently follows a viral infection (Schwartz, 1996).

Etiology

TEC is associated with temporary failure of erythropoiesis caused by probable viral suppression or as a result of an IgG-mediated autoimmune response.

Clinical Findings

HISTORY. TEC occurs mainly in previously healthy children between 6 months and 3 years of age. The child may have a history of preceding infection.

PHYSICAL EXAMINATION. Patients have symptoms of anemia, including pallor.

DIAGNOSTIC TESTS. The following are seen in TEC:

- Anemia (in which the hemoglobin content may be as low as 2.5 g/dl)
- Low reticulocyte count
- WBC count usually normal
- Platelets normal or elevated
- High serum iron level reflecting decreased utilization (Martin & Pearson, 1994)
- Bone marrow aspiration results indicating erythyroid hypoplasia

Differential Diagnosis

The syndrome can be differentiated from congenital hypoplastic anemia (Diamond-Blackfan syndrome) by the normal size of the RBCs (MCV, <80 fl). Reticulocytes are markedly decreased (Schwartz, 1996).

Management

TEC is self-limited, with recovery taking place 1 to 2 months after diagnosis. No specific treatment is indicated, although transfusions may be required for severe anemia.

Hemolytic Anemias

Hemolytic anemias can be classified as either hereditary or acquired. In particular, the hereditary and congenital anemias are manifested in infancy and early childhood. They may be due to a variety of hemoglobinopathies or to defects in the red cell membrane.

SICKLE CELL ANEMIA AND TRAIT

Etiology

Children who have sickle cell anemia or disease do not form the normal Hb A molecule but rather synthesize hemoglobin S (Hb S), which carries the amino acid valine instead of glutamic acid. Because of this change, Hb S tends to polymerize or come out of solution at low Pao_2, low pH, low temperature, and low osmolality. This process damages the RBC by giving it a "sickled" appearance and causes a chronic hemolytic anemia with associated ischemia and vaso-occlusive problems.

Incidence

Sickle cell disease has an autosomal recessive inheritance pattern. It is found most often in people of African descent but is also detected among ethnic groups from the Mediterranean, the Caribbean, and India. In the United States, sickle cell disease occurs in about 1 of every 400 black infants (Lane et al., 1999). Children with sickle cell trait who are heterozygous for the gene essentially have a benign clinical course. Their RBCs contain only 30 to 40% Hb S, and sickling does not occur under most conditions. It is only in rare instances of hypoxia, such as in shock, while flying in unpressurized aircraft, or at high elevations, that signs of vaso-occlusion can occur.

Clinical Findings

The diagnosis of sickle cell anemia can and should be made in the newborn period by taking a careful family medical history. Universal screening of all newborns for sickle cell disease is now recommended (Agency for Health Care Policy and Research [AHCPR], 1993).

PHYSICAL EXAMINATION. Symptoms begin to emerge in the second 6 months of life as the amount of Hb S increases, Hb F declines, and painful, vaso-occlusive crises occur. The following may be noted:

- Pale and slightly jaundiced appearance with splenomegaly
- Painful swelling of the hands and feet (hand–foot syndrome) caused by infarction of the small bones
- Low-grade fever
- Leukocytosis
- Painful involvement of the larger bones (in older patients)
- Diffuse abdominal pain
- Chest pain
- Sequestration crisis, which occurs when large amounts of blood are pooled in the abdominal organs and the spleen becomes enlarged

After the age of 5, splenomegaly usually disappears because of autoinfarction. Rates of height and weight gain are usually slowed after 7 years, and puberty may be delayed 3 to 4 years.

DIAGNOSTIC TESTS. The following laboratory results are seen in sickle cell disease:

- Hematocrit with percentages in the 20s and sickled cells, nucleated RBCs, and Howell-Jolly bodies on the peripheral smear (Platt, 1999)
- Reticulocyte count with percentages in the 20s
- Increased WBC and platelet count
- Hemoglobin electrophoresis (after infancy) showing a predominance of Hb S and no Hb A

Differential Diagnosis

Chronic hemolytic anemia should be included in the differential diagnosis. Other syndromes characterized by hemolytic anemia and vaso-occlusion are hemoglobin sickle cell disease and a combination of Hb S with α- or β-thalassemia. These diseases may be differentiated through electrophoresis and family testing if necessary.

Management

The following measures are instituted:

- Baseline laboratory data (CBC, reticulocyte count) monitored every few months.
- Pneumococcal vaccine given at age 2.
- Prophylactic penicillin (125 mg twice daily) given by 2 months of age and continued through the first 5 years of life (AHCPR, 1993; Platt, 1999).
- Folic acid supplementation may be indicated if the diet is low in green leafy vegetables.
- Aggressive treatment of infections and maintenance of hydration and body temperature are used to prevent hypoxia and acidosis; volume replacement may be necessary to prevent circulatory collapse.

Children with sickle cell disease are usually comanaged by specialists in hematology and their primary provider. Emergency admission or referral is necessary in the presence of:

- Fever (to rule out sepsis)
- Pneumonia
- Sequestration crisis (splenomegaly with decreased hemoglobin or hematocrit)
- Aplastic crisis (decreased hematocrit and reticulocyte count)
- Severe painful crisis
- Unusual headache, visual disturbances
- Priapism

Consultation is also necessary for the chronic sequelae of persistent bone pain, leg ulcers, and issues of pregnancy and contraception. Further information is contained in the clinical practice guideline *Sickle Cell Disease: Screening, Diagnosis, Management and Counseling in Newborns and Infants,* released by AHCPR (1993). See Resource Box 27-1.

Complications

Because of functional asplenia, the most worrisome manifestation is febrile illness indicating infection. In view of the serious threat of pneumococcal sepsis in children younger than 5 years, all complaints of fever, poor feeding, lethargy, and irritability should be evaluated in person rather than by telephone (Platt, 1999).

Education

The parents of children with sickle cell anemia need a great deal of support in raising a child with a genetically transmitted chronic disease. Clear patterns of communication should be established between the family and the provider. In particular, parents should be counseled about early signs of illness and should seek medical care even if the illness appears minor. Genetic counseling should be offered to the parents at the time of diagnosis, and siblings should also be tested to determine their carrier status.

Preventive Care

Preventive measures for infants and children include the following:

- Pneumococcal vaccine
- Prophylactic antibiotics
- Genetic counseling
- Support groups

THALASSEMIAS

The thalassemias are a group of approximately 100 types of hereditary, hypochromic anemias that are associated with the absence or decreased synthesis of the normal hemoglobin polypeptide chains—usually the α- and β-chains (Honig, 1996). They occur primarily in people of Mediterranean and Southeast Asian descent.

β-Thalassemias cover a broad clinical spectrum of disorders that are classified according to patterns of inheritance and the severity of the anemia. The heterozygous states are thalassemia minor and thalassemia minima, which is essentially a silent carrier state. Homozygous forms are thalassemia intermedia and thalassemia major, or Cooley anemia.

β-Thalassemia Minor

DESCRIPTION. β-Thalassemia minor disease or trait is associated with a mild, hypochromic, microcytic anemia in which hemoglobin levels are 2 to 3 g/dl below normal and the MCV averages 65 fl (Honig, 1996). It may be confused with iron deficiency or lead poisoning and can be differentiated by measuring serum iron or lead levels, transferrin saturation, or serum ferritin levels (Table 27-4). Thus it is particularly important to avoid long-term unnecessary administration of iron supplements that could result in iron overload. In thalassemia minor, the RDW coefficient is elevated. The primary diagnostic feature is the increased Hb A_2 (>3.5%) on electrophoresis.

CLINICAL FINDINGS. Clinically, most individuals with thalassemia trait are asymptomatic, although mild pallor and splenomegaly may be found. The degree of anemia may be exacerbated in concurrent illness or pregnancy.

MANAGEMENT. No specific treatment is known for β-thalassemia minor. Primary emphasis should be on education of all family members and genetic testing, and counseling should be offered.

T A B L E 27-4

Laboratory Findings in Anemia of Infants and Children

DIAGNOSIS	LABORATORY TEST	EXPECTED RESULTS
Iron deficiency	Serum ferritin	Low <25 µg/dl
	Serum iron and total iron-binding capacity	Low/high
	% Iron saturation	Low <15%
	Bone marrow iron stores	Absent
	Stool for occult blood	Absent
	Urine for blood, hemoglobin, or hemosiderin	Present (if renal loss)
	MCV/RBC ratio	>13
β-Thalassemia trait	Blood film	Basophilic stippling
	Hemoglobin electrophoresis	Increased A_2 or F hemoglobin
	Biosynthetic β/α-globin chain ratio	<1
	MCV/RBC ratio	<13
	Family studies	Hb/Hct decreased
		Blood film
		Anisocytosis
		Poikilocytosis
		Basophilic stippling
		MCV <70 fl/cell
Chronic inflammation	Nonspecific tests	
	Erythrocyte sedimentation rate	Increased
	Acute-phase reactants	Increased
	C-reactive protein	
	Fibrinogen	
	Haptoglobin	
	Serum ferritin	Increased
	Serum iron and total iron-binding capacity	Low/low
	% Iron saturation	Low
	Bone marrow iron stores	Increased
	Bone marrow sideroblasts	Decreased
Lead intoxication	Blood film	Basophilic stippling
	Erythrocyte protoporphyrin	Increased
	Blood lead	Increased

MCV = mean corpuscular volume; RBC = red blood cell; Hb/Hct = hemoglobin/hematocrit.
From Segel GB: Anemia. Pediatr Rev 10:77–88, 1988.

β-Thalassemia Major

DESCRIPTION. Homozygous β-thalassemia major (or Cooley anemia) is associated with severe anemia resulting from decreased or absent production of Hb A and hemolysis caused by the precipitation of excess α-chains in the RBCs.

CLINICAL FINDINGS. Affected infants usually become symptomatic in the first year of life and have pallor, failure to thrive, hepatosplenomeg-aly, and a severe anemia with an average hemoglobin of 6 g/dl and low MCV (60 to 70 fl). RBC morphology reveals significant microcytosis, poikilocytosis, hypochromia, target cells, and nucleated RBCs. Hb A and Hb F levels are elevated.

MANAGEMENT. Proper management of the child is in collaboration with a pediatric hematologist. Exchange transfusions are usually necessary every 4 to 5 weeks to maintain the hemoglobin level above 10 g/dl. Iron chelation therapy is indicated. Splenectomy and bone marrow transplants may be indicated as well (Honig, 1996).

COMPLICATIONS. If the condition is left untreated, the characteristic facies of frontal bossing and maxillary overgrowth will develop as a result of bone marrow expansion.

HEREDITARY SPHEROCYTOSIS (HS)

Description

HS is a hemolytic anemia characterized by a deficiency or abnormality of the RBC membrane protein spectrin, which reduces the RBC surface area. The RBCs assume a spherical shape and are more likely to be sequestered and destroyed in the spleen.

Incidence

HS occurs in 1 in 5000 persons of predominantly Northern European ancestry.

Clinical Findings

PHYSICAL EXAMINATION. Jaundice usually appears in the newborn period, and it may be difficult to differentiate HS from hyperbilirubinemia caused by ABO incompatibility. After age 2, splenomegaly is usually present. Chronic fatigue, malaise, and abdominal pain may also be noted.

DIAGNOSTIC TESTS. Laboratory findings in HS include the following:

- Chronic anemia (hemoglobin, 6 to 10 g/dl).
- Reticulocyte count ranging from 5 to 20%.
- On peripheral smear, a small proportion of the RBCs are spherocytic and smaller than normal and lack the central pallor of the usual biconcave disk-shaped cell.
- Osmotic fragility of the cells is increased, as is the rate of autohemolysis of incubated blood.

Management

The treatment of choice is splenectomy, which usually produces a clinical cure. Except

in severe cases, it should be deferred until 5 or 6 years of age because of the increased risk of infection before that age. Pneumococcal vaccine should be given before splenectomy.

Prophylactic penicillin therapy, 250 mg twice a day, is recommended. Because of increased hemolysis, children with HS should receive 1 mg folic acid daily until splenectomy (Poncz, 1997).

Complications

Aplastic crises (which can be indicated by fever, fatigue, abdominal pain, and jaundice) associated with parvovirus infections are the most serious complications during childhood. Febrile illnesses should be vigorously treated. A splenectomized child with a temperature over 101.5°F and without an obvious source of infection should be hospitalized and treated with intravenous antibiotics until blood cultures prove to be negative (Poncz, 1997).

GLUCOSE-6-PHOSPHATE DEHYDROGENASE SYNDROME

Description

G6PD syndrome is a drug-induced hemolytic anemia caused by deficiency of the G6PD enzyme in the RBC. Symptoms are generally associated with infections or exposure to oxidant metabolites of certain drugs that cause precipitation of hemoglobin, injury to the red cells, and rapid hemolysis.

Etiology and Incidence

G6PD syndrome is transmitted as an X-linked recessive trait. In the United States, about 10% of black males and 1 to 2% of black females are affected. It may also occur in a more severe form in Greeks, Italians, Arabs, Southeast Asians, and Chinese.

Clinical Findings

HISTORY. Patients generally have a history of recent infection or drug ingestion—specifically, antipyretics, sulfonamides, antimalarials, naphthaquinolones, and the fava bean. The degree of hemolysis is dependent on the amount of the drug ingested and the extent of enzyme deficiency.

PHYSICAL EXAMINATION. The patient may have pallor, jaundice, or dark urine after drug ingestion.

DIAGNOSTIC TESTS. Several dye reduction tests provide the diagnosis. Screening tests available to measure a deficiency of G6PD should be used in high-risk groups. After a hemolytic crisis, however, screening may produce a false-negative result because the younger blood cells that remain after hemolysis may show normal enzymatic activity. A more representative enzyme assay can be obtained 2 to 3 months after the episode.

Management

No specific treatment is available for this syndrome. Red cell transfusion and supportive therapy may be indicated in cases in which the anemia is severe.

Education

Patients and families should be taught to avoid the offending drugs—the most common being aspirin, sulfonamide antibiotics, and antimalarials.

Bleeding Disorders

Bleeding disorders should be ruled out in a child before undergoing extensive surgery. Bleeding disorders should also be considered in a child with petechiae, frequent nosebleeds, mucous membrane bleeding, and excessive bleeding from minor trauma. Evaluation of these complaints includes a family history of bleeding or platelet disorders and a history of drug or toxin exposure. Initial laboratory studies should include a CBC, platelet count, PT, and PTT. Among the diagnoses that may be differentiated with these tests are ITP, hemophilia, von Willebrand disease, and leukemia.

IDIOPATHIC THROMBOCYTOPENIC PURPURA

Description

ITP is the most common of the thrombocytopenic purpuras in childhood. It is believed to be an autoimmune response in which circulating platelets are destroyed and usually occurs after viral illnesses (Corrigan, 1996).

Incidence

Most cases occur between the ages of 2 and 5 years, and the incidence is increased in fair-skinned children.

Clinical Findings

ITP is essentially a clinical diagnosis and does not rest on any one diagnostic test. It is characterized by the following:

- Acute onset of petechiae, purpura, and bleeding in an otherwise healthy child; the bruising or bleeding may be most prominent over the legs.
- A viral illness 1 to 4 weeks before onset in 70% of cases.
- Hemorrhage of the mucous membranes, particularly the gums and lips.
- Nosebleeds that can be severe and difficult to control.
- The liver, spleen, and lymph nodes are not generally enlarged.

DIAGNOSTIC TESTS. Laboratory findings in ITP include

- Low platelet count ($<150,000/mm^3$) with an otherwise normal CBC
- Normal PT and PTT
- Megathrombocytes on the peripheral smear (Platt, 1999)

Differential Diagnosis

If the smear shows fragmented RBCs, blood urea nitrogen and creatinine levels should be measured to rule out *hemolytic–uremic syndrome*. If the PT and PTT are elevated with thrombocytopenia, disseminated intravascular coagulation is a possibility, and cultures should be taken to identify sources of infection. A prolonged PT and PTT with a normal platelet count suggest a coagulation factor deficiency. If the syndrome is complicated by prolonged thrombocytopenia, neutropenia, anemia, bone pain, or congenital anomalies, the child should be referred to a hematologist for possible bone marrow aspiration to rule out ALL and other disorders (Platt, 1999). In a sick, febrile child with isolated thrombocytopenia and petechiae, the major diagnosis to consider first is meningococcemia. Such children should also be referred, hospitalized, and treated for presumed sepsis.

Management

The prognosis for children with ITP is excellent, with spontaneous recovery in 75% of cases in the first 3 months (Corrigan, 1996). Most cases of ITP can be managed on an outpatient basis without any specific therapy. If the platelet count is greater than 50,000/mm³ and no bleeding is observed, children and parents should be taught to avoid contact sports and aspirin ingestion and to notify the practitioner of any bleeding. Epistaxis can be treated with local measures. In severe cases (platelets, <50,000/mm³) in which the diagnosis of leukemia is ruled out, a short course of corticosteroid therapy may reduce severity in the initial phases. A suggested dosage schedule for prednisone is 2 mg/kg per day for 10 days and then tapered over a period of 10 days (Platt, 1999).

Complications

The most serious complication is intracranial hemorrhage, which occurs in less than 1% of cases (Corrigan, 1996).

HEMOPHILIA

Description

Inherited deficiencies are known for each of the coagulation factors, with most of them resulting in abnormal bleeding. Hemophilia refers to a deficiency of factor VIII (hemophilia A) or factor IX (hemophilia B). In hemophilia A and B, absence or deficiency of the coagulation factor results in prolonged bleeding either spontaneously from small vessels or as a result of trauma.

In plasma, factor VIII is complexed with von Willebrand protein, which acts as a carrier protein. von Willebrand disease (also known as vascular hemophilia) is a deficiency of this protein that results in a bleeding disorder.

Etiology and Incidence

Because the genes for the coagulation factors are sex linked and recessive, the disease affects primarily males. In the United States, about 1 in 10,000 males is affected with hemophilia A, which is four times more common than hemophilia B (Manno, 1997).

Clinical Findings

The following are seen in hemophilia:

- A positive family history in 80% of cases (Corrigan, 1996)
- Excessive bruising
- Prolonged bleeding from mucous membranes after minor lacerations
- Hemarthroses characterized by pain and swelling in the elbows, knees, and ankles
- A greatly prolonged PTT

A specific assay for factor VIII activity confirms the diagnosis.

Management

Treatment consists of prevention of trauma and replacement therapy to increase factor VIII activity in plasma. Several products are available for replacement, including human plasma fraction concentrates (antihemolytic factors), cryoprecipitate, and desmopressin (DDAVP). Local measures include the application of cold and pressure to affected, painful joints. Aspirin should never be used, and drugs that interfere with coagulation should be used with caution (Corrigan, 1996).

Ideally, most children with hemophilia should be enrolled in a local hemophilia treatment center to facilitate a collaborative, interdisciplinary approach to management. The primary provider should remain central to the care of the child. All immunizations should be given subcutaneously with a 26-gauge needle, followed by firm pressure at the site for several minutes. Iron replacement may also be necessary in children with severe bleeding disorders.

A written treatment plan stating the dosage

of the replacement product for the location of the bleed should be in the chart and given to the parents to carry with them. The child should wear a medical alert bracelet or necklace.

Complications

Without factor replacement, bleeding persists, particularly in closed areas such as the joints. Continued hemorrhage results in anemia and eventually hypovolemic shock.

The use of therapeutic replacement materials derived from blood carries some inherent risk. Hepatitis infection was a problem in the past. Infection with human immunodeficiency virus (HIV) is unfortunately frequent in patients who were exposed to multiple donors before the revision of blood donor screening tests and the use of heat-treated concentrates.

LEUKEMIAS

Description

The leukemias represent a group of malignant hematological diseases in which normal bone marrow elements are replaced by abnormal, poorly differentiated lymphocytes known as blast cells. Leukemias are classified according to cell type involvement (i.e., lymphocytic or nonlymphocytic) and by cellular differentiation. ALL is characterized by predominantly undifferentiated WBCs.

Incidence

The leukemias are the most common form of childhood cancer and occur in nearly 4 in 100,000 children younger than 14 years. ALL accounts for about 75% of cases, with a peak incidence around 4 years of age (Crist & Pui, 1996). It occurs more frequently in boys than in girls and more commonly in blacks than in whites. Acute nonlymphocytic leukemia (ANLL) accounts for about 20% of all cases and occurs primarily in older children. Chronic myelogenous leukemia (CML) is an adult form of the disease seen in only about 3% of children (Heslop, 1996).

Etiology

As with all types of malignancy, the exact cause of leukemia is unknown. Several factors associated with increased risk have been identified, including infection, radiation, chemical and drug exposure, and genetic factors.

Clinical Findings

Most of the clinical signs and symptoms of leukemia are related to leukemic replacement of the bone marrow and the absence of blood cell precursors. The child may be anemic, pale, listless, irritable, or chronically tired and have the following:

- A history of repeated infections
- Bleeding episodes characterized by epistaxis, petechiae, and hematomas
- Lymphadenopathy and hepatosplenomegaly
- Bone and joint pain

All these symptoms may be rather vague or nonspecific, in which case it is important for the provider to have a high index of suspicion for cancer.

DIAGNOSTIC TESTS. The following are used to diagnose leukemia:

- CBC with differential WBC, platelet, and reticulocyte counts. Thrombocytopenia is present in up to 85% of cases, and anemia is also usually present.
- Peripheral smear, which may demonstrate malignant cells.
- Bone marrow examination, which shows an infiltration of blast cells replacing normal elements of the marrow. Further classification regarding cell type, morphological characteristics, and cell surface markers is generally made at the cancer treatment center to which the child is referred.

Management

The treatment program for most types of acute leukemia involves an induction phase (usually with vincristine, prednisone, and L-asparaginase), prophylactic central nervous system therapy, and a maintenance phase of therapy. Today, remission can be induced in 95% of patients, and 5-year leukemia-free survival rates may be as high as 70% (Needle & Lange, 1997). The role of the primary care provider is crucial in facilitating proper referrals and effective interdisciplinary communication and in assisting the family in their coping and adaptation processes.

Long-term sequelae of cancer therapy for ALL have been identified in research studies and include effects on cognition and neuropsychological functioning. Central nervous system irradiation has been linked to learning disabilities and impaired IQ, especially in children younger than 5 years who also received intrathecal therapy. As a result, cranial radiation dosages have been reduced and earlier neuropsychological testing is recommended. Other documented potential late effects of treatment are the following:

- Short stature, muscle wasting, and avascular necrosis of the bone caused by high-dose steroid therapy—more pronounced in young children.
- Obesity and gonadal dysfunction resulting from a neuroendocrine effect.
- Potential alterations in pubertal development and gonadal function if given high-dose alkylating agents, especially if given in puberty and to girls.
- Cardiomyopathy if given anthracyclines. Children given these drugs are at risk for this problem and need to be educated, just before their teen years, about avoiding alcohol, which increases the likelihood of cardiotoxicity, as well as cautioned about cigarette smoking.
- Malignant glioma associated with cranial irradiation.
- Second leukemias (usually AML) again associated with therapy with alkylating agents
- Infertility with alkylator therapy.
- Cystitis or bladder dysfunction with cyclophosphamide.
- Delayed recovery of normal immune function (may need readministration of immunization).
- Psychosocial effects associated with chronic illness.
- Relapse of ALL.

Risk-directed treatment based on high-risk

features at diagnosis, response to chemotherapy, and transplantation options has drastically improved cure rates in the past two decades. It is hoped that the incidence and severity of late-term effects will likewise diminish (Friebert & Shurin, 1998)

Lymphomas

NON-HODGKIN'S LYMPHOMA

Description

The non-Hodgkin's lymphomas (NHLs) are a diverse group of solid tumors of the lymphatic tissues. Different classification systems have been used. In pediatrics, the common types of NHL are Burkitt's lymphoma (small noncleaved cell lymphoma), lymphoblastic lymphoma, and large cell lymphoma (Needle & Lange, 1997).

Incidence

In children, these lymphomas usually occur before puberty or in early adolescence at a rate of 0.5 cases per 100,000 children, and they are more common in boys than in girls (Needle & Lange, 1997).

Clinical Findings

The most common site of origin is in the lymphoid structures of the intestinal tract. The most common manifestations in children are (1) acute abdomen, including abdominal pain, distention, fullness, and constipation, and (2) nontender lymph node enlargement.

Management

The diagnosis is confirmed by surgical biopsy, and the extent of the disease can be determined by scans, bone marrow aspiration, and lumbar puncture. Because of rapid developments in treatment and the importance of careful histological evaluation, these children should be referred to a major pediatric cancer center for care.

Lymphomas are sensitive to both chemotherapy and radiation. Maintenance therapy may be continued for 6 months to 2 years. The prognosis has improved dramatically over the past few years. For early-stage disease in which the disease is localized, 90% of patients can expect long-term disease-free survival. Patients with more extensive disease may have a 70 to 80% failure-free survival rate (Albano et al., 1999).

HODGKIN DISEASE

Description

Like the NHLs, Hodgkin disease is a malignancy of the lymph nodes. It usually originates in a cervical lymph node and spreads to other lymph node regions and, if left untreated, to organ systems. Unlike in NHL, involvement of the bone marrow and central nervous system is rare (Needle & Lange, 1997). Clinical and pathological staging of the disease is usually done by specialists according to what is known as the Ann Arbor staging criteria.

Incidence

Hodgkin disease represents 50% of the lymphomas of childhood. It is rare in children younger than 5 years. Sixty percent of children with Hodgkin disease are between the ages of 10 and 16 years (Albano et al., 1999).

Clinical Findings

The most common manifestation of Hodgkin disease includes the following:

- Painless enlargement of the lymph nodes, usually in the cervical area; the nodes may feel firm, are often matted together, and are nontender to palpation
- Chronic cough if the trachea is compressed by a large mediastinal mass
- Fever, decreased appetite, weight loss, and night sweats

DIAGNOSTIC TESTS. Hematological findings are often normal but may include:

- Anemia
- Elevated or depressed leukocytes or platelets
- Elevated sedimentation rate, serum copper level, and abnormal liver function test results

Management

The diagnosis is confirmed by histological examination of an excised lymph node, followed by bone marrow studies and gallium scans to determine the extent of the disease. The child should receive treatment at a pediatric oncology center in collaboration with the primary provider. Optimum results are obtained through irradiation and chemotherapy with numerous agents. Children with Hodgkin disease have a better response to treatment than do adults, with a 75% overall survival rate at more than 20 years' follow-up (Albano et al., 1999).

RESOURCE BOX 27-1

AHCPR—Sickle Cell Disease Guideline
Tel: (800) 358-9295
Website: www.ahcpr.gov

National Hemophilia Foundation (NHF)
Tel: (800) 424-2634

Sickle Cell Disease Association of America
Tel: (800) 421-8453, (310) 216-6363
Newsletter, informational materials, networking, referrals to local resources, local chapters. Fund research, maintain research registry.

REFERENCES

Agency for Health Care Policy and Research: Sickle Cell Disease: Screening, Diagnosis, Management and Counseling in Newborns and Infants. Silver Spring, MD, US Public Health Service, 1993, AHCPR Publication No. 93-0562.

Albano E, Stork L, Greffe B, et al: Neoplastic disease. *In* Hay W, Hayward JA, Levin M, et al (eds): Current Pediatric Diagnosis and Treatment, 14th ed. Stamford, CT, Appleton & Lange, 1999, pp 774–797.

American Academy of Pediatrics (AAP): Guidelines for Health Supervision III. Elk Grove Village, IL, American Academy of Pediatrics, 1997.

Bullock B: Hematology. *In* Bullock B (ed): Pathophysiology: Adaptations and Alterations in Function. Philadelphia, JB Lippincott, 1996, pp 367–423.

Centers for Disease Control: Preventing Lead Poisoning in Young Children. Washington, DC, US Department of Health and Human Services/Public Health Service, 1991.

Corrigan J: Hemorrhagic and thrombotic diseases. *In* Behrman R, Kliegman RM, Arvin A (eds): Nelson Textbook of Pediatrics, 15th ed. Philadelphia, WB Saunders, 1996, pp 1422–1438.

Crist W, Pui C: The leukemias. *In* Behrman R, Kliegman RM, Arvin A (eds): Nelson Textbook of Pediatrics, 15th ed. Philadelphia, WB Saunders, 1996, pp 1452-1456.

Friebert SE, Shurin SB: Acute lymphocyctic leukemia. Part 2: Treatment and beyond. Contemp Pediatr 15(3):39-54, 1998.

Guyton A, Hall J: Textbook of Medical Physiology, 9th ed. Philadelphia, WB Saunders, 1996.

Heslop H: Chronic myelogenous leukemia. *In* Behrman R, Kliegman RM, Arvin A (eds): Nelson Textbook of Pediatrics, 15th ed. Philadelphia, WB Saunders, 1996, pp 1456-1457.

Honig G: Hemoglobin disorders. *In* Behrman R, Kliegman R, Arvin A (eds): Nelson Textbook of Pediatrics, 15th ed. Philadelphia, WB Saunders, 1996, pp 1396-1405.

Lane RA, Nuss R, Ambruso DR: Hematologic disorders. *In* Hay WW, Hayward AR, Levin MR, et al (eds): Current Pediatric Diagnosis and Treatment, 14th ed. Stamford, CT, Appleton & Lange, 1999, pp 723-773.

Manno C: Hemophilia. *In* Schwartz M, Curry T, Sargent A, et al (eds): Pediatric Primary Care, 3rd ed. St Louis, CV Mosby, 1997, pp 595-600.

Martin P, Pearson H: The anemias. *In* Oski F, DeAngelis C, Feigin R, et al (eds): Principles and Practice of Pediatrics, 2nd ed. Philadelphia, JB Lippincott, 1994, pp 1657-1660.

Needle M, Lange B: Oncology. *In* Schwartz M, Curry T, Sargent A, et al (eds): Pediatric Primary Care, 3rd ed. St Louis, CV Mosby, 1997, pp 601-618.

Platt O: Hematologic problems. *In* Dershewitz RA (ed): Ambulatory Pediatric Care, 3rd ed. Philadelphia, Lippincott-Raven, 1999, pp 668-685.

Poncz M: Anemia. *In* Schwartz M, Curry T, Sargent A, et al (eds): Pediatric Primary Care, 3rd ed. St Louis, CV Mosby, 1997, pp 589-595.

Schwartz E: Anemias of inadequate production. *In* Behrman R, Kliegman R, Arvin A (eds): Nelson Textbook of Pediatrics, 15th ed. Philadelphia, WB Saunders, 1996, pp 1380-1390.

CHAPTER **28**

Neurological Disorders

Catherine E. Burns

INTRODUCTION

Neurological disorders in children are difficult for primary care providers to assess and manage. Central nervous system (CNS) problems can affect many systems, be manifested in many ways, and have profound effects on the lives of children and their families. No other body system has as much influence on development. The problems may be subtle or overwhelming. The nurse practitioner's (NP) work is important: screening and identifying neurological problems, referring to the appropriate healthcare resources, monitoring general health, serving as a case manager and patient advocate as school and long-term care issues arise, and supporting families as they deal with grief and caregiving issues.

ANATOMY AND PHYSIOLOGY

Anatomy

Any NP interested in the functional neurological capabilities of patients is well served by understanding neurological anatomy and physiology. The nervous system is divided into two parts, the CNS and the peripheral nervous system (PNS). The CNS consists of the brain and spinal cord. The PNS is made up of a network of afferent nerves and sense organs, which send information to the brain, and the efferent nerves, which send information out to the body for responses. Descending tracts from the brain to the gray matter of the spinal cord include the extrapyramidal tract, which conveys information from the cerebellum to the motor cells of the anterior column, and the pyramidal tract, which is the main motor pathway from the cerebral cortex to the spinal nerves and carries messages for voluntary movement. Most pyramidal tract fibers cross in the medulla, so the left half of the brain controls the right side of the body and vice versa. The anatomical units of the brain and their functions are found in Table 28-1 (see also Figs. 28-1 and 28-2).

AUTONOMIC NERVOUS SYSTEM

The autonomic nervous system (ANS) also involves CNS and PNS components. However, the sensory neurons and the efferent fibers that supply the organs, smooth muscles, and glands are sufficiently different to merit a separate classification. The ANS consists of the parasympathetic and sympathetic systems. The sympathetic system begins in the thoracolumbar area of the spinal cord and extends distally, whereas the parasympathetic system begins in the medulla and midbrain with relays to the thalamus and higher centers. The principal sympathetic system neurotransmitters are epinephrine and

T A B L E 28-1

Anatomical Units of the Nervous System and Functions

ANATOMICAL UNIT	FUNCTIONS
I. Central nervous system	
A. Brain	
1. Forebrain—cerebrum	
a. Cortex (gray matter)	Posterior—motor skills
1) Frontal area	Anterior—decision-making, emotions, memory, judgment, ethics, abstract thinking
	Broca's area—speech
2) Parietal area	Sensory integration, language, reading, writing, pattern recognition
3) Temporal area	Memory storage, auditory processing, olfaction, limbic system in deep temporal lobe—arousal
4) Occipital area	Visual processing
b. Diencephalon	
1) Thalamus	Receives and sorts sensory input, modulates motor impulses from cortex
2) Hypothalamus	Integrates autonomic functions
2. Midbrain	Connects brain with cerebellum, pons, medulla
3. Hindbrain	
a. Pons	Bridges cerebellum, medulla, midbrain. Cranial nerves V, VI, VIII arise here
b. Medulla	Proximal end of spinal cord. Contains reticular system—arousal. Cranial nerves IX–XII arise here
c. Cerebellum	Coordination and movement. Balance. Smooth movements
B. Cranial nerves	Sensory and motor components. Olfaction; vision; hearing; facial, tongue, pharyngeal, eye, shoulder movements
II. Spinal cord	
A. Dorsal roots	Afferent sensory fibers
B. Ventral roots	Efferent motor fibers
III. Protective layers	
A. Meninges	Protection of delicate nervous tissues
B. Ventricles	
C. Cerebrospinal fluid	

norepinephrine. The parasympathetic fibers produce acetylcholine. The two systems function in balance: one excites whereas the other inhibits (Table 28–2).

Physiology

Nerve impulses are transmitted along a nerve fiber through changes in polarization of the membrane, during which electrical activity is produced. Certain chemicals diffuse across the synapses between nerves and end-organs. The primary transmitter is acetylcholine; however, other transmitters, including norepinephrine and dopamine, are also important.

PATHOPHYSIOLOGY AND DEFENSE MECHANISMS

Pathophysiology

The nervous system is so intimately related to functioning of the entire body that problems in any system can have neurological implications. For example, seizures result from uncontrolled firing of cerebral neurons. Coma results from the inability of cerebral neurons to fire or the inability of the CNS to process stimuli and respond accordingly. Paralysis occurs when the peripheral nerves are unable to respond or do not receive signals through the pyramidal sys-

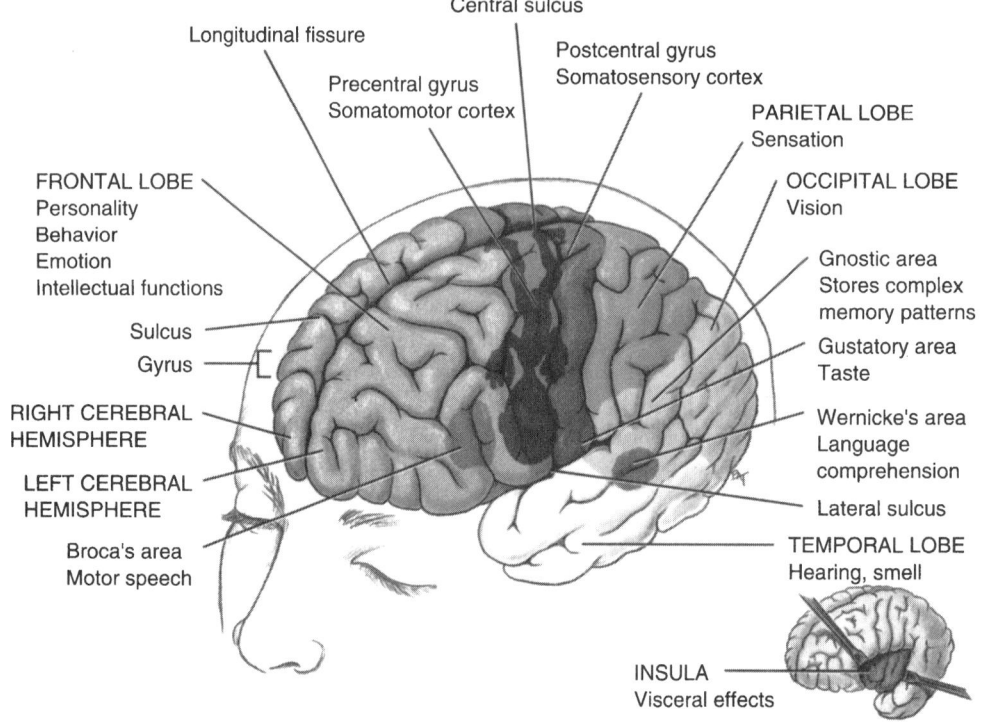

F I G U R E 28–1
Lobes and functional areas of the cerebrum. (From Polaski AL: Luckmann's Core Principles and Practice of Medical-Surgical Nursing. Philadelphia, WB Saunders, 1996, p 245.)

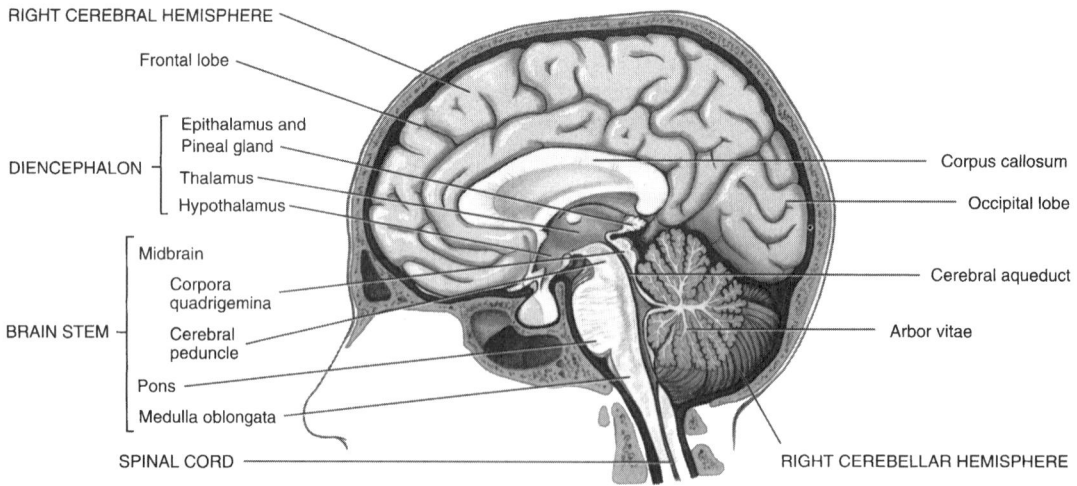

F I G U R E 28–2
Midsagittal section of the brain showing the major portions of the diencephalon, brain stem, and cerebellum. (From Polaski AL: Luckmann's Core Principles and Practice of Medical-Surgical Nursing. Philadelphia, WB Saunders, 1996, p 245.)

T A B L E 28–2

Autonomic Nervous System: Parasympathetic and Sympathetic Functions

PARASYMPATHETIC SYSTEM	SYMPATHETIC SYSTEM
Pupil constriction	Pupil dilation
Increased saliva	Decreased saliva
Lacrimal gland vasodilation	
Coronary vessel vasoconstriction	Coronary vessel vasodilation
Bronchial muscle constriction	Bronchial muscle relaxation
Stomach peristalsis	Stomach constriction
	Adrenaline secretion
Colon peristalsis	Colon relaxation
Sphincter relaxation	Sphincter constriction
Genitalia vasodilation	Genitalia vasoconstriction
Urinary bladder constriction	Urinary bladder relaxation
Skin vessel dilation	Skin vessel constriction

Data from Anderson P: Basic Human Anatomy and Physiology. Monterey, CA, Wadsworth, 1984.

tem of afferent and efferent nerves. Of course, more specific problems occur when special areas of the nervous system or individual nerves are damaged. Broad incapacity occurs with neurotransmitter problems.

SYSTEMIC PROBLEMS. The brain is extremely sensitive to changes in physiology anywhere in the body. Thus any metabolic change, from external or internal factors, affects the CNS. Examples include delirium from toxins and diabetic coma.

GENETIC PROBLEMS. All chromosomal defects are associated with some neurological effects because they are disorders involving many genes. Some of the single-gene defects may have direct neurological effects (such as neurofibromatosis), whereas others, typically inborn errors of metabolism, can have indirect effects via the abnormal metabolites released (e.g., phenylketonuria).

CONGENITAL DEFECTS. Because the CNS is structurally complex, there are many opportunities for defects to occur during fetal development. Hydrocephaly, spina bifida, and other problems can result.

INJURIES. Head and spinal cord injuries are common and can have long-term serious consequences for the child, especially since such complex neurological tissue has relatively little ability to heal.

Defense Mechanisms

Nerves can regenerate somewhat if conditions are right. When an axon is cut, the distal end degenerates. However, if the cut ends are reconnected with special attention to the myelin sheath, the axon stump begins to grow and the proximal and distal portions are united at a slow rate of about 1 to 2 mm/d (Gilman & Newman, 1992). The neurons that regenerate most rapidly are sympathetic fibers, followed by sensory fibers and finally motor neurons. First, skin color improves, followed by sensation to pressure and then pain and, finally, by return of motor function.

ASSESSMENT OF THE NERVOUS SYSTEM

Assessment of the nervous system requires a careful history and detailed physical examination. Imaging or laboratory studies may be required. For children with complex or severe neurological problems, daily living, developmental, and family issues need thorough exploration. See Chapter 2 for information regarding complete disease, daily living, and developmental history.

History

NEUROLOGICAL DISEASE HISTORY

A. History of present illness
   1. Onset. When did the very first symptoms appear? Was the onset insidious or sudden? Was it associated with any injury or strain? If yes, describe the trauma. Was the onset accompanied by any constitutional symptoms? How has the disorder evolved?
   2. Pain and headache. Location and charac-

ter, path of radiation, severity, extent of disability produced, effect of various activities or stimuli, relief measures, changes from day to night, effects of previous treatment, presence of pain or discomfort in other parts of the body.

3. Sensory deficits. Changes in hearing, vision, taste; loss of pain sensation; vertigo.

4. Injury. How, when (time and date), why, where, mechanism or manner in which the injury was produced. Immediate treatment provided.

5. Reflexive responses. Vomiting, coughing, primitive reflexes, tics.

6. Behavioral changes. Irritability, stupor, changes in appetite, lack of attention, random activity, emotional lability, changes in school performance.

7. Motor and balance changes. Ataxia, spasticity, increased or decreased tone.

B. Past medical history

1. Prenatal history: Maternal/paternal ages, alcohol, drug ingestion, radiation exposure, nutrition, prenatal care, injuries, hyperthermia, smoking, human immunodeficiency virus (HIV) exposure, maternal illness, bleeding, toxemia, diabetes, previous abortions and stillbirths.

2. Birth history and neonatal course: Complications, labor and delivery, resuscitation, trauma, congenital anomalies, feeding success, jaundice, convulsions, infection, gestational age.

3. Injuries or infections. Meningitis, encephalitis, head injuries, seizures—types, frequency, medications.

4. Cardiovascular or respiratory disorders.

5. Environmental or drug exposure. Consider lead exposure.

6. Metabolic disorders. Diabetes mellitus, thyroid disease. Hypoglycemia causes confusion, convulsion, loss of consciousness. Hyperglycemia causes lethargy, coma. Hyperthyroidism causes tremor. Hypothyroidism causes weakness, coma.

7. Past neurological disease and tests. Tics, hydrocephaly.

8. Psychiatric disorders. Hallucinations.

9. Drug ingestion.

10. Urinary tract disease. Uremic syndrome gives confusion, convulsions, coma.

11. Physical growth.

C. Family disease history

1. Family members with similar symptoms or genetic disorders.

2. Consanguinity.

3. Migraine history.

4. Mental functioning of family members.

D. Review of systems

1. Growth pattern. Height, weight, and head circumference.

2. Review *all* systems. Allergies, medications, hearing, vision, dental, skin integrity, behavior are all important areas to assess.

DEVELOPMENTAL HISTORY

Achievement of all developmental milestones—language, gross motor, fine motor, social, and cognitive—and school performance should be reviewed. Inquire about developmental changes, loss of skills, and lack of progression.

FUNCTIONAL HEALTH

Inquire about the effects of symptoms on all areas of health promotion and safety, nutrition, elimination, activity, communication, role relationships, values and beliefs, sexuality, sleep, coping and stress tolerance, temperament, and self-concept.

SOCIAL CONTEXT

Because neurological problems can have such profound consequences on the child and family, it is important to understand the social context of the child and family. Learn about the family composition, home environment, stressors, resources, financial issues, social supports, and community agencies involved with the family and child (Liptak, 1998).

Physical Examination

A complete physical examination is always important. The following should be noted:

• Abnormalities of the skin
• Anomalies

- Low-set ears
- Cardiovascular system
- Musculoskeletal system
- Hearing
- Vision; eye problems including cataract, corneal clouding, cherry-red spot
- Head circumference, growth measurements
- Tanner stage
- Hepatomegaly

COMPONENTS OF THE NEUROLOGICAL EXAMINATION

The provider conducting the neurological examination moves from the highest level of functioning to the lowest. Cerebral function is tested first; then cranial nerves, motor function, and sensory function; and finally, reflexes. In infants and children, watching them carefully while collecting the history and actively playing with them provides a great deal of neurological information.

BEHAVIOR AND MENTAL STATUS. Test the following cortical functions through evaluation of behavior and mental status.

- Responsiveness
- Judgment
- Language and speech (receptive, expressive, written)
- Memory
- General knowledge
- Ability to relate to others
- Mood and affect

The level of consciousness is also a CNS function and includes speech flow, voice quality, and organization of thoughts.

CRANIAL NERVES. Cranial nerves II through XII are tested.

MOTOR EXAMINATION. When conducting the motor examination, look for symmetry and quality of movement. Gait, posture, coordination, balance, strength, and tone are all aspects of this examination.

- Muscle strength and size. Look at muscle size and contour. Look for symmetry. Have the child stand from a lying position. Look for Gowers' sign (a child using the arms to push off from bent knees and gradually climbing the body and straightening up, which is common in children with muscular dystrophy). Ask the child to move extremities against resistance and to grip your fingers hard.
- Muscle tone. Muscle tone might be considered the resting strength of the muscle. Is the trunk or extremities floppy, rigid, or somewhat stiff when the child is resting? How difficult is it to move body parts passively? Remember that tone may be increased or decreased all over or differ between the legs and the trunk and arms.
- Fine motor coordination. Fine motor coordination is tested by having the child pick up small pellets, write, stack blocks, cut with scissors, turn book pages, or do other hand activities.
- Involuntary movements. Tremors are fine involuntary movements. Chorea or choreiform movements are large, irregular jerking and writhing movements. Athetoid movements are slow writhing movements, especially of the hands and feet. Dystonia is an uncontrolled change in tone with movement and a tendency to hyperextend the joints.
- The reflexes involve a combination of motor functioning and transmission of nerve impulses from various parts of the body to the spine and brain and back again. When a reflex is abnormal, the question is why. Did the impulse not go through or did the child have a problem in the ability to move responsively because of either efferent signals or problems of muscle tissue contractility? The reflexes and their testing are described later.

SENSORY EXAMINATION. Examine for pain sensation and stereognosis. This part of the examination is always limited in infants and young children. Use a light pinprick to check for mild pain sensation.

REFLEXES. The types of reflexes tested include deep tendon, superficial, and primitive reflexes.

- Deep tendon reflexes include the biceps, brachioradialis, triceps, patellar, and Achilles.
- Superficial reflexes include the upper ab-

dominal, lower abdominal, cremasteric, gluteal, and plantar.
- Primitive reflexes include sucking, rooting, asymmetrical tonic neck, grasp, trunk incurvation, stepping, and others found in Table 28–3.

CRANIUM EXAMINATION. The neurological examination should always include measurement of head circumference and inspection of the skull for symmetry and shape. Auscultation over the skull or above the eyes can reveal a cranial bruit. Percussion of the skull can give a sound resembling a cracked pot when the sutures are separated, as with increased intracranial pressure. The skull of the infant can be transilluminated to look for the absence of cortical tissue.

AUTONOMIC NERVOUS SYSTEM EXAMINATION. Alterations in blood pressure, sweating, or body temperature can be indicators of ANS problems.

MENINGEAL SIGNS. Signs of meningeal irritation such as with meningitis include Kernig and Brudzinski signs. Kernig sign is resistance and pain elicited on extension of the leg at the knee with the patient in the supine position and the hips flexed perpendicular to the trunk. Brudzinski sign consists of spontaneous flexion of the knee and hip provoked by passive flexion of the neck.

NEUROLOGICAL EXAMINATION OF THE INFANT. The neonate's neurological functioning is largely subcortical. Therefore, the examination is more limited than in an older infant or child. The cranium can be measured and transilluminated to look for structural or brain development problems. The primitive reflexes are all tested, although they can be absent or decreased in a satiated or sleepy infant. These reflexes include Moro, stepping and placing, sucking and rooting, and palmar and plantar grasp. Postural reflexes, including tonic neck, neck righting, and the Landau reflex, appear over the first few months of life. Tendon reflexes can be tested as in an older child. Babinski sign is not helpful in an infant. In older children and adults, it is an important sign of upper motor neuron disease.

Motor testing should include observation for symmetry of movements, consistent fisting of the hands, opisthotonos, scissoring, abnormal tone, and tremors. The infant's cry can be an indicator of several diseases: it is high pitched with increased intracranial pressure, resembles mewing in cri du chat syndrome, and is hoarse with hypothyroidism.

Cranial nerves can be tested. Vision (cranial nerve II) is indicated by blinking in response to a bright light. Cranial nerves III, IV, and VI can be tested by assessing the neonate's ability to track through the visual fields. Facial grimaces test for cranial nerves V and VII. Hearing (cranial nerve VIII) can be tested with a small bell. The gag reflex tests cranial nerves IX and X.

Diagnostic Studies

Radiographs have relatively little diagnostic value for the neurological system. Computed tomography (CT) scans display the soft tissues of the body and are often more helpful. Magnetic resonance imaging (MRI) can provide additional information related to the cellular activity of various parts of the neurological system.

Laboratory studies can provide indicators of systemic disease, infection, or inflammation. Laboratory studies are especially important for children receiving medication for seizures. Drug levels, liver function, and blood studies are done routinely.

Lumbar puncture provides a specimen of cerebrospinal fluid. The fluid provides information about metabolism, infections, and trauma within the CNS.

The electroencephalogram (EEG) provides information about the electrical activity of the CNS, which is important in assessing the function, not the structure, of the system.

Management Strategies

COUNSELING

Counseling for neurological problems involves several components. The family should understand the pathology, including possible etiologies, and the treatment plan. Parents also need information about the prognosis with and without treatment, as well as any genetic implications of the diagnosis. The latter can best be communicated through formal genetics counseling. Family members should have time to ask questions about all these issues.

Counseling also involves helping families cope with the diagnosis and its implications for the patient and family, both short term and long term. Congenital problems are often identified at birth or shortly thereafter. Families need to receive diagnoses truthfully, humanely, and promptly. Issues of etiology need to be addressed to relieve the guilt that some parents feel about causing the problem. A plan of care needs to be mutually agreed on by the family and care provider before the infant or child is discharged from the hospital or clinic.

ANTICIPATORY GUIDANCE

NEUROLOGICAL DEVELOPMENT. Families are sometimes concerned about problems that providers believe are within normal limits. In these situations, no neurology referral is necessary. The family needs to understand the predicted neurological development and be provided with time lines and markers that they can use to monitor their child's development. Misperceptions about the implications of minor variations need to be dealt with, and the family should always be given the opportunity to return for further assessment or discussion if concerns remain. The temperament of the child and the child's learned social behavior vs. pathological symptoms may need to be addressed (e.g., breath-holding vs. seizures).

EDUCATIONAL NEEDS. Many neurological problems in children affect learning, although neurological problems are not synonymous with mental retardation. Sensory problems affect the child's ability to receive the input necessary for learning. Motor problems can affect both the child's ability to interact with the environment and the child's ability to communicate or indicate understanding. Management should always consider the educational needs of the child. Special infant or preschool educational programs can assist the child to learn by using the most appropriate learning modalities. Teachers often need assistance in understanding the limitations and strengths of the child.

GENETICS COUNSELING. Many neurological conditions are genetic in origin. See Chapter 41 for a discussion of genetics assessment and management, including counseling.

PHYSICAL, OCCUPATIONAL, AND SPEECH THERAPY

Physical therapy can be very useful to help restore or maintain function or to teach new motor skills. The physical therapist should be accustomed to dealing with children. Occupational and speech therapy may also be essential to promote maximal development. Early intervention programs offer such assistance in many states and are generally free to qualifying patients.

SOCIAL SERVICES

Children with multiply handicapping conditions and their families frequently have ongoing issues of coping, as well as identification and management of medical and financial resources. Medical social workers can be a great help to these families.

MEDICATIONS

A variety of medications are used to control the effects of neurological problems. Most require time for the effects to become apparent, need dose adjustments, and are affected by the metabolism of the individual child. Thus blood levels are often needed. Side effects of medications need to be weighed against their beneficial effects. Many require tapering of dosages when treatment with the medication is to be discontinued. A variety of anticonvulsant medications are described in Table 28-6.

▒▒▒ SPECIFIC NEUROLOGICAL PROBLEMS OF CHILDREN

Cerebral Palsy

DESCRIPTION

Cerebral palsy (CP) is a handicapping disorder of motor function caused by a lesion in the brain. The condition is nonprogressive and nonhereditary. Depending on the area affected and the extent of damage, children with CP can also have mental retardation (50 to 66%), seizures (33 to 50%), neurosensory disorders, perceptual disorders, hyperkinesis, visual problems

T A B L E 28-3
Primitive Reflexes

REFLEX	AGE APPEARS	AGE DISAPPEARS	DESCRIPTION	RESPONSE	NOTES
NEWBORN REFLEXES					
Rooting	Birth	3–4 mo	Head midline, stroke perioral area	Infant opens mouth and turns head to stimulated side	Absence indicates severe CNS disease or depressed infant; sleeping infant may not respond
Sucking	Birth	3–4 mo	Place nipple or finger 3–4 cm into mouth	Suck should be strong: push finger up and back; note rate	Absence indicates CNS depression; satiated or sleeping baby may not respond well
Asymmetrical tonic neck (ATNR)	Birth	4–6 mo	With baby supine, rotate head to one side. Hold 15 s	Arm and leg extend on facial side; arm and leg on other side flex	Obligatory response when child cannot get out of position is abnormal; persistence beyond 4–6 mo indicates CNS lesion (e.g., CP)
Palmar grasp	Birth	3–6 mo	Place finger into infant's palm and press against palm	Infant flexes all fingers around examiner's finger	Grasp should be strong and symmetrical; tests cranial nerves VI and VIII
Trunk incurvation (Galant)	Birth	2 mo	Suspend baby prone; stroke 2–3 cm from spine with fingernail	Baby flexes toward stimulus	Asymmetry is significant; tests for spinal cord lesions. Should not persist after 6 mo
Stepping	Birth	6–8 wk	Infant is held as though weight bearing with feet on surface	Infant steps along, raising one foot at a time	Tests brain stem, spinal column; absence indicates paralysis or depressed baby

Reflex	Appears	Disappears	Procedure	Normal Response	Significance
Moro	Birth	4 mo	Present loud noise or allow infant's head to drop slightly	Arms spread and fingers extend and then flex; then arms come toward each other; cry is possible	Asymmetry indicates paralysis or fractured clavicle, absence indicates brain stem problem, usually severe; persistence also abnormal
Crossed extension	0–4 mo		Passively extend one leg and press knee to table; prick sole of that foot with pin	Other leg should slightly extend and adduct	
Plantar grasp	Birth	10 mo	Place finger firmly against base of toes	Toes should curl down	Tests S1–S2 spinal nerves. Suspect after 4 mo
LATER REFLEXES					
Landau	3 mo	15 mo–2 y	Suspend infant prone by supporting abdomen	Infant should lift both head and legs	Abnormal if arm tone increased with internal rotation, arm held at side, or arm does not lift as noted
Neck righting	6 mo	2 y	With infant supine, turn head to one side	Infant's trunk rotates in direction of head	Absent or decreased can indicate spasticity; can also rotate trunk and then look for head to follow; tests midbrain
Parachute	6–8 mo	Never	Suspend infant prone and lower quickly toward table	Infant should extend arms, hands, fingers	Response should be symmetrical as well as "protective"

CNS = central nervous system; CP = cerebral palsy.

(25%), hearing deficits, speech disorders, and other learning, emotional, and family problems (Davis, 1997a). Microcephaly occurs in about 25% of spastic quadriplegics and diplegics (Hay et al., 1997). CP can involve the trunk and extremities, but it also often involves the oral–motor region and affects speech, chewing, and swallowing.

The five main types of CP are spastic, dyskinetic, rigid, ataxic, and mixed (Taft, 1995). Children with spasticity are further described by the area of paralysis: diplegic, hemiplegic, or quadriplegic (sometimes called "tetraplegic"). Children with the dyskinetic types may be athetoid, dystonic, choreic, ballismic, or tremulous. To complicate the picture, some children may have mixed types, or the type may change over time (Table 28–4).

ETIOLOGY

The term *cerebral palsy* refers to motor deficits caused by a problem in the brain. Many etiologies are known. The condition is sometimes due to injury to the pyramidal or extrapyramidal tract or injury to both. The injuries can be vascular or traumatic, caused by metabolic events such as anoxia, or both. In the past, 85% of cases were thought to occur in utero or during labor and delivery. However, over half of children with CP in the 1981 Collaborative Perinatal Project had Apgar scores of 7 to 10 at 1 minute, and 75% had normal Apgar scores at 5 minutes (Nelson & Ellenberg, 1987). Neonates weighing over 2500 g were more likely to have CP if they had low Apgar scores plus signs of neonatal problems, including decreased activity after the first day of life, need for incubator care for 3 or more days, feeding problems, poor suck, respiratory difficulty, and/or neonatal seizure (Nelson & Ellenberg, 1987). This study is still cited as being important for understanding the etiology of the condition. Low birth weight and preterm babies are at greater risk for CP. Prematurity, prolonged labor, precipitous delivery, traumatic delivery, abnormal

T A B L E 28-4

Classification of Cerebral Palsy Types

TYPE	DESCRIPTION	COMMENTS
Spastic	Increased tone. Toe walks. Fisted hands and other signs	70–80% frequency. Diplegia most common in preterm babies. Usually hypertonic but may be hypotonic early or in some positions. Often shows after 4–6 mo
Diplegic	Affects both legs	
Quadriplegic	Affects all 4 extremities. Scissors	
Hemiplegic	Affects one side of the body. One hand fisted, toe walks on affected side	
Dyskinetic	Problems with voluntary movements	10–15% frequency
Athetoid	Continuous, writhing movements	
Dystonic	Problems with tone	
Choreic	Disorganized tone	
Ballismic	Violent, jerky movements	
Tremulous	Involuntary, rhythmic movements of opposing muscles	
Rigid	Stiffness	5% frequency. Associated with severe decerebrate lesions
Ataxic	Balance problems. Wide-based gait, clumsiness	1% frequency. Often not identified until child walks
Mixed		10–15% frequency

presentation, anoxia, intracranial hemorrhage, toxemia, preeclampsia, antepartal hemorrhage, postmaturity, fetal distress, and neonatal seizures are all considered risk factors (Barabas & Taft, 1986; Rosenbloom, 1995). Other etiologies included drug exposure, intrauterine infections such as cytomegalovirus, and congenital brain malformations. CP can also arise postnatally after meningitis, encephalitis, head trauma, and kernicterus.

INCIDENCE

The prevalence is 1 to 3 per 1000 live births across many studies. The incidence has not declined in many years and may be slowly increasing in the very low birth weight population because more of these babies are now surviving (Davis, 1997b).

CLINICAL FINDINGS

History

The history that should be obtained from a patient with CP in terms of pathology, development, and functional health patterns follows.

- Prenatal/natal history of risk factors as listed previously
- Seizures
- Hearing and vision or ocular problems such as strabismus, nystagmus, optic atrophy
- Muscle tone (can be hypotonic before 6 months, but then tone usually increases)
- Growth parameters, especially decreased head circumference
- Early head injury or meningitis

Development

- Milestones may be delayed but should still be attained; persistent primitive reflexes are common. Handedness before 1 year is suspect.

Functional Health Patterns

- Feeding history of regurgitating through the nose, inability to coordinate suck and swallow, inability to advance the diet to textured foods—in short, oral-motor coordination problems
- Irritability or depressed affect (including sleepiness) as a neonate
- Difficulty with movement, cuddliness, grasp and release, self-feeding, and head control to look around; inability to change position per developmental level
- Persistent primitive reflexes
- Communication problems, either language or speech proficiency

Physical Examination

SKIN. Dermatological signs of syndromes such as neurofibromatosis may be apparent.

ORTHOPEDIC EXAMINATION. Scoliosis, contractures, and dislocated hip may be present.

NEUROLOGICAL EXAMINATION. The following may be seen on the neurological examination:

- Deep tendon reflexes are increased.
- Tone is increased, although occasionally decreased; hypotonia before 6 months of age is common. Tone may also be mixed.
- Minimal muscle atrophy.
- No fasciculations.
- Persistent primitive reflexes, especially grasp, plantar grasp, Galant, asymmetrical tonic neck, crossed extension (Zafeiriou et al., 1995).
- Asymmetrical movement.
- Structural defects such as hydrocephaly or microcephaly are common.

HEARING AND VISION. Testing of both should be done.

Other Studies

DEVELOPMENTAL LEVEL. Assessment of motor, fine motor, language, and personal social skills is needed. The Denver Developmental Screening Test II (Denver II) can be used for initial screening. Also look at the quality of movements (e.g., smoothness of gait, grasping, clarity of speech). In children with CP, motor milestones are commonly delayed.

COMPUTED TOMOGRAPHY. A CT scan can be obtained to identify brain malformations.

CHROMOSOMAL AND METABOLIC STUDIES. These studies can be done to identify genetic disorders, especially single-gene defects.

FEEDING ASSESSMENT. A patient with CP can have a reversed swallow wave; uncoordinated suck and swallow; decreased tone of the lips, tongue, and cheeks; increased gag reflex; involuntary tongue and lip movements; increased sensitivity to food stimuli; poor occlusion; and delayed inhibition of the suck reflex. Evaluate the diet and the height and weight for adequate nutrition.

DIFFERENTIAL DIAGNOSIS

The first and main requirement is to differentiate central from peripheral disorders. CP is always central and is characterized by brisk deep tendon reflexes. Many other conditions can have CP/motor involvement features. These conditions include intrauterine infections, fetal alcohol syndrome, hydrocephalus, tumors, agenesis of the corpus callosum or other brain malformations, Tay-Sachs disease, phenylketonuria, Lesch-Nyhan syndrome, spinal cord injury, hypothyroidism, and many genetic and metabolic disorders. Also, mental retardation results in delayed milestones but should not include increased reflexes. Not every condition characterized by deterioration is CP. Neuromuscular disorders are associated with signs of weakness, muscle atrophy, and decreased deep tendon reflexes.

MANAGEMENT

The management of children with CP described here can serve as a model for the management of children with a variety of neurological problems.

REFERRAL OF SUSPECTED CASES. Children with CP should be evaluated and cared for at centers that provide interdisciplinary caregivers, including developmental pediatricians, orthopedists, neurologists, nurses, speech pathologists, physical and occupational therapists, education consultants and psychologists, and social workers. The care of children with CP may also involve an ophthalmologist, feeding clinic and nutritionist services, and genetics counseling.

FAMILY EDUCATION ABOUT THE DIAGNOSIS. Families need to understand the diagnosis and its nonprogressive but noncurable characteristics. They need to understand that the extent of brain damage is not always related to the extent of disability. Thus no one can predict what the future for a given child will be. It is known that children who receive special services and therapy have better outcomes than do children who are left to develop on their own. United Cerebral Palsy has educational materials and a variety of services available for affected children and their families (see Resource Box).

FAMILY SUPPORT. Generally, families grieve when given the diagnosis of CP and need support during this time. Support groups or opportunities to meet other families with affected children are often helpful. The emotional needs of siblings must not be overlooked either. The social worker can be very helpful to families trying to cope with complex health problems.

FINANCIAL AID. CP services are long term and expensive. Many children will be eligible for Supplemental Security Income or state program benefits for the severely handicapped. Respite care can be a benefit that is also available to families. Again, social workers can be very helpful in connecting families to appropriate services.

NUTRITION MANAGEMENT. Children with CP often have inadequate nutrition because of their problems with biting, sucking, chewing, swallowing, and self-feeding. Additionally, children with athetosis may need as much as 50 to 100% more calories to support their increased caloric needs because of their constant writhing movements. Children with spasticity, on the other hand, may need fewer calories because of their decreased movements. Occasionally, the problems are so severe that a gastrostomy is needed, sometimes with fundal plication to prevent reflux and aspiration. Special positioning, feeding therapy by a speech pathologist, and special feeding devices can help. High nutrient density is a key to providing a nutritious diet (i.e., getting more nutrients into the same volume of food). Feeding clinics are often helpful to plan management of nutrition.

ELIMINATION MANAGEMENT. Constipation is common because of lack of exercise, inadequate fluid and fiber intake, medications, poor positioning, low abdominal muscle tone, and other factors. Stool softeners such as docusate sodium may help. Laxatives such as senna concentrate (Senokot) or milk of magnesia may be useful.

Bladder control and urinary retention are also problems for children with CP. Most achieve bladder control between 3 and 10 years of age. Mental retardation makes toilet training difficult for some. Sensations regarding bladder fullness or emptiness, fluid restrictions, and reflux may all contribute to problems of urinary tract infection in children with CP (Nehring & Steele, 1996).

DENTAL MANAGEMENT. Orofacial muscle tone can contribute to malocclusion, and problems with oral mobility make daily dental hygiene difficult. Thus these children also have more gum disease and caries (Nehring & Steele, 1996). A careful dental care program is necessary.

DROOLING. Inability to manage oral secretions results in drooling. Social isolation, wet clothing, skin excoriation, malodorous breath, and discomfort can make these oral secretions a serious problem. Glycopyrrolate, 0.05 to 1.0 mg twice or three times daily, may help, but side effects may also be problematic. Surgical intervention is a last resort.

MOVEMENT AND MOBILITY MANAGEMENT. Positioning and seating, standing, transportation, bathing, dressing, mobility for play and getting to school, and oral hygiene are important to assess and manage. Occupational and physical therapists are essential to these aspects of care. Families need help incorporating various strategies into their homes and lifestyles. The goals of therapy are to improve physical conditioning and gain maximum independence in mobility, fine motor activities, self-care, and communication. Therapists try to promote efficient movement patterns, inhibit primitive reflexes, and achieve isolated extremity movements. Bracing, adaptive devices, and early intervention programs beginning in infancy are important. Children need to experience different environments for developmental growth. Wheelchairs and motorized wheelchairs can be beneficial in helping children explore their environment more efficiently. Furthermore, although the condition is not progressive in terms of the brain lesion, contractures, scoliosis, dislocated hips, and other deformities can develop if the child is allowed to maintain abnormal positions for long periods. Thus therapy for range of motion is a long-term need for many of these children. Orthopedic care may be necessary.

COMMUNICATION MANAGEMENT. With the combined problems of lack of oral–motor control and the high incidence of mental retardation, communication can be a real problem for children with CP. Speech therapy is important to achieve oral speech when possible or to use augmentative devices such as computers with voices to allow language development and communication of needs even without oral speech. Hearing deficits need to be identified and managed by an audiologist.

ADVOCACY. Families often need help accessing services through schools because children with CP may have special education needs. Some insurance companies try to avoid the costs of long-term care and therapy. The primary care provider is important to families as an advocate and resource.

SPECIAL EDUCATION. Early intervention programs and specialized educational programs through school systems are often beneficial.

COMPLICATIONS

Children who receive no intervention have poorer functional abilities than do children who have physical therapy, speech therapy, and other interventions. They make less progress developmentally and are at risk for unnecessary contractures and deformities. Gastroesophageal reflux with aspiration and chronic respiratory infections can be a serious complication.

Other associated problems can include

- Amblyopia or strabismus
- Seizures, which are managed according to the same guidelines used for other children with seizure disorders
- Retinopathy of prematurity or blindness
- Conductive or sensorineural hearing loss
- Hip subluxation, scoliosis, or contractures
- Drooling
- Growth disorders, nutrition deficits
- Constipation or encopresis
- Enuresis, urinary retention, or urinary tract infections
- Dental malocclusions or caries

- Pneumonias
- Decubitus ulcers
- Behavioral and/or attention deficit disorder
- Speech impairments

PREVENTION AND SCREENING

The incidence of CP can be decreased through good prenatal care. However, it is not a condition that can be directly prevented. On the other hand, early identification and intervention can significantly improve the outlook for children who are affected and their families.

Epilepsy and Seizure Disorders

DESCRIPTION

Seizures are due to misfiring of the neurons of the brain. Convulsive seizures occur when misfiring causes attacks of involuntary contraction of voluntary muscles. See Table 28-5 for

T A B L E 28-5
International Classification of Seizures

SEIZURE TYPE	AGE	PATTERN	COMMENTS

I. Partial seizures
  A. Simple partial
		Begin locally
		Consciousness not
		  impaired
			Affect one hemisphere
			Lasts 10–20 s

1. With motor symptoms	Any age	Any part of body:
		  includes jacksonian
		  seizures
			Birth trauma,
			  inflammation,
			  cerebrovascular
			  accident; tumor if new
			  or with progressive
			  neurological
			  symptoms

2. With sensory or
      somatosensory symptoms
	Any age	"Pins and needles,"
		  numb; auras include
		  lights, tastes, sounds	

3. With autonomic
      symptoms
	Any age	Recurrent abdominal
		  pain, headache,
		  sweat, laugh, cry,
		  tachycardia, dilated
		  pupils
			May have migraine
			  quality; family history
			  of migraine or seizures

4. Compound forms	Any age		

B. Complex partial	Any age; may
	  be hard to
	  recognize in
	  young child
		Consciousness
		  impaired; complex
		  symptoms and
		  interesting
		  automatisms
			Lasts 1–2 min

1. Impaired consciousness only		Staring spell	
2. With cognitive symptoms		May have confusion	
3. With affective symptoms		Aura of fear	

4. With "psychosensory"
      symptoms
		May have odd smell/
		  taste; visual or
		  auditory hallucination	

5. With "psychomotor"
      symptoms
		Automatisms; facial,
		  tongue, or swallow
		  movements	

6. Compound forms			

types of seizures. When seizures are recurrent and unrelated to fever, the disorder is called epilepsy. Seizures represent either brain dysfunction or significant underlying disorders.

ETIOLOGY

Different kinds of seizures arise from disorders in different parts of the brain. Seizures can result from a variety of causes, including congenital defects, metabolic disorders, trauma, tumors, genetic conditions, and toxins. By 1997, chromosomal loci had been located for seven genes related to epilepsy and three epilepsy syndromes (Haslam, 1997). Seizures can also be idiopathic. Most children with an unprovoked seizure will not have recurrences (Shinnar et al., 1996).

CLINICAL FINDINGS

History

The history of a patient with seizures should include the following:

- Description of the seizure: focal or generalized, loss of consciousness, aura, postictal sleep or lethargy, duration of the episode, and associated illness
- Underlying medical diagnosis: diabetes, renal disease, cardiovascular disorder
- Previous CNS infection or birth trauma
- Intrauterine infection, trauma, bleeding
- Toxic exposure or drug use
- Anticonvulsant medication stopped abruptly
- Recent head injury
- Family history of seizures

T A B L E 28-5

International Classification of Seizures Continued

SEIZURE TYPE	AGE	PATTERN	COMMENTS
C. Partial seizures secondarily generalized		Seizure begins in one part of body but then generalizes	Aura can let person seek safe position
II. Generalized seizures			No aura
A. Absence	4–8 y most common	Petit mal; 5–30-s lapses of consciousness; can have associated movements; no falling; no aura	Hyperventilation for 3–4 min can trigger; blinking lights can trigger
B. Myoclonic	Infancy	Head drops or sudden flexing; may cry out	Hypsarrhythmia on EEG with no normal background activity; difficult to treat
C. Clonic		Rhythmic jerking	
D. Tonic		Intense muscle contraction	
E. Tonic-clonic	Any age: most common type	Grand mal; begins with loss of consciousness; stiffens, then jerks violently; postictal phase of sleep and confusion; 15% incontinent	Aura in some; may have abdominal pain or headache; life-threatening if continues, producing hypercarbia, respiratory acidosis, lactic acidemia; some occur in sleep
F. Atonic		Similar to myoclonic	Child often falls

EEG = encephalogram; s = seconds.

Physical Examination

The following should be determined on physical examination:

- Focal abnormalities, weakness
- Seizures still occurring intermittently
- Hypertension (for renal disease)
- Systemic disease
- Cardiovascular disorder
- Neurocutaneous disease, café au lait spots of neurofibromatosis, ash leaf spots or adenoma sebaceum of tuberous sclerosis, facial hemangioma of Sturge-Weber syndrome
- Signs of head trauma

Other Studies

A complete blood count (CBC) and chemistry screen, including liver function studies, are useful for diagnostic purposes and/or a baseline before anticonvulsant therapy is started. An abnormal EEG supports the seizure diagnosis. However, a normal EEG when the child is not seizing does not rule out a seizure disorder. A CT scan is often useful to identify tumor, abscess, or an arteriovenous anomaly. MRI may also be useful in identifying temporal lobe and hippocampal atrophy and sclerosis. It should be used for children with complex partial seizures, those with a focal neurological deficit, and those with complex seizures of increasing frequency or severity and adolescents with a first seizure (Haslam, 1997).

DIFFERENTIAL DIAGNOSIS

Consider breath-holding, syncope, migraine headaches, gastroesophageal reflux, night terrors, metabolic problems, tumors or other CNS problems, or a cardiovascular problem. Vertigo has been confused with epilepsy. Tics (involuntary, spasmodic, nonrhythmic, repetitive movements) are stereotypic but not associated with impaired consciousness and at times can be suppressed by the patient. Pseudoseizures sometimes occur, especially in adolescent girls. Incest or sexual abuse must be addressed in these girls (Haslam, 1997).

MANAGEMENT

REFERRAL. A child with suspected seizures should be referred to a neurologist for diagnosis and initiation of treatment. Anticonvulsant drugs are usually prescribed, especially after the second seizure in 6 to 12 months. A fasting blood sugar and serum calcium levels are usually indicated if the history suggests hypoglycemia or hypocalcemia as a cause.

MANAGEMENT OF STABLE PATIENTS WITH DIAGNOSED SEIZURE DISORDERS. Some NPs monitor stable children with seizures. Such activity includes prescribing anticonvulsants, monitoring drug levels, and performing case management. Any change in status requires consultation with or referral to the neurologist.

DRUG MONITORING. All NPs working with patients receiving anticonvulsants should be familiar with the common drugs and their major side effects (Table 28–6). Helping with compliance issues is also a component of the monitoring role. Haslam (1997) recommends routine drug monitoring for children who experience a change in seizure type, patients with seizures despite adequate drug dosing based on weight and age, patients with renal or hepatic disease, children taking phenytoin or multiple anticonvulsants, those with mental or physical handicaps making monitoring of drug toxicity difficult, and patients and families who are noncompliant with the drug regimen. If toxic effects appear before the seizures are controlled, the dosage must be tapered while a new antiepileptic is slowly introduced with increasing dose (Valente & Valente, 1998).

ANTICONVULSANT MEDICATION WITHDRAWAL. After 2 years without seizures, consideration may be given to gradually withdrawing anticonvulsant therapy. Absence and generalized tonic-clonic seizures on awakening are associated with the best prognosis. Some evidence indicates that spike-and-wave paroxysmal features on EEG are a contraindication to drug withdrawal. Children with mental retardation, CP, focal motor deficits, age of onset younger than 2 years or older than 12 years, or juvenile myoclonic or benign rolandic epilepsy are not good weaning candidates. Weaning is supervised closely and occurs over 6 weeks to 4 to 6 months, with one drug removed at a time. Of children who have been seizure free for 2 years and have no risk factors, 70 to 75% remain seizure free without drugs. Most seizures that recur do so within the first 6 months of weaning (Haslam, 1997; Tennison, 1996).

KETOGENIC DIET. The ketogenic diet has recently reemerged as a treatment of epilepsy, especially in children who have not achieved good seizure control with antiepileptic drugs (Batchelor et al., 1997). The diet is very high in fat and low in carbohydrates and protein and thus has significant risks. It is best managed under very tight control with medical and dietician leadership. A prescreening process, including psychological testing to determine the child's and family's emotional functioning, coping, and problem-solving abilities, is recommended. A dietician should screen the child for nutrition and growth status. A nurse should interview the family for understanding and education about the protocol. The diet is started while the child is admitted to the hospital, where metabolic and neurological states can be monitored. For carefully selected and monitored children, 50% seizure reduction was achieved in 40% of children, with 25% seizure free (Batchelor et al., 1997; McDonald, 1997).

EPILEPSY SURGERY. Surgery has been successful in helping some children with partial seizures. However, as with the ketogenic diet, selection of appropriate children is done with great care. Surgery is currently used only in children with complex partial seizures who cannot achieve seizure control by any other method. A focal site of origin for the seizures must be demonstrable to the surgical team (Lannon, 1997). The main risk is hemiparesis (Valente & Valente, 1998).

COUNSELING. Older children need to understand the seizures they are experiencing and their significance. They also need to know about the anticonvulsant medications they are taking. Teenagers want to drive. Laws vary from state to state, but generally a teenager who has been seizure free for 2 years and has demonstrated good drug compliance should be allowed to drive. Parents need to understand the diagnosis, treatment, and necessary follow-up. They also need to understand the implications of seizure disorders and long-term prognoses. Negative attitudes continue to surround epilepsy and may need to be addressed. Epilepsy is not synonymous with mental retardation.

Children with epilepsy may experience social stigmas and problems with self-esteem. Other mental health problems may also occur in these children as they try to cope with a chronic disease. The primary care provider needs to monitor the child's and family's quality of life and coping (Valente & Valente, 1998).

SAFETY. Uncontrolled seizures can present safety hazards for an unsupervised child. The child and family need to consider the situations that the child will be in and be sure that someone knows what to do if a seizure occurs. School personnel need to be informed and prepared. Safety helmets worn at all times are sometimes warranted if falls and head injury occur frequently. Swimming alone is never recommended.

IMMUNIZATIONS. The decision to give pertussis vaccine to children with neurological seizures and/or other neurological conditions needs to be made on an individual basis. If used, DTaP is recommended. Children who will be in child care centers, special clinics, or residential care centers should be immunized if possible. Progressive neurological conditions with developmental delays are reason for deferral of pertussis vaccine. Infants and children with a personal history of seizures have been noted to have a sevenfold increase in post–diphtheria-pertussis-tetanus (DPT) immunization seizures. Thus DtaP and acetaminophen at the time of administration and every 4 hours for the first 24 hours is recommended. Other neurological conditions that predispose to seizures or neurological deterioration should result in consideration of deferral of pertussis immunization (American Academy of Pediatrics, 1997).

COMPLICATIONS

A child in status epilepticus, a grand mal seizure lasting more than 30 minutes, is at risk for brain damage and death. Lack of oxygenation, decreased cerebral perfusion, metabolic acidosis, hypoglycemia, hyperkalemia, lactic acidemia, increased temperature, and increased intracranial pressure can all result in significant morbidity and mortality. Mortality can be 10%

T A B L E 28-6

Anticonvulsant Medication Therapy for Children

DRUG	HALF-LIFE (h)	ORAL DOSE* (mg/kg/24 hr)	FREQUENCY (doses/24 hr)	BLOOD LEVELS (µg/ml)	SEIZURE TYPE	SIDE EFFECTS	LABORATORY MONITORING*
Carbamazepine (Tegretol)	6–20	10 to start; 20–30	2–3	4–12	Partial, tonic-clonic	Vertigo, diplopia, drowsiness, hepatotoxicity, anemia, leukopenia	CBC: baseline, at 6–12 wk, then annually Blood levels
Phenytoin (Dilantin)	10–40	4–8	1–2	10–20	Partial, tonic-clonic	Drowsiness, gum hyperplasia, rash, Stevens-Johnson syndrome, anemia, behavioral and cognitive problems, hirsutism	None recommended Blood levels
Phenobarbital	50–150	4–8	1–2	10–40	Partial, tonic-clonic	Sedation, irritability, hyperkinesis, ataxia, slurred speech, nystagmus, Stevens-Johnson syndrome, attention, memory, learning	None recommended
Ethosuximide (Zarontin)	20–60	10–20 to start; 20–50	2–3	50–100	Absence, myoclonic	Gastric upset, drowsiness, hematological problems	None recommended
Valproic acid (Depakene)	6–12	10 to start; 15–50	3–4	50–150	Partial, tonic-clonic, absence, myoclonic	Nausea/vomiting, weight gain, transient alopecia, tremor, hepatic failure, hematological problems	Baseline (and after 1 mo) AST, ALT, ammonia, prothrombin, partial thromboplastin

Drug	Serum half-life (hr)	Dose (mg/kg/day)	Number of doses	Therapeutic serum level	Seizure type	Side effects	Laboratory monitoring
Primidone (Mysoline)	6–18	1–2 to start; 5–10 maximum	3–4	5–12	Partial, tonic-clonic, myoclonic	Drowsiness, ataxia, vertigo, anorexia, nausea/vomiting, rash, aggression	None recommended
Vigabatrin	5–7	30–40 to start; 80–100 maximum	1–2	1.4–14	Partial, myoclonic, infantile spasms	Agitation, depression, drowsiness, abdominal pain, weight gain, dizziness, headache, ataxia	
Felbamate (Felbatol)	14–22	15–45	3–4	Not determined	Partial, Lennox-Gastaut syndrome	Drowsiness, lethargy, nausea, vomiting, aplastic anemia, hepatitis, anorexia, ataxia	ALT, AST, bilirubin, CBC with differential, platelet, reticulocyte count weekly
Gabapentin (Neurontin) (add-on therapy)	5–7	300 to start; 900–1200 maximum	3	Not monitored	Complex partial, secondarily generalized	Somnolence, dizziness, ataxia, headache, tremor, vomiting, nystagmus, fatigue	
Lamotrigine (add-on therapy)	7–45; up to 6 d with valproic acid	5–15, 1–5 with valproic acid	2	1–4	Lennox-Gastaut syndrome, partial tonic-clonic	Rash (Stevens-Johnson syndrome), drowsiness, headache, blurred vision, vomiting	

ALT = alanine aminotransferase; AST = aspartate aminotransferase; CBC = complete blood count.
*Data from Burg F, Ingelfinger J, Wald E, et al: Gellis & Kagan's Current Pediatric Therapy, 16th ed. Philadelphia, WB Saunders, 1999. Other data from Burg F, Ingelfinger J, Wald E: Gellis & Kagan's Current Pediatric Therapy, Philadelphia, WB Saunders, 1993; Haslam R: Nonfebrile seizures. Pediatr Rev 18:39–49, 1997. Russell J & Parles B: Anticonvulsant medications. Pediatr An 28:238–245, 1999. Calli J & Farrington E: Vigabatrin. Pediatr Nurs 24:357–361, 1998.
Consult a more specific reference for information on initial dosing, adult doses, and maximum doses.

or more. Adverse outcomes can include behavioral problems, mental retardation, and focal motor deficits.

PREVENTION AND SCREENING

Epilepsy cannot be prevented, but early diagnosis and intervention can often reduce the disabilities and risks associated with the condition.

Febrile Seizures

DESCRIPTION

Febrile seizures are brief, generalized, clonic or tonic-clonic attacks. Fever develops in most children at the time of the attack, and temperatures can range from 38 to 41°C. Little postictal confusion is associated with febrile seizures. Simple febrile seizures last less than 15 minutes and do not recur within a 24-hour period.

ETIOLOGY AND INCIDENCE

The etiology of febrile seizures is unclear and by definition excludes seizures that recur without concurrent illness or are related to an underlying CNS problem. They can occur at the height of the fever or as the fever begins to rise. Febrile seizures generally occur in children between the ages of 3 months and 7 years, with most (95%) occurring before 5 years and a peak incidence occurring at 23.2 months. Boys and girls are equally affected. Three percent to 4% of all children have a febrile seizure. The risk for subsequent febrile seizures is 30 to 50% (Burg et al., 1999; Behrman et al., 1996).

ASSESSMENT

HISTORY
The history of a patient with febrile seizures involves the following:

- Description of seizure duration, type (generalized or focal), frequency in 24 hours
- Relationship of the seizure to the febrile episode
- Abnormal neurological status before the seizure, which is not consistent with a febrile seizure
- Family history of afebrile seizures

- Maternal smoking in the perinatal period
- Prematurity or neonatal hospitalizations for more than 28 days
- Parents' impression of slow development

Day care for more than 20 hr/wk and frequent infections in the first 6 months increase the risk (Camfield & Camfield, 1993).

PHYSICAL EXAMINATION. The physical examination is the same as that described earlier for seizures.

LABORATORY STUDIES. Blood glucose and sodium levels may be appropriate if recent poor feeding or gastrointestinal fluid loss is noted. Other electrolytes provide little information. A white blood cell count may be helpful in evaluating the fever itself, but the count may be increased just as a result of the seizure. Neuroimaging studies are not usually indicated. An EEG is not necessary in an otherwise healthy child. If it is suspected that recurrent seizures without fever are occurring, EEG may be useful (Burg et al., 1999).

DIFFERENTIAL DIAGNOSIS

Consider meningitis, metabolic or toxic encephalopathies, hypoglycemia, anoxia, trauma, tumor, and hemorrhage. Febrile delirium and febrile shivering can be confused with seizures. Breath-holding spells can mimic febrile seizures; however, the former are always related to crying or tantrums. Febrile seizures come at unpredictable times during sleep, eating, play, or other generally calm times and are related to the onset of an illness. Epileptic seizures occur without concurrent illness and at unpredictable times.

MANAGEMENT

The following steps should be taken in the management of a febrile seizure:

- Protect the airway, breathing, and circulation if the seizure is still occurring. Place the child in a side-lying position to prevent aspiration or airway obstruction.
- Do not put anything in the child's mouth.
- Time the duration of the seizure, and observe whether it is focal or generalized.

- Reduce the fever with acetaminophen or ibuprofen.

The child should be seen shortly after the seizure. Advise transport to an emergency center if the seizure is lasting more than 10 minutes. A child younger than 1 year who is experiencing a first seizure should have a lumbar puncture; immediate referral is needed. Anticonvulsants are not recommended for febrile seizures.

The family should receive information about febrile seizures, their risks, and their management. Education should include information explaining the febrile seizure, reassurance that no long-term consequences are associated with febrile seizures, information that febrile seizures recur in some children and that nothing can be done to prevent the seizures, and first-aid information in case another seizure occurs at some time.

A follow-up phone call to the parents after 1 week is often helpful.

COMPLICATIONS

Deaths or persisting motor deficits do not occur in patients with febrile seizures. No indication has been found that intellect or learning is impaired. An affected child has an increased risk for the development of epilepsy (up to 10 or 15%) if the seizure is prolonged or unilateral and if the child has a prior neurological deficit, a family history of epilepsy, or both. Two thirds of patients who have had one simple febrile seizure will not have any more.

Headaches

DESCRIPTION

Headaches in children can be classified as vascular (migraine), muscle contraction (tension or psychogenic), or inflammatory (increased intracranial pressure) (Table 28–7).

Migraine is the most common cause of recurrent headache in children. Characteristics of classic migraine include nausea, abdominal pain, vomiting, unilateral pain, pulsating pain, relief with sleep, an aura, visual changes such as dark or blind spots, and a family history of headache. Infants and toddlers may be seen with irritability, sleepiness, pallor, and/or vomiting (Behrman et al., 1996). In preadolescents, common migraine symptoms are more likely. Nausea and vomiting might not occur, and the pain can be more frontal. Lethargy and sleep can follow. Visual changes are rare, and the pain quality is variable. Times between headaches are pain free.

Muscle contraction or tension headaches are also common. They have no prodrome, and the pain is dull and bifrontal or occipital, with nausea and vomiting occurring only rarely. They can last for days or weeks but do not interfere with activities. In children it can be difficult to differentiate migraine and muscle contraction headaches. Psychosocial stress seems to be a major factor in tension headaches in both children and adolescents.

Traction or inflammatory headaches are much more rare. They occur when a mass is causing inflammation or traction on the brain. The key point for these headaches is their increasing severity, often with accompanying neurological signs. Pain that is worse in the mornings (sometimes with vomiting), diplopia, increased pain with straining, sneezing, and coughing, occipital pain, association with neurological signs or symptoms, and edema of the optic disk all point toward a significant structural headache needing prompt referral (O'Hara & Koch, 1998; Robertson, 1998).

ETIOLOGY AND INCIDENCE

Pain fibers line the walls of the large intracranial blood vessels, the meninges, the muscles around the head and scalp as well as the jaw, and the sinuses and around the eyes. Finding the source of the pain and its cause can be difficult. As many as 82% of children experience headaches (Scheller, 1995). Almost 90% of school-aged children in another study reported headaches, although only 55% of their parents recognized their problem (Cady et al., 1996).

ASSESSMENT

HISTORY. The following is assessed in the history of a child with headache:

- Duration. Recent onset is worrisome.
- Frequency and triggers. Children with re-

T A B L E 28-7

Differential Diagnosis of Headaches

CHARACTERISTICS	VASCULAR (MIGRAINE)	TENSION	TRACTION AND INFLAMMATORY (INCREASED INTRACRANIAL PRESSURE)
Time, course	Acute, paroxysmal, recurrent	Chronic, recurrent, nonprogressive	Chronic or intermittent but with increasing frequency and severity
Prodrome	Yes; aura in older children	No	No
Description	Intense, pulsating, unilateral in older children; frontotemporal Infants: irritability, pallor, sleepiness, and/or vomiting	Diffuse, band-like, tight, dull, bifrontal or occipital; mild to moderate intensity	Diffuse, can be localized to one area (e.g., occipital)
Predisposing factors	Positive family history (75%), head trauma	Problems at home, school, or with peers common	No
Associated findings	Transient neurological signs, sleep relief, nausea/vomiting in older children; older children can have visual changes, abdominal pain	Depression, inadequacy, anxiety; school avoidance common. Sleep may help. Nausea/ vomiting rare	Positive neurological signs such as ataxia, weakness, lethargy, decreased intellectual functioning, visual disturbances, sensory abnormalities, behavior/ mood alterations. Papilledema, worse in morning (with vomiting); straining increases pain, diplopia

current headaches usually have fewer than one per week. A recurrent headache of more than 3 months' duration is rarely organic (Smith, 1995).

- Location. Occipital or consistently localized headaches can indicate underlying pathology. Facial pain might be sinusitis. Ocular motor imbalance can produce a dull periorbital discomfort, whereas temporomandibular joint pain tends to localize around the periauricular or temporal areas.
- Quality of pain and severity. Sharp, throbbing, or pounding pain is probably vascular (migraine). Dull and constant pain may be tension or organic. Severity can be assessed by asking how much activities are interfered with.

- Presence of an aura or other premonitory symptoms.
- Age of onset and progression of the headaches over time.
- Home management and medications used.
- Amount of school missed, limitation of activities.
- Self-coping activities.
- Associated symptoms. Nausea, vomiting, visual changes, dizziness, paresthesia, confusion, ataxia, pallor, photophobia, and phonophobia can occur with migraine. Changes in gait, personality, or behavior that do not occur at the same time as the headache are worrisome and merit further evaluation with medical referral.
- Head trauma. If associated with headache,

head trauma can represent a subdural hematoma or postconcussive syndrome.

- Psychological symptoms. Depression can occur with loss of a family member or friend. Deteriorating performance in school can be related to organic or psychological causes. Also consider stressors resulting from family and peer relationships, expectations as related to developmental stage, and community/environment conflict or danger (Smith, 1995).
- Family history. Most children with headache, especially migraine, have a family history of headaches.

PHYSICAL EXAMINATION. The physical examination is usually normal. The following areas must be assessed:

- Blood pressure
- Neurological examination
- Optic fundi
- Height and weight
- Pericranial muscles
- Sinuses
- Teeth
- Temporomandibular joints
- Thyroid gland
- Cranial bruits

OTHER STUDIES. Other studies are rarely indicated except if the history is not compatible with a known headache disorder, the history or physical examination indicates a possibility of serious pathology, a bruit is heard, no improvement is seen with appropriate medication, or the headache changes in character from a previous headache disorder (O'Hara & Koch, 1998). Recent behavioral changes, a drop in growth rate, reduced visual acuity, abnormalities on neurological examination, pain on awakening, coughing, straining or changing position, and frequent wakening at night are additional indications for neuroimaging studies (Smith, 1995).

DIFFERENTIAL DIAGNOSIS

The differential diagnosis consists of sinusitis, an intracranial mass, pseudotumor cerebri, sleep disorder, hyperthyroidism, hypertension, and temporomandibular joint dysfunction. Visual acuity is rarely a cause of headaches. Psychological/psychosocial problems may be a factor in tension headaches (Smith, 1995). Tumors are manifested as a nonpulsatile, deep ache. The pain may be intermittent, worse with activities or changes in position, and more severe in the morning or at night. The key is increasing severity over time.

MANAGEMENT

MEDICATIONS. Treatment can include general pain management, abortive therapy to interrupt migraine headaches, and prophylactic medications to prevent or reduce the frequency and severity of acute attacks (Table 28–8). Acetaminophen or ibuprofen is the drug of choice. For children with auras preceding the onset, give acetaminophen (10 to 15 mg/kg every 4 hours) or ibuprofen dosed at 30 to 70 mg/kg per day in three divided doses. Give acetaminophen no more than five times in 24 hours and for no longer than 5 consecutive days. Naproxen sodium may be more effective than acetaminophen or ibuprofen but has more gastrointestinal side effects.

Abortive therapy is used to interrupt migraine headaches after they have begun. Sumatriptan causes vasoconstriction and is helpful in many cases. It may be given as an injection or a tablet. A 5- or 20-mg single-dose nasal spray is also available. Experience is limited with younger children. Isometheptene and ergots also can interrupt migraines (O'Hara & Koch, 1998).

Prophylactic therapy is considered when headaches are frequent enough to interfere with activities. β-Blockers are usually tried first (propranolol, nadolol). Tricyclic agents such as nortriptyline and amitriptyline can be tried. Cyproheptadine can be helpful for migraines in younger children. Anticonvulsants are also used, especially if the child also has a seizure disorder. Calcium channel blockers may have mixed effectiveness in children (O'Hara & Koch, 1998).

REFERRAL. Refer all patients with organic (structural) headaches.

COUNSELING. For nonorganic headaches (no tumor, aneurysm, or metabolic or structural cause), reassure the parents and patient. The patient should be taught pain and stress management techniques. School attendance should

T A B L E 28-8

Medications for Migraine and Tension Headaches in Children

ANALGESIC DRUG	DOSAGE
Acetaminophen	10–15 mg/kg not to exceed 90 mg/d
NSAIDs:	
Ibuprofen (DOC)	5–10 mg/kg per dose (200–800 mg/dose q 6–8 h; maximum, 40 mg/kg per d)
Naproxen	10 mg/kg per d (250–500 mg bid)
Naproxen sodium (Anaprox, Aleve)	220–550 mg 1st dose; maximum dose, 825 mg/d
ABORTIVE PHARMACOLOGY FOR MIGRAINE HEADACHE	
Ergotamine tartrate	2 mg dose SL. Maximum, 6 mg/d or 10 mg/wk to avoid chronic ergotism, dependency, withdrawal symptoms
	Contraindications: heart disease, hypertension, pregnancy (uterine stimulant, teratogen)
Dihydroergotamine (DHE)	0.5–1.0 mg IM; can be repeated in 1 h
	No associated dependence/withdrawal symptoms
	Side effects: nausea/vomiting
	Contraindications: heart disease, hypertension, pregnancy (uterine stimulant, teratogen)
	Give metoclopramide or prochlorperazine as pretreatment for nausea
Metoclopramide (Reglan)	5–10 mg (up to 1 mg/kg)
	Side effects: sedation, dizziness, confusion
Prochlorperazine (Compazine)	2.5–5.0 mg/kg q 4 h (up to 0.1 mg/kg in younger children)
Sumatriptan (Imitrex)	6 mg SC, 100 mg PO, or 10–20 mg nasal spray. May repeat injection in 1 h
	Contraindications: do not give with ergotamine derivatives
	Side effects: irritation at site, flushing, tachycardia, disorientation, chest tightness for several minutes after parenteral administration
PROPHYLACTIC MEDICATIONS FOR MIGRAINE HEADACHE	
Propranolol (Inderal)	1–2 mg/kg/d in 2–3 divided doses; maximum, 320 mg/d
	Contraindications: asthma, arrhythmia, depression, diabetes
Amitriptyline (Elavil)	Adolescents: 0.1 mg/kg at bedtime (may be increased q 2 wk to 0.5–2 mg/kg)
	Contraindications: not recommended for children younger than 12 y
Cyproheptadine (Periactin)	Children: 0.2–0.5 mg/kg per d in 2–3 divided doses; 2–6 y: 12 mg/d; 7–14 y: 16 mg/d; adults: 32 mg/d
	Contraindications: none
Nortriptyline (Pamelor)	10 mg/d hs
	Contraindications: may cause sudden death with prolonged QT interval syndrome; less sedation than amitriptyline; not recommended for children younger than 12 y

DOC = drug of choice; hs = at bedtime; IM = intramuscularly; NSAIDs = nonsteroidal anti-inflammatory drugs; SC = subcutaneously; SL = sublingually.

From Graf W, Riback P: Pharmacologic treatment of recurrent pediatric headache. Pediatr Ann 24:477–484, 1995.

be mandatory, although a quiet rest period may be allowed at school if needed. School nurses can be helpful in developing a plan for school attendance. If the child remains home, activities should be restricted to bed and only homework done. The child should be returned to school if the pain improves during the school day. Minimize attention to the headache. Relaxation exercises or biofeedback training can be helpful. Trigger factors should be avoided.

COMPLICATIONS

Brain tumors in children are generally associated with ataxia, papilledema, intellectual changes, or behavioral changes. These changes are either present at the onset or within 2 months, and 88% of patients show neurological signs within 4 months (Barlow, 1986). Serious pathology is also indicated with headaches that interrupt sleep, increase in frequency and severity over a period of only a few weeks, occur on rising and then fade, are exacerbated by changes in position or with straining, persist at the occiput, or are related to personality, ataxic, or behavioral changes.

Head Injury

DESCRIPTION

Head trauma involves tissue damage to the brain and its surrounding structures. Closed head injuries cause more multifocal or diffuse damage, whereas open head injuries produce more focal injuries. Primary brain injuries are related to mechanical forces that tear connections within the brain and cause contusions where the brain hits the skull surfaces. Axons to distant areas, fibers in the corpus callosum connecting the two hemispheres, or both can be torn. Contusions and hemorrhage can occur. Secondary brain injuries result from hypoxia, ischemia, hypotension, and status epilepticus.

A study of the incidence of traumatic brain injuries in Colorado provides data that these injuries occur most often in young adults aged 20 to 24 years, followed by adolescents aged 15 to 19 years. Nineteen percent of the injuries were fatal (Gabella et al., 1997).

HEAD INJURY SEQUELAE

Immediate care of a head-injured patient is outside the scope of this chapter. More information is found in Chapter 40, including the Glascow Coma Scale, which is often used to measure the severity of head injury. However, the NP is likely to encounter post-trauma patients. Five percent to 10% of children with head injuries will have long-term mental or physical handicaps. The most important determinant of physical and intellectual recovery is the duration of coma. Recovery within 14 days gives the best hope. Seizures, hemiparesis, aphasia, cognitive problems, and behavioral disorders may occur after severe head injuries. Even relatively minor head trauma can result in symptoms of post-trauma syndrome, including hyperactivity, decreased attention span, temper outbursts, sleep disturbances, and headaches. The impact of mild to moderate head injury on school performance and adjustment should not be overlooked. A neuropsychological evaluation may be helpful to plan appropriate educational and behavioral management.

Concussions are commonly related to sports injuries. See Chapter 15 for information on post-trauma management of head injuries related to sports.

PREVENTION

Wearing of helmets by children using bicycles, skateboards, motorcycles, and in-line skates prevents many head injuries. Protection of children from falls in the home or from playground equipment is also important in reduction of head injuries. School-aged children and adolescents should have properly fitting headgear appropriate for their sports participation. Finally, adequate seat restraints can reduce the incidence of head injuries from motor vehicle accidents.

Prevention of secondary brain trauma from hemorrhage, edema, and other factors can be facilitated by prompt management of head trauma events.

Macrocephaly, Hydrocephaly, and Microcephaly

MACROCEPHALY

Macrocephaly is defined as a head circumference more than 3 SD above the mean for age and sex or one that increases too rapidly. It can be caused by hydrocephaly, chronic subdural hematoma, tumor, cystic defects, or other problems. Benign familial macrocephaly occurs as or can be related to a genetic syndrome such as Sotos syndrome (cerebral gigantism). Referral is necessary if a syndrome is suspected.

HYDROCEPHALY

Hydrocephaly is a condition in which an increased volume of cerebrospinal fluid causes progressive ventricular dilation. The etiology includes a wide variety of disorders, such as infection, tumor, hemorrhage, and congenital malformation. The patient can have a large head, an excessive rate of head growth, irritability, vomiting, loss of appetite, impaired upgaze and other extraocular movements, hypertonia, and hyperreflexia. Papilledema may not be present in an infant, whereas it does appear in older children with closed cranial sutures. In a neonate, the head can sometimes be transilluminated. Prompt referral and surgical treatment are necessary.

MICROCEPHALY

Microcephaly is defined as a head circumference 3 SD or more below the mean for age and sex or one that is increasing slower than normal. Microcephaly is an indicator of failure of brain development and can be due to many problems. Commonly, microcephalic children have delayed developmental milestones, neurological problems, and a poorly formed frontal area of the skull. Management of microcephaly is supportive and directed toward management of the resulting deficits. Protein–calorie malnutrition, craniosynostosis, and hypopituitarism are treatable causes of microcephaly. Referral to pediatrics or neurology should be made for diagnosis. Development of an interdisciplinary management plan may be useful.

Craniosynostosis

Craniosynostosis involves fusion of various skull bones across the sutures. Growth along whatever suture lines are open in craniosynostosis produces progressive skull deformity or increas-

ing intracranial pressure as the brain tries to grow within the confined space. The incidence is 1 per 2000 births (Behrman et al., 1996). The condition may be related to a genetic syndrome—Crouzon, Apert, Carpenter, Chotzen, Pfeiffer, and others. Treatment is surgical. If the condition is genetic, management will need to be planned according to the problems associated with the syndrome. Genetic counseling is important.

Central Nervous System Infections

DESCRIPTION

All the infections of the CNS have similar symptoms. These infections can be manifested acutely (over 1 to 24 hours) or chronically (over 1 to 7 days or more).

ETIOLOGY

Bacteria, viruses, and other microorganisms can all cause CNS infection. The meninges, superficial cortical structures, blood vessels, and brain parenchyma can be involved. *Toxoplasma,* mycobacteria, amoebae, spirochetes, and other microorganisms can produce CNS infection. By age, common microbes are as follows (Willoughby & Polack, 1998):

- 0 to 3 months: enteroviruses, group B streptococci, *Escherichia coli, Listeria monocytogenes, Streptococcus pneumoniae, Neisseria meningitides, Haemophilus influenzae* type B
- 3 months to 5 years: bacterial infections most common—*N. meningitides, S. pneumoniae*
- 6 to 18 years: *N. meningitides, S. pneumoniae,* enteroviruses, *Rickettsia rickettsii,* herpes simplex virus type 2 (HSV-2), HIV

CLINICAL FINDINGS

HISTORY. The following may be noted from the history:

- Recent head injury or neurosurgical procedure
- Immunodeficiency diseases
- Infections of the sinuses or other structures of the head

PHYSICAL EXAMINATION. Findings on physical examination include

- Systemic signs, including fever; malaise; impaired heart, lung, or kidney function
- CNS signs, including headache, stiff neck, fever or hypothermia, changes in mental status ranging from irritability to lethargy or coma, seizures, and focal or sensory deficits
- Presence of Kernig or Brudzinski sign of meningeal irritation (may be absent in a young infant)
- Bulging fontanel and increasing head circumference in a young infant
- Papilledema late in the course in older children or adolescents
- Cranial nerve palsies

By age, the most common findings are as follows:

- 0 to 3 months: fever, hypothermia, lethargy, irritability, poor feeding, apnea, focal seizures, enteric or respiratory symptoms. Nuchal rigidity and a bulging fontanel are infrequent.
- 3 months to 5 years: petechial rash, localized CNS signs as described earlier.
- 6 to 18 years: petechial rash, cranial nerve VII palsy (Lyme disease), sinusitis symptoms, genital lesions, localized CNS signs.

OTHER STUDIES. Blood cultures, CBC with differential, urinalysis, chemistry panel, and lumbar puncture for cerebrospinal fluid studies are done. Enterovirus meningitis and HSV rapid tests are available. EEGs, CT or MRI scan, and brain biopsy may be needed.

MANAGEMENT AND COMPLICATIONS

The NP needs to refer all children with potential CNS infection as rapidly as possible. Hypovolemia, hypoglycemia, hyponatremia, acidosis, septic shock, increased intracranial pressure, seizures, and other complications can occur quickly and need aggressive management. Hearing loss can occur in all forms of meningitis. Blindness, seizures, developmental delay, and paresis all occur in 15% of preschool meningitis survivors (Willoughby & Polack, 1998).

The Floppy Infant

A floppy infant should arouse suspicion. The range of causes is broad, and the conditions are serious. The baby might be *hypotonic,* which means that underlying tone in the alert infant is low. This assessment is subjective. Hypotonic infants can increase their tone over the first year of life and then demonstrate spastic CP. A baby can have low tone but still not lack strength when actively moving. The infant may also be *weak,* which means that its maximum effort lacks strength. Babies with Werdnig-Hoffmann disease are weak. An infant might also *fatigue* easily. Cardiac defects can cause fatigue, as can myasthenia muscle metabolism problems. Floppy infants with brisk reflexes almost certainly have a CNS disorder. All these babies need to be referred.

Reye Syndrome

DESCRIPTION AND ETIOLOGY

Reye syndrome is an encephalopathy that is decreasing in incidence. No etiological factor has been isolated; however, the decline has been associated with decreased use of salicylates in younger children. Some have theorized that the problem is related to mitochondrial damage by metabolites of salicylates in a viral infection environment.

CLINICAL FINDINGS

The clinical findings in Reye syndrome include

- Prodromal upper respiratory infection, influenza A or B, or chickenpox
- Lethargy, drowsiness progressing to semicoma
- Vomiting, irrational behavior, progressive stupor, coma
- Hyperpnea, irregular respirations
- Dilated and sluggish pupils
- Positive Babinski sign, hyperreflexia, decorticate posturing with increasing cerebral edema

MANAGEMENT

Immediate referral with admission to a hospital setting is essential. About 70% of patients survive, some with severe neurological sequelae.

Rett Syndrome

Rett syndrome is a recently described, but relatively common neurodegenerative disease that affects only females, with onset at about 1 year of age. Affected girls cease to gain developmental milestones. CNS irritability and withdrawal develop, and then these girls begin to lose skills, including speech and hand skills. Stereotypic hand movements, delayed head growth, and later seizures, scoliosis, and hypertonicity develop. The etiology is unknown. Physical therapy, occupational therapy, speech therapy, and seizure management are important to preserve functional abilities. As with all neurodevelopmental problems, families need significant support and social services.

Tic Disorders

Tic disorders are found in children and adults. Boys are two to three times more likely to be affected than girls. Ages 7 to 11 years are the most common time for onset. Four types of tic disorders are recognized: Tourette syndrome, transient tic disorder, chronic motor or vocal tic disorder, and unspecified type. Tourette syndrome is the most complex of these disorders. It is chronic, hereditary (autosomal dominant with varying levels of penetrance, which is gender related), and characterized by tics that vary in severity over time. Simple motor tics are gradually replaced with more complex motor and vocal tics. To meet the diagnostic criteria for Tourette syndrome, the tics must

- Be of several types
- Be repeated many times every day for more than a year with no tic-free periods of longer than 3 months
- Cause marked distress or impairment socially, occupationally, or otherwise
- Begin before the age of 18 years
- Not be related to some other medical condition or substance use (Diagnostic and Statistical Manual of Mental Disorders—IV, 1994).

Simple motor tics include eye blinks, eyebrow raising, nose flaring, head or arm jerking, kicking, toe curling, and other motor movements. More complex motor tics include head shaking, touching, hitting, jumping, smelling objects, repeating movements, self-mutilating activities such as lip biting, and other behavior. Vocal tics include sniffing, grunting, throat clearing, coughing, moaning, humming, and other vocal sounds. The more complex vocal tics include stammering, stuttering, muttering unintelligible words, repeating words, and swearing (Clarksean, 1998).

DIAGNOSIS

Consider hyperkinesis, choreiform or dystonic movements, genetic disorder such as Huntington or Wilson disease, obsessive–compulsive disorder, structural lesion in the brain, and pharmacological side effect. Vocal tics are less commonly related to neurological or medical diseases (Clarksean, 1998). Attention deficit hyperactivity disorder may be concurrent.

RESOURCES BOX 28–1

American Epilepsy Society
Tel: (860) 586–7505
Website: www.aesnet.org.

Brain Injury Association, Inc. (BIA)
Tel: (800) 444–6443, (202) 296–6443

Epilepsy Foundation of America
Tel: (800) 332–1000, (301) 459–3700

International Rett Syndrome Foundation
Tel: (800) 818–7388, (301) 856–3334

National Headache Foundation
Tel: (800) 843–2256, (312) 878–7715
Website: headaches.org.

National Spinal Cord Injury Association
Tel: (800) 962–9629, (617) 441–8500

Spina Bifida Association
Tel: (800) 621–3141, (202) 944–3285

Tourette Syndrome Association
Tel: (718) 224–2999
Website: www.tsa.mgh.harvard.edu/

United Cerebral Palsy Associations
Tel: (800) 872–5827
Website: ucpa.org.

MANAGEMENT

Pharmacological management of motor or vocal tics may include haloperidol (Haldol), pimozide (Orap), fluphenazine (Prolixin), thiothixene (Navane), clonazepam (Klonopin), and clonidine (Catapres). Fluoxetine (Prozac) and other drugs have also been used. Management must also involve the family and educational and other supportive measures. Children with the disorder may be depressed and suffer from social stigma (Hyde & Weinberger, 1995).

REFERENCES

American Academy of Pediatrics Committee on Infectious Diseases: 1997 Redbook: Report of the Committee on Infectious Diseases. Elk Grove Village, IL, American Academy of Pediatrics, 1997.

American Psychiatric Association: Diagnostic and Statistical Manual of Mental Disorders, 4th ed. Washington, DC, American Psychiatric Association, 1994.

Anderson P: Basic Human Anatomy and Physiology: Clinical Implications for the Health Professions. Monterey, CA, Wadsworth, 1984.

Barabas G, Taft L: The early signs and differential diagnosis of cerebral palsy. Pediatr Ann 15:203, 205-214, 1986.

Barlow C: Juvenile migraine. Resident Staff Physician 30:53, 1986.

Batchelor L, Nance J, Short B: An interdisciplinary team approach to implementing the ketogenic diet for the treatment of seizures. Pediatr Nurs 23:465-473, 1997.

Behrman R, Kliegman R, Arvin A: Nelson Textbook of Pediatrics, 15th ed. Philadelphia, WB Saunders, 1996.

Burg F, Ingelfinger J, Wald E, et al: Gellis & Kagan's Current Pediatric Therapy, 16th ed. Philadelphia, WB Saunders, 1999.

Cady R, Farmer K, Griesemer K, et al: Prevalence of headaches in children. Headache Q Curr Treat Res 7:312-318, 1996.

Calli J, Farrington E: Vigabatrin. Pediatr Nurs 24:357-361, 1998.

Camfield C, Camfield P: Febrile seizures: An RX for parent fears and anxieties. Contemp Pediatr 10:26-44, 1993.

Clarksean L: Tic disorders in children. Adv Nurs Pract 6(8):69-71, 1998.

Davis D: Review of cerebral palsy, part I: Description, incidence, and etiology. Neonat Network 16(3):7-12, 1997a.

Davis D: Review of cerebral palsy, part II: Identification and intervention. Neonat Network 16(4):19-25, 1997b.

Gabella B, Hoffman R, Marine W, et al: Urban and rural traumatic brain injuries in Colorado. Ann Epidemiol 7:207-212, 1997.

Gilman S, Newman S: Essentials of Clinical Neuroanatomy and Neurophysiology, 8th ed. Philadelphia, FA Davis, 1992.

Haslam R: Nonfebrile seizures. Pediatr Rev 18:39-49, 1997.

Hay W, Groothius J, Hayward A, et al: Current Pediatric Diagnosis & Treatment. E Norwalk, CT, Appleton & Lange, 1997.

Hyde T, Weinberger D: Tourette's syndrome: A model neuropsychiatric disorder. JAMA 273:498-501, 1995.

Lannon S: Epilepsy surgery for partial seizures. Pediatr Nurs 23:453-459, 1997.

Liptak G: The child who has severe neurologic impairment. Pediatr Clin North Am 45:123-144, 1998.

McDonald M: Use of the ketogenic diet in treating children with seizures. Pediatr Nurs 23:461-464, 1997.

Nehring W, Steele S: Cerebral palsy. In Jackson P, Vessey J (eds): Primary Care of the Child With a Chronic Condition, 2nd ed. St Louis, CV Mosby, 1996, pp 232-254.

Nelson K, Ellenberg J: The asymptomatic newborn and risk of cerebral palsy. Am J Dis Child 141:1333-1335, 1987.

O'Hara J, Koch T: Heading off headaches. Contemp Pediatr 15:97-116, 1998.

Robertson, P: Pediatric brain tumors. Primary Care 25, 323-339.

Rosenbloom L: Diagnosis and management of cerebral palsy. Arch Dis Child 72:350-354, 1995.

Scheller J: The history, epidemiology, and classification of headaches in childhood. Pediatr Neurol 2:102-108, 1995.

Shinnar S, Berg A, Moshe S, et al: The risk of seizure recurrence after a first unprovoked afebrile seizure in childhood: An extended follow-up. Pediatrics 98:216-225, 1996.

Smith M: Comprehensive evaluation and treatment of recurrent pediatric headache. Pediatr Ann 24:450-465, 1995.

Taft L: Cerebral palsy. Pediatr Rev 16:411-418, 1995.

Tennison M: Discontinuing antiepileptics: When and how. Contemp Pediatr 13:49-58, 1996.

Valente M, Valente S: Pediatric epilepsy: Primary care treatment and health care management. Nurse Pract 23:38-57, 1998.

Willoughby R, Polack F: Meningitis: What's new in diagnosis and management. Contemp Pediatr 15(9):49-70, 1998.

Zafeiriou D, Tsikoulas I, Kremenopoulos G: Prospective follow-up of primitive reflex profiles in high-risk infants: Clues to an early diagnosis of cerebral palsy. Pediatr Neurol 2:148-152, 1995.

CHAPTER 29

Eye Problems

Margaret MacDonald and Nancy Barber Starr

INTRODUCTION

Ocular disorders and visual impairments are relatively common in childhood. One of every 25 preschoolers has a vision problem that can result in a decrease in sight, and 1 in 4 school-aged children require some corrective treatment, with the two most common visual conditions being amblyopia and strabismus (Preller, 1998). A number of factors may be involved, including familial, prenatal/intrauterine, perinatal, and postnatal causes. Priorities of the nurse practitioner (NP) in caring for children with eye problems or concerns include promoting optimal growth and development of the ocular structures and maximizing visual acuity. To this end, NPs seek to maintain good vision and health, detect abnormalities, treat those conditions that fall within their scope of practice, refer patients with conditions requiring physician expertise, and provide education and reassurance to parents and children. In some cases, consultation with a pediatrician or family practice physician suffices to ensure optimal care. Other cases warrant direct referral to an ophthalmologist.

STANDARDS FOR VISUAL SCREENING AND CARE

Healthy People 2000: National Health Promotion and Disease Prevention Objectives for the Year 2000 (US Department of Health and Human Services, 1990) addressed issues of screening and prevention of visual problems for infants and children. The objective related to vision in the *Healthy People 2010 Objectives: Draft for Public Comment* (US Department of Health and Human Services, 1998) is to

- Increase the proportion of primary care providers who routinely refer or screen infants and children for impairments of vision, hearing, speech, and language and who assess other developmental milestones as part of well-child care.

The *Guide to Clinical Preventive Services* (US Preventive Services Task Force, 1997) clinical intervention states that

- Vision screening to detect amblyopia and strabismus is recommended once for all children before entering school, preferably between the ages of 3 and 4. Clinicians should be alert for signs of ocular misalignment when examining infants and children. Stereoacuity testing may be more effective than visual acuity testing in detecting these conditions. Evidence is insufficient to recommend for or against routine screening for diminished visual acuity among asymptomatic schoolchildren. Recommendations against such screening may be made on other grounds, including the inconvenience and cost of routine screening and the fact that refractive errors can be readily corrected when they produce symptoms.

The *Put Prevention into Practice: Clinician's Handbook of Preventive Services* (US Public Health Service, 1997) outlines recommendations from major authorities, including

- The American Academy of Pediatrics and Bright Futures—Visual acuity testing should first be performed at 3 years of age. If the child is uncooperative, retesting should occur 6 months later. Subsequent testing should occur at 4, 5, 10, 12, 15, and 18 years of age. Subjective assessment by history should occur at visits at all other ages. All infants should be examined by 6 months of age to evaluate fixation preference, alignment, and the presence of any eye disease. Children should again be medically evaluated for these problems by 3 to 4 years of age.
- The American Academy of Ophthalmology (AAO), American Association for Pediatric Ophthalmology and Strabismus (AAPOS), and the American Optometric Association (AOA)—Eye and vision screening should be performed at birth and approximately 6 months, 3 years, and 5 years of age. The AAO has published recommendations regarding screening methods and indications for referral to be used by primary care clinicians in screening preschool children (see Table 29-3 and 29-4) (AAO, 1997a and 1997b). The AAO and AAPOS recommend that screening after 5 years of age be carried out at routine school checks or after the appearance of symptoms. The AOA recommends optometric examinations every 2 years throughout school.
- For high-risk children, the AAO recommends that asymptomatic children have a comprehensive examination by an ophthalmologist if they are at high risk because of health and developmental problems that make screening by the primary care clinician difficult or inaccurate (e.g., retinopathy of prematurity [ROP] or diagnostic evaluation of a complex disease with ophthalmologic manifestations); a family history of conditions that cause or are associated with eye or vision problems (e.g., retinoblastoma, significant hyperopia, strabismus [particularly accommodative esotropia], amblyopia, congenital cataract, or glaucoma); or multiple health problems, systemic disease, or the use of medications that are known to be associated with eye disease and vision abnormalities (e.g., neurodegenerative disease, juvenile rheumatoid arthritis, systemic steroid therapy, systemic syndromes with ocular manifestations, or developmental delay with visual system manifestations).

DEVELOPMENT AND PHYSIOLOGY OF THE EYE

Development of the Ocular Structures

At 21 days of gestation the human embryo is one fifth of an inch in length, and the first recognizable ocular tissue is visible on each side of the head. Within 10 days the eyes become much more prominent and, by the end of the eighth week, have moved medially toward the front of the face. The eyelids are completely formed, and the edges of the upper and lower lids fuse and seal the eye while it develops. At 16 weeks of gestation the eyes are fully anterior, and over the ensuing weeks they continue to move closer to the bridge of the nose. By the seventh month of pregnancy the fetus can open its eyes.

Development of the eye as a visual organ is not complete at birth, yet newborns have the ability to fix their gaze, follow an object to midline, and react to a change in the intensity of light. Over the first 2 to 3 months of extrauterine life, the ability to focus at any range develops as the eyes become coordinated horizontally and vertically. By 3 months of age, infants can follow moving objects, and by 4 months, they can indicate visual recognition of familiar objects. The shape and contour of the eyeball change, and visual acuity and binocularity gradually increase with age. The size of the orbits doubles by the time that the child is 1 year of age and doubles again by 6 years of age.

When eye growth is completed at 10 to 12 years of age, the diameter of the eyeball is about 2.5 cm.

Anatomy and Physiology of the Eye

The eyeball consists of three layers of tissue: the fibrous tunic, the vascular tunic, and the inner tunic or retina (Fig. 29-1). The fibrous tunic consists of the sclera and the cornea. The vascular tunic, the middle layer, is composed of the choroid, the ciliary body, and the iris. All the structures of the eye are dedicated to accurate and efficient functioning of the innermost layer of the eyeball, the retina. The optic disk consists only of nerve fibers (no rods or cones), so no visual images are formed here. Thus it is referred to as the blind spot.

The inside of the eyeball consists of the anterior and posterior cavities. The anterior cavity is divided into anterior and posterior chambers. The anterior chamber lies between the cornea and the iris. The posterior chamber lies between the iris and the suspensory ligament. Aqueous humor circulates throughout these chambers to maintain intraocular pressure and link the circulatory system with the avascular lens and cornea. The other cavity within the eyeball, the posterior cavity, lies between the lens and the retina. The gelatinous vitreous humor found in this cavity contributes to the maintenance of intraocular pressure and holds the retina in place. The lens, which separates the cavities, hangs by the suspensory ligament. Six muscles guide movement of the globe. Four rectus muscles (superior, inferior, lateral, and medial) move the eyeball up, down, in, and out, respectively. Two oblique muscles (superior and inferior) rotate the eyeball on its axis. Cranial nerves III (oculomotor), IV (trochlear), and VI (abducens) innervate these muscles.

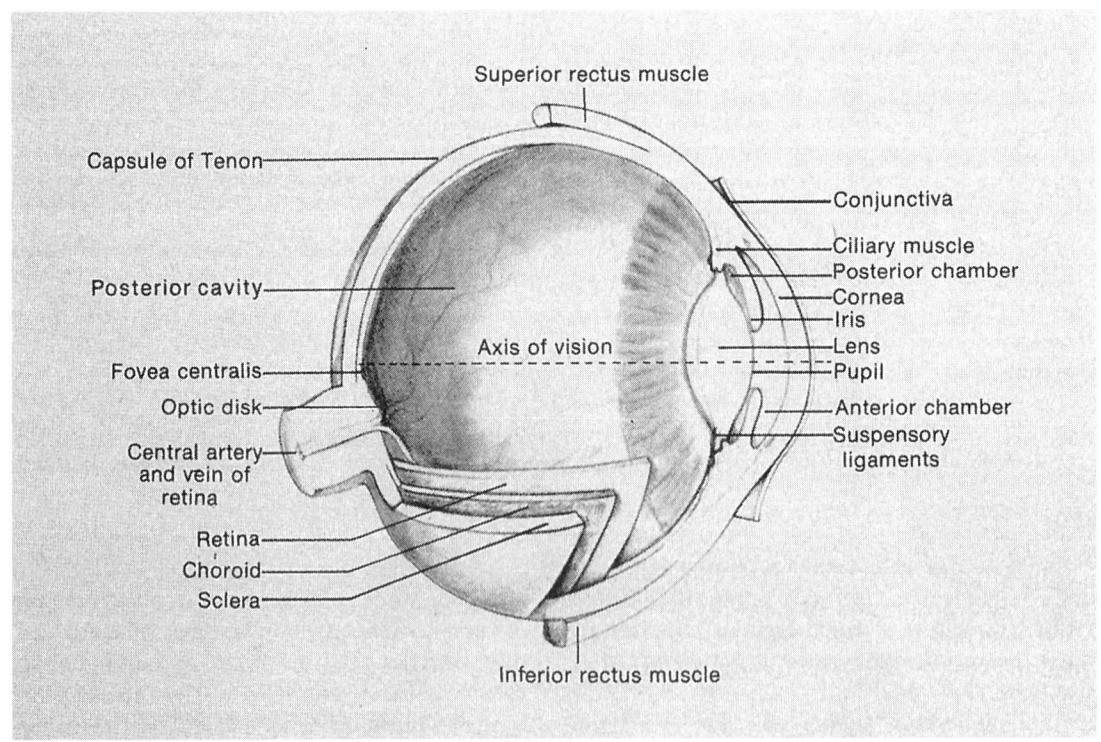

FIGURE 29-1
Structure of the eye, transverse section. (From Anderson PD: Basic Human Anatomy and Physiology: Clinical Implications for the Health Professions. Copyright 1984, Sudbury, MA: Jones & Bartlett Publishers. www.jbpub.com. Reprinted with permission.)

The focusing of light rays involves four basic processes: refraction of light rays, accommodation of the lens, constriction of the pupil, and convergence of the eyes. *Refraction* is the bending of light rays as they pass from one transparent medium (air) to another (cornea or lens). The lens modifies the degree of refraction to create the sharpest image on the retina. *Accommodation* is the ability of the lens to focus on close objects by increasing its curvature. The normal eye refracts light rays from an object 20 ft away to focus a clear image onto the retina; hence the fraction 20/20 is used to denote the accepted standard of normal vision. The circular muscle fibers of the iris, which contract in response to light, cause *constriction* of the pupil. Regulating the light entering the eye can also facilitate production of a precise image. To maintain single binocular vision, close objects require the eyes to rotate medially so that the light rays from the object hit the same points on both retinas. This rotation is called *convergence.* A normal neonate demonstrates disconjugate fixation, but convergence and accommodation normally develop by 3 to 4 months of age, with parallel alignment by 6 months of age without nystagmus or strabismus.

After an image is formed on the retina, light impulses are converted into nerve impulses and transmitted to the visual centers located in the occipital lobes of the cerebral cortex. Lesions in various places along the neural tracts from the eye to the cortex cause different types of loss of visual fields (Fig. 29–2).

PATHOPHYSIOLOGY OF THE EYES

Potential problems with the eyes or visual system can take the form of specific disorders, infections, or injuries to the eye. Two common disorders of the eye interfering with vision are refractive errors and strabismus. Other less common disorders are ptosis, nystagmus, cataracts, glaucoma, ROP, and retinoblastoma. Infection and injury are other potential problems that may be relatively minor and superficial or be critical and involve deep tissues of the eye. Certain systemic diseases (e.g., juvenile rheuma-

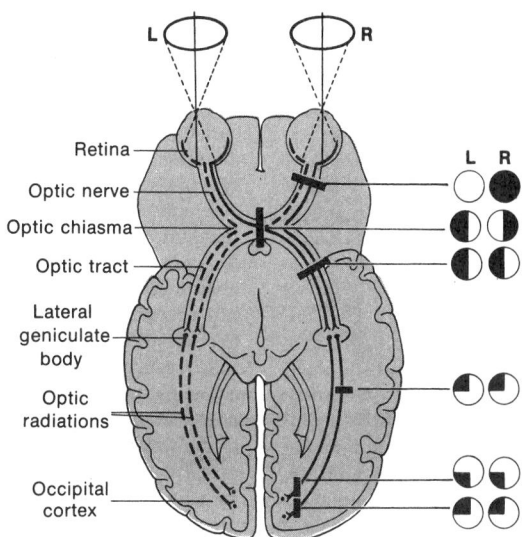

F I G U R E 29-2
Visual pathway. On the right are diagrams of the visual fields with areas of blindness darkened to show the effects of injuries in various locations. (From Anderson PD: Basic Human Anatomy and Physiology: Clinical Implications for the Health Professions. Copyright 1984, Sudbury, MA: Jones & Bartlett Publishers. www.jbpub.com. Reprinted with permission.)

toid arthritis) and medications (e.g., steroids) can affect the eyes and warrant extra assessment measures.

ASSESSMENT

Assessment of the eye, as with all body systems, requires a thoughtful history and careful physical examination, as well as certain specialized screening tests.

History

The history should include the following:

1. Past eye evaluations
   • Date (and results) of the last vision screening and/or visit to the ophthalmologist or optometrist
2. Symptoms of eye dysfunction or disease
   • Visual loss or change in vision such as blurring, diplopia, spots, and halos in older children; problems with fixing, tracking, squinting, head tilt, eye-hand co-

ordination, grasp, gait, balance, behavior, and changes in the ability to maintain eye contact in younger children

- Pain or sensitivity to light (photophobia) resulting in irritability and shielding or rubbing of the eyes
- Swollen eyelids, pruritus, excessive tearing or discharge, erythema, burning, eye fatigue, strabismus
- Constant blinking, chronic bulbar conjunctival injection
- History of trauma to the eye
- Whether the child wears prescription glasses or contacts

3. Past medical history
   - Past medical history or a family medical history of ocular disease (e.g., glaucoma)
   - History of surgery on the eyes
   - Past or present substance abuse
   - History of chronic systemic disease (e.g., inflammatory bowel disease, collagen diseases, diabetes, sickle cell hemoglobinopathies, or tuberculosis)
   - Presence of allergies—to what substances
   - Recent or current history of infection
   - Current medications (e.g., steroids)
   - Pregnancy or birth complications, gestational age, communicable diseases
   - Prescription and use of eyeglasses or contact lenses (Does the child have glasses that were prescribed? Are they used? If not, why?)
   - Use of sunglasses with ultraviolet (UV) protection and/or protective glasses

4. In case of injury
   - One or both eyes involved
   - Vision changes
   - Other symptoms (e.g., photophobia, visual field defect)

Physical Examination

The physical examination includes gross inspection of the external structures with special attention to the lids and conjunctiva, the lacrimal structures, and the size, symmetry, and reactivity of the pupils. In older children, funduscopic examination allows for visualization of the retina, choroid, fovea, macula, optic disk and cup, and the entry and exit of the vessels and nerves. In infants and young children, the red reflex is tested. Knowledge of visual developmental norms is also helpful in assessing a child's visual capabilities (Table 29-1).

Examination of the eye is sometimes facilitated by using a cotton-tipped applicator to evert the eyelid. Eyelid eversion is accomplished by having the patient look down while the examiner grasps the lashes with the thumb and index finger, places the applicator in the middle of the lid, pulls the eyelid down and out, and everts it over the applicator. Irrigation of the eye with normal saline is another technique useful in situations where removal of a foreign body or irritating substance is desired.

Screening Tests

CONDUCTING SCREENING TEST

Fatigue, hunger, anxiety, and environmental distractions can interfere with vision testing. Testing should always precede the administration of immunizations or any procedure that might cause discomfort. While testing, observe chil-

T A B L E 29-1
Normal Visual Developmental Milestones

Birth to 2 wk:	Infant sees and responds to change in illumination; refuses to reopen eyes after exposure to bright light; increasing alertness to objects; fixes on contrasts (e.g., black and white).
_2–4 wk:_	Infant fixes on an object.
_By 1 mo:_	Infant fixes on and follows an object.
_By 3–4 mo:_	Infant recognizes parent's smile; looks from near to far and focuses close again; beginning development of depth perception; follows 180-degree arc; reaches toward toy.
_By 4 mo:_	Color vision near that of an adult; tears are present.
_By 6–10 mo:_	Infant fixes on and follows toy in all directions.
_By 12 mo:_	Vision is close to fully developed.

dren for behavior indicating that they are having difficulty, such as straining, squinting, excessive blinking, head tilting or shaking, and thrusting of the trunk and head forward. The tendency to peek out from behind the eye shield may or may not reflect difficulty; the child may do so out of a desire to be successful and please the tester. The examiner should also resist the tendency to give the child nonverbal clues that can affect results when finger-pointing tests are used.

Children who have difficulty performing any of the vision tests in the primary care provider's office should be tested again at another time. An alternative to office testing is to teach the parents how to assess vision by using one of the aforementioned methods and to loan them the necessary supplies for use at home. Vision should then be retested in the office.

VISUAL ACUITY TESTING

Visual acuity testing (Tables 29–2 and 29–3), for both near and distance vision, should be performed on all children every time they come for a routine checkup, when problems with visual acuity are suspected, and when eye trauma occurs. It is important to obtain a visual acuity measurement with correction if the child wears eyeglasses or contact lenses.

COLOR VISION TESTING

Color blindness is an X-linked inherited disorder. It is more common in males and affects about 8% of white males, 4% of black males, and 0.4% of females (Jarvis, 1996). Several different forms of color blindness may occur. Significant color blindness can affect school performance. It also has safety implications in that the child may be unable to distinguish traffic or vehicle brake lights. Color vision is tested by using the Hardy-Rand-Rittler test (for preschoolers) or Ishihara's plates (for school-age children).

PERIPHERAL VISION TESTING

Examination of peripheral visual fields provides information with regard to retinal function, the neuronal visual pathway to the brain, and the function of cranial nerve II (optic nerve). In an infant, assessment is limited to a rough estimate of peripheral visual fields by watching the child's response to a familiar object (e.g., bottle, toy) or a threatening gesture as it is brought into each of the four quadrants. In children mature enough to cooperate, peripheral visual fields can be measured by confrontation or by finger counting. Peripheral visual fields should be approximately 50 degrees upward, 70 degrees downward, 60 degrees medially (toward the nose), and 90 degrees laterally.

TESTING FOR OCULAR MOTILITY AND ALIGNMENT

The *Hirschberg test* (also called the *corneal light reflex*) evaluates extraocular muscle function by projecting a small light source onto the cornea of the eye with the child looking straight ahead. A normal test reveals a small white dot symmetrically located in the same position of each eye (often slightly nasal of center). The *cover-uncover test* and the *alternating cover test* should be performed with the child fixating straight ahead first on a near point and then on a far point about 20 ft away (Fig. 29–3). The process is sometimes aided by asking the child questions about the object (e.g., "How many cows do you see?"). During the alternating cover test the examiner rapidly covers and uncovers the eye while shifting between the two eyes. Any movement is an indication of misalignment.

ASSESSMENT OF VISUAL LOSS

If significant visual disturbance is suspected, the following functional vision assessments

TABLE 29-2

Visual Acuity Norms

AGE	VISUAL ACUITY	VISUAL RANGE (degrees)
Birth	20/100	45
6 wk	20/100	90
4 mo	20/80	180
1 yr	20/40	180
3–4 yr	20/30	180
6 yr	20/25 or 20/20	180

T A B L E 29-3

Pediatric Eye Evaluation Screening Recommendations for Primary Care Providers, Nurses, Physician's Assistants, and Trained Lay Personnel

RECOMMENDED AGE FOR SCREENING	SCREENING METHOD	CRITERIA FOR REFERRAL TO AN OPHTHALMOLOGIST
Newborn to 3 mo	Red reflex* Inspection	Abnormal or asymmetrical Structural abnormality
6 mo to 1 yr	Fix and follow with each eye Alternate occlusion Corneal light reflex Red reflex* Inspection	Failure to fix and follow in cooperative infant Failure to object equally to covering each eye Asymmetrical Abnormal or asymmetrical Structural abnormality
3 yr (approximately)	Visual acuity† Corneal light reflex/cover-uncover Red reflex* Inspection	20/50 or worse or 2 lines of difference between eyes Asymmetrical ocular refixation movements Abnormal or asymmetrical Structural abnormality
5 yr (approximately)	Visual acuity† Corneal light reflex/cover-uncover Stereoacuity‡ Red reflex* Inspection	20/40 or worse or 2 lines of difference between eyes Asymmetrical/ocular refixation movements Failure to appreciate stereopsis Abnormal or asymmetrical Structural abnormality
Older than 5 yr	Visual acuity† Corneal light reflex/cover-uncover Stereoacuity‡ Red reflex* Inspection	20/30 or worse or 2 lines of difference between eyes Asymmetrical/ocular refixation movements Failure to appreciate stereopsis Abnormal or asymmetrical Structural abnormality

Note: These recommendations are based on expert opinion.
*Physician or nurse responsibility.
†Figures, letters, "tumbling E," or optotypes.
‡Optional: Random Dot E Game (RDE), Titmus Stereograms (Titmus Optical, Inc., Petersburg, VA), Randot Stereograms (Stereo Optical Company, Inc, Chicago).
    Reprinted with permission from the American Academy of Ophthalmology: Pediatric Eye Evaluations Preferred Practice Pattern®. © 1997, American Academy of Ophthalmology, Inc.

should be performed, the results documented, and the child referred immediately to an ophthalmologist:

- Shine a penlight into the eye from a lateral position and turn the light off and on several times to assess light perception. If the child can identify when the light is on or off, vision is described as "LP" (light perception).

- If hand movements can be seen 12 in. from the child's face, it is documented as "H/M at 1 ft." Indication of search and recognition should be seen as the hand is slowly moved back and forth with periodic cessation.
- Ask the child to count the number of fingers seen when one, two, or three fingers are held up 12 in. from the child's face. If the child is correct, document the vision as "C/F 1 ft."

CORNEAL LIGHT REFLEX

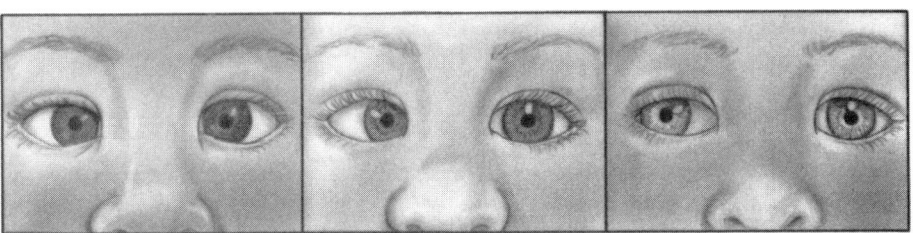

A   Pseudostrabismus   B   R Esotropia   C   R Exotropia

Symmetric Corneal Light Reflex

A. *Pseudostrabismus* has the appearance of strabismus due to epicanthal fold but is normal for a young child.

Asymmetric Corneal Light Reflex

Strabismus is true disparity of the eye axes. This constant malalignment is also termed tropia and is likely to cause amblyopia.
B. Esotropia—inward turn of the eye.
C. Exotropia—outward turn of the eye.

COVER TEST

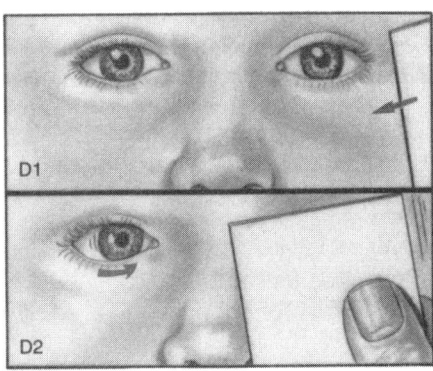

D   Right, uncovered eye is weaker

D. Uncovered eye—if it jumps to fixate on designated point, it was out of alignment before (i.e., when you cover the stronger eye, the weaker eye now tries to fixate).

Phoria—mild weakness, apparent only with the cover test and less likely to cause amblyopia than a tropia but still possible.

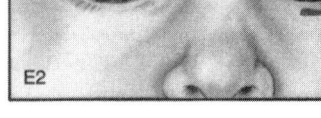

E   Left, covered eye is weaker

E. Covered eye—if this is the weaker eye, once macular image is suppressed it will drift to relaxed position.
As eye is uncovered—if it jumps to re-establish fixation, weakness exists.
Esophoria—nasal (inward) drift.
Exophoria—temporal (outward) drift.

F I G U R E 29-3
Extraocular muscle function testing (corneal light reflex and cover test). (From Jarvis C: Physical Examination and Health Assessment, 2nd ed. Philadelphia, WB Saunders, 1996, p 340.)

Diagnostic Studies

LABORATORY STUDIES

Studies such as a complete blood count (CBC), cultures, and Gram stain are done if identification of infection or particular organisms would be helpful in guiding management.

Ultrasound or radiographic studies such as computed tomography (CT) or magnetic resonance imaging (MRI) are sometimes useful in determining a diagnosis of orbital cellulitis, trauma, or tumor or substantiating concern about the central nervous system.

FLUORESCEIN STAINING

Fluorescein staining may be used to determine the extent of damage to the corneal epithelium as a result of trauma, infection, or exposure to a foreign body. Moisten a small strip of fluorescein tape and place it in the lower conjunctival sac. Allow the fluorescein to mix with tears, and then irrigate with sterile normal saline. After the eye has been well irrigated, examination with a cobalt blue filter light highlights the uptake of fluorescein stain and thereby identifies injury to the corneal epithelium.

VISUAL EVOKED RESPONSE TESTING

Visual evoked response testing, an electrical response after stimulation of the central nervous system by a specific stimulus, is used by an ophthalmologist to estimate visual acuity in infants and children who cannot cooperate with visual acuity testing.

PHOTOSCREENER

This new technique uses a portable camera with high-speed film and a flash to take a photograph of the pupillary reflex of the eye, which allows the examiner to measure refractive error and muscle balance abnormalities or other disease processes.

▉ MANAGEMENT STRATEGIES

Referral for Ophthalmological and Specialty Management

Many eye problems require referral to ophthalmologists or optometrists for management. See Table 29-4 for referral points. Although any child with eye pathology should be referred to an ophthalmologist, optometrists can be a valuable resource in caring for children with refractive errors or certain common eye conditions (e.g., corneal abrasions, foreign bodies). It is recommended that NPs acquaint themselves with the statutory guidelines for scopes of practice and prescription privileges as designated by the state boards of optometry within their state in order to optimize referral possibilities.

PATCHING. Covering one eye with a patch to improve amblyopia is a technique often used to treat strabismus.

CORRECTIVE LENSES. In children, eyeglasses are used to correct refractive errors. Contact lenses are occasionally recommended for older children (and frequently for adolescents) (Table 29-5). Keratorefractive surgery is rarely recommended for children.

The best eyeglasses for children are those with plastic frames (lightweight yet sturdy), spring hinges, and ear pieces that gently hug the back of the ear. Large bifocal segments are well tolerated by children, and tinted lenses are recommended for those with photosensitivity. In particular, children with aphakia (absence of the lens), congenital absence of the iris, and albinism benefit from glasses with UV light filters.

Glasses must be changed frequently in children because of head growth. Because the child may be reluctant to wear eyeglasses that hurt or pinch, parents should assess the fit of the eyeglasses on a monthly basis and watch for behavior (e.g., constantly removing glasses, rubbing at the frames or face) that indicates discomfort in a preverbal child.

Contact lenses, in addition to the cosmetic benefit, provide better refractive error correction than eyeglasses do and thereby enhance visual acuity and the total corrected field of

T A B L E 29-4

Indications for a Comprehensive Eye Evaluation by an Ophthalmologist

INDICATION	SPECIFIC EXAMPLES
Abnormalities on screening evaluations	Decreased visual attentiveness or acuity (monocular or binocular)* Strabismus Leukokoria or opacities of ocular media (emergency referral) Behavior indicating difficulty (straining, squinting)**
Signs or symptoms of eye problems by history or intuitive concerns of family members†	Defective ocular fixation development or visual interactions (bonding or contact) Misaligned eyes (strabismus) Light sensitivity Ocular discharge Persistent redness Tearing Nystagmus (shaking of eyes) Abnormal light reflex (including both the corneal light reflections and the "red" fundus reflection) Reading difficulty or complaints of eye fatigue, blurry vision**
General health problems, systemic disease, or use of medications that are known to be associated with eye disease and visual abnormalities	Diabetes present for 5 yr Juvenile rheumatoid arthritis Neurodegenerative disease Neurodevelopmental delay Prematurity (born at 28 wk or less gestational age or weighing 1500 g or less; first examination due at chronological age of 4–6 wk or at 31 to 33 wk postconceptional age)‡ Systemic steroid therapy Systemic syndromes with ocular manifestations
A family history of conditions that cause or are associated with eye or vision problems	Glasses in preschool children Strabismus Amblyopia Retinoblastoma Presenile cataract Infantile or childhood glaucoma Retinal dystrophy/degeneration Systemic syndromes with ocular manifestations
Health and developmental problems that make screening by the primary care physician difficult or inaccurate	Developmental delay

Note: These recommendations are based on expert opinion.

*Approximately 5% of school-age children have refractive errors.

†"Headache" is not included because it is rarely caused by eye problems in children. This complaint should first be evaluated by the primary care physician.

‡American Academy of Pediatrics, American Association for Pediatric Ophthalmology and Strabismus, American Academy of Ophthalmology: Screening Examination of Premature Infants for Retinopathy of Prematurity. Information Statement. San Francisco, American Academy of Ophthalmology, 1996.

**Inserted by authors.

Reprinted with permission from the American Academy of Ophthalmology: Pediatric Eye Evaluations Preferred Practice Pattern®. © 1997, American Academy of Ophthalmology, Inc.

TABLE 29-5

Recommendations for Use of Corrective Lenses

EYEGLASSES

Plastic frames, lightweight yet sturdy, with spring hinges, and rounded temporal pieces that hug the back of the ear are best.

In infants, the temples can be shortened and an elastic strap attached that goes around the back of the head to allow movement without dislodging the glasses.

Rolled or flared nose pads help prevent glasses from sliding down the nose.

Tinted lenses can be used for photosensitivity.

Remove eyeglasses with both hands.

Do not lay eyeglasses directly on any surface.

Clean glasses daily with liquid soap and a soft cloth. Do not use paper towels, toilet tissue, or facial tissues.

CONTACT LENSES

Child or adolescent is able to demonstrate ability to cleanse, insert, and remove lenses.

Protective gear should be worn when participating in contact sports.

Lenses should not be worn when eye is inflamed or when topical ophthalmic medications are being used.

Adapted from MacDonald MA: Refractive errors and corrective lenses in children and adolescents. J Pediatr Health Care 10(3):121–123, 1996.

vision. Contact lenses are appropriate for older children and adolescents when they can demonstrate the ability to manage lens hygiene, including insertion and removal of the lenses. They are particularly helpful in an aphakic child who would otherwise require very thick glasses that distort images. They are not indicated in individuals who have recurrent conjunctival or corneal infections, inadequate tears, severe allergies, or excessive exposure to dust or smoke. The NP can promote eye health by reinforcing instructions regarding proper contact lens care and reminding the patient that contact lenses should not be worn when the eye is inflamed or topical ophthalmic medications are being used.

Ophthalmic Medications

Caution and precision must be exercised when administering ocular medications to children because their smaller body mass and faster metabolism may potentiate the action of the drugs and result in adverse ocular and systemic side effects.

Topical ophthalmic medications such as antibiotics, mydriatics, and corticosteroids are frequently found in ointment or solution vehicles. These topical agents are primarily used for treating disorders affecting the anterior segment of the eye. Solubility is one of several factors that influence the absorption of topical ophthalmic medications. Those that are water soluble (e.g., anesthetics, steroids, and alkaloids) penetrate the corneal epithelium easily. Fat-soluble preparations (e.g., most antibiotics) do not penetrate the epithelium of the cornea unless it is inflamed.

TOPICAL ANTIBIOTICS. Prescription of topical antibiotics is frequently based on empirical evidence that infection exists. The best choice of a topical antibiotic is one that is not often prescribed for problems in other body systems. For example, topical ophthalmological preparations such as 10% sodium sulfacetamide, 4% sulfisoxazole, and broad-spectrum antibiotics are effective and rarely produce a hypersensitivity reaction. Topical penicillins, on the other hand, are to be avoided. Ophthalmic ointments are generally preferred over solutions for use in children because they last longer, do not sting, do not need to be given as often, and are less likely to be absorbed into the lacrimal passage. Ointments interfere with vision because they coat the eye, and they are more likely to cause contact dermatitis. Special care must be taken to ensure that the tip of the tube or dropper is not contaminated. Ophthalmic ointment should be transferred from the tube to moistened cotton swabs (one for each eye) and then rolled into the lower portion of each conjunctival sac (see Appendix A for ophthalmic drugs).

OPHTHALMIC CORTICOSTEROIDS. Although ophthalmic corticosteroids are effective in the treatment of numerous ocular disorders, a patient with a condition severe enough to warrant consideration of corticosteroid use should be referred to an ophthalmologist. Steroids are associated with numerous complications, such as an increased incidence of herpes simplex keratitis and corneal ulcers, glaucoma, slowed healing of corneal abrasions and wounds, and cataract formation. A child receiving long-term ophthalmological steroids should be assessed frequently for signs of adrenal suppression or other side effects. Encourage parents to keep scheduled tonometry appointments at 2- to 3-month intervals.

OTHER TOPICAL PREPARATIONS. Decongestants or antihistamines or a combination of the two, mast-cell stabilizers, and nonsteroidal anti-inflammatory drugs are all agents used in treating various ophthalmological conditions such as allergic conjunctivitis. Cycloplegic agents are used for iritis.

SYSTEMIC ANTIBIOTICS. In ocular disorders involving the posterior segment and the orbit, systemic preparations are necessary. A combination of topical and systemic antibiotics can also be used. In general, these conditions warrant referral to an ophthalmologist.

Eye Injury Prevention

Every year 24 million eye injuries occur in the United States, and 20,000 to 70,000 result in some loss of vision. Forty percent of injuries occur in people younger than 20 years, with a male-to-female ratio of 4:1. It is estimated that 90% of the injuries could be prevented (Hoffman, 1997).

Parental supervision and education of children regarding prevention of eye injury are essential to minimize these injuries. Prevention includes such fundamental concepts as the following:

- Do not run with or throw sharp objects.
- Store harmful chemicals and sharp objects out of the reach of small children.
- Limit and supervise the use of BB guns, air rifles, darts, and fireworks.
- Use protective eyewear when hammering or using power tools.
- Use eye wash fountains when indicated.
- Use orthodontic headwear that breaks away if force is applied.
- Do not shine laser pointers in eyes.

SUNGLASSES. UV radiation from the sun can damage the lens and retina of the eye and cause cataracts and other conditions harmful to vision later in life. Sunglasses should be used whenever a child is in the sun long enough to get a burn or tan, beginning in infancy. It is never too early to start wearing sunglasses. Wearing a hat with a wide (3-in.) brim is recommended in addition to sunglasses, and parents should be encouraged to set an example by wearing sunglasses. The greatest risk of eye injury occurs between 10 AM and 2 PM, at high altitude, with proximity to water or snow, and on the beach.

Sunglasses that have large-framed, wrap-around lenses with side shields provide the best protection. The lens and frame should be constructed of nonbreakable plastic. Neither dark lenses, mirrored lenses, nor polarized lenses alone offer the protection that is needed; protection comes from a chemical added to the lens (Wagner, 1995). One of the following labels indicates adequate UV protection: blocks 99% of UV rays, UV absorption to 400 nm, special purpose, meets ANSI (American National Standards Insititute) UV requirement.

SPORTS PROTECTION. Protective glasses or goggles are mandatory for all functionally one-eyed individuals or for any athlete who has had eye surgery or trauma or whose ophthalmologist recommends eye protection (American Academy of Pediatrics [AAP], 1996). Additionally, these children or adolescents should not participate in boxing, wrestling, or full-contact martial arts. Eye protection is recommended for any child or adolescent participating in sports that have a high eye injury rate. The greatest number of injuries occurs in basketball and baseball or softball. However, eye protection is also recommended for pool activities, racquet sports, football, soccer, hockey, lacrosse, and squash. Eye protection also should be used in shop class or labs or when working with high-velocity projectiles (e.g., hammer on metal, power tools or lawn mowers).

Protective glasses or goggles should be properly fitted with a 2- to 3-mm plastic-blend polycarbonate lens set deeply in a grooved frame with padding or rubber bridges around the nose. A headband or wraparound earpieces should be used to secure the glasses.

LASER POINTERS. The Food and Drug Administration (FDA) released a warning about the misuse of laser pointers (FDA, 1997). Although harmless when used as intended by lecturers, reports of eye injury when the pointers are used as toys have appeared. The light energy from the laser aimed at the eye can be more damaging than staring directly into the sun.

Vision Therapy, Lenses, and Prisms

Vision therapy, lenses, and prisms are controversial methods of treatment claimed by some to be effective therapy for learning disabilities and dyslexia. The NP should have a basic knowledge of this field to assist families in making decisions about what treatment to undertake.

Vision therapy as defined by the joint organizational policy for the AAO and the AOA is "the art and science of developing and enhancing visual abilities and remediating vision dysfunctions" (AAO & AOA, 1997). These interventions consist of (1) visual training, including muscle exercises, ocular pursuit, tracking exercises, or "training" glasses (with or without bifocals or prisms); (2) neurological organizational training (laterality training, crawling, balance board, perceptual training); and (3) wearing of colored lenses (AAP, 1998).

The AAO and AOA statement says "Learning is accomplished through complex and interrelated processes, one of which is vision." Visual function is defined as visual pathway integrity, visual efficiency, and visual information processing. Visual therapy is aimed at improving visual efficiency and processing; it "does not preclude any other form of treatment and should be a part of a multidisciplinary approach to learning disabilities."

The AAP, AAO, and AAPOS statement, *Learning Disabilities, Dyslexia and Vision: A Subject Review* (AAP, 1998), states that "Vision problems are rarely responsible for learning difficulties. No scientific evidence exists for the efficacy of eye exercises ('vision therapy') or the use of special tinted lenses in the remediation of these complex pediatric developmental and neurologic conditions." Indeed, a substantial body of research has shown that dyslexia is not caused by visual–perceptual problems (Gabriels, 1998). The AAP, AAO, and AAPOS statement concludes by stating specifically to "avoid remedies involving eye exercises, filters, tinted lenses, or other optical devices that have no known scientific proof of efficacy."

When counseling parents who inquire about vision therapy, the NP should be aware of the pressure that parents may be under from vision therapists and the divergent opinions held about this modality of treatment. Educating parents that learning disabilities are caused by the brain, not vision, and that no *scientific* evidence has proved any benefit to this treatment should be the goal of the NP.

■■■ COMMON EYE DISORDERS

Visual Disorders

REFRACTIVE ERRORS AND AMBLYOPIA

Description

Alterations in the refractive power of the eye include myopia, hyperopia, and astigmatism. In a normal eye, light from a distant object focuses directly on the retina. When variations in axial length of the eyeball or curvature of the cornea or lens exist, light focuses in front of or behind the retina. This abnormal focusing produces an alteration in the refractive power of the eye that results in a visual acuity deficit (see Table 29-6 for further definitions).

Etiology and Incidence

Refractive errors are the most common visual disorder seen in children (MacDonald, 1996). Myopia may be present at birth, but it is more likely to develop during the middle school years (8 to 10 years of age). Mild hyperopia is normal in a young child but should resolve spontaneously by 6 years of age. Amblyopia occurs in the general population at a rate of 2 to 4% (Zwaan, 1999; Bacal & Hertle, 1998).

Clinical Findings

The following may be noted:

- Squinting
- Fatigue
- Headaches
- Pain in or around eyes
- Dizziness

T A B L E 29-6
Descriptive Terms for Refractive Errors

Myopia, or nearsightedness, exists when the axial length of the eye is increased in relation to the eye's optical power. As a result, light from a distant object is focused in front of the retina rather than directly on it. A myopic child sees close objects clearly, but distant objects are blurry.

In *hyperopia,* or farsightedness, the visual image is focused behind the retina, and as a result, distant objects are seen clearly but close objects are blurry.

Astigmatism exists when the curvature of the cornea or lens is uneven; thus the retina cannot appropriately focus light from an object regardless of the distance, which makes vision blurry close up and far away. Rarely, astigmatism can be caused by an alteration in the corneal sphere caused by a soft tissue mass on the inner aspect of the eyelid, such as chalazion or hemangioma.

Anisometropia is a different refractive error in each eye. It may consist of any combination of refractive errors discussed above or it may occur with aphakia.

Amblyopia is a unilateral or bilateral developmental deficit in vision caused by inadequate or unequal visual stimulation that has progressed to a point that it is not correctable with eyeglasses or contact lenses. It may be caused by congenital nystagmus, corneal or lenticular opacities, retinal disorders, optic nerve abnormalities, central nervous system abnormalities, and severe myopia or hyperopia in infants. In older children, amblyopia is associated with long-standing, uncorrected refractive errors and strabismus. Amblyopia is described as the following types:

Deprivational—unilateral condition that obstructs vision, e.g., lid abnormalities or cataract
Strabismic—caused by strabismus of an eye
Refractive—caused by one of the refractive errors described above

---

- Mild nausea
- Developmental delay
- Tendency to cover or close one eye when concentrating
- Family history of refractive errors, strabismus, or amblyopia

A rule of thumb is that if the examiner cannot see into the eye (e.g., poor eye reflex), the patient cannot see out (amblyopia)

Management

Detection of visual problems in children at an early age is essential to prevent the development of otherwise avoidable permanent visual loss. The following steps are involved:

1. Refer to an ophthalmologist or optometrist for prescription corrective lenses.
2. Older children should have an annual refraction and eyeglass evaluation.
3. Patching may be recommended and, occasionally, surgery.
4. Extended-wear contact lenses may be prescribed in unilateral aphakia, severe anisometropia, corneal scarring with irregular astigmatism, and keratoconus.

5. Support and reassurance according to the child's developmental level are needed during the period of adjustment to contact lenses or eyeglasses.
   - Infants and toddlers need distraction, with replacement of glasses if removed.
   - Verbal children may be aided by the use of positive reinforcement such as sticker charts.
   - School-aged children and teenagers should participate in the selection of frames. If desired, contacts may be considered.
6. Claims of certain diets or exercises as means of correcting or preventing refractive errors have not been substantiated by research efforts. (See the discussion in Management Strategies earlier in the chapter.)

Complications

Amblyopia can cause strabismus.

STRABISMUS

Description

Strabismus is a defect in the position of the eyes in relation to each other, commonly called a lazy eye. In strabismus, the visual axes are not parallel because the muscles of the eyes are not coordinated; when one eye is directed straight ahead, the other deviates. As a result, one or both eyes appear crossed. In children, strabismus may be manifested as a phoria or a tropia (see Table 29-7). Pseudostrabismus is present when the sclera between the cornea and the inner canthus is obscured by closely placed eyes, a flat nasal bridge, or prominent epicanthal folds (see Fig. 29-3). Upper eyelid ptosis may accompany strabismus in some cases (Zwaan, 1999).

Etiology and Incidence

Affecting approximately 4% of children, strabismus usually develops before 3 to 4 years of age. Approximately 50% of cases develop over time; the other 50% are present at birth. Phorias are common before 6 years of age, become symptomatic when the child is ill or tired, and are rarely of clinical significance. Esodeviations are the most common type of strabismus and are visible when the child is looking at a near object. Exodeviations occur 25% of the time and are usually intermittent and more visible when the child is looking far away. Early-onset esotropia is evident by 2 to 12 months of age. Accommodative esotropia becomes evident later, usually between 6 months and 7 years of age. Both types of strabismus may be hereditary, the result of various eye diseases, or in rare

T A B L E 29-7
Descriptive Terms for Strabismus

A *phoria* is an intermittent deviation in ocular alignment that is held latent by sensory fusion.
A *tropia* is a consistent or intermittent deviation in ocular alignment. A child with a tropia is unable to maintain alignment on an object of fixation.
Phorias and tropias are classified according to the pattern of deviation seen:
  Hyper (up) and hypo (down) are used to classify vertical strabismus.
  Exo (away from nose) and eso (toward the nose) describe horizontal deviations.
  Cyclo describes a rotational or torsional deviation.

instances, the result of paralysis of the extraocular muscles (Burke, 1998; Preller, 1998; Calhoun, 1997; Castiglia, 1994; Catalano, 1990).

Clinical Findings

Clinical findings can involve the following:

- Intermittent esotropia may be seen in normal children younger than 4 years who are ill or tired or when they are exposed to flashes of light or with sudden changes from close to distant vision.
- When only one eye is affected, the child always fixates with the unaffected eye.
- When both eyes are affected, the eye that looks straight at any given time is the fixating eye.
- The angle of deviation may be inconsistent in all fields of gaze, actually changing in some forms of strabismus.
- Persistent squinting, head tilting, face turning, overpointing, awkwardness, or marked decreased visual acuity in one eye may be seen.
- Cataracts, retinoblastoma, anisometropia, and high refractive errors are found infrequently.

DIAGNOSTIC TESTING. The corneal light reflection technique and the cover-uncover and the alternating cover tests are assessments used to screen for strabismus. Asymmetry of light reflection on the cornea is indicative of a deviation in ocular alignment. The cover-uncover test is used to detect tropias, whereas the alternating cover test detects phorias (see Fig. 29-3). The photoscreener can also be used to detect strabismus.

Management

Management steps include the following:

1. Any deviation seen after 6 months of age is considered abnormal and the child should be referred. Hypertropia or hypotropia, exodeviation, or any fixed deviation is an indication for referral as soon as it is first observed.
2. The fixating eye is patched, which forces the child to use the deviating eye.
3. Surgical alignment of the eyes is often neces-

sary. It is usually done before 2 years of age and as early as 6 months of age.

4. Orthoptic exercises as a treatment modality are indicated only in certain forms of intermittent strabismus or when the visual axes are nearly aligned.
5. Corrective lenses may or may not be indicated, depending on the presence of refractive errors.
6. Annual follow-up with an ophthalmologist is needed for monitoring of visual acuity, refraction, alignment, and mobility if surgery was performed.
7. Assessment for amblyopia should be done at every visit, even after straightening the eyes, because changes in alignment can occur through the fifth year.
8. The ocular status of an affected child's siblings is monitored.
9. Research on the use of levodopa shows reversal of strabismus and improved vision secondary to the reestablishment of nerve connections.

Complications

Amblyopia occurs in 30 to 50% of children with strabismus (Castiglia, 1994), especially if eyes are not used alternately. Uncorrected strabismus can have a negative effect on self-esteem.

BLEPHAROPTOSIS

Description

Blepharoptosis or ptosis is drooping of the upper eyelids affecting one or both eyes. It can be congenital or acquired.

Etiology

Congenital ptosis caused by an abnormality in development of the levator muscles or cranial nerve III may be an autosomal dominant trait. Other possible etiologies include trauma to cranial nerve III during the birthing process, trauma to the eyelid in older children, chronic inflammation (particularly of the anterior segment of the eye), or a neurological disorder (Newell, 1996).

Management

Management involves the following steps:

1. Correction of any underlying systemic disease.
2. Evaluation for anisometropia (unequal refractive errors in each eye).
3. Referral to an ophthalmologist. If vision is compromised, surgery is performed in an effort to prevent amblyopia and developmental delay. If vision is not compromised, correction is usually delayed until the child is at least 3 years old.

NYSTAGMUS

Description

Nystagmus is the presence of involuntary, rhythmic movements that may be pendular oscillations or jerky drifts of one or both eyes. Movement is horizontal, vertical, rotary, or mixed.

Etiology

Nystagmus occurs in association with albinism, refractive errors, central nervous system abnormalities, and various diseases of the inner ear and the retina.

Clinical Findings

Oscillation in the newborn's eyes is common and exists for a short time during the neonatal period. Involuntary oscillation that persists or occurs beyond the initial weeks of life indicates pathology. The movements may be constant or varied, depending on the direction of gaze.

Management

Key principles in management are the following:

1. Treat any underlying systemic disorder.
2. Refer the patient to an ophthalmologist.
3. Acquired nystagmus is most worrisome and requires prompt evaluation.

CATARACTS

Description

Cataract, a partial or complete opacity of the lens affecting one or both eyes, is the most common cause of an abnormal pupillary reflex. Some cataracts are considered clinically significant, others insignificant.

Etiology

Cataracts may be congenital or a result of infection, trauma to the eye, or long-term use of systemic corticosteroids or ocular corticosteroid drops. They may also be seen in children who have other ocular abnormalities, such as strabismus or pendular nystagmus, and in children with trisomy 21, diabetes mellitus, galactosemia, atopic dermatitis, or Marfan syndrome. Prematurity and congenital rubella syndrome are also associated with cataracts.

Clinical Findings

The following history and physical examination findings are present:

- A history of maternal prenatal infection, drug exposure, or hypocalcemia is usually elicited.
- Cataract appears as a black dot or line surrounded by a red reflex, usually bilateral.
- Visual acuity deficits may vary.
- A pale red reflex in people of color should not be confused with a cataract.

Management

Key principles in management are the following:

1. Surgical removal of the lens optically clears the visual axis.
2. The resultant aphakic refractive errors are corrected with lenses.
3. Correct any sensory deprivation amblyopia.

Complications

Visual developmental delay (amblyopia), especially in neonates with bilateral congenital cataracts that are dense, has been reported.

Prognosis

The success of treatment depends on the cataract type. Visual outcomes tend to be better with unilateral than bilateral cataracts. Good results are more likely if cataracts are removed before 3 months of age.

GLAUCOMA

Description

Glaucoma is a disturbance in the circulation of aqueous fluid that results in an increase in intraocular pressure and subsequent damage to the optic nerve. It is classified according to age at time of its appearance and other associated conditions.

Etiology and Incidence

Infantile glaucoma, which occurs in the first 3 years of life, is a congenital abnormality of the structures that drain the aqueous humor. It is an anomaly of the drainage apparatus over 50% of the time (Nelson, 1996). It is also seen in association with other developmental anomalies such as neurofibromatosis, diffuse facial nevus flammeus (port-wine stain), or Sturge-Weber, Marfan, Hurler, or Pierre Robin syndromes. The incidence is 0.3%, with more males than females affected (Nelson, 1996). Secondary or juvenile glaucoma occurs between 3 and 30 years of age, when the drainage network for aqueous humor becomes obstructed after ocular infection, trauma, neoplasm, or long-term corticosteroid use.

Clinical Findings

Symptoms of infantile glaucoma (unilateral or bilateral) include the following:

- "Classic triad" of tearing, photophobia, and excessive blinking or blepharospasm (only one third of patients manifest this triad [Nelson, 1996]) caused by irritation
- Enlarged, hazy corneas
- Corneal edema, corneal and ocular enlargement, conjunctival injection, and visual impairment

Symptoms of secondary glaucoma include:

- Extreme pain
- Blurred vision
- Tunnel vision
- Pupillary dilation
- Erythema (often in only one eye)
- Change in configuration of optic nerve cupping, with asymmetry between the eyes and loss of vision over time

Management

Early diagnosis is important. The goal is normalization of intraocular pressure and prevention of optic nerve damage along with correction of associated refractive errors and amblyopia.

1. Refer to an ophthalmologist.
2. Primary treatment is surgery as early as possible (often multiple surgeries are required).
3. Medications may include topical β-blockers and carbonic anhydrase inhibitors.
4. Parent and patient education must emphasize the importance of medication compliance and discourage excessive physical or emotional stress and straining at stool.
5. A medical identification tag is worn at all times.
6. Routine tonometry and an ophthalmoscopic examination are needed for every member of the family every 2 years.

Complications

Stretching of the cornea and sclera and blindness can occur.

RETINOPATHY OF PREMATURITY

Description

ROP is a vascular disorder involving abnormal growth of the retinal vessels of both eyes. Previously, ROP was called retrolental fibroplasia. An international classification of ROP has been identified and is important both for understanding the disease and for predicting outcome. The classification system describes ROP according to site (zone), severity (stage), and extent (clock hours) (Phelps, 1995). ROP is

important because of the increasing incidence, the critical window of time for treatment, and the need for monitoring for late complications.

Etiology and Incidence

ROP is a multifactorial disease primarily caused by early gestational age and the use of supplemental oxygen. ROP can occur in full-term neonates, but it is primarily seen in premature infants, usually those weighing less than 1500 g. Infants born at less than 30 to 32 weeks of gestation or weighing less than 1250 grams are particularly vulnerable for more severe ROP. Exposure to supplemental oxygen for greater than 30 days is an additional risk (not causative) factor. The incidence of ROP is increasing because of survival of the very smallest babies. Infants weighing 1000 to 1250 g have a 40% incidence, infants under 1000 g have a 75% incidence, and infants under 750 g have a 90% incidence (Stevens, 1998). Forty percent of babies under 750 g have moderate to severe disease and 18% have severe disease (Phelps, 1995). An increased incidence of the disease is noted in whites vs. blacks (Stevens, 1998).

Clinical Findings

ROP is initially diagnosed by a pediatric ophthalmologist while the infant is in the nursery. Once the baby is discharged, the following may be seen as sequelae to ROP:

- Leukokoria (white fibrovascular tissue in the retrolental space)
- Vitreous hemorrhage
- Myopia
- Strabismus
- Cataracts

Management

The NP's role in managing ROP is to:

- Ensure that all premature infants receive initial and follow-up examinations as indicated by their gestational maturity and size
- Discuss with parents the implications of their child's disease
- Monitor for late sequelae to ROP (frequent assessment is needed to rule out strabis-

mus, amblyopia, and other potential complications quickly)

- Assist children who have sequelae to maximize their potential (see Wheeler et al., 1997)

Management of ROP is constantly evolving as long-term outcomes become available. Therefore, it is important to keep current on new recommendations (Schalij-Delfos et al., 1996). The current joint statement from the AAP, the AAPOS, and the AAO (1997) recommends the following:

- Ophthalmological examination should be performed on all infants born at less than 28 weeks of gestation or weighing 1500 g or less or more than 1500 g with an unstable course before leaving the hospital.
- Examination should be performed by a pediatric ophthalmologist experienced in the examination of preterm infants.
- Examination should be done at 4 to 6 weeks' chronological age or between 31 to 33 weeks' postconceptual age.
- The need for and frequency of follow-up examinations are determined during the initial examination by using the international classification of ROP. Cryosurgery, vitrectomy, or retinal detachment surgery may be needed.

Complications

Retinal detachment, amblyopia, serious myopia, strabismus, glaucoma, and cicatrix (residual retinal scars) leading to later vision loss are possible complications. Complete loss of vision occurs in 2 to 4% of infants with ROP (Phelps, 1995). Educational problems, including low IQ, poor social development, perceptual interpretation of the environment, motor skill development, and language acquisition; stereotypic behavior such as rocking or moving the head; and behavioral problems are possible (Wheeler et al., 1997).

Prevention

Minimizing or preventing ROP can be accomplished by decreasing the occurrence of premature births, minimizing the oxygen needed, us-

ing vitamin E to maintain physiological serum levels, and possibly, reducing exposure to high ambient and supplemental lights (an issue currently under study and debate).

RETINOBLASTOMA

Description

Retinoblastoma is a rare malignant tumor of the retina.

Etiology and Incidence

Retinoblastoma occurs as a genetic defect on the 13th chromosome. It is the most common childhood ocular malignancy and the most common primary intraocular tumor. It may be found as a single tumor in one eye or as multiple tumors in one or both eyes. Bilateral disease occurs 25 to 35% of the time and is usually recognized at about 12 months of age. Unilateral disease occurs two thirds of the time and is more commonly recognized at 24 months. The overall incidence is 1 in 17,000 to 1 in 30,000 live births, without race or sex preference. Both hereditary and nonhereditary forms may occur (Zwaan, 1999; West, 1998; Nelson, 1996).

Clinical Findings

The following may be seen:

- Positive family history
- Leukokoria (60% of cases; Abramson, 1998) is the initial sign
- Strabismus is the second most common finding (20% of cases; Abramson, 1998).
- Decreased visual acuity
- Possible inflammation, orbital cellulitis, hyphema, abnormal red reflex, nystagmus, glaucoma, hypopyon, or signs of global rupture

Management

1. Refer the patient to an ophthalmologist for diagnosis and management by a multidisciplinary team. Irradiation, chemotherapy, cryotherapy, and laser treatment are possible therapeutic modalities. Surgical removal of

the affected eye is sometimes necessary if the tumor is large or intraocular. An ocular prothesis for enucleation can be fitted 3 to 4 weeks after surgery.
2. Frequent follow-up (every 3 months until 6 or 7 years of age) to assess treatment and to monitor for recurrence is important. Examination of the eye may be done under anesthesia.
3. Refer the parents for genetic counseling.

Complications

Metastasis is possible if the diagnosis is delayed. Those who survive are at high risk for a secondary nonocular malignancy (often pinealoblastoma or sarcoma of the head or orbit) within 5 years of treatment; the metastasis is usually fatal.

Prognosis

The size and extent of the tumor determine the prognosis. If the orbit or optic nerve is involved, the prognosis is poor. Retinoblastoma is responsible for 1% of tumor deaths in children up to 15 years of age (Zwaan, 1999).

Infections

CONJUNCTIVITIS

Description

Conjunctivitis is an inflammation of the palpebral conjunctiva (the lining of the upper and lower eyelids) and occasionally the bulbar conjunctiva (layer of conjunctival tissue over the sclera).

Etiology and Incidence

Conjunctivitis is the most frequently seen ocular disorder in pediatric practice. Bacteria (most commonly *Haemophilus influenza*) are responsible for the infection greater than 50% of the time in children; conjunctivitis also occurs as a viral or fungal infection or as a response to allergens or chemical irritants (Yetman & Coody, 1997; Gigliotti, 1995; Wagner, 1993) (Table 29–8). Infectious conjunctivitis is often bilateral; unilateral disease suggests a toxic, chemical, mechanical, or lacrimal cause.

Differential Diagnosis

Blockage of the tear drainage system, injury, foreign body, abrasion or ulcers, iritis, herpes simplex, and infantile glaucoma are all in the differential diagnosis.

CONJUNCTIVITIS IN THE NEWBORN (OPHTHALMIA NEONATORUM)

Description

Conjunctivitis in the newborn, formerly known as ophthalmia neonatorum or neonatal blennorrhea, is a form of conjunctivitis that occurs in the neonatal period. In most states, conjunctivitis of the newborn is a reportable infectious disease.

Etiology and Incidence

The disorder occurs in 1.6 to 12% of newborns in the first month of life and is most commonly caused by *Chlamydia* or chemical irritation by prophylactic medication. *Staphylococcus, Streptococcus, Haemophilus, Neisseria gonorrhoeae,* and herpes simplex virus (HSV) can also be found. Chemical conjunctivitis usually occurs in the first day or two of life. Conjunctivitis caused by *Chlamydia* begins in the 5th to 14th day of life (Yetman & Coody, 1997; Gigliotti, 1995; Wagner, 1993).

Clinical Findings

- Maternal history of vaginal infection during pregnancy or current sexually transmitted disease (STD)
- Redness and swelling of the bulbar and palpebral conjunctiva
- Purulent exudate

LABORATORY STUDIES

- Gram stain, cultures, and antigen detection tests can be used. Gonorrhea should also be considered in any infant younger than 2 weeks.

T A B L E 29-8
Types of Conjunctivitis

TYPE	POPULATION AND ETIOLOGY	CLINICAL FINDINGS	DIAGNOSIS	MANAGEMENT
Ophthalmia neonatorum	Neonates *Chlamydia*, *Neisseria gonorrhoeae* (GC), herpes simplex virus (HSV) Silver nitrate reaction occurs in 10% of neonates	Erythema, chemosis, purulent exudate	Cultures Gram stain R/O GC, *Chlamydia*	Saline irrigation to eyes till clear, followed by erythromycin ointment GC: ceftriaxone or cefotaxime *Chlamydia*: erythromycin PO HSV: IV antivirals
Bacterial conjunctivitis	Preschoolers and sexually active teens *Haemophilus influenzae* (nontypable), *Streptococcus pneumoniae*, GC, enterococci	Erythema, chemosis, itching, burning, mucopurulent d/c, matted eyelashes	Cultures Gram stain Chocolate agar R/O pharyngitis, GC, AOM, URI, seborrhea	Sulfacetamide sodium 10% ophthalmic solution Chloramphenicol 1% ophthalmic ointment Erythromycin 0.5% ophthalmic ointment Augmentin oral suspension if concurrent AOM Warm soaks to eyes tid till clear No sharing towels, pillows No school until treatment begins

Condition	Etiology/Comments	Signs and Symptoms	Diagnostic Tests	Treatment
Chronic bacterial conjunctivitis	School-aged children and teens *Staphylococcus aureus*	As for bacterial conjunctivitis; foreign body sensation	Cultures R/O dacryostenosis, blepharitis	Gentamicin 0.3% ophthalmic solution/ointment Erythromycin 0.5% ophthalmic ointment Lacrimal duct massage tid–qid, 10 strokes Refer to M.D. if no improvement in 3 d
Inclusion conjunctivitis	Neonates and sexually active teens	Erythema, chemosis, clear or mucoid d/c, palpebral follicles	Cultures R/O sexual activity	Erythromycin PO for 2–3 wk Tetracycline PO (adolescents only)
Viral conjunctivitis	More common in children older than 6 yr Adenovirus 3, 4, 7, HSV, herpes zoster, enterovirus	Erythema, chemosis, tearing; HSV and herpes zoster: unilateral photophobia, fever Zoster: nose lesion	Cultures R/O corneal infiltration	Refer to ophthalmologist if herpes lesions or photophobia present Cool compresses tid–qid
Allergic and vernal conjunctivitis	Atopy sufferers, seasonal (warm)	Erythema, chemosis, clear or mucoid d/c, palpebral follicles, headache, rhinitis	Eosinophilia in exudate	Vasocon 0.1%, 0.012%, 0.03% ophthalmic solution Refer to allergist

AOM = acute otitis media; d/c = discharge; IV = intravenous; PO = oral; qid = four times a day; R/O = rule out; tid = three times a day; URI = upper respiratory tract infection.

Management

Irrigate the eyes with sterile normal saline until clear of exudate.

GONOCOCCAL CONJUNCTIVITIS IN THE NEWBORN. Hospitalization for a 7-day course of intravenous ceftriaxone or cefotaxime is needed.

NONGONOCOCCAL CONJUNCTIVITIS IN THE NEWBORN. A topical ophthalmic antibiotic preparation such as erythromycin 0.5% ointment (¼- to ½-in. strip to each eye) is applied two to four times a day. The eyes should be cleansed with water or saline on cotton balls before instillation of the ointment into the lower conjunctival sac.

CHLAMYDIAL CONJUNCTIVITIS IN THE NEWBORN. A 2-week course of systemic erythromycin ethylsuccinate (50 mg/kg per day) is prescribed. A second course is sometimes required.

HERPES SIMPLEX CONJUNCTIVITIS IN THE NEWBORN. Hospitalization and topical and systemic antivirals are needed.

CHEMICAL-INDUCED CONJUNCTIVITIS IN THE NEWBORN. This form of conjunctivitis resolves spontaneously within 3 to 4 days without specific treatment.

Prevention

Prophylactic administration of silver nitrate 1% ophthalmic solution (2 drops to each eye) or an ophthalmic antibiotic ointment such as 1% tetracycline or 0.5% erythromycin (¼ to ½ in. into each eye within 1 hour of delivery) is recommended (Centers for Disease Control and Prevention [CDC], 1998; AAP, 1997) and required by law in most states and territories to prevent gonococcal conjunctivitis in the newborn. It should be determined at the time of the first visit whether infants born at home have received this prophylaxis.

INCLUSION CONJUNCTIVITIS (*CHLAMYDIA*)

Etiology

Inclusion conjunctivitis is usually caused by *Chlamydia* and is most often seen in a neonate or sexually active adolescent.

Clinical Findings

- Maternal history of a sexually transmitted disease (STD) or a history of a sexual partner with an STD
- Conjunctival erythema and clear or mucoid discharge
- Follicular reaction (large, round elevations) in the conjunctiva of the lower eyelids
- Associated cervicitis or urethritis

Laboratory Studies

Culture or rapid screen of the exudate is done.

Management

The following treatment is recommended:

1. Erythromycin, 50 mg/kg per day in three to four divided doses or 500 mg twice a day for 10 to 14 days (infants or children younger than 9 years).
2. Tetracycline, 25 to 50 mg/kg per day in four divided doses or 250 mg four times a day for adolescents with all their secondary teeth for 10 to 14 days.
3. Doxycycline, 100 mg twice a day for 10 to 14 days for adolescents.
4. Topical treatment as well as oral is often recommended.
5. Partners of sexually active adolescents are examined and treated (CDC, 1998).

BACTERIAL CONJUNCTIVITIS

Description

Acute bacterial conjunctivitis is commonly called pinkeye.

Etiology and Incidence

Bacterial conjunctivitis is frequently caused by *Staphylococcus,* nontypable *H. influenzae* (especially in temperate climates), and *Streptococcus pneumoniae* (especially in cold weather). It is most common in the winter and in children younger than 6 years (Wagner, 1997).

Clinical Findings

The following may be noted:

- Erythema of one or both eyes (*key* finding)
- Burning, stinging, or itching of the eyes and a feeling of a foreign body
- Photophobia
- Petechiae on bulbar conjunctiva
- Sticky purulent or mucopurulent discharge, usually bilateral (*key* finding)
- Encrusted and matted eyelashes on awakening
- Symptoms of upper respiratory infection, otitis media, or acute pharyngitis

Laboratory Studies

Gram stain and culture can be done if the conjunctivitis is chronic, recurrent, or difficult to treat.

Management

Bacterial conjunctivitis is considered a self-limited disease (unless caused by gonorrhea) and usually resolves within 7 to 10 days. However, studies show that children who receive topical antibiotics demonstrate faster clinical improvement than do those left untreated (Zwaan, 1999; Wagner, 1997; Gigliotti, 1995).

UNCOMPLICATED CONJUNCTIVITIS. Sodium sulfacetamide 10% ophthalmic solution or ointment (1 to 2 drops or ¼ to ½ in. into each eye four times a day) or trimethoprim sulfate plus polymixin B sulfate ophthalmic solution (Polytrim, less irritating to the eye) is given for 5 to 10 days. Chloramphenicol 1% ophthalmic ointment (½ in. into each eye every 4 to 6 hours) or erythromycin 0.5% ophthalmic ointment (¼ to ½ in. into each eye four times a day) is recommended for patients with sulfa allergy. Other options are gentamicin or bacitracin. Newer antibiotic drops or ointments include tobramycin, ofloxacin, ciprofloxacin, and norfloxacin, which should be reserved for conjunctivitis that is nonresponsive to more conventional treatment. Neomycin is to be avoided because of possible sensitization.

CONJUNCTIVITIS–OTITIS SYNDROME. This syndrome is usually caused by a β-lactamase-resistant organism, often *H. influenzae* (74%; Gigliotti, 1995) and requires amoxicillin with clavulanic acid (Augmentin) at 40 to 90 mg/kg per 24 hours or another appropriate antibiotic for 10 days (Bodor, 1982 [classic article describing the syndrome]; Bodor, 1989; Lohr, 1993; Gigliotti, 1995).

CHRONIC BACTERIAL CONJUNCTIVITIS. Rule out nasolacrimal duct obstruction in infants and *Staphylococcus aureus* infection in older children. Gentamicin 0.3% ophthalmic solution (1 drop to each eye every 4 hours) or ointment (½ in. into each eye every 6 to 12 hours) or erythromycin 0.5% ophthalmic ointment (¼ to ½ in. into each eye four times a day) is recommended.

INFLAMMATION OF THE UVEAL TRACT. See the section on uveitis. Refer suspected cases to an ophthalmologist immediately.

Patient Education

If only one eye is involved, it is likely that the infection will spread within a day or two to involve both eyes. The patient (or parent) is instructed to:

- Cleanse the eyelashes several times a day with a weak solution of no-tears shampoo and warm water. The importance of wiping from the inner canthus outward and using a different cloth or cotton ball for each eye should be emphasized.
- Use warm soaks three to four times a day to relieve itching and burning.
- Instill prescription ophthalmic solutions or ointments into the lower conjunctival sac. A moistened cotton swab may be used to facilitate instillation of ointments.
- Wash hands frequently and avoid shared linens to limit spread of the infection.
- Also treat seborrheic dermatitis on the scalp and face if present.

Some day care centers exclude children with conjunctivitis until they have completed 1 to 2 days of treatment. Improvement in the child's condition should be seen within 48 hours. If medication compliance is not in question and improvement is not seen within 72 hours of administration, the parent should be instructed to return so that a smear of the exudate can be taken for culture and sensitivity testing.

Differential Diagnosis

Chronic bacterial conjunctivitis that is resistant to treatment requires ruling out nasolacrimal duct obstruction in infants and staphylococcal blepharitis in older children.

Complications

If vision is blurred or ophthalmoscopic examination reveals a bulging iris and a contracted, fixed pupil, suspect more serious inflammation of the uveal tract (iritis, cyclitis, or choroiditis) and refer immediately to an ophthalmologist.

VIRAL CONJUNCTIVITIS

Etiology and Incidence

Usually caused by an adenovirus, viral conjunctivitis can also be caused by herpes simplex, herpes zoster, or varicella virus. It is more common in children older than 6 years of age and in the summer (Wagner, 1997).

Clinical Findings

The following may be noted:

- Pharyngitis with enlarged preauricular nodes.
- Itchy, red, and swollen conjunctiva.
- Tearing and profuse clear, watery discharge.
- Fever, headache, anorexia, malaise, upper respiratory symptoms (pharyngitis-conjunctivitis-fever triad with adenovirus).
- Photophobia with measles or varicella rashes.
- Herpetic vesicles may be found on the eyelid margins and eyelashes (marginal blepharitis) or on the conjunctiva and cornea (keratoconjunctivitis).
  - Vesicles with superficial painful ulcerations, particularly on the tip of the nose, may be associated with herpes.

Management

1. Viral conjunctivitis is self-limited and should resolve in 7 to 14 days. Conjunctivitis is often difficult to distinguish from keratitis. If the NP has any question, referral for ophthalmological care is recommended.
2. Sodium sulfacetamide 10% ophthalmic solution or ointment (1 to 2 drops or ½ in. into each eye four times daily) or broad-spectrum antibiotic preparations may be used to prevent secondary bacterial infection.
3. Antihistamine or vasoconstrictive ophthalmic solutions may be used for symptomatic relief.
4. With HSV infection, immediate referral to an ophthalmologist should occur because of potential complications. Vidarabine or trifluridine (Viroptic) may be used in treatment. Topical corticosteroids should be avoided because they may worsen the course.
5. Molluscum requires referral for excision.
6. Cleansing and soothing measures are prescribed as described under general management of conjunctivitis.

Complications

Involvement of deeper layers of the cornea (keratitis) can occur and must be differentiated from conjunctivitis. Scarring of the cornea resulting in blindness is a significant complication of HSV infection.

ALLERGIC CONJUNCTIVITIS

Description

Four types of allergic conjunctivitis have been identified: (1) *hay fever–associated conjunctivitis* is characterized by mild injection and swelling; (2) *vernal conjunctivitis* is more severe and is more common in 3- to 12-year-olds and has an increased prevalence in warm weather; (3) *atopic keratoconjunctivitis* occurs with atopic dermatitis and is notable for significant itching; and (4) *giant papillary conjunctivitis* occurs most often in contact lens wearers allergic to the thimerosal in solutions. Individuals with atopic conjunctivitis have an increased susceptibility to herpes simplex infection (blepharitis or keratitis) (Raizman, 1998).

Etiology

Seasonal allergens, often unidentified, cause these types of conjunctivitis.

Clinical Findings

The following may be noted:

- Family history of seasonal allergies
- Other atopic disease—rhinitis, eczema, asthma
- Acute attacks precipitated by allergens (e.g., pollen, animals, dust, occasionally food)
- Severe itching and tearing
- Redness and swelling of the conjunctiva
- Follicular reaction of the conjunctiva
- Stringy, mucoid discharge
- Bilateral involvement most common
- Cobblestone papillary hypertrophy in the tarsal conjunctiva

LABORATORY STUDIES. Scrapings or smears of the conjunctiva reveal numerous eosinophils and may isolate the offending allergen.

Management

The following steps are taken:

1. Prevention is best. Avoidance of allergens gives 30% improvement (Finegold, 1998).
2. For mild cases, saline solution or artificial tears are administered along with cool compresses. Refrigerated eyedrops are more soothing.
3. The next step is decongestants and antihistamines—given topically or systemically.
   - Topical decongestants such as naphazoline hydrochloride (Naphcon or Vasocon) ophthalmic solution (1 to 2 drops every 3 to 4 hours) or combination (Naphcon-A or Vasocon-A) opthalmic solution (1 to 2 drops four times a day) can be used sparingly to reduce ocular congestion, irritation, and itching. To avoid rebound congestion, these drugs should not be used for more than 3 days or more frequently than recommended.
4. Topical mast cell stabilizers may be helpful

for maintenance therapy or vernal conjunctivitis.
   - Cromolyn sodium 4%, 1 to 2 drops four times a day for children older than 4 years.
   - Lodoxamine tromethamine (Alomide) 1%, 1 to 2 drops four times a day for children older than 2 years.
   - Olopatadine (Patanol) is a mast cell stabilizer combined with an antihistamine for children older than 3 years.
5. Nonsteroidal anti-inflammatory drugs can be used for late-phase treatment of itching and burning.
   - Ketorolac tromethamine (Acular) 0.5%, 1 drop four times a day up to 1 week in children older than 12 years.
6. Topical steroids are sometimes used in severe cases of allergy, but they must be used with caution because of possible side effects (increased intraocular pressure, potential for infection, contraindication with herpes, potential to cause cataracts, and poor corneal healing). At maximum they should be used for 1 week. If additional therapy is required, referral for ophthalmological care is necessary.
7. Refer to an allergist or ophthalmologist if unresponsive (corneal abrasions, impaired vision, need for corticosteroids, severe keratoconjunctivitis, or atypical manifestations).
8. Maintain a high threshold of suspicion for herpes-induced blepharitis or keratitis.

BLEPHARITIS

Description

Blepharitis is an acute or chronic inflammation of the eyelash follicles and meibomian glands of the eyelids (Table 29-9). It is usually bilateral.

Etiology

Blepharitis is commonly caused by contaminated makeup or contact lens solution. Poor hygiene and tear deficiency are also possible etiologic factors. The ulcerative form of blepharitis is usually caused by *S. aureus*. Nonulcerative blepharitis is occasionally seen in children with psoriasis, seborrhea, eczema, allergies, or lice infestation and in children with trisomy 21.

T A B L E 29-9

Common Eye Infections

CONDITION	CLINICAL FINDINGS	MANAGEMENT	PREVENTION
Blepharitis	Swelling, erythema of eyelid margins and palpebral conjunctiva, pruritus, flaking	Cleanse eyes, warm compresses, antibiotic drops or ointment	New eye makeup, clean contacts and glasses, hygiene
Hordeolum	Tender, red, swollen furuncle at eyelid margin	Warm compresses, remove eyelash, antibiotic drops or ointment	Hygiene
Chalazion	Initially, mild erythema and slight swelling; later, slow-growing, round painless mass	As for hordeolum plus treat cellulitis if present	Hygiene
Nasolacrimal duct obstruction (dacrostenosis)	Tearing or mucus, continuous or inter-mittent, blepharitis; express thin muco-purulent discharge from punctum	Daily massage, antibiotic ointment with inflammation or infection, normal saline for nasal congestion	Massage duct, minimize nasal congestion
Nasolacrimal duct infection (dacrocystitis)	Tenderness and swelling over lacrimal duct, edema and erythema of tear sac, excoriation of skin; express purulent discharge from punctum	Warm compresses, massage, oral antibiotic	As above
Periorbital cellulitis	Acute onset, pain, swelling and erythema; temperature >39°C, systemic symptoms	Outpatient systemic antibiotic therapy with close follow-up or hos-pitalization if moderate to severe infection, nonresponsive, or younger than 1 yr	HIB vaccine, hygiene, thorough cleansing of any skin disruption around eye, prompt treatment of sinusitis

HIB = *Haemophilus influenzae* type b.

Clinical Findings

The following can be seen in blepharitis:

- Swelling and erythema of the eyelid margins and palpebral conjunctiva.
- Pruritus and flaky or purulent discharge.
- Presence of lice.
- Ulcerative form: hard scales at the base of the lashes. If the crust is removed, ulcer-ation is seen at the hair follicles, the lashes fall out, and an associated conjunctivitis is present.

Management

The patient is instructed to perform the fol-lowing procedures:

1. Scrub the eyelashes and eyelids with a cot-ton-tipped applicator containing a weak (50%) solution of no-tears shampoo to main-tain proper hygiene and débride the scales.
2. Use warm compresses several times a day.
3. Apply sodium sulfacetamide 10% ophthalmic solution (1 to 2 drops into each eye twice a day) or erythromycin 0.5% ophthalmic oint-ment (¼ to ½ in. into each eye twice daily) until symptoms subside and for at least a week thereafter. Ointment is preferable to eyedrops because of increased duration of contact between the medication and ocular tissue (Baum, 1995).
4. Treat associated seborrhea, psoriasis, ec-zema, or allergies as indicated.

5. Remove contact lenses and wear eyeglasses for the duration of the treatment period. Sterilize or clean lenses before reinserting to avoid recurrence of infection.
6. Purchase new eye makeup to prevent recurrence.

HORDEOLUM

Description

Commonly called a stye, hordeolum is an infection of the sebaceous glands of the eyelash (external hordeolum) or posterior margin of the eyelid (internal hordeolum).

Etiology

The causative organism is *S. aureus.*

Clinical Findings

A tender, swollen, red furuncle is seen along the eyelid margin. The patient complains of a foreign body sensation. A hordeolum on the posterior of the eyelid margin can be inspected by rolling back the eyelid.

Management

1. Rupture often occurs spontaneously when the furuncle becomes large and a point develops. Removal of an eyelash near the furuncle frequently promotes rupture.
2. Warm, moist compresses three to four times daily, 15 minutes each time, facilitate the process of rupturing. Hygiene for the eye can be maintained by scrubbing the eyelashes and eyelids with a cotton-tipped applicator containing a weak (50%) solution of no-tears shampoo once or twice a day.
3. Sodium sulfacetamide 10% solution or ointment (1 to 2 drops or ¼ to ½ in. into each eye four times a day) or an antibiotic ophthalmic ointment (e.g., erythromycin, ¼ to ½ in. into each eye four times a day) until 2 to 3 days after resolution is effective treatment.
4. Refer for incision and drainage if the hordeolum does not rupture on its own after coming to a point.

CHALAZION

Description

Chalazion is a chronic inflammation of the eyelid resulting from obstruction of the meibomian glands that line the posterior margins of the eyelids.

Clinical Findings

- Initially, mild erythema and slight swelling of the involved eyelid are seen.
- After a few days the inflammation resolves, and a slowly growing, round, painless (*key* finding) mass remains.

Management

The following steps are taken:

1. Warm compresses are used three to four times a day for 15 minutes for 2 to 3 days. Hygiene for the eye can be maintained by scrubbing the eyelashes and eyelids with a cotton-tipped applicator containing a weak (50%) solution of no-tears shampoo once or twice a day.
2. Erythromycin ophthalmic ointment 0.5% (¼ to ½ in. into each eye four times a day) or sodium sulfacetamide 10% (1 to 2 drops or ¼ to ½ in. of ointment into each eye four times a day).
3. If cellulitis is present, erythromycin (30 to 50 mg/kg per 24 hours in divided doses every 6 to 8 hours) or cephalexin (20 to 40 mg/kg per 24 hours in divided doses every 8 hours) can be used.
4. Referral to an ophthalmologist for surgical incision or corticosteroid injections is made if the condition is unresolved after medical treatment.

Complications

Fragile, vascular granulation tissue called pyogenic granuloma that enlarges and bleeds rapidly can occur if a chalazion breaks through the conjunctival surface.

NASOLACRIMAL DUCT OBSTRUCTION: DACRYOSTENOSIS AND DACRYOCYSTITIS

Description

Nasolacrimal duct obstruction, formally known as dacryostenosis, is an abnormal stricture of the nasolacrimal duct or tear sac, usually at the nasal end. Dacryocystitis is an inflammation of the involved nasolacrimal duct.

Etiology

Nasolacrimal duct obstruction is fairly common in neonates (20% incidence in a Scottish study; Wagner, 1997). It is thought to be due to congenital failure of the duct to canalize, but it may also occur secondary to infection or trauma. Congenital failure of the duct to canalize may be unilateral or bilateral, and clinical signs appear 3 to 12 weeks after birth. When inflammation is seen, it is most commonly caused by *S. aureus,* and is often unilateral. Nasal polyps or dacrolithiasis can be the cause in older children (Darmstadt, 1997).

Clinical Findings

The following are seen:

- Continuous or intermittent tearing and mucoid discharge at the inner canthus that can become purulent
- Blepharitis in lids and lashes
- Occasional nasal obstruction and drainage
- Expression of thin mucopurulent exudate from the punctum lacrimale

The following additional symptoms may be noted if inflammation is present:

- Tenderness and swelling over the lacrimal duct
- Edema and erythema of the tear sac
- Excoriation of the surrounding skin
- Fever
- Expression of purulent material

Laboratory Studies

A white blood cell (WBC) count (elevated) and cultures are obtained if the inflammation is severe.

Management

Treatment of *dacrostenosis* is as follows:

1. Duct blockage usually resolves spontaneously, 80 to 90% by 9 to 12 months of age (Zwaan, 1999; Wagner, 1997). Treatment consists of minimizing stagnation in the tear duct and avoiding infection.
2. Daily massage may be performed to facilitate canalization of the duct by gently, but firmly stroking the skin over the medial aspect of the eyelids and lacrimal sac with 10 straight downward motions toward the nose four times daily.
3. A topical ophthalmic ointment such as 0.5% erythromycin may be prescribed (¼ to ½ in. into each eye four times a day) until the inflammation clears and at the first sign of infection.
4. Saline drops into the nose, followed by aspiration before feeding and at bedtime, helps relieve any concurrent nasal congestion.
5. Refer children with persistent nasolacrimal duct obstruction to an ophthalmologist for evaluation and possible duct probing. The timing of probing is controversial, with some ophthalmologists preferring as early as 4 months of age and others opting to wait until 9 to 12 months. The disadvantage of waiting is that general anesthesia may be required (Zwaan, 1999; Kassoff & Meyer, 1995).

If *dacrocystitis* occurs, the following actions are indicated:

1. Warm compresses four times a day
2. Continued lacrimal sac massage as described above
3. Topical antibiotics with the addition of an oral antistaphylococcal antibiotic that treats for β-lactamase resistance

Complications

Periorbital or orbital cellulitis is a complication of dacrocystitis.

PERIORBITAL CELLULITIS

Description

Periorbital cellulitis, or inflammation of the tissues surrounding the involved eye, is often associated with trauma or focal infection near the eye, bacteremia, or sinusitis.

Etiology

Most common in children younger than 2 years in conjunction with bacteremia, periorbital cellulitis also occurs with infected lacerations, abrasions, insect stings or bites, impetigo, or a foreign body. It may also be secondary to inflammation and edema from frontal, maxillary, and ethmoid sinusitis. The etiology is often unknown, but the bacterium most commonly responsible for periorbital cellulitis is *S. pneumoniae. S. aureus, Streptococcus pyogenes,* and *H. influenzae* type b are other bacterial possibilities (Zwaan, 1999; Powell, 1995; Malinow & Powell, 1993). The infection is usually unilateral (90 to 95%), although 5% of cases can be bilateral (Powell, 1995).

Clinical Findings

The following may be noted:

- Acute onset
- Swelling and erythema of tissues surrounding the eye
- Discomfort
- Temperature higher than 39°C if associated with bacteremia
- Deep red color of the eyelid or purple blue with *H. influenzae* infection
- Symptoms of bacteremia or sinusitis

LABORATORY STUDIES. Depending on the severity of the cellulitis, the following can be done:

- CBC with differential (WBC count usually >15,000 if bacteremic)
- Blood cultures and culture of purulent wounds near the eye
- Lumbar puncture (infants younger than 1 year)
- CT scan to rule out sinusitis, orbital cellulitis, abscess, or proptosis
- Visual acuity, extraocular movement, and pupillary reaction testing

Differential Diagnosis

Conjunctivitis (bilateral conjunctival inflammation), cavernous thrombosis, and orbital cellulitis (proptosis, limited extraocular movement, and reduced visual acuity) are the differential diagnoses.

Management

The child may be managed as an outpatient if the cellulitis is mild, the orbit is not involved, and the child is not in a toxic state. Otherwise, hospitalization and intravenous antibiotics are required.

1. Outpatient management begins with ceftriaxone (50 to 75 mg/kg [up to a maximum of 1 g] intramuscularly divided every 12 hours). The child is monitored daily until blood cultures are negative for 48 hours or clinical improvement is seen. Oral antibiotics may then be used to complete a 7- to 14-day course. Amoxicillin with clavulanic acid or cefaclor are first-line choices for treatment, with trimethoprim-sulfamethoxazole or erythromycin as alternatives (Loch-Donahue & Donahue, 1997). If a rapid clinical response is not seen, further evaluation and treatment should be done. Warm soaks to the periorbital area every 2 to 4 hours for 15 minutes may provide comfort and speed healing. The parent is advised to call immediately upon any change in condition.
2. Hospitalization and intravenous administration of nafcillin, chloramphenicol, or cefuroxime, followed by a 10-day course of oral antibiotics, are required for the following:
   - Moderate to severe cases of cellulitis.
   - A poor response to outpatient management.
   - A purulent wound near the eyelid.
   - Infants younger than 1 year.
   - Children with suspected meningitis.
3. Consultation is needed when proptosis, ophthalmoplegia, or changes in visual acuity occur; these conditions are suggestive of more extensive infection involving the orbit.

Complications

Complications include the following: orbital cellulitis or extension of the infection into the orbit, subperiosteal or orbital abscess, optic neuritis, retinal vein thrombosis, panophthalmitis, meningitis, epidural and subdural abscesses, and cavernous sinus thrombosis.

KERATITIS AND CORNEAL ULCERS

Description

Keratitis, or inflammation of the cornea, can cause a dramatic alteration in visual acuity and can progress to corneal ulceration and blindness. A corneal ulcer begins as a well-defined infiltration at the center or edge of the cornea and subsequently suppurates and forms an ulcer that may penetrate deep into the corneal tissue or spread to involve the width of the cornea. Involvement is usually unilateral.

Etiology and Incidence

The most common cause of keratitis is HSV-1, although other viruses, as well as bacteria and fungi, may be responsible (Baum, 1995). The most common risk factor for keratitis is trauma, although an allergic reaction, conjunctivitis, a systemic infection, and the use of corticosteroids are other less common causes (Clinch et al., 1994).

Clinical Findings

Symptoms vary in intensity according to the depth and extent of ulceration. The following are reported or seen:

- Exposure to an infected individual
- History of illness, eye trauma, foreign body, or the use of antibiotics
- Vesicles on the skin or eyelids and herpes lesions elsewhere on body
- Severe pain, sensation of a foreign body, and photophobia
- Tearing, erythema, and spasms of the eyelid
- Pus in the anterior chamber
- Loss of the anterior substance of the cornea (irregular surface) with surrounding opaque gray or white necrotic areas
- Area staining green with a fluorescein strip (if herpes, a dendritic ulcer is seen)

Management

When a corneal ulcer is suspected, the child should be referred immediately. Delay can re-

sult in loss of vision in the eye. A patch is never placed over an eye thought to have an infection.

1. Preliminary treatment of keratitis or mild superficial bacterial ulcers is bacitracin, 500 u/g (¼ to ½ in. into the lower conjunctival sac two to four times per day). Referral for ophthalmological care is necessary.
2. Steroids should never be used.
3. If herpes simplex is suspected, immediate referral is necessary. Treatment with antivirals such as trifluridine or vidarabine may be used to speed healing.

Complications

Corneal opacification, scarring, and loss of vision can occur if treatment is delayed.

INFLAMMATION OF THE UVEAL TRACT

Description

Inflammation of the uveal tract—the iris, the ciliary body, and the choroid—is often called uveitis. The inflammation may be anterior (affecting the iris, ciliary body, or both) or posterior (affecting the choroid). Adjacent ocular structures (retina, vitreous, and optic nerve) may also be involved.

Etiology

The etiology is often unknown, but viral or bacterial infection is a likely cause. Uveitis may also occur with ocular trauma and infection elsewhere in the eye, as well as with allergy, dental abscess, and systemic diseases such as juvenile or psoriatic arthritis, inflammatory bowel, Kawasaki syndrome, herpes zoster, tuberculosis, diabetes, and the collagen diseases (Siegel, 1995; Persaud et al., 1993). The inflammation may be acute or chronic.

Clinical Findings

The following may be noted:

- Acute onset of pain (*key* finding)
- Excessive tearing and eyelid edema

- Conjunctival erythema
- Photophobia and blurred or decreased vision (*key* findings)
- Circumcorneal injection
- Hypopyon (pus layer in the bottom of the anterior chamber)
- Cloudy appearance of the eye with a bulging iris and a contracted, irregular, or fixed pupil
- If chronic, no ocular pain, photophobia, redness, or tearing

Differential Diagnosis

Conjunctivitis is the differential diagnosis.

Management

1. Evaluate and treat any underlying systemic disease.
2. Refer the patient to an ophthalmologist. A definitive diagnosis is made by slit-lamp examination. The prognosis is improved with early treatment, and delay may result in scarring of the pupil with cataract formation or the development of glaucoma.
3. Cycloplegics and topical corticosteroids (depending on the cause of the inflammation) are often used in treatment. Mydriatics are used regularly to prevent posterior synechiae.
4. Nonsteroidal anti-inflammatory agents are used as an adjunct to treatment.

Complications

Anterior and posterior synechiae, changes in intraocular pressure, and corneal edema are possible complications.

TRACHOMA

Description

A chronic infectious disease of the eye, trachoma is characterized by follicular keratoconjunctivitis with neovascularization of the cornea.

Etiology and Incidence

Trachoma is caused by *Chlamydia trachomatis* and is endemic in hot, dry, poverty-stricken areas. It is rare in the United States but can cause blindness from local scarring (AAP, 1997).

Clinical Findings

The following are noted:

- Inflammation
- Pain
- Photophobia
- Excessive tearing
- Granulation follicles on the upper eyelids and eventual invasion of the cornea causing blindness

Management

1. Consult with an ophthalmologist because treatment is difficult and recommendations vary.
2. Treat with systemic tetracycline, erythromycin, or topical sulfacetamide ointment twice a day for 2 months or twice a day for the first 5 days of the month for 6 months (AAP, 1997).
3. Give oral doxycycline (if older than 9 years) or erythromycin for 40 days.
4. Reinforce frequent handwashing and careful cleansing of the eyes. Discourage sharing of towels and handkerchiefs.

Emergency Care of the Injured Eye

CORNEAL INJURY

Description

Damage to the epithelial lining of the cornea in the form of a corneal abrasion (Table 29-10) or tear is relatively common. Scratches from paper, brushes, fingernails, or a foreign body in the conjunctival sac are often responsible.

Clinical Findings

The following may be noted:

- Evidence and sensation of a foreign body
- Severe pain and photophobia
- Tearing and blepharospasm
- Decreased vision
- Conjunctival erythema

T A B L E 29-10
Common Eye Injuries

INJURY	CLINICAL FINDINGS	TREATMENT
Corneal injury (abrasion)	Sensation or evidence of foreign body, pain, photophobia, tearing and blepharospasm, decreased vision, positive fluorescein staining	Rest and patch for 24 hr, topical antibiotics and cycloplegics, oral analgesics, follow-up in 24 hr
Foreign body	Vertical striation on cornea, pain, tearing, sensation of foreign body, irregular or peaked pupil, perforating wound	*Do not* remove intraocular foreign body; irrigate eye to remove; topical antibiotic and patch for 5–7 d
Burns Chemical Thermal UV radiation	Pale, necrotic appearance to skin and eyelids, opaque cornea, visual impairment, photophobia, tearing, pain with UV injury only	*Chemical:* emergency; continuous irrigation for 20–30 min; to ophthalmologist with ongoing irrigation *Thermal:* as for abrasion *UV:* topical antibiotic, patch, analgesics; heal in 1–2 d
Hyphema	Pain, tearing, photophobia; blood in anterior chamber, hazy iris, or inability to detect red reflex; change in visual acuity	Refer to ophthalmologist; restrict intake, place eye shield; increased risk if child has sickle cell trait or disease

UV = ultraviolet.

OTHER STUDIES. Fluorescein staining with superficial uptake is indicative of a minor corneal abrasion. If the fluorescein staining goes deep into the cornea, subepithelial corneal damage (e.g., corneal ulceration or a corneal tear) is possible. Vertical striations on the cornea suggest a foreign body embedded under the eyelid.

Management

The following steps are taken:

1. Refer severe corneal injuries or possible subepithelial damage to an ophthalmologist.
2. Prescribe rest and patching for 24 to 48 hours for mild injuries. The patch should be snug to hold the eye closed. Reexamine in 24 hours and repatch if not healed.
3. Use elbow restraints for the infant to ensure that the patch remains in place.
4. Topical antibiotics (sulfacetamide, 10%, should be used three to four times a day for 5 days).
5. Topical cycloplegic (1% atropine) may be used with caution to decrease pain.
6. Oral analgesics may be used to ease the discomfort.
7. Repeated instillation of local anesthetic is

not recommended because it interferes with reepithelialization of the cornea.

8. Advise the patient to return daily for follow-up evaluation. If no improvement is seen after 48 to 72 hours or if symptoms worsen, refer to an ophthalmologist.

FOREIGN BODY

Description

A superficial foreign body in the eye is usually lodged in the surface of the eye or superficially in the cornea. It rarely results in serious trauma.

Etiology

Foreign bodies commonly occur in younger children during play and in older children during sports. Common foreign bodies include BB gun pellets and debris thrown up by a lawnmower or in shop class.

Clinical Findings

The following may be noted:

- Pain and foreign body sensation
- Tearing

- Irregular or peaked pupil
- Opaque lens
- Perforating wound to the cornea or iris

OTHER STUDIES. Fluorescence staining may be useful if no foreign body is visualized. Radiographs may be needed, depending on the foreign body and its location.

Management

Recommendations include the following:

1. Never remove an intraocular foreign body. Refer immediately to an ophthalmologist.
2. Remove an extraocular foreign body via irrigation with sterile saline (eversion of the eyelid facilitates visualization).
3. A moistened cotton swab is *not* recommended as a means to remove a foreign body from the surface of the cornea because it can cause considerable additional damage to the epithelial surface.
4. Use of a topical anesthetic facilitates patient cooperation.
5. If any difficulty is encountered when removing a foreign body from the eye, stop all efforts, patch the eye, and refer the patient immediately to an ophthalmologist.
6. After removal of the foreign body, an ophthalmic antibiotic solution is instilled and an eye patch applied for 5 to 7 days.

Complications

Sympathetic ophthalmia, a uveitis of the uninjured eye, can occur any time from 10 days to years after a penetrating injury of the globe.

BURNS

Etiology

Burns to the eyes and surrounding tissues can be thermal (caused by exposure to steam, intense heat, cinders, or cigarettes) or chemical (such as cleaning agents or laboratory products) or induced by UV light (such as from bright snow, laser pointers, or a sunlamp). The amount of damage to the eye is directly related to the length of exposure to the source of the burn. Chemical burns are true emergencies because of the progressive damage that can occur. Burns on the eyelids are classified and treated the same as burns elsewhere on the body.

Clinical Findings

The following may be noted:

- Pale or necrosed appearance of the surrounding skin and eyelids
- Opacity of corneal tissue
- Visual impairment (decreased acuity)
- Absence of complaints of pain, except in UV burns, where pain emerges about 6 hours after exposure
- Photophobia
- Tearing within 12 hours of exposure
- Swollen corneas
- Fluorescein stain revealing pinpoint uptake

Management

The following steps are taken:

1. *Chemical burns* require immediate, ongoing irrigation with a steady, gentle solution of saline, weak boric acid, or water for 20 to 30 minutes with the eyelids held apart. Topical anesthesia may be used to ease patient discomfort. Refer to an ophthalmologist after irrigation to determine the extent of damage. Do not patch the eye; allow tearing to continue to cleanse the eye. Cool compresses applied to the surrounding skin may be comforting. Hospitalization may be needed for sedation and analgesia.
2. *Thermal burns* are treated the same way as corneal injuries (see the earlier section): antibiotic ointment, saline soaks, and artificial tears.
3. *UV burns* are treated by using topical antibiotic prophylaxis, patches, and analgesics. Healing should occur in 1 to 2 days.

LACERATIONS

Management

Apply an eye shield to protect the eye. Refer the patient immediately to an ophthalmologist to rule out damage to the globe and surrounding structures and to a plastic surgeon for closure of the laceration.

HYPHEMA

Description

A hyphema is an accumulation of visible blood or blood products in the anterior chamber of the eye.

Etiology and Incidence

A hyphema is the result of blunt trauma to the globe, most often caused by balls, fists, and sticks. It may also occur secondary to birth trauma or in patients with abnormal hematological profiles such as sickle cell trait or disease (Hertle & Bacal, 1997; Behrman et al., 1996). Hyphema is the most common contusion injury to the eye seen in children. It is responsible for more hospitalizations than any other ophthalmological condition. Hyphema is the leading cause of permanent impairment in sports-related eye trauma (Hertle & Bacal, 1997) and occurs with other ocular injuries 25% of the time (Hoffman, 1997).

Clinical Findings

Vision, pupil motility, the lids and adnexa, the cornea and anterior segment, and the red reflex should all be assessed. The following may be noted:

- History of traumatic eye injury
- Somnolence (often associated with intracranial trauma)
- Blood in the anterior chamber on gross examination (hazy-appearing iris and/or an inability to detect a bilateral red reflex)
- Pain, photophobia, and tearing
- Visual acuity changes and impaired vision (light perception and hand motion perception)
- Abnormal pupillary reflex
- Need for slit-lamp examination

Management

The goals of treatment include resolving the hyphema, making the patient comfortable, and preventing complications; however, no consensus has been reached on how to best accomplish such treatment (e.g., hospitalization or not, systemic medication or not, which medications). However, the following steps should be taken:

1. Refer the patient immediately to an ophthalmologist.
2. Restrict oral intake until the child has been seen by an ophthalmologist.
3. Assume that any patient with a traumatic hyphema has a ruptured globe until proved otherwise (Hertle & Bacal, 1997). Place an eye shield (not a patch) over the eye—avoid pressure.
4. If a hematological disorder is detected, ensure quick intervention and close follow-up.
5. Reduce activity for several days (quiet indoor activities only) or hospitalize. Elevate the head of the bed to 35 degrees. Encourage the child to sleep in a supine position. Discourage reading or close eye work during this period.
6. Bilateral patching may be recommended.
7. Cycloplegic drops (1% atropine) may be prescribed to immobilize the ciliary body.
8. Steroids may be used to reduce the chance of glaucoma, rebleed, or corneal blood staining.
9. Acetaminophen (Tylenol) is the analgesic of choice; aspirin and nonsteroidal anti-inflammatory agents are to be avoided.
10. Prophylactic use of antifibrinolytic agents to reduce secondary hemorrhage is recommended by some.
11. Surgery may be necessary to remove the trapped blood from the chamber if it is causing an increase in intraocular pressure.
12. Close and long-term follow-up by an ophthalmologist is needed to monitor for traumatic cataract, retinal detachment, or glaucoma.

COMPLICATIONS. A second hemorrhage can occur within 5 to 7 days of the first (in 3 to 38% of cases; Hertle & Bacal, 1997; Hoffman, 1997). Glaucoma, amblyopia, or both can develop and result in visual loss. Patients with abnormal hematological profiles are more likely to rebleed and are more likely to have visual loss because of glaucoma (Hoffman, 1997).

RETINAL DETACHMENT

Description

Retinal detachment is detachment of the retina from its base within the globe.

Etiology

Frequently associated with severe ocular trauma or child abuse, retinal detachment also occurs as a congenital abnormality or with pronounced myopia, aphakia, cataracts, or ROP.

Clinical Findings

The following may be noted:

- Blurry vision that becomes progressively worse
- Dark cloud in one visual field, flashing lights, or a "shower of floaters"
- Darkening of retinal vessels on funduscopic examination
- Gray elevation at the site of detachment

Management

Instruct the patient not to eat, and refer the patient to an ophthalmologist for surgery to reattach the retina.

ORBITAL HEMATOMA/CONTUSION OF THE GLOBE

Clinical Findings

The following may be seen:

- Visual acuity changes
- Severe bruising of the eyelids and periorbital tissues
- Lens dislocation
- Retinal detachment or edema
- Vitreous, retinal, or choroid hemorrhage
- Rupture of the eyeball

Management

The following steps are taken:

1. Refer the patient immediately to an ophthalmologist.
2. Rule out closed head injury, damage to the skull, and facial bone fractures.
3. Prescribe cold compresses for the first 48 hours to reduce the swelling and bleeding.
4. Prescribe warm packs after 48 hours to promote reabsorption of extravasated blood.
5. Occasionally, surgery is needed for contusions of the globe.

ORBITAL FRACTURES

Description

A blowout fracture occurs when damage to the floor of the orbit causes the orbital contents to herniate and become entrapped in the area of the fracture.

Etiology

The usual cause of an orbital fracture is a blow or blunt trauma to the orbit with a ball or a fist (Coody et al., 1997).

Clinical Findings

The following may be noted:

- Pain, diplopia
- Loss of sensation along the path of the infraorbital nerve (upper lip and ipsilateral cheek)
- Ecchymosis of the lids, nosebleed, trouble chewing
- Limited ocular movement (especially upward) and weakness in downward movement
- Globe displacement with a sunken-eye appearance or a protruding eye
- Bony discontinuity or "step-off"
- Subcutaneous emphysema in surrounding tissues
- Enophthalmos

RESOURCE BOX 29-1

American Academy of Ophthalmology
Tel: (415) 561-8500
Website: www.eyenet.org
Pamphlets and other information, including "Eye safety for children: Prevention is the best medicine"

American Council of the Blind
Tel: (800) 424-8666, (202) 467-5081
Website: www.acb.org
Informational materials, referrals to local resources, local chapters

American Foundation for the Blind
Tel: (800) 232-5463, (212) 502-7600
Website: www.afb.org/
Newsletter, informational materials, referrals to local resources, local chapters, fund research

American National Standards Institute
11 West 42nd St
New York, NY 10036
Information on standards for eye protection

American Optometric Association
Tel: (800) 262-2210
www.aoanet.org

Blepharophimosis, Ptosis, Epicanthus Inversus Support Group
Tel: (509) 332-6628
Newsletter, networking; maintain research registry

Blind Children's Center
Tel: (800) 222-3566, (800) 222-3567 (CA only)
Website: www.blindcntr.org/bcc
Newsletter, information materials (including Spanish), referrals to local resources, networking

National Association for Visually Handicapped
Tel: (212) 889-3141
Website: www.navh.org
Information, referrals, catalog of large-print books to borrow and low-vision aids

National Eye Institute
Tel: (301) 496-5248
Website: www.nei.nih.gov
Speak with an eye specialist, order information including research updates, or visit a website with a searchable database and ongoing clinical trials information

National Organization of Parents of Blind Children
Tel: (410) 659-9314
Newsletter, informational materials, referrals to local resources, local chapters, advocacy

National Society to Prevent Blindness
Tel: (708) 843-2020
Brochure, poster, flyers, packets

The Lighthouse
Tel: (800) 334-5497
Information, referrals, catalog with large-print books and low-vision aids

---

Diagnostic Studies

CT is the best imaging modality

Management

1. An orbital fracture is an ophthalmologic emergency requiring immediate intervention. Diagnostic studies are performed to rule out injury to the skull and cranial contents. Open reduction may be necessary if any of the orbital bones are displaced or to rule out displacement of the globe or enophthalmos.
2. Icing the injury for 24 hours, followed by heat for 2 to 3 days, allows the swelling to subside before surgical repair. Surgery is often best done within 2 weeks of the injury.

3. Antibiotics are used if contamination from sinus contents is a possibility.

REFERENCES

Abramson DH: Retinoblastoma. *In* Finberg L (ed): Saunders Manual of Pediatric Practice. Philadelphia, WB Saunders, 1998.

American Academy of Ophthalmology: Indications for a comprehensive eye evaluation by an ophthalmologist. *In* Preferred Practice Patterns. San Francisco, American Academy of Ophthalmology, 1997a.

American Academy of Ophthalmology: Pediatric eye evaluation screening recommendations. *In* Preferred Practice Patterns. San Francisco, American Academy of Ophthalmology, 1997b.

American Academy of Optometry, American Optometric Association: Vision, learning and dyslexia. J Am Optom Assoc 68:284–286, 1997.

American Academy of Pediatrics: Learning disabilities, dyslexia, and vision: A subject review. Pediatrics 102:1217–1219, 1998.

American Academy of Pediatrics: 1997 Red Book: Report of the Committee on Infectious Diseases, 24th ed. Elk Grove Village, IL, American Academy of Pediatrics, 1997.

American Academy of Pediatrics: Protective eyewear for young adults. Pediatrics 98:311–313, 1996.

American Academy of Pediatrics, American Association of Pediatric Ophthalmology and Strabismus, American Academy of Ophthalmology: Screening examination of premature infants for retinopathy of prematurity. Pediatrics 100:273, 1997.

Anderson PD: Basic Human Anatomy and Physiology: Clinical Implications for the Health Professions. Boston, Jones & Bartlett, 1984.

Bacal DA, Hertle KW: Don't be lazy about looking for amblyopia. Contemp Pediatr 15(6):99–107, 1998.

Baum J: Infections of the eye. Clin Infect Dis 21:479–486, 1995.

Behrman RE, Kliegman R, Arvin AM (eds): Nelson Textbook of Pediatrics, 15th ed. Philadelphia, WB Saunders, 1996.

Bodor RR: Systemic antibiotics for the treatment of the conjunctivitis–otitis media syndrome. Pediatr Infect Dis J 8:287, 1989.

Bodor RR: Conjunctivitis–otitis syndrome. Pediatrics 69:695–698, 1982.

Burke MJ: Strabismus. *In* Finberg L (ed): Saunders Manual of Pediatric Practice. Philadelphia, WB Saunders, 1998, pp 953–955.

Calhoun JH: Eye examinations in infants & children. Pediatr Rev 18(1):28–31, 1997.

Castiglia PT: Strabismus. J Pediatr Health Care 8:236–238, 1994.

Catalano JD: Strabismus. Pediatr Ann 19:292, 292–297, 1990.

Centers for Disease Control and Prevention: 1998 Guidelines for the treatment of sexually transmitted diseases. MMWR Morb Mortal Wkly Rep 47(RR-1):1–111, 1998.

Clinch TE, Palmon FE, Robinson MJ, et al: Microbial keratitis in children. Am J Ophthalmol 117:65–71, 1994.

Coody D, Banks JM, Yetman RF, et al: Eye trauma in children: Epidemiology, management and prevention. J Pediatr Health Care 11:182–188, 1997.

Darmstadt GL: A guide to superficial strep and staph skin infections. Contemp Pediatr 14(5):95–116, 1997.

Finegold I: Successful management of ocular allergy with atopic diseases. Presented at the American College of Allergy, Asthma and Immunology meeting, Philadelphia, Nov 6–11, 1998.

Food and Drug Administration: FDA issues warning on misuse of laser pointers. http://www.fda.gov/bbs/topics/NEWS/NEW00609.html. Press release P97-45, Dec 18, 1997.

Gabriels R: Vision therapy: A controversial therapy for children with dyslexia. Personal communication, 1998.

Gigliotti F: Acute conjunctivitis. Pediatr Rev 16(6):203–207, 1995.

Hertle RW, Bacal D: Traumatic hyphema: Evaluation and management. Contemp Pediatr 14(1):51–68, 1997.

Hoffman RO: Evaluating and treating eye injuries. Contemp Pediatr 14(4):74–98, 1997.

Jarvis C: Physical Examination and Health Assessment, 2nd ed. Philadelphia, WB Saunders, 1996.

Kassoff J, Meyer DR: Early office-based vs late hospital-based nasolacrimal duct probing. A clinical decision analysis. Arch Ophthalmol 113:1168–1171, 1995.

Loch-Donahue J, Donahue SP: Orbital and peri-orbital cellulitis. *In* Finberg L (ed): Saunders Manual of Pediatric Practice. Philadelphia, WB Saunders, 1997, pp 957–959.

Lohr JA: Treatment of conjunctivitis in infants and children. Pediatr Ann 22:359–364, 1993.

MacDonald MA: Refractive errors and corrective lenses in children and adolescents. J Pediatr Health Care 10(3):121–123, 1996.

Malinow I, Powell K: Periorbital cellulitis. Pediatr Ann 22:241–246, 1993.

Nelson L: Disorders of the Eye. *In* Behrman RE, Kliegman RM, Arvin AM (eds): Nelson Textbook of Pediatrics, 15th ed. Philadelphia, WB Saunders, 1996, pp 1764–1803.

Newell FW: Ophthalmology Principles and Concepts. St Louis, CV Mosby, 1996.

Persaud D, Moss W, Munoz J: Serious eye infections in children. Pediatr Ann 22:379–383, 1993.

Phelps DL: Retinopathy of prematurity. Pediatr Rev 16(2):50–56, 1995.

Powell KR: Orbital and periorbital cellulitis. Pediatr Rev 16(5):163–167, 1995.

Preller MB: Super vision: How to make sure your child's eyesight develops according to the charts. Healthy Kids, 5(5):45–51, 1998.

Raizman M: Pathophysiology and differential diagnosis of ocular allergy. Presented at the American College of Allergy, Asthma and Immunology meeting, Philadelphia, Nov 6–11, 1998.

Schalij-Delfos NE, Zijlmans BL, Wittebol-Post D, et al: Screening for retinopathy of prematurity: Do former guidelines still apply? J Pediatr Ophthalmol Strabismus 33:35–38, 1996.

Siegel DM: Uveitis. Pediatr Rev 16(12):477–478, 1995.

Stevens JL: Retinopathy of prematurity. *In* Finberg L (ed): Saunders Manual of Pediatric Practice. Philadelphia, WB Saunders, 1998.

US Department of Health and Human Services: Healthy People 2010 Objectives: Draft for Public Comment: Child and Adolescent Focused Objectives. Washington, DC, US Department of Health and Human Services, 1998. http://web.health.gov/healthypeople.

US Department of Health and Human Services: Healthy People 2000: National Health Promotion and Disease Prevention Objectives for the Year 2000. Washington, DC, US Department of Health and Human Services, 1990.

US Preventive Services Task Force: Guide to Clinical Preventive Services, 2nd ed. Baltimore, Williams & Wilkins, 1996.

US Public Health Service: Put Prevention into Practice: The Clinician's Handbook of Preventive Services, 2nd ed. Germantown, MD, International Medical Publishing, 1997.

Wagner RS: Eye infections and abnormalities: Issues for the pediatrician. Contemp Pediatr 14(6):137-153, 1997.

Wagner RS: Why children must wear sunglasses. Contemp Pediatr 12(6):27-37, 1995.

Wagner RS: Do the eyes have it? Contemp Pediatr 10(1), 1993.

West CE: Retinoblastoma. *In* Finberg L (ed): Saunders Manual of Pediatric Practice. Philadelphia, WB Saunders, 1998, pp 967-968.

Wheeler LC, Griffin HC, Taylor JR, et al: Educational intervention strategies for children with visual impairment with emphasis on retinopathy of prematurity. J Pediatr Health Care 11(6):275-279, 1997.

Yetman RJ, Coody DK: Conjunctivitis: A practice guideline. J Pediatr Health Care 11:238-241, 1997.

Zwaan J (ed): Eye problems. *In* Dershewitz RA (ed): Ambulatory Pediatric Care, 3rd ed. Philadelphia, Lippincott-Raven, 1999, pp 526-565.

CHAPTER 30

Ear Disorders

Ann M. Petersen-Smith

INTRODUCTION

The ear provides the body with the ability to hear and maintain equilibrium. Appropriate functioning of the ear is essential for hearing, acquisition of speech, and the ability to maintain an upright position. The ear extends from the external to the inner ear structures. Malfunction of any of the structures of the ear can have an impact on both the ear and surrounding tissue. Additionally, ear dysfunction can cause systemic problems that can have a lifelong impact. Adequate hearing is important to learning, socialization, and language development. Caring for children with ear problems is an important role of the nurse practitioner (NP), and understanding of ear anatomy, physiology, and disorders allows the NP to thoughtfully assess the system and its functions.

STANDARDS FOR HEARING SCREENING

Universal detection of hearing loss before 3 months of age is endorsed by the American Academy of Pediatrics (AAP) Task Force on Newborn and Infant Hearing (AAP, 1999), Healthy People 2010 (US Department of Health and Human Services, 1998), the Joint Committee on Infant Hearing (1995), and the National Institutes of Health (NIH) (NIH Consensus Statement, 1993). This recommendation includes follow-up by 3 months of age and appropriate intervention by 6 months of age. Screening of newborns or infants can be done by using evoked otoacoustical emission testing or the auditory brain stem response. The *Guide to Clinical Preventive Services* (US Preventive Services Task Force, 1996), however, states that evidence is insufficient to recommend for or against routine screening of asymptomatic newborns, but it does agree with the need for predischarge screening of newborns who have one or more neonatal risk criteria.

During childhood, routine screening of asymptomatic children older than 3 years is debated. The *Guide to Clinical Preventive Services* (US Preventive Services Task Force, 1996) does not recommend screening beyond 3 years of age or in adolescence. However, the Joint Committee on Infant Hearing, the AAP, and Bright Futures all recommend pure tone audiometry at 3, 4, 5, 10, 12, 15, and 18 years of age, with subjective assessment at other ages (US Public Health Service, 1997). The American Speech-Language-Hearing Association recommends annual pure tone audiometry from age 3 to grade 3 (US Public Health Service, 1997). Screening of high-risk children including those with frequently recurring otitis media (OM), middle ear effusion, or both, or those with chronic exposure to loud noises, should include annual audiological screening and monitoring the development of communication skills.

DEVELOPMENT, ANATOMY, AND PHYSIOLOGY

Development

Development of the ear begins during the third week of gestation and is complete by the third month of embryonic life. Insult to the fetus during this time can cause irreparable damage to the ear. Ear development occurs at the same time as kidney development, so malformation or dysfunction in one system should alert the practitioner to problems in the other.

Anatomy and Physiology

The external ear is responsible for transmission of sound waves from outside the ear to the middle ear and for clearance of debris. The canal contains glands that secrete sweat, sebum, and cerumen, which help lubricate the hair follicles and aid in the removal of debris. Patency of the ear canal is imperative for proper functioning.

The tympanic cavity constitutes the middle ear. The tympanic membrane is at the proximal end of the external auditory canal and separates the external ear from the middle ear. The middle ear is a small chamber in the temporal bone that contains the ossicles—the malleus, incus, and stapes—which function to transmit sound waves from the external auditory canal to the inner ear. The malleus lies against the tympanic membrane, which vibrates when sound waves hit it. The stapes rests against the oval window, and its vibration causes the oval window to stimulate the fluids of the inner ear.

The eustachian tube has three physiological functions with respect to the middle ear: (1) ventilation of the middle ear to equalize air pressure in the middle ear with atmospheric pressure and to replace oxygen that has been absorbed; (2) protection from nasopharyngeal sound, pressure, and secretions; and (3) drainage of secretions from the middle ear into the nasopharynx.

The inner ear functions to transmit sound and aid in balance. Vibrations of the tympanic membrane, ossicles, and oval window set the inner ear fluids in motion. The fluid sound waves reach the cochlea, wherein lies the organ of Corti, which contains the hearing receptor hair cells. The hair cells transmit impulses to the cochlear nerve (cranial nerve II), which transmits stimuli to the auditory cortex of the temporal lobe in the brain. The equilibrium receptors lie in the semicircular canals and vestibule of the inner ear. The semicircular canals respond to changes in direction of movement. The vestibule contains receptors essential to the maintenance of equilibrium (Fig. 30-1).

PATHOPHYSIOLOGY AND DEFENSE MECHANISMS

Pathophysiology

The processes that negatively affect the ear are usually localized; however, ear pathology can be related to systemic dysfunction or disorders. Common localized pathology includes disruption of defense mechanisms; viral, bacterial, or fungal infections in the inner, middle, and outer ear; foreign bodies in the ear; and trauma. Neurological dysfunction, poor immunological competence, and congenital anomalies are common systemic disorders that can affect the ear and its functions. External influences such as excessive noise in the environment can cause irreparable damage to the ear's hearing function.

Defense Mechanisms

Debris formed by keratinizing cells in the ear is lubricated and extruded by the cilia in the external auditory canal. Maintenance of an acidic pH in the ear canal prevents the growth of pathogenic bacteria. Additionally, the surface lining of the external ear is water resistant and has ample blood and lymph supply. These characteristics, as well as the antibacterial properties of cerumen, help protect against invading microorganisms. In comparison to the distal end of the external auditory canal, the proximal end has fewer hair fibers, a thinner epithelial layer, and more nerve fibers that cause great

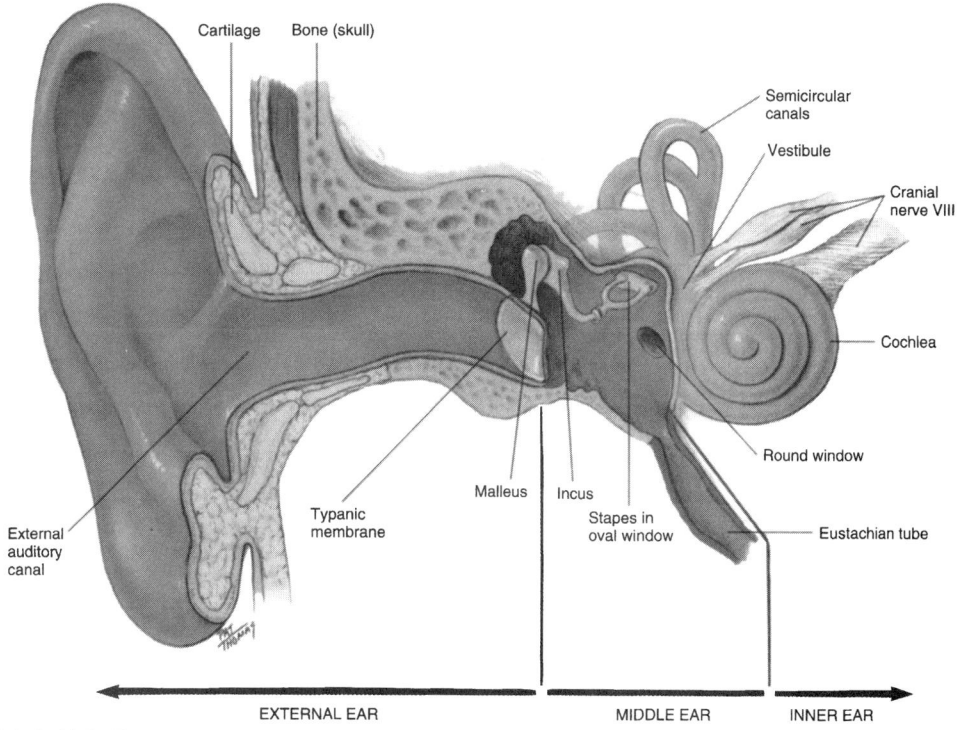

F I G U R E 30-1
Anatomy of the ear. (From Jarvis C: Physical Examination and Health Assessment, 2nd ed. Philadelphia, WB Saunders, 1996, p 365.)

discomfort when touched. This sensitivity to pain serves a protective function by deterring the insertion of foreign bodies into the ear, thus avoiding damage to the middle ear.

The inner ear is also well protected inasmuch as the structures for both hearing and equilibrium are set deep within the skull.

ASSESSMENT

History

The history of a patient with an ear disorder should include the following:

- Previous medical history significant for craniofacial abnormalities or syndromes associated with craniofacial anomalies
- Pain (onset, location, quality, duration, alleviating or aggravating factors)
- Associated symptoms such as fever, vom-

iting and diarrhea, nasal congestion, or other symptoms of upper respiratory infection
- Itching or discharge
- Tinnitus or hearing loss
- Past medical history pertinent to the ear
- Family history of ear dysfunction
- Craniofacial abnormality (cleft lip/palate) or syndrome associated with craniofacial abnormality (Down syndrome, Treacher Collins syndrome)
- Prematurity
- Exposure to risk factors: environmental tobacco smoke (ETS), bottle propping, day care, noise, swimming

Physical Examination

The physical examination includes:

- Inspection of the external structures of the ear for symmetry, skin abnormalities, discharge, or lesions. The inner and outer canthi of the eye should form a straight line with the superior portion of the pinna. If the pinna inserts below this line, the ear is said to be low set.

- Observation for developmental milestones related to hearing (Table 30–1).
- Palpation and rotation of the external ear for tenderness and inflammation; push on the tragus and apply pressure to the mastoid process.
- An otoscopic examination, which can be better accomplished in a young child at the end of the physical examination with the child on an examining table or seated on the parent's lap. Pulling the ear downward, outward, and backward can enhance visualization of the external auditory canal in infants and small children. In older children and adolescents, the external auditory canal is lifted upward and backward, slightly away from the head.

T A B L E 30-1

Developmental Milestones Used to Assess Hearing

Birth to 3 mo
  Startles (Moro reflex) to loud noise
  Awakens to sounds
  Blinks or widens eyes to noises
3–6 mo
  Quiets to parent's voice
  Stops activity to listen to new sound
  Looks for source of sound
  Reciprocates vocally and initiates sounds
6–12 mo
  Coos and gurgles with inflection
  Responds to simple phrases
  Turns to localize sound in any plane
  Responds to own name
12–18 mo
  Points to unexpected sound or familiar objects
    when asked
  Follows simple direction without cues
  Imitates some sounds, first words by 12–15
    mo
18–24 mo
  Points to body parts when asked
  Has expressive vocabulary of 20–50 words
  50% of speech intelligible to strangers

- Decreased tympanic membrane mobility secondary to effusion is noted through pneumatic otoscopy, tympanometry, or acoustical reflectometry.
- Examination of the canal for redness, edema, or discharge. Assess all 360 degrees of the tympanic membrane, the bony processes, and the cone of light. Use pneumatic otoscopy to note the position, color, gloss, and movement of the eardrum. Look for air-fluid level or bubbles behind the tympanic membrane. Note any retraction or perforation (see Color Fig. 3).

Common Diagnostic Studies

Evoked otoacoustical emission testing (EOAE) is the method of hearing screening being used for universal newborn screening. Dr. Kemp first described the phenomenon of otoacoustical emissions in 1978. The normal hearing ear emits detectable 20-dB sounds called spontaneous otoacoustical emissions. The normal ear also emits these sounds when given a stimulus. EOAE is very sensitive and easy to perform. It can be completed in less than 10 minutes. EOAE does not quantify hearing deficit but identifies whether the cochlea is functioning. It does have an approximately 10% false-positive result and may not identify a child with auditory nerve damage (Shuman, 1994).

Auditory brain stem response (ABR) measures the initiation of sound-induced electrical signals in the cochlea. The ABR is useful in identifying hearing loss in a young infant or in children unable to cooperate with audiometry. *Automated ABR* is now available as a screening device. It takes 10 to 15 minutes to perform, has a 5% false-positive rate, and can be administered in a noisy nursery (Shuman, 1994).

Audiometry, useful in assessing hearing loss in children, measures hearing threshold via bone or air conduction, or both, in decibels at varying frequencies (Table 30–2). Twenty decibels is about as loud as a whisper, 90 dB produces pain, and 40 dB is normal speaking loudness. The frequencies of normal speaking range from 250 to 4000 Hz. Hearing loss, especially in the higher frequencies (2000 to 6000 Hz), can cause significant problems in understanding speech. A screening audiogram that tests

T A B L E 30-2

Evaluation of Audiometric Results

AVERAGE THRESHHOLD AT 500–2000 Hz (dB)	DESCRIPTION	SIGNIFICANCE
−10 to +15	Normal	
16–25	Slight loss	Difficulty hearing faint speech, slight verbal deficit
26–40	Mild loss	Auditory learning dysfunction, language or speech problems
41–55	Moderate loss	Trouble hearing conversational speech, may miss 50% of class discussion
56–70	Moderately severe loss	
71–90	Severe loss	Educational retardation, learning disability, limited vocabulary
90+	Profound loss	

each ear at 20 dB and frequencies of 500, 1000, 2000, and 4000 Hz is a useful assessment tool in office pediatrics. If a more detailed audiogram is needed, a qualified audiologist should perform it.

Pneumatic otoscopy helps assess tympanic membrane mobility. A good seal with the speculum and otoscope before insufflation of air into the ear canal is required. Brisk movement of the membrane should be seen; altered mobility suggests middle ear effusion or possible perforation.

Tympanometry assesses movement of tympanic membranes by applying from −400 to 100 mm H_2O pressure to the ear canal. Movement of the tympanic membrane is translated into a graph called a tympanogram. The type A tympanogram has a compliance peak between ± 100 cm H_2O and reflects a normal tympanic membrane. The type B tympanogram generally has no peak or a flattened wave and suggests effusion, perforation, or the presence of a pressure-equalizing tube (PET). The type C tympanogram has a sharp peak between −100 and −200 cm H_2O and reflects negative ear pressure (Fig. 30-2). Tympanograms are helpful when otitis media with effusion (OME) is persistent or a question remains regarding the results of physical examination of the eardrum. Tympanograms are of little use in children younger than 7 months because their ear canals are hypercompliant in response to pressure from the tympanometer.

Acoustical reflectometry is a newer sonar technology that can be used in the primary care setting. The hand-held instrument detects the presence of middle ear effusion. This hand-held instrument consists of an acoustical transducer that has 44 different frequencies at 80 dB. A microphone records sound reflection back from the eardrum. A microprocessor measures the difference in frequency of the sound emitted and the sound returned. A fluid-filled middle ear space restricts vibration of the eardrum, so sound is intensified when returning to the device. The result is a spectral gradient angle that is displayed on a panel on the device. The angle size correlates with the likelihood of middle ear disease. It is a painless procedure, does not require an airtight seal, and does not pressurize the canal (Schuman, 1997).

Tympanocentesis with aspiration of middle ear fluid is helpful for the relief of pain and/or identification of persistent infecting organisms. It is rarely used in clinical pediatrics and is generally considered outside the scope of practice of the NP.

Laboratory tests of blood and urine are rarely indicated unless questions remain regarding perinatal infection, systemic illness, or concomitant kidney dysfunction.

▬ MANAGEMENT STRATEGIES

Medications

Medications are used only when indicated. Antibiotics and antifungals are necessary when in-

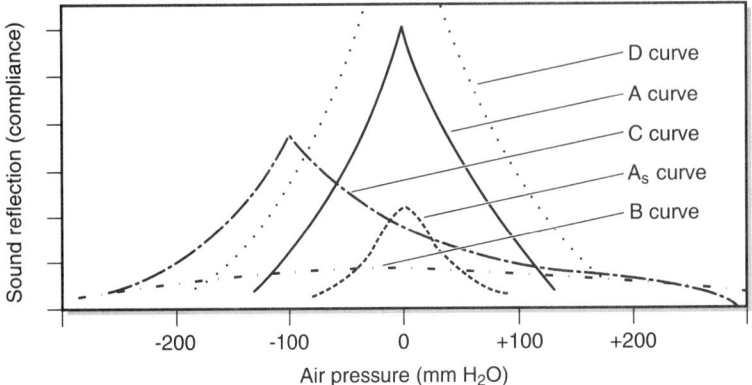

F I G U R E 30-2
Tympanogram. Five types of tympanogram curves. Generally, an *A* curve indicates a normal tympanic membrane, a *B* curve is abnormal, a *C* curve may be abnormal, and a *D* curve indicates hypermobility. An A_s curve may be normal in infants. (From Harrison CJ, Belhorn TH: Acute otitis media: Management and prophylaxis. Clin Rev, April 1992, p 55.)

fection is present. Principles for the judicious use of antimicrobial agents in pediatric patients have been identified by the AAP (see Chapter 24). The NP should be familiar with these recommendations and be aware of their role in the prevention of superinfections caused by the indiscriminate use of antibiotics. Oral steroids have been suggested for use with persistent middle ear effusion. However, current guidelines from the Agency for Health Care Policy and Research do not recommend the use of steroids because of limited scientific evidence of their effectiveness and possible adverse effects (US Department of Health and Human Services, 1994). Topical nasal steroids can be used to decrease inflammation in the eustachian tubes and upper respiratory tract. Antipyretics and analgesics are useful in treating fever and discomfort. Use of ceruminolytics or removal of the impaction is essential when excessive cerumen impedes examination of the ear or alters hearing. Acidic eardrops help maintain an environment in the external auditory canal that prevents the growth of fungi and bacteria.

Education and Counseling

Education and counseling of the patient and family regarding both the prevention of additional problems and the treatment course are important in the treatment of ear problems. Areas of particular importance include avoiding passive smoke exposure, avoiding bottle propping, minimizing exposure to other children with minor acute illnesses, and decreasing exposure to loud noises.

Prevention of Noise-Induced Hearing Loss

Firecrackers (especially Chinese ones), toy cap pistols, firearms, loud pop music, squeaking toys, snowmobiles, farm equipment, lawn mowers, and ill-fitted hearing aids have all been shown to cause some degree of hearing loss (Nash et al., 1997). The NP should actively educate patients and parents to avoid damaging sources of sound and use protective devices. Three types of protective devices are readily available at pharmacies or hardware stores: earmuffs, form-fitting foam earplugs, and premolded earplugs. Additionally, being aware of risk factors should lead the NP to early detection of cochlear damage and hearing loss.

Removal of Cerumen

Cerumen in the ear canal can be removed with the use of a cerumen scoop or by gently irrigating the ear. Before irrigation, 2 to 3 drops of docusate sodium (Colace) or mineral oil or other warm oil may be instilled to help soften the obstructive wax. Tap water irrigation alone is as effective as using a softener before irrigation. For dry, hardened wax, softeners may decrease the amount of irrigant required (Spiro, 1997). Irrigation is then accomplished by using a bulb syringe or "water pick." The irrigation solution can be warm water or hydrogen peroxide diluted 1:1 with warm water. Irrigation should be done on a low setting and not be attempted if the tympanic membrane is possibly perforated.

Follow-up and Referral

Close follow-up of infection and assessment for hearing loss are necessary to be aware of changes in hearing and recurrence of illness. Referral is necessary when the problem is beyond the scope of the NP's expertise. An otolaryngology referral is indicated for unusual ear conditions, when appropriate therapy for OM has failed, or if ongoing effusion or infection persists. Myringotomy and/or placement of pressure-equalization tubes (PETs) can help relieve discomfort and prevent further infection. Audiological referral is necessary if ear pathology is prolonged or when the child's ability to hear is questioned. Speech and language evaluations are imperative to resolve questions about whether the child's verbal development is delayed because of persistent or recurring ear problems. Chapter 32 addresses criteria for tonsillectomy and adenoidectomy.

Pressure-Equalizing Tubes

Indications for tympanostomy and the insertion of PETs are listed in Table 30–3. The procedure takes less than 15 minutes and is done with

T A B L E 30-3

Indications for Tympanostomy and the Insertion of Pressure-Equalizing Tubes

Otitis media with effusion lasting more than 3 mo or with language delay, hearing loss, severe retraction pocket, vertigo, tinnitus, or frequent superimposed acute otitis media
Recurrent otitis media (if the child has 2 or more infections despite prophylaxis, instead of prophylaxis if avoidance of long-term antibiotics is desired, or with language delay, hearing loss, or multiple drug allergies)
Severe eustachian tube dysfunction (persistent ear popping, pain, vertigo, tinnitus, or fluctuating hearing loss)
Complications of otitis media present or suspected (mastoiditis, facial nerve paralysis, brain abscess, labyrinthitis)

Adapted from Pizzuto MP, Volk MS, Kingston LM: Common topics in pediatric otolaryngology. Pediatr Clin North Am 45:973–991, 1998.

general anesthesia. The child is usually discharged after about an hour and is treated with otic drops for several days.

Insertion of PETs in a child with recurrent OM or prolonged middle ear effusion provides less discomfort with acute otitis media (AOM), appropriate ventilation of the middle ear space, and improved hearing (Isaacson & Rosenfeld, 1996). Additionally, there is evidence that the use of PETs may decrease the incidence of AOM in some children (Debruyne & Degroote, 1993).

The examiner can establish that the tube is functioning properly if the tube spans the eardrum, the lumen is unobstructed, and no middle ear effusion is present (Isaacson & Rosenfeld, 1996). If appropriate functioning of the tube cannot be established, pneumatic otoscopy or tympanometry may be useful. A flat (type B) tympanogram with large volume measurements confirms appropriate function of the PET. A normal (type A) tympanogram suggests a clogged or extruded tube.

Using ototopical drops for 5 to 7 days can occasionally clear clogged PETs. Otic suspensions, such as Pediotic, that are mildly acidic should be used because they are less irritating to middle ear mucosa. Water and ceruminolytics are contraindicated. If the child can taste the drops or complains of stinging, the drops are most likely reaching the middle ear space and indicate a functioning tube.

Generalized water precautions for children with PETs are controversial. Water does not enter the middle ear space via the PET during bathing, showering, or surface swimming. Diving and head dunking may allow water into the middle ear space. Chlorinated pools have few bacteria, and earplugs are most likely unnecessary. However, lakes, ponds, rivers, and bath water may have increased bacterial counts, so earplugs are recommended if head dunking may occur (Isaacson & Rosenfeld, 1996).

Viral myringitis or early AOM without otorrhea in a child with PETs will most likely resolve spontaneously because of increased middle ear ventilation. Antibiotics are not indicated. When a child with PETs has an upper respiratory infection and drainage is coming from the tube, the same bacterial pathogens seen in AOM are usually present in the fluid. In this case, treatment with oral antibiotics is appropriate. When otorrhea is unresponsive to oral antibiotics or if water contamination is involved, the most likely organisms are *Pseudomonas* or *Staphylococcus aureus,* and ototopical drops need to be added to the treatment plan. An otic suspension containing neomycin, polymixin B, and hydrocortisone with an acidic pH (Pediotic) or tobramycin or gentamicin ophthalmic can be used either until the drainage is gone or for up to 7 days (Isaacson & Rosenfeld, 1996). If the otorrhea is resistant to oral and ototopical agents, referral to an otolaryngologist is recommended.

Many PETs fall out well before their usefulness has been expended, with 20 to 50% of children requiring a second set (Pizzuto et al., 1998; Eden et al., 1996b). Once the PET has been extruded from the tympanic membrane, follow-up every 6 to 12 months is suggested until the tube falls out of the ear completely. For the rare set of PETs that remain in situ, surgical removal is suggested after 2 years. Complications of PETs include otorrhea, granuloma, cholesteatoma, PET obstruction, tympanic membrane perforation, and tympanosclerosis.

SPECIFIC EAR PROBLEMS IN CHILDREN

Otitis Externa

Description

Otitis externa (OE) is an inflammatory reaction of the external auditory canal. Inflammation is evidenced as (1) simple infection with edema, discharge, and erythema; (2) furuncles or small abscesses that form in hair follicles; or (3) impetigo or infection of the superficial layers of the epidermis. OE can also be classified as mycotic OE, caused by fungus, or as chronic external otitis, a diffuse low-grade infection of the external auditory canal (Table 30-4).

Etiology

OE is most frequently caused by retained moisture in the external ear canal, which changes the acidic environment of the external ear canal to a neutral or basic environment, thereby promoting bacterial or fungal growth.

T A B L E 30-4
Management of Otitis Externa

Clinical findings	Simple infection with edema, discharge, and erythema
	Furuncles or small abscesses in hair follicles
	Impetigo or infection of superficial layers
Treatment	Remove any foreign body
	Irrigate with saline or Burow solution
	Instill antibiotic with steroid drop—use wick if significant swelling
	Administer analgesics as needed
	If furuncle is present, lance
	If impetigo is present, clean with antiseptic and apply antibiotic ointment
	If mycotic infection is present, clean with 5% boric acid in ethanol solution, followed by antifungal cream
Prevention	Avoid water in ears
	Use acetic or boric acid and alcohol solutions after swimming
	Avoid scratching, persistent cleaning, or prolonged use of ceruminolytics

Chlorine in swimming pools adds to the problem because it kills the normal ear flora and allows the growth of pathogens. The most common pathogen in "swimmer's ear" is *Pseudomonas aeruginosa* (Jahn & Hawke, 1993).

Furunculosis of the external canal is generally caused by *S. aureus* and *Streptococcus pyogenes* carried by dirty fingers. Mycotic external otitis is usually caused by *Aspergillus, Trichophyton,* or *Candida* (Williams, 1999). Foreign bodies that disrupt the lining of the ear canal can also lead to OE.

Clinical Findings

HISTORY. The following can be found:

• Itching and irritation progressing to severe pain
• Pressure and fullness in ear and occasion-

ally hearing loss that can be conductive or sensorineural

- Rare systemic complaints and symptoms
- Rare hearing loss and otorrhea

PHYSICAL EXAMINATION. Findings on physical examination can include the following:

- Pain with movement of the tragus or on attempts to examine the ear with an otoscope
- Swollen external auditory canal with difficult visualization of the tympanic membrane
- Rare otorrhea
- Occasional regional lymphadenopathy
- Tragal tenderness with a red, raised area of induration that can be deep and diffuse or superficial and pointing, which is characteristic of furunculosis (Jahn & Hawke, 1993)
- Red crusty or pustular spreading lesions
- Black spots over the tympanic membrane, indicative of mycotic infection
- Dry-appearing canal with some atrophy or thinning of the canal and virtually no cerumen visible with chronic OE

LABORATORY STUDIES. Culturing the discharge from the ear is not customary but can be done if clinical improvement is not seen during or after treatment, or if chronic OE is suspected. Culturing requires a swab premoistened with sterile nonbacteriostatic saline or water.

Differential Diagnosis

AOM with perforation, dental infection, mastoiditis, posterior auricular lymphadenopathy, and eczema are differential diagnoses.

Management

The following steps are taken:

1. Remove any foreign body (see the next section).
2. If no perforation of the tympanic membrane exists, irrigate the canal with saline or Burow's solution. Burow's solution is soothing, decreases edema, and kills *Pseudomonas*. Instill an antibiotic with steroid

eardrops such as Cortisporin Otic eardrops (4 to 5 drops three to four times daily for 10 days) or Floxin Otic suspension (2 drops twice a day for 7 to 10 days). If significant swelling is present, insert a cotton wick soaked with the antibiotic eardrop solution. Avoid neomycin drops because of the risk of contact dermatitis in 1 in 1000 patients (Barkin & Rosen, 1999).
3. Oral or parenteral antibiotics are not needed except for systemic illness.
4. Avoid cleaning, manipulating, and getting water into the ear.
5. Acidic drops (diluted vinegar or diluted alcohol, 3 to 5 drops) can be used daily, especially after swimming, to prevent the recurrence of OE. Over-the-counter drugs such as VōSol Otic eardrops can be used (5 drops in each ear after swimming).
6. Administer analgesics for pain, as needed. Codeine works well for severe pain and is indicated for short-term use.
7. Lance a furuncle that is superficial and pointing with the end of a 14-gauge needle. If it is deep and diffuse, a heating pad or warm oil-based drops can speed resolution.
8. If impetigo is present, clear the canal by using half-strength hydrogen peroxide or other antiseptic solutions, followed by a warm-water rinse. Apply an antibiotic ointment (mupirocin) once or twice a day for 5 to 7 days. The child should avoid touching the ear. Fingernails should be short and hands cleansed with antibacterial soap. Systemic antibiotics are generally unnecessary.
9. A dermatology consultation is indicated if no improvement in symptoms is seen within 1 week.
10. Mycotic OE is treated with a solution of 5% boric acid in ethanol, which is antiseptic and promotes drying. Clotrimazole-miconazole cream can be used alone or with a topical antibiotic corticosteroid solution for 5 to 7 days.
11. A follow-up visit is necessary after 1 to 2 weeks for reevaluation of the OE and removal of debris.

Complications

Infection of surrounding tissues with impetigo, irritated furunculosis, and malignant OE with progression and necrosis caused by *Pseudomonas* infection are possible complications.

Prevention

The patient should be instructed to

1. Avoid water in the ear canals.
2. Use earplugs for swimming if susceptible.
3. Use over-the-counter acetic or boric acid and alcohol solutions routinely after swimming (1:1 white vinegar and water or 70% ethyl alcohol).
4. Avoid persistent scratching or cleaning of the external canal.
5. Avoid prolonged use of ceruminolytic agents.

Foreign Body in the Ear Canal

Description

A foreign body in the external ear canal is a problem frequently seen in pediatric patients.

Etiology

Foreign bodies are usually placed in the ear canal by the child. Insects can also be found in the canal.

Clinical Findings

HISTORY. The history can include the following:

- Child reports putting something into the ear
- Complaints of buzzing, fullness, or an object in the ear
- Ear pain or otorrhea

PHYSICAL EXAMINATION. A foreign body is visible with the naked eye or by otoscopic examination.

Management

The following steps are taken:

1. Straighten ear canal by pulling on the pinna and shake patient's head gently.

2. Bayonet forceps can be used to grasp the object, especially if it is irregularly shaped.
3. If the object is metal, try a magnet to retrieve it.
4. Kill insects by instilling 70% alcohol in the ear canal before flushing.
5. Irrigate the ear canal with water; if vegetable matter, use 70% alcohol.
6. Refer the patient to an otolaryngologist if you are unable to extract the object without causing discomfort or trauma to the canal wall.

Complications

Infection, perforation of the tympanic membrane, and damage to the ossicles are possible if the object is not removed.

Prevention

Educate children and their parents to not put objects in the ear.

Acute Otitis Media

Description

AOM is an infection of the middle ear that can be of several types (see Color Fig. 4, Table 30-5, and Fig. 30-3).

Etiology

AOM often follows eustachian tube dysfunction. When the eustachian tube is obstructed, negative pressure develops as air is absorbed in the middle ear (see Color Fig. 5). The negative pressure pulls fluid from the mucosal lining and causes an accumulation of sterile fluid. Bacteria pulled in from the eustachian tube lead to the accumulation of purulent fluid. *Streptococcus pneumoniae* (40 to 50%), *Haemophilus influenzae* (20 to 30%), and *Moraxella catarrhalis* (10 to 15%) are the most common infecting organisms (Dowell et al., 1999). *S. pneumoniae* causes the most cases of AOM, is the least likely bacterium to resolve without treatment, and is responsible for the increasing treatment failures because of the emergence of multiple drug resistance (drug-resistant *S. pneumoniae* [DRSP]) (Dowell et al., 1999).

TABLE 30-5

Types of Acute Otitis Media

TYPE	CHARACTERISTICS
AOM	Suppurative effusion of the middle ear
Bullous myringitis	AOM in which bullae form between the inner and middle layers of the tympanic membrane and bulge outward
Persistent otitis media	Initial AOM that has not resolved after 4–6 wk of treatment
Recurrent otitis media	Three separate bouts of AOM within a 6-mo period, six within a 12-mo period, or six episodes by 6 y of age

AOM = acute otitis media.

Young children have shorter, more horizontal, and more flaccid eustachian tubes that are easily disrupted by viruses, which predisposes them to AOM. Other predisposing factors include upper respiratory infection, allergies, Down syndrome, cleft palate, bottle propping

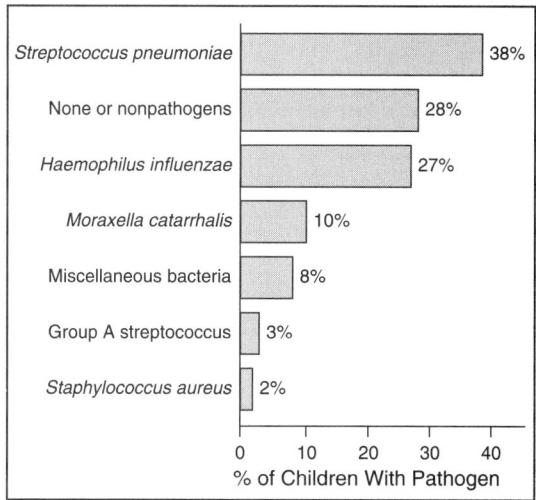

F I G U R E 30-3
Pathogens isolated from children with acute otitis media. (From Bluestone CD, Klein JO: Otitis Media in Infants and Children, 2nd ed. Philadelphia, WB Saunders, 1995.

during feedings, day care attendance, and passive cigarette smoke. Cigarette smoking leads to functional eustachian tube obstruction and decreases the protective ciliary action in the eustachian tube.

Incidence

Annual visits for AOM have more than doubled from 1975 to 1990 (Rosenfeld, 1996a). AOM develops in approximately 70% of children younger than 3 years (Pichichero & Cohen, 1997). It is the most common indication for antibiotic prescriptions in the United States (Kozyrskyj et al., 1998). The incidence of AOM is greater in males, white children, and Native Americans, including Eskimos. Approximately 20% of children have recurrent AOM (Eden et al., 1996a).

Clinical Findings

HISTORY. The following can be noted:

- Previous medical history significant for craniofacial anomalies or congenital syndromes associated with craniofacial anomalies, prematurity, or exposure to risk factors (ETS, bottle propping, and day care)
- Ear pain, manifesting in an infant or a young child as irritability, inability to sleep, or ear pulling; severe ear pain with bullous myringitis
- Lethargy, dizziness, tinnitus, and unsteady gait
- Diarrhea and vomiting
- Fever
- Sudden hearing loss
- Stuffy nose, rhinorrhea, and sneezing
- Rare facial palsy and ataxia

PHYSICAL EXAMINATION. The following can be apparent on physical examination:

- Tympanic membrane showing increased vascularity, erythema, bulging, and obscured or absent landmarks (see Color Fig. 4).
- Tympanic membrane that is red, yellow, or purple. Redness alone should not be used to diagnose AOM, especially in a crying child.

- Thin-walled, sagging bullae filled with straw-colored fluid are seen with bullous myringitis.
- Decreased tympanic membrane mobility secondary to effusion is noted with pneumatic otoscopy, tympanometry, or acoustical reflectometry (see Color Fig. 8).

LABORATORY FINDINGS. Tympanometry reflects effusion (type B pattern). Tympanocentesis to identify the infecting organism is helpful in the treatment of infants younger than 2 months. In older infants and children, tympanocentesis is rarely done and is useful only if the patient is in a toxic state or immunocompromised or in the presence of resistant infection or acute pain from bullous myringitis (Barkin & Rosen, 1999). If a tympanocentesis is warranted, refer the patient to an otolaryngologist for this procedure.

Differential Diagnosis

Otitis media with effusion (OME), mastoiditis, dental abscess, sinusitis, lymphadenitis, parotitis, peritonsillar abscess, trauma, eustachian tube dysfunction, impacted teeth, temporomandibular joint dysfunction, and immune deficiency are differential diagnoses.

Management

The following are issues to be considered when treating AOM (Fig. 30–4):

1. Currently, much controversy surrounds the use of antibiotics in the treatment of AOM. The main reason for the ongoing discussion is the increasing rate of antibiotic-resistant bacteria related to the injudicious use of antibiotics (see the earlier section on judicious use of antibiotics). Ample evidence has also been presented that as many as 60 to 90% of cases of AOM resolve without antibiotics (Pelton & Barnett, 1998; Maxson & Yamauchi, 1996), usually those caused by *H. influenza* or *M. catarrhalis* (Dowell et al., 1999). There seems to be some agreement that antibiotic treatment of a carefully diagnosed and documented AOM is appropriate. Diagnosis is made with pneumatic otoscopy, which can assess position, color, translucency, and mobility. Treatment is also recommended if the AOM is accompanied by clear local signs (bulging membrane with cloudy or yellow fluid, very red membrane, or otorrhea), if systemic signs (fever) are present, if more than three attacks of AOM have occurred in the past 18 months, or if the patient has a history of OME or PET use (Dowell et al., 1998; Pelton & Barnett, 1998).

2. Ten days of antibiotic therapy is suggested for AOM with perforation, in children with an underlying medical condition, or in children younger than 15 to 24 months. The risk of treatment failure is higher in younger children. Amoxicillin is still the first-line drug choice for AOM. Children with AOM who have high fever most likely have *S. pneumoniae* in the middle ear fluid and might benefit from high-dose amoxicillin therapy (80 to 90 mg/kg per day [Dowell et al., 1999] or 60 to 80 mg/kg per day [Fitzgerald, 1998]). Children at low risk for DRSP (no antimicrobial exposure in the previous 3 months, no day care attendance, older than 2 years) are still appropriate for the 40 to 45 mg/kg per day dosage (Dowell et al., 1999). Recommendations from the DRSP Therapeutic Working Group (Dowell et al., 1999) are amoxicillin-clavulanate (70 to 90 mg/kg per day divided in two doses, given twice daily, with the clavulanate component at ≤10 mg/kg per day); cefuroxime

FIGURE 30-4

Management of acute otitis media. See Tables 30–6 and 30–7 for medications. (From Eden AN, Fireman P, Stool SE: Managing acute otitis: A fresh look at a familiar problem. Contemp Pediatr 12: 80. Copyright © 1996 Medical Economics, Montvale, NJ. No part of this flow chart may be reproduced or extracted in any form without written permission.)

Your patient has recently had a viral upper respiratory tract infection and now has an earache, fever, and some degree of hearing loss. You suspect acute otitis media.

↓

Confirm the diagnosis with pneumatic otoscopy. Consider tympanometry as an adjunct to confirm the presence of fluid in the middle ear. If the diagnosis is uncertain or the child is seriously ill or toxic, consider tympanocentesis and culture of the exudate.

Is any statement true?
- The child has had six episodes by age 6.
- The child has had five episodes in 1 year.
- The child has had three episodes in 6 months.

NO →

YES ↓

Diagnose recurrent acute otitis media. Treat the current episode as indicated. Consider prophylaxis with amoxicillin or sulfisoxazole and examine regularly for an asymptomatic effusion. If the child is allergic to these drugs, prophylaxis fails to prevent recurrence, or hearing loss or other complications develop, consider tympanostomy tube insertion. Depending on age and individual circumstances, other options include adenoidectomy, pneumococcal vaccine, and influenza vaccine.

Is any statement true?
- You suspect or confirm a ß-lactamase-producing pathogen.
- The incidence of resistant strains in the community is high.
- The patient previously failed to respond to amoxicillin or ampicillin.

NO →

YES ↓

Consider a 10-day course of amoxicillin/clavulanate potassium if there is ß-lactam resistance. Other choices include cefaclor, cefuroxime axetil, cefixime, cefproxil, loracarbef, and cefpodoxime proxetil.

Is the chid allergic to penicillin?

YES →

NO ↓

Prescribe a 10-day course of amoxicillin or ampicillin.

Consider a 10-day course of erythromycin ethylsuccinate/sulfisoxazole acetyl. An alternative is trimethoprim/sulfamethoxazole (TMP/SMX).[†]

↓

Recommend warm compresses for the ear and an analgesic-antipyretic such as acetaminophen. Consider prescribing eardrops containing antipyrine and benzocaine for pain relief. Instruct the parent to return if symptoms do not significantly improve within 48–72 hr.

→

Has the infection resolved by the end of the antibiotic course?

YES ←

Do symptoms significantly improve within 48–72 hours?

NO ↓

Consider switching to another antibiotic. If amoxicillin or ampicillin was used, consider amoxicillin/clavulanate potassium, cefaclor, or another suitable cephalosporin. If a cephalosporin was used, consider switching to a different one.[†] Cephalosporins should be used cautiously in children with penicillin sensitivity because of cross-hypersensitivity among ß-lactam antibiotics. Consider also tympanocentesis and culture of the exudate.

NO ←

Consider tympanocentesis and culture of the exudate. Consider switching to another antibiotic. Examine the child every 2 to 4 weeks until the infection resolves. Monitor for suppurative complications and concurrent infection such as meningitis.

YES ↓

Schedule a follow-up visit for 2 to 3 weeks afterward to confirm that the infection has resolved and most of the fluid has dissipated.

*TMP/SMX is associated with rare but severe adverse reactions, including Stevens-Johnson syndrome, toxic epidermal necrolysis, fulminant hepatic necrosis, agranulocytosis, and aplastic anemia and other blood dyscrasias.

[†]Recommendations from the Drug-Resistant Streptococcus Pneumoniae (DRSP) Working Group supersede these recommendations.

FIGURE 30-4
See legend on opposite page

axetil and intramuscular ceftriaxone (50 mg/kg daily as a single dose or three daily doses) are useful alternative agents for clinical treatment failure. Treatment failure is defined as "lack of clinical improvement in signs and symptoms such as ear pain, fever and tympanic membrane findings of redness, bulging or otorrhea after 3 days of therapy" (Dowell et al., 1999). The NP is cautioned to keep current on updated recommendations for the treatment of AOM because of the rapid changes in resistance patterns and newly developed treatments. Table 30-6 lists the current antibiotics approved by the Food and Drug Administration for the treatment of AOM.

T A B L E 30-6

Medications Approved by the Food and Drug Administration to Treat Acute Otitis Media as of 1999

DRUG	DOSE	COMMENTS
Amoxicillin	40–90 mg/kg per d given t.i.d.	First choice unless contraindicated
TMP-SMX	0.5 ml/kg per d given b.i.d.	Potent side effect profile
Erythromycin-sulfisoxazole (Pediazole)	50 mg/kg per d and 150 mg/kg per d given t.i.d. or q.i.d.	Broad spectrum of activity but a higher cost than for amoxicillin or TMP-SMX
Clarithromycin (Biaxin)	15 mg/kg per d given b.i.d.	Children older than 6 mo
Azithromycin (Zithromax)	10 mg/kg per d on day 1, then 5 mg/kg per d on days 2–5 given q.d.	Children older than 6 mo, 5-d treatment course
Cefaclor (Ceclor)	40 mg/kg per d given b.i.d. or t.i.d.	Broad spectrum but poor *Haemophilus influenzae* coverage and costly; risk of erythema multiforme; 2nd generation; not recommended; rarely used
Amoxicillin–clavulanate (Augmentin)	40–90 mg/kg per d given b.i.d. with clavulanate < 10 mg/kg per d	Good β-lactamase coverage; costly and more likely to cause diarrhea
Cefixime (Suprax)	8 mg/kg per d given q.d. or b.i.d.	Good β-lactamase coverage but poor *Streptococcus pneumoniae* coverage and very costly; 3rd generation
Cefuroxime (Ceftin)	30 mg/kg per d given b.i.d. 125 mg b.i.d. if younger than 2 y 250 mg b.i.d. if 2–12 y old 250–500 mg b.i.d. if older than 12 y	Broad spectrum of coverage, costly; 2nd generation
Cefprozil (Cefzil)	30 mg/kg per d given b.i.d.	Broad spectrum of coverage, cost similar to that of other cephalosporins; 2nd generation
Cefpodoxime (Vantin)	10 mg/kg per d given b.i.d.	Broad spectrum of coverage, costly; 3rd generation
Loracarbef (Lorabid)	30 mg/kg per d given b.i.d.	Broad spectrum of coverage, costly; 2nd generation
Ceftibuten (Cedax)	9 mg/kg per given q.d.	Children older than 6 mo; active against β-lactamase; 3rd generation
Ceftriaxone (Rocephin)	50–75 mg/kg per d IM in 1 dose (may be given q.d. up to 5 d)	Costly; 3rd generation

IM = intramuscularly; TMP-SMX = trimethoprim-sulfamethoxazole.

3. Five- to 7-day treatment regimens may be appropriate for other groups of children not heretofore mentioned (e.g., children older than 2 to 6 years, with a mild episode, few previous infections) (Pelton & Barnett, 1998). The child's symptoms should improve after 24 to 48 hours. If no clinical improvement is seen in this time frame, changing to an antibiotic with broader microbial coverage is indicated.

4. Bullous myringitis should be treated with an erythromycin/sulfa combination for *H. influenzae* and *Mycoplasma* coverage.

5. Persistent OM occurs when antibiotic therapy has been completed and evidence of AOM is still present or AOM recurs within days of treatment (Eden et al., 1996b). Retreatment with a broader-spectrum antibiotic is suggested. OME should not be considered treatment failure and should be expected in up to 70% of cases (Dowell et al., 1999).

6. Recurrent AOM (being "otitis prone") is present when more than three bouts of AOM have occurred in 6 months or six in 12 months (Shutze & Jacobs, 1994). Children with recurrent AOM are more likely to have a family history of AOM in the father and have other ear, nose, and throat (ENT) diseases (Stenstrom & Ingvaarson, 1996). The use of prophylactic antibiotics in the treatment of recurrent AOM is a highly debated issue. Antibiotic-resistant bacteria are the key concern. Prophylaxis should be reserved for children who suffer frequent, severe bouts of AOM. When used, prophylaxis is thought to decrease recurrent infection, which can lead to chronic OME and potential hearing loss and have a detrimental effect on language and cognition. Treatment has traditionally been once daily with amoxicillin or sulfisoxazole (preferable because it is no longer routinely used to treat AOM) in half the therapeutic dose, with treatment limited to fall, winter, and early spring (Blumer, 1998; Pizzuto et al., 1998) (Table 30–7). Reexamine the child at 2-month intervals, watch community resistance patterns, and treat breakthrough infections (Klein, 1994).

T A B L E   30-7

Medications for Prophylaxis of Otitis Media

Amoxicillin	20 mg/kg per d
Sulfisoxazole (Gantrisin)	50–75 mg/kg per d

7. Decongestants and antihistamines are not helpful.

8. Antimicrobial ototopical drops (Pediotic or Cortisporin) or ophthalmic drops (tobramycin or gentamicin) are indicated if the tympanic membrane is perforated or the child has otorrhea.

9. Analgesic eardrops (Auralgan Otic) are helpful for pain relief in the absence of perforation or PETs.

10. Oral antipyretics and analgesics should be given as needed: acetaminophen (10 to 15 mg/kg every 4 to 6 hours) or children's ibuprofen (5 to 10 mg/kg every 6 to 8 hours).

11. A follow-up appointment needs to be scheduled 14 to 21 days after the initial diagnosis.

Complications

Persistent AOM, persistent OME, tympanic membrane perforation (see Color Fig. 6), OE, mastoiditis, cholesteatoma, tympanosclerosis (see Color Fig. 7), hearing loss of 25 to 30 dB for several months, ossicle necrosis, pseudotumor cerebri, and cerebral thrombophlebitis are possible complications.

Prevention and Education

Patients and parents should be instructed regarding the following:

1. *H. influenzae* type b vaccine is not helpful because the *H. influenzae* responsible for AOM is usually nontypable.

2. Bottle propping, feeding infants lying down, and passive smoke exposure should be avoided.

3. Breastfeeding until at least 4 months of age is protective against single and recurrent episodes of AOM (Duncan et al., 1993).

4. The importance of keeping follow-up appointments should be stressed.
5. Educate regarding the problem of drug-resistant bacteria and the need to avoid the use of antibiotics unless absolutely necessary.
6. If antibiotics are used, the child needs to complete the entire course of the prescription.
7. If the child is in day care, another less populated day care environment may need to be considered.

Otitis Media With Effusion

Description

OME, also referred to as middle ear effusion, secretory, nonsuppurative, or serous OM, is characterized by an accumulation of fluid in the middle ear and a decrease in mobility of the tympanic membrane with pneumatic otoscopy (see Color Fig. 8).

Etiology and Incidence

OME usually begins with eustachian tube dysfunction (ETD) caused by viral illness, anatomical abnormalities, barotrauma, allergies, or a combination of these conditions. ETD changes the middle ear mucosa in the following sequence: (1) the mucosa becomes secretory with increased mucus production, (2) the mucus becomes viscous as the mucosa absorbs water, and (3) fluid becomes stuck behind the tympanic membrane (Williams, 1999).

In another process, ETD causes OME, which then becomes AOM. OME is a natural consequence of both treated and untreated AOM (Rosenfeld, 1996a). Ninety percent of effusions of less than 2 to 3 months in duration resolve without treatment within a few months. OME that lasts longer than 2 to 3 months has only a 15 to 30% resolution rate even when monitored for 30 months (Rosenfeld, 1996b).

Thirty percent of children with OME have bacteria (nontypable *H. influenzae, M. catarrhalis,* and *S. pneumoniae*) in their middle ear effusions. OME is the most common cause of hearing loss in children.

Clinical Findings

HISTORY. The following features may be noted in the affected child:

- Often asymptomatic, afebrile, and without complaints of otalgia
- Fullness in the ear or the feeling of "talking in a barrel"
- Complaint of hearing loss in older children
- Dizziness or impaired balance
- Chronic vomiting with failure to thrive, which can be related to chronic OME (Granot et al., 1990)

PHYSICAL EXAMINATION. An abnormal-appearing tympanic membrane, often described as dull, varying from bulging and opaque with no visible landmarks to retracted and translucent with visible landmarks and an air-fluid level, may be seen (see Color Fig. 9). Pneumatic otoscopy reveals decreased tympanic membrane mobility. Head and neck structures should be examined for abnormalities.

LABORATORY FINDINGS. The tympanogram is flat—type B. The audiogram can show hearing loss of 15 to 31 dB.

Differential Diagnosis

Differential diagnoses include all causes of hearing loss and anatomical abnormalities, including AOM; unilateral OME can indicate nasopharyngeal carcinoma.

Management

Treatment of OME is controversial and varied. The Agency for Health Care Policy and Research issued guidelines for the treatment of OME in 1994 (Fig. 30–5).

1. Current treatment guidelines suggest that OME does not need treatment with antibiotics (Dowell et al., 1998; Eden et al., 1996b; Rosenfeld, 1996b). For OME lasting longer than 3 months, a hearing evaluation and a course of antibiotics might prove useful. PETs should be considered if OME is bilateral for more than 4 months and hearing loss has been documented. PETs would also be considered for OME that is unilateral and lasts longer than 6 months.

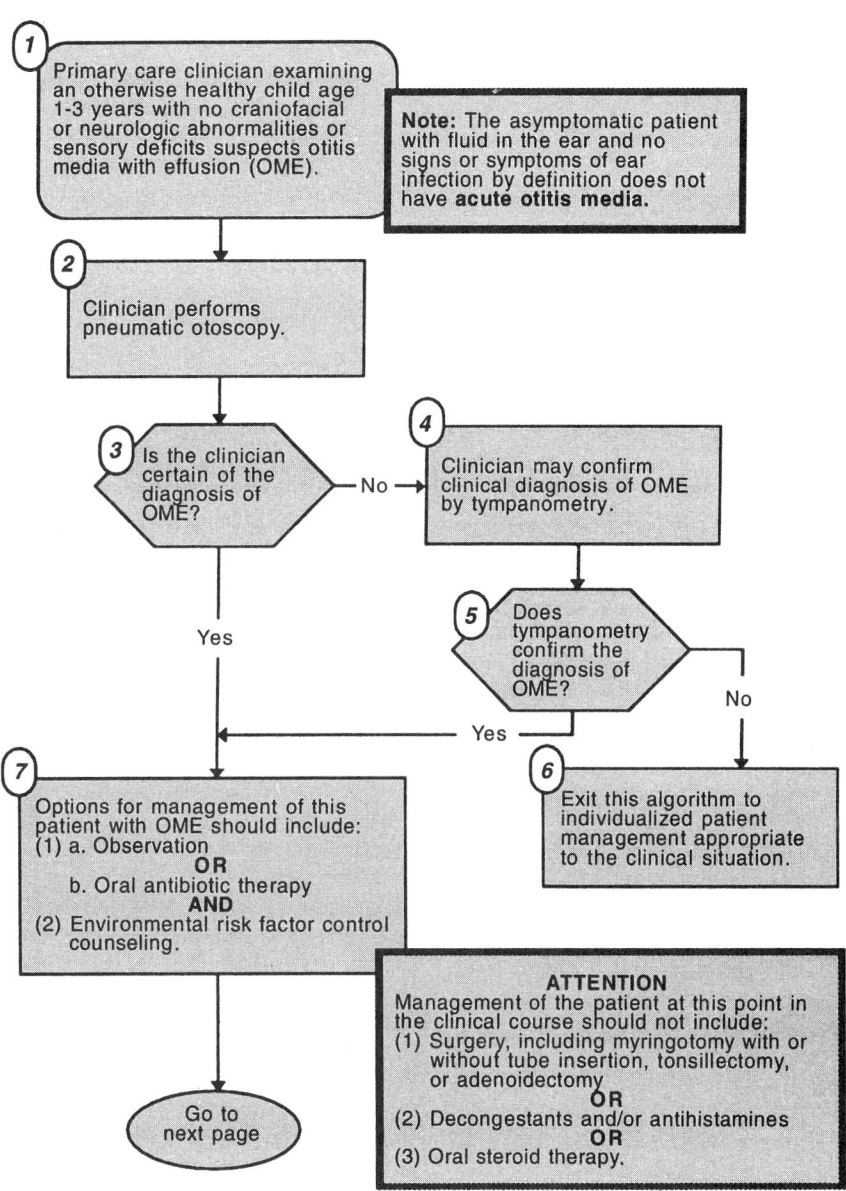

F I G U R E 30-5

Management of otitis media with effusion. (From Agency for Health Care Policy and Research: Quick Reference Guide for Clinicians: Managing Otitis Media With Effusion in Young Children, Rockville, MD, Agency for Health Care Policy and Research, 1994, AHCPR Publication No. 94-0623).

Illustration continued on following page

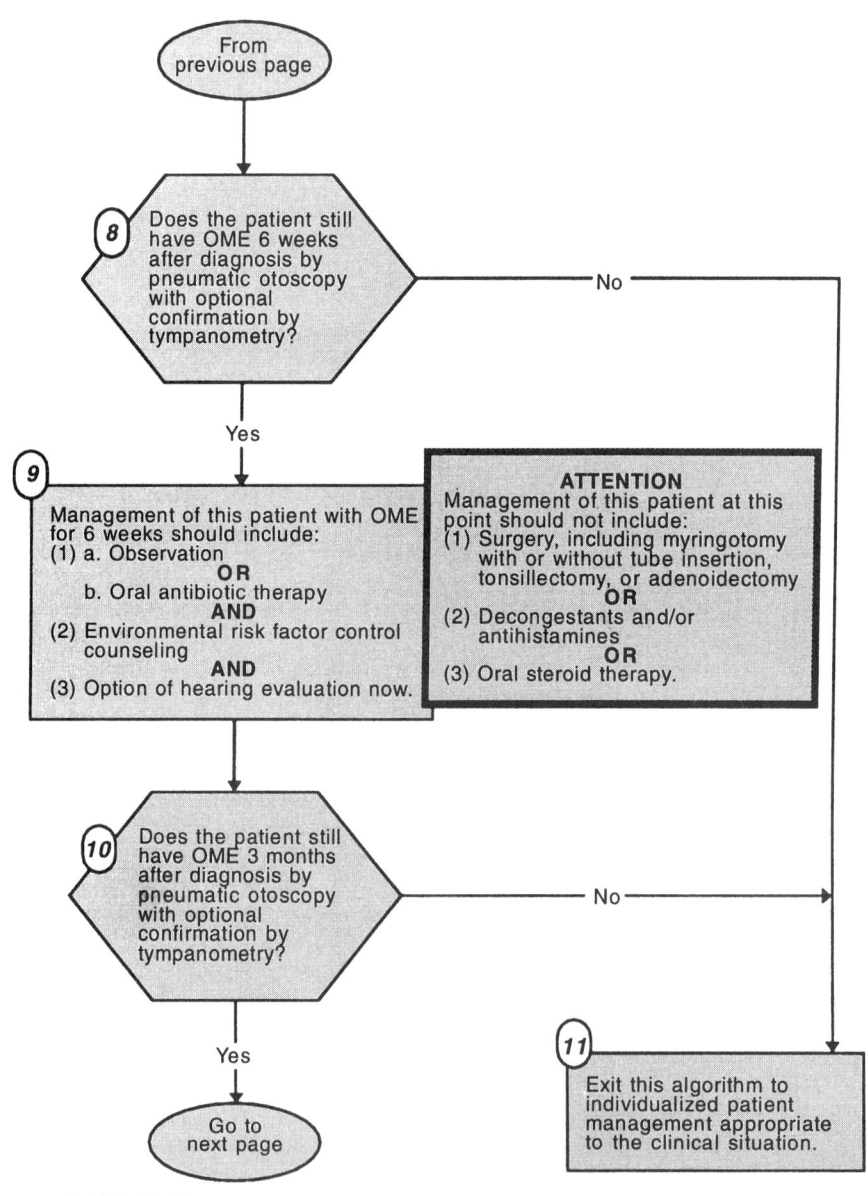

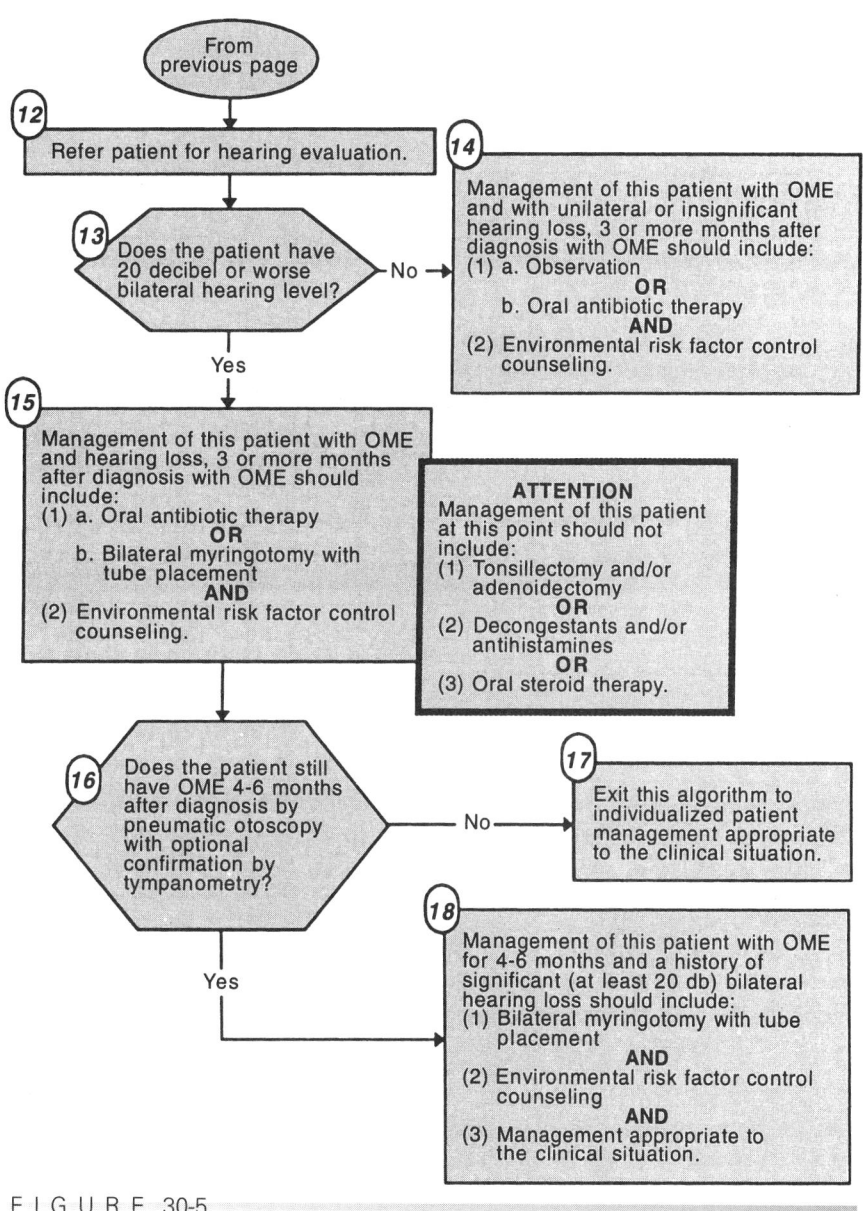

F I G U R E 30-5
Continued

2. Evaluate relevant risk factors and recurrence.
3. Follow up every 4 to 8 weeks.
4. Oral corticosteroids are not recommended for children younger than 3 years, but they can be used selectively in older children as a last resort before surgery. Corticosteroids (1 mg/kg per day for 1 week) should be given in conjunction with a second-line antibiotic. Be certain that the child has not had an exposure to varicella for 3 weeks before the initiation of steroid therapy (Rosenfeld, 1996a).
5. Antihistamines and decongestants are not helpful unless the child has nasal allergies (see Chapter 25).
6. Nasal corticosteroids can be helpful in conjunction with antibiotics if nasal congestion or allergy symptoms are present (Williams, 1999).
7. Recommend that the child be given preferential seating in school and be spoken to face to face.
8. After 3 months of persistent OME, refer to an otolaryngologist for evaluation. If persistent hearing loss or speech delay is apparent, refer to an audiologist and speech therapist for evaluation and treatment.

Complications

Complications include recurrent AOM, speech delay, and hearing loss.

Prevention and Education

1. Stress the importance of follow-up until the tympanic membrane and hearing are normal.
2. Advise parents of the length of time (weeks to months) required for resolution of OME.
3. Encourage parents to decrease background noise, speak louder than usual, and focus on the child's face when speaking because of the mild, transient hearing loss.

Cholesteatoma

Description

Cholesteatoma is an epidermal inclusion cyst of the middle ear or mastoid consisting of des-

quamated debris from the keratinizing, squamous epithelial lining of the middle ear (see Color Fig. 10). If the condition is untreated, bone destruction and chronic infection may occur and may lead to hearing loss, facial nerve paralysis, and vertigo.

Etiology and Incidence

Cholesteatomas can be congenital or acquired. Varied theories explaining their formation include the following: an inflammatory process, perforation of the tympanic membrane, and failure of desquamated tissue to clear from the middle ear. The incidence rate is unknown.

Clinical Findings

HISTORY. The history can include

- Chronic OM with malodorous purulent otorrhea
- Vertigo and hearing loss (Sie, 1996)

PHYSICAL EXAMINATION. A pearly white lesion is present on or behind the tympanic membrane. Aural polyps are considered cholesteatomas unless proved otherwise.

Differential Diagnosis

Aural polyps is the differential diagnosis.

Management

Accurate diagnosis and immediate otolaryngological referral for surgical excision are needed.

Complications

Complications include irreversible structural damage, permanent bone damage, facial nerve palsy, hearing loss, and intracranial infection.

Mastoiditis

Description

Mastoiditis is suppurative infection of the mastoid cells.

Etiology and Incidence

Mastoiditis may accompany OM. The muco-periosteal lining of the mastoid air cells becomes inflamed, with subsequent progressive swelling and obstruction of drainage from the mastoid. Common organisms identified include *S. pneumoniae*, group A streptococci, *S. aureus*, *H. influenzae*, and *Mycobacterium tuberculosis* (rare).

Incidence

Mastoiditis is uncommon but potentially life threatening.

Clinical Findings

- Concurrent AOM.
- Fever and otalgia.
- Postauricular swelling. Infants may have swelling above the ear, displacing the pinna inferiorly or laterally. In older children, the swelling pushes the ear lobe superiorly and laterally.
- Persistent OM unresponsive to antibiotic therapy.

LABORATORY STUDIES

- Radiography (may show coalescence of mastoid air cells and loss of bony trabeculation)
- Computed tomography (CT) (can provide definitive anatomical information)
- Tympanocentesis (culture and Gram stain help identify offending organism) (Barkin & Rosen, 1999)

Management

Urgent ENT referral is imperative. Hospitalization and intravenous antibiotics are usually required.

Sensorineural and Conductive Hearing Loss

Description

Hearing loss is defined as bilateral pure tone hearing loss of 40 dB or more at frequencies of 500, 1000, and 2000 Hz in the better ear (Centers for Disease Control and Prevention, 1997). Three types of hearing loss are recognized—sensorineural, conductive, and central—although there may also be a combined type. Either or both ears may be involved. The average age at detection of hearing loss is somewhere between 14 and 24 months if profound and up to 48 months for lesser degrees (AAP, 1999; Bachmann & Arvedson, 1998).

Sensorineural hearing loss (SNHL) occurs because of damage to the cochlear structure of the inner ear or to fibers of the auditory nerve. SNHL may be mild or severe and is permanent and not usually treatable. Noise-induced hearing loss (NIHL) is a preventable type of SNHL that is permanent and incurable and affects cognitive, social, emotional, and psychological functioning (Nash et al., 1997).

Conductive hearing loss results from blocked transmission of sound waves from the external auditory canal to the inner ear (e.g., AOM, OME). Bone conduction is usually normal with decreased air conduction. Conductive hearing loss is usually in the range of 15 to 40 dB (mild to moderate) and is not permanent (Castiglia, 1998; Stewart & Downs, 1993). Middle ear effusions result in an average hearing loss of 27 to 31 dB.

Etiology

SNHL and conductive hearing loss can be caused by craniofacial anomalies (e.g., aural atresia, cleft lip/cleft palate, external ear deformity without atresia, dysmorphic facies without external ear deformity), genetic aberrations/congenital deformities (e.g., white forelock, café au lait spots, family history of SNHL, metabolic abnormalities), or environmental exposure (e.g., ototoxic drugs, bacterial or viral meningitis, loud noises, head trauma). NIHL occurs when hair cells in the cochlea are injured by exposure to excessive noise over a variable period. SNHL can also come from prenatal and perinatal exposure (e.g., intrauterine infections, toxic chemicals, erythroblastosis fetalis). Conductive hearing loss can also be caused by AOM and OME with or without perforation, tumors, cerumen impaction, or idiopathic causes (e.g., otosclerosis).

Incidence

SNHL occurs in 1 to 3 per 1000 infants in well-baby nurseries and in 2 to 4 per 1000 infants in the intensive care unit. Fifty percent of cases are genetically linked, 20 to 25% are from environmental factors, and 25 to 30% are from an uncertain cause. Hereditary SNHL accounts for 20 to 50% of all cases of severe to profound SNHL. SNHL occurs in 10.3% of children with meningitis (Williams, 1999; Bachmann & Arvedson, 1998; Castiglia, 1998; Brookhouser, 1996).

Conductive hearing loss occurs in 15% of school-aged children (Williams, 1999). Congenital deformities causing conductive hearing loss occur in 1 in 10,000 to 20,000 live births (Stewart & Downs, 1993).

Clinical Findings

HISTORY. Hearing loss is often a "silent disease" (Williams, 1999). Both SNHL and conductive hearing loss can be accompanied by a history of:

- Failure to learn to speak at the appropriate age or failure to respond to auditory stimuli, speech that sounds like baby talk or is monotone and difficult to understand, avoidance of speaking
- Parental observation of an inappropriate response to auditory stimuli (e.g., lack of eye blinking, eye widening, startle, or head turning; inability to locate sounds) or parental concern about lack of appropriate speech development or failure to follow instructions; parents tend to be about 12 months ahead of care providers in identifying hearing loss in the child (Bachmann & Arvedson, 1998)
- Family history of any hearing loss
- Failed school screening audiogram; decreased note taking; seeming to misunderstand, ignore, confuse, or miss what is being said
- Increased volume of TV
- Aggression, increased physical complaints, difficulty in school and social situations
- History of any of the aforementioned causes of hearing loss (e.g., perinatal infection, meningitis, ototoxic drugs)

SNHL can also be associated with a history of:

- Birth weight less than 1500 g
- Hyperbilirubinemia requiring exchange transfusion or causing kernicterus
- Severe depression at birth (e.g., Apgar score of 0 to 3 at 5 minutes, failure to initiate a response by 10 minutes, or hypotonia up to 2 hours of age)
- Prolonged mechanical ventilation for greater than 10 days
- History of neurodegenerative disorders
- Environmental exposure to firecrackers, toy cap pistols, firearms, loud music, squeaking toys, and machines (e.g., snowmobiles, farm equipment, lawn mowers)

Conductive hearing loss can also occur in children with a history of:

- Kidney malformation
- Recurrent bouts of AOM or acute OE bilaterally for more than 3 months

PHYSICAL EXAMINATION. The following may be found in children with SNHL and conductive hearing loss:

- Presence of craniofacial anomalies (see Etiology).
- Presence of genetic stigmata associated with SNHL (see Etiology).
- Abnormal hearing screening during routine well-child care visits or other office visits. For children younger than 6 months, an ABR test is recommended. Behavioral testing using a conditioned response or an ABR is appropriate for children older than 6 months.

A complete physical examination with special attention to the eyes, skin, and skeletal and nervous systems is needed.

- Ears—preauricular pits, auricular malformation or appendage, abnormal tympanic membrane integrity, or impaired mobility with pneumatic otoscopy.
- Eyes—cataracts, corneal opacities, coloboma, blindness, nystagmus, exophthalmos, night blindness, heterochromia iridis, or blue sclerae (associated with genetic disorders that can cause SNHL).

DIAGNOSTIC TESTS. Audiometry is often the first testing performed. In younger children, an ABR or EOAE may be ordered. For SNHL, tests are ordered as indicated by the history and physical findings:

- Urinalysis, serum blood urea nitrogen, and creatinine to rule out renal disease.
- Complete blood count, TORCH (toxoplasmosis, rubella, cytomegalovirus, herpes simplex) screen, sickle cell screen.
- CT as indicated to rule out inner ear malformation.

For conductive hearing loss, a tympanogram can show decreased mobility of the tympanic membrane. Tympanometry is used as the confirmatory test after suspected decreased mobility is noted with pneumatic otoscopy.

Differential Diagnosis

Included is mixed SNHL with conductive hearing loss.

Management

The following should occur for any child with suspected hearing loss:

1. Refer any child with suspected hearing loss, including symptoms, history or physical findings, or known diagnosis associated with hearing loss, to an audiologist, otolaryngolo-

---

R E S O U R C E B O X 30-1

Agency for Health Care Policy and Research
Tel: (800) 358-9295 (publication clearing house)
Website: www.ahcpr.gov
E-mail: info@ahcpr.gov

Alexander Graham Bell Association for the Deaf
Tel: (202) 337-5220 (voice/TTY)
Fax: (202) 337-3814
Website: www.agbell.org
E-mail: agbell2@aol.com

American Academy of Otolaryngology–Head and Neck Surgery
Tel: (703) 836-4444

American Society for Deaf Children
Tel: (800) 942-2732 (voice/TTY)
Tel: (916) 641-6084 or 6085
E-mail: asdcl@aol.com

American Speech-Language-Hearing Association
Tel: (800) 638-8255
Tel: (301) 897-5700
Website: www.asha.org

Auditory-Verbal International
Tel: (703) 739-1049 (voice)
TTY: (703) 739-0874
Fax: (703) 739-0395

Center for Advancement of Deaf Children
Tel: (562) 430-1467 (voice/TTY)
Fax: (562) 430-6614

Cochlear Implant Club International
Tel: (716) 838-4662 (voice/TTY/fax)

EAR Foundation
Tel: (800) 545-4327
Tel: (615) 329-7807
Website: www.theearfound.com

Hear Now
Tel: (800) 648-4327, (303) 695-7797 (voice/TTY)
Fax: (303) 695-7789

Hearing Aid Helpline
Tel: (800) 521-5247

National Association of the Deaf
Tel: (301) 587-1788
TTY: (301) 587-1789
Fax: (301) 587-1791
E-mail: NADINFO@NAD.ORG

National Institute of Deafness and Other Communication Disorders
Tel: (301) 496-4000
Website: www.nih.gov/nidcd

Telecommunications for the Deaf
Tel: (301) 589-3789
TTY: (301) 589-3006
Fax: (301) 589-3797

gist, or both for full evaluation as soon as possible.
2. Encourage the use of amplification devices as appropriate. They may be personal (e.g., hearing aids) or group (e.g., teacher microphone). Cochlear implants with an external speech processor are sometimes used for profound SNHL.
3. Recommend special school and teaching strategies such as front-of-room placement and focusing on the child when speaking.
4. Evaluate and treat AOM and OME if present (see the AOM and OME sections).
5. Screen for hearing loss if bilateral middle ear effusion is present for 3 or more months.
6. Ensure a family-centered approach in making decisions regarding interventions for the child (e.g., PL 99-457).
7. Refer to Chapter 17 for discussion of children who are deaf.

Complications

Significant hearing loss impedes speech, language, cognitive development, and social interaction skills (AAP, 1999; Castiglia, 1998).

Prevention

- Recommend avoidance of environmental factors associated with hearing loss.
- Avoid ototoxic drug use.
- Immunize against mumps, rubella, varicella, *H. influenzae* type b, and other diseases that can cause SNHL through central nervous system damage.
- Treat prenatal and perinatal infections promptly.
- Provide $Rh_0(D)$ immune globulin to prevent erythroblastosis fetalis in susceptible women.

REFERENCES

American Academy of Pediatrics Task Force on Newborn and Infant Hearing: Newborn and infant hearing loss: Detection and intervention. Pediatrics 103:527-530, 1999.

Bachmann KR, Arvedson JC: Early identification and intervention for children who are hearing impaired. Pediatr Rev 19(5):155-165, 1998.

Barkin R, Rosen P (eds): Emergency Pediatrics: A Guide to Ambulatory Care, 5th ed. St Louis, CV Mosby, 1999.

Blumer J: Traditional management of acute otitis media. *In* Otitis Media: Management Strategies for the 21st Century. Bala Cynwyd, PA, Meniscus Educational Institute, 1998.

Brookhouser P: Sensorineural hearing loss in children. Pediatr Clin North Am 43:1195-1217, 1996.

Castiglia PT: The young child with hearing loss. J Pediatr Health Care 12:265-267, 1998.

Centers for Disease Control and Prevention: Serious hearing impairment among children aged 3-10 years. MMWR Morb Mortal Wkly Rep 46:1075-1076, 1997.

Debruyne F, Degroote M: One-year follow up after tympanostomy tube insertion for recurrent acute otitis media. J Otolaryngol 55:226-229, 1993.

Dowell SF, Butler JC, Giebink GS, et al: Acute otitis media: Management and surveillance in an era of pneumococcal resistance—a report from the Drug-Resistant Streptococcus Pneumonia Therapeutic Working Group [published erratum appears in Pediatr Infect Dis J 1999 Apr; 18(4):341]. Pediatr Infect Dis J 18:1-9, 1999.

Dowell S, Marcy M, Phillips W, et al: Otitis media—principles of judicious use of antimicrobial agents. Pediatrics 101:165-171, 1998.

Duncan B, Ey J, Holberg CJ, et al: Exclusive breast-feeding for at least 4 months protects against otitis media. Pediatrics 91:867-872, 1993.

Eden A, Fireman P, Stool S: Managing acute otitis: A fresh look at a familiar problem. Contemp Pediatr 13(3):64-85, 1996a.

Eden A, Fireman P, Stool S: Otitis media with effusion: Sorting out the options. Contemp Pediatr 13(3):85-93, 1996b.

Fitzgerald M: Reducing antibiotic angst. Ensuring that your therapy choice is effective. Adv Nurse Pract 6(3):43-46, 1998.

Granot E, Matoth I, Feinmesser R: Chronic middle ear effusion—a possible cause of protracted vomiting and failure to thrive in infancy. Clin Pediatr (Phila) 29:722-724, 1990.

Isaacson G, Rosenfeld R: Care of child with tympanostomy tubes. Pediatr Clin North Am 43:1183-1193, 1996.

Jahn A, Hawke M: Infections of the external ear. *In* Cummings CW (ed): Otolaryngology—Head and Neck Surgery. St Louis, CV Mosby, 1993, pp 2787-2808.

Joint Committee on Infant Hearing: Joint Committee on Infant Hearing 1994 position statement. Pediatrics 95:152-156, 1995.

Klein J: Preventing recurrent otitis: What role antibiotic. Contemp Pediatr 11:44-60, 1994.

Kozyrskyj A, Hildes-Ripstein G, Longstaffe S, et al: Treatment of acute otitis media with a shortened course of antibiotics. JAMA 279:1736-1742, 1998.

Maxson S, Yamauchi T: Acute otitis media. Pediatr Rev 17(6):191-195, 1996.

Nash D, Schochat E, Rozycki A, et al: When loud noises hurt. Contemp Pediatr 14(6):97-109, 1997.

National Institutes of Health: Early identification of hearing impairment in infants and young children. NIH Consensus Statement 11(1):1-24, 1993.

Pelton SI, Barnett ED: New strategies for the treatment of AOM. *In* Otitis Media: Management Strategies for the 21st Century. Bala Cynwyd, PA, Meniscus Educational Institute, 1998.

Pichichero M, Cohen R: Shortened course of antibiotic therapy for acute otitis media, sinusitis and tonsillopharyngitis. Pediatr Infect Dis J 16:680–695, 1997.

Pizzuto MP, Volk MS, Kingston LM: Common topics in pediatric otolaryngology. Pediatr Clin North Am 45:973–991, 1998.

Rosenfeld R: An evidence-based approach to treating otitis media. Pediatr Clin North Am 43:1165–1181, 1996a.

Rosenfeld R: How can meta-analysis help in treatment of otitis media? Presented at the Sixth International Symposium on Recent Advances in Otitis Media. 1996b.

Schuman A: Best new products for pediatrics: 1997. Contemp Pediatr 14(12):61–76, 1997.

Schuman A: The challenge of universal newborn hearing screening. *In* Contemporary Pediatrics Pediatricians Product Guide 1994, pp 15–24.

Schutze G, Jacobs R: Antimicrobial prophylaxis. Pediatr Rev 15:377–382, 1994.

Sie K: Cholesteatoma in children. Pediatr Clin North Am 43:1245–1253, 1996.

Spiro S: A cost effectiveness analysis of ear wax softeners. Nurse Pract 22(8):28–32, 1997.

Stenstrom C, Ingvaarson L: Otitis-prone and healthy children—what makes the difference? Presented at the Sixth International Symposium: Recent Advances in Otitis Media. 1996.

Stewart J, Downs M: Congenital conductive hearing loss: The need for early identification and intervention. Pediatrics 91:355–359, 1993.

US Department of Health and Human Services: Managing Otitis Media With Effusion in Young Children. Rockville, MD, US Department of Health and Human Services, 1994, AHCPR Publication No. 94-0623.

US Department of Health and Human Services: Healthy Children 2000: National Health Promotion and Disease Prevention Objectives for the Year 2000. Washington, DC, US Government Printing Office, 1990.

US Department of Health & Human Services: Healthy People 2010. Objectives: Draft for Public Comment: Child and Adolescent Focused Objectives. 1998, http://web.health.gov/healthypeople.

US Preventive Services Task Force: Guide to Clinical Preventive Services, 2nd ed. Baltimore, Williams & Wilkins, 1996.

US Public Health Service: Put Prevention Into Practice: The Clinician's Handbook of Preventive Services, 2nd ed. Germantown, MD, International Medical Publishing, 1997.

Williams MA: Hearing loss. *In* Dershewitz RA (ed): Ambulatory Pediatric Care, 3rd ed. Philadelphia, Lippincott-Raven, 1999, pp 467–472.

CHAPTER 31

Cardiovascular Disorders

Jan Freitas-Nichols

▨▨ INTRODUCTION

Most cardiovascular problems in the pediatric population are due to congenital heart disease (CHD). CHD is present in 0.8 to 1% of all live births and is more common in the premature infant population. More than half of cases of CHD are detected within the first 6 weeks of life. Less than 15% of conditions remain undetected after the first year of life (Brooks, 1998). Close to half of all congenital heart defects are relatively insignificant, whereas the other half may be critical (Brooks, 1998). Defects such as small ventricular septal defects (VSDs) or a bicuspid aortic valve cause little or no disability to an infant or child, although the diagnosis itself can cause great concern for parents and caregivers.

Today it is possible to make an accurate diagnosis noninvasively in almost every case. Evaluation and diagnosis can occur as early as 20 weeks' gestation with the help of fetal echocardiography (Williams et al., 1994). Early detection of CHD is important in decreasing the morbidity and mortality associated with undiagnosed, complex problems of the heart.

The nurse practitioner (NP) must maintain a high index of suspicion regarding small signs and symptoms of cardiovascular disease. Such suspicion allows early identification and referral of infants and children with potential cardiovascular problems. Additional roles that the NP

offers include provision of support to families and children once a diagnosis is made and education of families about prevention of acquired heart disease. This chapter presents information on both congenital and acquired heart disease in the pediatric population that should assist the NP in assessment, management, family support, and referral.

▨▨ STANDARDS OF CARE

The *Guide to Clinical Preventive Services* (US Preventive Services Task Force, 1996) recommendations related to cardiovascular health are as follows:

- Measurement of blood pressure (BP) during office visits is recommended for children and adolescents. This recommendation is based on proven benefits from the early detection of treatable causes of secondary hypertension; evidence is insufficient to recommend for or against routine periodic BP measurement to detect essential (primary) hypertension in this age group. Sphygmomanometry should be performed in accordance with the recommended technique for children, and hypertension should only be diagnosed on the basis of readings at each of three separate visits. In children, criteria defining hypertension vary with age. Age-, sex-, and height-specific BP nomograms for US children and adolescents have been published.

- Routine counseling to promote physical activity and a healthy diet for the primary prevention of hypertension is recommended.

The *Put Prevention into Practice: Clinician's Handbook of Preventive Services* (US Public Health Service, 1997) outlines recommendations from major authorities including the following:

- American Academy of Pediatrics (AAP) and Bright Futures—BP should be measured in children at 3, 4, 5, 6, and 8 years of age and annually beginning at 10 years of age.
- National Heart, Lung, and Blood Institute Task Force on Blood Pressure Control in Children—BP pressure should be measured annually beginning at 3 years of age.

ANATOMY AND PHYSIOLOGY

Fetal Circulation

Knowledge of the fetal circulation is essential for understanding the circulatory changes that occur in the newborn at delivery (see Fig. 31-1). The fetal circulation has four unique features that differ from the postnatal circulation:

- Oxygenation of the blood occurs in the placenta, not the lungs.
- Fetal pulmonary vascular resistance is high and systemic vascular resistance is low (high pressure on the right side of the heart, low pressure on the left side).
- The foramen ovale, the opening in the septum between the two atria, permits a portion of the blood to flow from the right atrium directly to the left atrium.
- A patent ductus arteriosus (PDA) is a vessel connection between the pulmonary artery and the aorta that allows blood to flow from the pulmonary artery to the aorta and bypass the fetal lungs.

Oxygen is diffused into the fetal circulation from the maternal uterine arteries in the placenta. From the placenta, oxygenated blood flows through the umbilical vein and is diverted through the liver to the inferior vena cava by the ductus venosus. When this well-oxygenated blood reaches the right atrium, it flows preferentially toward the atrial septum, through the foramen ovale, and into the left atrium. This oxygenated blood then flows into the left ventricle and out the aorta. Approximately two thirds of the blood from the aorta flows toward the head and neck to ensure that the fetal brain constantly receives well-oxygenated blood.

Venous blood returns from the head and upper extremities through the superior vena cava to the right atrium. This blood preferentially flows toward the tricuspid valve into the right ventricle. From the right ventricle, the blood enters the pulmonary artery. Because pulmonary vascular resistance is high and systemic resistance is low, most blood in the pulmonary artery flows through the ductus arteriosus into the descending aorta to supply oxygen and nutrients to the trunk and lower extremities. Only a small amount of blood flows into the pulmonary circuit to perfuse the lungs.

The fetal circulation is best described as two parallel circuits, with the left ventricle supplying blood to the upper extremities and the right ventricle serving the lower extremities and the placenta. At the time of transition to extrauterine life, these separate blood flows become a serial circuit.

Neonatal Circulation

A number of complex events occur at birth that rapidly shift the fetal circulation toward a neonatal circulation. Clamping of the umbilical cord and subsequent removal of the placenta as the oxygenating organ causes an immediate circulatory change in which the lungs are the new source of oxygenation. This change causes an increase in systemic vascular resistance (systemic BP). With the first breath, mechanical inflation of the lungs and an increase in oxygen saturation bring about a dramatic fall in pulmonary vascular resistance and, consequently, increased pulmonary blood flow. This activity leads to beginning constriction of the ductus arteriosus. As the pressures within the heart become relatively higher on the left side and

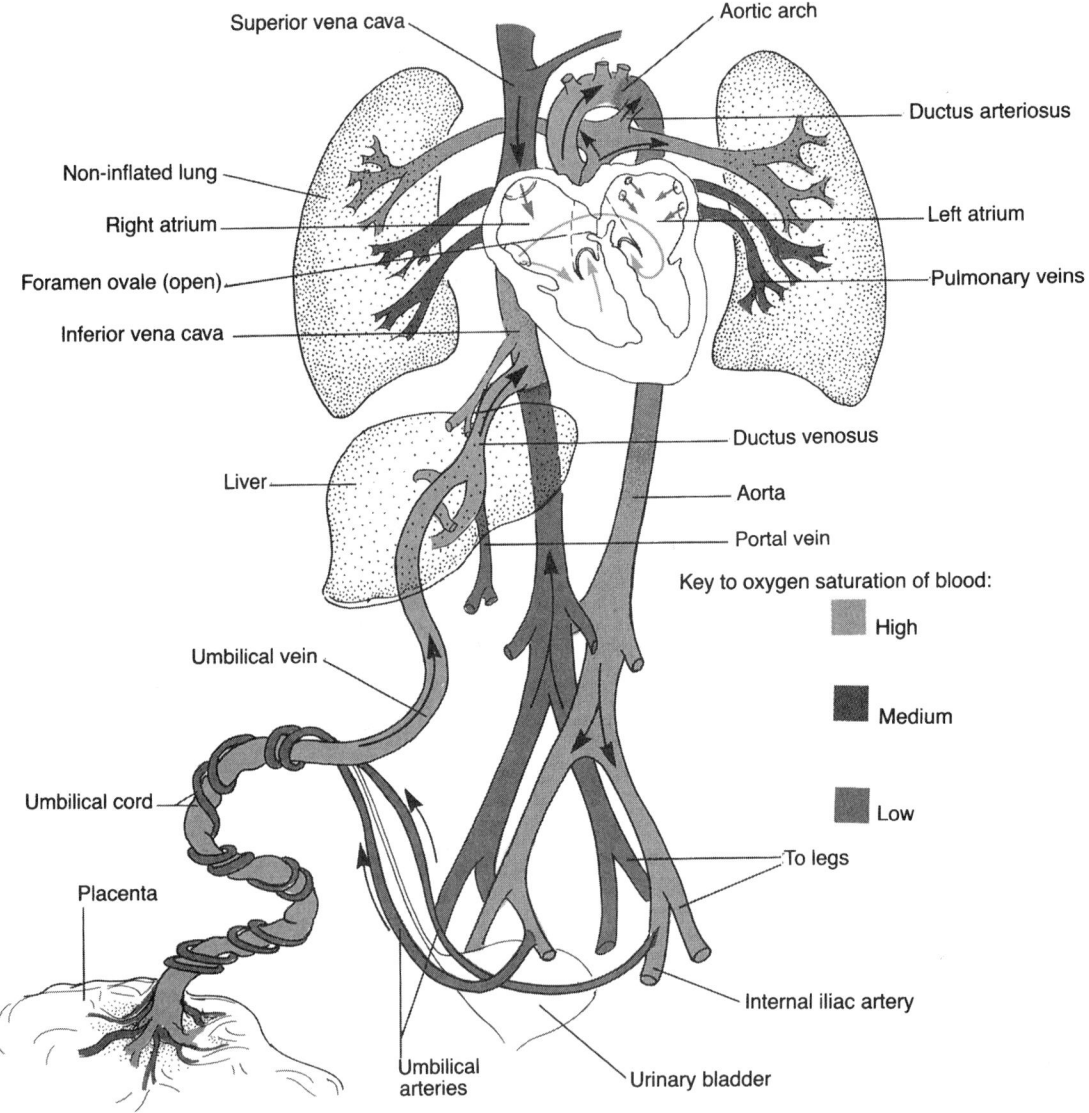

FIGURE 31-1
Fetal Circulation. (From Gorrie TM, McKinney ES, Murray SS. Foundations of Maternal-Newborn Nursing. Philadelphia, WB Saunders, 1994.)

lower on the right, the foramen ovale closes. Functional closure of the ductus arteriosus and foramen ovale usually occurs within the first hours to days of life, and a serial circuit forms out of the once-parallel pulmonary and systemic circulation.

The transition toward complete anatomical closure, or obliteration of fetal structures by tissue growth or constriction, is more gradual. Pulmonary vascular resistance drops gradually over the first 6 to 8 weeks of life, which may protect the pulmonary circulation against volume overload in some congenital heart anomalies. Shunt murmurs or symptoms of congestive heart failure (CHF) gradually become apparent as the infant approaches 8 weeks of age. At this time, resistance to flow is less, and shunting to the pulmonary bed is increased.

Conditions that cause persistence of fetal shunts, thus allowing unoxygenated blood to flow from the right side of the heart to the left, may cause cyanosis. Any murmur or cyanosis in a newborn should be carefully monitored and evaluated to detect cardiac abnormalities.

Normal Cardiac Structure and Function

The heart is a muscular, four-chambered organ located in the mediastinum, the space in the chest between the lungs. The four chambers are divided into two larger muscular pumping chambers, the ventricles, and two smaller receiving chambers, the atria. The right side of the heart receives blood low in oxygen returning from the systemic circulation by way of the inferior and superior venae cavae. The blood enters the right atrium and passes through the tricuspid valve to the right ventricle. It is then pumped through the pulmonic valve into the pulmonary artery and from there to the lungs, where it is oxygenated. Blood returning from the lungs enters the left atrium by way of the pulmonary veins and then passes through the mitral valve into the left ventricle. It is next pumped through the aortic valve into the aorta to provide oxygenated blood for the systemic circulation.

The heart valves are one-way valves that open and close because of pressure changes within the heart. The valvular system of the heart controls the flow of blood from chamber to chamber. The tricuspid valve, which controls flow between the right atrium and ventricle, has three cusps held in place by the chordae tendineae. The pulmonary valve directs blood flow from the right ventricle into the pulmonary artery, which bifurcates into right and left arteries to allow flow into both lungs. The pulmonary veins entering the left atrium contain no valves, so blood can flow freely from the lungs into the atrium. The mitral valve controls flow from the left atrium into the left ventricle. The aortic valve controls flow from the high-pressure left ventricle out to the body (see Fig. 31-2).

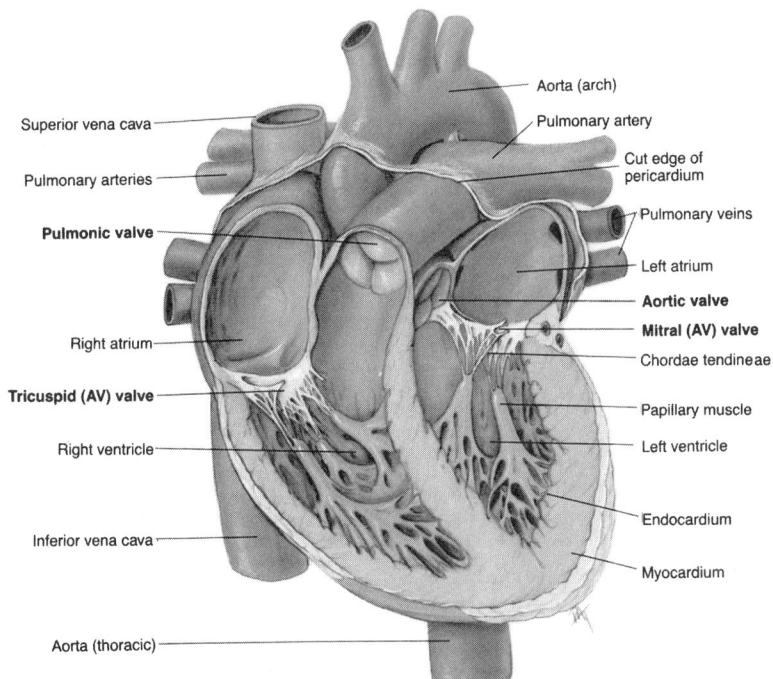

F I G U R E 31-2
Diagram of the heart. (From Jarvis C: Physical Examination and Health Assessment, 2nd ed. Philadelphia, WB Saunders, 1996.)

Superior vena cava

Pulmonary arteries

Pulmonic valve

Right atrium

Tricuspid (AV) valve

Right ventricle

Inferior vena cava

Aorta (thoracic)

Aorta (arch)

Pulmonary artery

Cut edge of pericardium

Pulmonary veins

Left atrium

Aortic valve

Mitral (AV) valve

Chordae tendineae

Papillary muscle

Left ventricle

Endocardium

Myocardium

Conduction System

Myocardial contraction is stimulated by electrical depolarization along the conduction tract within the heart. Depolarization begins at the sinoatrial node, which is high in the wall of the atrium. This node acts as the pacemaker of the heart by regularly beginning the depolarizing impulses of each heartbeat. The wave of depolarization travels from the sinoatrial node throughout the atria and produces contraction of the atrial muscle. The impulses reach the atrioventricular (AV) node, which is located in the lower portion of the right atrium at the junction of the atrium and ventricle. From the AV node, the depolarization wave passes through the bundle of His, the fibers extending from the AV node along the intraventricular septum. Depolarization spreads through the left and right branches of the bundle of His and from there through the Purkinje fibers extending into the ventricular muscle. Impulses then spread throughout the ventricles and cause contraction. The electrocardiogram (ECG) can demonstrate this pattern of changing electrical impulses.

Heart Sounds

Heart sounds are a reflection of the heart's functioning, although the intensity varies with age, thickness of the chest wall, and cardiac output. At the time of ventricular contraction, the beginning of systole, the mitral and tricuspid valves close and produce the first heart sound (S_1). S_1 is the "lubb" of lubb-dupp. Although the left side of the heart reacts slightly before the right side, closure of the mitral and tricuspid valves occurs so closely together that S_1 appears as a single sound. S_1 is best heard at the apex of the heart and is synchronous with the apical and carotid pulses.

After the blood has been ejected, the heart relaxes, the mitral and tricuspid valves open, and the aortic and pulmonary valves close to keep the blood from rushing back into the ventricles. This closure results in the second heart sound (S_2). S_2 reflects the onset of diastole and is the "dupp" of lubb-dupp.

▰▰▰ PATHOPHYSIOLOGY

The term *congenital heart disease* implies only that a cardiovascular malformation is present at birth. It does not indicate the etiology or cause of the malformation. When CHD is diagnosed in an infant or child, parents may assume that they are somehow responsible for the child's defect. Health care professionals must be clear about what is and what is not known about CHD to spare parents needless worry and guilt.

Most CHD is due to a complex interaction of genetic and environmental or intrauterine factors, a pattern called *multifactorial inheritance*. The heart develops primarily between the fourth and seventh weeks of fetal life, a time when the fetus is most susceptible to infectious or teratogenic exposure or to predisposing genetic or chromosomal factors (Moore & Persaud, 1998).

Although several factors can be *associated* with CHD, very few agents are known to *cause* cardiac defects. The only well-documented teratogens include maternal thalidomide, diazepam, corticosteroids, phenothiazine, and alcoholism. Paternal use of cocaine is frequently implicated in cases of CHD (Clark, 1995).

CHD has been associated with infectious exposure in the first 8 weeks of gestation, especially to cytomegalovirus, mumps, or rubella. A woman who contracts rubella during this phase of pregnancy has a 50% risk of having a baby with congenital rubella syndrome, which can include PDA and/or pulmonary artery branch stenosis. CHD, including hypertrophic cardiomyopathies and great vessel abnormalities, develops in approximately 10% of infants born to mothers with insulin-dependent diabetes (Friedman, 1996; Clark, 1995).

Genetic risk factors are most significant for children who have a family history of CHD. The incidence is between 4 and 14% and depends on the type of defect and familial relationship. The single greatest risk factor is a parent or sibling with a congenital heart abnormality. The risk is highest when the defect occurs in the mother or sibling and lowest when the defect is in the father (Clark, 1995).

The association of CHD with certain chromosomal abnormalities or syndromes (e.g., infants with Down syndrome [trisomy 21] have a 30 to 50% incidence of CHD) has been well documented (Mulhern, 1998) (Table 31–1). Additionally, up to 25% of children with CHD have extracardiac abnormalities (Ardinger, 1997).

T A B L E 31-1

Congenital Heart Defects Associated With Genetic or Chromosomal Abnormalities

SYNDROME	DEFECT
Trisomy 13,18	Patent ductus arteriosus, ventricular septal defect, atrial septal defect
Trisomy 21 (Down)	Endocardial cushion defect, ventricular septal defect, patent ductus arteriosus, atrial septal defect, tetralogy of Fallot
Turner syndrome	Coarctation of the aorta, pulmonary stenosis, aortic valve stenosis, hypoplastic left heart
Marfan syndrome	Aortic stenosis, mitral valve stenosis, total anomalous pulmonary venous return, aortic aneurysm, mitral valve prolapse
Williams syndrome	Aortic stenosis, partial anomalous venous return, pulmonary stenosis
DiGeorge syndrome	Interrupted aortic arch, atrial septal defect, truncus arteriosus, tetralogy of Fallot
Neurofibromatosis	Pulmonary stenosis

ASSESSMENT OF THE CARDIOVASCULAR SYSTEM

Cardiac assessment includes a comprehensive history, physical assessment, and a variety of diagnostic tests.

History

Review of the family, maternal, fetal, neonatal and infant medical history, as well as growth and development, is helpful in the cardiac evaluation of a newborn or child with a suspected cardiac abnormality (see Table 31–2 for risk factors).

Physical Examination

Physical assessment in a child with suspected CHD should be geared toward the age of the child (Table 31–3). It is not always possible to follow the same pattern of assessment with each child evaluated. It is important to be flexible, yet thorough in any evaluation and include all aspects of the physical examination in an order that best suits the comfort and needs of the infant or child. Emphasis should be on a developmental approach to cardiac assessment.

VITAL SIGNS

Heart rate, respiratory rate, and BP vary considerably throughout childhood. Measurements of vital signs must be obtained on each visit with the child at rest because crying and exercise affect results. The normal ranges for various age groups and gender are available for comparison.

- *Heart rate* (see Table 31–23). Heart rates should always be obtained by auscultation of the heart in children younger than 10 years. Assessment should include rate and rhythm variations. An increased heart rate can be caused by excitement, anxiety, hyperthyroidism, heart disease, anemia, or fever. Rhythm is assessed for regularity.
- *Pulses.* Pulses should be checked in the upper and lower extremities and evaluated for character (strength) and variation between the different sites. A bounding pulse may indicate PDA. Weak or thready pulses indicate CHF or an obstructive lesion such as severe aortic stenosis. Good brachial pulses in conjunction with weak, "thready," or absent femoral pulses indicate coarctation of the aorta.
- *BP* (see Tables 31–19 and 31–20). Assessment should begin at 3 years of age or younger if heart disease is suspected. It is important to always use a BP cuff that is appropriate for the child's size. For arm pressure, the width of the cuff should be two-thirds the size of the arm measured from the axilla to the anticubital space. A cuff that is too narrow or does not fit around a chubby arm may cause an erroneously high reading. Initial evaluation should compare the pressure in all four

T A B L E 31-2

Risk Factors for Congenital Heart Disease

Perinatal risk factors
 Maternal infections and exposures (CMV, rubella, other viral syndromes)
 Maternal use of tobacco, alcohol, street drugs, or prescription drugs
 Maternal health diseases (CHD, lupus, diabetes)
 Maternal age at child's birth (increase in chromosomal abnormalities after 40 y of age)
 Maternal pregnancy history (excessive weight gain, history of gestational diabetes)
Neonatal risk factors
 Fetal or newborn distress (aspiration, hypoxia, cyanosis)
 Prematurity (increased incidence of CHD in premature infants)
 Presence of associated anomalies (genetic or chromosomal abnormalities or syndromes)
 Neonatal infections (group A β-hemolytic streptococci)
 Birth weight (term infants, <2500 g; SGA, <2 SD from the mean for gestational age)
Newborn risk factors
 Murmur at birth or early infancy
 Hypertension (at birth or beyond)
 Feeding difficulty (SOB, easily fatigued, diaphoresis, poor intake)
 Poor weight gain (failure to regain birth weight by 2 wk, continued poor growth)
 Cyanosis (increase with crying, feeding, exertion)
 Tachypnea (persistent, with crying, feeding)
Toddler, school-aged, or teenage risk factors
 Deviation from normal growth and development (normal milestone development, following own
  growth curve)
 Deviation from activity level appropriate for chronological age (keeps up with peers; able to run,
  ride bike)
 Frequent respiratory tract infections (pneumonia, URIs that last longer than normal)
 Prior murmurs, blue spells
 Documented GABHS infection
 Hypertension (documented on a minimum of 3 separate visits)
 Chest pain with exertion
 SOB with exertion (beyond normal peers)
 Syncope or dizziness (especially associated with noted heart rate change)
 Tachycardia or bradycardia (fluttering in chest, racing heart)
 Diet (excessive caffeine usage, obesity)
 Alcohol, drug, or tobacco use
 Other health factors (disease state, general health status)
Family history risk factors
 CHD (especially siblings, parents, first-degree relatives)
 Sudden death or premature myocardial infarction (before age 50)
 Hypertension
 Rheumatic fever
 Genetic syndromes
 Hypercholesterolemia

CHD = congenital heart disease; CMV = cytomegalovirus; GABHS = group A β-hemolytic streptococcus; SGA = small for gestational age; SOB = shortness of breath; URIs = upper respiratory infections.

T A B L E 31-3

Developmental Approach to Cardiac Assessment

INFANTS	TODDLERS	SCHOOL AGED	ADOLESCENTS
Complete the assessment with the infant in the parent's arms to keep the infant quiet and cooperative. Perform uncomfortable aspects of the exam after auscultation to ensure a quiet listen. Keep the infant covered and warm to minimize discomfort and physiologic changes associated with chilling. Observe color, respiratory effort, and general effort level while the baby is quiet.	Approach the child quietly, calmly, and slowly. Loud boisterous greeting may frighten the toddler. Complete the assessment wherever the child is most comfortable—sitting on the floor, in the parent's lap, on the exam table. Allow the child to handle a stethoscope while the history is being taken. Have a toy or distraction item available during the exam. Consider "listening" to the parent first to improve comfort with the exam.	Clearly explain the plan and expectations before the exam. Answer the child's questions honestly. Talk about topics of interest (school, sports) during the exam. School-aged children may be modest and prefer to keep a gown on during most of the exam. School-aged children may be helpful in discussion of symptoms and events surrounding current concerns.	Questions should be directed at the adolescent and parent. Communicate in a manner that conveys honesty, professionalism, and interest in their concerns. Ensure privacy related to both the physical exam and information sharing. Provide a choice of having a parent present for any or all aspects of the history and exam. Adolescents are very "body aware" and need reassurance that their concerns are valid, even when the symptom is within normal limits.

extremities. Pressure in all extremities should be equal, with pressure in the legs being slightly higher (10 to 20 mm Hg) in a child who walks. In a child 2 to 10 years of age, the average systolic blood pressure is determined by a simple equation:

$$90 + (2 \times \text{age in years})$$

The pulse pressure (difference between systolic and diastolic pressure) is normally 20 to 50 mm Hg throughout childhood. A wide pulse pressure caused by an unusually high systolic reading can be due to an increased heart rate. If it is due to an abnormally low diastolic pressure, it may be an indication of PDA, aortic regurgitation, or other cardiac pathology.

• *Respiratory rate.* Evaluation of the respiratory system includes the respiratory rate, assessment of effort, and breath sounds in all five lobes of the lungs. It is important to evaluate the respiratory rate in a quiet infant or child. A stethoscope should be used to listen for breath sounds while counting the rate. A respiratory rate above 40 in a young child or 60 in a newborn who is quiet, resting, and afebrile warrants further evaluation. Ease or difficulty of respiratory effort and adventitious sounds such as rales, rhonchi, or wheezing should be assessed. An infant with cyanotic CHD may be tachypneic but not show significant signs of dyspnea; the use of accessory muscles for breathing results in intercostal retractions, nasal flaring, and/or tracheal pulling. An infant or child with CHF demonstrates significant tachypnea, as well as dyspnea.

GENERAL APPEARANCE

- Observation of an infant is best accomplished before any other part of the physical examination occurs so that the observer can get a true picture of the appearance, general nutritional state, respiratory effort, color, physical abnormalities, and distress or discomfort level before the child has been disturbed. It is important to validate with the caregiver the child's comfort level to assess any variation from normal.

- During this observation period one should notice unusual facial characteristics (e.g., malformed ears, wide-spaced eyes, noticeable anomalies) or extracardiac anomalies (e.g., cleft lip or palate, polydactyly, microcephaly) that may be associated with a syndrome or chromosomal abnormalities. Children may have obvious stigmata such as Down syndrome, Marfan syndrome (unusually tall with an arm span wider than the head-to-toe height), Turner syndrome (webbed neck, pixie-like facies), or fetal alcohol syndrome (microcephaly and pinched facies), all of which are associated with CHD (Clark, 1995).

- Overall skin color should be assessed for signs of mottling or central cyanosis while the infant is at rest. Cyanosis caused by heart disease is recognized as a pale blue or ruddy red color of the mucous membranes (lips, tongue, nail beds). Peripheral cyanosis or acrocyanosis, a blueness or pallor noted around the mouth and on the hands or feet, can be a normal variant, especially if it intensifies when the child is cold or crying. Clubbing of the fingers and toes may be seen in children with long-standing cyanosis.

- Signs of peripheral or periorbital edema should be noted. Edema or puffiness around the eyes may be evident in an infant with CHF even in the absence of peripheral edema of the hands or feet. True

pitting edema of the feet is an unusual finding in an infant with CHF.

- Diligent measurement of height and weight, accurate plotting on standardized charts, and continued analysis of growth and development are important tools that should be included at each assessment. Although many children with CHD fall within the normal ranges of height, weight, and development, a large number of infants and children with heart disease experience poor weight gain, less than normal linear growth, and delays in achieving developmental milestones.

PALPATION

- Palpation of the chest should include assessment of all five areas, including the aortic, pulmonic, tricuspid, and mitral areas and Erb's point (Fig. 31–3). Chest palpation is best accomplished by using the open palm of the hand near the base of the fingers. The hand should be gently moved from location to location across the chest to assess abnormal precordial activity, including pulsations, lifts, heaves, or thrills, and to determine the location of the apical impulse. The apical impulse is used to determine the size of the heart and is the most lateral point at which cardiac activity can be palpated. In infants and children, the impulse is normally palpated at the apex of the heart in the fourth intercostal space just to the left of the midclavicular line. At approximately 7 years of age the point shifts to the fifth intercostal space. In the presence of cardiomegaly, the apical impulse is shifted laterally or downward.

- Thrills are characterized by a palpable vibration caused by turbulent blood flow through abnormal structures or defects in the heart. The turbulent flow may be due to valvular narrowing or stenosis or defects such as VSD.

- Peripheral pulses (radial, brachial, carotid, dorsalis pedis, and posterior tibial) should be assessed for amplitude and intensity. Symmetry between the upper and lower extremity pulses is important for assess-

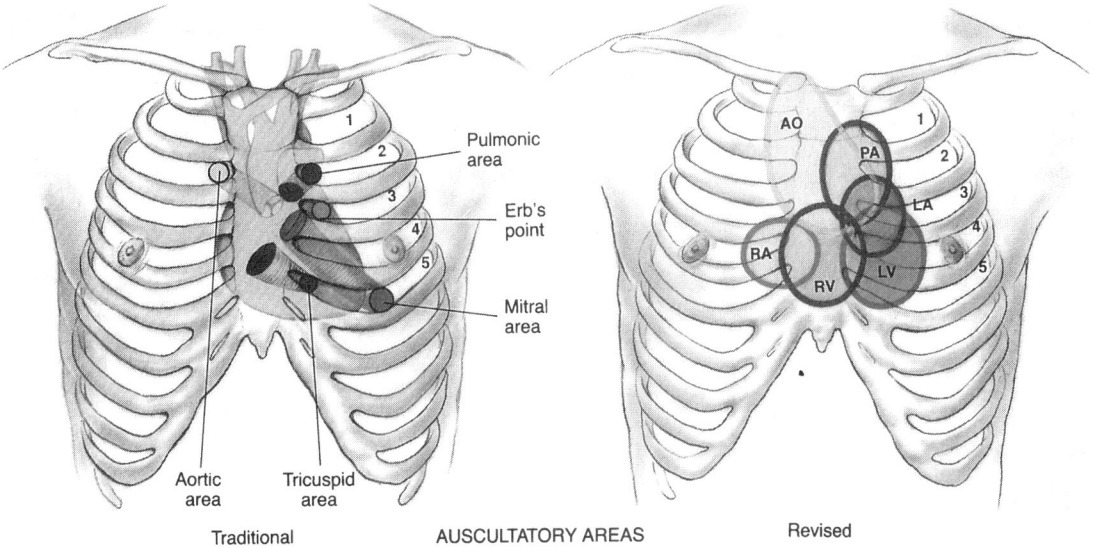

F I G U R E 31-3
Auscultatory areas. AO = aorta; LA = left atrium; LV = left ventricle; PA = pulmonary artery; RA = right atrium; RV = right ventricle. (From Jarvis C: Physical Examination and Health Assessment, 2nd ed. Philadelphia, WB Saunders, 1996.)

ment of obstructed blood flow as in coarctation of the aorta.

- The liver and spleen should be assessed for enlargement. A liver more than 1 cm below the right costal margin may indicate hepatomegaly and is an important finding in the assessment of a child with suspected heart disease. Infants may have a palpable liver edge as a normal finding.

AUSCULTATION OF HEART SOUNDS

- Auscultation of the heart should be approached in the same manner for every child. The practitioner can start either at the top of the heart and move downward toward the apex or mitral area or move in reverse as long as the same method is followed each time. It is important to try to assess heart sounds in a quiet environment with a cooperative child to ensure a thorough and accurate assessment.
- Determination of heart rate and rhythm followed by identification of heart sounds and detection of murmurs should occur in each of five previously noted areas of the heart (see Fig. 31-3).

- Heart sounds represent various events in the cardiac cycle. Four individual **heart sounds** can be heard: S_1, S_2, S_3, and S_4 (Table 31-4). S_1 and S_2 represent normal heart sounds, whereas the presence of S_3 or S_4 may indicate cardiac enlargement or volume overload. At each area of examination the evaluator should accurately identify the first (S_1) and second (S_2) heart sounds. S_1 is the more dominant sound at the apex of the heart; S_2 is best evaluated at the second left intercostal space. The stethoscope should be slowly moved up to the chest to other auscultatory locations. As the location changes, the intensity of the two heart sounds varies.
- Clicks: Ejection and nonejection clicks may be appreciated as an extra heart sound. Ejection clicks are evident early in systole, immediately after S_1 and give the impression of a split first heart sound. Pulmonic ejection clicks are heard best at the upper left sternal border, are high in frequency, and generally do not vary with respiration. This variation is evident in pulmonic stenosis. An aortic ejection click, heard best at Erb's point, has the sound of a "snap" or a

T A B L E 31-4

Characteristics of Heart Sounds

FIRST HEART SOUND (S₁)

The first heart sound is heard in the beginning of systole and indicates closure of the atrioventricular valves (mitral and tricuspid). Normally S_1 is a single heart sound and is the "lubb" of the lubb-dupp in the cardiac cycle. The first heart sound may be differentiated from early systolic clicks by the low frequency of the sound, as opposed to clicks, which have a higher frequency. The first heart sound is heard best at the apex of the heart.

SECOND HEART SOUND (S₂)

The second heart sound is heard at the end of systole and indicates closure of the aortic and pulmonic valves. S_2 is normally split as the aortic valve closes slightly before the pulmonic valve. This sound is the "dupp" of the cycle. The importance of accurately assessing the second heart sound cannot be overemphasized. Normally, in children and infants beyond a few weeks of age, the second heart sound widens with inspiration and narrows or becomes singular with expiration. This pattern is best assessed at the upper left sternal border in the pulmonic area. Pulmonary hypertension causes earlier closure and accentuation of the pulmonic component of S_2, which may sound like a loud single second heart sound. Wide splitting of the second heart sound without completely becoming single with expiration may indicate increased pulmonary flow, characteristic of an atrial septal defect.

THIRD AND FOURTH HEART SOUNDS (S₃ AND S₄)

A third heart sound (S_3) is associated with rapid ventricular filling and may be heard in a quiet infant or child with a rapid heart rate. If present, an S_3 "gallop" is heard best at the apex with the bell of the stethoscope during early diastole and, when put together with the first and second heart sounds, gives an impression of the word "Kentucky." A fourth heart sound (S_4) is always pathological and represents increased force of atrial contraction and ventricular distention. An S_4 gallop, which sounds like the word "Tennessee," is heard in late diastole just before S_1. It is low pitched and heard best at the apex with the bell of the stethoscope.

"click." This sound may be due to valvular aortic stenosis or a dilated aortic root. Non-ejection clicks are heard best in midsystole, or midway between S_1 and S_2 in the cardiac cycle. These clicks are best heard in upright or standing patients, vary with respirations, and are due to mitral valve prolapse.

MURMURS

A murmur is an extra sound that may be detected during examination of the heart and may be heard in 50 to 90% of children at some point (Feit, 1997; Smith, 1997; Harris, 1994). Less than 5% of murmurs denote pathology. A murmur alone is not a diagnosis. It may be caused by normal blood flow through normal cardiac structures (innocent or physiologic murmur) or by turbulent blood flow caused by a defect or abnormal cardiac structures. Murmurs may also be due to normal transitional physiological processes and may be intensified by anything that increases cardiac output (e.g., anemia, fever, exercise).

Innocent or Functional Murmurs

Functional or innocent cardiac murmurs are quite common in children and can be evident in newborns. These murmurs are asymptomatic and are usually classic in quality (Table 31–5). Innocent or functional murmurs are not caused by abnormal cardiac structures but are due to transitional flow or mildly turbulent flow through a normal heart. Table 31–6 describes common innocent murmurs.

Families and older children should be reassured that nothing is wrong with the heart. They should be told that this murmur may come and go and may be louder at times of fever, anxiety, pain, or exercise but in no way

TABLE 31-5
Characteristics of Innocent Murmurs

Usually grade I–II/VI in intensity and localized
Changes with position (sitting to lying)
May vary in loudness or presence from visit to visit
May increase in loudness (intensity) with fever, anemia, exercise, or anxiety
Musical or vibratory in quality
Systolic in timing except for venous hum, which is continuous
Duration is short
Best heard in LLSB or pulmonic area (except for venous hum)
Rarely transmitted
May disappear with Valsalva maneuver, position, or gentle jugular pressure
Vital signs are normal
ECG is normal
General health status is good

ECG = electrocardiogram; LLSB = left lower sternal border.

represents cardiac pathology. Families should be reminded that activities need not be limited and that special precautions are not necessary.

Assessment of a Heart Murmur

All cardiac murmurs should be thoroughly evaluated to determine an accurate diagnosis. Every murmur is assessed according to the criteria listed in Table 31–7. Types of murmurs are listed in Table 31–8. Characteristics of pathological murmurs are listed in Table 31–9. It is important to note that the presence of a murmur causes great anxiety for a family while waiting for a diagnosis. All murmurs should have a second opinion from a pediatric colleague or pediatric cardiologist unless it is definitely clear that the sound is innocent in nature.

Common Diagnostic Studies

- Chest radiograph. Radiography provides the following information: cardiac size and size of specific chambers and great vessels, cardiac contour, status of pulmonary blood flow, and status of the lungs and other surrounding tissue (Fig. 31–4).
- ECG. ECG monitors the electrical activity of the heart from different locations and in different planes of the body (Fig. 31–5).
- Echocardiogram. Echocardiography uses reflected sound waves to identify intracardiac structures and their motion. The types of recordings include two-dimensional, M-mode, contrast, and Doppler studies (Fig. 31–6).
- Cardiac catheterization. An opaque catheter is introduced into the heart chambers via the large peripheral vessels. The dye introduced through the catheter is ob-

TABLE 31-6
Common Innocent Heart Murmurs

Still's murmur is the most common type of innocent murmur heard. It is a systolic ejection murmur that is vibratory or musical in quality and heard best at the apex or the lower left sternal border. The murmur is of low frequency and grade I–II/VI and may change with respiration or position.

Pulmonary flow murmur is commonly heard in a newborn but may also be heard in children. This murmur is a soft, blowing systolic murmur that is grade I–II/VI in intensity. It is heard best in the pulmonic area or the upper left sternal border and is related to high velocity of flow in the pulmonary artery. An important characteristic of this murmur is that it disappears with the Valsalva maneuver.

Venous hum is a murmur consisting of a soft, low-frequency, continuous sound heard best at the upper left or right sternal borders or clavicles and may be mistaken for a patent ductus arteriosus. This murmur is caused by turbulent flow in the veins draining the superior vena cava. It is loudest in the sitting position and should disappear when lying down. It may also disappear with very light, gentle pressure on the right or left external jugular vein. Turning the head to "flatten" the vessels can also decrease the sound.

Peripheral pulmonic stenosis is a short systolic murmur heard best in the axillae and back that usually disappears during infancy as the pulmonary arteries enlarge.

T A B L E 31-7

Assessment of a Heart Murmur

1. Intensity or grade. Murmurs are reported as I/VI, II/VI, etc. Intensity of the murmur does not necessarily indicate severity of the problem. Intensity may be altered with position change from supine to sitting:
   Grade I: Barely audible. Heard faintly after a period of attentive listening
   Grade II: Soft but easily audible
   Grade III: Moderately loud, no thrill
   Grade IV: Loud, thrill present
   Grade V: Loud, audible with stethoscope barely on the chest
   Grade VI: Loud, audible without stethoscope
2. Timing within the cardiac cycle:
   Systolic
   Diastolic
   Continuous
3. Location defines area on chest where the murmur is loudest:
   Aortic
   Pulmonic
4. Transmission or radiation to other locations:
   To back
   To apex
   To carotids
5. Quality:
   Musical
   Vibrating
   Harsh
   Blowing
6. Duration: point of onset and how much of systole and diastole murmurs last
7. Pitch:
   Low
   Middle
   High

served via fluoroscopy and provides information about cardiac output, vascular resistance, and the response of the heart to exercise and medications.

• Arterial blood gases. Determination of arterial blood gas content assesses blood levels of oxygen and carbon dioxide. Respiratory acidosis occurs with pulmonary disease, and metabolic acidosis occurs with cardiac disease.

• Hyperoxia test. Supplementation of 100% oxygen results in "pinking" and increased arterial oxygen saturation when the disease is primarily pulmonary; minimal or no color improvement indicates that the disease is cardiac.

• Magnetic resonance imaging. This technique uses a strong magnetic field to cause movement of nuclei to yield an image of the heart structures.

▐ MANAGEMENT STRATEGIES

Referral

Practitioners in primary care settings are likely to identify infants, children, and adolescents with suspected cardiac disease. Early detection and prompt referral with appropriate follow-up early in life can greatly reduce the morbidity and mortality associated with CHD. Whom to refer and when and where to refer are important aspects of any practice (Lott, 1998).

Findings suggestive of cardiac disease are the presence of cyanosis, symptoms of CHF, a nonfunctional murmur, or a difficult-to-differentiate

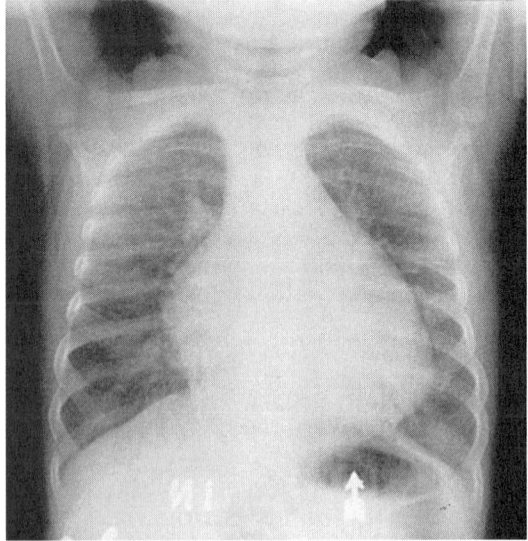

F I G U R E 31-4

Chest radiogram of a 3-month-old with ventricular septal defect and congestive heart failure. Cardiomegaly with increased pulmonary vascular markings from pulmonary venous congestion is visible.

T A B L E   31-8
Types of Heart Murmurs

SYSTOLIC MURMURS

Most murmurs are systolic and occur between S_1 and S_2. Systolic murmurs are either regurgitation murmurs, as with the holosystolic murmur of a VSD, or ejection murmurs caused by flow of blood through narrowed or stenotic areas, as in aortic stenosis. Systolic ejection murmurs are best heard at the second left or right intercostal space and begin after S_1 and end before S_2. Regurgitant murmurs begin with S_1 and generally continue throughout systole (Talner, 1995). Innocent or physiologic murmurs are always systolic murmurs.

DIASTOLIC MURMURS

Diastolic murmurs occur between S_2 and the return to S_1 and are graded I–IV (e.g., I/IV, II/IV). Diastolic murmurs are always due to cardiac pathology. A murmur that starts with S_2 and has a decrescendo quality is most commonly due to aortic or pulmonic regurgitation. A mid-diastolic "rumble," a short low-pitched rumble heard best at the apex of the heart, is commonly due to atrioventricular valve stenosis or increased flow across a nonstenotic valve because of a volume-overloaded ventricle as seen with a large VSD or PDA.

CONTINUOUS MURMURS

A continuous murmur starts at S_1 and goes completely through systole and diastole. The most common cause of such a murmur is a PDA. Continuous murmurs should be differentiated from the coexistence of separate systolic and diastolic murmurs (Van Hare, 1994).

PDA = patent ductus arteriosus; VSD = ventricular septal defect.

---

murmur in the presence of poor growth and development. A murmur alone in a child who is otherwise doing well should be referred to a pediatric cardiologist for further evaluation in a timely but not urgent time frame (2 to 4 weeks). An infant with suspected disease who has a murmur, symptoms of CHF, cyanosis, or poor feeding should be evaluated as soon as possible by a pediatric cardiologist. Newborns should be evaluated within a day or 2 of noticeable signs. An older child with dizziness, chest pain with dysrhythmia, dyspnea, syncope, signs of CHF, or abnormal vital signs should also be referred as soon as possible.

It is important for the practitioner to establish a relationship with a pediatric cardiologist who has diagnostic capabilities immediately available and can proceed with intervention should it prove necessary.

Family Support

Families with infants or children in whom a cardiac problem has been diagnosed may feel fearful, confused, and even guilty. The severity of the cardiac illness or disorder, the type of treatment needed, and the prognosis of the child dictate the kind of support that a family requires. Families need the support of their primary care provider to help them understand the diagnosis, to cope with the short- and long-term consequences, and to advocate for them within the referral center, which may be an overwhelming site.

Parents and their designated support people should clearly understand the diagnosis and have diagrams of the defect and general information to take away with them for future reference. Should medication be necessary, parents should understand the reason for the treatment, as well as the regimen for administration and side effects. They should have a good understanding of the signs and symptoms of deterioration (e.g., CHF) and clear information regarding how to proceed should they develop. Infant cardiopulmonary resuscitation certification is critical for anyone caring for a child with a heart condition.

Support of a family with a new diagnosis or a critical diagnosis is time consuming but necessary. When an infant or child must be seen frequently in a tertiary care center, routine primary care with well-child information and normal counseling may be neglected. It is im-

T A B L E 31-9

Characteristics of Pathological Murmurs That Merit Referral

Significant history
Loud, harsh quality or continuous murmur
Diastolic or late systolic murmur
Holosystolic or pansystolic murmur
Associated abnormalities in cardiac findings (e.g., loud single S_2 gallop, decreased femoral pulses, ejection click, cyanosis)
Associated failure to thrive, congestive heart failure, other systemic illness
Murmur not changing or diminishing in different positions and possibly becoming more intense (e.g., mitral valve murmur intensifying in the squatting position)

Data from Feit LR: The heart of the matter: Evaluating murmurs in children. Contemp Pediatr 14:97–122, 1997; Smith KM: The innocent heart murmur in children. J Pediatr Heath Care 11:207–214, 1997; McCrindle BW, Shaffer KM, Kan JS, et al: Cardinal clinical signs in the differentiation of heart murmurs in children. Arch Pediatr Adolesc Med 150:169–174, 1996.

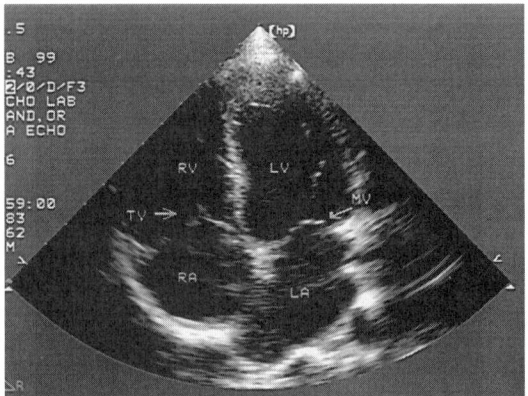

F I G U R E 31-6
Echocardiogram of a 2-year-old with atrial septal defect.

portant to encourage families to schedule regular appointments with the primary care provider for routine care and assessment of normal growth and development. The family needs to understand the importance of ongoing subspecialty care with the pediatric cardiologist. The importance of keeping appointments should be emphasized.

Every opportunity to connect with a family and provide reassuring information is usually welcomed and helpful. The NP helps the family understand the diagnosis and treatment plan, provides an opportunity for family members to express their feelings and concerns, and coordi-

F I G U R E 31-5
Normal electrocardiogram of a 1-year-old.

nates necessary community-based interventions.

Primary Health Care for Children With Cardiovascular Diseases

The goals of primary health care for a child with cardiovascular disease include the following (Uzark, 1996):

- Adequate nutritional intake and optimal growth
- Optimal psychosocial development and functioning
- Enhancement of self-esteem, social support, and coping
- Provision of comprehensive health care
- Promotion of compliance
- Prevention or identification of cardiac complications

As with any child, anticipatory guidance regarding ongoing preventive care and health maintenance emphasizing normal aspects of the child's growth and development enhance the family's coping. Specific areas that may need additional attention at various ages are listed in Table 31–10. Providing more detailed information regarding the following areas may be helpful to these families.

- Lifestyle and stress management. Discuss with the family the need to treat the child as normally as possible. Encourage the family to contact health care providers when they have questions or need reassurance. Direct parents to support groups that provide informational and emotional support for families. Discuss lifestyle changes regarding dietary practices, exercise patterns, and stress management for the patient and the family. Prevention of respiratory infections through good handwashing should be emphasized. All caregivers must understand that respiratory infections require prompt evaluation and treatment.
- Exercise and sports participation. Reassure the parents that the child generally "self-limits" activity according to ability. Exercise tolerance studies should be completed before entrance into sports or any activities

that require strenuous physical exertion. Parameters for sports participation for children with carditis, hypertension, CHD, dysrhythmias, mitral valve prolapse, and heart murmurs are discussed in Chapter 15.
- Diet and nutrition. Depending on the child's condition, the family may need help in modifying the diet to provide maximum calories or limit various types of foods. Nutritional referral may at times prove helpful (see Chapter 12 for more detailed information).

Prevention of Bacterial Endocarditis

Although uncommon, bacterial endocarditis (also called subacute bacterial endocarditis [SBE] or infectious endocarditis) has a high

---

T A B L E 31-10

Key Areas of Primary Health Care for Children With Cardiovascular Disease

INFANCY (BIRTH–2 Y)
Growth and development
Nutrition
Immunizations
Attention to siblings

PRESCHOOL YEARS
Development
Discipline
Dental care
Endocarditis prophylaxis

SCHOOL AGE (6–12 Y)
School program
Activity recommendations and sports
Endocarditis prophylaxis

ADOLESCENCE
Sexuality concerns, contraception, and pregnancy
Delayed puberty
Genetic counseling
Athletics/exercise
Vocational counseling
Endocarditis counseling

Adapted from Uzark K: Recognition and management of congenital heart disease in the neonate. Presented at the National Association of Pediatric Nurse Associates and Practitioners 17th Annual Conference. San Diego, CA, 1996.

morbidity and mortality rate (see later) and warrants primary prevention whenever indicated. Current recommendations for prophylaxis, updated by consensus in 1997, identify how the practitioner can (1) stratify risk categories into high, moderate, or negligible; (2) identify procedures for which prophylaxis is and is not recommended; and (3) simplify treatment regimens (Tables 31-11 to 31-15). Prophylaxis is recommended by the American Heart Associa-

T A B L E 31-11
Cardiac Conditions for Which Prophylaxis Is or Is Not Recommended

ENDOCARDITIS PROPHYLAXIS RECOMMENDED

High-risk category
  Prosthetic cardiac valves, including bioprosthetic and homograft valves
  Previous bacterial endocarditis
  Complex cyanotic congenital heart disease (e.g., single ventricle states, transposition of the great arteries, tetralogy of Fallot)
  Surgically constructed systemic-pulmonary shunts or conduits
Moderate-risk category
  Most other congenital cardiac malformations (other than above and below)
  Acquired valvar dysfunction (e.g., rheumatic heart disease)
  Hypertrophic cardiomyopathy
  Mitral valve prolapse with valvar regurgitation and/or thickened leaflets

ENDOCARDITIS PROPHYLAXIS NOT RECOMMENDED

Negligible-risk category (no greater risk than the general population)
  Isolated secundum atrial septal defect
  Surgical repair of atrial septal defect, ventricular septal defect, or patent ductus arteriosus (without residua beyond 6 mo)
  Previous coronary artery bypass graft surgery
  Mitral valve prolapse without valvar regurgitation
  Physiologic, functional, or innocent heart murmurs
  Previous Kawasaki disease without valvar dysfunction
  Previous rheumatic fever without valvar dysfunction
  Cardiac pacemakers (intravascular and epicardial) and implanted defibrillators

From American Heart Association Committee on Rheumatic Fever, Endocarditis, Kawasaki Disease. Prevention of bacterial endocarditis. JAMA 277:1794–1801, 1997. Copyright 1997, American Medical Association.

T A B L E 31-12
Dental Procedures for Which Prophylaxis Is or Is Not Recommended

ENDOCARDITIS PROPHYLAXIS RECOMMENDED

Dental extractions*
Periodontal procedures, including surgery, scaling and root planing, probing, recall maintenance
Dental implant placement and reimplantation of avulsed teeth
Endodontic (root canal) instrumentation or surgery only beyond the apex
Subgingival placement of antibiotic fibers/strips
Initial placement of orthodontic bands but not brackets
Intraligamentary local anesthetic injections
Prophylactic cleaning of teeth or implants when bleeding is anticipated

ENDOCARDITIS PROPHYLAXIS NOT RECOMMENDED

Restorative dentistry† (operative and prosthodontic) with/without retraction cord‡
Local anesthetic injections (nonintraligamentary)
Intracanal endodontic treatment; postplacement and buildup
Placement of rubber dams
Postoperative suture removal
Placement of removable prosthodontic/orthodontic appliances
Taking of oral impressions
Taking of oral radiographs
Fluoride treatments
Orthodontic appliance adjustment
Shedding of primary teeth

*Prophylaxis is recommended for patients with high- and moderate-risk cardiac conditions.
†Including restoration of decayed teeth (filling cavities) and replacement of missing teeth.
‡Clinical judgment may indicate antibiotic use in selected circumstances that may create significant bleeding.
From American Heart Association Committee on Rheumatic Fever, Endocarditis, Kawasaki Disease. Prevention of bacterial endocarditis. JAMA 277:1794–1801, 1997. Copyright 1997, American Medical Association.

tion (AHA) (Dajani et al., 1997) for *all* nonrepaired defects with the exception of a small isolated ASD. PDA and VSD require prophylaxis until 6 months after repair. Prophylaxis is initiated shortly before the procedure and given perioperatively. A high index of suspicion for bacterial endocarditis should be maintained if any unusual clinical findings (e.g., petechiae, fever) are present after any procedure.

TABLE 31-13

Prophylactic Regimens for Dental, Oral, Respiratory Tract, or Esophageal Procedures (No Follow-up Dose Recommended)

SITUATION	AGENT	REGIMEN*
Standard general prophylaxis	Amoxicillin	Adults: 2.0 g; children: 50 mg/kg PO 1 hr before procedure
Unable to take oral medications	Ampicillin	Adults: 2.0 g IM or IV; children: 50 mg/kg IM or IV within 30 min before procedure
Penicillin allergic	Clindamycin *or*	Adults: 600 mg; children: 20 mg/kg PO 1 hr before procedure
	Cephalexin† or cefadroxil† *or*	Adults: 2.0 g; children: 50 mg/kg PO 1 hr before procedure
	Azithromycin or clarithromycin	Adults: 500 mg; children: 15 mg/kg PO 1 hr before procedure
Penicillin allergic and unable to take oral medications	Clindamycin *or*	Adults: 600 mg; children: 20 mg/kg IV within 30 min before procedure
	Cefazolin†	Adults: 1.0 g; children: 25 mg/kg IM or IV within 30 min before procedure

IM = intramuscularly; IV = intravenously; PO = orally.

*The total children's dose should not exceed the adult dose.

†Cephalosporins should not be used in individuals with an immediate-type hypersensitivity reaction (urticaria, angioedema, or anaphylaxis) to penicillins.

From American Heart Association Committee on Rheumatic Fever, Endocarditis, Kawasaki Disease. Prevention of bacterial endocarditis. JAMA 277:1794–1801, 1997. Copyright 1997, American Medical Association.

Primary Prevention

Immunization schedules should be maintained into and throughout adulthood to prevent potential complications of these preventable diseases. Genetics counseling is recommended for parents with significant family histories of CHD (Ardinger, 1997). Early prenatal care and education are essential, and women should be counseled regarding the avoidance of teratogens during pregnancy.

CONGENITAL HEART DISEASES

An infant or child with heart disease may have a variety of disease manifestations. Signs and symptoms in infants with CHD depend on the type of cardiac defect, the timing of PDA closure, and the fall in the pulmonary vascular resistance. Cyanosis and CHF are more obvious signs. Some infants and older children may simply have a murmur without symptoms. In older children, chest pain or syncope is often the chief complaint. The NP must be open to all diagnostic possibilities.

Congestive Heart Failure

CHF is the most common emergency in children with heart disease and the major reason, other than elective procedures, for hospitalization of these children. Seventy-five percent to 80% of cases of CHF in children occur before their first birthday, most commonly in the first 2 months of life (Lamb, 1994).

CHF refers to a set of clinical signs and symptoms that indicate myocardial (heart muscle) dysfunction. This dysfunction results in cardiac output that is insufficient to meet the metabolic demands of the heart and body and requires additional work from the heart to maintain adequate cardiac output. Excessive volume or pressure load on the heart and poor myocardial function are the most common causes. VSD and PDA are examples of increased myocardial

T A B L E 31-14

Prophylactic Regimens for Genitourinary/Gastrointestinal (Excluding Esophageal) Procedures

SITUATION	AGENT(S)*	REGIMEN†
High-risk patients	Ampicillin plus gentamicin	Adults: ampicillin, 2.0 g IM/IV, plus gentamicin, 1.5 mg/kg (not to exceed 120 mg) within 30 min of starting procedure. Six hr later, ampicillin, 1 g IM/IV, or amoxicillin, 1 g PO Children: ampicillin, 50 mg/kg IM or IV (not to exceed 2.0 g), plus gentamicin, 1.5 mg/kg within 30 min of starting procedure. Six hr later, ampicillin, 25 mg/kg IM/IV, or amoxicillin, 25 mg/kg PO
High-risk patients allergic to ampicillin/amoxicillin	Vancomycin plus gentamicin	Adults: vancomycin, 1.0 g IV over 1–2 hr, plus gentamicin, 1.5 mg/kg IV/IM (not to exceed 120 mg). Complete injection/infusion within 30 min of starting procedure Children: vancomycin, 20 mg/kg IV over 1–2 hr, plus gentamicin, 1.5 mg/kg IV/IM. Complete injection/infusion within 30 min of starting procedure
Moderate-risk patients	Amoxicillin *or* ampicillin	Adults: amoxicillin, 2.0 gm PO 1 hr before procedure, *or* ampicillin, 2.0 g IM/IV within 30 min of starting procedure Children: amoxicillin, 50 mg/kg PO 1 hr before procedure, *or* ampicillin, 50 mg/kg IM/IV within 30 min of starting procedure
Moderate-risk patients allergic to ampicillin/amoxicillin	Vancomycin	Adults: vancomycin, 1.0 g IV over 1–2 hr. Complete infusion within 30 min of starting procedure Children: vancomycin, 20 mg/kg IV over 1–2 hr. Complete infusion within 30 min of starting procedure

IM = intramuscularly; IV = intravenously; PO = orally.
*No second dose of vancomycin or gentamicin is recommended.
†The total children's dose should not exceed the adult dose.
From American Heart Association Committee on Rheumatic Fever, Endocarditis, Kawasaki Disease. Prevention of bacterial endocarditis. JAMA 277:1794–1801, 1997. Copyright 1997, American Medical Association.

workload caused by excessive volume secondary to shunting of blood. Structural or valvular abnormalities (e.g., coarctation or aortic stenosis) impede the normal flow of blood through cardiac structures and thereby increase the pressure load on the heart. Any condition that decreases the effectiveness of myocardial function (e.g., myocarditis, anemia, dysrhythmia) can also result in failure of the heart to maintain adequate cardiac output (Table 31–16).

Alterations in cardiac function occur because the cardiac muscle is overtaxed and compensation mechanisms are activated in an attempt to maintain adequate cardiac output. Ventricular dilation and hypertrophy are early indicators of the heart's reaction to increased workload. Tachycardia is an adaptive mechanism to in-

crease cardiac output and promote delivery of oxygen to the heart and body. If demands on the heart are increased past the point of maximal effectiveness, the result is decreased cardiac output, pulmonary and systemic congestion, and associated clinical manifestations (Table 31–17).

Acyanotic Congenital Heart Disease (Left-To-Right Shunts)

Acyanotic lesions have a communication between the two sides of the heart through which extra blood shunts from the high-pressure, left side of the heart to the low-pressure, right side of the heart. The result is an increase in pulmonary blood flow (see Fig. 31–7).

T A B L E 31-15

Other Procedures for Which Prophylaxis Is or Is Not Recommended

ENDOCARDITIS PROPHYLAXIS RECOMMENDED
Respiratory tract
  Tonsillectomy and/or adenoidectomy
  Surgical operations that involve respiratory
    mucosa
  Bronchoscopy with a rigid bronchoscope
Genitourinary tract
  Prostatic surgery
  Cystoscopy
  Urethral dilation
Gastrointestinal tract*
  Sclerotherapy for esophageal varices
  Esophageal stricture dilation
  Endoscopic retrograde cholangiography
    with biliary obstruction
  Biliary tract surgery
  Surgical operations that involve intestinal
    mucosa

ENDOCARDITIS PROPHYLAXIS NOT RECOMMENDED
Respiratory tract
  Endotracheal intubation
  Bronchoscopy with a flexible bronchoscope, with or
    without biopsy†
  Tympanostomy tube insertion
Gastrointestinal tract
  Transesophageal echocardiography†
  Endoscopy with or without gastrointestinal biopsy†
Genitourinary tract
  Vaginal hysterectomy†
  Vaginal delivery†
  Cesarean section
  In uninfected tissue:
    Urethral catheterization
    Uterine dilatation and curettage
    Therapeutic abortion
    Sterilization procedures
    Insertion or removal of intrauterine devices
Other
  Cardiac catheterization, including balloon angioplasty
  Implantation of cardiac pacemakers, implanted
    defibrillators, and coronary stents
  Incision or biopsy of surgically scrubbed skin
  Circumcision

*Prophylaxis is recommended for high-risk patients, optional for medium-risk patients.
†Prophylaxis is optional for high-risk patients.
From American Heart Association Committee on Rheumatic Fever, Endocarditis, Kawasaki Disease. Prevention of bacterial endocarditis. JAMA 277:1794–1801, 1997. Copyright 1997, American Medical Association.

Atrial Septal Defect

Description

An ASD is a defect or hole in the atrial septum. Of the three types of ASD, the most common involves the midseptum in the area of the foramen ovale and is called an ostium secundum-type defect (Fig. 31-8). Defects of the sinus venosus type are high in the atrial septum, near the entry of the superior vena cava, and are frequently associated with anomalous pulmonary venous return. A primum ASD is in the lower portion of the septum and may be seen in children with Down syndrome.

Incidence

ASD is one of the most commonly recognized congenital cardiac anomalies in adults.

ASD of the ostium secundum variety is twice as common in females. The incidence of ASD is 20% in patients with Down syndrome and Ellis-van Creveld syndrome (Vick & Titus, 1994).

Clinical Findings

HISTORY

- Often completely asymptomatic.
- May fatigue easily or have exertional dyspnea.
- May be somewhat underdeveloped physically.
- May have a history of frequent upper respiratory tract infections or pneumonia.

PHYSICAL EXAMINATION

- Typically, a murmur may not be noticed until the child is 2 to 3 years of age, when

TABLE 31-16

Conditions That Can Lead to Congestive Heart Failure in Children

AGE	CONDITION
Premature infant Birth–1 wk	Patent ductus arteriosus Hypoplastic left heart syndrome Coarctation of the aorta Critical aortic stenosis Interrupted aortic arch Arteriovenous malformations Tachycardia Cardiomyopathy
1 wk–3 mo	Ventricular septal defect Truncus arteriosus Atrioventricular canal (endocardial cushion defect) Total anomalous pulmonary venous return Coarctation Tachycardia Patent ductus arteriosus Aortic stenosis Tricuspid atresia
Over 1 y	Bacterial endocarditis Rheumatic fever Myocarditis

examination of a quiet child can be performed.

- The heart may be hyperactive.
- S_1 is normal or split, with accentuation of the tricuspid valve closure sound.
- S_2 is split widely and is relatively fixed in relation to respiration in patients with normal pulmonary pressure.
- A grade I–III/VI, widely radiating, rough or harsh systolic ejection murmur is heard best at the pulmonic area. If the shunt is large, increased blood flow across the tricuspid valve is responsible for a mid-diastolic, rumbling murmur at the left lower sternal border (LLSB).
- Arterial pulses are normal and equal.
- In older patients (teenage or older), the pulmonic and the tricuspid murmurs decrease in intensity and the second heart sound may be single and accentuated. A

diastolic murmur of pulmonic incompetence can appear.

DIAGNOSTIC TESTS

- Chest radiography reveals cardiac enlargement. The main pulmonary artery can be dilated and the pulmonary vascular markings increased.
- The ECG shows right axis deviation with right atrial enlargement.
- The echocardiogram identifies the specific location of the defect in the atrial septum and shows chamber enlargement.
- Cardiac catheterization is rarely necessary unless pulmonary hypertension is suspected from the echo (Park, 1996).

Management

Management of ASD includes the following:

1. Small defects found in infancy may close on their own.
2. Larger defects require surgical intervention, usually between 2 and 4 years of age or when the defect is identified in an older child. Such intervention can be planned electively to prepare the infant's family and child for surgery. Surgical closure may involve a patch placed over the defect or primary suture closure for smaller defects. Technology is advancing rapidly in the area

TABLE 31-17

Signs and Symptoms of Congestive Heart Failure

INFANTS	CHILDREN
Tachypnea	Tachypnea
Tachycardia	Tachycardia
Rales/wheezing	Rales/wheezing
Cardiomegaly and hepatomegaly	Cardiomegaly and hepatomegaly
Periorbital edema	Orthopnea
Poor feeding	Shortness of breath or dyspnea with exertion
Poor weight gain	Peripheral edema
Diaphoresis	Poor growth and development

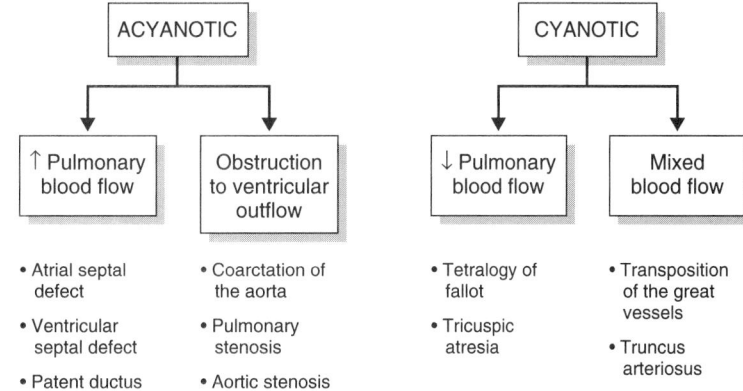

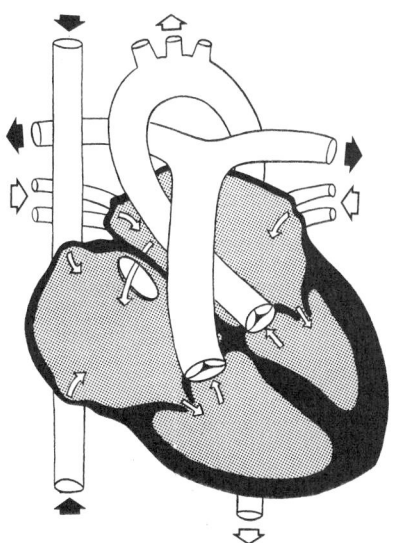

F I G U R E 31-7
Classification of congenital heart disease.

F I G U R E 31-8
Atrial septal defect. (Used with permission of Ross Products Division, Abbott Laboratories, Columbus, OH 43216. From Clinical Education Aid No. 7. Copyright 1970 Ross Products Division, Abbott Laboratories.)

of nonsurgical repair of ASDs, allowing the defect to be closed by a device in the cardiac catheterization laboratory.

3. An ECG every 3 to 5 years is necessary to rule out any late-occurring conduction abnormalities.

4. No SBE prophylaxis precautions are necessary if the defect is small and isolated (AHA, 1997).

5. Long-term outcome is excellent for patients after ASD repair.

Ventricular Septal Defect

Description

The ventricular septum is made up of four components: the membranous septum, the inlet septum, the trabecular septum, and the outlet or infundibular septum. A VSD is a hole or defect in one of these areas of the ventricular septum. Most commonly, defects occur in the region of the membranous septum and are referred to as perimembranous defects because they are larger than the membranous septum itself. Other defects occur in the trabecular or muscular portion of the septum (Fig. 31-9).

Incidence

VSD is the most common cardiac defect seen in childhood. Defects result from a deficiency in fetal growth or a failure of alignment or fusion of component parts. Close to 75% of muscular defects close by 5 years of age (Gumbiner, 1994).

Clinical Findings

HISTORY

- A murmur that may not have been evident at birth is noticed at 2 to 6 weeks of life as pulmonary vascular resistance falls.

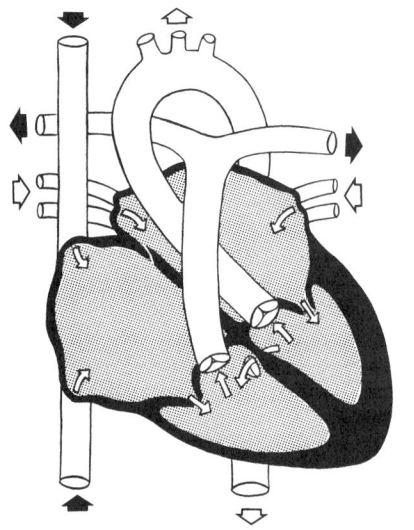

F I G U R E 31-9
Ventricular septal defect. (Used with permission of Ross Products Division, Abbott Laboratories, Columbus, OH 43216. From Clinical Education Aid No. 7. Copyright 1970 Ross Products Division, Abbott Laboratories.)

small shunts have normal heart size and pulmonary vascular markings that are just beyond the upper limits of normal. Patients with large shunts have cardiac enlargement involving both the left and right ventricles and a left atrium with pulmonary vascular markings that are significantly increased. (See Fig. 34–4.)

- The ECG is normal in patients with small defects and may show cardiac enlargement and left ventricular hypertrophy (LVH) with large shunts.
- The echocardiogram provides visualization of defects in most cases and usually pinpoints the exact anatomical location. In "pinhole" VSDs, a murmur may be present; however, a defect may not be visualized on the echocardiogram.
- Cardiac catheterization may be necessary to assess pulmonary artery pressure if pulmonary hypertension is suspected (Park, 1996).

- Signs of CHF may be present (e.g., poor weight gain, feeding difficulty, effort intolerance and fatigue, diaphoresis with crying or feeding).
- Small defects may be completely asymptomatic.

PHYSICAL EXAMINATION

- Small VSD
  - Harsh, high-pitched, grade II–IV/VI holosystolic murmur at the LLSB.
  - All other findings within normal limits.
- Large VSD
  - Low-pitched, grade II–V/VI holosystolic murmur at the LLSB.
  - A VSD murmur that becomes higher pitched over time indicates that the defect is becoming smaller.
  - Diastolic rumble at the apex.
  - A "thrill" along the left sternal border.
  - Signs of progressing CHF after the first weeks of life.
  - An S_3 or S_4 gallop if CHF is present.

DIAGNOSTIC TESTS

- Chest radiography findings vary depending on the size of the shunt. Patients with

Management

1. Infants with small defects and no symptoms of CHF are monitored closely throughout the first year of life and then biannually to assess for closure of the defect. Some defects may never close but cause no difficulty. The only precaution is SBE prophylaxis at the time of high-risk surgical or dental procedures.
2. Larger defects with signs of CHF are managed as follows:
   - Digoxin and/or diuretics may be helpful.
   - Adequate caloric intake to enhance growth must be ensured.
   - Families must be taught the signs and symptoms of developing or progressing CHF.
   - If no improvement is seen over weeks or months, surgery is indicated.
   - Surgical repair consists of closure of the defect with a Dacron patch.
   - ECG is necessary every 3 to 5 years to rule out any late-occurring conduction abnormalities.
   - SBE prophylaxis precautions are necessary until 6 months after repair (AHA, 1997).

- Long-term outcome is excellent after VSD repair.

Patent Ductus Arteriosus

Description

The ductus arteriosus, which should close in the first hours to days after birth, remains patent in some infants and leaves a connection between the aorta and the pulmonary artery. As pulmonary vascular resistance falls, aortic blood is shunted back into the pulmonary artery and recirculates through the lungs (Fig. 31–10).

Incidence

PDA is a common defect and accounts for 12% of all cases of CHD. The incidence in females outnumbers that in males 2:1. In intensive care nurseries with premature infants weighing less than 1500 g, the frequency of PDA is as high as 20 to 60% (Mullins, 1994).

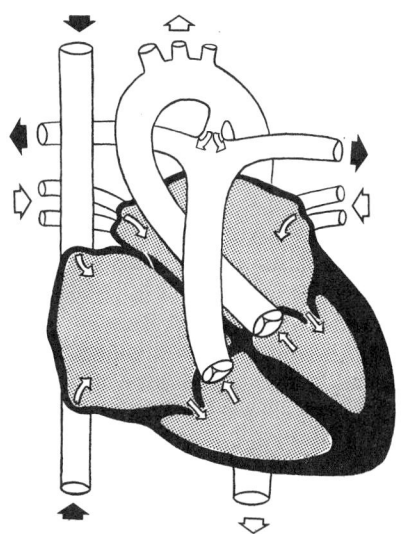

FIGURE 31-10
Patent ductus arteriosus. (Used with permission of Ross Products Division, Abbott Laboratories, Columbus, OH 43216. From Clinical Education Aid No. 7. Copyright 1970 Ross Products Division, Abbott Laboratories.)

Clinical Findings

HISTORY

- PDA is asymptomatic in term newborns.
- If the PDA is small, it may remain asymptomatic.
- Increasing signs of CHF may appear in the first weeks of life.

PHYSICAL EXAMINATION

- In the immediate postnatal period, the murmur is soft, systolic only, and heard along the left sternal border, under the left clavicle, and in the back.
- After the first weeks of life, a typical grade II–V/VI, harsh, rumbling, continuous "machinery murmur" is heard in the left infraclavicular fossa and pulmonic area.
- Physical findings of CHF (e.g., hepatomegaly, rales, respiratory distress, failure to thrive) may be present with a large shunt.

DIAGNOSTIC TESTS

- Chest radiography findings depend on the size of the shunt. With a small to moderate shunt, the heart is not enlarged. If the shunt is large, evidence of both left atrial and ventricular enlargement is apparent. In both cases, the aorta is prominent, as is the main pulmonary artery segment. Pulmonary vascular markings may be increased.
- ECG reveals LVH if the shunt is large.
- Echocardiograms show enlargement of the left atrium. This clue is important for detecting the presence of CHF and is especially useful in diagnosing PDA in a premature infant. The echocardiogram also shows directional shunting through the ductus.
- Cardiac catheterization is not necessary except for catheter closure of the ductus (Park, 1996).

Differential Diagnosis

See Table 31–18.

Management

1. Pharmacological management of a preterm infant with PDA depends on the magnitude

Congenital Heart Disease: Differential Diagnosis of Cardiac Defects

FEATURE	ATRIAL SEPTAL DEFECT	VENTRICULAR SEPTAL DEFECT	PATENT DUCTUS ARTERIOSUS	TRANSPOSITION OF THE GREAT VESSELS	TETRALOGY OF FALLOT	TRICUSPID ATRESIA	AORTIC STENOSIS	PULMONIC STENOSIS	COARCTATION OF THE AORTA
Incidence of total CHD	10%, 2:1 female to male	20%	10%	5%, 3:1 male to female	8%	2%	5%, 4:1 male to female	8%	5%
Age at initial presentation	Variable; may be asymptomatic into adulthood	Variable depending on size. Large by 4–8 wk. Small by 6 mo	Neonate to 3 mo	Immediately at birth	Usually by 6 mo	Usually newborn	Depends on severity; critical in newborn.	Depends on severity. Newborn to school-age children	First weeks of life or 3–5 y
Clinical findings	Murmur on preschool exam	CHF or murmur	CHF or murmur	Cyanosis	Cyanosis	Cyanosis	Murmur, CHF; older child, chest pain	Cyanosis or murmur	CHF in newborn; hypertension in pre-schooler
Auscultation	Midsystolic murmur at ULSB with wide-split 2nd heart sound	Holosystolic murmur at LLSB	Continuous murmur under left clavicle, refers to back	Usually no murmur	Early systolic ejection murmur at 2nd left intercostal space; holosystolic murmur at LLSB	ASD murmur may be associated with PDA	Systolic ejection murmur at URSB, constant systolic click at apex with bicuspid valve	Late systolic ejection murmur at ULSB, intermittent systolic ejection click	Systolic ejection murmur in left intra-clavicular region with transmission to back

Radiological findings Pulmonary vasculature	May have mild cardiomegaly Normal to slightly increased	Normal or cardiomegaly Normal or increased	Cardiomegaly Increased markings	Egg-shaped heart May have increased markings or be normal	Boot-shaped heart Decreased pulmonary vascularity	Cardiomegaly Decreased pulmonary markings	Normal Normal	Normal Decreased in severity	Rib notching Normal
ECG	May have RsR1 in V₁, right atrial enlargement	Combined ventricular hypertrophy	Combined ventricular hypertrophy	RV hypertrophy	RV hypertrophy	Right atrial enlargement, absent RV voltage	Left ventricular hypertrophy	RV hypertrophy	RV hypertrophy
Associations	Holt-Oram syndrome, Down syndrome in PAPVR, mitral valve prolapse	Associated with many defects	Associated with many defects	VSD, PDA, coronary artery anomalies	Down syndrome	VSD, PDA, ASD	Marfan syndrome, Turner syndrome, Williams syndrome	Turner syndrome, Williams syndrome, neurofibromatosis	Turner syndrome, neurofibromatosis, PDA
Treatments	Surgical closure	Observation, digoxin and/or diuretics; if large, surgical closure	Surgical closure if large	Newborn PGE, septostomy, arterial switch (Jatene)	Tetralogy repair, BT shunt	Shunt and surgical repair	Catheter valvulotomy or surgical repair	Catheter valvuloplasty or surgery	Surgical repair or balloon dilation

ASD = atrial septal defect; BT = Blalock-Taussig; CHF = congenital heart failure; ECG = electrocardiogram; LLSB = left lower sternal border; PAPVR = partial anomalous pulmonary venous return; PDA = patent ductus arteriosus; PGE = prostaglandin E; RV = right ventricular; ULSB = upper left sternal border; URSB = upper right sternal border; VSD = ventricular septal defect.

of the shunt. Indomethacin, a prostaglandin inhibitor that constricts and closes the ductus, may be given to preterm infants to effect closure.

2. Surgical intervention in an asymptomatic infant with a small left-to-right shunt is unnecessary because a small PDA usually undergoes spontaneous closure by the age of 2 years. Patients with large shunts and/or infants with pulmonary hypertension should have their PDA surgically closed within the first few months of life to prevent the development of progressive pulmonary vascular obstruction. Surgical ligation of the ductus is a low-risk procedure because cardiopulmonary bypass is not necessary. Cardiac catheterization techniques are commonly used to close the shunt. PDA is one of the few defects that is effectively "cured" by surgical intervention.

3. Families should be reassured that their children will live an active normal life.

4. SBE prophylaxis precautions are recommended 6 months after the repair (AHA, 1997).

Cyanotic Congenital Heart Disease (Right-To-Left Shunts)

Cyanotic CHD (see Fig. 31-7) represents 10 to 18% of all congenital heart lesions (Brooks, 1998). Cardiac cyanosis is due to obstruction of pulmonary blood flow or mixing of oxygenated and unoxygenated blood. Visible cyanosis is present when greater than 3 to 5 g/dl of desaturated hemoglobin is present. Cyanosis, given a constant hemoglobin oxygen saturation, is more readily apparent with polycythemia and less readily apparent with anemia or the presence of fetal hemoglobin, which shifts the oxygen–hemoglobin saturation curve. With cyanotic lesions, desaturated blood enters the systemic arterial circulation, regardless of whether cyanosis is clinically evident. Polycythemia approaching 60% is a compensatory mechanism to increase the oxygen-carrying capacity (Mair et al., 1995). Common heart conditions causing cyanosis in the immediate newborn period include tetralogy of Fallot (TOF), transposition of the great arteries (TOA), truncus arteriosus, and tricuspid atresia.

Transposition of the Great Arteries (TGA)

Description

TGA is the result of incomplete septation and migration of the truncus arteriosus during fetal development. In TGA, the aorta arises from the right ventricle and the pulmonary artery arises from the left ventricle. The aorta receives the unoxygenated systemic venous blood and returns it to the systemic arterial circuit. The pulmonary artery receives oxygenated pulmonary venous blood and returns it to the pulmonary circulation (Fig. 31-11).

Incidence

TGA accounts for 5% of all cases of CHD and is three times more common in males (Neches et al., 1994).

Clinical Findings

HISTORY

- Cyanosis is immediately evident at birth with or without CHF.

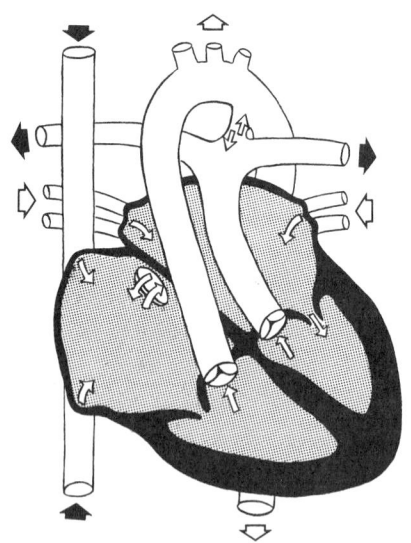

F I G U R E 31-11
Complete transposition of the great vessels. (Used with permission of Ross Products Division, Abbott Laboratories, Columbus, OH 43216. From Clinical Education Aid No. 7. Copyright 1970 Ross Products Division, Abbott Laboratories.)

- Symptoms of CHF are present.
- Affected infants are often large for gestational age with retardation of growth and development after the neonatal period.

PHYSICAL EXAMINATION

- Infants may have no murmur at birth or may have a murmur characteristic of associated lesions such as VSD, ASD, or PDA.
- S_2 is loud and single.

DIAGNOSTIC TESTS

- Chest radiography findings show cardiomegaly, and the heart may appear egg shaped.
- ECG findings show right axis deviation and right ventricular hypertrophy.
- Echocardiography is diagnostic and shows the pulmonary artery arising from the left ventricle and the aorta arising from the right (Park, 1996)

Management

1. Immediate referral and transfer to a pediatric cardiac center are necessary. Correction of electrolyte and acid-base imbalance may be necessary.
2. Pharmacological management may include oxygen administration and intravenous prostaglandin E_1 (PGE_1, 0.05 to 0.2 μg/kg per min) to delay closure of the ductus arteriosus.
3. A balloon atrial septostomy may be performed in the catheterization laboratory to promote mixing of oxygenated and unoxygenated blood in the atria.
4. The most common surgical repair is the Jatene procedure, also known as the arterial switch, and is usually performed in the first few days of life.
5. The long-term outcome of this procedure is still unknown, but the Jatene procedure appears to minimize complications associated with the Mustard or Senning procedures (Kirklin et al., 1996). These patients are monitored closely throughout life with annual echocardiogram follow-up. Families require information and support as their child develops.
6. SBE prophylaxis precautions are indicated.

Prognosis

In recent years, surgical and follow-up care advancements have improved the life expectancy for children with TGA. In the decades before the 1980s, survival into the third decade of life was essentially unheard of, but today, patients with these lesions are expected to live well into adulthood (Neches et al., 1994).

Tetralogy of Fallot

Description

The tetralogy of Fallot, often referred to as TOF or TET, is a combination of four anatomical cardiac defects resulting in right ventricular outflow tract obstruction. These defects include (1) pulmonary valve stenosis, (2) right ventricular hypertrophy, (3) VSD, and (4) an aorta that overrides the ventricular septum (Fig. 31-12). A pink TET (without evident signs of cyanosis) occurs when the valvular stenosis is mild. A blue TET occurs when the right-to-left shunting increases across the VSD because of increased right-sided pressure secondary to constriction of the right ventricular outflow tract.

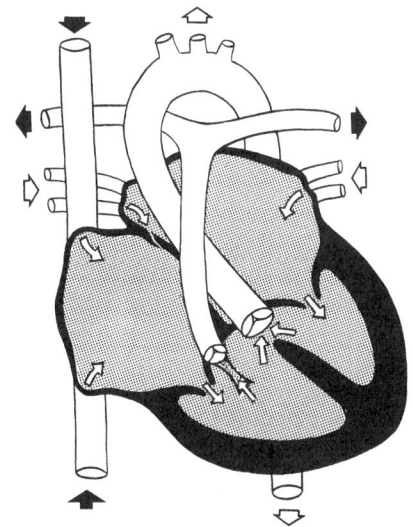

F I G U R E 31-12
Tetralogy of Fallot. (Used with permission of Ross Products Division, Abbott Laboratories, Columbus, OH 43216. From Clinical Education Aid No. 7. Copyright 1970 Ross Products Division, Abbott Laboratories.)

Incidence

TOF, the most common cyanotic lesion, accounts for 6% of all cases of CHD (Neches et al., 1994).

Clinical Findings

HISTORY

- The severity of symptoms depends on the degree of right ventricular outflow obstruction.
- With mild obstruction, the cyanosis may be so slight that it is not initially evident. These infants have a VSD murmur and possibly a pulmonary stenosis murmur.
- Severe obstruction results in cyanosis at birth.
- Most affected infants are cyanotic by 4 months of age, fatigue easily with crying or feeding, and demonstrate dyspnea.
- Hypercyanotic episodes or TET spells, in which the infant becomes intensely cyanotic and extremely dyspneic and appears to be unable to get air, are induced by crying, defecating, or feeding and occur during the first 2 to 3 months of life.
- Poor weight gain is common.
- Older children can have dyspnea on exertion or squatting, poor appetite, poor growth, increasing cyanosis, and alterations in consciousness from irritability to syncope.

PHYSICAL EXAMINATION

- Cyanosis of the mucous membranes and dyspnea may be evident.
- A grade III–V/VI, harsh systolic ejection murmur is heard at the second intercostal space along the left sternal border with a palpable thrill and a holosystolic murmur at the LLSB.
- Observable sternal lift secondary to right ventricular hypertrophy may be present.
- Usually no diastolic murmurs are heard.
- A loud aortic closure can be heard at the left sternal border.

DIAGNOSTIC TESTS

- Chest radiography shows a boot-shaped heart with decreased pulmonary vascular markings.
- ECG shows right ventricular hypertrophy and may show a conduction delay in V_1.
- Echocardiography is diagnostic in that it shows the extent of the pulmonary obstruction and demonstrates the anatomy of the overriding aorta and VSD.
- Cardiac catheterization may be necessary only before surgery (Park, 1996).

Management

1. In neonates with severe pulmonary obstruction, patency of the ductus arteriosus is critical and can be accomplished with PGE_1 as described in management of TGA.
2. For hypercyanotic, or TET, spells, the child should be cradled in chest position until the spell subsides. This maneuver increases systemic resistance, decreases right-to-left shunting, and increases pulmonary blood flow, thus alleviating symptoms. Immediate intervention is required for infants who are "spelling."
3. A Blalock-Taussig shunt is performed between birth and 4 months of age to increase oxygen saturation and pulmonary flow. A complete repair involving closure of the VSD and relief of the pulmonary outflow tract obstruction is performed when the child weighs 10 kg or by 9 to 12 months of age.
4. These children are routinely monitored for life because they may demonstrate outflow tract obstruction or a late arrhythmia may develop many years after the initial repair. Intensive family education and support are necessary. Parents must understand the signs of deterioration and be able to immediately recognize and treat TET spells (Van Hare, 1994).
5. SBE prophylaxis precautions are indicated.

Tricuspid Atresia

Description

Pulmonary atresia results in the absence of communication between the right ventricle and the pulmonary artery. The atresia can be at the level of the main pulmonary artery or the pulmonary valve. Atresia of the pulmonary valve is the most common type (Fig. 31–13).

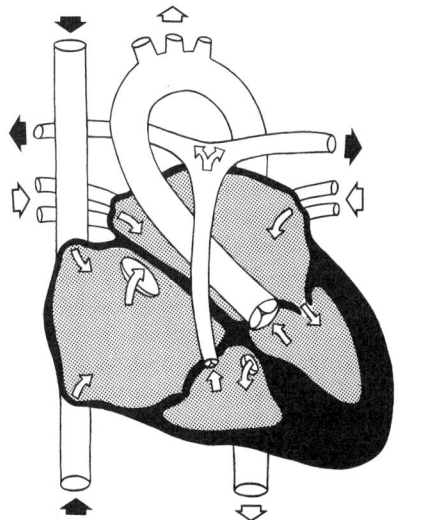

F I G U R E 31-13
Tricuspid atresia. (Used with permission of Ross Products Division, Abbott Laboratories, Columbus, OH 43216. From Clinical Education Aid No. 7. Copyright 1970 Ross Products Division, Abbott Laboratories.)

The right ventricle may be hypoplastic with ventricular hypertrophy. The presence of a PDA, ASD, or patent foramen ovale to allow mixing of blood is crucial for survival.

Incidence

One percent to 2% of all children with CHD have tricuspid atresia (Zuberbuhler, 1995).

Clinical Findings

HISTORY

- Cyanosis in the newborn period with dyspnea on exertion
- Fatigue with the effort of crying or feeding
- Occasional hypoxic episodes
- Failure to thrive (poor weight gain)

PHYSICAL EXAMINATION

- Grade III–V/VI, harsh pansystolic murmur along the middle left sternal border with a single S_2

DIAGNOSTIC TESTS

- Chest radiography shows cardiomegaly and decreased markings.

- ECG shows LVH with small or absent right ventricular voltage.
- Echocardiography is diagnostic and shows the specifics of the atresia (Park, 1996).

Management

1. Palliative shunts and eventual total surgical repair, usually with a staged Fontan procedure (multiple surgical interventions), are required.
2. Close follow-up is indicated because ventricular failure may develop later in life in these patients. Families require much support throughout the child's life. Frequent surgeries and hospitalizations can interfere with normal social development. Early recognition and intervention for developmental delays are important to the child's future.
3. SBE prophylaxis precautions are indicated (Zuberbuhler, 1995).

Obstructive Cardiac Lesions

AORTIC STENOSIS

Description

Normally, the aortic valve opens to allow oxygenated blood to flow from the left ventricle to the aorta. Stenosis may be valvular, subvalvular, or supravalvular, with valvular being the most common. Valvular stenosis is usually characterized by a bicuspid valve. Stenosis causes increased pressure load on the left ventricle leading to LVH and, ultimately, ventricular failure. Obstruction of the aortic valve may cause a decrease in coronary artery blood flow. Unless severe, congenital aortic stenosis is often not diagnosed until early adulthood. (Fig. 31–14).

Incidence

Aortic stenosis accounts for 5% of all cases of CHD and is four times more common in males (Park, 1996).

Clinical Findings

HISTORY

- Aortic stenosis may be asymptomatic, depending on the severity of the defect.

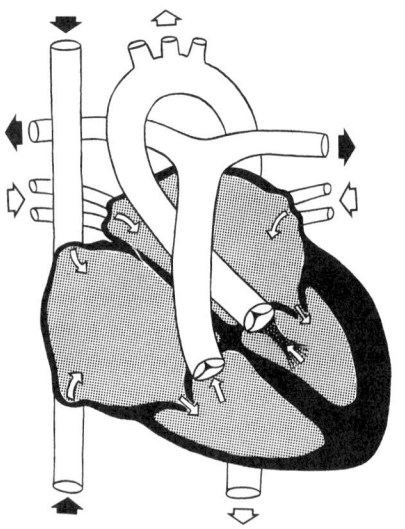

F I G U R E 31-14
Subaortic stenosis. (Used with permission of Ross Products Division, Abbott Laboratories, Columbus, OH 43216. From Clinical Education Aid No. 7. Copyright 1970 Ross Products Division, Abbott Laboratories.)

- Symptoms may develop or increase with age.
- Activity intolerance, chest pain, or syncope can develop.
- With severe aortic stenosis in a neonate, CHF may be evident in the first days of life.

PHYSICAL EXAMINATION

- BP may reveal a narrow pulse pressure or a high systolic pressure in the right arm.
- A grade III–IV/VI, harsh systolic ejection murmur may be heard at the upper right sternal border.
- If the lesion is valvular, an opening snap or "click" can be heard.
- In most severe lesions the S_2 is paradoxically split.
- A thrill may be present at the suprasternal notch.
- Poor peripheral pulses with poor cardiac output are seen in severe obstruction (Park, 1996).

DIAGNOSTIC TESTS

- Chest radiographs are usually normal with a dilated aortic knob in some cases.

- ECG can be normal or reveal LVH and inverted T waves.
- Echocardiography can demonstrate the anatomy of the valve (Park, 1996).

Management

1. The timing of treatment depends on the severity of the obstruction. Treatment is not usually necessary unless the stenosis is moderate to severe. However, aortic stenosis tends to progress with age.
2. Treatment can include surgical excision of the stenotic area, valvuloplasty, or balloon dilation of the stenotic valve in the catheterization laboratory. Aortic valvulotomy has a high mortality rate during the neonatal period.
3. Avoidance of high-risk sports is often recommended because of the risk of sudden death. Families should be counseled to encourage their children to avoid competitive athletics. Golf is a good sport to encourage from an early age.
4. Aortic stenosis has the highest complication rate for bacterial endocarditis; therefore, SBE prophylaxis is always necessary (Mair et al., 1995).

PULMONIC STENOSIS

Description

Normally, the pulmonary valve opens to allow the flow of blood from the right ventricle into the pulmonary artery, which carries blood to the lungs to receive oxygen. Pulmonic stenosis is characterized by narrowing or noncompliance of the pulmonic valve as blood is ejected through it. Right-sided pressure is increased as the ventricle pumps against the obstruction. Right ventricular hypertrophy occurs as a result of this increased load. Pulmonary stenosis can also occur in the pulmonary arterial system and cause mild to severe obstruction to pulmonary blood flow. Mild pulmonic stenosis is usually identified on routine examination.

Incidence

Isolated pulmonic stenosis makes up approximately 7% of all cases of CHD. It is seen in 20%

of all patients with CHD when associated with other cardiac defects (Cheatham, 1994).

Clinical Findings

HISTORY

- Pulmonic stenosis is usually asymptomatic, with a murmur noted on routine physical examination.
- Cyanosis from obstruction to pulmonary blood flow may be evident with severe pulmonic stenosis in infancy.

PHYSICAL EXAMINATION

- A grade II–IV/VI, harsh, mid-to-late systolic ejection murmur is heard at the upper left sternal border over the pulmonic region, with transmission along the left sternal border and into both lung fields.
- An intermittent systolic ejection click may be evident in the pulmonic area.
- Cyanosis and symptoms of right CHF can occur in severe cases.

DIAGNOSTIC TESTS

- Chest radiographs are within normal limits in mild pulmonic stenosis. Right-sided cardiac enlargement and decreased peripheral pulmonary vascular markings may be evident in moderate to severe cases of pulmonic stenosis.
- ECG shows right atrial and ventricular hypertrophy.
- The echocardiogram is helpful in confirming the diagnosis, identifying the gradient, and monitoring progression of the stenosis (Park, 1996).

Management

1. Valvuloplasty is completed in the catheterization laboratory.
2. With mild stenosis, families need to be encouraged to treat their children normally and not limit their activity.
3. SBE prophylaxis is necessary in those with moderate to severe stenosis.

COARCTATION OF THE AORTA

Description

Coarctation of the aorta is a narrowing of a small or long segment of the aorta (Fig. 31–15). Coarctation may occur as a single defect caused by a disturbance in the development of the aorta or may be secondary to constriction of the ductus arteriosus. The severity of the coarctation, its location, and the degree of obstruction determine the effect of the coarctation. A preductal coarctation may go unnoticed until the ductus begins to close and causes obstruction of blood flow to the lower part of the body. Systolic and diastolic hypertension exists in vessels above the area of narrowing. Hypotension is present in vessels below the area of narrowing.

Incidence

Coarctation of the aorta is not always apparent until 7 to 14 days after birth once the ductus closes. It occurs twice as often in males. Patients with Turner syndrome have close to a 20% incidence of coarctation (Morriss & McNamara, 1994).

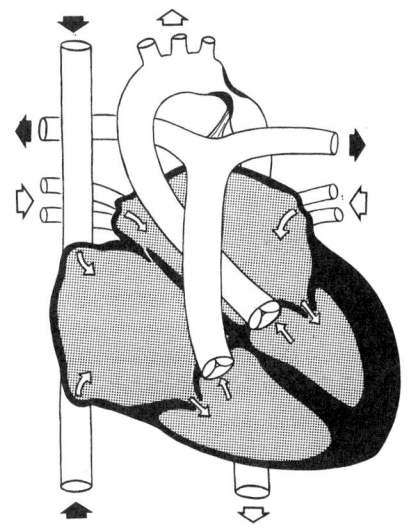

F I G U R E 31-15
Coarctation of the aorta. (Used with permission of Ross Products Division, Abbott Laboratories, Columbus, OH 43216. From Clinical Education Aid No. 7. Copyright 1970 Ross Products Division, Abbott Laboratories.)

Clinical Findings

HISTORY

- In older children, coarctation may go unnoticed until BP is checked at the time of a preschool physical examination and mild hypertension is noted in the upper extremities.
- Retrospectively, children with coarctation may have had complaints of leg pain or headaches.
- Early signs of CHF may be noted soon after birth in infants with severe coarctation.

PHYSICAL EXAMINATION

- Upper extremity hypertension with lower extremity hypotension is present, though milder cases may present with only a minimal gradient between upper and lower extremity blood pressures. In severe cases, poor lower extremity perfusion may be noticed with lower body mottling or pallor.
- Absent or weak femoral and other distal pulses in an infant.
- Bounding brachial, radial, and carotid pulses.
- Signs of CHF may be evident.
- Systolic ejection murmur in the left infraclavicular region with transmission to the back.

DIAGNOSTIC TESTS

- Chest radiography can reveal a normal or slightly enlarged heart.
- ECG findings depend on the severity of the lesion and the age of the patient. In infants, variant right ventricular hypertrophy can be seen; in older children, left ventricular changes are found secondary to hypertension.
- Echocardiography is helpful in confirming the diagnosis and location of the constricted aortic segment. It may also show associated cardiac abnormalities.

Management

1. In critical or severe coarctation, initial management is aimed at maintaining the ductus arteriosus to keep blood flowing to the lower part of the body. PGE_1 may be used.

2. Surgical repair is completed either as an emergency during the neonatal period or electively at 2 to 4 years of age. The most common surgical intervention involves resection of the constricted area with an end-to-end anastomosis of the upper and lower portions of the aorta. Other procedures, including bypass grafting, may be necessary with unusually long coarcted segments. Balloon dilation of the coarcted area may be performed in recoarctation or in the case of isolated mild coarctation.
3. Monitoring of hypertension postoperatively is imperative. In older children with long-standing hypertension, antihypertensive medication may be required for several months after repair.
4. Competitive sports should be restricted until the hypertension has resolved.
5. SBE prophylaxis precautions are necessary (Morriss & McNamara, 1994).

ACQUIRED HEART DISEASE

Chest Pain

Description

Chest pain in the pediatric population is a common complaint and does not usually represent a serious cardiovascular problem. Chest pain of any kind can cause great anxiety for children, adolescents, and their parents. It is important to thoroughly evaluate the complaint, including performance of a careful history (especially a family history of sudden death or early cardiac disease), physical examination, ECG, and other laboratory tests that may be indicated by the findings. Reassurance is of the utmost importance in each case.

Etiology and Incidence

The most frequent cause of chest pain is musculoskeletal in origin. Costochondritis is frequently seen in growing preadolescents and adolescents. It is often related to sports or casual athletic activity. Chest pain secondary to a pulmonary (asthma, pneumonia, embolism, pneumothorax) or gastrointestinal problem (reflux esophagitis, esophageal foreign body) is part of any evaluation. Chest wall pain, particularly with exercise, may indicate exercise-induced asthma but rarely indicates cardiac disease. Chronic chest pain that is vague and occurs over many months in a variety of circumstances, particularly around stressful events, may be psychogenic (anxiety or hyperventilation). Most concerning is chest pain suggestive of cardiac disease, that is, pain associated with syncope, exertional dyspnea, or irregularities in heart rhythm. Usually, children or adolescents who have true cardiac pain describe a very specific history with details that are consistent from event to event.

The incidence was found to be 6 per 1000 visits in one urban clinic, and chest pain occurred equally in males and females. The mean age at initial evaluation was 12 years. Young children are more likely to have a cardiorespiratory cause, whereas adolescents may be more likely to have a psychogenic cause (Selbst, 1997).

Clinical Findings

HISTORY

- Family history of sudden death or heart disease
- Heart disease or condition, asthma, Marfan syndrome, sickle cell disease
- Casual or sports activities, trauma, muscle strain
- Relation of pain to exercise
- Syncope, exertional dyspnea
- Burning, substernal pain worse with reclining and with spicy food (gastrointestinal etiology)
- Awakening because of pain (more likely organic)
- Fever or other systemic symptoms
- Recent major stressful events
- Use of oral contraceptives (embolism)
- Foreign body ingestion or choking

PHYSICAL EXAMINATION

- Complete chest (lungs and heart) and abdominal examination
- Cardiac murmur, rubs, or clicks
- Point tenderness of one or more costochondral joints exaggerated with physical activity or breathing (costochondritis)

- Irregular heart rhythm (cardiac disease)
- Sternal pain (exercise-induced asthma)
- Rales, wheezing, tachypnea, decreased breath sounds (pulmonary disease)

DIAGNOSTIC TESTS

- Chest radiograph if febrile or cardiac or pulmonary condition suspected
- Pulmonary function testing with exercise if exercise-induced asthma is suspected
- Twenty-four-hour Holter monitor and/or stress test if cardiac disease is suspected
- ECG to evaluate for signs of CHD, pericarditis, or myocarditis

Differential Diagnosis

Musculoskeletal, respiratory, psychogenic, and gastrointestinal disorders, as discussed earlier, as well as miscellaneous entities such as sickle cell crisis, aortic abdominal aneurysm (Marfan syndrome), pleural effusion (collagen-vascular disorders), and shingles, are in the differential diagnosis.

Management

1. When chest pain has no clear-cut cause, the child appears well, and all aspects of the evaluation are normal, reassurance may be the most important treatment. Frequently, when reassured that the pain has no organic cause, the pain subsides or becomes less of an issue for the child.
2. In cases in which pulmonary, gastrointestinal, or cardiac disease is a concern, treatment, referral, and/or evaluation is necessary.
   - Costochondritis is usually responsive to nonsteroidal anti-inflammatory treatment and rest.
   - Antacids may be tried if esophagitis is suspected; see Chapter 33.
   - See management of foreign body ingestion in Chapter 33.
   - See Chapters 25 and 32 for management of asthma and respiratory diseases.
3. Follow-up is indicated to ensure that no new findings have emerged and that the child is participating in normal activities, and to

monitor potential psychoemotional problems.

Hypertension

Definition

Hypertension is defined as a systolic and/or diastolic BP in the 95th or higher percentile for age, sex, and height on at least three consecutive occasions. High-normal BP is defined as average systolic or diastolic BP in the 90th percentile or higher but less than the 95th percentile. Normal BP is defined as systolic and diastolic BP below the 90th percentile for age, sex, and height (National High Blood Pressure Education Program [NHBPEP], 1996).

Etiology and Incidence

Hypertension is a significant problem in children and young adults and results from the interaction of genetic and environmental factors. Increasingly, children are found to have high BP associated with obesity, sedentary lifestyles, and stress. It is estimated that the etiology is genetic in 60% of cases (AAP, 1997). Hypertension occurs in 1.3% of children and teens (Jones, 1998). African Americans and Asians have higher BP levels than do whites (NHBPEP, 1996). Primary hypertension is most common after 6 years of age. Secondary hypertension is common before 6 years of age (Daniels, 1997). Underlying causes of secondary hypertension, usually with systolic and diastolic levels well above the 95th percentile, are due to renal causes 74% of the time, coarctation of aorta 15% of the time, and renovascular disease 7% of the time (Hohn, 1997).

Clinical Findings

HISTORY

- Diet, activities, and other habits (e.g., smoking, drinking)
- Medications taken, including oral contraceptives, cold medications, steroids
- Chronic illness, especially renal or diabetes
- Headache, chest pain, dyspnea, muscle weakness, palpitations
- Family history of a first-degree relative with

myocardial infarction, especially before 50 years of age, stroke, hypertension, diabetes, hyperlipidemia, sudden cardiac death, or obesity

PHYSICAL EXAMINATION

- Body habitus, especially obesity.
- Edema, pallor, flushing.
- Pulses in all extremities.
- Fundi, thyroid gland, abdominal mass, flank bruit.
- BP. Accurate BP measurement is essential. An appropriately sized cuff must be used with the cubital fossa supported at the heart level. The right arm is preferred for comparison with normative charts, but right thigh measurement is also recommended if elevated pressure is suspected. The child or adolescent should be seated and have been resting in that position for 3 to 5 minutes. Deflation should be controlled at 2 to 3 mm Hg/s. Systolic pressure is recorded at the onset of tapping sounds; diastolic pressure is recorded at the disappearance (not the muffling) of sounds. Some authorities recommend recording the pressure twice on each occasion and using an average of each to record.

Management

See Figure 31-16 for an algorithm to identify children with high BP. Early identification and prompt evaluation of these children are critical.

1. BP measurements should be done annually on all children 3 years and older, with baseline and serial measurements documented carefully in the child's record. Standardized measurements are available (Tables 31-19 and 31-20).
2. *High normal BP.* At least two follow-up BP measurements should be taken within 1 to 2 months of the initial reading to determine whether this high reading is a single, isolated event. If subsequent readings fall below the 95th percentile, the child should continue with routine BP checks during annual visits.
3. *Sustained elevated BP.* A history and physical examination with laboratory evaluation to include a complete blood count (CBC),

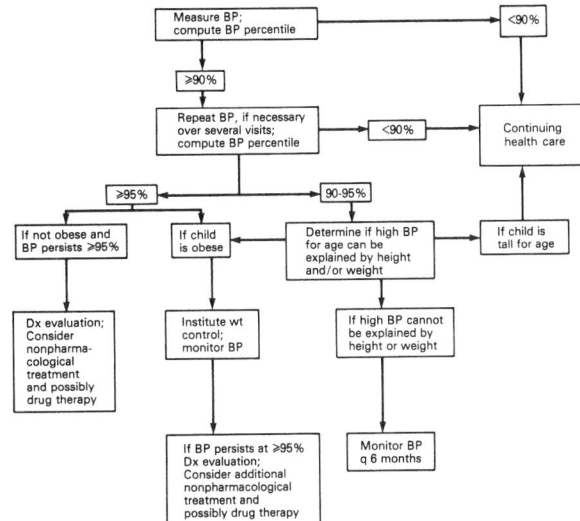

F I G U R E 31-16

Algorithm for identifying children with high blood pressure (BP). Note: Whenever BP measurement is stipulated, the average of at least two measurements should be used. (Reproduced by permission of Pediatrics, Vol. 79, p 7, copyright 1987.)

erythrocyte sedimentation rate (ESR), fasting serum lipids, urinalysis and culture, electrolytes, blood urea nitrogen, creatinine, uric acid (a marker for hypertension in young people; Hohn, 1997), glucose, ECG, and chest radiograph are needed. Abnormalities in a child or young adult who is not overweight should be referred for evaluation.

4. Hypertension secondary to obesity can be as serious as hypertension secondary to other organic disease and should be treated as such. Diet and weight management should be used in conjunction with antihypertensive therapy. Again, referral is necessary.

5. General measures
   • Dietary intervention to control/reduce obesity includes ingestion of a low-fat, high-fiber diet with lots of fresh fruits and vegetables; elimination of foods high in sodium and salt added to foods; adequate calcium (1200 mg/d); and adequate potassium from fruits and beans.
   • Increased physical exercise and sports participation balanced with relaxation techniques. Aerobic exercise is recommended, not static or isometric exercise. Other techniques that are helpful are pairing with family or friends for exercise and maintaining a diary or log of exercise.
   • Avoidance of smoking, caffeine, drinking, and drug consumption.

• Drug therapy (in conjunction with appropriate referrals) is considered if no change is seen after 6 to 12 months of diet and exercise therapy (Sardegna & Loggie, 1996). The goal is to reduce BP below the 95th percentile. Antihypertensives, diuretics, and β-blockers are drugs that are used.
• Periodic echocardiograms may be recommended to evaluate LVH.

Complications

Atherosclerotic lesions and coronary artery calcifications are possible complications.

Prevention

1. Because much of hypertension is genetic in origin, prevention through optimal health promotion and maintenance is essential. Regular health maintenance, including evaluation of BP and health education regarding risk factors, is essential. Counseling should emphasize the following (Cornell, 1997):
   • Healthful nutrition
   • Prevention of obesity
   • Decrease in dietary fat and sodium
   • Aerobic exercise every other day for a period of at least 20 minutes
   • Stress management
   • Avoidance of caffeine and tobacco use and

T A B L E 31-19

Blood Pressure Levels for the 90th and 95th Percentiles of Blood Pressure for Girls Aged 1 to 17 y by Percentiles of Height

AGE	BP*	SYSTOLIC BP (mm Hg) AT HEIGHT PERCENTILE† OF							DIASTOLIC BP (mm Hg) AT HEIGHT PERCENTILE† OF						
		5%	10%	25%	50%	75%	90%	95%	5%	10%	25%	50%	75%	90%	95%
1	90th	97	98	99	100	102	103	104	53	53	53	54	55	56	56
	95th	101	102	103	104	105	107	107	57	57	57	58	59	60	60
2	90th	99	99	100	102	103	104	105	57	57	58	58	59	60	61
	95th	102	103	104	105	107	108	109	61	61	62	62	63	64	65
3	90th	100	100	102	103	104	105	106	61	61	61	62	63	63	64
	95th	104	104	105	107	108	109	110	65	65	65	66	67	67	68
4	90th	101	102	103	104	106	107	108	63	63	64	65	65	66	67
	95th	105	106	107	108	109	111	111	67	67	68	69	69	70	71
5	90th	103	103	104	106	107	108	109	65	66	66	67	68	68	69
	95th	107	107	108	110	111	112	113	69	70	70	71	72	72	73
6	90th	104	105	106	107	109	110	111	67	67	68	69	69	70	71
	95th	108	109	110	111	112	114	114	71	71	72	73	73	74	75
7	90th	106	107	108	109	110	112	112	69	69	69	70	71	72	72
	95th	110	110	112	113	114	115	116	73	73	73	74	75	76	76
8	90th	108	109	110	111	112	113	114	70	70	71	71	72	73	74
	95th	112	112	113	115	116	117	118	74	74	75	75	76	77	78
9	90th	110	110	112	113	114	115	116	71	72	72	73	74	74	75
	95th	114	114	115	117	118	119	120	75	76	76	77	78	78	79
10	90th	112	112	114	115	116	117	118	73	73	73	74	75	76	76
	95th	116	116	117	119	120	121	122	77	77	77	78	79	80	80
11	90th	114	114	116	117	118	119	120	74	74	75	75	76	77	77
	95th	118	118	119	121	122	123	124	78	78	79	79	80	81	81
12	90th	116	116	118	119	120	121	122	75	75	76	76	77	78	78
	95th	120	120	121	123	124	125	126	79	79	80	80	81	82	82
13	90th	118	118	119	121	122	123	124	76	76	77	78	78	79	80
	95th	121	122	123	125	126	127	128	80	80	81	82	82	83	84
14	90th	119	120	121	122	124	125	126	77	77	78	79	79	80	81
	95th	123	124	125	126	128	129	130	81	81	82	83	83	84	85
15	90th	121	121	122	124	125	126	127	78	78	79	79	80	81	82
	95th	124	125	126	128	129	130	131	82	82	83	83	84	85	86
16	90th	122	122	123	125	126	127	128	79	79	79	80	81	82	82
	95th	125	126	127	128	130	131	132	83	83	83	84	85	86	86
17	90th	122	123	124	125	126	128	128	79	79	79	80	81	82	82
	95th	126	126	127	129	130	131	132	83	83	83	84	85	86	86

*Blood pressure percentile determined by a single measurement.
†Height percentile determined by standard growth curves.

T A B L E 31-20

Blood Pressure Levels for the 90th and 95th Percentiles of Blood Pressure for Boys Aged 1 to 17 y by Percentiles of Height

AGE	BP*	SYSTOLIC BP (mm Hg) AT HEIGHT PERCENTILE† OF							DIASTOLIC BP (mm Hg) AT HEIGHT PERCENTILE† OF						
		5%	10%	25%	50%	75%	90%	95%	5%	10%	25%	50%	75%	90%	95%
1	90th	94	95	97	98	100	102	102	50	51	52	53	54	54	55
	95th	98	99	101	102	104	106	106	55	55	56	57	58	59	59
2	90th	98	99	100	102	104	105	106	55	55	56	57	58	59	59
	95th	101	102	104	106	108	109	110	59	59	60	61	62	63	63
3	90th	100	101	103	105	107	108	109	59	59	60	61	62	63	63
	95th	104	105	107	109	111	112	113	63	63	64	65	66	67	67
4	90th	102	103	105	107	109	110	111	62	62	63	64	65	66	66
	95th	106	107	109	111	113	114	115	66	67	67	68	69	70	71
5	90th	104	105	106	108	110	112	112	65	65	66	67	68	69	69
	95th	108	109	110	112	114	115	116	69	70	70	71	72	73	74
6	90th	105	106	108	110	111	113	114	67	68	69	70	70	71	72
	95th	109	110	112	114	115	117	117	72	72	73	74	75	76	76
7	90th	106	107	109	111	113	114	115	69	70	71	72	72	73	74
	95th	110	111	113	115	116	118	119	74	74	75	76	77	78	78
8	90th	107	108	110	112	114	115	116	71	71	72	73	74	75	75
	95th	111	112	114	116	118	119	120	75	76	76	77	78	79	80
9	90th	109	110	112	113	115	117	117	72	73	73	74	75	76	77
	95th	113	114	116	117	119	121	121	76	77	78	79	80	80	81
10	90th	110	112	113	115	117	118	119	73	74	74	75	76	77	78
	95th	114	115	117	119	121	122	123	77	78	79	80	80	81	82
11	90th	112	113	115	117	119	120	121	74	74	75	76	77	78	78
	95th	116	117	119	121	123	124	125	78	79	79	80	81	82	83
12	90th	115	116	117	119	121	123	123	75	75	76	77	78	78	79
	95th	119	120	121	123	125	126	127	79	79	80	81	82	83	83
13	90th	117	118	120	122	124	125	126	75	76	76	77	78	79	80
	95th	121	122	124	126	128	129	130	79	80	81	82	83	83	84
14	90th	120	121	123	125	126	128	128	76	76	77	78	79	80	80
	95th	124	125	127	128	130	132	132	80	81	81	82	83	84	85
15	90th	123	124	125	127	129	131	131	77	77	78	79	80	81	81
	95th	127	128	129	131	133	134	135	81	82	83	83	84	85	86
16	90th	125	126	128	130	132	133	134	79	79	80	81	82	82	83
	95th	129	130	132	134	136	137	138	83	83	84	85	86	87	87
17	90th	128	129	131	133	134	136	136	81	81	82	83	84	85	85
	95th	132	133	135	136	138	140	140	85	85	86	87	88	89	89

*Blood pressure percentile determined by a single measurement.
†Height percentile determined by standard growth curves.

prescription or over-the-counter medications that can exacerbate high BP (e.g., cold medications with ephedrine or phenylephrine, steroids)

- Monitoring of BP if oral contraceptives are used

2. Children and adolescents with systemic hypertension may have significant rise in BP during exercise. This rise in systolic pressure puts young athletes at risk for complications such as cerebrovascular accidents (AHA, 1997). The AAP recommends the following (AAP, 1997):
   - The presence of significant hypertension in the absence of target organ damage or concomitant heart disease should not limit a person's eligibility for competitive athletics. Athletes with significant hypertension should have their BP measured regularly (every 2 months) to monitor the impact of exercise on BP.
   - Youth who have severe hypertension need to be restricted from competitive sports and highly static (isometric) activities until their hypertension is under adequate control and they have no evidence of target organ damage. Because cardiovascular conditioning may be less strenuous than competitive athletics, complete restriction of exercise may not be necessary for those with severe hypertension.
   - When hypertension and other cardiovascular diseases coexist, eligibility for participation in competitive athletics is usually based on the type and severity of the other cardiovascular disease.
   - A young athlete with hypertension, regardless of degree of severity, should be strongly encouraged to adopt healthy lifestyle behavior, including the avoidance of exogenous androgens, growth hormone, drugs of abuse (especially cocaine), alcohol, use of tobacco (by all routes), and high sodium intake. In addition, the athlete should be advised that the use of diuretic drugs and β-blockers has been prohibited by some athletic governing bodies. In these instances, other types of medication may need to be considered.

Kawasaki Disease

Description

Kawasaki disease (also known as mucocutaneous lymph node syndrome or infantile polyarteritis) is characterized by an acute generalized systemic microvasculitis occurring throughout the body in the first 10 days of the disease. During this initial stage, inflammation of the arterioles, venules, and capillaries of the heart can occur and later progress to the formation of a coronary artery aneurysm in some children.

Etiology and Incidence

Although the etiology of Kawasaki disease remains unconfirmed, clinical evidence supports a viral infectious cause. It exhibits geographical and seasonal outbreaks, with cases predominantly reported in the late winter and early spring (Feit, 1995). Person-to-person spread is not a characteristic of this disease. Approximately 2000 children per year contract Kawasaki syndrome (Castiglia, 1996). Although children of all racial groups are susceptible, the incidence is as much as 6 times higher in Asian children and 1.5 times higher in black children compared with caucasians, with a 1.5:1 male-to-female ratio. More than 80% of cases occur in children younger than 5 years, with a peak incidence in the toddler age group. It is rare in children older than 8 years (Fredriksen, 1998; Melish, 1996).

Clinical Findings

Diagnostic criteria are listed in Table 31–21. Children younger than 6 to 12 months may have atypical findings. The three phases of the disease are acute, subacute, and convalescent.

- The *acute phase*, which lasts 8 to 12 days, begins with an abrupt onset of high fever that is unresponsive to antipyretics or antibiotics.
  - Typically, significant irritability, bilateral conjunctival inflammation, erythema of the oropharynx, dryness and fissuring of the lips, "strawberry tongue," cervical lymphadenopathy, and a polymorphous rash are noted.

T A B L E 31-21
Diagnostic Criteria for Kawasaki Disease

The child must exhibit fever plus 4 of the 5 other criteria *OR*, if fewer than 4 conditions, coronary vessel involvement:

1. Fever for 5 or more d
2. Bilateral conjunctival injection without exudate
3. Polymorphous rash that may be urticarial or pruritic
4. Inflammatory changes in the lips and oral cavity
5. Changes in the extremities such as peripheral edema, erythema of the palms and soles, or desquamation of the hands and feet (convalescent period)
6. Cervical lymphadenopathy that is often unilateral (least constant finding; Melish, 1996)

○ Laboratory findings include an elevated ESR and platelet count (>480,000 in 50% by day 10 [Melish, 1996]), mild anemia, polymorphonuclear leukocytosis, hypoalbuminemia, thrombocytosis, increased liver enzymes, and sterile pyuria.
- The *subacute phase*, which lasts 10 to 14 days, begins with resolution of the fever and lasts until all other clinical signs have disappeared.
  ○ Irritability may be prolonged throughout this phase.
  ○ Desquamation of the fingers and toes occurs.
  ○ The greatest risk for development of a coronary artery aneurysm occurs in this period.
- During the *convalescent phase*, all clinical signs of Kawasaki disease have resolved, but the laboratory values may not have returned to normal. This phase is complete when all blood values are normal (6 to 10 weeks from onset). Throughout this phase children may have less energy and general malaise that gradually improves and is normal by the end of the eighth week (Dajani, 1993).
- A fourth, *chronic phase* with coronary

complications that can persist into adulthood is identified by some.

Differential Diagnosis

Measles, scarlet fever, drug reactions, Stevens-Johnson syndrome, juvenile arthritis, leptospirosis, and mercury poisoning are in the differential diagnosis.

Management

Early diagnosis is essential to prevent cardiac complications. Goals of treatment include (1) evoking a rapid anti-inflammatory response, (2) preventing coronary thrombosis by inhibiting platelet aggregation, and (3) minimizing long-term coronary risk factors by exercise, diet, and smoking prevention.

1. Current treatment includes
   - Gamma globulin therapy (a single dose of 2 g/kg intravenously over a period of 10 to 12 hours in the first 10 days of the illness) is effective in reducing the incidence of coronary artery abnormalities (Dajani et al., 1994).
   - High-dose aspirin is given for its anti-inflammatory properties (80 to 100 mg/kg per day in four divided doses every 6 hours initially). Once the fever resolves, aspirin is continued at an antiplatelet dose (3 to 5 mg/kg per day) in patients without ECG evidence of coronary artery changes until the ESR and platelet count have returned to normal (6 to 8 weeks). If coronary artery abnormalities do develop, aspirin therapy is used indefinitely, with warfarin (Coumadin) sometimes added for very large aneurysms.
2. An echocardiogram is the only way to diagnose and monitor the progression of coronary artery abnormalities. An echocardiogram should be obtained as soon as the diagnosis is established as a baseline study, with subsequent studies done in the subacute and convalescent phase. If no evidence of coronary artery dilation is seen by week 8, a final study should be performed 4 to 6 months after the acute onset for final confirmation (Pahl, 1997).

3. If varicella or influenza develops, aspirin treatment should be stopped during the course of illness to minimize the risk of Reye's syndrome (Fredriksen, 1998).
4. Live virus vaccines should be delayed until 6 months after administration of intravenous gamma globulin.
5. Patients with no coronary or cardiac changes on echocardiography at any stage require no activity restrictions, no medication beyond 4 to 6 weeks after the illness, and minimal if any long-term follow-up (Pahl, 1997).
6. Patients with small aneurysms should be maintained on low-dose acetylsalicylic acid (aspirin) and minimal to no exercise restrictions; patients with giant (>8 mm) aneurysms require close surveillance and limited activity (Pahl, 1997).

Complications

The acute disease is self-limited; however, if left untreated, significant cardiac sequelae will develop in 18 to 25% (Melish, 1996; Dajani et al., 1994). The process of aneurysm formation and subsequent thrombosis or scarring of the coronary artery may be seen as late as 6 months after the initial illness. Possible complications include recurrence (1 to 2%; Feit, 1995) coronary aneurysm (10%; Pahl, 1997), CHF, massive myocardial infarction leading to death in 1 to 2% (Fredriksen, 1998), myocarditis, pericarditis, pericardial effusion, mitral valve insufficiency, and coronary vessel stenosis.

Prognosis

Kawasaki syndrome is self-limited, and the risk of coronary aneurysm is reduced to 3% in patients older than 1 year if intravenous immune globulin is given within 10 days of the illness. Aneurysm regression is common by 1 year after the illness, but vessels do not return to normal elasticity and diameter. Patients with coronary artery abnormalities are at risk for myocardial infarction, sudden death, and myocardial ischemia for at least 5 years after the illness. Prompt treatment of chest pain, dyspnea, extreme lethargy, or syncope is essential (Pahl, 1997; Melish, 1996).

Rheumatic Fever

Description

Rheumatic fever (RF) is an inflammatory disease affecting the heart, joints, central nervous system, and subcutaneous tissue. The most significant sequela of RF is rheumatic heart disease, which can cause significant damage and scarring of the mitral valve (see Chapter 25 for more information).

Etiology and Incidence

In the 1950s and early 1960s, RF and its major complication, valvular heart disease, were significant problems worldwide. During the late 1960s and 1970s, the disease almost disappeared in the United States and western Europe, only to resurge in the mid-1980s. The reason for this resurgence remains unknown (Kaplan, 1998). It occurs most commonly in school-aged children 5 to 15 years old.

The relationship between upper respiratory tract infection, group A β-hemolytic streptococcal (GABHS) infection, and the subsequent development of RF is well established. This disease classically occurs after a latent period of 10 to 20 days following streptococcal pharyngitis or tonsillitis. Progression of symptoms is evident within 2 to 6 weeks of a streptococcal infection that has usually been untreated or only partially treated.

Clinical Findings

The diagnosis of RF is based on a set of guidelines recommended by the AHA (1994). These guidelines are known as the Jones criteria (Table 31–22). The presence of two major or one major and two minor criteria with evidence of a preceding GABHS infection indicates a high probability of RF. Children with fewer manifestations can also have RF.

Management

See Chapter 25 for further discussion of RF.

1. Treatment and prevention of GABHS infection.

TABLE 31-22

Jones Criteria for Rheumatic Fever*

EVIDENCE OF PRECEDING GABHS INFECTION
Positive throat culture or rapid streptococcal
  antigen test result
Elevated or rising streptococcal antibody titer

MINOR MANIFESTATIONS
Arthralgia
Fever
Elevated acute-phase reactants
Elevated erythrocyte sedimentation rate
Elevated C-reactive protein

MAJOR MANIFESTATIONS
Carditis
  Tachycardia out of proportion to degree of fever
  Cardiomegaly
  New murmurs or change in pre-existing
    murmurs
  Muffled heart sounds
  Precordial friction rub
  Precordial pain
  Changes in electrocardiogram (especially
    prolonged PR interval)
Polyarthritis
  Swollen, hot, red, painful joint(s)
  After 1 to 2 d, affects different joints
    (migratory)
  Favors large joints—knees, elbows, hips,
    shoulders, wrists

MAJOR MANIFESTATIONS Continued
Erythema marginatum
  Erythematous macules with clear center and
    wavy, well-demarcated border
  Transitory
  Nonpruritic
  Primarily affects trunk and extremities (inner
    surfaces)
Chorea
  Sudden, aimless, irregular movements of
    extremities
  Involuntary facial grimaces
  Speech disturbances or emotional lability
  Muscle weakness (can be profound)
  Muscle movements exaggerated by anxiety and
    attempt at fine motor activity; relieved by
    rest
Subcutaneous nodes
  Nontender swelling
  Located over bony prominence
  May persist for some time and then gradually
    resolve

*The presence of two major or one major and two or more minor criteria with evidence of preceding group A β-hemolytic streptococcal (GABHS) infection indicates a high probability of rheumatic fever.
  From American Heart Association Committee on Rheumatic Fever, Endocarditis, and Kawasaki Disease of the Council on Cardiovascular Disease in the Young: Guidelines for the diagnosis of rheumatic fever: Jones criteria, 1992 (update). Circulation 89:915–922, 1994. By permission of The American Heart Association.

2. Use of anti-inflammatory agents to control clinical manifestations of the disease.
3. Supportive therapy, including treatment of CHF.
4. Compliance with drug regimens, including ongoing antibiotic prophylaxis, is essential. Compliance may require monthly penicillin injection in a patient who is unable to comply with the twice-a-day oral regimen.
5. Prevention of recurrence can be achieved with prompt identification and treatment of future GABHS infections.

Bacterial Endocarditis

Description

Bacterial or infective endocarditis, also referred to as subacute bacterial endocarditis (SBE), is a condition in which a bacterial or fungal infection invades the endocardial surface of the heart, most commonly the cardiac valves. SBE usually occurs in children (average age, 12) or adults with underlying structural cardiac abnormalities, but it may rarely be seen in those without structural heart disease. Such an infection carries a high morbidity and mortality rate (20 to 30%) and can lead to destruction of heart valves or disseminated sepsis. The importance of prevention in patients who are at risk, as well as the importance of early diagnosis and treatment, cannot be overemphasized (Friedman & Starke, 1994a; Danilowicz, 1995).

Etiology

The disease is thought to involve the introduction of pathogens into the bloodstream. The most common portal of entry is oral from the release of bacteria *(Streptococcus viridans)* during dental work or oral surgery. SBE is also seen after cardiac catheterization or surgery, in patients with indwelling catheters, or in those who are at risk because of structural abnormalities of the heart. The microorganisms that are released into the blood at the time of mild or severe bacteremia grow on the endocardium and form vegetation, fibrin deposits, and platelet thrombi. The lesion may invade surrounding tissues, such as heart valves, or may break off and embolize in other organs such as the lungs, kidney, spleen, or brain.

Clinical Findings

HISTORY AND PHYSICAL EXAMINATION

- *Acute manifestation*: short duration of illness, high fever, and signs of progressive CHF secondary to valve destruction
- *Serious embolization*: hematuria, acute onset of respiratory distress, stroke or peripheral emboli
- *SBE*: prolonged period of illness, low-grade fever, signs of glomerulonephritis, arthritis, or skin rash
- *Cardiac disease*: may demonstrate a new murmur of valvular insufficiency

DIAGNOSTIC TESTS

- The diagnosis is based on clinical findings and results of blood cultures. The presence of a persistent low-grade fever in a patient with known cardiac abnormalities should be evaluated immediately with four to six blood cultures from different sources before the administration of empirical antibi-

otic therapy. When three to four cultures are positive for the same organism, SBE must be considered and treatment instituted.
- The ESR and white blood cell count are elevated in the acute stage.
- Echocardiography, although not a diagnostic modality in itself, may be helpful in patients who have evident vegetation, new valvular insufficiency, or obvious damage to a valve (Dajani et al., 1997).

Management

1. Treatment should begin as soon as SBE is suspected in order to decrease the subsequent morbidity and mortality associated with untreated bacteremia.
2. High doses of appropriate antibiotics are given intravenously for 4 to 6 weeks.

Prevention

Infective endocarditis in those at risk because of structural heart disease is prevented by administering prophylactic antibiotic therapy before procedures known to increase the risk of SBE (Dajani et al., 1997; AHA, 1997). Such procedures include dental work and manipulation of the respiratory, genitourinary, or gastrointestinal tract (see the management strategies section on prevention of bacterial endocarditis and Tables 31–11 to 31–15).

Myocarditis

Description

Myocarditis refers to active inflammation of the *myocardium*, or the muscular walls of the heart. Myocarditis may go unrecognized in many children whose infective illness resolves spontaneously, or it may lead to fulminant disease with rapid progression resulting in chronic cardiomyopathy.

Etiology and Incidence

Symptoms of myocarditis, which are secondary to reduced myocardial function, are caused by interstitial inflammation or damage. As a result, muscle function decreases and causes enlargement of the heart with decreased contractility. As this process progresses, cardiac function decreases and symptoms of CHF become evident.

Although rare, myocarditis is often caused by viral infections, most commonly coxsackievirus A and B (Friedman & Starke, 1994b). Echovirus, influenza, and rubella are other viral causes. Nonviral infections, various medications, autoimmune or inflammatory disorders (e.g., RF), and toxic reactions to infectious agents or other disorders (e.g., Kawasaki disease) may also be etiological agents; however, the etiology is often unknown. Myocarditis may occur as a seasonal outbreak, usually in infants in association with coxsackievirus B (Towbin, 1998; Zales & Wright, 1997; Steeg, 1994).

Clinical Findings

HISTORY
Infants
- Fever, irritability or listlessness, episodes of pallor, diaphoresis
- Tachypnea or respiratory distress
- Poor appetite and vomiting

Children and Adolescents
- Recent flu-like or gastrointestinal viral illness (10 to 14 days previously)
- Lethargy, low-grade fever, pallor
- Decreased appetite and abdominal pain
- Respiratory distress (late finding)

PHYSICAL EXAMINATION

- Pallor, mild cyanosis, skin cool and mottled with poor perfusion
- Rapid laborious respirations, grunting
- Tachycardia, gallop rhythm, muffled heart sounds, apical systolic murmur, weak pulses
- Hepatomegaly

DIAGNOSTIC TESTS

- Chest radiography shows cardiomegaly and prominent pulmonary markings.
- ECG shows a sinus tachycardia and possibly conduction disorders or arrhythmias.
- Echocardiography shows a dilated and dys-

functional left ventricle, pericardial effusion, mitral regurgitation.
- CBC, ESR, cardiac and liver enzymes, viral titers, blood cultures, metabolic studies (e.g., thyroid and carnitine).

Differential Diagnosis

Asthma, recurrent vomiting, and chronic viral illness are in the differential.

Management

1. The diagnosis is often difficult, and many forms of myocarditis have a subclinical manifestation. However, any child with unexplained CHF or ventricular tachycardia should be evaluated for myocarditis.
2. Treatment is supportive with bed rest, and medications such as digitalis, diuretics, and angiotensin-converting enzyme blockers are used as signs and symptoms indicate. Occasionally, anticoagulation and antiarrhythmia medications may be used. Many experimental therapies are under study, including the use of intravenous gamma globulin (McNamara et al., 1997). Severe cases may require hospitalization for mechanical ventilation and inotropic support.
3. Recovery often takes 2 to 3 months.

Complications

Pericardial effusion and pericarditis can occur concurrently. Scarring of the myocardium may occur and cause persistent heart failure and ventricular arrhythmias.

Prognosis

Cardiomyopathies may result in a need for cardiac transplantation (Canter & Strauss, 1995). Approximately 30 to 50% of neonates die, whereas 20 to 30% have a chronic cardiomyopathy. Eighty percent of children and adolescents show full clinical improvement; a "significant percentage" die or have end-stage dilated cardiomyopathy (Towbin, 1998; Steeg, 1994).

Pericarditis

Description

Pericarditis refers to an inflammation or other abnormality of the *pericardium*, the sac that surrounds the heart. Excess fluid accumulates in the pericardial space and causes the normally compliant pericardium to distend. If the volume is increased slowly, no hemodynamic compromise occurs. If the pericardium is required to distend rapidly, however, as in tamponade or a severe infectious process, it may become less compliant and cause a rapid increase in pressure. As intrapericardial pressure increases, the heart becomes compressed and its ability to fill is limited. Thus pericarditis is a serious illness that may have rapidly fatal consequences if not diagnosed and treated in a timely manner.

Etiology and Incidence

Pericarditis may be seen in individuals without a prior history of cardiac disease. Viral infection (usually coxsackievirus or adenovirus) is the most common cause of pericarditis, but other infectious agents, trauma, hypersensitive reactions to medication, collagen-vascular diseases, Kawasaki disease, postsurgical complications, and complication of systemic infection are also etiological agents. Pericarditis is most common in children younger than 2 years and demonstrates equal sex distribution (Towbin, 1998; Zales & Wright, 1997).

Clinical Findings

HISTORY

- Chest pain altered by respiration or position
- Lethargy, loss of appetite, abdominal pain
- Fever, irritability
- Tachypnea, tachycardia, and precordial pain with respiration or cough (reported in 15 to 20%; Towbin, 1998)

PHYSICAL EXAMINATION

- Distended neck veins
- Tachycardia, pericardial friction rub (an early sign heard best along the left sternal border with the patient leaning forward), or muffled heart sounds (if the effusion is large)
- Kussmaul sign
- Pulsus paradoxus—change in BP of greater than 10 mm Hg during inspiration
- Hepatomegaly

DIAGNOSTIC STUDIES

- CBC with elevated leukocytosis and elevated ESR, blood cultures; viral cultures may be done.
- Chest radiography shows a globular (water bottle)-shaped heart with increased pulmonary vascular markings.
- ECG may be normal or show ST elevation or depression with T-wave inversion and a low-voltage QRS complex.
- Echocardiography demonstrates effusion and detects tamponade (essential if effusion is suspected).

Management

1. The combination of sepsis with an enlarged heart should immediately suggest *bacterial pericarditis* in someone who has no history of CHD. In patients with a history of CHD, bacterial endocarditis is a possibility and rapid confirmation with an echocardiogram is necessary. Blood cultures should be obtained before initiation of broad-spectrum antibiotic therapy. If any signs of cardiac tamponade are seen (e.g., pulsus paradoxus or hemodynamic deterioration), immediate pericardiocentesis is mandatory. Hemodynamic support is provided as necessary.

2. In the case of *viral pericarditis* or pericarditis caused by *collagen-vascular disease* (e.g., lupus), the manifestation and course are usually less severe. Patients with large amounts of fluid in the pericardial sac should be observed closely and prepared for therapeutic pericardiocentesis if early signs of tamponade become evident. Management with nonsteroidal anti-inflammatory agents alleviates symptoms and may slow the accumulation of pericardial fluid.

3. In the case of *postoperative* patients or patients who have sustained a *traumatic blow or wound* to the chest, a cardiac tear or

perforation may be present and allow rapid blood accumulation in the pericardial space. This development is usually a hemodynamic emergency requiring immediate drainage, often by sternotomy or thoracotomy, to control the intrapericardial bleeding.

Complications

Cardiac tamponade can occur with large or rapid effusion.

Prognosis

Most children recover fully within a 3- to 4-week period.

CARDIAC ARRHYTHMIAS

Description

Abnormal heart rates (see Table 31–23) or rhythms, also called arrhythmias or dysrhythmias, that the NP should be familiar with include the following:

- Sinus arrhythmias—variable heart rate that increases with inspiration and decreases with expiration
- Bradycardia or slow heart rate (less than 60 bpm in newborns, 40 in children)
  - Sinus bradycardia
  - Complete atrioventricular block
- Tachycardia, or a rate that exceeds the upper limits of normal (220 bpm in newborns, 190 in older children)
- Conduction disturbances

T A B L E   31-23

Normal Heart Rates (bpm) in Infants and Children

AGE	RESTING (AWAKE)	RESTING (ASLEEP)	EXERCISE/ FEVER
Newborn	100–180	80–160	Up to 220
1 wk–3 mo	100–220	80–200	Up to 220
3 mo–2 y	80–150	70–120	Up to 200
2 y–10 y	70–100	60–90	Up to 200
10 y–adult	55–90	50–90	Up to 200

- AV block (first-, second-, and third-degree block)
- Premature atrial contractions—depolarization may or may not be conducted through the AV node
- Premature ventricular contractions—premature QRS complex with a prolonged duration or morphological difference from the preceding QRS

Etiology and Incidence

Most abnormal heart rhythms in children with entirely normal hearts are benign, but an arrhythmia in a child with a cardiac abnormality can be lethal. As more and more children survive complex congenital heart surgery, conduction system abnormalities are becoming more evident as a late complication (Garson, 1994).

The most commonly seen bradycardia in an otherwise normal child is a *sinus bradycardia*. This arrhythmia may be caused by hypoxia, acidosis, increased intracranial pressure, abdominal distention, hypothermia, or hypoglycemia. It may also be caused by drugs such as β-blockers or digoxin. Mild slowing may be due to increased vagal tone or cardiac conditioning (e.g., athletes) (Brooks, 1998). A *complete AV block* (complete heart block) can either be congenital, as seen in infants of mothers with an autoimmune disease such as lupus erythematosus, or may be acquired after cardiac surgery. This conduction abnormality is also seen postoperatively in patients who have had surgery in the area of the septum (ASD, VSD) or the AV (tricuspid or mitral) valves (Brooks, 1998). The hemodynamic effect of a slow heart rate depends on how different it is from the patient's usual heart rate.

Sinus tachycardia can be caused by any factor that increases cardiac output, including fever, anxiety, dehydration, pain, or anemia. It also can be a symptom or hyperthyroidism. The most common pathological tachycardia is *supraventricular tachycardia* (SVT), which can be seen in infants and young children, as well as young adults (Robinson et al., 1996).

Premature contractions can be seen in an infant or child with an otherwise normal heart. It is not unusual to see multiple *premature atrial contractions* on the ECG of a newborn.

Occasional *premature ventricular contractions* are also seen in otherwise normal infants. Premature ventricular contractions that are uniform in appearance, which means that they have the same QRS complex appearance every time, are usually of no consequence.

Clinical Findings

HISTORY

- Bradycardia with a sudden decrease in heart rate can cause syncope or severe dizziness.
- SVT onset is sudden and its duration is variable.
  - Infants tolerate several hours of SVT with rates up to 250 bpm before demonstrating evidence of poor feeding, irritability, or pallor that can eventually lead to CHF if not converted.
  - Older children may feel quite ill after a few minutes and have complaints of "butterflies" in the chest, dizziness, and nausea

PHYSICAL EXAMINATION

- Slow or fast heart rate
- Rhythm—regular, irregular, or regularly irregular

DIAGNOSTIC STUDIES

- ECG is the basic screening tool.
- Twenty-four-hour Holter monitor or event monitor if symptoms are sporadic and the ECG is normal.

Differential Diagnosis

Heart rates that are elevated or slowed because of exercise, physical conditioning, or other physiological reasons are included in the differential diagnosis.

Management

Identification of an arrhythmia can be challenging.

1. Sinus arrhythmia requires no treatment.
2. Sinus bradycardia:
   - If asymptomatic, watch.

- If symptomatic, correct the cause (e.g., acidosis or hypoxia require immediate intervention). If persistently low, pacemaker implantation may be required.
3. AV block—if first degree and asymptomatic, may observe.
4. SVT—initial treatment is aimed at using vagal maneuvers to convert the SVT:
   - Infant—apply ice to the face.
   - Child—have the child hold breath and bear down or gag.
   - If persistent—may need to be seen in the emergency department or office and treated with adenosine.
   - Referral to a cardiologist is indicated if recurrent or in the presence of structural heart disease or Wolff-Parkinson-White syndrome; long-term digoxin therapy may be used.
   - If SVT is persistent and frequent, radiofrequency ablation can be used to obliterate the accessory pathway that is causing the SVT.
5. Premature atrial contractions:
   - In a stable infant without cardiovascular compromise, premature atrial contraction is often a normal variant and will be gone on a 2-week repeat ECG.
   - Observe unless persistent and frequent; then refer to a cardiologist.
6. Premature ventricular contractions:
   - If uniform in appearance, of no consequence.
   - In an older child (heard on examination), have the child race down the hall and back and check for recurrence. Usually the premature beats disappear with exercise. If not, further evaluation is necessary.
   - If the premature ventricular contraction is multiformed or has more than one QRS appearance, referral is indicated because such may be seen in long QT syndrome, cardiomyopathy, or CHD (before or after surgery).
7. Conduction abnormalities or irregular rhythm after open heart surgery:
   - Annual surveillance with a Holter monitor.
   - If an AV block or premature contractions are present, drug treatment or pacer placement may be indicated.

8. Referral to a cardiologist is always indicated for the following:
   - Abnormal ECG.
   - History of unusual heart rhythm.
   - History of syncope or dizziness with palpitations.

Complications

Death can occur with some arrhthymias if left untreated.

Education/Prognosis

- Recurrent SVT—the child or parent should be taught to monitor the heart rate and use vagal manuevers to break the spell.
- Most arrhythmias in children with normal hearts are benign. Such is not the case for children with an abnormal heart. Arrhythmia in a child with a cardiac abnormality can be lethal.

RESOURCE BOX 31-1

RESOURCES FOR INFORMATION FOR FAMILIES

Mended Hearts—a support group through the American Heart Association (AHA)
Website: www.mendedheart.org

Children's Health Information Network
Website: www.tchin.org

The Heart of a Child: What a Family Needs to Know About Heart Disorders in Children
By Catherine Neill et al.
Johns Hopkins University Press, 1992.

American Heart Association
Tel: (800) 242-8721, (214) 373-6300
Website: www.amhrt.org
Informational materials (inc. Spanish), networking, referrals to local resources, local chapters, advocacy, fund research, maintain research registry

High Blood Pressure Line
National Heart, Lung and Blood Institute
Website: www.nhlbi.nih.gov
Tel: (800) 575-WELL

REFERENCES

Allen HD, Golinko RJ, Williams RG: Heart murmurs in children: When is a workup needed? Contemp Pediatr 11:29–52, 1994.

American Academy of Pediatrics: Task force report on blood pressure control in children (update). Pediatrics 99:637–638, 1997.

American Heart Association Committee on Rheumatic Fever, Endocarditis, and Kawasaki Disease of the Council on Cardiovascular Disease in the Young: Prevention of bacterial endocarditis: Recommendations by the American Heart Association. JAMA 277:1794–1801, 1997.

American Heart Association Committee on Rheumatic Fever, Endocarditis, and Kawasaki Disease of the Council on Cardiovascular Disease in the Young: Guidelines for the diagnosis of rheumatic fever: Jones Criteria, 1992 (update). Circulation 89:915–922, 1994.

American Heart Association Committee on Rheumatic Fever, Endocarditis, and Kawasaki Disease of the Council on Cardiovascular Disease in the Young: Kawasaki disease: Recommendations by the American Heart Association. Circulation 89:915–922, 1994.

Ardinger RH: Genetic counseling in congenital heart disease. Pediatr Ann 26:99–104, 1997.

Brooks MM: The cardiovascular system. *In* Behrman RE, Kliegman RM (eds): Nelson Essentials of Pediatrics, 3rd ed. Philadelphia, WB Saunders, 1998, pp 497–544.

Canter CE, Strauss AW: Cardiomyopathies—when to think of congenital causes. Contemp Pediatr 12:25–40, 1995.

Castiglia PT: Kawasaki syndrome. J Pediatr Health Care 10:124–126, 1996.

Cheatham JP: Pulmonary stenosis. *In* Oski FA, DeAngelis CD, Feigin RE, et al (eds): Principles and Practice of Pediatrics, 2nd ed. Philadelphia, JB Lippincott, 1994, pp 1567–1571.

Child JS: Risks for and prevention of infective endocarditis. Cardiol Clin 14:327–343, 1996.

Clark EB: Epidemiology of congenital cardiovascular malformations. *In* Emmanouilides GC, Allen H, Riemenschneider T, et al (eds): Moss and Adams Heart Disease in Infants, Children and Adolescents, 5th ed. Baltimore, Williams & Wilkins, 1995, pp 60–69.

Coody DK, Yetman RJ, Portman RJ: Hypertension in children. J Pediatr Health Care 9:3–11, 1995.

Cornell S: Rethinking hypertension in children. Adv Nurse Pract 5:39–42, 1997.

Dajani A: Diagnosis and therapy of Kawasaki disease in childhood. Pediatric Consultant: A Publication for the Medical Community. Winter:199–201, 1993.

Dajani, AS, Taubert KA, Takahasi M: Guidelines for long-term management of Kawasaki disease. Circulation 89:916–922, 1994.

Dajani AS, Taubert KA, Wilson W, et al: Prevention of bacterial endocarditis: Recommendations by the American Heart Association. JAMA 277:1794–1801, 1997.

Daniels SR: The diagnosis of hypertension in children: An update. Pediatr Rev 18:131–135, 1997.

Danilowicz D: Infective endocarditis. Pediatr Rev 16:148–154, 1995.

Feit LR: The heart of the matter: Evaluating murmurs in children. Contemp Pediatr 14:97–122, 1997.

Feit LR: Keeping up with Kawasaki syndrome. Contemp Pediatr 12:37–49, 1995.

Fredriksen M: An infant with persistent fever. Clin Rev 8:129–136, 1998.

Friedman RA, Starke JR: Infective endocarditis. *In* Oski FA, DeAngelis CD, Feigin RE, et al (eds): Principles and Practice of Pediatrics, 2nd ed. Philadelphia, JB Lippincott, 1994a, pp 1614–1625.

Friedman RA, Starke JR: Myocarditis. *In* Oski FA, DeAngelis CD, Feigin RE, et al (eds): Principles and Practice of Pediatrics, 2nd ed. Philadelphia, JB Lippincott, 1994b, pp 1240–1243.

Friedman WF: Congenital heart disease in infancy and childhood. *In* Brunwald D (ed): Heart Disease: A Textbook of Cardiovascular Medicine, 5th ed. Philadelphia, WB Saunders, 1996.

Garson A: Abnormalities of cardiac rate and rhythm. *In* Oski FA, DeAngelis CD, Feigin RE, et al (eds): Principles and Practice of Pediatrics, 2nd ed. Philadelphia, JB Lippincott, 1994, pp 1641–1645.

Gumbiner C: Ventricular septal defect. *In* Oski FA, DeAngelis CD, Feigin RE, et al (eds): Principles and Practice of Pediatrics, 2nd ed. Philadelphia, JB Lippincott, 1994, pp 1561–1564.

Harris JP: Evaluation of heart murmurs. Pediatr Rev 15:490–493, 1994.

Hohn AR: Diagnosis and management of hypertension in childhood. Pediatr Ann 26:105–110, 1997.

Jones AK: The numbers game. Adv Nurse Pract 6:63–65, 1998.

Kaminer SJ, Strong WB: Cardiac arrhythmias. Pediatr Rev 15:437–439, 1994.

Kaplan EL: Rheumatic fever. *In* Finberg L (ed): Saunders Manual of Pediatric Practice. Philadelphia, WB Saunders, 1998, pp 596–599.

Kirklin JW, Colvin EV, McConnell ME, et al: Complete transposition of the great arteries: Treatment in the current era. Pediatr Clin North Am 37:171–177, 1996.

Lamb F: Heart failure. *In* Oski FA, DeAngelis CD, Feigin RE, et al (eds): Principles and Practice of Pediatrics, 2nd ed. Philadelphia, JB Lippincott, 1994, pp 1561–1564.

Lott J: Assessment and management of cardiovascular dysfunction. *In* Kenner C, Lott JW, Flandermeyer AA (eds): Comprehensive Neonatal Nursing: A Physiologic Perspective, 2nd ed. Philadelphia, WB Saunders, 1998, pp 306–335.

Mair DD, Edward WM, Julsrud PR: Aortic stenosis. *In* Emmanoulides GC, Allen H, Riemenschneider T (eds): Moss and Adams Heart Disease in Infants, Children and Adolescents Including the Fetus and Young Adult, 5th ed. Baltimore, Williams & Wilkins, 1995, pp 1026–1041.

McCrindle BW, Shaffer KM, Kan JS, et al: Cardinal clinical signs in the differentiation of heart murmurs in children. Arch Pediatr Adolesc Med 150:169–174, 1996.

McNamara D, Rosenblum WD, Janosko KM, et al: Intravenous immune globulin therapy in myocarditis. Circulation 19:2476–2478, 1997.

Melish ME: Kawasaki syndrome. Pediatr Rev 17:153–162, 1996.

Moore K, Persaud TVN: The Developing Humans, 6th ed. Philadelphia, WB Saunders, 1998.

Morriss MJ, McNamara DG: Coarctation of the aorta. *In* Oski FA, DeAngelis CD, Feigin RE, et al (eds): Principles and Practice of Pediatrics, 2nd ed. Philadelphia, JB Lippincott, 1994, pp 1575–1580.

Mulhern K: Marfan syndrome. *In* Oski FA, DeAngelis CD, Feigin RE, et al (eds): Principles and Practice of Pediatrics, 2nd ed. Philadelphia, JB Lippincott, 1994, pp 1561–1564.

Mullins CE: Patent ductus arteriosus. *In* Oski FA, DeAngelis CD, Feigin RE, et al (eds): Principles and Practice of Pediatrics, 2nd ed. Philadelphia, JB Lippincott, 1994, pp 1561–1564.

National High Blood Pressure Education Program (NHBPEP) Working Group in Hypertension Control in Children and Adolescents: Update on the 1987 task force report on high blood pressure in children and adolescents: A working group report from the National High Blood Pressure Education Program. Pediatrics 98:649–658, 1996.

Neches WH, Park SC, Ettedgui J: Transposition of the great arteries. *In* Oski FA, DeAngelis CD, Feigin RE, et al (eds): Principles and Practice of Pediatrics, 2nd ed. Philadelphia, JB Lippincott, 1994, pp 1528–1531.

Pahl E: Kawasaki disease: Cardiac sequelae and management. Pediat Ann 26(2):112–115, 1997.

Park MK: Pediatric Cardiology for Practitioners, 3rd ed. St Louis, CV, Mosby, 1996.

Robinson B, Anisman P, Eshaghpour E: Is that fast heartbeat dangerous (and what should you do about it?). Contemp Pediatr 13:52–85, 1996.

Sardegna KM, Loggie JMH: Hypertension in teens. Contemp Pediatr 13:96–112, 1996.

Selbst SM: Chest pain in children. Pediatr Rev 18:169–173, 1997.

Smith KM: The innocent heart murmur in children. J Pediatr Health Care 11:207–214, 1997.

Steeg CN: Myocarditis. Pediatr Rev 15:120–121, 1994.

Talner NS: Heart failure. *In* Emmanoulides GC, Allen H, Riemenschneider T, et al (eds): Moss and Adams Heart Disease in Infants, Children and Adolescents Including the Fetus and Young Adult, 5th ed. Baltimore, Williams & Wilkins, 1995, pp 1746–1772.

Towbin JA: Myocarditis and pericarditis. *In* Finberg L (ed): Saunders Manual of Pediatric Practice. Philadelphia, WB Saunders, 1998, pp 581–587.

US Preventive Services Task Force: Guide to Clinical Preventive Services, 2nd ed. Baltimore, Williams & Wilkins, 1996.

US Public Health Service: Put Prevention Into Practice: The Clinician's Handbook of Preventive Services, 2nd ed. Germantown, MD, International Medical Publishing, 1997.

Uzark K: Recognition and management of congenital heart disease in the neonate. Presented at the 17th Annual National Association of Pediatric Nurse Associates and Practitioners (NAPNAP) Conference. San Diego, CA, 1996.

Van Hare GF: Circulation: Congenital heart disease. *In* Abraham R, Kamei RK (eds): Fundamentals of Pediatrics. E Norwalk CT, Appleton & Lange, 1994, pp 499–536.

Vick GW, Titus J: Atrial septal defect. *In* Oski FA, DeAngelis CD, Feigin RE, et al (eds): Principles and Practice of Pediatrics, 2nd ed. Philadelphia, JB Lippincott, 1994, pp 1553–1555.

Williams RG, Kennedy TL, Moller JH: Pediatric cardiology for the '90's. J Am Coll Cardiol 23:977–980, 1994.

Zales VR, Wright KC: Endocarditis, pericarditis & myocarditis. Pediatr Ann 26:116–121, 1997.

Zuberbuhler JR: Tricuspid atresia. *In* Emmanoulides GC, Allen H, Riemenschneider T, et al (eds): Moss and Adams Heart Disease in Infants, Children and Adolescents Including the Fetus and Young Adult, 5th ed. Baltimore, Williams & Wilkins, 1995, pp 998–1017.

CHAPTER 32

Respiratory Disorders

Mark H. Goodman and Margaret A. Brady

INTRODUCTION

Respiratory problems are a leading cause of illness in children and a major reason for health care visits. Viral upper respiratory tract infections (URIs) and otitis media are common diagnoses seen every day by practitioners. Guiding parents in the appropriate management of upper respiratory disorders is often a challenge for health care providers seeking to treat such problems as the common cold, otitis media, rhinitis, tonsillopharyngitis, and sinusitis. Parents seeking to relieve their child's upper respiratory tract symptoms are often tempted to use a variety of over-the-counter medications readily available to them or to pressure the nurse practitioner (NP) to prescribe needless antibiotics. In contrast, a child with a lower respiratory tract disorder such as asthma or bacterial pneumonia can experience a potentially life-threatening illness that demands prompt attention. NPs who ask key questions about the history of the respiratory symptoms, do a systematic and complete examination of the upper and lower airways, including the sinuses, and if indicated, order specific laboratory tests and radiographic examinations can determine an accurate diagnosis and develop a successful treatment plan in most cases. When children have complicated problems, they can be referred with baseline information to the appropriate medical specialist for additional studies and treatment.

ANATOMY AND PHYSIOLOGY

Upper Respiratory Tract

The upper respiratory tract includes the nostrils, nasopharynx, larynx, upper part of the trachea, eustachian tubes, and sinuses. Air is warmed and humidified as it travels down the nasal passages, and particles are filtered out by coarse nasal hairs. A blanket of mucus covers the surface epithelium of the nasal mucosa. Nasal secretions contain lysozymes and secretory immunoglobulin A (IgA) to defend against microbial invasion. Similarly, the paranasal sinuses are lined with ciliated, mucus-secreting epithelium. The maxillary and ethmoid sinuses are the earliest sinuses to develop and can be visualized on plain radiographs by 1 to 2 years of age. The sphenoid and frontal sinuses become visible on radiographs at approximately 5 to 6 years of age. The sinuses become clinically significant sites of infection as follows:

- Maxillary and ethmoid sinuses as early as infancy
- Sphenoid sinuses around the 3rd and 4th year of life

- Frontal sinuses around the 6th to 10th year of life

The sinuses continue to grow through adolescence.

Lower Respiratory Tract

The right lung has three lobes, the upper and middle being separated by a minor fissure. The left lung has two lobes separated by a major fissure. The upper left lobe has an area called the lingula that corresponds to the right middle lobe. The right main stem bronchus is shorter and wider and forms a smaller angle away from the trachea than the left bronchus does. This anatomical variation explains why foreign bodies usually end in the right main stem bronchus. Although the body surface and the number of respiratory airways and alveoli increase 10-fold from birth to adult life, the tissue available for gas exchange increases approximately 20-fold. The newborn's chest is cylindrically shaped and has relatively horizontal ribs. The shape of the chest changes during the first few years of life because of greater transverse growth of the lower part of the chest wall. This differential growth results in the ribs being positioned lower anteriorly than posteriorly. The change in positioning of the ribs adds rigidity to the thorax of older children.

The diaphragm is the main muscle of respiration, and the intercostal, sternocleidomastoid, spinal, neck, and abdominal muscles are accessory muscles that can be used to increase effort. Normal exhalation occurs from elastic recoil of the lung.

Primitive airways appear around the 4th week of gestation. At approximately the 16th week of gestation, the number of bronchial branches equals that in adults. Subsequent growth continues by increasing the length of the respiratory tract. During the 16th to the 26th week of gestation, vascularization of the future respiratory portion of the lung occurs. Cartilage, glands, and muscles of the airways and type II alveolar cells are formed by the 28th week. Type II cells allow the fetus to produce surfactant. The airways continue to grow, and terminal sac formation occurs. Around the 36th week, the terminal sacs divide and alveoli are formed. Approximately 50 million primitive alveoli are present at birth.

After birth, the alveolar ducts branch off the third respiratory bronchioles. Alveoli continue to form and number 100 to 200 million in older children and 200 to 600 million in adolescents. The alveolar sacs continue to increase in size. The adult lung contains approximately 300 million alveoli.

Other structures important for gas exchange and pulmonary function are present at birth and include cartilage, mucous glands, goblet cells, and ciliated cells of the conducting airways. Smooth muscle is also present; therefore, even very young infants can have bronchospasm.

Airway resistance is higher in newborns and young children than in adults. The airways of young infants and children are easily obstructed by inflammation, foreign bodies, or mucus secretion. The maximal inspiratory pressure generated by an infant is equal to that of an adult. However, the chest wall and supporting structures are softer and more flexible, so chest wall retraction is greatest in young infants (Behrman et al., 1996).

PATHOPHYSIOLOGY INVOLVED IN LOWER AIRWAY DISEASE

All lung disorders eventually result in some form of airway obstruction. Narrowing of the lumen of the airway results from one or more of the following:

- Presence of intraluminal material (e.g., secretions, tumors, or foreign matter)
- Mural thickening (e.g., edema and hypertrophy of the glands or mucosa)
- Contraction of smooth muscle (e.g., spasm)
- Extrinsic compression

These factors rarely occur in isolation and cause pulmonary malfunction by impairing tracheobronchial hygiene and impeding normal airflow. Even small blockages in an infant's or young child's airway can lead to severe airway obstruction.

The two major types of airway obstruction

are complete and partial. In complete obstruction, neither airflow nor drainage of secretions occurs. Such occlusion leads to lobar atelectasis after the residual gas diffuses into the pulmonary circulation. In partial obstruction, flow of air and drainage of secretions occur but are impaired. Partial obstruction can be further divided into two separate classifications. The first consists of a bypass valve obstruction caused by narrowing of the lumen. Although resistance to flow is increased, air can still flow in during inspiration and out during expiration. The second is a check-valve obstruction; air entry is possible, but during expiration the lumen is completely occluded so that escape of air is impossible.

High airway obstruction occurs above the level of the secondary bronchi and generally interferes more with inspiration than expiration. If the obstruction is complete and above the bifurcation of the trachea, asphyxia and death can result. Partial obstruction may result in severe dyspnea, stridor (a harsh, low-pitched *inspiratory* sound), and subcostal retractions. Coughing is the mechanism to remove non-fixed, high airway obstruction. Poor inspiratory airflow limits the effectiveness of coughing. The sound produced by coughing can help detect the level of obstruction and assists in making a diagnosis. Obstructions next to the larynx produce a cough that sounds croupy or barking; obstructions in the trachea or major bronchi produce a brassy sound.

Low airway obstructions are caused by peripheral lesions that are usually diffuse in location and involve bronchioles less than 3 mm. The usual mechanism of narrowing is spasm, accumulation of secretions, edema of the mucous membrane, extrinsic compression, or any combination of these factors. Complete obstruction causes atelectasis. A large percentage of the lung volume needs to be involved before symptoms become apparent; small atelectatic changes do not produce obvious clinical manifestations.

The primary clinical manifestation of lower airway obstruction is *expiratory*-phase symptoms. Wheezing is the principal sound patients make if the obstruction allows enough air to pass through the narrowed lumen. Chest excursion is diminished, and the expiratory phase is prolonged. Increased airway resistance during exhalation results in overinflation of the lungs, which in turn eventually increases the anteroposterior diameter of the chest. Chronic overinflation results in the "barrel chest" typical of a patient with chronic lung disease such as occurs with emphysema. The accumulation of fluids and inflammation in the lower airways usually result in a repetitive hacking, ineffectual cough. On physical examination, percussing an overinflated chest elicits hyperresonance.

The more marked the obstruction, the more symptoms induced. The body attempts to compensate by using accessory muscles to assist in breathing. Dyspnea can result, often in association with orthopnea, and exercise tolerance is limited. Cyanosis is an ominous sign that can suggest impending death.

Fine crackles or rales also indicate respiratory pathology and are short crackling sounds heard during inspiration. These sounds are not cleared by coughing and are caused by airways suddenly opening after having been previously closed. The gas pressure between the compartments equalizes and creates the crackling sound.

DEFENSE SYSTEMS

The respiratory defense system includes the upper airway structures of the nose, paranasal sinuses, and pharynx. Approximately 75% of inspired air is warmed as it passes through the nose, pharynx, larynx, and upper portion of the trachea. Final warming and humidifying of the air stream take place in the trachea and large bronchi. Heat and moisture are removed during the expiratory phase of respiration. The nose has a large surface area on which particles larger than 6 mm are impacted and filtered to prevent them from entering the lower airways. The larynx is a narrow tube with cartilaginous rings and is easily obstructed by inflammation in children. In very young children, hyperextension of the neck or external pressure can cause laryngeal obstruction. The trachea and bronchioles are lined with various defensive cells and mucous glands. Goblet cells secrete the mucous layer that lies on the tip of cilia.

The respiratory system's defenses include:

- Filtering of particles
- Warming and humidifying of inspired air
- Absorption of noxious gases in the vascular upper airway

Particles entering the conducting airway are quickly cleared by the mucociliary defenses. Those reaching the alveoli can take days to months to clear. These particles can be phagocytized by alveolar macrophages, cleared from the lung by the mucociliary system, or carried by lymphocytes into regional lymph nodes or the blood. Coughing can propel particles, but in young infants and children, coughing is often unproductive in expectorating mucus.

The temporary cessation of breathing, reflex shallow breathing, laryngospasm, and even bronchospasm are compensatory efforts aimed at stopping foreign matter from further entry into the lower respiratory tract. However, these respiratory efforts offer limited protection and have significant drawbacks.

Phagocytosis aided by the secretory immunoglobulins IgA, IgM, and IgG, plus interferon, lysozyme, and lactoferrin, is the principal antimicrobial defense. Phagocytic ability is reduced by many substances, including ethanol ingestion and cigarette smoke. Hypoxemia, starvation, chilling, corticosteroids, nitrogen dioxide, ozone, increased oxygen, narcotics, and some anesthetic gases also impair phagocytosis. Recent acute viral infections can reduce antibacterial killing capacity.

Damage to epithelial cells is caused by a variety of substances and gases such as sulfur, nitrogen dioxide, ozone, chlorine, ammonia, and cigarette smoke. Hypothermia, hyperthermia, morphine, codeine, and hypothyroidism can adversely alter mucociliary defenses. Dry air from mouth breathing during periods of nasal obstruction, tracheostomy placement, or inadequately humidified oxygen therapy results in dryness of the mucous membrane and slowing of the cilia beat. Cold air is also irritating to the lower airways. Damage from infection and chemical irritants may or may not be reversible (Behrman et al., 1996).

ASSESSMENT OF THE RESPIRATORY SYSTEM

History

1. History of the present illness
   - Onset. Was the onset acute or insidious and/or preceded by the common cold?
   - Key signs/symptoms. Has the child had symptoms or signs of a daytime or nighttime cough, fever, rhinorrhea, sore throat, lesions in the mouth, retractions, cyanosis, dyspnea, or increased respiratory effort? See Table 32–1 for key characteristic and causes of cough.
   - Progression. Are the respiratory signs or symptoms increasing in severity, lessening, or about the same? Is the child easily fatigued, less active, and/or having trouble sleeping?
   - Associated symptoms. Has there been a decrease in appetite or feeding? Any rashes, headache, or abdominal pain?
   - Contacts. Are any family members or close contacts (day care, school) ill with similar signs and symptoms?
   - Similar illnesses in the past. Does the child have a history of respiratory tract infections, allergies, or asthma? How many similar past infections (e.g., croup, pneumonia, sinusitis, streptococcal tonsillopharyngitis, frequent colds)?
   - Treatment. Have any over-the-counter or prescription drugs been used? Have any other treatment modalities been used, including folk cures or home remedies?
2. Family history
   - Do others in the family have a history of allergies or asthma? Is there any family history of ear-nose-throat or respiratory problems that could be familial or genetic diseases such as cystic fibrosis (CF)?
3. Review of systems
   - Note any infections, constitutional diseases, or congenital problems that might have a respiratory component.
4. Environment
   - Does anyone in the family or in the day care setting smoke? Does the child live in an urban or industrial area subject to air

T A B L E 32-1

Key Characteristics of Cough, Common Causes, and Questions to Ask in a Pediatric History

Purpose	A cough is a protective reflex to ensure airway patency
Characteristics	
Age factor	Infants have a weak, nonproductive cough
Quality	Staccato-like, brassy, barking (LTB), whooping (pertussis), weak, honky (psychogenic)
Duration	Acute (most causes are infectious), recurrent (associated with allergies and asthma), or chronic (e.g., cystic fibrosis); continuous or intermittent. A chronic cough is defined as coughing that lasts more than 3 to 4 wk
Productive	Mucus producing or nonproductive
Timing	During the day, night (associated with asthma), or both
Associated symptoms	Fever—may indicate bacterial infection
	Rhinorrhea, sneezing, wheezing, atopic dermatitis—associated with asthma and allergic rhinitis
	Malaise, sneezing, watery nasal discharge, mild sore throat, no or low fever, not ill appearing—typical of URI
	Tachypnea—pneumonia or bronchiolitis in infants (infants may not have a cough)
Causes	
Congenital anomalies	Tracheoesophageal fistula, laryngeal cleft, vocal cord paralysis, pulmonary malformations and tumors, tracheobronchomalacia, congenital heart disease, congestive heart failure
Infectious agents	Viral (respiratory syncytial virus, adenovirus, parainfluenza, HIV), bacterial (tuberculosis, group A β-hemolytic streptococci, pertussis), fungal, and others (*Chlamydia* and *Mycoplasma*)
Allergic conditions	Allergic rhinitis, asthma
Other	Foreign body aspiration, gastroesophageal reflux, psychogenic cough, environmental triggers (air pollution, tobacco smoke, wood smoke, glue sniffing, volatile chemicals), cystic fibrosis, drug induced

HIV = human immunodeficiency virus; LTB = laryngotracheobronchitis; URI = upper respiratory infection.
Adapted from Noble JE: Cough. *In* Berkowitz C (ed): Pediatrics: A Primary Care Approach. Philadelphia, WB Saunders, 1996, pp 226–239; Guilbert TW, Taussig LM: Chronic cough. Contemp Pediatr 15:155–172, 1998.

pollution (e.g., near a major highway or industrial plant)?

Physical Examination

Chapter 2 covers physical examination of the respiratory system. Additional information pertinent to the physical examination of a child with suspected respiratory disease includes:

1. Measurement of vital signs and observation of general appearance
   - A normal respiratory rate is age dependent and, if elevated, is a key indicator of lower respiratory involvement.
   - The level of anxiety, nasal flaring, and position of comfort are useful indicators of respiratory distress.
2. Inspection of
   - The nose for rhinorrhea—clear, mucoid, mucopurulent; foreign bodies, erosion, polyps, lesions, bleeding; and color of the mucous membrane.
   - The throat, pharynx, and tonsillar areas for lesions, vesicles, exudate, enlargement of any structure, or other abnormalities. *If epiglottitis is a consideration, do not inspect the mouth.*
   - The chest for the depth, ease, symmetry, and rhythm of respiration. These elements

are key indicators of lower respiratory tract involvement. The use of accessory muscles and the presence of retractions should be noted. A prolonged expiratory phase is associated with respiratory obstruction in the lower airways.

3. Palpation and/or percussion of
   - The paranasal and frontal areas to check for signs of sinus tenderness.
   - The chest for signs of dullness or hyperresonance caused by consolidation, fluid, or air trapping.

4. Auscultation of the chest
   - Upper tract involvement frequently causes rhonchi or referred breath sounds.
   - Lower tract involvement is suggested by fine crackles or rales (interrupted abnormal breath sounds) or by wheezing.

5. Determination of respiratory distress
   - Based on physical findings—consider the anxiety level, respiratory rate and rhythm, use of accessory muscles, color, breath sounds, and pulse oximetry.

Diagnostic Procedures

Diagnostic procedures used to evaluate respiratory illness in children managed as outpatients include:

- Monitoring oxygenation by pulse oximetry and blood gases.
  - Pulse oximetry can be used to continuously measure peripheral oxygen saturation. Results generally correlate well with simultaneous arterial saturation (Sao_2). The equation to determine Pao_2 is $Pao_2 = Fio_2 (Ba - Ph_2o) - 1.2Paco_2)$. The partial pressure of H_2O is constant at 47 and that of CO_2 is usually 45. This dependence on barometric pressure (Ba) is the limiting factor: the higher the altitude at which one lives, the more hypoxic one becomes (e.g., the Pao_2 on room air at sea level $= 0.21(760 - 47) - 1.2 \cdot 45 = 95.73$). If Ba falls 50 mm Hg, the resultant Pao_2 in room air changes drastically (e.g., $Pao_2 = 0.21(710 - 47) - 1.2 \cdot 45 = 85$). People living in higher altitudes suffer from chronic hypoxia (Maggi, 1998). When

first arriving at a high elevation, many individuals will experience a transient mountain sickness with symptoms that include headache, insomnia, irritability, breathlessness, nausea, and vomiting. This phenomenon can last approximately 1 week before acclimatization begins to occur. The affected person begins to increase production of red blood cells. Changes in hemoglobin result in decreased O_2 affinity, which makes more O_2 available to the cells. Finally, a functional nonpathological right ventricular hypertrophy takes place. These effects last as long as the person remains at high altitude (Maggi, 1998).

- Blood gas studies can help the NP in assessing possible respiratory collapse. A rising $Paco_2$ is an ominous sign. Table 32-2 lists normal values for blood gases at sea level.

- Radiographic imaging, including radiographs, ultrasonography, magnetic resonance imaging (MRI), and computed tomography (CT) of the sinuses, soft tissues of the neck, and chest. Fluoroscopy is useful in the evaluation of stridor and abnormal movement of the diaphragm. Contrast studies are useful for patients with recurrent pneumonia, persistent cough, or suspected fistulas.

- Pulmonary function tests are discussed in Chapter 25 under asthma.

- Other specialized tests, including cultures and blood work, are addressed under the specific illness.

- Other imaging studies that might be

T A B L E 32-2

Normal Blood Gas Values at Sea Level

Normal Pao_2: 90–100 mm Hg
Normal $Paco_2$: 38–42 mm Hg
Capillary Po_2: roughly one half the arterial
Capillary Pco_2: the same as arterial
Hypoventilation: $Paco_2$ >45 mm Hg; as $Paco_2$ rises, the risk of respiratory failure increases
Hyperventilation: $Paco_2$ <35 mm Hg (usually need a respiratory rate >60/min)

needed to assess these children include bronchograms (useful in delineating the smaller airways), pulmonary arteriograms (evaluation of the pulmonary vasculature), and radionuclide studies (evaluation of the pulmonary capillary bed). Endoscopy, bronchoscopy, percutaneous tap, lung biopsy, sweat testing, and microbiology studies are other helpful diagnostic procedures if used appropriately. Children who are significantly ill or have unusual signs and symptoms that require such procedures should be referred to medical specialists.

BASIC RESPIRATORY MANAGEMENT STRATEGIES

General Measures

General management measures include the following:

- Fluid. Hydration is important to keep mucous membranes and secretions moist. Intake of fluids should be encouraged and parents of young children given guidelines regarding the amount of fluids that their child should take and the frequency of feedings.
- Humidification. For a child with laryngotracheobronchitis (LTB), taking the child out into the cold night air, opening a freezer door, or turning on the shower at home is often beneficial. A cold-mist vaporizer helps provide moisture to the nares and oropharynx; the vaporizer must be cleaned daily so that it will not become a source of infection. To prevent the growth of organisms, nebulizers and humidifiers should be cleaned first with soapy water, rinsed thoroughly, soaked for one-half hour in a solution of 1 part vinegar to 2 or 3 parts distilled water, and then air-dried. Control 3 is a commercial product that can be substituted for vinegar. However, it is expensive.
- Bulb syringe. Because infants are obligate nose breathers, parents should be instructed on use of the bulb syringe to relieve obstruction of the infant's nares with mucus. Use the bulb syringe gently and

intermittently because improper use can cause irritation, inflammation, and respiratory obstruction from tissue damage. Be sure to obstruct one nostril while suctioning the other.
- Normal saline nose drops or spray. Use before feedings and when mucus is thick or crusted. Follow by suctioning the nares with a bulb syringe; remember that the naris not being suctioned must be occluded.

Children who are significantly ill or have unusual manifestations need referral to or consultation with a pediatrician.

Medications

The following pharmacological agents may be needed to treat various respiratory illnesses:

- Antibiotics. Specific agents are discussed in the section on individual illnesses. If an antibiotic is prescribed, the drug should be taken until completed.
- Analgesics and antipyretics. Acetaminophen and ibuprofen may be prescribed for relief of pain or fever.
- Decongestants and antihistamines. The use of decongestants, antihistamines, or both is controversial. Often they do not shorten the course of a disease but can provide relief of nasal symptoms. Use these agents with caution, especially in children younger than 9 months to 1 year.
- Expectorants. Water is one of the most effective expectorants. Over-the-counter agents provide some symptomatic relief but do not shorten the course of respiratory illnesses. Use with care in children younger than 1 year.
- Cough medication. Cough suppressant medications should be prescribed judiciously because coughing is a protective mechanism to clear secretions. Prescribing a cough suppressant at bedtime can help the child and parent sleep. Use very carefully in infants younger than 1 year.

Principles identified in the American Academy of Pediatrics (AAP) guidelines for the judicious use of antimicrobial agents in pediatric patients with common respiratory illnesses such as otitis media, pharyngitis, sinusitis, and cough/bronchitis are discussed in Chapter 24. The NP should be familiar with the recommendations listed in this chapter. All health care providers must be cognizant of their role in the prevention of superinfections caused by the indiscriminate use of antibiotics.

Patient and Parent Education

Parents should be educated about assessment and management of changes in the child's condition. Include the following:

- Indications for immediate reevaluation of the child
  - Signs and symptoms of respiratory distress
  - Other indicators of worsening of the illness (e.g., toxic appearance, malaise, feeding difficulty)
- Information on when to expect improvement in the child's symptoms and, if symptoms do not improve as expected, what to do next
- Clear instructions about medications— how much to give, when to give, side effects to watch for, how long to give, and the necessity of completing the course of antibiotics
- Infection control information if needed
- Instructions on the next return visit

■■■ INDICATIONS FOR TONSILLECTOMY AND ADENOIDECTOMY

The only two absolute indications for tonsillectomy are suspicion of tumor and severe aerodigestive tract obstruction (Behrman et al., 1996). For any other indication, the risk–benefit ratio of the procedure must be weighed. Significant morbidity and mortality are associated with this procedure. One percent to 5% of tonsillectomies result in postoperative hemorrhage. One in 1500 tonsillectomies ends in significant nasopharyngeal stenosis (Wilner, 1998). Quite a few indications for adenoidectomy exist and include the following: chronic persistent upper airway

problems manifested by obstructive sleep apnea, chronic persistent otitis media (especially if accompanied by conductive hearing loss), persistent mouth breathing, nasal speech, adenoid facies (narrow high arched palate and elongated mandible), and persistent or chronic nasopharyngitis (if related to chronic hypertrophied infected adenoid tissue). The morbidity and mortality connected with this procedure are not as high as with tonsillectomy. This procedure may often be accompanied by tonsillectomy.

■■■ UPPER RESPIRATORY TRACT DISORDERS

Nasopharyngitis (The Common Cold or Upper Respiratory Tract Infection) and Tonsillopharyngitis

Description

Nasopharyngitis and tonsillopharyngitis are frequent problems seen in pediatric practice. Young children have, on average, six to eight URIs, or colds, per year. (See Table 32-3 for a differential diagnosis of URI from sinusitis and purulent rhinitis.) When tonsillar involvement is significant, the term *tonsillopharyngitis* or *tonsillitis* is used; when tonsillar involvement is minor, the term *nasopharyngitis* is used. Nasopharyngitis is most often caused by a viral agent.

Management

Only supportive care is needed for a URI as addressed in the sections entitled General Measures and Patient Education under Basic Respiratory Management Strategies. Antibiotics are not appropriate treatment. The use of antipyretics, analgesics, decongestants, antihistamines, and cough medication is controversial but can help alleviate the distress caused by URI symptoms if used cautiously.

ACUTE VIRAL PHARYNGITIS AND TONSILLITIS

Etiology

Viral infection is the leading cause of nasopharyngitis and tonsillopharyngitis. Adenovirus

Differentiation of Common Upper Respiratory Infections in Children

SITE OF INFECTION	SYMPTOMS	DURATION OF SYMPTOMS (d)	ETIOLOGICAL AGENT	MANAGEMENT	DURATION OF TREATMENT	COMMENTS
The common cold (viral URI)	Malaise, sneezing, watery nasal discharge, mild sore throat, may have a fever, not ill appearing	0–10	Rhinoviruses (cause 40% of URIs), RSV, parainfluenza, enteroviruses, adenoviruses	No antibiotics; symptomatic Rx, e.g., saline nose drops, increased fluids; for infants, bulb-syringe the nose before meals and bedtime; for older children, cough suppression at night if unable to sleep; humidifier		If lasts longer than 10–14 d, consider other diagnosis (e.g., sinusitis)
Acute purulent rhinorrhea	Thick, yellow nasal discharge (often associated with URI)	>3	Part of the natural history of URI; superinfection by *Streptococcus pneumoniae*, *Haemophilus influenzae*, β-hemolytic streptococci	Symptomatic care; a wait-and-see approach for antibiotics; if >10- to 14-d duration, treat with amoxicillin or dicloxacillin if staphylococci suspected	Best approach, *wait and see*; if a persistent cycle of symptoms is seen in an occasional child, consider a 3-d course of amoxicillin (Abbasi & Cunningham, 1996)	Avoid indiscriminate and frequent use of antibiotics (development of antibiotic resistance)
Acute purulent sinusitis	Persistent nasal symptoms for more than 10 d with URI, nasal drainage, cough, recalcitrant asthma	10–30	*S. pneumoniae*, *Moraxella catarrhalis*, nontypable *H. influenzae*	Amoxicillin, trimethoprim-sulfamethoxazole, or amoxicillin-clavulanate	10–14 d	By 7 d should be asymptomatic; change antibiotics 48–72 hr after start of treatment if no response
Subacute sinusitis	Same as above but persistent for at least 30 d	30–120	Same as above; may be β-lactamase producing	Amoxicillin-clavulanate		Initial acute infection did not clear; need to switch antibiotics
Chronic/recurrent sinusitis	Malaise, easy fatigability, unilateral or bilateral nasal discharge, postnasal discharge, nasal obstruction if middle turbinate significantly obstructed	>120	Same as above plus α-hemolytic streptococci and *Staphylococcus aureus*	Amoxicillin-clavulanate, azithromycin, cefixime, clindamycin	3–6 wk	May need endoscopic sinus surgery if chronic sinusitis does not respond to prolonged medical management, including antibiotic prophylaxis; investigate differential diagnoses

RSV = respiratory syncytial virus; Rx = medication; URI = upper respiratory infection.

is the most common cause of viral pharyngitis and tonsillitis. The enteroviruses (coxsackievirus, echovirus), herpesvirus, and Epstein-Barr virus are also common. Although not a virus, *Mycoplasma pneumoniae* is a frequent cause of pharyngitis and tonsillitis in school-age children. Viral infections occur year-round, and it is helpful to know what agents are currently infecting children in the community. It can be difficult to differentiate viral from bacterial infections because of overlapping symptoms. However, hoarseness, cough, coryza, and conjunctivitis are classic features of a viral infection (Pitetti & Wald, 1998).

Clinical Findings

HISTORY. The following may be reported:

- Gradual onset
- Prominent nasal symptoms of rhinorrhea (key finding)
- Sore throat and dysphagia
- Mild cough
- Low-grade fever

PHYSICAL EXAMINATION. Virus-specific findings include the following:

- Epstein-Barr virus can produce exudate on the tonsils, soft palate petechiae, and diffuse adenopathy.
- Adenovirus can produce exudate on the tonsils and cervical adenopathy.
- Enteroviruses can produce vesicles or ulcers on the tonsillar pillars and posterior fauces; coryza, vomiting, and/or diarrhea may be present.
- Herpesvirus produces ulcers anteriorly and marked adenopathy.

DIAGNOSTIC TESTS. If a diagnosis of viral infection is in doubt, a culture should be done. Cultures are useful in differentiating viral from group A β-hemolytic streptococci (GABHS). If infectious mononucleosis is suspected, a heterophil antibody test and complete blood count (CBC) can be helpful in confirming the diagnosis.

Management

For viral infection, only supportive care is needed, including fever and sore throat pain relief with acetaminophen or ibuprofen. Fluid intake should be encouraged (Gaebler, 1998).

ACUTE BACTERIAL PHARYNGITIS AND TONSILLITIS

Etiology

The three most common bacterial causes of pharyngitis and tonsillitis in children and adolescents are GABHS, *Neisseria gonorrhoeae*, and *Corynebacterium diphtheriae*. GABHS accounts for less than 10% of infections in children with sore throat and fever. *N. gonorrhoeae* pharyngitis is a sexually transmitted disease that can mimic GABHS pharyngitis or can run a subclinical course. *C. diphtheriae* causes diphtheria and is discussed later in this chapter. The latter two organisms are rare causes of tonsillopharyngitis.

Clinical Findings

HISTORY. The following characterize GABHS infection:

- Less commonly seen in children younger than 2 years; most commonly found in 5- to 11-year-old children
- Abrupt onset without nasal symptoms
- Fever, malaise, sore throat, dysphagia
- Nausea, abdominal discomfort, vomiting, headache

PHYSICAL EXAMINATION. The following may be seen:

- Petechiae, beefy-red uvula, red tonsillopharyngeal tissue
- Tonsillopharyngeal exudate (frequently)
- Tender anterior cervical lymph nodes
- Scarlatiniform rash

DIAGNOSTIC TESTS. A positive throat culture confirms the diagnosis and is still the test of choice; however, a positive culture can also identify a carrier state. Some rapid streptococcal identification tests are not as sensitive as culture in picking up GABHS; therefore, a negative rapid test must be followed by culture. The specificity of the rapid streptococcal test is very good (95%); therefore, if the rapid test is positive, the diagnosis of GABHS is confirmed. The

Strep A Optical Immuno Assay (rapid streptococcal test) reportedly has a sensitivity better than routine throat culture does. Documentation of past GABHS infection is obtained by antibody titer to various streptococcal enzymes such as antistreptolysin O.

Management

The goal of antibiotic therapy is to prevent the development of rheumatic fever, the spread of illness to others, and the development of suppurative complications. Antibiotics also shorten the course of the illness and the severity of symptoms. The management plan includes:

- Antimicrobial therapy (based on clinical need)—one of the following (AAP, 1997):
  - Benzathine penicillin G intramuscularly (600,000 U if <60 lb; 1.2 million U for larger children and adults).
  - Potassium penicillin V orally (250 mg two to three times a day for 10 days in children; 500 mg two to three times a day for 10 days in adolescents).
  - Erythromycin estolate (20 to 40 mg/kg per day in two to four divided doses for 10 days) or erythromycin ethyl succinate (40 mg/kg per day in two to four divided doses) if allergic to penicillin. Resistance to erythromycin is being reported in Finland but is not yet a significant problem in the United States.
  - A 10-day course of a narrow-spectrum (first generation), orally administered cephalosporin is now acceptable, particularly if the child is allergic to penicillin. However, about 15% of patients allergic to penicillin also are allergic to the cephalosporins (AAP, 1997).
  - If evidence of penicillin resistance is present, a β-lactamase–resistant antibiotic can be used such as amoxicillin-clavulanate or dicloxacillin.
- Supportive care—antipyretics, fluids, rest.
- Reculture is not generally needed except in situations in which it is necessary to ensure eradication of the organism.
- If the child *continues to have symptoms* of streptococcal pharyngitis and a positive

culture for streptococcus, this child may represent an actual treatment failure or have a new infection with a different serological type of streptococcus.
- Noncompliance with pharmacological therapy can explain treatment failure, and in these instances an injection of benzathine penicillin is recommended.
- For a compliant patient with treatment failure, treat with any of the following drugs: erythromycin, a penicillinase-resistant penicillin, amoxicillin-clavulanate, a cephalosporin, dicloxacillin, or other macrolides (AAP, 1997).
- If clinical relapse occurs, a second course of antibiotic is indicated, as discussed earlier. If recurrent infection is a problem, culturing of the family for the chronic carrier state is advised. Toothbrushes or orthodontic devices may harbor GABHS.
- Children can return to school when they are afebrile and have been taking antibiotics for at least 24 hours.

Complications

Major late complications caused by GABHS are rheumatic fever and acute glomerulonephritis. Suppurative complications include cervical adenitis, sinusitis, otitis media, pneumonia, and retropharyngeal or peritonsillar abscess. Recurrent GABHS tonsillopharyngitis can also be a problem.

Acute Purulent Rhinitis

Description

Acute purulent rhinitis often represents a superinfection of a common cold or purulent sinusitis. Remember that thick, yellow discharge is a common sequela of an uncomplicated URI.

Etiology

Likely organisms involved in the superinfection are pneumococci, *Haemophilus influenzae*, β-hemolytic streptococci, and *Staphylococcus aureus*.

Clinical Findings

HISTORY. Complaints of URI with characteristic symptoms and a profuse and continuous, purulent, yellow to green nasal discharge for more than 3 days are reported.

PHYSICAL EXAMINATION. A yellow to green nasal discharge is seen.

Differential Diagnosis

A nasal foreign body and sinusitis are the differential diagnoses. The mucopurulent discharge associated with the common cold (acute viral rhinitis) is intermittent and worse in the early morning on awakening. Allergic rhinitis is discussed in Chapter 25.

Management

Controversy surrounds the appropriateness of early intervention with antibiotic therapy (antibiotics were prescribed for a minimum of 10 days) if the only major symptom is a purulent nasal discharge. The following approaches may be considered:

- Take a wait-and-see plan.
- Advise symptomatic treatment because the discharge may be only a symptom of an uncomplicated URI.
- Prescribe a short course of antibiotics (10 days) if a child has a history of persistent cycles of symptoms (Abbasi & Cunningham, 1996). The following antibiotics may be considered.
  - Oral amoxicillin (40 mg/kg per day in two or three divided doses) or trimethoprim-sulfamethoxazole (6 to 10 mg/kg per day in two divided doses) for 10 days.
  - Dicloxacillin if staphylococcus is suspected.
- Removal of purulent material—may need to instill saline into the nares and use a bulb syringe or do saline washes.

Sinusitis

Description

Inflammation and secondary infection of the paranasal sinuses can be either an acute or a chronic problem. Sinusitis is a complication of approximately 5 to 10% of URIs in children. Persistence of URI symptoms for longer than 10 days without improvement separates a simple URI from sinusitis. The maxillary and ethmoid sinuses are most frequently involved. Inflammation and edema of the mucous membranes lining the sinuses cause obstruction and set up an ideal situation for bacteria to invade the sinus cavities. Certain conditions predispose children to chronic sinus infections, including allergies, nasal deformities, CF, nasal polyps, and human immunodeficiency virus (HIV) infection.

Differentiation of acute from chronic sinusitis is based on the duration of respiratory symptoms. In acute sinusitis, respiratory symptoms last more than 10 days but less than 30 days (Wald, 1994). When respiratory symptoms persist more than 30 days and do not improve, a diagnosis of subacute sinusitis is made. If symptoms last more than 120 days, a diagnosis of chronic sinusitis is appropriate. Remember that sinus inflammation is part of the natural history of a cold or allergic rhinitis. Thick, yellow discharge is a common and normal finding with a URI. Therefore, the NP must be cautious to not overdiagnose sinusitis and subsequently indiscriminately use antibiotics (Abbasi & Cunningham, 1996).

Etiology

The common bacterial organisms responsible for superinfections are *Streptococcus pneumoniae, H. influenzae, Moraxella catarrhalis*, and GABHS. The role of viruses in sinusitis is not clear. Anaerobic and staphylococcal agents are implicated in chronic sinusitis. The various sinuses develop, aerate, and become clinically important at different times during childhood. Ethmoiditis can occur after 6 months of age, in contrast to frontal sinusitis, which is first seen around 10 years of age. Cases of recurrent and chronic sinusitis are often caused by recurrent viral URI associated with day care attendance, smoking in the home, older siblings at home who reinfect the child, or certain predisposing conditions such as allergies, immunodeficiency disorders, or CF.

Clinical Findings in Acute Sinusitis

HISTORY. The following may be reported:

- URI more severe or prolonged than usual
- Coughing during the day, often worse at night, and rhinorrhea lasting more than 10 days
- Fever—low grade or temperature higher than 39°C
- Clear or mucopurulent rhinorrhea or post-nasal drip
- Facial pain
- Sore throat, bad breath, headache (Finberg & Bergelson, 1998)

PHYSICAL EXAMINATION. The nasal mucosa is often reddened or swollen, and sometimes peri-orbital edema is apparent.

Clinical Findings in Chronic Sinusitis

HISTORY. The following may be reported:

- Protracted respiratory symptoms (>30 days)
- Nasal congestion and discharge
- Cough (day and night)
- Malaise, fatigue, anorexia
- Fever (rare but can be low grade)
- Sore throat (frequent complaint)

PHYSICAL EXAMINATION. The following are frequently seen:

- Nasal discharge, either unilateral or bilateral, that varies from day to day
- Postnasal discharge
- Swelling of the middle turbinates, which can result in nasal obstruction
- Allergic rhinitis manifestations (Behrman et al., 1996)

DIAGNOSTIC TESTS. If the clinical findings suggest sinusitis, radiographs are not needed. Facial swelling, acute sinusitis unresponsive to 48 hours of antibiotics and a child with a toxic appearance, chronic or recurrent sinusitis, and chronic asthma are indications for imaging studies, including either sinus radiographs, ultra-sonograms, or CT scanning. A Waters view is usually sufficient to demonstrate sinusitis on a radiograph. Nasal cultures are not useful.

Differential Diagnosis

Viral upper respiratory tract illness, allergic rhinitis, and other causes of headache are the differential diagnoses.

Management

Antimicrobial therapy should be prescribed for a course of 10 days in acute sinusitis or, if responding slowly but not symptom free, an additional 7 days of medication. Most children show dramatic improvement in 3 to 4 days (Wald, 1994; Berman & Chan, 1999). The course of therapy may be up to 21 days in acute sinusitis and up to 6 weeks in chronic sinusitis.

In uncomplicated sinusitis in children:

- Amoxicillin (40 mg/kg per day in three divided doses) is the desirable therapy (Finberg & Bergelson, 1998). Other sources treat with amoxicillin at 60–80 mg/kg per day divided into three doses. If the child is allergic to penicillin:
  - Trimethoprim-sulfamethoxazole (0.5 ml/kg twice daily or 6 to 10 mg trimethoprim per kilogram per day in divided doses every 12 hours).
  - Erythromycin-sulfamethoxazole (based on erythromycin, 10 mg/kg per dose three to four times a day).

If a β-lactamase–positive organism is suspected (e.g., failure to improve with treatment or residence in a geographical area that has a high prevalence of β-lactamase–producing *H. influenzae*) or for chronic sinusitis:

- Amoxicillin-clavulanate—for children less than 40 kg: 20 to 40 mg (amoxicillin component) per kilogram per day divided every 8 hours or 25 to 40 mg (amoxicillin component) per kilogram per day divided every 12 hours.
- Trimethoprim-sulfamethoxazole, a third-generation cephalosporin, a newer macrolide, or erythromycin plus sulfamethoxazole.

Failure to improve in 48 hours suggests a resistant organism or complications. If improvement is seen but the child is still symptomatic, antibiotic therapy should be continued for an additional week.

Additional management considerations include the following:

- The use of decongestants, antihistamines, or both in the treatment of acute sinusitis is controversial and has not proved effective (Finberg & Bergelson, 1998). They can be useful in recurrent or chronic sinusitis, especially if allergic manifestations are present (see the management section for allergic rhinitis). See Chapter 25 for information on the use of decongestants and antihistamines.
- Children with complications or signs of invasive infection should be referred to the appropriate medical specialist. Surgical drainage by an otolaryngologist, treatment of allergies and control of allergic rhinitis by an allergist, or both may be necessary.
- Comfort measures include the use of acetaminophen, ibuprofen, or codeine for severe pain. A humidifier helps relieve the drying of mucous membranes associated with mouth breathing. Increase oral fluid intake; saline irrigation of the nostrils is recommended by some allergists.
- Diving is contraindicated with sinusitis.

Complications

Chronic or recurrent sinusitis can become a problem often needing referral to an otolaryngologist or allergist. Orbital cellulitis secondary to ethmoiditis, manifested by swelling and erythema of the eyelids, proptosis, decreased extraocular movements, and altered vision, is a serious, life-threatening complication that is a medical emergency. Intracranial complications such as cavernous sinus thrombosis, subdural empyema, and brain abscess can also occur. Chronic sinusitis is also associated with intractable wheezing in children with asthma (Behrman et al., 1996; Wald, 1994).

Diphtheria

Description

Diphtheria occurs as an acute infection of the upper respiratory tract, the trachea, or both. Diphtheria can cause membranous obstruction of the upper airway. It also produces a neurotoxin. Although only about five cases of diphtheria are reported annually in the United States, it remains an important and dangerous disease.

Etiology

C. diphtheriae is a gram-positive rod with three strains that can be either toxigenic or nontoxigenic. Transmission results from intimate contact with an infected person or carrier. Discharge from the nose, throat, eye, and skin lesions can produce infection. Although rare, fomites can act as a vehicle of transmission, and foodborne outbreaks have been reported. The incubation period averages from 2 to 5 days; communicability lasts for 2 weeks or less in untreated cases. Chronic carriage can occur even with antimicrobial therapy.

Clinical Findings

Characteristic signs and symptoms follow.

PRIMARY INFECTION

- Low-grade fever
- Grayish, adherent pseudomembrane found in either the nasopharynx, pharynx, or trachea
- Sore throat, serosanguineous nasal discharge, hoarseness

TOXIN PRODUCTION

- The ability of a strain of *C. diphtheriae* to produce toxin or not is unrelated to colony type but rather to bacteriophage infection of the bacterium.
- Toxin production is more lethal than the primary infection and can induce:
  - Myocarditis
  - Motor paralysis
  - Guillain-Barré–type paralysis

DIAGNOSTIC TESTS. A confirmatory diagnosis is based on a positive culture of *C. diphtheriae*. Specimens should be obtained from the nose, throat, any skin lesions, and either beneath the membrane or from a portion of the membrane. A special culture medium is needed, and toxigenicity tests are performed if *C. diphtheriae* is confirmed. Culture results take 8 to 48 hours; treatment begins when diphtheria is suspected.

Do not wait for laboratory confirmation. Results of the CBC may be normal or show a slight leukocytosis and thrombocytopenia.

Differential Diagnosis

Acute streptococcal pharyngitis and infectious mononucleosis are included in the differential diagnosis of pharyngeal diphtheria. A nasal foreign body or purulent sinusitis can resemble nasal diphtheria; epiglottitis and viral croup can also cause obstruction, as does laryngeal diphtheria.

Management

Children with diphtheria require hospitalization. Treatment consists of:

• Antitoxin administration and antimicrobial therapy with erythromycin or penicillin G
• Supportive care for respiratory, cardiac, and neurological complications as appropriate
• Immunization of the child after recovery because disease does not necessarily confer immunity

Prevention

Universal immunization against diphtheria with regular booster injections is the only effective method of control. Infection can occur in immunized or partially immunized children, but the severity of the disease is greatly diminished. Disease generally occurs in nonimmunized children; the frequency of severe life-threatening complications in this group is high. Care of a child exposed to diphtheria is individualized and based on immunization status, likelihood of follow-up, and compliance with antimicrobial therapy. The AAP Committee on Infectious Diseases (1997) lists specific guidelines that should be followed for the care of exposed children.

Pertussis

Description

Pertussis is commonly known as whooping cough because of the high-pitched inspiratory whoop that is characteristic of this illness in young children. It is an acute, highly communicable infection that produces a toxin responsible for the severe symptoms associated with pertussis. If this disease occurs in unvaccinated infants younger than 1 year, it is often associated with pneumonia, seizures, and encephalopathy. Pertussis in older children and vaccinated children produces a milder respiratory illness (Behrman et al., 1996).

Etiology

Pertussis is caused by *Bordetella pertussis*, *Bordetella parapertussis*, and *Bordetella bronchiseptica*. Transmission of these gram-negative pleomorphic bacilli is via aerosol droplets from close contact with infected individuals, who generally have mild or atypical illness that is not recognized as pertussis. The incubation period is between 6 and 20 days; the period of communicability is greatest during the catarrhal stage until before or during the early paroxysmal stage of coughing. Cases of pertussis occur in adults, who constitute a reservoir for the disease.

Clinical Findings

Manifestations of this disease vary by age group, stage of disease, and whether the child has received any immunization against pertussis.

Characteristics of the disease in infants and young children include the following:

• Catarrhal stage—1 to 3 weeks
  ○ Mild cough, coryza, sneezing, and fever to 101°F
• Paroxysmal stage—2 to 4 weeks
  ○ Persistent staccato, paroxysmal cough ending with an inspiratory whoop
  ○ Vomiting at the end of paroxysmal coughing and whoop
  ○ Cyanosis, sweating, prostration, and exhaustion after coughing
• Convalescent stage—2 to 3 weeks
  ○ Waning of paroxysmal coughing episodes

Specific findings in *infants younger than 6 months* are

• Apnea (common)
• No inspiratory whoop

Findings in *older children* include:

- Persistent irritating cough but no inspiratory whoop
- Low-grade fever
- Highest incidence of mortality (1.3%) (AAP, 1997)

DIAGNOSTIC TESTS. Culturing for *B. pertussis* requires special media and takes 7 days for incubation. The organism is found most frequently during the catarrhal or early paroxysmal stage. A positive culture from the nasopharynx is diagnostic; however, false-negative results do occur. Leukocytosis (20,000 to 30,000/ml) with 70 to 80% lymphocytes is a common finding in young children and appears around the end of the catarrhal stage.

Management

The following steps are involved:

- Young infants and children with severe respiratory symptoms require hospitalization.
- Erythromycin (40 to 50 mg/kg per day [maximum, 2 g/d] in four divided doses for 14 days) can improve symptoms if given in the catarrhal stage. However, in 1995, reports of erythromycin-resistant pertussis were documented (Centers for Disease Control and Prevention, 1994).
- Antimicrobial therapy given in the paroxysmal stage does not alter the course of pertussis per se, but administration of erythromycin limits spreading of the organism.
- Corticosteroids and albuterol are currently under investigation regarding their usefulness in relieving paroxysmal coughing (Behrman et al., 1996).

CARE OF EXPOSED CHILDREN. The AAP Redbook (1997) lists specific guidelines for the care of exposed children and adults, including:

- Immunization coverage with diphtheria-tetanus-pertussis (DTP) or diphtheria-tetanus-acellular pertussis (DTaP), depending on the child's prior history of immunization
- Chemoprophylaxis with erythromycin (40 to 50 mg/kg per day [maximum, 2 g/d] orally in four divided doses for 14 days) for all household and close contacts, including children in day care, irrespective of their immunization status
- Close monitoring of respiratory symptoms for 14 days after last contact with an infected individual

Complications

Secondary bacterial pneumonia, seizures, epistaxis, subconjunctival hemorrhage, encephalopathy, and death can occur. Activation of tuberculosis is associated with pertussis infection.

Prevention

Active immunity follows natural pertussis; reinfections are mild and may not be noticed. Young infants are at greatest risk for pertussis. The recommended guidelines for giving the initial series of DTP vaccines and booster doses should be followed. Remember that just one DTP or DTaP immunization can reduce the severity of symptoms in an infant infected with pertussis. Universal immunization of children younger than 7 years is crucial to control of this disease.

Only children with valid contraindications to receiving pertussis vaccine, as identified in Chapter 24, should be excluded from receiving the vaccine. Immunity from pertussis immunization wanes over time, and the vaccine does not confer active immunity. Pertussis in older children, adolescents, and adults is a mild, often unrecognized disease that, if transmitted to an unimmunized infant, can result in life-threatening illness.

Recurrent Epistaxis

Etiology and Incidence

Recurrent epistaxis is commonly seen in children living in dry climates or during the winter months when artificial heating is used. The cause is often benign and due to mechanical trauma to the area (e.g., nose picking). Other factors that can also cause mucosal irritation that results in bleeding include allergies, neoplasms (e.g., polyps, hemangiomas), chronic rhinitis, chronic use of nasal sprays or drying agents such as decongestants, and viral or bacterial infections of nasal tissue. In adolescents, the use of recreational drugs such as cocaine and cannabis also causes local mucosal irritation. The anterior portion of the nasal septum, Kiesselbach area, is the usual site of involvement (Edelstein, 1997; Inkelis, 1996).

Clinical Findings

HISTORY. The following may be reported:

- Tarry stools
- Frequent nose bleeds
- Recent URI
- Allergic rhinitis

PHYSICAL EXAMINATION. Bleeding from the nares can often be seen, and the anterior aspect of the nares is red and raw with or without fresh clots or old crusts. The nasal mucosa may be dry or cracked.

DIAGNOSTIC TESTS. A baseline hematocrit may be indicated in severe or chronic epistaxis. It can reveal iron deficiency anemia secondary to the bleeding.

Differential Diagnosis

A bleeding disorder or nasal tumor is characterized by epistaxis that is severe, prolonged, and recurrent. Be suspicious of epistaxis in a child younger than 2 years of age, evidence of bleeding at other sites, and bleeding that lasts longer than 20 minutes. If these abnormalities occur and a coagulopathy is suspected, order a CBC, platelet count, prothrombin time (PT), and partial thromboplastin time (PTT).

Management

The following steps are taken:

- Have the child sit upright and lean forward to avoid swallowing the blood.
- Apply pressure to the nose (pinch the nares at the bony structure) for 10 minutes.
- Packing and topical vasoconstrictor drugs are occasionally needed.
- Use a bedside humidifier to moisten the air in dry climates or in winter with forced air heating.

Prevention

Use of a vaporizer and normal saline nose drops and application of petroleum jelly (Vaseline), a topical antibiotic (Neosporin), or hydrocortisone cream to the inside of the nares are preventive measures.

Nasal Foreign Body

Description

It is not uncommon for young children to insert all types of foreign bodies into any body orifice. Nasal foreign bodies can be noted immediately by the parent or lie undetected until symptoms appear.

Clinical Findings

HISTORY. A persistent or recurrent *unilateral* purulent nasal discharge is reported.

PHYSICAL EXAMINATION. A foreign body may be seen with a purulent, foul-smelling nasal discharge.

Differential Diagnosis

Nasal polyps, purulent rhinitis, adenoiditis, sinusitis, and nasal tumors are conditions that are also associated with either bilateral or unilateral discharge.

Management

Management involves the following:

- Detection of a foreign body in the nasal cavity, which secures the diagnosis.
- Removal of the nasal foreign body, depending on its location, composition, and the skill of the practitioner.
- Use of alligator forceps, suction with narrow tips, cotton-tipped applicators with collodion, and topical vasoconstrictor drugs if needed to remove the object, depending on its size and consistency. Good lighting is essential.
- Referral to an otolaryngologist for young children who cannot cooperate or when the foreign body is extremely difficult or dangerous to remove, such as paper clips

or staples (Dolitsky & Ward, 1997; Kelley, 1999).

![icon] EXTRATHORACIC AIRWAY DISORDERS

Laryngotracheobronchitis—Infectious Croup

Description

LTB is a rapid, acute, upper airway obstruction at the larynx characterized by a harsh, barking cough and inspiratory stridor.

Etiology

Viral agents are responsible for most cases of croup, with the parainfluenza viruses being the leading viral organisms, followed by the adenoviruses, respiratory syncytial virus (RSV), and rubeola. *M. pneumoniae* has been implicated in a small percentage of croup illnesses (Larsen et al., 1999). Other bacterial agents include *H. influenzae* type b, GABHS, pneumococcus, and staphylococcus. These organisms are infrequent causes of croup but cause very serious illness. Viral croup is common in children between 3 months and 5 years of age and occurs most often in the cold season of the year. Males are affected more often than females. Recurrent croup and recurrent laryngitis can develop in children until 6 years of age. A positive family history has been noted in 15% of children in whom croup develops.

Clinical Findings

Clinical manifestations depend on the type of infectious agent responsible for the croup and the area of the upper airway affected.

HISTORY. The history includes the following:

- URI symptoms of rhinitis, conjunctivitis, or both are sometimes present before stridor.
- Intermittent stridor—mild to moderate.
- Gradual onset of symptoms (1 to 2 days).
- Symptoms worse at night.
- Most children with viral croup improve within a few hours.

PHYSICAL EXAMINATION. The following can be seen:

- Slight dyspnea, retractions.
- Mild, brassy, or barking cough.
- Temperature elevated to 104°F.
- Decreased breath sounds bilaterally with rhonchi and crackles.

DIAGNOSTIC TESTS. Usually the diagnosis is evident clinically. Radiography of the soft tissues of the neck and chest displays a classic pattern of subglottic narrowing. Microbiology studies can be helpful in selected cases.

Differential Diagnosis

The differential diagnoses include acute epiglottitis; acute spasmodic croup (no signs of infection); aspiration of a foreign body; retropharyngeal abscess; extrinsic compression from tumors, trauma, or congenital malformations; angioedema (anaphylaxis) or early asthmatic attack; infectious mononucleosis; and psychogenic stridor.

Table 32-4 differentiates acute infectious LTB from other common causes of stridor.

Management

Therapy depends on the cause, severity, and location of the disease. The aim of therapy is to provide adequate respiratory exchange.

- If bacterial infection is present, treat with an antibiotic that is likely to eradicate the suspected organisms, which are *S. aureus* and *H. influenzae*.
- Symptomatic relief of mild croup can be provided with the judicious use of steam from a hot shower or bath or "cold" steam from a humidifier. These measures usually terminate the laryngeal spasm. Often a ride in a car at night with the windows down accomplishes the same result. Occasionally, vomiting also relieves the spasm.
- Cough and cold medicines sometimes help, especially if the child has URI symptoms.
- If bronchospasm is also suspected, the use of bronchodilators in the usual doses prescribed for relief of asthma as discussed in Chapter 25 may be advantageous.

T A B L E 32-4

Differentiating Common Respiratory Diseases That Can Cause Stridor or Similar Signs

CHARACTERISTIC	LTB	EPIGLOTTITIS	BACTERIAL TRACHEITIS	DIPHTHERIA	FOREIGN BODY
Peak age Onset	3-60 mo Gradual, acute onset at night	2-7 y Rapid	≤12 y Acute	Any age/unimmunized Gradual onset	Toddlers Acute symptoms or gradual onset
Common findings	URI, seal-bark cough, mild-moderate dyspnea, symptoms worse at night	Sore throat, drooling, aphonia, looks toxic, dysphagia, tripod position	URI, may have cough, looks toxic, purulent sputum	Pharyngeal membrane, sore throat, nasal discharge, hoarseness	Coughing/choking episode, dyspnea, wheezing, cyanosis, signs and symptoms of secondary infection
Respiratory efforts	Rate generally <50	Marked distress	Marked distress	Minor to signs and symptoms of obstruction	Minor to significant distress
Fever CBC	Common—low grade Generally normal	High (39°C) High, left shift	High (>39°C) High, left shift	Low grade Normal to slight leukocytosis, decreased thrombocyte count	Normal to low grade Normal unless secondary infection
Organism(s)	Usually viral: parainfluenza, adenovirus, RSV	Usually *Haemophilus influenzae* type b	Usually *Staphylococcus aureus*	*Corynebacterium diphtheriae*	
Specific laboratory tests	None	None	None	Positive culture	None
Radiographic view/findings	Lateral or AP of neck/subglottic narrowing	Lateral of neck/ thumb sign	Lateral of neck/subglottic narrowing	Signs of obstruction in severe cases	May see localized hyperinflation, mediastinal shift, atelectasis
Treatment	Humidification, corticosteroids in selected cases	Hospitalization, cefuroxime, corticosteroids	Hospitalization, *Staphylococcus* coverage	Hospitalization, erythromycin/penicillin, antitoxin	Removal of foreign body, treatment of secondary infection/bronchospasm
Intubation	Rare	Usually necessary	Frequently necessary	May be necessary	Endoscopy to remove foreign body
Prevention	None	Immunization	None	Immunization	Education on child-proofing home and monitoring child

AP = anteroposterior; CBC = complete blood count; LTB = laryngotracheobronchitis; URI = upper respiratory tract infection.

Corticosteroids as part of outpatient management of LTB are controversial but gaining in use. Corticosteroids reduce inflammatory edema and prevent destruction of ciliated epithelium. No substantial evidence has suggested any adverse effect of corticosteroid treatment (Behrman et al., 1996). Children hospitalized with LTB are those whom primary care practitioners were unable to treat effectively as outpatients. Including corticosteroids in the management of children in whom traditional courses of therapy are ineffective could prevent some of these admissions. A one-time dose of dexamethasone 0.6 mg/kg can be given as part of outpatient management.

INDICATIONS FOR HOSPITALIZATION. Children in distress with respiratory rates in the 70s to 80s should be hospitalized. A child with a temperature higher than 102.2°F should be carefully evaluated; hospitalization may be necessary if other worrisome symptoms are also present. Racemic epinephrine by aerosol (a 2.25% solution diluted 1:8 with water in doses of 2 to 4 ml/15 min) may help. Corticosteroid use is becoming commonplace in hospital settings and widely accepted (Finberg & Bergelson, 1998); a short course of high-dose corticosteroid (one to three doses of dexamethasone, 1 mg/kg every 6 hours) is generally beneficial.

Complications

Increasing obstruction of the airways causes continuous stridor, nasal flaring, and suprasternal, infrasternal, and intercostal retractions. With further obstruction, air hunger and restlessness occur and are quickly followed by hypoxia, weakness, decreased air exchange, decreased stridor, an increased pulse rate, and eventual death from hypoventilation. Anything that taxes the child's respiratory efforts such as crying or feeding causes more respiratory distress. Examination of the nasopharynx with a tongue depressor may result in sudden respiratory compromise. Severely ill children should be evaluated for acute epiglottitis.

Acute Spasmodic Croup

Description

Some children are prone to recurrent episodes of acute LTB. The term *acute spasmodic croup* is used to describe this condition. Recurrent croup may be related to airway hypersensitivity or allergy. The clinical manifestations and treatment plan are the same as indicated for acute LTB. The causes of spasmodic croup cannot be differentiated from the usual causes of croup; most likely a viral agent triggers the airway reaction.

Epiglottitis

Etiology

Epiglottitis occurs in children between 2 and 7 years of age. *H. influenzae* type b is usually the cause of this illness. Use of *H. influenzae* type b vaccine beginning at 2 months of age has resulted in a drastic decline in the number of children with invasive infections caused by this organism. Group A streptococcus is a rare cause of epiglottitis (Finberg & Bergelson, 1998).

Clinical Findings

HISTORY. An affected child has a sudden escalating course of fever, sore throat, and dyspnea and looks sick.

PHYSICAL EXAMINATION. Findings include:

- Inspiratory and sometimes expiratory stridor
- Drooling, aphonia, and high fever
- Rapidly progressive respiratory obstruction and prostration
- Flaring of the alae nasi and retraction of the supraclavicular, intercostal, and subcostal spaces
- Child assuming a position of hyperextension of the neck
- In older children, one may find
  - Complaints of sore throat and dysphagia
  - Stridor, brassy cough, irritability, and restlessness
  - Child assuming a "tripod" position with mouth open and tongue hanging out

A rare, unusual finding is that of just a hoarse cough and a cherry-red epiglottis. No attempt should be made to examine the posterior of the pharynx because stimulation of the area can induce spasm and obstruction of the epiglottis and lead to respiratory arrest.

DIAGNOSTIC TESTS. Blood cultures should be ordered. If the possibility of epiglottitis is thought to be remote in a patient with croup, a lateral neck radiograph may be obtained before the physical examination is undertaken. Absence of the "thumb" sign on the radiograph rules out the condition. A health care professional capable of supporting the airway and skilled in intubation must accompany the child to the radiology department and back.

Management

The time from the onset of symptoms until death may be only a matter of hours. *Acute epiglottitis is a pediatric emergency!* If epiglottitis is suspected, do not examine the throat. The child should *not* be placed in the supine position and should be immediately transported to the hospital. The child should be examined in the operating room by someone who can do an emergency tracheostomy. An airway must be established, either a nasotracheal airway or a tracheostomy. The diagnosis is confirmed in the operating room by depressing the tongue to view the swollen cherry-red epiglottis. Such children have a risk of reflex laryngospasm and acute and complete airway obstruction.

Begin the following treatments:

- Intravenous antibiotics that cover β-lactamase–producing *H. influenzae* in a septic dose schedule. Ceftriaxone sodium, 150 mg/kg per day in two divided doses, or and equivalent cephalosporin is given (Larsen et al., 1999).
- Oxygen.
- Corticosteroids to reduce the swelling.

The acute infection rarely lasts more than 48 to 72 hours. As improvement occurs, the child can be extubated, but antibiotic therapy should be continued for 10 days. Patients heal completely. Untreated or undertreated, patients have a significant mortality rate. Remember that the time from the onset of symptoms to death can be a matter of hours. If *H. influenzae* is identified as the causative agent, rifampin prophylaxis (20 mg/kg in a single dose [maximum, 600 mg] for 4 days) should be given to all family contacts with children younger than 4 years and all child contacts younger than 4 years.

Prevention

Routine immunization against *H. influenzae* type b, the leading cause of epiglottitis, is the primary means of prevention.

Bacterial Tracheitis

Etiology

Bacterial tracheitis is an acute, potentially dangerous bacterial infection of the upper airway that does not involve the epiglottis. This condition occurs in younger children, usually younger than 3 years. *S. aureus* is the most common organism cultured. *H. influenzae* and *M. catarrhalis* have also been implicated as causative agents. Bacterial tracheitis usually follows a viral respiratory infection (generally parainfluenza virus type 1). No sexual differentiation has been noted in the incidence or severity of symptoms (Behrman et al., 1996).

Clinical Findings

HISTORY. A brassy cough as part of a "typical viral LTB or URI" and a high fever may be reported.

PHYSICAL EXAMINATION. Copious purulent sputum is seen in older children. Inspiratory stridor develops and the child begins to look "toxic."

DIAGNOSTIC TESTS. The diagnosis is based on confirming a bacterial upper airway infection. The white blood cell count will be elevated. Bacterial tracheitis can be differentiated from epiglottitis by its slower clinical course and a normal-appearing epiglottis on examination. The "classic" features of acute epiglottitis are absent (e.g., no thumb sign on a lateral neck film).

Management

Management issues include the following:

- The usual treatments for croup are ineffective, and hospitalization is necessary.
- Intubation or tracheostomy is usually necessary to bypass the swelling that develops at the level of the cricoid cartilage and to manage the copious purulent secretions.

- Antibiotics that cover staphylococcus are administered.
- Oxygen and airway support are necessary.
- Most patients become afebrile in 48 to 72 hours; the child is weaned from the artificial airway and usually does quite well.

INTRATHORACIC AIRWAY DISORDERS

Foreign Body Aspiration

Description

The symptoms and physical findings associated with aspiration of a foreign body depend on the nature of the material aspirated plus the location and degree of the obstruction. The cough reflex protects the lower airways, and most aspirated material is immediately expelled with coughing. Onset of a sudden episode of coughing without a prodrome or signs of respiratory infection should make the provider suspicious of foreign body aspiration.

Etiology

Objects that are either too large to be eliminated by the mucociliary system or not expelled by coughing eventually lead to some form of respiratory symptomatology. Obviously, a large foreign body occluding the upper airway can cause suffocation. A small object in the lower respiratory tree may not produce symptoms for days to weeks. Obstruction results from either the foreign body itself or edema associated with its presence. Hot dogs are one of the most common causes of fatal aspiration.

LARYNGEAL FOREIGN BODY

Clinical Findings

HISTORY. A rapid onset of hoarseness and the development of a croupy cough with aphonia are reported.

PHYSICAL EXAMINATION. The child can also have hemoptysis, dyspnea, wheezing, and cyanosis.

DIAGNOSTIC TESTS. Because most foreign objects are not radiopaque, radiographs may not be useful in the diagnosis. If the history suggests foreign body aspiration, bronchoscopy must be undertaken. Direct laryngoscopy might reveal the presence of foreign matter.

TRACHEAL FOREIGN BODY

Clinically, the child has a history of cough, hoarseness, dyspnea, and possibly cyanosis. The most characteristic signs of tracheal foreign body aspiration are the asthmatic wheeze and the audible slap and palpable thud sound produced by the momentary expiratory impact of the foreign body at the subglottic level.

BRONCHIAL FOREIGN BODY

The initial clinical findings are similar to those seen in either tracheal or laryngeal foreign body aspiration. Blood-streaked sputum may be expectorated. Children aspirating a metallic object often complain of a "metallic taste" in their mouths. If the object is nonobstructive and nonirritating, few or no initial symptoms may be seen. A small object can act as a bypass valve, and wheezes can be heard; emphysema or atelectasis can develop as the result of a large obstruction caused by a bronchial foreign body. The child may have limited chest expansion, decreased vocal fremitus, atelectasis, or emphysema-like changes with resulting hyporesonant or hyperresonant changes. Diminished breath sounds are often found. Crackles, rhonchi, and wheezes can be present if air movement is adequate. Most objects are aspirated into the right lung. A careful medical history may reveal a forgotten episode of choking.

Clinical Findings

HISTORY. An initial episode of coughing, gagging, and choking is described. Hemoptysis rarely occurs as an early symptom but, on rare occasion, does occur as an initial symptom months or years after the aspiration event took place.

PHYSICAL EXAMINATION. If the acute episode is missed or not appreciated, a latent period of mild "wheezing" or cough may be seen. Lobar pneumonia, intractable wheezing, and status asthmaticus can develop.

DIAGNOSTIC TESTS. Clinical suspicion is the clue to this diagnosis! Inspiratory and forced expiratory chest radiographs or chest fluoroscopy are useful in identifying radiolucent foreign bodies (Fig. 32–1).

Management

If the object is removed via bronchoscopy before permanent damage occurs, recovery is usually complete. Secondary lung infections and bronchospasms should be treated as suggested in the section on management of pneumonia and asthma.

Complications

If the foreign body is vegetable matter, vegetal or arachidic bronchitis can occur. This severe condition can be characterized by sepsis-like fever, dyspnea, and cough. If the material has been there for a long time, suppuration can occur.

Bronchitis

Description

The diagnosis of acute bronchitis is often made by practitioners; however, it probably does not exist as a single pathological entity in children. Rather, inflammation of the main stem bronchus exists in combination with either concurrent upper or lower respiratory tract infections. Bronchitis can be divided into three subgroupings. The first is asthmatic bronchitis, an infection with associated bronchospasm. The second is acute LTB and has already been described. The third is chronic bronchitis, which is characterized by a productive cough lasting for more than 3 months that is usually a symptom of another chronic disorder (e.g., allergies, CF, cigarette smoking).

Etiology

This condition is usually preceded by a viral URI. Although a virus is the most common cause of true bronchitis, weakened tissue can

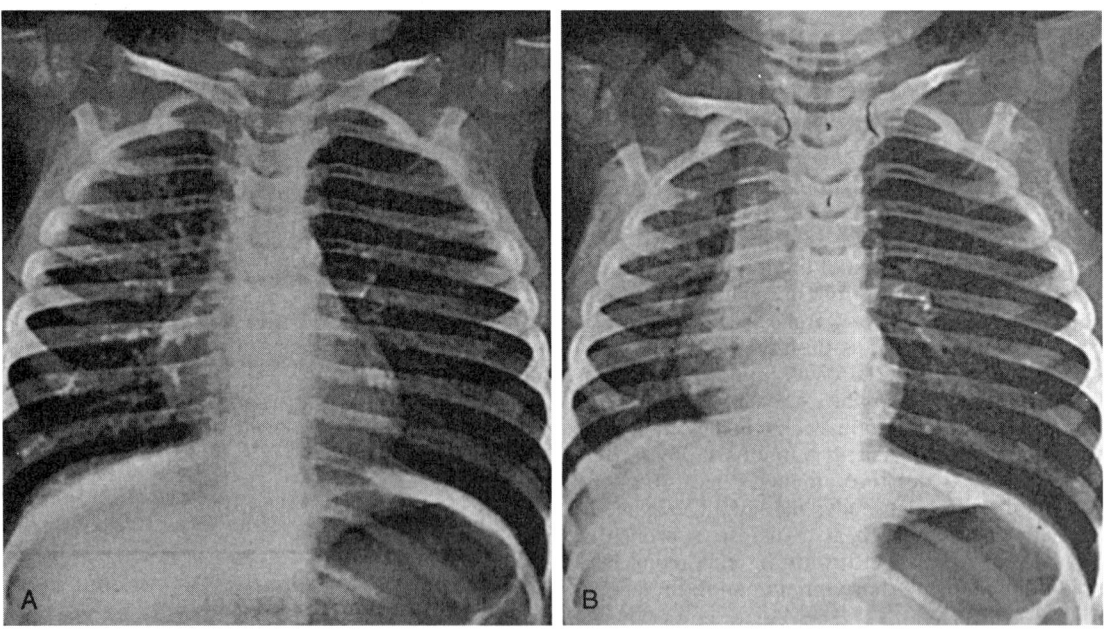

F I G U R E 32-1
Obstructive overinflation due to a peanut fragment in the left mainstem bronchus. *A,* Inspiration. *B,* Expiration. (From Orenstein D: Foreign bodies in the larynx, trachea, and bronchi. *In* Behrman R, Kliegman RM, Arvin AM (eds): Nelson Textbook of Pediatrics, 15th ed. Philadelphia, WB Saunders, 1996, p 1207.)

succumb to a secondary bacterial infection. *S. pneumoniae, M. catarrhalis,* and *H. influenzae* are the most commonly cultured bacterial organisms.

Clinical Findings

HISTORY. The following are reported:

- A dry, hacking, unproductive cough begins a few days after the onset of rhinitis.
- Complaints of low substernal discomfort or burning chest pain aggravated by coughing are made.
- The cough becomes productive after a few days, and shortness of breath can occur.

PHYSICAL EXAMINATION. Findings can vary and include:

- Low-grade or no fever
- Signs of nasopharyngeal infection, conjunctivitis, and rhinitis (common)
- Coarse breath sounds and coarse to fine moist rales
- The presence of rhonchi, which can be high pitched and resemble wheezes (sibilant)

Differential Diagnosis

Children with recurrent acute bronchitis must be evaluated for underlying pathology. Respiratory tract anomalies, foreign body aspiration, bronchiectasis, immunodeficiency, allergy, sinusitis, tonsillitis, exposure to air pollutants, adenoiditis, and CF must be considered in the differential diagnosis. Check for tobacco or marijuana use in teenagers.

Management

No specific therapy is known, and most patients require none. Care is primarily supportive. Postural drainage and the use of a humidifier can be helpful. Cough suppressants should be prescribed judiciously. Antihistamines should not be used because of their excessive drying effect; these drugs tend to only prolong the symptoms. If evidence of a bacterial infection such as high fever and crackles is observed, antibiotics may be considered. Mucus generally thins in 5 to 10 days, and the cough decreases.

Complications

In normal, healthy children, the condition is not serious; however, malaise continues for another week or so after the cough lessens. In undernourished or chronically ill children, otitis, sinusitis, and pneumonia are common.

Bronchiolitis

Description

Bronchiolitis is a common disease of the lower respiratory tract that causes inflammation leading to obstruction of the small respiratory airways. In mild cases, symptoms can last for 1 to 3 days. In severe cases, cyanosis, air hunger, retractions, and nasal flaring with symptoms of severe respiratory distress within a few hours may be seen.

Etiology

Bronchiolitis is a viral illness, with RSV responsible for more than 50% of cases. Parainfluenza virus (type 3), mycoplasma, or adenoviruses generally cause the remainder of cases. Adenovirus and RSV can cause long-term complications. Bronchiolitis commonly occurs in young children from infancy to 2 years of age. The source of infection is an older family member with a "mild" URI. Older children and adults have larger airways and tolerate the swelling associated with this infection better than infants do.

Clinical Findings

HISTORY. The following are reported:

- URI symptoms lasting for several days
- Moderate fever to 102°F
- Decrease in appetite
- Gradual development of respiratory distress

PHYSICAL EXAMINATION. Findings include:
- Paroxysmal wheezing
- Very high respiratory rate ranging around 60 to 80/min
- Varying signs of respiratory distress and pulmonary involvement (e.g., nasal flaring,

retractions, cyanosis, prolonged expiration)
- Palpable liver and spleen because of their being pushed down by hyperinflated lungs

DIAGNOSTIC TESTS. A chest radiograph displays hyperinflation of the lungs and increased anterior–posterior diameter. Some infants may have scattered areas of consolidation caused by atelectasis or inflammation of the alveoli. Early bacterial pneumonia can be difficult to detect and cannot be ruled out by radiographs. Immunofluorescence analysis of nasal washings is needed to detect RSV.

Differential Diagnosis

Making the diagnosis is not usually a problem. In mild afebrile cases, bronchial asthma can be confused with bronchiolitis. A successful challenge with bronchodilators favors the diagnosis of asthma. Less than 5% of cases of recurrent bronchiolitis have a virus as their cause. Other, rarer conditions to be ruled out include congestive heart failure, tracheal foreign body aspiration, organophosphate poisoning, CF, and bronchopneumonia with generalized obstructive emphysema.

Management

Most infants with mild signs of respiratory distress can be treated as outpatients.

- Supportive care consists of adequate hydration and use of antipyretics.
- Careful instructions must be given to parents regarding:
  ○ Management of rhinitis (use of saline drops)
  ○ Signs of increasing respiratory distress or dehydration that call for hospitalization
  ○ Indications for the use of antipyretics
  ○ Guidelines for feeding an infant with signs of mild respiratory distress (amount of fluid needed per 24 hours; smaller, more frequent feedings; monitoring of the respiratory rate; and guarding against vomiting)

Infants younger than 2 months and older infants with signs of severe respiratory distress should be hospitalized. Signs that suggest increasing respiratory distress include:

- Progressive stridor
- Stridor at rest
- Increasing respiratory rate
- Restlessness
- Hypoxia (recorded by either blood gas or pulse oximetry)
- Rising P_{CO_2} (recorded by blood gas)
- Pallor
- Cyanosis
- Depressed sensorium

In-hospital management focuses on supportive care and includes oxygen and elevation of the child to a sitting position at a 30- to 40-degree angle. The infant's neck should be extended to 30 to 40 degrees. Intravenous fluids are frequently needed because respiratory distress interferes with nursing or bottle feeding. Ribavirin (Virazole) can be used in documented RSV infection in young children with underlying diseases such as congenital heart lesions and bronchopulmonary dysplasia, in infants younger than 6 weeks, and in those with severe disease. Ribavirin is expensive and a known teratogen in rats. Bronchodilators can be tried if it is suspected that the child has reactive airway disease rather than bronchiolitis. Epinephrine (Sus-Phrine) may be helpful. The use of corticosteroids and bronchodilators is controversial (Bergelson & Finberg, 1998).

Both LTB and bronchiolitis can cause significant respiratory tract damage. Occasionally, a hospitalized child may not be quickly weaned back to room air. Home management of these patients is very difficult and should be undertaken only by someone with excellent pulmonary skills and consultation with a pediatrician or pediatric pulmonologist. The child should have an O_2 saturation study before discharge to help determine the O_2 requirements at rest, feeding, play, and sleep. A pneumogram to rule out apnea may also be indicated. Strict outpatient follow-up is mandatory for as long as the child is receiving home O_2.

Complications

The first 48 to 72 hours after the onset of cough is the most critical. Apneic spells are common in an infant. The child can be desperately ill but gradually improves. The fatality rate associated with bronchiolitis is less than 1%. Prolonged apnea, uncompensated respiratory acidosis, and profound dehydration secondary to loss of water from tachypnea and an inability to drink are the factors leading to death in young infants with bronchiolitis. A significant number of children in whom bronchiolitis developed during infancy suffer from reactive airway disease later in life.

Prevention

RSV immune globulin is used to protect high-risk infants from RSV. Vaccine research and development are in progress to prevent this disease (Bergelson & Finberg, 1998). Palwizumab (Synagis) is an RSV-specific monoclonal antibody used for high-risk infants (see Chapter 25).

Pneumonia

Description

Pneumonia is a disease marked by inflammation of the parenchyma of the lung. Several subclassifications of pneumonia are recognized: bacterial, viral, other infectious agents, mycotic, aspiration, and a few other rare syndromes. Table 32–5 differentiates the various forms of pneumonia commonly found in infants, children, and adolescents.

BACTERIAL PNEUMONIA

Description

Primary bacterial infection is less common in childhood than secondary bacterial infection after a viral infection. Viral infection affects the lung defenses by altering normal secretions, inhibiting phagocytosis, modifying the normal bacterial flora, and disrupting the epithelial layer. Thus the many childhood viruses set the stage for secondary bacterial infection. Children with immunological problems or chronic illnesses are prone to primary bacterial pneumonia and experience recurrent pneumonias or fail to clear the initial infection completely.

Etiology

The usual cause of bacterial pneumonia is *S. pneumoniae*. It causes more than 90% of cases of childhood bacterial pneumonia. Pneumococcal pneumonia occurs most commonly in the late winter and early spring, after the cycle of viral URIs. Asymptomatic carriers play a more important role in dissemination of disease than do sick contacts. Children younger than 4 years suffer the highest attack rate. Other, less common organisms are:

- GABHS, seen most frequently in children 3 to 5 years old.
- Group B β-hemolytic streptococcus, a cause of pneumonia in neonates and infants.
- *S. aureus*, a very serious infection more common in infants than in older children.
- Gram-negative organisms, which cause a very small percentage of childhood pneumonias. These bacteria include *H. influenzae* (type b), *Klebsiella pneumoniae*, and *Pseudomonas aeruginosa*. They usually have significant morbidity and mortality rates. Altered host resistance is often associated with some of these infections.

Clinical Findings in Infants and Young Children

HISTORY. The following may be reported:

- History of a mild URI for a few days and then an abrupt high fever to temperatures of 104°F and above
- Cough, usually not severe
- Restlessness, shaking chills, apprehension

PHYSICAL EXAMINATION. Findings include:

- Nasal flaring, grunting, retractions
- Tachypnea (may be the only clue), tachycardia, air hunger, cyanosis
- Fine crackles, dullness, diminished breath sounds
- Presence of a pleural effusion and signs of congestive heart failure
- Abdominal distention, downward displacement of the liver or spleen
- Nuchal rigidity without meningeal infec-

T A B L E 32-5

Differentiating Various Forms of Pneumonia in Infants, Young Children, and Adolescents

CHARACTERISTIC	BACTERIAL	VIRAL	MYCOPLASMAL	CHLAMYDIAL
Common age	All ages	All ages	>5 y	3–19 wk
Onset	Acute; gradual	Acute; gradual	Slow	Gradual
Clinical findings	Depend on age; starts with URI, cough, dyspnea, tachypnea, rales, decreased breath sounds, grunting, retractions, toxic look	Depend on age; cough, coryza, hoarseness, crackles, wheezing	Persistent cough, malaise, headache	Tachypnea, staccato cough, crackles, wheezing rare, 50% have signs or history of conjunctivitis
Fever	Acute onset of fever (≥39°C)	Present	>39°C	Afebrile
CBC	WBCs often elevated >15,000/µl	Normal/slight elevation	Normal	Eosinophilia in 75% of cases
Organism(s)	90% caused by *Streptococcus pneumoniae*	RSV, parainfluenza, influenza (types A and B)	*Mycoplasma pneumoniae*	*Chlamydia trachomatis*
Radiographic findings	Lobar consolidation	Transient lobar infiltrates	Varies, interstitial infiltrates	Hyperinflation, infiltrates
Treatment	Depends on bacteria; penicillin, methicillin, cefuroxime, gentamicin, vancomycin	Supportive care	Erythromycin/clarithromycin	Erythromycin

CBC = complete blood count; RSV = respiratory syncytial virus; URI = upper respiratory infection; WBCs = white blood cells.

tion resulting from involvement of the right upper lobe

Clinical Findings in Children and Adolescents

HISTORY. The patient can have:

- Sudden onset of shaking chills, followed by a high fever, cough, chest pain
- Intermittent periods of drowsiness, restlessness, rapid respiration
- Dry, hacking, unproductive cough

PHYSICAL EXAMINATION. The following may be seen:

- Retractions, decreased tactile and vocal fremitus, and diminished breath sounds
- Dullness plus fine and crackling rales on the affected side
- Splinting of the affected side to minimize pleuritic pain or lying on the side in a fetal position—helps compensate for decreased air exchange and improves ventilation
- Progression to delirium, circumoral cyanosis, and posturing

DIAGNOSTIC TESTS. Usual findings in a bacterial infection include the following:

- The white blood cell count is elevated with a left shift, and arterial blood gases are consistent with hypoxia.
- The organism may be found by culture of nasopharyngeal scrapings, tracheal aspirates, blood (only 30% of cases are positive), lung tap fluid.
- Counterimmunoelectrophoresis results are positive.
- Radiographs are consistent with lobar or segmental consolidation. Staphylococcal pneumonia involves the right lobe 65% of the time. Pneumatoceles are common in staphylococcal pneumonia (Behrman et al., 1996; Bergelson & Finberg, 1998).

Differential Diagnosis

Other types of pneumonia, bronchiolitis, allergic bronchitis, congestive heart failure, acute bronchiectasis, aspiration of a foreign body, pulmonary abscess, and endotracheal tuberculosis are included in the differential diagnosis. Also, right lower lobe pneumonia can be confused with appendicitis. Right upper lobe pneumonia can often closely resemble meningitis.

Management

Management consists of appropriate antibiotic coverage, adequate fluid intake, and respiratory therapy (humidified oxygen) if needed. Older children with pneumococcal pneumonia can usually be treated safely at home if not in severe respiratory distress. Most children who are moderately ill and can be treated at home respond to amoxicillin. If resistant pneumococcus is suspected, clindamycin should be considered (Bergelson & Finberg, 1998). Common pharmacological therapy is based on the infecting organism as outlined:

1. *S. pneumoniae* and β-hemolytic streptococcus:
   - Penicillin G (100,000 U/kg per 24 hours)—usually given as one 600,000-U intramuscular injection followed by oral penicillin.
   - Erythromycin and trimethoprim-sulfamethoxazole can be used in children with mild to moderate disease who are allergic to penicillin.
   - Third-generation cephalosporins are also used.
2. *S. aureus* (Behrman et al., 1996; Bergelson & Finberg, 1998):
   - Semisynthetic penicillinase-resistant penicillin (oxacillin, vancomycin, or nafcillin) should be used.
   - Third-generation cephalosporins are also used.
   - A chest tube may be needed if significant empyema is present.
3. *H. influenzae*:
   - Third-generation cephalosporins are used.
   - Cefuroxime (100 mg/kg per 24 hours divided every 8 hours).
4. *K. pneumoniae* and *P. aeruginosa*:
   - A third-generation cephalosporin and an aminoglycoside at the appropriate doses may be administered.

Complications

By the second to third day, auscultation reveals a change in respiratory sounds as the infection begins consolidation. Increased fremitus, tubular breath sounds, and the disappearance of crackles may be noted. As resolution occurs around the seventh day (the day of crisis in untreated cases involving children and adolescents), crackles can recur. Empyema is common in staphylococcal and GABHS infections.

VIRAL PNEUMONIA

Description

Viral pneumonia often involves both the conducting airways and the alveoli. This type of pneumonia is a common problem in young children and can result in serious illness in a young infant.

Etiology

Viruses commonly causing pneumonia in children, particularly infants, are RSV, adenoviruses, parainfluenza virus (types 1, 2, and 3), and enterovirus. Influenza virus, rhinovirus, and herpes simplex virus are less likely causative agents.

Clinical Findings

HISTORY. The onset of illness caused by viral pneumonia is similar to that caused by bacterial pneumonia—history of an initial URI. However, the progression of respiratory symptoms is slower in viral illnesses than in bacterial pneumonia.

PHYSICAL EXAMINATION. Findings may include:

- Tachypnea, cough, retractions
- Rales, wheezing, decreased breath sounds, cyanosis
- Other symptoms specific to the individual viral organism

DIAGNOSTIC TESTS. The typical radiograph shows patchy (diffuse infiltrates) bronchopneumonia. Hyperinflation (hyperexpansion of the lungs) is a common radiographic finding (Fig. 32–2).

Management

Management of children with viral pneumonia is similar to that of children with bacterial pneumonia. Most children are managed as outpatients with:

- General supportive measures consisting of hydration and antipyretics.

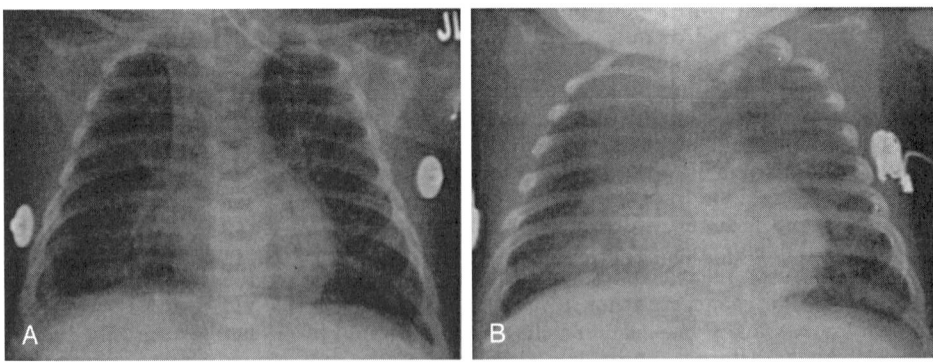

F I G U R E 32-2
Six-month-old infant with rapid respirations and fever. An anteroposterior radiograph of the chest shows hyperexpansion of the lungs with bilateral fine air space disease and streaks of density, indicating the presence of both pneumonia and atelectasis. (From Prober CG: Pneumonia. *In*: Behrman R, Kliegman RM, Arvin AM (eds): Nelson Textbook of Pediatrics, 15th ed. Philadelphia, WB Saunders, 1996, p 717.)

- Antibiotics only if secondary bacterial infection is diagnosed.
- Humidified oxygen, vigorous pulmonary therapy, and intubation. These measures may be necessary for children in severe distress; such children require hospitalization.

Complications

Secondary bacterial pneumonia can be a frequent problem. Premature and young infants with chronic diseases and severe cases of pneumonia caused by RSV often require hospitalization and may need ribavirin therapy (Behrman et al., 1996; Larsen et al., 1999).

MYCOPLASMAL PNEUMONIA

Description

Mycoplasmal pneumonia or primary atypical pneumonia is the most common cause of pneumonia in children older than 5 years through the young adult years. This disease is usually mild and self-limited.

Etiology

M. pneumoniae, an organism without a cell wall, is responsible for this form of pneumonia. It is transmitted from one symptomatic patient to another by droplet spread. The incubation period is 2 to 3 weeks, and asymptomatic carriage after infection can last for weeks.

Clinical Findings

HISTORY. Upper respiratory tract symptoms, fever (temperature >39°C), and dry cough, often associated with chills, headache, sore throat, and malaise, are frequently reported.

PHYSICAL EXAMINATION. Minimal changes or harsh breath sounds and rhonchi may be heard on auscultation.

DIAGNOSTIC TESTS. Chest radiograph findings are nonspecific and reveal bronchovascular markings with areas of atelectasis.

Management

Erythromycin is the drug of choice for children younger than 9 years. Clarithromycin (15 mg/kg per day divided in two doses with 1 g/d maximum) is better tolerated than erythromycin. Tetracycline can be used in children 9 years of age or older.

Complications

Most children have an uneventful recovery, but it is important to inform parents that their child's cough can last for several weeks. *M. pneumoniae* can spread to the blood, central nervous system, heart, skin, or joints. A child with sickle cell disease and mycoplasmal pneumonia has more severe pulmonary disease than the average child does.

CHLAMYDIAL PNEUMONIA OF INFANCY

Description

This type of pneumonia is transmitted from the infected genital tract of the mother to the infant. It does not become apparent until 3 to 19 weeks of age.

Etiology

Chlamydia trachomatis is an organism that has many subtypes within the species. Approximately 50% of infants born to infected mothers acquire this infection, but only 5 to 20% are at risk for chlamydial pneumonia. The incidence of this disease is increasing; the disease in untreated infants can linger and recur (AAP, 1997).

Clinical Findings

HISTORY. The infant is afebrile. A prior, concurrent, or no history of inclusion conjunctivitis is reported.

PHYSICAL EXAMINATION. Findings include:

- Repetitive, staccato cough with tachypnea
- Cervical adenopathy
- Crackles and tachypnea, rarely wheezing
- Hyperinflation noted on chest radiography

DIAGNOSTIC TESTS. The diagnosis is often based on clinical signs and symptoms, as well as chest radiographic findings of hyperinflation and bilateral diffuse infiltrates. An eosinophil count of 300 to 400/mm³ or greater and elevated serum IgG and IgM concentrations are indirect evidence of infection. An elevated serum titer of *Chlamydia*-specific IgM is diagnostic of the disease, but this test is not available in all laboratories. The organism may be cultured.

Differential Diagnosis

Other forms of bacterial, viral, or parasitic pneumonias or pertussis are included in the differential diagnosis.

Management

Most infants can be treated as outpatients; those with severe respiratory distress need hospitalization. Oral erythromycin (50 mg/kg per day in four divided doses for 14 days) is the treatment of choice (AAP, 1997).

Prevention

Identification and treatment of pregnant women with *C. trachomatis* in their genital tract are necessary for prevention.

Tuberculosis

Tuberculosis is discussed in Chapter 24.

Cystic Fibrosis

Description

CF is a multisystemic congenital disorder manifested by chronic obstructive pulmonary disease (COPD), gastrointestinal disturbances, and exocrine dysfunction.

Etiology and Incidence

CF is an autosomal recessive genetic disorder. It occurs in approximately 1 in 3000 white births. Although not common, it does occur in 1 in 17,000 black births and 1 in 90,000 Asian births. The basic insult is an inability to clear mucoid secretions and inadequate salt and water secretion on the cellular level. The endobronchial spaces are not cleared of their mucoid secretions, which leads to colonization by

bacteria with resulting chronic inflammation and infection. Inadequate water secretion also causes desiccation of mucoid and proteinaceous secretions and, consequently, pulmonary and exocrine duct obstruction and tissue damage (Behrman et al., 1996).

Clinical Findings

CF is a multisystemic illness. Clinical manifestations include the following:

- *Pulmonary.* CF is a major cause of severe chronic lung disease in children. The pulmonary system manifestations run the clinical spectrum from dry, frequent cough to COPD. Bronchitis, bronchiolitis, bronchiolectasis, and pneumonia are frequent. Bronchospasm resembling acute or chronic asthma may be present. The airways become colonized with *S. aureus*, *H. influenzae,* and finally, *P. aeruginosa. Burkholderia cepacia* is a slower-growing organism found in children with CF. Pulmonary disease usually becomes progressive and leads to COPD, cor pulmonale, respiratory failure, and death. Other respiratory problems associated with CF include recurrent acute sinusitis and nasal polyps.
- *Gastrointestinal tract.* Meconium ileus develops in up to 15% of newborns born with CF. A meconium ileus syndrome equivalent can also develop in older patients, with desiccated fecal material causing gastrointestinal obstruction. Eighty-five percent of affected children have failure to thrive because of pancreatic enzyme insufficiency. These children have thick, fat-laden stools, poor muscle mass, and delayed maturation. Please note that infants with CF who are fed soy-based formulas do very poorly, and severe hypoproteinemia and anasarca quickly result. Other gastrointestinal problems associated with CF include intussusception, duodenal inflammation, gastroesophageal reflux, bile reflux, rectal prolapse, and vitamin E and K deficiencies with resulting bleeding diathesis.
- *Hepatobiliary tract.* Biliary cirrhosis occurs in 2 to 3% of children affected with

CF and is characterized by jaundice, ascites hematemesis from esophageal varices, and splenomegaly. Adolescent patients experience biliary colic and cholelithiasis.

- *Pancreas.* Recurrent acute pancreatitis is not uncommon. Diabetes mellitus develops in 8% of such patients, usually in the second decade of life.
- *Genitourinary tract.* Affected children have delayed sexual development. Ninety-five percent of males have fertility problems. The incidence of inguinal hernia, hydrocele, and undescended testes is higher. Females experience secondary amenorrhea, cervicitis, and decreased fertility. A pregnancy is usually carried to term if pulmonary function is not severely compromised.
- *Sweat glands.* Excessive salt loss can lead to hypochloremic alkalosis, especially in warm weather or after gastroenteritis. Children with CF often taste salty because of elevated amounts of NaCl lost in endogenous sweat.

DIAGNOSTIC TESTS. The diagnosis of CF is based on an abnormal sweat test. Sweat tests should be done at a laboratory that regularly deals with children and routinely does these tests. Fifty to 100 mg of sweat should be collected to ensure accuracy and precision of the sweat test. A result of greater than 60 mEq/L of chloride is considered diagnostic of CF. Forty to 60 mEq/L is suggestive of CF, and less than 40 mEq/L is negative. Children with hypoproteinemia may elicit false-negative sweat test results.

Pancreatic function tests include 3-day stool collection to measure fat balance (a cumbersome test) and quantification of trypsin and chymotrypsin activity in a fresh stool sample (patients with CF have decreased stool trypsin and chymotrypsin activity). Glycosylated hemoglobin levels may be elevated in older children (Behrman et al., 1996).

Pulmonary function tests usually follow the clinical course.

Prenatal diagnosis has a 90% sensitivity for detecting a CF gene mutation on the long arm of chromosome 7. Newborn screening for immunoreactive trypsinogen is positive in 95% of cases. Routine screening of all newborns is not recommended.

Treatment

Children with CF have very complicated treatment regimens and should be monitored by a multidisciplinary team. Pulmonary, nutritional, physical, and pharmacological (antibiotic and anti-inflammatory) therapy and psychological counseling must be individualized for each child at each stage of the illness.

Syncope

A child with a syncopal episode requires a thoughtful approach. Many possible etiologies can produce syncopal episodes, including autonomic causes, cardiac dysrhythmias, obstructive cardiac lesions, anomalous coronary arteries, and a group of other miscellaneous problems such as psychogenic causes, seizures, vestibular diseases, and drug use (Hardy, 1994; Lauer, 1998).

A detailed history and careful physical examination should be performed on all children with syncope. If warranted, the NP may order some initial screening diagnostic tests. Appropriate referral to pediatric specialists for further evaluation and diagnostic testing is suggested for children whose history, physical examination, or diagnostic tests suggest a potential pathological problem that is outside the range of practice for the NP. See Chapter 31 for discussion about cardic etiologies.

The initial approach to the assessment and management of syncope includes a thorough history and analysis of the symptom, a physical examination, and selected screening tests if indicated.

HISTORY. Important information to obtain about the syncopal incident includes whether the child had:

- A triggering factor such as exercise, pain, or an emotional event
- A prior incident or incidents of syncope or fainting
- An associated injury, clonic-tonic movements, or vertigo
- A family history of sudden death
- The possibility of pregnancy or the use of drugs
- A history of exercise-induced reactive airway disease or respiratory distress

- A known psychological stress or stressors at home or school or in social environments

PHYSICAL EXAMINATION. A detailed neurological examination is needed if the syncopal episode suggests a seizure disorder. Careful evaluation of the head, eyes, ears, nose, and throat is done if vestibular disease is likely. A cardiovascular examination is always important.

DIAGNOSTIC SCREENING TESTS. For possible cardiac causes of syncope, a 12-lead electrocardiogram (ECG) is performed and a 24-hour ambulatory monitor is used (if concerned with intermittent cardiac arrhythmia). If a seizure disorder is suspected, appropriate neurological evaluation is done as outlined in Chapter 28. Note that a CBC, random glucose test, and glucose tolerance test have low yields and are not recommended as routine tests for a syncopal episode.

Pectus Excavatum

Description

Pectus excavatum, or funnel chest, is an abnormality of the skeleton and chest wall. Midline narrowing of the thoracic cavity and restriction in chest wall movement are characteristic.

Etiology and Incidence

Children with upper airway obstruction have a higher incidence, but about 86% of children with this defect are identified at birth or within the first year of life. The cause of pectus excavatum in these instances is often unknown. About 79% of cases occur in males, and a positive family history of chest wall deformity is found in about 37% of cases.

Clinical Findings

HISTORY. The parent may note a depression in the chest wall. A positive family history of chest wall deformity may be elicited.

PHYSICAL EXAMINATION. Findings include posterior depression of the sternum and costal cartilage.

DIAGNOSTIC TESTS. Diagnostic tests include:

- Chest radiography
- Exercise testing if substantial pectus deformity is present
- Other cardiac (echocardiogram) and pulmonary function studies as suggested by the degree of deformity and symptomatology

Management

If the deformity is the result of a pulmonary disease, early treatment of the underlying pulmonary problem occasionally resolves the skeletal deformity. Surgical repair depends on the severity of the defect, demonstration of a decrease in pulmonary function, progression of the defect on serial radiographs, or sometimes the patient's and parents' wish for cosmetic repair. If the patient is male with an associated scoliosis or has a severe defect, evaluate for Marfan syndrome.

Complications

Pectus excavatum can also affect cardiopulmonary function.

RESOURCE BOX 32-1

Cystic Fibrosis Foundation
Tel: (800) 344-4823
Website: http://www.cff.org
E-mail: info@cff.org
Refer to Chapter 25 for resources related to respiratory conditions.

REFERENCES

Abbasi S, Cunningham AS: Are we overtreating sinusitis? Contemp Pediatr 13:49-62, 1996.

American Academy of Pediatrics Committee on Infectious Diseases: 1997 Red Book: Report of the Committee on Infectious Diseases, 24th ed. Elk Grove Village, IL, American Academy of Pediatrics, 1997.

Behrman R, Kliegman R, Arvin AM, et al (eds): Nelson Textbook of Pediatrics, 15th ed. Philadelphia, WB Saunders, 1996.

Bergelson J, Finberg R: Lower respiratory infection. *In* Finberg L (ed): Saunders Manual of Pediatric Practice. Philadelphia, WB Saunders, 1998, pp 315-318.

Berman S, Chan K: Ear, nose and throat. *In* Hay WW, Hayward AR, Levin MR, et al (eds): Current Pediatric Diagnosis and Treatment, 14th ed. E Norwalk, CT, Appleton & Lange, 1999.

Centers for Disease Control and Prevention: Erythromycin resistant *Bordetella pertussis*—Yuma County, Arizona, May-October 1994. JAMA 273:13-14, 1994.

Dolitsky JN, Ward RF: Foreign bodies of the ear, nose, airway and esophagus. *In* Hoekelman RA, Friedman SB, Nelson NM, et al (eds): Primary Pediatric Care, 3rd ed. St Louis, CV Mosby, 1997, pp 1300-1303.

Edelstein DR: Epistaxis. *In* Hoekelman RA, Friedman SB, Nelson NM, et al (eds): Primary Pediatric Care, 3rd ed. St Louis, CV Mosby, 1997, pp 936-939.

Finberg R, Bergelson J: Upper respiratory infection. *In* Finberg L (ed): Saunders Manual of Pediatric Practice. Philadelphia, WB Saunders, 1998, pp 311-314.

Gaebler J: Pharyngitis and tonsillitis. *In* Finberg L (ed): Saunders Manual of Pediatric Practice. Philadelphia, WB Saunders, 1998, pp 624-627.

Guilbert TW, Taussig LM: Chronic cough. Contemp Pediatr 15:155-172, 1998.

Hardy CE: Syncope and chest pain: To worry, or not? Contemp Pediatr 11:19-42, 1994.

Inkelis SH: Nosebleeds. *In* Berkowitz C (ed): Pediatrics: A Primary Care Approach. Philadelphia, WB Saunders, 1996, pp 191-194.

Kelley PE: Foreign bodies in the nose and pharynx. *In* Burg FD, Ingelfinger JR, Wald ER, et al (eds): Gellis & Kagan's Current Pediatric Therapy, 16th ed. Philadelphia, WB Saunders, 1999, pp 503-504.

Larsen GL, Abman SH, Fan LL, et al: Respiratory tract and mediastinum. *In* Hay WW, Hayward AR, Levin MR, et al (eds): Current Pediatric Diagnosis and Treatment, 14th ed. E Norwalk, CT, Appleton & Lange, 1999, pp 418-464.

Lauer RM: Symptoms of cardiovascular disorders. *In* Finberg L (ed): Saunders Manual of Pediatric Practice. Philadelphia, WB Saunders, 1998, pp 532-533.

Maggi C: Director Critical Care and Pulmonary Medicine, Miller Children's Hospital, Long Beach, CA. Private correspondence, 1998.

Noble JE: Cough. *In* Berkowitz C (ed): Pediatrics: A Primary Care Approach. Philadelphia, WB Saunders, 1996, pp 226-239.

Pitetti RD, Wald ER: Strep throat: Weighing the diagnostic options. Contemp Pediatr 15:68-74, 1998.

Wald ER: Sinusitis. Pediatr Rev 14:345-351, 1994.

Wilner A: Associate Professor of Medicine, University of California Irvine School of Medicine. Private correspondence, 1998.

CHAPTER 33

Gastrointestinal Disorders

Ann M. Petersen-Smith

INTRODUCTION

The gastrointestinal (GI) system functions to ingest and absorb nutrients and discard waste products. Appropriate functioning of the system is essential for normal growth and development and maintenance of other organ systems.

The nurse practitioner (NP) plays an integral role in the care of children with GI dysfunction. An understanding of the anatomy, physiology, and common disorders of the system allows NPs to thoughtfully assess and treat problems. This chapter focuses on GI disorders that involve organic pathology. Functional problems of the GI system such as obesity, anorexia, bulimia, encopresis, and constipation that can best be managed by changes of habit are discussed in Chapters 12 and 14.

ANATOMY AND PHYSIOLOGY

The GI system begins to develop during the third week of gestation. The primitive gut is initially formed and then divides into the foregut, midgut, and hindgut. The structures further develop in an intricate and complex fashion to become the digestive tract and accessory organs.

The GI tract extends from the mouth to the anus. It includes the organs of digestion and accessory organs such as the liver, pancreas, and gallbladder. The system provides the following functions:

- Ingestion of food
- Movement of food from the mouth toward the rectum
- Mechanical dissolution of food
- Chemical dissolution of food
- Absorption of nutrients
- Expulsion of waste products

The mouth serves as the site for ingestion, chewing, and mixing of food with saliva. The tongue senses the texture and taste of foods, which initiates salivation and release of gastric juices in the stomach.

The esophagus transports food from the mouth to the stomach by peristalsis, the sequential contraction and relaxation of the musculature in the esophagus. The upper esophageal sphincter prevents air from being swallowed while breathing. The lower esophageal sphincter (LES) prevents food from being regurgitated from the stomach, which is important because intra-abdominal pressure exceeds intrathoracic and atmospheric pressure.

The stomach serves as a reservoir for ingested foods. It secretes digestive juices, mixes food with the gastric fluids, and propels the liquid material into the small intestine.

The small intestine's primary function is absorption of nutrients (carbohydrates, fats, proteins, minerals, and vitamins) into the systemic circulation. Absorption occurs through villi, which cover the mucosal folds and serve as the functional unit of the intestine. Each villus contains an artery, vein, and lymph vessel, which serve to transport nutrients from the intestine into the systemic circulation. The villi are covered with enterocytes, whose major role is the digestion of carbohydrates and proteins. Enterocytes secrete proteins and enzymes known as brush border enzymes, which assist in digestion.

Carbohydrates must be converted to monosaccharides before their absorption is possible. This process begins in the mouth, where the salivary enzyme amylase breaks down complex starches into disaccharides. The brush border enzymes convert disaccharides into monosaccharides (sucrose to glucose and fructose, lactose to glucose and galactose, and maltose to glucose). When this process is hindered, disaccharides remain osmotically active and can cause diarrhea.

Fat absorption, which occurs mainly in the jejunum, is accomplished through the addition of lipases secreted by the pancreas. Lipases break down fats into particles that are easily absorbed by the villi. Fats then rely on the lymphatic system for absorption.

Proteins are converted to amino acids by pancreatic enzymes. The resulting amino acids are further divided into smaller amino acid particles that are absorbed via the brush border into the systemic circulation. After appropriate absorption of nutrients, the small intestine is left with the initial fecal liquid. This liquid is then propelled by peristalsis into the large intestine.

The large intestine removes water from the fecal liquid and allows for short-term storage. The fecal mass, which consists of waste products, bacteria, intestinal secretions, and shed cells, is pushed into the sigmoid colon.

Entry of feces into the rectum stimulates the defecation reflex. This reflex stretches the rectal wall, relaxes the internal anal sphincter, and thereby creates the need to defecate. If this urge is ignored, further fluid resorption occurs as the stool is retained.

PATHOPHYSIOLOGY

The GI tract can be affected by illness, injury, or generalized problems that prevent it from functioning normally. Dysfunction can be localized or systemic. Categories of dysfunction include:

- Disorders of motility
- Infection
- Malabsorption syndromes
- Impairment of digestion, absorption, and nutrition
- Congenital malformations
- Genetic syndromes
- Metabolic disorders
- Behavioral problems
- Injuries and trauma

ASSESSMENT

History

The history assesses the following:

- Family history of gallbladder disease, ulcers, or allergy to any food product
- Past medical history related to the GI system (e.g., illnesses, surgeries, anatomical problems such as cleft lip/palate, esophageal atresia)
- Presence of pain (location, type, quality)
- Bowel habits (frequency, times per week, consistency, associated pain, aids such as medications or enemas)
- Constipation and diarrhea (patient's definition of each, how often they occur, treatment tried thus far)
- Changes in appetite
- Thirst level (increased or decreased)
- Food intolerance or allergy (what foods, symptoms, treatment)
- Belching and flatulence
- Vomiting
- Heartburn
- Feeding habits and nutrition history or current diet (what, when, how often, what tolerated)
- Apnea (in infants with gastroesophageal reflux [GER])

Physical Examination

When assessing a suspected GI problem, a head-to-toe physical examination is frequently indicated.

- Plot growth parameters, including weight for height, to establish proportionality of the patient and exclude certain growth aberrations from the diagnosis.
- Determine the patient's hydration status (skin turgor, mucous membranes, peripheral pulses, tears).
- Inspect the abdomen for visible peristalsis, rashes, lesions, asymmetry, masses, enlarged organs, and pulsations.
- Auscultate for frequency of bowel sounds (normal is 5 to 20 per minute).
- Percuss for density and to measure organs.
- Palpate both lightly and deeply.
- Assess peritoneal irritation:
  - Have the patient walk standing straight up or cough.
  - Have the patient stand on tiptoes and fall onto the heels.
  - Palpate for rebound tenderness.
  - Check for the obturator sign: a supine patient flexes the right thigh at the hip with the knee bent and internally rotates the hip. The sign is positive when it induces abdominal pain.
  - Check for the psoas sign: the patient lies on the left side and extends and then flexes the right leg at the hip. A positive sign is one that induces abdominal pain.
- Perform a rectal examination when intra-abdominal, pelvic, or perirectal disease is suspected. This examination includes external inspection and internal palpation for masses, stool, or irregularities. The index finger should be used because of its increased sensitivity. Insert a gloved, lubricated finger into the rectum. Place the other hand on the abdomen for a bimanual examination.
  - Young pediatric patients should be supine with their feet held together and knees and hips flexed over the abdomen.
  - Adolescent males can be lying on their side or standing with the hips flexed and the upper part of the body on the examination table.
  - Adolescent females can be lying on their side or, if a concurrent pelvic examination is to be done, in the lithotomy position.
- Perform a gynecological examination if pelvic pathology is suspected (see Chapter 36).

Common Diagnostic Studies

Laboratory tests are performed as indicated by the history, initial symptoms, and physical examination and include:

- Urinalysis (UA) and urine culture
- Complete blood count (CBC) with differential
- Serum chemistry screen, liver profile, lipid profile, erythrocyte sedimentation rate (ESR), C-reactive protein (CRP), thyroid function
- Pregnancy test
- Stool examination for ova and parasites, culture, blood, white blood cells, pH, Clinitest for reducing substances
- Fecal fat collection for 72 hours to rule out fat malabsorption
- Radiological examination, including abdominal radiographs, abdominal and pelvic ultrasonography, chest radiographs (referred pain with pneumonia), upper and lower GI series, and radionuclide studies with scintiscan, depending on the suspected pathology
- Bone age to assess suspected growth abnormalities
- Papanicolaou smear and vaginal cultures and smears if pelvic pathology is suspected
- Additional, more specialized tests can be ordered after consultation with a physician:
  - Duodenal aspirate to identify existing infection
  - Esophageal pH probe to establish GER, with a pH of less than 4 representing a reflux episode
  - Breath hydrogen test if lactose intolerance is suspected
  - Sweat chloride test if cystic fibrosis is suspected

MANAGEMENT STRATEGIES

Medications

Many common medications are used to treat various GI disorders:

- Antibiotics may be necessary for bacterial or fungal infection.
- Antiemetics can be used to treat nausea or vomiting.
- Antidiarrheals are occasionally appropriate for persistent diarrhea or diarrhea associated with chronic disease, but they are never appropriate with acute diarrheal diseases because toxins need to be excreted from the body.
- Stool softeners, laxatives, and cathartics are useful in the acute treatment and long-term management of constipation and encopresis.
- Medications that alter GI motility or tone can be used to treat GER.
- Oral steroids, parenteral steroids, and other immunosuppressants may be indicated in the treatment of inflammatory bowel disease.
- Pain medication and antispasmodics may occasionally be used in some acute and chronic GI conditions.
- Medications that alter gastric acidity can be used to treat GER and ulcer disease.
- Iron supplementation may be needed as supportive therapy for chronic disease.

Nutrition

Normal nutrition that meets the recommended daily needs should be encouraged to promote normal GI function, growth, and development. Intake of fluids to ensure hydration is equally important. Dysfunction of the GI tract can be either short or long term and can require alterations in dietary intake. Consultation with a registered dietitian is important in designing an adequate diet for a child with a long-term GI problem. See Chapter 12 for more detail.

Activity

Age-appropriate activity should be encouraged on a regular basis to help maintain normal GI function. Some GI maladies require short-term rest, but generally the system functions better when activity is regular and consistent.

Counseling and Education

It is important to spend time assessing and planning for the unique needs of a child with GI dysfunction. Helping the family understand the disease or disorder and its course, prognosis, and management is essential. Planning for specific needs related to medication, diet, and activity assists the family to normalize life for the child.

▨ UPPER GASTROINTESTINAL TRACT DISORDERS

Dysphagia

Description

In dysphagia, younger children are unable to swallow and older children can have an awareness that something is wrong with their swallowing ability.

Etiology

True dysphagia is never psychogenic, and these patients must be evaluated. Pharyngeal, laryngeal, and esophageal lesions, foreign bodies, anatomical malformations, physiological dysfunction, neurological dysfunction, and tumors can be responsible for symptoms.

Clinical Findings

HISTORY. The following may be reported:

- Progressive dysfunction
- Symptoms such as discomfort with swallowing or a sense of food getting stuck
- Picky eating, for example, a child preferring liquids to solids and refusing feedings

PHYSICAL EXAMINATION. Observe a feeding and the child's ability to swallow. Look for choking, vomiting, or regurgitation. Carefully palpate the neck to feel for masses.

DIAGNOSTIC TESTS. Diagnostic tests include:

- Lateral neck films
- Barium swallow
- Fluoroscopy

Differential Diagnosis

Obstructive and compressive lesions usually cause trouble only with solids. Physiological dysfunction is usually associated with systemic disease, and the patient has trouble with liquids and solids.

Management

Referral and treatment of the cause are needed.

Vomiting and Dehydration

Description

Vomiting is the forceful emptying of gastric contents. The type of emesis may assist in determining the cause (Murray & Christie, 1998):

- Nonbilious vomit is generally caused by infection, inflammation, or metabolic, neurological, psychological, or obstructive problems.
- Bilious vomit is generally caused by an obstructive lesion.
- Bloody vomit accompanies active bleeding in the GI tract.

Etiology and Incidence

Inflammation of the GI tract secondary to viral or bacterial organisms, eating disorders, stretching of an organ or membrane (e.g., overfilled stomach), vestibular reflex, protein intolerance, urinary tract infection (UTI), otitis media, medications, pregnancy, Reye syndrome, pneumonia, increased intracranial pressure, meningitis, and tumors can cause vomiting. It is one of the most common symptoms in childhood.

Clinical Findings

HISTORY. The history should assess the following:

- Onset and duration of vomiting, quality and quantity, presence of blood or bile, odor
- Relationship of vomiting to meals, time of day, or activities
- Vomiting early in the morning
- History of trauma
- Presence of associated symptoms: diarrhea, fever, ear pain, UTI symptoms, vision changes, headache, seizures, high-pitched cry, polydipsia, polyuria, polyphagia, anorexia
- Symptoms of dehydration (Table 33-1)

PHYSICAL EXAMINATION. The following are needed:

- Assessment of dehydration (see Table 33-1)
- Neurological examination: nuchal rigidity, level of consciousness, behavioral changes, which can include irritability or lethargy

DIAGNOSTIC STUDIES. Diagnostic studies are performed as indicated by the probable diagnosis.

- CBC with differential, blood culture, liver function tests, glucose, ammonia, electrolytes
- UA and urine culture
- Stool for culture and occult blood
- Pregnancy test
- Abdominal radiograph, abdominal ultrasonogram, or both
- Barium swallow, enema, or both
- Esophageal pH probe analysis
- Computed tomography (CT) scan
- Electroencephalogram (EEG)

Differential Diagnosis

The differential diagnosis includes organic lesions, chronic problems, and eating disorders (weight loss); overfeeding (weight gain); esophageal disorders, achalasia, and stricture (undigested food in the vomitus); metabolic disease and increased intracranial pressure (early-morning vomiting); psychogenic or peptic ulcer disease (PUD) (vomiting after meals); hepatobiliary or pancreatic dysfunction (if vomiting does not relieve pain); obstruction (bilious vomiting); volvulus and malrotation (intermittent vomiting); and gastroenteritis (concurrent diarrhea).

Management

The following steps are taken:

1. Determine the degree of dehydration and treat the cause.

T A B L E 33-1
Estimation of Dehydration

CHARACTERISTIC	EXTENT OF DEHYDRATION			
	Mild	Moderate	Severe	Shock
Weight loss—infants (%)	3–5	5–10	10–15	>15
Weight loss—children (%)	3–4	6–8	10	
Pulse	Normal	Slightly increased	Very increased	Rapid and weak
Blood pressure	Normal	Normal to orthostatic, >10-mm Hg change	Orthostatic to shock	
Behavior	Normal	Irritable, more thirsty	Hyperirritable to lethargic	Difficult to awaken/ unresponsive. Too weak to stand; very dizzy
Thirst	Slight	Moderate	Intense	
Mucous membranes*	Normal	Dry	Parched	
Tears	Present	Decreased	Absent; sunken eyes	
Anterior fontanel	Normal	Normal to sunken	Sunken	
External jugular vein	Visible when supine	Not visible except with supraclavicular pressure	Not visible even with supraclavicular pressure	
Skin* (S & S less useful in children >2 yr of age)	Capillary refill >2 s	Slowed capillary refill, 2–4 s (decreased turgor)	Very delayed capillary refill (>4 s) and tenting; skin cool, acrocyanotic, or mottled*	Capillary refill time >4 s. Cold/ acrocyanotic
Urine production	Slight decrease	>8 hr infants >12 hr children; oliguria	Very decreased or absent	Anuria
Urine specific gravity	>1.020	>1.020; oliguria	Oliguria or anuria	

S & S = signs & symptoms.
*These signs are less prominent in patients who have hypernatremia.
From Jospe N, Forbes G: Fluids and electrolytes: Clinical aspects. Pediatr Rev 17:395–403, 1996.

2. Rehydrate (Table 33-2). After 1 to 2 hours with nothing by mouth, introduce an appropriate rehydration solution. Avoid plain water, apple juice, soda, milk, and sports drinks as none of these liquids provide appropriate replacement of sugars and electrolytes (Tables 33-3 and 33-4). Begin with small amounts (as little as 5 to 10 ml) of clear liquids offered frequently. Breastfed infants should continue to breastfeed more frequently for shorter periods.
3. Resume maintenance fluid levels (see Table 33-2).
4. Avoid solids for 4 to 6 hours, and then reintroduce age-appropriate bland solids slowly as tolerated. Bland solids might include complex carbohydrates, bananas, applesauce, pretzels, and rice or rice cereal.
5. Prescribe antiemetics cautiously (promethazine [Phenergan], 0.5 to 1 mg/kg per dose per rectum every 6 hours) if vomiting is excessive, dehydration imminent, and GI pathology excluded.
6. Monitor urine output.
7. Treat fever.
8. Refer if the child has a toxic appearance or moderate to severe dehydration, projectile vomiting, abnormal examination, vomiting for greater than 12 hours, or vomiting of blood, bile, or fecal matter.

T A B L E 33-2

Treatment of Dehydration

REHYDRATION (with increased sodium concentration)

Mild	ORS	40–50 ml/kg over 4 hr (10 ml/kg per hr)
Moderate	ORS	60–100 ml/kg over 4–6 hr (20 ml/kg per hr)
Severe	IV fluids	Ringers lactate or normal saline, 20-ml/kg bolus over 1 hr; may repeat bolus if needed (until pulse, perfusion, mental status are normal)
		Follow with 5% dextrose with NaCl and KCl added (once the child has voided) for maintenance fluids and abnormal loss replacement (see later); if severe dehydration, give ½ amount over 8 hr, the other ½ over the next 16 hr; include bolus amounts in the 24-hr total
		Begin ORS as soon as possible

MAINTENANCE

Total water volume	0–10 kg	100 ml/kg per 24 hr
	10–20 kg	1000 ml + 50 ml/kg for each kg over 10 kg/24 hr
	>20 kg	1500 ml + 20 ml/kg for each kg over 20 kg/24 hr

May give up to 150 ml/kg in first 24 hr

REPLACEMENT OF FLUID LOSSES (if continued, heavy losses)
10 ml/kg or 4–8 oz of ORS for each diarrhea stool (1 to 1½ times the amount of stool)

REFEEDING
Reintroduce age-appropriate diet within 24 hr. Avoid fatty foods and foods high in simple sugars
Encourage complex carbohydrates, lean meats, yogurt, bananas, and applesauce
Formula-fed infants should have full-strength formula. If that is not tolerated, use lactose-free or soy formula
Breastfeeding infants should continue to breastfeed with shorter duration and more frequent feedings
Use regular milk for older children

IV = intravenous; ORS = oral rehydration solution.

Data from Lasche J, Duggan C: Managing acute diarrhea, Contemp Pediatr 16(2):74–83, 1999; Jospe N, Forbes G: Fluids and electrolytes: Clinical aspects, Pediatr Rev 17(11):395–403, 1996; Northrup RS, Flanagan TP: Gastroenteritis: Pediatr Rev 15(12):461–472, 1994.

T A B L E 33-3
Rehydration Solutions

SOLUTION	SODIUM*	CHLORINE*	POTASSIUM*	BASE Type	BASE Concentration*	CARBOHYDRATE Type	CARBOHYDRATE Concentration (g/L)	OSMOLALITY
STOOL								
Pediatric diarrheal stool	50–100	75–90	25–35	HCO$_3$	25–40	—	—	250–300
ORAL REHYDRATION SOLUTIONS								
Recommended:								
WHO ORS	90	80	20	Citrate	30	Glucose	20	300
WHO recommendations for ORS solutions	60–90	50–80	20–30	Citrate	25–35	Glucose	20	<300
Pedialyte (Ross)	45	35	20	Citrate	30	Glucose	25	264
Rehydralyte (Ross)	75	65	20	Citrate	30	Glucose	25	327
Cereal-based ORS	60–90	—†	—†	—†	—†	Starch‡	50	200–225
Infalyte (Mead-Johnson)	50	45	25	Citrate	34	Rice syrup solids	30	
Home sugar–salt solution	30–60	30–60	—	—	—	Sucrose	40	170–230
Other solutions:								
Soft drinks, cola, etc.	2	(—)§	0.1	HCO$_3$	13	F/G	50–150	550
Apple juice	3	(—)§	32	—	0	F/G/S	63	700
Chicken broth	250	(—)§	5	—	0	—	0	450
Gatorade	20	(—)§	3	HCO$_3$	3	G/others	45	330
INTRAVENOUS SOLUTIONS								
Recommended:								
Ringer lactate	135	90	4	Lactate	49	—	—	278
Normal saline	135	135	0	—	0	—	—	270
5% Dextrose in saline	135	135	0	—	0	Glucose	50	545
Not recommended:								
5% Dextrose in water	0	0	0	—	0	Glucose	50	275

F = fructose; G = glucose; ORS = oral rehydration solution; S = sucrose; WHO = World Health Organization.
*In millimoles or milliequivalents per liter.
†Variable.
‡From various cereals: rice, wheat, sorghum, etc.
§Value not reported.
From Northrup RS, Flanagan TP: Gastroenteritis. Pediatr Rev 15(12):461–472, 1994.

T A B L E 33-4
Rehydration Solutions (Homemade)*

Option 1†	½ cup dry precooked baby rice cereal
	2 cups water
	¼ teaspoon salt (level measure)
Option 2‡	200 ml water
	2 teaspoons sugar
	⅛ teaspoon salt

*Caution: Having parents prepare their own rehydration solution is discouraged because of concern about accurate measurement.

†Data from Meyers A: Modern management of acute diarrhea and dehydration in children. Am Fam Physician 51:1103–1113, 1995.

‡From Northrup RS, Flanagan TP: Gastroenteritis. Pediatr Rev 15:461–472, 1994.

Gastroesophageal Reflux

Description

GER refers to the passage of gastric contents into the esophagus from the stomach through the LES. It can be a normal phenomenon. Three classifications of GER are recognized (Armentrout, 1995):

- Physiological: infrequent, episodic vomiting
- Functional: painless, effortless vomiting with no physical sequelae
- Pathological: frequent vomiting with alteration in physical functioning (e.g., failure to thrive [FTT], aspiration pneumonia)

Etiology

The etiology is unclear and probably multifactorial. The LES is influenced by intra-abdominal pressure, hormones, neurological control, and age. LES tone is normal in infants and children with GER. Inappropriate relaxation of the LES may be responsible for many instances of GER (Cucchiara & Bartolotti, 1993). Animal studies suggest that newborn and infant gastric musculature may function differently from the gastric musculature of adults (Hillemeier, 1996). Young infants have increased intra-abdominal pressure because of their inability to sit upright.

Alterations in swallowing, pharyngeal coordination, and esophageal motility and delayed gastric emptying are also potential factors related to GER. Children with neurodevelopmental disability commonly have GER. Increased muscle tone, chronic supine positioning, and altered GI motility exacerbate GER (Roberts, 1996).

Incidence

Up to 70% of infants less than 1700 g have pathological GER. Forty percent have symptomatic improvement by 3 months of age, and 70% are symptom free by 18 months (Armentrout, 1995).

Clinical Findings

HISTORY. Important historical information to elicit includes:

- Careful birth, medical, and social history
- Concerns about feeding difficulty, pulling from the bottle or breast, crying, choking, coughing/wheezing, apnea, weight loss, irritability, recurrent pneumonia, and bloody emesis in younger children
- Sandifer syndrome, abnormal behavior and posturing with the tilting of the head to one side and bizarre contortions of the trunk (Hillemeier, 1996)
- Heartburn, painful belching, headache, dyspnea, abdominal pain, stool pattern changes, and/or recurrent pneumonia in older children
- A 24-hour diet history and discussion of feeding circumstances

PHYSICAL EXAMINATION. Findings can include:

- Signs of FTT
- Torticollis
- Tooth erosion due to destruction of enamel by gastric acids is caused by frequent vomiting
- Rash, recurrent diarrhea, persistent vomiting, or early morning vomiting (symptoms of other primary disease with GER as a secondary problem)

DIAGNOSTIC TESTS. The following are obtained as indicated in consultation with a physician or a pediatric gastroenterologist:

- CBC with differential to rule out anemia and infection
- UA and urine culture
- Stool for occult blood
- Abdominal ultrasonography to rule out pyloric stenosis if age appropriate
- Barium swallow—examination of choice
- Endoscopy to rule out esophagitis if deemed necessary
- Esophageal pH monitoring, with a pH lower than 4 indicating reflux
- Radionucleotide scan with scintiscan

Differential Diagnosis

Included in the differential diagnosis are anatomical obstruction, antral or esophageal webs, masses, malrotation, otitis media, UTI, gastroenteritis, formula intolerance, inborn errors of metabolism, brain tumors, increased intracranial pressure, Reye syndrome, obstructive uropathy, pancreatitis, and hepatobiliary problems (Chang, 1999).

Management

1. For infants, use small, frequent feedings, frequent burping during feedings, continued breastfeeding, avoidance of formula changes, and 1 tablespoon of rice cereal per ounce of formula. It is also helpful to have the head of the bed elevated or to have the child lie on the right side.
2. For older children, avoid chocolate, caffeine, high-fat foods, spicy foods, alcohol, and bedtime snacks.
3. See Table 12-19 for feeding strategies in patients with GER.
4. Medications can be helpful when the aforementioned measures have failed to give relief (Table 33-5).
5. A combination of an H_2 inhibitor and agent that promotes gastric emptying is often an effective regimen.
6. Close follow-up of growth parameters to ensure adequate weight gain is important.
7. Refer for Nissen fundoplication or similar surgical procedures if the GER is severe, not well managed medically, or causing significant secondary morbidity.

Complications

Complications include FTT, aspiration, recurrent pneumonia, apnea, asthma, esophagitis with pain, bleeding and formation of strictures, weight loss, irritability, malnutrition, and developmental delays. GER has been implicated in sudden infant death syndrome.

Patient Education

- Assure parents that GER is usually self-limiting and that symptoms improve as the child grows.
- Remind parents that GER may be temporarily worse during illness.
- Review medication information, including doses and side effects.

Peptic Ulcer Disease

Description

PUD consists of a group of disorders. With duodenal ulcers, mucosal defects penetrate the duodenal mucosa and submucosa. Gastric ulcers result from gastric mucosal defects that penetrate the mucosa and submucosa.

Etiology

Primary ulcers have no underlying cause. Secondary ulcers are associated with known ulcerogenic events (Mezoff & Balistreri, 1995). Ulceration in children is commonly associated with stressful situations and critical illness. Stress ulcers account for 80% of peptic disease in infancy and childhood (Mezoff & Balistreri, 1995). A strong familial predisposition for PUD has been noted. There is no evidence that diet plays a role in the formation of ulcers. Chronic aspirin therapy and nonsteroidal anti-inflammatory drugs (NSAIDs) cause gastric mucosal damage but are not associated with ulcer formation. Smoking can cause duodenal ulcers and decreases the rate of healing.

Primary gastric ulcers are about seven times

T A B L E 33-5

Medications Used in the Treatment of Gastroesophageal Reflux

DRUG	DOSAGE	COMMENT
Ranitidine (Zantac)	1.5–2.3 mg/kg per dose bid	Inhibits histamine at H_2-receptor sites and decreases gastric acid secretion
Cimetadine (Tagamet)	20–40 mg/kg per d qid	Inhibits histamine at H_2-receptor sites and decreases gastric acid secretion
Metoclopramide (Reglan)	0.1 mg/kg per dose, up to qid	Hastens gastric emptying High range of side effects
Cisapride (Propulsid)	0.2 mg/kg per dose tid or qid	Give 30 min before meals Increases muscle contractions in GI tract Give with caution with antidepressants, macrolide antibiotics, antifungals, and HIV medications
Bethanechol	0.1–0.2 mg/kg per dose, up to qid	Give 30 min before meals Questionable effectiveness in GER

bid = twice daily; GER = gastroesophageal reflux; GI = gastrointestinal; HIV = human immunodeficiency virus; qid = four times daily; tid = three times daily.

less likely to occur in children than duodenal ulcers are. Cytomegalovirus (CMV) and *Helicobacter pylori* are associated with PUD in children. The incidence of *H. pylori* infection is 10% in children. Colonization rates have been suggested to be 8 to 63%. *H. pylori* is transmitted person to person, most likely by fecal–oral contamination. It induces a chronic inflammation in the stomach/duodenal mucosa and destroys the protective mucosal layer (Preud'-Homme & Mezoff, 1996). No correlation between *H. pylori* infection and recurrent abdominal pain (RAP) has been found in children.

Incidence

PUD is more common in children who are living in lower socioeconomic surroundings or are institutionalized, African American, Chinese, eastern Indian, or Mexican (Preud'-Homme & Mezoff, 1996). The male-to-female ratio is about 2 to 3:1. Most children with duodenal ulcers have a positive family medical history (key finding).

Clinical Findings

HISTORY
- Positive family history
- Can be asymptomatic

- Symptoms possibly waxing and waning
- Infants: poor feeding, GI bleeding, vomiting, intestinal perforation
- Toddlers/preschoolers: poorly localized abdominal pain, vomiting, GI bleeding
- School-aged children and adolescents: poorly localized epigastric or right lower quadrant (RLQ) pain, dyspepsia (Preud'-Homme & Mezoff, 1996).
- Predisposing factors: alcohol, smoking, aspirin, NSAIDs, or corticosteroids
- Pain (onset, location, duration, severity) with eating, awakens from sleep (key finding)
- Vomiting

PHYSICAL EXAMINATION
- Height, weight, head circumference, and percentiles
- Complete physical examination (which may be normal)

LABORATORY FINDINGS
- Stool for blood
- Upper GI series
- Endoscopy (especially if pain persists more than 3 months)
- Tissue biopsy or rapid urease test
- Polymerase chain reaction from tissue biopsy for *H. pylori*
- Serum gastrin level (especially if considering Zollinger-Ellison syndrome)

- Serum IgG antibody for *H. pylori* (level greater than 500 [normal, 0 to 200]) (many argue that this test alone should not be the basis for starting therapy)
- Urea breath test (not available for children)

Differential Diagnosis

All other causes of abdominal pain (Table 33–6), GER, and GI bleeding are included in the differential diagnosis.

Management

For PUD not related to *H. pylori*, the following treatment may be helpful:

1. Antacids: any liquid preparation, 0.5 ml/kg, given between 1 and 3 hours after eating and before bed.
2. H_2-receptor antagonists may include one of the following:
   - Cimetidine, 7 mg/kg every 6 to 8 hours
   - Ranitidine, 1.5 to 2.3 mg/kg per dose every 12 hours
   - Famotidine, 40 mg/d in one dose (for young adults)
3. Proton pump inhibitors:
   - Omeprazole, 20 mg/d in one dose (for young adults)
4. Cytoprotective agents:
   - Sucralfate, 1 g four times daily (for young adults)
5. Empirical therapy for suspected *H. pylori* is not recommended. Once *H. pylori* has been identified, the treatment regimen will consist of the following:
   - For younger children:
     ◦ H_2-receptor antagonist (see earlier), *and*
     ◦ Metronidazole, 35 to 50 mg/kg per day in three divided doses, *and*
     ◦ High-dose amoxicillin, 40 to 60 mg/kg per day in three divided doses
     ◦ Treat for 14 days. Shorter courses have a high failure rate and longer courses result in poorer compliance (Preud'-Homme & Mezoff, 1996; Bujanner et al., 1996)
   - For older adolescents and young adults:
     ◦ Bismuth subcitrate (Pepto Bismol) added to the regimen

   ◦ Metronidazole, 250 mg orally four times daily, *and*
   ◦ Tetracycline, 25 to 50 mg/kg per day in two to four divided doses (if older than 9 years), *or* clarithromycin, 15 mg/kg in two divided doses
   ◦ Treatment duration: 14 days

Complications

Recurrence, hemorrhage, perforation, gastric outlet obstruction, and gastric malignancy are possible complications.

Patient Education/Prevention/ Prognosis

- Stress the importance of completing the drug regimen.
- Avoid spicy foods, caffeine, and chocolate.
- This area of pediatric primary care is being actively studied, and NPs must be aware of ongoing changes in recommendations for therapy.

LOWER GASTROINTESTINAL TRACT DISORDERS

Infantile Colic

Description

Infantile colic is characterized by persistent crying in infants younger than 3 months. The average infant cries for 2 to 3 hours per day. An infant with colic usually cries for more than 4 hours a day.

Etiology

No specific cause of colic has been identified, although both physical and psychosocial factors may play a role. Certain physical factors have been implicated and include sensitivity to diet (e.g., cow's milk), excessive gas, swallowed air during feeding, inadequate burping, hypermotile bowel, and cigarette smoke in the infant's environment. Psychosocial factors can include the perception of a stressful pregnancy,

Text continued on page 909

T A B L E 33-6
Differential Diagnosis of Gastrointestinal Causes of Abdominal Pain in Children

DISEASE	MAJOR SYMPTOMS	SIGNS	EXCRETA	TESTS	AGE OF ONSET
Anal fissure	Constipation, crying with defecation, bright red blood on stool or in diaper	Small tears in anal mucosa	Constipation with bloody streaks	Stool occult blood	Any
Appendicitis	Fever, anorexia, vomiting; process evolves over 12 hr	Diffuse then localized to right-sided (RLQ) tenderness, guarding, maximal pain over McBurney point	Constipation or diarrhea, rare blood and pus	CBC: increased neutrophils UA: pyuria Abdominal radiograph: *may* show fecalith Ultrasonography: *may be* abnormal	Frequency increases with age, peaking between 15 and 30 y
Colic	Persistent crying in infant	Duration of crying >4 hr/d for 3 or more d/wk	Normal	Stool: r/o blood, mucus	<3 mo
Constipation	Poor appetite, soiling, straining with stools	Possible tenderness over colon and small bowel, rectal fissures, encopresis, fewer than 3 stools per week	Hard or soft, may have blood on outer surface of stool	Abdominal radiograph Barium enema if unresponsive to intervention	Peaks between 2–4 y
Foreign body	Children may be asymptomatic *or* Coughing, choking, gagging, pain in throat or chest, anorexia, pain with swallowing	May have increased salivation, refusal to swallow, respiratory symptoms Normal abdominal exam	May see passage of FB	Chest radiograph if respiratory symptoms Abdominal radiograph if FB not seen to pass in stool or signs of abdominal pain/obstruction present	Highest incidence between 14 mo and 6 y
Gastroenteritis, viral or bacterial	Vomiting, diarrhea	General abdominal tenderness	Watery, bilious (green) vomitus, may or may not have blood in stool	Stool: *may* show bacteria, WBCs, blood, mucus	Any

Disorder	History/Symptoms	Physical Findings	Stool/Other	Diagnostic Evaluation	Age
Gastroesophageal reflux (chalasia)	Regurgitation, vomiting, irritability, recurrent pain after bedtime	Infants: gastric distention, effortless regurgitation during or after feedings; FTT, stridor, apnea, recurrent pneumonia, bronchospasm. Older children: vomiting, sour taste in mouth, abdominal pain, burning sensation in substernal area; chronic nocturnal cough, wheezing, pneumonia; dysphagia, nausea, FTT	Rare hematemesis	Barium swallow with fluoroscopy; 24-hr esophageal pH probe study. Esophageal manometry. Endoscopy for esophageal biopsy	Commonly 0–24 mo with 60–80% spontaneous resolution; can occur in specific disorders and in older children and adolescents
Hepatitis	Nausea, anorexia	Tender liver with or without spenomegaly, jaundice	Pale stools, diarrhea	Elevated ALT and AST. Mild elevations of LDH and alkaline phosphatase. Elevated bilirubin (direct and indirect). May have mild lymphocytosis. Hepatitis panel may show active or carrier status	Any–dependent on type of hepatitis
Hernia (strangulated)	Vomiting, crying	Distention, bulge in inguinal area	Fecal vomitus	None—refer for immediate surgical evaluation	70% occur in first year
Hirschsprung's disease	Failure to pass stool within 24 hr in an infant or rectal stimulation required to pass stools; history of constipation since infancy in children	FTT, abdominal distention, palpable stool throughout abdomen but empty rectal ampulla	May have diarrhea, bilious (green) vomiting	Abdominal radiograph. Barium enema. Rectal exam: absence of stool in rectal ampulla. Electrolytes, CBC	Infancy to adult
Inflammatory bowel diseases: Crohn	Umbilical or RLQ pain, diarrhea, weight loss, anorexia	Short stature, tender abdominal mass, fever, arthralgias or arthritis, perianal lesions	Loose and usually nonbloody stools unless anal fissures present	CBC, total protein, albumin, ESR, CRP. Stool for blood and WBCs. Bone age. Refer for endoscopy	Childhood and adolescence with peak at 20–30 y

Table continued on following page

T A B L E 33-6

Differential Diagnosis of Gastrointestinal Causes of Abdominal Pain in Children *Continued*

DISEASE	MAJOR SYMPTOMS	SIGNS	EXCRETA	TESTS	AGE OF ONSET
Ulcerative colitis	Weight loss, abdominal pain	Tender colon	Bloody stools	Same as above	Peak incidence at 16–20 y
Intestinal obstruction	Vomiting, abdominal distention; failure to pass feces in newborn after 24 hr; acute or gradual onset of periumbilical or lower abdominal pain	Alternating crampy and quiescent periods of periumbilical to lower abdominal pain; increased bowel sounds, obstipation	Bilious (green) emesis	Abdominal radiograph (flat, upright views)	Neonates; if occurs after 2 mo, usually due to intussusception or other causes
Intussusception	Episodic, cyclical abdominal pain with vomiting alternating with calm periods	Tender, sausage-shaped mass in RUQ, distension, legs drawn up at time of pain followed by periods of lethargy, absence of bowel sounds in RLQ. These "classic" symptoms occur in <50% of cases	Blood-tinged mucus ("currant jelly" stool); this occurs as a late sign	Abdominal ultrasound 100% reliable (abdominal radiography misses diagnosis in 33–55% of cases) Barium enema	70% <2 y old with peak incidence at 5 mo and 3 y. As age of onset increases, further pathology is often present
Irritable bowel	Recurrent, intermittent, dull, crampy abdominal pain, diarrhea or constipation	Intense thirst, fluctuating abdominal distension, increased bowel sounds; history of others in family with recurrent abdominal pain especially with social stimulation, travel, holidays, trauma; healthy appearance; borborygmus and flatus in school-age and older children; vague tenderness in RLQ, LLQ, and epigastrium; pain usually not related to eating or defecation; occasional pallor and nausea	Watery, malodorous stools; first stool of day may be formed, followed by 3 + watery stools through the day	CBC, ESR, UA, stools for O&P and occult blood Abdominal ultrasonography Upper GI series with small bowel follow-through	5–15 y

Lactose intolerance	Bloating, gaseousness, crampy abdominal pain	Pain and diarrhea within hours of lactose ingestion; may have history of recent severe viral gastroenteritis. In infants: vomiting, distention, abdominal pain after lactose-containing formula or bovine milk ingestion by breastfeeding mother	Acidic diarrhea	Breath hydrogen test after lactose challenge; Reducing substances in stool; Lack of normal increase in blood glucose after ingestion of lactose	5–15 y, rare in infancy; prominent in some ethnic groups
Mesenteric lymphadenitis	Fever, vomiting	Right-sided (RLQ often) or diffuse tenderness		Abdominal ultrasonography may show mesenteric adenitis	
Meckel diverticulum	Painless rectal bleeding	Anemia, periumbilical or lower abdominal pain may be manifested similar to appendicitis or volvulus	Bloody stools	CBC; Stools for occult blood; Refer for surgical consultation	65% incidence in children <5 y old with peak at 2 y
Necrotizing enterocolitis	Feeding intolerance; abdomen distended, tense, and tender	Possible palpable abdominal mass and cellulitis of abdominal wall, GI bleeding, shock		CBC, chemistry panel; Abdominal radiograph/ultrasound	Premature and term infants
Parasites	Parasite dependent: possibly diarrhea, bloating, distention, flatulence	Parasite dependent: rectal itching, weight loss, malaise, cough, hepatomegaly, vague abdominal pain, anemia	May or may not have diarrhea, which may be bloody, greasy, or foul smelling; visible worms in stool or vomitus	Stools for O&P; CBC: may show increased eosinophils	Any

Table continued on following page

T A B L E 33-6

Differential Diagnosis of Gastrointestinal Causes of Abdominal Pain in Children *Continued*

DISEASE	MAJOR SYMPTOMS	SIGNS	EXCRETA	TESTS	AGE OF ONSET
Peptic ulcer disease	Poor appetite, weakness, epigastric pain with or without nausea	Vague abdominal pain or RLQ localization; epigastric tenderness, which can occur at night; vomiting	Black stools or coffee-ground vomitus	CBC Stool for occult blood Upper GI series Serum IgG antibody for *Helicobacter pylori* Urea breath test	Any, usually above 8 y
Recurrent abdominal pain	At least 3 episodes of abdominal pain over 3-mo period	Periumbilical to generalized abdominal pain, sometimes sharp or dull and lasting 1–3 hr; occasional nausea/ vomiting	Normal	CBC, ESR, chemistry screen UA and urine culture Stool O&P, culture, pH, reducing substances	Usually between 6 and 19 y with peak at 9 y
Volvulus or malrotation	Bilious (green) vomiting	Abdominal distention, GI bleeding, palpable epigastric mass, dehydration, lethargy, shock	May be bloody	CBC Abdominal radiograph Barium enema Upper GI series Refer immediately for surgical consultation	First month of life

Table developed by Catherine Blosser with information from Burg F et al (1996); Teitelbaum SJ et al (1999); Behrman RE, Kliegman RM (1998); Finberg L (1998); Irish MS et al (1998); Kaye R et al (1988).

ALT = alanine aminotransferase; AST = aspartate aminotransferase; CBC = complete blood count; CRP = C-reactive protein; ESR = erythrocyte sedimentation rate; FB = foreign body; FTT = failure to thrive; GI = gastrointestinal; LDH = lactate dehydrogenase; LLQ = left lower quadrant; O&P = ova and parasites; RLQ = right lower quadrant; r/o = rule out; RUQ = right upper quadrant; UA = urinalysis; WBCs = white blood cells.

negative childbirth experience, unsatisfying interactions among family members, and overstimulation. The parents' inability to accurately read and respond to the infant's cries may contribute to colic. The infant may become overstimulated, underfed, or overfed. Colicky babies have a low sensory threshold (Carey, 1972). The stress created by a crying baby contributes to ineffective parental interventions and can exacerbate the problem.

Incidence

Colic has been estimated to occur in about one third of all infants. A study that defined colic as "paroxysms of crying for 3 or more hours per day for 3 days or more per week during a period of at least 3 weeks" found an incidence of 13% (Lehtonen & Korvenranta, 1995).

Clinical Findings

HISTORY. Parents or caregivers report that the infant is less than 3 months old and cries 3 or more hours a day for 3 or more days per week (Fleisher, 1998). Additional findings include the following:

- Demands frequent feeding and is often fussy while feeding
- Has excessive gas
- Is inconsolable or is comforted for short periods only
- Is "tense" or "tight" and keeps the legs stiff and fists clenched tightly

PHYSICAL EXAMINATION. If possible, see the family during a crying time. A thorough examination must be completed to rule out other pathology and should include:

- Evaluation of growth parameters
- Abdominal examination for masses, tenderness, and bowel sounds
- Stool for blood or mucus

Differential Diagnosis

All other causes of abdominal pain are in the differential diagnosis (see Table 33-6).

Management

1. No cure is known for infantile colic. The goal of treatment is to manage the situation until the colic resolves itself. Parents and providers who are flexible, creative, and persistent in seeking solutions are most likely to be successful. See Table 33-7 for management strategies.
2. Medications (e.g., simethicone) are ineffective in treating colic. Sedation for either the parent or the child is sometimes indicated in extreme cases (Behrman et al., 1996). It

T A B L E 33-7
Management Strategies for Infantile Colic

Acknowledge the importance of the concern.
Provide support for the parents.
Affirm the baby's good health.
Remind the parents that colic is temporary.
Reinforce parents' efforts to comfort their infant.
Encourage parents to take time off from child care by finding assistance from family or friends.
Inform parents that the stress they feel is sensed by the infant, which may cause more crying.
Allow parents to express feelings of anger, guilt, and frustration.
Inform parents of equipment sold to soothe babies (vibrating infant seats and cribs).
Share anecdotal reports of using noise from hair dryers or vacuum cleaners or a ride in the car to calm the infant.
Implement strategies to calm the infant (decrease in environmental stimulation, swaddling the infant, carrying the infant, firm and gentle pressure to the abdomen, rocking, swinging).
Ensure proper feeding (e.g., correct latch-on, frequent burping, avoidance of early addition of solids, change in diet if lactose intolerance or milk allergy is a problem).
Have the parents keep a diary of the baby's crying for analysis by the health-care provider; a diary may assist in identifying patterns that can lead to interventions.

Data from Dihigo S: New strategies for the treatment of colic: Modifying the parent/infant interaction, J Pediatr Health Care 12(5):256–262, 1998; Fleisher D: Coping with colic. Contemp Pediatr 15(6):144–156, 1998; Cervisi J, Chapman M, Niklas B, et al: Office management of the infant with colic, J Pediatr Health Care 5:184–190, 1991.

may also give the parents "something to do," but it can potentiate the myth of a physical cause.

Complications

Stress created by a crying baby can contribute to parental feelings of hostility, anger, and guilt, ultimately leading to poor parent–child interaction. Parents may be driven to physical or emotional abuse.

Acute Abdominal Pain

Description

The location and character of abdominal pain can be helpful in identifying the disease process. Visceral pain is generally dull and diffuse. Visceral pain fibers are located in the muscular wall of hollow viscera and the capsule of solid viscera. Visceral nerves are stimulated by tension and stretching. Parietal pain is usually sharp, localized, and stimulated by inflammation in the parietal peritoneum. The shared innervation of many abdominal organs leads to poor localization of pain.

Epigastric pain usually indicates pain from the liver, pancreas, biliary tree, stomach, and upper part of the small bowel.

Periumbilical pain is generated from the distal end of the small intestine, cecum, appendix, and ascending colon.

Suprapubic discomfort indicates distal intestine, urinary tract, and pelvic organ dysfunction.

Referred pain is usually sharp, localized pain felt in remote areas innervated by the same nerves as the affected organ. When visceral pain is overwhelming, referred pain occurs. ·

Acute, continuous pain is more indicative of an acute process.

Etiology

Primary GI causes of abdominal pain include appendicitis, viral and bacterial enteritis, inflammatory bowel disease, intussusception, pancreatitis, cholecystitis, and liver dysfunction.

Primary extragastrointestinal causes of abdominal pain include ovarian cyst, salpingitis, sexually transmitted diseases, otitis media, pneumonia, pharyngitis, UTI, Henoch-Schönlein purpura, rheumatic fever, sickle cell disease, pleurisy, kidney pain, rectal or uterine disease, and hernia. Referred pain in the shoulder can be generated from pneumonia, subphrenic abscess, pleurisy, pancreatitis, and the spleen, gallbladder, and liver. Testicular pain occurs with kidney disease and appendicitis. Back pain can also accompany retroperitoneal hematoma, pancreatitis, and rectal or uterine disease (Barkin & Rosen, 1999; Caty & Azizkahn, 1997).

Clinical Findings

HISTORY. The history should assess the following:

- Family history of gallbladder disease, hernia, kidney or liver disease, and so forth
- Past medical history of illnesses/surgeries
- History of trauma or abuse
- Pain: onset, location, duration, distribution, quality, radiation; shifting, awakening from sleep
- Activity level
- Appetite and food intake
- History of recent infection
- Fever (high fever usually not associated with acute abdomen)
- Nausea, vomiting, diarrhea, or constipation
- Aggravating/alleviating factors
- Hematuria, dysuria, frequency, incontinence
- Menstrual history and last period, vaginal discharge, sexual activity, birth control, and penile discharge

PHYSICAL EXAMINATION. Adolescents should be examined with parents out of the room (for privacy and to elicit a complete history). The following are needed for all children:

- Complete physical examination
- Weight and vital signs (temperature, heart rate, respiratory rate, and blood pressure)
- Abdominal examination, including rectal examination, psoas and obturator signs, rebound tenderness, decreased bowel sounds

- Pelvic examination as indicated
- Repeated examinations as necessary to observe for changes
- See Differential Diagnosis for specific findings; also see section on Appendicitis and Intussusception

DIAGNOSTIC TESTS. The following are performed as indicated:

- CBC with differential, serum electrolytes, ESR, amylase, pregnancy test (as indicated by the history and examination)
- UA and urine culture
- Stool for occult blood
- Pelvic examination—gonococcal and/or chlamydial culture, Papanicolaou smear, vaginal smears
- Abdominal radiograph
- Chest radiograph, anteroposterior and lateral as indicated to rule out pneumonia
- Abdominal or pelvic ultrasonography or both

Differential Diagnosis

See Table 33-6 and Figure 33-1.

Management

Treatment involves the following:

1. Consultation and referral, including surgery as indicated
2. No sedatives or pain medication until the diagnosis is made
3. Intravenous rehydration and gastric decompression as necessary
4. Treatment of the cause

Complications

Complications include ruptured viscera, intra-abdominal bleeding, strangulation leading to ischemia of the gut, and shock leading to death.

Appendicitis

Description

Appendicitis is inflammation of the appendix.

Etiology

Initiated by obstruction of the appendiceal lumen by a fecalith, lymphoid tissue, tumor, parasite, foreign body, or inspissated cystic fibrosis secretions, the appendix becomes distended and subject to ischemia and necrosis. Peritoneal inflammation around the infected appendix causes the characteristic symptoms.

Incidence

Appendicitis is the most common reason for abdominal surgery in childhood. Frequency increases with age, and the peak incidence is between 15 and 30 years. Children younger than 8 years have twice the perforation rate of those older than 8 years (Irish et al., 1998).

Clinical Findings

HISTORY. The following may be reported:

- Diffuse abdominal pain leading to RLQ pain
- Anorexia, vomiting, diarrhea, or constipation
- Low-grade fever
- Evolution of the process over 12 hours, with the potential for infants and young children to become sick much more quickly
- Most comfortable position on the side with the legs flexed
- Infants demonstrating irritability, pain with movement, flexed hips
- Child possibly becoming quiet because crying hurts

PHYSICAL EXAMINATION. A complete physical examination is necessary. Reexamination may be needed in 4 to 6 hours. The following can be found:

- Presence of guarding, rebound tenderness, maximal pain over the McBurney point (1½ to 2 in. from the iliac crest, along a line between the iliac crest and umbilicus) on abdominal examination
- Tenderness and possibly a mass on the right side on rectal examination
- Inability to stand straight or climb stairs
- Psoas and/or obturator signs positive

Differential Diagnosis

Accidental Injury
Accidental Ingestion
Anaphylactoid Purpura
Appendicitis
Child Abuse
Constipation

Ectopic Pregnancy
Food Intolerance
Gastroenteritis
Hemolytic Uremic Syndrome
Mechanical Obstruction
Mononucleosis

Pneumonia
Renal Stones
Sickle Cell Anemia
Tortion of Ovary or Testicle
Trauma
Urinary Tract Infection
Viral Syndrome

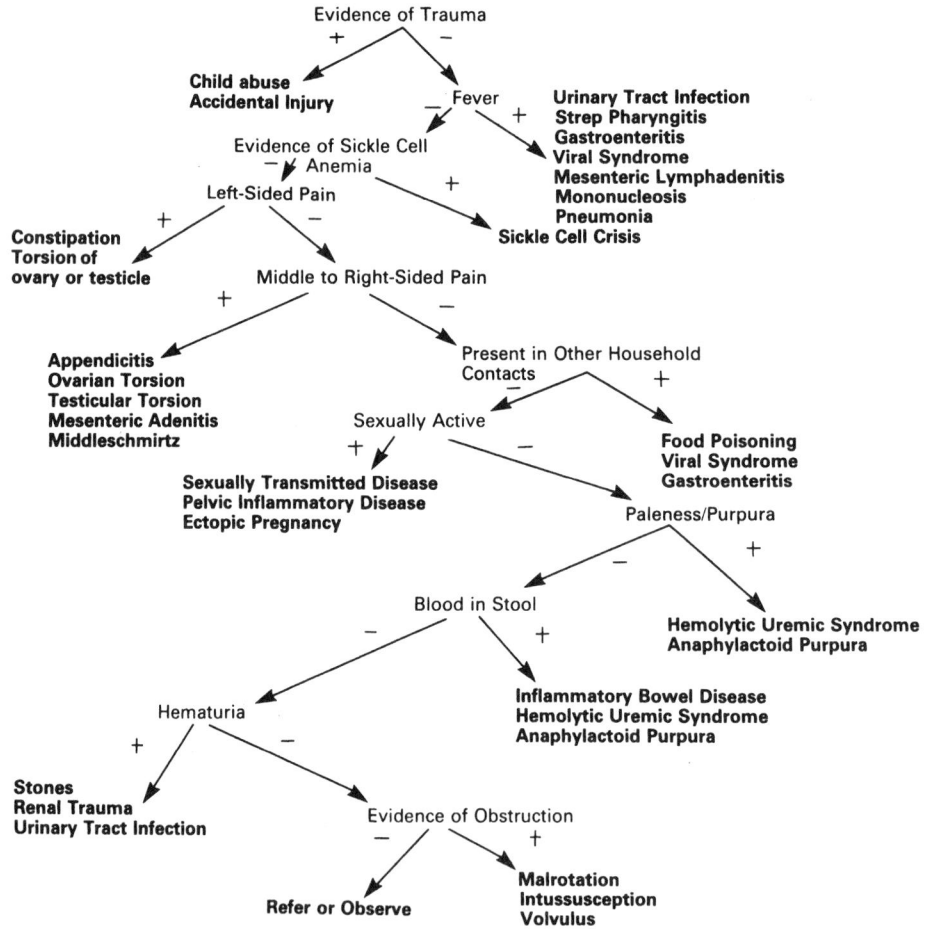

F I G U R E 33-1

Decision tree for differential diagnosis of acute abdominal pain. (From Schwartz MW, Curry TA, Sargent AJ, et al [eds]: Pediatric Primary Care: A Problem-Oriented Approach, 3rd ed. St Louis, CV Mosby, 1997.)

DIAGNOSTIC TESTS. The following may be noted with appendicitis:

- CBC with differential shows increased neutrophils ($>$10,000/mm^3).
- UA can show pyuria.
- Examination of stool may demonstrate blood and pus (rare finding).
- Abdominal radiographs can show a fecalith, especially if rupture has occurred.
- Ultrasonography demonstrates abnormality.

Differential Diagnosis

The differential diagnosis includes viral gastroenteritis (fever and crampy abdominal pain with vomiting, diarrhea, or both), constipation, UTI (fever, chills, and urinary symptoms), pelvic inflammatory disease or organ pathology, pneumonia, duodenal ulcer (gnawing and burning), intestinal obstruction (crampy pain), peritonitis (worse pain when jumping or coughing), and intussusception (child younger than 2 years with a RUQ mass).

Management

1. A surgical consultation for an appendectomy is needed.
2. Intravenous and preoperative antibiotics are given if perforation is suspected.
3. Patients should be seen in follow-up 2 to 4 weeks after surgery. If appetite, bowel function, energy, and activity level are normal, no pain or fever is present, findings on physical examination are normal, and the wound is well healed, the child can resume unrestricted activity.
4. If at the 2- to 4-week follow-up the child has signs of delayed infection, abnormal bowel function, or unexplained weight loss, refer back to the surgeon (Irish et al., 1998).

Complications

Perforation, peritonitis, pelvic abscess, ileus, obstruction, sepsis, shock, and death can occur.

Intussusception

Description

The invagination of bowel begins proximal to the ileocecal valve and is usually ileocolic, but it can be ileoileal or colocolic. Swelling, hemorrhage, incarceration, and necrosis of the bowel requiring bowel resection may occur (Irish et al., 1998).

Etiology

The cause is not generally apparent. Polyps, Meckel diverticulum, Henoch-Schönlein purpura, constipation, lymphomas, lipomas, parasites, rotavirus, adenovirus, and foreign bodies can be predisposing factors. Intussusception may be a complication of cystic fibrosis.

Incidence

Intussusception is the most common cause of intestinal obstruction in the first 2 years of life, with males predominating by a 3:2 ratio. The peak incidence is between 5 and 9 months of age. The incidence is increased in the spring, summer, and the middle of winter (Irish et al., 1998).

Clinical Findings

HISTORY. The following can be reported:

- Paroxysmal, episodic abdominal pain with vomiting every 5 to 30 minutes
- Screaming with drawing up of the legs
- Periods of calm or lethargy between episodes
- Stool possibly diarrheal in nature with blood ("currant jelly")
- Fever sometimes present
- Possible severe prostration

PHYSICAL EXAMINATION
- Observe the baby's appearance and behavior over a period of time.
- A sausage-like mass in the RUQ of the abdomen may be felt (in 85%) (Irish et al., 1998).
- The abdomen is often distended and tender to palpation.

DIAGNOSTIC TESTS

- An abdominal flat plate radiograph can appear normal (Fig. 33-2).
- A barium enema is diagnostic and frequently therapeutic (80 to 90%) (Irish et al., 1998)
- Abdominal ultrasonography may be helpful.

Differential Diagnosis

The differential diagnosis includes incarcerated hernia, testicular torsion, acute gastroenteritis, appendicitis, colic, and intestinal obstruction.

Management

The following steps are taken:

1. Emergency management and intervention with a pediatric surgical consultation
2. Barium enema
3. Surgery if perforation is suspected or barium enema fails
4. Intravenous antibiotics with suspected perforation

Complications

Perforation, sepsis, shock, and reintussusception (5 to 10% in nonoperative reduction) (Irish et al., 1998) can all occur.

Recurrent Abdominal Pain

Description

RAP is defined as a minimum of three episodes of abdominal pain occurring over a 3-month period. It is differentiated from chronic abdominal pain in that each episode of RAP is distinct and separated by periods of wellness (Pearl et al., 1998).

Etiology

The cause of the pain remains unclear, but it is a genuine pain. A localized increase in intraluminal pressure may cause stretching of the intestinal wall leading to functional abdominal pain. Intestinal dysmotility can prevent normal movement of intestinal contents and cause local distention, which is perceived as pain. The term *biopsychosocial dysfunctional pain* has been applied to children with RAP.

Affected children have an involuntary predisposition for the development of physiologic pain (e.g., a family history of RAP). Temperament and personality can make the child more vulnerable to environmental stressors (often minor) that precipitate the sensation of pain. Children who are perfectionists or dependent or who have low self-esteem may be more likely to experience RAP. Maternal depression, overprotectiveness, and poor conflict resolution in the household are also contributing factors. Occasionally a precipitating event occurs, but commonly none is found. Positive and negative reinforcement of the pain can modify the RAP (Nurko, 1999b; Poole et al., 1995).

Incidence

RAP occurs in 10 to 15% of children between the ages of 4 and 16 years. Males and females are affected equally until the age of 9, and then the incidence in males decreases (Boyle, 1997). Approximately 10% of children with RAP have an organic etiology (Pearl et al., 1998).

Clinical Findings

HISTORY. The history can include the following:

- Complete review of systems
- Careful psychosocial history (home, school, parents, friends)
- Episodes described as vague and paroxysmal
- Periumbilical, generalized, sharp or dull, constant or intermittent pain reported
- Pain occurring on a daily basis and lasting 1 to 3 hours with complete recovery between episodes
- Nighttime pain rare
- Pain often accompanied by a dramatic reaction (clutching abdomen, doubling over, or throwing self to ground)
- School attendance affected
- Slight or no fever, nausea, and vomiting
- Bowel habits rarely affected

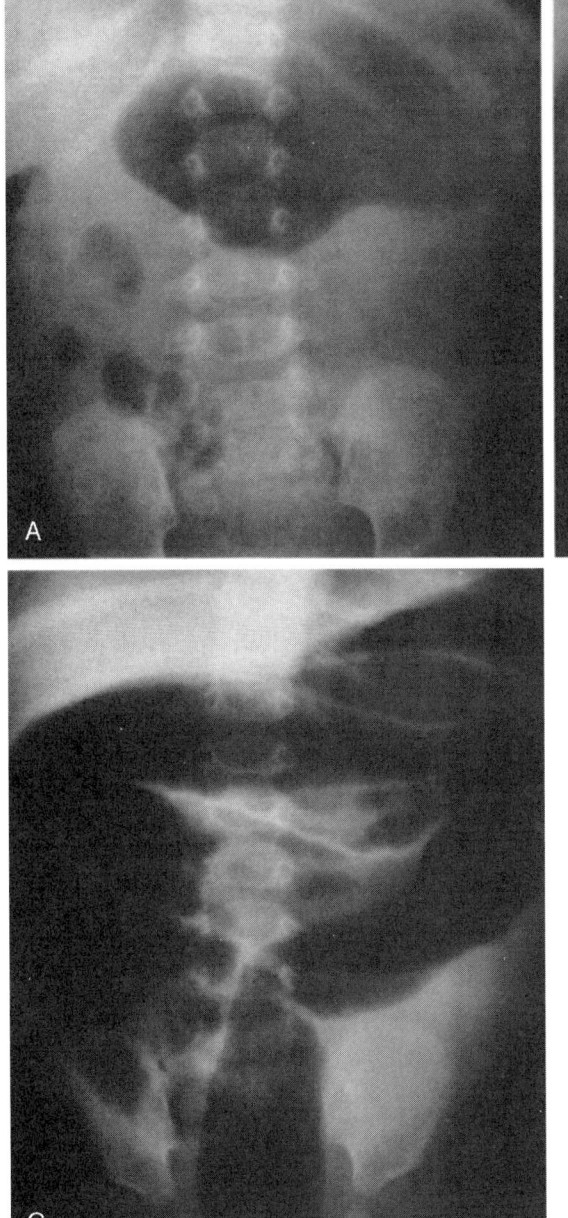

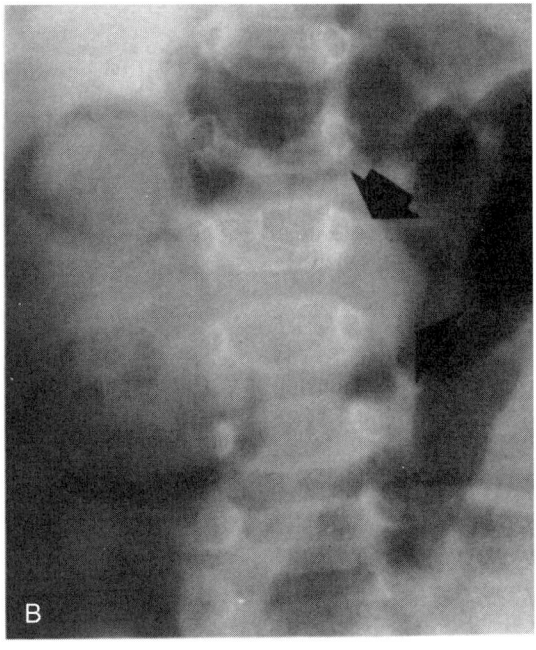

FIGURE 33-2

Intussusception. *A*, Plain abdominal radiograph demonstrating a gas-filled stomach and relatively little gas in the distal end of the bowel. This baby had typical clinical features of intussusception and a palpable upper abdominal mass. Therefore, an enema with air was performed. *B*, The intussusception *(arrows)* is outlined by air. *C*, Reduction is proved by air refluxing into loops of small bowel. (From Burg FD, Ingelfinger JR, Wald ER, et al [eds]: Gellis & Kagan's Current Pediatric Therapy, ed 15. Philadelphia, WB Saunders, 1999.)

- Complex rituals—hot pads, repositioning, gentle rubbing by parent—the only providers of relief (Nurko, 1999b)
- Parental history of recurrent abdominal pain
- Medication taken for pain does not alleviate pain
- Illicit drug use
- Sexual activity or abuse and possibility of pregnancy
- Functional or autonomic symptoms (nausea, vomiting, pallor, perspiration, flushing, palpitations, headache)

PHYSICAL EXAMINATION. The physical examination is usually normal but should include the following:

- Abdominal examination: presence of pain, rebound tenderness, masses
- Perianal and rectal examination
- Weight and height plotted on growth curves
- Vital signs (temperature, heart rate, respiratory rate, blood pressure)
- Complete neurological examination
- Pelvic examination as indicated
- Examination of skin and joints for lesions, swelling, discoloration
- Reexamination during an acute episode
- Complete reexamination with each recurrent visit

DIAGNOSTIC TESTS. The following are ordered as indicated:

- CBC with differential, ESR, albumin, liver and renal function tests if question of organic cause or systemic illness
- UA and urine culture to rule out infection
- Stool for occult blood, pH, reducing substances, culture, and ova and parasites
- Breath hydrogen testing if concerned about carbohydrate malabsorption (lactose intolerance)
- See Table 33-8.

Differential Diagnosis

See Figure 33-3. The following are included in the differential diagnosis:

- All organic causes of abdominal pain, including urinary tract, GI tract, and extraabdominal causes

TABLE 33-8

Diagnostic Criteria for Recurrent Abdominal Pain

Documentation of chronicity
Compatible age range, age of onset
Characteristic features of abdominal pain
Evidence of physical or psychological stressful stimuli
Environmental reinforcement of pain behavior
Normal physical examination (including rectal examination and stool guaiac)
Normal laboratory evaluation (complete blood count, sedimentation rate, urinalysis, urine culture, stool ovum and parasites)

From Boyle JT: Recurrent abdominal pain: An update. Pediatr Rev 18:314, 1997.

- Lactose intolerance (usually involving diarrhea, belching, flatulence, and bloating)
- Organic causes of abdominal pain (pain at night, weight loss, and recurrent fever)
- Abdominal pain associated with depression (usually includes social isolation, decreased activity and attention span, difficulty sleeping, and irritability)
- School avoidance (usually associated with severe pain and anxiety on weekday mornings only)
- Irritable bowel syndrome (usually has onset of pain after age 14)

Management

Functional disorders and organic diseases are managed as follows:

1. Functional disorder:
   - Suggest that the pain can be functional (inorganic) early in the visit. Assure the patient and family that the symptoms are real and that they will not be ignored.
   - Reassure the patient and family that no organic cause is present, which is good, and that the child is in no physical danger.
   - Discuss how stressful events and emotional issues might affect the pain.
   - Encourage return to school, normalization of lifestyle, and deemphasis on pain episodes.

Differential Diagnosis

Bacterial enteritis
Collagen vascular disease
Constipation
Enteritis

Functional
Inflammatory bowel disease
Lactase deficiency
Pancreatitis

Tumor
Ureteropelvic obstruction
Urinary tract infection

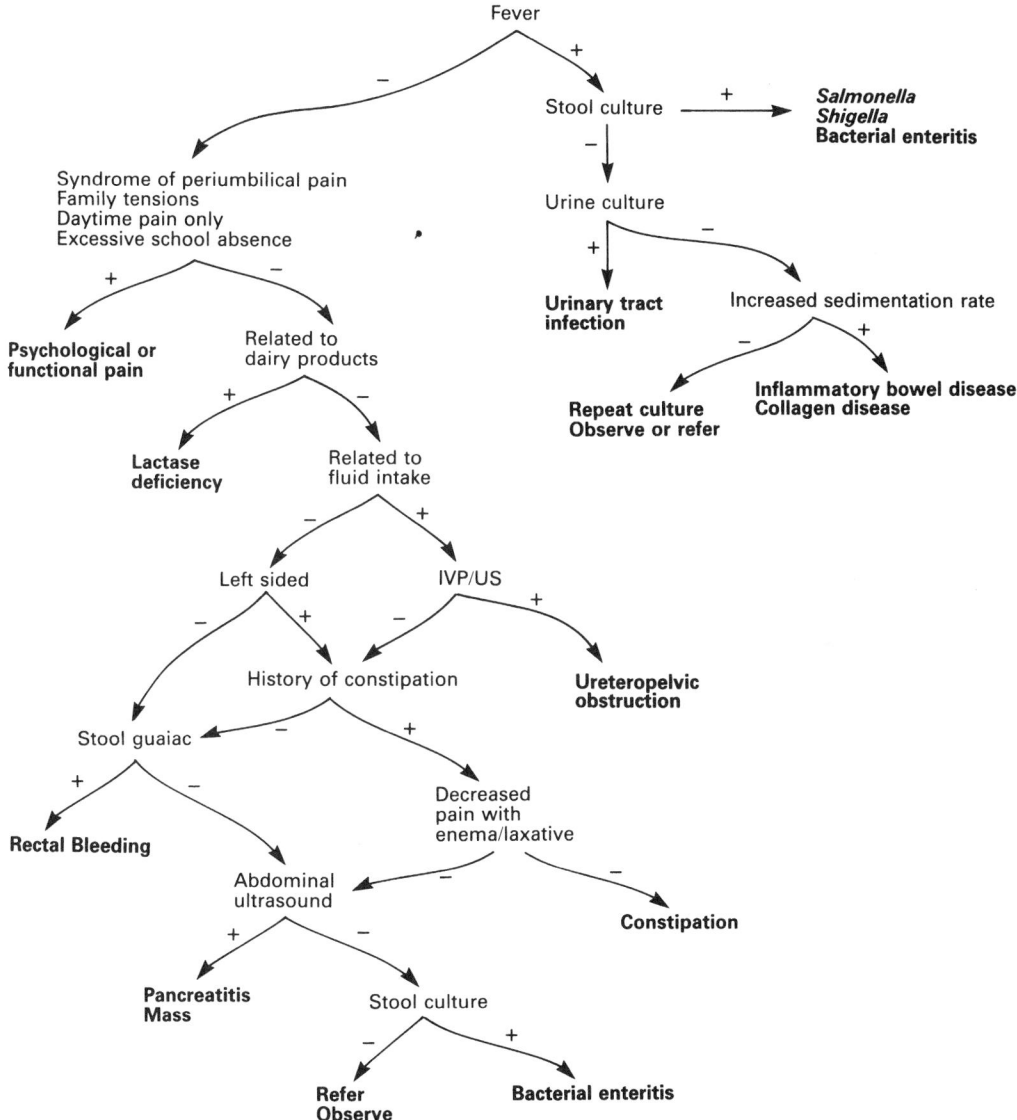

FIGURE 33-3
Decision tree for the differential diagnosis of chronic abdominal pain. (From Schwartz MW, Curry TA, Sargent AJ, et al [eds]: Pediatric Primary Care: A Problem-Oriented Approach, 3rd ed. St Louis, CV Mosby, 1997.)

- Recommend increased dietary fiber if constipation is an issue.
- Inform parents and child that medications generally do not help.
- Refer for psychological dysfunction (maladaptive behavior, conversion reaction, depression, anxiety).
- Discuss "red flags" (Table 33-9) so that the parents/child can identify changes in status and illness.
2. Organic disease:
- Refer for organic problem or breath hydrogen testing.
- Establish regular follow-up.

T A B L E 33-9

"Red Flags" to Consider in Recurrent Abdominal Pain

Positive family history of GI problems (not recurrent abdominal pain)
No stressful life events
No school absences
No evidence of need to be high achiever
Anorexia
Diarrhea
Pain related to mealtimes
Vomiting/bloody emesis
Extraintestinal symptoms (rash, joint pain, dysuria)
Sleepiness following pain
Night awakening
Change in bowel habits, dysuria, polyuria, menstrual problems
Sexual activity
Weight loss
Growth deceleration
Child keeping eyes open during examination
Localized pain away from umbilicus
Anemia
Elevated ESR
Abnormal UA/UC
Blood in stool

ESR = erythrocyte sedimentation rate; UA = urinalysis; UC = urine culture.
Data from Pearl RH, Irish MS, Caty MG, et al: The approach to common abdominal diagnoses in infants and children, part 2, Pediatr Clin North Am 45:1287–1326, 1998; Boyle JT: Recurrent abdominal pain: An update, Pediatr Rev 18(9): 310–320, 1997; Pierce C: What not to do for a child with recurrent abdominal pain, Pediatr News March 25, 1995.

Malabsorption Syndromes

Description

The inability to digest or absorb dietary nutrients leads to malabsorption syndromes. Children can be nearly asymptomatic or suffer from severe malnutrition and FTT.

Etiology and Incidence

Malabsorption syndromes are not disease entities themselves but, rather, manifestations of other problems. Improperly absorbed carbohydrates act as osmotic laxatives that pull fluid and electrolytes into the intestine. Carbohydrates are fermented in the bowel and produce abdominal distention and excessive flatus. Fats and proteins can also be malabsorbed and cause symptoms. Lactose malabsorption is the most common malabsorption syndrome.

Malabsorption secondary to infection may occur. Postinfectious diarrhea is most common in children. Prolonged infection or damage to the intestinal mucosa from the infecting organism may prolong the diarrhea for weeks. The damaged intestine is unable to absorb nutrients appropriately, which causes an osmotic pull of fluid into the intestine, decreased reabsorption of bile acids, and fermentation leading to the diarrhea (Lencer & Wolf, 1999; Taluson-Soriano & Lake, 1996).

Clinical Findings

HISTORY. The history can include the following:

- Symptoms that vary by cause
- Chronic diarrhea with frequent, large, foul-smelling, pale stools
- May not have diarrhea
- Excessive flatus with abdominal distention
- Increased appetite
- Growth failure (a common symptom of nutritional deficiency and malabsorption)
- Pallor, fatigue, hair and dermatological abnormalities, dizziness, cheilosis, glossitis, peripheral neuropathy (symptoms of vitamin deficiency seen with malabsorption)

A complete dietary history is needed to distinguish between undernutrition and malabsorption. Aversions occur to foods that precipitate symptoms. Note that delayed puberty can coexist with malabsorption. Past surgical and trauma history is needed.

PHYSICAL EXAMINATION. The following should be included:

- Growth parameters and percentiles
- Skinfold thickness and lean body mass
- Tanner stage
- Examination for delayed growth and puberty, which can be seen with significant malabsorption

DIAGNOSTIC TESTS. The following are ordered as indicated:

- Stool assessment for occult blood, ova and parasites, white blood cells, and culture; liquid stool for pH and reducing substances; 72-hour fecal fat collection or Sudan stain for stool fat
- CBC with differential, serum calcium, phosphorus, alkaline phosphatase, total protein, ferritin, folate, and liver function tests
- Lactose and sucrose breath hydrogen testing
- Bone age

Differential Diagnosis

FTT, short stature, chronic diarrhea, CF, immune deficiency, hepatic disease, inflammatory bowel disease, and celiac disease are included in the differential diagnosis.

Management

1. Treat persistent enteric infection.
2. Identify and avoid offending foods. If malabsorption is a primary problem, lifelong food avoidance may be necessary. If it is a secondary problem, retrial of the food at intervals can be attempted.

Foreign Bodies in the Gastrointestinal Tract

Description

Most swallowed foreign bodies pass through the GI tract without difficulty. Some objects get lodged at points of narrowing (cricopharyngeal muscle, the carina, Schatzki ring, cardioesophageal junction, ligament of Treitz). Anything 3 to 5 cm or larger might have trouble passing the ligament of Treitz.

Etiology and Incidence

The cause is a swallowed foreign body, with the highest incidence occurring between 6 months and 6 years of age (Muñiz & Jaffe, 1997). Foreign body ingestion occurs equally in boys and girls, with developmentally delayed children at higher risk. Common items include coins (most commonly pennies), food, toys, marbles, buttons, and batteries.

Clinical Findings

HISTORY
- No history of swallowing a foreign body is in up to 40% of cases (Muñiz & Jaffe, 1997).
- Initially the child might have experienced a coughing, choking, or gagging episode (although this episode might not have been observed by the parents).
- Subsequent symptoms can include discomfort in the throat or chest, refusal to eat, increased salivation, vomiting, pain with swallowing, and respiratory difficulty (Karjoo, 1998).

PHYSICAL EXAMINATION
- Most children are asymptomatic (Muñiz & Jaffe, 1997).
- GI examination is normal.
- Respiratory symptoms may be found if the foreign body is lodged in the esophagus and pressing on the trachea.

DIAGNOSTIC TESTS
- If symptoms of obstruction persist, radiographic studies are ordered to rule out a foreign body. A dime is 17 mm, a penny is 18 mm, a nickel is 20 mm, and a quarter is 23 mm.
- A contrast study or forced expiratory film is needed if a foreign body is suspected but is not radiopaque.
- Abdominal radiographs can be ordered if an object has not been seen in the stool

and symptoms of distress or obstruction are present.
- An alternative to radiography is a hand-held metal detector.

Management

1. If asymptomatic or if the foreign body is in the stomach or intestine, no intervention is necessary and the family can be reassured. Smooth objects, buttons, and most coins can remain in the intestines for months without symptoms. The exception is new, mostly zinc pennies, which can cause a chemical reaction and poisoning. Watch for fecal passage and report any new associated symptoms. Follow-up radiography is indicated after 2 weeks if a coin has not been identified in stool.
2. If symptomatic, the child is given nothing by mouth until a decision is made. Consultation with the physician and pediatric surgeon is necessary. Generally, foreign bodies remaining in the esophagus longer than 3 hours or in the small intestine longer than 5 days need to be removed. Open safety pins or sharp objects, wooden toothpicks, and small batteries also need to be removed. Removal is often accomplished via a Foley catheter technique or by gastroesophagoscopy.

Complications

Perforation or stricture formation can occur in up to 10% of children.

Prevention

Parent education, anticipatory counseling, and careful supervision of children are needed. Avoid ear piercing in children younger than 2 years because earrings are easily ingested.

Anal Fissure

Description

Anal fissures are small tears in the anal mucosa.

Etiology and Incidence

The usual cause of an anal fissure is passage of frequent or hard stools. Anal stenosis and other trauma can also be causative factors. Anal fissures are the most common cause of rectal bleeding in all pediatric groups.

Clinical Findings

HISTORY. The following can be reported:

- Crying with stooling
- Bright red streaks of blood in the stool or diaper
- Withholding of stool

PHYSICAL EXAMINATION. With the patient in the knee–chest position and the anus slightly everted, small tears in the anal mucosa can be visible. An otoscope with a large speculum is needed if the external fissures are not readily visible. A digital anal examination with the fifth finger rules out anal stenosis (Muñiz & Jaffe, 1997).

Differential Diagnosis

Other sources of lower intestinal hemorrhage such as infection, formula intolerance, necrotizing enterocolitis, intussusception, juvenile polyps, hemolytic-uremic syndrome, Henoch-Schönlein purpura, irritable bowel disease, and vascular lesions are included in the differential diagnosis.

Management

1. Treat the cause.
2. Local wound care should include sitz baths twice a day and application of 0.5% hydrocortisone cream or K-Y jelly to the anus.

Complications

Recurrence of fissures is common (e.g., constipation causes a fissure, which leads to a retention–constipation cycle) (Sondheimer & Silverman, 1997).

Prevention

Preventive measures include the following:

- Avoid constipation.
- Encourage regular toileting habits.
- Avoid the use of laxative medications and enemas.

▆ INFLAMMATORY BOWEL DISEASES

Crohn Disease

Description

Crohn disease is a chronic inflammatory disease with exacerbations and remissions involving any portion of the intestinal tract. Areas of intestine that are unaffected are called skip areas.

Etiology and Incidence

The cause is largely unknown. The disease is probably a genetically determined response that is immunologically mediated. Crohn disease has a multifactorial basis (heredity, diet, immunological aberrations, and ineffective mucosal integrity) that is probably influenced by environmental factors (Israel, 1999). The disease occurs in 16 of every 100,000 individuals, affects males and females equally, and is more common in white people. Twenty-five percent to 40% of cases are diagnosed in childhood and adolescence. Siblings are 17 to 35 times more likely to get Crohn disease than the general population is (Winesett, 1997; Hyams, 1996).

Clinical Findings

HISTORY. The following can be reported:

- Fever
- Weight loss (average of 5 to 7 kg)
- Delayed growth
- Arthralgias/arthritis in large joints, occasional joint destruction
- Obstructive symptoms associated with meals
- Pain in the umbilical region and RLQ; may awaken at night
- Anorexia
- Malabsorption and lactose intolerance
- Bloody diarrhea and pain with stooling
- Mouth sores, especially during exacerbations of the illness

PHYSICAL EXAMINATION. An abdominal examination is performed while observing for RLQ tenderness and a mass. Perianal skin tags, deep anal fissures, and perianal fistulas strongly suggest Crohn disease. Clubbing of digits may be present. Erythema nodosum is common.

DIAGNOSTIC TESTS. The following are ordered as needed:

- CBC, total protein, albumin, ESR, CRP
- Stool for culture, ova, parasites, and *Clostridium difficile* (with recent antibiotic use)
- Stool for blood and white blood cells
- Bone age (usually delayed by 2 years)

Differential Diagnosis

Rheumatoid arthritis, systemic lupus erythematosus, hypopituitarism, acute appendicitis, peptic ulcer, intestinal obstruction, and intestinal lymphoma are included in the differential diagnosis (Sondheimer & Silverman, 1997).

Management

The goals of therapy are to (1) control the disease and induce a lasting remission; (2) prevent relapses; and (3) achieve normal nutrition, growth, and lifestyle. Treatment is pharmacological, nutritional, surgical, and psychosocial (Mascarenas & Altschuler, 1997). The following management steps are taken:

1. Refer for endoscopy, definitive diagnosis, consultation, and follow-up care, which can include the following:
   - Steroids orally, rectally, or intravenously for acute exacerbations. Not intended for use in remission
   - Aminosalicylates (sulfasalazine, olsalazine, and mesalamine) given topically (enema) or orally
   - Immunomodulatory agents (azathioprine, 6-mecaptopurine, methotrexate, and cyclosporine)
   - Antibiotics for acute exacerbation (ampicillin, gentamicin, clindamycin, or metronidazole)

- Metronidazole (Flagyl) prophylaxis (15 mg/kg per day) for perianal disease until the patient has mild to no disease symptoms
2. Severe disease can require hospitalization, total parenteral nutrition, a nasogastric tube for decompression, and surgery. Seventy percent of patients eventually require surgery (Lifshitz et al., 1991).
3. Monitor growth.
4. If the small bowel is involved, an ophthalmological examination is needed to rule out underlying ophthalmological manifestations of the disease.
5. Refer for nutritional therapy to help induce remission, prevent/correct malnutrition, and maintain and promote growth. See Table 12–17 for specific nutritional recommendations.
6. Refer for psychosocial therapy as indicated. Depressive disorders are common.

Complications

Growth failure, fistula formation, intestinal obstruction, and malnutrition can occur. Abscesses, perforation, and hemorrhage are rare. Cholelithiasis, nephrolithiasis, pancreatitis, pericarditis, and peripheral neuropathy are other complications of Crohn disease (Winesett, 1997).

Prevention

Follow recommended therapy to avoid sequelae.

Ulcerative Colitis

Description

Ulcerative colitis is characterized by recurring bloody diarrhea with acute and chronic inflammation limited to the colon. Patients with ulcerative colitis have significant weight loss secondary to chronic caloric insufficiency.

Etiology and Incidence

The cause is largely unknown but is probably a genetically determined response that is immunologically mediated. It is thought to be an altered immunological response in the intestinal mucosa. The disease has a multifactorial basis (heredity, diet, immunological aberrations, and ineffective mucosal integrity) influenced by environmental factors (Israel, 1999). The overall incidence is 2 cases per 100,000, with the peak onset occurring among 16- to 20-year-olds. Approximately 20% occur in children younger than 20 years (Snyder, 1998; Winesett, 1997).

Clinical Findings

HISTORY. The following can be reported:

- Fever
- Weight loss (average of 4 kg)
- Delayed growth and sexual maturation
- Arthritis/arthralgias of the large joints
- Anorexia
- Diarrhea
- Lower abdominal cramping, left lower quadrant pain
- Pain increased before stooling and passing flatus
- Stool with bright red blood and mucus
- Oral ulcers possible with active disease
- Skin lesions (erythema nodosum, pyoderma gangrenosum, and diffuse papulonecrotic eruptions)

PHYSICAL EXAMINATION. Weight and height are recorded. Abdominal examination can reveal rebound tenderness if the disease is severe.

DIAGNOSTIC TESTS. The following are ordered as needed:

- CBC with differential, iron-binding capacity, total protein, albumin, ESR, CRP, platelet count
- Stool for white blood cells, blood, and culture
- Bone age (usually delayed up to 2 years)

Differential Diagnosis

Shigella, Salmonella, Yersinia, Campylobacter, Escherichia coli, C. difficile, irritable bowel syndrome, and Crohn disease are the differential diagnoses.

Management

The goals of therapy are to (1) control the disease and induce a lasting remission; (2) prevent relapses; and (3) achieve normal nutrition, growth, and lifestyle. Treatment is pharmacological, nutritional, surgical, and psychosocial (Mascarenas & Altschuler, 1997). Management involves the following:

1. Refer for endoscopy, definitive diagnosis, consultation, and follow-up care, which may include the following:
   - Aminosalicylates (sulfasalazine, mesalamine) orally or rectally
   - Parenteral or oral steroids for moderate to severe disease, tapered doses for remission
   - Immunomodulatory agents (azathioprine or 6-mecaptopurine) to wean off steroids (Kirshner, 1996)
   - Hydrocortisone rectal preparation for tenesmus
   - Antispasmodics before meals
   - Iron supplementation to correct anemia
   - Diet high in protein and carbohydrate, normal amount of fat, and decreased roughage. Poor toleration of lactose (Sondheimer & Silverman, 1997)
   - Parenteral/enteral nutritional supplements (60 to 70 calories/kg per day)
2. Refer for surgery as indicated (can be curative).
3. Monitor growth.
4. Refer for ophthalmological examination to rule out ophthalmological manifestations of the disease (Kirshner, 1996).
5. Refer for nutritional therapy to prevent/correct malnutrition and maintain and promote growth. See Table 12–17 for nutritional recommendations.
6. Refer for psychosocial therapy as indicated. Depressive disorders are common.

Complications

The following can occur: growth failure, toxic megacolon, intestinal perforation, sepsis, colitis (children with pancolitis experience a much more severe course), cancer of the colon (can be long-term sequela—1 to 2% per year after 10 years of disease), arthritis, uveitis, and malnutrition (Sondheimer & Silverman, 1997).

Prevention

Follow the recommended therapy to avoid complications.

FAILURE TO THRIVE (ORGANIC)

Description

FTT is described as inadequate weight gain as determined by standardized growth charts. The diagnosis is based on a child's weight being below the 3rd to 5th percentile or falling more than two major percentile groups or becoming flat. Weight almost always falls before height and head circumference do.

Etiology

FTT can be associated with multiple medical conditions and psychological factors (Table 33–10). The purpose of this section is to discuss the assessment, laboratory findings, and differential diagnosis related to medical/organic causes of FTT.

Incidence

Ten percent of children seen for primary care have signs of growth failure, with 15 to 30% seen in inner-city emergency departments (Zevel, 1997).

Clinical Findings

A thoughtful approach to the history, physical examination, and laboratory evaluation of children with FTT includes the following (Lopez, 1997; Yetman & Coody, 1997; Frank et al., 1993):

HISTORY
- Careful family history of weight, height, growth patterns, and chronic health conditions
- Collection and interpretation of growth data for the child's measurements, percentiles, height for weight
- General parental concerns about the child's weight and FTT
- Prenatal factors: drug, alcohol, and tobacco exposure; length of gestation; illnesses; weight gain; nutrition; TORCHES (toxoplasmosis, rubella, cytomegalovirus, herpes, syphilis) exposure
- Perinatal factors: birth weight, Apgar

T A B L E 33-10

Major Organic Causes of Failure to Thrive

SYSTEM	CAUSE
Gastrointestinal	Gastroesophageal reflux, celiac disease, pyloric stenosis, cleft palate/cleft lip, lactose intolerance, Hirschsprung disease, milk protein intolerance, hepatitis, cirrhosis, pancreatic insufficiency, biliary disease, inflammatory bowel disease, malabsorption
Renal	Urinary tract infection, renal tubular acidosis, diabetes insipidus, chronic renal insufficiency
Cardiopulmonary	Cardiac diseases leading to congestive heart failure, asthma, bronchopulmonary dysplasia, cystic fibrosis, anatomical abnormalities of the upper airway
Endocrine	Hypothyroidism, diabetes mellitus, adrenal insufficiency or excess, parathyroid disorders, pituitary disorders, growth hormone deficiency
Neurological	Mental retardation, cerebral hemorrhage, degenerative disorders
Infectious	Parasitic or bacterial infections of the gastrointestinal tract, tuberculosis, human immunodeficiency virus disease
Metabolic	Inborn errors of metabolism
Congenital	Chromosomal abnormalities, congenital syndromes (e.g., fetal alcohol syndrome), perinatal infections
Miscellaneous	Lead poisoning, malignancy, collagen-vascular disease, recurrently infected adenoids and tonsils

From Behrman RE, Kliegman R, Arvin AM (eds): Nelson Textbook of Pediatrics, 15th ed. Philadelphia, WB Saunders, 1996.

scores, complications, length of stay in the hospital, congenital anomalies, neurological insults

- General health history: hospitalizations, medications, surgeries, accidents
- Nutrition history: caloric intake; feeding behavior; feeding cues; cues to hunger and satiety; ability to suck, swallow, chew; progression to solids; frequency of feedings; amount taken per feeding; preparation of formula (overdilution)
- Psychological information: caregiving environment, day care, family support, finances, parent–child relationship, parenting attitudes, typical day
- Careful review of systems

PHYSICAL EXAMINATION

- Weight, height, and head circumference (in those younger than 2 years) plotted on standardized growth curves and percentiles
- Skinfold measurements
- Vital signs (temperature, pulse, respiratory rate, blood pressure)

- Evidence of abuse or neglect
- Presence of dysmorphic features
- Upper and lower segment measurements (Fig. 33–4) to rule out dwarfism
- Skin, hair, nails, and mucous membranes
  - Scaling skin seen with zinc deficiency
  - Rough or hard skin with hypothyroidism
  - Edema with protein deficiency
  - Alopecia with hypervitaminosis or syphilis
  - Spoon-shaped nails with iron deficiency or GI diseases
  - Cyanosis with heart disease
  - Labial fissures with vitamin deficiency
- Oral findings: dental caries, tonsillar hypertrophy, submucous cleft palate or tongue enlargement
- Lymphadenopathy and splenomegaly, with malignancy and immune deficiency
- Endocrine: thyroid enlargement, precocious or ambiguous sexual development
- Disproportionate somatic growth (dwarfism)

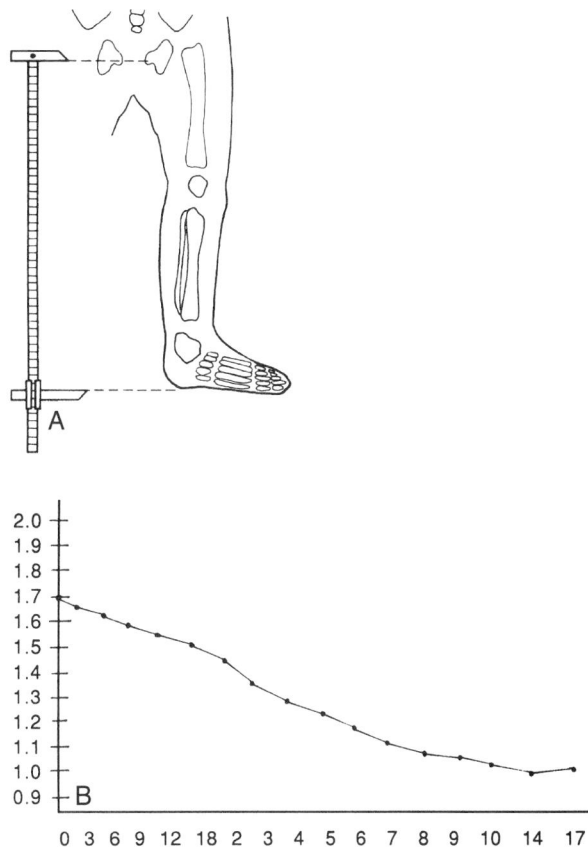

F I G U R E 33-4
Upper:lower segment ratios.
  A, To calculate upper:lower segment ratios use the following formula:

$$\frac{\text{upper segment}}{\text{lower segment}} \times \frac{\text{height-lower segment}}{\text{lower segment}}$$

  B, Upper:lower segment ratios.
  (From Siberry GK, Iannone R [eds]: The Harriet Lane Handbook, 15th ed. St Louis, CV Mosby, 2000, p 278.)

DIAGNOSTIC TESTS. Appropriate use of laboratory tests is indicated by the history and physical examination.

- UA and urine culture
- CBC, differential and platelets, ESR
- Serum electrolytes (make sure to get total CO_2)
- Lead level
- Purified protein derivative (PPD) with *Candida* control
- Human immunodeficiency virus (HIV) screening
- Serum protein, albumin, alkaline phosphatase, blood urea nitrogen (BUN), and creatinine
- Growth hormone and thyroid functions
- Stool studies for fat, reducing substances, ova and parasites, and culture

- Bone age
- Chest radiograph
- Renal ultrasonography and voiding cystourethrography
- Developmental testing

Differential Diagnosis

(Table 33-10).

Management

1. Manage treatable causes
2. Nutritional support: vitamin supplementation with iron, zinc, and minerals; calorically enriched formula and foods (up to 150 calories/kg per day). See Chapter 12 for further information related to FTT.
3. Parent education and support

4. Referrals as needed
5. Close follow-up

LOWER GASTROINTESTINAL TRACT INFECTIONS

Acute Diarrhea

Description

Acute diarrhea is excessive loss of fluid and electrolytes in the stool. Significant stool losses are defined as greater than 10 g/kg per day in infants and greater than 200 g/d in children (Nurko, 1999a; Vanderhoof, 1998).

Etiology and Incidence

Five causes of diarrhea are recognized (Nurko, 1999a; Vanderhoof, 1998):

- Osmotic diarrhea results when osmotically active particles are present in the intestine; this condition occurs with dumping syndrome, lactase deficiency, overfeeding, malabsorption syndromes, and excess ingestion of hypertonic juices.
- Secretory diarrhea occurs in the presence of inhibition of ion absorption or stimulation of ion excretion, as seen in the presence of bacterial endotoxins.
- Motility disorders cause diarrhea but not malabsorption. Bile salt and pancreatic enzyme deficiency can cause diarrhea by deletion or inhibition of the normal absorption process.
- Inflammatory processes such as bacterial invasion, celiac sprue, and irritable bowel syndrome or surgical procedures can change the anatomy and functional ability of the intestine. Abnormal peristalsis for any reason can result in acute diarrhea.
- Diarrhea can be caused by various viral and bacterial agents, including the following:
  - *Campylobacter jejuni* is a gram-negative rod found in contaminated food and water. It is usually acquired by toddlers and children from household pets, which serve as reservoirs. *C. jejuni* is less common after the age of 7 to 8 years, although neonates are susceptible. It is most common in the summer months.

- *C. difficile* is a gram-positive anaerobic bacillus. Asymptomatic carriers of *C. difficile* who take antibiotics (usually ampicillin, clindamycin, and cephalosporins) experience increased growth of the organism. *C. difficile* intestinal colonization rates in healthy neonates and young infants can be as high as 50% but are usually less than 5% in children older than 2 years and adults (AAP, 1997).
- *Yersinia enterocolitica* is a gram-negative rod found in contaminated food (uncooked pork and unpasteurized milk) and water. It produces an enterotoxin that causes secretion of fluid and electrolytes into the bowel. *Y. enterocolitica* causes diarrhea in children of all ages.
- *Salmonella* is a gram-negative rod found in contaminated, improperly cooked poultry, eggs, dairy products, and sausage. It is spread by human-to-human contact. *Salmonella* is most common in children younger than 5 years and adults older than 70 years. The peak incidence is in the first year of life (AAP, 1997). Invasive disease is more common in children with underlying chronic illness (AAP, 1997).
- *Shigella* is a gram-negative rod found in contaminated food and water. Humans are the host and reservoir, and the organism is spread by the fecal–oral route. The organism multiplies and releases cytotoxin, which causes epithelial damage and ulceration. *Shigella* is most common in children 6 months to 3 years of age.
- Enterohemorrhagic *E. coli* strains are associated with diarrhea, hemorrhagic colitis, hemolytic-uremic syndrome, and postdiarrheal idiopathic thrombocytopenic purpura. *E. coli* O157:H7 is the prototype that can cause mild to severe, profuse, and bloody diarrhea. The disease can be transmitted from infected persons, carriers, or food and water contaminated by human feces. *E. coli* O157:H7 has been found in undercooked ground beef, raw fruit and vegetables, and unpasteurized fruit juices. Incubation is from 10 hours to 6 days; *E. coli* O157:H7 infec-

tion usually lasts 3 to 4 days and can be fatal.

○ Viruses (human rotavirus, Norwalk-like virus, and small round viruses) invade the intestinal mucosa and leave a decreased surface area and decreased absorptive capacity. This type of diarrhea is the most common.

Acute diarrhea accounts for approximately 20% of acute care visits in children younger than 2 years. It is the cause of 8 in 1000 hospitalizations in children younger than 1 year and is the reason for 10% of preventable deaths in the United States. Acute diarrhea is responsible for 500 deaths per year in the United States for children 1 to 4 years of age. Poor access to care and poverty are correlated with increased mortality from diarrhea.

Clinical Findings

HISTORY. The following should be included:

- Dietary record, changes in diet that might correlate with increased stooling
- Family members with similar illness or other GI diseases
- Day care or school illness patterns and contacts
- Travel history
- Previous growth pattern
- Number of wet diapers in the past 24 hours and approximate time of last voiding
- Signs and symptoms associated with infectious diarrhea: bloody stool, abdominal pain, vomiting, or fever (Table 33-11)

PHYSICAL EXAMINATION. See Table 33-11. Assess:

- Vital signs
- Hydration status (see Table 33-1)
- Weight and height
- State of alertness
- Anterior fontanel if still open

DIAGNOSTIC TESTS. The following are ordered as indicated:

- Stool examination (color, consistency, blood, mucus, pus, odor, volume)
- Stool pH, Clinitest, and heme test

- Stool for ova and parasites, white blood cells, and culture
- Specific laboratory findings (Table 33-12)

Differential Diagnosis

Numerous causes, including infection (bacterial or viral), medication ingestion, parasitic infestations, anatomical abnormalities, dietary intolerances, and appendicitis, may be responsible for acute diarrhea.

Management

The following steps are taken:

1. Restore and maintain hydration. Oral rehydration with an oral electrolyte solution should be attempted. Appropriate rehydration solutions include Pedialyte and Infalyte. It is inappropriate to use fruit juices, Kool-Aid, sports drinks, or soda. If the child is not vomiting, oral rehydration can be accomplished quickly (<4 hours) (see Tables 33-2, 33-3 and 33-4). For formula-fed infants, returning to full-strength formula as quickly as possible is recommended. If the child is unable to tolerate full-strength formula, a diluted formula (one fourth to half strength) can be used for a short time (4 to 6 hours) as tolerated. The child's regular formula can be used initially as long as it is tolerated. If not tolerated, use soy or hydrolysate formula. Breastfed infants should continue to breastfeed more frequently for shorter periods.

2. For children who are taking solids, it is important to introduce bland, soft foods within the first 24 to 48 hours of rehydration. An age-appropriate diet with avoidance of fatty foods and foods high in simple sugars is recommended. Complex carbohydrates, lean meat, yogurt, fruit, and vegetables are well tolerated and assist in firming up the stool (AAP, 1996).

3. Prescribe medications as indicated (see Table 33-11).

4. Antidiarrheals are not generally recommended because the offending organism must be excreted. If diarrhea persists beyond the initial infection, cautious use of these agents in older children is acceptable.

T A B L E 33-11

Infectious Diarrhea: Signs, Symptoms, and Treatment

CAUSE	DIARRHEA	BLOODY STOOL	ABDOMINAL PAIN	VOMITING	FEVER	OTHER	TREATMENT
Campylobacter jejuni	+++ Foul smelling		+	+	+		Erythromycin, 40 mg/kg per d in 3 divided doses for 5–7 d. Decreases fecal excretion in 24–48 hr. Illness lasts 7–12 d
Clostridium difficile	++	+	+				Discontinue offending antibiotic Metronidazole, 30 mg/kg per d in 4 divided doses for 7–10 d, or Vancomycin, 40 mg/kg per d in 4 divided doses for 7–10 d Cholestyramine helps bind the toxin and decrease diarrhea
Yersinia entercolitica	+ Green/ malodorous	+	+ RLQ pain		+		Usually resolves spontaneously in 3–4 d. If septic, TMP-SMZ, 8 mg TMP/kg per d in 2 divided doses for 7–10 d, or Chloramphenicol, 50–75 mg/kg per d in 4 divided doses for 7–10 d, or Tetracycline, 25–50 mg/kg per d in 4 divided doses for 7–10 d (older teens only)

Organism							Treatment
Salmonella	+ +	+	+ Rebound tenderness	+	+	Sepsis Bacteremia	No treatment if uncomplicated. Usually resolves spontaneously Antibiotics can prolong the carrier state Antibiotics indicated for children younger than 1 y who are at risk for bacteremia and for patients who are immunosuppressed, have cardiac or valvular disease, lymphoproliferative diseases, sickle cell disease, or hemolytic anemias If indicated, use amoxicillin, 40 mg/kg per d in 3 divided doses for 7–10 d, *or* TMP-SMZ, 8 mg TMP/kg per d for 7–10 d in 2 divided doses, or Chloramphenicol, 50–75 mg/kg per d in 4 divided doses for 7–10 d Steroids and prostaglandins may be necessary for severe illness
Shigella	+ + + (initially) + (after 1–3 d)	+	+	+	+	Irritability Listlessness Patulous rectum	Need susceptibility information Resistance is common TMP-SMZ, 8 mg TMP/kg per d in 2 divided doses for 5 d, *or* Cefixime, 8 mg/kg per d for 5 d
Escherichia coli	+ +	+	+ Cramps and abdominal pain	–/+	+	Hemolytic-uremic syndrome	TMP-SMZ, 8 mg TMP/kg per d in 2 divided doses for 7–10 d if diarrhea is moderate to severe Do CBC, platelets, and kidney function tests
Virus	+ + + Watery	+	+ Cramps	+	+		Symptomatic treatment and maintenance of fluids

CBC = complete blood count; RLQ = right lower quadrant; TMP-SMZ = trimethoprim-sulfamethoxazole.

T A B L E 33-12

Laboratory Findings Associated With Infectious Diarrhea

CAUSE	BLOODY STOOL	WBCs IN STOOL	STOOL CULTURE	CBC	OTHER
Campylobacter jejuni	+ Gross	+	+	↑ WBC	Darting and motility on microscopy
Clostridium difficile	+ Gross	+	+ For toxin	Slightly ↑ WBCs ESR nl	
Yersinia enterocolitica	+ Gross or occult	+	+		
Salmonella	+ Gross	+	+	↓, nl, or slightly ↑ WBCs with left shift	
Shigella	+ Gross	+	+	nl or slightly ↑ WBCs with left shift	
Escherichia coli	+ Gross	−	+		Hemolytic-uremic syndrome as a complication
Virus	−	−	± *		

CBC = complete blood count; ESR = erythrocyte sedimentation rate; nl = normal; WBCs = white blood cells; + = present; − = not a clinical finding.

*If virus suspected, consider studying stool for reducing substances, Clinitest, heme test, and pH. Can test stool using enzyme-linked immunosorbent assay (ELISA) and latex agglutination assay for rotavirus.

5. Administer parenteral hydration if necessary for:
   - Impaired circulation and possible shock.
   - Weight less than 4 to 5 kg or a child younger than 3 months.
   - Intractable diarrhea, lethargy, anatomical anomalies.
   - Failure to gain weight or continued weight loss despite oral fluids.
6. Use telephone follow-up as indicated.

Complications

Chronic diarrhea and/or dehydration leads to acidosis causing cardiovascular collapse and possible death.

- *C. jejuni* can lead to hemorrhagic necrosis of the jejunum, reactive arthritis, seizures, pseudotumor in the mesenteric lymph nodes, and hemolytic-uremic syndrome.
- *C. difficile* can cause pseudomembranous colitis, toxic megacolon, colonic perforation, relapse, intractable proctitis, and death in debilitated children.

- *Y. enterocolitica* can result in septicemia and acute ileitis syndrome.
- *Salmonella* can cause bacteremia, focal infection, and a carrier state.
- *Shigella* can lead to toxic megacolon, cholestatic hepatitis, hemolytic-uremic syndrome, Reiter syndrome, and bacteremia.
- *E. coli* O157 can cause hemolytic-uremic syndrome.

Prevention

Preventive measures include:

- Good handwashing by the child and care providers. Liquid soap and paper towels are recommended at day care centers.
- Good sanitation and appropriate removal of soiled clothing and diapers. The diapering area should be cleaned after changing each baby at day care centers.
- Avoiding contaminated sources; meat should be properly cooked.
- With *Shigella*, culture all symptomatic con-

tacts and treat those with positive stool cultures.

Chronic Diarrhea

Description

Chronic diarrhea is defined as one or more liquid to semiliquid stools passed per day for 14 or more days.

Etiology

Causes include the following:

- Iatrogenic causes: excessive fluids (>150 ml/kg per day) (including juices) and a diet in which less than 25% of the total calories is from fat (Gryboski, 1993)
- Infants: formula protein intolerance (50% crossover between cow's milk and soy formulas)
- Toddlers: chronic nonspecific diarrhea— usually appears in 6-month- to 30-month-old children and resolves by the age of 5 years (Huffman, 1999; Vanderhoof, 1998; Liacouras & Baldassano, 1998; Judd, 1996)
- Children/adolescents: acquired lactose intolerance, short-bowel syndrome, Crohn disease, ulcerative colitis, intestinal lymphangiectasia, secretory tumors, irritable bowel
- Viral or bacterial agent
- Overfeeding, malabsorption (disaccharide intolerance)
- Carbohydrate intolerance (sorbitol, fructose, etc.)
- Intractable diarrhea of infancy
- Radiation therapy
- Severe combined immunodeficiency syndrome

Clinical Findings

HISTORY. The following should be assessed:

- Occurrence of more than one liquid stool per day for 2 or more consecutive weeks
- Dietary history (especially the ingestion of large amounts of fruit juices)
- Stool consistency, blood, mucus, pus, particles of food

- Stool incontinence
- Day care exposure
- Teething
- Treatment by parents (any dietary manipulation, drug or home treatments)
- Recent travel

PHYSICAL EXAMINATION. Look for physical findings associated with the underlying pathology (see Differential Diagnosis). The physical examination includes:

- Hydration status
- Weight and height measurements, skinfold thickness
- Skin and hair condition, color of skin and conjunctivae
- Vital signs (heart rate and blood pressure)
- Palpation of the thyroid
- Abdominal examination

DIAGNOSTIC TESTS. The following are ordered as indicated:

- Stool for culture, ova and parasites, pH, Clinitest (for reducing substances), heme test, fat stain
- CBC with differential, ESR, and serum electrolytes and albumin
- Sweat chloride test
- Lactose tolerance test
- Urinalysis and urine culture

Differential Diagnosis

The differential diagnosis includes allergy (the patient usually has other systemic symptoms), hyperthyroidism (enlarged thyroid, increased heart rate), malabsorption (weight loss and growth retardation), iatrogenic causes (dietary history includes excessive fluids and insufficient dietary fat), toddler's chronic nonspecific diarrhea (food particles in stool, loose mucoid stools, exacerbated by environmental stressors), CF (clubbing, respiratory symptoms), celiac disease, Crohn disease, and nonacute UTI.

Management

The following steps are taken:

1. Treat the underlying cause.
2. Provide enteral or parenteral support if the

patient is unable to maintain adequate intake orally.

3. Treat toddler's diarrhea (chronic nonspecific diarrhea) as follows:
   • Normalize the diet.
   • Decrease excess intake of juice or fluids (100 ml/kg per day).
   • Give half of fluid as milk (whole or 2%).
   • Increase fat in the diet to a total of 4 g/kg per day.
   • Increase fiber.
4. Refer the following patients to a gastroenterologist:
   • Newborns with diarrhea in first hours of life
   • Patients with abnormal growth delay/failure or abnormal physical findings (anorexia, abdominal pain, chronic bloating, vomiting, or weakness)
   • Those with severe illness

Complications

Malnutrition and growth failure can occur.

Intestinal Parasites

Description

Multiple organisms cause parasitic infestation in the GI tract. *Giardia lamblia, Enterobius vermicularis* (pinworm), *Ascaris lumbricoides* (roundworm), and *Taenia* (tapeworm) are some of the most common intestinal parasites that affect pediatric patients.

Etiology and Incidence

G. LAMBLIA. G. lamblia is a flagellate protozoan generally found in contaminated mountain water sources, municipal water supplies, and food. Person-to-person spread is via the fecal-oral route, often in day care and industrial settings. The organism resides in the small intestine, and encystation occurs as feces dehydrate in transit. Cysts can be excreted for months or years and are resistant to chlorine (AAP, 1997). An increased incidence is seen in homosexuals and children. Seventy-six percent of infected individuals are asymptomatic.

E. VERMICULARIS. Pinworms are 1 cm long,

white, and threadlike and live in the colon and rectum. The female lays eggs in the perianal area and dies. The eggs come from contaminated fomites and the anus, fingers, and mouth. They survive in bedding, clothing, and house dust for 2 weeks. The eggs are ingested, hatch, and become larvae in the small intestine; they migrate, once mature, to the rectum (AAP, 1997). Eggs are easily transmitted within families, day care settings, and institutions. It is the most common parasite in children in the United States.

A. LUMBRICOIDES. Roundworm comes from fecal contamination of soil and contaminated vegetables. Ingested eggs hatch, and the larvae penetrate the wall of the small intestine and enter the pulmonary system via the circulatory system. They break out of blood vessels into the lungs, are coughed up and then swallowed, and become adult worms in the small intestine. The process takes 2 months. The worms can grow to 30 cm in length and survive cold, drying, and chemicals. They can penetrate the liver or perforate the intestine. Found in the rural southern part of the United States, they are most common in children younger than 10 years. A 50% prevalence has been noted in some tropical areas.

TAENIA. Tapeworm, also known as "beef" or "pork" tapeworm, comes from the consumption of raw or undercooked beef or pork with encysted parasites. The larval form of pork tapeworm causes cysticercosis, with space-occupying lesions in the viscera, brain, and muscle. The incidence is unknown.

Clinical Findings

(Table 33–13 and 33–14).

Differential Diagnosis

The differential diagnosis includes all other causes of infectious and noninfectious diarrhea; pinworms, in particular, can be associated with "pinworm neurosis" after successful therapy or as a fantasy infestation in unaffected contacts (Lerman, 1999).

T A B L E 33-13

Intestinal Parasite Infestation: Signs, Symptoms, and Treatment

PARASITE	GI SYMPTOMS	DIARRHEA	WEIGHT LOSS	OTHER	TREATMENT
Giardia lamblia	+ Abdominal cramps, flatulence, bloating	+ + Rarely bloody, watery, greasy, foul smelling	+		Treat *all* positive stool cultures with Furazolidone, 5–8 mg/kg per d in 4 divided doses for 7–10 d, *or* Metronidazole, 40 mg/kg per d in 3 divided doses for 7–10 d Can repeat either if treatment fails
Enterobius vermicularis (pinworms)	—	—	—	Perirectal/ vaginal itching	Mebendazole, 100-mg tablet for 1 dose, then repeat in 2 wk, *or* Pyrantel pamoate, 11 mg/kg (max, 1 g) for 1 dose, then repeat in 2 wk Simultaneously treat family members Vaginitis is self-limiting
Ascaris lumbricoides (roundworm)	Worms in stool or vomit Bowel or biliary obstruction	—	+ Malnutrition		Pyrantel pamoate, 11 mg/kg for 1 dose (max, 1 g), *or* Mebendazole, 100-mg tablet per d for 3 d If intestinal obstruction present, piperazine citrate, 75 mg/kg per d (max, 3.5 g) for 2 d; makes worms flaccid and easier to pass
Taenia (tapeworm)	Worms in stool, abdominal pain, excessive appetite	—	—		Praziquantel, 20 mg/kg per d in 4 divided doses for 1 d

T A B L E 33-14

Laboratory Findings Associated With Intestinal Parasite Infestation

PARASITE	STOOL FINDINGS	STOOL FOR OVA AND PARASITES	STOOL CULTURE	CBC	DUODENAL ASPIRATE	OTHER
Giardia lamblia		−	+ Three cultures over 1 wk		± May be necessary	EIA for Giardia
Enterobius vermicularis (pinworm)						Transparent tape test during night
Ascaris lumbricoides (roundworm)	Worms in stool	+	−	Marked eosinophilia		
Taenia (tapeworm)		+ Ova in stool				

CBC = complete blood count; EIA = enzyme immunoassay; + = present; − = negative.

Management

See Table 33-13.

Complications

The following can occur:

- *G. lamblia* can lead to malabsorption, weight loss, and FTT.
- *E. vermicularis*, even untreated, is self-limited.

RESOURCE BOX 33-1

American Pseudo-Obstruction and Hirschsprung's Disease Society
Tel: (800) 394–2747, (508) 685–4477
Website: www.tiac.net/users/aphs

Newsletter, informational materials (inc. Spanish), networking, referrals to local resources, local chapters, advocacy, fund research, maintain research registry

CCFA: Crohn's and Colitis Foundation of America
Tel: (800) 932–2423 or (800) 343–3637
Tel: (212) 685–3440
Website: ccfa.org

Newsletter, informational materials (inc. Spanish), referrals to local resources, local chapters, advocacy, fund research

Cyclic Vomiting Syndrome Association
Tel: (414) 784–6842
Website: beaker.iupui.edu/cvsa

Newsletter, informational materials, networking, referrals to local resources, local chapters, fund research, maintain research registry

IFFGD International Foundation for Functional Gastrointestinal Disorders
Tel: (414) 964–1799
Website: www.execpc.com/iffgd

Newsletter, informational materials, referrals to local resources, advocacy

National Digestive Diseases Information Clearinghouse
Tel: (301) 654–3810

National Institute of Diabetes and Digestive and Kidney Diseases
Tel: (301) 496–3583

- *A. lumbricoides* can lead to Löffler syndrome (fever, respiratory symptoms, pulmonary infiltrates, excessive serum eosinophilia) caused by an allergic response as the larvae migrate to the lungs.
- *Taenia* can cause systemic cysticercosis.

Prevention

Most parasitic infestations can be prevented by good handwashing and good sanitation. The following parasites can be avoided or eliminated:

- *G. lamblia*: Treat questionable water with iodine or boiling for 20 minutes. Exclude symptomatic children from school/day care until asymptomatic.
- *E. vermicularis*: Avoid scratching. Wash sheets and clothing in hot water and detergent.
- *A. lumbricoides*: Appropriate food preparation is necessary to prevent infection.
- *Taenia*: Avoid raw or undercooked beef or pork.

REFERENCES

American Academy of Pediatrics: Report of the Committee on Infectious Diseases, 24th ed. Elk Grove Village, IL, American Academy of Pediatrics, 1997.

American Academy of Pediatrics Provisional Committee on Quality Improvement, Subcommittee on Acute Gastroenteritis. Practice parameter: The management of acute gastroenteritis in young children. Pediatrics 97:424-436, 1996.

Armentrout D: Gastroesophageal reflux in infants. Nurse Pract 20:54-63, 1995.

Barkin R, Rosen P: Emergency Pediatrics: An Approach to Ambulatory Care, 4th ed. St Louis, CV Mosby, 1999.

Behrman RE, Kliegman RM: Nelson Essentials of Pediatrics, 3rd ed. Philadelphia, WB Saunders, 1998.

Behrman RE, Kliegman R, Arvin AM (eds): Nelson Textbook of Pediatrics, 15th ed. Philadelphia, WB Saunders, 1996.

Boyle JT: Recurrent abdominal pain: An update. Pediatr Rev 18(9):310-320, 1997.

Bujanner Y, Reif S, Yahar J: *Helicobactor pylori* and peptic ulcer disease in the pediatric patient. Pediatr Clin North Am 43:213-233, 1996.

Burg F, Ingelfinger J, Wald E, et al (eds): Gellis & Kagan's Current Pediatric Therapy, 15. Philadelphia, WB Saunders, 1996.

Carey WB: Clinical applications of infant temperament measurements. J Pediatr 81:823-828, 1972.

Caty M, Azizkahn G: Acute surgical conditions of the abdomen. Pediatr Ann 23:192-201, 1997.

Cervisi J, Chapman M, Niklas B, et al: Office management of the infant with colic. J Pediatr Health Care 5:184-190, 1991.

Chang T: Gastroesophageal reflux. _In_ Dershewitz RA (ed): Ambulatory Pediatric Care, 3rd ed. Philadelphia, JB Lippincott, 1999, pp 570-573.

Cucchiara S, Bartolotti M: Fasting and postprandial mechanisms of gastroesophageal reflux in children with gastroesophageal reflux disease. Dig Dis Sci 1:86-92, 1993.

Dihigo S: New strategies for the treatment of colic: Modifying the parent/infant interaction. J Pediatr Health Care 12(5):256-262, 1998.

Finberg L: Saunders Manual of Pediatric Practice. Philadelphia, WB Saunders, 1998.

Fleisher D: Coping with colic. Contemp Pediatr 15(6):144-156, 1998.

Frank PA, Silva M, Neeldeman R: Failure to thrive: Mystery, myth and method. Contemp Pediatr 10(2):114-133, 1993.

Gryboski J: The child with chronic diarrhea. Contemp Pediatr 10(5):71-97, 1993.

Hillemeier A: Gastroesophageal reflux: Diagnostic and therapeutic approaches. Pediatr Clin North Am 43:197-212, 1996.

Huffman S: Toddler diarrhea. J Pediatr Health Care 13(1):32-33, 1999.

Hyams J: Crohn's disease in children. Pediatr Clin North Am 43:255-277, 1996.

Irish MS, Pearl RH, Caty MG, et al: The approach to common abdominal diagnoses in infants and children. Pediatr Clin North Am 45:729-772, 1998.

Israel E: Inflammatory bowel disease. _In_ Dershewitz RA (ed): Ambulatory Pediatric Care, 3rd ed. Philadelphia, JB Lippincott, 1999, pp 593-597.

Jospe N, Forbes G: Fluids and electrolytes: Clinical aspects. Pediatr Rev 17(11):395-403, 1996.

Judd RH: Chronic nonspecific diarrhea. Pediatr Rev 17(11):379-384, 1996.

Karjoo M: Caustic ingestion and foreign bodies in the gastrointestinal system. Curr Opin Pediatr 10:516-522, 1998.

Kaye R, Oski F, Barness L: Core Textbook of Pediatrics. New York, JB Lippincott, 1988.

Kirschner B: Ulcerative colitis in children. Pediatr Clin North Am 43:235-254, 1996.

Lasche J, Duggan C: Managing acute diarrhea. Contemp Pediatr 16(2):74-83, 1999.

Lehtonen L, Korvenranta H: Infantile colic: Seasonal incidence and crying profiles. Arch Pediatr Adolesc Med 149:533-536, 1995.

Lencer W, Wolf AA: Malabsorption syndrome and chronic diarrhea. _In_ Dershewitz RA (ed): Ambulatory Pediatric Care, 3rd ed. Philadelphia, JB Lippincott, 1999, pp 589-593.

Lerman S: Common intestinal parasites. _In_ Dershewitz RA (ed): Ambulatory Pediatric Care, 3rd ed. Philadelphia, JB Lippincott, 1999, pp 994-998.

Liacouris CA, Baldassano RN: Is it toddler's diarrhea? Contemp Pediatr 15(9):131-144, 1998.

Lifshitz F, Finch N, Lifshitz J: Children's Nutrition. Boston, Jones & Bartlett, 1991.

Lopez RF: Clinical health problem: Failure to thrive. J Am Acad Nurse Pract 9(10):490-493, 1997.

Mascarenas MR, Altschuler SM: Treatment of inflammatory bowel disease. Pediatr Rev 18(3):95-98, 1997.

Meyers A: Modern management of acute diarrhea and dehydration in children. Am Fam Physician 51:1103-1113, 1995.

Mezoff A, Balistreri W: Peptic ulcer disease in children. Pediatr Rev 16(7):257-265, 1995.

Muñiz AE, Jaffe MD: Foreign bodies: Ingested and inhaled. Contemp Pediatr 14(12):78-103, 1997.

Murray KF, Christie DL: Vomiting. Pediatr Rev 19(10):337-341, 1998.

Northrup RS, Flanigan TP: Gastroenteritis. Pediatr Rev 15(12):461-472, 1994.

Nurko S: Acute diarrhea. _In_ Dershewitz RA (ed): Ambulatory Pediatric Care, 3rd ed. Philadelphia, JB Lippincott, 1999a, pp 582-589.

Nurko S: Recurrent abdominal pain. _In_ Dershewitz RA (ed): Ambulatory Pediatric Care, 3rd ed. Philadelphia, JB Lippincott, 1999b, pp 578-582.

Pearl RH, Irish MS, Caty MG, et al: The approach to common abdominal diagnoses in infants and children, part 2. Pediatr Clin North Am 45:1287-1326, 1998.

Pierce C: What not to do for a child with recurrent abdominal pain. Pediatr News March 25, 1995.

Poole S, Schmitt B, Mauro R: Recurrent pain symptoms in children: A streamlined approach. Contemp Pediatr 12(1):47-77, 1995.

Preud'Homme D, Mezoff A: _Helicobacter pylori_: A pathogen for all ages. Contemp Pediatr 13(11):27-49, 1996.

Roberts K: Gastroesophageal reflux in infants and children who have neurodevelopmental disabilities. Pediatr Rev 17(6):211-212, 1996.

Schwartz MW, Curry TA, Sargent AJ, et al (eds): Pediatric Primary Care: A Problem Oriented Approach, 3rd ed. St Louis, CV Mosby, 1997.

Siberry GK, Iannone R (eds): The Harriet Lane Handbook, 15th ed. St. Louis, CV Mosby, 2000.

Snyder JP: Inflammatory bowel disease: Ulcerative colitis and Crohn disease. _In_ Finberg L (ed): Saunders Manual of Pediatric Practice. Philadelphia, WB Saunders, 1998, pp 510-513.

Sondheimer J, Silverman A: Gastrointestinal tract. _In_ Hathaway WE, Groothuis JR, Hay WW, et al (eds): Current Pediatric Diagnosis and Treatment. E Norwalk, CT, Appleton & Lange, 1997.

Talusan-Soriano K, Lake A: Malabsorption in children. Pediatr Rev 17(4):135-142, 1996.

Teitelbaum SJ, Leichtner AM, Tunnessen WW: "Read my lips": Abdominal pain in a 14 year old. Contemp Pediatr 16(3):31-41, 1999.

Vanderhoof JA: Chronic diarrhea. Pediatr Rev 19(12):418-422, 1998.

Winesett M: Inflammatory bowel disease in children and adolescents. Pediatr Ann 26(4):227-234, 1997.

Yetman R, Coody D: Failure to thrive: A clinical guideline. J Pediatr Health Care 11(3):134-137, 1997.

Zevel JA: Failure to thrive: A general pediatrician's perspective. Pediatr Rev 18(11):371-378, 1997.

CHAPTER 34

Dental and Oral Diseases

Charles Poland III and Jeffrey A. Dean

INTRODUCTION

The focus of ambulatory care in the pediatric setting is directed toward keeping the child well and minimizing the impact of disease, developmental problems, and disturbances in behavior to which every child is susceptible. This concept of care places a major emphasis on prevention, early intervention, and anticipatory guidance to minimize the effects of developmental, psychological, and chronic disease in children.

Pediatric dentists use these same strategies to achieve their successes. The primary focus of pediatric dentistry is to establish preventive dental health habits that successfully guide the child and parent through childhood into adulthood free of dental disease. Although nearly every human disease may have oral manifestations, dental caries, periodontal disease, and malocclusions are the primary oral diseases. The caries process that leads to dental cavities is most often initiated early in the life of a child, whereas periodontal disease is primarily a disease of adults. Both diseases are entirely preventable if modern preventive dental strategies are instituted or early intervention in the disease process is accomplished. Most malocclusions are genetically induced, result from premature tooth loss, or are a result of digit or pacifier habits. Implementation of preventive measures, as well as definitive treatment of mal-

occlusion, enhances the child's physical and psychosocial growth and development.

Because of the unique trust that parents have in their child's primary care provider, nurse practitioners (NPs) can have a profound impact on the outcomes of children's oral health. By providing early oral health counseling and encouragement to establish a "dental home" for the child at 12 months of age, before the processes of oral diseases are initiated or out of control, NPs are using the same principles of ambulatory care that they use every day in their clinical practice to prevent other diseases.

Unfortunately, most pediatric practitioners have not applied this same standard of care to pediatric oral health. Some pediatric practitioners have failed to recognize that optimal oral health is an integral part of total body health. Others do not believe that dental health is a significant issue in children. Often, however, lack of understanding about the basic disease processes of caries and periodontal disease is responsible for the delay in providing dental health counseling or referring for professional dental care at the appropriate age. Failure to significantly reduce the incidence of caries in young children demands a better understanding of the basic disease processes by all pediatric health professionals. The dental profession alone cannot eliminate the present prevalence of caries in young children by drilling and filling teeth with "cavities," but as oral health supervisors focused on prevention and early intervention of the disease processes, optimal oral health can be provided for every child.

STANDARDS OF CARE

A 1995 United States (US) Public Health Service review on *Healthy People 2000: Objectives for oral health* (US Department of Health and Human Services, 1995) noted that substantial progress was not being made on these goals. The percentage of children aged 6 to 8 years with untreated dental caries increased from 24 to 31%, and the percentage of 15-year-old children with untreated dental caries remained at 24%. The proportion of people receiving optimally fluoridated water remained at 61%, and the proportion of children receiving protective sealants increased only to 25%. Particularly disappointing was the finding that the overall percentage of children who had received an oral examination before entering school decreased from 66 to 63%, a movement away from the Year 2000 Objectives. The percentage of black and Hispanic students who had not had a dental examination was significantly higher, thus identifying a major access-to-care issue for these populations. The projected goals for *Healthy People 2010* are found in Appendix D.

Consensus on dental and oral health issues for children and parents that should be addressed routinely by primary care clinicians includes the following:

- Counseling patients about regular dental care, (including visiting a dental care provider on a regular basis, flossing daily, brushing teeth daily with fluoride toothpaste, using fluoride and chemotherapeutic mouth rinses)
- Educating parents to eliminate bottles in bed with infants and children and to use appropriate dietary fluoride supplements
- Counseling patients to discontinue the use of tobacco and to limit the consumption of alcohol
- Remaining alert for obvious signs of oral disease when examining the oral cavity, and remaining alert to signs and symptoms of oral cancer and premalignancy in persons who use tobacco or regularly use alcohol

Additionally, most authorities recommend that a child's first dental visit should occur at 6 months of age or when the first tooth erupts, whichever comes later, but no later than 1 year of age. The dentist should determine frequency of subsequent visits (US Public Health Service, 1997; US Preventive Services Task Force, 1996; Elster & Kuznets, 1994).

Bright Futures: Guidelines for Health Supervision of Infants, Children, and Adolescents (Green, 1994) has detailed oral health anticipatory guidance guidelines for each health supervision visit from infancy through adolescence. *Bright Futures in Practice: Oral Health* guidelines (Casamassimo, 1996) and quick reference cards (Casamassimo, 1997) provide the clinician with a detailed and comprehensive reference to current standards of dental care.

The American Academy of Pediatric Dentistry in its *Special Issue: Reference Manual 1999–2000* (1999) outlines dental health objectives for the year 2000, oral health policies, and guidelines for pediatric dentistry. The manual emphasizes the need to start professional dental care at 12 months of age.

The caries prevalence in preschool children remains very high, particularly in minority and underserved children. A study from the Office of the Inspector General (US Department of Health & Human Services, 1996) found that only one in five children receiving Medicaid assistance was seen for dental screening despite a program requirement that children have annual dental screening and follow-up care. Most state dental Medicaid programs are so poorly funded and filled with bureaucratic red tape that few providers participate in these programs. Other barriers to care continue to be transportation and patient compliance with appointments and preventive dental principles.

ANATOMY AND PHYSIOLOGY

The oral cavity consists of the gingiva (gums), mucosa, tongue, hard and soft palate, and teeth. Tooth development is described in four stages:

initiation, calcification, eruption, and shedding. Initiation refers to initial development of the tooth follicle, which occurs in the first trimester in utero. All 20 primary teeth begin hard tissue formation by 4 to 6 months' gestation. The first permanent molars and lower incisors are the first permanent teeth to develop and begin to calcify just before or soon after birth. Calcification refers to the deposition of inorganic mineral crystals of enamel and dentin on the teeth and affects the color, texture, and thickness of the tooth. Teeth begin to erupt at about 6 to 7 months of age (primary dentition), and all 20 teeth are usually present by the end of the third year. Permanent teeth begin erupting around 6 years of age, and all 32, except the third molars, are in place by 13 to 14 years of age (Table 34-1). The ages of eruption given in Table 34-1 are guidelines and vary by as much as 6 months or more. It is not unusual to see the mandibular lateral incisors delayed in their eruption until the mandibular cuspids erupt. The clinician should not be overly concerned about delayed eruption of teeth as long as the child is achieving other normal growth parameters. When related to chronological age, the timing of tooth eruption is one of the most variable milestones. The clinician should, however, be concerned with contralateral asymmetrical eruption patterns that persist more than 3 to 4 weeks and refer the child to a pediatric dentist for evaluation. Several multiple congenital disorders and syndromes are associated with delayed eruption and missing teeth, but these issues are normally secondary and can be dealt with when the "dental home" is established.

PATHOPHYSIOLOGY AND DEFENSE MECHANISMS

Disruption in Formation, Eruption, or Shedding of Teeth

Genetic defects, infection, malnutrition, trauma, and fluorosis are the most common causes of abnormal tooth development. Enamel hypoplasia is caused by a disturbance in the formation of enamel matrix and is the most common defect. Enamel hypoplasia can appear as a simple opacity, severe discoloration of the

T A B L E 34-1
Eruption Sequence

PRIMARY DENTITION	AGE AT ERUPTION (mo)
MAXILLARY	
Central incisor	71/2
Lateral incisor	9
Cuspid	18
First molar	14
Second molar	24
MANDIBULAR	
Central incisor	6
Lateral incisor	7
Cuspid	16
First molar	12
Second molar	20

PERMANENT DENTITION	AGE AT ERUPTION (yr)
MAXILLARY	
Central incisor	7–8
Lateral incisor	8–9
Cuspid	11–12
First bicuspid	10–11
Second bicuspid	10–12
First molar	6–7
Second molar	12–13
MANDIBULAR	
Central incisor	6–7
Lateral incisor	7–8
Cuspid	9–10
First bicuspid	10–12
Second bicuspid	11–12
First molar	6–7
Second molar	11–13

Adapted from Logan WHG, Kronfeld R: The chronology of human dentition. J Am Dent Assoc 20:1933 (slightly modified by McCall & Schour).

enamel, or a misshapen tooth devoid of much of its enamel (Fig. 34-1). Hypocalcification defects of enamel are rare and usually associated with metabolic diseases such as rickets and parathyroid deficiency. Alterations in the size and shape of teeth include microdont (small tooth) or macrodont (large tooth). Fusion is a single enlarged tooth or joined "double" tooth in which the tooth count reveals a missing tooth when the anomalous tooth is counted as one (Fig. 34-2). Hypodontia refers to the ab-

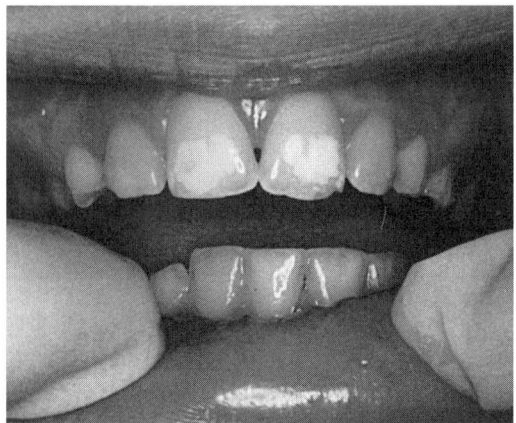

F I G U R E 34-1
Enamel hypoplasia of the two central incisors. Note, fluorosis or a febrile illness would have affected other teeth during time of similar development.

sence of one or more teeth and is common in the permanent dentition. The third molars, second bicuspids, and maxillary lateral incisors are the most frequently missing teeth in the permanent dentition. Congenitally missing teeth in the deciduous dentition are much rarer but do occur, with the lateral incisors and cuspids most frequently missing. When deciduous teeth are congenitally missing, the permanent successor is also frequently missing.

Hyperdontia, the presence of supernumerary teeth, can occur in any location within the dental-alveolar areas but is most commonly found in the anterior maxilla. Such teeth need

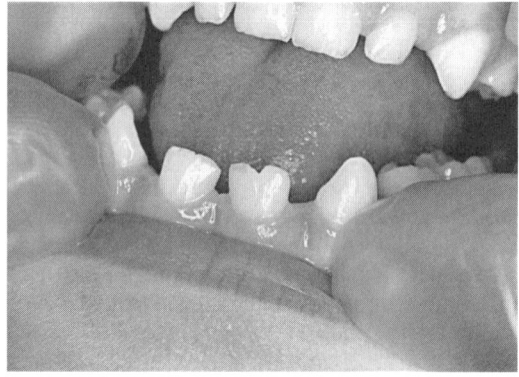

F I G U R E 34-2
Fusion of deciduous incisors.

to be identified and the tooth occasionally removed to prevent asymmetrical or delayed eruption of the permanent maxillary incisors.

Premature loss of deciduous teeth not associated with infection should alert the clinician to other growth disturbances or inborn errors of metabolism. Exfoliation of deciduous teeth occurs as the permanent successor erupts into the mouth, and the timing of this event is as variable as the eruption of deciduous teeth. Eruption of the permanent tooth normally stimulates the deciduous tooth root to be resorbed. When the deciduous tooth root is not resorbed properly, the permanent tooth can be diverted from its normal eruption path and forced into an abnormal position requiring orthodontic repositioning. Most pediatric dentists observe an over-retained deciduous tooth for a period of 2 to 3 weeks in the hope that the tooth will exfoliate before putting the child through an extraction procedure.

Dental Caries

THE CARIES PROCESS

The caries process is a chronic, infectious, bacterial disease initiated by the introduction of mutans streptococci (*Streptococcus mutans* [SM]) and maintained by these and other related bacteria. The caries process is also multifactorial in that nutritional modifiers and host resistance play an important role in progression of the disease. "Dental cavities" are the end-result of the caries process when the tooth structure finally breaks down and cavitates. Cavitation of the tooth from the caries process can occur within months or may not occur for years, depending on the virulence of the process. For young children, this process can begin shortly after eruption of the first tooth (6 to 9 months) and, if not adequately addressed, continues throughout the life of the child. Acquisition of SM is necessary but, alone, is not sufficient to promote the caries process. The course of the disease, similar to other infectious diseases, is modified by the virulence of the infecting organism and host resistance. In the caries process, host resistance is defined as resistance of the tooth surface to demineralization, the capacity to remineralize tooth structure, dietary modifiers, and oral hygiene habits. Parents should be counseled that genetic and developmental factors play a very limited role in progression of the caries process, and they should not be permitted to believe that "soft teeth just run in the family."

BACTERIAL COMPONENT OF THE CARIES PROCESS

The infectious and transmissible nature of dental caries was initially described by Keyes (1960). Kohler (1983) identified SM as the important pathogen in initiation of the caries process and demonstrated that transmission of SM to the child could be delayed or prevented by reducing SM reservoirs in the child's mother, an approach that has successfully prevented other infectious diseases. More recent studies have identified a discrete "window of infectivity" that occurs between 19 and 33 months (26 months on average), when the introduction of SM and related cariogenic organisms is most likely to occur (Caufield et al., 1993). The presence of caries in children 12 to 18 months of age, however, indicates that there is opportunity for an earlier "window." *Streptococcus sanguis* is known to be associated with an earlier "window" (9 to 12 months), but its influence on SM activity is not clearly identified (Caufield, 1997). The main source of these bacteria is direct transmission from the mother or close caregiver to the child (e.g., kissing, wetting a pacifier in the mouth). The acquisition of specific strains of SM from the mother to the child is known to be as high as 88%, with race, gender, ethnic population, and virulence of the organism being variables (Li & Caufield, 1995). Mothers' salivary SM colony counts correlate with their young children's salivary SM counts, and a young child's caries experience tends to correlate with that of the mother. Before blaming mothers for early transmission of all SM, over 40% of older adults aged 55 to 75 years have active root caries and are known to have high reservoirs of SM (Shay, 1996). A loving kiss from a grandparent may not be completely harmless if the grandparent's dental health is not good. The mother or close caregiver's history of recent caries, the presence of active caries, poorly adapted or broken dental restora-

tions, poorly coalesced biting surface, pits and fissures on molar teeth, and SM activity during the child's 6- to 33-month age period are the most critical risk factors.

For optimal oral health, introduction and colonization of the enamel with SM during this "window of infectivity" must be prevented until the other normal flora of the mouth can be established. As with other viral or bacterial diseases, young preschool children can "catch cavities" from adults with whom they interact, thus the phrase *"cavities are catching."* All children are likely to acquire and harbor some SM as part of their oral flora, particularly as they get older. If the caries process is initiated in older children or adults, it is from an as yet undiscovered second "window" or the takeover of normal oral flora by cariogenic bacteria rather than colonization by one predominant organism. The caries process can be modified by the influence of diet, fluoride exposure, virulence of the bacteria, capacity to remineralize enamel, and plaque control (brushing and flossing). Whether the caries process was initiated during an early "window of infectivity" or later in the child's life, once the caries process is initiated, dental decay prevalence increases at an alarming rate through the adolescent years (Fig. 34-3).

A risk assessment to identify parents with high reservoirs of SM can be easily done by taking a simple dental history from an expectant or new mother (Table 34-2).

In addition, tongue blade examination of the mother's teeth and gums reveals oral hygiene practices and the presence of decay or broken fillings. Mothers or close caregivers who are in need of dental care or who do not seek preventive dental services are at risk for high SM reservoirs and should be counseled regarding the risk that they pose for their young children.

THE DEMINERALIZATION–REMINERALIZATION PHASE

The eruption of teeth signals the time that SM can be introduced and will begin to colonize the infant's mouth. Once colonization of the infant's mouth has occurred, the caries process proceeds as a back-and-forth process of demineralization and remineralization of enamel. Den-

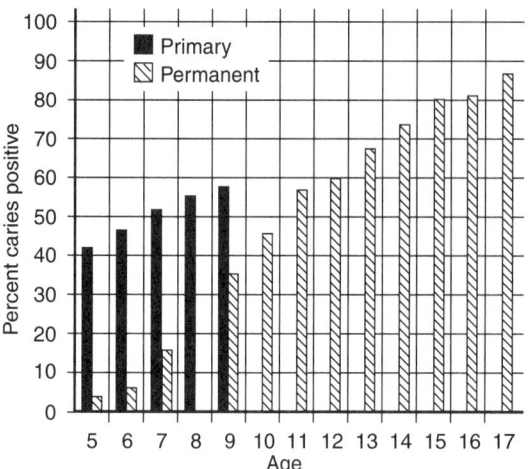

F I G U R E 34-3
Percentage of children with caries in primary and permanent teeth, National Institute of Dental Research (NIDR, 1986–1987). Caries prevalence in children steadily progresses. Caries prevalence appears low in ages 6–9 years as carious primary teeth are shed. (From Edelstein SL, Douglas CW: Dispelling the myth that 50% of US schoolchildren have never had a cavity. Public Health Rep 110:522–530, 1995.)

tal enamel is a permeable structure composed of an organic matrix and an inorganic hydroxyapatite crystal. The organic matrix permits exchange of the basic composition of the hydroxyapatite crystal with salivary calcium, phosphates, fluorides, and other dietary minerals. When the pH or ion concentration in the oral environment is altered, demineralization or remineralization *will* occur. Fluorides support the remineralization process. When in contact with the enamel surface, fluorides hasten the

remineralization process, reduce the solubility of enamel crystal, enhance the nucleation of calcium phosphate in the enamel crystal, and accelerate maturation of the enamel surface. Newly erupted teeth, particularly deciduous teeth, are highly susceptible to caries. When fluorides are applied during the immediate posteruptive period, fluoride penetration into enamel is increased by five times and significantly reduces enamel solubility and demineralization when compared with enamel that matures without fluoride exposure. Parents should be instructed to use very small amounts of fluoride toothpaste on children as soon as teeth appear in the mouth to reduce enamel solubility, promote the remineralization process, and enhance the enamel maturation process. Many health professionals have mistakenly advised parents to not use fluoride toothpaste on young children for fear of enamel fluorosis. Small amounts of a fluoride toothpaste (less than one fourth of the size of a pea) brushed daily on the child's newly erupted teeth and then wiped out with a cloth afford these susceptible young teeth the opportunity to resist demineralization and enhance remineralization.

The acid attack produced by cariogenic bacteria and carbohydrate substrate does not produce cavitation directly on the enamel surface but rather produces the cycle of demineralization–remineralization of subsurface enamel (Fig. 34-4). Advanced subsurface lesions may appear as white chalky lesions commonly found along the gingival margin of deciduous anterior teeth. Early subsurface lesions are not visible but may be present on most tooth surfaces. Subsurface lesions may be reversible with fluoride therapy and other preventive measures (see Color Fig. 11). In dynamic equilibrium, the

T A B L E 34-2

Parental Dental History for Risk Assessment

When was the last time you had a cavity filled?
Do you have any untreated cavities or broken fillings in your mouth?
When was the last time you visited a dentist?
Do you see your dentist on a regular one- or two-times-a-year schedule for preventive dental services?

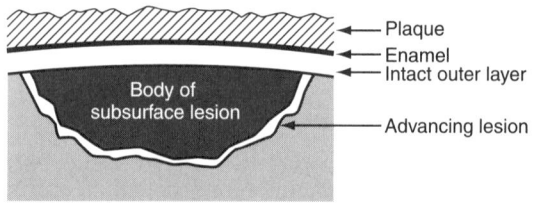

F I G U R E 34-4
Caries process proceeds as a subsurface lesion beneath an intact layer of enamel.

caries process continues without destruction of enamel, but when the process reaches disequilibrium, enamel structure weakens to a point that cavitation occurs.

NUTRITIONAL MODIFIERS

As carbohydrate substrate is introduced into the mouth, bacterial plaque pH will fall within 2 to 3 minutes and initiate the demineralization process. Demineralization occurs when plaque pH falls below 5.5. Over the next 25 to 30 minutes, saliva will neutralize and buffer the plaque pH and support the remineralization process. Parents should be counseled that a child's eating habits will have a more significant influence on the caries process than will restricting any one food or snack. The uncontrolled frequent ingestion of sugars, natural and refined, as well as cooked starches, maintains low plaque pH over a sustained time interval and promotes the demineralization process. Children who are "nibblers and sippers" have a higher risk for caries than do children who eat the same foods but are "wolfers and gobblers." The most significant modifiers of the caries process in young children are the milk bottle in bed or used as a pacifier (behavior purposes, not nutritional) and the uncontrolled use of a sippy cup containing milk or fruit juice. Parents who practice inappropriate feeding/behavior practices *may* have children at high risk for early childhood caries (ECC) and should be counseled and referred to a pediatric dentist as early as possible.

Even with the knowledge that caries is caused by an infectious bacterial disease, bottle and nursing habits have been the focus of caries control in young children. While acknowledging that the bottle or improper nursing habit is a major modifier of the disease, the clinician should recognize that the bacterial component transmitted from a caregiver is the basic etiology of the caries process in young children and is key to an accurate risk assessment to prevent caries in preschool children. This point was confirmed in a study of Head Start children: 86% of children with caries were reported to have taken the bottle to bed, whereas 69% of children with no caries also reported similar use of the bottle in bed (Tinanoff & O'Sullivan,

1997). Understanding the timing of infectivity and the mechanism of demineralization-remineralization should clarify the rationale to initiate early preventive dental strategies and repair subsurface lesions before cavitation occurs. Figure 34-5 illustrates the dynamic nature of the caries process and control strategies.

Malocclusions

Dental malocclusions are best defined as crowded, irregular, or protruding teeth that interfere with dental-oral function or dental-facial aesthetics or increase the likelihood of injury to the teeth. When severe, malocclusions may produce a functional disturbance that interferes with mastication, swallowing, speech, and normal function of the temporomandibular joint. Less severe malocclusions often require some physiological compensation for the anatomical deformity to allow for adequate function.

Impaired dental-facial aesthetics can have a profound effect on a child's psychosocial development and, if extreme, should be considered a social handicap. Different cultures, families, and individuals have different views on dental-facial aesthetics, and these individual views should be respected. However, as unfortunate as it is, dental-facial aesthetics has become a factor in how children feel about themselves and how others view them. This fact should not be ignored, especially when a child's self-image is being affected by malposed teeth.

Protruding incisor teeth have twice the chance of receiving some sort of trauma resulting in dental fractures or devitalization of the pulp (Andreasen, 1994). Minimizing the risk of dental trauma to anterior teeth through interceptive or definitive orthodontic treatment is considered a part of comprehensive preventive dental care.

DESCRIPTION AND INCIDENCE OF OCCLUSION

The Angle orthodontic classification system is based on Edward H. Angle's classification established in the early 1900s and continues to be the standard to describe dental and facial-skeletal occlusion. This classification system

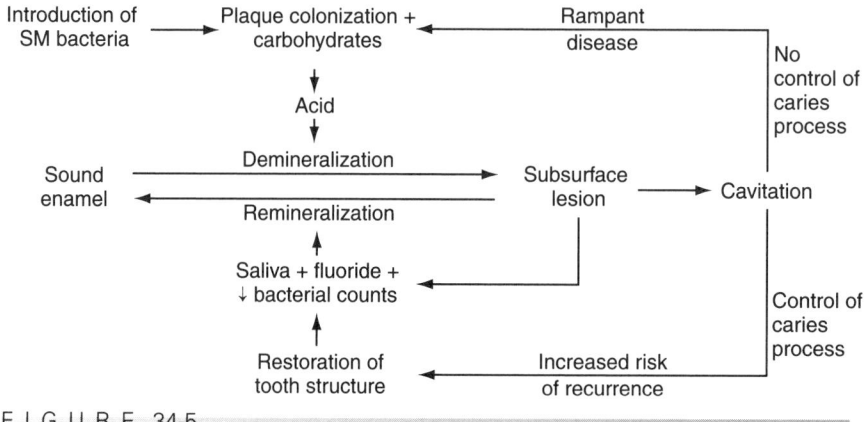

F I G U R E 34-5
The dynamic process of caries formation and control. SM = *Streptococcus mutans.*

uses the maxillary and mandibular permanent first molars and their relationship with each other to describe the anterior–posterior relationship of the dentition. Class I normal occlusion is described as follows:

The maxillary first permanent molar interdigitates into the mandibular first permanent molar. When the crown and root angulation of these molar teeth are in proper alignment, as well as being in a Class I relationship, the premolars and canines of the dentition can fully interdigitate with each other. It is essential that this Class I or normal occlusion be established for proper overjet and overbite to occur.

Classes I, II, and III malocclusion are illustrated and defined in Figure 34-6.

This classification system has been expanded to describe not only the specific tooth-to-tooth relationships of the dental arches but also the skeletal relationships of the maxilla and mandible (Table 34-3 and Figs. 34-7 and 34-8). As an example, a patient with a prognathic maxilla and/or a retrognathic mandible would have a Class II skeletal occlusion.

The reported incidence of dental–facial malocclusions varies with the defining criteria used by different investigators. Using Grainger's Treatment Priority Index, the US Public Health Service reports that approximately 25% of children aged 6 to 11 years have nearly ideal occlusion but, by 12 to 17 years of age, only 12% have nearly ideal occlusion (Grainger, 1967). Crowding and malaligned teeth account for

40% of malocclusions in 6- to 11-year-old children and 85% of malocclusions in children 12 to 17 years old.

CHRONOLOGICAL STAGES OF OCCLUSAL DEVELOPMENT

Pediatric dentists and orthodontists refer to three stages to identify milestones of dental development related to timing and growth of the oral-facial structures (Table 34-4).

As the occlusion develops from the primary dentition through the transitional (or mixed dentition) to the permanent dentition, the sequence of events should occur in an orderly, symmetrical, and timely fashion. This arrangement results in a functional, aesthetic, and stable occlusion. When this sequence is disrupted, final occlusion of the permanent dentition is affected. The most common factors initiating abnormal development of occlusion are:

- Genetic control of the size, shape, and position of the maxilla and mandible within the facial structure and the direction of growth of both bones
- Genetic control of tooth size, shape, development, and eruption
- Abnormal oral musculature
- Digit/pacifier habits
- Premature loss of deciduous teeth, particularly the second deciduous molar
- Over-retained deciduous teeth

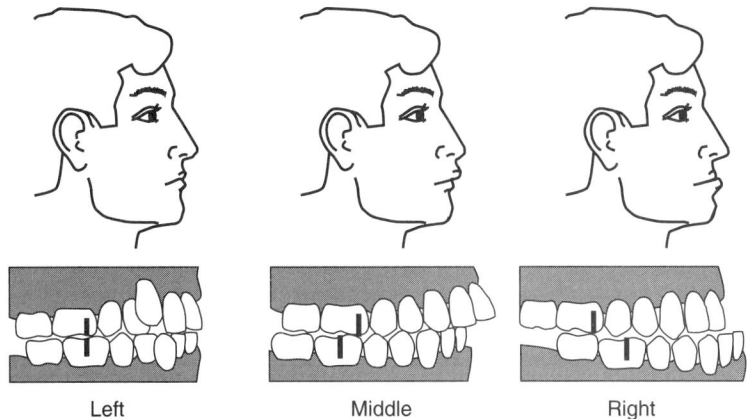

| Left | Middle | Right |

FIGURE 34-6
Orthodontic Classification System

Left: Class I facial relationship and dental malocclusion: The molar relationship is the same as in normal occlusion; however, some other problem with alignment of the teeth exists, such as crowding in one section or throughout the entire dental arch.

Middle: Class II facial relationship and dental malocclusion: This classification refers to any positioning of the maxillary molars more anterior to the Class I position, the mandibular molars more posterior to the Class I position, or a combination of the two.

Right: Class III facial relationship and dental malocclusion: This classification is the opposite of Class II, the Class III classification being any positioning of the maxillary molars more posterior to the Class I position, the mandibular molars more anterior to the Class I position, or a combination of the two.

When such disruptions do occur, appropriate corrective measures are needed to restore normal occlusal development. Such corrective procedures may require some type of passive space maintenance, active tooth guidance, or a combination of both.

Gingivitis and Periodontal Disease

Red swollen gingiva that easily bleeds is caused and perpetuated by bacterial plaque accumulations under the gingival crevice (Fig. 34-9). Gingivitis is a sign of poor oral hygiene and

bacterial plaque control that leads to increased caries activity. Advanced periodontal disease rarely develops in young children, but older teenagers with poor oral hygiene do show early signs of periodontal disease (an extension of the infection and inflammation into deeper structures of the periodontium) that becomes more difficult to control with increasing age. Other risk factors include tobacco or other drug use and children with special health needs or a disability that interferes with oral hygiene (e.g., systemic diseases that compromise immune function or require medication such as phenytoin or antineoplastics).

FIGURE 34-7
Dental Bite Relationships
Left: Anterior openbite (also called negative overbite)
Middle: Anterior deepbite (overbite)
Right: Posterior and anterior crossbite

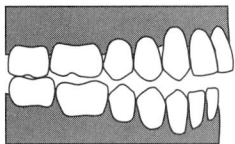
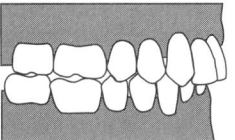
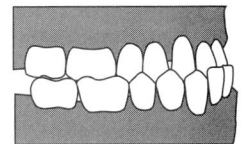

| Left | Middle | Right |

T A B L E 34-3

Classifications of Skeletal Relationships of the Maxilla and Mandible*

Overbite: Overbite is the amount of overlap of the maxillary incisors over the mandibular incisors. It is measured from the incisal edge of the maxillary teeth to the incisal edge of the mandibular teeth. In addition, it can describe a negative overbite, which is actually an _open bite_ in which the anterior teeth or incisors do not overlap each other at all (Ngan & Fields, 1997). A 2-mm space from incisal edge to incisal edge in a vertical direction between the incisors would be described as a negative 2-mm overbite or a 2-mm open bite.

Overjet: Overjet is an anterior–posterior relationship description. It describes how far the maxillary incisors are in front of or behind the mandibular incisors and is described in millimeters. An overjet is measured from the lingual surface of the incisal edge of the maxillary incisors to the facial surface of the incisal edge of the mandibular incisors. Parents often refer to an excessive overjet as a "bad overbite" when describing their child's occlusion. These two terms should not be confused because they may have different treatment consequences.

Crossbite: In normal occlusion, the maxillary dentition occludes a half-tooth outside or lateral to the posterior mandibular teeth and in front of the mandibular incisor teeth.

In an anterior crossbite, the maxillary anterior teeth are behind (lingual) the mandibular anterior teeth. A _complete anterior crossbite_ can indicate a skeletal growth problem and developing class III malocclusion. Anterior crossbite of one or more of the permanent incisors (see Fig. 34–8), however, may be evidence of a localized discrepancy, which in most cases should be treated as soon as it is discovered. Delayed treatment can lead to serious complications.

A _posterior crossbite_ can be two different types. In the most common type, the maxillary posterior teeth are lingual or medial to their normal position with the mandibular posterior teeth. In the second, less common type of posterior crossbite, the maxillary posterior teeth are lateral to the mandibular posterior teeth such that the entire maxillary tooth is not in contact with the biting surface of the lower tooth. Posterior crossbites result from skeletal, dental, or functional causes, or a combination of all three.

A _skeletal crossbite_ results from a discrepancy in the structure of the mandible or maxilla. A basic discrepancy in the width of the arches may be noted, especially a narrow maxillary or wide mandibular arch.

A _posterior crossbite_ in the primary dentition involving the second molar or even all the teeth anterior to it occurs in 3% to 7% of all children (McDonald and Avery, 1999).

A _dental crossbite_ results from a faulty eruption pattern in which one or more of the posterior teeth erupt into a crossbite relationship. There may be no irregularity in the basal bone. After the teeth erupt, the occlusion locks them into position and drives them even further into a crossbite relationship.

A _functional crossbite_ results from the mandible shifting into an abnormal, but often more comfortable, position. Occlusal interference and the resultant functional shift of the mandible into a crossbite relationship can develop into a true skeletal defect with mandibular asymmetry, if untreated.

*See also Figures 34–7 and 34–8.

Trauma

Injury can occur to the supporting structures (the jawbones), the soft tissues, or the teeth. Traumatic injuries to a child's mouth and teeth are common (e.g., toddlers learning to walk, preschoolers on mobile toys and in the park, older children on the playground and participat-ing in sports). Additionally, all children are at risk while riding in a motor vehicle. Children with poor coordination or a lack of protective reflexes are also at risk. These injuries are not usually severe but require attention.

The teeth and oral soft tissues are susceptible to injury from other causes as well. The re-peated vomiting that occurs in bulimia deminer-

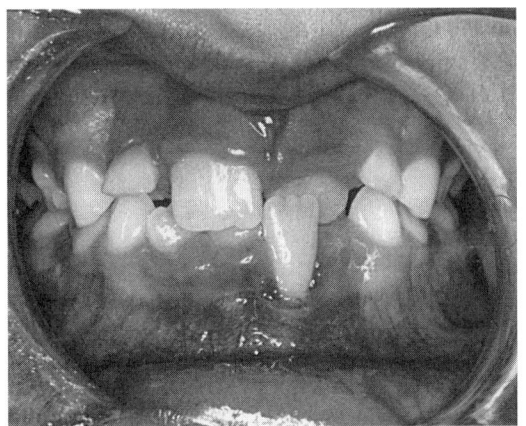

F I G U R E 34-8

Anterior crossbite involving maxillary left central incisor and mandibular left central incisor. Note stripping of gingiva from facial of lower incisor as a result of this traumatic occlusion.

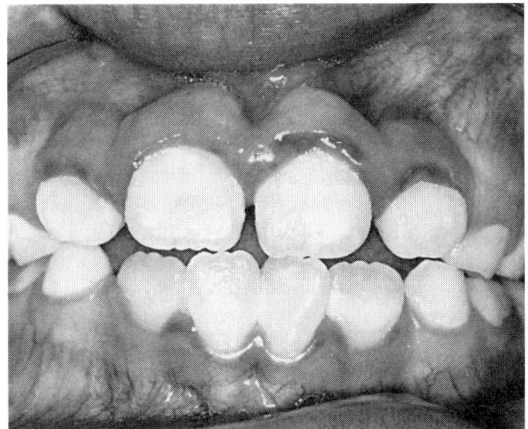

F I G U R E 34-9

Gingivitis. Gingival inflammation is caused and perpetuated by plaque accumulation under the gingival crevice. Proper oral hygiene can correct this common condition. (Photo courtesy of Berg and Jones.)

T A B L E 34-4

Stages of Dental Development

1. *Primary Dentition*—By 3 years of age all 20 primary teeth should be erupted or erupting. It is preferable to have some spacing between the primary teeth even after full eruption to allow for the size of the permanent teeth. A 3- or 4-year-old child with no spacing between the deciduous teeth (primate space) is most likely to have crowding and require orthodontic treatment when the permanent teeth erupt.

2. *Transitional Dentition*—This term applies to a "mixed dentition" of primary and permanent teeth and generally includes ages 6 to 12 years. Two stages of development occur during this period. Stage 1 occurs early in the transitional dentition and involves exfoliation of the primary central and lateral incisors and eruption of the permanent central and lateral incisors, as well as the permanent first molars. Stage 2 occurs late in the transitional dentition. It involves exfoliation of the primary canines and molars and eruption of the permanent canines and premolars (bicuspids). This time frame is often referred to as the "Ugly Duckling" period because of the spaces commonly seen between the newly erupted permanent incisors.

3. *Early Permanent Dentition*—This stage includes the time from exfoliation of the last primary tooth until full eruption allows for complete occlusion of all the permanent teeth, except for the third molars (wisdom teeth). The age range is usually from 12 to 16 years old.

alizes tooth enamel and causes a unique type of trauma. Tobacco use in either smoke or spit (chewing tobacco or snuff) form damages oral tissue and predisposes the user to oral cancer. Approximately one in three adolescents uses tobacco (Casamassimo, 1996; Johnson & Squier, 1993).

Injuries about the head, neck, and face occur in about half of all child abuse cases. Many of these children also have accompanying dental involvement, so this diagnosis must be kept in mind when evaluating injury to the mouth and oral cavity.

ASSESSMENT

History

The history should include the following:

- Parental dental history for risk assessment (see Table 34-2)
- Assessment of risk factors for early childhood caries (Table 34-5)
- Family history of caries, craniofacial deformities, malocclusion, periodontal disease
- Pattern of tooth eruption
- Fluoride content of the primary water supply
- Fluoride supplementation
- Use of toothbrush, toothpaste, and floss
- Age at the first dental visit and periodicity of subsequent preventive dental visits
- Whether a "dental home" has been established

- Traumatic injuries
- Other age-related factors:
  - Infants and toddlers up to 3 years of age: feeding/behavioral habits, including the frequency and types of feedings/meals/snacks (e.g., nibblers and sippers) and the use of breast, bottle, or cup for behavioral purposes, not just nutrition
  - Preschool children 3 to 5 years of age: oral habits—finger sucking, pacifier use
  - School-age children and adolescents: oral habits, orthodontic and orthopedic corrections, activities and sports participation
  - Children with an increased susceptibility to surgically induced bacteremias (e.g., cardiac defects) and the need for antibiotic prophylaxis with some dental procedures. (Many dental procedures are not as traumatic to gingival tissue as daily toothbrushing and may not require antibiotic prophylaxis. Advising a patient or parent to take an antibiotic before having any "dental work" oversimplifies the variety of dental procedures available that a patient may require and leads to overuse of antibiotics and the risk of acquiring resistant bacteria.) (See Chapter 31 for specific information.)

Physical Examination

POSITIONING

INFANTS. The infant's mouth is best examined with the child lying on the lap of the

T A B L E 34-5
Risk Factors for Early Childhood Caries

Active caries in the mother or close caregiver	History of poor family oral health
High SM counts in the mother	Previous ECC
High SM counts in the child	Inadequate systemic fluoride
Visible decalcified lesions	High sugar intake
Inappropriate bottle use	Poor oral hygiene
Frequent snacks	Oral dysfunction
Physical handicaps	Children in free or reduced lunch programs
Poverty	Children with special health care needs
Frequent use of medicines containing sucrose	Cultural customs
Complicated pregnancy	

ECC = early childhood caries; SM = *Streptococcus mutans.*

parent and examiner or on an examination table with the hands and arms held above the baby's head by the parent. This position stabilizes the head and enables the examiner to look into the mouth with only overhead illumination. Talking throughout the examination eases the anxiety of both the parent and the child.

TODDLERS, PRESCHOOLERS, AND OLDER CHILDREN. Examination of a toddler's mouth is accomplished with the toddler lying with legs around the parent's waist and head in the examiner's lap and the parent holding the child's hands and lower torso. Alternatively, the child stands between the examiner's legs, facing the same direction as the examiner, opens the mouth and tilts the head back. The examiner's crossed legs help hold the child and enable both the parent and the examiner to view the child's mouth. This method is also excellent for parents to use when brushing and flossing the child's teeth. Examining an older child's mouth can be performed with the child in the standing, sitting, or prone position (with a tongue blade and good lighting).

EXAMINATION

Physical examination assesses the following:

- Facial symmetry, jaw size
- Mouth—moistness, color, odor, lesions, frenulum
- Lips—cracking, scaling, maceration, lesions
- Gums—color, texture, bleeding, lesions, overgrowth, plaque
- Mucosa—color, lesions, hydration
- Tongue—color, texture, fissured, geographical, coated
- Hard and soft palate—intact, cleft, bifid uvula
- Teeth—number, size, shape, color, crowding, pits, fissures, caries, staining, interarch occlusion (best examined with the child's mouth closed and the lips lifted with a tongue blade)

▄▄▄ MANAGEMENT AND PREVENTIVE DENTAL STRATEGIES

Establishing the Dental Home

All children should have a dental home where comprehensive, continuously accessible and af-

fordable care is available and delivered or supervised by qualified pediatric dental specialists (adapted from the medical home concept, American Academy of Pediatrics [AAP], 1992). Referring the child for dental care at 12 months of age establishes the child's "dental home" and provides an opportunity to implement preventive dental health habits that keep the child free of dental/oral disease. The "dental home" should be expected to provide:

- An accurate risk assessment for dental diseases.
- An individualized preventive dental health program based on the risk assessment.
- Anticipatory guidance about growth and development issues (e.g., teething, digit or pacifier habits).
- A plan for emergency dental trauma.
- Information about proper care of the child's teeth and gingiva.
- Information about proper nutrition practices.
- Pit and fissure sealants.
- Restorative and surgical dental care when necessary that meets the parents' and child's psychological needs.
- Interceptive orthodontic and facial orthopedic care for children with developing malocclusions.
- A special place for the child and parent to establish a positive attitude about dental health without acquiring the classic dental phobias that are still common in many adults.
- Referrals to other dental specialists such as endodontists, periodontists, oral surgeons, and orthodontists when care cannot be directly provided within the "dental home."
- Comprehensive dental care in accordance with accepted guidelines and periodicity schedules for pediatric dental health. Table 34-6 outlines the periodicity schedule for comprehensive pediatric preventive dental care as recommended by the American Academy of Pediatric Dentistry (AAPD). Standards for performing dental radiographs as recommended by the US Food and Drug Administration (FDA) and all professional dental organizations can be found in the AAPD reference manual (1999).

T A B L E 34-6

Recommendations for Preventive Pediatric Dental Care

Because each child is unique these recommendations are designed for the care of children who have no important health problems and are developing normally. These recommendations will need to be modified for children with special health care needs or if disease or trauma manifests variations from normal. The Academy emphasizes the importance of very early professional intervention and the continuity of care based on the individualized needs of the child.

Age[1]	Infancy 6–12 Months	Late Infancy 12–24 Months	Preschool 2–6 Years	School-Aged 6–12 Years	Adolescence 12–18 Years
Oral Hygiene Counseling[2]	Parents/Guardians/ Caregivers	Parents/Guardians/ Caregivers	Child/Parent/ Caregivers	Child/Parent/ Caregivers	Patient
Injury Prevention Counseling[3]	•	•	•	•	•
Dietary Counseling[4]	•	•	•	•	•
Counseling for Non-nutritive Habits[5]	•	•	•	•	•
Fluoride Supplementation[6,7]	•	•	•	•	•
Assess Oral Growth & Development[8]	•	•	•	•	•
Clinical Oral Exam	•	•	•	•	•
Prophylaxis and Topical Fluoride Treatment[9]		•	•	•	•
Radiographic Assessment[10]					
Pit & Fissure Sealants			If indicated on primary molars	1st permanent molars as soon as possible after eruption	2nd permanent molars and appropriate pre-molars as soon as possible after erup-tion

Treatment of Dental Disease/Injury

Assessment and Treatment of Developing Malocclusion

Substance Abuse Counseling

Assessment and Removal of 3rd Molars

Referral for Regular and Periodic Dental Care

Anticipatory Guidance[11]

1. First exam at the eruption of the 1st tooth and no later than 12 months.
2. Initially, responsibility of parent; as child develops jointly with parents; then when indicated only child.
3. Initially play objects, pacifiers, car seats; then when learning to walk; and finally sports and routine playing.
4. At every appointment discuss the role of refined carbohydrates; frequency of snacking.
5. At first discuss the need for additional sucking; digits vs. pacifiers; then the need to wean from the habit before the eruption of the first permanent front teeth. For school-aged children and adolescent patients, counsel regarding any existing habits such as fingernail biting, clenching, or bruxism.
6. As per AAP/ADA Guidelines and the water source.
7. Up to at least 16 years.
8. By clinical examination.
9. Especially for children at high risk for caries and periodontal disease.
10. As per AAPD Radiographic Guidelines.
11. Appropriate discussion and counseling; should be an integral part of each visit for care.

From the American Academy of Pediatric Dentistry Reference Manual, Chicago, 1999.

Dental care for most children is provided in a quiet, nonthreatening environment, particularly when professional dental care is started early in a child's life. Pediatric dentists have considerable training in child psychology and accept the responsibility to guide and manage the child's behavior in the dental office environment. Pediatric dentists are teachers and want the child's undivided attention in order to guide and mold the child's attitude and behavior related to dental care. Frequently, the child is separated from the parent during dental visits. At other times, the pediatric dentist may request that the parent help manage the child, particularly if the child is very young or noncommunicative. Very young children who require considerable treatment, children with overt behavior problems, or children with developmental delay may require sedation, general anesthesia, or physical stabilization (restraints). Some pediatric deaths have been associated with the improper use of sedation or anesthesia. The NP should be familiar with the indications for sedation and anesthesia in children undergoing dental procedures and with the levels of sedation and monitoring requirements that are recommended for these children in order to counsel parents seeking advise about dental work for their children. Guidelines related to sedation and anesthesia have been established and are available from the AAPD. Similar guidelines on the use of restraints and behavior modification can also be obtained from the AAPD (see Resource Box).

The NP should be aware of the child's treatment needs and behavior challenges and the accepted guidelines of care used by pediatric dental providers. NPs should feel comfortable consulting with the pediatric dentist and be able to help support and counsel the family to receive the best possible dental care.

Oral Health Counseling and Risk Assessment

The NP should include oral health counseling and caries risk assessment as part of well-child care.

INFANTS 6 TO 12 MONTHS OF AGE

During this first year, the NP should:

- Complete a risk assessment for the trans-

mission of SM from the mother or close caregivers to the child. If necessary,
  - Counsel the parents about the risk they pose to their child.
  - Refer the parents for dental care.
  - Prescribe chlorhexidine (0.12%) mouth rinse to reduce SM reservoirs in the parent.
- Complete a risk assessment for the child to acquire ECC (see Table 34-5).
- Refer the child for professional preventive dental care and establish the "dental home" at 6 to 18 months of age, depending on the risk assessment for ECC. All authorities recommend that the first dental visit occur on or near the first birthday (12 months of age) for first-born children, unless the risk assessment indicates a higher susceptibility for ECC and thus a need for an earlier time for the first dental visit.
- Implement appropriate systemic fluoride therapy.
- Teach the parents proper oral hygiene care for their infant shortly after birth. A hands-on demonstration should be done to show the parent that the procedure will not hurt the child. Wiping the inside of an infant's mouth with a moistened washcloth cleans the oral mucosa and begins to desensitize the infant to oral manipulation. As soon as teeth erupt, the parent should begin to use a wide-bristled soft toothbrush to brush the child's teeth at least one time per day. Toothbrushing for infants is best accomplished in bed or in the child's bassinet from behind the child. A very small amount of toothpaste (less than one fourth the size of a pea) should be used and then wiped from the infant's mouth. Removing bacterial plaque from the newly erupting teeth not only reduces the chance of SM colonization but also prevents the bacterial gingivitis that accounts for much of teething pain.
- Discuss appropriate feeding and behavior guidance practices. Parents need to be taught appropriate feeding practices and cautioned about the risks that come from inappropriate breastfeeding intervals or bottle use. They should also be given guidance on managing a crying or fussy child.

Although not approved by all pediatric authorities, the use of a pacifier does not disturb normal growth and development of the oral–dental structures at this age.

- Examine the child's teeth and gums during well-child visits for signs of demineralization or decay and adequate plaque removal at the gum line of erupted and erupting teeth. Providing anticipatory guidance about dental development helps the parent understand the changes that occur within the child's mouth with growth. Referral to a pediatric dentist should be made quickly if abnormalities in development arise or areas of demineralization of enamel are visualized.
- Identify children with special health care needs because they have a much higher risk of caries and periodontal disease. Their "dental home" should be established during the second 6 months of life.

CHILDREN 12 TO 24 MONTHS OF AGE

During the second year, the NP should do the following:

- Continue oral health assessment.
- Examine the child's teeth and gums as described earlier.
- Ensure that the "dental home" is established and confirm that the child is receiving timely appropriate dental care and appropriate systemic fluoride therapy. For younger siblings from low-risk families, delaying the first dental visit until the child is 15 to 18 months old may be permitted because the "dental home" for that family is established.
- All children should be seen in a dental office by 18 months of age to receive their first dental prophylaxis, topical fluoride treatment, and initial behavior guidance experience.
- Review proper oral hygiene techniques, appropriate feeding, and behavior guidance practices with the parents as necessary.
- Reinforce injury prevention, including the use of a car seat, belts for shopping carts, and gates.

CHILDREN 24 MONTHS TO 5 YEARS OF AGE

During health supervision visits, the NP should be alert to identify any signs of poor oral hygiene, abnormal growth and development of the teeth, malocclusion, or signs of dental trauma, including nonvital teeth. In addition, the NP should:

- Confirm that the child is receiving timely preventive dental care and appropriate systemic fluoride therapy.
- Ascertain who the child's primary care dentist is and how often the child sees the dentist.
- Examine the child's teeth and gums for signs of demineralization or decay and adequate plaque removal at the gum line of erupted and erupting teeth.
- Identify nonvital dark deciduous teeth (Fig. 34-10). Deciduous teeth that appear dark have been subjected to enough trauma that the dental pulp tissue has undergone necrosis and lost its vitality. Nonvital deciduous teeth have the potential for peripheral root resorption, chronic apical granulomas, and infection that can damage the underlying developing permanent tooth bud or spread to other tissues. Prompt endodontic treatment improves the prognosis for retention of the tooth until it exfoliates at the normal age.
- Reinforce supervised oral hygiene home care. Oral hygiene for a preschool child

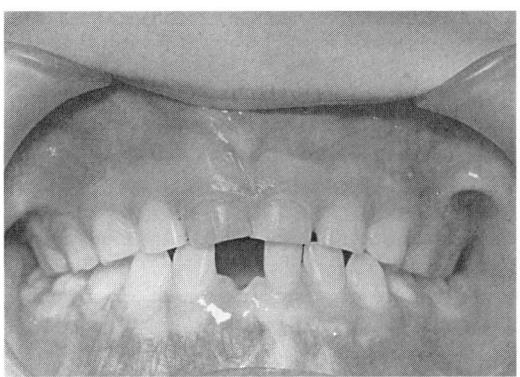

F I G U R E 34-10
Dark, nonvital tooth indicating necrotic pulp.

needs to be performed at least one time a day by a parent or caregiver. The family habit of sending children to brush after meals or before bedtime unsupervised is not successful. Parents need to understand that the objective of toothbrushing is to remove bacterial plaque from the gum line and from in between the teeth, not just to remove food.

- ○ Preschool and school-age children who do not yet have sufficient fine motor coordination to write their name in cursive require daily help from a parent. In addition to the oral hygiene provided by the parent, these children should be provided a soft-bristled toothbrush with a large handle and wide bristle head and asked to brush their own teeth two times per day to practice their skills and develop personal hygiene habits. Children should be encouraged to use the gross motor (back and forth) scrub brush technique until fine motor skills have matured (12 to 14 years).
- ○ Dental flossing (to remove the bacterial plaque that accumulates between the teeth, where the toothbrush is ineffective) is a very difficult skill to master. Flossing should be performed by the parent at least three to four times per week in children older than 3 years until they have the coordination to do their own teeth (at 8 years of age).
- Reinforce appropriate injury prevention, including the use of seat belts and helmets for bicycling and rollerblading.
- Review with parents the importance of fluoride treatments, use of dental sealants, oral development, and tooth eruption.
- Educate parents about handling dental emergencies.

CHILDREN 5 TO 10 YEARS OLD

During these years, the NP should continue to use all the aforementioned information and, in addition, should:

- Identify and counsel children regarding the need for a sports mouthguard or face protector.

- Reinforce proper nutritional practices with particular reference to frequent ingestion of sugars. Excessive ingestion of soda and gum chewing are frequent contributors to increased caries activity as school-age children and teenagers become more independent of parental controls.

ADOLESCENTS

During adolescence, the NP should use the information just presented and, in addition, should:

- Reinforce proper oral hygiene procedures to teenagers, including brushing twice a day and flossing daily.
- Teach the adolescent to identify signs of gingivitis and gingival bacterial plaque accumulation.
- Educate the child and parent regarding the dangers of using tobacco (smoke and spit) and other drugs.

Controlling the Caries Epidemic

Many health professionals have been misled into believing that dental caries is no longer a major health issue for children and that fluoridated water has been the solution. Yet, 50% of schoolchildren have decay by 7 years of age. By 17 years of age, 84% of teenagers have eight carious or filled teeth (Edelstein & Douglass, 1995) (see Fig. 34-5). Recent studies continue to find decay prevalence clustering between 6 and 30% in preschool children younger than 3 years, and in some underserved and indigent segments of our society, decay prevalence as high as 85% is reported (Bolden et al., 1993).

The Centers for Disease Control and Prevention now defines dental caries as "perhaps the most common infectious disease in the US population." It accounts for more than 50 million hours of school time lost annually because of dental problems or dental visits. Furthermore, a terminology change from Baby Bottle Tooth Decay to Early Childhood Caries (ECC) to identify a specific dental disease found in young children is now suggested so that the name of the disease is not confused with a potential disease modifier (see Color Fig. 12). Clearly, a different strategy to prevent the caries process, the resultant destruction of teeth, and the pattern of decay throughout childhood must be developed and implemented.

Historically, primary medical care providers have assumed responsibility for the oral care of children younger than 3 years or ignored the need for dental care and waited until a child was 3 or 4 years of age before suggesting that the parents seek professional dental care. Often, parents were told to wait until all the "baby teeth erupt" or until the child could cooperate. If decay was identified, referral to a pediatric dentist was made. This concept of dental care:

- Ignores the reservoirs of bacteria that infect young children.
- Permits the infectious bacterial process to spread.
- Addresses only the modifiers of the caries process (the bottle or breast).
- Ignores the availability of fluoride vehicles to increase host resistance to the caries process.
- Treats with surgical or restorative dentistry the ravages of the disease instead of concentrating on prevention.
- Ignores the relationship of ECC to the systemic health of the child. Acs and associates (1992) reported that children with ECC have weights significantly lower than children without ECC and that the mean age of low-weight patients with ECC was significantly greater than that of patients at or above their ideal weights, thus indicating that progression of ECC may affect growth adversely.

Most pediatric dentists are not confident that the high caries prevalence in preschool children will ever be reduced without initiating earlier professional preventive dental care. Simply stated, it is no longer "best practice" to delay the timing of the first dental visit until after the caries process has begun or a cavity is detected, but rather, a risk-based assessment of the child's liability to the caries process should be completed before bacterial colonization has begun. This assessment is a prerequisite to determine appropriate preventive or treatment options for dental care.

Fluoride supplementation and pit and fissure sealants are two successful and readily available preventive strategies. Fluoride supplementation is indicated for all children 6 months to 16 years of age who are living in areas without optimally fluoridated community water, for breastfed infants older than 6 months, and for children who drink only fluoride-free bottled or osmotically purified water as their primary water source. Systemic fluoride reduces dental decay by nearly 50% and is considered to be a significant part of successful preventive dental strategies (AAP, 1995; McDonald & Avery, 1994). The incidence of mild and moderate dental fluorosis is increasing (Fig. 34-11). Most fruit juices and sodas are reconstituted or made with fluoridated water. This practice is reported to be partially responsible for the increase in the ambient level of fluoride in a child's diet. Other sources of excessive ingestion of fluoride include young children swallowing too much fluoride toothpaste and fluoride supplementation when the primary water source contains optimal or high levels of fluoride. The clinician should always analyze the fluoride content of the child's primary water source (unless the water comes from a known community fluoride source) and review the child's ECC risk assessment before prescribing fluoride supplements. Recommended supplemental fluoride doses are listed in Table 34-7 and should be accurately prescribed.

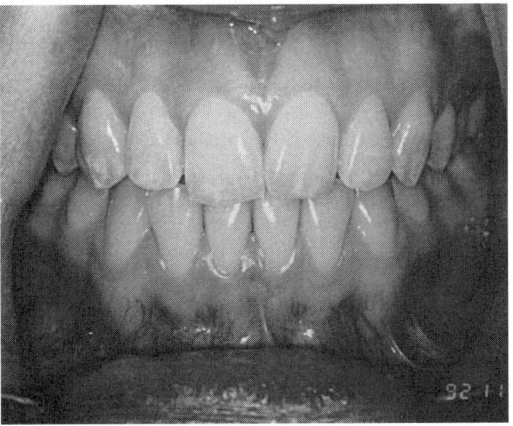

F I G U R E 34-11
Mild dental fluorosis.

T A B L E 34-7

*Fluoride Supplementation Regimen**

AGE	CONCENTRATION OF FLUORIDE IN WATER		
	<0.3 ppm (mg)	0.3–0.6 ppm (mg)	>0.6 ppm (mg)
Birth–6 mo	0	0	0
6 mo–3 yr	0.25	0	0
3–6 yr	0.50	0.25	0
6 yr up to at least 16 yr	1.0	0.50	0

*Recommended daily dosage of fluoride in milligrams per day; 1 mg of fluoride is equivalent to 2.2 mg of sodium fluoride. Fluoride is available in the following formulations: drops, 0.5 mg/ml; oral solution, 2.5 mg/ml; tablets (dissolve or chew), 0.25, 0.5, and 1 mg; in combination with multivitamins
From American Academy of Pediatric Dentistry: Special Issue: Reference Manual 1999–2000. 21(6), 1999.

Pit and fissure sealants provide one of the most beneficial and cost-effective preventive treatments available. Sealants involve the application of protective resin coatings that bond to the biting (occlusal) surfaces of molars and premolars (Fig. 34-12). Most molars and premolars are susceptible to decay in the poorly formed grooves on the biting surface. Some of the pits, fissures, or grooves are so deep and narrow that even the bristle of the toothbrush cannot effectively remove plaque and food debris. This inaccessibility allows caries to occur even in the presence of impeccable oral hygiene. Children with deep grooves on their posterior teeth should have sealants placed soon after eruption.

Preventing and Treating Malocclusion

Evaluation of the child's developing occlusion is the first step in preventing and treating malocclusion. If malocclusion is recognized, referral for a comprehensive evaluation in the primary or early mixed dentition stage identifies abnormalities that if addressed early in a child's dental development often prevent major orthodontic treatment later. Orthodontic treatment provided by the pediatric dentist or orthodontist may be preventive, interceptive, or comprehensive.

PREVENTIVE TREATMENT

Space maintenance and control of oral habits (bruxism, non-nutritive sucking that interferes with normal growth and development, and abnormal tongue and swallowing habits) are the two main orthodontic treatments that prevent the oral neuromuscular complex from developing into an abnormal physical relationship (malocclusion).

F I G U R E 34-12
Sealants. Pit and fissure sealants are the most underutilized preventive regimen in dentistry. They can prevent carious lesions from forming in the occlusal (biting) surfaces of most teeth with susceptible deep grooves. (Photo courtesy of Berg and Jones.)

Space Maintenance

When a primary or permanent tooth is lost prematurely, the forces that hold that tooth in space three-dimensionally are no longer in equilibrium. It is not unusual for the teeth anterior and posterior to the lost tooth to tip into the newly opened space. By placing a space maintainer, these three-dimensional forces are held in balance. Space maintainers are either fixed (unilateral or bilateral) or removable. Unilateral fixed spacers are the most common (Fig. 34-13).

Bruxism

Bruxism is nonfunctional grinding or gnashing of teeth and occurs in approximately 15% of adult and child patients. The habit usually occurs at night and, if continued over a prolonged period, can result in abrasion of the permanent teeth. In adolescents, the habit is usually associated with stress and may lead to temporomandibular joint disturbances. The treatment of choice for adolescents is a nighttime mouthguard to prevent wear of the teeth and encourage oral–facial muscle relaxation. Younger children rarely continue to grind their teeth on a consistent enough basis to abrade their teeth or produce temporomandibular joint disturbances. Childhood night grinding has been shown to have association with chronic middle ear congestion but is not related to stress or emotional disturbances. The disorder is self-limited and rarely of any consequence, but it should be addressed by the dental home provider.

Non-nutritive Sucking

Thumb/finger sucking and pacifier use are common practices that should not be allowed to complicate or interfere with normal growth and development of the oral–facial structures. Non-nutritive sucking is a normal activity in most children younger than 2 years, with many parents encouraging this habit for behavioral control. Any attempts to change this habit before the age of 24 to 30 months usually proves difficult and unnecessary. However, if continued beyond this age (depending on the frequency, duration, and intensity of the habit), the position of the teeth, as well as growth and function of the mandible, can be altered. The most commonly observed changes from these habits are flaring of the maxillary incisors (bucked teeth), development of an anterior open bite, or development of a posterior crossbite with a functional shift of the mandible.

Flaring of the maxillary deciduous incisors and persistence of a small open bite will have no abnormal effect on the position of the permanent incisors if the habit is stopped before appearance of the erupting permanent incisors. Severe flaring of the deciduous maxillary incisors or a large anterior open bite, particularly when combined with a retrognathic mandible, can interfere with speech development and mastication and should receive attention. The presence of a posterior crossbite (maxillary canines or molars inside the mandibular teeth) accompanied by a shift of the mandible laterally when the child bites the teeth together signals a

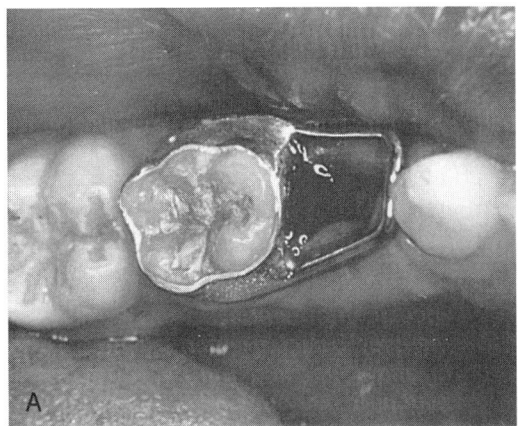
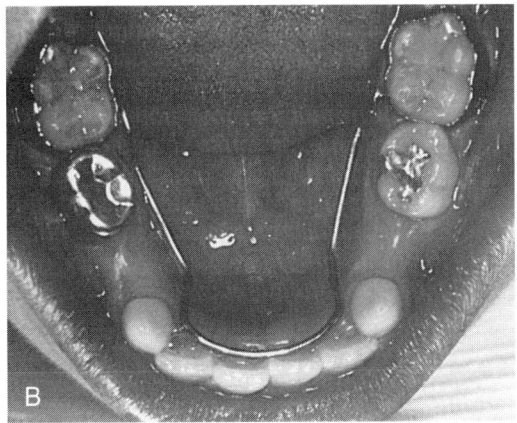

FIGURE 34-13
Fixed space maintainers: *A,* unilateral; *B,* bilateral.

potentially serious developmental disturbance. These functional shifts of the mandible should be referred and treated as early as possible (between 3 and 4 years of age) to prevent asymmetrical growth of the temporomandibular joint and excessive unilateral growth of the mandible causing lower facial asymmetry.

Various and conflicting theories explain the cause of thumb/finger sucking in children, and equally conflicting recommendations have been presented for its correction. Many children suck their thumbs or fingers for short periods during infancy or early childhood. Although the habit may be considered normal during the first 2 years of life, many children never have a digit-sucking habit. Parents should be advised to observe the child, and if the sucking gradually diminishes, it is probable that the child will stop without intervention. However, if the child shows no inclination to stop the habit, it becomes a problem that should be addressed by the dental home provider.

Corrective appliances for oral habits are indicated when the child reaches 4 to 5 years of age and when the child wants to discontinue the habit and needs only a reminder to accomplish the task. If an appliance is used, it should not be painful or a punishment or interfere with occlusion; instead, it should merely be a reminder. A retainer with a series of smooth loops placed lingual to the incisors has proved successful in helping children overcome maladaptive oral habits.

Some dentists have practiced an entirely different approach when it is evident that a child wants to discontinue the habit. This approach involves cooperation by the parents and their consent to disregard the habit and not mention it to the child. In private conversation with the child, the dentist discusses the problem and its effect. The child is asked to keep a daily record on a card of each episode of thumb sucking and to call the dentist each week and report on progress in stopping the habit. A decrease in the number of times that the habit is practiced is evidence of progress and indicates that the child will discontinue the habit. The parents' role in the correction of an oral habit is important. Parents are often overanxious about the habit and its possible effects and are tempted to use negative reinforcement, which is rarely effective. This anxiety may result in nagging or punishment and often creates greater tension and intensifies the habit. Painting the child's thumb or fingers with a noxious-tasting substance is also ineffective.

Correction of Tongue and Swallowing Habits

Abnormal tongue position and deviation from the so-called normal movement of the tongue during swallowing have long been associated with anterior open bite, protrusion of the maxillary incisors, and in some cases, lisping. Normal infants position the tongue anteriorly in the mouth at rest and during swallowing. The first physiological priority at birth is establishment of an airway so that respiration can begin. Accomplishment of this priority requires holding the tongue forward and down. The set of postural relationships of the oral and pharyngeal structures established in the first few minutes of life in response to respiratory requirements is maintained thereafter.

An infant's normal swallow is characterized by strong lip activity to seize the nipple, place the tongue tip against the lower lip beneath the nipple, and relax the elevator muscles of the mandible so that the mouth is wide open. As oral function matures, the elevator muscles of the mandible are gradually activated and the mandible is brought up toward what ultimately will be occlusal contact of the teeth. This act occurs while the tongue tip is still placed against the lower lip. The physiological transition in swallowing begins during the first year of life and normally continues over the next several years. A mature swallow pattern is characterized by relaxation of the lips, placement of the tongue behind the maxillary incisors, and elevation of the mandible until posterior teeth contact; this sequence is not usually observed before a child is 4 or 5 years of age. Myofunctional therapy for tongue thrusting or a deviated swallow is sometimes considered for children in the normal transitional stages of swallow maturation, but this procedure should be seriously questioned. Some preschool children with a forward tongue position have not yet learned to follow the adult pattern and with time will correct the problem. Dental open bite and abnormal tooth position are more likely caused by the influence of the resting position of the tongue rather than thrusting of the tongue while swallowing.

INTERCEPTIVE TREATMENT

Interceptive orthodontic treatment is designed to enhance the child's occlusal function and aesthetics at an early age and to minimize occlusal abnormalities that worsen with growth and as permanent teeth erupt. Typically, interceptive orthodontics involves correction of transverse (arch width) abnormalities, arch development to prevent dental crowding, anterior-posterior skeletal and dental relationships, and alignment of the eight incisors. An almost endless list of therapeutic tools are used in the dental profession to modify abnormally developing occlusions. Most of these tools are either fixed or functional appliances. Table 34-8 describes some of the more common ones.

COMPREHENSIVE TREATMENT

Comprehensive orthodontic treatment provides for diagnosis and treatment of the patient's entire oral-facial complex from early childhood through the completion of dental-facial growth. If financial resources are a problem for the family, help may be sought through special health care needs financing, Medicaid, or other funding sources.

It is best to look at comprehensive orthodontic care in terms of the three chronological stages of occlusal development. The objective of early treatment in the first two stages is to establish normal relationships of the dentition and the skeletal components of the face. It is sometimes possible, however, to establish such a harmonious relationship of the dental and skeletal units that further treatment is unnecessary once the full permanent dentition has erupted.

- *Primary Dentition.* When children are treated during this stage, normal patterns of growth and development can be established and, it is hoped, maintained throughout growth of the child. This objective is important not only from the perspective of the individual teeth but also for development of the entire oral-facial complex, including the temporomandibular joint. Abnormal dental and skeletal relationships that are perpetuated through the primary dentition become increasingly difficult to correct as the child becomes older. Orthopedic treatments are most commonly used during this stage (e.g., use of reverse headgear to protract the maxilla in Class III skeletal cases).
- *Mixed Dentition.* Early intervention during the mixed dentition stage is also designed to put the patient back into a normal occlusal and orthopedic relationship to enhance the probability that the patient will grow and develop with a normal oral-facial complex. Specific dental tooth corrections can be accomplished with fixed edgewise appliances (orthodontic bands and brackets) and functional appliances or headgear therapy. This phase of treatment lasts from 9

T A B L E 34-8

Fixed and Functional Appliances for Modifying Abnormally Developing Occlusions

Fixed Appliances primarily affect tooth position. Traditional orthodontic braces or bracketing systems consist of a metal band that wraps around the molar, a bracket bonded to the tooth, and arch wire to level and align the teeth with each other. Rubber bands or headgear can be used in combination with these brackets. Rubber bands are used to correct anterior-posterior relationships of the arches; headgear is used to correct skeletal and dental relationships.

Functional Appliances are removable appliances that cause skeletal changes in the oral-facial complex. The basic tenet of functional appliance therapy in a growing patient is to modify abnormal neuromuscular patterns so that the skeletal components and the dental units grow and develop into a more desirable Class I relationship.

to 18 months, at which time the patient goes through a rest phase until full eruption of the permanent dentition is achieved around 12 to 14 years of age.

* *Early Permanent Dentition Treatment.* This phase includes both orthopedic and orthodontic components. If a patient has undergone an earlier phase of comprehensive orthodontic treatment, this phase of treatment might take as little as 12 to 18 months. However, if this phase is the start of comprehensive care, 24 months is the normal length of treatment time.

Preventing Trauma to the Teeth and Mouth

During the early years of life, a focus on injury prevention facilitates protection of the mouth and oral cavity. Preventive measures include the use of gates at the top and bottom of stairs, avoidance of walkers, use of safety seats and seat belts when in motor vehicles, and use of bike helmets.

As children become older and more involved in organized sports, the incidence and severity of oral/dental trauma increase. Fortunately, many of these injuries can be prevented through the use of dental mouthguards. During health supervision visits or sports physical examinations, the NP should stress to the child and parent the importance of mouthguard protection.

Although "boil and bite" mouthguards are available from retail stores, custom-fitted mouthguards afford the best protection and allow for better speech, breathing, and retention. Because they are more comfortable, compliance is rarely the problem that it is with the more bulky retail mouthguards. Mouthguards were first developed in the 1950s to prevent chronic brain concussion in football players before the use of facemasks was made mandatory. Although prevention of concussion continues to be the primary objective of mouthguards, they also protect the lips, gingiva, and teeth by:

* Keeping the lips away from the teeth and preventing lip lacerations
* Preventing violent contact of the upper and lower teeth with resultant tooth and jaw fracture

* Holding the jaws apart, acting as a shock absorber to minimize energy transfer through the maxilla and condylar fossa to the cranial bones, and thereby preventing concussion
* Spreading the forces of the blow throughout the dentition rather than being directed at any one tooth or segment of bone to prevent tooth fractures and avulsions

Mouthguards should be recommended for all sports that involve heavy physical contact with another player or an object such as a hardball or softball (which is really as hard as a hardball, only bigger). Most football and hockey organizations mandate the use of mouthguards, and few oral injuries are seen in these sports. However, soccer, basketball, wrestling, and baseball/softball are the sports that the dental community now associates with oral/dental sports injuries. Mouthguards are also beneficial in activities such as skateboarding and in-line skating. All pediatric health professionals should recommend that mouthguards be required for these sports.

Discouraging the Use of Tobacco

Because of the recognized hazards of tobacco use (smoke and spit forms), it is important for the NP to educate children and adolescents about the hazards of tobacco use and discourage their starting any form of the habit. Additionally, NPs should encourage and counsel those who are already using tobacco to stop, which may include treating them or referring them for further treatment.

Prevention of Bacterial Endocarditis

Although uncommon, bacterial endocarditis (also called subacute bacterial endocarditis or infectious endocarditis) has a high morbidity and mortality rate and warrants primary prevention when indicated. The current recommendations, updated by consensus in 1997, are discussed in Chapter 31. Tables 31–11 to 31–15 outline the categories and indications for prophylaxis. Not every dental procedure requires prophylaxis. A simple guideline is that if the procedure causes no more trauma than daily toothbrushing, antibiotic coverage is not needed.

SPECIFIC DENTAL AND ORAL PROBLEMS

Infants

NATAL AND NEONATAL TEETH

Description

Natal teeth are present at birth and neonatal teeth erupt within the first 30 days of life (Fig. 34-14). They are usually in the mandibular incisor area, and a large majority are primary incisors. Only a small percentage are supernumerary teeth.

Etiology

Natal or neonatal teeth occur in 1 in 2000 births. A 15 to 20% familial occurrence has been noted.

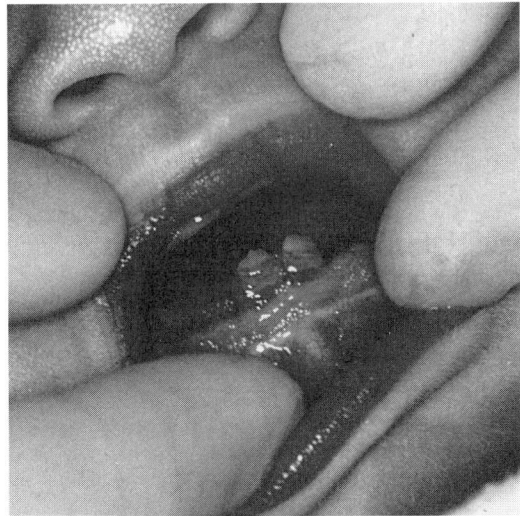

F I G U R E 34-14
Natal teeth. Natal teeth are distinguished from neonatal teeth in that they are present at birth. These teeth are extracted if they present a risk of aspiration. (Photo courtesy of Berg and Jones.)

Management

- If the tooth is extremely loose, it should be extracted before the infant is discharged from the nursery to prevent aspiration.
- If the tooth is not excessively loose, it should be evaluated by a pediatric dentist before the child leaves the hospital or within the first few days of life. Extracting a neonatal tooth on the basis that the tooth will interfere with breastfeeding is not warranted because children routinely breastfeed after 6 months of age, when teeth are present. A lactation nurse should be consulted if the mother has discomfort adjusting to the infant's suckling; use of a breast pump and bottling of mother's milk should be considered.

Complications

Aspiration of the tooth, pain, refusal to feed, and maternal discomfort with breastfeeding can occur.

TEETHING DISCOMFORT

Description

The inflammation and sensitivity that can be present in gingival tissue as deciduous teeth erupt is commonly referred to as "teething."

Assessment

The following are noted:

- Actively erupting deciduous teeth
- Irritability and fussiness
- Gingival inflammation
- Eruption hematoma or eruption cysts
- Bacterial plaque accumulation

Management

The following steps can be taken:

- Thorough daily toothbrushing of the erupting deciduous teeth should be done to prevent the gingival inflammation and infection that occur with dental bacterial plaque accumulation.
- A cold liquid-filled teething ring provides

an object that slightly anesthetizes the gums and allows the baby to chew and apply pressure to the gums. A hard rubber ring and/or beads also help without running the risk of aspirated fluid from a ruptured ring.

- A non–aspirin-containing analgesic can help.
- Topical creams or oil of clove should be avoided.
- If the parents report that the child has a fever, look for other systemic infections because tooth eruption does not cause a fever. Fever speeds up selected metabolic processes and may stimulate accelerated tooth eruption.

ERUPTION HEMATOMA (ERUPTION CYSTS)

Description

An eruption hematoma is a bluish lesion on the gums preceding eruption of a tooth. These lesions are not true cysts but result from bleeding into the dental follicular space of the erupting tooth as it emerges through the alveolar bone beneath the alveolar mucosa.

Assessment

The 5- to 10-mm lesion is a well-circumscribed, dome-shaped, fluctuant bluish swelling located over an erupting tooth.

Management

The enlargement ruptures spontaneously and the tooth erupts. Rarely does an eruption hematoma cause the child discomfort requiring analgesics.

Complications

If the gum appears infected, refer the patient to a pediatric dentist for excision of the overlying gingival tissue.

ORAL CANDIDIASIS

Description

Pseudomembranous candidiasis (thrush) is commonly manifested as adherent white plaques that resemble curdled milk and is sometimes mistaken for formula remaining in the mouth (Fig. 34–15).

Etiology

Candida albicans (a common inhabitant of the oral cavity) may be present in the normal oral flora in 30 to 50% of the population (Neville et al., 1995). Other forms of candidiasis are rare in children but may be seen as red macules or red areas with white patches. The organisms multiply rapidly when host resistance is lowered, after exposure to broad-spectrum antibiotics, or in association with immunosuppression or systemic disease. Neonatal candidiasis is contracted during passage through the vagina and appears during the first 2 weeks of life.

Assessment

The following are seen:

- Decreased feeding, fever, and lymphadenopathy
- Raised, furry, white patches or red lesions combined with white patches on the buccal mucosa, tongue, and palate that bleed when scraped with a tongue blade

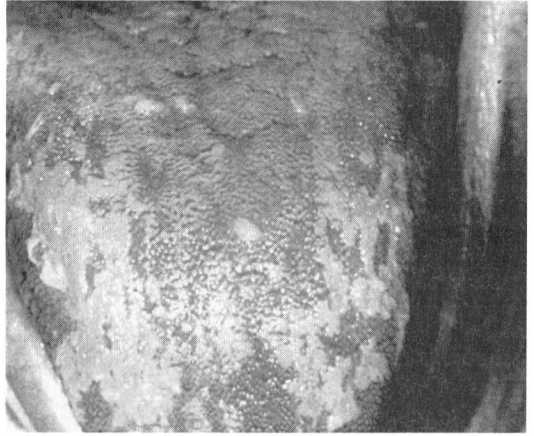

F I G U R E 34-15
Oral candidiasis. White patches on the intraoral soft tissues that rub off, exposing an underlying bleeding tissue, are often *Candida* lesions. (Photo courtesy of Berg and Jones.)

Management

Oral candidiasis is often self-limited. The following steps are taken if necessary to clear the lesions:

- Rub nystatin oral suspension (1 ml [1 million U]) into the lesions after feeding and cleaning the mucosa or hold a gauze pad moistened with nystatin on the child's buccal mucosa for 1 to 2 minutes four times a day until the lesions are cleared. Sterilize nipples and pacifiers if the baby is bottle-fed. Apply nystatin cream to the mother's nipples if breastfeeding.
- If recurrent, look for other causes such as conditions associated with immunosuppression.
- Systemic antifungal agents are not recommended for children unless associated with immunosuppression or multiorgan involvement.

Toddlers

HYPERPLASTIC MAXILLARY FRENUM

Description

The wedge-shaped tissue connecting the upper lip to the area of the gum between the two central incisor teeth is called the maxillary frenulum or frenum. Many parents are concerned with an abnormally large frenum causing a diastema (spacing) between the teeth.

Etiology

No etiology is known for this condition. A hyperplastic maxillary frenum is considered an aspect of normal variation. Ideally, primary teeth have wide spacing to allow room for the permanent teeth. As the primary teeth are exfoliated, the maxilla grows downward and forward; the maxillary frenum does not grow with the rest of the maxilla and becomes smaller in comparison.

Management

If a space is still present between the two front teeth after all six of the permanent upper incisor teeth have erupted (at around 12 years of age), the frenum may need to be excised in conjunction with orthodontic treatment for either occlusion or cosmetic purposes.

Complications

Early excision can result in scar tissue that is more dense and fibrous than the original tissue.

MANDIBULAR LABIAL FRENUM

Description

The wedge-shaped tissue connecting the lower lip to the area of the gum in front of the two central incisor teeth is called the mandibular labial frenulum or frenum.

Etiology

On occasion the mandibular labial frenum attaches into the marginal gingiva instead of the fixed gingival tissues and causes gingival recession on the labial surface of one or both incisors.

Assessment

- Observe for premature or asymmetrical gingival recession on the labial surface of the lower incisors.

Management

Refer to a pediatric dentist for evaluation and treatment. A gingival autograft surgical procedure is often necessary to prevent alveolar bone resorption and advanced periodontal disease in the area of gingival recession.

Complications

Without surgical intervention, periodontal disease and tooth loss will occur.

MANDIBULAR LINGUAL FRENUM (TONGUE-TIE)

Description

A short fibrous strand of connective tissue that originates along the anterior ventral surface and tip of the tongue to the lingual mandibular gingiva is known as a mandibular lingual frenum, or tongue-tie.

Etiology

No etiology is known. A mandibular lingual frenum is considered to be a normal variation.

Assessment

Determine the ability to produce normal articulation sounds. Most speech pathologists believe that children will have no problem making normal speech sounds if the child can extend the tongue over the lower incisor teeth and touch the lower lip.

Management

Referral to a speech pathologist and pediatric dentist for evaluation of any restriction of tongue movement or if the clinician or parent is concerned. Historically, lingual frenectomies were common and many times unnecessary. Consequently, many pediatric practitioners do not approve of any surgical intervention or even evaluation of the condition.

Complications

Stripping or recession of the lingual gingiva may accelerate periodontal disease and tooth loss. Surgical scarring and damage to Wharton ducts can occur as a result of surgical intervention.

HERPES SIMPLEX VIRUS

Description

Primary infection with herpes simplex virus type 1 (HSV-1) usually occurs as acute gingivostomatitis. The virus then becomes dormant in certain nerve cells until reactivated by triggering factors such as stress, menses, illness, and fatigue. Recurrent infection occurs as herpes labialis infection, commonly called cold sores or fever blisters. See Chapters 24 and 37 for more information (Table 34–9).

Etiology

See Chapters 24 and 37.

Assessment

Findings include:

1. Gingivostomatitis
   - Erythema of the soft mucosa of the mouth
   - Yellow or white liquid-filled vesicles that rupture and form painful oral ulcers 1 to 3 mm in diameter and covered with a whitish gray membrane
   - Cervical lymphadenopathy
   - Friable gingiva that bleeds easily
   - Fever, irritability, headache
   - Weight loss and dehydration
2. Herpes labialis
   - Cluster of small, clear vesicles with an erythematous base that become weepy and ulcerated and progress to crustiness, usually only on one side of the mouth

Management

Lesions heal spontaneously in 1 to 2 weeks. The following steps can be taken:

- Oral hygiene is performed with a soft toothbrush, cotton-tipped applicator, or cloth.
- Encourage fluids, especially cold ones, and a soft diet.
- Oral analgesics (acetaminophen or ibuprofen) may be used for control of pain.
- An equal mixture of diphenhydramine and Maalox applied topically provides symptomatic relief.
- Some clinicians recommend acyclovir (Zovirax), 20 to 40 mg/kg per day given in 5 doses for up to 5 days for children older than 1 year with severe gingivostomatitis, especially if at risk for dehydration.
- Small children who cannot control their secretions should be excluded from day care during the initial course.

Complications

It is not uncommon to have herpetic whitlow (see Chapters 24 and 37).

Differentiating Oral Herpes Simplex Infection, Gingivitis, and Aphthous Ulcers

	ETIOLOGY AND AGE	CLINICAL FINDINGS	TREATMENT
Herpes simplex (HSV)	HSV type 1 primary infection is gingivostomatitis, which usually occurs before 5 y of age; recurrent infection is herpes labialis and occurs at any age	Gingivostomatitis—erythematous soft mucosa of the mouth with vesicles that ulcerate and form white plaques on mucous membranes. Herpes labialis—burning, itching cluster of small clear vesicles with an erythematous base that become crusty, usually near the mouth	Lesions heal spontaneously. Encourage fluids. Oral analgesics, oral anesthetics in older children. Occasional use of acyclovir (Zovirax) in severely ill children. Exclusion from day care if drooling
Gingivitis	Retention of bacterial plaque in the soft tissue of the neck of the tooth; most prevalent in young children because of poor hygiene	Early—mild erythema and inflammation at the margins of gum tissue. Moderate—red, glazed bleeding gums. Severe—spontaneously bleeding gums, fetid breath, enlarged gums	Antibacterial mouth rinses with chlorhexidine, 0.12%, if the child can expectorate. Improved oral hygiene. Refer to a dentist if severe
Aphthous ulcers	Idiopathic in origin, precipitated by trauma, stress, sun, allergies, and certain chronic disorders; most common in adolescents	Tingle or burn before lesion occurs, pain with the lesion. Single or multiple small circular lesions with an erythematous halo and pale center on the alveolar and buccal mucosa, tongue, soft palate, and floor of the mouth	Resolves spontaneously. Oral analgesics, topical anesthetics, antibacterial rinse as above. Topical steroids if severe. Refer to a dentist if duration >14 d

Prevention

Contact with the mouth and sharing of food and utensils should be avoided until the lesions have resolved.

Preschool and School-Age Children

GEOGRAPHICAL TONGUE (ERYTHEMA MIGRANS)

Description

An irregular circinate lesion on the dorsal surface of the tongue with a red, smooth, erythematous central area surrounded by a thin, yellowish white line or band is called a geographical tongue (Fig. 34-16).

Etiology

The etiology of this anomaly is unknown. Desquamation of the filiform papillae on the dorsum of the tongue is responsible for the appearance of the lesion, which characteristically changes shape with time before it spontaneously resolves.

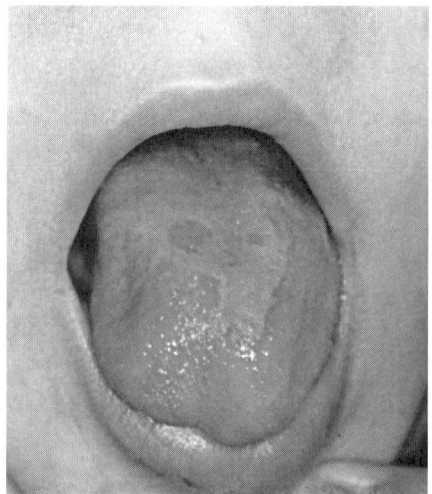

FIGURE 34-16
Geographical tongue in an 18-month-old child.

Assessment

None is required.

Management

Reassure the concerned parent that the condition is commonly seen in children (14% prevalence; McDonald & Avery, 1994), is self-limited, and requires no treatment.

GINGIVITIS

Description

Gingivitis is an inflammation of the marginal (meaning margin of the gum or the gum line) and the interdental papillary portion of the periodontium (see Table 34-9).

Etiology

Gingivitis is the most prevalent lesion of the oral soft tissues in young children, with estimates varying from 80 to 90% of children (Carranza & Newman, 1996). Gingivitis results from retention of bacterial plaque in the soft tissue crevice around the neck of the tooth and causes significant inflammation. Poor oral hygiene is the most common cause of gingivitis (see Fig. 34-9).

Assessment

The following are seen:

- Early—mild erythema and inflammation of the marginal gum tissues
- Moderate—red, glazed gums that bleed with manipulation
- Severe—red, enlarged gums covering more tooth than normal, spontaneous bleeding, fetid breath

Management

Treatment includes the following:

- Mouth rinses of chlorhexidine (0.12%) as a topical antibactericidal if the child is old enough to rinse and expectorate.
- Improved brushing and flossing tech-

niques. Oral hygiene procedures may need to be provided by a caregiver if the child is unable or unwilling to successfully improve technique.

- Referral to a pediatric dentist if the condition is severe, especially if calculus is found on the surfaces of teeth above or below the gingival margins.

Complications

Chronic gingivitis is the precursor to periodontal disease, which leads to periodontal bone loss, tooth mobility, and tooth loss.

PARULIS (GUMBOIL)

Description

A parulis is a chronic mass of granulation tissue localized on the gingiva that is the external portion of a draining apical dental abscess.

Etiology

Extensive decay or pulpal necrosis from a traumatic injury produces an apical dental abscess that drains through the labial periodontal tissues.

Assessment

The following are reported:

- Facial pain
- Gingival swelling, erythema, abscess, fistula, granuloma (localized infection)
- Lymphadenopathy, fever (cellulitis)

Management

Management involves the following:

- Referral for tooth extraction, pulpectomy, or endodontics.
- If infection is localized, antibiotic therapy is not usually indicated.
- If cellulitis is present, antibiotic therapy is given before or along with endodontic therapy or extraction (penicillin VK, 125 to 250 mg four times a day for 7 to 10 days, or erythromycin). Referral to a pediatric dentist for follow-up care is necessary.

TRAUMA

Etiology and Incidence

Falls account for most dental trauma in children 1 to 5 years old. In children 6 to 12 years old, bicycle accidents, sports, and being struck by an object account for most injuries. Bicycle accidents and sports are the most common causes of dental trauma in 13- to 17-year-old adolescents, with fights, sports, and vehicle accidents accounting for most dental injuries in young adults. Motor vehicle accidents are responsible for oral trauma at all ages. At least 50% of children experience one injury involving their teeth by 14 years of age, and children with protrusion of the front teeth have twice the risk for anterior dental trauma (Casamassimo, 1996; Andreasen, 1994; Liew & Daly, 1986).

Clinical Findings

HISTORY. Recording when, where, and how the injury took place helps identify any suspicions of child abuse.

PHYSICAL EXAMINATION. Examining a child with an oral/dental injury can be a challenge if the child is crying or agitated. Nevertheless, the examination must be thorough and complete to identify injuries that require immediate treatment. Examine for:

- Facial asymmetry, bruising, and a full range of motion of the mandible
- Any injury to the lips, frena, tongue, soft palate, gingiva, and other mucosal surfaces
- Soft tissue injury such as puncture wounds, foreign bodies, torn tissue that exposes underlying bone, or lacerations over 2 mm long that would require suturing
- Alignment of the teeth within the dental arch and alignment with the opposing dental arch
- Mobility in both a labial and palatal (lingual) direction while noting any teeth that exhibit more than 2 mm of movement
- Fractured teeth, with the extent of the fracture into dentin noted and whether any pulp tissue is exposed

DIAGNOSTIC TESTS. When a missing tooth or tooth fragment cannot be found and identified, lateral soft tissue neck and thoracoabdominal radiographs for foreign bodies (teeth or tooth fragments) in the airway must be taken.

Management

Immediate management of trauma seeks to prevent the aesthetic disfigurement of tooth loss, future pain or infection, or expensive dental treatment.

- Advice over the telephone is often requested and should be avoided other than recommending an immediate dental referral or office visit for evaluation.
- The need for a tetanus booster should be considered.
- When the child arrives at the office, it is most important to take a careful history to ensure that the child has no special health care needs that would alter routine dental care. Table 34-10 identifies dental injuries that require immediate dental intervention. Table 34-11 identifies dental injuries that are of concern but can be dealt with by a dental professional within 1 to 3 days.
- A follow-up appointment should be made with a pediatric dentist for all types of dental trauma to ensure that the child has no detrimental effects of pulp necrosis, subsequent infection, or peripheral root resorption from the injury.

ORAL ASPECTS OF CHILD ABUSE

Because pediatric medical clinicians receive little training in oral diseases, detection of dental injuries, treatment, and the sequela of dental trauma, collaboration with a pediatric dentist or a dentist with training in forensic oral pathology should be done when oral abuse is suspected.

Blunt trauma injuries are most commonly inflicted with an instrument, eating utensils, hands, or fingers. Contusions, lacerations, punctures, fractured teeth, or displaced or avulsed teeth are the common physical injuries of the oral cavity. The oral cavity is a frequent site of sexual abuse, and the clinician should be alert for oral signs of gonorrhea or syphilis and confirm the diagnosis through cultures.

When bite marks are observed, the intercuspid distance should be measured to identify whether a child or adult is responsible for the bite. Bite marks with an intercuspid distance of 3.0 mm or more are most likely caused by an adult. The physical findings of child abuse should be photographed for later documentation. A pediatric dentist or forensic oral pathologist can often record bite marks with either photography or dental impressions of the bite marks.

DENTAL NEGLECT

The AAPD defines "dental neglect" as the willful failure of a parent or guardian to seek and follow through with treatment necessary to ensure a level of oral health essential for adequate function and free from pain and infection (AAPD, 1999). Indicators of dental neglect include:

1. Untreated rampant caries easily detected by a layperson
2. Untreated pain, infection, bleeding, or trauma affecting the oral-facial region
3. A history of a lack of follow-through for care when pathology is identified to a parent or guardian

Many factors influence a family to not seek dental care for their children. Ignorance, cultural values, lack of perceived health value, lack of finances, or geographical isolation are the most common reasons. The NP should first be certain that the parent or guardian thoroughly understands the significance of dental pathology and the potential for life-threatening infections if left untreated. Once such understanding is established, a place for the child to receive dental care should be identified. If the parent continues to be negligent, referral to social services may be warranted.

Adolescent

PERIODONTAL DISEASE

Description

Periodontal disease is a bacterial inflammatory disease of the gingiva and supporting alveolar bony structures.

T A B L E 34-10

Traumatic Dental Injuries That Require Immediate Attention by a Dental Professional

INJURY	CLINICAL FEATURES	TREATMENT ACTION
Fractured jaw	Facial asymmetry, swelling, pain, limitation of movement	Radiographic diagnosis, immobilization
Dental alveolar bone fracture	Mobility of segments of teeth rather than individual teeth	Radiographic diagnosis, intra-arch stabilization
Dental crown fractures involving exposure of pulpal tissue	Pulp tissue visible in the tooth fracture site	Pulp capping and coverage of the fracture to prevent bacterial infection of pulp, dental abscess, and endodontics
Root fractures	Mobility of one or more teeth more than 2 mm in any direction	Radiographic diagnosis, intra-arch stabilization
Intruded tooth	Tooth completely or partially intruded or jammed into its socket	Radiographic diagnosis Primary tooth—allowed to reerupt, followed by pulpotomy Permanent tooth—requires orthodontic repositioning and endodontics
Partial avulsions (extrusions)	Tooth dislodged from its socket and will not remain stable or has >2-mm mobility	Radiographic diagnosis to rule out root fracture Primary teeth—extract if severely mobile or intra-arch stabilization and pulpotomy Permanent tooth—intra-arch stabilization and endodontics
Complete avulsion	Entire tooth displaced from the dental socket intact	Radiographic confirmation Primary tooth—stop bleeding; do not reimplant Permanent tooth—gently clean root surface, reimplant immediately, intra-arch stabilization; transport the tooth in saline, milk, or cold water to the dental office if necessary
Toothache accompanied by swelling	Cellulitis or localized facial erythema Broken or carious tooth	Confer with a pediatric dentist about antibiotic choice Start antibiotic therapy

From American Academy of Pediatric Dentistry: Special Issue: Reference Manual 1999–2000. 21(6), 1999.

Etiology

Oral hygiene neglect that allows subgingival colonization by bacteria initiates or exacerbates many forms of periodontal disease. Inadequate nutrition also contributes to this disease. Adolescent periodontal disease is a common finding in individuals with systemic diseases that alter the body's defense mechanisms to infection such as juvenile diabetes and various forms of immunosuppression. Otherwise, it is not common in adolescent children.

Clinical Findings

The following may be seen:

- Bleeding gums, fetid breath, and pain in gingival tissue

T A B L E 34-11

Traumatic Dental Injuries That Require Attention by a Dental Professional Within 1 to 3 Days

INJURY	CLINICAL FEATURES	TREATMENT ACTION
Bumped deciduous incisors	Dark discolored anterior deciduous or permanent tooth	Radiographic diagnosis, pulpectomy, endodontics
Toothache not accompanied by swelling	Painful carious or fractured tooth often accompanied by mobility or a draining fistula	Start antibiotics/analgesics, insist on professional dental follow-up
Simple crown fractures	Fractures of enamel and/or dentin that do not expose the pulp	Restore the tooth to function and aesthetics as convenient
Broken braces, wires, dental appliances	Dental appliances loose or irritating to the child	Dental appointment as soon as possible; remove the appliance
Minor bumps	Teeth slightly loosened in their sockets with <2-mm mobility and stable in the dental arch	Insist on professional dental follow-up

- Tooth mobility even when the gingiva appears normal
- Severely stained teeth, cavitation of teeth, obvious signs of intraoral neglect
- Inflammation especially noticeable around first permanent molars and lower incisors

Diagnostic Studies

- Dental radiographs are needed to evaluate periodontal bone loss.

Management

- Refer the patient to a dentist for diagnosis, professional oral prophylaxis, oral hygiene instructions, and follow-up care.
- Prevention is proper oral hygiene.
- Children with juvenile diabetes or children who are immunosuppressed should be identified as being at high risk for periodontal disease and receive close preventive dental supervision.

Complications

Resorption of alveolar bone, lateral periodontal abscesses, and tooth loss can occur.

SMOKELESS TOBACCO USE

Description

Smokeless tobacco is chewed, held between the cheek and gum, or sniffed through the nose. Adolescents who use chewing tobacco or snuff have blood nicotine levels equal to those of smokers.

Etiology and Incidence

Adolescent males, especially those participating in recreational team sports, are at greatest risk. The incidence is greater in the Southwest, in rural areas, and among Native Americans. An estimated 25 to 30% of adolescent males use smokeless tobacco (Casamassimo, 1996; Harris & Christen, 1995).

Assessment

- Erythema of isolated intraoral soft tissue areas is seen.
- White patches (leukoplakia) or oral ulceration may also develop on the gingiva or buccal mucosa.

Management

Management involves the following:

- Periodic oral cancer screening
- Preventive dental care as required

- Referral to a dentist for biopsy of *any* changes in the oral mucosa
- Education and counseling regarding smokeless tobacco use and its health implications (see Resource Box)
- Referral to cessation groups for assistance

Complications

Smokeless tobacco use is associated with dental caries, discolored teeth, gingivitis, localized gum recession, soft tissue changes, and elevated cholesterol levels, blood pressure, and heart rate. Smokeless tobacco users have an increased risk of oral cancer, including epithelial dysplasia, carcinoma in situ, and squamous cell carcinoma.

RECURRENT APHTHOUS ULCERS

Description

Recurrent aphthous ulcers are commonly called canker sores (Fig. 34-17). They recur frequently and are sometimes confused with herpetic lesions (see Table 34-9).

Etiology and Incidence

An aphthous ulcer is considered idiopathic in origin but can be precipitated by trauma, stress, sun, allergies, and endocrine or hematological disorders. Onset may be in childhood but often occurs in adolescence with a prevalence rate of about 20% (Neville et al., 1995). Occasionally, these patients have underlying iron, vitamin B_{12}, or folate deficiency or celiac disease.

Assessment

The following can be seen:

- Tingling or burning preceding appearance of the lesions and pain once the lesions are visible
- Single or multiple small, circular to oval lesions with an erythematous halo and a pale to yellow center
- Occurrence on the alveolar mucosa, ventral surface of the tongue, soft palate, buccal mucosa, and floor of the mouth
- Lack of systemic symptoms

Differential Diagnosis

The differential diagnosis includes herpes simplex or herpes zoster lesions, herpangina (coxsackievirus A), trauma, hand-foot-and-mouth disease, and chemical burns. Severe persistent lesions are associated with juvenile diabetes and inflammatory bowel syndrome.

Management

Aphthous ulcers spontaneously resolve in 1 to 2 weeks. The following steps can be taken:

- Palliative treatment with oral analgesics, topical anesthetics, diphenhydramine (Benadryl) elixir, and attapulgite (Kaopectate) in a 50–50 mixture (for children older than 6 years) or a viscous lidocaine (Xylocaine) solution (for children older than 12 years). Children should not swallow solutions.
- Antibacterial rinses to mitigate secondary bacterial infection. Tetracycline elixir applied topically or used as a 2-minute rinse shortens the disease course.
- Topical steroid rinses or triamcinolone acetonide (Kenalog in Orabase) can provide some relief for severe ulcerations.
- Silver nitrate cauterization has been used to provide pain relief but delays healing.
- Referral to an oral surgeon or pediatric

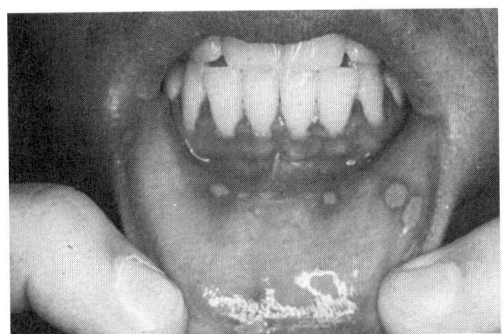

F I G U R E 34-17
Apthous ulcers, also called "canker sores," are vesicles at first; they become small round ulcers with a white base surrounded by a red halo.

RESOURCE BOX 34-1

Academy of Sports Dentistry
c/o Dr. Dave Kumamoto
Tel: (312) 792–1354

American Academy of Pediatric Dentistry
Tel: (312) 337–2169
Website: www.aapd.org

American Dental Association
Tel: (800) 947–4746 or (312) 440–2500
Website: www.ada.org

American Dental Hygienists' Association
Tel: (312) 440–8900
Website: www.adha.org

American Society of Dentistry for Children
Tel: (312) 943–1244
E-mail: asdckids@aol.com

Bright Futures in Practice: Oral Health & Quick Reference Guidelines
National Center for Education in Maternal and Child Health
Tel: (703) 524–7802
Website: www.brightfutures.org

Federation of Special Care Organizations
Academy of Dentistry for Persons with Disabilities
Tel: (312) 440–2661

National Cancer Institute Smokeless Tobacco Educational Program
Office of Cancer Communication
National Institute of Dental and Craniofacial Research
Tel: (301) 496–4261
Website: www.nider.nih.gov

National Foundation of Dentistry for the Handicapped
Tel: (303) 298–9650

National Institute of Dental Research
Tel: (301) 496–4261
Website: www.nidr.nih.gov

National Oral Health Information Clearinghouse
Tel: (301) 402–7364
Website: www.aerie.com/nohicweb/ohurap.html
Produces and distributes patient and professional educational materials, including fact sheets, brochures, and information packets for patients with special oral health needs.

Prevent Abuse and Neglect through Dental Awareness (PANDA)
Lynn Douglas Mouden, DDS, MPH
Tel: (314) 751–6247

---

dentist for biopsy if the condition lasts more than 14 days.

SEXUALLY TRANSMITTED DISEASES

Assessment

- Palatal petechia, focal ulcerations, and mucosal erythema may identify sexually active adolescents engaging in oral sex. These individuals should be examined for lesions associated with sexually transmitted diseases such as infection with *Candida, Trichomonas,* herpes, *Chlamydia, Neisseria gonorrhoeae,* and human immunodeficieny virus (HIV) (Neville et al., 1995). (See Chapters 24 and 36 for more information.)

Management

- Diagnosis and treatment of the disease
- Referral to an oral surgeon or pediatric dentist for any unusual lesions or a lesion that does not resolve by 14 days

REFERENCES

Acs G, Lodolini G, Kaminsky S, et al: Effect of nursing caries on body weight in a pediatric population. Pediatr Dent 14(55):302–305, 1992.

Adair SM, Milano M, Lorenzo I, et al: Effects of current and former pacifier use on the dentition of 24 to 59 month old children. Pediatr Dent 17:437–444, 1995.

American Academy of Pediatric Dentistry: Special Issue: Reference Manual 1999-2000. 21(6), 1999.

American Academy of Pediatrics: Policy statement on medical home. Pediatrics 90:774, 1992.

American Academy of Pediatrics Committee on Nutrition: Fluoride supplementation for children. Pediatrics 95:777, 1995.

Andreasen JO: Textbook and Color Atlas of Traumatic Injuries to the Teeth, 3rd ed. St Louis, CV Mosby, 1994.

Angle EH: Treatment of Malocclusion of the Teeth and Fractures of the Maxillae, Angle's System, 6th ed. Philadelphia, SS White Dental Manufacturing Company, 1900.

Behrman RE, Kliegman R, Arvin AM: Nelson Textbook of Pediatrics, 15th ed. Philadelphia, WB Saunders, 1996.

Bolden AJ, Henry JL, Allukian A: Implications of access, utilization, and need for oral health care by low-income groups and minorities on the dental delivery system. J Dent Educ 57:888-889, 1993.

Carranza FA, Newman MG: Clinical Periodontology, 8th ed. Philadelphia, WB Saunders, 1996.

Casamassimo P: Bright Futures in Practice: Oral Health. Arlington, VA, National Center for Education in Maternal and Child Health, 1996.

Casamassimo P: Bright Futures in Practice: Oral Health Quick Reference Cards. Arlington, VA, National Center for Education in Maternal and Child Health, 1997.

Caufield PW: Dental caries—a transmissible and infectious disease, revisited, a position paper. Pediatr Dent 19:491-498, 1997.

Caufield PW, Cutter GR, Dasanayake AP: Initial acquisition of mutans streptococci by infants: Evidence for a discrete window of infectivity. J Dent Res 72:37-45, 1993.

Edelstein BL: Case planning and management according to caries risk assessment. Dent Clin North Am 39:721-737, 1995.

Edelstein BL, Douglass CW: Dispelling the myth that 50% of US schoolchildren have never had a cavity. Public Health Rep 110:522-530, 1995.

Elster AB, Kuznets NJ: AMA Guidelines for Adolescents Preventive Services (GAPS). Baltimore, Williams & Wilkins, 1994.

Grainger RM: Orthodontic Treatment Priority Index. PHS Publication No. 1000, Series 2, No 25. Washington, DC, National Center for Health Statistics, 1967.

Green M (ed): Bright Futures: Guidelines for Health Supervision of Infants, Children, and Adolescents. Arlington, VA, National Center for Education in Maternal and Child Health, 1994.

Harris NO, Christen A (eds): Primary Preventive Dentistry, 4th ed. Paramount, Norwalk, CT, 1995, pp 259-287.

Johnson GK, Squier CA: Smokeless tobacco use by youth: A health concern. Pediatr Dent 15(3):169-174, 1993.

Keyes PH: The infectious and transmissible nature of experimental dental caries. Arch Oral Biol 1:304-320, 1960.

Kohler B: Preventive measures in mothers influence the establishment of the bacterium *Streptococcus mutans* in their infants. Arch Oral Biol 25:221-231, 1983.

Li Y, Caufield PW: The fidelity of initial acquisition of mutans streptococcus by infants from their mothers. J Dent Res 74:681-685, 1995.

Liew VP, Daly CG: Anterior dental trauma treated after-hours in Newcastle, Australia. Community Dent Oral Epidemiol 14:362-366, 1986.

Logan WHG, Kronfeld R: The chronology of human dentition. J Am Dent Assoc 20, 1933.

McDonald RE, Avery AD: Dentistry for the Child and Adolescent, 6th ed. St Louis, CV Mosby, 1994.

Neville BW, Damm DD, Allen CM, et al: Oral and Maxillofacial Pathology. Philadelphia, WB Saunders, 1995.

Ngan P, Fields HW: Open bite: A review of etiology and management. Pediatr Dent 19:91-98, 1997.

Peretz B, Kafka I: Baby bottle tooth decay and complications during pregnancy and delivery. Pediatr Dent 19(1):34-36, 1997.

Shay K: Root caries in the elderly, an update for the next century. J Indiana Dent Assoc 96(4):37-43, 1996.

Tinanoff N, O'Sullivan DM: Early childhood caries: Overview and recent findings. Pediatr Dent 19:12-16, 1997.

US Department of Health and Human Services: Healthy People 2010 Objectives: Draft for Public Comment: Child and Adolescent Focused Objectives. Washington, DC, 1998, http://web.health.gov/healthypeople.

US Department of Health and Human Services: Office of the Inspector General. Children's Dental Services Under Medicaid—Access and Utilization. OEI-09-93-00240, Washington, DC, 1996.

US Department of Health and Human Services: Report for the Healthy People 2000 Objectives. Washington, DC, 1995, http://odphp.osophs.dhhs.gov/pubs/hp2000/progrvw/ORAL.HTM.

US Department of Health and Human Services: Healthy People 2000: National Health Promotion and Disease Prevention Objectives for the Year 2000. Washington, DC, US Government Printing Office, 1995.

US Preventive Services Task Force: Guide to Clinical Preventive Services, 2nd ed. Baltimore, Williams & Wilkins, 1996.

US Public Health Service: Put Prevention Into Practice: The Clinician's Handbook of Preventive Services, 2nd ed. Germantown, MD, International Medical Publishing, 1997.

Weddell JA, Klein AI: Socioeconomic correlation of oral disease in six to thirty-six month old children. Pediatr Dent 3:306-310, 1981.

CHAPTER 35

Genitourinary Disorders

Nancy Barber Starr

INTRODUCTION

The genitourinary system is responsible for maintaining an optimal environment for metabolism, including regulation of water and electrolytes (sodium, potassium, chloride, calcium, phosphate, and magnesium), excretion of waste products (urea, creatinine, poisons, and drugs), acid–base regulation, and hormonal secretion (vitamin D, renin, erythropoietin, and prostaglandins). The male system has both reproductive and excretory functions. Genitourinary problems in children and adolescents range from commonly occurring, easily treated diseases to significant congenital or acquired conditions. Pediatric primary care providers play a significant role in working with children, adolescents, and families to identify problems, manage disorders, maintain optimal function, and provide education and support related to genitourinary function. Referral to and collaboration with pediatric urologists and nephrologists are also important components of patient management. However, first-line assessment and management, as well as provision of continuity of care, are important responsibilities of the nurse practitioner (NP).

Discussion of related functional health problems—enuresis and dysfunctional voiding—is included in Chapter 14.

STANDARDS OF CARE

The *Guide to Clinical Preventive Services,* second edition (US Preventive Health Services Task Force, 1996), does not recommend any urine screening for asymptomatic bacteriuria in any child of any age.

The *Put Prevention Into Practice: Clinician's Handbook of Preventive Services,* 2nd edition (US Public Health Services, 1997), lists the following recommendations from major authorities:

- American Academy of Pediatrics—Urinalysis (UA) should be performed once at 5 years of age. Also, dipstick leukocyte esterase testing to screen for sexually transmitted diseases (STDs) should be performed once in adolescence, preferably at 14 years of age.
- American Medical Association and Bright Futures—Sexually active adolescents should be screened yearly for gonorrhea and chlamydia by urinalysis with a dipstick leukocyte esterase test.

If a UA is done, it should be done on a first morning urine to establish a baseline (Kaplan et al., 1997).

ANATOMY AND PHYSIOLOGY

The renal system is composed of two kidneys, two ureters, a bladder, and a urethra. The kidneys are positioned posteriorly on the abdominal wall. The main features of the kidney are the cortex, the medulla, and the collecting system. The renal medulla and nephrons are present at birth, but the peripheral tubules are small and immature. By adolescence, the kidneys are of adult size and weight. The ureters are muscular tubes that convey urine from the kidneys to the bladder by peristaltic contractions. The bladder is a muscular reservoir to collect the urine. It lies close to the anterior abdominal wall in early childhood. With growth, it descends into the pelvis and changes shape from cylindrical to pyramidal. The urethra extends from the bladder to allow for the discharge of urine. The male urethra is significantly longer than the female urethra.

Physiologically, the kidneys serve to filter, clear, reabsorb, and secrete substances essential to the body's metabolism. The urinary system begins forming and excreting urine at 3 months of gestational age. Glomerular filtration and renal blood flow begin to increase at birth and become stable by 1 to 2 years of age. In infants, total extracellular fluid volume is significantly greater than that of adults, and fluid composition tends to have a lower bicarbonate concentration. Normal urine excretion is 1.5 to 3 ml/kg per hour. Because the kidneys are still maturing throughout infancy and early childhood, urine is also more dilute than in adulthood. Concentrating capacity reaches adult values at 6 to 12 months.

PATHOPHYSIOLOGY AND DEFENSE MECHANISMS

Pathophysiology

Problems in the urinary system occur in either the upper or the lower urinary tract and can be relatively silent in appearance or noticeably present at birth. Additional problems can arise in the male reproductive system. The main mechanisms can be classified as follows:

- Infection
- Inflammatory response
- Congenital malformation or condition
- Abnormalities acquired from injury, infection, or malfunction within the system

Defense Mechanisms

The urinary tract is normally a sterile system. The mucosal lining of the bladder serves as the first line of defense and provides inhibition of bacterial growth and adherence. The acid pH of the urine also protects the urinary system by inhibiting bacterial growth. Finally, actual flow of urine out of the bladder provides mechanical defense by its flushing action. If these defenses are compromised, the body initiates an inflammatory response.

ASSESSMENT OF THE GENITOURINARY SYSTEM

History

The following information should be obtained:

1. History of the present illness
   - Onset and pattern of symptoms
   - Fever, abdominal pain, or both
   - Preceding injury or illness, especially streptococcal infection
   - Vomiting
   - Voiding pattern—stream force and direction, any dribbling or discharge
   - Color, odor, frequency, and volume of urine, dysuria, urgency; enuresis or incontinence
   - Sexual activity or abuse
2. Family history
   - Any familial history of renal disease, deafness, high blood pressure (BP), structural abnormalities, or syndromes involving the genitourinary system
3. Past history of urinary tract infection (UTI), hematuria, proteinuria, or any other related finding

Physical Examination

Pertinent findings include the following:

- Growth parameters—failure to thrive (FTT) can be associated with UTI in infants; increased weight can be associated with nephrotic syndrome.
- BP—often elevated with nephritis and nephrotic syndrome.
- Edema, pallor, dehydration.
- Ear position and formation—if low set or abnormal, may have concurrent renal involvement.

- Abdominal masses, ascites, flank or suprapubic tenderness.
- Costovertebral tenderness.
- External genitalia abnormalities.

Diagnostic Studies

Diagnostic studies are ordered as indicated. The proper collection, transport, and storage of urine are essential to obtain accurate results. Most tests on urine, unless otherwise indicated, are best done on a first morning void. A second morning void, collected before the ingestion of large amounts of fluid, is recommended for microscopic examination (Linshaw & Gruskin, 1997). This practice collects fresh urine and increases the likelihood of seeing cellular casts, which can dissolve within 10 to 30 minutes. Urine should be evaluated within 30 minutes and, if stored, kept below 4°C.

1. UA. The efficacy and cost efficiency of routine UA is much debated. The method of collection of urine is an important factor to note when interpreting UA results. Bag collection is considered reliable only if the results are negative. The clean-catch method increases reliability, but sterile catheterization and suprapubic tap provide the most accurate results.
   - Physical characteristics. Color, clarity, odor, specific gravity, and osmolality are noted.
   - Chemical characteristics. Urine dipsticks are available and widely used to determine pH, glucose, ketones, protein, bile pigments, hemoglobin, nitrites, and leukocyte esterase. For correct results, strips must remain in their original containers and not be exposed to moisture, light, cold, or heat until used. Urine must be fresh, warmed if refrigerated, and read at correct intervals for each test strip (Table 35-1).
     - A dipstick positive for blood indicates the presence of hemoglobin. Intact erythrocytes cause spotty changes on the dipstick, whereas free hemoglobin or myoglobin causes uniform changes of color.
     - The nitrite test is an indirect measure of bacteria in the urine. Common urinary pathogens contain enzymes that reduce nitrate in urine to nitrite. However, the urine should have been in the bladder at least 4 hours to show accurate results. Urine culture should be done on any urine sample positive for nitrites for confirmation of infection.
   - Microscopic examination of urine. Urine can be spun by centrifuge and the sediment examined, or it can be examined unspun. When evaluating results, consideration must be given to which method was used, and repeated examination is recommended. Urine should be examined under the microscope for red blood cells (RBCs), white blood cells (WBCs), bacteria, casts, and crystals. Microscopic examination of a fresh specimen is essential if blood or protein is found on the dipstick or urinary tract symptoms are present (see earlier comments).
     - RBCs—the number of RBCs per high-power field (hpf) that are thought to be abnormal varies, but in general, more than 2 to 5/hpf ($\times$40) in unspun urine or more than 2 to 10/hpf in spun urine is thought to be abnormal (Roy, 1998; Finberg, 1998; Cruz & Spitzer, 1998; Feld, et al., 1997; Opas, 1998; Fitzwater & Wyatt, 1994; Yadin, 1994). If cells are dysmorphic, the origin of the blood is most likely the kidney (Fig. 35-1).
     - WBCs—fewer than 2 WBCs/hpf should be seen. More than 10 WBCs often accompany a symptomatic infection. If between 2 and 10 WBCs/hpf are seen, urine culture or other workup should be performed (Fig. 35-2).
     - Bacteria and leukocytes seen in an *unspun* sample are associated with colony counts on culture of 100,000 (Fig. 35-3).
     - Casts—RBC, hyaline, waxy, epithelial, leukocyte, or fatty casts are seen in various disease states (Fig. 35-4).
     - Crystals, if amorphous, are not unusual. Calcium oxalate, cystine, tyrosine, leucine, cholesterol, or sulfa crystals are abnormal.
2. Gram stain. A Gram stain of the urine can be helpful in identifying organisms.
3. Urine culture and sensitivities. Urine culture

T A B L E 35-1

Chemical Characteristics of Urine

CONSTITUENT	POSITIVES INDICATE	FALSE POSITIVES CAUSED BY	FALSE NEGATIVES CAUSED BY
Glucose	Metabolic problem (e.g., diabetes), recent high glucose intake, galactosemia	Antibiotics, delay in reading, myoglobin, oxidizing contaminants	Ascorbic acid intake, ketones, high specific gravity
Ketones	Dehydration, starvation, strenuous exercise, stress, fever, metabolic problems (e.g., diabetes)		If urine left standing, acetone evaporates
Protein	Renal disease, orthostatic proteinuria	Exercise, fever, dehydration, alkaline or concentrated urine (SG >1.020), semisynthetic penicillin, oxidizing cleansing agents	Dilute or acidic urine
Blood (hemoglobin)	If microscopic examination is negative for RBCs: Free hemoglobin secondary to chemicals, illness, or drugs; myoglobin secondary to burns, muscle trauma, physical child abuse, myositis, strenuous exercise If microscopic examination is positive for RBCs: Renal problems	Menses, oxidizing cleansing agents, dilute urine	Ascorbic acid
Nitrite	Bacteria causing urinary tract infection	Rare	Common; urine should be in bladder at least 4 hr
Leukocyte esterase	Pyuria (WBCs in urine); inflammation from irritation or infection of vulva, vagina, or urethra; inflammation of bladder or kidneys with or without infection	Oxidizing agents	Immunocompromised status

RBCs = red blood cells; SG = specific gravity; WBCs = white blood cells.

is easily done by standard culture methods or with a dipslide incubated overnight at room temperature. Urine should be cultured immediately or refrigerated. Doubling of pathogens occurs in as little as 20 minutes (Woodhead, 1999). Bacterial identification and sensitivities need only be performed in complicated or nonresponsive cases.

4. A 24-hour urine collection. Collecting a 24-hour sample of urine is done to determine calcium excretion, the calcium-creatinine ratio, and quantification of protein.

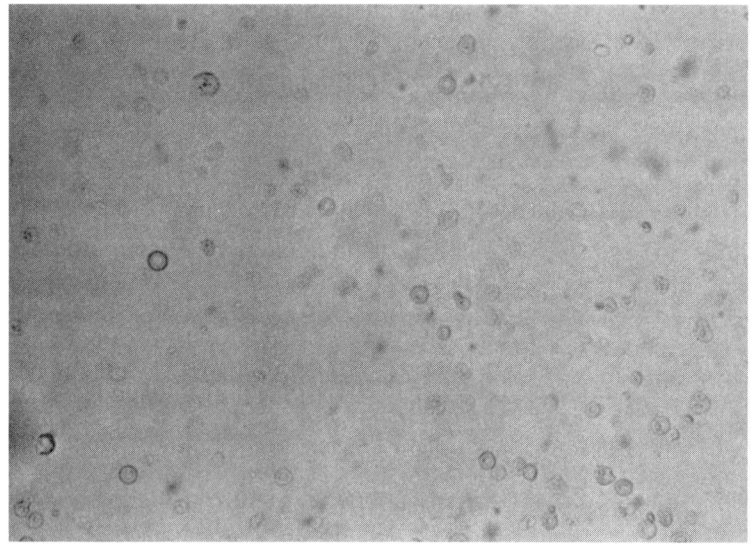

FIGURE 35-1
Red blood cells (RBCs) may originate from any part of the renal system. The presence of large numbers of RBCs suggests pathology. (From Graff SL: A Handbook of Routine Urinalysis. Philadelphia, JB Lippincott, 1983.)

5. Blood work.
   • Serum or blood urea nitrogen (BUN) estimates the urea concentration in serum or blood and is a measure of toxic metabolites that can cause uremic syndrome.
   • Serum creatinine in combination with creatinine clearance is used to estimate the glomerular filtration rate (GFR) or kidney function.
   • Serum electrolytes and acid–base status can detect renal tubular abnormalities.
6. Ultrasonography. Ultrasonography of the renal system provides noninvasive structural information and is useful as a first-line evaluation of the renal system.
7. Voiding cystourethrogram (VCUG). A VCUG is the most accurate test to evaluate reflux of urine from the lower tract to the upper tract.

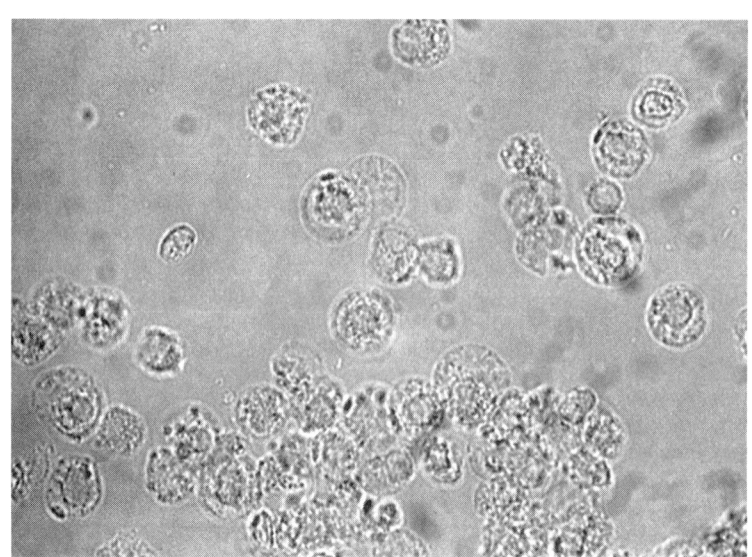

FIGURE 35-2
White blood cells (WBCs) in the urine (pyuria) may originate from any part of the renal system. The presence of more than 5 WBCs per high-power field (HPF) suggests pathology. (From Graff SL: A Handbook of Routine Urinalysis. Philadelphia, JB Lippincott, 1983.)

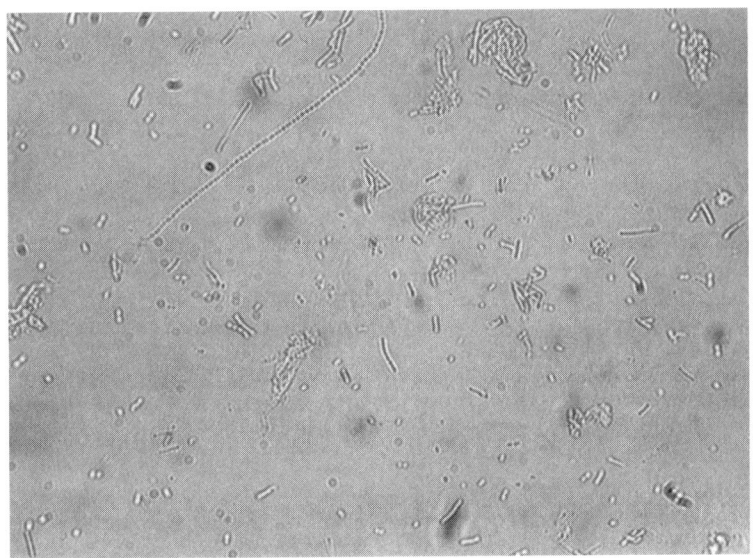

F I G U R E 35-3
Bacteria (rods, cocci, and chains). (500×). (From Graff SL: A Handbook of Routine Urinalysis. Philadelphia, JB Lippincott, 1983.)

8. Intravenous pyelogram (IVP). IVPs are readily available and provide structural and functional information about the renal system.

9. Nuclear imaging scans. These scans provide less structural and functional detail than an IVP but involve less radiation exposure. Nuclear scans are especially helpful in the early identification of pyelonephritis and parenchymal scarring and in monitoring reflux.

MANAGEMENT STRATEGIES

Education and Counseling

Education and counseling are essential components in the management of genitourinary tract disorders. Parents and children must be informed about the pathology, etiology, treatment, and prognosis with and without treat-

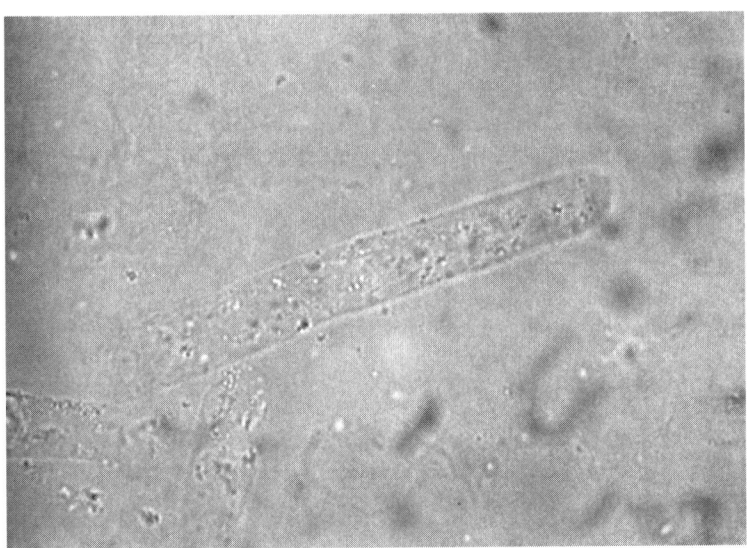

F I G U R E 35-4
Hyaline casts. Viewed with an 80A filter (400×). (From Graff SL: A Handbook of Routine Urinalysis. Philadelphia, JB Lippincott, 1983.)

ment. A plan of care that the family, as well as the care provider, is comfortable with must be decided on and initiated. Urinary problems can occur as early as the newborn period or any-time throughout childhood or adolescence. They vary in severity and chronicity. The NP must modify appropriate strategies for each individual situation.

Medication, Diet, and Activity

Common medications include antibiotics and steroids (see discussion of specifics later). Diet and activity may need to be modified in some chronic renal conditions. These modifications are usually carried out in consultation with appropriate specialists.

Referral

Referral to a pediatric urologist, nephrologist, and/or surgeon may be required. When a referral is made, the primary care provider retains the essential role of serving as case manager for the child and providing continuity of care over time. The primary care provider is often the one whom the family best knows and is most comfortable with in discussing concerns, potential plans, and longer-term management.

▓▓▓ UPPER GENITOURINARY TRACT DISORDERS

Renal Tubular Acidosis

Description

Dysfunction of renal tubule transport capability results in a condition known as renal tubular acidosis (RTA). Three distinct types of RTA have been identified. When the defect occurs in the proximal tubules, it is known as proximal RTA (pRTA), type II, or bicarbonate-wasting RTA. Type I, classic or distal RTA (dRTA), occurs when the defect is in the distal tubule. Type IV, also known as hyperkalemic RTA, occurs with problems in the functioning of aldosterone. A type III has been proposed but is thought to be a variant of type I.

Etiology and Incidence

The dysfunction in the transport capability of the renal tubules affects either the reabsorp-

tion of filtered bicarbonate, excretion of hydrogen ion, or both and results in a metabolic acidosis. RTA is often an isolated and primary problem with unknown cause, but diseases or intoxication can cause it. It is seen most typically in children evaluated for growth failure and is often revealed when illness, dehydration, or starvation stresses a child. RTA is more common in males than females, with pRTA being the more common form seen in children.

The proximal tubule, which normally absorbs 85% of bicarbonate, is only able to reabsorb 60% of bicarbonate from filtered urine in patients with pRTA (Bergstein, 1996). The distal tubule continues to function and reabsorbs approximately 15% of the bicarbonate, and the urine is acidified (pH < 5.5). However, a large amount of bicarbonate is wasted. As the body adapts, a new threshold for serum bicarbonate is set, usually around 14 to 16 mEq.

A defect in the ability of the distal renal tubule to excrete hydrogen is the cause of dRTA. This defect causes complete loss of reabsorption of the final 15% of bicarbonate and an inability to acidify urine (pH > 5.5). Type IV RTA is characterized by a deficiency in the production or responsiveness of aldosterone and impaired ammonia production. Type IV RTA is often associated with an obstructive uropathy or other transient phenomenon in infancy (Alon, 1998; Friedman, 1998).

Clinical Findings

HISTORY. The following information is often reported:

- Failure to gain weight (especially) and height—the most common symptom (Lum, 1997)
- Polyuria and polydipsia
- Muscle weakness
- Irritability before eating, satiation after eating, vomiting, diarrhea or constipation in dRTA
- Preference for liquids over solid foods, poor appetite, or anorexia, especially with type IV

PHYSICAL EXAMINATION. Findings can include:

- Arrested growth curve toward the end of the first year with consistent growth before that

- Normal physical examination and development

LABORATORY STUDIES. The following studies are recommended when the child is well:

- Serum electrolytes, including CO_2, renal function tests (BUN, creatinine), calcium, phosphorus, alkaline phosphatase, and UA (first morning void) to test for glucose and pH
- A 24-hour creatinine clearance to establish the normal GFR
- Renal ultrasonography to determine the anatomy and rule out nephrocalcinosis, nephrolithiasis, hydronephrosis, and parenchymal damage

Differential Diagnosis

The diagnosis depends on a combination of clinical features, laboratory values, and response to treatment. RTA is suggested by a serum carbon dioxide level below 20, especially if the anion gap is normal (12 $\pm$ 4 mEq/L). Anion gap = $Na^+ - (Cl^- + HCO_3^-)$. Hypokalemia and hyperchloremia are present in pRTA and dRTA. Hyperkalemia is found in type IV. If total serum CO_2 is below 16 and urine pH is less than 5.5, pRTA is likely; if urine pH is greater than 5.5, dRTA is likely. Fanconi syndrome is an uncommon and more complex form of pRTA with associated glycosuria, phosphaturia, aminoaciduria, and a defect in vitamin D metabolism manifested as nausea, anorexia, intermittent vomiting, and possibly rickets. Primary RTA must be differentiated from secondary RTA, which can be due to many disease states or conditions. The differential diagnosis must include other causes of growth failure (FTT) and systemic acidosis.

Management

Goals of management include correcting the acidosis and maintaining normal bicarbonate (>20 mEq/L), thereby restoring growth and minimizing complications.

1. Oral alkalizing medications given to achieve these goals include:
   - Bicitra (sodium citrate and citric acid),

which equals 1 mEq bicarbonate per milliliter and is relatively pleasant tasting.
- Polycitra (sodium and potassium citrate and citric acid), which equals 2 mEq bicarbonate per milliliter and is less palatable. Giving it in juice, water, or formula may ease its administration. Polycitra is especially useful if the child is hypokalemic or requires an excess quantity or if compliance is an issue.
- $NaHCO_3$ tablets are available in 325-mg strength (4 mEq bicarbonate) and 650-mg strength (8 mEq bicarbonate).
- Eight ounces of baking soda mixed with 2.65 L of distilled water equals 1 mEq/ml bicarbonate.
- Dosing is determined by the type of RTA. Distal RTA requires low doses, often between 2 and 5 mEq/kg per day. Proximal RTA requires high doses, often between 5 and 15 mEq/kg per day and sometimes as high as 20 mEq/kg per day. The dose must be titrated to the child's response as determined by weight and laboratory results (CO_2 and electrolytes). Initiate medication at 3 mEq/kg per day and check laboratory results in a few days. Titrate the dose until a serum bicarbonate level of 20 to 22 mEq/L is achieved.
- To maintain as normal a bicarbonate level as possible, doses should be given frequently throughout the day (with meals) and as late as possible at night (at bedtime).
- The response to medication helps confirm the diagnosis and type of RTA. dRTA has a rapid response to treatment, and normal bicarbonate levels are maintained with little difficulty. pRTA requires higher doses to normalize bicarbonate and is less easily maintained. Type IV RTA requires mineralocorticoid treatment if aldosterone is deficient.

2. Maximizing caloric intake to enhance growth can be accomplished by:
   - Giving solid foods first at meals and snacks and avoiding water and noncaloric foods.
   - Providing nutritional supplements.
3. Meticulous follow-up is imperative.
   - Weight and laboratory results should be monitored biweekly to monthly until

weight gain is established and CO_2 is stabilized. Weighing on the same scale and by the same person is essential.
4. Pseudoephedrine should be avoided because it is minimally excreted in alkalinized urine and associated with a risk of intoxication.

Complications

It is rare to have complications with pRTA. Hypercalciuria leading to nephrocalcinosis, nephrolithiasis, renal parenchymal destruction, and occasionally renal failure can occur with dRTA. Rickets are sometimes found in type IV RTA.

Patient Education, Prevention, and Prognosis

Isolated pRTA responds quickly to treatment, with children showing catch-up growth and obtaining normal maximal height. pRTA resolves spontaneously without recurrence of symptoms, often within 1 to 2 years but at worst over the first decade of life (Petersen-Smith, 1995; Bergstein, 1996; Soriano, 1996). dRTA usually lasts a lifetime, and type IV resolves with correction of the underlying problem.

Wilms Tumor

Description

Wilms tumor, the most common malignancy of the genitourinary tract, is typically recognized as a firm smooth mass in the abdomen or flank. It is staged according to the National Wilms Tumor Study as follows. Stage I is limited to the kidney and can be completely excised with the capsular surface intact (35%). Stage II extends beyond the kidney but can still be completely excised (30%). Stage III has postsurgical residual nonhematogenous extension confined to the abdomen (20%). Stage IV has hematogenous metastasis, most frequently to the lung (12%). Stage V is bilateral kidney involvement (3 to 5%) (Steinhurz, 1998; Abelson, 1998).

Etiology and Incidence

This malignancy is manifested as a solitary growth in any part of either or both kidneys. Two forms are recognized, heritable (less than 1%) and nonheritable. An important feature of Wilms tumor is the occurrence of associated congenital anomalies in 15% of children, including renal abnormalities such as cryptorchidism, hypospadias, duplication of the collecting system, ambiguous genitalia (4.4%), hemihypertrophy (2.9%), aniridia (1.1%), cardiac abnormalities, and Beckwith-Wiedemann, Drash, and Perlman syndromes. Wilms tumor will develop in 15 to 20% of children with neurofibromatosis. It occurs with equal frequency in both sexes and has a 3:1 black:white incidence. Fifty-five percent occur on the left side. The incidence of Wilms tumor is 1 per 10,000 children younger than 15 years per year, or about 400 to 500 cases annually, with 80% being diagnosed before 5 years of age. The peak incidence and median age at diagnosis are both 3 years (Steinhurz, 1998; Miser, 1996; Shearer & Wilimas, 1996; Warner, 1996).

Clinical Findings

HISTORY
- The most frequent finding is increasing abdominal size or an actual palpable mass.
- Pain is reported if the mass has undergone rapid growth or hemorrhage (25 to 50%).
- Fever, dyspnea, diarrhea, vomiting, weight loss, or malaise may be reported.

PHYSICAL EXAMINATION
- A firm, smooth abdominal or flank mass that does not cross the midline may be noted.
- BP is elevated if renal ischemia is present (rare).
- A left varicocele is found in males if the spermatic vein is obstructed.
- A careful examination is needed to rule out congenital anomalies.

LABORATORY STUDIES
- Chest and abdominal radiography is performed to differentiate neuroblastoma, which is usually calcified.
- Abdominal ultrasonography is used to dif-

ferentiate a solid from a cystic mass or hydronephrosis and multicystic kidney.

- UA demonstrates hematuria in 25 to 33%.
- A complete blood count (CBC), reticulocyte count, and liver and renal chemistry studies are performed.
- A computed tomographic (CT) scan of the chest, abdomen, and pelvis to stage the disease and bone marrow is often done by the oncology team.

Differential Diagnosis

Neuroblastoma is the main differential diagnosis (the mass often crosses the midline). Multicystic kidney, hydronephrosis, renal cyst, or other renal malignancies are other conditions to consider.

Management

Diagnostic workup is the initial urgent priority, with subsequent timely referral to a pediatric cancer center for treatment. Surgery is scheduled to remove the affected kidney and possibly the ureter and adrenal gland; combined chemotherapy and radiotherapy are instituted if the disease is advanced or histological findings are unfavorable. Close follow-up after the initial treatment should be coordinated with the cancer team.

Complications

The lungs and liver are the most common sites of metastasis. High BP is possible because of renal ischemia and will occasionally lead to cardiac failure. Scoliosis resulting from radiation therapy is uncommon because the radiation is carefully controlled.

Patient Education, Prevention, and Prognosis

The prognosis is determined by the histology of the neoplasm, by the patient's age (the younger the better), the size of the tumor, positive nodes, and most significantly, the extent or stage of the disease. If the child has favorable histological parameters, the 4-year survival rate according to the Third National Wilms Tumor Study is as follows: 97% if stage I, 92% if stage II, 87% if stage III, and 73% if stage IV. Forty-five percent of relapses occur within 6 months, 28% more within 12 months (Steinhurz, 1998).

Hematuria

Description

Hematuria refers to blood in the urine that may be persistent, recurrent, or transient. It is detected by dipstick, by microscopic examination, or with the naked eye (macroscopic). Hematuria is a symptom of disease or injury to the urinary system, although a few RBCs can be normal in a pediatric patient. The number of RBCs/hpf considered to be abnormal varies and ranges from any to more than 5/hpf ($\times 40$) in unspun urine to more than 5 to 10/hpf in spun urine (Fitzwater & Wyatt, 1994; Feld et al., 1997; Opas, 1998; Roy, 1998; Finberg, 1998; Yadin, 1994). For management purposes, hematuria in this text is defined as more than 2/hpf in unspun or 5/hpf in spun urine.

Etiology and Incidence

RBCs arise from any point in the urinary tract. The term "gross hematuria" is related to the concentration of RBCs rather than to the location or significance of the disorder. The causes of macroscopic hematuria are as follows: UTI, 49%; trauma/irritation, 25%; glomerulonephritis (GN), 9%; coagulopathy/hemoglobinopathy, 3%; stones, 2%; and unknown, less than 9%. Hydronephrosis, tumor, cystitis cystica, or epididymitis are characterized by macrohematuria less than 1% of the time (Opas, 1998). Brownish, tea-colored urine with casts or protein is usually glomerular in origin; clots and red to pink urine with isomorphic RBCs but no protein usually originate from the lower tract. The incidence of hematuria is 0.5 to 2% when confirmed with repeat UA (Langman, 1999; Kaplan et al., 1997; Cruz & Spitzer, 1998; Finberg, 1998; Feld et al., 1997; Roy, 1998; Fitzwater & Wyatt, 1994; Yadin, 1994).

Clinical Findings

HISTORY. The following information is obtained:

- Previous medical history of cystic kidney disease, sickle cell, lupus, malignancy
- Family or previous history of hematuria, nephrolithiasis, cystic kidney, hemoglobinopathy, sickle cell disease or trait, systemic lupus erythematosus (SLE), hypertension, congestive heart disease, malignancy, deafness, renal failure
- Onset, duration, pattern, and timing of episodes
- Color of urine
- Presence of pain—back, abdominal, or flank, with voiding
- Straining or squatting with urination (tumor)
- Preceding illness—viral or streptococcal pharyngitis or impetigo
- Strenuous exercise or trauma (including bladder catheterization)
- Enuresis
- Trauma, foreign body, or sexual activity or abuse
- Current menstruation or medication
- Edema, rash, pallor, or arthralgias
- Drug ingestion, especially nonsteroidal anti-inflammatory drugs (NSAIDs), aspirin, or antibiotics
- Symptoms related to chronic renal disease (Table 35-2)

PHYSICAL EXAMINATION. Findings include

- FTT or falling growth curves (chronic renal insufficiency or long-standing acidosis)
- Malformed ears (congenital renal disease)
- Oliguria/anuria, edema, hypertension, and proteinuria, which are suggestive of glomerular disease
- Dysuria, urgency, frequency, and/or flank pain, which are suggestive of a lower tract disorder
- Abdominal or flank mass, which suggests an obstruction such as Wilms tumor, cystic disease, or posterior valves
- External genitalia—bleeding, foreign body, abuse

LABORATORY STUDIES. The following studies are essential:

- UA.
  - Color—a tea or smoky color indicates a

T A B L E 35-2

Seven Red Flags for Chronic Renal Failure

1. Failure to thrive (poor growth, fatigue, anorexia, nausea, gastroesophageal reflux, vomiting)
2. Chronic anemia (normochromic, normocytic), nonresponsive to medication
3. Complicated enuresis (daytime frequency, urgency, incontinence, chronic constipation, encopresis, infrequent voiding, straining to void, recurrent urinary tract infection)
4. Prolonged, unexplained vomiting or nausea (especially in the morning), anorexia, weight loss without diarrhea
5. Hypertension
6. Unusual bone disease (rickets, valgus deformity, fracture with minor trauma)
7. Poor school performance (headache, fatigue, inattention, withdrawal from family activity)

Adapted from Vogt BA: Identifying renal disease: Simple steps can make a difference. *Contemp Pediatr* 14(3): 115–127, 1997.

nephrological disorder; red indicates a urological disorder.
  - If greater than 1+ by dipstick (which equals 3 RBCs/hpf or 0.02 mg/dl hemoglobin) for blood, microscopic examination for RBCs is needed to differentiate hemoglobin or myoglobin from RBCs.
  - If protein is present, refer to the section on proteinuria and nephritis for further workup. *Note*: The most significant differentiating factor is the presence of proteinuria. If present, rapid evaluation and early referral to a nephrologist are essential.
- Microscopic examination for RBCs, including size and shape, casts, crystals, and WBCs.
  - A few RBCs/hpf can be normal in a pediatric patient (see description of hematuria).
  - Distorted, misshapen RBCs of different size suggest glomerular disease.
  - A negative microscopic examination occurs in dilute urine because RBCs undergo lysis as a result of the hypotonicity of urine.

- Urine culture (approximately 33% are positive).
- UA on first-degree relatives.
- Some nephrologists recommend a CBC with platelets, electrolytes, BUN, creatinine, sickle cell screen, complement component C3, and Streptozyme test at this point (Roy, 1998).
- Ultrasonography is performed if any concerns remain, although "renal ultrasound, voiding cystourethrogram, cystoscopy and renal biopsy are not indicated in the workup of microscopic hematuria" (Feld et al., 1998).
- If results show isolated, transient hematuria, monitor every year with UA, growth performance, and BP.

Differential Diagnosis

Five patterns of hematuria have been identified and may be helpful when considering the differential diagnosis of hematuria (Boineau & Lewy, 1989):

Type 1—microscopic and persistent
Type 2—microscopic and intermittent
Type 3—persistent macroscopic
Type 4—intermittent or recurrent macroscopic
Type 5—intermittent or recurrent macroscopic with persistent microscopic

Types 1 and 2 account for most cases of hematuria in pediatrics. Type 3 is common in urological and nephrological disorders such as UTI, GN, hemoglobinopathies, renal stones, and trauma. Types 4 and 5 occur with immunoglobulin A (IgA) nephropathy, hypercalciuria, and benign recurrent hematuria.

Other differential diagnoses to consider include the following:

- *Pseudohematuria* occurs when a false-positive dipstick reading is noted but no RBCs are found on the microscopic examination. The two most common causes are myoglobinuria and hemoglobinuria (see Table 35-1).
- *Extrarenal hematuria* is common with systemic bleeding disorders and is evidenced by macroscopic and microscopic hematuria.

- The presence of RBC casts, proteinuria, or both is a manifestation of *glomerular hematuria,* such as acute or chronic GN.
- *Idiopathic hypercalciuria* is an inherited tubulointerstitial disorder with excessive urinary calcium excretion in the presence of macroscopic and microscopic hematuria. It represents the most frequently seen isolated cases of hematuria in children and occurs more commonly in the southeastern United States and southern Canada. It occurs in 5% of healthy white children and accounts for 30% of cases of hematuria (Roy, 1998; Fitzwater & Wyatt, 1994). The diagnosis is made by laboratory examination of urine. The calcium-creatinine ratio done on a random urine sample is elevated (>0.18 to 0.21 mg/dl). Elevated 24-hour calcium excretion (>4 mg/kg per 24 hours) confirms the diagnosis. Idiopathic hypercalciuria and Berger disease (see the section on nephritis) are responsible for 50% or more of cases of isolated hematuria in children.
- Although rare, *renal stones (nephrolithiasis) or calcification (nephrocalcinosis)* can occur. If suspected, a renal ultrasonogram can be included as part of the workup.
- *Exercise-induced hematuria* occurs when hematuria is present after vigorous exercise, but not at other times.
- Hematuria caused by *viral or bacterial illnesses* is not uncommon, with adenovirus known to cause hemorrhagic cystitis (Cruz & Spitzer, 1998).

Management

A progressive approach to evaluating hematuria should be undertaken with the goal of not overlooking serious, treatable progressive conditions while avoiding unnecessary studies.

1. *Macroscopic hematuria* without proteinuria or casts (Fig. 35-5).
   - Urine culture is done initially to rule out UTI.
   - Ultrasonography may be done to evaluate for renal stones, an obstructive lesion, or tumor; IVP or VCUG is performed as indicated.

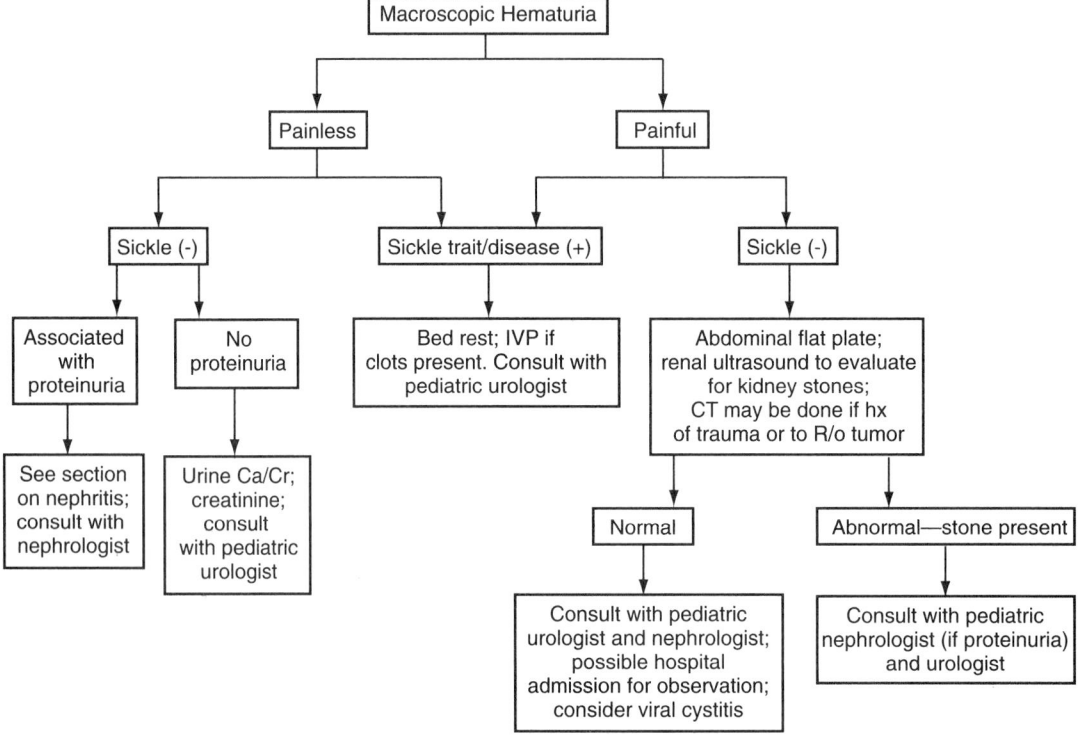

FIGURE 35-5

Management of macroscopic hematuria. Ca/Cr = calcium/creatinine ratio; CT = computed tomography; hx = history; IVP = intravenous pyelogram; R/O = rule out. (Adapted from Dershewitz RA (ed): Ambulatory Pediatric Care, 3rd ed. Philadelphia, Lippincott-Raven, 1999.)

- Type 4 or 5 hematuria may need an immunological workup—antistreptolysin O (ASO), C3, antinuclear antibody (ANA), anti-DNA, BUN, creatinine.
- Consultation or referral to a nephrologist or urologist may be necessary, depending on the findings.
2. *Microscopic hematuria.* Initially, three first morning urine samples should be examined within 7 to 14 days to confirm the presence of hematuria (Fig. 35–6).
   - If exercise-induced hematuria is suspected, recheck the urine after refraining from exercise for 72 hours.
   - If repeated urine specimens are negative, recheck the urine in 1 month and again in 6 months.
   - If protein or casts are found in the urine (a red flag), suspect glomerular hematuria and see the section on nephritis.

- If urine culture is positive, see the section on UTI.
- If the calcium-creatinine ratio is greater than 0.18 to 0.21, suspect idiopathic hypercalciuria.
  - Increase fluid to dilute the calcium concentration.
  - Refer to a nephrologist.
  - Perform ultrasonography if nephrolithiasis is suspected.
  - Monitor BP.
- If asymptomatic microscopic hematuria is suspected,
  - Perform microscopic examination of family members' urine.
  - Consultation with or referral to a nephrologist may be warranted.
  - Monitor UA, BP, and growth every 6 to 12 months.
3. Refer to a nephrologist for persistent micro-

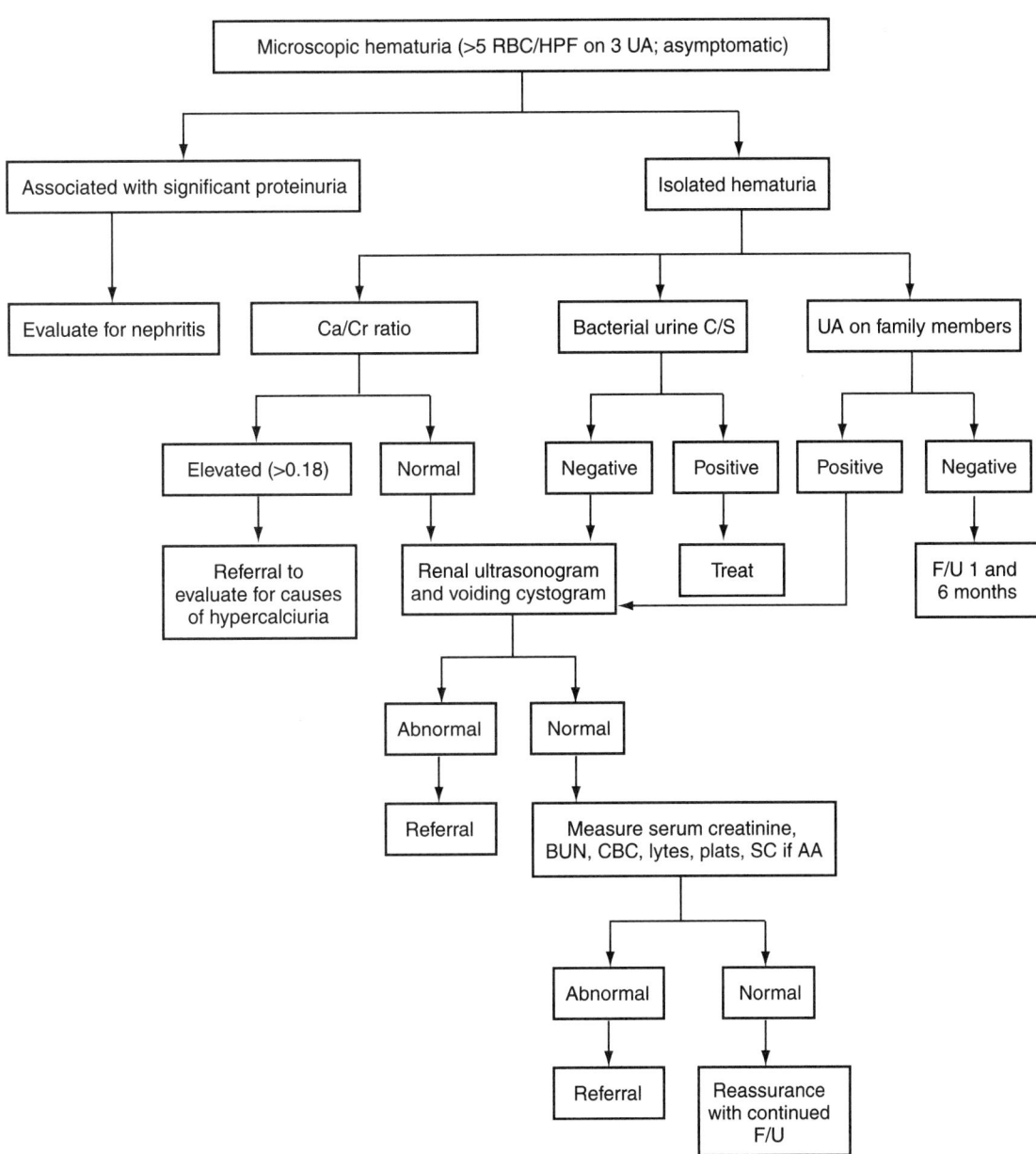

F I G U R E 35-6

Management of asymptomatic microscopic hematuria. AA = African American; BUN = blood urea nitrogen; CBC = complete blood count; Ca/Cr = calcium/creatinine ratio; C/S = culture/sensitivity; F/U = follow-up; lytes = electrolytes; plats = platelets; RBC/HPF = red blood cells per high-power field; SC = sickle cell; UA = urinalysis. (Adapted from Dershewitz RA (ed): Ambulatory Pediatric Care, 3rd ed. Philadelphia, Lippincott-Raven, 1999.)

hematuria, recurrent gross hematuria, proteinuria, RBC or other casts detected by UA, family history, or any signs of renal failure.

Prognosis

Microscopic hematuria is a benign finding in the vast majority of patients (Feld et al., 1998).

Proteinuria

Description

Protein in the urine is commonly detected by dipstick tests. It may be transient, recurrent, or fixed. Proteinuria can be a symptom of disease, or it can reflect a benign, self-limited condition. The quantity of protein and the timing of its presence determine its significance. Qualitative protein in urine, as tested by dipstick, is considered positive if it registers 1+ (30 mg/dl) or more in urine with a specific gravity of less than 1.015. Quantitative protein is tested by measuring a timed urine. A level of less than 4 mg/m^2 per hour is considered normal, 4 to 40 mg/m^2 per hour is abnormal, and greater than 40 mg/m^2 per hour is nephrotic.

Etiology and Incidence

Proteinuria originates from problems with glomerular filtration, tubular reabsorption or secretion, or both. The child is often asymptomatic. If proteinuria is significant enough to cause hypoproteinemia, edema is present.

The incidence of proteinuria is cited at 5 to 10% in school-age children. It drops to 2% if a criterion of 1+ is used and to 0.1% if greater than 2+ is used. Its peak incidence (2%) occurs in adolescence (16 years for boys, 13 for girls) (Langman, 1999; Cruz & Spitzer, 1998; Finberg, 1998; Kaplan, 1997; Ettenger, 1994).

Clinical Findings

HISTORY
- Family history of deafness, visual problems, and renal disease
- Recent strenuous exercise or febrile illness
- Polydipsia or polyuria

- Vague symptoms such as malaise, fatigue, or pallor
- Symptoms related to chronic renal disease (see Table 35–2)

PHYSICAL EXAMINATION
- BP (hypertension), pulse, respiratory rate
- Growth and development parameters (poor weight gain or FTT with chronic disease; weight gain with nephrotic syndrome)
- Edema, especially periorbital edema, or symptoms of fluid retention
- Abdominal examination for a mass, enlarged kidney, fluid, tenderness

LABORATORY STUDIES. The following are done as indicated:

- UA (repeated three times over 1 to 2 weeks), preferably done on a first-voided specimen
  - A 1+ protein (30 mg) is significant if the specific gravity is less than 1.015; 2+ protein (100 mg) is significant if the specific gravity is greater than 1.015.
  - At least 75% of asymptomatic patients with proteinuria in a single urine specimen have normal urine on repeated testing.
  - False-positive results occur in highly concentrated or alkaline urine. False-negative results occur in dilute or acidic urine.
- Microscopic urine
  - RBCs and/or WBCs, casts, bacteria, oval fat bodies, or other abnormalities are present in most pathological conditions.
- The protein-to-creatinine ratio on a random daytime urine sample is elevated. Normal values are less than 0.5 for a child 6 months to 2 years of age, less than 0.2 to 0.25 for a child older than 2 years, and less than 0.1 to 0.2 mg/dl for an adult; greater than 2 mg/dl is considered nephrotic.
- A 12- or 24-hour timed urine collection for creatinine (normal, 10 to 15 mg/kg per 24 hours) and protein excretion (normal, <4 mg/m^2 per hour) is elevated. A back-to-back collection (e.g., bedtime to arising, arising to bedtime) is done to compare active or upright and resting levels.
- If protein in urine is greater than 4 mg/m^2

per hour, check the CBC, electrolytes, BUN, creatinine, albumin/total protein, C3, C4, cholesterol, liver function tests, and urine culture. Perform an ultrasonogram, VCUG, and radionuclide scans as indicated. Evaluate for systemic disease as indicated (e.g., ANA, ASO, Streptozyme, hepatitis B, human immunodeficiency virus [HIV], tuberculosis).

Differential Diagnosis

Four groups of proteinuria exist: isolated, transient or functional, glomerular, and tubulointerstitial.

- Orthostatic proteinuria and persistent asymptomatic proteinuria, which are members of the first group, termed isolated proteinuria, are the most common.
  - *Orthostatic proteinuria* accounts for up to 60% (75% in adolescents) of cases of proteinuria (Finberg, 1998; Opas, 1998). In this condition, the child excretes abnormal amounts of protein when upright but normal amounts when lying down. Orthostatic proteinuria is demonstrated by collecting a urine sample immediately on arising and comparing it with a specimen collected after several hours of activity. The child must have voided before sleep to obtain accurate results. A typical result yields negative to trace amounts on overnight specimens but 1+ or greater on daytime specimens. If the result is equivocal, back-to-back urine samples (from arising to bedtime and bedtime to arising) to quantitate protein are evaluated.
  - *Persistent asymptomatic proteinuria* is a common, transient phenomenon in which an otherwise healthy child, with normal clinical and laboratory workup, has an abnormally high level of protein in the urine.
- The second group of proteinuria is transient or functional proteinuria and is caused by some type of stress.
  - *Exercised-induced proteinuria* is documented by collecting a urine sample, having the patient exercise vigorously for several minutes, and then collecting another sample. The postexercise sample is usually strongly positive.
  - *Fever-induced proteinuria* can accompany any febrile state and usually subsides with resolution of the fever. Other stress-related causes include cold exposure, infection, congestive heart failure, and seizures. This type of proteinuria usually resolves in 1 to 2 weeks and does not require any workup.
- The third and fourth groups, glomerular proteinuria, which is typified by GN, and tubulointerstitial proteinuria, are least common and are characterized by high levels of proteinuria. Some authorities believe that persistent proteinuria in childhood, even at low levels, should be placed in these groups with a high index of suspicion for an underlying, progressive renal disorder.
- *Pseudoproteinuria* can be caused by semisynthetic penicillins or benzalkonium chloride.

Management

The persistence, quantity, and presence of other abnormalities (e.g., hematuria) are key to evaluating proteinuria.

1. If protein by dipstick is trace or 1+ and specific gravity is greater than 1.015,
   - Offer reassurance.
   - Do monthly recheck of urine for 4 to 6 months.
     - If protein is persistent, refer the patient to a nephrologist.
2. If protein by dipstick is greater than 1+, see Figure 35-7. To evaluate for orthostatic proteinuria, collect urine immediately after arising.
   - If protein is negative to trace, orthostatic proteinuria is confirmed.
3. If protein is 1+ or 2+, perform a quantitative 12- to 24-hour urine protein excretion test.
   - If less than 4 mg/m^2 per hour, reassure.
   - If greater than 4 mg/m^2 per hour, proceed as in Figure 35-7.
4. If protein by dipstick is greater than 2+,

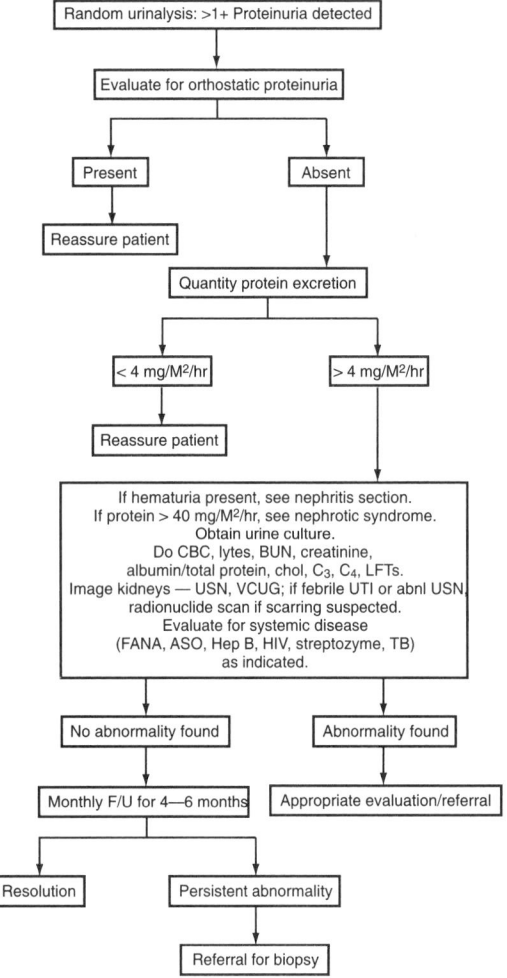

F I G U R E   35-7
Evaluation of proteinuria. abnl = abnormal; alb/TP = albumin/total protein; ANA = antinuclear antibody; ASO = antistreptolysin O; BUN = blood urea nitrogen; C_3 = complement 3; C_4 = complement 4; CBC = complete blood count; chol = cholesterol; Cr = creatinine; FANA = fluorescent antinuclear antibody; F/U = follow-up; Hep B = hepatitis B; HIV = human immunodeficiency virus; LFTs = liver function tests; lytes = electrolytes. (Adapted from Dershewitz RA (ed): Ambulatory Pediatric Care, 3rd ed. Philadelphia, Lippincott-Raven, 1999.)

    evaluate for nephrotic syndrome (see later section).

5. If hematuria is present, evaluate for nephritis (see later section).

6. Follow-up is important to monitor for any change in status.

7. Refer the following to a nephrologist: persistent unexplained nonorthostatic proteinuria, any hematuria or RBC or WBC casts, polyuria or oliguria, nephrotic levels of protein, elevated BUN or creatinine, elevated BP, or a child with a family history of renal failure, GN, sensorineural hearing loss, kidney transplantation, or systemic complaints (joint pain, rashes, or arthralgias).

Prognosis

Orthostatic proteinuria with a 10-year follow-up showed resolution in 50% and the remainder with a normal GFR.

Nephritis or Glomerulonephritis

Description

Nephritis is a noninfectious, inflammatory response of the kidneys characterized by varied degrees of hypertension, edema, proteinuria, and hematuria that can be either microscopic or macroscopic with dysmorphic RBCs and casts. Nephritis is classified as acute, intermittent, or chronic. Primary GN occurs when the original and predominant structure impaired is the glomerulus. Secondary GN occurs when renal involvement is secondary to systemic disease, (e.g., lupus, Henoch-Schönlein purpura [HSP], primary vasculitis, Goodpasture syndrome, or drug hypersensitivity reactions). Involvement can be in the glomerulus or the interstitium and either localized in one part of the kidney or generalized throughout. GN refers to inflammation primarily in the glomeruli; interstitial nephritis refers to inflammation in the interstitium primarily caused by drug reactions. Poststreptococcal GN (PSGN) is the classic form of GN.

    Pyelonephritis, discussed later in the UTI section, is inflammation of the renal parenchyma, calyces, and pelvis caused by bacteria.

Etiology and Incidence

The inflammatory response of the kidneys results from infection, an immunological response, a drug or toxin, and vascular or systemic disorders. PSGN is an immune response by the host to a nonrenal group A β-hemolytic streptococcal infection, whereas acute postinfectious GN (APGN) can be caused by bacterial, fungal, viral, parasitic, or rickettsial agents.

PSGN is the most common form of nephritis in childhood, occurs more often in males (2:1), peaks at 7 years of age, and is unusual in children younger than 3 years or in adults. The incidence of APGN is difficult to determine because of the large number of patients with subclinical cases, most younger than 5 to 10 years (Blowey, 1998; Simckes & Spitzer, 1995).

Clinical Findings

HISTORY. The following may be reported:

- Streptococcal skin (more likely) or pharyngeal infection within the past 2 to 3 weeks (PSGN). Classically, a latent period of 7 to 10 days elapses between infection and the onset of symptoms; if less than 5 days or more than 14 days, consider other causes.
- Abrupt onset of gross hematuria.
- Reduced urine output.
- Lethargy, anorexia, nausea, vomiting, abdominal pain.
- Chills, fever, backache (pyelonephritis).
- Medication taken in the last few weeks.

PHYSICAL EXAMINATION. Findings to look for include:

- Hypertension (60 to 80% in PSGN; Simckes & Spitzer, 1995) that is transient and resolves in 1 to 2 weeks
- Edema, especially periorbital edema, of abrupt onset with weight gain
- Ear malformations
- Flank or abdominal pain or a mass (in polycystic kidney or malignancy, e.g., Wilms tumor)
- Costovertebral angle tenderness (in pyelonephritis)
- Circulatory congestion—dyspnea, cough, pallor, pulmonary edema if severe
- Oliguria, with diuresis in 5 to 7 days
- Rashes or arthralgias (with SLE, HSP, or impetigo)
- Evidence of trauma or abuse

LABORATORY STUDIES. The following are done as indicated:

- UA with microscopic examination—tea color, elevated specific gravity, macrohematuria and microhematuria, proteinuria not exceeding the amount of hematuria, pyuria in PSGN; granular, hyaline, WBC, or RBC casts and dysmorphic RBCs
- Serum C3/C4 (low early in disease, back to normal in 6 to 8 weeks), total protein and albumin (elevated)
- CBC, erythrocyte sedimentation rate (ESR), ASO titer (elevated), Streptozyme test (positive), anti-DNAseB titer
- Electrolytes, BUN, creatinine, and cholesterol
- Fluorescent antinuclear antibody (lupus), hepatitis titers, sickle cell or hemoglobin electrophoresis, tuberculin purified protein derivative (PPD), and fluorescent treponemal antibody absorption (syphilis)

Differential Diagnosis

Acute nephritis most commonly occurs as PSGN, which is characterized by a history of streptococcal infection within the last 2 weeks and an acute onset of edema, oliguria, hypertension, and gross hematuria. Consider an alternative diagnosis if the following findings are present:

- Nephrotic levels of protein
- Lack of evidence for a postinfection mechanism
- Rapidly deteriorating renal function
- Clinical or laboratory findings suggesting other forms of GN, for example, rash, positive ANA

Intermittent gross hematuria and *proteinuria syndromes* include the following:

1. *IgA nephropathy*, or *Berger disease*, is the most common chronic GN in children of European-Asian descent and uncommon in blacks; it has a 2:1 male preponderance (Roy, 1998; Cruz & Spitzer, 1998; Andreoli, 1995). It is an immunological entity causing recurrent gross and microscopic hematuria and often proteinuria and is present in about 15% of cases of hematuria lasting more than a year (Fitzwater & Wyatt, 1994). It is often precipitated by viral infections or strenuous exercise, and each episode lasts less than 72

hours. BP is normal, no edema is present, and C3 is normal. Definitive diagnosis is made by biopsy. The prognosis is good in the absence of elevated serum creatinine or nephrotic-range proteinuria, although progression to chronic renal insufficiency can occur (25 to 30%; Fitzwater & Wyatt, 1994; Andreoli, 1995; Roy, 1998). Berger disease and idiopathic hypercalciuria (see the section on hematuria) are responsible for 50% or more cases of isolated hematuria in children.

2. *Hereditary or familial nephritis* involves many disorders, but the best known is *Alport syndrome*. More common and severe in males, with onset before 15 years of age in 75% of children, this condition is inherited as an X-linked dominant trait. The initial manifestation is isolated, persistent microscopic hematuria with intermittent macrohematuria and variable proteinuria occurring with an upper respiratory infection or exercise. Laboratory abnormalities are variable; biopsy verifies the diagnosis. Extrarenal abnormalities, including neurogenic deafness (hearing loss in 50% with females often spared), ocular abnormalities (30%), and macrothrombocytopenia, are often found (Fouser, 1998). Vision and hearing screening is essential, with referral for any abnormalities. Severe forms of the disease can lead to end-stage renal disease, which is often heralded by hypotension.

3. *Familial or benign recurrent nephritis,* now also called *thin-basement-membrane disease*, is a disorder inherited as an autosomal dominant trait with unknown etiology. Macroscopic and microscopic hematuria and mild proteinuria, often precipitated by upper respiratory tract infection, characterize episodes. Laboratory values other than the UA are normal. The diagnosis is confirmed by biopsy, which may not be needed if the disease is mild and confirmed in relatives. In the absence of notable proteinuria, deafness, ocular defects, and renal failure and with normal biopsy findings, the prognosis is excellent.

Chronic nephritis, most commonly known as membranoproliferative GN (MPGN) and hav-

ing four types based on biopsy, can be found after acute nephritis or when investigating non-specific complaints such as anorexia, intermittent vomiting, and malaise. It is manifested by diminished renal function associated with detrimental effects on other organ systems. Types I and II may respond to steroids, but the overall prognosis is guarded.

Acute nephritis also occurs as part of systemic illnesses such as SLE, HSP, hemolytic-uremic syndrome, vasculitis, or as a reaction to a drug or irradiation.

Management

See Figure 35–8. Consultation with a nephrologist is recommended in all cases.

1. *PSGN* treatment is supportive because resolution occurs spontaneously 90% of the time within 6 to 24 months. The course does not seem to be affected by corticosteroids, immunosuppression, or other treatment modalities. During the peak of oliguria and hypertension in the first few days of illness, hospitalization may be required with fluid and sodium limitation and diuretic, antihypertensive, and antibiotic treatment if cultures are positive. Resolution occurs once diuresis begins. Gross hematuria persists for 1 to 2 weeks, urine can be abnormal for 6 to 12 weeks, and microscopic hematuria can persist for up to 2 years. Complement levels return to normal in 3 to 6 weeks.

2. *Acute nephritis*—possible hospitalization with treatment as just described.

3. *IgA nephropathy*—annual follow-up with BP, UA, and determination of renal function.

4. *Benign familial or hereditary nephritis*—perform audiometry and review family medical history. Hereditary markers are being developed for this disease.

5. *Benign recurrent nephritis*—monitor UA and renal function every 1 to 2 years.

6. *Chronic nephritis*—a team approach is required to adequately provide care.

Complications

Prolonged oliguria and renal failure can occur if acute nephritis progresses. Hypertensive

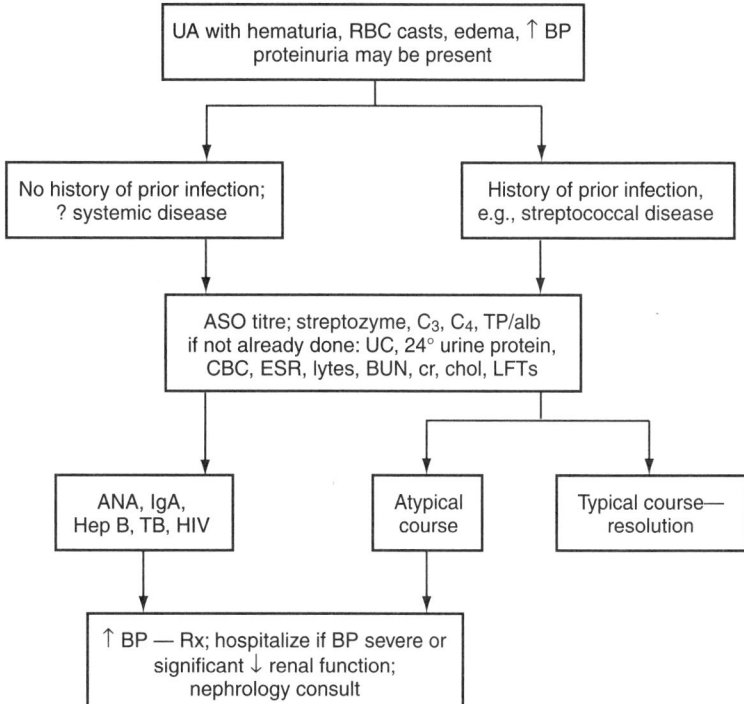

F I G U R E 35-8
Evaluation of nephritis. alb = albumin; ANA = antinuclear antibody; ASO = antistreptolysin O; BP = blood pressure; BUN = blood urea nitrogen; C_3 = complement 3; C_4 = complement 4; CBC = complete blood count; chol = cholesterol; cr = creatinine; ESR = erythrocyte sedimentation rate; HepB = hepatitis B; HIV = human immunodeficiency virus; IgA = immunoglobulin A; LFT = liver function test; RBC = red blood cells; Rx = prescribe; TB = tuberculosis; TP = total protein; UA = urinalysis.

encephalopathy and/or congestive heart failure can occur secondary to PSGN. Irreversible parenchymal damage causes hypertension and renal insufficiency.

Prognosis

Patients with PSGN may have macrohematuria or microhematuria for up to 6 to 12 months, but the long-range outcome is excellent. Thin-basement-membrane disease has a good outcome. IgA nephropathy with severe histological findings has a poor outcome, especially if the child is black.

Nephrotic Syndrome

Description

Nephrotic syndrome is due to excessive excretion of protein in urine. The "classic" definition of nephrotic syndrome is massive proteinuria (>40 mg/m^2 per hour and a protein-creatinine ratio on spot urine of greater than 1.0), hypoalbuminemia (<2.5 g/dl), edema, and hyperlipid-

emia. The latter two findings may not be present in all cases or at all times. The main mechanism of the massive protein loss is increased glomerular permeability. The loss can be selective (albumin only) or nonselective (including most serum proteins), and such selectivity is an important distinction in diagnosis. With protein loss, the liver increases its synthesis of protein and thereby causes concurrent hyperlipidemia and lipiduria. Nephrotic syndrome is a chronic disease characterized by periods of remission (urinary protein excretion and serum albumin normalize) and relapses (recurrence of proteinuria and hypoalbuminemia after complete remission). Most children are steroid responders, with remission subsequent to treatment with steroids. Of the remainder, most are steroid resistant and show no response to steroids. A small number are partial responders with minimal response to steroids or are steroid dependent and require high doses of prednisone with frequent relapses.

The classification of nephrotic syndrome as described by the International Collaborative

Study of Kidney Diseases in Children (Warshaw, 1994) is as follows:

1. Primary nephrotic syndrome, unrelated to systemic disease, is also called minimal change nephrotic syndrome (MCNS) or idiopathic nephrotic syndrome, lipoid nephrosis, or nil disease. Histopathological examination shows glomerular lesions without inflammation and mild to no morphological abnormality. This type occurs in 80 to 90% of cases and is usually characterized by resolution of symptoms in response to steroids.

2. Secondary nephrotic syndrome occurs in association with or secondary to systemic disorders (e.g., SLE, HSP), infectious processes (e.g., syphilis, hepatitis B, HIV, or malaria), drug toxicities (e.g., NSAIDs, mephenytoin), allergens, or other renal disorders (e.g., IgA or congenital nephritis). Histopathological examination shows moderate to severe morphological abnormality. This type occurs in 10% of cases.

Etiology and Incidence

Nephrotic syndrome occurs as a result of immune, systemic, nephrotoxic, allergic, infectious, malignant, vascular, or idiopathic processes. The actual mechanism of nephrotic syndrome has been extensively studied, and the understanding of its histopathology is better than the understanding of its pathogenesis. At this point, the primary mechanism is believed to be immunological rather than renal (Warshaw, 1994).

The incidence of nephrotic syndrome is 1.2 to 2.3 per 100,000, with a 15 times greater incidence in children than in adults. Sixty-six percent to 80% of cases are MCNS, with a peak incidence at 2 to 6 years. Eighty-five percent of patients are steroid responders. In early childhood, the male-to-female ratio is 2:1; however, by midadolescence, the rate of occurrence is equal.

Clinical Findings

HISTORY. The following may be reported:

- Edema, which is a cardinal clinical feature, especially periorbital edema, in dependent areas (tight shoes or underwear) and lax tissues (puffy eyes)
- Low urine production
- Gastrointestinal symptoms: anorexia, paleness, listlessness, diarrhea, vomiting, abdominal pain (right upper quadrant)
- Recent prodromal infection
- Respiratory difficulties secondary to ascites, effusion, pneumonia, if advanced disease

PHYSICAL EXAMINATION. Findings include

- Edema—periorbital in the morning, dependent in the evening
- Hypertension, normal BP if hypovolemic
- Chronically ill appearing
- Muscle wasting, malnourishment, growth failure if prolonged
- If the disease is progressive, hydrothorax with respiratory difficulty or ascites with labial edema

LABORATORY STUDIES. The following are ordered as indicated:

- UA and microscopic examination, which reveal protein of 2+ or greater, hyaline and fine granular casts, microhematuria in 33%, elevated specific gravity, fat bodies, and casts in urine
- Quantitative urine protein excretion (24-hour collection or protein-creatinine ratio on a random first morning urine)
- CBC; electrolytes, BUN, creatinine (normal); calcium; serum albumin (<2 g/dl), total protein; liver enzymes; triglycerides, lipoproteins, cholesterol (elevated); C3 and C4 (normal); ANA
- Consideration of VDRL, hepatitis B surface antigen, HIV, malaria, PPD as indicated by history
- Kidney biopsy is recommended in the following circumstance:
  - If criteria for MCNS are not met
  - If systemic disease is present
  - In the presence of hypertension *and* hematuria
  - With hypocomplementemia or nonselective proteinemia
  - If the patient is older than 7 years or an adolescent
  - If the patient is nonresponsive to steroids
  - If relapses are frequent

Differential Diagnosis

Minimal change disease is characterized by the following:

- Age 1 to 7 years (strongest factor)
- Normal vascular volume despite edema (normal BP, normal heart size)
- Absence of gross hematuria or urinary casts
- Absent or transient microhematuria
- Normal serum creatinine, complement components, ANA

Infants (newborn to 1 year) usually have congenital renal problems, children 7 years and older are likely to have focal glomerulosclerosis or mesangial proliferative GN, and teens have membranous nephropathy. The differential diagnosis includes hypoproteinemia from starvation, liver disease, and protein-losing enteropathy; none of these conditions has associated proteinuria. GN should also be considered in the differential diagnosis.

Management

Nephrotic syndrome is a complex, often chronic disorder that responds to careful management with a gratifying long-term outcome. A major goal is to control edema while awaiting definitive remission. Management involves the following:

1. The diagnosis is made with 95% certainty on clinical impressions.
2. Referral to a nephrologist; initial hospitalization if severe.
3. Prednisone (2 mg/kg per day; maximum, 60 mg) to induce remission, which can occur as early as 14 days as evidenced by diuresis. Steroids are continued for at least 4 to 6 weeks. A crushed or quartered pill is economical and often easier to give than liquid. Once remission occurs, steroid therapy is tapered and weaned over several months. Relapses are treated with a short course of steroids and the patient weaned as soon as the proteinuria resolves. Consultation with a nephrologist is important because of the constantly changing strategies for managing these children.
4. Activity and diet recommendations. No limi-tation is placed on activity. During active disease, salt may be restricted. At other times, a diet appropriate for age is recommended. A high-protein, low-salt/no-salt diet with less than 35% fat and less than 300 mg cholesterol per day is sometimes recommended (Kelsch & Sedman, 1993).
5. Diuretics and albumin replacement are sometimes used in the acute phase. Monitoring of BP at home is sometimes recommended.
6. Proteinuria testing at home is recommended to monitor the child and identify exacerbations as soon as possible. Relapses begin with persistent proteinuria of greater than 2+ every day for 3 days.
7. Routine immunizations, including varicella vaccine, should be given during remissions and at least 3 months after immunosuppressive drugs, especially live vaccines. Pneumococcal and influenza vaccines are recommended for these children.
8. Monitoring and prompt treatment of infection are essential. Exposure to varicella zoster requires that varicella zoster immune globulin be given within 72 hours of exposure. Sepsis workup should be done with any fever and broad-spectrum antibiotics given until the organism is identified. Although some experts recommend that penicillin be given as a prophylactic measure, most experts state that prophylaxis is of no benefit (Mendoza & Tune, 1995).

Complications

Children with nephrotic syndrome are susceptible to pneumococcal, *Escherichia coli*, *Pseudomonas*, and *Haemophilus influenzae* infection because of stasis of fluid; such infection is seen as peritonitis, pneumonia, cellulitis, or septicemia. Hypertension or hypotension is a possibility. Because the child is in a hypercoagulable state, thromboembolism is possible. Protein losses and compromising edema are also potential complications.

Patient Education/Prognosis

The prognosis is good in steroid responders, with resolution by adolescence without any residual renal dysfunction (Burg et al., 1996). Families must know that relapses are the rule. An understanding of the disease process, side effects of steroids, recognition of infection, and the importance of monitoring proteinuria for relapses is crucial. If chronic steroid treatment is needed, the child and family must understand the side effects of the medication.

LOWER GENITOURINARY TRACT DISORDERS

Urinary Tract Infection

Description

Not only are UTIs frequently seen in primary care, but they are also the most commonly seen serious bacterial infection in young febrile children without an obvious source of infection. Because young children have limited symptoms, a high degree of suspicion must be maintained to diagnose UTI. Inflammation and infection can occur at any point in the urinary tract, so a UTI must be identified according to location. Bacteriuria is bacteria in the urine without other symptoms and is notable as a marker for possible underlying anatomical abnormality. Cystitis is infection of the bladder that produces lower tract symptoms. Pyelonephritis is the most severe type of UTI involving the renal parenchyma or kidneys and must be identified because of its potential for causing renal damage. Clinical signs thought to indicate pyelonephritis are a febrile infant with no other sign of infection or an older child with significant bacteriuria, systemic symptoms, or renal tenderness. UTIs may also be differentiated according to the type of infection. A UTI may be symptomatic or asymptomatic. It may also be complicated or uncomplicated. A complicated UTI is defined both as a UTI with fever, toxicity, dehydration, and poor compliance or occurring in a child younger than 3 to 6 months and as a UTI associated with a structural or functional abnormality such as vesicoureteral reflux (VUR), obstruction, voiding dysfunction, instrumentation, or pregnancy. Additionally, a UTI must be identified as a *first occurrence*, *recurrent* (within 2 weeks with the same organism or any reinfection with a different organism), or *chronic* (ongoing, unresolved, often caused

by an abnormality or resistant organism). Finally, age at the time of occurrence and gender of the child are important factors in determining the course of treatment. (*Note*: Pyelonephritis, although an upper tract disorder, is discussed in this section because it can be an infection ascending from the lower tract.)

It should be noted that evaluation and treatment of UTIs have changed dramatically over the last 30 years because of new knowledge regarding the pathogenesis of infection, especially kidney damage, but also because of new imaging technologies and treatment. Therefore, the practitioner must remain alert to new information as it becomes available.

Etiology and Incidence

The organism most commonly associated with UTI is *E. coli* (75 to 95%), although other organisms such as *Enterobacter, Klebsiella, Pseudomonas,* and *Proteus* can be found. Several factors are believed to contribute to the etiology of UTIs. Most UTIs are thought to be ascending—that is, the infection begins with colonization of the urethral area and ascends the urinary tract. If the infection progresses to the kidney, intrarenal reflux deep into the kidneys can lead to scarring. This damage to the kidney occurs in the composite papillae, which have wide and gaping openings allowing intrarenal reflux. Simple papillae have slit-like openings at an angle that resist intrarenal reflux (Fig. 35-9). The composite papillae are located in the upper and lower poles of the kidney, which is the usual site of scarring.

Host resistance factors and bacterial virulence factors are also important in the etiology of UTIs. Host resistance factors include the presence of a structural abnormality or dysplasia (such as VUR, obstruction, or any other anatomical defect) or the presence of functional abnormalities (such as dysfunctional voiding or constipation). Other factors affecting resistance include female gender (having a short urethra), poor hygiene, irritation from bubble baths, sexual activity or sexual abuse, and pinworms.

Several bacterial factors are known, but the two most important ones are adherence and virulence of the bacteria. Bacteria that have fimbriae or pili are able to anchor or adhere to

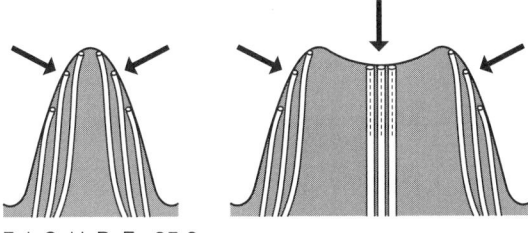

F I G U R E 35-9

Most renal papillae are conical, with papillary ducts that open obliquely into the renal pelvis (left). These do not allow intrarenal reflux. But some kidneys have compound papillae, formed by the fusion of conical papillae (right). These have papillary ducts with gaping openings at right angles to urine flow and do permit intrarenal reflux. (From Ransley PG: Intrarenal reflux: Anatomical, dynamic and radiological studies—part I. Urol Res 5, 61–69, 1977.)

the surface of the bladder mucosa. This adherence allows the bacteria to resist the bladder's defensive cleansing flow of urine and causes tissue inflammation and cell damage. Adherence may also play a role in bacteria ascending the urinary tract. Virulence refers to the toxicity of substances released by bacteria. The greater the virulence, the greater the damage to the urinary tract. Both these factors enhance colonization of the urinary tract and aid in the persistence and impact of the bacteria.

The incidence of UTI in newborns is 1 to 1.4%, with a greater frequency in males, especially if uncircumcised, and in premature and low birth weight infants. After the first year of life it is more common to find a UTI in females

(8.8%) than in males (2.5%) (Hellerstein, 1995; Todd, 1995). The incidence in infants and children is 4.1 to 7.5%. Symptomatic UTI is found in 3 to 7.8% of females and 1.1% of males (Rushton, 1997; Hoberman & Wald, 1997). By 11 years of age, 3% of girls and 1% of boys will have had a UTI (Finberg, 1998). The incidence of UTI is often increased in adolescents girls as they become sexually active. Recurrence is common, often within the first year after the initial infection.

Clinical Findings

HISTORY
- See Table 35–3 for age-related symptoms.
- The following information should be elicited:
  - Previous infection? How diagnosed? Workup done? Results?
  - Hygiene habits
  - Voiding and bowel patterns: frequency, completeness, dribbling, daytime enuresis, and weak stream
  - Irritants such as bubble bath, nylon underwear, or clothing (spandex, tight pants or shorts that rub)
  - Masturbation, sexual activity, or sexual abuse
  - Family history of VUR or recurrent UTI
  - Other infection: pinworms, diaper rash

PHYSICAL EXAMINATION
- BP, temperature, and general appearance (toxic appearing?)

T A B L E 35-3

Clinical Findings of Urinary Tract Infection in Children of Various Ages

NEONATES	INFANTS	TODDLERS AND PRESCHOOLERS	SCHOOL AGE AND ADOLESCENTS
Jaundice	Malaise	Altered voiding pattern	"Classic dysuria" with frequency, urgency, and discomfort
Hypothermia	Irritability	Malodor	
Failure to thrive	Difficulty feeding	Abdominal/flank pain*	
Sepsis	Poor weight gain	Enuresis	Malodor
Vomiting or diarrhea	Fever*	Vomiting or diarrhea*	Enuresis
Cyanosis	Vomiting or diarrhea	Malaise	Abdominal/flank pain*
Abdominal distention	Malodor	Fever*	Fever/chills*
Lethargy	Dribbling	Diaper rash	Vomiting or diarrhea*
	Abdominal pain/colic		Malaise

*Findings especially likely with pyelonephritis.

- Growth parameters—growth may be decreased with chronic UTI or renal insufficiency
- Flank pain or tenderness in the costovertebral angle
- Abdominal examination—suprapubic tenderness, bladder distention or a flank mass (obstructive signs), mass from fecal impaction
- Genitalia—vaginal erythema, edema, irritation, or discharge; labial adhesions; uncircumcised male, urethral ballooning; weak, dribbling, thread-like stream
- Neurological examination (if voiding is dysfunction)—perineal sensation, lower extremity reflexes, sacral dimpling, or cutaneous abnormality

LABORATORY STUDIES. The method used to collect urine has an impact on the interpretation of results. Urine collected in a bag, because of the high degree of contaminants, is accurate only if negative. Voided midstream clean-catch specimens are somewhat more accurate, especially if collected as a first morning specimen and kept refrigerated until analysis. Suprapubic tap or sterile catheterization obtains the most accurate specimen. Refer to the Diagnostic Studies section in the first part of this chapter to review other pertinent information.

- UA has limited value in diagnosing UTI because it can be negative even with a positive culture. It should be used only to raise or lower suspicion. Suspicious findings include foul odor, cloudiness, alkaline pH, proteinuria, hematuria, pyuria, and bacteriuria.
- Nitrite chemical tests are reliable on overnight urine specimens when gram-negative bacteria are present and when the urine has been in the bladder for 4 or more hours. False-positive results are rare, whereas false-negative results are common.
- Leukocyte esterase chemical tests detect pyuria, but pyuria may arise from causes other than UTI.
- Microscopic evaluation of uncentrifuged urine is helpful if bacteria are seen.
- Gram stain is helpful if bacteria are identified.
- Urine culture by standard culture methods

or by dipslide is essential to confirm the diagnosis. See Table 35–4 for evaluation of culture results. If culture growth is 10,000, repeat the culture unless the sample was collected by suprapubic aspiration or catheterization.
- Bacterial identification and determination of sensitivities are necessary in patients who appear toxic or could have pyelonephritis, have relapses or recurrent UTI, or are nonresponsive to medication.
- Blood culture should be done if sepsis is suspected or in infants younger than 1 year.
- CBC (elevated WBC count), ESR, C-reactive protein, BUN, and creatinine should be done if pyelonephritis is suspected.
- A limulus lysate assay done on a urine sample can detect endotoxin from gram-negative organisms, which helps identify pyelonephritis (Heldrich, 1995).
- An enhanced UA done with a Neubauer hemocytometer has a positive predictive value of 93% vs. 81% by standard UA (Hoberman & Wald, 1997). See the Resource Box for further information.

Differential Diagnosis

The differential diagnosis includes a foreign body, urethritis, vaginitis, viral cystitis, reflux, sexual abuse, dysfunctional voiding, dysuria-pyuria syndrome, abdominal pain or diarrhea from appendicitis, pelvic abscess, and pelvic inflammatory disease. Any child with fever without focus, with FTT, or with recurrent abdominal pain should be evaluated for UTI.

Management

A. Goals of treatment are to quickly identify the extent and level of infection, to treat appropriately to eradicate infection and provide symptomatic relief, to find and correct anatomical or functional abnormalities, and to prevent recurrence and new or progressive renal damage. When deciding on a treatment plan, the child's age, sex, and symptoms and the suspected location of the UTI must be kept in mind.

B. Bacteriuria. Whether asymptomatic bacteri-

T A B L E 35-4

Criteria for Diagnosis of Urinary Tract Infections

METHOD OF COLLECTION	COLONY COUNT (PURE CULTURE)	PROBABILITY OF INFECTION (%)
Suprapubic aspiration	Any organism	>99
Catheterization	>10^5	95
	10^4–10^5	Infection likely, especially if obstruction or if frequent voider
	10^3–10^4, single organism	Suspicious, repeat
	<10^3	Infection unlikely
Clean voided		
Boy	>10^4, single organism	Infection likely
Girl	Three specimens >10^5	95
	Two specimens >10^5	90–95%
	One specimen >10^5	80–90%
	5×10^4–10^5	Suspicious, repeat
	10^4–5×10^4	Symptomatic; suspicious, repeat
	10^4–5×10^4	Asymptomatic; infection unlikely
	<10^4	Infection unlikely

Modified from Feld LG, Greenfield SP, Ogra PL: Urinary tract infections in infants and children, Pediatr Rev 11:72, 1989; updated from Rushton HG: UTI in children: Epidemiology, evaluation & management, Pediatr Clin North Am 44:1139–1169, 1997; Hoberman A, Wald ER: UTI in young children: New light on old questions, Contemp Pediatr 14(11):140–156, 1997; Heldrich FJ: UTI diagnosis: Getting it right the first time. Contemp Pediatr 12(2):110–133, 1995; Opas LM: UTI: Burning issues (unpublished manuscript), Los Angeles, CA, 1998.

uria should be treated is controversial. Those who advocate treatment do so with the intent of preventing further infection or sequelae and identifying any underlying abnormalities.

C. Cystitis (Fig. 35-10):

1. Antibiotic treatment for 10 days. Single-dose or 3-day treatment for adolescent girls with uncomplicated UTI is occasionally considered. First-line drugs are as follows:
   - Trimethoprim-sulfamethoxazole (6 to 12 mg/kg trimethoprim plus 30 to 60 mg/kg per day sulfamethoxazole in two divided doses if older than 2 months); a 15% rate of resistance has been noted in some communities (Hoberman & Wald, 1997).
   - Amoxicillin (40 mg/kg per day in two or three divided doses) if no resistance is found in the community.

   Also recommended are the following:
   - Sulfisoxazole (120 to 150 mg/kg per day in three or four divided doses if older than 2 months).
   - Nitrofurantoin (4 to 8 mg/kg per day four times a day if older than 1 month).
   - If allergic to the drugs just mentioned or a broader spectrum is needed:
     - Cefixime (8 mg/kg per day in one dose).
     - Cephalexin (50 mg/kg per day in three or four divided doses).
     - Cefpodoxime (10 mg/kg per day in two divided doses).

2. Follow-up urine culture should be done 48 to 72 hours after initiating treatment, especially if symptoms persist or organism resistance is found in the community.
   - If the culture is sterile, continue antibiotic therapy.
   - If the culture is not sterile or if no clinical improvement is seen, urine should be sent for bacterial identification and sensitivity studies, and an alternative broad-spectrum antibiotic

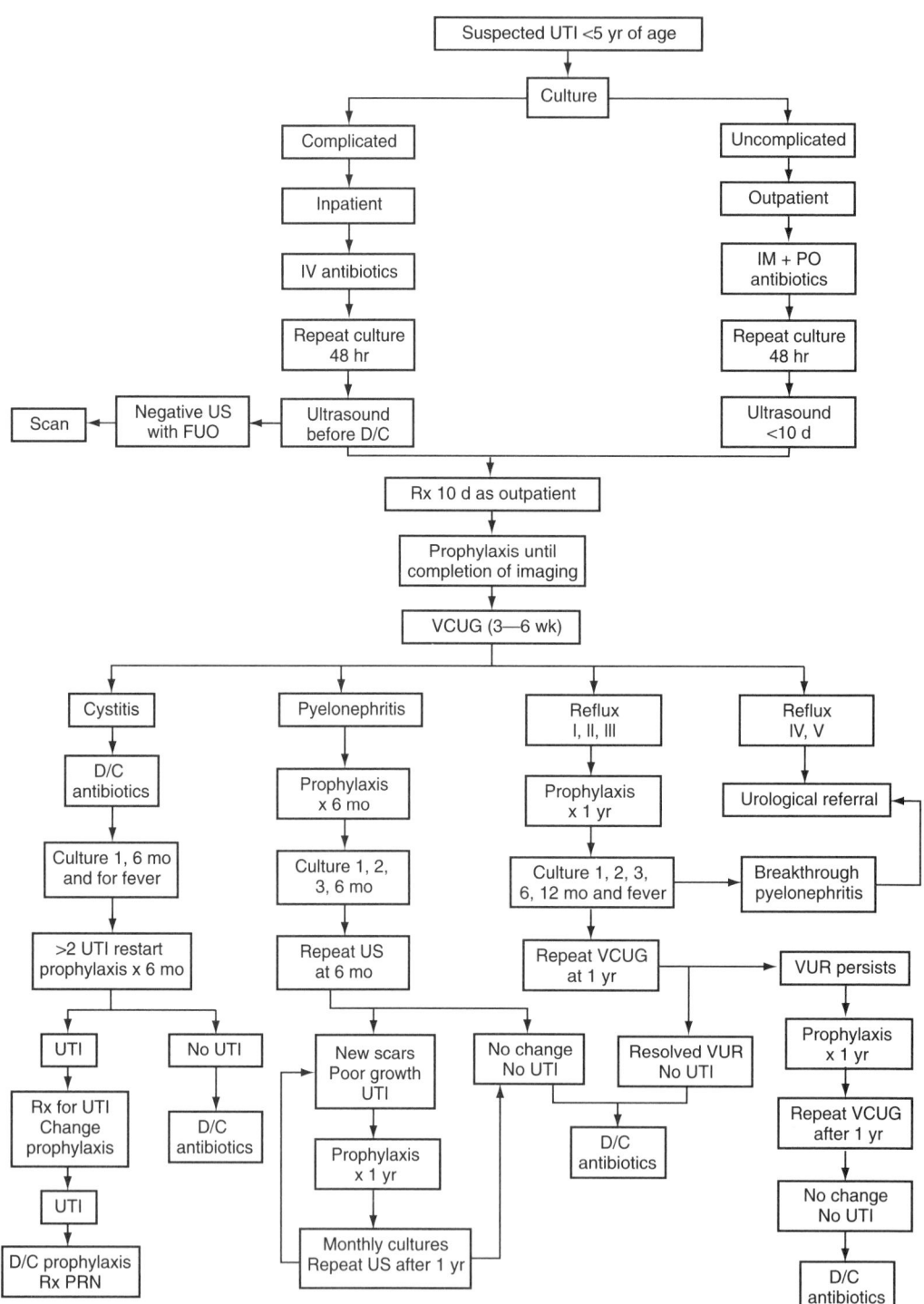

F I G U R E 35-10

Evaluation of urinary tract infection (UTI). Reproduced with permission from Opas LM: Urinary Tract Infections—Burning Issues 1998. D/C = discharge; FUO = fever of unknown origin; IM = intramuscular; IV = intravenous; PO = oral; Rx = prescribe; US = ultrasonogram; VCUG = voiding cystourethrogram; VUR = vesiculoureteral reflux.

should be used pending those results. Culture should be repeated after 48 to 72 hours and, if sterile, antibiotic therapy continued.

3. Follow-up cultures should be obtained 3 to 4 days after finishing antibiotic treatment.

4. Repeat urine culture should be done with any fever, illness, dysuria, or frequency. Because recurrent UTI is so common, monitoring urine culture at 1 and 6 months is often recommended.

5. If child is younger than 5 years, once a sterile urine is obtained, low-dose prophylaxis should be continued until radiological workup is completed (see section E).

6. If adolescent, a 3- to 5-day course of antibiotics is adequate (Montgomery et al., 1998).
   - Phenazopyridine (Pyridium), 100 to 200 mg twice daily for dysuria may be given.

D. Febrile UTI. Because fever is often an indicator of pyelonephritis, treatment must be initiated promptly to prevent or minimize sequelae (see Fig. 35-10).

1. Uncomplicated (not seeming to be ill, tolerating oral fluids and medicine, mildly dehydrated, with good compliance):
   - Third-generation cephalosporin administered intramuscularly for the first 24 hours or until afebrile with a normal ESR and sterile culture.
     - Ceftriaxone, 75 mg/kg per dose, is often used
     - Cefotaxime, 150 mg/kg in three to four divided doses
     - Ceftazidime, 150 mg/kg in three or four divided doses
     - Gentamicin, 7.5 mg/kg per day in three divided doses if unable to tolerate the above drugs
     - Cefixime at 16 mg/kg the first 24 hours, followed by 8 mg/kg for 13 days, is in clinical trials
   - Oral antibiotics (see the section on cystitis) to follow intramuscular therapy for a total of 10 to 14 days, followed by prophylaxis until the radiological workup is complete; if pyelonephritis

is the final diagnosis, continue prophylactic antibiotics for 6 months.
- Repeat urine culture after 48 hours of antibiotic therapy and 1, 2, 3, and 6 months after infection.
- Ultrasonography may be performed within 10 days, VCUG within 3 to 6 weeks. If pyelonephritis is the final diagnosis, repeat the ultrasound 6 months after the infection.

2. Complicated (high fever, toxic, persistent vomiting, moderate to severe dehydration, poor compliance, younger than 3 to 6 months):
   - Inpatient treatment consisting of intravenous antibiotics until afebrile for 24 to 36 hours with a normal ESR and sterile culture.
   - The remainder of treatment is as presented earlier.

E. Radiological workup:

1. Table 35-5 lists criteria for the radiological workup of children with UTI; Table 35-6 details radiological studies that can be done.

2. In a child is older than 5 years with an uncomplicated UTI and no voiding dysfunction before the UTI, no further workup is needed at this time.

3. Renal and bladder ultrasonography should be done during hospitalization or within 10 days in any child younger than 5 years, any child with a complicated UTI, or any child with a history of dysfunctional voiding.
   - If the ultrasonogram is normal,
     - In a child older than 5 years but with complicated UTI or in a child with previous dysfunctional voiding, start prophylaxis and perform VCUG.
     - In a child younger than 5 years, start prophylaxis and perform VCUG.
     - In a child younger than 5 years with complicated UTI, start prophylaxis and perform VCUG and a nuclear scan.
   - If the ultrasonogram is abnormal, start prophylaxis and perform VCUG. Depending on the abnormality, the child may need referral to a urologist.

4. VCUG should be done after the infection

T A B L E 35-5

Radiological Workup and Prophylaxis for Urinary Tract Infections

WHY DO A WORKUP?
1. To identify any structural or functional abnormality of the urinary tract
2. To identify any renal scarring or damage

WHO REQUIRES A WORKUP?
Recommendations vary among experts. Those who recommend the most aggressive workup (all children after any infection) do so to identify scarring early and prevent further damage
1. Infants or any child <5 yr old (Opas, 1998)
2. Any child <8 y with *acute* symptoms, especially fever or toxicity (at least 50% have reflux or obstructive lesions)
3. Any child with pyelonephritis
4. Males with a first infection; females after a second infection if no other criteria are met
5. Any child with suspicious factors (e.g., high blood pressure, abnormal urine stream, poor growth) or with a positive family history of UTI or abnormal voiding patterns
6. Adolescents with pyelonephritis or after a second UTI with documented culture and no history of recent sexual activity

WHAT SHOULD BE DONE?
1. Renal and bladder ultrasonography: done initially in all children.
2. Voiding cystourethrogram: done if ultrasound is abnormal, if child is <5 y old, or if voiding dysfunction was present before UTI
3. Nuclear imaging scan: done to detect renal scars or parenchymal inflammation
4. Intravenous pyelogram: done if further definition of structure or function of the kidney is needed

WHEN SHOULD IT BE DONE?
1. Ultrasonography: during hospitalization or within 10 d in any child <5 y old or with complicated UTI
2. VCUG: after urine has become sterile and the patient is asymptomatic. Some authorities recommend 4–6 wk after the diagnosis of UTI
3. As follow-up for pyelonephritis and vesicoureteral reflux

WHEN SHOULD PROPHYLAXIS BE USED?
1. After resolution of UTI and before radiological workup
2. To suppress recurrent UTI after radiological workup

WHAT SHOULD BE USED FOR PROPHYLAXIS?
Approximately 1/3 to 1/2 the treatment dosage of antibiotic should be given at bedtime (Sheldon & Wacksman, 1995)
1. Nitrofurantoin (1 to 2 mg/kg qd or bid if >2 mo of age); expensive
2. TMP (2 mg/kg) + SMX (10 mg/kg) qd if >2 mo of age; TMP (1 mg/kg) + SMX (5 mg/kg) bid (can be used if bedwetting is a problem). A yearly CBC should be done to monitor for neutropenia
3. Sulfisoxazole (50 mg/kg bid if >2 mo of age)
4. Penicillin or ampicillin can be used for a newborn or premature infant

---

bid = twice daily; CBC = complete blood count; qd = every day; SMX = sulfamethoxazole; TMP = trimethoprim; UTI = urinary tract infection; VCUG = voiding cystourethrography.

is treated, once the patient is asymptomatic with sterile urine culture. Waiting until 4 to 6 weeks after infection is often recommended to allow any inflammatory changes to subside (Baskin, 1998; Ortigas & Cunningham, 1997).

- Prophylaxis should be continued until the workup is complete.
5. Nuclear scans (dimercaptosuccinic acid [DMSA] or technetium-labeled diethylenetriamine pentaacetic acid [Tc-DTPA]) can be performed to diagnose acute py-

elonephritis and to evaluate for scarring. These tests are especially helpful in neonates and in children with fever of unknown origin. However, they are the most expensive test available (>$1000 in 1999) and should be ordered only as indicated.
   • Any evidence of acquired kidney damage requires suppression.
F. Recurrent infection (two or more in 1 year):
   1. Initial treatment as for cystitis.
   2. Radiological workup if not previously done.
   3. Once urine is sterile, prophylactic antibiotics and monitoring of urine cultures for 6 to 12 months. See Figure 35–10 and Table 35–5.

Complications

Recurrent infection, chronic UTI, FTT, and irreversible renal scarring (the most significant complication) can occur. Major risk factors for renal damage are delay in treatment of pyelonephritis, age younger than 1 year, anatomical or neurogenic obstruction, severe reflux, and dysplasia. The same acute inflammatory process responsible for eradication of bacteria is also responsible for damage to renal tissue and subsequent scarring.

Patient Education and Prevention

1. Clear explanation of the etiology, potential complications, and overall treatment plan, including both short- and long-term plans.
2. Frequent and complete voiding and increased quantities of fluids, especially water. Sometimes, scheduled voiding times or double voiding can be helpful. An antispasmodic may be used if bladder spasms are present.
3. Proper hygiene and avoidance of irritants such as bubble baths and perfumed soaps. Treat perineal inflammation to help avoid UTI.
4. Sexually active females should be encouraged to drink water before intercourse and void immediately afterward.
5. Home monitoring of urine with nitrite sticks on first morning urine is helpful. If positive

or questionable or the child is symptomatic, a culture must follow.
6. Decrease intake of bladder irritants such as the 4 c's (caffeine, carbonated beverages, chocolate, citrus) and aspartame (Nutra-sweet), alcohol, and spicy foods.
7. Avoid constipation. Stool softeners and timed defecation may be helpful.
8. Three-day rule. To avoid delay in treatment, no infant or young child with unexplained fever should go longer than 3 days without examination of urine.

Vesicoureteral Reflux

Description

Regurgitation of urine from the bladder up the ureter to the kidney is called VUR. Primary VUR is the most common type and is typified by a congenital, abnormally short ureter and ineffective valve. Secondary VUR is due to bladder outlet obstruction and can be functional or structural. It is graded according to an international classification (Fig. 35–11). Grades I, II, and III (low grade) describe reflux to the renal pelvis with little or no distention. Grades IV and V (high grade) include definite distention of the ureters and renal pelvis and can include hydronephrosis or reflux into the intrarenal collecting system.

Etiology and Incidence

Reflux occurs because of congenital abnormalities and can persist with recurrent infection. VUR is the most common anatomical abnormality found in children with documented UTI, with an incidence of 20 to 50% (Rushton, 1997; Heldrich, 1995; Sheldon & Wacksman, 1995). The incidence in the general population is 1% (Sheldon & Wacksman, 1995). Reflux provides a route for bacteria to ascend to the kidney and cause pyelonephritis. A high occurrence (up to 45%; Shalaby-Rana et al., 1997) in siblings, a slightly higher incidence in white children, and an 85% rate of occurrence in females (Sheldon & Wacksman, 1995) have been noted.

T A B L E 35-6
Radiological Studies Done for the Evaluation of Urinary Tract Infection

STUDY	COST	ADVANTAGES	DISADVANTAGES	USE
USN	Least expensive	Shows structure, shape, and growth Detects structural abnormality, obstruction, pyelonephritis, large scars Pain, low risk, no radiation, noninvasive, available	Does not detect small scars or VUR Poor visualization of ureters Does not measure renal function or transient injury to kidney	Initial evaluation and follow-up
VCUG, radiographic	Least expensive	Detects and grades VUR—if high or low pressure, high or low bladder volumes, during voiding, during early or late bladder filling Visualize bladder and urethra (esp. in males) and diverticula	Does not detect obstruction, pyelonephritis, scars Risk of urethral trauma from catheterization Greater radiation than with scan	Initial evaluation In infants and children younger than 5 yr with abnormal USN or dysfunctional voiding
VCUG, nuclear	More expensive	Visualize bladder and reflux Constantly monitors for transient reflux Less radiation	Discomfort of catheterization No urethral visualization Unable to grade reflux	Follow-up of VUR To evaluate siblings of child with VUR Follow-up of surgery
IVP	Less expensive	Detects obstruction, pyelonephritis, large scars, stones, nephrocalcinosis Details pelvicaliceal system, shows ureters Estimates renal function Readily available	Does not detect small scars or VUR Risk of allergic reaction, acute renal failure, pain of injection, radiation Requires good renal function Only identifies structural damage	Better define level of obstruction Not used very often

Test	Cost	Advantages	Disadvantages	Indications
Nuclear scans DMSA Tc-DTPA	Most expensive	Detects acute inflammation, scars, and obstruction Earlier detection of parenchymal damage—large or small scars, permanent or focal—than with IVP (1–3 y) Good in neonates Shows renal outline, estimates renal and tubular function, measures changes Less radiation	Does not detect VUR or measure renal function Does not evaluate calyces, ureters, bladder, or urethra	Follow-up Fever of unknown origin and negative USN in neonates To diagnose APN To detect renal scars
CT scan (contrast)	Expensive	Detects obstruction, pyelonephritis, large scars	Does not detect small scars or VUR Risk of allergic reaction, acute renal failure	Trauma

APN = acute pyelonephritis; CT = computed tomography; DMSA = dimercaptosuccinic acid; IVP = intravenous pyelography; Tc-DTPA = technetium-labeled diethylenetriamine pentaacetic acid; USN = ultrasound; VCUG = voiding cystourethrography; VUR = vesicoureteral reflux.

Data from Feld LG, Greenfield SP, Ogra PL: Urinary tract infections in infants and children. Pediatr Rev 11:71–77, 1989; Rushton HG: UTI in children: Epidemiology, evaluation & management. Pediatr Clin North Am 44:1133–1169, 1997; Hoberman A, Wald ER: UTI in young children: New light on old questions. Contemp Pediatr 14(11):140–156, 1997; Heldrich FJ: UTI diagnosis: Getting it right the first time. Contemp Pediatr 12(2):110–133, 1995; Opas LM: UTI: Burning issues (Unpublished manuscript). Los Angeles, CA, 1999.

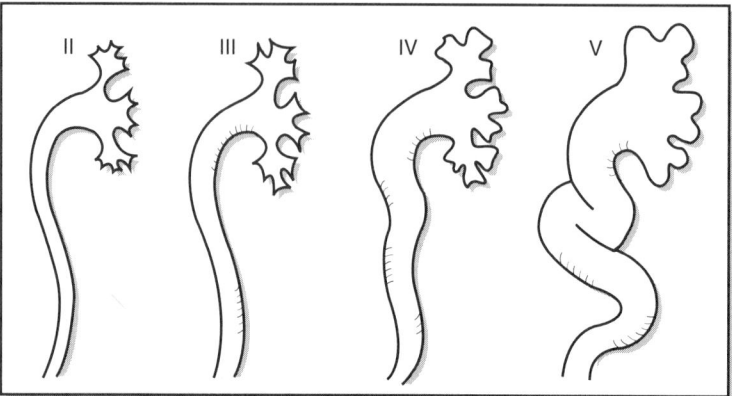

F I G U R E 35-11
International reflux grading. Grade I: ureter only. Grade II: ureter, pelvis, and calyces; no dilatation, normal calyceal fornices. Grade III: mild or moderate dilatation and/or tortuosity of ureter, and mild or moderate dilatation of renal pelvis but no or slight blunting of the fornices. Grade IV: moderate dilatation and/or tortuosity of ureter and moderate dilatation of renal pelvis and calyces. Complete obliteration of sharp angles of fornices but maintenance of papillary impressions in majority of calyces. Grade V: gross dilatation and tortuosity of ureter; gross dilatation of renal pelvis and calyces; papillary impressions are no longer visible in majority of calyces. (From International reflux grading. From the International Reflux Study in Children. International system of radiographic grading of vesicoureteral reflux. Pediatr Radiol 15:105, 1985.)

Clinical Findings

HISTORY. The history assesses for a previous UTI, voiding pattern or dysfunction, and asymptomatic or UTI symptoms.

LABORATORY STUDIES. The following, if not already done, are ordered as indicated to identify obstructive uropathy and dysplasia.

- Ultrasonography
- VCUG—establishes the presence of reflux, determines the grade, and gives high detail
- Nuclear scan—uses less radiation to identify VUR but gives less detail (no grading) and requires someone skilled in interpretation; most helpful in long-term follow-up and with neonates
- IVP—may be done if the VCUG is positive because it gives more defined structural and functional information
- Ultrasonography and IVP possibly normal even in the presence of reflux

Management

Management involves the following:

The goal of treatment is the prevention of infection and subsequent scarring. Early identi-fication and appropriate treatment of infection achieve this goal.

1. **Grades I, II, and III reflux.** Most children outgrow their reflux and should be left to do so. Grades I and II VUR resolve spontaneously in up to 85% of children (Opas, 1998; Sheldon & Wacksman, 1995). Primary VUR resolves spontaneously in 85%; secondary VUR resolves with correction of the underlying problem.

   a. Prophylactic antibiotics to prevent UTI (see Table 35-5) should be continued until the child has been infection-free over a 6- to 12-month period as documented by urine culture and no reflux as documented by two negative VCUGs done 1 year apart. If antibiotics are not taken or the child has recurrent infection, surgery may be needed.

   b. Interval urine cultures are performed as indicated and with symptoms or unexplained illness (see Fig. 35-10).

   c. Radiological studies—ultrasonography, VCUG, and/or renal scan—every 6 to 12 months to monitor reflux, renal growth, and scarring.

   d. CBC, BUN, and creatinine annually to monitor renal function.

2. Grades IV and V reflux are managed medically or surgically by a pediatric urologist.
3. Adolescents may need surgery because reflux in this age group is rarely outgrown.
4. Surgery is indicated for progressive renal injury and breakthrough infection (especially acute pyelonephritis) or with associated anatomical abnormalities.
5. Nephrology consultation is indicated in the presence of notable scarring, a solitary or atrophic kidney, hypertension, elevated creatinine, or evidence of abnormal kidney function.

Complications

Pre-existing renal damage may be present, and new renal scarring can occur. These complications can lead to ongoing renal disease, atrophy, growth failure, elevated BP, and decreased renal functioning.

Patient Education and Prevention

1. VUR does not cause scarring, infection does—but VUR is a risk factor for pyelonephritis and subsequent scarring.
2. Screening ultrasonography should be done on an infant born to parents with VUR or on any young siblings of a child with VUR and on any older siblings with any history of UTI.
3. Management, prevention of UTIs, and compliance must be understood by families. The necessity of routine urine culture should also be emphasized. The potential for untreated, chronic UTI leading to chronic renal disease must be explained. Other points to emphasize include the following:
   • Prompt treatment of UTI should be instituted.
   • Prophylactic medicines are best given at night because of urinary stasis while asleep.
   • BP and growth should be monitored.
   • Measures as discussed in the Patient Education and Prevention section of UTIs should be followed.

▓ COMMON GENITOURINARY CONDITIONS IN MALES

Hypospadias

Description

Hypospadias is a common congenital abnormality in which the urethral opening is on the ventral surface (underside) of the penis. Chordee, a ventral bowing of the penis, occurs when a tight band of fibrous tissue pulls on the penis. Torsion refers to rotation of the penis to the right or left.

Etiology and Incidence

The etiology of hypospadias is unclear. It is believed that the endocrine system probably has an important role, but what that role is remains unclear. A relatively new hypothesis is that hypospadias is actually a deformity, not a malformation (Zaontz & Packer, 1997). The primitive gonad in the eighth week of embryonic development differentiates into male or female. As the genital tubercle enlarges, developmental arrest occurs along the line of urethral fusion and causes hypospadias.

Hypospadias occurs in 8.2 per 1000 live births (Zaontz & Packer, 1997), or in 1 in 300 infant boys (Langer & Coplen, 1998). If minor degrees are also included, the rate increases to 1 in 125. Risk is increased if family members have hypospadias: 8% if the father, 14% if a sibling, and 21% if two family members. Hypospadias occurs more commonly in whites than in African-Americans, in Italians and Jews, and in winter conceptions (Duckett, 1989). Nine percent of boys with hypospadias also have undescended testicles, inguinal hernia, or hydrocele.

Clinical Findings

HISTORY
• A family history of a male relative with genitourinary problems is reported.
• The child sits to void or holds his penis to direct the stream.

PHYSICAL EXAMINATION. In a newborn, the classic finding is a dorsally hooded foreskin. It is essential to visualize the urethral meatus. Pulling the ventral shaft skin in a downward and outward direction facilitates visualization. Anatomical classification is made by location:

- Anterior (70%), glanular, coronal, or anterior penile
- Middle (10%)
- Posterior (20%), scrotal, penoscrotal, or posterior penile

Other findings include

- Urinary stream that aims downward rather than straight
- Inguinal hernia or undescended testicles (9%; Langer & Coplen, 1998)
- Chordee

Differential Diagnosis

The differential diagnosis includes intersex abnormalities.

Management

Circumcision must *not* be done because the foreskin is used in the surgical repair. Referral should be made to a urologist at birth for evaluation. Surgery to correct hypospadias is best done around 6 to 12 months of age. Repair is usually accomplished in a one-stage outpatient procedure unless it is a complex defect.

Complications

Peer taunting of boys with unrepaired hypospadias and problems with erections if chordee is not repaired are possible complications. Intersex abnormalities are possible if associated with cryptorchidism (Gill & Kogan, 1997). Fistulas and urethral or meatal stenosis are potential complications of surgery.

Patient Education

Hypospadias is usually an isolated anomaly that does not require further workup. Education and reassurance regarding cause, repair, and outcome should be provided.

Undescended Testes—Cryptorchidism

Description

Cryptorchidism describes a testis that does not reside in nor can be manipulated into the scrotum (Gill & Kogan, 1997). A retractile testis is out of the scrotum but can be brought into the scrotum and remains there. A gliding testis can be brought into the scrotum but returns to a high position in the scrotum once released (Pillai & Besner, 1998). An ectopic testis lies outside the normal path of descent. An ascended testis is one that has fully descended but has spontaneously reascended and lies outside the scrotum. A trapped testis is one dislocated after herniorrhaphy. Any testis that is not in the scrotum is subject to progressive deterioration. Undescended testes are a common disorder that often causes great anxiety for parents.

Etiology and Incidence

Testes develop in the abdomen and descend in the seventh fetal month to the upper part of the groin, subsequently progressing through the inguinal canal into the scrotum. Failure of the testes to descend can be caused by mechanical lesions or can be secondary to hormonal, chromosomal, enzymatic, or anatomical disorders.

The incidence of cryptorchidism is 0.2 to 1.8% in young adults, 0.5 to 0.8% in 1-year-olds, 2.5 to 4% in term infants, 20 to 30% in premature infants, over 60% if infant birth weight is under 1500 g, and near 100% in 900-g neonates (Boschert, 1998; Gill & Kogan, 1997; Rabinowitz & Hulbert, 1994). A great majority of undescended testes resolve spontaneously by 6 months to 1 year of age. The frequency of bilateral occurrence is 10 to 25%, and unilateral involvement (55 to 66%) is more likely to be right-sided. Retractile testes are bilateral and most common in boys 5 to 6 years of age (Pillai & Besner, 1998).

Clinical Findings

HISTORY. The history can include the following:

- Family history of undescended testes or testicular malignancy

- Testes sometimes felt during the infant's bath
- Associated urinary problems
- Prematurity
- Risk factors (Gill & Kogan, 1997): first-born, cesarean section, toxemia, hypospadias, congenital subluxation of the hip, low birth weight, winter conception
- Other congenital, endocrine, chromosomal, or intersex disorders

PHYSICAL EXAMINATION. Having the child sit cross-legged or frog-legged, squat, or stand can facilitate testicle descent and palpation. Findings include:

- Scrotal rugae less full
- Bilateral or unilateral absence of a testicle
- Retractile testes, which move between the scrotum and external ring but can be manipulated to the lower part of the scrotum and remain there; especially common with stimulation or cold between the ages of 3 months and 7 years
- Gliding testes, which lie between the scrotum and external ring and can be manipulated to the lower part of the scrotum but return to the high position
- Location:
  - Prescrotal (at the external inguinal ring), 25%
  - Canalicular, high or low (between the external and internal rings), the most common type, 40%
  - Ectopic (superficial inguinal, femoral, or perineal), 25%
  - Intra-abdominal (above the internal inguinal ring), not palpable, occurring in less than 15% of males with undescended testes
  - Indirect inguinal hernia, 90% (Pillai & Besner, 1998)

LABORATORY STUDIES. None are indicated except in newborns with potential sex abnormalities, hypopituitarism, or congenital adrenal hyperplasia. The risk of intersex abnormality is 27% if hypospadias and unilateral or bilateral cryptorchidism are present.

Differential Diagnosis

Retractile testes, anorchism, and chromosomal abnormalities are the differential diagnoses.

Management

The goals of treating undescended testes are to improve fertility outcome, decrease malignancy potential, and minimize the psychological stress associated with an empty scrotum (Gill & Kogan, 1997). Management has come full circle from an initial recommendation for surgery, to treatment with hormonal therapy, and back to early surgical intervention. Both forms of treatment are still options.

1. If the testes are undescended by 6 months of age with the peak of postnatal testosterone, they are unlikely to descend spontaneously. The American Academy of Pediatrics Action Committee of the Urology Section (1996) issued a statement recommending orchiopexy by 1 year of age if performed by a skilled pediatric urologist or surgeon with an attendant skilled pediatric anesthesiologist. Surgical repair can be done by inguinal incision, laparoscopy, or the intra-abdominal route, depending on placement of the testes.
2. Hormonal therapy can be used to differentiate a retractile testis from a true cryptorchid one. Human chorionic gonadotropin (hCG) by the intramuscular route is the only approved method in the Unites States, although intranasal gonadotropin-releasing hormone (GnRH) is used overseas.
3. In a child younger than 1 year, regular examination to assess the position of the testes should be performed with every well-child care. If the testes remains undescended, referral to a pediatric urologist or surgeon should occur by 1 year of age.
4. If undescended testes are found after 1 year of age, the child should be immediately referred to a pediatric urologist or surgeon for treatment.

Complications

Reascent, poor development, infertility, malignancy, vulnerability to trauma, testicular torsion, and inguinal hernia are possible complications.

Patient Education

Families and patients should be informed of the following:

1. Histological changes have been shown in an undescended testis as early as 6 months of

age, with irreversible changes shown by 2 years of age contributing to infertility and playing a role in malignancy.

2. Infertility as a complication of cryptorchidism has been reported in as many as 32 to 40% of men with unilateral undescended testes and in 59 to 70% if bilateral (Boschert, 1998; Gill & Kogan, 1997).

3. Testicular malignancy in males with cryptorchidism is reported to have a 3 to 18% incidence rate, or 1 in 45,000 males—a 20- to 40-fold greater incidence than in the general population (Pillai & Besner, 1998; Gill & Kogan, 1997). Malignancy is more common with an intra-abdominal testis. A progressive increase in the incidence of testicular tumor as the age at orchiopexy increases has been observed. A testicular neoplasm in one child mandates examination of his male siblings.

4. No evidence has indicated that undescended testes resolve with puberty; retractile testes generally settle into the scrotum by puberty.

5. Open discussion of the problem, management, and potential complications is essential both initially and over time.

Hydrocele

Description

A common cause of painless, scrotal swelling is a hydrocele, a collection of serous fluid in the scrotal sac. A noncommunicating hydrocele has a collection of fluid only in the scrotum. If the processus vaginalis remains patent so that fluid moves from the abdomen to the scrotum, it is called a communicating hydrocele and is more likely to be associated with a hernia (Fig. 35–12).

Etiology

Incomplete closure of the processus vaginalis through which the testes descend into the scrotum allows a hydrocele to develop.

Clinical Findings

HISTORY. The history includes the following:

- Intermittent or constant bulge or lump in the scrotum, often more distally placed.

Scrotal size increases with activity and decreases with rest.

- No distress, no vomiting, and present for more than 8 hours.

PHYSICAL EXAMINATION. Findings include:

- Asymmetry or a scrotal mass present; if swelling is present in the inguinal area, a hernia is probable
- Testes descended
- Usually unilateral swelling
- Translucent on transillumination (pink or red glow)
- Noncommunicating hydrocele—scrotal sac tense, slightly blue tinged, fluctuant, and does not reduce; no swelling in the inguinal region
- Communicating hydrocele—fluid in the scrotal sac comes and goes (probably flat in the morning, swollen later in the day)

Differential Diagnosis

Hernia, undescended testicle, retractile testicle, and inguinal lymphadenopathy are the differential diagnoses.

Management

The following steps are taken:

1. Noncommunicating hydrocele—fluid is generally absorbed spontaneously; no treatment is indicated unless the hydrocele is so large that it is uncomfortable or persists longer than 1 year.

2. Communicating hydrocele—can resolve, but more likely to develop a true hernia requiring surgical repair. Refer if persistent after 1 year of age.

3. Surgery is usually done on an outpatient basis.

Patient Education

Reassurance is needed that the increased size of the scrotal sac will resolve, usually by 1 year of age, and involves no danger. Signs of hernia must be explained, and parents must be alerted to observe and report any abnormal findings.

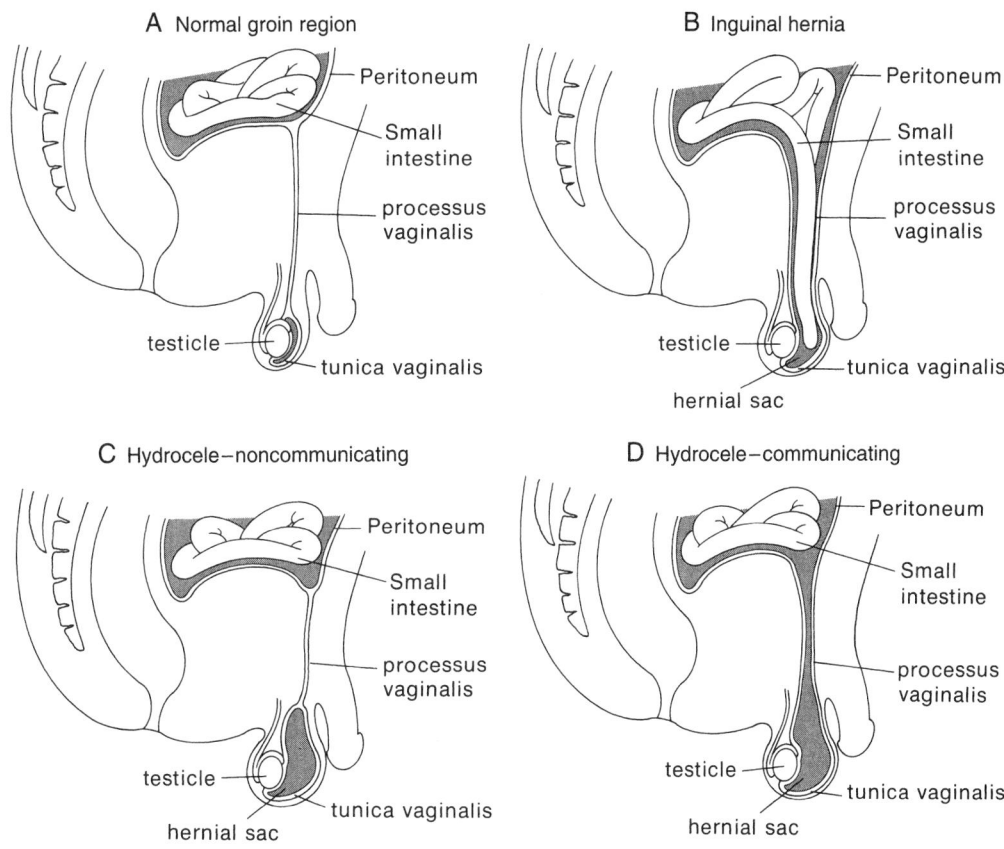

F I G U R E 35-12
Hydroceles and hernias. A, Groin region of the normal male infant. B, An inguinal hernia is the protrusion of bowel into the groin region. C, A hydrocele is a collection of fluid within the processus vaginalis. In a noncommunicating hydrocele, the scrotal swelling does not change in size or shape because there is no connection with the abdominal cavity. D, In a communicating hydrocele, the processus vaginalis remains open from the scrotum to the abdominal cavity, and scrotal swelling may vary in size during the course of an infant's day. (From Betz CL, Hunsberger M, & Wright S: Family-centered nursing care of infants, 2nd ed. Philadelphia: WB Saunders, 1994.)

Spermatocele

Description

A painless scrotal mass containing sperm is called a spermatocele.

Etiology and Incidence

A spermatocele is a benign cyst on the head of the epididymis or testicular adnexa. It is an uncommon finding but, when found, is usually in the neonatal period, late childhood, or early adolescence and peaks at 14 years (Skoog, 1997).

Clinical Findings

HISTORY
- Scrotal swelling but asymptomatic otherwise

PHYSICAL EXAMINATION
- Mobile cystic nodule usually less than 1 cm in size, superior and posterior to the testicle that transilluminates

- No change with the Valsalva maneuver

Differential Diagnosis

A varicocele or an epididymal cyst (identical in appearance, but not containing sperm) are the differential diagnoses.

Management

No treatment is required unless the cyst is large and painful. Refer to a urologist if needed.

Patient Education, Prevention, and Prognosis

Any pain or discomfort should be reported.

Varicocele

Description

A varicocele is a painless scrotal mass that feels like a "bag of worms"; it is usually found on the left side.

Etiology and Incidence

The etiology of varicoceles is probably multifactorial, with the physiologic changes associated with puberty playing some role. A varicocele is caused by valvular incompetence of the spermatic vein resulting in dilated or varicose veins. Varicoceles are rare before 10 years of age, may be indicative of malignancy, and occur in 10 to 15% of adolescent males (Skoog et al., 1997; Mandell, 1996). Up to 95% arise on left side, and 22% occur bilaterally (Pillai & Besner, 1998).

Clinical Findings

HISTORY
- Usually a painless swelling is noted in the left side of the scrotum, occasionally a "dull ache" or "heavy" feeling if large.
- Pain can occur with strenuous physical activity.
- Scrotal swelling with prolonged standing causes pain; swelling and pain resolve upon reclining.

PHYSICAL EXAMINATION
- In the standing position, a "bag of worms" can be felt posterior and superior to the testis that collapses upon lying and enlarges with the Valsalva maneuver.
- Measure and compare the size of both testes (length, width, and depth).
- Grade 1 varicoceles are larger than 2 cm and easily visualized; grade 2 varicoceles are 1 to 2 cm in diameter and are easily visualized; and grade 3 varicoceles are the most common, very small, and difficult to palpate (the Valsalva maneuver may help).

LABORATORY STUDIES
- Serial ultrasonography to measure testicular size every 6 to 12 months
- Ultrasonography to rule out malignancy in children younger than 10 years

Differential Diagnosis

Varicoceles must be differentiated from other testicular masses such as lipoma, hernia, hydrocele, spermatocele, and tumors.

Management

1. Ultrasonographic monitoring of testicular size can be done every 6 months if the varicocele is small and asymptomatic. Any change in comfort level should be reported.
2. Referral to a surgeon or urologist should be made if a varicocele is painful, if the difference in testicular volume is marked (greater than 2 mm by ultrasound), if the varicocele is right sided or bilateral, or if testicular growth becomes retarded over a 6- to 12-month period.
3. Treatment by spermatic vein embolization or ligation may be attempted in adolescents. Ligation is the usual procedure and has few complications; embolization is a 3-hour procedure with a high complication rate (Pillai & Besner, 1998).

Complications

Atrophy or testicular growth arrest as noted by a discrepancy in testicular size can occur. Lower fertility rates with decreased sperm concentration and motility have been noted.

Patient Education, Prevention, and Prognosis

A varicocele is the most common cause of infertility. Subsequent correction of testicular atrophy and an improved sperm count and fertility have been noted in 80 to 90% of those undergoing surgery early in adolescence. A persistent or recurrent varicocele occurs in 9 to 16% of adolescents after surgery (Skoog et al., 1997).

Inguinal Hernia

Description

A scrotal or inguinal swelling (or both) that includes abdominal contents is an inguinal hernia (see Fig. 35–12). In females, inguinal hernias cause swelling in the inguinal area and labia majora.

Etiology and Incidence

Incomplete closure of the processus vaginalis through which the testes descend into the scrotum allows the presence of abdominal contents in the inguinal canal (labia majora) or scrotum and thus the development of a hernia. Males who are obese or weight lifters or have a family history of undescended testes are at high risk for hernias (Moser, 1995).

Inguinal hernias occur in 1 to 5% of boys, with a progressive increase up to 50% seen in premature infants. Inguinal hernias are much more common in males (6:1), except during the first year of life. Over 50% of hernias are diagnosed during the first year of life, with the peak incidence in the first 3 months of life. Bilateral hernias are common (10 to 20%). Unilateral hernias are more likely to occur on the right side (50 to 60%) than the left (30%) (Gill, 1998; Ziegler, 1994). Indirect hernias are a congenital condition and are the most common type in children younger than 3 years. Direct hernias increase in incidence after 3 years and are usually acquired.

Clinical Findings

HISTORY
- A family history of undescended testes is reported.

- A swelling is noted in the inguinal area, scrotum, or both that comes and goes and increases with crying or straining.
- Weight lifting or obesity.
- Prematurity.

PHYSICAL EXAMINATION. Findings include the following:

- Swelling is found in the inguinal area, scrotal area (labia majora in females), or both.
- The hernia is reducible with pressure on the distal end.
- Transillumination does not occur unless the bowel is filled with fluid.
- Direct hernias push outward through the weakest point in the abdominal wall.
- Indirect hernias push downward at an angle into the inguinal canal.
- The child is fussy and has a distended abdomen if the hernia is incarcerated.
- Silk glove sign—a sensation of two surfaces rubbing against each other while one palpates the spermatic cord as it crosses the pubic tubercle.

LABORATORY STUDIES. An abdominal radiograph can be helpful if air is present below the inguinal ligament. Ultrasonography can differentiate a hernia from a hydrocele and is especially helpful if an incarcerated hernia is suspected.

Differential Diagnosis

Hydrocele, undescended testes (coexist in 15%), and inguinal lymphadenopathy are included in the differential diagnosis.

Management

Even if no swelling is seen at the visit but is elicited by the history, refer the patient to a surgeon or urologist for repair within 1 to 2 weeks. Inguinal hernias do not resolve spontaneously. Premature infants can be deferred until 42 weeks' gestation if the hernia is reducible. If the hernia is not easily reduced, if it is painful, or if a hard, tender or red mass is present, refer immediately. If reduction is difficult, observation for bowel ischemia after reduction can require hospitalization with surgical repair within 24 to 48 hours.

Complications

Incarceration and strangulation of a hernia cause pain, irritability, erythema, vomiting, and abdominal distention. Two thirds occur in patients younger than 1 year and are rare after 5 years of age (Kapur et al., 1998). Either of these conditions should be treated as a surgical emergency.

Patient Education

Because of the 40 to 60% contralateral occurrence of hernias in children, bilateral exploration is usually done at the time of surgery in infants younger than 1 year. If surgery is deferred, parents must be aware of the signs and symptoms of incarceration (tenderness, redness, crying, nausea, vomiting, abdominal distention) and be cautioned to seek immediate evaluation by a medical provider should they occur.

Testicular Masses

Description

A mass located on the testicle is most often a malignancy.

Etiology and Incidence

Testicular tumors are most common between 15 and 35 years of age but can be found anytime after 14 years.

Clinical Findings

HISTORY
- There may be no history because testicular masses cause little or no pain and are often small.

PHYSICAL EXAMINATION
- A hard, painless lump the size of a pea is palpated on the testis. Note the character and extension of the mass.
- The mass does not transilluminate.
- A hydrocele is present in 10% of malignancies.
- The abdomen and supraclavicular areas should be assessed for any palpable nodes.

LABORATORY STUDIES
- Levels of α-fetoprotein and the β-unit of hCG.
- Scrotal sonography to establish the exact location of the mass and differentiate a cystic from a solid mass
- CT scan to evaluate for metastasis

Differential Diagnosis

Intratesticular masses, which are almost always malignant, must be differentiated from extratesticular masses such as hernia, varicocele, hydrocele, or spermatocele.

Management

Any child or adolescent with a testicular mass must be referred immediately for further evaluation. Treatment is dependent on the stage and type of tumor and can include orchiectomy, irradiation, and chemotherapy.

Complications

Metastasis may have occurred before the initial tumor is noticed.

Patient Education, Prevention, and Prognosis

Early detection and therapeutic intervention can lead to a 90% survival rate. Ninety percent of relapses occur in the first 12 months after treatment (Moser, 1995). Testicular examination must not only be routinely done during physical examinations but must also be taught to adolescent males.

Phimosis and Paraphimosis

Description

Phimosis refers to a foreskin that is too tight to be retracted over the glans penis. Physiologic phimosis occurs between 3 and 5 years of age when the glans has not completely separated from the epithelium (Brown et al., 1997). Pathological phimosis occurs when the foreskin cannot be retracted after previously being retracted or after puberty (Brown et al., 1997). Paraphimosis is the opposite, a retracted foreskin that cannot be reduced to the normal position.

Etiology and Incidence

Phimosis can be congenital or acquired from infection and inflammation under the foreskin. Paraphimosis occurs if the foreskin does not return to its normal position after retraction. Constriction of the penis results in edema of the glans, pain, and possible necrosis.

Paraphimosis is most common in adolescents and can follow masturbation, sexual abuse, or forceful retraction.

Clinical Findings

HISTORY

- Infection or inflammation of the penis (phimosis)
- Retraction of the foreskin with an inability to reduce it (paraphimosis)
- Pain and dysuria

PHYSICAL EXAMINATION

- Phimosis—a tight, pinpoint opening of the foreskin with minimal ability to retract the foreskin; foreskin flat and effaced
- Pathological phimosis—thickened rolled foreskin
- Paraphimosis—edema and bluish discoloration of the glans and foreskin

Management

Management includes the following:

1. Phimosis
   - Normal cleansing with gentle stretching of the foreskin until resistance. Most foreskins are retractable by 5 years of age. Never forcefully retract the foreskin.
   - Circumcision is indicated if urinary obstruction or infection is present (Langer & Coplen, 1998).
   - Topical application of nonsteroidal anti-inflammatory ointment is advocated by some (Atilla et al., 1997).
2. Paraphimosis
   - A trial of ice may be done to reduce the swelling and allow reduction of the foreskin. Reduction may be accomplished by

using the index and third fingers to hold the penis with gauze proximal to the foreskin and by pushing the glans penis back with the thumbs (Brown et al., 1997).
- If this technique is not successful, surgical release of the constricting band must be done to prevent necrosis of the glans.
- Severe paraphimosis is a surgical emergency.
- Investigation of events leading to the paraphimosis is needed to rule out sexual abuse.

Complications

Infection, urinary obstruction, and reflux can occur with phimosis. Necrosis of the penis is possible with paraphimosis.

Patient Education

A tight foreskin in uncircumcised males is normal and usually resolves by 5 years of age. It is not an indication for circumcision. The foreskin of infants and children should never be forced back.

Balanitis and Balanoposthitis

Description

Balanitis is an inflammation of the glans; balanoposthitis is an inflammation of the foreskin and glans penis occurring in males with phimosis or in uncircumcised males.

Etiology

Accumulation of debris under the foreskin, probably resulting from poor hygiene, irritates the foreskin and glans and leads to infection. Skin flora are the usual causes of infection, but gram-negative bacteria can be involved. Occasionally, trauma or allergy can be the cause (Langer & Coplen, 1998).

Clinical Findings

HISTORY. A fussy infant and pain and dysuria in an older child are reported.

PHYSICAL EXAMINATION. Edema and inflammation are found.

Management

Antibiotics and warm soaks in the bathtub are prescribed.

Complications

Paraphimosis can occur.

Patient Education

A review of proper hygiene and the removal of irritants is needed. Occurrence is not an indication for circumcision.

Scrotal Trauma

Description

Trauma to the scrotum most often occurs as a result of sports participation or play.

Etiology and Incidence

Direct blows to the scrotum or a straddle injury are the most common causes of trauma. In a prepubertal child, the testicle is often spared damage because of the small size and mobility of the testes. Damage can occur when the testicle is forcibly compressed against the pubic bones. Significant injury (swelling, discoloration, and tenderness) from minor trauma suggests an underlying tumor.

Clinical Findings

HISTORY
- Pain after some type of injury
- Swelling, discoloration

PHYSICAL EXAMINATION
- Swelling, discoloration, and tenderness of the scrotum
- Transillumination if a hematoma is present

LABORATORY STUDIES
- A radionuclide scan may be useful to differentiate the degree and type of injury.

Differential Diagnosis

Urethritis, epididymitis, orchitis, and prostatitis should all be included in the differential diagnosis. Degrees of injury include

- Traumatic epididymitis—inflammation, but no infection. Pain and tenderness with scrotal erythema and edema and a tender indurated epididymis develop within a few days after injury. UA and Doppler ultrasonographic findings are normal. The course is usually acute, but short lived.
- Intratesticular hematoma.
- Hematocele with contusion and ecchymosis of the scrotal wall with severe scrotal injury.
- Testicular torsion.

Management

1. NSAIDs, cool compresses, scrotal support or elevation, and bed rest are modalities used to help relieve pain.
2. An enlarging scrotum merits immediate surgical exploration.

Complications

On rare occasion, testicular rupture can occur and be manifested by massive swelling and ecchymosis.

Patient Education, Prevention, and Prognosis

An athletic cup should be worn when participating in any sport where injury could occur. A testicular hematoma should be considered cancer until proved otherwise.

Testicular Torsion

Description

Testicular torsion, a severely painful condition of acute onset in which interruption of the blood supply to the testis causes subsequent ischemic injury, results in an emergency surgical situation.

Etiology and Incidence

Normal fixation of the testis is absent, so the testis can rotate and block lymphatic and then blood flow. Torsion can occur after physical exertion or trauma or on arising.

Torsion occurs at any age but most commonly in adolescence, with a peak between 12 and 18 years (1 in 4000 males younger than 25 years and a cluster in infancy) (Doody & Ryan, 1999; Pillai & Besner, 1998; Kass & Landzk, 1997; Palmer, 1994). The left side is twice as likely to be involved because of the longer spermatic cord.

Clinical Findings

HISTORY. The following may be reported:

- Unilateral pain that starts acutely and gradually and progressively worsens (the cardinal symptom); it can be scrotal or testicular and may worsen if elevated.
- Minor trauma, physical exertion, or onset of acute pain upon arising is possible.
- Prior episodes of transient pain are reported in up to 50% of patients (Pillai & Besner, 1998).
- Nausea, vomiting, or anorexia.
- May be described as abdominal or inguinal pain by the embarrassed child.
- Minimal or absent fever.

PHYSICAL EXAMINATION. Findings include the following:

- Ill-appearing and anxious male resisting movement.
- Gradual, progressive swelling of involved scrotum with redness, warmth, and tenderness.
- The ipsilateral scrotum can be edematous, erythematous, and warm.
- Testis swollen larger than opposite side, elevated, lying transversely, exquisitely painful.
- Spermatic cord thickened, twisted, and tender.
- Slight elevation of the testis increases pain (in epididymitis it relieves pain).
- Transillumination can reveal a solid mass.
- The cremasteric reflex is absent on the side with torsion.

- Neonate—hard, painless, nontransilluminating mass with edema or discolored scrotal skin.

LABORATORY STUDIES. Potential studies to consider include

- CBC (possible elevated WBC count) probably not useful
- UA (usually normal)
- Radiographic imaging (color ultrasonography or nuclear scintigraphy) to measure intratesticular blood flow if the diagnosis is in question

Differential Diagnosis

Torsion of the testicular or epididymal appendage, acute epididymitis (mild to moderate pain of gradual onset), orchitis, trauma (pain is better within an hour), hernia, hydrocele, and varicocele are included in the differential diagnosis.

Management

Testicular torsion is a surgical emergency, and identification with prompt surgical referral must occur immediately. Occasionally, manual reduction can be performed, but surgery should follow within 6 to 12 hours to prevent retorsion, preserve fertility, and prevent abscess and atrophy. Contralateral orchiopexy may be done because of a 40% occurrence of torsion in nonfixed testes. Rest and scrotal support do not provide relief.

Complications

Testicular atrophy, abscess, or decreased fertility and loss of the testis as a result of necrosis can occur if the torsion persists more than 24 hours.

Epididymitis

Description

Epididymitis is an inflammation of the epididymis that is painful and acute.

Etiology and Incidence

Epididymitis is commonly caused by *Neisseria gonorrhoeae* or *Chlamydia*, with infection already existing in the urethra or bladder. However, it can also be caused by a viral, coliform bacterial, or tubercular infection; by anomalies of the genitourinary tract; or by dysfunctional voiding (Tennenbaum & Kim, 1996).

Epididymitis is rare before puberty except with genitourinary tract abnormalities and occurs primarily in sexually active adolescents. In children younger than 2 years, it can be secondary to urogenital anomalies.

Clinical Findings

HISTORY. The following may be reported:

- Sexual encounters within 45 days
- Painful scrotal swelling, gradual or acute in onset
- Dysuria and frequency
- Fever

PHYSICAL EXAMINATION. Findings include the following:

- Scrotal edema and erythema are noted.
- The epididymis is hard, indurated, enlarged, and tender; the spermatic cord is tender.
- The testis has normal position and consistency.
- The cremasteric reflex is normal (not present in older adolescents).
- Prehn's sign—elevation of testis relieves pain (in torsion it increases pain)—can be elicited.
- Hydrocele may be present as a reaction to inflammation.
- Urethral discharge may be present, purulent in gonorrhea, scant and watery in chlamydial infection if associated with urethritis.
- Rectal examination reveals prostate tenderness and can produce a urethral discharge.

LABORATORY STUDIES. The following are done as indicated:

- UA (pyuria and occasional bacteria may be present) and Gram stain and culture for gonococci and chlamydia on first morning urine
- CBC (elevated WBC count)
- Urethral culture and Gram stain (nucleic acid amplification tests may be done for gonococci and chlamydia)
- Testing for other STDs if the epididymitis is due to sexual activity
- Doppler ultrasonography or radionuclide imaging to differentiate torsion of the testis
- Follow-up VCUG, ultrasonography, or both in younger children and those who deny sexual activity to rule out urogenital problems

Differential Diagnosis

The differential diagnosis includes testicular torsion of the spermatic cord or appendix testis, hernia, hydrocele, trauma, tumor, or concomitant urethritis.

Management

Management is directed toward symptom relief and treatment of a causative organism if found. The following steps are taken:

1. Bed rest, scrotal support, and elevation; ice packs as tolerated.
2. Analgesics or NSAIDs to relieve pain.
3. Antibiotic treatment (Centers for Disease Control and Prevention [CDC], 1998):
   a. First line: ceftriaxone (250 mg intramuscularly one time) *plus* doxycycline (100 mg twice a day for 10 days)
   b. Alternative treatments: ofloxacin (300 mg twice a day for 10 days)
4. Referral to a urologist is indicated if a solitary testicle is involved, if a prompt response to treatment does not occur, or if a question about the diagnosis remains.
5. Treatment of sexual partner(s) from the last 60 days is indicated if caused by an STD. Intercourse should be avoided until cured.
6. If prepubertal, a sonogram and voiding cystogram are needed to rule out structural problems.
7. Follow-up is needed within 3 days if no improvement is seen or if symptoms recur after treatment.

Complications

Infertility, abscess formation, testicular infarction, and late atrophy are possible.

Patient Education

Because epididymitis is an STD, partners must be evaluated and treated. Patients must understand the sexually transmitted nature of this disease. Pain and edema usually resolve within 1 week.

Urethritis

Description

An inflammation or infection of the urethra may be symptomatic or asymptomatic.

Etiology and Incidence

N. gonorrhoeae or *Chlamydia trachomatis* (23 to 55%) are the most common pathogens. *Ureaplasma urealyticum* and *Mycoplasma genitalium* cause one third of nongonococcal urethritis (CDC, 1998). *Trichomonas vaginalis* and herpes simplex virus are the other common causative agents.

Clinical Findings

HISTORY
- Often asymptomatic
- Urethral discharge
- Burning with urination

PHYSICAL EXAMINATION
- Purulent or mucopurulent urethral discharge

LABORATORY STUDIES
- UA with positive leukocyte esterase or more than 10 WBCs/hpf
- Gram stain (>5 WBCs/oil immersion field)
- Microscopic examination and culture recommended
- Nucleic acid amplification test on first morning urine (positive)

Differential Diagnosis

Epididymitis is the main differential diagnosis.

Management

1. Nongonococcal urethritis:
   - Azithromycin, 1 g orally in a single dose *or*
   - Doxycycline, 100 mg orally twice a day for 7 days
   - Alternative: Erythromycin base, 500 mg orally four times a day for 7 days *or*
   - Erythromycin ethylsuccinate, 800 mg orally four times a day for 7 days *or*

RESOURCE BOX 35-1

American Association of Kidney Patients
Tel: (800) 749-2257
Website: www.aakp.org
Newsletter, informational materials, networking, advocacy, maintain research registry

American Kidney Fund
Tel: (800) 638-8299, (301) 881-3052
Website: www.arbon.com/kidney
Newsletter, informational materials (inc. Spanish), fund research

NIH Cancer Information
Website: Cancernet.nic.nih.gov/clinpdq/soa/wilms'_tumor_physician.html

IgA Nephropathy Support Network
Tel: (215) 884-9038
Newsletter, informational materials, networking, referrals to local resources, maintain research registry

National Institute of Diabetes and Digestive and Kidney Disease
Tel: (301) 496-3583

National Kidney Foundation
Tel: (800) 622-9010, (212) 889-2210
Website: kidney.org
Newsletter, informational materials, referrals to local resources, local chapters, fund research

National Kidney and Urologic Disease Information Clearinghouse
Tel: (301) 654-4415

Universal Health Communications
Tel: (800) 229-1842
Video available on performing enhanced UA with Neubauer hemocytometer

- Ofloxacin, 300 mg orally twice a day for 7 days (CDC, 1998).
2. If gonococci or chlamydia are identified, see the section in the gynecological chapter for more details.
3. If sexually active, treat any partners within the last 60 days.
4. A return visit is necessary if symptoms persist or recur after treatment.
5. Abstain from sexual intercourse until 7 days after treatment.
6. Report identifiable disease to the state health department.

Complications

Epididymitis or Reiter syndrome are possible complications.

REFERENCES

Abelson HT: Wilms tumor. *In* Behrman RE, Kliegman RM (eds): Nelson Essentials of Pediatrics, 3rd ed. Philadelphia, WB Saunders, 1998, pp 600-603.

Action Committee Report of the Urology Section, American Academy of Pediatrics: Timing of elective surgery on the genitalia of children with particular reference to the risks, benefits and psychological effects of surgery and anesthesia. Pediatrics 97:590-594, 1996.

Alon US: Renal tubular acidosis. *In* Finburg L (ed): Saunders Manual of Pediatric Practice. Philadephia, WB Saunders, 1998.

Andreoli SP: Chronic glomerulonephritis in childhood. Pediatr Clin North Am 42:1487-1503, 1995.

Atilla MK, Dundaroz R, Odabas O, et al: A nonsurgical approach to the treatment of phimosis: Local nonsteroidal anti-inflammatory ointment application. Urology 158:196-197, 1997.

Baskin LS: Know all the facts before ordering a VCUG. Contemp Pediatr 15(3):23, 184, 1998.

Bergstein JM: Renal tubular acidosis. *In* Behrman RE, Kliegman RM, Arvin AM (eds): Nelson Textbook of Pediatrics, 15th ed. Philadelphia, WB Saunders, 1996, pp 1504-1506.

Betz CL, Hunsberger M, Wright S: Family-Centered Nursing Care of Children. Philadelphia, WB Saunders, 1994, p 1458.

Blowey DL: Acute glomerulonephritis. *In* Finburg L (ed): Saunders Manual of Pediatric Practice. Philadephia, WB Saunders, 1998.

Boineau FG, Lewy JE: Evaluation of hematuria in children and adolescents. Pediatr Rev 11(4):101-107, 1989.

Boschert S: Undescended testis may decrease fertility later. Pediatr News Feb:7, 1998.

Brown MR, Cartwright PC, Snow BW: Common office problems in pediatric urology and gynecology. Pediatr Clin North Am 44:1091-1115, 1997.

Burg FD, Ingelfinger JR, Wald ER, et al: Gellis & Kagan's Current Pediatric Therapy 15. Philadelphia: WB Saunders, 1996.

Centers for Disease Control and Prevention: 1998 Guidelines for treatment of sexually transmitted diseases. MMWR Morb Mortal Wkly Rep 47(RR-1):1-111, 1998.

Cruz CC, Spitzer A: When you find protein or blood in the urine. Contemp Pediatr 15(9):89-109, 1998.

Dershewitz RA (ed): Ambulatory Pediatric Care, 3rd ed. Philadelphia, JB Lippincott, 1999.

Doody EP, Ryan DP: Genital pain. *In* Dershewitz RA (ed): Ambulatory Pediatric Care, 3rd ed. Philadelphia, JB Lippincott, 1999, pp 644-648.

Duckett JW: Hypospadias. Pediatr Rev 11(2):37-42, 1989.

Ettenger RB: The evaluation of the child with proteinuria. Pediatr Ann 23(9):486-494, 1994.

Feld LG, Meyers KEC, Kaplan BS, et al: Limited evaluation of microscopic hematuria in pediatrics. Pediatrics 102(4):E42, 1998.

Feld LG, Waz WG, Perez LM, et al: Hematuria: An integrated medical and surgical approach. Pediatr Clin North Am 44:1191-1210, 1997.

Fitzwater DS, Wyatt RJ: Hematuria. Pediatr Rev 15(3):102-108, 1994.

Finberg L: Saunders Manual of Pediatric Practice. Philadelphia, WB Saunders, 1998.

Fouser L: Familial nephritis/Alport syndrome. Pediatr Rev 19(8):265-267, 1998.

Friedman AL: Renal tubular acidosis. *In* Behrman RE, Kliegman RM (eds): Nelson Essentials of Pediatrics, 3rd ed. Philadelphia, WB Saunders, 1998, pp 627-629.

Gill FT: Umbilical hernia, inguinal hernias, and hydroceles in children: Diagnostic clues for optimal patient management. J Pediatr Health Care 12(5):231-235, 1998.

Gill B, Kogan B: Cryptorchidism: Current concepts. Pediatr Clin North Am 44:1211-1227, 1997.

Graft SL: A Handbook of Routine Urinalysis. Philadelphia, JB Lippincott, 1983.

Heldrich FJ: UTI diagnosis: Getting it right the first time. Contemp Pediatr 12(2):110-133, 1995.

Hellerstein S: UTI: Old and new concepts. Pediatr Clin North Am 42:1433-1457, 1995.

Hoberman A, Wald ER: UTI in young children: New light on old questions. Contemp Pediatr 14(11):140-156, 1997.

Kaplan RE, Springate JE, Feld LG: Screening dipstick urinalysis: A time to change. Pediatrics 100:919-921, 1997.

Kapur P, Caty MG, Glack PL: Pediatric hernias and hydroceles. Pediatr Clin North Am 45:773-791, 1998.

Kass EF, Landzk B: The acute scrotum. Pediatr Clin North Am 44:1251-1266, 1997.

Kelsch RC, Sedman AB: Nephrotic syndrome. Pediatr Rev 14(1):30-38, 1993.

Langer JC, Coplen DE: Circumcision and pediatric disorders of the penis. Pediatr Clin North Am 45:801-812, 1998.

Langman CBL: Hematuria and proteinuria. *In* Dershewitz RA (ed): Ambulatory Pediatric Care, 3rd ed. Philadelphia, JB Lippincott, 1999, pp 631-638.

Linshaw MA, Gruskin AB: The routine UA: To keep or not to keep: That is the question. Pediatrics 100:1031-1032, 1997.

Lum GM: Kidney and urinary tract. *In* Merenstein GB, Kaplan DW, Rosenberg AA (eds): Handbook of Pediatrics, 18th ed. Stamford, CT, Appleton & Lange, 1997, pp 584-600.

Mandell J: Penis, spermatic cord and testes. *In* Burg FD, Ingelfinger JR, Wald ER, et al (eds): Gellis & Hagan's Current Pediatric Therapy 15. Philadelphia, WB Saunders, 1996, pp 390-391.

Mendoza SA, Tune BM: Management of the difficult nephrotic patient. Pediatr Clin North Am 42:1459-1468, 1995.

Miser JS: Malignant tumors of the kidney. *In* Burg FD, Ingelfinger JR, Wald ER, et al (eds): Current Pediatric Therapy 15. Philadelphia, WB Saunders, 1996.

Montgomery DF, Parks DK, Yetman RJ: Managing urinary tract infections in children. J Pediatr Health Care 12(5):268-270, 1998.

Moser R: Genitourinary problems in adolescent boys. Adv Nurse Pract Aug:3-39, 1995.

Opas LM: UTI: Burning issues (Unpublished manuscript). Los Angeles, CA, 1999.

Ortigas AP, Cunningham AS: Three facts to know before you order a VCUG. Contemp Pediatr 14(9):69-79, 1997.

Palmer LS: Testicular torsion. Pediatr Rev 15(11):155-156, 1994.

Petersen-Smith AM: Renal tubular acidosis: When kids won't grow. J Pediatr Health Care 9(3):131-133, 1995.

Pillai SB, Besner GE: Pediatric testicular problems. Pediatr Clin North Am 45:813-830, 1998.

Rabinowitz R, Hulbert WC: Cryptorchidism. Pediatr Rev 15(7):272-274, 1994.

Ransley R: Intrarenal reflux: Anatomical, dynamic and radiological studies—part I. Urol Res 5(2):61-69, 1977.

Roy S: Hematuria. Pediatr Rev 19:209-212, 1998.

Rushton HG: UTI in children: Epidemiology, evaluation & management. Pediatr Clin North Am 44:1133-1169, 1997.

Shalaby-Rana E, Lowe LH, Balsk AN, et al: Imaging in pediatric urology. Pediatr Clin North Am 44:1065-1089, 1997.

Shearer PD, Wilimas JA: Neoplasms of the kidney. *In* Behrman RE, Kliegman RM, Arvin AM (eds): Nelson Textbook of Pediatrics, 15th ed. Philadelphia, WB Saunders, 1996, pp 1463-1464.

Sheldon CA, Wacksman J: Vesicoureteral reflux. Pediatr Rev 16(1):22-27, 1995.

Simckes AM, Spitzer A: Poststreptococcal acute glomerulonephritis. Pediatr Rev 16(7):278-279, 1995.

Skoog SJ: Benign and malignant pediatric scrotal masses. Pediatr Clin North Am 44:1229-1250, 1997.

Skoog SJ, Roberts KP, Goldstein M, et al: The adolescent varicocele: What's new with an old problem in young patients? Pediatrics 100:112-122, 1997.

Soriano JR: Renal tubular disorders. *In* Burg FD, Ingelfinger JR, Wald ER, et al (eds): Current Pediatric Therapy 15. Philadelphia, WB Saunders, 1996, pp 450-451.

Steinhurz PG: Wilms tumor. *In* Finburg L (ed): Saunders Manual of Pediatric Practice. Philadephia, WB Saunders, 1998, pp 462-466.

Tennenbaum S, Kim D: Acute epididymitis and orchitis in children. Pediatr Rev 17(12):424-425, 1996.

Todd JK: Management of UTI: Children are different. Pediatr Rev 16(5):190-196, 1995.

US Preventive Health Services Task Force: Guide to Clinical Preventive Services, 2nd ed. Baltimore, Williams & Wilkins, 1996.

US Public Health Service: Put Prevention Into Practice: The Clinician's Handbook of Preventive Services, 2nd ed. Germantown, MD, International Medical Publishing, 1997.

Vogt BA: Identifying kidney disease: Simple steps can make a difference. Contemp Pediatr 14(3):115-127, 1997.

Warner BW: Wilms tumor. Pediatr Rev 17(10):371-372, 1996.

Warshaw BL: Nephrotic syndrome in children. Pediatr Ann 23(9):495-504, 1994.

Woodhead JC: Urinary tract infections. *In* Dershewitz RA (ed): Ambulatory Pediatric Care, 3rd ed. Philadelphia, JB Lippincott, 1999, pp 619-627.

Yadin O: Hematuria in children. Pediatr Ann 23(9):474-485, 1994.

Zaontz MR, Packer MG: Abnormalities of the external genitalia. Pediatr Clin North Am 44:1267-1297, 1997.

Ziegler MM: Diagnosis of inguinal hernia and hydrocele. Pediatr Rev 15(7):286-288, 1994.

CHAPTER 36

Gynecological Conditions

Nancy Barber Starr

INTRODUCTION

Gynecological concerns or problems in the child or adolescent provide the nurse practitioner (NP) varied and interesting challenges regarding health and medical matters as well as psychosocial interventions. Sensitivity to the patient and family and comfort with these issues aid the NP in working with the child or adolescent and the parent. Educating children and adolescents about their bodies as they mature is essential. Approaching issues that may be considered personal or embarrassing openly and directly allows more comprehensive care and anticipatory guidance. Establishing and maintaining a good relationship with both parents and adolescents helps ease the transition during which adolescents take an increasingly larger role in determining their own care.

Gynecological issues range from normal transitions that are perceived as abnormal to serious systemic diseases or abnormalities. The practitioner is required to have a high level of suspicion in all cases in order not to miss any significant signs. At the same time, most conditions are normal and can be easily addressed, reassuring the child or adolescent that all is well and that she is normal, healthy, and gynecologically intact.

STANDARDS OF CARE

An interim progress report on the goals related to decreasing the incidence of sexually transmitted diseases (STDs) from *Healthy Children 2000 National Health Promotion and Disease Prevention Objectives for the Year 2000* (United States [US] Health and Human Services, 1994) reported overall decreases in the incidence of gonorrhea, syphilis, and chlamydia. One of the goals of *Healthy Children 2010: National Health Promotion and Disease Prevention Objectives for the Year 2010* (US Department of Health and Human Services, 1998) (see Appendix D) is "A society where healthy sexual relationships, free of infection as well as coercion and unintended pregnancy are the norm."

The *Guide to Clinical Preventive Services, 2nd ed.* (US Preventive Services Task Force, 1996) recommends routine screening for syphilis (all pregnant women and persons at increased risk of infection) and for asymptomatic infection with *Chlamydia trachomatis* (all sexually active female adolescents, high-risk pregnant women, and other asymptomatic women at high risk of infection). Routine screening for genital herpes simplex virus (HSV) infection is not recommended. Further recommendations include counseling all adolescent patients about risk factors for infection with human immunodeficiency virus (HIV) and other STDs and offering testing for syphilis, gonorrhea, hepatitis B, HIV, and chlamydial infection.

The American Academy of Pediatrics, the American Nurses Association, and the American Medical Association (AMA) Guidelines for Adolescent Preventive Services (GAPS) recommend as a routine part of health supervision that adolescents (both male and female) be asked annually about sexual health behavior and that sexually active adolescents be screened for STDs. Adolescents should receive counseling about responsible sexual behavior including using contraception and condoms to prevent infection with STDs and HIV, abstention from intercourse as the surest way to prevent STDs and pregnancy, and the benefit of postponing future sexual relationships. Providers should be involved in making these objectives a major priority within community health practice, with a special emphasis in school health settings and school-based clinics (US Public Health Service, 1997; Elster & Kuznets, 1994).

ANATOMY AND PHYSIOLOGY

During the first 8 weeks of gestation, male and female fetuses are sexually undifferentiated, both having one pair of gonads and a pair of ducts. At 8 weeks, the male gonad produces testosterone and antimüllerian hormone (AMH), which causes the gonads to become testes and the tubules to become the vas deferens. In the female, the gonads do not produce testosterone or AMH, so ovaries are formed from the gonads and the ducts become the uterus and fallopian tubes. External genital structures are also undifferentiated until 8 weeks of gestation, at which time the presence or lack of testosterone causes the external genitalia to develop as either male or female. By 9 months of gestation, all internal and external genital structures are present.

In the first few weeks of life, maternal estrogen thickens and enlarges the genital structures, sometimes causing a physiological discharge or bleeding in females. Between 8 weeks and 7 years of age, without maternal or endogenous estrogens, the labia majora are flat, the labia minora are thin, and neither offer protection to the genitalia. Between 6 and 8 years of age, sexual maturation is triggered by the presence of adrenal androgens and then estrogen in females and testosterone in males. In the female, this causes labial thickening and enlargement

and sometimes a physiological leukorrhea. The ovaries contain the lifetime number of immature ova at birth, with the ova maturing generally one per cycle from puberty to menopause. In the male, the production of sperm by the testes begins and continues throughout the life span.

The structure and function of the reproductive system are controlled by the hypothalamic-pituitary-ovarian (HPO) axis (also called the hypothalmic-pituitary-gonadal axis). This complex process begins in the neurological system (the hypothalamus), involves the endocrine system (the anterior pituitary), and completes its cycle with the gonads (ovaries or testes). The hypothalamus releases gonadotropin-releasing hormone, which stimulates the anterior pituitary to release the gonadotropins, luteinizing hormone (LH), and follicle-stimulating hormone (FSH). These, in turn, stimulate the gonads to release the sex hormones. See Figures 9-1 and 9-2. Initially, this cycle causes sexual maturation, and, once that is completed, the ongoing release of hormones controls the menstrual cycle, pregnancy, and lactation. The primary female hormones are estrogen and progesterone, with small amounts of androgens (Fig. 36-1).

PATHOPHYSIOLOGY AND DEFENSE MECHANISMS

Pathophysiology

The primary disorders of the gynecological system can be classified as menstrual cycle disorders, inflammatory reactions, infection, and reproductive problems.

MENSTRUAL CYCLE DISORDERS

Commonly seen menstrual problems are mittelschmerz, dysmenorrhea, abnormal uterine bleeding, endometriosis, and amenorrhea. The three most important disorders are delayed thelarche and menarche, amenorrhea, and anovulatory cycles or short luteal phase cycles that appear as irregular cycles (Gidwani, 1997). The female athlete is especially prone to exercise-related menstrual problems. However, considering the complexity of the HPO axis, many other

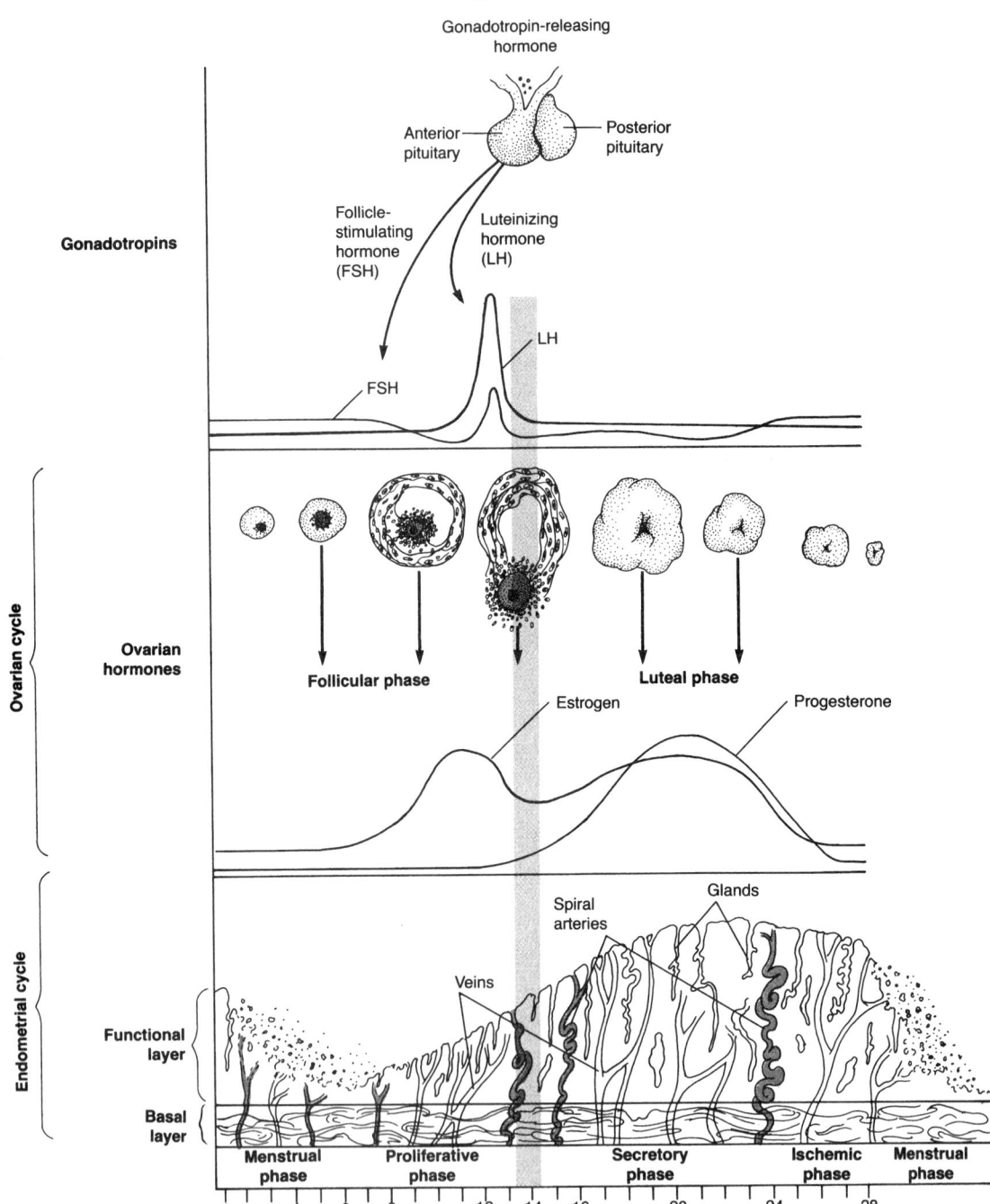

F I G U R E 36-1
Female reproductive cycle showing changes in hormone secretion and in the ovary, and the uterine endometrium. (From Gorrie T, McKinney E, Murray S: Foundations of Maternal Newborn Nursing, 2nd ed. Philadelphia, WB Saunders, 1998.)

neurological, endocrine, and reproductive problems can present initially as deviations or problems with menstruation.

INFLAMMATORY REACTIONS

An inflammatory response can occur in either the external or internal genitalia. Local reactions involve the external genitalia and can be caused by dermatological disorders or skin irritation from such factors as normal leukorrhea, chemical or allergic reactions, or nonspecific causes. Internal inflammation caused by infection is not always obvious.

INFECTIONS

The warm, moist environment that the reproductive tract provides an ideal place for infection. Viral pathogens, such as HSV and human papilloma virus (HPV) or fungal infection can present as a vulvitis or vaginal infection. Trichomonas, a protozoan infection, colonizes the vaginal vault. By contrast, the bacterial infections chlamydia and gonorrhea ascend into the upper genital tract where pelvic inflammatory disease (PID) or tubal damage can occur.

REPRODUCTIVE PROBLEMS

Reproductive problems occur in the adolescent as a result of structural, hormonal, or endocrine disorders or as sequelae of infection. Refer to an obstetrical text for further information.

Defense Mechanisms

The gynecological system has both anatomical and physiological defense mechanisms. The labia majora and the pubic hair provide a barrier that serves as the first line of defense. The vagina, serving as an exit for mucosal secretion, menstrual fluids, and products of conception, also provides a means of defense with its natural downward and outward flow of secretions.

Additionally, with increasing estrogen exposure, the vaginal epithelial tissue thickens and an acid pH develops, discouraging infection. The small external cervical os, a thick mucous plug, and the downward flow of cervical secretions provide barriers to entry to the uterus. A

chemical barrier is also established by the cervical enzymes and antibodies.

ASSESSMENT OF THE GYNECOLOGICAL SYSTEM

History

The history must include assessment of the following:

- Family history: maternal age of menarche, dysmenorrhea or endometriosis, diabetes mellitus, thyroid, bleeding disorders, malignancy, diethylstilbestrol (DES) exposure, ovarian cysts, genetic disorders
- Menstrual history: age of menarche, length of cycles, duration of flow, estimated blood loss, last menstrual period, dysmenorrhea
- Sexual history: sexual activity (voluntary or forced); type of activity (oral, vaginal, anal, and heterosexual, homosexual, bisexual); age of first intercourse, number of sexual partners in previous 60 days, 12 months, lifetime; exposures to infection; previous infections; previous STDs (see Chapter 20)
- Contraceptive history: type, duration, and frequency of use, problems
- Pregnancy as well as obstetrical, and gynecological history, as appropriate.
- Review of systems: vaginal, urinary, abdominal or pelvic, general

Physical Examination

When a gynecological examination is performed, the child or adolescent should maintain a feeling of being in control. It is important to establish rapport, preserve modesty, and obtain consent to examine. An adolescent often wishes to have an adult, usually her mother, present (Baldwin & Landa, 1995). A good light and a hand mirror for patient use are often helpful.

PREPUBERTAL CHILD

- Position: The lithotomy position with stirrups can be used. However, having the patient lie supine in the frog-leg (with heels together, knees flat on table) or knee-chest (chest prone, weight on knees, buttocks in air) position is more comfortable for the child and provides for a better examination. The traction maneuver, gripping the labia and pulling forward and laterally, gives better visualization. An otoscope often provides the light and magnification needed to examine the vagina.

• Examine
  ○ Breasts, abdomen, and inguinal area.
  ○ Presence and distribution of pubic hair.
  ○ State of hygiene.
  ○ Size of clitoris (approximately 3×3 mm).
  ○ Signs of estrogenization (pubertal vaginal mucosa—moist, thin, and red, whereas post-pubertal vaginal mucosa—moist and dull pink).
  ○ The hymen, normally smooth and continuous, can be described as crescent-shaped, annular, or redundant (Fig. 36–2). The significance of the diameter of the hymenal opening as a diagnostic finding is debated. Both transverse and anteroposterior diameter are dependent on age, relaxation, method of examination, and type of hymen. In general, the older and more relaxed the child, the larger the opening. It is also larger with retraction and in the knee-chest position. In the 3- to 6-year-old, range of normal findings for the transverse diameter is 1 to 6 mm and for the anterior-posterior diameter is 1 to 7 mm. Obesity in young children is associated with hymenal openings larger than average for age (e.g., a 2-year-old with a 4-mm opening when average is 2 mm).
  ○ Sexual maturity rating (SMR) or Tanner staging is discussed in Chapters 9 and 20. See Figures 9–3 and 9–4.
  ○ Anus for cleanliness, excoriation, or erythema.

ADOLESCENT

• Examine the breasts.
• Inspect the external genitalia and determine Tanner staging.
• If the adolescent is sexually active, has gynecological complaints, was exposed to DES, or is 18 years of age, visualize the vagina and cervix through speculum examination. Palpate the uterus and adnexa rectoabdominally.

Diagnostic Studies

The following studies can be ordered as appropriate for history and examination. Collection of specimens, especially in children, must be done with care. Techniques that may be helpful include using a small amount of saline as a

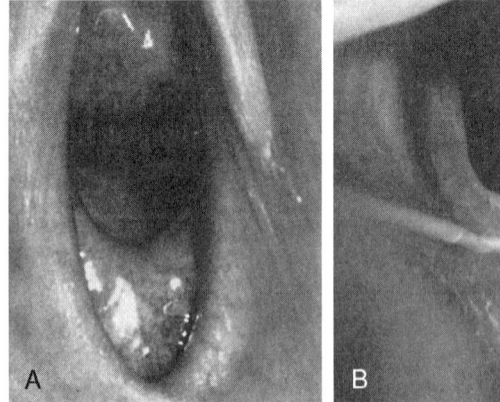
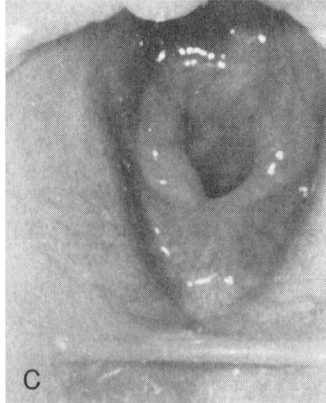

FIGURE 36-2
Types of hymens, photographed through a colposcope. *A,* Crescentic hymen. *B,* Annular hymen. *C,* Redundant hymen with crescent appearance after retraction. (From Emans S, Laufer M, Goldstein D: Pediatric and Adolescent Gynecology, 4th ed. Philadelphia, Lippincott-Raven, 1998.)

vaginal wash, using a soft plastic eyedropper or feeding tube, or using a moistened cotton or Calgiswab.

- Cultures for gonorrhea, *Chlamydia*, or *Monilia*: The laboratory should be notified if the specimen is from a prepubertal child. The specimen to test for yeast can be taken from anywhere in the vaginal canal and tested on Biggy agar culture. Chlamydia sampling is most accurate when taken from areas of columnar epithelium (e.g., urethra, endocervical opening).
- Serological studies such as Venereal Disease Research Laboratories (VDRL) or rapid plasma reagin (RPR) test, fluorescent treponemal antibody absorption (FTA-ABS) test, or microhemagglutination test for *Treponema pallidum* (MHA-TP).
- Vaginal smear of cells from the upper lateral wall of the vagina to determine estrogenization.
- Examination of dried cervical mucus for ferning that occurs late in the menstrual cycle (does not occur in the presence of progesterone).
- Wet preparations. A saline slide of secretions prepared for microscopic examination shows motile trichomonads, clue cells (bacteria attached to epithelial cells), and occasional white blood cells (WBCs). Mixing this with potassium hydroxide (KOH) can cause a fishy odor (positive whiff test) in the presence of certain bacteria. Microscopic examination of the KOH slide can show pseudohyphae and yeast forms (Fig. 36-3).
- pH of vaginal mucus (neutral, prepubescent; <4.5, pubertal; >4.5 with *Trichomonas* and bacterial vaginosis).
- Gram's stain for increased polymorphonuclear leukocytes (*Chlamydia*, herpes, *Trichomonas*) or gram-negative diplococci (gonorrhea).
- Rapid detection tests: Many new tests are available. Direct immunofluorescent antibody (DFA), enzyme immunoassay (EIA), and DNA probes have been used for some years but are not relied upon in situations involving possible abuse or prepubertal children. Newer ligase chain reduction

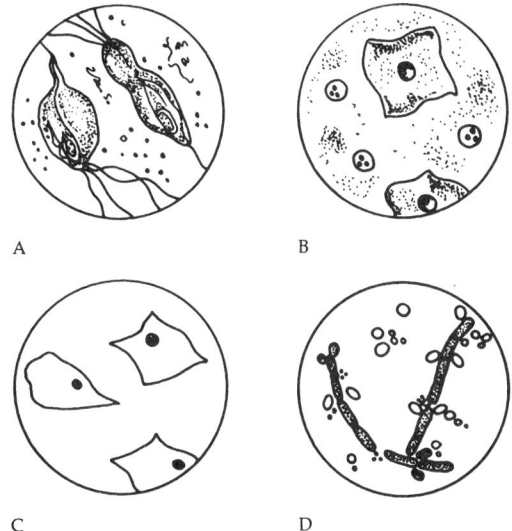

F I G U R E 36-3
Fresh vaginal smear showing *A*, trichomonas; *B*, clue cells of bacterial vaginosis; *C*, leukorrhea; *D*, candida. *A*, *B*, and *C* are saline preparations; *D* is a potassium hydroxide (KOH) preparation. (From Emans S, Laufer M, Goldstein D: Pediatric and Adolescent Gynecology, 4th ed. Philadelphia, Lippincott-Raven, 1998.)

(LCR) and polymerase chain reaction (PCR) genetic amplification tests for *Neisseria gonorrhoeae* and chlamydia can be performed on urine, vaginal, or cervical samples and have sensitivities greater than 98% (Shafer, 1998). Transcription mediated amplification (TMA) is another test. None of these are readily available and have yet to be accepted as documentation in abuse cases or with prepubertal children. Standarized cultures are still recommended.

- Papanicolaou (Pap) smear in sexually active females at 18 years of age or with any exposure to HPV allows early identification of cell abnormalities and precancerous conditions.
- Pregnancy test by urine or serum methods.
- Progesterone challenge for primary or secondary amenorrhea.
- Ultrasonogram of pelvic and renal systems (cysts, tumors, PID, pregnancy, pelvic abnormalities).

• Biggy agar culture for suspected yeast infection.

MANAGEMENT STRATEGIES

Anticipatory Guidance

Anticipatory guidance related to gynecological issues is important to both the child or adolescent and parents. Good genital hygiene can help avoid some potential problems. The transition to puberty and establishment of menses may be eased with appropriate education. With the advent of puberty and the increasing interest in sexuality, much guidance is needed before initiation of sexual activity. Guidance should continue as the teenager contemplates or initiates sexual activity. See Chapters 9 and 20 for further discussion of these topics.

Counseling and Education

Counseling and education related to disorders of the gynecological system need to be tailored to the child or adolescent and the parents. Confidentiality is a matter to be established with both the parents and the adolescent. Some states have specific laws that allow the NP to treat for obstetrical and family planning conditions in adolescents without parental knowledge or consent. Additional team members can be involved, depending on the diagnosis. Coordination, interpretation, and follow-up of these details are important tasks. The resources in the box at the end of the chapter offer the NP additional information.

Medications

Medications play an important role in some disorders of the gynecological system.

- Nonsteroidal anti-inflammatory drugs (NSAIDs) contain *prostaglandin inhibitors* that are used primarily in dysmenorrhea. Ibuprofen, naproxen, naproxen sodium, and mefenamic acid are commonly used for menstrual cramps.
- *Oral contraceptives* (OCs) are used for dysmenorrhea, dysfunctional uterine bleeding, or to prevent conception (see Chapter 20). Low-dose estrogen (20 to 35 μg) in combination with progesterone is most commonly used. The estrogen is either mestranol or ethinyl estradiol. The progesterone can be any one of the numerous progestins (synthetic progesterones). Some progestins include norethindrone, levonorgestrel, norgestrel, norgestimate, norethindrone acetate, ethynodiol diacetate, desogestrel, norethynodrel, or gestodene. New progestins regularly emerge from clinical trials.
- *Progesterone* is used in dysfunctional uterine bleeding or in the evaluation of primary amenorrhea. It is given by either oral or intramuscular route.
- *Antibiotics*, *antivirals*, and *antifungals* are used in topical, oral, vaginal insert, intramuscular, or intravenous form to treat infection.
- *Creams* and *ointments* such as estrogen cream or hydrocortisone can be used for therapeutic or curative measures.

SPECIFIC GYNECOLOGICAL PROBLEMS OF CHILDREN AND ADOLESCENTS

Labial Adhesions

Description

The fusion of tissue between the labia minora that appears to cover the vaginal opening is a common, benign condition in infants and prepubertal girls. It is also called agglutination, synechia vulvae, or vulvar adhesion if only the lower half of the labia minora is involved (Fig. 36–4).

Etiology and Incidence

Before puberty, the vaginal tissues are in a hypoestrogenized state and are prone to inflammation and denudation. As the tissues heal, adhesion of the labia occurs. Mechanisms for the initial insult are irritation, infection, and trauma. The most common precipitant is an asymptomatic, nonspecific vulvovaginitis caused by poor hygiene. There is debate about whether lack of hygiene, masturbation, fond-

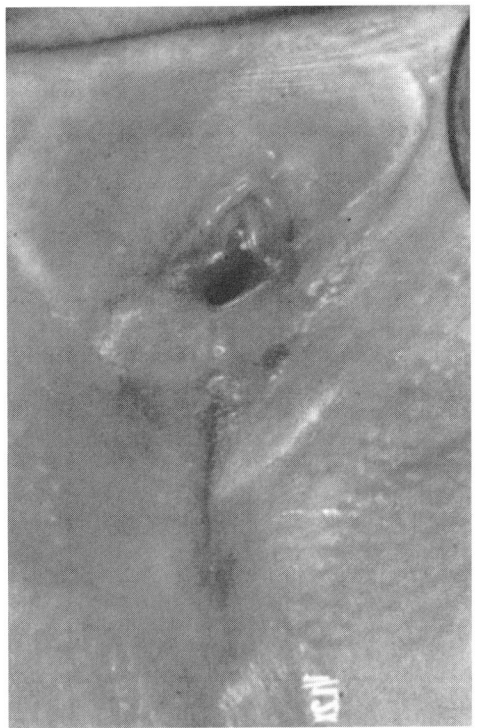

Labial adhesions that are thinned and almost translucent inferiorly following topical estrogen therapy. (From Craighill MC: Pediatric and adolescent gynecology for primary care pediatricians. Pediatr Clin North Am 45: 1668, 1998.)

ling, and subsequent irritation from sexual abuse in older females are potential causes (Emans et al., 1998).

Labial adhesions occur primarily in girls 3 months to 6 years of age but can persist until puberty (Emans et al., 1998; Brown et al., 1997). Ten percent to 20% of all females have some adhesion before 1 year of age (Howard, 1992).

Clinical Findings

HISTORY. The history can include the following:

- Concern about rash in genital area
- Parental concern about vaginal opening
- Dysuria, difficult voiding, or local discomfort

PHYSICAL EXAMINATION. Physical examination reveals thin, flat membrane of varying length from the posterior fourchette to the clitoris. The degree of opening near the clitoris varies. The vulva appears flat with a central line of fusion. The urethra may or may not be visualized, and there may be urinary dribbling.

Differential Diagnosis

Scarring, imperforate hymen, clitoral hypertrophy, and intersex problems are the differential diagnosis.

Management

The treatment of labial adhesions is somewhat controversial; Table 36-1 outlines steps that are generally accepted. It may be necessary to emphasize that no treatment is the best treatment and to give much reassurance. Forceful separation is always contraindicated because it may result in both trauma to the child and recurrence of adhesions.

Complications

Urinary tract infections and readhesion following mechanical lysis can occur.

Patient Education

Premarin cream can cause breast tenderness and transient enlargement and vulvar pigmentation or erythema, that resolves with discontinuation of the cream.

Mittelschmerz

Description

Pelvic pain that occurs at the time of ovulation, midway between menstrual periods, is referred to as mittelschmerz (middle pain) (Table 36-2).

Etiology and Incidence

Exact etiology of the pain is unclear but is probably caused by rapid enlargement of the

T A B L E 36-1

Treatment of Labial Adhesions

DEGREE OF INVOLVEMENT	TREATMENT	PROGNOSIS
No urinary tract infection, no obstruction, no parental concern.	No treatment. Reassure and observe.	Resolution with puberty and estrogenization of tissue.
Opening ensures urinary and vaginal drainage, but treatment desired.	Apply ointment (e.g., A & D or Vaseline) nightly with cotton tipped swab with gentle pressure. Following separation, maintain good hygiene and mild ointment, e.g., Vaseline, nightly for 6–12 mo.	Separation within 8 weeks. If not, double check technique to ensure gentle pressure is being applied. If persists, see use of estrogen cream below.
Urinary and vaginal drainage impaired.	Apply estrogen-containing 1% cream, e.g., Premarin, qd or b.i.d. for 2–3 wk with cotton-tipped swab. Use gentle pressure until separation occurs. Following separation, use Vaseline nightly as outlined above. Alternate treatment is to use transdermal estrogen patch (Climara or FemPatch [change weekly], Alora or Vivelle [change twice a week] or Estraderm [cannot be cut]). Other patches may be cut to alter dosage. Apply near labial adhesions. Continue use for 1 month following separation (Craighill, 1998).	Separation usually occurs within 8 weeks (80–90%) (Emans et al., 1998). If not, check technique to ensure pressure is being applied. If unresponsive, may treat with 5% Xylocaine ointment or EMLA cream and gentle teasing of adhesions with a swab. Always avoid forceful separation.

follicle just before follicular rupture. Incidence is unknown, although some ultrasonographic studies have detected fluid in 40% of normal women's midmenstrual cycle.

Clinical Findings

HISTORY

- Midway between menstrual cycles
- Recurrent discomfort at same time in each cycle
- Dull, aching lower abdominal pain lasting from a few minutes to several hours; occasionally severe and crampy, persisting up to 3 days
- Occasional slight vaginal bleeding

PHYSICAL EXAMINATION

- Pain to palpation of either or both sides of the lower quadrants of the abdomen, overlying the ovaries

Differential Diagnosis

Included in the differential diagnosis are appendicitis, torsion or rupture of an ovarian cyst, and ectopic pregnancy.

Management

1. The benign nature of the pain must be explained to the adolescent.
2. A heating pad may provide some relief.
3. Analgesics, especially prostaglandin inhibitors (ibuprofen, naproxen), may be used. Table 36-3 lists dosages.
4. Rarely oral contraceptives may be prescribed for relief. See Chapter 20.

Patient Education

- Reassurance and comfort measures as outlined in the management section.
- The adolescent should be encouraged to

T A B L E 36-2

Evaluation and Treatment of Menstrual Disorders

	ETIOLOGY	HISTORY	PHYSICAL EXAMINATION & LABORATORY TESTS	MANAGEMENT
Mittelschmerz	Pain caused by rapid enlargement of dominant follicle before follicular rupture	Pain midway between cycles; dull, achy pain in lower abdomen lasting few minutes to several hours	Pain to palpation in either or both sides of lower abdomen overlying ovaries	Explain benign nature; heating pad; analgesics, especially PG inhibitors; follow up if pain changes
Dysmenorrhea	Primary: caused by exaggerated production of PGs; Secondary: caused by infection, abnormality, or intrauterine device	Onset 6–24 mo after menarche; pain begins with menses, lasts less than 2 days; mild to severe cramping in lower midabdominal area radiating to back, thighs	Normal PE except for pain with examination of lower abdomen; may be pale	PG inhibitors at onset of menses for duration of pain; follow up by phone or if pain changes; refer for gynecological care if fails to respond after 6 mo
Endometriosis	Bleeding from ectopic endometrial tissue outside pelvic cavity causes pain, irritation of nerve endings, and uterine contractions	Progressive dysmenorrhea; onset before menses continuing for several days; unresponsive to OC or PG inhibitors in moderate to severe forms; irregular or excessive bleeding; bowel and bladder dysfunction; chronic pelvic pain; first-degree relative with endometriosis	Small papules on labia, vagina clear to red; limited or fixed uterine mobility; enlarged ovaries; adnexal masses; pelvic tenderness; uterosacral ligament nodules or tenderness with movement	*Mild to moderate:* PG inhibitors, OC or progestin treatment; recheck 1–3 mo; refer if symptoms persist after 3–6 mo. *Severe:* refer for laparoscopy
Dysfunctional Uterine Bleeding	Defect in the maturation of negative feedback system of estrogen and follicle-stimulating hormone causing disorderly endometrial shedding	Bleeding that may be excessive in quantity or duration, irregular in occurrence	Normal PE except pale if HgB is low; possible petechiae, bruising; observe for androgen excess, galactorrhea; rule out pregnancy, STD	*HgB > 12 g:* PG inhibitor or OC; iron supplement; menstrual calendar; reevaluate in 3 mo; *HgB 10–12 g:* as above, OC preferred; folic acid supplement; reevaluate monthly

HgB = hemoglobin; OC = oral contraceptive; PE = physical examination; PG = prostaglandin; STD = sexually transmitted disease.

T A B L E 36-3

Common Prostaglandin Inhibitors Used to Treat Adolescent Menstrual Disorders

Ibuprofen (Advil, Motrin): 400–800 mg every 4–6 hr; loading dose of 800 mg

Naproxen: 500 mg at onset followed by 250–375 mg every 6–8 hr

Naproxen sodium (Aleve, Anaprox): 550 mg at onset followed by 275 mg every 6 hr; max dose 1375 mg per 24 hr

Mefenamic acid: 500 mg at onset followed by 250 mg every 6 hr

Flurbiprofen: 50 mg every 6 hr; 100 mg every 8–12 hr

Meclofenamate: 100 mg initially; 50–100 mg every 6 hr

return if the pain worsens or changes, or if the adolescent is concerned.

Dysmenorrhea

Description

Painful menstruation with cramping in the lower abdomen or pelvis is the most common gynecological problem seen in adolescence. Primary dysmenorrhea has no pelvic pathology identified, whereas secondary dysmenorrhea is due to a pelvic abnormality.

Etiology and Incidence

Primary dysmenorrhea is painful menses caused by an exaggerated production of, or response to, prostaglandins, causing uterine hypercontractility, tissue ischemia, and nerve hypersensitivity (Braverman & Sondheimer, 1997; Polaneczky & Slap, 1992b). Secondary dysmenorrhea may be prompted by endometriosis, abortion, complications of pregnancy, outflow obstruction, ovarian cysts, fibroids, or other uterine abnormalities, infection, or intrauterine device.

Dysmenorrhea is present in more than 50% of female adolescents and is the leading cause (>10%) of absenteeism from school (Emans et al., 1998; Braverman & Sondheimer, 1997).

Clinical Findings

HISTORY. The history should assess the following:

Primary Dysmenorrhea
- Family history of cramps or endometriosis.
- Menstrual history.
- Onset of pain (usually 6 months to 2 years after menarche).
- Sexual activity.
- Number of days of school or activities missed.
- Timing, location, and character of pain. Pain varies from mild to severe and is in the lower midabdominal area. Radiation to lower back, labia majora, and inner thighs can occur. Pain begins near the onset of menses and lasts less than 2 days.
- Systemic symptoms associated with prostaglandin release such as nausea, vomiting, headache, fatigue, nervousness, dizziness, urinary frequency, lower back or thigh pain.
- Medication or treatments used.

Secondary Dysmenorrhea
- History of infection, menorrhagia, intermenstrual bleeding, or abnormal vaginal discharge
- Onset (with menarche or later than 2 to 3 years after)
- Pelvic pain at times other than menstruation (worsens over time)
- Character of pelvic pain (dull and constant rather than crampy)
- Dyspareunia

PHYSICAL EXAMINATION. A complete physical examination is recommended. A pelvic and rectovaginal examination is deferred only if the adolescent is not sexually active, if the dysmenorrhea does not interfere with daily activities and is mild, or if the dysmenorrhea is responding to treatment.

LABORATORY STUDIES. The following are ordered as indicated:

- Complete blood count (CBC) and sedimentation rate if PID is suspected
- Pap smear and pregnancy test
- Cervical cultures for gonorrhea and chlamydia

- Pelvic ultrasonogram if abnormalities are suspected
- Renal ultrasonogram and intravenous pyelography if uterine malformation found

Differential Diagnosis

Endometriosis, acute and chronic PID, intrauterine contraceptive device, obstructive malformations or other pathology of the reproductive tract, and psychogenic etiology are included in the differential diagnosis.

Management

The following steps are recommended:

1. Primary dysmenorrhea
   - Prostaglandin synthetase inhibitors provide relief in 75 to 90% of patients (Emans et al., 1998; Braverman & Sondheimer, 1997). They should be administered at onset of menses or, if cramping precedes menses, at onset of symptoms. Treat the patient for the duration of the pain, usually 1 to 2 days. The trial period should extend for three cycles; if no relief is experienced, an alternate prostaglandin inhibitor should be tried. See Table 36–3 for specific prostaglandin inhibitors. For patients with severe symptoms, naproxen sodium is a good choice because it is quickly absorbed.
   - Oral contraceptives are effective in 90% of patients by reducing endometrial growth and, thus, total prostaglandin production. Achieving optimal effect can take several months. A combination 20- to 35-μg estrogen-progestin pill is used for a 3- to 6-month trial if prostaglandin inhibitors are not successful. Oral contraceptives can be continued if contraception is needed.
   - Depot medroxyprogesterone and implantable levonorgestrel are also useful.
   - Follow-up by telephone or visit to adjust dose or change medication as needed. The adolescent should be seen again in 3 to 4 months.
   - If there is failure to respond after 6 months of treatment or if pain worsens over time, the patient should be referred for gynecological care to rule out endometriosis or other etiology.

2. Secondary dysmenorrhea
   - Requires referral for gynecological care.
   - Explain that the pain is not "in the patient's head" and can be managed.
   - Assist with stress control to alleviate pain.

Patient Education and Prevention

- Encourage exercise and stress reduction to help control pain.
- A well-balanced diet with ample amounts of fiber and water are useful to control dysmenorrhea. Some herbal teas, fruits, and vegetables may also help.
- Taking NSAIDs with food helps to avoid abdominal complaints.
- Application of heat provides short-term relief. Pelvic exercise, biofeedback, relaxation therapy, or transcutaneous electronic nerve stimulation (TENS) as adjunct therapies can also provide relief.
- Oral contraceptives (OCs) offer many noncontraceptive advantages, including protection from endometrial and ovarian cancer, decreased symptoms of PID, decreased iron deficiency, and slowed progress of endometriosis.

Endometriosis

Description

Endometriosis is the proliferation of ectopic endometrial tissue outside the pelvic cavity. It is primarily manifested by dysmenorrhea that progressively worsens. It is the most common cause of chronic pelvic pain in adolescents who do not have PID.

Etiology and Incidence

Several theories have been developed to explain the possible cause of endometriosis, including retrograde menstruation; coelomic metaplasia; lymphatic, vascular, and iatrogenic dissemination; genetic factors; and immunological or hormonal problems or defects (Craighill, 1998; Zivnuska, 1995; Durinzi & DeLeon, 1993; Hurd & Adamson, 1992). Dysmenorrhea occurs as the endometrial lesions bleed into the adjacent closed cavity, causing pressure, irritating nerve endings, and stimulating uterine contractions.

The incidence rate in adolescents is difficult to obtain because endometriosis has only recently been studied in this age group. Estimates of 7% in the population with a first-degree relative with endometriosis, and 1% otherwise, are reported. Average age of onset is 14.7 years of age, 2.9 years after menarche (Emans et al., 1998; Hurd & Adamson, 1992). Approximately 50% of adolescents with chronic pelvic pain who have a laparoscopic examination have endometriosis (Braverman & Sondheimer, 1997).

Clinical Findings

HISTORY. The history can include the following:

- First-degree relative with endometriosis
- Deep uni- or bilateral pain described as sharp or dull
- Dysmenorrhea that is acquired and progressive, starting before menses and continuing for several days, and unresponsive to prostaglandin inhibitors or oral contraceptives
- Irregular or excessive bleeding
- Chronic pelvic pain that is acyclic and mildly to severely disabling, disrupting routine and causing missed school days or emergency department visits without definitive diagnosis
- Bladder and bowel dysfunction; rectal pain
- Dyspareunia

PHYSICAL EXAMINATION. The following may be seen:

- Small papules on labia, vagina, or cervix that are clear to red in color in adolescents (in young women they become bluish to brownish)
- Fixed uterus or limited mobility
- Tender, enlarged, or fixed ovaries
- Adnexal masses, thickening, or tenderness
- Pelvic tenderness
- Uterosacral ligament nodules or tenderness with movement

Differential Diagnosis

Primary dysmenorrhea, PID, chronic anovulation with cystic ovaries, eating disorders, lactose intolerance, irritable bowel syndrome, chronic constipation, and depression are included in the differential diagnosis.

Management

The goal in treating endometriosis is to control pain by interrupting the menstrual cycle. Decreasing circulating estrogen decreases the proliferation of endometrial tissue.

1. For mild to moderate symptoms, mobile uterus, no pelvic nodularity or adnexal mass:
   - Prostaglandin inhibitor therapy should be prescribed for pain, then oral contraception or progestin therapy or both to decrease endometrial tissue proliferation (see Table 36–3 and Chapter 20). High-dose contraceptive therapy may be helpful in recalcitrant cases (Craighill, 1998).
   - See at 1- to 3-month intervals to provide support and reevaluate.
   - Refer for laparoscopy if symptoms persist after 3 to 6 months.
   - Avoid dairy, wheat, sugar, and caffeine products (Craighill, 1998).
   - Diet and exercise are important aspects in coping with chronic pain. Stress reduction techniques are also helpful.
2. For severe symptoms, fixed uterus, nodular pelvis, or pelvic mass:
   - Refer for diagnostic laparoscopy and treatment, which can include surgery and alternative medications. Androgen therapy (Danazol) and the synthetic analogues of GnRH (e.g., Lupron or Synarel) are most commonly used.

Complications

Miscarriage and infertility can occur. Endometriomas are encapsulated implants attached to the ovaries that become cysts. Gastritis that may be treated with H_2-blockers is seen frequently (Craighill, 1998).

Prognosis and Prevention

Endometriosis is a chronic disease, and remission and exacerbation are to be expected. Stressful events often cause exacerbation. The goals of treatment are to control pain and prevent infertility. The patient should be counseled to plan for pregnancy at an early age.

Dysfunctional Uterine Bleeding

Description

Dysfunctional uterine bleeding (DUB) refers to abnormal menstrual bleeding that is excessive, prolonged, or unpatterned (Table 36-4). The bleeding is unrelated to structural or systemic disease and commonly occurs during anovulation. DUB is a diagnosis of exclusion, so any other causes of pathology must first be ruled out. DUB can be classified as mild, moderate, or severe based on hemoglobin level, duration of cycle, and quantity of bleeding.

Etiology and Incidence

The mechanism of DUB appears to be a delay in the maturation of the negative feedback cycle and is not related to structural pathology or medical illness (Emans et al., 1998). Estrogen production continues without the balancing decrease in FSH, which would suppress estrogen: this results in abnormal endometrial thickening. The abnormal endometrium then sheds in a disorderly manner manifested by heavy, irregular, and/or prolonged bleeding. There is great variation in what is considered to be a normal mensis, especially in adolescents. Normal can range from 21 to 45 days between periods, with duration of flow from 3 to 7 days and 30 to

TABLE 36-4

Types of Dysfunctional Uterine Bleeding

Oligomenorrhea: More than 35 days between menses or 4–9 periods per year
Polymenorrhea: Less than 21 days between menses
Menorrhagia: Excessive flow or duration of menses
Metorrhagia: Irregular frequency of cycles with bleeding in between cycles
Menometorrhagia: Excessive amount of bleeding with irregular frequency
Amenorrhea: Absence of bleeding

40 ml of blood loss (10 to 15 soaked tampons or pads) per cycle. Periods that last longer than 8 to 10 days or blood loss in excess of 80 ml are considered excessive (Emans et al., 1998).

Anovulation is the most common cause of DUB and occurs in approximately 50% of females in the first 2 years of their menstrual cycles. However, up to 33% of adolescents can have anovulatory cycles in the fifth year after menarche (Hillard, 1995). Adolescents with sustained anovulation (e.g., eating disorders, weight fluctuations, competitive athletes, chronic illness, or endocrine disease) have an increased incidence of DUB. Anovulation can also be due to stress or illness, thus appearing in adolescents after several years of regular cycles. DUB persists for up to 2 years in 60% of patients, 4 years in 50%, and 10 years in 30% (Emans et al., 1998; Mehring, 1997; Polaneczky & Slap, 1992b).

Clinical Findings

HISTORY. The history should assess the following:

- Family history of bleeding disorders or dyscrasias, thyroid dysfunction, diabetes mellitus, or DES exposure
- Menstrual history: onset, pattern, duration, quantity and color; last menstrual period; breakthrough bleeding; dysmenorrhea; number of tampons, pads, or sponges used
- Sexual activity and contraception used
- Previous infection or STDs
- Galactorrhea, hirsutism (endocrine disease), or other chronic disease
- Bleeding gums, nosebleeds, bruises, hemorrhage (bleeding disorders)
- Recent stressors, athletic events, medications, or illicit drug use
- Weight, eating patterns, and weight fluctuations
- Genital trauma

PHYSICAL EXAMINATION. The physical examination should include the following:

- Height, weight, body type, blood pressure, and fat distribution
- Observation for acne, hirsutism, clitoromegaly (evidence of androgen excess)

- Thyroid palpation
- Observation for petechiae, bruising, pale color
- Breast examination for galactorrhea
- Abdominal examination for mass or tenderness
- Pelvic examination, including digital examination for foreign bodies (e.g., missed tampon)
- Bimanual and rectoabdominal examination

LABORATORY STUDIES. The following are ordered as indicated:

- Pregnancy test
- Complete blood count (CBC) with differential, platelet count, reticulocyte count
- Sedimentation rate (if infection or inflammation is suspected)
- Coagulation studies: prothrombin time, partial thromboplastin time, bleeding time (if bleeding disorder is suspected)
- Thyroid function test, blood sugar, prolactin level (if systemic disease is suspected)
- Wet preparations and culture for gonorrhea, chlamydia, *Trichomonas* if patient is sexually active
- Pap smear if patient is pregnant
- Ultrasonogram of pelvis if mass is palpated, anomaly is suspected, bimanual examination cannot be completed, or condition is unresponsive to treatment

Differential Diagnosis

The differential diagnosis includes pregnancy or pregnancy-related complications (postabortion, ectopic pregnancy); stress; excessive participation in athletics; eating disorders including obesity; drug use; systemic diseases such as blood dyscrasias (20% of patients with coagulation defects have excessive menstrual bleeding); infection (e.g., STDs or PID); trauma including forceful intercourse or rape; foreign bodies including intrauterine device; tumors; anomalies; endometriosis; endocrine disorders (e.g., thyroid disorder, diabetes mellitus); debilitating or chronic diseases (especially hepatic or renal diseases); reproductive tract disorders; medications or irregular use of oral contraceptives, progesterone implants (Mehring, 1997; Hillard, 1995; Pinsonneault, 1993).

Management

The goals in managing DUB include controlling bleeding, preventing endometrial hyperplasia, preventing and treating anemia, restoring quality of life, and preventing recurrence.

1. Mild DUB: a shortened cycle or menses longer than normal with flow slightly to moderately increased or unpredictable; hemoglobin greater than 12 g/dl:
   - Observe and reassure.
   - Have patient start and maintain a menstrual calendar.
   - Prescribe iron supplementation to prevent anemia.
   - Use prostaglandin inhibitors to reduce heavy bleeding (see Table 36–3).
   - Consider OCs for 3 to 4 months to decrease menorrhagia and stabilize menses (see Chapter 20).
   - Reevaluate every 3 months.
2. Moderate DUB: shortened (1 to 3 weeks), irregular cycle with moderate to heavy bleeding, hemoglobin between 10 and 12 g/dl:
   - Prescribe OCs, initially 35 to 50 µg monophasic, subsequently mono- or triphasic for 3 to 6 cycles.
   - Alternatively, prescribe a progestin such as medroxyprogesterone acetate (5 to 10 mg every day for 10 to 14 days started on the 14th day of cycle for 1 to 2 months).
   - Have patient start and maintain a menstrual calendar.
   - Prescribe iron supplementation with 1 mg folic acid.
   - Reevaluate at least monthly until condition is stable.
   - Reassess after 6 months. If contraception is not needed, a trial of medication can be made.
3. Severe DUB: irregular, prolonged, heavy bleeding; hemoglobin less than 10 g/dl:
   - Hospitalize if actively bleeding; treatment may include transfusion, intravenous (IV) hormonal therapy, and dilatation and curettage.

- Manage as moderate DUB if not actively bleeding.

Complications

Anemia, profuse bleeding, shock, and side effects of OCs can occur. A long history of anovulatory cycles and DUB increases the risk of infertility and endometrial carcinoma.

Patient Education and Prognosis

Encourage teen to keep a calendar of bleeding days and amounts. This includes keeping track of the number of pads or tampons used in order to increase accuracy. If medroxyprogesterone is prescribed, know that depression is a side effect and be alert for signs. Prognosis is excellent if DUB is due to anovulation following onset of menses.

Amenorrhea

Description

Amenorrhea is lack of menstruation and is described as either primary or secondary. Primary amenorrhea is defined as any one of the following (Prose et al., 1998; Emans et al., 1998; Braverman & Sondheimer, 1997; Gidwani, 1997; Polaneczky & Slap, 1992a):

- Absence of menarche by 16 years of age with normal pubertal growth and development
- Absence of any pubertal development (breast budding is initial sign in most females) by 13 years of age (14 years if thin, chronically ill, or athlete)
- Absence of menarche 2 to 3 years after beginning puberty, especially if Tanner stage 4 or 5
- Absence of menarche 1 year after age of onset in other female family members (Committee on Sports Medicine, 1989)

Secondary amenorrhea (also called postmenarchal amenorrhea) is defined as the absence of menstruation for at least three cycles or more than 6 months in females who have an established menstrual pattern.

Etiology and Incidence

There are multiple etiologies for primary and secondary amenorrhea. Conditions to be considered include pregnancy; hormonal contraception; immature HPO axis; eating disorders including anorexia nervosa, obesity, and weight fluctuations; poor nutrition; stress; systemic illness (diabetes mellitus, hypothyroidism, tuberculosis); STD; medications; smoking more than one pack of cigarettes per day; extreme exercise; central nervous system, endocrine, or genetic disorders; or structural abnormalities of the genital tract. Risk factors specific for secondary amenorrhea include binging and purging, weight loss or weight gain of more than 4.5 kg, or both weight loss and gain, smoking more than one pack of cigarettes per day, and being less than 1 year postmenarche (Emans et al., 1998).

Primary amenorrhea is uncommon (<3 in 100 females) and is often due to simple constitutional delay (Emans et al., 1998; Blythe et al., 1991) or Turner syndrome. The two most common causes of secondary amenorrhea are pregnancy and stress, with changes in environment, changes in weight, and eating disorders being the next most common (Emans et al., 1998; Castiglia, 1996).

Clinical Findings

HISTORY. The history should assess the following:

Primary Amenorrhea
- Maternal and sibling age of menarche
- Any prenatal exposure to hormones
- Pubertal development
- Chronic systemic disease or illness or previous surgery, radiation, or chemotherapy
- Nutrition, including eating habits, dieting, weight fluctuations
- Exercise patterns, including amount and intensity, level of participation, weigh-ins, or standards for weight that must be kept
- Family history of genetic abnormalities

Secondary Amenorrhea
- Family history of menstrual irregularities, miscarriage, eating disorders, diabetes, or thyroid disease

- Menstrual calendar (last menses, number and pattern of cycles, age at menarche)
- Sexual activity, contraceptive use
- Stress, recent change in environment, or depression
- Nutrition, including caloric intake, weight fluctuation, dieting, or any eating disorder
- Exercise patterns; amount, intensity, involvement in competitive athletics; stress fractures
- Systemic or chronic illness
- Bowel patterns or abdominal pain
- Headache or visual change
- Galactorrhea, hirsutism, acne
- Medication or drug use (contraceptives, phenothiazines, antihypertensives) or illicit drug use

PHYSICAL EXAMINATION. The physical examination should include the following:

Primary Amenorrhea
- Height, weight, nutritional status, blood pressure
- Sexual maturation rating
- Complete neurological examination including smell, funduscopic examination, and visual fields
- Midline facial defects or other congenital anomalies or stigmata of Turner syndrome
- Palpation of thyroid, dry skin, pitted nails
- Breast examination with attempt to elicit galactorrhea (elevated prolactin)
- Palpation of abdomen and groin for masses
- Examination of skin, hair, and genitalia for signs of virilization
- External genital examination for estrogenization of vaginal mucosa (indicates ovarian function), vaginal and hymenal patency, and clitoromegaly (androgen excess)
- Digital vaginal examination and speculum examination if any abnormality is suspected
- Bimanual examination

Secondary Amenorrhea
- Height, weight, body habitus, blood pressure, and pulse
- Sexual maturity rating
- Cachexia, lanugo, parotid enlargement, bradycardia, hypotension, hypothermia (anorexia nervosa)

- Funduscopic examination, gross visual fields, cranial nerves (pituitary lesion)
- Palpation for thyroid gland
- Breast examination with attempt to elicit galactorrhea
- Observation for hirsutism (thorax, midline, inner abdomen), severe acne, obesity, and clitoromegaly (androgen excess)
- Palpation for abdominal tenderness or mass (pregnancy)
- Rectal examination for fissure, fistula, skin tags, or occult blood
- Pelvic examination, and bimanual and rectovaginal examination to evaluate size of the uterus and to screen for masses

LABORATORY STUDIES. The following may be indicated. See text for specific indications.

- Pregnancy test
- Smear for vaginal estrogenization
- Thyroid function studies
- Serum prolactin (elevated in pituitary adenoma)
- LH, FSH (elevated in ovarian failure), estradiol
- Chromosomes by buccal smear (Turner syndrome most common)
- DHEA-S (dehydroepiandrosterone sulfate), testosterone, and 17-hydroxyprogesterone if there are signs of androgen excess
- Assessment of body fat percentage
- Bone age (marked delay equals less than 75% chronological age)
- Ultrasound (to determine normal anatomy)
- Magnetic resonance imaging (MRI) or computed tomography (CT) scan (intracranial lesion)

Differential Diagnosis

Table 36–5 lists the differential diagnosis of primary amenorrhea. An important marker of hypogonadotropic hypogonadism is the female athlete triad of amenorrhea, eating disorder, and osteoporosis (American College of Sports Medicine, 1992; Nattiv & Lynch, 1994; Emans et al., 1998). Especially common in gymnasts, figure skaters, ballet dancers, and long distance runners at elite or highly competitive levels, amenorrhea may first be noted with stress fractures or skeletal problems.

T A B L E 36-5

Differential Diagnosis of Primary Amenorrhea

AMENORRHEA WITH DELAYED PUBERTAL DEVELOPMENT

Hypergonadotropic hypogonadism due to ovarian failure causes hypoestrogenic state, e.g., Turner syndrome or XY gonadal dysgenesis. Elevated follicle-stimulating hormone (FSH) is almost diagnostic. Elevated luteinizing hormone (LH) and low estradiol are also present.

Hypogonadotropic hypogonadism (or hypothalamic amenorrhea) due to dysfunction at level of hypothalamus (tumor or syndrome) or pituitary gland or other endocrinopathies (chronic disease, undernutrition). Normal to low LH, FSH, and estradiol.

AMENORRHEA WITH NORMAL PUBERTAL DEVELOPMENT

Pregnancy, acquired abnormality of ovaries or pituitary (e.g., chemotherapy), thyroid disease, hypothalamic suppression (stress, athletic, eating disorder, chronic or systemic illness, hormonal contraception).

GENITAL TRACT ABNORMALITY

Agenesis, imperforate hymen, obstruction, testicular feminization (androgen insensitivity).

AMENORRHEA WITH VIRILIZATION OR HYPERANDROGENIC ANOVULATION

Polycystic ovary syndrome, late-onset congenital adrenocortical hyperplasia, tumor.

In secondary amenorrhea, the differential diagnosis includes pregnancy; stress or change in environment; weight fluctuations, including obesity, eating disorders, inadequate nutrition or low body fat, excessive exercise, or involvement in competitive sports; cigarette smoking; hypothyroidism; pituitary adenoma; irregular OC use; chronic illness; or drug use. With signs of androgen excess, polycystic ovarian syndrome, ovarian tumors, congenital adrenal hyperplasia, adrenal tumors, and Cushing syndrome are possibilities.

Management

Goals in assessing amenorrhea include ruling out pregnancy, thyroid disease, and prolactin-secreting adenomas; distinguishing hypo- from hypergonadotropic conditions; and determining estrogen status. If physical examination reveals absent or abnormal vagina or uterus, checking karyotype and testosterone should be the first step with referral based upon findings. If genital examination is normal, proceed as follows and in Figure 36–5:

Primary Amenorrhea

- If growth and pubertal development are normal, educate, reassure, and follow-up (Blythe et al., 1991).

- If any of the criteria listed in the definition of amenorrhea are met, initiate workup by reviewing growth charts, checking thyroid-stimulating hormone (TSH), FSH, and LH levels, vaginal estrogenization, and possibly a CBC, sedimentation rate, and blood chemistry panel. Bone age radiographs, a prolactin level, and a thyroid level may be ordered if central cause is suspected.

- If FSH and LH levels are elevated, proceed with karyotype determination. Once results are known, appropriate specialty care or consultation can be sought.

- If FSH and LH levels are low to normal, exclude systemic disease, poor nutrition, central nervous system disorder, or other endocrinopathy. Seeking consultation at this point is appropriate.

Secondary Amenorrhea

- When considering whom to evaluate, the following guidelines may be helpful: abrupt cessation of menses for 4 months after regular cycles have begun; persistent oligomenorrhea after 2 years; persistent amenorrhea 6 months after OC use or 12 months after Depo-Provera; if there is no obvious cause; or if any signs of estrogen deficiency or androgen excess are present (Emans et al., 1998) (see Fig. 36–4).

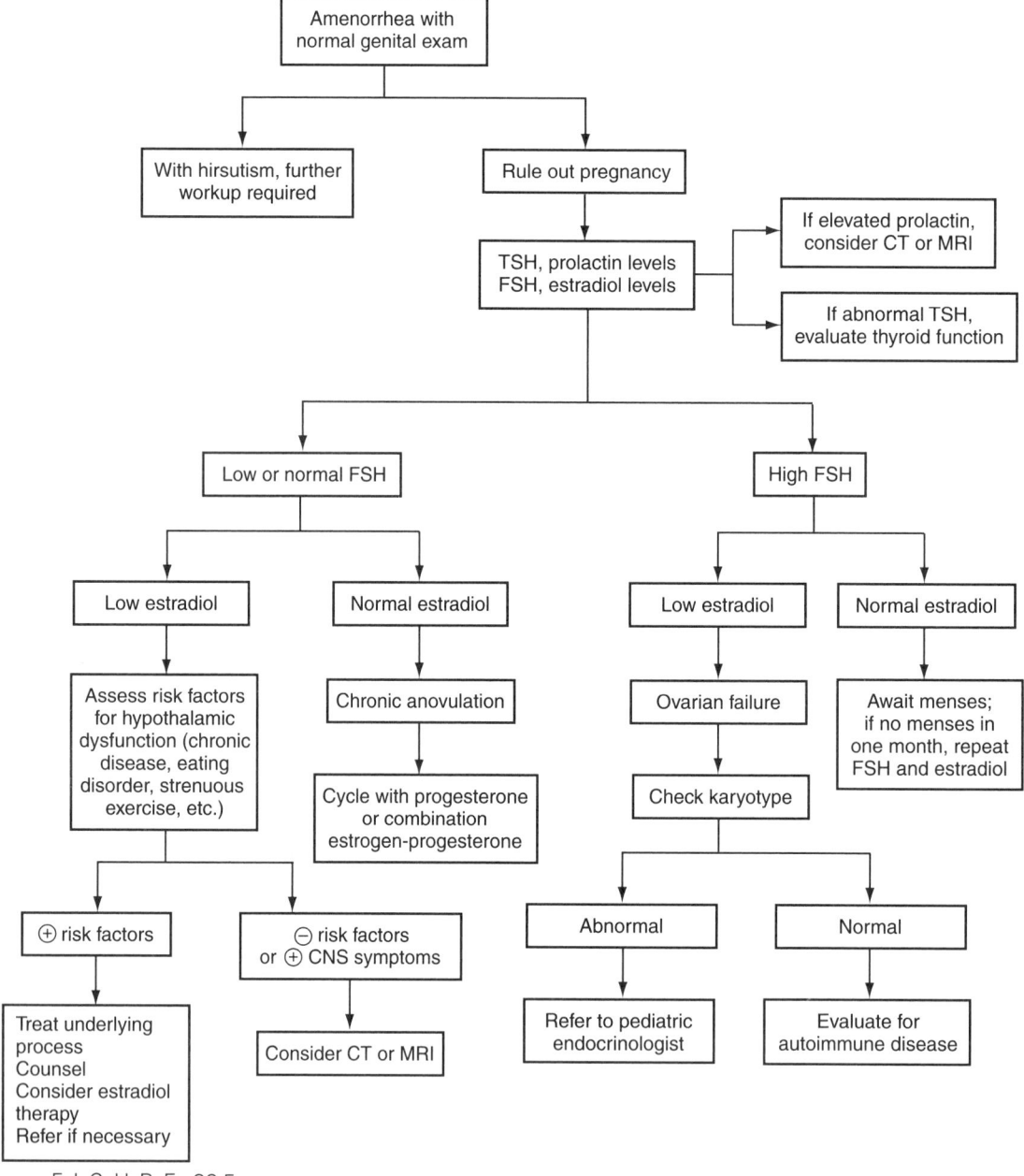

F I G U R E 36-5
Evaluation of amenorrhea with a normal genital tract. TSH = thyroid-stimulating hormone; FSH = follicle stimulating hormone; CNS = central nervous system. (From Prose C, Ford C, Lovely L: Evaluating amenorrhea: The pediatrician's role. Contemp Pediatr 15:106, 1998.)

- Performing a pregnancy test should be the initial evaluation. Some recommend measuring T4, TSH, prolactin level, FSH, and estradiol level at this point; others recommend a progesterone challenge first.
- If pregnancy test is negative, a progesterone challenge is done with medroxyprogesterone (10 mg every day for 5 to 10 days, or 50 to 100 mg progesterone in oil intramuscularly one time). This indicates adequate ovarian production of estrogen to produce an endometrium. A smear for vaginal estrogenization can also be done at this time.
  - ○ If withdrawal bleeding occurs within 7 to 10 days, a normal HPO axis and estrogen-primed uterus can be assumed; amenorrhea is secondary to anovulatory cycles: (1) Cycle with medroxyprogesterone acetate (10 mg every day for 14 days) every 6 weeks to 3 months as needed to reduce risk from endometrial hyperplasia; (2) if menses have been present for more than 3 years, treatment with OCs or Depo-Provera (100 mg intramuscularly every 3 months) is recommended, because normal ovulatory cycles should already be established; (3) if oligomenorrhea is persistent, measure FSH, LH, prolactin, TSH levels. Consider androgen levels (testosterone, free T, DHEA-S). Refer as indicated.
  - ○ If there is no withdrawal bleeding, measure TSH, LH, FSH, estradiol, and prolactin levels if not done previously (see Fig. 36-4): (1) If FSH level is high and estradiol is low, do karotype (most likely causes of elevated FSH level are genetic or iatrogenic; e.g., chemotherapy, or radiation). (2) If FSH is low to normal, follow diagram and seek consultation as indicated.
- Counseling regarding diet and exercise should be geared to the individual. Some authorities recommend estrogen supplementation (e.g., hormonal contraceptive) if the athlete is older than 16 years and is 3 years beyond menarche. Dietary considerations include calcium supplementation to 1500 mg per day and increased protein.

The possibility of decrease in the intensity of exercise should also be considered.

Vulvovaginitis and Vaginal Discharge

Description

Vulvovaginitis refers to inflammation, often with discharge, from infection or irritating substances. Vulvitis alone refers to erythema and pruritus; vaginitis refers to discharge with pruritus and irritation that may be secondary to the vulvitis.

Etiology and Incidence

Age is important in differentiating the etiology of vulvovaginitis. In prepubescent children, several factors make vulvovaginitis a common problem. The lack of estrogen stimulation leaves the vulvar skin thin, the vaginal mucosa atrophic, and minimal vaginal secretions with neutral pH. At puberty, the pH changes from 7 to 4.5, vaginal mucosa thickens, acidogenic bacteria predominate, and lactobacillus stabilizes the environment, all offering protection from infection. The lack of pubic hair and labial fat pads diminish barrier protection, and the proximity of the vaginal opening to the anus predisposes prepubertal females to irritation and infection of the vulva and vagina. Poor hygiene, including wiping technique and lack of handwashing, and irritants such as bubble bath, soaps, sand from playtime, or tight-fitting clothing provide additional insults. Prepubescent vulvovaginitis most commonly is nonspecific (up to 80%). Other causes include monilia, foreign bodies (most often toilet paper), bacterial infection (often group A β-hemolytic *Streptococcus*) or pinworms (Emans et al., 1998; Barron, 1998; Megglio, 1998; Dodds, 1997; Farrington, 1997; Boynton et al., 1994; Smith & Lohr 1993).

Adolescent vulvovaginitis is most often due to a specific cause, often secondary to sexual contact. Normal physiological leukorrhea occurs 6 to 12 months before puberty. *Monilia*, group A β-hemolytic streptococci or other infections, foreign bodies (most often a tampon), and pinworms are possible causes. Bacterial vaginosis (Selleck, 1997), *Trichomonas*, or other STDs (discussed later in this chapter) must also be considered. Up to one half of female gynecological complaints are related to vulvovaginitis, with bacterial vaginosis, candida, *Trichomonas*, or mixed infections being the most common (Preminger & Pokorny, 1998).

Clinical Findings

The clinical findings pertaining to vaginitis are found in Table 36-6.

HISTORY. The history can include the following:

Prepubertal Child and Adolescent
- Previous occurences and treatment used
- Genital irritation, itching, pain, and inflammation
- Vaginal discharge—note onset, quantity, color, type (bloody, mucoid), odor, consistency, and duration
- Urinary complaints, including dysuria and enuresis
- Recent medications, especially antibiotics
- Perineal hygiene or anal pruritus
- Underlying illnesses (e.g., *Streptococcus* infection, dermatosis, diabetes, immunosuppression)
- Possible trauma, foreign body, or sexual abuse

Prepubertal Child
- Use of harsh soaps or bubble baths
- Tight-fitting or nylon underwear or clothing
- Nighttime perianal itching

Adolescent
- Menstrual and sexual history
- Exposures to STDs
- Use of contraception

PHYSICAL EXAMINATION. A good light and magnifying glass may aid in the physical examination. Prepubertal examination includes inspection, possible vaginal otoscopy in frog-leg or knee-chest position, and rectal examination. Adolescent examination may also include pelvic and bimanual examination. See Table 36-6 for physical examination findings.

LABORATORY STUDIES. The following should be considered:

- Urinalysis for WBCs, yeast, or trichomonads
- pH of vaginal secretions
- Wet preparation with saline for WBCs; pseudohyphae or yeast buds; motile, pear-shaped, flagellated clue cells or epithelial cells sprinkled with bacteria; bacteria; wet preparation with 10% KOH for whiff test and better visualization of monilia (branching pseudohyphae and spores)
- Gram's stain
- Rapid antibody tests for *Streptococcus* or *Trichomonas*
- Culture of *Monilia*, *Streptococcus*, or *Trichomonas*
- Pinworm eggs visualized on tape slide under microscope
- Papanicolaou smear

Differential Diagnosis

Atopic dermatitis, psoriasis, seborrhea, or other dermatosis; labial adhesions; polyps or tumors; systemic diseases such as Kawasaki or Crohn; other STDs; and sexual abuse are included in the differential diagnosis.

Management

General treatment measures for any type of vulvovaginitis are listed in Table 36-7. Specific recommendations include:

1. Prepubertal nonspecific etiology
   - If persistent, prescribe antibacterial cream at night (e.g., Bactroban, Sultrin, or clindamycin) for 2 weeks.
   - If persistent after 3 weeks, rule out pinworms, then prescribe a trial of amoxicillin, Augmentin, or one of the cephalosporins.
   - If symptoms still persist, prescribe estrogen cream at bedtime for 2 to 3 weeks, then every other night at bedtime for 2 weeks to thicken vulvar epithelium.
   - If recurrent vulvovaginitis appears, a 1- to 2-month course of low-dose cephalexin or trimethoprim–sulfamethoxazole (TMS/SMX) at bedtime should be tried.

- If a specific infection is found, treat as outlined herein or refer to appropriate section.
- If therapy fails, refer to a gynecologist.
- If an STD is found in a child, a complete workup for sexual abuse is indicated.
2. Contact dermatitis
   - Topical steroids and hormonal cream can be used to thicken vaginal skin and minimize irritation.
3. Foreign body
   - Prepubertal: irrigate with warm normal saline with a small feeding tube at the hymenal opening with the child seated over a pan.
   - Adolescent: do a pelvic examination followed by irrigation and cultures as indicated.
   - A broad-spectrum antibiotic, such as amoxicillin or a cephalosporin, may be indicated if infection is apparent.
4. Bacterial infection
   - Obtain cultures and prescribe appropriate treatment: (1) penicillin (125 to 250 mg in three or four divided doses for 10 days) *or* (2) erythromycin (30 to 50 mg/kg per day in three or four divided doses for 10 days).
5. Monilial infection
   - There are multiple preparations, but the "azole" drugs are recommended as being more effective than nystatin. There are many preparations, some obtainable over the counter, in single-dose to 7-day dose cream or suppository (Centers for Disease Control and Prevention, 1998; Emans et al., 1998). For sexually active adolescents, many of these preparations are oil based and may weaken latex condoms or diaphragms.
   - Butoconazole 2% cream (5 g, 1 applicator) intravaginally for 3 days.
   - Clotrimazole 200-mg vaginal tablet for 3 days *or* l00-mg vaginal tablet for 7 days *or* 1% cream (5 g, 1 applicator) intravaginally for 7 to 14 days *or* 500-mg vaginal tablet in single application.
   - Miconazole 200-mg vaginal suppository for 3 days *or* 100-mg vaginal suppository for 7 days *or* 2% cream (5 g, 1 applicator) intravaginally for 7 days.
   - Terconazole 80-mg vaginal suppository for

3 days *or* 0.4% cream for 7 days *or* 0.8% cream for 3 days.
   - Tioconazole 6.5% ointment (5 g, 1 applicator) intravaginally 1 time.
   - Nystatin 100,000-unit vaginal tablet for 14 days.
   - Fluconazole 150 mg orally one time *or* 5.5 mg/kg suspension in single dose.
   - Ketoconazole and itraconazole may be effective treatments, but are avoided because of side effects.
   - Treatment failure or recurrence may occur because of increasing resistance of organisms.
   - If appropriate, evaluate for STDs.
   - Complicated candidal infections (severe local, recurrent in abnormal host) require documentation by culture, workup for predisposing conditions, longer duration of treatment, and treatment of partners.
   - Complementary medicine recommendations include intravaginal garlic for 10 to 12 hours; decreasing foods high in simple carbohydrates; avoiding foods with yeast or mold; increasing fiber, garlic, ginger, cinnamon; live lactobacillus (1 to 2 billion live organisms per day) and acidophilus in diet.
6. Pinworms
   - Mebendazole (100-mg tablet, repeated in 2 weeks).
   - Handwashing is important to minimize the spread of infection.
   - See Chapter 33 for further discussion.
7. Bacterial vaginosis
   - If asymptomatic, treatment is not recommended.
   - If symptomatic, the following drugs are recommended except in pregnancy (Centers for Disease Control and Prevention, 1998): metronidazole 500 mg orally two times a day for 7 days *or* Clindamycin vaginal cream 2% at bedtime for 7 days *or* metronidazole gel 0.75% once or twice a day vaginally 5 days.
   - Treatment of partners is not recommended, but evaluation for other STDs may be indicated.
   - Recurrence is not uncommon.
   - Latex in condoms may be weakened by clindamycin vaginal cream. Abstain from

T A B L E 36-6
Evaluation and Treatment of Vaginitis

	SIGNS AND SYMPTOMS	VAGINAL DISCHARGE	ETIOLOGY	LABORATORY DATA	TREATMENT
Nonspecific vaginitis	Itching burning; dysuria; varied vulvitis	Scant to copious; brown to green; mucoid; foul smelling	Irritation from contact with various substances; poor hygiene	pH variable; no odor on whiff test; micro: leukocytes, bacteria, debris; normal UA	Refractory cases may need topical estrogen or antibiotics
Physiologic leukorrhea	None or minimal itch or burn; minimal vulvitis; 6–12 mo before menarche; small hymenal opening; possible mild erythema	Scant to moderate; clear to white; odorless; nonirritating	Endogenous hormones 6–12 mo before menarche	pH <4.5; no odor on whiff test; micro: epithelial cells, lactobacilli; normal UA	No treatment needed; explain and reassure
Chemical or mechanical	Itch, erythema, vulvar inflammation, dysuria	Scant amount yellow to white	Bubble bath, perfumed soap, lotion; tight-fitting clothes, sand or dirt from playground	pH < 4.5; no odor on whiff test; micro: leukocytes, epithelial cells	Remove irritant; topical steroids
Foreign body	Dysuria, discomfort, bleeding, minimal vulvar excoriation; history of foreign body in other orifices	Purulent, persistent, dark brown, foul smelling (18%), bloody (82%)	Toilet paper (prepubescent); tampons (adolescent); condoms or object used for masturbation	pH > 4.5; odd odor on whiff test; micro: WBCs, epithelial cells with bacteria and debris; UA normal	Remove foreign body with forceps or by irrigating with saline and small feeding tube; knee-chest position may work best
Bacterial	Acute respiratory, enteric or skin infection	Green color, foul, copious with possible bleeding	*Streptococcus* (most common), *Escherichia coli, Enterococcus, Shigella, Staphylococcus* or other bacteria	Strep test positive; culture positive	Penicillin, erythromycin, amoxicillin, broad-spectrum cephalosporin or other antibiotic as indicated

Condition	Symptoms	Discharge	Etiology	Diagnosis	Treatment
Candidiasis	Itching, burning, vulvar inflammation, dysuria, dyspareunia; history of antibiotic or steroid use	Thick, white, curdy cottage cheese adherent, odorless; vulva red, edematous with satellite lesions	Recent antibiotic or steroid use; diabetes or immunodeficiency; *Candida albicans*; pregnancy	pH < 4.5; no odor on whiff test; micro: fungal hyphae and buds or spores; culture positive for *monilia*; UA with WBCs	Imidazoles or triazoles topically or intravaginally; ketoconazole orally
Pinworms	Recent exposure to pinworms; perineal itching especially at night; anal excoriation, erythema and lesions from scratching	No discharge	Enterobius vermicularis spread from anus	Normal UA; tape test reveals eggs	Mebendazole 100 mg once; repeated in 2 weeks; treat family members
Bacterial vaginosis (need 3 of 4* findings to diagnose)	Foul odor, especially after menses or intercourse; often asymptomatic; no inflammation; abdominal pain or irregular, prolonged bleeding	Homogenous, thin milky white discharge adherent* to vaginal walls and pools in posterior fornix; increased amount	*Gardnerella vaginalis* and anerobic bacteria; caused by replacement of normal vaginal flora; may or may not be sexually transmitted	pH > 4.5*: fishy odor on whiff test*; micro: clue cells,* few lactobacilli, gram-negative rods, no WBCs	May resolve without treatment. Treat only if symptomatic with metronidazole for 7 days or clindamycin; increased risk for PID
Trichomonas	Lower abdominal discomfort, dysuria, symptoms worse before and after menses; history of sexual contact; vulvar itching and erythema	White to yellow-grey, frothy, foul odor, profuse, purulent, slightly watery; vaginal mucosa erythematous, cervix friable with petechiae	*Trichomonas vaginalis*, flagellated protozoa, primarily sexually transmitted	pH > 4.5, frequently has fishy odor on whiff test; micro: motile, flagellated organisms, WBC > 10/hpf on UA	Metronidazole for 7–10 days; prepubertal 15 mg/kg in three divided doses or 40 mg/kg in single dose; postpubertal 2 g in single dose

hpf = high-power field; micro = microscopic exam; UA = urinalysis; WBC = white blood cells.

T A B L E 36-7

General Treatment Measures for Vaginitis

1. Hygiene
   • Wipe front to back
   • Change underwear everyday
   • Wash hands frequently
   • Blow dry perineal area with cool to warm air (especially if overweight)
2. Clothing
   • Wear absorbent white underwear, changing once or twice daily; do not wear underwear at night
   • Wear loose clothing—no pantyhose or tight jeans
   • Avoid spandex and sleeper pajamas
   • Change out of swim suit after swimming
3. Comfort and healing measures
   • Take sitz bath with thorough drying
   • Blow dry for 10–15 min once or twice daily with cool to warm air or pat dry with towel
   • Apply hydrocortisone cream 1% once or twice daily for itching
   • Use oral diphenhydramine or hydroxyzine if itching is severe
4. Protective measure
   • Avoid bubble baths and perfumed lotions or powder
   • Use mild soap, e.g., Dove, Basis, Neutrogena
   • Avoid shampoo in bath water
   • Use protective ointment twice a day, e.g., Vaseline, A&D, Aquaphor
   • Avoid bleach or fabric softener in wash, double rinse
   • Urinate with knees spread apart to minimize urinary reflux

consuming alcohol while taking metronidazole.

8. Trichomonas in adolescents
   • Oral metronidazole 2-g dose once *or* 500 mg twice a day for 7 days.
   • Recurrent disease: 500 mg twice a day for 7 days. If repeated failure: 2 g daily for 3 to 5 days.
   • Clotrimazole intravaginal cream may give symptomatic relief.
   • Testing for other STDs is needed; treat sexual partners.
   • Abstinence from sexual activity is required until treatment is complete and partners are asymptomatic. Latex in condoms may be weakened by medications.
   • If prepubertal, workup for sexual abuse is necessary.
   • Abstain from consuming alcohol while taking medication.
9. Gonorrhea or chlamydia in prepubescent children needs to be evaluated and treated as child abuse. See the following section, Chapter 19, and the 1998 *Guidelines for*

Treatment of Sexually Transmitted Diseases (Centers for Disease Prevention and Control, 1998) for more details.

Complications

Labial adhesions can occur. Bacterial vaginosis can contribute to cervical neoplasm, PID, endometritis, postsurgical infection (therapeutic abortion), abnormal Pap results, and pregnancy complications. Trichomonas is associated with adverse pregnancy outcomes, especially premature rupture of membranes and preterm delivery.

Patient Education, Prognosis, and Prevention

• See Table 36-7 for general treatment measures.
• Follow up in 5 days if there is no improvement.
• Recurrence is common, especially with

poor hygiene, in obese girls, and during upper respiratory infection.

- Protective measures for the sexually active adolescent include recommending not using diaphragm or condom until 3 days after treatment with topical vaginal cream or tablet.
- Recommend frequent change of tampons and use of a pad at night.

Sexually Transmitted Diseases

Description

Multiple organisms are responsible for STDs in children and adolescents. Gonorrhea (GC), syphilis, chlamydia, HSV, and human papilloma virus (HPV) are the most common STDs affecting the lower female reproductive tract. *Trichomonas* (discussed in previous section), hepatitis B, and HIV infections also are recognized as STDs. See Chapter 24 for discussion of hepatitis B and HIV (systemic STDs). The term *sexually transmitted infection* is sometimes used to refer to asymptomatic infection. Diagnosis can also be made in terms of the location of the infection (e.g., vaginitis, cervicitis, or urethritis).

STDs are a significant public health problem, placing a heavy financial health burden on society, having a tremendous impact on individuals' lives, and playing an important role in the transmission of HIV. The past 40 years have brought progress in treating STDs, with historic low incidence rates for GC and syphilis. However, the highest STD rates in the industrial world still occur in the United States.

Etiology and Incidence

Considered an epidemic, STDs have the highest rates in adolescents, documented as 3 million of the 12 million reported cases per year or one case in every eight 13- to 19-year olds. Minorities, especially African Americans, are disproportionally affected. More than 1 million teenage girls with STDs become pregnant, raising concerns about perinatal transmission (Centers for Disease Control and Prevention, 1998; Bonny & Biro, 1998).

Factors contributing to this epidemic (Table 36-8) are the increasingly early age and frequency of sexual activity, inconsistent use of contraceptive and protective devices, the physiological characteristics that predispose adolescents to infection, adolescents' lack of access to and use of health care, and societal influences. Another factor that may be increasing the reported numbers of STDs comes with increasing access to treatment, allowing earlier identification.

STDs must be reported, and the NP must be aware of each state's specific rules. All 50 states allow adolescents to be evaluated and to receive treatment for STDs without parental consent. The etiology and incidence for specific

T A B L E 36-8

Risk Factors for Sexually Transmitted Diseases

1. Adolescent younger than 15 years of age
2. Sexually active adolescent, especially with two or more casual partners in 6 months, high frequency of intercourse, or high rate of new partners
3. Use of drugs or alcohol, or other high-risk behaviors
4. Pregnancy or abortion
5. Homosexual
6. Victim of abuse, rape, or incest
7. Incarcerated, runaway, homeless, in group shelter or detention home
8. Clients in sexually transmitted disease (STD) clinics or with any other STD or previous history of STD
9. Lack of family availability; low level of parental support and monitoring
10. Beliefs about normative behaviors among peers
11. Inappropriate health-care behaviors (e.g., not seeking medical care, not adhering to treatment regimen, failure to recognize symptoms, delay in notifying partners, nonuse of barrier contraceptive)

Data from Biro FM, Rosenthal SL: Adolescent STDs: Diagnosis, developmental issues, and prevention. J Pediatr Health Care 9:256–262, 1995; Bonny AE, Biro FM: Recognizing & treating STDs in adolescent girls. Contemp Pediatr 15:119–143, 1998; Emans S, Lauter MR, Goldstein D: Pediatric and adolescent gynecology, 4th ed. Philadelphia, Lippincott-Raven, 1998.

STDs follow (Centers for Disease Control and Prevention, 1998; Bonny & Biro, 1998; Sung & MacDonald, 1998a & 1998b; Emans et al., 1998; Darville, 1998; American Academy of Pediatrics, 1997; Patel, 1998; Coles & Hipp, 1996):

- Gonorrhea, caused by *Neisseria gonorrhoeae*, a nonmotile, gram-negative diplococcus, is often found in carriage with chlamydia. Incidence was 150 per 100,000 in 1995. This represented a declining rate, but less so for adolescents; the highest rate occurred in the 15- to 19-year-old group. GC is reportable in every state. It can progress to PID and persists perinatally up to 6 months. There are more reported cases of GC in African Americans (40:1) compared with Caucasians.
- Syphilis, caused by *Treponema pallidum*, is a spirochete with a declining rate of infection (26.5 per 100,000 in 1995). The highest rate occurs in adolescents, inhabitants of the southern United States, and blacks (12:1) compared with Caucasians. It is reportable in every state. Co-infection with HIV exists in up to 15% of cases.
- *C. trachomatis* infection is the most frequently reported infectious disease and the most common STD, with 4 million new cases per year. Chlamydia is present in 8 to 40% of sexually active teenage females. Adolescent patients aged 15 to 19 years old have 46% of chamydial infections, whereas 20- 24-year-olds represent 33%. Chlamydia is reportable in many states and in *all* prepubescent children. It persists up to 3 years perinatally and can progress to PID. Even with treatment of reported partners, reinfection is common.
- HSV types 1 and 2 are DNA viruses. There are 200,000 to 500,000 new cases per year with a 2–3:1 black to white occurrence. A 30% increase has been reported over the past 20 years, especially in white adolescents (one in five are infected with HSV-2). About 20% of all adolescents are infected with HSV-2. Type 2 is reportable in prepubescent children in some states.
- HPV is a small DNA virus. A wart visible on inspection is called a condyloma acuminatum, whereas subclinical infection is condyloma planum. Twenty of the 70 different types infect the genital tract. HPV-6 and -11 cause visible warts; types 16, 18, 31, 33, and 35 cause anogenital warts. The highest rates of HPV are in teenagers, affecting 15 to 38% of adolescent females. Eleven percent of HPV infections are detected by virapap and 1% by gross visualization. They are a significant finding because of their link to cervical cancer.

Clinical Findings

HISTORY. The history should assess the following:

- Type of sexual activity (including oral, vaginal, anal) and contraceptive use.
- Number of sexual partners over 60 days, 12 months, and lifetime; heterosexual and/or homosexual activity.
- Known exposure or previous STDs.
- Use of drugs or alcohol.
- Chapter 20 for further details on obtaining history

Many patients are asymptomatic. The following can be reported:

- Vaginal: discharge (amount, color, odor), pruritus, irregular or painful bleeding, dysmenorrhea, dyspareunia.
- Urinary: dysuria, urgency, frequency.
- Abdominal or pelvic pain.
- Skin rashes or lesions, ulcers, warts (Clayton & Krowchuk 1997).
- Systemic symptoms: fever, malaise, headache.
- See Table 36–8 for risk factors for STDs

PHYSICAL EXAMINATION. The physical examination should include the following:

- General examination—skin rashes and lesions, lymphadenopathy. If there is a question about whether a lesion is HPV, wetting the lesion with acetic acid turns it white.
- Abdominal examination—hepatic or splenic enlargement or tenderness in right upper quadrant.
- Pelvic examination—inspection of external genitalia and vaginal mucosa, vaginal pH and discharge, cervical erythema, friability

and mucopus, bimanual examination for motion tenderness, uterine size, adnexal tenderness.

- Rectal examination.
- Colposcopy of cervix, vagina, and vulva—recommended on all patients with evidence of HPV infection or any suspicion of sexual abuse.

LABORATORY STUDIES. In deciding the types of studies to order, the NP needs to know the difference in types and accuracy of tests. Methods that are sufficiently accurate for adolescents (presumptive tests) are not for children who are being evaluated for possible abuse and who need definitive tests (Emans et al., 1998; Judson & Ehret, 1994).

- Gonorrhea. Both Gram stain of vaginal discharge that shows gram-negative diplococci in polymorphonuclear leukocytes and culture on selective media with determination of penicillin resistance are definitive tests for gonorrhea. Rapid tests such as DFA, EIA, or DNA probes may be used in adolescents but are not used in children. Culture, including swabs from rectum and pharynx, should be done if abuse is suspected.
- Syphilis. Direct visualization with dark-field microscopy or DFA test is definitive. Serological nontreponemal tests (VDRL, RPR, or automated reagin test) correlate with disease activity, decline after treatment, and are used to monitor disease progress. Treponemal tests (FTA-ABS or MHA-TP) are confirmatory, but once positive, they usually remain so for years.
- Chlamydia. Culture is the only acceptable method to diagnose possible sexual abuse cases; DFA, EIA, or DNA probes are acceptable in adolescents, especially in high prevalence populations. PCR, LCR, and transcription-mediated amplification are more sensitive than culture but are not always available.
- Herpes. Culture of scraped vesicle or ulcer is most accurate. Tzanck stain, DFA, and EIA are quicker but less sensitive. Blood tests are being studied but are not routinely used because they are not readily available.

- Human papillomavirus. Virapap is the specific test. Pap smear can show koilocytosis; dysplasia, atypia, or cervical intraepithelial neoplasia is suspicious. Biopsy for histological and cytological microscopic evaluation and typing by DNA hybridization are more specific but rarely needed.

Differential Diagnosis

Chancroid, lymphogranuloma venereum, cytomegalovirus, hepatitis, granuloma inguinale, and molluscum are included in the differential diagnosis.

Management

The guidelines identified in this section are those recommended by the American Academy of Pediatrics Committee on Infectious Diseases (1997) and the Centers for Disease Control and Prevention *1998 Guidelines for Treatment of Sexually Transmitted Diseases* (1998) for uncomplicated, initial treatment of STDs. Other recommendations and options for children weighing less than 45 kg and for recurrent and complex cases can also be found in this literature or in adolescent gynecology or child abuse literature.

The goals of treatment include making a prompt diagnosis, determining the mode of acquisition, instituting appropriate treatment, preventing complications, contacting appropriate authorities, ensuring appropriate follow-up, and educating the adolescent and partner about risk reduction. All adolescents in the United States can consent to confidential diagnosis and treatment of STDs.

Several options for treatment are given for each disease (see Table 36–9). When determining appropriate treatment, consideration should be given to the site of infection, the resistance patterns in the community, concurrent infections, side effects of the medication, and cost. See Table 36–10 for general treatment measures for STDs.

1. Gonorrhea (uncomplicated, patient >45 kg)

   - Prescribe ceftriaxone 125 mg intramuscularly one time *or* cefixime 400 mg orally one time *or* ciprofloxacin 500 mg orally

T A B L E 36-9
Evaluation and Treatment of Sexually Transmitted Disease

	HISTORY	PHYSICAL EXAMINATION	ETIOLOGY	LABORATORY DATA	TREATMENT (See Table 36–10 and text for alternative medication)
Gonorrhea (GC)	Often asymptomatic (33%); dysuria; vaginal discharge or bleeding; dyspareunia	Profuse, thick, green discharge, urethritis, cervicitis; Skene's or Bartholin's gland abscess; exudative pharyngitis	*Neisseria gonorrhoeae*; gram-negative diplococcus; often co-infected with chlamydia (15–20%) and other sexually transmitted diseases (STDs)	Gram's stain; culture; DNA probe for adolescent; rectal and pharyngeal swab if abuse suspected	Ceftriaxone 125 mg (IM) *plus* doxycycline 100 mg b.i.d. for 7 days; treat also for chlamydia; test for other STDs including HIV and hepatitis B; report to state health
Chlamydia	Often is asymptomatic (30–70%); spotting, vaginal discharge; dysuria, pyuria; mild abdominal pain or foreign body sensation in eyes possible	Clear to white or yellow discharge, mucopurulent cervicitis with edema, erythema, hypertrophy; Fitz-Hugh-Curtis syndrome (right upper quadrant pain); conjunctivitis	*Chlamydia trachomatis*; often co-infected with (GC) and other STDs; autoinoculation of eyes	Cell cultures; DNA probe in adolescent especially if part of high-prevalence population; direct fluorescent antibody (DFA) or enzyme immunoassays (EIA), polymerase chain reaction (PCR) or LCR, or TMA	Doxycycline 100 mg b.i.d. for 7 days *or* azithromycin 1 g single dose; test for other STDs; report to state health

Disease	Signs and symptoms	Etiology	Diagnosis	Treatment
Syphilis	*Primary:* vaginal, anal, or oral chancre. *Secondary:* copper-penny rash especially on palms and soles, adenopathy, alopecia	Single painless papule with serous discharge, smooth base, raised edges; painless regional lymphadenopathy	*Treponema pallidum*, a motile spirochete	Dark-field microscopy, DFA; nontreponemal tests; venereal disease research laboratory (VDRL), rapid plasma reagin (RPR), automated reagin test (ART) to follow disease activity; treponemal tests: fluorescent treponemal antibody resorption (FTA-ABS), microhemagglutination assay *Treponema pallidum* (MHA-TP) to confirm	Penicillin G IM 2.4 million units; refer if secondary to tertiary disease; follow with nontreponemal tests every 6–12 mo; test for other STDs; report to state health
Herpes simplex (HSV)	Painful rash, blisters and ulcers; HSV-1 of mouth and face; burning and irritation 24 hours before; dysuria; other systemic complaints	Clear to white to yellow discharge; vesicles on erythematous base that become ulcers in 1–3 days; extragenital lesions	HSV types 1 and 2, DNA virus from direct contact	Culture; Tzanck stain or DFA are presumptive	Acyclovir, famciclovir, or valacyclovir for 7–10 days; sitz bath, dry heat, lidocaine jelly 2%; candida often accompanies or follows
Human papilloma virus (HPV)	Asymptomatic or subclinical unrecognized; can be painful	Warts, friable and or pruritic; moist, cauliflower-like anogenital and inguinal 4–6 wk after exposure	Small DNA virus, 20 types can infect genital tract; visible warts: types 6 and 11; anogenital warts: 16, 18, 31, 33, 35	Virapap; Papanicolaou smear (koilocytosis, squamous atypia, squamous intraepithelial lesions); biopsy rarely needed; DNA/PCR screen	*Patient applied:* Podofilox or imiquimod; *Provider applied:* cryotherapy, podophyllin resin, trichloroacetic acid or bichloroacetic acid, or surgical removal

T A B L E 36-10

General Treatment Measures for Sexually Transmitted Diseases

1. Have patient abstain from sexual intercourse until patient and partner are cured (treatment complete and symptoms resolved). Consequences of untreated sexually transmitted diseases (STDs) should be explained.
2. Test for other STDs, including human immunodeficiency virus, bacterial vaginosis, and trichomonas.
3. Notify, examine, and treat all partners of patient for any STD identified or suspected.
4. Report STDs (include gonorrhea and syphilis in every state, and chlamydia in most states). Check with the health department. Reporting to appropriate authorities is important to identify those at risk, recognize new strains, and assess extent of infection in community and the effect of prevention efforts.
5. Provide regular sex health assessment including Papanicolaou smears, vaginal examination, and testing for STDs.
6. Give hepatitis B vaccine if not done already.
7. Discuss safer sex practices including abstinence and use of condoms.
8. Educate and counsel about complications and transmission of STDs as well as perinatal consequences.

one time if patient is older than 10 years *or* ofloxacin 400 mg orally one time if patient is younger than 10 years *or* spectinomycin 2 g IM one time
- *Plus* azithromycin 1 g orally in single dose *or* doxycycline (100 mg orally twice a day for 7 days if patient is older than 9 years).
- Treat for chlamydia, because it is documented in 45% of gonorrhea cases.
- Test for syphilis, chlamydia, HIV, and hepatitis.
- Do culture and sensitivities 2 weeks after treatment if symptoms persist.
- Evaluate and treat all partners in previous 30 to 60 days, and treat last sexual partner if more than 60 days since last intercourse.

2. Syphilis, primary or secondary

- Prescribe benzathine penicillin G 2.4 million units intramuscularly, *or*, if penicillin allergy: (1) doxycycline 100 mg orally twice a day for 14 days, *or* (2) tetracycline 500 mg orally four times a day for 14 days, *or* (3) erythromycin 500 mg orally four times a day for 14 days (less effective, but safe in pregnancy).
- Do follow-up examination and RPR or VDRL at 6 and 12 months. The same laboratory studies and tests should be used. RPR or VDRL should decrease four-fold by 6 months and become nonreactive at 1 year after treatment in primary cases. If still reactive after 12 months, re-evaluate for HIV.
- Treat all partners during symptomatic period and for the 3 months prior to onset of infection.
- An acute febrile reaction (Jarisch-Herxheimer reaction) with myalgia, headache, and other symptoms can occur within 24 hours after treatment.
- Test for GC, chlamydia and HIV at time of infection and in 3 months.
- Refer if symptoms of secondary or tertiary syphilis are present.
- Re-treat if symptoms persist, recur or if non-treponemal titer does not decrease four-fold in 1 year.

3. Chlamydia, uncomplicated genital infection

- Prescribe doxycycline 100 mg orally twice a day for 7 days *or* azithromycin 1 g orally in single dose.
- Alternate medications: (1) erythromycin 500 mg orally four times a day for 7 days, *or* (2) erythromycin ethylsuccinate 800 mg orally four times a day for 7 days, *or* (3) ofloxacin 300 mg orally twice a day for 7 days if patient is 18 years or older.
- Treat last partner, any partner within the 30 days before the onset of symptoms, and any partner within 60 days of asymptomatic index case.
- Test for syphilis, GC, hepatitis, and HIV.
- Do follow-up cultures 3 weeks after treatment only if symptoms persist.

4. Genital herpes. No treatment eradicates the disease. Treatment or prevention of acute outbreaks is the goal of therapy.

- Prescribe acyclovir 200 mg orally five times

daily for 7 to 10 days (primary) or for 5 days (recurrent) *or* acyclovir 400 mg three times a day for 7 to 10 days (primary) or for 5 days (recurrent) *or* famciclovir 250 mg three times a day for 7 to 10 days (primary) or 125 mg twice a day for 5 days (recurrent) *or* valacyclovir 1 g twice a day for 7 to 10 days (primary) or 500 mg twice a day for 5 days (recurrent). (No pediatric data are available on famciclovir and valacyclovir.)

- Use daily *suppressive* treatment if episodes occur 6 times or more in a year. This reduces the frequency of episodes by more than 75%. One of the following is used no more than 1 year: (1) acyclovir 200 mg orally three to five times a day *or* 400 mg twice a day for 6 to 12 months, *or* (2) famciclovir 250 mg orally twice a day, *or* (3) valacyclovir 500 mg once a day *or* 1000 mg once a day.
- Recommend sitz baths, dry heat, and lidocaine jelly 2% for relief.
- Treat candidal vaginitis that often accompanies or follows herpes.
- Test for other STDs as indicated.
- Counsel to abstain from sexual activity when active lesions are present.
- Stress the risk of perinatal infection and follow pregnancies closely.
- Educate regarding course of disease, self-inoculation, transmission, and asymptomatic viral shedding.
- Suggest dietary modifications including increased intake of vitamin C, B-complex and B6 vitamins, zinc, and calcium to boost the immune system. A diet high in lysine and low in arginine (e.g., eating fish, chicken, cheese, most fruits and vegetables, and avoiding chocolate, peanuts, and white and wheat flour) may be helpful (Andrist, 1997).

5. Human papillomavirus. No treatment eradicates this disease. The goal should be to remove visible warts and reduce symptoms. Patient preference and treatment availability should guide treatment course.

- Use 3% to 5% acetic acid (vinegar) on the skin to cause some lesions to blanch (not definitive diagnosis).
- Recommend patient-applied treatment

with (1) podofilox 0.5% solution or gel twice a day for 3 days, no treatment for 4 days, for a total of four cycles (contraindicated in pregnancy) *or* (2) imiquimod 5% cream applied with finger at bedtime three times a week for up to 16 weeks. Wash treated area with mild soap and water 6 to 10 hours after application. Warts should clear after 8 to 10 weeks. Safety in pregnancy is not determined, and there are no published data for adolescents younger than 18 years of age.

- Treat external visible warts with (1) cryotherapy with liquid nitrogen *or* cryoprobe every 1 to 2 weeks, (2) 10% to 25% podophyllin resin in benzoin washed off in 1 to 4 hours to decrease local irritation, repeated weekly (contraindicated in pregnancy), (3) trichloroacetic acid (TCA) or bichloroacetic acid (BCA) applied in small amounts, dried to frosting consistency, followed by powder or baking soda to remove unreacted acid, repeated weekly, or (4) surgical removal with scissor, shave, curette or electrosurgery.
- Change treatment if there is no response after three patient-applied treatments or six provider-applied treatments.
- Use only one treatment modality at a time to avoid increased complications (Centers for Disease Control and Prevention, 1998).
- Advise patient that an inflammatory reaction is common before resolution. After cryotherapy, pain, necrosis, and blistering are common.
- Refer patients with cervical warts, suspected abuse, or extensive lesions in difficult areas for gynecological treatment. Intralesional interferon or laser surgery may be necessary in severe cases.
- Do serological testing for syphilis.
- Perform regular Papanicolaou smears.
- Advise patient that recurrence is common, most often in the first 3 months following treatment.
- Remember that latent perinatal transmission of virus can be present for 1 to 3 years.

Complications

In general, perinatal transmission, disseminated infection, and increased risk for chronic hepatitis are possible. PID, ectopic pregnancy, and infertility are possible sequelae to GC and chlamydia. With each episode of PID, there is an increased risk of infertility (8% with one episode, 19.5% with two, and 40% with three). Tertiary disease is a risk with syphilis. An increased incidence of HIV infection occurs with syphilis and HSV infection. HPV infection is linked with cervical dysplasia.

Patient Education and Prevention

Prevention occurs at a variety of levels and in a variety of ways. The following approaches are recommended (Bonny & Biro, 1998; Stevens-Simon, 1998; Biro & Rosenthal, 1995):

- Primary prevention seeks to reduce the number of new cases of STDs. This best occurs before sexual debut, focusing on delaying initiation of sexual intercourse and avoiding exposure if the intent is to become sexually active. These topics must be addressed specifically, using knowledge, attitudes, and behaviors to guide education. Developmental needs, cultural values, misperceptions, and social skills are areas to be addressed.
- Hepatitis B and possibly hepatitis A immunizations are recommended.
- Secondary prevention seeks to reduce the numbers of existing cases by early detection and treatment through well-woman care, Papanicolaou smears, and STD screening recommended every 6 months for those at risk. Access to health care for treatment and follow-up, monitoring for sequelae, partner notification, and evaluating risk behaviors are important aspects to successful secondary prevention.
- Tertiary prevention seeks to minimize the psychological and biological sequelae of STDs. This includes minimizing perinatal complications and infant morbidity and mortality, and reducing the frequency of PID and its complications. Identifying coping strategies and means of increasing self-esteem are also important aspects.
- Treatment of any STD in a child should be coordinated with the laboratory, child protective services, and the state authorities.

- Important family factors that reduce risk behaviors include
  - Perceived parental support
  - Degree of family closeness
  - Communication among family members
  - Parenting style
  - Parental supervision and monitoring

Pelvic Inflammatory Disease

Description

Considered an ascending infection, PID refers to infection and inflammation involving the upper genital tract (uterus, fallopian tubes, ovaries, and/or peritoneal tissue). PID is either acute (less than 3 weeks' duration) or chronic. The classic picture is acute salpingitis that presents as lower abdominal pain, vaginal discharge, and fever with an onset after menses.

Etiology and Incidence

PID is considered a polymicrobial infection with a mean of 4.5 different types of organisms involved per infection. Gonorrhea (50% of first infections) and chlamydia (33% of first infections) are the two most common STDs causing PID. Other aerobic and anaerobic organisms, group B streptococcus, genital mycoplasmas, and gram-negative bacteria also are implicated (Pletcher & Slap, 1998).

There are 1 million new cases of PID every year, with 16 to 30% of them occurring in adolescents (Bonny & Biro, 1998; Emans et al., 1998; Pletcher & Slap, 1998). The two risk factors considered to be most significant among teenagers are multiple sexual partners and the high prevalence of STDs in this age group. Other risk factors include increased susceptibility of adolescents to infection, cervical ectopy and thinner cervical mucus, recent instrumentation or intrauterine device use, previous PID, history of lower genital tract infection (including trichomonas and bacterial vaginosis), and nonuse of contraceptives of any type. Use of oral contraceptives decreases the incidence of PID seven-fold (Pletcher & Slap, 1998).

Clinical Findings

PID in adolescents is often subtle and can go undiagnosed, contributing to the inflammatory sequelae. See Table 36–11 for criteria for diagnosing PID.

HISTORY

- Lower abdominal pain or tenderness (acute onset with gonorrhea, subtle with chlamydia)
- Temperature greater than 38°C
- Abnormal vaginal or cervical discharge
- Intermenstrual bleeding
- Sexual history, including number of partners and type of activity
- Last menstrual period, contraceptive use, and previous STD or PID
- Malaise, dysuria, nausea, vomiting, chills, dyspareunia

T A B L E 36-11

Criteria for Diagnosing Pelvic Inflammatory Disease

Minimum criteria for treating pelvic inflammatory disease (PID) in sexually active adolescents with no other cause for illness identified:
Lower abdominal tenderness
Adnexal tenderness
Cervical motion tenderness

Additional criteria that support a diagnosis of PID:
Oral temperature >101°F
Abnormal cervical or vaginal discharge
Elevated erythrocyte sedimentation rate
Elevated C-reactive protein
Laboratory documentation of cervical infection with gonorrhea or chlamydia

Definitive criteria for diagnosing PID, warranted in selected cases:
Histopathological evidence of endometritis on endometrial biopsy
Transvaginal sonography or other imaging techniques showing thickened fluid-filled tubes with or without free pelvic fluid or tubo-ovarian complex
Laparoscopic abnormalities consistent with PID

Adapted from Centers for Disease Control and Prevention: Guidelines for treatment of sexually transmitted diseases. MMWR Morb Wkly Rep 47(RR–1)i–116; 1998; and American Academy of Pediatrics Committee on Infectious Diseases: 1997 Red Book: Report of the Committee on Infectious Diseases, 24th ed. Elk Grove Village, IL, American Academy of Pediatrics, 1997.

PHYSICAL EXAMINATION

- Abdominal examination—bilateral lower quadrant tenderness (most common presenting symptom) and possibly right upper quadrant pain (Fitz-Hugh-Curtis syndrome: inflammation of liver capsule); occasional peritoneal signs
- Speculum examination—mucopurulent discharge
- Bimanual examination—cervical and fundal motion tenderness and adnexal tenderness (may be unilateral) and possible mass

LABORATORY STUDIES

- Urinalysis and culture if symptoms of pyelonephritis or cystitis
- CBC (WBCs >10,000), erythrocyte sedimentation rate (>15 mm/h), C-reactive protein (elevated)
- Microscopic examination of cervical discharge (>5 WBCs)
- Gram stain of cervical mucus (gonorrhea)
- Direct immunofluorescence antibody or polyclonal enzyme-linked immunoassay test (chlamydia)
- Serologic test for syphilis
- Pregnancy test (ectopic)
- Pelvic ultrasound (if adnexal enlargement or tubo-ovarian abscess suspected)
- Culdocentesis (pus)

Differential Diagnosis

Acute appendicitis, ectopic pregnancy, twisted ovarian cyst, ruptured corpus luteum cyst, salpingitis, tubo-ovarian abscess, endometriosis, acute pyelonephritis, gastroenteritis, vaginitis, and functional pain are included in the differential diagnosis.

Management

Goals of treatment include the relief of acute discomfort and prevention of infertility and other sequelae. More than one diagnosis is possible. Treatment should be initiated as soon as possible with broad-spectrum coverage to minimize long-term sequelae. Hospitalization is recommended in the following situations: surgical emergency cannot be excluded; pregnancy;

lack of response to oral antibiotics; inability to tolerate oral antibiotics; severe illness with nausea, vomiting or high temperature; tubo-ovarian abscess; or immunodeficiency (Centers for Disease Control and Prevention, 1998; American Association of Pediatrics Committee on Infectious Diseases, 1997).

1. Parenteral treatment—choose either Regimen A *or* B
   - REGIMEN A
     - Cefoxitin 2 g intravenously every 6 hours *or* cefotetan 2 g intravenously every 12 hours *plus*
     - Doxycycline 100 mg orally or intravenously every 12 hours, both continued until 48 hours after improvement
   - REGIMEN B
     - Clindamycin 900 mg intravenously every 8 hours *plus*
     - Gentamicin 2 mg/kg intravenous or intra-

muscular loading dose followed by 1.5 mg/kg every 8 hours, both continued until 48 hours after improvement
   - AT DISCHARGE
     - Doxycycline 100 mg twice a day for a total of 14 days from time medication was initiated *or* clindamycin 450 mg orally four times a day for a total of 14 days

2. Oral treatment—choose either Regimen A *or* B
   - REGIMEN A
     - Cefoxitin 2 g intramuscularly *plus* probenecid 1 g orally once *or*
     - Ceftriaxone 250 mg intramuscularly once *plus* doxycycline 100 mg orally twice a day for 14 days
   - REGIMEN B (>18 years)
     - Ofloxacin 400 mg orally twice a day for 14 days *plus*

RESOURCE BOX 36-1

NATIONAL RESOURCES FOR PEDIATRIC AND ADOLESCENT GYNECOLOGY

American College of Obstetricians & Gynecologists (ACOG) (pamphlets)
Tel: (202) 638-5577
Tel: (800) 762-2264
Website: www.acog.com

American Social Health Association (pamphlets)
Tel: (800) 783-9877

CDC STD Hotline
Tel: (800) 227-8922

ETR Associates (pamphlets)
Tel: (800) 321-4407

Focus on the Family (videos on "No Apologies: The Truth About Life, Love & Sex"; "Sex, Lies and ... the Truth")
Tel: (800) 232-6459

Medical Institute for Sexual Health (medical data)
Tel: (512) 328-6268

National Abstinence Clearinghouse
Tel: (888) 577-2966

National Herpes Hotline
Tel: (919) 361-8488

National STD Hotline
Tel: (800) 227-8922 or
Tel: (809) 765-1010

North American Society for Pediatric & Adolescent Gynecology (NASPAG)
Tel: (215) 955-6331

Planned Parenthood Federation of America
Tel: (800) 669-0156

Project Reality, Choosing the Best Abstinence Program
Tel: (847) 729-3298
Website: www8.pair.com/abcvisn

Sex Information & Education Council of the U.S. (SIECUS)
Tel: (212) 819-9770

SHARE (abstinence presentation, speaker training materials)
Tel: (425) 644-3312

Society for Adolescent Medicine
Tel: (816) 224-8010

Teen Aid, Inc. (abstinence curricula)
Tel: (800) 357-2868

- Clindamycin 600 mg orally three times a day for 14 days *or* metronidazole 500 mg orally twice a day for 14 days
- FOLLOW-UP
  - Follow-up in 72 hours. If no response, reevaluate diagnosis and treatment. Parenteral therapy should be started and continued until defervescence, evidenced by decreased abdominal tenderness, and decreased uterine, adnexal, and cervical motion tenderness.
3. Other recommendations
   - Treatment of any sexual partners within 60 days of onset of symptoms is imperative. No intercourse until partners treated.
   - Screen for syphilis.
   - Follow-up 7 to 10 days after treatment.
   - Rescreen for chlamydia and GC 4 to 6 weeks after treatment.
   - HIV screening should be offered.

Complications

Infertility (15 to 30% attributable to PID, higher with subsequent episodes), tubo-ovarian abscess, ectopic pregnancy (50% of cases), chronic pelvic pain (18% of cases), dyspareunia, repeated PID, tubal scarring, and extrapelvic infection are possible complications (Centers for Disease Control and Prevention, 1998; Pletcher & Slap, 1998; Sung & MacDonald, 1998 a & b).

Prevention

- PID is considered a "sentinel infection"—a marker for other STDs, recurrent STDs, potential HIV exposure, cervical dysplasia, or unplanned pregnancy (Paradise & Grant, 1992). Appropriate measures should be taken.
- Decrease prevalence and transmission of STDs by promoting abstinence (Bond, 1998) and barrier methods (condoms, diaphragms, cervical caps, spermicidal foams). Screen sexually active adolescents for gonorrhea and chlamydia every 6 months.

REFERENCES

American Academy of Pediatrics Committee on Infectious Diseases. 1997 Red Book: Report of the Committee on Infectious Diseases, 24th ed. Elk Grove Village, IL, American Academy of Pediatrics, 1997.

American College of Sports Medicine: The female athlete triad: Disordered eating, amenorrhea, osteoporosis: Call to action. Sports Medicine Bulletin 27:4, 1992.

Andrist LC: Genital herpes: Overcoming the barriers to diagnosis and treatment. Am J Nurs 97:16AAA–16DDD, 1997.

Baldwin DD, Landa HM: Pediatric gynecology: Evaluation and treatment. Contemp Pediatr 12:35-60, 1995.

Barron SA: Index of suspicion, case 3. Pediatr Rev 19(2): 51-53, 1998.

Biro FM, Rosenthal SL: Adolescent STDs: Diagnosis, developmental issues, & prevention. J Pediatr Health Care 9:256-262, 1995.

Blythe M, Carter C, Orr D: Common menstrual problems. Part 2: Amenorrhea & oligomenorrhea. Adolesc Health Update 4:1-8, 1991.

Bond KG: Abstinence education: How parents are making it happen. Focus Fam 22:12-12, 1998.

Bonny AE, Biro FM: Recognizing & treating STDs in adolescent girls. Contemp Pediatr 15:119-143, 1998.

Boynton RW, Dunn ES, Stephens GR: Vulvovaginitis in the Prepubertal Child. *In* The Manual of Ambulatory Pediatrics. Philadelphia, JB Lippincott, 1994.

Braverman PK, Sondheimer, SJ: Menstrual disorders. Pediatr Rev 18:17-25, 1997.

Brown MR, Cartwright PC, Snow BW: Common office problems in pediatric urology & gynecology. Pediat Clin North Am 44:1091-1115, 1997.

Castiglia PT: Amenorrhea. J Pediatr Health Care 10:226-227, 1996.

Centers for Disease Control and Prevention: Guidelines for treatment of sexually transmitted diseases. MMWR Morbid Mortal Wkly Rep 47(RR-1):i-116, 1998.

Clayton BD, Krowchuk DP: Skin findings and STDs. Contemp Pediatr 14:119-137, 1997.

Coles, FB, Hipp SS: Syphilis among adolescents. Contemp Pediatr 13:47-62, 1996.

Committee on Sports Medicine: Amenorrhea in adolescent athletes. Pediatrics 84(2):394, 1989.

Craighill MC: Pediatric and adolescent gynecology for the primary care physician. Pediatr Clin North Am 45(6):1659-1688, 1998.

Darville T: Chlamydia. Pediatr Rev 19(3):85-91, 1998.

Dodds ML: Vulvar disorders of the infant & young child. Clin Obstet Gynecol 40(1):141-152, 1997.

Durinzi M, DeLeon F: Endometriosis in the adolescent and teenage female. Adolesc Pediatr Gynecol 6:3-7, 1993.

Elster A, Kuznets N: AMA Guidelines for Adolescent Preventive Services (GAPS). Baltimore, Williams & Wilkins, 1994.

Emans S, Lauter MR, Goldstein D: Pediatric and Adolescent Gynecology, 4th ed. Philadelphia, Lippincott-Raven, 1998.

Farrington PF: Pediatrics vulvovaginitis. Clin Obstet Gynecol 40(1):135-140, 1997.

Gidwani GP: Menstruation & the athlete. Contemp Pediatr 14:27-48, 1997.

Gorrie TM, McKinney ES, Murray SS: Foundations of Maternal Newborn Nursing, 2nd ed. Philadelphia, WB Saunders, 1998.

Hillard PA: Abnormal uterine bleeding in adolescents. Contemp Pediatr 12(1)79-90, 1995.

Howard BJ: Labial adhesions. *In* Hoekelman RA, Blatman S, Friedman S, et al (eds): Primary Pediatric Care, 2nd ed. St. Louis, CV Mosby, 1992, pp 1339-1340.

Hurd A, Adamson G: Pelvic pain: Endometriosis as a differential diagnosis in adolescents. Adolesc Pediatr Gynecol 5:3-7, 1992.

Judson FN, Ehret J: Laboratory diagnosis of sexually transmitted infections. Pediatr Ann 23:361-369, 1994.

Megglio GD: Genital foreign bodies. Pediatr Rev 19:34, 1998.

Mehring P: Dysfunctional uterine bleeding. Adv Nurse Prac 5:27-32, 1997.

Nattiv A, Lynch L: The female athlete triad: Managing an acute risk to long term health. Physician Sports Med 22:60-68, 1994.

Paradise JE, Grant L: Pelvic inflammatory disease in adolescents. Pediatr Rev 13:216-223, 1992.

Patel K: Sexually transmitted diseases in adolescents: Focus on gonorrhea, chlamydia, and trichomonas—Issues and treatment guidelines. J Pediatr Health Care 12:211-215, 1998.

Pinsonneault D: Menstrual problems. *In* Dershewitz R (ed): Ambulatory Pediatric Care, 2nd ed. Philadelphia, JB Lippincott, 1993, pp 467-471.

Pletcher JR, Slap GB: Pelvic inflammatory disease. Pediatr Rev 19(11):363-367, 1998.

Polaneczky M, Slap G: Menstrual disorders in the adolescent: Amenorrhea. Pediatr Rev 13:43-48, 1992a.

Polaneczky M, Slap G: Menstrual disorders in the adolescent: Dysmenorrhea and dysfunctional uterine bleeding. Pediatr Rev 13:83-87, 1992b.

Preminger MK, Pokorny SF: Vaginal discharge—A common pediatric complaint. Contemp Pediat 15:115-122, 1998.

Prose CC, Ford CA, Lovely LP: Evaluating amenorrhea: The pediatrician's role. Contemp Pediatr 15:83-110, 1998.

Selleck CS: Identifying & treating bacterial vaginosis. Am J Nursing 97:16AAA-16DDD, 1997.

Shafer M: Urine based STD testing. J Adolesc Health 23:63-73, 1998.

Smith DE, Lohr JA: Vulvovaginitis. *In* Dershewitz R (ed): Ambulatory Pediatric Care, 3rd ed. Philadelphia, JB Lippincott, 1999, pp 651-655.

Stevens-Simon C: Providing effective reproductive health care and prescribing contraceptives for adolescents. Pediatr Rev 19(12):409-417, 1998.

Sung L, MacDonald NE: Gonorrhea: A pediatric perspective. Pediatr Rev 19(1): 13-16, 1998a.

Sung L, MacDonald NE: Syphilis: A pediatric perspective. Pediatr Rev 19(1): 17-22, 1998b.

US Department of Health and Human Services: Healthy People 2010 Objectives. http://web.health.gov/healthypeople, 1998.

US Department of Health and Human Services: Healthy People 2000: Progress report for sexually transmitted diseases. 1994. http://odphp.osophs.dhhs.gov/pubs/hp2000/progvw/STD.HTM

US Preventive Services Task Force: Guide to Clinical Preventive Services. 2nd ed. Baltimore, Williams & Wilkins, 1996.

US Public Health Service: The Clinician's Handbook of Preventive Services, 2nd ed. Baltimore, Williams & Wilkins, 1997.

Wiener D: Labial adhesion. Pediatr Rev 15(3):87-88, 1994.

Zivnuska J: Endometriosis: An overview of diagnosis & treatment. Adv Nurse Practitioners 3:15-17, 1995.

CHAPTER 37

Dermatological Diseases

Nancy Barber Starr

INTRODUCTION

The skin is the body's largest organ and one of its most important. The condition of the skin reflects physical and emotional health, plays a major role in defining identity and supporting survival, and often gives clues to underlying conditions. Skin functions are multiple. Beauty is often defined by the appearance of the skin. Emotions are expressed by blushing and sweating. Skin conveys many impressions through its sensory functions, including reaction to touch, heat, cold, pressure, and pain. Additionally, the skin provides a protective physiological covering, the first line of defense against injury from chemical, physical, and microorganic invaders. Homeostasis is maintained through fluid regulation as well as thermoregulation.

Disruptions in the skin account for 20 to 30% of all pediatric office visits (Hurwitz, 1993). The primary care provider plays an essential role in maintaining skin integrity, identifying and minimizing skin disruptions, maximizing healing, and educating parents and children in care of their skin.

SKIN DEVELOPMENT

Skin development is constant from embryogenesis throughout life. During the embryonic period (the first 2 months of gestation), the skin differentiates into several layers. During the fetal period (four stages spanning from 9 weeks' gestation until birth), appendages (hair, nails, and sebaceous, apocrine, and eccrine glands) develop and all skin layers continue to mature. Neonatal skin continues to change and develop throughout childhood and adolescence, achieving adult skin thickness and characteristics in the late teenage years. Melanin in the skin reaches adult levels by 1 year of age. Vascularization is well developed by the end of the second year of life. Cutaneous nerves develop until puberty and beyond. Sebaceous glands cease production between 6 and 12 months of age but become active again around 7 years of age. Eccrine sweat function begins between 2 and 18 days of age, although full function is not in place until 2 or 3 years of age. The apocrine glands become active at puberty. Hair goes through three stages: growth (anagen), rest (telogen), and regression (catagen), with approximately 1 cm of growth per month. Nails, formed in the fifth fetal month, are spoon-shaped and thin from infancy until 2 to 3 years of age.

ANATOMY AND PHYSIOLOGY

The skin, covering the entire surface of the body, is composed of three layers: the epider-

1059

mis, the dermis, and the subcutaneous layer (Fig. 37-1). Skin thickness varies from 0.5 mm on the eyelids to 3 to 4 mm on the palms and soles.

The epidermis, the thinner outer layer, comprises five layers of stratified squamous epithelium. The outer horny layer is responsible for much of the barrier protection (against microorganisms and irritating chemicals and impeding the exchange of fluids and electrolytes with the environment) and strength of the skin. Melanin serves to protect DNA from damage by ultraviolet (UV) light irradiation. It is produced in the basal layer of the epidermis and contributes to the color of the skin, eyes, and hair. The water content of the environment influences the epidermal barrier with either excess or inadequate amounts contributing to micro- and macroscopic breaks.

The thicker middle layer, the dermis, contributes strength, support, and elasticity to the skin. It also regulates heat loss, provides host defenses of the skin, and aids in nutrition and other regulatory functions. The dermis is primarily composed of fibrous connective tissue,

with some elastic fibers and a mucopolysaccharide gel. It includes mast cells, inflammatory cells, and blood and lymph vessels, as well as cutaneous nerves that elicit sensations (touch, pain, itch, warmth, and cold).

Underlying the dermis is subcutaneous tissue primarily composed of adipose tissue. Networks of arteries lie here and branch into the dermis as small arterioles. The subcutaneous tissue is an insulator, a cushion against trauma, and a source of energy and hormone metabolism (see Fig. 37-1).

Skin appendages include the hair, nails, sweat glands, and sebaceous glands. Hair follicles are found over the entire body except for the palms, soles, knuckles, distal and interdigital spaces, lips, glans and prepuce of the penis, and areolae and nipples. Two types of hair can be found on the body. Terminal hair is thick and visible and found on the scalp, axillae, and pubis. Very fine vellus hair is found over the remainder of the body. The visible portion of the hair is the shaft. The root of the hair is embedded in the dermis as a pilosebaceous unit, consisting of a hair follicle and a sebaceous

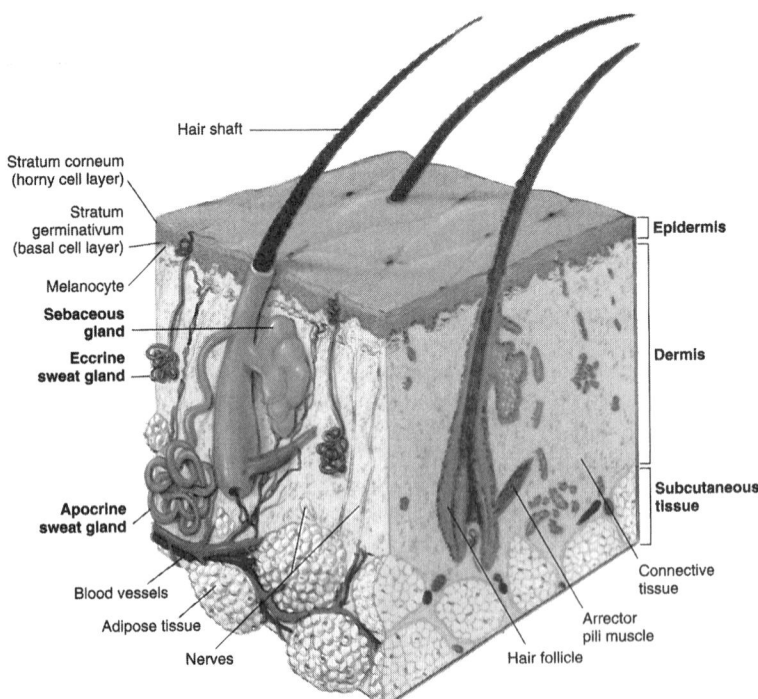

Hair shaft

Stratum corneum
(horny cell layer)

Stratum
germinativum
(basal cell layer)

Melanocyte

**Sebaceous
gland**

**Eccrine
sweat gland**

**Apocrine
sweat gland**

Blood vessels

Adipose tissue

Nerves

Epidermis

Dermis

Subcutaneous
tissue

Connective
tissue

Arrector
pili muscle

Hair follicle

F I G U R E 37-1
Structure of the skin. (From Jarvis C: Physical Examination and Assessment, 2nd ed. Philadelphia, WB Saunders, 1996, p 214.)

gland. The hair shaft may be straight, wavy, helical, or spiral. Following an acute febrile illness or stress, many hairs convert from anagen to telogen stage, resulting in a noticeably thinned amount of hair for several months.

Nails are epidermal cells converted to keratin that grow continually. The body of the nail (or nail plate) is visible. The nail bed, underneath the nail plate, is composed of layers of epidermis and dermis, which serve as structural support. The root of the nail lies just under the epidermis.

Sweat glands can be grouped into three categories: eccrine, ceruminous, and apocrine. Eccrine glands are numerous and are distributed over the entire body. The coiled bodies of the eccrine glands lie in the dermis and empty onto the surface of the skin, helping maintain fluid and electrolyte balance and body temperature as well as providing some excretory function. Ceruminous glands, thought to be modified sweat glands, are located in the external ear canal and secrete a waxy pigmented substance, cerumen. Apocrine glands, located primarily in the axillary, genital, and periumbilical areas, are larger coils than eccrine glands. They open into hair follicles, require androgens to stimulate their secretions, and are thought to be responsible for body odor.

Sebaceous glands, found in conjunction with hair follicles, are distributed over the entire body except the soles, palms, and dorsa of the feet. These glands secrete sebum (oil) when stimulated by androgen and function to prevent excessive water evaporation, minimize heat loss, and lubricate hair.

DERMATOLOGICAL CONSIDERATIONS IN CHILDREN WITH DARK SKIN OR FROM DIVERSE CULTURAL OR ETHNIC GROUPS

A knowledge of the normal variations in children with different levels of pigmentation of the skin and from diverse ethnic or cultural groups is important in assessing and treating dermatological conditions (Smith & Burns, 1999; Dinulos & Graham, 1998). Skin reaction to injury and inflammation of the skin, to common skin conditions, or to cultural practices is varied. A wise clinician listens to parents, because they are often the first to detect subtle changes in color or texture of the skin.

Cutaneous Reaction Patterns

Children with dark skin may have an exaggerated cutaneous response to common disorders of the skin. Three identified patterns are pigment lability, follicular response, and mesenchymal response (Dinulos & Graham, 1998). Pigment lability manifested as postinflammatory hypo- or hyperpigmentation is common. If superficial, with changes in the epidermis only, normal pigmentation returns in about 6 months (e.g., in diaper rash, seborrhea, tinea, pityriasis alba). If dermal changes occur, dermal tattooing may occur, causing permanent changes or changes that last for years (e.g., excoriated acne, impetigo, varicella, contact dermatitis). The exaggerated follicular response can be seen in prominent papules and follicles, especially with atopic dermatitis, pityriasis rosea, or tinea versicolor. The mesenchymal response causes hypertrophic scars and keloids (which extend beyond the edge of the scar), often following varicella, ear piercing, burns, or any surgical procedure. Other exaggerated responses include lichenification and vesicular or bullous reaction to bites or staphylococcal infection.

Normal Variations and Common Problems

The following are normal variations or common problems in children with darker skin:

- Variation in color and texture of skin from one part of the body to another
- Pigmentation of gingiva, mucous membranes, sclerae, and nails correlates with degree of cutaneous pigmentation
- Increased areas of melanin in thicker-skinned areas (elbow, knee)
- Futcher's (Voigt's, Ito's) lines—vertical lines separating hyperpigmented extensor surfaces from less pigmented ventral surfaces (upper arms, chest, abdomen)
- Mongolian spots and increased numbers of café-au-lait spots (see discussion later in chapter)

- Normal exfoliation produces a fine layer of gray scales, discoloring alcohol wipes when used
- Color alterations (jaundice, anemia, cyanosis)—difficult to assess
- Kinky, wooly, tightly curled hair with closely knit growth that tangles when dry and mats when wet
- Tinea versicolor (see section on fungal disorders), initially papular with hypo- or hyperpigmentation, occurring only on the face
- Atopic dermatitis (see Chapter 24) with prominent follicular pattern with pityriasis alba and postinflammatory hypopigmentation
- Pityriasis rosea (see section on papulosquamous disorders) often confused with tinea, primarily follicular, inverse distribution (face, neck, extremities, and torso)

Conditions occuring more commonly in dark-skinned children include tinea capitis, tinea versicolor, papular urticaria, infantile acropustulosis, dermatosis papulosa nigra, lichen nitidus, lichen spinulosis, pseudofolliculitis barbae, transient neonatal pustular melanosis, and acanthosis nigricans. Lichen planus is more severe and keloids are more frequent.

Cultural or Ethnic Practices

Grooming, cosmetic, or healing practices of cultural or ethnic groups contribute to various conditions that may be seen. These include:

- Hair pomade—acne
- Bleaching creams—discoloration and erythematous nodules
- Chemical or thermal hair straighteners—alopecia, fragile hair shaft, scalp contact dermatitis
- Coining—petechiae and ecchymoses, especially on chest and back
- Cornrowed hair or tight ponytails—traction alopecia
- Cupping—circular ecchymoses on neck, chest, back, and arms
- Henna—orange discoloration of skin, increased bilirubin in infants if applied topically
- Scars or tattoos from decorative practices

- Healing practices used during significant illness that produce burns—circular 1- to 2-cm scars on chest, periumbilicus, wrists, ankles, or back

PATHOPHYSIOLOGY AND DEFENSE MECHANISMS

Disruption of the skin and subcutaneous tissue occurs through a variety of assaults. These include:

- Bacterial, fungal, and viral infections
- Allergic and inflammatory reactions
- Infestations
- Vascular reactions
- Papulosquamous and bullous eruptions
- Congenital lesions
- Hair and nail disorders

The skin's outer layers provide the body's first line of defense from chemical, physical, and microorganic injury. The epidermis provides a functional barrier, the dermis provides strength and protection through the cutaneous nerves, and the subcutaneous tissue ensures insulation, cushion from injury, energy source, and hormonal metabolism. These layers, in turn, protect the other body systems. The water content of the skin enhances the protective barrier of the skin. If the skin becomes too dry or too wet, breaks in the barrier occur, eliciting an inflammatory response. As a continuously growing system, the skin not only heals itself but controls growth or colonization of microorganisms by continual shedding.

ASSESSMENT OF THE SKIN AND SUBCUTANEOUS TISSUE

History

The history should assess the following:

- History of present illness
  - Pruritus, scaling, and cosmetic appearance are the three most common presenting concerns (Weston et al., 1996)
  - Three key questions to ask (Nicol, personal communication, 1993): How long

have you had it? Does it itch? What have you used to treat it?
- ◦ Rash, lesions, discharge
- ◦ Associated systemic symptoms: fever, malaise
- ◦ Exposures or allergies: Medication, foods, animals, plants? Known allergens? New substances? Persons with similar symptoms or illness?
- ◦ All medication taken over the last few days, including creams, ointments, powders, or lotions (it is often helpful to have patients bring medications they have used to the appointment)
- ◦ Onset and length of present illness? Treatment used and effect?
- ◦ Prior incidents of similar rash
- ◦ What soaps, shampoos, and detergents are used
- Family history
- ◦ Similar symptoms
- ◦ Skin disorders or allergies
- Thorough review of systems and medical history, especially the following:
- ◦ Usual state of health and recent illnesses
- ◦ Skin, hair, and nails: skin type, recent and long-term changes, previous incidence of skin disease
- ◦ Eyes, ears, nose, and throat: swelling, itching, crusting, discharge or circles around eyes, nasal mucus discharge, patency or irritation, dry mouth, lesions, or pain
- ◦ Chest: wheezing, coughing, or respiratory difficulty

Physical Examination

A key question is, "Does the patient appear ill?" This clinical impression is important to differentiate the few serious illnesses from the majority of the remaining dermatological conditions. The entire body needs to be examined, not just exposed skin. Attention should be given to the eyes, nose, mouth, lymph nodes, and lungs because a skin disorder may be a cutaneous manifestation of other disease. The dermatological examination includes a thorough look at the skin, scalp, hair, palms and soles, nails, and anogenital region.

Special techniques for examination of the skin are discussed below. Good light (daylight is best) is essential to a good examination. A source of direct light, such as a gooseneck lamp, is the best alternative. Other helpful tools include a magnifying glass, a ruler, a glass slide, and a Wood's lamp (UV light). A glass slide gently pressed on the skin (diascopy) allows viewing of the skin with and without capillary filling. A Wood's lamp is used to examine fluorescent-positive fungal infections and depigmenting skin disorders such as vitiligo.

Identification of the type of lesion and correct use of terminology are essential to good dermatological care. Essential documentation includes the following:

- Location and type of lesion
- Color, size, and shape
- Arrangement (e.g., isolated, zosteriform)
- Pattern (e.g., sun-exposed, symmetry)
- Distribution of lesion (e.g., regional, generalized)
- Border (e.g., indistinct, well circumscribed)
- Consistency (e.g., firm, soft, mobile)

Primary skin lesions (Table 37–1) include changes that arise from previously normal skin. *Secondary* skin lesions (Table 37–2) result from changes in primary lesions. *Vascular* skin lesions (Table 37–3) involve the blood supply. Other useful descriptive terms are listed in Table 37–4.

Diagnostic Studies

A few simple laboratory tests are helpful in making or excluding dermatological disorders. Proper procurement of the sample is important. Scraping of lesions can be done with a scalpel or a toothbrush, and scales or debris placed on a glass slide or in culture material. It is important to scrape under any scabs to get the organisms. Moistening the lesion may facilitate this. Scrapings can be obtained from the edges of skin lesions; from plucked hair, including the root; from the nail plate; or from subungual debris. One rule is, "if it scales, scrape it" (Goldgeier, 1996). Laboratory tests that can be used include the following:

- Microscopic examination of skin scrapings
- ◦ Potassium hydroxide (KOH) can be used

T A B L E 37-1

Primary Skin Changes to Lesions

Macule—flat, nonpalpable, discolored lesion
  ≤1 cm
Patch—macule >1 cm
Papule—solid, raised lesion of varied color with
  distinct borders ≤1 cm
Plaque—solid, raised, flat-topped lesion with
  distinct borders >1 cm
Nodule—raised, firm, movable lesion with
  indistinct borders and deep palpable portion
  ≤2 cm
Tumor—large nodule, may be firm or soft
Wheal—fleeting, irregularly shaped, elevated,
  itchy lesion of varied size, pale at center,
  slightly red at borders
Vesicle—blister filled with clear fluid
Bulla—vesicle >1 cm
Cyst—palpable lesion with definite borders filled
  with liquid or semisolid material
Pustule—raised lesion filled with pus, often in hair
  follicle or sweat pore
Comedo—plugged, dilated pore; open
  (blackhead), closed (whitehead)

T A B L E 37-2

Secondary Skin Changes to Lesions

Crusting—dried exudate or scab of varied color
Scaling—thin, flaking layers of epidermis
Desquamation—peeling sheets of scale
Lichenification—thickening of skin with deep
  visible furrows
Excoriation—abrasion or removal of epidermis;
  scratch
Fissure—linear, wedge-shaped cracks extending
  into dermis
Erosion—oozing or moist, depressed area with
  loss of superficial epidermis
Ulcer—deeper than erosion; open lesion
  extending into dermis
Atrophy—thinning skin, may appear translucent
Scar—healed lesion of connective tissue
Keloid—healed lesion of hypertrophied connective
  tissue
Striae—fine pink or silver lines in areas where
  skin has been stretched

to examine for fungal disorders (hyphae or spores; Fig. 37-2). Add a drop of KOH 20% to dissolve debris and cover with a coverslip. Let sit for 20 to 30 minutes or heat gently (do not boil). Use ×10 magnification to examine.

○ Wright, Giemsa, or Gram stain is used to examine for bacteria or herpes simplex (HS) or herpes zoster (HZ) giant cells. Allow scrapings to air-dry, then stain with Wright or Giemsa stain. Use ×40 magnification to examine for bacteria.

○ Tzanck's smear for herpes, varicella, or zoster.

• Microbial culture of lesions for bacteria, viruses, or fungi. Simple, inexpensive culture methods for fungal organisms (Dermatophyte Test Medium or InTray CCD [includes *Candida*]—see Resource Box 37-1) can be done at room temperature. Skin or nail scrapings or hairs, including the root, are applied so that they break the agar surface. A color change is noted in 1 to 5 days.

• Patch or skin testing for allergic or contact reactions is usually done by dermatologists or allergists.

• Skin biopsy following local anesthesia may be done by punch or shave method for any tumor, palpable purpura, persistent dermatitis, or blister that is not otherwise definitively diagnosed. Such procedures often require referral to a dermatologist.

• Complete blood count (CBC) and erythrocyte sedimentation rate (ESR) may be done to evaluate infection or inflammation.

T A B L E 37-3

Vascular Skin Lesions

Angioma or hemangioma—papule made of blood
  vessels
Ecchymosis—bruise, purple to brown in color,
  macular or papular, varied in size
Hematoma—collection of blood from ruptured
  blood vessel >1 cm
Petechiae—pinpoint, pink to purple macular
  lesions 1–3 mm that do not blanch
Purpura—purple macular lesion >1 cm
Telangiectasis—collection of macular or raised,
  dilated capillaries

▰ MANAGEMENT STRATEGIES

Hydration and Lubrication

Maintenance of skin hydration is essential to prevention and treatment of skin conditions. If the skin is overhydrated, the bonds between cells at the stratum corneum loosen and the barrier is broken. If the skin is too dry, it cracks, again breaking the barrier.

BATHING

Although less frequent bathing is often recommended, especially with dry skin or in dry cli-

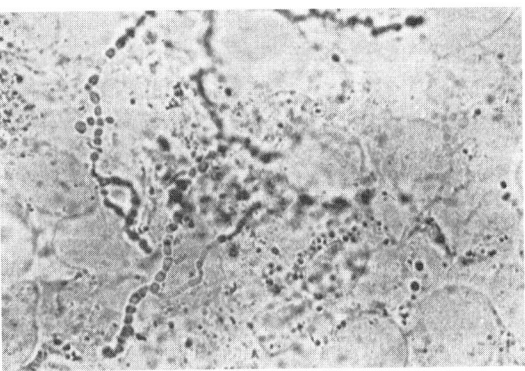

F I G U R E 37-2
Fungal elements (hyphae) as seen on microscopic examination of a potassium hydroxide preparation. (From Hurwitz S: Clinical Pediatric Dermatology, 2nd ed. Philadelphia, WB Saunders, 1993, p 374.)

T A B L E 37-4

Descriptive Terms for Dermatological Lesions

Acral—involving extremities (hands, feet, ears, etc.)
Annular—ring-shaped
Arcuate—arc-shaped
Circinate—circular
Confluent—running together
Contiguous—touching or adjacent
Discrete—distinct and separate
Diffuse or generalized—scattered, widely distributed
Eczematous—referring to vesicles with oozing crust
Grouped—arranged in sets
Guttate—small, drop-like
Herpetiform—referring to grouped vesicles resembling those of herpes
Iris—arranged in concentric circles, one inside the other
Linear—arranged in a line
Localized—in a limited area
Nummular—coin-shaped
Pedunculated—having a stalk
Polycyclic—oval with more than one ring
Reticular—net-like
Serpiginous—snake-like, creeping
Symmetrical—balanced on both sides
Telangiectatic—referring to dilated terminal vessels
Umbilicated—depressed or shaped like a navel
Verrucous—wart-like
Zosteriform—resembling shingles, following a nerve root or dermatome

mates, proper bathing can enhance addition and retention of water in the skin and is not contraindicated. Lukewarm, not hot, water should be used. The bath should not last long enough for skin to become supersaturated. In general, mild soaps such as Dove, Neutrogena, Aveeno, or Purpose should be used. Soap substitutes include Cetaphil and Purpose Gentle Cleansing Wash. Bubble-bath solutions are especially irritating and should be avoided. Soaping and shampooing should be done at the end of the bath followed by thorough rinsing. The skin should be gently dried and a lubricating agent applied immediately. Refer to Chapter 25 for further information on lubricating baths. Baths including baking soda or Aveeno colloidal ointment may be helpful to relieve pruritus. Tar baths can be used for psoriasis (e.g., Zetar, Polytar, or Balnetar). It is worth noting that bathing and other heat exposures can make a rash seem worse temporarily.

ENVIRONMENTAL CONSIDERATIONS

Because water is essential to skin integrity, environmental humidity also plays a role. Excessive humidity (>90%) or deficient humidity (<10%) can cause disruption of the skin. Macerated skin, for example, benefits from less humidity (e.g., wet dressings enhance evaporation and relieve symptoms). Itching from excessively dry skin is often relieved by increased humidity provided by humidified heating in winter or a vaporizer or humidifier. In hot temperatures, itching can be alleviated by cool air conditioning.

FLUID INTAKE

Water consumption also plays a role in maintaining proper skin hydration, and children should be encouraged to drink plenty of water.

SKIN CARE AGENTS

Soaps, Oils, and Colloids

Mild soaps include Dove, Aveeno, Neutrogena, Basis, Alpha Keri, Oilatum, and Lubriderm. Cetaphil lotion and Purpose Gentle Cleansing Wash are soap substitutes. Bath oils include Alpha Keri and Domol. Colloids include Aveeno.

Moisturizers and Lubricants

Moisturizers and lubricants treat chronic dryness and inflammation of the skin by retaining water in the skin. Composed of petrolatum or a mixture of petrolatum and lanolin, moisturizers and lubricants are most effective when applied to damp skin. Petrolatum-based lubricants include Moisturel, Purpose, Dermasil cream, Vaseline Pure Petrolatum Jelly, and Vaseline Dermatology Formula Lotion. Petrolatum and lanolin combinations include Aquaphor ointment, Eucerin cream and lotion, Lubriderm lotion, and Keri Creme.

Sunscreens and Sunblocks

Sunscreens and sunblocks protect the skin from UV light and are graded by their ability to provide sun protection. A fragrance-free sunscreen with a minimum of 15 SPF (sun protection factor) is recommended. Sunscreens that act by absorbing UV light in the B range include *para-aminobenzoic acid* (PABA) or PABA esters, cinnamates, salicylates, benzophenones, and anthranilates. Only benzophenones protect from UV rays in the longer UVA range. Sunblocks, including titanium dioxide, zinc oxide, and talc, scatter light and are especially useful on the nose, ears, and lips (see Table 37–17).

WET DRESSINGS

When skin is in an acute stage of oozing, crusting, or itching, wet dressings are useful to help dry the skin, decrease itching, and remove crusts. Thin cloths such as diapers, handkerchiefs, or strips of sheets make the best wet dressings. Dressings should be wet with lukewarm water and applied for 10 to 20 minutes 4 to 6 times daily for 48 to 72 hours. During the treatment, dressings must be kept wet either by removing and rewetting or by applying water. Alternative solutions include saline (1 tsp salt with 1 pt of water) or Burow solution (one Domeboro [aluminum acetate; calcium acetate] tablet with 1 pt of water). Creams or ointments applied following wet dressings enhance absorption of the medication in the cream. A slightly more intense technique includes applying a steroid ointment or cream to the skin, followed by a wet dressing and then a dry dressing (e.g., a sleeper, pajamas, or long johns are wetted and put on, and covered with a dry sleeper or long johns) (Weston et al, 1996). The dressing is changed every 6 hours for 24 to 72 hours or is used overnight for 5 to 10 nights. Care must be taken to avoid excessive steroidal absorption using this technique by applying steroid only to areas needing it, especially in infants and young children.

OCCLUSIVE DRESSINGS

Occlusive dressings decrease evaporation of water from the skin and enhance hydration and absorption of topical medications. Plastic wrap is placed over the affected area after hydrating the skin and applying cream or ointment; these dressings should not be left on longer than 8 hours. Ointments, oils, urea compounds, and propylene glycol used alone are occlusive. Skin folds serve as naturally occurring occlusive areas. Lichen simplex chronicus, dyshidrotic eczema, and psoriasis are skin conditions that benefit from occlusion.

OTHER CONSIDERATIONS

Irritants and sensitizing agents such as wool, sweat, and saliva should be avoided.

Allergens and foods that most commonly

T A B L E   37-5

Preparations of Topical Medications

SHAMPOOS
Liquid soaps or detergents for cleaning the hair, e.g., tar for psoriasis or seborrhea

POWDERS
Absorb moisture and reduce friction, provide cooling, decrease itching, increase evaporation

PASTES
Made of a combination of powder and oil, which makes them somewhat difficult to apply and remove, but effective in providing dryness and protection for skin

LOTIONS
Mixtures of powder and water, useful for drying, cooling, and soothing actions. *Emulsion lotions* contain some oil, so are not as drying as lotions. Lotions come in suspension or solution

GELS
Alcohol-based, provide good penetration of skin, but can burn on application. Primarily used for acne and in hairy areas

CREAMS
Contain more water than oil and therefore are less occlusive. Better used with less-dry skin, in high-humidity areas, in summertime, and on parts of body that naturally cause occlusion (body folds). Often accepted better by patient but must be applied every 2–3 h

OINTMENTS
Best used with dry skin. Composed primarily of oil with little or no water. Provide most potent concentration of medication because of their occlusive action on skin. Generally need to be used only every 12 hr. Tend to leave a greasy feeling and can cause heat retention from decreased evaporation. Come as water in oil, absorbent, or water repellent

OILS
Fluid fats that hold medication to the skin as barriers or occlusive agents

cause skin reactions include milk, eggs, wheat, tomato, citrus, chocolate, fish, and nuts.

Medications

Topical therapeutics are most commonly used for dermatological conditions. Topical therapy can achieve the following goals:

- Restore hydration
- Alleviate symptoms
- Reduce inflammation
- Protect the skin
- Reduce scale and debris
- Cleanse and debride
- Eradicate causative organisms

Thought must be given not only to the medication used in treating skin conditions but also to its preparation (Table 37-5) and vehicle (Fig.

37-3), including stabilizers, preservatives, and perfumes. Sensitization, and thus aggravation rather than relief of symptoms, is occasionally caused by the medication vehicle or its preparation. Common agents causing sensitization include ethylenediamine, lanolin, parabens, thi-

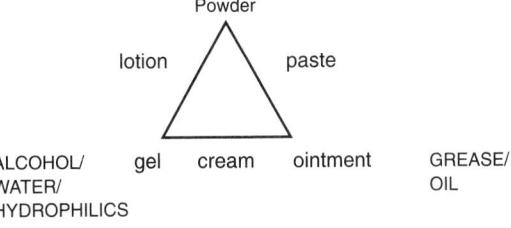

F I G U R E   37-3
Vehicles for dermatologic therapy. See Table 37–5 for description.

merosal, diphenhydramine, "caines," and neomycin. The following guidelines for use of preparations may be helpful:

- Acute inflammation—wet dressings, powders, suspension lotions, alcohol- or water-based lotions, or aerosols
- Chronic inflammation—creams, oil-based lotions or gels, ointments
- Patient's tolerance for and willingness to use certain vehicles
- Patient's environment (dry or humid)

All preparations of topical medication except powders have enhanced absorption if applied to skin immediately after it has been saturated with water. Absorption is also enhanced by occlusion (skin folds or plastic wraps; see above). Application of the topical medication is best done in one direction, preferably along the hair follicles, without rubbing, applied with a single motion. Use an adequate, but not excessive amount.

General categories of medication used for skin care include the following:

ANTIBACTERIAL AGENTS

Topical antiseptics, soap, and antibacterial soap reduce the number of bacteria on the skin and provide thorough cleansing. Examples of antiseptics include povidone-iodine (Betadine), chlorhexidine gluconate (Hibiclens), and pHisoDerm. Topical antibiotics such as mupirocin (Bactroban), applied directly to the skin, are used to treat minor skin infections. Neomycin should be avoided because of the high incidence of contact sensitization. Oral antibiotics used to treat more significant bacterial infections include penicillins, erythromycin, cephalosporins, and tetracycline.

ANTIFUNGAL AGENTS

Antifungal agents are used to treat *Candida, Malassezia (Pityrosporum)*, and dermatophyte infections. Many topical antifungals are over-the-counter medications. Oral antifungals are used for hair and nail infections or refractory skin infections. They are used with caution in children, not only because of the side effects but also because the newer agents are not Food

and Drug Administration (FDA) approved for children, or the experience in children is minimal. The traditional drugs are usually the first line of treatment. Antifungal agents are listed in Table 37-9 in the section on fungal infections.

ANTIVIRAL AGENTS

Topical antivirals are used to control cutaneous herpes infections. Oral antivirals, such as acyclovir for herpes infections, are used in more complicated or extensive cases.

Wart therapy agents destroy keratinocytes. These include salicylic acid and lactic acid collodion, salicylic plaster, salicylic solution, liquid nitrogen, cantharidin, podophyllum, and trichloroacetic acid.

ANTIACNE AGENTS

Topical keratolytics are used in acne to relieve follicular obstruction by promoting peeling of the skin and inhibition of bacteria. Benzoyl peroxide and retinoic acid are two main agents. Topical antibiotics have few side effects and are most effective in maintaining control of acne. Common ones used include clindamycin, erythromycin, and meclocycline. Systemic antibiotics are effective in inflammatory acne. Tetracycline and erythromycin are the most commonly used. Oral retinoid (isotretinoin), effective in nodulocystic acne not responding to other treatment, is contraindicated in pregnancy because of its teratogenic effects (see Table 37-14).

ANTI-INFLAMMATORY AGENTS

Topical glucocorticoids are frequently used to reduce inflammation, decrease itching, and for vasoconstriction without having the widespread systemic effects of oral steroids. They are subdivided into three categories: low-potency, moderate-potency, and high-potency (Table 37-6).

High-potency steroids should not be used in children. Only low-potency agents should be used on the face, in the diaper area, and in young children, and only for short periods of time. Steroids are also classified as fluorinated or nonfluorinated. Nonfluorinated steroids are

T A B L E   37-6

Topical Steroid Preparations

DRUG (BRAND NAME)	DOSAGE FORM
LOW POTENCY	
Aclometasone dipropionate (Aclovate)	0.05% cream, ointment
Desonide (DesOwen, Tridesilon)	0.05% cream, ointment
Fluocinolone acetonide (Fluonid, Synalar)	0.01% solution, cream
Fluorometholone (Oxylone)	0.02% cream
Hydrocortisone (Hytone, Nutracort, Cort-Dome, Synacort)	0.5% cream, ointment
	1% cream, ointment, lotion, solution
	2.5% cream, ointment
MODERATE POTENCY	
Betamethasone valerate (Valisone)	0.01% cream
	0.1% cream, ointment, lotion
Clocortolone pivalate (Cloderm)	0.1% cream
Desoximetasone (Topicort)	0.05% gel
Fluocinolone acetonide (Synalar, Fluonid)	0.025% cream, ointment
	0.1% cream
Flurandrenolide (Cordran)	0.05% cream, lotion, ointment
Halcinonide (Halog)	0.025% cream
Hydrocortisone valerate (Westcort)	0.2% cream, ointment
Triamcinolone acetonide (Kenalog, Aristocort)	0.025%, 0.1% cream, ointment, lotion
HIGH POTENCY	
Amcinonide (Cyclocort)	0.1% cream, ointment
Betamethasone dipropionate (Diprosone)	0.05% cream, lotion, ointment
Betamethasone dipropionate; clotrimazole (Lotrisone)	0.05% betamethasone; 1% clotrimazole cream
Desoximetasone (Topicort)	0.25% cream, ointment
Diflorasone diacetate (Florone)	0.05% cream, ointment
Fluocinolone acetonide (Synalar-HP)	0.2% cream
Fluocinonide (Lidex)	0.05% cream, solution, gel, ointment
Halcinonide (Halog)	0.1% cream, ointment, solution
Halobetasol propionate (Ultravate)	0.05% cream, ointment
Triamcinolone acetonide (Kenalog, Aristocort)	0.5% cream, ointment

less potent and have fewer side effects; fluorinated steroids are rarely used in pediatrics.

Oral glucocorticoids (prednisone) are used only in acute situations and are limited to short courses. Intralesional steroid injections may be used by the dermatologist to control localized eczema, lichen planus, or psoriasis.

A key to using steroids is to be familiar with a few low-, medium-, and high-level steroids and use them consistently. Use the lowest possible potency that has the desired effect, and with the least possible frequency. Brand name preparations often have a more consistent base and potency. Only low- or medium-low-potency steroids (in severe cases) should be used on the face, groin, and axillae. Remember that ointments are more potent than creams, and lotions are better in hairy areas. Absorption is enhanced in areas that are traumatized or denuded. Side effects are possible when using topical steroids, especially with prolonged use or more potent preparations. Common side effects are skin atrophy, striae, increased fragility of the skin, hypopigmentation, secondary infection, acneiform eruption, folliculitis, miliaria, hypertrichosis, telangiectasia, and purpura.

ANTIPRURITIC AGENTS

Antihistamines are used for both sedation and to relieve itching. The most commonly used antihistamines are hydroxyzine and diphenhydramine. Topical antihistamines, especially diphenhydramine HCl (Benadryl) and "caine" medications, should be avoided because of the possibility of contact sensitization. Menthol and pramoxine are topical anesthetics that do not cause sensitization (Paller, 1999). Nonsteroidal anti-inflammatory agents (NSAIDs) are used for relief of pain and in the treatment of sunburn. Ibuprofen and indomethacin are the two mainstays.

SCABICIDES AND PEDICULOCIDES

These agents are toxic to mites and lice. Crotamiton (Eurax), permethrin (Elimite, Nix), pyrethrin plus piperonyl butoxide, and lindane (Kwell) are commonly used. Lindane must be used with caution in pregnancy and in young infants.

HAIR AND SCALP PREPARATIONS

Antimicrobial, tar, keratolytic, and detergent shampoos are agents used on the hair and scalp.

OTHER MEDICATIONS AND TREATMENTS

Other medications and treatments used in dermatological care include retinoids, topical tars, anthralin, calcipotriene (a vitamin D analog), masking preparations, agents to relieve excessive sweating (aluminum chloride or chlorohydrate), cytotoxic and immunosuppressive agents, and phototherapy.

Counseling and Anticipatory Guidance

Essential to the successful management of skin and subcutaneous disorders is time spent with the patient and parents discussing the child's skin condition and the family's concerns and needs. Education regarding the disease, plan of treatment, and potential risks and benefits should be provided. Because disorders of the skin are so visible, time must be spent discussing the short- and long-term prognoses as well as potential plans to prevent complications, recurrence, and spread.

Ideas for preventive care for the dark-skinned patient should be implemented in routine care. The following are initial areas to consider:

- Avoiding acne or contact dermatitis
- Avoiding traction alopecia
- Varicella vaccine to prevent scarring
- Insect repellents to minimize insect bite reactions
- Early treatment of pruritic or inflammatory conditions (acne, eczema) and infections
- Moisturizing agents and elimination of soaps for dry, itchy skin
- Oral antipruritics for dry, itchy skin
- Avoiding topical medications, especially high-potency steroids, benzoyl peroxide, and isotretinoin
- Avoiding trauma and any procedures that can induce keloids

▰▰▰ BACTERIAL INFECTIONS OF THE SKIN AND SUBCUTANEOUS TISSUE (Table 37–7)

Impetigo

Description

Impetigo is a bacterial infection of the superficial layers of the skin. Nonbullous impetigo usually follows some type of skin trauma (e.g., bites, abrasions, varicella) or other skin disease (most commonly atopic dermatitis). Bullous impetigo develops on intact skin and is caused by *Staphylococcus aureus* toxin production (see Color Fig. 14).

Etiology and Incidence

Impetigo is the primary bacterial infection of the skin in children, accounting for 1% of all pediatric visits, 10% of all skin problems, and 50 to 60% of all bacterial skin infections (Kronemeyer, 1997; Darmstadt, 1997; Shriner et al., 1995). Nonbullous impetigo accounts for more than 70% of cases. Bullous impetigo occurs sporadically and is more common in infants and young children. *S. aureus*, the primary pathogen responsible for 70 to 85% of impetigo cases, usually spreads from hands, nasal discharge, or droplets. *Streptococcus pyo-*

T A B L E 37-7

Diagnosis and Treatment of Common Bacterial Infections

INFECTION	CAUSATIVE ORGANISM	PRESENTATION	AREA OF INVOLVEMENT	TREATMENT	PREVENTION
Impetigo	*Staphylococcus aureus* or *Streptococcus*	Honey-colored crust on erythematous base, or blisters that rupture, leaving varnish-like coat	Superficial layers of skin	Topical antibiotic if minor, oral antibiotics if more significant infection	Moisturize skin; thorough cleansing of any break in skin
Cellulitis	Most commonly *Streptococcus*	Erythema, swelling, tenderness	Dermis and subcutaneous tissue	Oral antibiotic depending on likely organism; often penicillin or dicloxacillin	Same as above
Folliculitis	*S. aureus*	Pruritus, erythematous papule or pustule at hair follicle	Hair follicle	Warm compresses, topical kerato-lytics, topical antibiotics, or antistaphylococcal antibiotic if severe	Same as above; good hygiene and antibacterial soap

genes, responsible for 30 to 40% of cases, is found most commonly in preschool children and is uncommon under 2 years of age on open skin. Both organisms may be found in an impetiginous lesion. Impetigo occurs more frequently with poor hygiene, during the summer months, in warm, humid climates, and in lower socioeconomic groups (Darmstadt, 1997; AAP, 1997; Weston et al., 1996).

CLINICAL FINDINGS

HISTORY

- Pruritus, spread of the lesion to surrounding skin, and earlier skin disruption at the site
- Recent sore throat
- Weakness, fever, diarrhea may accompany bullous impetigo

PHYSICAL EXAMINATION. The following can be found:

- Nonbullous, classic, or common impetigo—begins as macules that progress to vesicles

or pustules which rupture, leaving moist, honey-colored, crusty lesions on mildly erythematous, eroded skin; less than 2 cm in size; little pain but rapid spread
- Bullous impetigo—large, superficial, annular or oval pustular blisters that rupture, leaving thin varnish-like coating or scale
- *S. aureus* lesions—usually on the face, trunk, extremities; superficial blisters that rupture, leaving the skin with a scalded appearance
- *S. pyogenes* lesions—on traumatized skin, lower extremities; punched-out ulcers with crusts
- Lesions most common on face, extremities, or perineum; satellite lesions near the primary site, although they can be found anywhere on the body
- Lymphadenopathy in up to 95% (Darmstadt, 1997)

LABORATORY STUDIES. Gram stain and culture are ordered if identification of the organism is needed.

Differential Diagnosis

Herpes simplex, varicella, nummular eczema, contact dermatitis, tinea, kerion, and scabies are included in the differential diagnosis.

Management

Management involves the following:

1. Topical antibiotics may be used if the impetigo is superficial, nonbullous, or localized to one or two lesions. Topical treatment alone provides clinical improvement but may prolong the carrier state (Weston et al., 1996). Mupirocin ointment (as effective as cephalexin; Bass et al., 1997) or bacitracin (AAP, 1997) is used 3 times a day for 7 to 10 days. If there is no improvement in 3 days oral antibiotics should be started.
2. Oral antibiotics. Treatment for *S. aureus* and *S. pyogenes* is usually recommended because coexistence is common.
   - Cephalexin 40 mg/kg/d for 10 days.
   - Dicloxacillin 15 to 50 mg/kg/d for 10 days.
   - Cloxacillin 50 to 100 mg/kg/d for 10 days.
   - Erythromycin 40 mg/kg/d for 10 days; note that there is increasing resistance in some communities, up to 10 to 52% (Kronemeyer, 1997; Bass et al., 1997).
   - If streptococcus is cultured, treat with penicillin V 125 to 250 mg 4 times a day for 10 days.
3. For widespread infection with constitutional symptoms and deeper skin involvement, use oral antibiotic active against β-lactamase-producing strains of *S. aureus* such as dicloxacillin, cloxacillin, or cephalexin.
4. If an infant has bullous impetigo, use parenteral β-lactamase-resistant antistaphylococcal penicillin such as methicillin, oxacillin, or nafcillin.
5. If there is failure to respond in 7 days, swab beneath the crust, do Gram stain, culture, and sensitivities.
6. If there is recurrence, evaluate with nasal culture and treat with topical mupirocin to the nares twice a day for 5 days to eradicate staphylococcus carriage (Kronemeyer, 1997).
7. Local care of lesions before applying ointment may be helpful. Soak with Burow solution compresses to remove crusts and cleanse with soap.
8. Educate regarding cleanliness, handwashing, and spread of disease.
9. Exclude from day care or school until treated for 24 hours.
10. Follow-up appointment in 48 to 72 hours if not improved, and in 10 to 14 days.

Complications

- Cellulitis in up to 10% of cases (Darmstadt, 1997); ecthyma, erysipelas.
- Lymphangitis, suppurative lymphadenitis, guttate psoriasis, scarlet fever, acute rheumatic fever, or glomerulonephritis may occur following infection with some strains of streptococcus.
- *Staphylococcal scalded skin syndrome (SSSS)* results from circulating toxin. Unusual over 5 years of age, SSSS presents abruptly with fever, malaise, and tender erythematous skin, especially in the neck folds and axillae, rapidly becoming crusty around the eyes, nose, and mouth. The Nikolsky sign (peeling of skin with a light rub to reveal a moist red surface) is a key finding. Treatment with oral dicloxacillin, avoidance of steroids, minimal handling, and use of ointments as the skin heals results in quicker healing without scarring over 10 to 14 days (Darmstadt, 1998; Pollack & Adam, 1996; Weston et al., 1996; Hurwitz, 1993). Severe cases are dealt with as burn victims.

Patient Education and Prevention

- Thorough cleansing of any breaks in the skin helps prevent impetigo.
- Postinflammatory pigment changes can last weeks to months.

Cellulitis

Description

Cellulitis is a localized bacterial infection often involving the dermis and subcutaneous layers of the skin commonly seen following a disruption of the skin surface from an insect or animal bite, trauma, or a penetrating wound. Periorbital cellulitis is discussed in Chapter 29.

Etiology and Incidence

In children, cellulitis is often facial (one cheek), perivaginal, or perianal, or involves a joint or an extremity. Most cases of cellulitis are caused by streptococci, although *Haemophilus influenzae* (especially in children under 2 years of age) and *S. aureus* (increasing incidence) are also found. Seventy percent of cases of perianal cellulitis are found in males 6 months to 10 years of age. Cellulitis of the cheek is most common in 6-month- to 3-year-olds (Weston et al., 1996).

Clinical Findings

HISTORY

- A previous skin disruption at the site
- Fever, malaise, irritability, anorexia, vomiting, and chills can be reported
- Recent sore throat or upper respiratory infection
- Anal pruritus, blood-streaked stools, and stool retention (perianal cellulitis)

PHYSICAL EXAMINATION. The following can be seen:

- Erythematous, tender, swollen, warm areas of skin with irregular borders
- Blue to purple tinge to the skin, often produced when the causative organism is *H. influenzae* (in 3-month- to 3-year-olds)
- Lymphadenitis proximal to the site
- Bright erythema 2 to 3 cm around anus, superficial, well-marginated, not indurated "ring around the anus" (perianal cellulitis)

LABORATORY STUDIES. A CBC and blood culture are done if the child appears ill or toxic. Gram stain and culture of the area can also be done.

Differential Diagnosis

Early erythema nodosum, subcutaneous fat necrosis, giant urticaria, contact dermatitis, and panniculitis are included in the differential diagnosis.

Management

Immediate antibiotic therapy is needed.

1. Significant infection: An initial intramuscular (IM) dose of antibiotic chosen according to suspected organism (systemic penicillin if Streptococcus is suspected) or a third-generation cephalosporin such as ceftriaxone 50 mg/kg IM every 12 hours. Hospitalization may be required if the child is very young, febrile, and acutely ill or has facial, orbital, or periorbital cellulitis.
2. Oral antibiotics:
   - Dicloxacillin 50 to 100 mg/kg per day for 10 days if Staphylococcus is suspected.
   - Penicillin 30 to 60 mg/kg per day for 10 days if Streptococcus is suspected (usually perianal).
   - Amoxicillin 40 to 50 mg/kg per day for 10 days if *H. influenzae* is suspected, unless a β-lactamase-producing strain is a possibility; then use Augmentin (amoxicillin trihydrate; clavulanate potassium) or methicillin or a third-generation cephalosporin.
3. Followup in 24 hours to assess response, observe toxicity. Continue daily visits until child is recovering.

Complications

Recurrent perianal streptococcal infection, septicemia, necrotizing fasciitis, and toxic shock syndrome are possible complications.

- *Necrotizing fasciitis*, commonly called "flesh-eating strep," is an acute, rapidly progressing necrotic invasion of group A streptococcus through the skin and subcutaneous tissue to the fascial compartments. It is found when local resistance is decreased, general debilitation is present, or perforating trauma has occurred. Necrotizing fasciitis occurs most commonly in children as a complication of varicella (AAP, 1997); the peak incidence is in December through March (Working Group on Prevention of Invasive Group A Streptococcal Infections, 1998). Children with diabetes who are in ketoacidosis and immunosup-pressed children are most susceptible (Weston et al., 1996). Necrotizing fasciitis begins as cellulitis (usually on the leg, or on the abdomen in infants) with severe pain, edema, fever, and bullae on an ery-thematous surface. It quickly progresses to ulcer, eschar, and gangrene within 2 days. Prompt treatment (surgical debridement and prolonged antibiotic treatment) may be lifesaving, as overall mortality is as high as 15 to 20% (Working Group on Preven-tion of Invasive Group A Streptococcal In-fections, 1998).

- *Toxic shock syndrome (TSS)* is an acute febrile illness that presents with significant fever, diarrhea, engorged mucous mem-branes, hypotension, a diffuse macular or sunburn-like rash, and multiple organ sys-tem involvement. Either staphylococcal (more common) or streptococcal (more se-vere disease) organisms can cause TSS. Ini-tially recognized in menstruating adoles-cents, TSS is also found in males and younger children. When streptococcus is the causative organism, it is usually associ-ated with bacteremia or focal tissue inva-sion that is rapidly progressive and charac-terized (85%) by sudden, severe, localized pain out of proportion to physical findings. Treatment is intensive, requires hospitaliza-tion, and consists of fluid management, an-tibiotics, and other supportive measures. Mortality of up to 10% has been reported (Darmstadt, 1998; AAP, 1997; Weston et al., 1996). See Chapter 24 and Table 24–13 for the Centers for Disease Control and Prevention (CDC) case definition of strep-tococcal TSS.

Prevention

- Thorough cleansing of any break in the skin helps prevent cellulitis.
- Perianal spread can occur through shared bath water.

Folliculitis and Furuncle

Description

A superficial bacterial inflammation of the hair follicle is called folliculitis; a deeper infec-tion with involvement of the base of the follicle and deep dermis is called a furuncle (boil) (Fig. 37–4).

Etiology and Incidence

Obstruction of the follicular orifice is the most important factor contributing to the devel-opment of folliculitis, but a moist environment, maceration, poor hygiene, occlusive emollients, and prolonged submersion in contaminated wa-ter are also factors. *S. aureus* is the most com-mon causative organism, except for *Pseudomo-nas aeruginosa*, which causes hot-tub folliculitis. These infections are more common in males than in females.

Clinical Findings

HISTORY. The following can be reported:

- Pruritus with folliculitis; tenderness with furuncle

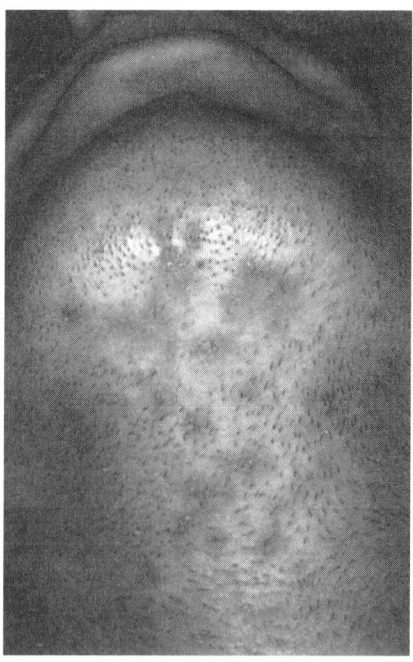

F I G U R E 37-4
Folliculitis. Superficial infection of hair follicles. Multiple pustules, "whiteheads," with hair visible at center and erythematous base. Usually on arms, legs, face, and but-tocks. (From Jarvis C: Physical Examination and Assess-ment, 2nd ed. Philadelphia, WB Saunders, 1996, p 263.)

- Hot-tub exposure
- Irritating surface agent
- Occasional fever, malaise, or lymphadenopathy

PHYSICAL EXAMINATION. The child often is asymptomatic, but the following can be seen:

- Discrete, erythematous 1 to 2-mm papules or pustules centered around a hair follicle
- Involvement of face, scalp, extremities, buttocks, and back
- Nodules with larger areas of erythema and tenderness (furuncle)
- Pruritic papules, pustules, nodules deep red to purple in color, most dense in areas covered by swimming suit 8 to 48 hours after exposure (hot-tub folliculitis)

LABORATORY STUDIES. Gram stain and culture are occasionally ordered.

DIFFERENTIAL DIAGNOSIS

Candida infection, tinea, acne pustules, and chemical folliculitis constitute the differential diagnosis.

Management

The following steps are taken:

1. Warm compresses after washing with soap and water several times a day.
2. Topical keratolytics such as benzoyl peroxide 5 to 10% (twice a day for 5 days), especially if chronic or recurrent.
3. Topical antibiotic cleansers (chlorhexidine or hexachlorophene) or ointments such as erythromycin or clindamycin (twice a day for 5 days).
4. Antistaphylococcal, β-lactamase-resistant antibiotics such as dicloxacillin 25 to 50 mg/kg per day twice a day for 7 to 10 days or cephalexin 40 mg/kg/d for 7 to 10 days in severe or widespread cases.
5. Review of good personal hygiene habits.
6. Follow-up in 1 week for folliculitis, in 1 day for furuncle or abscess, which may need incision and drainage done.
7. Identify and eliminate predisposing factors.
8. If recurrent, look for nasal or skin carrier state.

Complications

Deep abscess formation or carbuncles can occur. Sycosis barbae occurs on the chin, upper lip, and jaw, especially in adolescent black males.

Patient Education and Prevention

Good personal hygiene and an antibacterial soap minimize spread to other household members. Hot-tub folliculitis resolves in 5 to 14 days but can recur up to 3 months after exposure.

FUNGAL INFECTIONS OF THE SKIN (Table 37–8)

Candidiasis

Description

Candidiasis is a fungal infection of the skin or mucous membranes commonly called a yeast infection or thrush. See Chapters 34 and 36 for discussion of oral and vaginal candidiasis.

Etiology and Incidence

Candida albicans is commonly found on skin and oral, vaginal, and intestinal mucosal tissue. Although *Candida* is part of the normal flora, overgrowth and penetration of inflamed skin can occur on the skin or mucous membranes. Candidiasis is more common in infants, obese children, adolescents, and chronically ill or immunocompromised children. It also is often seen as a secondary infection in persistent diaper rashes, or with antibiotic, oral steroid, or oral contraceptive use.

Clinical Findings

HISTORY. The history often includes antibiotic or steroid use over the previous weeks and occurrence of a rash in a moist, warm area.

PHYSICAL EXAMINATION. The following can be seen:

- Mouth—white plaques on an erythematous base that adhere to mucous membranes tightly and bleed when scraped; outer lips cracked (cheilitis)

T A B L E   37-8

Diagnosis and Treatment of Common Fungal Infections

INFECTION	CAUSATIVE ORGANISM	CLINICAL FINDINGS	MANAGEMENT	COMPLICATIONS
Candidiasis	*Candida albicans*	Moist, bright-red diaper rash with sharp borders, satellite lesions; associated white spots in mouth, mucous membranes, or corner of mouth	Topical or oral antifungal, generally nystatin; diaper area hygiene	Paronychia or onychomycosis
Tinea corporis	*Trichophyton tonsurans, Microsporum canis, Epidermophyton floccosum*	Pruritic, slightly erythematous circular lesion with a slightly raised border and central clearing; well demarcated	Topical antifungals; identify and treat source; exclude from day care until treated	Tinea incognita from steroid treatment
Tinea cruris	Same as for tinea corporis	Raised-border, scaly lesion on upper thighs and groin; penis and scrotum spared; symmetrical	Same as for tinea corporis; loose clothes, absorbent powder	Possible secondary infection
Tinea pedis	Same as for tinea corporis	Vesicles and erosions on instep; fissure between toes with scaling and erythema; diffuse scaling on weight-bearing surfaces with exaggerated scaling in creases; pruritus	Same as for tinea corporis; absorbent powder; cotton socks; open-toed shoes; moisturize	Reinfection common
Tinea versicolor	*Malassezia furfur* or *Malassezia ovalis*	Multiple scaly, discrete oval macules on neck, shoulders, upper back, and chest; hypo- to hyperpigmented areas; fail to tan in summer	Selenium shampoo; topical imidazoles	50% recurrence rate

Data from Hurwitz S: Clinical Pediatric Dermatology, 2nd ed. Philadelphia, WB Saunders, 1993, pp 372–400.

- Corners of mouth—fissured and inflamed (perlèche or angular cheilitis)
- Intertriginous areas (neck, axillae, or groin)—bright erythema in flexural folds
- Diaper area—moist, beefy-red macules and papules with sharply marked borders and satellite lesions; erosions may also be present
- Vulvovaginal area—thick, cheesy, yellow discharge; erythema; edema; and itching

LABORATORY STUDIES. If treatment failure or questionable diagnosis, KOH-treated scrapings of satellite lesions or mucosa reveal yeast cells and pseudohyphae (see Fig. 37–2).

Differential Diagnosis

The differential diagnosis includes erythema toxicum, miliaria, staphylococcal pustulosis, transient neonatal pustulosis, neonatal herpes simplex, and congenital syphilis.

Management

The following steps are taken:

1. Skin infection: topical antifungals (Table 37–9) such as nystatin, miconazole, clotrimazole, ketoconazole, cyclopiroxolamine, and econazole applied to skin result in improvement within 3 to 5 days. These may be used at every diaper change for 2 to 3 days until improvement begins.
2. Oral infection: nystatin oral solution 4 times a day swabbed onto mucous membranes for 5 to 14 days, and gentian violet 1 to 2% aqueous solution applied twice a day, or clotrimazole troches 10 mg tablet dissolved slowly in the mouth 5 times a day for 14 days in children over 3 years of age. If breastfeeding, the mother should put solution on her nipples to eliminate reinfection. A second course is sometimes needed to clear the infection.
3. If inflammation is present, alternate nystatin cream and 1% hydrocortisone for a day or two.
4. If recalcitrant infection or nail involvement, oral ketoconazole, fluconazole, or itraconazole may be recommended.
5. Keep area dry and cool. Minimize skin irritation:

- Frequent diaper changes.
- Leave diaper area open to air.
- Blow-dry with warm air for 3 to 5 minutes at diaper change (especially helpful in intertriginous areas in infants and obese children).
- Avoid rubber pants.
- Use mild soap and water; rinse well; avoid diaper wipes.
- Avoid other powders and medications, especially antibiotics and steroids.
- Discontinue oral antibiotics and steroids when possible.
- Discard or sterilize pacifiers.

6. Cold milk compresses (if child is not allergic to milk): Mix equal parts skim milk and water with ice cubes in a bowl; saturate cloth and apply repeatedly until warm for 5 to 10 minutes 3 times a day in conjunction with hydrocortisone and antifungal creams (Weinberg, 1998).

Complications

Chronic mucocutaneous candidiasis due to immunological deficit can occur. Paronychia may occur with thumb-sucking.

Patient Education

Treatment failure is usually due to lack of compliance.

Tinea Capitis

See later section on alopecia.

Tinea Corporis

Description

Tinea corporis, commonly called ringworm, is a superficial fungal skin infection found on the face or body. It is also identified by the part of the body affected, for example, tinea manuum (hand), tinea faciei (face) (see Color Fig. 15).

Etiology

Tinea corporis is caused by the dermatophytes *Microsporum canis, Trichophyton ton-*

T A B L E 37-9

Antifungal Medications

DRUG (TRADE NAME)	STRENGTH AND FORMULATION	APPLICATION	INDICATIONS/SIDE EFFECTS
TOPICAL MEDICATIONS			
Imidazoles			
Clotrimazole (Lotrimin)	1% C, L, S, Su	bid	Erythema, stinging, blistering, peeling, edema, pruritus, hives, burning
Econazole nitrate (Spectazole)	1% C	qd/bid	Burning, pruritus, stinging, erythema; may have antibacterial effects
Ketoconazole (Nizoral)	2% C, Sh	qd	Irritation, pruritus, stinging
Miconazole nitrate (Micatin, Monistat)	2% C, P, S, Su	qd/bid	Irritation, dermatitis, pruritus; economical
Oxiconazole nitrate (Oxistat)	1% C, S	qd	Pruritus, burning, irritation, erythema, folliculitis
Sulconazole nitrate (Exelderm)	1% C, S	qd/bid	Pruritus, burning, stinging
Allylamines			
Butenafine HCl (Mentax)		qd	Fungicidal
Naftifine HCl (Naftin)	1% C, G	qd/bid	Burning, stinging, erythema, pruritus, irritation; fungicidal
Terbinafine HCl (Lamisil)	1% C	qd/bid	Pruritus, irritation, burning; fungicidal
Ethanolamine			
Cyclopirox olamine (Loprox)	1% C, L	bid	Irritation, erythema, burning; fungicidal
Others			
Gentian violet	1–2% S	bid	Staining
Nystatin (Mycolog-II,* Mycostatin, Nilstat, Mytrex*)	100,000 U/g C, L, P, O, Su	bid/tid	Rare adverse reactions; effective against yeast only
Selenium sulfide (Excel; Head & Shoulders Intensive Treatment Dandruff Shampoo; Selsun Blue)	1% Sh, 2.5% L, Sh	qd	For tinea capitis (reduces transmission), tinea versicolor (shampoo may be used as lotion)
Sodium thiosulfate; salicylic acid (Tinver)	25% L	qd/bid	For tinea versicolor
Tolnaftate (Desenex, Tinactin)	1% C, P, S	bid	Rare adverse reactions
Calcium undecylenate (Caldesene, Cruex)	10–20% P, C, O, L	bid	Irritation

T A B L E 37-9
Antifungal Medications Continued

DRUG (TRADE NAME)	STRENGTH AND FORMULATION	APPLICATION	INDICATIONS/SIDE EFFECTS
ORAL MEDICATIONS			
Clotrimazole	10 mg tab	1 tab 5 times a day dissolved slowly in mouth	Treatment of oral candidiasis
Fluconazole	10–40 mg/ml; 50, 100, 150, 200 mg capsules	3–6 mg/kg/d in single dose	Approved for pediatric use for oropharyngeal, esophageal, or disseminated candidiasis; possible drug interactions
Griseofulvin	Ultramicrosized Microsized	5–10 mg/kg in single dose; 10–20 mg/kg/d given qd or bid	Mainstay of therapy; fungistatic; excellent safety profile and extensive use; monitor CBC, LFTs, renal function at 4 wk and every 4–8 wk; possible drug interactions
Itraconazole	Liquid Su not recommended; 100 or 200 mg capsules	Dose not established for children; 3–16-y-olds treated with 100 mg/d or 3–5 mg/kg/d	Not approved for pediatric use; used in treatment failures or for onychomycosis by some; monitor monthly LFTs; pulse doses used in adults; broadest spectrum; possible drug interactions
Ketoconazole	100 mg/tsp Su 200 mg tab	3.3–6.6 mg/kg/d in single dose	Less effective than griseofulvin and higher risk of hepatotoxicity
Nystatin	100,000 U/ml	2 ml qid after meals	Treatment of oral candidiasis
Terbinafine	250 mg tab	< 20 kg, ¼ tab; 20–40 kg, ½ tab; >40 kg, 1 tab	Not approved for pediatric use; no studies in children; costly; possible drug interactions

C = cream; G = gel; L = lotion; O = ointment; P = powder; S = solution; Sh = shampoo; Su = suspension; CBC = complete blood count; LFTs = liver function tests.
*Nystatin; triamcinolone acetonide.
Data from American Academy of Pediatrics: Topical drugs for superficial fungal infections and recommended doses of parenteral and oral antifungal drugs. *In* 1997 Red Book: Report of the Committee on Infectious Diseases, 24th ed. Elk Grove, IL, American Academy of Pediatrics, 1997, pp. 628–629, 632–633; Cross JT, Hickerson SL, Yamauchi T: Antifungal drugs. Pediatr Rev 16:123–129, 1995; Friedlander SF, Suarez S: Pediatric antifungal therapy. Dermatol Clin 16:527–537, 1998; Stein DH: Tineas—Superficial dermatophyte infections. Pediatr Rev 19:368–372, 1998.

surans, and *Epidermophyton floccosum*. Transmission comes as the stratum corneum is invaded following direct contact with infected humans, animals, or fomites. The exact mechanism is unknown but is probably due to a toxin causing an inflammatory response.

Clinical Findings

HISTORY. Contact with a person or animal with ringworm is sometimes reported.

PHYSICAL EXAMINATION

- Flat, scaling, mildly erythematous circular patches with raised borders
- Spread peripherally and clear centrally or may be inflammatory throughout with superficial pustules
- Often prominent over hair follicles

LABORATORY STUDIES. If treatment failure or questionable diagnosis:

- KOH-treated scrapings of border of lesion reveal hyphae and spores (see Fig. 37-2).
- Fungal culture.
- Wood's lamp is helpful but does not fluoresce all tinea infections.

Differential Diagnosis

Pityriasis rosea, nummular eczema, psoriasis, seborrhea, contact dermatitis, tinea versicolor, granuloma annulare, and Lyme disease are the differential diagnosis.

Management

Management involves the following:

1. Topical antifungals (see Table 37-9) such as miconazole or clotrimazole are applied 3 times a day until 1 to 2 weeks after tinea is resolved, usually a minimum of 4 weeks (AAP, 1997). Prescriptive antifungals (e.g., econazole, ciclopirox) penetrate the skin more effectively but are more expensive.
2. Extensive infection, or tinea unresponsive to topical treatment, may be treated orally with griseofulvin (see Table 37-9) for 4 to 8 weeks; it must be taken with fatty foods and can cause headache, nausea, diarrhea, or crampy abdominal pain. Monitor CBC, liver function tests (LFTs), and possibly renal function tests if treatment duration is longer than 3 months; obtain initial laboratory panel at 4 weeks, repeat every 4 to 8 weeks (McDonald & Smith, 1998; Goldgeier, 1996; Schwartz & Janniger, 1995).
3. Identification and treatment of contacts.
4. Education about communicability of lesions and length of treatment.
5. Exclusion from day care or school until treatment has begun.
6. Follow up in 2 weeks or sooner if lesions are not responding. If unresponsive, diagnosis is incorrect or resistance is possible. Culture to confirm diagnosis and change class of antifungal used.

Complications

Tinea incognito occurs when tinea has been treated with hydrocortisone; signs and symptoms of infection are minimized, but the infection persists.

Patient Education

Find the source of infection and treat or eliminate it to prevent recurrence. Treat skin and 1-cm area beyond the border. Keep skin dry following application of antifungal

Tinea Cruris

Description

Tinea cruris, commonly called "jock itch," is a superficial fungal skin infection found on the groin, thighs, and intertriginous folds.

Etiology and Incidence

Caused by the dermatophyte *E. floccosum* or, occasionally, *Trichophyton rubrum* or *Trichophyton mentagrophytes*, tinea cruris rarely occurs before adolescence and is more common in males, obese individuals, or those experiencing chafing from tight clothes or moisture. It is extremely common and often occurs with tinea pedis (AAP, 1997; Hurwitz, 1993).

Clinical Findings

HISTORY

- Hot, humid weather, tight clothing, or contact sport such as wrestling
- Often associated with tinea pedis

PHYSICAL EXAMINATION

- Bilateral, symmetrical, scaly, erythematous to slightly brown, sharply marginated lesions with a raised border
- Occurs on inner thighs and inguinal creases; penis and scrotum spared

LABORATORY STUDIES. If treatment failure or questionable diagnosis:

- KOH scraping reveals hyphae and spores
- Fungal culture

Differential Diagnosis

Psoriasis, candidiasis, contact dermatitis, seborrhea, intertrigo, and erythrasma are in the differential diagnosis.

Management

Management is the same as for tinea corporis. Duration of treatment is usually 4 to 6 weeks. If griseofulvin is required, a treatment course of 2 to 6 weeks is usually indicated (see Table 37-9). Additionally:

1. Advise the patient to wear cotton underwear and loose clothing and to use absorbent powder.
2. Maintain good hygiene following a wrestling event (e.g., bathing, sole use of towel).
3. Do not use steroids because of risk of atrophy and striae.

Tinea Pedis

Description

Tinea pedis is a superficial fungal skin infection found on the feet, commonly called "athlete's foot." There are three clinical forms: (1) vesicles and erosions on the instep of one or both feet; (2) an occasional fissure between the toes with surrounding scale and erythema; (3) rare diffuse scaling on the weight-bearing surface of the foot with exaggerated scaling in creases (moccasin foot).

Etiology and Incidence

Caused by the dermatophytes *T. rubrum* and *E. floccosum* or *T. mentagrophytes*, tinea pedis rarely occurs before adolescence and is more common in males (AAP, 1997; Weston et al., 1996). It often occurs with tinea cruris.

Clinical Findings

HISTORY. The following are sometimes reported:

- Sweaty feet
- Use of nylon socks or nonbreathable shoes
- Exposure in family or at school
- Itching, stinging, foul odor
- Microtrauma to feet—cracks, abrasions, nicks, cuts
- Contact with damp areas (e.g., swimming pools, locker room, showers)

PHYSICAL EXAMINATION. Findings include the following:

- Red, scaly, cracked rash on soles or interdigital spaces and instep, especially between the third, fourth, and fifth toes
- Infection initially white, peeling lesions becoming erythematous, vesicular, macerated, or fissured, and scaly
- Dorsum of foot remains clear
- Chronic infection manifested by a moccasin pattern with diffuse scaling and erythema

LABORATORY STUDIES. These are the same as for tinea corporis.

Differential Diagnosis

Contact dermatitis, atopic dermatitis, dyshidrotic eczema, psoriasis, and juvenile plantar dermatosis (red, dry fissures of weight-bearing surface) are the differential diagnosis.

Management

Management is the same as for tinea corporis. Antifungal medication should be applied

1 in. beyond the borders of the rash for 7 days after clearing. Usual treatment is 3 to 6 weeks. If griseofulvin is required, treatment for 6 to 8 weeks is usually recommended. Additionally:

1. Advise patient to keep feet dry, use absorbent powder and cotton socks, avoid scratching, and wear shoes that allow the feet to breathe or go barefoot when home.
2. Rinse feet with plain water or water and vinegar; dry carefully, especially between the toes. Moisturize and protect feet to prevent splitting and cracking.
3. Aluminum chloride (Drysol) may be used for hyperhidrosis.
4. Tennis shoes may be washed in the machine with soap and bleach.
5. Physical education or sports may be continued, as tinea pedis is not so common.
6. Follow up in 2 to 3 weeks or sooner if lesions are not responding.

Complications

A secondary bacterial infection, indicated by foul odor, can occur. An allergic reaction to fungus, called an id response, is manifested by a vesicular eruption on the palms and sides of fingers, and occasionally on the trunk and extremities.

Tinea Versicolor

Description

Tinea versicolor is a superficial fungal infection, also called pityriasis versicolor, that tends to be persistent and occurs predominantly on the trunk. The lesions do not tan in the summer and become relatively darker in winter months.

Etiology and Incidence

This infection is caused by a yeast-like organism, *Malassezia furfur*, and occurs more commonly in adolescents than in younger children, in chronically ill and immunocompromised children, and in warmer seasons and humid climates (AAP, 1997; Weston et al., 1996).

Clinical Findings

HISTORY. The infection is associated with warm, humid weather. Occasional mild itching may occur.

PHYSICAL EXAMINATION. Multiple, annular, scaling, discrete macules ranging from hypo- to hyperpigmented (salmon-colored to brown) are seen on the neck, shoulders, upper back and arms, chest midline, and face (especially in children).

LABORATORY STUDIES. KOH scrapings, though not necessary, reveal short curved hyphae and circular spores ("spaghetti and meatballs"). Scrapings fluoresce yellow-orange under Wood's lamp if not cleansed recently.

Differential Diagnosis

Pityriasis alba, pityriasis rosea, vitiligo, postinflammatory hypo- or hyperpigmentation, seborrhea, and secondary syphilis are included in the differential diagnosis.

Management

The following steps are taken:

1. Selenium 2.5% lotion or 1% shampoo is considered the treatment of choice, applied from face to knees. There are several options for application including overnight once a week for 4 weeks; 10 to 30 minutes every day for 7 to 14 days; or daily for 1 week, then weekly for 1 month. Following one of the above routines, selenium should be used prophylactically once a month for 3 months. Sodium hyposulfite or thiosulfate can also be used.
2. Topical imidazoles (clotrimazole, miconazole, econazole, haloprogin, ketoconazole, or naftifine) for 2 to 4 weeks can be used instead of selenium (see Table 37–9).
3. Resistant cases or tropical climates are sometimes an indication for oral antifungal treatment such as with ketoconazole or fluconazole or itraconazole.
4. Education:
   • Fifty percent have recurrences within 1 to 10 years.
   • Sun exposure makes lesions appear hypopigmented as the surrounding skin tans.

- Repigmentation takes several months.
- If the patient is taking oral antifungal medication, encourage exercise to induce sweating because this may enhance concentration of medication in the skin.
- Skin irritation occurs with overnight application.
- Absence of flaking when skin is scraped is a sign of effective treatment.

▉▉▉ VIRAL INFECTIONS OF THE SKIN

Herpes Simplex

Description

In the active state, herpes simplex virus (HSV) causes contagious infections of the skin and mucous membranes ranging from mild to life-threatening. Primary infection with HSV type 1 (HSV-1) usually occurs as acute gingivostomatitis (see Chapter 34). The virus then becomes dormant in certain nerve cells until reactivated by triggering factors such as stress, menses, illness, and fatigue. HSV-1 causes recurrent herpes labialis infection, commonly called cold sores or fever blisters (see Color Fig. 16). HSV-2 infection commonly occurs as a neonatal infection (see Chapter 39) or herpetic vulvovaginitis (see Chapter 36) or progenitalis. Type 1 can also be found in the genital area; type 2 on the lips and mouth. Herpetic keratoconjunctivitis is discussed in Chapter 29; other information may be found in Chapter 24.

Etiology and Incidence

HSV-1 is transmitted by close contact with skin, mucous membranes, and body fluids, often through a break in the skin or by autoinoculation. Lesions occur in children of all ages, are contagious as long as they are present, and have an incubation period of 2 to 12 days. HSV is more common in lower socioeconomic groups (lower, 50 to 60%; middle, 35%; upper, 10 to 20%; Annunziato & Gershon, 1996). Primary lesions usually occur before 5 years of age, are more painful and extensive, and last longer. HSV-1 is responsible for gingivostomatitis, herpes labialis, and hand and finger infec-

tions. HSV-2 infection occurs most commonly in adolescents as a sexually transmitted disease and in infants from transmittal during delivery; in children, the possibility of sexual abuse must be considered.

Clinical Findings

HISTORY. In primary herpes, fever, malaise, sore throat, and decreased fluid intake can occur. In recurrent HSV infection, there is often a painful prodrome of burning, tingling, and itching at the involved site. Recent acute febrile illness or sun exposure may also be reported.

PHYSICAL EXAMINATION. The following are seen on physical examination:

HSV-1

- Gingivostomatitis—pharyngitis with grouped erythematous-based vesicles that ulcerate and form white plaques on mucosa, gingiva, tongue, palate, lips, chin, and nasolabial folds; lymphadenopathy and halitosis are present
- Herpes labialis—cluster of small, clear vesicles with an erythematous base that become weepy and ulcerated, progressing to crustiness, usually only on one side of the mouth
- Hand or fingers—deep-appearing vesicles
- Common sites of involvement: lips, hand, fingers, nose, cheek, forehead, and eyes; can also occur in the genital area

HSV-2

- Grouped vesicopustules and ulceration with edema
- Primary lesions on vaginal mucosa, labia, or perineum in females and on the penile shaft or perineum in males; oral lesions are possible
- Recurrent lesions on labia, vulva, clitoris, or cervix in females and on the prepuce, glans, or sulcus in males
- Regional lymphadenopathy

LABORATORY STUDIES. A Tzanck smear can be done on fluid from the lesions to identify epidermal giant cells. Viral cultures are the gold standard for definitive diagnosis. Direct fluorescent antibody (DFA) tests, enzyme-linked immunosorbent assay (ELISA) serology, and polymerase chain reaction (PCR) tests can be done but are usually only used with severe forms of HSV infection.

Differential Diagnosis

The differential diagnosis includes aphthous stomatitis, hand-foot-and-mouth disease, varicella, impetigo, folliculitis, and erythema multiforme.

Management

Management can be guided by considering the host (e.g., age, area and extent of involvement, and immune status), the organism (is it definitely HSV?), and the drug needed (Nelson & Demmler, 1996) (see Table 37–10).

1. Burow solution compresses 3 times a day to alleviate discomfort.
2. Acyclovir 20 to 40 mg/kg/d orally 5 times a day for 5 days *or* 200 mg every 4 hours 5 times a day for 7 to 10 days may be indicated to help shorten the course and alleviate symptoms for children with the following conditions:
   - Any underlying skin disorder (e.g., eczema)

- A severe case
- An immunocompromised disease
- Systemic symptoms with primary genital infection
- Occasionally for initial severe gingivostomatitis (Trizna & Tyring, 1998; Annunziato & Gershon, 1996).
3. Antibiotics for secondary bacterial (usually staphylococcal) infection:
   - Mupirocin topically 3 times a day for 5 days
   - Erythromycin 40 mg/kg/d for 10 days
   - Dicloxacillin 12.5 to 50 mg/kg/d for 10 days.
4. Oral anesthetics for comfort; use with caution in children (children should be able to rinse and spit).
   - Viscous lidocaine (xylocaine) 2% topical
   - Liquid diphenhydramine alone or combined with Maalox (aluminum hydroxide; magnesium hydroxide) as a 1:1 rinse (maximum of 5 mg/kg/d diphenhydramine in case it is swallowed). It can also be applied with Q-tips to the lesions.
5. Consult with or refer to an appropriate provider any newborn infant, immunosuppressed child, child with infected atopic dermatitis, or child with a lesion in the eye or on the eyelid margin.

T A B L E 37-10

Diagnosis and Treatment of Herpes Simplex (HS) and Herpes Zoster (HZ)

	PRESENTATION	CLINICAL FINDINGS	TREATMENT	EDUCATION
HS	Gingivostomatitis as primary infection; herpes labialis or herpes facialis as recurrent infection	Pharyngitis with erythematous vesicles on/in mouth; small, clear vesicles on erythematous base progressing to crusting	Burow solution; acyclovir in primary case or underlying disorder; antibiotics if secondary infection; oral anesthetics; supportive care	Degree and duration of contagion; triggers to infection
HZ	Reactivation of latent varicella virus, especially after mild cases or in infants <1 y of age or immunocompromised host	2–3 clustered groups of vesicles on erythematous base, especially over thoracic or lumbosacral dermatomes	Burow solution; antihistamine; drying lotions; possible acyclovir; silver sulfadiazine (Silvadene cream); antibiotics if secondary infection	New vesicles occur for up to 1 wk; take 2–3 wk to resolve; contagious for varicella; varicella vaccine to prevent

6. Offer supportive care such as antipyretics, analgesics, hydration, and good oral hygiene.
7. Exclude from day care only during the initial course (gingivostomatitis) and if the child cannot control secretions.
8. Recurrent, frequent and severe HSV infection may be treated with 6 months of prophylaxis with acyclovir.

Complications

Herpetic whitlow, occurring on a finger or thumb, is a swollen, painful lesion with an erythematous base and ulceration resembling a paronychia. It occurs on fingers of thumb-sucking children with gingivostomatitis or adolescents with genital HSV infection. Therapy with oral acyclovir 200 mg 5 times a day for 5 to 10 days may speed healing. *Eczema herpeticum* or *Kaposi's varicelliform eruption* is discussed in Chapter 24. HSV has also been implicated as a possible cause of erythema multiforme and Stevens-Johnson syndrome.

Patient Education, Prognosis, and Prevention

Recurrence of infection, possible triggering factors, and avoidance measures should be discussed. Triggers can include physical and psychological stress, trauma, fever, exposure to UV light, illness, menses, and extreme weather. Contagiousness of lesions and oral secretions must be understood. Explanation of the course of primary disease, with fever lasting up to 4 days and lesions taking at least 2 weeks to heal, is important. Famciclovir and perciclovir are in clinical trials for use in children. Vaccines are under development to decrease transmission and minimize recurrence.

Herpes Zoster

Description

Herpes zoster (HZ) is a recurrent varicella infection commonly called shingles (Fig. 37-5).

Etiology and Incidence

Caused by reactivation of the latent varicella infection, HZ occurs in 10 to 20% of all persons,

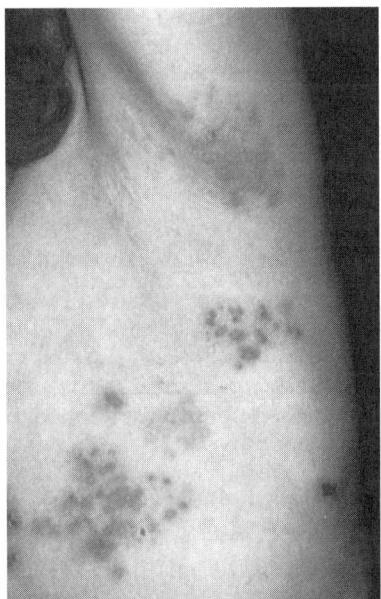

F I G U R E 37-5
Herpes zoster. Typical segmented papulovesicular eruptions on an inflammatory base occur in an interrupted band with dermatomal distribution. (From Hurwitz S: Clinical Pediatric Dermatology, 2nd ed. Philadelphia, WB Saunders, 1993, p 325.)

is rare in childhood, and occurs more frequently with increasing age (3 times more common in adolescents than preschoolers). HZ is more common following mild cases of varicella, following varicella prior to 1 year of age (3- to 20-fold increased risk), and in immunocompromised children. Occurrence of HZ more than once is rare (Fisher & Edwards, 1998).

Clinical Findings

HISTORY. Burning, stinging, or tingling precedes eruption by about 1 week, though this is less common in children. The lesions can be extremely itchy and painful.

PHYSICAL EXAMINATION. Findings include the following:

• Two or three clustered groups of macules and papules progressing to vesicles on an erythematous base. These vesicles become pustular, rupture, ulcerate, and crust.

- Lesions develop over 3 to 5 days and last 7 to 10 days
- Commonly seen on thoracic (50 to 70%), lumbosacral (20%), and fifth cranial nerve (10%) dermatomes with scattered lesions outside borders (Fisher & Edwards, 1998; Weston et al., 1996)
- Lesions do not cross midline (key to diagnosis)
- Lymphadenopathy

LABORATORY STUDIES. The Tzanck smear or viral culture can be done to distinguish from HSV infection. Bacterial culture or Gram stain can be used to distinguish from impetigo.

Differential Diagnosis

Local cutaneous HSV infection and impetigo are in the differential diagnosis.

Management

Management steps include the following:

1. Burow solution compresses 3 times a day to alleviate discomfort.
2. Antihistamines for itching, analgesics for discomfort.
3. Lotions like calamine help dry lesions and decrease itching.
4. Antiviral medications:
   - Acyclovir 800 mg orally every 4 hours 5 times a day for 7 to 10 days helps shorten the course and alleviate symptoms in immunocompromised or significantly ill children. Acyclovir has not been fully studied in children under 2 years of age.
   - Famciclovir 500 mg every 8 hours for 7 days at the earliest sign of HZ or within 48 to 72 hours of onset *or* valaciclovir 1 g orally 3 times a day for 7 days at the earliest sign of HZ or within 48 hours of onset has been approved for adults but not for children with HZ (Trizna & Tyring, 1998).
5. Silver sulfadiazine (Silvadene) cream to provide comfort and speed healing of lesions (Kurtz, 1993).
6. Antibiotics for secondary bacterial (usually staphylococcal) infection:
   - Mupirocin topically twice a day

   - Dicloxacillin 12.5 to 25 mg/kg/d for 7 to 10 days.
7. Refer for immediate ophthalmological examination if eyes, forehead, or nose is involved.

Complications

These are rare except in immunocompromised children. Occasionally, HZ is the initial finding in acquired immunodeficiency syndrome (AIDS), especially if more than one dermatome is involved (Marrazzo, 1998).

Patient Education, Prevention, and Prognosis

1. New vesicles appear for up to 1 week and take 2 to 3 weeks to resolve. Illness is usually mild.
2. The child is contagious for varicella until lesions are crusted and should be excluded from day care until this occurs. However, if the lesions can be covered, the child may return to child care (AAP, 1997).
3. The varicella vaccine has reduced the incidence of HZ from 77 per 100,000 to 18 per 100,000 (Fisher & Edwards, 1998).

Molluscum Contagiosum

Description

A benign, common childhood viral skin infection with little health risk, molluscum contagiosum often disappears on its own in a few weeks to months and is not easily treated (Fig. 37–6).

Etiology and Incidence

This highly contagious poxvirus that attacks skin and mucous membranes is spread by direct contact, by fomites, or by autoinoculation. It is commonly found in children and adolescents (AAP, 1997; Prasad, 1996). Three types are identified. Lesions found on the extremities, neck, and head are usually type 1; genital lesions are usually type 2 or 3. The incubation period is about 2 months; the child is contagious as long as lesions are present.

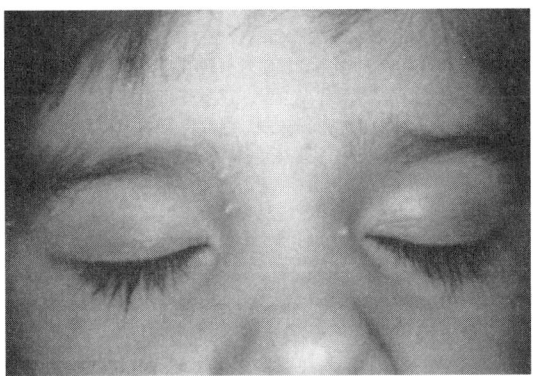

F I G U R E 37-6
Molluscum contagiosum. Discrete, flesh-colored, dome-shaped papules on the nasal area of a 3-year-old girl. (From Hurwitz S: Clinical Pediatric Dermatology, 2nd ed. Philadelphia, WB Saunders, 1993, p 338.)

Clinical Findings

HISTORY

- Itching at the site
- Possible exposure to molluscum contagiosum

PHYSICAL EXAMINATION. Findings include the following:

- Very small, firm, pink to flesh-colored discrete papules 1 to 6 mm in size (occasionally up to 15 mm), progressing to become umbilicated papules with a cheesy core; keratinous contents may extrude from the umbilication.
- Face, axillae, antecubital, trunk, crural, and extremities are the most commonly involved areas; palms, soles, and scalp are spared.
- Few in number, usually 2 to 20.
- Sexually active or abused children can have genitally grouped lesions.
- Children with eczema or immunosuppression can have severe cases; those with HIV infection or AIDS can present with hundreds of lesions.

Differential Diagnosis

Warts, closed comedones, small epidermal cysts, blisters, folliculitis, and condyloma acuminatum are included in the differential diagnosis.

Management

1. Lesions resolve spontaneously if left untreated. Mechanical removal of the central core is often done to prevent spread and autoinoculation. Use of EMLA cream (lidocaine; prilocaine) 30 to 45 minutes before the procedure is helpful.
2. Curettage is done with a sharp blade to remove the papule. Piercing the papule and expressing the plug can also be done but is painful.
3. Nightly application of surgical tape (Scotch or adhesive tape can be used) for 1 month followed by removal of lesions.
4. Medications that may prove beneficial follow. Recheck the patient in 1 to 2 weeks to determine need for retreatment.
   - Liquid nitrogen applied for 2 to 3 seconds (easiest but also painful).
   - Trichloroacetic acid 25 to 50% applied by dropper to the center of the lesion, followed by alcohol.
   - Cantharidin 0.7% in collodion applied by dropper to the center of the lesion, followed by alcohol. Salicylic or lactic acid or podophyllin can also be used.
   - Podofilox (Condylox) 0.5% topical solution may be used.
   - Tretinoin cream applied to lesion nightly.
   - Silver nitrate, iodine 7 to 9%, or phenol 1% applied for 2 to 3 seconds.
5. Cimetidine 30 to 40 mg/kg per day in three divided doses orally for 2 months (Friedlander, 1997).
6. Sexual abuse of children with genitally grouped lesions should be suspected and evaluated.
7. Evaluate for HIV infection if hundreds of lesions are found.

Complications

Molluscum dermatitis, a scaly, erythematous, hypersensitive reaction, can occur in 10% of cases (Prasad, 1996); inflammation of the eyes or conjunctiva; scarring can occur.

Patient Education and Prevention

Patients are contagious, but there is no need to exclude them from day care or school. Children with impaired immunity, atopic dermatitis, or traumatized skin are at greater risk for broader spread. Severe inflammation is possible several hours after application of cantharidin. Scarring is unusual.

Warts

Description

A common childhood skin infection characterized by a proliferation of the epidermis, warts are benign, usually self-regressing papillomas that are more of a bother and cosmetic concern than a serious health problem.

Etiology and Incidence

Occurring in approximately 5 to 10% of children 5 to 10 years of age, warts account for one in five pediatric visits for a skin problem and more than 5 million visits per year (Cohen, 1997; Siegfried, 1996). Most commonly transmitted from person to person, warts are caused by one of various subtypes of the human papillomavirus, with certain subtypes related to sexual transmission. Viral and host factors, such as quantity of virus, location of warts, preexisting skin injury, and cell-mediated immunity determine how contagious warts are. Although most warts resolve spontaneously in 12 to 24 months, there is a high incidence of recurrence.

Clinical Findings

HISTORY. The history can include exposure to someone with warts.

PHYSICAL EXAMINATION. Warts are common in areas of trauma, especially the dorsal surface of the face, hands, periungual areas, elbows, knees, and feet. The genital or perianal area may also be involved.

- *Common* warts (verruca vulgaris) are usually elevated, flesh-colored single papules with scaly, irregular surfaces and occasionally black pinpoints, which are thrombosed blood vessels. They are usually asymptomatic and multiple in number and are found anywhere on the body, although most commonly on the hands, nails, and feet (Fig. 37-7).

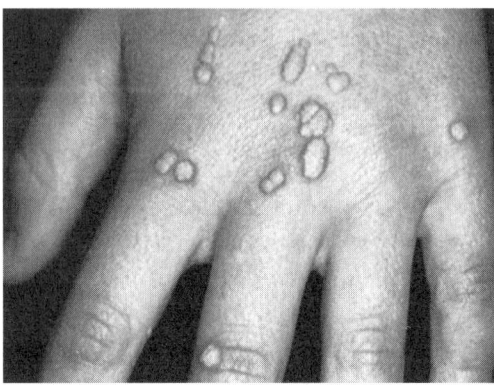

F I G U R E 37-7
Multiple common warts (verruca vulgaris). (From Hurwitz S: Clinical Pediatric Dermatology, 2nd ed. Philadelphia, WB Saunders, 1993, p 329.)

- *Periungual* warts are common warts occurring around the cuticles of the fingers or toes.
- *Plantar* warts (mosaic) are common warts found on weight-bearing surfaces of the feet. Their surface, although irregular, is even with the skin surface. Found alone or grouped, plantar warts grow inward and disrupt skin markings.
- *Filiform* warts project from the skin on a narrow stalk and are usually seen on the face, lips, nose, eyelids, or neck.
- *Flat* warts (verruca plana or juvenile warts) appear multiply, most commonly on the face and extremities, and are small (1 to 3 mm), subtle, flesh-colored, flat, and round.
- *Condylomata acuminata* on genital mucosa and adjacent skin are multiple, confluent warts with irregular surfaces, light in color, and cauliflower-like in appearance. See Chapter 36 for more detail.
- The Koebner phenomenon describes the occurrence of warts in areas previously injured or irritated.

Differential Diagnosis

The differential diagnosis is calluses, corns, foreign bodies, and moles.

Management

No treatment is needed if warts are asymptomatic, as most warts disappear over time (67 to 75% in 3 years) (Cohen, 1997; Siegfried, 1996). "Benign neglect" is often the treatment of choice. The decision to treat should be based on location, discomfort, and how long the wart has been present (>2 years). There is no treatment that guarantees resolution or prevents recurrence. If genital warts are found in a young child or an adolescent who is not sexually active, suspicion of sexual abuse must be raised. Chemical or physical destruction is the method used (Table 37–11). Follow up in 2 to 3 weeks to evaluate response.

Complications

Scarring from removal can occur. Immunocompromised hosts can have extensive involvement.

Patient Education

A blister, sometimes hemorrhagic, may form 1 to 2 days after freezing. Redness and itching may herald regression of a wart. Parents and patients must be warned that multiple or prolonged treatment is often necessary.

▨ INFESTATIONS OF THE SKIN (See Table 37–12)

Pediculosis

Description

Pediculosis, commonly called "lice infestation" affects the head, body, or pubic area. Pediculosis capitis (head) is most common, pediculosis corporis (body) is uncommon, and pediculosis pubis (pubic) is considered a sexually transmitted disease.

Etiology and Incidence

Lice infestation is caused by two subspecies of *Pediculus humanus* (head and body) or by *Phthirus pubis* (pubic). The adult female louse, which survives by sucking human blood, deposits 6 to 10 eggs per day at the base of the hair shaft within a waterproof, glue-like substance. The eggs mature in 7 to 10 days, and begin laying eggs in another 7 to 10 days. Typically,

no more than 12 to 24 head lice infest a child at a time (Brainerd, 1998), though in a 30-day life span, one louse can lay 150 to 300 eggs. Transmission of pediculosis occurs by direct or indirect contact, often by sharing hairbrushes, caps, clothing, or linen or through close living quarters, poor hygiene, or sexual activity (pubic lice).

Pediculosis capitis is considered an epidemic in the United States, with estimates ranging from 6 to 12 million cases per year (CDC, 1998; Connolly, 1998; AAP, 1997). All socioeconomic groups are affected, but lice are most common in school-aged white females, with the peak season occurring from August to November. Lice are uncommon in blacks, with a ratio of 1:34 whites (Weston et al., 1996). Pediculosis corporis is uncommon in childhood. If pediculosis pubis is found in a child, sexual abuse must be considered.

As with other medications, lice appear to have a growing resistance to available treatment options. Both European and Israeli scientists have documented this resistance, and it is being studied in the United States. The National Pediculosis Association (NPA, 1998a) states it receives over 50 calls a day reporting medication failure. This has led to the trial of many alternative treatment options.

Clinical Findings

HISTORY. The following may be elicited:

- A history of infestation in a family, friend, or day care contact
- Dandruff-like substance in the hair
- Itching of the scalp, scratching, and irritability if infestation has been present for a few weeks

PHYSICAL EXAMINATION. Findings include the following:

Head Lice

- Mites can be visualized; the nits or eggs can be seen as small, white oval cases attached to a hair shaft (Fig. 37–8).
- Common sites are the back of the head, nape of neck, and behind the ears; eyelashes can be involved.
- Scalp excoriations and occipital or cervical adenopathy can be present.

T A B L E 37-11

Treatment Options for Warts

Keratolytics eliminate the wart by causing topical peeling and an inflammatory response. They are often available over-the-counter, cause little pain, and are low in cost and risk, but are slow to work.

  Salicylic acid paints with a concentration of >20% are applied with a toothpick once or twice a day for 4–6 wk. On thick skin, a combination of 16.7% salicylic acid and 16.7% collodion is more effective. This method is useful for common or periungual warts and is not effective with warts >5 mm in diameter.

  Salicylic acid plasters with 40% concentration are cut to size and taped in place for 3–5 d. After the plaster is taken off, the area should be soaked for 45 min and the dead epidermis removed. A new plaster is then applied. Treatment can last 3–6 wk. This method is useful for plantar warts.

  Retinoic acid cream 0.025–0.05% applied once or twice daily brings resolution in 4–6 wk. This method is useful for flat warts, but does not work for common, plantar, or periungual warts.

  Occlusion with tape for 6½ days, off ½ day followed by scraping of epidermis, is painless, easy, and inexpensive (Siegfried, 1996).

  Hyperthermia treatments (a 30-min water bath, 3 times a week at 45°C) has produced improvement within 3 wk (Siegfried, 1996).

Destructive agents eliminate the wart by causing necrosis and blister formation. Most techniques are painful and require patient cooperation.

  Cryotherapy. Liquid nitrogen or CO_2 snow (dry ice) is applied for 10–30 s after an area 1–3 mm beyond the wart turns white or patient complains of pain. This is the treatment of choice for common warts and an alternative for venereal warts. It should not be used with periungual or plantar warts, or in warts >7 mm in size, because of the chance of scarring. Retreatment is often necessary.

  Cantharidin 0.7% applied directly to wart with a toothpick and covered with tape for 24 h. This creates a blister in 2–3 d, which is sloughed after 7–14 d. This method is useful for periungual and some plantar warts.

  Podophyllum 25% solution in alcohol applied to wart with a toothpick; may be repeated in 1 wk. Podofilox, available over-the-counter for home use, is applied twice a day for 3 d. After a 4-d rest period, the 3-d cycle may be repeated as necessary. This technique is useful for common or genital warts.

  Surgery by snipping with scissors, not scalpel, is useful for filiform warts.

  Electrocautery, CO_2 or pulsed laser, and bleomycin injections are other options but require anesthesia, are expensive, are more likely to scar, and often have recurrences.

Immunotherapy modalities stimulate an immune response to HPV. These newer treatment modalities do not have controlled studies evaluating their effectiveness.

  Contact sensitization and interferon injection are methods used by dermatologists, usually in adult patients.

  Cimetidine is a painless, low-risk, moderate-cost option with questionable efficacy used for common and plantar warts. A dose of 30–40 mg/kg/d orally in three divided doses for 2 mo has been used in clinical trials. This is usually used in conjunction with another method and often used for resistant cases (Friedlander, 1997; Siegfried, 1996).

HPV = human papillomavirus.

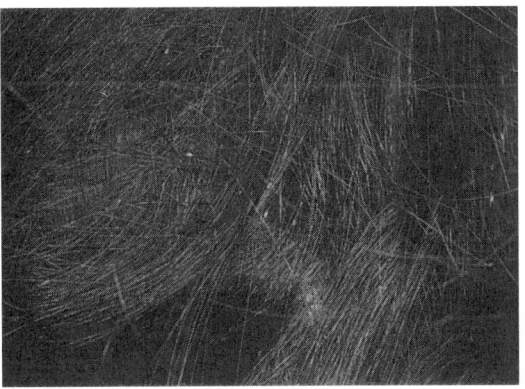

F I G U R E 37-8
Pediculosis capitis. Oval, grayish to yellowish white nits are present in the hair of the scalp. (From Hurwitz S: Clinical Pediatric Dermatology, 2nd ed. Philadelphia, WB Saunders, 1993, p 418.)

Body Lice

- Excoriated macules or papules.
- Belt line, collar, and underwear areas are common sites.
- A hemorrhagic pinpoint macule is seen where the louse extracted blood.
- Axillary, inguinal, or regional lymphadenopathy can be present.

Pubic Lice

- Excoriation and small bluish macules and papules.
- Eyelashes can be involved; spread to other short-haired areas (thighs, trunk, axillae, beard).
- Rule out sexual abuse.

LABORATORY STUDIES. The following can be helpful:

- Nits fluoresce under a Wood lamp.
- Microscopic examination of a hair shaft can more clearly identify nits.
- Test for other sexually transmitted diseases, especially gonorrhea and syphilis, with pubic lice.

Differential Diagnosis

Scabies, dermatitis herpetiformis, and necrotic excoriations are the differential diagnosis (see Table 37-12).

Management

Treatment options are varied, from standard pharmaceutical products, to many alternatives, to actually dangerous substances. Treatment failures are common but may be due to poor technique rather than medication resistance (Nopper, 1998; NPA, 1998b, 1998d; Hansen, 1998). The key to delousing a child is "parent power" (NPA, 1998d), the meticulous removal of nits, and surveillance to ensure a cure is achieved.

1. The *first step* is application of a pediculocide. Proper technique is key to success. If the hair is to be shampooed, do not use a shampoo containing conditioner or cream rinse. Shampoo the child's hair over a sink, not in the tub or shower. Keep the pediculocide out of the eyes. If applying solution to damp hair, make sure it is damp, not wet (dilutes the pediculocide). Do not rewash the hair for 1 or 2 days following treatment. Retreatment is recommended in 7 to 10 days. If the child is younger than 2 years of age, do not use pediculocide, but only manual removal (CDC, 1998). A reminder to follow package instructions is important, as pediculocides are pesticides and can easily be toxic to a child.
   - Permethrin 1% cream rinse (Nix), also called pyrethrum, is the current treatment of choice for head lice because of its safety, efficacy, and 10-day residual. Hair should be shampooed and towel-dried, permethrin applied and left on for 10 minutes, then rinsed. Hair should not be rewashed for at least 24 to 48 hours. Retreatment is advised in 7 to 10 days.
   - Lindane kills mites, nits, and ova effectively, but safety is a concern because of potential central nervous system (CNS) effects on the child and potential environmental effects through ineffective removal from wastewater. It is contraindicated for pregnant women and infants. The NPA, Consumer Reports, the Cancer Prevention Coalition, and the Public Citizen Health Research Group have all issued statements calling for a ban on lindane (NPA, 1998c; Consumer Reports, 1998). Eighteen countries outside of the United States have

T A B L E 37-12

Diagnosis and Treatment of Pediculosis and Scabies

	CLINICAL FINDINGS	TREATMENT
Pediculosis (head lice)	History of infestation; itchy scalp, scratches; postoccipital nodes; occasional visualization of mites or nits (small white oval cases), commonly on back of head, nape of neck, behind ears, possibly eyelashes	*Key* to treatment is proper technique! *First step* is pediculocide (permethrin or pyrethrin) *Second step* is removal of nits by combing hair with fine-toothed comb in 1-in. sections with special attention to nape of neck and behind ears *Third step* is to cleanse the environment: check family, friends, day care/school contacts; clean sheets, towels, clothing, headgear; store other things in plastic for 2 wk; vacuum; soak brushes and combs; follow up in 2 wk with daily recheck at home; return to school after treatment
Scabies	*Key finding:* itching, worse at night, and complaints more significant than findings; fitful sleep, crankiness; curving burrows, especially in webs of fingers, sides of hands, folds of wrist, armpits, forearms, elbows, belt line, buttocks, proximal half of foot and heel; may be <10 lesions total; secondary excoriation; infants may have lesions on palms, soles, scalp, face, posterior auricle and axilla, folds, red-brown in color, dozens in number	Pharmacological treatment with permethrin 5%, repeated in 1 wk; antihistamine, hydrocortisone, nonsteroidal anti-inflammatory drugs for itching; simultaneously treat family members (even if asymptomatic), friends, school/day care contacts; cleanse environment: linens and clothing, vacuum, store anything else in plastic bags for 1 wk; rash and itch persist for up to 3 wk after treatment; return to school 24 h after treatment

banned it. The CDC (1998) has stated that it "is probably safe if used as directed, but overuse, misuse, or swallowing is toxic to the CNS."

For head lice, a 1% shampoo is used for 4 minutes, rinsed, and repeated 1 week later. For body lice, cream or lotion is applied for 8 to 12 hours, then rinsed. For pubic lice, a 1% shampoo is used for 10 minutes, then rinsed and repeated in 1 week.

- Pyrethrin is a natural extract from the chrysanthemum plant. It is effective as a pediculocide but not as an ovicide. Commonly found as RID, A-200, Pronto, or Triplex, it is usually a 10-minute shampoo, with repeat application in 7 to 10 days. It

is contraindicated in children with allergy to ragweed.

- Malathion lotion 0.5% has a pine needle oil base and is a potent lice killer that binds to the hair shaft for 4 weeks. It has been withdrawn from the US market twice and currently is not available in the United States, though calls for its reintroduction have been made. The drug is flammable and must be used with caution. The potential for toxicity is still being investigated.

- Ivermectin in topical 0.8% solution (not available in the United States) or orally as a 200 μg/kg single-dose tablet (available, but not approved as a pediculocide nor for use in children younger than 5 years of age) is sometimes used to treat apparently resistant lice. Further clinical studies may place this medication on the list of available drugs.

2. The *second step* is ensuring removal of nits. Again, proper technique is the key to success. Covering hair with a warm, damp towel for 30 minutes before nit removal may help loosen nits. A good light, a magnifying glass, and tweezers are useful. A wide-toothed comb may be used initially to straighten the hair.

   - A proper comb has fine teeth. Most pediculocides include a nit-removal comb. The Lice-Meister comb from the NPA (see Resource Box 37-1) has been developed to efficiently remove nits. The correct technique in combing the hair is also essential. A minimum of 20 to 30 minutes should be spent combing damp hair. Working from the top of the scalp down, 1-in. sections should be divided out and combed. Special attention should be paid to the nape of the neck and behind the ears.
   - Some products claim to dissolve the substance (cement) that attaches the nit to the hair to facilitate removal. A 1:1 vinegar-to-water solution applied to the scalp for 30 minutes, covered with a warm, moist towel, may also help.
   - If eyelashes are involved, coat with petroleum jelly (Vaseline) 2 to 3 times a day for 8 to 14 days.
   - Comb-outs and inspection should be repeated every night for 2 to 3 weeks to ensure cure.

3. The *third step* is thorough cleansing of the environment.

   - Examination of family members, friends, school, and day care contacts is essential. Treatment of family members, even if nothing is found, is sometimes recommended to prevent recurrent infection, though this practice is now being discouraged due to the emergence of resistant lice.
   - Cleansing of sheets, towels, clothing, and headgear by hot-water washing and machine-drying on hot cycle for 20 minutes, ironing, or dry-cleaning is essential.
   - Any item that cannot be washed or dry-

cleaned should be stored in a plastic bag for 2 weeks.
   - Hot ironing or vacuuming of play areas, floors, rugs, and furniture is an important step in cleansing.
   - Brushes, combs, and hair accessories should be soaked in pediculocide, alcohol, or Lysol for an hour, followed by hot-water rinse.
   - Spraying or fumigating the house is not recommended.

4. *Alternative treatments* include such products as olive oil, pine oil, tea-tree oil, margarine, mayonnaise, dog shampoo, and petroleum jelly, all of which are said to suffocate and thereby kill the lice. No reliable studies have been done on these methods, except for a current study using olive oil overnight after having used a pediculocide (Connolly, 1998). Certain recommendations are definitely to be avoided, including wrapping the hair in plastic and putting the child under a hair dryer or washing the hair with gasoline or kerosene.

5. *Treatment failure* is not unusual. Common mistakes include the following:

   - Improper use of pediculocide
   - Dilution of pediculocide by applying to wet hair, not damp hair
   - Use of a shampoo with conditioner or cream rinse (decreases adherence of the pediculocide to the hair shaft)
   - Inadequate combing techniques
   - Not cleansing personal care items
   - Not screening and treating family and close contacts

6. Recommendations for dealing with potential *resistance* are varied. Neither formal recommendations nor FDA approval regarding any of these methods has yet been made. The bottom line to remember might be: "Mechanical removal is the common denominator for success. There's more to treating head lice than killing the bugs!" (NPA, 1998d). Some methods for treating resistant lice currently discussed include:

   - Using Nix creme rinse for 4 to 8 hours instead of 10 minutes
   - Using Nix creme rinse under a shower cap overnight

- Using Elimite cream (5 times stronger than Nix) overnight
- Using trimethoprim-sulfamethoxazole to kill symbiotic bacteria that lice survive on
- Using oral ivermectin 0.2 mg/kg as a single dose; if moving lice are present after 24 hours, repeat dose (Bell, 1998)

7. Nix creme rinse has received FDA approval for *prophylaxis* for "institutional use when 20% of the population is infested" or for use in immediate household members.

Patient Education and Prevention

Items for discussion include the following:

1. Follow-up visits in 10 to 14 days are helpful in individual cases to ensure complete resolution of infestation. However, daily to weekly checks for lice or nits should be carried out at home.
2. Educate family members about the following:
   - The expected course
   - Lice infestation is not a social disease
3. Educate family members about the need to avoid excessive or unnecessary retreatment because of the toxic hazard of medications. Do not use extra amounts; do not treat more than 3 times with the same medication without being seen by a care provider; do not mix pediculocides.
4. The child can return to school following initial treatment. The "no nits" policy has no documented effectiveness in controlling pediculosis outbreaks (AAP, 1997). However, close contacts in the neighborhood or at school, camp, or child care should be informed and checked for infestation.
5. The NPA has educational materials and information (see Resource Box 37–1).

Complications

Secondary bacterial infection can occur.

Scabies

Description

Scabies is caused by the itch mite, *Sarcoptes scabiei*, which burrows under the skin and causes intense itching. There are many different forms of presentation (see Color Fig. 17).

Etiology and Incidence

Scabies is a highly contagious infestation spread through close contact and shared clothing or linen. The female mite burrows into the skin, laying up to three eggs a day as she travels. The eggs hatch in about 2 weeks, and the new mites repeat the process. Sensitization, which causes intense itching, occurs approximately 3 weeks after infestation. Incubation is 1 to 2 months following contact.

Scabies occurs in all socioeconomic groups, and in all age groups. However, infestation of African Americans is rare (Peterson & Eichenfield, 1996; Rasmussen, 1994).

Clinical Findings

HISTORY. The following can be reported:

- *Key finding*: Itching, worse at night, initially mild but progressively more intense
- Fitful sleep, crankiness, or rubbing of hands and feet (infants)

PHYSICAL EXAMINATION. Findings include the following:

- Complaints are significantly greater than examination findings.
- Characteristic lesions include curving burrows, especially on webs of fingers and sides of hands, folds of wrists and armpits, forearms, elbows, belt line, buttocks, genitalia, or proximal half of foot and heel.
- Secondary lesions include itchy papules that can be excoriated, urticarial papules with excoriation, nodules from inflammatory response, and crusting and excoriation (signs of secondary infection).
- Infants classically have lesions on palms, soles, scalp, face, posterior auriculae, and axillae, concentrated in the folds; head and neck lesions typically are red-brown vesiculopustules or nodules. However, any child younger than 2 years of age can have an unusual manifestation.
- Infants classically have dozens of lesions; older children may have fewer than 10.

LABORATORY STUDIES. The following are done as indicated:

- Microscopic examination of scrapings from an unscratched burrow in saline or mineral oil can reveal an eight-legged mite, eggs, or feces. Do not use KOH because it dissolves the mites, eggs, and feces.
- Burrow ink test. Apply a drop of ink or washable felt-tipped pen to suspected burrow. Wipe off excess ink, and examine with magnifying glass for an ink-stained burrow.

Differential Diagnosis

Papular urticaria, atopic dermatitis, contact dermatitis, insect bites, folliculitis, lichen planus, and dermatitis herpetiformis are included in the differential diagnosis.

Management

Management involves the following:

1. Pharmacological treatment begins with applying a thin layer of scabicide to the entire body, excluding the eyes. Areas of special importance are under the fingernails, the scalp, behind the ears, all folds and creases, and the feet and hands. In general, the scabicide should be reapplied in 7 days on all symptomatic patients.
   - Permethrin 5% cream (Elimite) is the drug of choice for treating scabies because of its safety and efficacy (Hansen, 1998). It can be used on infants as young as 2 months of age. Apply for 8 to 14 hours and rinse. Re-treat in 1 week. In infants, special application is needed to head, postauricular area, and hands and feet.
   - Lindane 1% cream is effective but has potential CNS effects. It is contraindicated in children less than 6 months (some say under 2 years) of age, in pregnancy or breastfeeding, and in children who have seizures. (See discussion of lindane under Pediculosis.) The CDC (1998) recommends an alternative scabicide (usually permethrin) in children under 10 years of age. When lindane is used, it is applied and left on for 8 to 12 hours before wash-

ing off. Repeat application is recommended in 1 week.
   - Crotamiton 10% cream (Eurax) applied to the whole body has been used in infants, but it is not as effective as permethrin or lindane (Stavish, 1998). It must be applied daily for 5 days or to the whole body for 48 hours, rinsed, and repeated. Re-treatment in 2 weeks is suggested.
   - Sulfur cream or ointment 5 to 10% is an old treatment that is not highly effective, is smelly, and stains. However, it may be used in pregnant women, infants, and young children; it is applied nightly for 3 nights and washed off 24 hours after the final application.
   - Ivermectin orally or topically has not been approved as a scabicide. It is not approved for use in children under 5 years of age, but may be a new treatment on the horizon.
2. Antihistamines (hydroxyzine or diphenhydramine), topical 1% hydrocortisone, and nonsteroidal antipruritics such as Sarna Anti-Itch lotion (camphor; methol) and PrameGel (pramoxine HCl; menthol) can be helpful.
3. Simultaneous treatment of family members, friends, and school and day care contacts, even if asymptomatic, is essential.
4. At time of treatment, linens and any clothing worn over the last 48 hours should be washed with hot water, put in a hot dryer for 20 minutes, or dry-cleaned. The house should be vacuumed.
5. Nonwashable items should be stored in sealed plastic bags for 1 week.
6. A follow-up visit in 2 weeks can be scheduled to determine success of treatment.
   - Reasons for treatment failure include wrong diagnosis, medication not applied to the whole body, not treating all members of the household, or use of crotamiton. In addition, the child may develop postscabetic eczema that is not indicative of treatment failure.
   - Although resistance has been reported, it is not common and is often due to treatment failure rather than resistance (Schwade, 1999).

Complications

A secondary bacterial infection is possible. Postscabetic syndrome is common, with visible lesions and pruritus persisting for days to weeks following treatment, and nodular lesions persisting for weeks to months. Norwegian scabies is a nonpruritic crusted, scaling infestation with thousands to millions of mites occurring in immunosuppressed or institutionalized patients.

Patient Education, Prognosis, and Prevention

- Educate the family about the course of disease. Rash and itching persist for up to 3 weeks following treatment. Avoid overbathing and further irritation of the skin.
- The child should not be infectious 24 hours after treatment and may return to school or day care.

ALLERGIC AND INFLAMMATORY REACTIONS OF THE SKIN

Acne

Description

Acne is a disorder of the sebaceous follicle in which excess sebum, keratinous debris, and bacteria accumulate, producing microcomedones. The microcomedones may be noninflamed or inflamed lesions. Although rarely a serious medical disorder, acne occasionally heralds underlying disease. It is often of significant concern to the adolescent, having a serious effect on social development (see Color Fig. 18).

Etiology and Incidence

Four mechanisms are believed to contribute to the sebaceous follicle disorder: (1) follicular plugging with keratinous material; (2) bacterial colonization with overgrowth of anaerobic organisms deep in the follicle, primarily *Propionibacterium acnes*; (3) sebum overproduction and increased androgen production with an expansion of the follicle; and (4) inflammation due to trapping of *P. acnes* and sebum (Kristal & Silverberg, 1998). Acne is a common skin disease, occurring in up to 80 to 85% of all persons 12 to 24 years of age and appearing as early as 8 to 10 years of age in the form of a microcomedo (Krowchuk, 1998; Peters, 1997; Leyden, 1997; Weston et al., 1996; Bergfield, 1995). It is more common in females than in males but appears earlier in males. Acne tends to improve in the summer and worsen with menses and stress.

Clinical Findings

HISTORY. Information to obtain includes the following:

- Family history of acne
- Stage of pubertal development and menstrual history
- Facial products used, especially occlusive products or pomades
- Oral and prescription medication, especially oral contraceptives, antibiotics, or steroids
- Any current or previous acne treatment and results
- Sports participation, especially if wearing football pads or other protective devices
- Jobs such as cooking at a fast-food grill or working at a gas station
- Other medical conditions

PHYSICAL EXAMINATION. Lesions most commonly are found on the face, back, and chest.

- Noninflammatory lesions:
  - Open comedo (blackhead)—a noninflammatory lesion or papule, firm in consistency, caused by blockage at the mouth of the follicle and occurring on the face, upper back, shoulders, and chest. The black color comes from oxidized melanin.
  - Closed comedo (whitehead or microcomedo)—a noninflammatory lesion, semisoft in consistency, caused by blockage at the neck of the follicle.
- Inflammatory lesions occur secondary to rupture of noninflamed lesions into the dermis.
  - Papule—a "bump" in the follicle caused by bacterial overgrowth and rupture of the follicle wall
  - Pustule—raised, superficial, exudate-filled lesion

○ Excoriation and crusting of lesions—caused by manipulation
○ Nodule—firm, erythematous, and deeper in location, caused by rupture of a plug
○ Cyst—raised, large lesion, soft in consistency without erythema, formed from multiple ruptures and reencapsulations
○ Scar—red or purple hue initially, depressed or close to the skin
○ Sinus tracts—confluent nodules likely to cause scarring
• The severity of acne is determined by the quantity, type, and spread of lesions. It is helpful to use a diagram of the face or a grading graph to identify the number and type of lesions present. This allows more precise follow-up of the patient. If only open and closed comedones are found, the disorder is called *comedonal* acne. Most adolescents have a combination of comedones, red papules, and pustules called *papulopustular* acne, which can be mild or severe. *Nodulocystic* acne is the most severe form and requires more intensive intervention. Specific types of acne include *frictional*, occurring from rubbing of bras, tight clothes, or headbands; *pomadal*, along the temple and forehead, due to pomades or oil-based cosmetics; *athletic*, on forehead, chin, or shoulders, due to helmets and pads; and *hormonal*, with a beard distribution.

Differential Diagnosis

Cosmetic, mechanical, environmental, or drug-induced acne; rosacea; flat wart; milia; and folliculitis are included in the differential diagnosis.

Management

The goals of acne management are (1) to counteract the excess production of sebum, (2) to counteract the abnormal desquamation of epithelial cells, and (3) to decrease the proliferation of *P. acnes*. Choice of treatment depends on the extent, severity, duration of disease, type of lesions, and psychological effects the adolescent is experiencing (Tables 37-13 and 37-14).

1. *Education* is the first priority. The adolescent must have realistic expectations and an understanding of the pathophysiology and the process of treatment, including the fact that the acne often worsens before improving.
   • Wash face twice a day with a mild soap such as Neutrogena or Aveeno Cleansing bar. Scrubbing, rubbing, picking, and squeezing should be avoided. Medication should be applied lightly; do not rub in.
   • A comedo extractor can be used, but the face must be washed before and after use. Hot soaks applied to pustules may help their resolution.
   • If makeup is used, a nonacnegenic makeup is best.
   • Identify aggravating substances such as oil-based cosmetics, hair spray, mousse, and face creams.
   • Identify possible aggravating factors such as menses; stress; hot, humid weather; jobs involving frying oil or grease.
   • Reassure patient that no scientific evidence indicates that any particular foods adversely affect acne; however, a well-balanced diet is important to maintaining healthy skin.
   • Discuss psychosocial concerns and provide support.
   • Remind patient that results take months and that adherence to treatment is essential to improvement.
   • Sun exposure helps clear acne for some adolescents but may worsen it for others. Use of sunscreen is recommended, and caution about sun exposure should be given if using medication that increases photosensitivity.
2. *Topical keratolytic* or *comedolytic agents* are used to minimize follicular obstruction and break up microcomedones. Four to 6 weeks of treatment is required before improvement, but these agents control 80% of acne (Weston et al., 1996). Many strengths and forms are available, the most effective being the gels, if tolerated. A general rule is to start low (in strength) and slow (in frequency), and advance as tolerated or needed. There are three classes: retinoids (tretinoin, adapalene, tazarotene), benzoyl

T A B L E 37-13

Treatment of Acne

TYPE OF ACNE	LESIONS	INITIAL TREATMENT	IF NOT IMPROVING
Comedonal	Open or closed comedones	Benzoyl peroxide 5% qd (if mild) *or* Tretinoin (Retin A) 0.025% cream qd (if moderate)	Combine benzoyl peroxide with tretinoin *or* Increase strength to 0.05%
Mild papulopustular	Red papules, few pustules	Benzoyl peroxide 5–10% qd *or* Azelaic acid bid (if mild) *or* Topical antibiotic bid *or* Erythromycin 3% with 5% benzoyl peroxide qd–bid (if moderate)	Increase benzoyl peroxide to bid *or* Combine benzoyl peroxide with tretinoin (for comedones) Substitute topical antibiotic bid (for inflammatory)
Moderate to severe papulopustular	Red papules, many pustules	Benzoyl peroxide 5% *and* tretinoin 0.025% *or* Azelaic acid (if comedonal) *or* Topical antibiotic bid (if no comedones) *and* oral antibiotic bid	Increase strength of treatment *or* Refer to dermatologist
Nodulocystic, scarring, or unresponsive	Red papules, pustules, cysts, and nodules	Oral antibiotics bid *and* tretinoin 0.05% qd *and* benzoyl peroxide 10% gel bid (if comedonal)	Refer to dermatologist for oral isotretinoin

peroxide, and salicylic acid. Each works by a different mechanism so they can be used together as well as interchangeably. Dryness, erythema, irritation, and scaling can occur with these products, and the strength and frequency of use must be adjusted for this.

- Tretinoin (Retin-A, Avita) is considered the best available topical treatment. A pea-sized application should be made 20 minutes after washing the face. Initially it is used every other night, advancing to every night. If the skin is very sensitive, applications of 15 to 30 minutes just before bedtime may be used, with the duration gradually advanced.
- Adapalene (Differin) is a newer formulation with less irritation, more activity, and less photosensitivity.
- Tazarotene (Tazorac gel) is another newer agent, active against psoriasis, that is te-

ratogenic and causes irritation. Use with caution.

- Benzoyl peroxide is used once or twice a day, depending on the severity of acne and dryness of skin; it is also considered antibacterial by some.
- Salicylic acid is an over-the-counter agent.

3. *Topical antibiotics* are used to control the inflammatory process, usually most helpful in moderate inflammatory acne. Additionally, they are used as maintenance to control acne after initial treatment with oral antibiotics. Topical antibiotics are applied to the entire skin surface, not just to problem areas. The solution should not be applied until 30 minutes after shaving.

- Clindamycin is used twice a day.
- Erythromycin is used twice a day.
- Erythromycin with benzoyl peroxide (Benzamycin gel) is a combination product that

TABLE 37-14

Medications Commonly Used in Treating Acne

TOPICAL KERATOLYTIC OR COMEDOLYTIC AGENTS (3 CLASSES)
Retinoids
 Tretinoin (Retin A, Avita) 0.01–0.025% gel; 0.025–1.0% cream; 0.05% liquid; 0.1% microsphere
 Adapalene (Differin) 0.1% gel or solution
 Tazarotene (Tazorac) 0.05–1% gel
Benzoyl peroxide 2.5–20% gel, 5% and 10% cream, 5–20% lotion or wash
Salicylic acid up to 2% in various formulations

TOPICAL ANTIBIOTICS
Clindamycin 1% solution, lotion, gel, pledget
Erythromycin 1–2% solution, 3% gel or swabs
Erythromycin 3% with benzoyl peroxide 5% gel (Benzamycin)
Azelaic acid (Azelex) 20% cream

ORAL ANTIBIOTICS
Tetracycline 500–2000 mg given in 1–4 divided doses
Erythromycin 500–2000 mg given in 1–4 divided doses
Minocycline 50–200 mg given in 1–2 divided doses
Doxycycline 50–200 mg given in 1–2 divided doses
Trimethoprim with sulfamethoxasole is used but is not an FDA-approved indication

is more effective than either drug alone, has less resistance from *P. acnes*, and requires refrigeration. It is especially effective in mild to moderate inflammatory acne or as an adjunct to oral therapy.

- Azelaic acid (Azelex) is antibacterial and anticomedonal. Used twice a day it is a newer agent that is useful in individuals with sensitive or dark skin.

4. *Oral antibiotics* are used in addition to topical keratolytics and topical antibiotics to decrease the concentration of *P. acnes* and to decrease the degree of inflammation if there is no response to topical agents. Antibiotics are taken from 1 to 6 months and often require 3 to 4 weeks to see improvement (Savin & Donofrio, 1996; Hurwitz, 1994).

Once improvement is noted, dose should be tapered to daily dose and then discontinued. Tetracycline and erythromycin are the antibiotics most commonly used, but minocycline, doxycycline, and trimethoprim with sulfamethoxazole are also used.

- Tetracycline should be taken 1 hour before or 2 hours after eating with 8 oz of water. Tetracycline should not be used by pregnant or breastfeeding adolescents or in children under 9 years of age. Photosensitivity reactions can occur, but it has been used for over 40 years and is a favorite of many clinicians.
- Erythromycin can be taken with food.
- Minocycline can be taken with food and achieves a higher concentration in the follicles. However, side effects include blue-black discoloration in scars and photosensitivity and hypersensitivity reactions.
- Doxycycline also can be taken with food but has the highest rate of photosensitivity reactions.
- Trimethoprim with sulfamethoxasole has not been approved for this use but is sometimes tried before isotretinoin.

5. *Oral retinoids* are used for severe, resistant nodulocystic acne. Isotretinoin (Accutane) is contraindicated in pregnancy and usually requires evaluation by a dermatologist prior to use. The usual course is 20 weeks, there are many side effects, and CBC, LFTs, cholesterol, triglycerides, and urinalysis must be monitored every month while the patient is on the medication (Ruiz-Maldonado et al., 1998). Roche Pharmaceutical Company, the maker of Accutane, provides at no cost *Pregnancy Prevention Program for Women on Accutane*.

6. *Oral contraceptives* (Ortho Tri-Cyclen is the only one approved by the FDA for treatment for acne), antiandrogens (spironolactone), and intralesional steroid therapy are sometimes used in unresponsive cases. Erythromycin-zinc combination is used in Europe and Russia with success but has not been approved in the United States.

7. Follow-up visits should occur at least every 4 to 6 weeks until control is established. Control is indicated by clearing of lesions or the appearance of only a few new lesions

every 2 weeks. Referral to a dermatologist should be made for nonresponsive or severe cases.

Complications

Failure is usually due to lack of patient motivation or education, initial treatment that was too strong, or expectations of a quick fix. Psychological effects are real and include decreased self-esteem and poor body image, problems with interpersonal relationships, self-consciousness, embarrassment, depression, and decreased athletic participation, especially in gymnastics, swimming, and wrestling (Savin & Donofrio, 1996; Hurwitz, 1995; Koo, 1995). Resistance of *P. acnes* to tetracycline, erythromycin, and minocycline is increasing.

Atopic Dermatitis

See Chapter 25.

Contact Dermatitis

Description

Contact dermatitis is an acute or chronic inflammation due to a hypersensitivity reaction to a substance. The causative agents are either irritants or allergens. Common types of contact dermatitis are the following:

- *Dry skin dermatitis* due to extremely low humidity (less than 30%) or use of excess soaping or cleansing creams
- *Nickel dermatitis* from contact with jewelry, belts, snaps, or eyeglasses
- *Lip-licker dermatitis* due to constant lip-licking, most often in dry, cold weather
- *Phytophotodermatitis* occurs with sun exposure following contact with plants or juices such as limes, lemons, carrots, celery, figs, parsnips, or dill; presents as a blistered lesion on an erythematous base and may be confused with a burn
- *Plant oleoresins* such as poison ivy, oak, or sumac
- *Juvenile plantar dermatosis*, manifested as dryness, cracking, and erythema of weight-bearing surfaces of the feet, initially the big toes, mimicking tinea pedis, often

found in children with atopic dermatitis (see Chapter 25)
- *Latex dermatitis*

Etiology and Incidence

Irritant dermatitis, the most common form, occurs when a substance has a toxic effect on the skin. The severity of the rash depends on the length of exposure and the concentration of the irritant. Substances such as saliva, urine, or feces; baby wipes; bubble bath; or overbathing often cause irritation. Diaper dermatitis is the most common form (see section below). Allergic reactions occur as an immunological response to an antigen penetrating the skin. Common causes are contact with shoes, nickel, clothes with woolen or rough textures, topical medications (e.g., neomycin and lanolin), perfumed soaps or cosmetics, preservatives, or poison ivy, oak, or sumac. Sometimes the cause is obvious; often no specific cause can be identified. Occurring at any age, contact dermatitis (mostly irritant) is extremely common in children, with an incidence of 5 to 20% of all cases of dermatitis (Friedlander, 1997; Weston et al., 1996).

Clinical Findings

HISTORY. The following information should be sought:

- Contact with any new or unusual substances
- Repeated exposure to any substance or item
- Diarrhea or infrequently changed diapers
- Rash localized to specific area(s)

PHYSICAL EXAMINATION. The area of involvement offers clues to the causative agent. Often the rash is localized to one area and has sharp borders. Common examples include a linear-type rash secondary to wearing a necklace or bracelet, circular areas from snaps on clothing, or involvement of the earlobes from jewelry or the toes and dorsum of the foot from shoes. The duration and concentration of exposure also affect the intensity of the rash. Minimal contact may only produce mild erythema, while prolonged or concentrated contact may produce significant erythema, edema, and blistering with possible crusting and secondary infection. Irritant reactions tend to be immediate, whereas allergic ones are delayed.

- A chafed appearance with shiny, mild to severely erythematous, peeling, or dry, fissured skin may be seen if the reaction is due to an irritant.
- In the diaper area around the anus, the rash is often due to diarrhea; if the skin is affected but the folds are spared, urine is often responsible.
- Erythema, vesicles, and weeping may be present in the acute stage of allergic contact dermatitis.
- Hyperpigmentation and lichenification are seen in chronic conditions.

Differential Diagnosis

The differential diagnosis includes atopic dermatitis, impetigo, herpes simplex, psoriasis, and seborrhea.

Management

Appropriate skin care, recognizing and eliminating offending agents, and treatment of inflammation are the keys to managing contact dermatitis successfully.

1. Identify and avoid the substance causing dermatitis.
2. For dermatitis in the diaper area, change diapers frequently, keep the area dry and cool (use air-drying as much as possible), and avoid rubber pants. Hydrocortisone 1% may be used cautiously for a period of no more than 5 days. Secondary infection with *Candida* is often present and must be treated with an antifungal agent such as nystatin.
3. Burow solution soaks or oatmeal baths and cool compresses applied for 20 minutes every 4 to 6 hours soothe vesicular rashes.
4. Apply water and either petrolatum-based or lanolin-and-petrolatum–based emollients to the skin to restore moisture to areas of dryness and chafing.
   - Petrolatum-based emollients include di-
methicone (Moisturel), white petrolatum, and Vaseline Dermatology Formula.
   - Lanolin-and-petrolatum–based emollients include Aquaphor, Eucerin, Lubriderm, and Alpha Keri. Avoid use if there is inflammation.
5. Topical corticosteroids used 2 to 3 times daily give relief in 2 or 3 days, although it may take 2 or 3 weeks for complete healing. Occasionally, oral corticosteroids are used for short periods of time (10 to 14 days, tapered the last 7 days) if the area of involvement exceeds 10% of the skin surface.
6. Oral antihistamines are helpful if itching and scratching are problems.
7. Resolution may take 2 to 3 weeks. Referral to a dermatologist or allergist for patch testing may be indicated if the dermatitis worsens, fails to respond, or recurs.

Diaper Dermatitis

Description

Diaper dermatitis is most commonly an inflammatory disorder of the skin due to irritation causing breakdown of the skin's natural barrier (Table 37–15).

Etiology and Incidence

Factors contributing to diaper dermatitis include the following:

- Improper hygiene and cleansing methods
- Chemical irritation due to prolonged contact with skin products, urine, feces, or breakdown products
- Mechanical irritation from diapers, rubber pants, or skin folds
- Other skin dermatoses aggravated by wearing diapers (e.g., seborrhea, atopic dermatitis, or psoriasis)

Diaper rash is most commonly due to irritation from the wetness of urine, combined with friction and occlusion from diapers, and the byproducts of feces. The initial rash is *irritant contact diaper dermatitis*. A variation of this is called *tidewater* or *tidemark dermatitis* and is found at the diaper edges due to either chafing or irritation from talcum powder. *Jacquet's der-*

T A B L E 37-15

Diagnosis and Treatment of Diaper Dermatitis

TYPE	CAUSE	PRESENTATION AND LOCATION	OTHER CHARACTERISTICS	TREATMENT
Irritant contact dermatitis	Related to wearing diapers; contact with urine and feces	Chapped, shiny, erythematous, parchment-like skin with possible erosions on convex surfaces; creases spared	Peak at 9–12 mo; may progress to involve creases; skin may be dry	Frequent diaper changes, gentle cleansing; greasy lubricant; sitz bath, air-dry; hydrocortisone for inflammation
Candidiasis	Related to wearing diapers; a superinfection with *Candida*	Shallow pustules, fiery-red scaly plaques on convex surfaces, inguinal folds, labia, and scrotum	Satellite lesions, oral thrush; recent antibiotic or diarrhea; occurs at any age	Antifungal cream plus same measures as for contact dermatitis
Miliaria or intertrigo	Related to wearing diapers; due to heat and occlusion	Discrete vesicles or papules (miliaria); erythematous, scaly, maceration in folds of skin	Sweat retention or friction associated	Self-limited (miliaria); avoid precipitating factors; care as for contact dermatitis
Seborrhea	Exaggerated by wearing diapers; overgrowth of *Malassezia* yeast in areas of sebaceous gland activity	Greasy, erythematous scales, well circumscribed in creases of skin, groin; spared convex surfaces	Onset at 3–4 wk of age; also occurs on face or body; often super-infected with *Candida*	Ketoconazole is treatment of choice, or hydrocortisone
Atopic dermatitis (AD)	Exaggerated by wearing diapers; exact cause unknown	Increased number of lines in skin; areas of excoriation in folds and convex surfaces and buttocks; less widespread	AD in other areas; usually begins in first year of life; scratches skin with diaper change	Skin care as for contact dermatitis and as indicated for AD (see Chapter 25)
Psoriasis	Exaggerated by wearing diapers; psoriasis evolves as response to chronic trauma	Erythematous, well-defined sharp, scaly plaques on convex surfaces and inguinal folds; less widespread	Psoriasis affects other places; rare occurrence, if found, usually at 6–18 mo	Treatment often required for weeks or until toilet trained; steroids; ketoconazole if *Candida* present
Bacterial dermatitis	Usually due to staphylococcal or streptococcal infection	Red, denuded areas or fragile blisters; crusting and pustules in suprapubic area and periumbilicus	Usually in newborn, can occur anywhere	Econazole or ketoconazole cream if yeast present as well; mupirocin if minimal; cephalexin or erythromycin if extensive

matitis, a severe form manifested by punched-out lesions or erosions primarily on the labia and buttocks, is especially prone to secondary infection.

Approximately 50% of infants develop diaper rashes, less than 2% of which are serious, usually between 9 and 12 months of age (Friedlander, 1997; Hansen et al., 1998; Armsmeier & Paller, 1997).

Clinical Findings

HISTORY. The following should be assessed:

- Type of diapers and diaper covering used; any recent change in brand
- Frequency of diaper changes and methods of cleansing used
- Any new baby care products used
- Frequency of wet diapers and stools
- Medication taken and/or used on rash
- Present or recent use of antibiotics

PHYSICAL EXAMINATION. Findings can include the following:

Chemical Causes
- Shiny, peely, erythematous macular or papular rash confluent in the diaper area, sparing folds
- Head of penis erythematous and dry
- Erythema primarily on buttocks and around anus (fecal irritation)

Mechanical Causes
- Erythematous, macerated (acute) or dry (chronic), hyperpigmented area prominent along edges of diaper or plastic pants
- Erythematous, macerated folds due to overlapping skin

Hygiene Problems
- Any presentation listed above
- Poor hygiene in general

Differential Diagnosis

Differential diagnosis includes contact dermatitis; bacterial, viral, or monilial infection; atopic dermatitis; psoriasis; seborrhea; scabies; and congenital syphilis.

Management

The best treatment is prevention!

1. Keep diaper area dry, clean, and aerated:
   - Frequent diaper changes are essential; every 1 to 2 hours is recommended with one change at night and a minimum of eight changes in a 24-hour period. Cleanse the area well with water at every diaper change and use mild soap, rinsing well following a stool. Avoid vigorous cleansing as this can worsen matters. Avoid using wipes.
   - Use a greasy lubricant if skin is dry.
   - Use a protective barrier ointment or cream such as Desitin (cod liver oil with zinc oxide), A and D ointment, petrolatum, or zinc oxide at first sign of irritation.
2. Proper use of diapers:
   - Frequent changes are essential.
   - Use thick or absorbent diapers to pull wetness away from skin.
   - Avoid use of rubber or plastic pants.
   - Cloth diapers should be soaked, pre-rinsed, washed in a mild soap, double-rinsed with ¼ cup of vinegar, and dried in the sun if possible.
   - Disposable diapers must be large enough not to bind and should never be worn with rubber pants.
3. Treatment of diaper rash:
   - Sitz baths in warm water for 10 to 15 minutes 4 times a day.
   - Expose diaper area to air by leaving diaper off or by blow-drying with low heat 3 or 4 times a day.
   - Burow solution soaks or compresses 4 times a day if skin is weepy.
   - Undecylenic acid (Desenex) or calcium undecylenate (Caldescene) powder to decrease the friction and moisture in tidewater dermatitis.
   - Hydrocortisone 0.5% or 1% three times a day for no more than 5 days, especially if skin is dry, for moderate to severe diaper dermatitis. Do not use fluorinated steroids.
   - Increased fluids to dilute urine. In older infants, 2 to 3 oz of cranberry juice acidifies the urine.
   - If the rash has been present for more than 3 days, or if there is no response to the

above measures, add a topical antifungal cream such as clotrimazole or miconazole. If there is still no response, a trial of oral antifungal is indicated (see section on monilial dermatitis).
- Any recalcitrant rash should be referred to a dermatologist.
- Follow up by phone in 1 to 2 days. If not improved, reassess within a week.

Complications

Secondary infection with bacteria, viruses, or fungi can occur (see previous sections). *Red flags*: severe erosions or ulcers; bullae or pustules; large papules or nodules, purpura, or petechiae; and redness or scaliness over entire body.

Seborrhea

Description

Seborrhea is a chronic inflammatory dermatitis commonly called "cradle cap" in infants or dandruff in adolescents.

Etiology and Incidence

The condition appears related to overproduction of sebum, because it commonly occurs in areas with large numbers of sebaceous glands. It may be an abnormal reaction to *Malassezia ovalis (Pityrosporum ovale)* (a saprophytic yeast), which is present on everyone's body. Seborrhea occurs most often in early infancy and adolescence, is associated with blepharitis, and is more common in spring and summer.

Clinical Findings

HISTORY. Note age of onset (infancy or adolescence).

PHYSICAL EXAMINATION. In infants, erythematous, flaky to thick crusts of yellow, greasy scales occur predominantly on the scalp but also on the face, behind the ears, on the neck and trunk, and in the diaper area.

In adolescents, there are mild flakes with some erythema yellow, greasy scales on the scalp, forehead, and eyebrows, and behind the ears, on the face and flexural surfaces, and in intertriginous areas.

Differential Diagnosis

Atopic dermatitis, psoriasis, *Candida* infection, contact dermatitis, tinea, scabies, and pityriasis rosea are included in the differential diagnosis.

Management

Seborrhea in infants may be self-limited. However, in adolescents, it is usually chronic and recurring. The following measures are helpful in either age group:

1. Shampoo or wash areas daily with a mild soap. In more resistant cases, use antiseborrheic shampoos (e.g., Sebulex, Selsun, Head & Shoulders) every other day for infants or daily for adolescents. Tar shampoos can be used for adolescents if needed. Shampoo should be left on the scalp 5 to 10 minutes before scrubbing crusts and then rinsing.
2. Mineral oil, baby oil, or petroleum jelly placed on thick crusts 10 to 15 minutes prior to washing softens them, followed by gentle brushing during shampooing to remove crusts.
3. If inflammation is marked, low-potency steroid creams can be applied twice a day to face or 3 times a day to other body areas for several days and then weaned. A low to moderate steroid solution can be applied to the scalp if inflammation is present.
4. Oral biotin can sometimes improve the condition.
5. Educate parents about the etiology, control measures, and the need to continue treatment a few days after resolution.
6. Follow up in 1 to 2 weeks.

Complications

Secondary infection with bacteria or *Candida* can occur. Severe, generalized seborrhea is found in up to 83% of persons infected with HIV.

Sunburn

Description

Sunburn represents an injury to the skin occurring from overexposure of the skin to the UV rays of the sun. There is an increasing incidence of skin cancer due to overexposure to the sun.

Etiology and Incidence

Excessive sun exposure causes a change in the skin's blood flow, cell kinetics, and pigment products. Damage to the skin by sun (primarily ultraviolet B [UVB]) includes erythema, pigmentary or texture changes, and potential carcinogenesis. Injury to the skin begins as quickly as 30 minutes after exposure, peaks at 24 hours, and may last for 72 hours. Other factors that contribute to sun sensitivity are medications (especially griseofulvin, NSAIDs, oral contraceptives, tetracycline, topical diphenhydramine, and tretinoin) and some illnesses.

Children are at increased risk for sunburn because of the greater amount of time they spend outdoors. Most people receive 80% of their lifetime exposure to sun by the time they are 18 to 21 years of age (Kim et al., 1997; Weston et al., 1996). Blistering sunburns before 20 years of age more than double the chance of skin cancer. Factors contributing to the degree of burn include the coloring of skin and hair (Table 37–16) and amount of previous sun exposure. Burns are less common in children with darker hair and skin because of their increased amount of melanin. Timing of sun exposure, latitude, and altitude affect skin sensitivity, as UV rays are strongest between 10 AM and 2 PM, at higher altitudes, and nearer the equator. Sunburn can occur on cloudy days, and reflection from sand, water, snow, and concrete increases the risk.

Clinical Findings

HISTORY

- Length and time of sun exposure
- Previous sunburns, especially blistering ones
- Any medications currently taken
- Chills, headache, and fatigue with moderate to severe burn
- Family history of melanoma or other skin cancer

PHYSICAL EXAMINATION. Findings include the following:

- Mild or first-degree burns are evidenced by erythema, tenderness, and mild pain.
- Moderate or second-degree burns involve a greater degree of erythema, increased pain, edema, and blisters.
- Severe or third-degree burns involve greater areas of skin and include systemic symptoms of headache, fever, and fatigue.
- Erythema and tenderness are evident from 30 minutes to 4 hours after exposure; 2 to 7 days later, affected layers of the epidermis are shed.

Differential Diagnosis

The differential diagnosis includes photosensitization from medication, xeroderma pigmentosum, lupus erythematosus, viral exanthem, dermatomyositis, and porphyrias.

Management

The degree of burn helps determine which of the following strategies are most appropriate. Prevention is the best intervention (see section below).

T A B L E 37-16

Skin Types and Protection Needs

Fair (Celtic)—always burns, never tans; sun protection factor (SPF) 15+
Fair (white)—easily burns, minimally tans; SPF 15
Lightly pigmented (dark white)—sometimes burns, gradually tans; SPF 8–10
Pigmented (Mediterranean, Asian, Hispanic)—minimally burns, always tans; SPF 6–8
Moderately pigmented (American Indian, Hispanic, Mideastern)—rarely burns, profusely tans; SPF 4
Heavily pigmented (American and African black)—rarely burns, tans deeply; no or low SPF needed

1. Cool water, saline compresses, or ice packs at least 4 times a day to ease pain and reduce swelling. Baking soda or cornstarch baths help to cool skin. White vinegar or milk compresses help initiate healing.
2. Prostaglandin inhibitors such as ibuprofen 5 to 10 mg/kg per dose given as soon as possible and every 6 to 8 hours for the next 2 to 3 days or acetaminophen for fever and pain relief.
3. Low-dose cortisone creams 0.5% or 1%, used with caution because of the increased absorption due to damaged skin, 2 to 3 times a day help reduce inflammation and pain.
4. Local anesthetic sprays or first-aid creams with benzocaine are contraindicated because of the risk of sensitization.
5. Skin emollients such as aloe vera gel or moisturizer are helpful if skin is dry. Jojoba oil and vitamin E creams are sometimes helpful. Avoid petrolatum, butter, or any occlusive ointment as their occlusive properties intensify the burn.
6. Extra fluid intake prevents dehydration and restores natural moisture balance.
7. If blisters break, dead skin needs to be trimmed and an antibiotic ointment such as Polysporin (polymyxin B sulfate; bacitracin zinc) applied.

Complications

Photoaging, including telangiectasia and actinic keratosis, cataracts, retinal damage, heat stroke, and a change in immune response (Kim et al., 1997) are possible complications of sunburn.

The incidence of skin cancer (basal cell carcinoma, squamous cell carcinoma, and malignant melanoma) and resultant death is increasing rapidly, with 1 million cases diagnosed annually; 2% occur in children (Kim et al., 1997; Orlow, 1995). Risk factors include fair skin, history of multiple blistering sunburns, presence of multiple atypical moles, development of new nevi, and family history of melanoma. Basal and squamous cell carcinomas are slow-spreading cancers, directly linked with chronic exposure to UV light. Basal cell carcinomas present in varied forms, as nodular, pearly, pigmented lesions often on the hand, neck, or

head. Squamous cell carcinomas present as quickly growing, firm indurated nodules with or without ulceration on sun-exposed areas, especially the rim of the ear, face, lips, and mouth. Malignant melanomas account for 5% of skin cancers but 75% of deaths (Kim et al., 1997). Melanomas present as new lesions, or as changes in existing moles. There is a link to multiple severe, blistering sunburns, but family history is a more important factor. The majority of melanomas are found in sun-exposed areas in white adolescents (Orlow, 1995). Any change in a mole, especially with rapid asymmetrical growth, crusting, ulceration, or color variation, needs immediate evaluation. Treatment consists of surgical removal and histological evaluation. All school-age children and adolescents should be taught to do a monthly skin evaluation (see Table 37-18).

Patient Education and Prevention

These include the following:

1. Remember that a tan is not a sign of good health, but of skin injury. There is no such thing as a healthy tan. Never seek a tan; seek the shade. Avoid tanning devices or parlors (Clore, 1995).
2. Know your skin type and protection needs (see Table 37-16).
3. Avoid the sun between 10 AM and 2 PM. Learn the "shadow rule"—seek shade if your shadow is shorter than you are tall. Most newspapers print in the weather section the predicted index of UV exposure (1 to 10) as prepared by the National Weather Service.
4. Cover up with hats, sunglasses, and clothing.
   - Hats with a wide (3 in.) brim are recommended.
   - Sunglasses should be worn beginning in infancy. Large-framed, wraparound lenses provide the best protection. UV protection is provided by a chemical added to the lenses and is indicated by one of the following labels: UV absorption to 400 nm, special purpose, meets ANSI (American National Standards Institute) UV requirements (Wagner, 1995).
   - Tight-weave, long-sleeved, long-pants clothing with sunscreen applied to the

skin underneath provides maximum protection. Color, weight, stretch, wetness, and quality of material all affect the amount of protection offered. *Solumbra* and *SunSkins* offer clothes that provide 30+ SPF and block 97% of UV rays. *Shades* offers clothes that provide 81% UV protection. *Stingray* offers swimwear that blocks 99% of the sun's rays (see Resource Box 37-1).

5. Use sunscreen (Table 37-17).
6. Teach sun protection early on, by example, as well as words. "Block the Sun, Not the Fun" is a program with curricula, family support materials, and educational posters sponsored by the American Academy of Dermatology (AAD) and Coppertone to educate elementary school–aged children to reduce sun exposure and increase protective behavior. See AAD in Resource Box.
7. Do monthly skin checks (Table 37-18).

Drug Eruptions

Description

Drugs taken systemically can result in a variety of skin reactions or rashes. The three most common types found in children are (1) morbilliform (measles-like) rash, (2) urticaria, and (3) erythema multiforme rash (Table 37-19). Urticaria and erythema multiforme are discussed in the section on vascular reactions below. Other reactions not discussed here include acute generalized exanthematous pustulosis, erythema nodosum, leukocytoclastic vasculitis, fixed drug eruption, allergic contact dermatitis, photosensitivity, acneiform eruptions and pigmentary changes.

Etiology and Incidence

The morbilliform rash, also called an exanthematous rash, is the most common allergic

T A B L E 37-17

Sunscreen Recommendations

Sunscreens block the rays of the sun to help prevent sunburn. Sun protection factor (SPF) is the length of time an individual can be exposed to sun without burning if sunscreen is used appropriately. The substantivity of a sunscreen describes its adherence. Sweat resistant (effective for up to 30 min of heavy continuous perspiration), water resistant (effective for up to 40 min of swimming), and waterproof (effective for up to 80 min of immersion) are different types of substantivity. Specific recommendations include the following:

Use at least a 15 SPF, nonalcohol base, without lanolin, paraben, or fragrance. Use a waterproof product when in water but reapply every 80 min with continuous water exposure.

Apply at least 30 min before exposure to sun; reapply at least every 2 h while in the sun, and after swimming, toweling, or heavy perspiration.

Apply liberally (1 oz for an adult) and, for better coverage, use cream instead of lotion.

Pay special attention to eyelids, nose, cheeks, ears, neck, scalp, shoulders, hands, and feet. Use a lip balm with SPF of 15.

Do not use sunscreen on infants <6 mo of age, but keep baby out of the sun completely, using shade, brimmed hat, and protective clothing.

Use sunscreen daily in summer or in warm climates. Use even on overcast or cloudy days.

Extra protection is needed with increasing altitude, closer location to the equator, sand, snow, concrete, or water reflection.

Set an example by using sunscreen.

Sunscreens are available in various chemical combinations (e.g., *para*-aminobenzoic acid, [PABA], PABA esters, cinnamates, benzophenes, salicylates, octocrylene, dibenzoylmethane) and vehicles (e.g., emollient for dry skin, gel or lotion for oily skin, noncomedogenic for acne-prone skin). If a child is sensitive to one, try a sunscreen with different ingredients. A PABA-free sunscreen is recommended for children. Dibenzoylmethane provides the most protection from ultraviolet A.

Sunblocks scatter and reflect light. Zinc oxide, titanium oxide, or a combination product such as Sportz Bloc is useful for especially sensitive areas such as the nose or previously burned areas.

T A B L E 37-18
Monthly Skin Examination

The ABCDEs of skin examination:
  Asymmetry
  Border irregularity or notching
  Color variation especially if multicolored
  Diameter >6 mm
  Elevation, especially if asymmetrical
Note any new growths, itchy patches, nonhealing
  sores, changes in size, irritability, or different
  sensation in any moles
Process of skin examination. Use a full-length
  mirror, a hand mirror, and a brightly lit room,
  Examine the following areas:
    Front and back, right and left sides with arms
      raised
    With elbows bent, forearms, back of arms
      and palms
    Back of legs and feet, toes and soles
    Back of neck and scalp
    Back and buttocks

skin reaction to a drug, occurring in at least 50% of cases (Vanderhooft, 1998). The rash may be an immunological or nonimmunological reaction to the drug. The most common drugs causing reactions are the penicillins; sulfonamides; cephalosporins, especially cefaclor; erythromycin; NSAIDs; barbiturates; isoniazid; carbamazepam; and phenytoin (Richards, 1999; Goldstein & Adams, 1998; Vanderhooft, 1998). Onset of a rash often is within a week of starting the medication but can be as late as 2 or more weeks and can occur after the medication has been stopped. Incidence is between 8 and 11% for all courses of antibiotics (Richards, 1999).

Clinical Findings

HISTORY. The following can be reported:

- Medication taken within the last 3 weeks
- Intense itching
- Rash worsens even after medicine is discontinued for up to 5 days
- Possible systemic symptoms—fever, arthralgia, arthritis, lymphadenopathy, edema

PHYSICAL EXAMINATION. Findings include the following (see Color Fig. 19):

- Often begins as a fairly symmetrical, macular erythematous rash that becomes papular and confluent.
- Patches of normal skin scattered throughout areas of involvement.
- Rash begins on the trunk, where it is brighter red, more confluent, and extends distally to the extremities, including the palms and soles.
- The face often has confluent areas of erythema.

LABORATORY STUDIES. The following are ordered if necessary for differential diagnosis:

- CBC, Monospot test, C-reactive protein (CRP), antinuclear antibodies, cold agglutinins
- Chest radiograph

Differential Diagnosis

Viral exanthem; measles; toxic erythema such as in scarlet fever, staphylococcal scarlatina, or Kawasaki's disease; and morbilliform rash (if the patient has mononucleosis and is taking amoxicillin); toxic shock syndrome; roseola; and erythema infectiosum are included in the differential diagnosis.

Management

Decisions about whether a drug is to be implicated are dependent upon the patient's previous history of taking the drug, the experience of the general population with the drug, the morphology and timing of the rash, and other possible explanations for the rash (e.g., viral illness). The following steps are taken:

1. Discontinue the suspected drug.
2. Label the patient's medical record with the potential allergen.
3. Prescribe antihistamines if itching is present; recommend a lubricant and antipruritics as adjuncts.
4. Prescribe prednisone 1 to 2 mg/kg per day for 5 to 7 days if significant reaction.
5. Schedule follow-up visit as determined by severity of reaction and other illness.

T A B L E 37-19

Differentiating Drug Eruptions, Urticaria, and Erythema Multiforme

	ETIOLOGY	CLINICAL FINDINGS	TREATMENT
Drug eruption	Reaction to medication, especially penicillin, cephalexin, erythromycin, sulfa drugs, NSAIDs, barbiturates, isoniazid, carbamazepam, phenytoin	Symmetrical, macular, erythematous to papular, confluent morbilliform rash; intense itching; patches of normal skin throughout; begins on trunk, extends distally, including palms and soles; face with confluent erythema	Stop drug and label as allergen to the child; antihistamine, antipruritics, lubricate skin; prednisone if severe; rash can last 7–14 d; medical alert bracelet
Urticaria	Hypersensitive reaction; immunological antigen-antibody response to release of histamines; often unknown cause; possible reaction to food, drug, insect bite/sting, pollen; possible reaction to infection, especially strepto-coccal, sinus, mononucleosis, hepatitis	Family history of hives; rapid onset; possible atopy; intense itching; mild erythema, annular, raised wheals with pale centers; lesions scattered or coalesced; *key finding:* appear suddenly, fade from 20 min to 24 h; blanch with pressure; associated edema of eyelids, lips, tongue, hands, feet	Quick resolution; identify and remove or treat offending agent if possible; stop antibiotic; give oral antihistamines; topical antipruritics; epinephrine or prednisone if anaphylactic, angioedema, or refractory; refer if >6 wk duration
Erythema multiforme (minor)	Immune-mediated hypersensitivity reaction often to infection, especially HSV, also to many other agents	History of infection, especially herpes labialis; variety of lesions on skin and mucous membranes—macules, papules, vesicles, early lesions like urticaria; *key finding:* target or iris lesions; *key finding:* lesions fixed, symmetrical, typical distribution on hands, feet, elbows, knees, also face, neck, trunk; possible oral mucous membrane involvement	Identify, treat, discontinue trigger if possible; treat infection; supportive measures for hydration, prevention of secondary infection, relief of pain; oral antihistamines, cool compresses; oral lesions—mouthwash, topical anesthetics; lesions last 5–7 d, recur in batches over 2–4 wk, resolve without scarring or sequelae

NSAIDs = nonsteroidal anti-inflammatory drugs; HSV = herpes simplex virus.

6. Refer to allergist for skin testing to confirm allergy if there are limited or no alternative medications, for desensitization, to clarify drug allergy, for severe parental anxiety, or if symptoms were severe and life-threatening.

Complications

Body heat and water loss can occur if the rash is severe. Progression of the rash if medicine is continued can lead to toxic epidermal necrolysis or Stevens-Johnson syndrome (see section on erythema multiforme), or allergic interstitial nephritis.

Patient Education and Prevention

These should include the following:

1. The rash can last 7 to 14 days with itching present and worsening before getting better.
2. There is potential risk from further exposure to that drug or related ones; alternative therapies should be explained.
3. Identification and communication of the child's allergy are imperative. In life-threatening allergies, wearing a medical alert bracelet or necklace is essential.

▮▮▮ VASCULAR REACTIONS OF THE SKIN

Urticaria

Description

Urticaria is a hypersensitivity reaction commonly called hives (see Color Fig. 20). Transient or acute urticaria lasts less than 6 to 8 weeks; chronic, recurrent, or persistent urticaria lasts more than 6 to 8 weeks. Papular urticaria occurs in reaction to mosquito or flea bites. Physical causes of urticaria include dermatographism, cholinergic reactions (e.g., response to heat, exercise, hot baths), pressure, water, and cold.

Etiology and Incidence

Urticaria is caused by a complex interplay of immunologically mediated antigen-antibody responses to the release of histamine from mast cells. Vasodilation and increased vascular permeability cause erythema and the characteristic wheal. Onset is usually rapid, and resolution occurs within a few days of onset. The cause often remains a mystery (idiopathic). Possible causative factors include:

- Reactions to foods (e.g., nuts, eggs, shellfish, strawberries, tomatoes), drugs (salicylates and penicillins are the two most common), animal stings (e.g., bees, wasps, scorpion, spider, jellyfish), or pollen
- Response to bacterial, viral, or fungal infections, especially streptococcal or sinus infection (Moon, 1998), mononucleosis, hepatitis, adeno- and enteroviruses, or parasites
- Response to physical stimuli (e.g., heat or cold, sun or water, tight clothing, vibrations) or stress
- Genetic origin
- Concurrent with inflammatory systemic diseases (e.g., collagen-vascular or inflammatory bowel disease)

Between 16 and 25% of the population will have at least one attack of urticaria (Vanderhooft, 1998). Of all cases of urticaria, only 3 to 5% are IgE or allergy mediated. Fifteen percent are physical urticarias, and the remainder are idiopathic (Weston & Badgett, 1998; Presser, 1997). Portals of entry include infection (most common), ingestion, injection, inhalation, immunological (rare), and idiopathic.

Clinical Findings

HISTORY. The following should be assessed:

- Family or previous history of hives, angioedema, connective tissue disease, juvenile arthritis
- Possibility of atopy
- Intense itching
- Ingestion (within 4 hours) of nuts, shellfish, chocolate, berries, spices, egg white, milk, fish, sesame
- Ingestion or injection of medicines (penicillin, sulfa drugs, sedatives, diuretics, analgesics, acetylsalicylic acid), additives, or preservatives

- Injection of diagnostic agents, vaccine, insect venom, blood, medicine
- Infection with upper respiratory infectious agent, virus, streptococcus, mononucleosis; hepatitis; parasites
- Inhalation of animal danders, pollen, dust, smoke, or aerosols
- Cold, heat, exercise, sun, water, pressure, or vibration

PHYSICAL EXAMINATION. Location of lesions may help determine the cause (e.g., a lesion around the mouth or tongue is likely due to an ingested agent). Findings can include the following:

- Mildly erythematous, annular, raised wheals or welts with pale centers from 2 mm to 20 cm in diameter
- Lesions scattered or coalesced but generalized
- Lesions appear suddenly and fade in anywhere from 20 minutes to less than 24 hours, reappearing in other areas later; if fixed more than 48 hours, it is not urticaria
- Lesions blanch with pressure
- Heat seems to intensify the presentation
- Associated edema of eyelids, lips, tongue, hands, feet, and genitalia
- Wheals after rubbing or stroking the skin (dermatographism)
- Papulovesicular lesions with central punctate lesion and wheals most common in toddlers (papular urticaria)
- Large, blotchy erythematous lesions with 1 to 3 mm central wheals (cholinergic urticaria)

LABORATORY STUDIES. If urticaria with possible anaphylaxis from an insect bite is suspected, referral to an allergist for testing and hyposensitization is needed. If fever is present, evaluation for underlying disease can be useful.

Differential Diagnosis

Contact dermatitis, atopic dermatitis, scabies, erythema multiforme (lesions are fixed with dusky centers and appear within 72 hours), mastocytosis, reactive erythemas, vasculitis, psoriasis, and juvenile arthritis are also included in the differential diagnosis.

Management

The following steps are taken:

1. Identify and remove the offending substance if possible. Stop all antibiotics. Avoid any possible food or environmental trigger.
2. Test for dermatographism by stroking the skin, for cholinergic urticaria by applying heat or observing immediately after exercising, for cold urticaria by applying cold packs, for pressure urticaria by applying weighted bands for several minutes, and for water urticaria by applying wet compresses.
3. Administer medications as indicated:
   - Oral antihistamines such as diphenhydramine 5 mg/kg per d or hydroxyzine 2 to 4 mg/kg per d every 4 to 6 hours until itching and urticaria are resolved. Nonsedating antihistamines are less effective, but if needed, astemizole, cetirizine, or loratadine are best. Urticaria is less likely to recur if the antihistamine is continued for 1 to 2 weeks after resolution.
   - Topical antipruritics may be helpful.
   - Aqueous epinephrine 1:1000 (subcutaneously 0.01 ml/kg up to 0.3 ml) may be needed if anaphylaxis or significant angioedema with swelling of mucous membranes and airway is present.
   - Prednisone 1 to 2 mg/kg/d for 1 week with rapid taper only if refractory to other measures or if angioedema is present with swelling of lips and face.
4. Follow-up visit if not improved within 48 hours.
5. Chronic urticaria persisting longer than 6 weeks needs evaluation for infection or systemic causes or referral for further evaluation.

Complications

Angioedema or anaphylaxis occurs by the same mechanism as urticaria.

- Anaphylactic symptoms require emergency intervention.
- Angioedema is an extension of the reaction into the subcutaneous tissue. It occurs in 50% of children with urticaria at some time during the episode and involves the face

(especially the eyes), the hands, and feet 85% of the time (Weston & Badgett, 1998). Angioedema is gradual in onset and often involves reaction to medication (Wolf, 1999). Pseudoephedrine as an adjunct to antihistamine may be helpful. Hereditary angioedema is rare (0.4%; Weston & Badgett, 1998); however, it is life-threatening and usually presents in adolescence, often following trauma (e.g., dental work, surgery, accident). It is manifested by repeated episodes of swelling of the extremities (75%), face, and throat (30%), accompanied by abdominal pain (52%) that becomes progressively more severe (Weston & Badgett, 1998). Severe airway edema, if untreated, is often the cause of death.

- Serum sickness begins with hives but has other systemic symptoms, for example, fever, arthralgias, malaise, lymphadenopathy, proteinuria.
- If urticaria is from a drug reaction, rechallenge with the drug is more likely to cause anaphylaxis.

Patient Education and Prevention

The following are needed:

- Explanation of causes, course, and treatment. The cause often cannot be found, and control of symptoms is the main goal of treatment. The entire episode usually resolves in 24 to 48 hours, rarely extending beyond 3 to 4 weeks. Further evaluation is needed only if the hives lasts longer than 6 weeks.
- Papular urticaria hypersensitivity often declines within 6 to 12 months.
- Physical urticarias last 2 to 4 years in most cases, but occasionally persist into adulthood.
- Occasionally macular blue-brown lesions are found upon resolution of urticaria.
- Avoidance of allergen if known; medical alert bracelet if severe reaction; hyposensitization if life-threatening symptoms occur.
- Carry an anaphylactic kit if indicated.

Erythema Multiforme

Description

Erythema multiforme (EM) minor is a self-limited, immune complex hypersensitivity reaction characterized by skin and mucous membrane involvement in response to a variety of agents (see Color Fig. 21). EM major is a separate entity with two variants, Stevens-Johnson syndrome (SJS) and toxic epidermal necrolysis (TEN). Four major types of erythema multiforme have been identified (Weston et al., 1996):

1. Typical SJS with macules and blisters, and mucous membrane involvement on less than 10% of the body surface
2. An overlap of SJS and TEN with 10 to 30% of the body surface involved
3. A TEN with large confluent areas of the face and trunk involving more than 30% of the body surface
4. TEN with "spots," or many red macules with blisters involving more than 10% of the body

Etiology and Incidence

Although not clearly understood, EM minor is thought to be an immune-mediated hypersensitive reaction with lesions similar to a graft-versus-host reaction. Infection is the primary precipitating event in EM minor in children and adolescents, most notably due to herpes simplex virus (HSV, 80%; Weston, 1996), Epstein-Barr virus (EBV), orf, histoplasmosis, and mycoplasma. EM major is more commonly related to medications (specifically anticonvulsants, sulfa drugs, penicillins, NSAIDs, and salicylates). Infection, immunizations, foods, and systemic disease also have been implicated. Early recognition and immediate discontinuation of any drug involved shortens the course and prevents serious complications (Vanderhooft, 1998; Weston et al., 1996; Rauch & Adam, 1996; Cohen, 1994).

Erythema multiforme occurs in healthy individuals of any age, but the highest incidence is in 20- to 40-year olds. However, 20 to 50% of all cases are seen in children, most commonly in adolescents. EM is more common in males and in the winter months. Recurrence occurs in approximately 33% of cases (Rauch & Adam, 1996; Weston et al., 1996; Cohen, 1994). TEN occurs most commonly after 10 years of age as a complication of a drug, most commonly a sulfonamide, penicillin, NSAID, anticonvulsant, or barbiturate (Paller, 1999).

Clinical Findings

HISTORY. The following are sometimes reported:

- Recent or current infection with a viral (HSV, EBV), bacterial (mycoplasma), fungal, or protozoal agent; 50% of cases have a history of herpes labialis within 7 to 10 days prior to onset of rash (Weston, 1996)
- Recurrence, especially with herpes simplex (EM minor) or mycoplasmal pneumonia (EM major)
- Use of sulfa drugs, penicillin, salicylates, anticonvulsants, or barbiturates
- Prodrome to EM major includes fever, malaise, sore throat, cough, headache, vomiting, diarrhea, chest pain, myalgia, and arthralgia in 33% of cases (Rauch & Adam, 1996)
- Exposure to UV light or trauma to area

PHYSICAL EXAMINATION. Lesions vary from patient to patient, within a single episode, and with recurrence.

EM Minor
- A variety of lesions on skin and mucous membranes, including macules, papules, vesicles of varying size; early lesions often mistaken for urticaria; lesions may fuse to form large annular plaques.
- A diagnostic clue is the presence of target lesions (a distinct dark central area with possible blistering or necrosis and an outer ring of erythema) or iris lesions (with a central blister or whitish area, a middle dusky zone, and an outer erythematous ring).
- Lesions are fixed (another diagnostic clue), tend to be symmetrical, and have a typical distribution predominantly on the hands, feet, elbows, and knees, but also on the face, neck, and trunk.
- Mucous membranes are usually spared, but

a single surface, usually lips and mouth, may be involved, including blisters, crusted swollen lips, and tongue lesions.

EM Major (SJS or TEN)
- Sudden, widespread onset with high fever and weakness; child or adolescent appears ill
- Involvement of at least two mucous membranes, including the oral mucosa and bulbar conjunctiva, genitalia, rectum, nasopharynx, esophagus, respiratory, or gastrointestinal mucosa
- Extensive blisters, bullae, crusts, erosions, ulcerations; rash begins on trunk and disseminates to extremities; often no target lesions are present, and there are areas of skin that are spared
- The TEN rash has rapidly coalescing target lesions and widespread bullae that become full-thickness epidermal peeling within 24 hours

LABORATORY STUDIES. The following are ordered as indicated by the clinical condition of the child:

- Chest radiograph to screen for mycoplasmal pneumonia
- Tzanck's preparation to screen for herpes
- CBC and urinalysis to screen for leukocytosis and renal involvement
- Other studies may be indicated if EM major is suspected

Differential Diagnosis

Urticaria can be differentiated by lack of itching, lability of lesions, and shorter-lasting hives that are pale centrally, not target or iris lesions. Viral exanthems are more centrally located, confluent, and less erythematous. Purpura is present in vasculitis. In staphylococcal scalded skin syndrome, the skin peels superficially (not full-thickness) and is significantly red. Also included in the differential diagnosis are Kawasaki's disease and lupus erythematosus.

Management

Care for EM minor is generally supportive, as the condition is self-limited. Children with EM major require hospitalization and intensive support and intervention.

EM Minor

1. Identify, discontinue, or treat the stimulus, if possible.
2. Treat precipitating infection as appropriate.
   - If HSV, a 5-day course of oral acyclovir 400 mg/d at the onset of each episode, or if recurrent, a 6-month course
3. Supportive measures to maintain hydration, prevent secondary infection, and relieve pain.
   - Mild analgesics, cool compresses, and oral antihistamines such as diphenhydramine
   - Soothing mouthwashes or topical anesthetics such as Kaopectate or Maalox mixed in equal parts with diphenhydramine
   - Topical intraoral anesthetics, such as dyclonine liquid or viscous lidocaine, are sometimes used with caution in older children and adolescents
   - Debridement of oral lesions with half-strength hydrogen peroxide
   - Intravenous fluids if oral hydration is not adequate
4. The role of steroids in treating EM is controversial. Some believe they may be helpful in recurrent cases or early in the course of the disease to moderate symptoms. In evolving SJS or TEN, however, steroids may increase the risk of secondary infection and delay wound healing (Vanderhooft, 1998; Rauch & Adam, 1996; Weston et al., 1996).

EM Major

EM major can be life-threatening and requires hospitalization, burn care, and daily ophthalmological care.

Complications

Dehydration from reduced oral intake is the most common complication. With EM major there is a mortality rate of 5 to 70%, with morbidity including pneumonitis, renal disease, keratitis, and other ophthalmological disorders (Vanderhooft, 1998; Weston et al., 1996; Rauch & Adam, 1996).

Patient Education and Prevention

EM minor lesions last 5 to 7 days, recur in batches over 2 to 4 weeks, but resolve without scarring or sequelae, except for transient desquamation, scaling, or hyperpigmentation. Recurrence of EM minor is common, often once or twice a year (Weston, 1996).

PAPULOSQUAMOUS ERUPTIONS OF THE SKIN

Pityriasis Rosea

Description

Pityriasis rosea (PR), meaning rose-colored flaking, is a common, mild, self-limited papulosquamous disease (see Color Fig. 22).

Etiology and Incidence

PR is believed to be viral in origin, though no specific organism has been isolated. It is minimally contagious and occurs most commonly in the fall, early winter, and spring months in temperate climates. Though it occurs in all age groups, the greatest incidence is in 10- to 35-year-olds (Hebert & Goller, 1996; Bloomfield, 1994).

Clinical Findings

HISTORY. Although there is usually no prodrome, mild symptoms of malaise and fever prior to onset of rash are sometimes reported.

PHYSICAL EXAMINATION. Findings include the following:

- Herald spot—1- to 10-cm solitary, ovoid, slightly erythematous lesion that enlarges quickly with central clearing, usually occurring 1 to 30 days prior to the onset of rash *(key finding)*
- Generalized, symmetrical, small macular to papular, thin, round to oval lesions, thin scale centrally with thicker scale peripherally, pale pink in color, more common on trunk and proximal extremities from neck to knees but also found on face and neck 7 to 15 days after the herald spot

- Christmas tree pattern—rash, especially on back, follows skin lines with oval lesions running parallel
- Oral lesions have punctate hemorrhages, erosions or ulcerations, erythematous macules, or annular plaques
- In blacks, 2- to 3-mm papular lesions are more common on the neck, proximal extremities, inguinal and axillary areas, less common on trunk
- Atypical disease may have urticarial, purpuric, or lichenoid variants or absence of herald patch (10 to 15% of cases; Bloomfield, 1994)

LABORATORY STUDIES. If needed, a skin scraping to rule out tinea; a VDRL to rule out secondary syphilis.

Differential Diagnosis

Psoriasis, scabies, tinea (especially the herald patch), secondary syphilis, drug eruptions, or viral exanthems should be ruled out in the differential diagnosis.

Management

The following steps are taken:

1. Application of calamine, tepid baths with Aveeno, antihistamines, emollients, or mild topical steroids as needed for itching.
2. Minimal sun exposure can help lesions resolve more quickly. Avoid sunburn.
3. For oral lesions, triamcinolone acetonide (Kenalog in Orabase) in dental paste may be applied, or in patients over 8 years of age, mouthwash with tetracycline and diphenhydramine.

Patient Education and Prevention

PR is a benign, self-limited, and noncontagious disease that has three cycles (emerging, persisting, and fading) with resolution spontaneously in 4 to 12 weeks. There is a 2% chance of recurrence (Hebert & Goller, 1996). Transient pigmentary changes can occur, especially in blacks.

Psoriasis

Description

Psoriasis, a chronic skin disorder with spontaneous remissions and exacerbations, is characterized by thick silvery scales, its distribution pattern, and an isomorphic (Koebner's phenomenon) response (see Color Fig. 23). Types of psoriasis include guttate psoriasis (following a streptococcal infection), psoriasis vulgaris, napkin psoriasis (occurring in the diaper area), inverse psoriasis (limited to areas that are normally spared), localized pustular psoriasis, generalized pustular or psoriatic erythroderma, and psoriatic arthritis.

Etiology and Incidence

Though the cause is unknown, there is a familial predisposition, and probable polygenic inheritance pattern. An accelerated epidermal proliferation of keratinocytes and dermal vascular abnormalities contribute to the characteristic look of the lesions. Trigger factors including infection, local trauma, stress, and certain drugs (corticosteroids, lithium, NSAIDs) play a role in psoriasis.

Psoriasis occurs in 1 to 3% of the population, with 25 to 45% of cases appearing before 10 to 16 years of age. It is more common in whites than in blacks and in males than in females. Guttate psoriasis is the first sign of psoriasis in 15 to 34% of children (Paller, 1999; Arbuckle & Hartley, 1998; McDonald & Smith, 1998; Vernon, 1997; Hebert & Goller, 1996; Weston et al., 1996).

Clinical Findings

HISTORY. The following may be reported:

- Family history in approximately one third of cases
- Streptococcal pharyngitis prior to onset
- Trauma prior to onset

PHYSICAL EXAMINATION. Findings include the following:

- The scalp (encircling the hairline and external ears), elbows, knees, and buttocks (especially the diaper area in infants) are the most common sites of involvement. In children, the face may also be involved. Lesions are often found around areas of trauma (e.g., genitalia, palms, soles).

- Discrete, initially erythematous, symmetrical, well-marginated rash becoming papular with silver scales that may be trivial to widespread.
- *Acute guttate (teardrop) psoriasis.* Widespread, symmetrical, round, or oval, 0.5- to 2-cm lesions occurring primarily on the trunk and proximal extremities, occasionally on the face, and rarely on the palms or soles. There is less scaling than in psoriasis vulgaris.
- *Psoriasis vulgaris.* Well-circumscribed, erythematous plaques with silvery-white scales concentrated on elbows, knees, scalp, and hairline, but also seen on eyebrows, around ears, and in intergluteal fold and genital area.
- *Koebner's phenomenon (isomorphic response).* The occurrence of psoriasis 1 to 3 weeks after trauma (e.g., bites, scratch, abrasion, sunburn, pressure) (45% of cases; Weston et al., 1996).
- *Auspitz's sign.* Bleeding occurs when a scale is removed.
- *Nail signs.* Nails have "ice pick" pits and ridges, are thick and discolored, and can have splinter hemorrhages and be separated from the nail bed; present in 15% of cases (Weston et al., 1996).
- *Napkin psoriasis.* Appears eczematous, affecting inguinal and gluteal folds.

LABORATORY STUDIES. The following are to be considered:

- Streptococcal throat culture if presenting with guttate pattern
- KOH and culture to rule out fungal infection
- VDRL to rule out secondary syphilis

Differential Diagnosis

Pityriasis rosea, seborrhea, *Candida* infection, contact or irritant dermatitis, atopic dermatitis, tinea, dyshidrosis, secondary syphilis, and other nail pitting conditions are included in the differential diagnosis.

Management

In children, treatment should be as conservative as possible. Medications and treatments should be rotated for best effectiveness. The following are options for management:

1. Sun exposure in moderate amounts alleviates lesions. Avoid sunburn.
2. Emollient cream for dry skin can minimize trauma and subsequent psoriasis and may improve psoriasis by 40% (Arbuckle & Hartley, 1998).
3. Topical steroids, moderate or strong and sometimes fluorinated, applied 2 to 3 times a day for 2 to 3 weeks. They should be used intermittently but not discontinued spontaneously, as worsening can occur. Monitoring of the patient during use is important. Small localized lesions can be treated with topical, fluorinated steroids. A moderate-potency steroid can be used on thick plaques and larger areas. Severe plaques on the elbow and knees may need a higher-potency steroid (see Table 37–6). Systemic steroids are not indicated and may worsen the condition. Consultation with a dermatologist is often indicated.
4. Tar or keratolytic shampoos (ketoconazole [Nizoral], anthralin, salicylic acid [P & S]) can be used on the scalp. Tar preparations can also be used on the skin alone or in combination with UV light treatment.
5. Mineral or olive oil and warm towels to soak and remove thick plaques.
6. Keratolytic agents such as sulfur 3% or salicylic acid 3 to 6% to reduce thick, unresponsive plaques.
7. Anthralin ointment for plaques that are resistant to steroids and tar. In high strengths (1% and higher), apply ointment for 10 to 30 minutes once a day and then wash off. In lower strengths, leave ointment on for 8 hours. Strength used is determined by tolerance. Anthralin stains skin and clothing and can irritate skin.
8. Vitamin D analog (Calcitrol) produces improvement in 60% of patients (Paller, 1999) but is approved for use only in children over 12 years of age.
9. Follow up every 2 weeks until psoriasis is

controlled and during exacerbations, and then as needed.

10. Refer to a dermatologist if psoriasis is not responsive. Other treatment options include UV light treatment, psoralens, intralesional steroids, retinoids (Ruiz-Maldonado et al., 1998), cyclosporine, or immunotherapy.

Complications

The following complications are possible:

- *Candida* infection as a secondary infection in the diaper area.
- *Pustular psoriasis.* Unusual in childhood. Generalized or local multiple 1- to 2-mm pustules with erythema and scaling also involving palms and soles. Accompanied by malaise, fever, and leukocytosis. Should be referred to a dermatologist.
- *Exfoliative erythroderma.* Rare presentation, including desquamation and loss of hair and nails with previous history of psoriasis. Should be referred to a dermatologist.
- *Psoriatic arthritis.* An inflammatory arthritis that is rare (1%) but increasing in frequency, most common in females aged 9 to 12 years (Paller, 1999; Weston et al., 1996). Rheumatoid factor is negative, cutaneous symptoms mild or absent. Prognosis is good.

Patient Education and Prevention

Emotional support and education are the most important aspects in dealing with psoriasis. Areas for discussion include the following:

1. Psoriasis is chronic and involves spontaneous remission and exacerbations. Control and relief are sought, but cure is not available at this time. Treatment may require up to a month to determine effectiveness.
2. Guttate psoriasis often resolves with antibiotic treatment for streptococcal infection. Psoriasis vulgaris may persist for months to years.
3. Lifestyle changes help prevent recurrence. These include avoidance of cutaneous injury, streptococcal infection, sunburn, stress, itch-

ing, bites, tight clothes and shoes, some medications (e.g., oral steroids, NSAIDs), and occlusive dressings. Good skin care, including regular use of emollients, may improve psoriasis and minimize recurrences.
4. Tends to improve during summer and with pregnancy.
5. Psoriasis is considered stable if there are either no new plaques or if existing plaques are not enlarging.

▇ CONGENITAL LESIONS OF THE SKIN

Vascular and Pigmented Nevi

Description

Nevi are a common finding in children. The two most common types are vascular nevi (vascular malformations and hemangiomas) and pigmented nevi (mongolian spots, café-au-lait spots, acquired melanocytic nevi, acanthosis nigricans, and lentigines).

Etiology and Incidence

Vascular nevi are caused by a structural abnormality (malformations) or by an overgrowth of blood vessels (hemangiomas), and are flat, raised, or cavernous (Fishman & Mulliken, 1998). Flat lesions or vascular malformations include salmon patches (also called macular stains), an innocent malformation occurring in 30 to 70% of newborns, and port-wine stains, occurring in 1 to 3 per 1000 newborns. Raised or cavernous lesions, also called hemangiomas, are present in up to 10% of newborns. Hemangiomas occur more commonly in females (75%) and in 22 to 30% of premature infants weighing less than 1500 g (Fishman & Mulliken, 1998; Paller, 1999; Weston et al., 1996; Castiglia, 1994; Wahrman & Honig, 1994).

Pigmented nevi are caused by an overgrowth of pigment cells. Pigmented nevi most commonly seen are mongolian spots (up to 90% in blacks, 81% in Asians, 70% in Hispanics, and East Indians, <10% in whites), café-au-lait spots (12 to 22% in blacks, 0.3 to 19% in whites), and acquired nevi, the most common tumor of childhood, 2% of which are atypical (Paller,

1999; Dinulos & Graham, 1998; Weston et al., 1996).

Clinical Findings

HISTORY. The following should be noted:

- Presence from birth, or age first noted
- Progression of lesion
- Familial tendencies for similar nevi

PHYSICAL EXAMINATION. Findings include the following (Table 37–20):

- Vascular malformations or flat vascular nevi are present at birth, and grow commensurate with the child's growth.
- Hemangiomas are classified as superficial, deep, or mixed. They are not present at birth, but usually emerge by 1 month of age. They may present as a pale macule, a telangiectatic lesion, or a bright-red nodular papule. Involution occurs spontaneously, often between 12 and 15 months of age, heralded by gray areas in the lesion followed by flattening from the center outward. Most are flat by 5 years of age, the remainder by puberty.
- Pigmented nevi may be present at birth or may be acquired during childhood.

Differential Diagnosis

Hematomas or ecchymoses of child abuse are occasionally confused with some nevi. Non–insulin-dependent diabetes mellitus (NIDDM) often presents with acanthosis nigricans.

Management

1. Flat vascular nevi:
   - Salmon patches
     - Fade with time, usually by 5 or 6 years of age
   - Port-wine stains
     - A permanent defect that grows with the child, so cosmetic covering is often used.
     - Refer to a dermatologist for possible pulsed dye laser and corrective cosmesis.
     - If forehead and eyelids are involved, there is potential for multiple syndromes,

including Sturge-Weber, Klippel-Trenaunay-Weber, and Parkes-Weber. Neurodevelopmental and ophthalmological follow-up is needed.
   - Angiomatous papules and underlying soft tissue hypertrophy develop over years.
2. Hemangiomas:
   - Reassure and educate the family about the nature and course of this nevus. A word that there is no relationship to anything the mother did during pregnancy is often appreciated.
   - Frequent follow-up, especially during the growing phase. Sequential photographs are helpful.
   - If the lesions are strategically placed (eye, lip, oral cavity, ear, airway, diaper area), very large, or grow very quickly, prompt referral is indicated as early treatment is most effective.
   - If treatment is required during the proliferative stage, steroids (1 to 4 mg/kg/d) are prescribed until growth is stabilized, then tapered over 4 to 6 weeks, with a 30 to 90% success rate. Patients should be followed every 2 weeks while on therapy. Indications for steroid treatment are interference with physiological functions (e.g., breathing, hearing, eating, vision), recurrent bleeding or ulceration, high-ouput congestive heart failure, Kasabach-Merritt syndrome, rapid growth that distorts facial features, or presence in the diaper area (Morelli, 1996; Wahrman & Honig, 1994).
   - Treatment by surgery, cryotherapy, radiation, or injecting sclerosing agents often leads to scarring.
   - Danger of cardiovascular complications, disseminated intravascular coagulation, or compression of internal organs with large, deep lesions.
   - Regression occurs in 25% of cases by 2 years of age, in 40 to 50% by 4 years of age, in 60 to 75% by school age, and in 95% by adolescence. Scarring may be present if ulceration has occurred; loose skin and telangiectasis follow in 30 to 50% of cases (Paller, 1999; Morelli, 1996; Cohen, 1998; Wahrman & Honig, 1994).

T A B L E 37-20

Common Vascular and Pigmented Nevi

I. Vascular malformations or flat vascular nevi
  A. Salmon patch or nevus flammeus
    1. Light-pink macule of varying size and configuration
    2. Commonly seen on the glabella, back of neck, forehead, or upper eyelids
  B. Port-wine stain or nevus flammeus
    1. Purple-red macules that occur unilaterally, tend to be large
    2. Usually occur on face, occiput, or neck, although they may be on extremities
II. Hemangiomas
  A. Superficial (strawberry) hemangiomas are found in the upper dermis of the skin and account for the majority of hemangiomas
  B. Deep cavernous hemangiomas are found in the subcutaneous and hypodermal layers of the skin; although similar to superficial hemangiomas, there is a blue tinge to their appearance
    1. With pressure, there is blanching and a feeling of a soft, compressible tumor
    2. Variable in size, they can occur in places other than skin
  C. Mixed hemangiomas have attributes of both superficial and deep hemangiomas
III. Pigmented nevi
  A. Mongolian spots
    1. Blue or slate-gray, irregular, variably sized macules
    2. Common in the presacral or lumbosacral area of dark-skinned infants; also on the upper back, shoulders, and extremities
    3. The majority of the pigment fades as the child gets older and the skin darkens
    4. Solitary or multiple, often covering a large area
  B. Café-au-lait spots
    1. Tan to light-brown macules found anywhere on the skin; oval or irregular in shape; increase in number with age
  C. Acquired melanocytic nevi are benign, light brown, to dark brown, to black, flat, or slightly raised, occurring anywhere on the body, especially on sun-exposed areas, above the waist
    1. *Junctional nevi* represent the initial stage, with tiny, hairless, light brown to black macules
    2. *Compound nevi*—a few junctional nevi progress to these more elevated, warty, or smooth lesions with hair
    3. *Dermal nevi* are the adult form, dome-shaped with coarse hair
    4. *Atypical nevi* usually appear at puberty, have irregular borders, variegated pigmentation, are larger than normal nevi (6–15 mm); usually found on trunk, feet, scalp, and buttocks
    5. *Halo nevi* appear in late childhood with an area of depigmentation around a pigmented nevus, usually on trunk
  D. Acanthosis nigricans is velvety brown rows of hyperpigmentation in irregular folds of skin, usually the neck and axilla; tags may also be present
  E. Lentigines are small brown to black macules 1–2 mm in size appearing anywhere on the body in school-age children

3. Pigmented nevi. Educate family about the nature of these lesions:
- *Mongolian spots*: document to distinguish from bruise; fade with time, usually to traces by adulthood.
- *Café-au-lait spots*: if six or more lesions larger than 0.5 cm in diameter are present, or if axillary freckling or tumors are also present, refer child to rule out neurofibromatosis.
- *Acquired melanocytic nevi*
  ○ Giant nevi (e.g., bathing trunk nevus) need referral to a dermatologist.
- *Atypical nevi* need regular follow-up because of increased risk for melanoma. However, melanoma often presents with new lesions rather than from transformation of current ones. (See section on sunburn complications.)
- *Acanthosis nigricans*: a decrease in weight

sometimes results in resolution of lesions; can also be a presentation of NIDDM in children.

- *Lentigines*: may fade or disappear with time but are also associated with various syndromes.

Complications

Ulceration, infection, platelet trapping, airway or visual obstruction, or cardiac decompensation can occur with large vascular nevi. Kasabach-Merritt syndrome occurs when thrombocytopenic hemorrhage occurs in a large, deep hemangioma.

Vitiligo and Hypopigmentation

Description

Lack of pigment in the skin causing white or light-colored areas can be either hypopigmentation or vitiligo. Two types of vitiligo have been identified: type A has a generalized, acral symmetrical distribution; type B, a segmental, dermatome distribution.

Etiology and Incidence

Vitiligo, presumed to be an immune disorder, occurs in 1 to 2% of the US population, with 50% of cases beginning before 20 years of age. It appears more commonly in children with various systemic or immune disorders (Weston et al., 1996; Hurwitz, 1993). Hypopigmentation follows inflammation or injury to the melanocytes in the skin resulting from diseases such as atopic dermatitis, psoriasis, or pityriasis rosea, or from abrasions, burns, injury from liquid nitrogen, or severe sunburn.

Clinical Findings

HISTORY. The following should be elicited:

- Family history of vitiligo, halo nevi, traumatic depigmentation of skin, or markedly premature graying of the hair is present in 30% of cases (Hurwitz, 1993)
- Onset of depigmentation (birth or more recent)
- Presence of any systemic or skin diseases
- Any recent trauma to the skin

PHYSICAL EXAMINATION. Findings include the following:

Vitiligo
- Flat, milk-white macules or papules with scalloped, distinct borders of varied size
- Symmetrical or asymmetrical, possibly following a nerve segment
- Few to multiple, seen most commonly on face and trunk

Hypopigmentation
- Macules and patches with irregular mottling and borders
- Linear or patterned
- Possibly associated hyperpigmented areas

LABORATORY STUDIES. For vitiligo, a skin biopsy and CBC, fasting glucose, thyroid function and antithyroid antibodies, early-morning serum cortisol, and VDRL are sometimes indicated.

Differential Diagnosis

Pityriasis rosea, pityriasis alba, tinea versicolor, and albinism (eye color affected and onset at birth) are included in the differential diagnosis.

Management

The following steps are taken:

Vitiligo
- Broad-spectrum sunscreens are used to decrease the tanning of normal skin.
- Cover-up agents such as skin dyes and walnut oil.
- Mild to moderate steroids may show success in some patients.
  - Triamcinolone 0.1% twice a day to skin for 4 to 6 months
  - Hydrocortisone 1% twice a day to face for 4 to 6 months
- Refer for treatment with psoralens. May be used in combination with UVA radiation (best used in children under 9 years of age).
- Family should be encouraged to be in a support group since this is a very disfiguring condition, especially for those with dark complexion.

Hypopigmentation

- Reassure family that repigmentation will occur. Hypopigmentation is self-limited and lasts only a few months.

Complications

With vitiligo, complications include thyroid disease, diabetes mellitus, pernicious anemia, Addison disease, uveitis, alopecia areata, and severe sunburn.

▨▨▨▨ HAIR AND NAIL DISORDERS

Alopecia, hair loss from areas of skin normally producing hair, can be limited to one area or scattered over the scalp, and can be complete or leave residual hairs of differing lengths. The three main causes of hair loss are tinea capitis, traumatic alopecia, and alopecia areata (Table 37–21).

Tinea Capitis

Description

Ringworm of the scalp and hair may be seen in four different presentations: (1) diffuse fine scaling without obvious hair breaks and with subtle to significant hair loss; (2) discrete areas of hair loss with stubs of broken hairs (black-dot ringworm) (see Color Fig. 24); (3) "classic" patchy hair loss and scaly lesions with raised borders; and (4) scaly, pustular lesions, or kerions. Tinea capitis occurs in a noninflammatory stage for 2 to 8 weeks, then becomes inflammatory.

Etiology and Incidence

The fungus invades the scalp and hair shaft, causing an inflammatory response and fragile hair shaft. *T. tonsurans* is the causative organism 90 to 95% of the time, and the infection is near epidemic in the United States, but *M. canis* or other species can be responsible (McDonald & Smith, 1998; Stein, 1998; AAP, 1997; Vasiloudes et al., 1997; Weston et al., 1996). Tinea capitis is transmitted by humans sharing hats, combs, and brushes, or by cats, dogs, or rodents. Tinea capitis is the most common dermatophyte infection, occurring primarily in children 2 to 10 years of age (Friedlander, 1998; AAP, 1997; Weston et al., 1996). It is more common in boys (5:1) than in girls (Hurwitz, 1993), and in blacks (>90% of cases; McDonald & Smith, 1998).

Clinical Findings

HISTORY. Hair loss, itching, and contact with another person or pet with ringworm are sometimes reported.

PHYSICAL EXAMINATION. Findings include the following:

- Scaling, erythema, or crusting
- Bald patches or areas of broken hairs
- Occipital or posterior cervical adenopathy may be significant
- *Microsporum* species leaves the hair broken and lusterless with a fine gray scale on the scalp
- *T. tonsurans* presents as black-dot tinea, with tiny black dots that are the remainder of hair that has broken off at the shaft; no scalp scale is present (most common)
- A boggy, inflamed mass filled with pustules (kerion) is a delayed allergy reaction; cervical lymphadenopathy, fever, and leukocytosis may be present
- The inflammatory stage is noted by widespread pustules, suppuration, and kerion formation

LABORATORY STUDIES. Examination of hair scrapings as follows:

- Wood's light fluoresces yellow-green (positive with *M. canis*, negative with *T. tonsurans*)
- KOH examination of scraped hair; wait 20 to 40 minutes after application of KOH to examine; if Wood's light is positive, outer surface of hair is coated with tiny mats of spores; if Wood's light is negative, hyphae and spores are present in hair shaft
- Fungal culture of a plucked hair is most reliable

T A B L E 37-21

Diagnosis and Treatment of Alopecia

	ETIOLOGY	CLINICAL FINDINGS	TREATMENT
Tinea capitis	*Trichophyton tonsurans* 90–95%; *Microsporum canis*; others	Fine diffuse scaling without obvious hair breaks and subtle to significant hair loss; hair loss discrete with stubs of broken hair; patchy hair loss with scaling and raised borders to lesions; scaly, pustular lesions or kerions	Griseofulvin taken with fatty food until 2 wk after negative culture; monitor CBC, LFTs, renal function at 4 wk and every 4–8 wk; prednisone if kerion present; culture family members; sporicidal shampoo; keep from school 1 wk; follow-up in 2 wk; launder sheets, clothes, vacuum house
Traumatic alopecia	Chemical, thermal, traction (hair-styling), friction (trichotillomania)	*Traumatic:* incomplete hair loss with varying lengths; *Traction:* erythema and pustules, thins and breaks in certain areas, especially linear; *Trichotillomania:* circumscribed hair loss with irregular borders and broken hair of varied lengths, no erythema or scarring, especially frontal, parietal, or temporal	*Traction:* avoid hairstyles that precipitate; mild shampoo, gentle brushing; short course of antibiotics if pustules *Trichotillomania:* discussion with parents, oil at night, counseling if entrenched, other interventions if significant
Alopecia areata	Autoimmune mechanism	Family history; single or multiple round or oval patches of complete or near-complete hair loss; no erythema or scaling, scalp smooth with fine new hair growth, usually frontal or parietal; "exclamation hairs" present; nail ridging or pitting; occasional loss of body or pubic hair	Discussion and support; often self-limited course; if extensive, refer to dermatologist for alternative treatments; supportive care—Rx for wig, refer to National Alopecia Foundation

CBC = complete blood count; LFTs = liver function tests.

Differential Diagnosis

Traumatic alopecia, alopecia areata, hypo- and hyperthyroid hair loss, seborrhea, atopic dermatitis, psoriasis, impetigo, and folliculitis are included in the differential diagnosis.

Management

The following steps are taken:

1. Griseofulvin 10 to 20 mg/kg/d, occasionally up to 25 mg/kg per d if no response, once daily with fatty food such as ice cream to enhance absorption. Treatment should be continued until 2 weeks after resolution, a minimum of 4 to 12 weeks (Friedlander, 1998; McDonald & Smith, 1998; AAP, 1997; Vasiloudes et al., 1997; Goldgeier, 1996). Topical antifungals are ineffective.

2. If a long-standing kerion with severe inflammation is present, prednisone 1 to 2 mg/kg/d for 5 to 14 days. Antibiotic treatment is not indicated.

3. Family members and pets should be checked

for infection by fungal culture and treated if positive. More than 50% are positive (Weston et al., 1996), so do not rely on lack of symptoms. Asymptomatic carriers are common.

4. Shampooing with selenium sulfide 2.5% or econazole or ketoconazole 2% (2 times per week for 4 weeks) decreases spore viability and keeps other household members from being infected.

5. Child should be kept out of school for 1 week.

6. A follow-up visit should be scheduled after 2 weeks to evaluate response to treatment. Medication should be continued until 2 weeks after culture is negative. Follow-up should be continued every 2 to 4 weeks until new hair growth is evident.

7. Monitoring of CBC, LFTs, and possibly renal function tests is recommended at 4 weeks and every 4 to 8 weeks thereafter if griseofulvin is continued for more than 3 months (McDonald & Smith, 1998; Goldgeier, 1996; Schwartz & Janniger, 1995).

8. If resistance to griseofulvin is encountered, oral itraconazole, terbinafine, fluconazole, and ketoconazole have been used but are not approved for use in children.

Complications

An id reaction is a hypersensitivity reaction to the fungus, not to the medication it is being treated with. It presents either as a red, superficial edema or as scaly, red plaques and papules and is treated with 1 to 2 weeks of topical or systemic steroids. Permanent hair loss and scarring can occur with an untreated kerion.

Patient Education and Prevention

1. Sites and modes of transmission are identified (*M. canis*, animal source; *T. tonsurans*, human source) and treated.

2. Side effects of medication should be explained and monitored.

3. Hair regrowth is slow (3 to 12 months) and, if a kerion was present, hair loss can be permanent.

4. Laundering sheets and clothes in a hot-water wash or hot dryer cycle and vacuuming may decrease spread in the family.

5. Grooming practices (e.g., hair traction, greasy pomades, infrequent shampooing) may be predisposing factors.

6. There is a high rate of asymptomatic carriers; culture is the only definitive means of identification.

Traumatic Alopecia

Description

Traumatic hair loss can be due to chemical or thermal traction or friction. The most common forms are traction alopecia and trichotillomania.

Etiology and Incidence

Traction alopecia, commonly seen in black females, is due to hair styling. Common causes are cornrows, ponytails, or braids; tight curlers; or excessive brushing.

Trichotillomania occurs in 1% of the population, with age of onset before 8 years in males and 12 years in females. Five to 10% of cases may be due to an emotional trauma such as divorce or death in the family (Vasiloudes et al., 1997). It is often seen in children with other obsessive-compulsive habits such as thumb-sucking or nail-biting, although some authorities consider it an entity of its own rather than a symptom of a psychiatric disorder.

Clinical Findings

HISTORY. The history can include the following:

- Various methods of hair styling with tight pull on hair
- Habits such as nail-biting, finger-sucking, or hair-twirling
- Any recent life changes or stressors
- Medications (anticonvulsants, antithyroids, beta blockers, isotretinoin, lithium, oral contraceptives, vitamin A supplements, warfarin)
- Excess time spent lying in supine position

PHYSICAL EXAMINATION. The following findings are present:

Traumatic Alopecia
- Incomplete hair loss with hair of varying lengths

Traction Alopecia
- Possible erythema and pustules
- Thinning and breaking in certain areas, tending to occur in a linear pattern related to hairstyle

Trichotillomania
- Circumscribed hair loss with irregular borders and broken hairs of varied length
- No erythema or scaling of the scalp
- Commonly found on frontal, parietal, and temporal areas with peripheral sparing

Differential Diagnosis

The differential diagnosis includes tinea capitis, alopecia areata, neonatal occipital alopecia, rub alopecias in atopic dermatitis, and child abuse (make sure no one but the child is pulling out the hair).

Management

The following steps are taken:

Traction Alopecia
- Avoid any hairstyle or device that causes traction on the hair, including cornrows, ponytails, braids, and curlers.
- Use only mild shampoo, shampoo infrequently, use wide-toothed combs with rounded ends, and brush gently.
- A short course of antibiotics is prescribed if pustules are present.

Trichotillomania
- A straightforward discussion and ongoing support of the child and parents are essential. Remember that 1% of children are trichotillomaniacs. Attempt to find means to relieve stress and cope with any traumatic events.
- Applying oil to the hair at night makes it slippery and harder to pull.
- Referral for counseling is needed if the habit is entrenched.

- Medication, behavior therapy, habit reversal, relaxation, and hypnosis are modalities sometimes used.

Complications

Trichobezoars (hairballs) in the child with trichotillomania can cause gastrointestinal symptoms.

Patient Education and Prevention

The cause of the hair loss must be discussed and support offered to resolve issues. New hair growth can take 3 to 6 months.

Alopecia Areata

Description

Alopecia areata is an asymptomatic, complete hair loss occurring primarily in frontal or parietal areas (Fig. 37-9).

Etiology and Incidence

The cause of alopecia areata is unknown, but is thought to be an autoimmune mechanism. It is unusual under 2 years of age but can be seen anytime throughout childhood. There is a 10 to 20% familial occurrence (Vasiloudes et al., 1997).

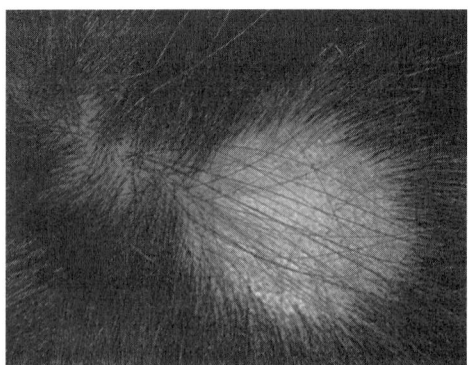

FIGURE 37-9
Alopecia areata with sharply defined oval patches of hair loss. (From Hurwitz S: Clinical Pediatric Dermatology, 2nd ed. Philadelphia, WB Saunders, 1993, p 486.)

Clinical Findings

HISTORY. The history can include other family members with alopecia areata.

PHYSICAL EXAMINATION. Findings include the following:

- Single or multiple (up to three) round or oval patches of complete or nearly complete hair loss without erythema or scaling. Scalp is smooth with fine new hair growth.
- The frontal and parietal areas are involved 90% of the time (Vasiloudes et al., 1997).
- "Exclamation hairs" are narrower at the base, short, and broken off.
- Nail ridging or pitting (a helpful distinguishing factor).
- Occasional loss of body or pubic hair, or eyelashes or eyebrows.
- Possible atopic dermatitis or vitiligo.

LABORATORY STUDIES. The following are sometimes performed:

- KOH examination or fungal culture to rule out tinea
- Skin biopsy

Differential Diagnosis

Tinea capitis vs. traumatic alopecia is the differential diagnosis.

Management

No pharmacological intervention for this condition has proved helpful. The following steps should be taken:

1. Open discussion and support of the child and parents. If only one or two patches are present, reassure that regrowth will occur.
2. If extensive involvement, refer to a dermatologist for potential treatment options. These include potent topical steroids, intralesional steroids, minoxidil, anthralin, or contact sensitization.
3. Recommend wearing a wig, depending on the severity of involvement; prescribing the wig as a medical treatment helps defray the cost.

Complications

Self-esteem issues are common. *Ophiasis* is a form of alopecia areata that begins in the frontal or occipital hairline and spreads along the hair margins. *Alopecia totalis* is a loss of all the hair on the scalp. *Alopecia universalis* is a loss of all the hair on the body.

Patient Education, Prognosis, and Prevention

All families should be put in touch with the National Alopecia Areata Foundation (see Resource Box 37-1). The condition is self-limited in most (95%) school-aged children and adolescents (McDonald & Smith, 1998; Vasiloudes et al., 1997). Full recovery, often within a year, is more likely if three or fewer areas are involved and if onset is in late childhood. However, the greater the hair loss, the longer it takes for regrowth. Prognosis is guarded in infants and toddlers. One third of patients will have a recurrence within months to years, with a worsening prognosis with each episode (Vasiloudes et al., 1997).

Onychomycosis

Description

A fungal infection of the nail(s) with tinea or *Candida* is called onychomycosis (Fig. 37-10). One or two nails are often involved. The infec-

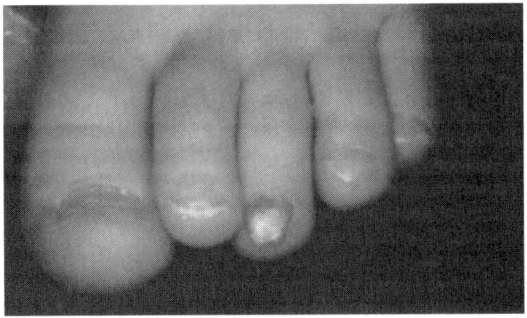

F I G U R E 37-10
Onychomycosis (tinea unguium). Thickening and discoloration on the toe of a 4½ year-old-child caused by tinea infection. (From Hurwitz S: Clinical Pediatric Dermatology, 2nd ed. Philadelphia, WB Saunders, 1993, p 386.)

tion may be superficial, hypertrophic (ony-chauxic), or cause separation of the nail plate from the tissue (onycholytic).

Etiology and Incidence

The infecting organism invades the nail, proliferates, and destroys the nail integrity, causing separation of the nail plate from the nail bed. The infection originates at the distal edge of the nail. It is uncommon during the first two decades of life, with a worldwide prevalence from 0 to 2.6%, limited almost exclusively to adolescents. Often there is concurrent tinea pedis or tinea manuum. There may be a relation to the use of occlusive shoes. The causative organisms include *Trichophyton rubrum, Trichophyton mentagrophytes, E. floccosum,* and *Candida albicans.* However, 50% of the time another condition is responsible for dystrophic nail (Stein, 1998; Friedlander, 1998; Krusinski, 1997).

Clinical Findings

HISTORY. The adolescent may report a thickened, discolored nail.

PHYSICAL EXAMINATION

- Opaque white or silvery nail that becomes thick, yellow, with subungal debris
- Toenails are involved more often than fingernails with tinea
- Fingernails are involved more often than toenails with *Candida*
- Seldom symmetrical; it may be one to three nails on one extremity

LABORATORY STUDIES
- KOH preparations and fungal cultures of the material under the nail are helpful in confirming diagnosis

Differential Diagnosis

Psoriasis (involves all nails and includes pitting), hereditary nail defects, dystrophy secondary to eczema or chronic paronychia, lichen planus, and trauma are the differential diagnoses.

Management

1. Griseofulvin and ketoconazole are the established medications to treat onychomycosis, but their side effects, length of treatment, and the high recurrence rate following treatment make successful management uncommon. Only 17.5% of cases respond to 6 to 12 months of griseofulvin therapy (Weston et al., 1996).
2. Newer triazole medications—terbinafine, itraconazole (the recommended drug; Friedlander, 1998), and fluconazole—are less costly and safer, with cure rates of 65 to 94% and relapse rates of 15 to 20% at 2-year follow-up (Krusinski, 1997). Safety and efficacy studies have not been completed in children, however, nor has FDA approval for children been granted (Weston et al., 1996; Goldgeier, 1996).
   - The FDA-approved drugs and dose for older children follow:
     ○ Itraconazole 100 mg 2 times a day for 12 weeks for toenails
     ○ Terbinafine 250 mg/d for 12 weeks for toenails
   - Pulse regimens are used but not FDA approved the following (Paller, 1999; Krusinski, 1997):
     ○ Itraconazole 200 mg twice a day for 7 days a month for 3 to 5 months for toenails or for 7 days a month for 2 months for fingernails
     ○ Fluconazole 150 mg once a week for 6 to 9 months for toenails
     ○ Terbinafine 250 mg twice a day for 7 days a month for 3 to 4 months for toenails
   - Suggested pediatric dosages are as follows (Stein, 1998):
     ○ Itraconazole 3 to 5 mg/kg/d for 4 to 6 weeks (available in liquid form) or until clearing followed by 4 weeks off therapy with close follow-up and additional treatment as needed
     ○ Terbinafine 3 to 6 mg/kg/d for 4 to 6 weeks (limited pediatric experience)
3. If triazoles are used, a careful review of current medications must be taken as there are many interactions. Baseline and every-6-weeks monitoring of CBC and hepatic func-

tion are recommended if continuous therapy is used.

4. *Candida* infection is treated with topical application of ketoconazole (Nizoral) under occlusion (plastic glove covered by a cotton sock at bedtime) for 2 to 4 weeks.

Patient Education, Prognosis, and Prevention

The unfortunate truth to communicate is that cure is difficult to obtain and relapse is common.

Paronychia

Description

Chronic or acute inflammation and infection around a fingernail or toenail is called paronychia.

Etiology and Incidence

Infection of a nail with bacteria (often *S. aureus*, occasionally *Streptococcus* or *Pseudomonas*), *Candida* (in infants with thrush or thumb-sucking or when hands are immersed in water a lot), or herpes is common in school-aged children and adolescents. It is more common with tight shoes or when nails are malaligned, cut with rounded edges, or too short.

Clinical Findings

HISTORY. Tenderness and drainage are reported, as well as discomfort, especially with walking.

PHYSICAL EXAMINATION. Findings include the following:

- Proximal nail fold erythematous, swollen, and tender; if chronic, may not be tender
- Purulent exudate expressed
- Cuticle broken or absent
- Nontender erythema and edema with thickened, disrupted nail (*Candida* infection, often with secondary bacterial infection)

LABORATORY STUDIES. A culture of the exudate is occasionally done.

Differential Diagnosis

Herpetic whitlow (grouped vesicules on an erythematous base) and eczematous inflammation should be ruled out.

Management

Management includes the following:

1. Antistaphylococcal oral antibiotic if acute infection
2. If *Candida* is suspected, nystatin cream under occlusion (a plastic glove covered by a cotton stocking) every night for 3 to 4 weeks
3. If purulent area is full, loosen cuticle from nail with a No. 11 blade to allow exudate to escape
4. Frequent warm soaks, after which cotton pledgets are inserted beneath the nail to lift it up
5. Instruction on proper trimming of nails and care of toenails
   - Wear wide-toed shoes
   - Trim nails straight across and not too short
6. If condition is recurrent, referral for surgical removal of lateral portion of nail

Complications

Recurrent infection is possible.

BODY ART

Tattoos and Body Piercing

Description

A tattoo is an indelible mark fixed on the body by insertion of pigment under the skin. Body piercing is the creation of a hole anywhere in the body (typically the ear, eyebrow, lip, naris, tongue, navel, nipple, or genitalia) to insert jewelry. Both tattoos and piercing are considered forms of body art or embellishment of one's appearance that have been practiced throughout the ages in many cultures as rites of passage, as means of showing status or membership in a particular group, or as proof of virility.

Etiology and Incidence

A tattoo is accomplished by injection of an insoluble ink via a uniform series of punctures into the dermal layer of the skin. Piercing is accomplished by inserting a sharp implement through the skin. Most tattoos or piercings are done in unregulated, unlicensed tattoo parlors, though some adolescents may tattoo or pierce themselves or their peers. Some states have legislation preventing tattooing of minors or requiring parental consent.

Questioned as to why they obtained tattoos, 81% of adolescents in one study related it to "personal identity, be myself; I don't need to impress people any more" (Armstrong & Murphy, 1998). Four reasons given by adolescents for body piercing are as follows: "it is a form of body art," "it is fashionable," "it makes a personal statement," and "it is daring" (Armstrong, 1996). Piercing is considered less permanent than a tattoo.

The media tend to classify these behaviors as carefree and risqué (Armstrong et al., 1994). Adults and parents may see piercing or tattooing as a deviant behavior, a strange new trend, a fetish, fad, or fashion (Armstrong et al., 1994; Muldoon, 1997). Both tattooing and piercing have an increased incidence in the United States, especially in the adolescent population. The average age at first tattoo is 14 years; the average age at first piercing is 15 years (Armstrong & Murphy, 1998; Armstrong et al., 1994).

Clinical Findings

HISTORY. Questions to discuss include the following:

- When and where was the body art obtained?
- Where is it located and what care is being given?
- Were there any complications?

Physical Examination

- Any symptoms of infection—erythema, crusting, or scabs?

Differential Diagnosis

Branding, the burning of the skin aimed at creating a permanent scar in a desired design via blowtorch or wire coat hanger in hot oil, is one differential diagnosis. *Self-mutilation*, a self-directed violence that ranges from altering physical appearance (e.g., ear piercing) to extreme forms (e.g., amputation), is another consideration. Some forms are considered normal, but deviant forms are physically damaging, done in response to crisis, demonstrating disconnectedness and alienation from others (Dallam, 1997).

Management

1. Aftercare for tattoos (Grief & Hewitt, 1998)
   - Basic wound care, including not touching for 24 hours
   - Oozing and local swelling is normal for 48 hours
   - Scab should be left alone except for the application of ointment
   - Protect from rough surfaces that can traumatize; protect from sunburn
   - Review signs and symptoms of infection
2. Aftercare for body piercings (Grief & Hewitt, 1998)
   - Wash hands before touching; wash area with soap twice daily
   - Some oozing and swelling is normal; if crusts appear, remove with wet swab
   - Tongue
     - Use ice to minimize swelling
     - Rinse mouth 10 to 12 times a day with half-strength Listerine, twice a day with carbamide peroxide (Gly-Oxide)
     - No deep kissing for 48 hours; once healed, use dental dams for dental work and avoid smoking
   - Navel
     - Slowest to heal, most likely to reject jewelry
     - Cleanse twice a day with antibacterial soap
     - Avoid handling; avoid clothing that rubs for up to 1 year
   - Nipples and genitalia
     - Cleanse with antibacterial soap twice a day
     - Avoid manipulation and tight garments; cotton clothes are ideal
     - Latex barriers must be used with sexual activity

TABLE 37-22
So You Are Thinking About Getting a Tattoo or Body Piercing

KNOW THE FACTS: MAKE AN INFORMED DECISION

Unsterile tattooing and piercing equipment and needles can spread serious infections, hepatitis, or possibly even human immunodeficiency virus (HIV).

The law in many states prohibits the tattooing of minors.

Asking a friend to apply a tattoo may ruin a friendship if the tattoo doesn't look like you thought it would.

Tattoos and permanent makeup are not easily removed and in some cases may cause permanent discoloration. Think carefully before getting a tattoo.

Tattoo removal is very expensive. A tattoo that costs $50 to apply may cost over $1000 to remove.

Blood donations cannot be made for a year after getting a tattoo, body piercing, or permanent makeup.

BEFORE YOU GET A TATTOO OR BODY PIERCING

First: Talk to your friends or others who have been tattooed or pierced.

Ask them about their experience, the cost, pain, healing time, etc.

Ask them what they would do if they had a chance to do it over again.

Second: Understand that you do not have to tattoo or pierce your body to belong.

Remember that you are directly involved in decisions that affect your health and body.

You can always change your mind or wait if you are not sure.

Third: Because of potential complications, if you decide to get a tattoo or body piercing, never tattoo or pierce your own body or let a friend do it.

HEALTH RISKS TO CONSIDER BEFORE YOU ACT

Both tattooing and piercing involve puncturing the skin to introduce a foreign material, jewelry, or ink, and the procedures carry similar risks. The primary health concern is introducing bloodborne germs or viruses into your body.

Blood-borne illnesses: hepatitis B and C, tetanus, tuberculosis, and HIV infection can lead to very serious health problems or death.

Localized infections: *Staphylococcus* or *Pseudomonas* infection can lead to illness, deformity, and scarring.

Tattoo troubles: Tattoos are open wounds that may become infected. The new tattoo must be kept clean. It must also be kept moist with an ointment to prevent a scab from forming. If you are allergic to the inks in the tattoo, the site will not heal properly and scarring may occur.

Piercing problems: Complications depend on where the body has been pierced. Navel infections are the most common; it takes a year for navel piercings to heal. Ear cartilage heals slowly. Tongue piercings may lead to tooth damage from biting on the jewelry, partial paralysis if the jewelry pierces a nerve, and extreme inflammation during the first few days.

SELECTING A TATTOO ARTIST OR PIERCER

Visit several piercers or tattooists. The work area should be kept clean and have good lighting. If they refuse to discuss cleanliness and infection control with you, go somewhere else.

Consent forms (which the customer must fill out) should be handled before tattooing. Reputable piercing and tattoo studios will not serve a minor without signed consent from parents. Check the laws in your state about tattooing of minors if you are under 18.

The tattooist or piercer should have an autoclave—a heat sterilization machine used to sterilize equipment between customers.

Packaged, sterilized needles should be used only once and then disposed of in a biohazard container.

Immediately before tattooing or piercing, the tattooist or piercer should wash and dry his or her hands and wear latex gloves. These gloves should be worn at all times during the tattoo or piercing procedure. If the tattoo artist or piercer leaves the procedure or touches other objects, such as the telephone, new gloves should be put on before the procedure continues.

A piercing gun should not be used because it cannot be sterilized properly. Only jewelry made of a noncorrosive metal such as surgical stainless steel, niobium, or solid 14-karat gold, is safe for a new piercing.

Leftover tattoo ink should be disposed of after each procedure. Ink should never be poured back into the bottle and reused.

Table by Barbara Freyenberger from data from Armstrong ML: You pierced what? Pediatr Nurs 22:236–238, 1996.
Data from Armstrong ML, Murphy KP: Adolescent tattooing. Prev Researcher 5(3):1–4, 1998.

R E S O U R C E   B O X   37-1

American Academy of Dermatology
Tel: 800-462-DERM or (312)-856-8888
Website: www.aad.org or www.coppertone.com
Block the Sun, Not the Fun program available

Association of Professional Piercers
519 Castro Street, Box 120
San Francisco, CA 94114

Cancer Research Institute or Cancer Care, Inc. (Melanoma Initiative)
Tel: (800)-813-HOPE
Website: www.cancercareinc.org

Cancer Research Foundation of America
Tel: (703)-836-4412
Website: www.prevent cancer.org/kids

Dermatology Nurses Association
North Woodbury Road, Box 56
Pitman, NJ 08071

Dermatology Online Atlas/Erlangen University
Website: www.derma.med.uni-erlangen.de/bilddb/
Extensive online image database with more than 500 diagnoses; search engine for diagnosis

Dermatology Online Journal
Website: Matrix.ucdavis.edu/DOJ.html/
Printed journal format with editorials, articles, case reports, and original articles

Dermatophyte Test Medium
Available from
Acuderm
Tel: 800-327-0015
Baker/Cummins
Tel: (305)-590-2282

The Electronic Textbook of Dermatology
Website: Telemedicine.org/stamfor1.htm/
From the Internet Dermatology Society

FIRST: Foundation for Ichthyosis and Related Skin Types
Tel: (800)-545-3286
Tel: (610)-789-3995
Newsletter, informational materials (incl. Spanish), networking, referrals to local resources, advocacy, fund research, maintains research registry

Hemangioma Hope
c/o Cindy Dougan
Tel: (814)-898-1054
Newsletter, informational materials, networking

Internet Dermatology Society
Website: Telemedicine.org/ids.htm/
An overview of resources and links to an assortment of sites and mailing lists.

InTray CCD
Alpha Tec Systems
Tel: (360)-260-2779

Koala Konnection
Tel: (888)-GO-KOALA
Website: www.suninfo@koala.com
Products include a sunhat called "legionnaire's hat"

Loyola University Dermatology Medical Education Web Site
Website: www.meddean.luc.edu/lumen/MedEd/medicine/dermatology/melton/title.htm/
Mix of materials for clinician and educator, pictorial representations, quiz, skin cancer atlas and benign tumor image atlas, and other links

National Alopecia Areata Foundation
Tel: (415)-456-4644
Newsletter, informational materials (incl. Spanish), networking, local chapters, advocacy, fund research

National Organization for Albinism and Hypopigmentation
Tel: (800)-473-2310
Website: www.albinism.org/
Newsletter, informational materials, chapters, advocacy, research

National Pediculosis Association (NPA)
Tel: (718)-449-NITS or 6487
Website: www.npa@headlice.org
Recorded messages, news, reporting registry, patient handouts

National Psoriasis Foundation
Tel: (503)-244-7404
Website: www.psoriasis.org
Newsletter, informational materials, networking, referrals to local resources, advocacy, fund research, maintains research registry

National Vitiligo Foundation
Tel: (903)-534-2925
Website: http://nvfi.org

Continued on next page

3. Healing times are variable and should be considered. A tattoo may take 2 to 3 weeks to heal. Body piercing, depending on the site, can take from 4 to 8 weeks for ears, to 6 to 12 months for navel and genital piercings.
4. Infection can be treated with dicloxacillin 500 mg 4 times a day for 10 days. Whether or not to remove jewelry should be decided by whether it will provide a drain, become an obstacle to healing, or be an ongoing source of infection.

Complications

The most common complications of tattooing or body piercing include infections, allergic reactions to the dyes or jewelry, and the transmission of blood-borne diseases, primarily hepatitis B and C, and, potentially, HIV. Other reported complications of tattoos include skin neoplasms, syphilis, leprosy, cutaneous tuberculosis, tetanus, hyperplasia, and granuloma annulare. Complications of piercings also include excessive bleeding, nerve damage, keloids, dental fracture, soft tissue damage, and speech impediments.

Patient Education, Prognosis, and Prevention

Providing information and encouraging teenagers to thoroughly research and consider the idea of getting a tattoo or body piercing is an important area of education. Table 37-22 is a helpful handout that covers much of the important information to be discussed. Maintaining an open, nonjudgmental attitude in discussing the options and in caring for adolescents who have body art is also essential.

REFERENCES

American Academy of Pediatrics (AAP). 1997 Red Book: Report of the Committee on Infectious Diseases, 24th ed. Elk Grove Village, IL, American Academy of Pediatrics, 1997.

Annunziato PW, Gershon A:. Herpes simplex virus infections. Pediatr Rev 17:415–423, 1996.

Arbuckle HA, Hartley AH: Psoriasis. Pediatr Rev 19:106–107, 1998.

Armsmeier SL, Paller AS: Getting to the bottom of diaper dermatitis. Contemp Pediatr 14(11):115–139, 1997.

Armstrong ML: You pierced what? Pediatr Nurs 22(3):236–238, 1996.

Armstrong ML, Ekmark E, Brooks B: Body piercing: Promoting informed decision making. J School Nurs 11(2):20–25, 1994.

Armstrong ML, Murphy KP: Adolescent tattooing. Prev Researcher 5(3):1–4, 1998.

Bass JW, Chan DS, Creamer KM, et al: Comparison of oral cephalexin, topical mupirocin and topical bacitracin for treatment of impetigo. Pediatr Infect Dis J 16:708–709, 1997.

Bell TA: Ivermectin and the LiceMeister Comb in the treatment of resistant pediculosis. Pediatr Infect Dis J 17:923, 1998.

Bergfield WF: Evaluating and managing acne. Skin 1:17–21, 1995.

Bloomfield D: Pityriasis rosea. Pediatr Rev 15:159-160, 1994.

Brainerd E: From eradication to resistance: Five continuing concerns about pediculosis. J School Health 68(4):146-150, 1998.

Castiglia PT: Hemangiomas. J Pediatr Health Care 8(3):130-131, 1994.

Centers for Disease Control and Prevention (CDC): Treating head lice. 1998. http://www.cdc.gov/ncidod/dod/lice.htm.

Clore ER: Natural and artificial tanning. J Pediatr Health Care 9(13):103-108, 1995.

Cohen B: The many faces of erythema multiforme. Contemp Pediatr 11:19-39, 1994.

Cohen BA: Warts and children: Can they be separated? Contemp Pediatr 14:128-149, 1997.

Cohen BA: What's your diagnosis? Contemp Pediatr 15:23-27, 1998.

Connolly J: Olive oil treatment may be effective method for killing head lice. Infect Dis Child 11:12-13, 1998.

Consumer Reports: A modern scourge. Consumer Reports, 62-63, 1998.

Cooley S, Atkinson P, Parks D, et al: Management of acne vulgaris. J Pediatr Health Care 12:38-40, 1998.

Cross JT, Hickerson SL, Yamauchi T: Antifungal drugs. Pediatr Rev 16:123-129, 1995.

Dallam SJ: The identification and management of self-mutilating patients in primary care. Nurse Pract 22(5):151-164, 1997.

Darmstadt GL: A guide to superficial strep and staph skin infections. Contemp Pediatr 14(5): 95-116, 1997.

Darmstadt GL: Scarlet fever and its relatives. Contemp Pediatr 15(2):44-63, 1998.

Dinulos JG, Graham EA: Influence of culture and pigment on skin conditions in children. Pediatr Rev 19(8):268-275, 1998.

Fisher RG, Edwards KM: Varicella-zoster. Pediatr Rev 19:62-67, 1998.

Fishman SJ, Mulliken JB: Vascular anomalies: A primer for pediatricians. Pediatr Clin North Am 45:1455-1477, 1998.

Friedlander SF: Pediatric exanthems. Presented at the 55th Annual Meeting of the American Academy of Dermatologists, San Francisco, March 21-26, 1997.

Friedlander SF: Update on fungal infections in childhood. Presented at the 56th Annual Meeting of the American Academy of Dermatologists. Orlando, FL, February 27-March 4, 1998.

Friedlander SF, Suarez S: Dermatol Clin 16:527-537, 1998.

Goldgeier MH: Fungal infections: Tips from a dermatologist. Contemp Pediatr 13(9):21-50, 1996.

Goldstein H, Adams HM: Drug sensitivity. Pediatr Rev 19:33, 1998.

Grief J, Hewitt W: The living canvas: Health issues in tattooing, body piercing and branding. Adv Nurse Pract 6:26-82, 1998.

Hansen RC. Update in managing cutaneous infections. Contemp Pediatr (suppl):9-10, 1998.

Hansen RC, Krafchik BR, Lane AT, et al: Dealing with diaper dermatitis. Contemp Pediatr 5-14, 1998.

Hebert AA, Goller MM: Papulosquamous disorders in the pediatric patient. Contemp Pediatr 13:69-88, 1996.

Hurwitz S: Clinical Pediatric Dermatology, 2nd ed. Philadelphia, WB Saunders, 1993.

Hurwitz S: Acne vulgaris: Pathogenesis and management. Pediatr Rev 15:47-52, 1994.

Hurwitz S: Acne treatment for the 90's. Contemp Pediatr 12:19-32, 1995.

Jarvis C: Physical Examination and Assessment, 2nd ed. Philadelphia, WB Saunders, 1996.

Kim HJ, Ghali FE, Tunnessen WW: Here comes the sun. Contemp Pediatr 14(7): 41-69, 1997.

Koo J: The psychosocial impact of acne: Patients' perceptions. J Am Acad Dermatol 32:526-530, 1995.

Kristal L, Silverberg, N: Acne: simplifying a complex disorder. Contemp Pediatr (suppl):3-10, 1998.

Kronemeyer B: Mupirocin helpful in treating impetigo and recurring staphylococcal infections. Infect Dis Child 10:23, 1997.

Krowchuk DP: Treating acne: A practical guide for pediatricians. Adolesc Health Update 11:1-10, 1998.

Krusinski P: New treatments for onychomycosis. Clin Lett Nurse Pract 1:8, 1997.

Kurtz ML: Treatment of herpes zoster. Personal communication, June 6, 1993.

Leyden JJ: Therapy for acne vulgaris. N Engl J Med 336:1156-1162, 1997.

Marrazzo JM: A new rash, sharp pain and small blisters. Clin Advisor 1(2):40-42, 1998.

McDonald LL, Smith ML: Diagnostic dilemmas in pediatric/adolescent dermatology: Scaly scalp. J Pediatr Health Care 12(2):80-84, 1998.

Moon MA: Sinus infection often at root of cutaneous urticaria. Pediatr News 32:36, 1998.

Morelli JG: Hemangiomas and vascular malformations. Pediatr Ann 25:91-96, 1996.

Muldoon KA: Body piercing in adolescents. J Pediatr Health Care 11:298-301, 1997.

National Pediculosis Association (NPA): Resistant lice? 1998a www.headlice.org/FAQ/

National Pediculosis Association (NPA): 10 tips for manual removal of head lice and nits. 1998b. www.headlice.org/FAQ/

National Pediculosis Association (NPA): NPA position statement on lindane. 1998c. www.headlice.org/news/mad.html

National Pediculosis Association (NPA): Lice and nits—Hold the mayo. 1998d. www.headlice.org/FAQ/

Nelson CT, Demmler GJ: Superficial HSV infection: How serious is it? What should you do? Contemp Pediatr 13(5):96-111, 1996.

Nicol N: Assessing skin disruptions (personal communication, 1993).

Nopper AJ: Out, out, darned nit. Pediatr Primary Care 12:35-36, 1998.

Orlow SJ: Melanomas in children. Pediatr Rev 16:365-369, 1995.

Paller A: Dermatologic problems. In Dershewitz RA (ed): Ambulatory Pediatric Care, 3rd ed. Philadelphia, Lippincott-Raven, 1999, pp 392-449.

Peters S: Saving face: Treating adolescents affected by acne vulgaris. Adv Nurse Pract, 5:43-64, 1997.

Peterson CM, Eichenfield LF: Scabies. Pediatr Ann 25(2):97-100, 1996.

Pollack S, Adam HM: Staphylococcal scaled skin syndrome. Pediatr Rev 17:18, 1996.

Prasad SM: Molluscum contagiosum. Pediatr Rev 17:118–119, 1996.

Presser R: Urticaria: A NP's approach. J Am Acad Nurse Pract 9:437–443, 1997.

Rasmussen JE: Scabies. Pediatr Rev 15(3):110–114, 1994.

Rauch D, Adam HM: The spectrum of erythema multiforme. Pediatr Rev 17(2):63–64, 1996.

Richards CA: Some antibiotics are commonly associated with skin rashes. Infect Dis Child 12(2):24–25, 1999.

Ruiz-Maldonado R, Tamayo-Sanchez L, Orozco-Covarrubias MLL: The use of retinoids in the pediatric patient. Dermatol Clin 16:553–569, 1998.

Savin RC, Donofrio LM: Aggressive acne treatment: As simple as one, two, three? Physician Sports Med 24(9):41–51, 1996.

Schwade S: Reports of resistant scabies out of proportion. Pediatr News 33:21, 1999.

Schwartz RA, Janniger CK: Tinea capitis. Cutis 55:29–32, 1995.

Shriner DL, Schwartz RA, Janniger CK: Impetigo. Cutis 56:30–32, 1995.

Siegfried EC: Warts on children: An approach to therapy. Pediatr Ann 25:79–90, 1996.

Smith W, Burns C: Managing the hair and skin of African American pediatric patients. J Pediatr Health Care 13(2):72–78, 1999.

Stavish S: Persistent scabies due to one of five causes. Pediatric News 32(4):38, 1998.

Stein DH: Tineas—Superficial dermatophyte infections. Pediatr Rev 19:368–372, 1998.

Trizna A, Tyring SK: Antiviral treatment of diseases in pediatric dermatology. Dermatol Clin 16:539–552, 1998.

Vanderhooft SL: Is the rash a drug reaction? Contemp Pediatr 15(5):118–137, 1998.

Vasiloudes P, Morelli JG, Weston WL: Bald spots: Remember the "big three." Contemp Pediatr 14:76–91, 1997.

Vernon P: The heartbreak of psoriasis: No laughing matter. J Pediatr Health Care 11(1):32–33, 1997.

Wagner RS: Why children must wear sunglasses. Contemp Pediatr 12:27–37, 1995.

Wahrman JE, Honig PJ: Hemangiomas. Pediatr Rev 15:266–271, 1994.

Weinberg S: Secondary infection often occurs with diaper dermatitis. Infect Dis J, 11:42–43, 1998.

Weston WL: What is erythema multiforme? Pediatr Ann 25:106–109, 1996.

Weston WL, Badgett JT: Urticaria. Pediatr Rev 19:240–244, 1998.

Weston WL, Lane AT, Morelli JG: Color Textbook of Pediatric Dermatology, 2nd ed. St Louis, Mosby-Year Book, 1996.

Wolf RL: Urticaria, angioedema, anaphylaxis, and serum sickness. In Dershewitz RA (ed): Ambulatory Pediatric Care, 3rd ed. Philadelphia, Lippincott-Raven, 1999.

Working Group on Prevention of Invasive Group A Streptococcal Infections: Prevention of invasive group A streptococcal disease among household contacts of case-patients. JAMA 279:1206–1210, 1998.

CHAPTER **38**

Musculoskeletal Disorders

Catherine E. Burns and Margaret A. Brady

INTRODUCTION

Orthopedic conditions in children are disruptions to the major structural system of the body. A variety of conditions can present with orthopedic findings; even family problems or child abuse may present with bone or muscle complaints. There also can be iatrogenic deformities that result from cultural practices such as binding the feet or using a cradleboard. Disorders of the musculoskeletal system present unique problems, because growth and development of this system contribute to the evolution of pathology over time. For example, untreated developmental dysplasia of the hip results in derangement of the hip socket with limping and eventual wearing away of the femoral head. Limited mobility, pain, and deformity interfere with the lifestyle of the child. The disabled child may not be able to participate in some activities with peers and family or have access to all occupations. The child faces challenges to self-esteem. Primary care providers seek to help children and their families avoid these problems.

The nurse practitioner (NP) plays a significant role in the management of children with orthopedic problems, although, in many cases, specialists manage specific conditions. The provider assesses development of the musculoskeletal system, identifies problems for early intervention, focuses on lifestyle and injury prevention, monitors the long-term outcomes of orthopedic care, and helps the family to integrate orthopedic care with the daily living patterns of home and school. Assisting the family to cope with the issues of disability, deformity, and long-term care is also an important role.

ANATOMY AND PHYSIOLOGY

Ossification of the fetal skeleton begins during the fifth month of gestation. The clavicles and skull bones are the first to ossify, followed by the long bones and spine. Bone age, measured by radiographs of the wrists, is used to determine general growth. In adolescents, the skeletal growth spurt begins at about Tanner stage 2 in girls and Tanner stage 3 in boys. It is at its peak around stage 4 and then ends with stage 5. The growth spurt lasts longer in boys than in girls. The pelvis widens early in pubescent girls. In both sexes, the legs usually lengthen before the thighs broaden. Next, the shoulders widen and the trunk completes its linear growth. Bone growth ends when the epiphyses close.

Long bones have a growth plate, or physis, at each end, which separates the epiphysis from the diaphysis or shaft. Openings through this plate allow blood vessels to penetrate from the epiphysis. In the growth plate, chrondrocytes produce cartilage cells, dead cells are absorbed, and the calcified cartilage matrix is converted into bone. The entire growth plate area is weaker than the remaining bone, because it is less calcified. Because the blood supply to the growth plate comes primarily through the epiphysis, damage to epiphyseal circulation can jeopardize the survival of the chondrocytes. If chondrocytes stop producing, growth of the bone in that area stops (Fig. 38-1).

The length of long bones comes from growth at the epiphyseal plates. The diameter of long bones increases as a result of deposition of new bone on the periosteal surface and resorption on the surface of the medullary cavity. Growth of the small bones, hip, and spine comes from one or more primary ossification centers in each bone. Apophyses are the sites for connection of tendons to bone. In children, these sites, similar to epiphyses, allow for growth and are weaker than bone. They can be sites for inflammation with stress.

The development of bones and muscles is influenced by use. Thus, in infants and toddlers, the legs straighten and lengthen with the stimulus of weight bearing and independent walking. The infant is born with the full complement of muscle fibers. Growth in muscle length results from lengthening of the fibers, and growth in bulk comes from hypertrophy. Length of muscles is related to growth in length of the underlying bone. If a limb is not used, it grows minimally. Furthermore, if the use is abnormal, such as in spastic diplegia, the forces for development tend to stimulate growth in abnormal patterns. Thus, scoliosis can develop or bowlegs may increase in severity. Muscle contractures occur if muscles are not used regularly through their full range of motion. The growth of fibrous tissue, tendons, and ligaments is also dependent on mechanical demands.

PATHOPHYSIOLOGY AND DEFENSE MECHANISMS

Pathophysiology

Muscles and bones can be affected by localized or systemic problems. Thus, the presenting orthopedic problem can be symptomatic of a larger problem.

SYSTEMIC PROBLEMS

Systemic problems can include chronic conditions such as hemophilia, sickle cell disease, rheumatoid diseases, neurological problems such as cerebral palsy, and various cancers in-

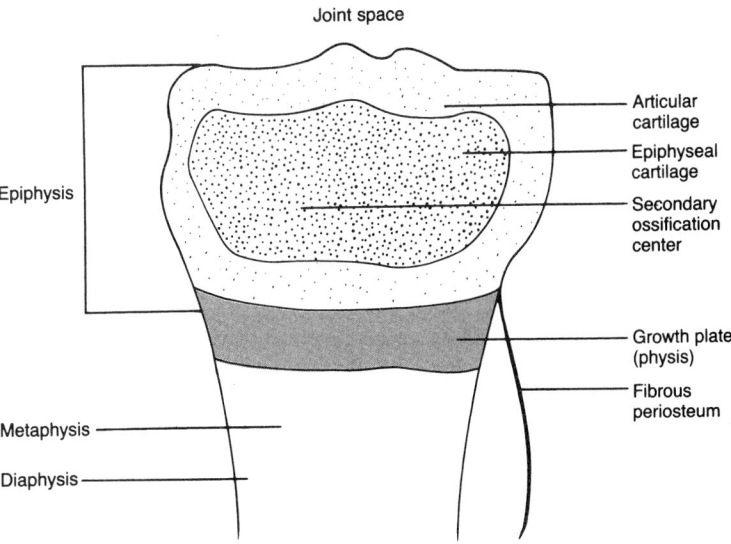

F I G U R E 38-1
Anatomy of long bones. (Modified from Shapiro F: Epiphyseal disorders. N Engl J Med 317:1702–1710, 1987.)

cluding osteosarcomas and leukemias. Children with metabolic problems such as vitamin D–resistant rickets have bony deformities. Acute systemic problems can also affect the musculoskeletal system. For example, viruses and bacteria can infect joints and bones. In developing countries, tubercular infections of bones are common and devastating. Thus, the NP must assess patients from a broad perspective, asking questions about other body systems and ordering appropriate laboratory studies that might reflect systemic problems.

GENETIC PROBLEMS

Many genetic problems have an orthopedic component. Osteogenesis imperfecta is well known. Children with Down syndrome are more likely to have hip problems. Children with Marfan syndrome have defective connective tissue, have disproportionately long limbs, and may develop scoliosis or dislocate a patella. Severe scoliosis may develop in children with neurofibromatosis. Mucopolysaccharidosis disorders and other syndromes can result in affected children having short stature.

Many orthopedic problems have a multifactorial inheritance pattern. Thus, if one child in a family has a dislocated hip or scoliosis, the risks increase for other children and offspring. The NP needs to understand the genetic disorder in order to monitor related orthopedic problems, consider the genetic implications, and provide families with appropriate genetic information or refer them for genetic counseling (see Chapter 41).

UTERINE PACKING DEFORMATIONS

The developing fetus moves its body parts frequently, and this movement influences musculoskeletal development. When the baby fills the uterine space, movements are restricted and body parts begin to assume the shape in which they are fixed. Because much of the bony structure is cartilaginous, molding occurs with relative ease. Thus, the tibia are normally bowed. Occasionally, a foot is turned awkwardly, the legs might be fixed straight up with the feet near the ears, or the neck may be tipped to one side. The outcomes are deformities in various

degrees. The longer the position is maintained, the more severe the problems are. In general, there is a tendency for bowing and late deformations to straighten. More severe deformities need to be referred to orthopedists as soon as they are found because a softer skeleton is easier to alter in a positive direction.

INJURIES

Ligamentous injuries can produce joint instability. Unstable joints should always be referred to an orthopedist. The most common injuries to muscles produce bleeding in the muscle, at the muscle-tendon junctions, or at tendon insertion points. Muscle hematomas generally heal in 3 weeks, but significant muscle bleeding can lead to scarring. Injuries sufficient to produce significant soft tissue damage also can damage the underlying bone.

Trauma to the bone can cause a fracture, dislocation of the epiphysis (an orthopedic emergency), or damage to the periosteum covering the bone, with bleeding in the space between the two tissues. The effects of fractures through the growth plates of long bones is discussed later in this chapter. Fractures that are misaligned generally have related soft tissue damage. Damage to the nerves and vascular supply must be carefully assessed. Management of traumatic injuries is discussed in Chapter 40.

The possibility of child abuse should always be considered when orthopedic injuries, especially fractures, are present. The rule of thumb is that the injury history should match the appearance of the problem and be consistent with the child's developmental capabilities. Certain injuries, such as spiral fractures of the long bones, are especially suspect, because few independent activities of the child can produce these injuries. They occur with wrenching motions such as when a child's arm or leg has been jerked. Multiple fractures in various stages of healing must be considered evidence of child abuse until proved otherwise.

Defense Mechanisms

FRACTURE HEALING

Fractures heal by the creation of a callus at the fracture site. The process is the same in children as in adults. When the fracture occurs, there is damage to the blood vessels, destruction of bone matrix, and death of bone cells adjoining the fracture site. The body reabsorbs the clot and dead cells, while the periosteum responds by producing new fibroblasts that invade the fracture site. Immature bone is formed with irregular trabeculae, creating the callus. Normal stresses then cause the bone to remodel into the optimal shape, and the callus bone is gradually replaced by lamellar bone.

Growth Plate Fractures

Fractures of the long bones can produce permanent deformities in children if the fracture occurs through the growth plate. The outcomes depend on the fracture location and type, the age of the child, the status of the blood supply to the physis, and the treatment. Epiphyseal fractures have been classified by Salter and Harris into five types (Fig. 38–2). The number is a guide to the frequency of that type of fracture as well as an indicator of the prognosis for further epiphyseal growth. Thus, type I is the most frequent type of epiphyseal injury and has a good prognosis; type V is the

rarest type of epiphyseal fracture and has the worst prognosis because it results in premature closure of the growth plate.

Fracture types I and II occur when there is a shearing force applied to the epiphysis and metaphysis. For both types, part of the perichondrium is preserved, and the blood supply to the growth plate is maintained. With no disruption to the growth plate, there will be no permanent, worsening deformity as the child grows. Type I and II fractures do not require perfect anatomical alignment to heal with a good functional prognosis. Closed reduction is generally the treatment for type I and II fractures; a type II fracture of the distal femur, however, requires anatomical alignment by either open or closed reduction.

Types III and IV are more serious fractures that must be promptly realigned, usually with open reduction, to prevent growth arrest. The prognosis for types III and IV is fair and depends on the severity of the injury and the accuracy in achieving anatomical alignment through open reduction. Growth arrest and progressive deformities can result from these fractures.

Type V fractures are rare but have serious

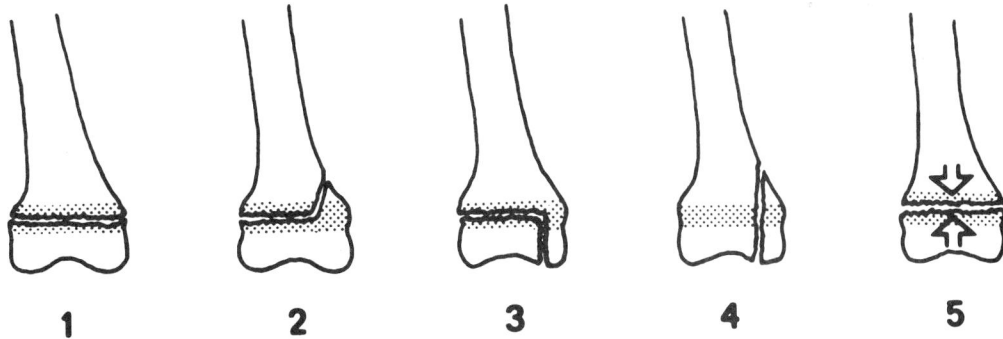

1   2   3   4   5

F I G U R E 38-2
Salter fracture types. Salter-Harris classification of epiphyseal fractures. Type I: The epiphysis separates from the metaphysis. The germinal cells remain with the epiphysis, usually uninjured. Healing is rapid and growth is seldom arrested. Type II: Similar to type I, except that a small piece of metaphysis breaks free to remain with the epiphysis. Healing is rapid, and growth is usually normal. Types I and II are the most common. Type III: Separation passes a variable distance along the growth plate and then enters the joint. Accurate reduction of the intra-articular fracture is necessary to prevent lateral traumatic arthritis. Open reduction may be needed. Growth disturbances are not usually a problem. Type IV: The fracture extends from the joint across the growth plate and into the metaphysis. This usually requires open reduction to prevent unilateral growth arrest and traumatic arthritis from malposition. Type V: This is a crushing injury that leads to death of the germinal cells of the epiphyseal cartilage and arrest of growth. This type is rare. (From Behrman R [ed]: Nelson Textbook of Pediatrics, 14th ed. Philadelphia, WB Saunders, 1992.)

effects when they occur. This fracture results from a crush injury to the physis, often from a fall from a height, and the growth plate cells are crushed. No further growth occurs at that growth plate unless the epiphyseal blood supply was preserved. Sometimes this fracture is missed on radiographic study because no fracture line can be discerned (Behrman & Kliegman, 1998; Staheli, 1998).

Shaft Fractures

There is a tendency for the long bones to remold into the most normal position possible when they are fractured in places along the shaft. Young children may not fracture bones all the way across (the greenstick fracture). As with adults, young children can experience complete fractures or stress fractures.

◼◼◼ ASSESSMENT OF THE ORTHOPEDIC SYSTEM

See Table 38-1 for orthopedic terminology.

History

1. History of present illness
   - Onset: appearance of first symptoms; insidious or sudden; association with injury or strain; accompanied by any constitutional symptoms or sign (e.g., fever, malaise, ecchymosis)
   - Pain: location and character, course of radiation, severity, extent of disability produced, effect of various activities including weight bearing, relief measures, changes from day to night or from day to day, child's refusing to move the painful part or assuming a pain-relieving position, effects of previous treatment, presence of pain or discomfort in other parts of the body
   - Deformity: character (swelling, inflammation, contracture, stiffness, appearance); first appearance and who noted it; association with injury or disease; rate of change; extent of disability; a cosmetic problem or a cause of embarrassment
   - Injury: how, when (time and date), why,

and where; mechanism or manner in which injury was produced
   - Altered function: weakness, limp, decreased range of motion
2. Family history
   - Any family members with musculoskeletal problems; many orthopedic problems have a genetic component
3. Past medical history
   - Pregnancy history and birth history: breech delivery, shoulder presentation, multiple births
   - Development history: milestones met at appropriate age such as first walking and sitting
4. Review of systems
   - Any infections, constitutional diseases, or congenital problems that might have an orthopedic component

Physical Examination

Special orthopedic examination techniques are described in the following paragraphs.

RANGE-OF-MOTION EXAMINATION

Passive range of motion, in which the examiner moves the joint, provides information about joint mobility and stability. It can also provide information about the limits of tendons and muscles that are contracted. It is necessary to find the bony limits of movement. An excessive range of motion can indicate an unstable joint. Active range of motion, in which the child moves the joint, provides information about both muscle and bony structures working together for functional movement. To assess such problems as developmental dysplasia of the hip, passive range of motion must be used. Note pain, stiffness, limitations or deviations, and rigidity. The normal values of joint motion are age related, which must be kept in mind (e.g., external hip rotation is greatest in early infancy).

GAIT EXAMINATION

Observe the child walking without shoes and with only minimal covering. Inspect from the front, side, and back as the child walks nor-

T A B L E 38-1

Orthopedic Terminology

TERM	DEFINITION	TERM	DEFINITION
DESCRIPTIVE TERMS FOR POSITIONS		**DESCRIPTIVE POSITIONS FOR PARTS OF LONG BONE**	
Abduction	Movement away from midline.	Apophysis	Insertion point of tendon on long bone.
Adduction	Movement toward midline.	Diaphysis	Shaft or middle part of long bone.
Dorsiflexion	Movement of toes/foot or fingers/hand toward dorsal surface (up).	Epiphysis	Distal side of growth plate, a secondary ossification center separated from parent bone.
Eversion	Same as pronation. Palmar surface turned away from midline.	Metaphysis	Proximal side of growth plate, on edge of parent bone.
External rotation	Turning anterior surface of limb outward or away from midline.	Perichondrium	Membrane of fibrous connective tissue surrounding cartilage.
Internal rotation	Turning anterior surface of limb inward or toward midline.	Physis	Growth plate.
Inversion	Same as supination. Palmar surface turned toward midline.	**DESCRIPTIVE TERMS FOR FEET**	
Luxation	Dislocation.	Calcaneus	Ankle fixed in position of dorsiflexion (foot up).
Plantarflexion	Movement of toes/foot or fingers/hand toward plantar surface (down or toes pointed).	Malleolus	Medial or lateral bony prominence of ankle.
		Pes cavus	Foot with a high arch.
		Pes planus	Flatfoot.
Pronation	Palmar surface turned downward or toward posterior surface of body.	Pronation	Foot where center of weight lies over medial side of foot rather than being centered—foot sags toward center. Often associated with flatfoot.
Subluxation	Partial dislocation.		
Supination	Palmar surface turned upward or toward anterior surface of body.		
Valgus	Deviation away from midline, a >< shape of the two legs, for instance.	Talipes equinovarus	Clubfoot.
Varus	Deviation toward midline, a <> shape of the two legs, for instance.		

mally, on his or her toes, and then on heels. The gait should be smooth, rhythmic, and efficient. The gait cycle includes the heel-strike, foot-flat, toe-off, and swing phases. Ankle, knee, and hip movements should be symmetrical and full with little side-to-side movement of the trunk.

The smaller child has a faster gait than the larger child, but less distance is covered with each stride. This is related to the smaller child's poorer balance. With a short, quick stride, each

leg is off the ground for less time. The feet are spread wider and, in the toddler, the arms may be held up to increase balance. The mature pattern develops by about age 3 years.

Antalgic gaits (gaits to avoid pain) serve to reduce stress or pain at the affected area. For example, the toe-off phase is restricted if the toe is sore. A Trendelenburg gait indicates hip disease and might or might not be painful, because it also involves muscle weakness around the hip joint.

POSTURE

To assess posture adequately, the child should be undressed to his or her underwear. The examiner needs to look at the child from the front, side, and back.

1. Pelvis and hips should be level. Place hands on the iliac crest to test for a pelvic tilt caused by limb length discrepancy.
2. Legs should be symmetrical in shape and size. The patellae should be straight ahead.
3. The feet should point straight ahead, with an imaginary line from the center of the heel through the second toe. There should be an arch (except in babies, in whom a fat pad obscures the arch) and straight heel cords.
4. The spine should be straight, and the back should look symmetrical, with shoulder and scapula heights and waist angles equal. There should be slight lordotic curves at the cervical and lumbar areas.

▓▓▓▓ SPECIAL EXAMINATIONS

Hip Examinations

GALEAZZI MANEUVER

The Galeazzi maneuver includes flexing the hips and knees while the infant or child lies supine, placing the soles of the feet on the table near the buttocks, and then looking at the knee heights for equality (Fig. 38-3). The Galeazzi sign is positive if the knee heights are unequal.

BARLOW MANEUVER

Barlow maneuver dislocates a dislocatable hip posteriorly. The hip is flexed, and the thigh is brought into an adducted position. From that position, the femoral head drops out of the acetabulum or can be gently pushed out of the socket. The dislocation should be palpable as it occurs. The maneuver needs to be done gently in a noncrying neonate in order to keep from damaging the femoral head. The hips should be examined one at a time.

ORTOLANI MANEUVER

Ortolani maneuver can be done after Barlow maneuver or separately. The Ortolani maneuver reduces a posteriorly dislocated hip. Again, it is not done forcefully. The hip is flexed 90 degrees and then abducted while pushing up with the fingers located over the trochanter posteriorly. A clunk and a palpable jerk are obtained as the femur is relocated. A mild clicking sound is not a positive Ortolani sign. These are common and normal sounds that are fine, of short duration, and high pitched. Of note, the hip may be dislocated easily only during the first month or two of life. The examiner should not still be charting "no hip click" on examinations at 6 months of age. Dislocation can occur late in infancy. However, if this occurs, the NP will note limited abduction on the side of the dislocation (Fig. 38-4).

TRENDELENBURG SIGN

The Trendelenburg sign is elicited by having the child stand and then raise one leg off the ground. If the pelvis drops on the raised leg side, the sign is positive and indicates weak hip abductor muscles on the side that is bearing the weight. Normally, the muscles around a stable hip are strong enough to maintain a level pelvis if one leg is raised (see Fig. 38-3).

MEDIAL ROTATION (INTERNAL ROTATION)

The child is placed prone, and the knees are flexed 90 degrees. Medial rotation is measured as the legs are allowed to fall apart as far as possible, using gravity alone or with light pressure. The angle between vertical (0 degree) and the leg position is the medial rotation. It is measured for each leg (Fig. 38-5). Asymmetrical hip rotation is abnormal.

LATERAL ROTATION (EXTERNAL ROTATION)

Lateral rotation is measured by allowing the legs to cross while the child is still prone. The angle between vertical and the leg position is

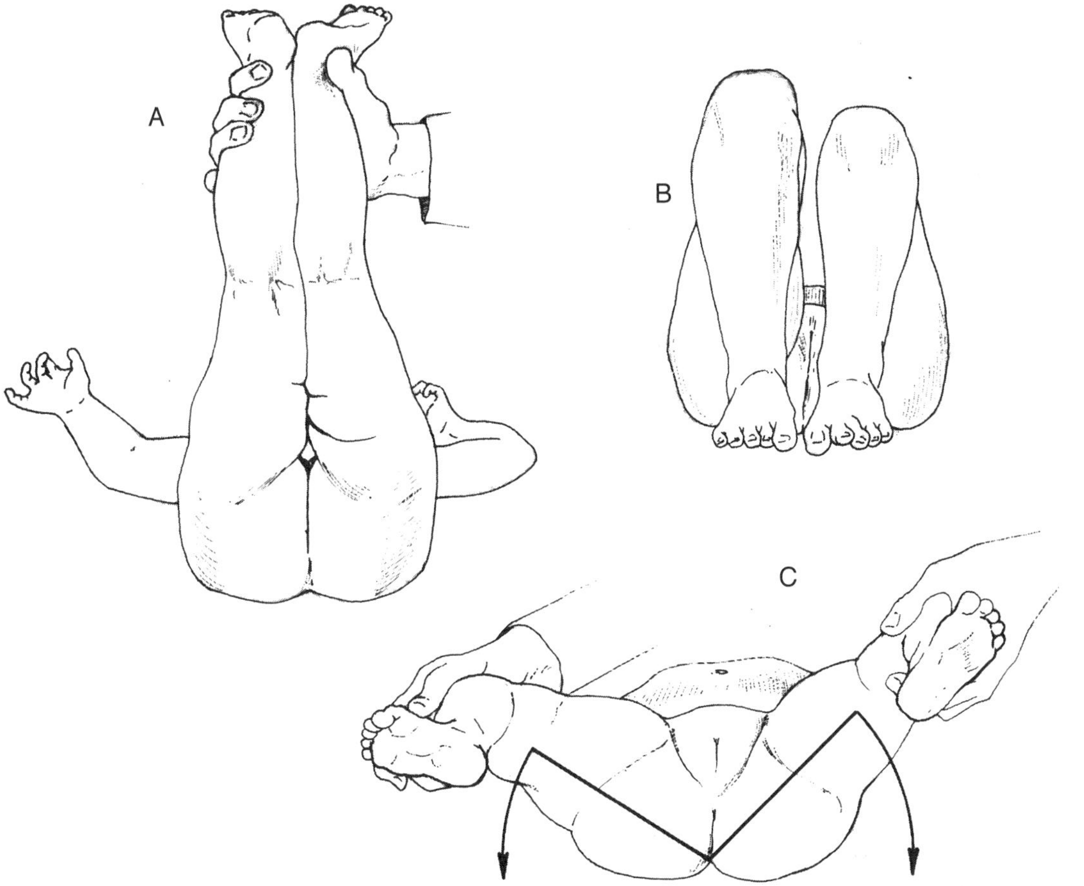

A

B

C

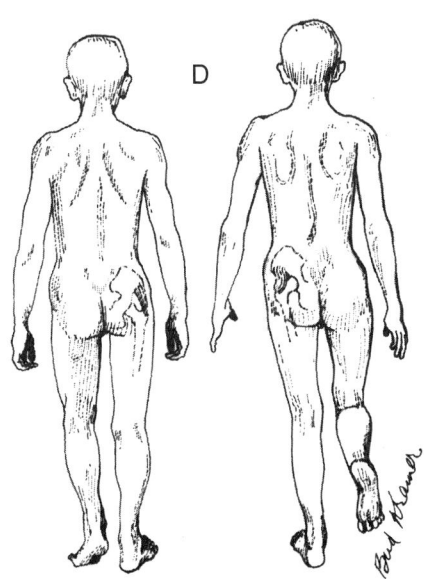

D

F I G U R E 38-3

Physical findings in congenital hip dislocation. *A,* Thigh fold asymmetry is often present in infants with unilateral hip dislocation. An extra fold can be seen on the abnormal side. The finding is not diagnostic, however. It may be found in normal infants and may be absent in children with hip dislocation or dislocatability. *B,* Leg length inequality is a sign of unilateral hip dislocation (Galeazzi sign). It is not reliable in children with dislocatable but not dislocated hips or in children with bilateral dislocation. *C,* Limitation of hip abduction is often present in older infants with hip dislocation. Abduction of greater than 60 degrees is usually possible in infants. Restriction or asymmetry indicates the need for careful radiologic examination. *D,* Trendelenburg sign. In single-leg stance, the abductor muscles of the normal hip support the pelvis. Dislocation of the hip functionally shortens and weakens these muscles. When the child attempts to stand on the dislocated hip, the opposite side of the pelvis drops. When bilateral dislocation is present, a wide-based Trendelenburg limp will result. (From Scoles P: Pediatric Orthopedics in Clinical Practice, 2nd ed. St. Louis, Mosby–Year Book, 1988.)

ABDUCTION TEST

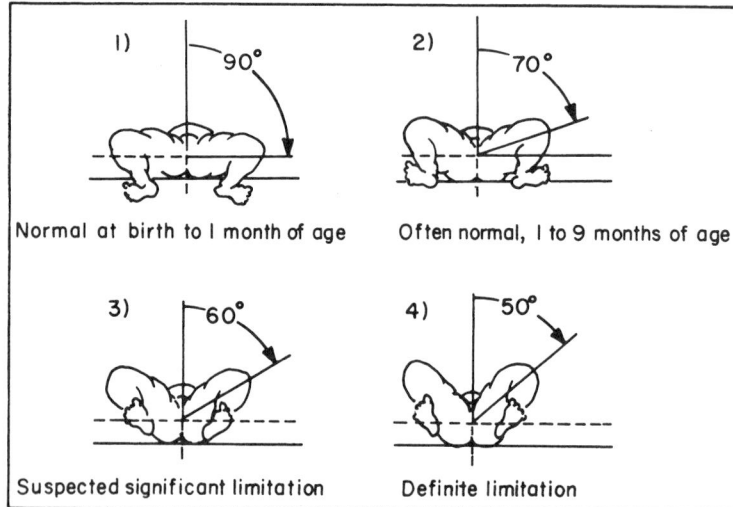

1) 90°
Normal at birth to 1 month of age

2) 70°
Often normal, 1 to 9 months of age

3) 60°
Suspected significant limitation

4) 50°
Definite limitation

F I G U R E 38-4
Hip abduction test. The child is placed supine, the hips are flexed 90 degrees, and fully abducted. Although the normal abduction range is quite broad, one can suspect hip disease in any patient who lacks more than 35 to 45 degrees of abduction. (From Chung SMK: Hip Disorders in Infants and Children. Philadelphia, Lea & Febiger, 1981.)

measured for each leg (see Fig. 38–5). Again, asymmetrical hip rotation is abnormal.

Back Examination

ADAM POSITION OR THE FORWARD BENDING POSITION

This position allows for evaluation of structural scoliosis. The child bends at the waist to a position of 90 degrees back flexion with straight legs, ankles together, and arms hanging freely or with palms together but not touching the toes or floor (Fig. 38–6). The back is inspected for asymmetry of the height of the curves on the two sides. The examiner should be seated in front of the child to best visually scan each level of the spine. If a rib hump is present, a scoliometer, if available, can be used to measure the angular tilt of the trunk. Other characteristics of scoliosis to look for include unequal scapula heights, unequal waist angles, asymmetry of the elbow to flank distance, and some deviation of the spine from a straight head-to-toe line. Looking primarily at the straightness of the spine, however, can be misleading, because scoliosis involves both rotation and misalignment of the vertebrae. Adam's position accentuates the rotational deformity of scoliosis.

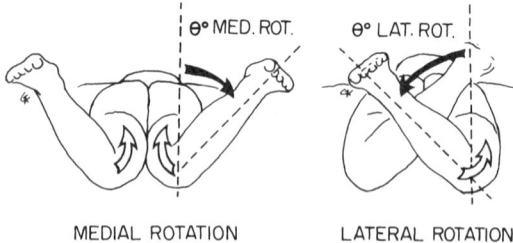

θ° MED. ROT.   θ° LAT. ROT.

MEDIAL ROTATION   LATERAL ROTATION

F I G U R E 38-5
Medial and lateral rotation measurement. With the patient lying prone and the knees flexed 90 degrees, the femurs are examined for their range of motion at the hips in extension. (From Behrman R [ed]: Nelson Textbook of Pediatrics, 14th ed. Philadelphia, WB Saunders, 1992.)

DIAGNOSTIC STUDIES

Radiographs are an important diagnostic tool for the musculoskeletal system. Views of both sides of the body or both extremities are usually ordered so that comparisons can be made. Generally, two views are needed to analyze the anatomical structures. Computed tomography (CT) scans augment radiographs to detail specific areas of the body, especially in identification of soft tissue lesions. Magnetic resonance imaging (MRI) can provide additional information such as the degree of bone demineraliza-

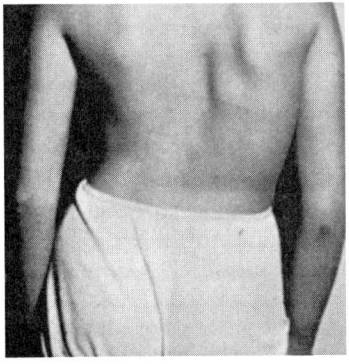

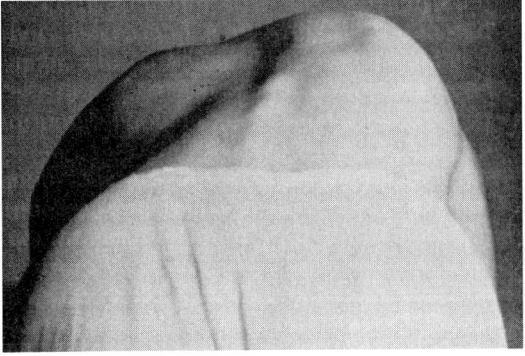

F I G U R E 38-6
Adam's position with rib hump of structural scoliosis. Lateral curvature of thoracic and lumbar segments of the spine, usually with some rotation of involved vertebral bodies. Functional scoliosis is flexible; it is apparent with standing and disappears with forward bending. It may be compensatory for other abnormalities such as leg-length discrepancy. Structural scoliosis is fixed; the curvature is visible both on standing and on bending forward. Note rib hump with forward flexion. At greatest risk are females aged 10 through adolescence. (From Delp MH, Manning RT: Major's Physical Diagnosis: An Introduction to the Clinical Process, 9th ed. Philadelphia, WB Saunders, 1981.)

tion before the tissue loss is radiographically apparent; whereas, 30 to 50% of bone density must be reduced to show a change on conventional radiography. Ultrasonography also provides information about cartilaginous areas or tissues not visible on radiograph. Bone scans (scintigraphy) demonstrate abnormal uptake earlier than conventional radiographs and are useful in detecting causes of obscure skeletal pain because this study is more sensitive than radiographs. The amount of radiation that the child is exposed to during scintigraphy is equiv-

alent to skeletal survey radiography (Staheli, 1998).

It is important to remember that false-negative imaging studies can occur in early stages of disease (e.g., osteomyelitis) or conditions (developmental hip dysplasia of the newborn). Also, in those circumstances in which a child will most likely be referred to a specialist, it may be more prudent to defer to the specialist to order imaging studies rather than expose the child to unnecessary radiation.

Various laboratory studies can indicate systemic disease, infection, or inflammation. They also can provide an understanding of muscle metabolism (e.g., lactic acid, pyruvates, carnitine).

Some bony lesions may need to be biopsied for diagnosis, and muscle tissue frequently needs to be sampled to determine specific disease pathology.

MANAGEMENT STRATEGIES

Counseling

Counseling for orthopedic problems involves several components. The family should understand and have time to ask questions about all the following issues:

- The pathology, including possible etiologies
- The treatment plan
- The prognosis with and without treatment
- Any genetic implications of the diagnosis

Counseling also helps families cope with the diagnosis and its short-term and long-term implications. Congenital problems are often identified at birth or shortly thereafter. Families need to be given the diagnosis truthfully, humanely, and as soon as possible. Issues of etiology need to be discussed to address parents' feelings of guilt for causing the problem and to discuss genetic implications if any. A plan of care that is mutually agreed on by the family and care provider must be developed before the infant is discharged from the hospital or clinic.

Exercise

All children need exercise to promote their growth and development. Even children with disabling conditions can exercise in some way. Exercise for children should be fun and perceived as play, not work. Often, physical therapists or the child's orthopedist can provide ideas for safe, therapeutic play or sports activities. At school, children with orthopedic problems should engage in physical activities that are as much a part of the regular physical education class as possible.

Anticipatory Guidance: Musculoskeletal Development

Families are sometimes concerned about problems that providers believe are within normal limits and do not require an orthopedic referral. The NP should provide the child's family with a description of the child's predicted musculoskeletal development. Timelines and markers that parents can use to monitor their child's development are particularly helpful in allowing families to understand their child's pattern of growth. Misperceptions about the implications of minor variations need to be clarified, and the family should always be given the opportunity to return for further assessment or discussion if concerns remain.

Shoes

The use of therapeutic shoes to correct orthopedic problems is controversial. Recent studies confirm that therapeutic shoes do very little to correct deformities. Shoes for the average child should keep the feet warm and protected from injury. Shoes should be selected to fit properly and comfortably with room for growth. High-top shoes for toddlers may have the advantage of staying on pudgy little feet better, but they do not provide additional support. Toddler feet do not need extra support.

Shoe modifications may be needed in certain conditions. Shoe lifts are needed if limb length differences exceed 2.5 cm. Orthotics also can be used in certain orthopedic situations to more evenly distribute pressure on the sole of the foot and facilitate function.

Care of Children in Casts

Children in casts need special attention, and their parents need instructions for care and monitoring for problems. If a plaster cast is used, the major concern is wetness—urine, feces, or environmental substances. The cast absorbs it all. Therefore, attention needs to be given to protecting the cast (including a fiberglass cast) from moisture at all times. If the cast becomes wet, a hair dryer can be used for drying small areas; for big casts, drying may affect only the surface. Good pediatric nursing texts can provide ideas for caring for infants in spica casts—the most difficult to manage. For all casts, openings should be inspected and smelled to help identify pressure sores inside the casted areas. The heel is particularly vulnerable to pressure sores.

The child's cast should be kept cool, clean, and dry. Cover the cast with plastic wrap or a plastic bag when the child bathes or is in a situation in which the cast may get wet.

A child in a cast needs to have developmental stimulation, physical contact, changes in environment, and opportunities to make choices and control his or her care within limits, just as any other child does.

Splints and Braces

Splints and braces need to be monitored for good fit and correct use. Splints are useful to provide temporary immobilization and reduce hygiene problems.

Genetics Counseling

See Chapter 41.

Physical Therapy

Physical therapists can help restore or maintain function or teach new motor skills. The physical therapist should be accustomed to dealing with children. Their work is especially important to prevent deformities, teach new motor skills, and rehabilitate injuries.

SPECIFIC ORTHOPEDIC PROBLEMS OF CHILDREN

Brachial Plexus Injuries

DESCRIPTION

Brachial plexus injuries are conditions in which innervation to the arm is disrupted, resulting in paralysis. They represent stretch or traction injuries. Superior brachial palsy (C5 and C6) affects the shoulder and arm muscles and is commonly known as Erb palsy. Inferior brachial palsy (C8, T1), or Klumpke palsy, is rare; it affects the wrist and hand. Complete brachial palsy (both superior and inferior injuries) is the most serious, resulting in a flaccid extremity, and is known as Erb-Duchenne-Klumpke palsy. Phrenic nerve palsy (C3, C4, C5) also occurs in approximately 5% of brachial plexus injuries, affecting diaphragm innervation and respirations.

ETIOLOGY

Brachial palsies generally occur through traumatic stretching of the neck and shoulder during birth, producing damage to the brachial plexus. Erb palsy accounts for 80% of the cases of brachial plexus palsy. Incidence is about 0.5 in 1000 births (Sawyer & Esterhai, 1999; Piecuch, 1998).

CLINICAL FINDINGS

History

There may be a history of a traumatic delivery, often of a large baby.

Physical Examination

Findings include the following:

- Neonate has affected limb adducted, internally rotated at the shoulder, pronated at the elbows, flexed at the wrist and fingers; however, grasp reflex is present (Erb palsy)
- Limp wrist and hand with absent grasp reflex (Klumpke palsy)
- Moro reflex absent or incomplete on affected side

Traumatic delivery causing brachial plexus injury also can cause the following associated injuries:

- Rupture of intra-abdominal structures, especially liver and spleen
- Fracture of the skull or clavicle
- Damage to the sternocleidomastoid muscle with resulting limitation of neck movement (a "sternocleidomastoid tumor" indicates the injury, which results in torticollis if prompt and vigorous physical therapy is not initiated)
- Impaired respiratory effort
- Horner syndrome (ptosis, miosis, enophthalmos, delayed pigmentation of the iris if the sympathetic fibers of C8 are injured)

Diagnostic Studies

Electromyographic studies and radiographs of the clavicle and cervical spine are ordered as indicated.

DIFFERENTIAL DIAGNOSIS

Consider dislocation, fracture of the arm or clavicle, cerebral lesions, and cervical column lesions.

MANAGEMENT

The following steps are taken:

1. Refer to an orthopedist for immobilization for the first 2 weeks, followed by physical therapy and splints to prevent contractures.
2. Physical therapy may be necessary to maintain a full range of motion.
3. Counsel the family, including explanation of the injury, its prognosis, and its management. The child should be held and cared for as any other baby.

COMPLICATIONS

Paralysis can be permanent. Contractures can occur if regular physical therapy is not started and continued for as long as the paralysis lasts. Physical findings are important to rule out concurrent injuries from traumatic delivery.

PROGNOSIS

Recovery may or may not be complete and requires time, 18 months in mild cases. Improvement is generally seen in the first few days to weeks, with 80 to 90% resolving spontaneously during the first year of life. If there has been no improvement by 2 to 3 months of age, the infant needs evaluation for nerve root avulsion and possible surgery. The prognosis for complete recovery of upper brachial plexus injury is excellent, with a more guarded prognosis for lower brachial plexus injury.

Clavicle Fracture

ETIOLOGY

In neonates, this fracture occurs during the birth process, especially in large babies. Because the clavicle is the first bone to ossify, it is the bone most frequently fractured at birth and is generally a greenstick fracture involving the middle third of the clavicle. Childhood fractures of the clavicle are related to trauma.

CLINICAL FINDINGS

History

In the neonate, assess the following:

- History of difficult delivery—large baby and shoulder dystocia
- Irritability when infant is moved or lifted
- Decreased movement of arm on affected side, including during Moro reflex

In the older child, assess the following:

- History of fall or trauma

Physical Examination

In all children, look for the following:

- Pain occurring with shoulder movement
- Decreased arm movement or absent Moro reflex
- Swelling and crepitus elicited over fracture site
- Callus felt over fracture site within a few days

- Spasm of sternocleidomastoid muscle on affected side
- An associated Erb palsy

Radiographic Studies

These are usually not necessary. Clavicle shaft fractures can be difficult to see radiographically in children but are clinically identifiable. Radiographs can be helpful in identifying a fracture near the shoulder joint.

DIFFERENTIAL DIAGNOSIS

Brachial palsy, shoulder dislocation, or other bony problem should be considered.

MANAGEMENT

Management involves the following:

1. Immobilization of the shoulder is an option. Generally, the neonate is just moved gently without undue stress to the arm and shoulder until a callus forms.
2. For the older child, sling immobilization for comfort is often sufficient.
3. A figure-eight clavicle brace is used if displacement results in a decreased shaft length. However, it is uncomfortable to wear.
4. Protection for 4 to 5 weeks is generally sufficient in that union requires about 4 weeks of healing.
5. An older child may need analgesics or nonsteroidal anti-inflammatory drug (NSAID) for pain.

PROGNOSIS

The prognosis is excellent. Often the injury in neonates is identified only at later primary care visits, when the callus lump is palpated. The child may be irritable until the fracture is stable. Parents need information and emotional support. The infant is usually asymptomatic within 7 to 10 days.

Rib Problems—Costochondritis

DESCRIPTION

Costochondral disease (costochondritis) is a benign disorder marked by pain that is localized at the costosternal or costochondral junction where the sternum, ribs, and costal cartilages connect. It is a common complaint.

ETIOLOGY

Trauma to the area and unaccustomed physical effort (lifting heavy objects or coughing) are factors known to cause costochondritis.

CLINICAL FINDINGS

History

Pain localized to the costosternal or costochondral junction is the major symptom. Characteristics of the pain include

- Acute or gradual onset
- Sharp, darting, or dull quality
- Short duration of hours or lasting days
- Occasional complaints of a feeling of tightness caused by muscle spasm
- No exacerbation of pain with respiratory or mild movements

Physical Examination

The major clinical finding on examination is localized tenderness of one or more costochrondral joints with palpation of the costal cartilage. The presence of pain, swelling with or without redness, and tenderness at the costal cartilage is referred to as Tietze syndrome.

Diagnostic Studies

No diagnostic studies are needed because history and physical findings are the key to the diagnosis.

DIFFERENTIAL DIAGNOSIS

Rib fractures are the key differential if pain is associated with an injury. Childhood rheumatic diseases also can have complaints similar to costochondritis but generally have other characteristic physical findings. Costochondritis is one of the differential diagnoses of pediatric chest pain (see Chapter 31).

MANAGEMENT

Treatment consists of the use of mild analgesia to relieve discomfort and avoidance of strenuous activity. Parents and children need to be reassured that this is a benign condition and is not related to cardiac disease (Schaller, 1996).

Back Problems

SCOLIOSIS

Description

Scoliosis is a lateral curvature of the spine. It involves significant transverse and sagittal plane rotations. There are six classifications of scoliosis:

1. Secondary
2. Congenital
3. Neuromuscular
4. Constitutional
5. Idiopathic that has an infantile (0 to 3 years), juvenile (4 years to puberty), or adolescent (puberty to maturity) presentation
6. Miscellaneous

Structural scoliosis is the general term used to indicate a true deformity of the vertebrae rather than a postural problem (secondary or functional scoliosis). Approximately 10% of the population has mild truncal asymmetry. However, curves greater than 15 degrees in children are abnormal and can progress to significant curves in the growing child (Staheli, 1998).

Etiology

The etiology of scoliosis varies by its classification. Secondary or functional scoliosis, when there is the appearance of a lateral curvature but no structural change in the vertebral column, is due to such secondary problems as leg length inequality, poor posture, or muscle spasm. Congenital scoliosis is due to bony deformity caused by failure in formation or segmentation of vertebrae during fetal development (e.g., neural tube disorders). Neuromuscular scoliosis is caused by myopathies, upper or lower neuron diseases (e.g., muscular dystrophy, cerebral palsy, and polio). Constitutional scoliosis is associated with syndromes (e.g.,

Marfan syndrome or diastrophic dwarfism). Miscellaneous scoliosis has numerous etiologies including trauma, infection, tumors, and thoracoplasty. Idiopathic is the most common type of scoliosis. Its etiology is unknown but often has a familial pattern. Females with this type of scoliosis are more likely than males to have lateral curvatures that progress. The most common type of idiopathic scoliosis is found in adolescents and is the major focus of the remaining discussion (Staheli, 1998).

Most scoliotic curves do not increase significantly after skeletal growth is complete. Double curves and more severe curves are more likely to progress during the growth years. For a given child, however, the ability to predict progression is difficult because even small curves can progress to severe deformity. Thus, regular monitoring of the curve is important.

Incidence

Idiopathic scoliosis is found in children from around the world. Small curves (<10 degrees) of the spine occur in 2 to 4% of the adolescent population, and only 0.1 to 0.3% of these adolescents progress to have significant curves (>20 degrees). The female-to-male ratio is equal but jumps to 5:1 for curves greater than 21 degrees (Bennett, 1998).

Clinical Findings

HISTORY. A painless and insidious onset is typical. Generally there is no significant history. The NP should assess:

- Family history of scoliosis
- Etiological factors related to the various causes of structural scoliosis

The presence of pain with a lateral curvature of the spine suggests an inflammatory or neoplastic lesion as the cause of the scoliosis.

PHYSICAL EXAMINATION. The predominant features in the child who is standing with weight equally on both feet, legs straight, and arms hanging loosely at the sides include the following, although the location of the curve affects the findings:

- Painless lateral curvature of the spine with greater than 10 degrees of rotation.

- The curve can have one turn ("C curve") or may include two compensating curves ("S curve").
- Lateral deviation and rotation of each vertebra is accentuated by looking at the ribs as well as the spinal column itself.
- Unequal shoulder heights.
- Congenital scoliosis may be visible in the infant lying prone; is sometimes more prominent if the infant is suspended prone.
- Unequal scapula prominences and heights. (Note that the muscle masses may be somewhat unequal, especially if the child uses one shoulder more than the other as in carrying books. Look for bony, not muscular prominence.)
- Unequal waist angles.
- Unequal rib prominences and chest asymmetry.
- Unequal rib heights when the child stands in the Adam forward bend position (see Fig. 38-6).

The physical examination should also include the following:

- Observation for equal leg lengths
- Examination of the skin for hairy patches, nevi, café au lait spots, lipomas, dimples
- Neurological examination
- Cardiac examination for Marfan syndrome

RADIOGRAPHIC STUDIES. The clinical diagnosis is always confirmed by radiograph, although some newer techniques of curve measurement are being studied. If a scoliometer is used to measure the tilt of the rib hump, readings greater than 5 degrees indicate the need for radiographs. The anteroposterior (AP) and lateral standing views are recommended with shielding; however, a single AP view is an adequate screening or baseline radiograph for referral to an orthopedist (Staheli, 1998). The radiograph identifies the degrees of curvature and is the only way to assess the status of the back accurately. In infants, the rib vertebral angle difference (RVAD) is an important measurement for orthopedists.

The radiograph is an important baseline study, in that the rate of change of the curve determines the severity of the problem and appropriate treatment. The curves of idiopathic adolescent scoliosis are classified radiographically as thoracic, double major, thoracolumbar, double thoracic, and lumbar. The Risser sign is an iliac apophysis maturation index of bone growth and is useful in determining the likelihood of curvature progression.

Differential Diagnosis

Structural scoliosis must be differentiated from functional scoliosis. The latter disappears when the child is placed in Adam's position, whereas the former is enhanced in this position. Persistent functional scoliosis to one side in a child with a neuromotor problem can eventually become structural and must be managed with physical therapy or other means to prevent progression.

Consider systemic problems such as neurofibromatosis, cerebral palsy, multiple sclerosis, Rett syndrome, rickets, tuberculosis, and tumor.

Management

The goal of treatment is to prevent increasing deformity, not full correction of the deformity.

1. Refer to an orthopedic surgeon. Because most treatment relies on growth to assist in correcting the problem, referrals need to be made as early as possible. Most curves require only observation; however, bracing and surgical correction of large curves may be necessary.
2. For congenital scoliosis, constitutional, neuromuscular, or miscellaneous scoliosis, treatment depends on the etiology and severity of the curve and the rate of its progression. Bracing may be tried, is controversial, and is generally not effective. Bracing may help to reduce compensatory curves in congenital scoliosis. Rapidly increasing curves need early operative treatment (e.g., spinal fusion and instrumentation) (Bennett, 1998; Staheli, 1998). Supervision needs to be maintained until growth is complete. Exercises are not helpful.
3. For idiopathic scoliosis, treatment varies depending on age at presentation. Infantile sco-

liosis often involves a left thoracic curvature in males and resolves spontaneously in 90% of children. Nonresolving and progressive infantile curves are treated with bracing. Juvenile scoliosis is more likely seen in females, is generally progressive, and commonly is a right thoracic curvature that requires treatment with bracing. Adolescent scoliosis has a 3:2 female to male ratio and can resolve, remain static, or increase. Mild curves need observation and reassurance only; curves greater than 25 degrees need brace management (e.g., Milwaukee brace) and observation; curves greater than 45 degrees or curves expected to progress to that range in children who are not candidates for bracing need surgical intervention—instrumentation and fusion. Bracing and casting after surgery may be necessary (Staheli, 1998).
4. Monitoring, treatment, or both, until growth is complete is necessary.
5. Support must be given to the child and family through the diagnostic and treatment phases, considering school and peer factors. Assist the child with psychological adjustment issues that arise if casting, bracing, or surgery is recommended and instituted. Some specific concerns of the child can include self-esteem problems, managing hostility and anger, learning about the disease and its care, wondering about the long-term prognosis, and concerns about clothing and participation in sports and other activities.

Parents often worry about the long-term prognosis and finances to cover care, experience guilt for possibly causing the problem (if it is thought to be genetic) or not identifying the problem earlier, and feel concern about the possible pain and treatment that the child will experience.

Complications

Progressive scoliosis can result in a severe deformity of the spinal column. Severe deformities can result in impairment of respiratory and cardiovascular function as well as limitation of physical activities and decreased comfort. The psychological consequences of an untreated scoliosis deformity can be severe.

Prevention

Prevention is not possible; however, early identification of children with scoliosis can help them avoid more expensive, invasive care and prevent the long-term consequences of the disorder. School screening clinics, recommended by the American Academy of Orthopedic Surgeons and the Scoliosis Research Society, have been instituted in many parts of the country to help identify affected children as early as possible. Several studies conducted in the 1960s and 1970s demonstrated that, when children had been screened at school, a trend toward fewer curves requiring surgery and an overall decrease in the magnitude of curves being treated were seen. Screening is effective, however, only if identified children are referred for care. Their parents must be notified, a referral arranged, and follow-up ensured.

KYPHOSIS

Description

Kyphosis is an AP curve of the thoracic spine with the apex posterior (i.e., the back is prominent). The most common clinical type of kyphosis is usually postural (postural round back). Scheuermann disease is a common pathological form of kyphosis that is a familial osteochondrosis and involves wedging of multiple thoracic vertebrae. Kyphosis in children can be secondary to congenital deformity, tumor, trauma, infection, or such problems as achondroplasia. A radiograph can be useful to identify nonpostural causes. The radiograph shows narrowed disk space, loss of normal anterior height of the involved vertebrae, and other findings.

Management

Postural kyphosis needs to be managed by referral to a physical therapist. Activities such as dancing or swimming, which require a full range of motion of the shoulders, back, and arms, can be helpful. If the problem is structural and not functional, a referral to an orthopedic surgeon is warranted. If pain is a problem, immobilization of the back in a brace or fiberglass jacket for several weeks is an option. For mild curves, observation and bracing are the usual options. For severe and congenital kyphosis (>65 degree curves), surgery with instrumentation and fusion is the appropriate management strategy (Bennett, 1998; Staheli, 1998).

LUMBAR LORDOSIS

Description

Lumbar lordosis or hyperlordosis is an AP curve of the lumbar area of the spine (i.e., the child stands with the abdomen and buttock protuberant). It sometimes occurs with kyphosis. Lordosis can be a secondary result of a hip problem in which full extension is limited by hip flexion contractures or from lumbosacral deformities. Physiological lordosis is commonly seen in families, certain racial groups, and just before onset of puberty. Physiological lordosis is not a fixed deformity.

Management

If the NP suspects lumbar lordosis, have the child bend forward. If the lumbar spine flattens and the lordosis disappears in the forward bending position, it indicates that the spine is flexible and the lordosis is only physiological. This child should be seen for follow-up in 6 to 12 months. If the lordosis persists in the forward bending position, this indicates a fixed structural deformity and needs referral to an orthopedist. Lordosis resulting from hip flexion contractures is absent while sitting and commonly seen in children with cerebral palsy, spina bifida, and developmental dysplasia of the hip.

Hip Problems

DEVELOPMENTAL DYSPLASIA OF THE HIP

Description

Developmental dysplasia of the hip (DDH), formerly congenital dislocated hip, is the term used to describe a variety of disorders resulting in abnormal development of the hip joint. These disorders include partial subluxation or complete dislocation of the femoral head out of the pelvic acetabulum and failure of the hip to deepen. The disorder may have occurred congenitally or developed in infancy or childhood.

Etiology

The etiology of DDH is multifactorial, with mechanical, environmental, and physiological factors and a genetic predisposition for the condition. Physiological factors include the hormonal effect of maternal estrogen and relaxin on joint laxity that can contribute to DDH in the neonatal period. Mechanical factors include uterine packing stresses (e.g., breech position), especially during the last trimester if the fetal pelvis becomes locked in the maternal pelvis. Sometimes the condition is found at birth, but frequently the actual dislocation occurs postnatally, even after some months. In cultures that swaddle infants in an extended position or place them on cradleboards, the incidence of DDH is greater than normal because of such neonatal positioning.

The mechanism for dislocation is considered to be related to distention of the joint capsule, which allows the femoral head to disengage from the acetabulum. If the head is relocated soon after birth, the soft tissues tighten around the joint within a few weeks.

The hip can dislocate noncongenitally in children with neurological disorders that affect the use of the lower extremities, such as cerebral palsy or myelomeningocele. Dislocation results from the abnormal use of the extremity over time.

Incidence

The incidence of DDH is estimated to be 10 per 1000 live births with a 6:1 ratio of females to males. It is found more commonly with breech births. A positive family history increases risk 10-fold. Other risk factors seen in infants that are associated with DDH include torticollis (10 to 20% association) as well as foot and knee deformities (Bennett, 1998; Staheli, 1998).

Clinical Findings

HISTORY. The history may include a positive family history, associated neck, knee, and foot

deformities noted at or shortly after birth, and breech delivery.

PHYSICAL EXAMINATION. Findings include the following:

- Limited abduction of the affected hip. Normal abduction with comfort is 70 to 80 degrees bilaterally. Limited abduction includes those cases with less than 60 degrees abduction or unequal abduction from one side to the other (see Fig. 38-4).
- Asymmetry of inguinal or gluteal folds (thigh-fold asymmetry is not related to the disorder [see Fig. 38-3]).
- Unequal leg lengths, shorter on the affected side.
- Unequal knee heights (Galeazzi sign [see Fig. 38-3]).
- Positive Ortolani or Barlow sign, or both, in infants up to 2 to 3 months of age. After this time, limited abduction and shortening of the thigh become well established and must be relied on as the primary sign in the older infant (see Fig. 38-4).

In the ambulatory child, the following might also be noted:

- Short leg with toe-walking on the affected side
- Positive Trendelenburg sign (see Fig. 38-3)
- Marked lordosis
- Limping or waddling gait

If the hips are dislocated bilaterally, asymmetries are not observed. Limited abduction is the primary indicator in this situation (see Fig. 38-4). Also, in the subluxed hip (not frankly dislocated), limited abduction again is the primary indicator that there is hip dysplasia.

RADIOGRAPHIC STUDIES. Radiological evaluation of the newborn to detect DDH is unreliable, because so much of the hip joint is cartilaginous in young infants. Also, the dislocation may be so recent that pathological changes in addition to the loose capsule may not yet have developed. Ultrasound study provides useful information, especially in neonates with suspicious findings or when hip risk factors are present. If an infant's hip is unstable by examination, the diagnosis is made. By 2 to 3 months of age, radiography is reliable. A single AP view is adequate.

Differential Diagnosis

The condition is relatively unique.

Management

The goal of management is to restore the articulation of the femur within the acetabulum.

1. Refer to an orthopedist promptly while the infant is still in the newborn nursery, if possible. Any child with subluxed, dislocatable, and dislocated hips needs to be referred. The earlier treatment is begun, the better the prognosis is for functional development of the acetabulum. A Pavlik harness is fitted to hold the hip in flexion and abduction until stable, permitting flexion motion. If the harness fails or diagnosis is delayed past about 6 months of age, traction or open reduction is necessary to bring the femoral head into place. A femoral and pelvic osteotomy is the treatment of choice in children 18 months of age or older with DDH. Surgery is done to bring the acetabulum down over the femoral head when the possibility of further positive development of the joint ceases.
2. Triple diapering is not helpful, because the musculoskeletal forces far outweigh the force that can be exerted by the diaper material.
3. Continue long-term monitoring of hip development if neonatal hip instability was noted at birth. About 0.5 to 1% of infants are noted to have hip instability at birth, vs. the 1% of infants with classic DDH. The majority of neonatal hip instability resolves spontaneously. Close observation of these children is recommended, and some providers treat even instability (no DDH findings) with a Pavlik harness (Staheli, 1998).
4. The child with a Pavlik harness should be seen weekly to ensure that it fits properly. It is worn until a normal pelvic radiograph is obtained.
5. Support the child and family through the treatment phases. Explain management goals clearly. Caring for a child in a Pavlik harness or spica cast requires special knowledge. Cast care, skin care, and car safety when the child cannot easily be placed in a car seat are all issues to be addressed. (One way to provide for child safety restraints is to cut out the sides of the car seat to accommodate the frog position.) Also see Chapter 10 for reference to safety restraints for children with special conditions. Furthermore, the child needs special attention to maintain developmental stimulation while immobilized. For Pavlik harness instructions for families, see Speers and Speers (1992).

Complications

The long-term outcomes depend on the age at diagnosis, the severity of the joint deformity, and the effectiveness of therapy. Untreated cases may result in a permanent dislocation of the femoral head so that it lies just under the iliac crest posteriorly. Clinically, the child has limited mobility of this artificial joint and related short leg. Forceful reduction can result in avascular necrosis of the femoral head with permanent hip deformity. Redislocation or persistent dysplasia can occur. Adult degenerative arthritis is associated with acetabular dysplasia.

Prevention

The condition cannot be prevented, but early identification resulting in early treatment significantly reduces the long-term consequences of the problem. Screening of all neonates and infants should include full hip abduction, examination for unequal folds and unequal leg lengths, and Barlow, Ortolani, and Galeazzi maneuvers at every examination. The hip can dislocate at any point in early development, even up to the point of first ambulation. In older children, limited abduction, gait, and standing position, including the Trendelenburg position, add important information. Charting should always include notation about hip findings because these can change at subsequent visits.

LEGG-PERTHES (OR LEGG-CALVÉ-PERTHES) DISEASE

Description

Legg-Calvé-Perthes (LCP) disease is idiopathic, juvenile avascular necrosis of the femoral head.

Etiology

There is an initial ischemic episode of unknown etiology interrupting vascular circulation to the capital femoral epiphysis. A familial predisposition is reported (Dyment, 1999). The articular cartilage hypertrophies, and the epiphyseal marrow becomes necrotic. The area revascularizes, and the necrotic bone is replaced by new bone. There is a critical point in these dual processes when the subchondral area becomes weak enough that fracture of the epiphysis occurs. At this time, the child becomes symptomatic. With fracturing, further reabsorption and replacement by fibrous bone occurs, and the shape of the femoral head is altered. Articulation of the head in the hip joint is interrupted. The bone reossifies with or without treatment, but the femoral head flattens and enlarges, causing joint deformity (Warren, 1998b; Staheli, 1998).

Incidence

The disorder occurs primarily in boys in a ratio of boys to girls of 4 to 5:1, most commonly between the ages of 4 and 8 years. It occurs bilaterally in approximately 10 to 12% of cases. A familial tendency may be a predisposing factor. Approximately 10% of children with LCP have a history of breech delivery, low birth weight, or abnormal birth presentations; 17% have a history of preceding trauma. LCP in girls tends to be a more serious problem with a poor prognosis (Warren, 1998b; Staheli, 1998).

Clinical Findings

HISTORY. There can be an acute or chronic onset with or without a history of trauma to the hip such as jumping from a high place.

Acute Onset
- Sudden onset of pain in the groin or knee often presenting at night with pain on weight bearing or stiffness
- May have little restriction in motion of the hip

Chronic
- Recurring pain (mild or aching) at the hip or referred to the knee, anterior thigh, or groin for days to weeks and limp

- Insidious limping generally in the morning and after activities
- Stiffness in the morning or after rest

PHYSICAL EXAMINATION. Findings may include

- Antalgic gait (usually the first sign) with a component of shortening and positive Trendelenburg sign
- Muscle spasm
- Decreased abduction, internal rotation, and extension of the hip
- Pain on rolling the leg internally
- Short stature if bone age is delayed

RADIOGRAPHIC STUDIES. AP and frog-leg lateral views of the pelvis are used. Alterations in the roundness of the epiphysis, subluxation, and other features as well as changes in the epiphysis margin are discerned by the orthopedist and radiologist (Fig. 38–7). However, there may be no radiographic findings early in the disease. Bone scans and MRI are helpful in recognizing early disease but are of limited value in assessing the extent of involvement or following disease progression.

Differential Diagnosis

Sepsis, dislocation, sickle cell disease, toxic synovitis, and slipped capital femoral epiphysis are other hip problems that may occur with similar features. Generally, slipped capital femoral epiphysis occurs in obese preadolescent and adolescent boys.

Management

The following steps are taken:

1. Refer to an orthopedist immediately and ensure access to care for the child and family. Initial bed rest and possible femoral abduction traction may be used to reduce hip irritability (1 to 2 weeks). Physical therapy may then be needed to reduce residual stiffness. The orthopedist works to prevent extrusion and collapse of the femoral head and attain or maintain a round shape using nonoperative or operative procedures, or both. Containment of the femoral head within the acetabulum is important. Milder cases of LCP may just require monitoring.

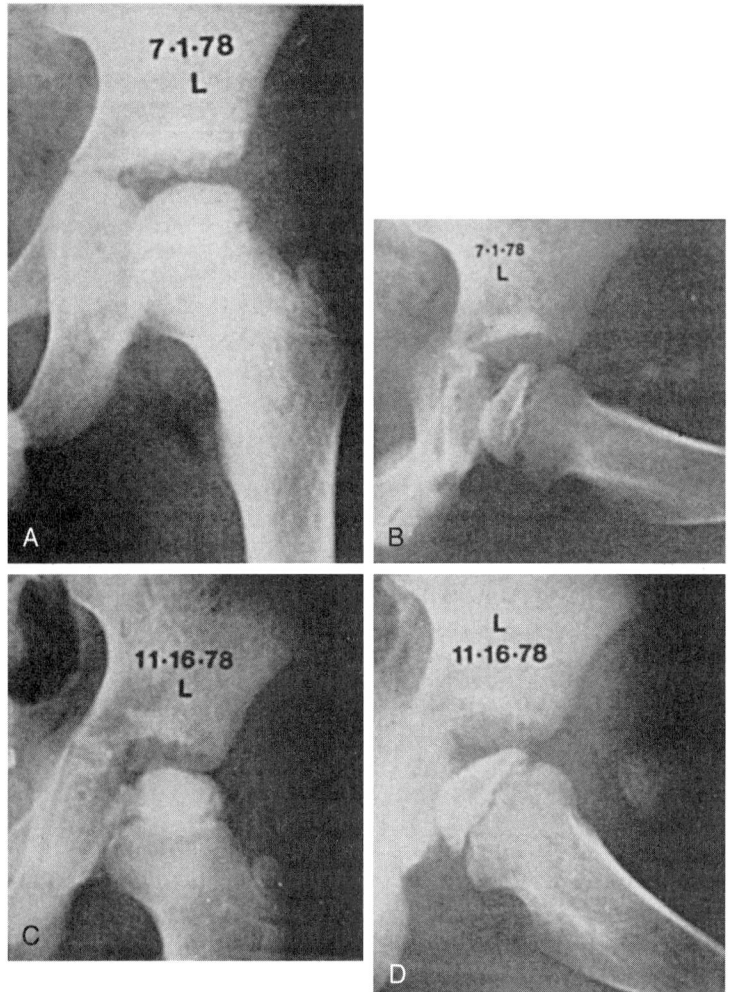

FIGURE 38-7
Radiologic evolution of Legg-Calvé-Perthes disease. *A,* Anteroposterior view of left hip in a 7-year-old boy with hip pain of 4 weeks duration. No abnormality is obvious. *B,* Frog-leg lateral view demonstrates area of microfracture and compaction of the anterolateral portion of the secondary ossification center of the proximal femur. Treatment with an abduction brace was started. *C,* Four months later, increased radiodensity is noted in the infarcted segment. *D,* Slight collapse of the infarcted area has occurred but no further extension into the remainder of the epiphysis has taken place.

For moderate to severe cases, bracing and surgical intervention are the treatment options. Bracing is continued for 12 to 16 months. Operative treatment is generally used in older children, for those who are not satisfactory candidates for bracing, or for those with extensive necrosis of the femoral head.

2. Educate the family regarding the condition and its management and the risk for development of the condition on the other side.

3. Support and monitor the child throughout treatment and recovery, including during interruption of school or other activities. The management of LCP often involves several years of treatment and monitoring.

Complications

Osteoarthritis related to femoral head deformity and decreased use of the hip joint may occur, depending on the femoral head remodeling status. Older children have a poorer prognosis owing to the decreased opportunity for femoral head remodeling in the remaining growth period (Staheli, 1998).

Prevention

The condition is not preventable, but early identification and treatment reduce the long-term complications of the disorder such as premature degenerative arthritis in early adult life.

SLIPPED CAPITAL FEMORAL EPIPHYSIS

Description

Slipped capital femoral epiphysis (SCFE) is a condition in which the upper femoral epiphysis gradually slips from its functional position in the hip joint, and the femoral neck assumes a more varus angle. During the process, the physis of the femur (the growth plate area) becomes less competent, resulting in a weakening of the perichondrial ring. This weakening allows the epiphysis to slip posteriorly and distally. Because the blood supply to the epiphysis crosses the weakened area, the epiphysis is at risk for avascular necrosis. The condition resolves when the growth plate closes with whatever position the epiphysis has taken in relation to the femoral shaft.

Etiology and Incidence

The etiology is unknown and thought to be multifactorial. Possible causes include mechanical susceptibility or vulnerability of the hip, endocrinopathies (e.g., hypothyroidism, hypopituitarism, hypogonadism, and chronic renal failure), trauma resulting from repetitive shear stress (for a minority of cases), inflammatory changes, and familial association (Warren, 1998c). Obesity increases the shear forces across the femoral head and growth plate.

Genetic, racial, and geographical factors are associated with the incidence of SCFE. The problem occurs more commonly in males in a male to female ratio of 2 to 3:1, especially those who are skeletally immature and obese. Affected males are generally between 10 and 12 years of age and females are between 11 and 12 years of age (before menarche), but the condition can occur anywhere from 9 to 15 years of age. African-American males and females have a higher incidence, and about 5% have a positive family history. Bilateral involve-

ment occurs in 20 to 25% of cases. The majority of children are above the 90th percentile for weight (Warren, 1998c).

Clinical Findings

The findings are similar to those of younger children with Legg-Perthes disease.

HISTORY. The following may be reported:

- Acute (symptoms within 3 weeks) or chronic (>3 weeks) hip or knee pain
- Sometimes a history of mild trauma to the hip area

PHYSICAL FINDINGS. Findings include

- Pain in the groin or diffusely over the knee or anterior thigh
- Pain and limited range of motion when the leg is rolled internally
- Antalgic limp with short leg component
- External rotation of the leg when walking
- External rotation of the thigh when the hip is flexed
- Thigh atrophy
- Limited abduction and extension

RADIOGRAPHIC STUDIES. AP and frog-leg lateral views of the pelvis are obtained. Radiographic findings include flattening of the epiphyseal prominence, widening or irregularity of the growth plate, and narrowing of the area if the epiphysis has slipped posteriorly. The varus angle between the femoral head and the shaft is also assessed (Fig. 38–8).

Differential Diagnosis

LCP disease, sepsis of the hip joint, and osteoarthritis should be considered.

Management

The following steps are taken:

1. Refer immediately to an orthopedic surgeon because there is risk of an acute and more devastating slip, which can occur at any time. Assist the family to attain prompt intervention. Immediate hospitalization is needed once the diagnosis is made.
2. Place the patient on non–weight-bearing

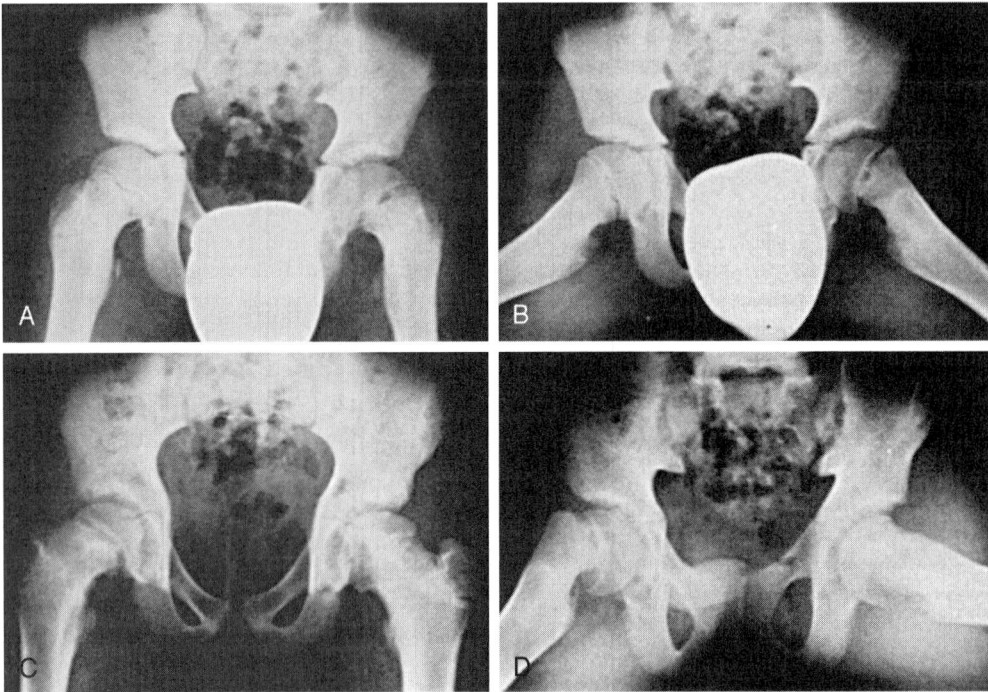

F I G U R E 38-8
Acute slipped capital femoral epiphysis in a 10-year-old boy with acute left hip and thigh pain. *A,* Anteroposterior views of both hips. A line drawn along the superior surface of the femoral head, as seen on the right side should intersect a corner of the femoral head. The left femoral head has slipped inferiorly. *B,* Frog-leg lateral roentgenograms of both hips demonstrate the mild displacement of the left femoral head more clearly. There is no evidence of remodeling in this acute slip. *C,* The left hip was treated by open epiphysiodesis; the bone graft placed across the growth plate is evident and the left growth plate has closed. At this time, 2 years after the onset of left hip pain, the patient had slight right hip pain of 3 months' duration. *D,* Lateral roentgenograms demonstrate moderate to severe slip of the right femoral head.

crutches until admitted to the hospital. Wheelchair sitting is not advised, because acute flexion can cause further slippage. Adequate instruction should be given so that the child will not fall on the crutches, another risk factor for an acute slip.

3. For mild to moderate slips, fixation of the epiphysis to the femur with a metallic screw or pins is the accepted treatment of choice. The screw or pins are removed after the growth plate closes. For very severe slippage, osteotomy is sometimes required.

4. Inform the family about the condition and its management and the risk for slippage on the other side if only one side is treated.

5. Support and monitor the child throughout the treatment phase, which includes interruption of school and activities during the

recovery period. Contact sports are usually restricted by the orthopedist until growth is complete.

Complications

Avascular necrosis of the femoral head (rare) or chondrolysis of the cartilage lining the hip joint with narrowing of the hip joint is possible. A bilateral slip may have occurred on the other side at the time of diagnosis or can occur at a later time (Warren, 1998c).

Prevention

SCFE is not a preventable condition. However, identification of the condition during the preslip period, when complaints of hip or referred knee pain, loss of motion, or weakness in the hip are present, allows early intervention that can prevent deformity and long-term sequelae such as premature degenerative arthritis in early adult life.

FEMORAL ANTEVERSION

Description

Everyone has some degree of femoral anteversion. By age 10 to 12 years, the normal angle of anteversion is 10 to 15 degrees. Younger children have a somewhat wider angle. Increased femoral anteversion (>2 SD from the mean) is called femoral torsion and can be either medial or lateral. Medial femoral torsion or medial antetorsion generally presents around 2 to 3 years of age and lasts until about 5 years of age. It is a condition in which the head and neck of the femur are rotated at an increased angle anteriorly in relation to the femoral shaft.

Etiology

A family history is often identified, and it occurs more commonly in girls. "W" sitting can increase the deformity. Physiologically, the condition produces an intoeing gait because the anteriorly directed femoral neck internally rotates to a more neutral position and the head of the femur fits neatly into the acetabulum. This results in internal rotation of the lower femur and leg with the feet intoeing. Increased femoral anteversion generally is more severe between ages 4 and 6 years and resolves as the child grows and the tibia rotate laterally and the angle of anteversion decreases.

Clinical Findings

HISTORY. The following may be reported:

- Intoeing gait, perhaps more severe with fatigue
- Runs awkwardly (looks like an "egg beater")
- Possible family history
- Usually a history of W sitting (TV squat)

PHYSICAL EXAMINATION. Findings include

- Intoeing gait with patellae medial
- Medial rotation normally less than 70 de-

grees. A mild deformity is 70 to 80 degrees, moderate between 80 and 90 degrees, and severe greater than 90 degrees (Staheli, 1998) (see Fig. 38-5).
- Lateral rotation decreased (−10 degrees lateral is abnormal)
- Knees medially rotated ("kissing patella") when standing

RADIOGRAPHIC STUDIES. Radiographs are not merited unless surgery is contemplated.

Differential Diagnosis

Consider other rotational deformities such as internal tibial torsion or metatarsus adductus. Cerebral palsy with a "scissoring gait" might be mistaken for severe femoral anteversion.

Management

Observation of the child and referral to an orthopedist if medial rotations are significant (no external rotation of the hip in extension) or child or family has significant concerns. Nonoperative management strategies such as shoe modifications, twister cables, and night splints have all been found ineffective. Operative correction is successful but carries the risk of complications. Osteotomy is done only in the older child (older than 8 years) with significant cosmetic and functional deformity. The natural history of the condition is for the medial rotation to decrease, giving some improvement (Staheli, 1998).

Complications

Studies have shown that the condition does not cause flatfoot, bunions, knee problems, back difficulties, difficulties in running, or degenerative arthritis of the hip in adults (Staheli, 1998). It is primarily a cosmetic problem unless severe enough to interfere with activities. Self-esteem can be affected.

Prevention

The condition cannot be prevented, but its aggravation can be minimized by discouraging W sitting, which places the weight of the upper body directly on the femoral neck, thus increasing the molding in the abnormal direction. Ballet lessons or activities such as skating or skiing can help mildly affected children learn to point their feet straight ahead, but such activities do not modify the bony structures (Eilert & Georgopoulos, 1999).

Knee Problems

GENU VARUM

Description

Genu varum or bowing of the legs can be a physiological or developmental variation of normal or a pathological condition. The term bowlegs is used to describe physiological variations of the normal knee angle resulting in bowing of the legs that is seen in children until the age of 3 years. Knee angle variations that fall 2 SD beyond the mean are outside the normal range of varus and are considered pathological. The typical pattern of normal bowing seen in children is lateral bowing of the tibia in the first year followed by bowlegs in the second year.

Etiology

The angle between the tibia and femur is in pronounced varus (up to 15 degrees) in normal children before 1 year of age. This is considered a uterine packing effect. The angle approaches neutral by 18 months and then proceeds to a valgus angle, with an average angle of 12 degrees from 2 to 3 years of age. The angle then gradually decreases to 8 degrees in females and 7 degrees in males by adulthood. If the varus angle is greater than 15 degrees in infants, does not begin to decrease in the second year, is asymmetrical, is associated with short stature, or is rapidly progressing, the condition is considered pathological. Increasing pathology may represent Blount disease, rickets, tumor, neurological problems, infection, or other conditions. A Salter fracture through the tibial growth plate can result in later genu varum as growth across the plate progresses unevenly (Staheli, 1998; Kling, 1987).

Blount disease (tibia vara) is seen more frequently in the African-American, Hispanic, and Scandinavian populations. It is associated with obesity and early walkers, and a positive family history. Blount disease can occur at any age in a growing child or adolescent.

Clinical Findings

HISTORY. The NP should assess

* Progression since birth; increasing deformation is problematic
* Risk factors such as metabolic disease

PHYSICAL EXAMINATION. Findings include

* Tibial-femoral angle greater than 15 degrees.
* Associated internal tibial torsion, common
* Intercondylar (knees) distance with the ankles together—measurement greater than 4 to 5 inches suggestive of the need for additional evaluation (Mankin & Zimbler, 1997)

RADIOGRAPHIC STUDIES. Radiographs are not necessary for physiological bowlegs. Metaphyseal dysplasia is usually apparent radiographically in pathological genu varum.

Differential Diagnosis

Physiological and pathological genu varum must be differentiated. Metabolic (rickets) or neurological problems, Blount disease, infections, tumor, osteochondrodysplasias, or internal tibial torsion should be ruled out.

Management

In physiological genu varum (no increasing deformity):

1. No active treatment. Denis Browne sleeping splints, corrective shoes, and passive exercises have not proved useful.
2. Reassure parents, provide information about the natural progression of the problem.
3. Observe child's condition over time (in 3 to 6 months) to be sure the problem is resolving, especially during the second year of life. Photographs of the legs for the chart can be helpful.

In pathological genu varum (increasing deformity):

1. Refer to an orthopedist. Blount disease may be treated with a Blount brace in the early stages of the disease because the bowing is reversible. In later stages of the disease, in older children, or if the disease is progressing, osteotomy is the treatment of choice. Other conditions need to be treated according to the etiology (Staheli, 1998).
2. Monitor to be sure braces are used consistently with good fit.
3. Observe to be sure the problem is not worsening.

Complications

Knee degeneration and deformity result if pathological genu varum is not treated.

Prevention

Early identification and referral reduce the complexity and expense of treatment as well as the residual deformities.

GENU VALGUM

Description

Genu valgum is "knock-knees." Females tend to have a somewhat higher degree of valgus knee posture than males. Physiological genu valgum tends to be most severe around 3 and 3½ years.

Etiology

The condition can be considered developmental or physiological in children starting anywhere from 2 to 4 years of age. It can be pathological in the following situations: found in child older than 6 to 7 years; tibial-femoral angle greater than 15 degrees valgus; increasing in severity; and found in the presence of asymmetry, short stature, or obesity (Warren, 1998a). Causes of pathological genu valgum include rickets, osteochondrodysplasias, trauma, congenital defect, osteogenesis imperfecta, and juvenile arthritis of the knee.

Clinical Findings

HISTORY. The NP should assess

- Progression of the deformity
- Risk factors as listed under etiology
- Joint pains

PHYSICAL EXAMINATION. Findings include

- Bilateral tibial-femoral angle less than 15 degrees of valgus in the child up to 7 years of age is considered normal and can be safely ignored; a valgus angle greater than 15 degrees is outside the range of normal.
- Unilateral deformity.
- Awkwardness of gait.
- Subluxing patella.
- Intermalleolar (ankles) distance with the knees together—measurement greater than 4 to 5 inches suggest the need for additional evaluation (Mankin & Zimbler, 1997).

RADIOGRAPHIC STUDIES. No radiographic studies are needed unless pathological condition is suspected.

Differential Diagnosis

Rule out pathological conditions of genu valgum as listed.

Management

Management is the same as for physiological and pathological genu varum. However, for pathological genu valgum, the type of braces prescribed are different, as are the surgical procedures.

Prevention

This is the same as for genu varum.

OSGOOD-SCHLATTER DISEASE

Description

This condition is caused by inflammation of the tibial tubercle, an apophysis site.

Etiology and Incidence

The problem occurs when the infrapatellar ligament of the quadriceps muscle is not well anchored to the tibial tubercle, so excessive activity of the quadriceps results in repetitive microtrauma, causing pain and swelling at the insertion area (the apophysis). With the end of growth, the apophysis fuses to the shaft of the tibia and pain diminishes. Thus, the incidence declines in late adolescents and adults.

This is a common problem of adolescents who engage in active sports. It is most often unilateral and occurs in males between the ages of 10 and 15 years and in girls between 8 and 13 years.

Clinical Findings

HISTORY. The following may be reported:

*   Recent physical activity such as playing track, soccer, or football; surfboarding commonly produces the condition.
*   Pain increases during and immediately after the activity and decreases when the activity is stopped for a while.

PHYSICAL EXAMINATION. Findings include

*   Point tenderness over the tibial tubercle
*   Possible redness and swelling at this point

Differential Diagnosis

Other knee derangements, tumors, and hip problems with referred pain should be considered. The referred pain of hip problems is diffuse across the distal femur without point tenderness at the tibial tubercle.

Management

The following steps are taken:

1. Decrease activity until the inflammation subsides; often 4 to 8 weeks is sufficient.
2. Applying ice to the site after activity may help.
3. Try hamstring and quadriceps stretching exercises before sports.
4. Use of nonsteroidal anti-inflammatory drugs (NSAIDs) is recommended by some but

thought ineffective by others. Because this condition may last up to 12 to 18 months, chronic use of NSAIDs may be problematic.
5. Apply a knee immobilizer if pain is severe and persistent.

Complications

In the postpubertal child, a residual ossicle in the tendon next to the bone may cause persistent pain. Surgical removal is indicated and will relieve the pain.

Prevention

The condition cannot be prevented, but earlier management may decrease the length of disability and the discomfort associated with it. Avoid overuse and encourage balanced training and adequate warm-up before exercise or sports participation.

TIBIAL TORSION

Description

Tibial torsion is the twisting of the long bone along its long axis. Tibial version is the term used to describe the normal variation in tibial rotation. At birth, the tibias have a mean lateral rotation of 2.2 degrees and rotate laterally over time, with an adult mean lateral tibial rotation of about 23 degrees. Tibial torsion describes those rotations that are outside the range of normal. Medial tibial torsion (MTT) consists of abnormal medial rotation, resulting in intoeing of the feet; lateral tibial torsion (LTT) consists of abnormal lateral rotation resulting in out-toeing.

Etiology

Tibial torsion may be congenital, developmental, or acquired.

Incidence

MTT is the most common cause of intoeing during the second year of life and is often noted around 6 to 12 months of life. Lateral tibial torsion is a cause of out-toeing in late childhood.

Clinical Findings

PHYSICAL EXAMINATION. The thigh-foot angle (TFA) is used to assess tibial rotation. With the patient prone and the knees flexed 90 degrees, the foot and thigh are viewed from directly above. The foot should be relaxed. MTT exists if the TFA is negative by more than 5 degrees (Staheli, 1998). Intoeing is expressed in negative values (Fig. 38–9).

RADIOGRAPHIC STUDIES. These are usually not necessary.

Differential Diagnosis

Genu varum in which the problem originates at the knee with a tibial-femoral angle, femoral torsion (femoral anteversion), adducted great toe, and metatarsus adductus also produce intoeing gaits. Adducted great toe (the searching toe) is a benign condition that resolves spontaneously. Lateral femoral torsion also causes an out-toeing gait.

Management

1. Treatment of tibial version (the normal variation in tibial rotation) is observation and monitoring of the child.

2. MTT should be referred to an orthopedist if the problem is significant (greater than −20 by age 3 years). Stretching exercises or external rotational splints may be recommended. Surgical intervention may be needed for severe cases that persist into late childhood and cause significant functional problems.

3. Shoes have been shown to be ineffective for the treatment of MTT. The avoidance of certain postures (e.g., sleeping in the knee-chest position and sitting with the feet tucked under the buttocks) thought to exacerbate MTT is controversial.

4. LTT with TFA greater than 30 degrees should be referred to an orthopedist. It usually worsens with growth. Medial femoral torsion with pain also should be referred (Dise, 1998; Staheli, 1998).

Complications

There are no complications with normal tibial versions and no interference with activities. Tibial torsion (the TFA is outside the acceptable range of normal) can lead to significant functional problems in severe cases.

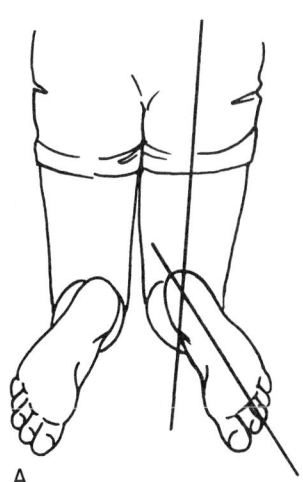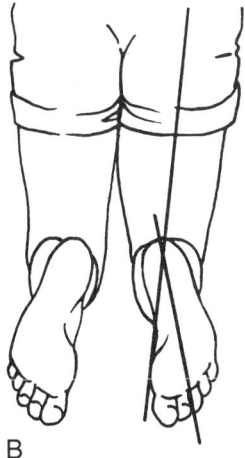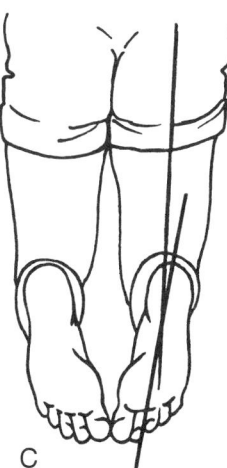

F I G U R E 38-9
Thigh-foot angle. With the child in the prone position and the knees flexed and approximated, the long axis of the foot can be compared with the long axis of the thigh. The long axis of the foot bisects the heel and the second toe or lies between the second and third toes. External tibial torsion, *A*, produces excessive outward rotation. Normal alignment, *B*, is characterized by slight external rotation. Internal tibial torsion produces inward rotation of the foot and is a negative angle, *C*. (From Thompson GH: Gait disturbances. *In* Kliegman RM, Nieder ML, Super DM [eds]: Practical Strategies in Pediatric Diagnosis and Therapy. Philadelphia, WB Saunders, 1996.)

POPLITEAL CYSTS

Description

Popliteal or Baker cysts are synovial lesions that result from herniation of the synovium of the knee joint into the popliteal space. In children, they are benign cysts and are not associated with intra-articular defects.

Clinical Findings

The major findings are swelling behind the knee with or without mild discomfort.

DIAGNOSTIC STUDIES. Ultrasonography, transillumination of cyst, and diagnostic aspiration of synovial fluid are usual diagnostic studies.

Management

Observation is the treatment of choice because the majority of these cysts resolve on their own in a year or two. The rare, large, painful, and persistent cyst should be referred to an orthopedic surgeon.

Foot Problems

PES PLANUS

Description

Physiological pes planus (flatfoot) is commonly seen in neonates and toddlers and is due to a fat pad in the arch that makes the appearance of the arch seem flat. This generally resolves by 2 to 3 years of age but in a small percentage of cases can persist into adulthood. Flexible flatfoot is often familial, common, and benign. The arch is seen when the foot is suspended but flattens with weight bearing. Rigid flatfoot is pathological.

Etiology

Flatfoot is the result of soft tissue laxity, muscular weakness, or a tight Achilles tendon. There is often a familial tendency toward the problem. Flatfoot also is associated with certain syndromes (Marfan and Down syndromes), myelodysplasia, cerebral palsy, and obesity.

Clinical Findings

HISTORY. Onset is noticed with weight bearing. The flexible flatfoot is usually painless.

PHYSICAL EXAMINATION. The NP should assess the following:

- Is there an arch in the suspended foot or when the child toe-stands?
- Can an arch be molded with pressure by the examiner's fingers?
- Is the Achilles tendon tight?
- Is there abnormal shoe wear on the inner side?

Differential Diagnosis

Congenital vertical talus should be considered if the foot is rigid and no arch can be molded or if the foot has a rocker-bottom appearance. Calcaneovalgus foot might be considered also.

Management

Management involves the following:

- Only symptomatic feet and rigid flatfoot should be treated; refer to an orthopedist.
- For painful, flexible flatfoot, a longitudinal arch support may be recommended by the orthopedist.
- If the Achilles tendon is tight, passive stretching may be helpful.

Complications

Flatfoot should be considered a variation of normal unless there is pain or rigidity. Congenital vertical talus is difficult to treat and should not be missed. Some cases of flatfoot are symptomatic in adulthood, and, in severe cases, the bones of the feet adapt to abnormal position with pronation and possible development of bunions.

Patient Education

Parents need to understand that special shoes do not cure the problem and arch supports do not help the foot to "grow" an arch.

The so-called Thomas heel is considered ineffective as a treatment.

METATARSUS ADDUCTUS

Description

Metatarsus adductus (MA) is a condition in which the hindfoot is straight but the forefoot is adducted, giving the foot a curved, intoeing shape.

Etiology and Incidence

When the foot is flexible, the condition is usually considered a result of uterine packing, with some tightness of the soft tissues in the area of the arch. A nonflexible foot, especially with heel valgus, or persistence may indicate a more serious problem.

Flexible MA is very common (1 in 1000 births). In 10% of cases, it is associated with DDH (Sawyer & Esterhai, 1999).

Clinical Findings

HISTORY. There can be a family history.

PHYSICAL EXAMINATION. Findings include the following:

- The lateral border of the foot has a convex shape. Normally, this border should look straight. Sometimes spreading of the toes is noted with a wider space between the first and second toes.
- The foot should normally be straight. If one draws a line from the middle of the heel it should pass through the second toe or between the second and third toes (Mankin & Zimbler, 1997). In metatarsus adductus, the forefoot has an increased angle (>15 degrees) or resists stretching (Fig. 38–10).
- To determine whether the foot is flexible or rigid, the heel is grasped with one hand while the forefoot is abducted with the other hand. In flexible MA, the forefoot can be abducted past midline.

RADIOGRAPHIC STUDIES. Radiographic studies need to be ordered if the foot is not flexible or MA persists beyond 6 months of age.

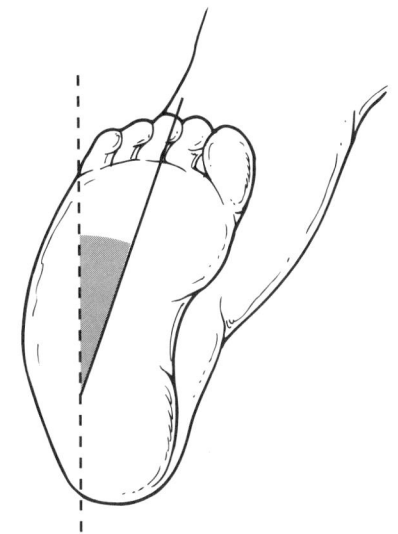

F I G U R E 38-10
Metatarsus adductus angle. An angle created by the intersecting lines that is greater than 15 degrees indicates metatarsus adductus.

Differential Diagnosis

Consider congenital vertical talus, which will be rigid, or clubfoot, in which the foot will also be inverted, and the foot is in the pointed-toe position.

Management

Management involves the following:

1. For the flexible foot that can be brought past midline, the soft tissues can be stretched by the parents with each diaper change. Stretching is done as described under physical examination when the examiner determines whether the foot is flexible. Instruct the parents to hold the stretch to the count of five and repeat five times. The soft tissues should blanch with each stretch. Be sure that the parent is not just pushing on the great toe. If no improvement is evident by 6 months of age, casting is appropriate.
2. For the nonflexible foot:
   - Refer to an orthopedist when the problem is identified.
   - Educate the family that the treatment for infants may include serial short-leg casts

or braces to stretch the foot (2 or 3 casts for 2 weeks per cast) or other management if the bones of the foot are more severely affected. If the child is older than 2 to 3 years of age, surgery may be needed to correct the problem.

3. Corrective shoes or night splints are not helpful for flexible metatarsus adductus.

Complications

Early intervention can prevent more intensive therapeutic measures to correct the deformity.

TALIPES EQUINOVARUS

Description

Talipes equinovarus (clubfoot) has three elements: the ankle is in equinus (the foot is in a pointed-toe position), the sole of the foot is inverted as a result of hindfoot varus or inversion deformity of the heel, and the forefoot has the convex shape of metatarsus adductus. The foot cannot be manually corrected to a neutral position with the heel down.

Etiology

The etiology of clubfoot may be idiopathic (which tends to be hereditary), neurogenic as seen with myelomeningocele, or associated with certain syndromes such as arthrogryposis and Larsen syndrome. It varies in severity with uterine positioning a factor in mild clubfoot. The incidence is 1:1000 live births with approximately 50% of cases being bilateral. The problem is congenital and can be identified in neonates (Eilert & Georgopoulos, 1999; Staheli, 1998).

Clinical Findings

HISTORY. Clubfoot is present at birth.

PHYSICAL EXAMINATION. The foot appears as described above.

RADIOGRAPHIC STUDIES. AP and lateral standing or simulated weight-bearing studies are obtained.

Management

The following steps are taken:

1. Refer to an orthopedist as early as possible, ideally in the newborn nursery, because the joints are most flexible in the first hours and days of life. The foot can become rigid in a matter of days. The orthopedist may begin with weekly long-leg casting, but surgical correction is commonly required.

2. Monitor throughout childhood, as the condition can recur. Postcorrection night splinting may be needed.

Complications

With growth, the abnormality can become increasingly distorted, making correction more difficult. Calf hypoplasia and a shorter than normal foot can occur even with correction.

OVERRIDING TOES

Overriding toes are generally identified at birth. Efforts to tape them into a correct position or otherwise modify their position are usually futile. Overriding of the second, third, and fourth toes generally resolves with time. Occasionally, if severe, they can be surgically improved. Shoe fit can be a problem.

INTOEING AND OUT-TOEING ROTATIONAL PROBLEMS

When a child has an intoeing or out-toeing gait, the degree of rotation and source of the rotational deformity must be assessed. These include internal femoral torsion (femoral anteversion), internal tibial torsion, and metatarsus adductus. The causes of intoeing usually are physiological, are related to age, and resolve as the child grows (Table 38–2). In addition, intoeing in children can vary with activities and from step to step.

Clinical Findings

HISTORY. The NP assesses

• Onset of problem
• Increasing or decreasing deformity

T A B L E 38-2

Typical Cause of Intoeing and Out-Toeing Rotational Problems

	CAUSE	TYPICAL FINDING	AGE OF PRESENTATION
INTOEING	Equinovarus	Plantar foot flexion, forefoot adduction, and hindfoot varus	At birth
	Metatarsus adductus	Curved foot—refer if not flexible	Birth to 6 mo
	Abducted great toe	Searching toe—resolves spontaneously	Toddler period
	Medial tibial torsion	Refer if − 20 degree thigh-foot angle (TFA)	12–18 mo
	Medial femoral torsion	Refer if 70 degrees + medial and 10 degrees lateral hip rotation	2–5 yr
OUT-TOEING	Physiological infantile out-toeing	Feet may turn out when infant positioned upright—resolves spontaneously	Early infancy
	Lateral tibial torsion	Refer if TFA > +30 degrees	Late childhood
	Lateral femoral torsion	Refer if >2 SD of the mean	Late childhood

- Treatments used to date
- Degree of interference with activities
- Effects on self-image for older children
- Neurological history

PHYSICAL EXAMINATION. The physical examination involves the following:

- Observe the gait. Note that the slightly older child may consciously or unconsciously improve or worsen the gait for the examiner. Asking the child to run may also be helpful.
- Lay the child prone on the examining table.
- Examine for femoral anteversion (medial and lateral rotations).
- Examine for internal or external tibial torsion (TFA).
- Examine for MA or other deformity.
- The child may have a combination of any or all of the aforementioned problems.

Management

See the individual diagnoses for management strategies.

OTHER COMMON MUSCULOSKELETAL SYSTEM FINDINGS NEEDING ATTENTION

Toe-Walking

DESCRIPTION

Consistent toe-walking is frequently associated with neurological problems such as cerebral palsy. Autistic children or those with early muscular dystrophy may toe-walk. Children with tight heel cords may toe-walk. Unilateral toe-walking can be associated with a short leg, as found with a dislocated hip. Toe-walking also can be a habit, especially in children who used walkers. In these children, toe-walking generally resolves before the age of 3 years and is not associated with any musculoskeletal deformity.

CLINICAL FINDINGS

History

The NP should assess

- Onset
- Severity
- Neurological history

Physical Examination

The NP should

- Look at shoe wear to assess extent of toe-walking. For example, is the heel worn?
- Assess for tight heel cords. The foot should be brought beyond a 90-degree angle.
- Conduct a neurological assessment.
- Measure leg lengths and examine hips.

Management

Management depends on the etiology. Orthopedic management is needed for tight heel cords, unequal leg lengths, and hip problems.

Growing Pains or Leg Aches of Childhood

DESCRIPTION

Transient aches are common complaints during childhood that have been reported to occur in 15 to 30% of normal children, usually involving the lower extremities (Staheli, 1998). The term *growing pains* has been used to describe this discomfort but not without controversy, because musculoskeletal growth has never been proved to be the cause of these aches or pains. Their cause is unknown; genetic, functional, or structural (hypermobility) factors have been implicated. Differentiating benign leg aches of childhood from more serious pathology is important. Onset is common at 3 to 5 years of age and again at 8 to 12 years of age.

CLINICAL FINDINGS

History

Pain or leg aches are typically described as

- Occurring characteristically at night
- Poorly localized and bilateral
- Transient and occurring over a period of time as long as several years
- Not associated with a limp or disability

Physical Examination

Normal physical examination with no tenderness, guarding, or reduced range of joint motion.

Diagnostic Studies

Radiographs and blood work are not necessary if a classic history is given and there are no physical findings.

DIFFERENTIAL DIAGNOSIS

Neoplastic lesions, leukemia, sickle cell anemia, and subacute osteomyelitis must be ruled out.

MANAGEMENT

Reassure the parents that these are common complaints that are benign. Symptomatic treatment with heat and analgesic may be of benefit. Stress the need for parents to bring the child in for reevaluation if there is a change in symptoms or other signs emerge.

Limps

Children limp for reasons including pain, deformity, or weakness. Limps must always be carefully assessed and managed. Limps may be of several types.

DESCRIPTION

1. *Antalgic.* This is a gait caused by pain that increases with the normal stresses of walking. The child tries to get weight off the affected side quickly; thus, the normal walking cadence is off with a shortened stance phase. Examples of antalgic gaits: The child with a sore knee walks with a fixed knee, whereas the child with a sore toe tries not to roll off the toe at the toe-off phase of the stride. A child with appendicitis may also have an antalgic gait, with a slight slumping posture and a shortened stride on the right resulting from psoas muscle irritation.
2. *Trendelenburg gait or abductor lurch.* This gait is caused by a hip problem such as hip dysplasia. The child tilts over the affected hip with each stride to decrease the mechanical stresses while the opposite side is off the ground during the swing-through phase of the gait.
3. *Equinus or toe to heel gait.* This is caused by lack of neurological coordination, creating an unsteady, wide-based gait. For example, children with cerebral palsy often exhibit this characteristic toe-to-heel sequence

during the stance phase of their gait because of heel-cord contractures.

4. *Circumduction.* This gait allows a functionally longer leg to progress forward using a circular swing motion. Children with leg length inequality and painful foot or ankle conditions use this gait.

CLINICAL FINDINGS

History

A careful history is needed, including

- Onset
- Location of pain
- Changes in limp or pain during the day or since onset
- Interference with activities
- Past medical history including injury or illness
- Review of systems

Physical Examination

The NP should do the following:

- Identify the type of limp from the gait
- Examine the hips, legs, feet, and back for range of motion, asymmetry, changes in tissues, signs of infection
- Complete a neurological examination, including strength, reflexes, balance, coordination
- Assess Trendelenburg sign for hip stability

Radiographic Studies and Laboratory Tests

Studies are ordered appropriate to the findings and history. Knee pain and limp may be referred from the hip.

DIFFERENTIAL DIAGNOSIS

Age is an important factor in diagnosing the many causes of limping. Fracture, congenital dislocated hip, Legg-Perthes disease, slipped capital femoral epiphysis, tumor, infection, juvenile arthritis, and others should be considered (Table 38-3).

MANAGEMENT

Refer the patient to an orthopedist immediately unless the etiology is a mild strain or a local lesion that can be managed conservatively by the primary care provider.

Overuse Syndromes of Childhood and Adolescence

DESCRIPTION

Overuse syndrome is caused by repetitive movement injury that causes microtrauma. Osgood-Schlatter disease, discussed earlier, is a classic example of an overuse injury commonly seen in children aged 10 to 14 years. Other typical overuse injuries of childhood are varus overload of the elbow ("Little League elbow"), proximal humeral epiphysiolysis ("Little League shoulder"), patellofemoral pain syndrome, shin splints, and stress fractures (Table 38-4).

MANAGEMENT

Treatment often involves resting and icing the extremity or joint, doing retraining and strengthening exercises, gradually reintroducing activities, and using analgesics. NSAIDs help to reduce the inflammatory component of the trauma. Patient and parent education is important to prevent further injury and disability and to allow the child to return to safe sport participation (Sawyer & Esterhai, 1999).

Muscle Diseases

DESCRIPTION

Muscle diseases in children are rare. However, there are many types of problems that can affect muscle metabolism or function. It can be difficult to discern whether the lack of good muscular function is due to problems of enervation or an inability of the muscle to contract efficiently.

CLINICAL FINDINGS

History

The following may be reported:

- Failure to achieve motor milestones
- Loss of motor skills such as the ability to climb stairs easily

T A B L E 38-3

Differential Diagnosis of Limping

CONDITION	AGE	PAIN +/−	HISTORICAL FINDINGS	CLINICAL FINDINGS	CAUSATIVE FACTORS
Developmental dysplasia of the hip	T, C, A	−	Breech delivery; metatarsus adductus; torticollis; poor treatment outcomes if not diagnosed at birth or shortly afterward	Limited abduction; + Trendelenburg; + radiography at 2–3 mo; shortening of leg; acetabular dysplasia	Familial; joint laxity, positioning, maternal hormones
Leg length inequality	T, C, A	−	None	Circumduction gait; joint contracture; >1 cm discrepancy in leg lengths	Congenital; neurogenic; vascular; tumor; trauma; infection
Neuromuscular (NM) disease	T, C, A	−	Depends on cause	Depends on cause; equinus or abductor gait	Cerebral palsy, muscular dystrophy, and other NM diseases
Discitis	T, C, A	+	Varied: fever, malaise, unwilling to walk, backache	Stiff back, ↑ ESR; + x-ray 2–3 wk; early bone scan +	Bacterial infection in disc space (*Staphylococcus aureus*) or inflammatory response
Septic arthritis	T, C, A	+ +	Moderate to high fever, malaise, arthralgias; irritability; progressive course	Redness, warmth and swelling of joint—knee or hip; limited hip motion; >ESR 25 mm/hr	*S. aureus* likely organism
Osteomyelitis	T, C, A	+	Fever	Refusal to walk or move limb; point tenderness; 7–10 days to see radiographic bony changes	*S. aureus* likely organism
Neoplastic	T, C, A	+	Depends on type of neoplasm	Varied	Neoplasm—benign or malignant

T A B L E 38-3

Differential Diagnosis of Limping *Continued*

CONDITION	AGE	PAIN +/−	HISTORICAL FINDINGS	CLINICAL FINDINGS	CAUSATIVE FACTORS
Trauma	T, C, A	+	Depends on type (fractures, strains, sprains)	Varied	Varied
Occult trauma: toddler fracture	T	+	Well child	Commonly spiral fracture of tibia; refusal to walk, mild soft tissue swelling; + radiograph	Trauma
Transient synovitis	3–8 yr	+	Mild to moderate fever, mild irritability; resolves within 1 wk	Limited hip motion; ESR <25 mm/hr	Inflammatory reaction; unknown etiology; often URI (50%) prior
Juvenile arthritis (JA)	Childhood until 16 yr	+	Fever, rashes, ↑ WBC; some iritis; joint stiffness and swelling; S & S >3 mo	Mono/polyarticular arthropathy; +ANA (25–88%); ↑ ESR in moderate/severe JA	Unknown; genetic (HLA) or environmental
Slipped capital femoral epiphysis	9–15 yr	+	>90 percentile weight; African-American; male	Limited abduction and extension; external rotation of thigh if hip flexed	Multifactorial: mechanical; endocrine; trauma; familial
Legg-Calvé-Perthes	4–8 yr	+	Acute/chronic onset; pain in hip, groin, knee; stiffness; male	+ Trendelenburg, shortening; ↓ abduction, internal rotation, hip extension; + radiographs but not early	Familial; breech birth; prior trauma (17%)

T = toddler (1–3 yr); C = childhood (4–10 yr), A = adolescent (≥11 yr); ESR = erythrocyte sedimentation rate; S & S = signs and symptoms; URI = upper respiratory infection; WBC = white blood cell; HLA = human leukocyte antigen; ANA = antinuclear antibody.

Adapted from Behrman R, Kliegman RM, Arvin AM (eds): Nelson Textbook of Pediatrics, 15th ed. Philadelphia, WB Saunders, 1996; Staheli L: Fundamentals of Pediatric Orthopedics, 2nd ed. Philadelphia, Lippincott-Raven, 1998.

T A B L E 38-4

Overuse Injuries of Childhood: Characteristic Features and Their Treatment

CONDITION	CLINICAL FINDINGS	TREATMENT	COMMENTS
Patellofemoral pain syndrome	Anterior knee pain	Rest, nonsteroidal anti-inflammatory drugs (NSAIDs), retraining, and strengthening of quadriceps muscles	Arthroscopic surgery only if recurring problems
Proximal humeral epiphysiolysis "Little League shoulder"	Shoulder pain—gradual onset; pain ↑ with throwing especially curve ball	Modify activity; gradual restart but limit intensity and frequency of throwing with retraining	Seen in skeletally immature children; + radiographs—widening proximal humeral physis
Shin splints	Pain along medial border of tibia; child does prolonged running	NSAIDs; ice after running; retraining and muscle strengthening after inflammation ↓; gradual return to running	Associated with poor running technique, hard running surface, muscle weakness; inadequate running shoes; sudden increase in running; is an inflammatory response
Stress fractures	Tenderness and swelling at site	Reduce or eliminate activity that caused injury for 10–14 days; may need to cast	Due to microtrauma; most commonly seen in active teens but can occur during childhood; proximal tibia most common site
Varus overload of the elbow "Little League elbow"	Elbow pain with activity; locking and ↓ extension of elbow; medial humeral epicondyle tenderness	Rest; NSAIDs; ice; when pain-free, gradual return to activity with retraining; surgery if elbow instability	Leads to osteochondral lesions and stress fractures if severe; radiographs—widening proximal physis; also seen in gymnasts

- Easy fatigue with physical activity
- A history of good days and bad days with relation to ability to accomplish physical activities
- Increasing difficulties with motor activities

Physical Examination

Findings include

- Fibrotic or "doughy" feel to the muscles.
- Muscle hypertrophy, especially of the calf muscles.
- Muscle wasting.
- Fibrillations or fasciculations.
- Positive Gowers sign. This is obtained by asking the child to get up off the floor without help. The sign is positive if the child uses his or her arms to push off from the legs, gradually standing in a segmented fashion.
- Muscle contractures.
- Weakness.

MANAGEMENT

Referral is necessary. These conditions may need to be handled by an interdisciplinary team with orthopedic, metabolic, and physical therapy, social service, and nursing care. Genetics counseling may be necessary, depending on the diagnosis. The muscular dystrophies, for instance, are autosomal dominant and can appear in several children in a family.

Patient and family support is needed. Muscle diseases are chronic, debilitating, and sometimes fatal conditions. Helping the child to lead as normal a life as possible while coping with his or her condition is a major task. The family may need help maintaining caregiving and coping with the implications of the diagnosis.

REFERENCES

Behrman R (ed): Nelson Textbook of Pediatrics, 14th ed. Philadelphia, WB Saunders, 1992.

Behrman RE, Kliegman RM: Nelson Essentials of Pediatrics, 3rd ed. Philadelphia, WB Saunders, 1998.

Behrman R, Kliegman RM, Arvin AM: Nelson Textbook of Pediatrics, 15th ed. Philadelphia, WB Saunders, 1996.

Bennett J: Scoliosis and kyphosis. *In* Finberg L (ed): Saunders Manual of Pediatric Practice. Philadelphia, WB Saunders, 1998, pp 999–1001.

Dise TL: Flatfleet and tibial torsion. *In* Finberg L (ed): Saunders Manual of Pediatric Practice. Philadelphia, WB Saunders, 1998, pp 994–995.

Dyment PG: The hip. *In* Burg FD, Ingelfinger JR, Wald ER, et al (eds): Gellis and Kagan's Current Pediatric Therapy 16th ed. Philadelphia, WB Saunders, 1999, pp 934–937.

Eilert RE, Georgopoulos G: Orthopedics. *In* Hay WW, Hayward AR, Levin MJ, et al (eds): Current Pediatric Diagnosis & Treatment, 14th ed. East Norwalk, CT, Appleton & Lange, 1999, pp 695–714.

Kling T: Angular deformities of the lower limbs in children. Orthop Clin North Am 18:513–527, 1987.

Mankin KP, Zimbler S: Gait and leg alignment: What's normal and what's not. Contemp Pediatr 14(11):41–70, 1997.

Piecuch S: Birth injuries. *In* Finberg L (ed): Saunders Manual of Pediatric Practice. Philadelphia, WB Saunders, 1998, pp 59–64.

Sawyer JR, Esterhai JL: Orthopedic problems of the extremities. *In* Burg FD, Ingelfinger JR, Wald ER, et al (eds): Gellis & Kagan's Current Pediatric Therapy, 16th ed. Philadelphia, WB Saunders, 1999, pp 922–930.

Schaller JG: Nonrheumatic conditions mimicking rheumatic diseases of childhood. *In* Behrman R, Kliegman RM, Arvin AM (eds): Nelson Textbook of Pediatrics, 15th ed. Philadelphia, WB Saunders, 1996, pp 689–690.

Scoles P: Pediatric Orthopedics in Clinical Practice, 2nd ed. St. Louis, Mosby–Year Book, 1988.

Speers A, Speers M: Care of the infant in a Pavlik harness. Pediatr Nursing 18:229–232, 1992.

Staheli L: Fundamentals of Pediatric Orthopedics, 2nd ed. Philadelphia, Lippincott-Raven, 1998.

Warren FH: Genu varum and genu valgum. *In* Finberg L (ed): Saunders Manual of Pediatric Practice. Philadelphia, WB Saunders, 1998a, pp 994–995.

Warren FH: Legg-Calvé-Perthes disease. *In* Finberg L (ed): Saunders Manual of Pediatric Practice. Philadelphia, WB Saunders, 1998b, pp 996–997.

Warren FH: Slipped Capital Femoral Epiphysis. *In* Finberg L (ed): Saunders Manual of Pediatric Practice. Philadelphia, WB Saunders, 1998c, pp 991–993.

CHAPTER 39

Perinatal Conditions

Deborah K. Parks, Diane Montgomery, and Robert J. Yetman

INTRODUCTION

The neonatal period is a highly vulnerable time for the infant. In the United States, two thirds of all deaths in the first year of life occur among infants less than 28 days of age (Behrman et al., 1996). Mortality is highest during the first 24 hours of life. Because serious health problems can arise for the infant in the hours after the initial transition to extrauterine life, the nurse practitioner (NP) must be prepared to manage these problems while providing psychosocial support and education for the families. An understanding of the physiology of fetal development, risk factors for potential problems, and pertinent physical findings prepares the NP to assist the newborn's transition to extrauterine life effectively.

STANDARDS OF CARE

The *Healthy Children 2000 National Health Promotion and Disease Prevention Objectives for the Year 2000* guidelines (United States [US] Department of Health and Human Services, 1990) set goals related to reducing infant mortality, increasing the proportion of newborns screened by state-sponsored programs for genetic disorders and other disabling conditions, and increasing the proportion of newborns test-

ing positive for disease who receive appropriate treatment.

The *Healthy People 2010: National Health Promotion and Disease Prevention Objectives for the Year 2010* (US Department of Health and Human Services, 1998a) related to maternal, infant, and child care are included in Appendix D. The overall goal of these objectives is to:

Improve maternal health and pregnancy outcomes and reduce rates of disability in infants, thereby improving the health and well-being of women, infants, children, and families in the United States. The health of a population is reflected in the health of its most vulnerable members. A major focus of many public health efforts, therefore, is improving the health of pregnant women and their infants, including reductions in rate of birth defects, risk factors for infant death, and death of infants and their mothers.

The *Guide to Clinical Preventive Services* (US Preventive Services Task Force, 1996) recommends the following preventive services for neonates:

Neonatal screening for sickle hemoglobinopathies is recommended to identify infants who may benefit from antibiotic prophylaxis to prevent sepsis. . . . All screening efforts must be accompanied by comprehensive counseling and treatment services.

Screening for congenital hypothyroidism with thyroid function tests on dried blood spot specimens is recommended for all newborns during the first week of life.

Screening for phenylketonuria (PKU) by measurement of phenylalanine level on a dried blood spot is recommended for all newborns prior to discharge from the nursery. Infants who are tested before 24 hours of age should receive a repeated screening test by 2 weeks of age.

The *Put Prevention Into Practice*: *Clinician's Handbook of Preventive Services* (US Public Health Services, 1997) outlines recommendations from major authorities, including:

American Academy of Pediatrics and *Bright Futures*—Newborn screening should be performed according to each state's regulations.

Specific recommendations regarding screening for hypothyroidism, PKU, and hemoglobinopathies are detailed in this handbook.

Bright Futures: *Guidelines for Health Supervision of Infants, Children, and Adolescents* (Green, 1994) has detailed anticipatory guidelines for the newborn, first-week, and 1-month health supervision visits.

Guidelines for Perinatal Care from the American Academy of Pediatrics and American College of Obstetricians and Gynecologists (Hauth & Merenstein, 1997) is another thorough compendium of standards of caring for the newborn.

ANATOMY AND PHYSIOLOGY

Intrauterine-to-Extrauterine Transition

The infant's intrauterine-to-extrauterine transition requires many biochemical and physiological changes. In utero, the placenta provides metabolic functions for the fetus. Oxygenated blood from the placenta arrives to the fetus through the umbilical vein. Because of high pulmonary vascular pressure, this blood is shunted from the right to the left side of the heart through the foramen ovale, or to the systemic circulation through the ductus arteriosus. At birth, the umbilical cord is severed. Simultaneously, the infant begins to breathe and the high pulmonary vascular pressure drops, allowing blood flow to the lungs for oxygenation. The foramen ovale and ductus arteriosus are no longer necessary and close after birth.

The newborn becomes dependent on gastrointestinal tract function to absorb nutrients, renal function to excrete wastes and maintain chemical balance, liver function to metabolize and excrete toxins, and the functions of the immunological system to protect against infection. Many of the newborn's problems are related to poor adaptation following birth owing to asphyxia, premature birth, congenital anomalies, or adverse effects of delivery.

A predictable series of changes or reactivities in vital signs and clinical appearance takes place after the delivery of most normal infants (Desmond et al., 1966) (Fig. 39–1). The first period of reactivity includes changes at the sympathetic level such as tachycardia, rapid respirations, transient rales, grunting, flaring and retractions, a falling body temperature, hypertonus, and alerting exploratory behavior. Parasympathetic system changes during the first period of reactivity include the initiation of bowel sounds and the production of oral mucus.

After an interval of sleep, the infant enters the second period of reactivity. During this time the oral mucus again becomes evident, the

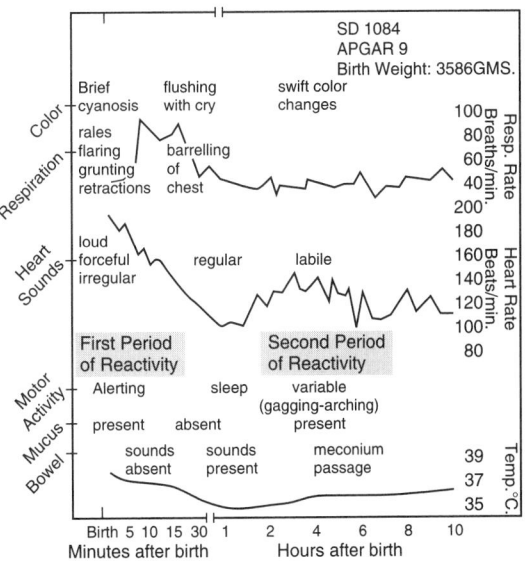

F I G U R E 39-1
Summary of normal transition. (From Desmond MM, Rudolph AJ, Phitaksphraiwan P: The transitional care nursery. Pediatr Clin North Am 13:651–668, 1966.)

heart rate become labile, the infant becomes more responsive to endogenous and exogenous stimuli, and meconium is often passed.

PATHOPHYSIOLOGY

High-Risk Pregnancy

High-risk pregnancies are defined as those in which factors exist that increase the chances of abortion, fetal death, premature delivery, intrauterine growth retardation, fetal or neonatal disease, congenital malformations, mental retardation, and other handicaps. Identification of high-risk pregnancies is the first step toward prevention of neonatal problems (Table 39-1). Comprehensive and frequent prenatal visits for high-risk pregnancies are aimed at preventing complications in the newborn.

Acquired Health Problems

In utero exposure to poor nutrition, alcohol, drugs, viruses or bacteria, and maternal conditions such as hypertension and diabetes can result in prematurity and abnormalities at birth. The risk of neonatal problems increases with maternal age younger than 16 years and older than 40 years.

Genetic Problems

The presence of chromosomal abnormalities, congenital anomalies, inborn errors of metabolism, mental retardation, and familial diseases increases the risk of the same condition in the infant. Since many conditions are not easily identifiable on physical examination, it is important to explore family histories to determine if a newborn is at risk for any inheritable diseases. Anticipation of potential problems associated with various inherited conditions leads to their early identification and management.

Perinatal Complications and Injuries

Perinatal complications occur immediately before or during birth. Prolonged or dysfunctional labor increases the risk of fetal distress. Pro-longed rupture of the membranes and chorioamnionitis increase the risk of infection in the infant, and ruptured placenta previa increases the risk of blood loss in the infant. Cesarean deliveries, the use of forceps or vacuum extraction, and the type of maternal anesthesia used also pose risks. The term "birth injury" includes mechanical and anoxic trauma incurred by an infant during labor and delivery. The incidence of birth injuries has been estimated at 2 to 7 per 1000 live births; these injuries represent 2 to 3% of infant deaths. Predisposing risk factors include macrosomia, prematurity, cephalopelvic disproportion, dystocia, prolonged labor, and breech presentation (Behrman et al., 1996). Birth injuries include caput succedaneum, cephalhematoma, subcutaneous fat necrosis of the face or scalp, fractures of the skull, subconjunctival and retinal hemorrhages, intracranial hemorrhage, peripheral nerve palsies (brachial, phrenic, facial), fractured clavicle or humerus, ruptured liver or spleen, and hypoxic-ischemic insults. Proper steps to monitor and treat an infant with perinatal complications and injuries must be undertaken immediately after birth. The NP must be familiar with perinatal conditions that subject the newborn to a higher risk and be prepared to intervene quickly based on the available perinatal information.

ASSESSMENT OF THE NEONATE

History

The history includes the following:

- Past maternal history
- Past obstetrical history
  - Number of previous pregnancies, number born alive
  - Number of elective or spontaneous abortions, preterm and term deliveries
  - Health status of living children; if deceased, age and cause of death
  - Cesarean deliveries and indications for them
- Family history
  - Genetically acquired conditions, birth defects, mental retardation, or other diseases

T A B L E 39-1
High-Risk Infants

DEMOGRAPHIC SOCIAL FACTORS
Maternal age <16 or >40 yr
Developmentally delayed mother
Illicit drug, alcohol, cigarette use
Poverty
Unmarried
Emotional or physical stress

PAST MEDICAL HISTORY
Diabetes mellitus
Hypertension
Asymptomatic bacteriuria
Rheumatological illness (SLE)
Chronic medication

PRIOR PREGNANCY
Intrauterine fetal demise
Neonatal death
Prematurity
Intrauterine growth retardation
Congenital malformation
Incompetent cervix
Blood group sensitization, neonatal jaundice
Neonatal thrombocytopenia
Hydrops
Inborn errors of metabolism

PRESENT PREGNANCY
Vaginal bleeding (abruptio placentae, placenta
   previa)
Sexually transmitted diseases (colonization:
   herpes simplex, group B streptococcus)
Multiple gestation
Preeclampsia
Premature rupture of membranes
Short interpregnancy time
Poly- or oligohydramnios
Acute medical or surgical illness
Inadequate prenatal care

LABOR AND DELIVERY
Premature labor (<37 wk)
Postdates (>42 wk)
Fetal distress
Immature L/S ratio: absent
   phosphatidylglycerol
Breech presentation
Meconium-stained fluid
Nuchal cord
Cesarean delivery
Forceps delivery
Apgar score <4 at 1 min

NEONATE
Birthweight <2500 or >4000 g
Birth before 37 or after 42 wk of gestation
SGA, LGA growth status
Tachypnea, cyanosis
Congenital malformation
Pallor, plethora, petechiae

SLE = systemic lupus erythematosus; SGA = small for gestational age; LGA = large for gestational age; L/S = lecithin-sphingomyelin ratio.
   From Behrman RE, Kliegman RM, Arvin AM (eds): Nelson Textbook of Pediatrics, 15th ed. Philadelphia, WB Saunders, 1996, p 440.

- ○ Hypertension, hyperlipidemias, heart disease, or familial cancers
- ○ Age and health status of other living relatives
- ○ Causes of death of family members
- Current obstetrical history
- Medical history
  - ○ Age of mother
  - ○ Prenatal care
  - ○ Infections, illnesses, medications during pregnancy
  - ○ Hypertension or glucose intolerance
  - ○ Duration of labor, duration of ruptured membranes, and presentation and route of delivery
  - ○ Polyhydramnios (excessive fluid) or oligohydramnios (little to no fluid)
  - ○ Infant meconium stained or amniotic fluid foul-smelling
  - ○ Forceps used
  - ○ Fever
- Social history
  - ○ Emotional stressors during pregnancy
  - ○ Unplanned or unwanted pregnancy
  - ○ Financial and emotional support
  - ○ Alcohol, cigarettes, or drugs used during pregnancy
  - ○ Educational background of parents
  - ○ Father's anticipated involvement in raising infant

Physical Examination

IMMEDIATELY AFTER BIRTH

APGAR SCORE. Immediate evaluation of the newborn infant at 1 and 5 minutes of age is a valuable routine procedure. An Apgar score is assigned to the baby based on the criteria in Table 39–2.

- Apgar score 8 to 10
  - ○ Vigorous, pink, and crying
  - ○ Requires only warming, drying, gentle stimulation
  - ○ Occasionally requires oxygen for a short period of time
- Apgar score 5 to 7
  - ○ Cyanotic
  - ○ Slow, irregular respirations
  - ○ Good muscle tone and reflexes
  - ○ Responds to bag-and-mask ventilation
- Apgar score 4 or less
  - ○ Limp, pale, or blue
  - ○ Apneic, slow heart rate
  - ○ Maximal resuscitative efforts with bag and mask, chest compressions, intravenous volume expansion, and drug therapy

The 5-minute Apgar score is an indication of how well the resuscitation efforts have succeeded. Caution must be exercised when using the Apgar score to predict long-term outcomes of mortality and developmental delay. Only when combined with other factors such as fetal status, umbilical cord or scalp blood pH, evidence of organ injury, or seizures can the Apgar score be useful in determining long-term outcome (Goodwin, 1997).

GESTATIONAL AGE. Assessment of an infant's gestational age is based on the physical examination. The assessment is:

- Done promptly after birth to confirm maternal factors (Fig. 39–2)

T A B L E   39-2
Apgar Scores

SIGN	SCORE		
	0	1	2
Heart rate (bpm)	Absent	Slow (<100)	>100
Respiratory effort	Absent	Weak cry; hypoventilation	Good; strong cry
Muscle tone	Limp	Some flexion of extremities	Well flexed
Reflex irritability (response of skin stimulation to feet)	No response	Some motion	Cry
Color	Blue; pale	Body pink; extremities blue	Completely pink

From Apgar V: Evaluation of the newborn infant. Second report. JAMA 168:1985, 1958.

MATURATIONAL ASSESSMENT OF GESTATIONAL AGE (New Ballard Score)

NAME _____ SEX _____

HOSPITAL NO. _____ BIRTH WEIGHT _____

RACE _____ LENGTH _____

DATE/TIME OF BIRTH _____ HEAD CIRC. _____

DATE/TIME OF EXAM _____ EXAMINER _____

AGE WHEN EXAMINED _____

APGAR SCORE: 1 MINUTE _____ 5 MINUTES _____ 10 MINUTES _____

NEUROMUSCULAR MATURITY

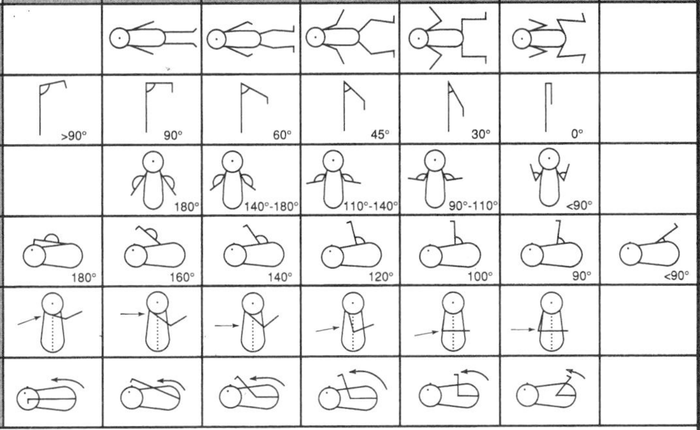

NEUROMUSCULAR MATURITY SIGN	SCORE							RECORD SCORE HERE
	-1	0	1	2	3	4	5	
POSTURE								
SQUARE WINDOW (Wrist)	>90°	90°	60°	45°	30°	0°		
ARM RECOIL		180°	140°-180°	110°-140°	90°-110°	<90°		
POPLITEAL ANGLE	180°	160°	140°	120°	100°	90°	<90°	
SCARF SIGN								
HEEL TO EAR								

TOTAL NEUROMUSCULAR MATURITY SCORE

SCORE
Neuromuscular _____
Physical _____
Total _____

MATURITY RATING

score	weeks
-10	20
-5	22
0	24
5	26
10	28
15	30
20	32
25	34
30	36
35	38
40	40
45	42
50	44

GESTATIONAL AGE (weeks)
By dates _____
By ultrasound _____
By exam _____

PHYSICAL MATURITY

PHYSICAL MATURITY SIGN	SCORE							RECORD SCORE HERE
	-1	0	1	2	3	4	5	
SKIN	sticky friable transparent	gelatinous red translucent	smooth pink visible veins	superficial peeling &/or rash, few veins	cracking pale areas rare veins	parchment deep cracking no vessels	leathery cracked wrinkled	
LANUGO	none	sparse	abundant	thinning	bald areas	mostly bald		
PLANTAR SURFACE	heel-toe 40-50 mm:-1 <40 mm:-2	>50 mm no crease	faint red marks	anterior transverse crease only	creases ant. 2/3	creases over entire sole		
BREAST	imperceptible	barely perceptible	flat areola no bud	stippled areola 1-2 mm bud	raised areola 3-4 mm bud	full areola 5-10 mm bud		
EYE/EAR	lids fused loosely: -1 tightly: -2	lids open pinna flat stays folded	sl. curved pinna; soft; slow recoil	well-curved pinna; soft but ready recoil	formed & firm instant recoil	thick cartilage ear stiff		
GENITALS (Male)	scrotum flat, smooth	scrotum empty faint rugae	testes in upper canal rare rugae	testes descending few rugae	testes down good rugae	testes pendulous deep rugae		
GENITALS (Female)	clitoris prominent & labia flat	prominent clitoris & small labia minora	prominent clitoris & enlarging minora	majora & minora equally prominent	majora large minora small	majora cover clitoris & minora		

TOTAL PHYSICAL MATURITY SCORE

Reference
Ballard JL, Khoury JC, Wedig K, et al: New Ballard Score, expanded to include extremely premature infants. J Pediatr 1991; 119:417-423. Reprinted by permission of Dr Ballard and Mosby-Year Book, Inc.

FIGURE 39-2
Classification of newborns by intrauterine growth and gestational age. (From Ballard JL, Khoury JC, Wedig K, et al: New Ballard Score, expanded to include extremely premature infants. J Pediatr 119:417–423, 1991.)

- Based on the mother's menstrual history, obstetrical milestones achieved during pregnancy, and prenatal ultrasonograms

An infant's length, weight, and fronto-occipital head circumference are measured and plotted on growth curves based on gestational age (Fig. 39-3). Infants whose weights fall above the 90th percentile for age are classified as large for gestational age (LGA); those whose measurements fall below the 10th percentile for age are classified as small for gestational age (SGA). Those whose measurements fall between the 10th and 90th percentiles are classified as appropriate for gestational age (AGA).

TEMPERATURE. Body surface of the newborn infant is approximately 3 times that of the adult relative to weight. Estimated rate of heat loss in the newborn is 4 times that of an adult (Behrman et al., 1996). Body temperature falls precipitously in a cool environment unless adequate precautions are taken.

- Towel-dry infant after birth to prevent evaporative heat loss
- Use radiant warmer
- Wrap infant in warm blankets and cover head to reduce heat loss when baby is to be held by parents

LUNGS. During a vaginal delivery, the squeezing action on an infant's chest as it passes through the pelvis and vagina results in expulsion of amniotic fluid from the lungs. Further expulsion of amniotic fluid from the lungs and reversal of high pulmonary vascular resistance ensue with an infant's first large breaths. Careful bulb suctioning assists in clearing the amniotic fluid from the oropharynx. An infant born by cesarean delivery does not experience the squeezing action of a vaginal birth and is dependent on respiratory efforts and appropriate bulb suctioning to adequately clear the amniotic fluid. Auscultation of the newborn's lungs reveals bronchovesicular or bronchial breath sounds. Fine crackles can be present during the first few hours of life.

UMBILICAL CORD. The normal umbilical cord contains two thick-walled arteries and a single thin-walled vein. Vessel numbers other than this are abnormal and can be associated with congenital anomalies. The umbilical cord is clamped using sterile technique to avoid infection and bleeding.

AFTER STABILIZATION

A more complete physical examination is completed after stabilization (Table 39-3 and Fig. 39-4). When performing the physical, the infant's stage of transition must be considered.

Diagnostic Studies

NEWBORN SCREENING

All states require screening of infants for a variety of congenital abnormalities, although the tests done vary from state to state. Screening panels may include PKU, congenital hypothyroidism, galactosemia, hemoglobin type, homocystinuria, tyrosinemia, maple syrup urine disease, and congenital adrenal hyperplasia. Other testing, such as for cystic fibrosis and the organic acidemias, is being considered by some states. The ideal timing of these tests is usually after the infant is older than 24 hours of age to ensure the baby's feeding and production of metabolites. Early discharge often necessitates repeating some tests (Table 39-4). Two screenings are required in selected states.

SPECIAL SCREENING

Although most infants require no special screening tests, some are at risk for complications in the newborn period. Infants born to mothers with poorly controlled diabetes and LGA or SGA infants are at higher risk for hypo-

Text continued on page 1185

F I G U R E 39-3
Newborn maturity rating and classification. (From Ross Hospital Formula System, Ross Products Division, Abbott Laboratories, Columbus, Ohio; adapted from Battaglia FC, Lubchenco LO: A practical classification of newborn infants by weight and gestational age. J Pediatr 71:159–163, 1967; and Lubchenco LO, Hansman C, Boyd E: Intrauterine growth in length and head circumference as estimated from live births at gestational ages from 26 to 42 weeks. Pediatrics 37:403–408, 1966.)

CLASSIFICATION OF NEWBORNS (BOTH SEXES)
BY INTRAUTERINE GROWTH AND GESTATIONAL AGE [1,2]

NAME_____   DATE OF EXAM_____   LENGTH_____

HOSPITAL NO._____   SEX_____   HEAD CIRC._____

RACE_____   BIRTH WEIGHT_____   GESTATIONAL AGE_____

DATE OF BIRTH_____

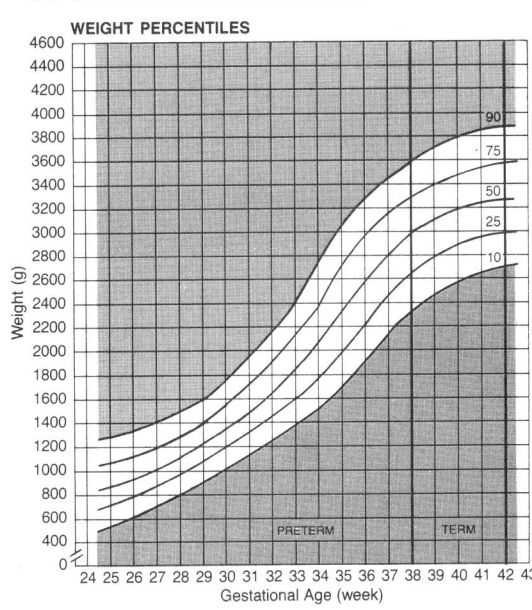

WEIGHT PERCENTILES

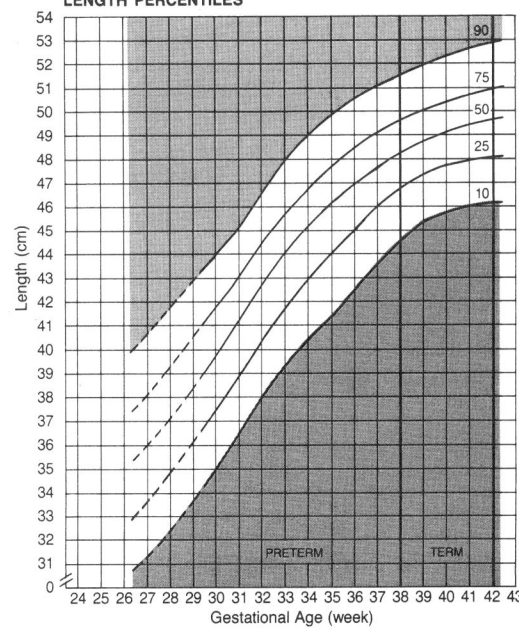

LENGTH PERCENTILES

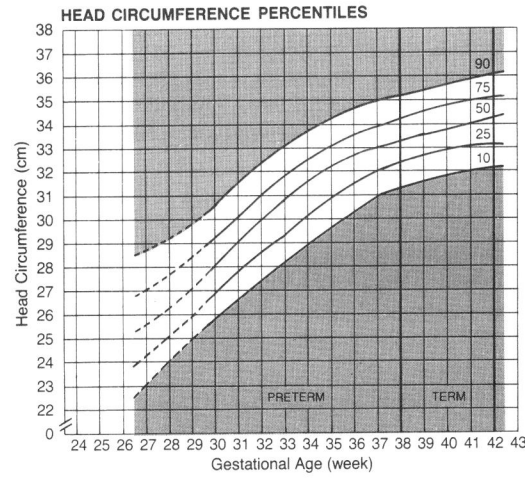

HEAD CIRCUMFERENCE PERCENTILES

CLASSIFICATION OF INFANT*	Weight	Length	Head Circ.
Large for Gestational Age (LGA) (>90th percentile)			
Appropriate for Gestational Age (AGA) (10th to 90th percentile)			
Small for Gestational Age (SGA) (<10th percentile)			

*Place an "X" in the appropriate box (LGA, AGA or SGA) for weight, for length and for head circumference.

References
1. Battaglia FC, Lubchenco LO: A practical classification of newborn infants by weight and gestational age. J Pediatr 1967; 71:159-163.
2. Lubchenco LO, Hansman C, Boyd E: Intrauterine growth in length and head circumference as estimated from live births at gestational ages from 26 to 42 weeks. Pediatrics 1966; 37:403-408.

Reprinted by permission from Dr Battaglia, Dr Lubchenco, Journal of Pediatrics and Pediatrics.

A service of **SIMILAC® WITH IRON** Infant Formula

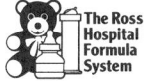

The Ross Hospital Formula System

A5860(0.05)/JULY 1993

ROSS PRODUCTS DIVISION
ABBOTT LABORATORIES
COLUMBUS, OHIO 43215-1724

LITHO IN USA

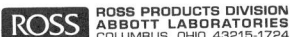

FIGURE 39-3
See legend on opposite page

T A B L E 39-3

Physical Examination Findings

SYSTEM	FINDINGS
Vital signs and measurements	• Check vital signs frequently in the first hours after birth, then every 6 to 8 h when stable • Evaluate ability to maintain temperature above 97°F after transition to extrauterine environment. *Failure to maintain temperature* requires evaluation for other problems, particularly sepsis • Respirations should remain between 30 and 60 breaths/min • Heart rate should remain between 120 and 160 bpm • Significant molding of the head requires repeated measurements to verify size • Daily weight losses of up to 100 g or so in the first 2–3 days of life are not abnormal, as normal infants excrete a large amount of water in the first days of life. *Weight loss of greater than 10%* is abnormal and often due to poor intake or excessive losses
Skin	• Lanugo and vernix. Lanugo is fine dark hair, prominent over the trunk and shoulders. It is seen in infants born prematurely, becoming less prominent as the gestation approaches term. Thick, greasy, white vernix is more common on prematurely born infants' skin • Dry and cracked skin. This is normal over the first several days of life. If associated with thin subcutaneous fat (parchment-like), it is suggestive of a postmature infant, fetal growth retardation, or both (Behrman et al., 1996) • *Cyanosis.* Acrocyanosis, bluish changes in the color of the hands and feet, and generalized mottling of the skin are frequently noted in the first several days of life when an infant loses body heat. *Central cyanosis* beyond the first few moments of life is abnormal and can represent a significant problem with oxygenation • *Pallor.* Many perinatal events can result in pallor, indicating a significant disruption of the infant's circulatory system. Specific causes include anemia, sepsis, cold stress, hypoglycemia, and seizures • Plethora. An excessively reddish discoloration to the skin can be caused by polycythemia or hyperthermia. Infants born to diabetic mothers can be plethoric • *Meconium staining.* Stress prior to birth can cause the first stool to pass in utero. If this greenish-black meconium remains in the amniotic fluid for a prolonged period, staining of the infant's skin and fingernails results • *Jaundice.* See the discussion of jaundice in the text under Hematological Conditions
Head	• Sutures and molding. Vaginally delivered infants demonstrate some degree of molding, usually elongation of the anteroposterior diameter of the skull; if delivered by cesarean method, there are minimal alterations to the shape of the head • Fontanels. The anterior fontanel is usually about 2–3 cm in diameter; the posterior fontanel is about 1 cm in diameter. Both are usually slightly depressed (see Fig. 39–4)
Face	• Symmetrical structures of the face should be apparent, although unilateral facial edema as a result of delivery conditions can occur normally • Overall view of the face may reveal maxillary or mandibular hypoplasia, distortion, or hemifacial hypoplasia
Eyes	• Size, shape, and position of eyes. Too small or large, too widely spaced, or abnormal upward or downward slanting of palpebral fissures should alert the practitioner to potential congenital problems • Uncoordinated eye movements. Intermittent uncoordinated eye movements (disconjugate gaze) during the first weeks after birth are common, improving by 2 to 4 mo of age and resolving by 6 mo of age. *Fixed disconjugate gaze* is abnormal, even in the neonate

T A B L E 39-3

Physical Examination Findings *Continued*

SYSTEM	FINDINGS
Eyes *Continued*	• Conjunctivae. Reddening in the first 24–48 hr of life due to chemical irritation of the eyes from silver nitrate drops or erythromycin ointment is normal. *Purulent discharge* in the first days or weeks of life can be associated with gonococcus, chlamydia, or herpes. Conjunctival hemorrhages secondary to delivery resolve spontaneously over the first weeks of life • Sclerae. Yellowing is associated with hyperbilirubinemia. Small hemorrhages secondary to delivery resolve spontaneously over the first weeks of life. Thinning of the sclera, common in blacks, is manifested by dark blue or black patches. Blue sclerae are associated with osteogenesis imperfecta • Red reflex. Shining an ophthalmoscope white light through the pupil reveals the "red reflex," a disc ranging from pearly gray to orange in color. *Absence of a red reflex* may indicate the presence of lens opacities secondary to cataracts, congenital infection (rubella), or calcium metabolism abnormality. A *white reflex* can indicate retinoblastoma. Absence of the expected red reflex indicates the need for an immediate ophthalmological evaluation
Ears	• Identify normalcy in the size, rotation, shape, position, and patency of external auditory canal • Presence of low-set ears should prompt careful examination for other dysmorphic features • Abnormalities in shape require thorough physical examination, especially of the genitourinary system • Assessment of hearing is done by noting a startle response to a loud noise, avoiding any tactile sensations such as a wind current on the face due to clapping near the ear. Auditory brain response testing should be ordered for any infant in whom a question of hearing exists • Screening for universal detection of infants with hearing loss is encouraged by the American Academy of Pediatrics (AAP, 1995b). When universal screening is not available, screening of high-risk infants is recommended (e.g., family history, in utero infection, craniofacial anomalies, etc.) • Preauricular skin tags or significant pits should be noted (can be a genetic red flag). See text section on skin dimpling
Nose	• Patency of the nasal passages can be tested by closing the mouth and one nostril at a time or by passing a small catheter into the nasopharynx to see if the passage is clear • Nasal flaring is a sign of respiratory distress that can be caused by any number of abnormalities, including mechanical obstruction, parenchymal lung disease, or acidosis

Mouth	• Size and symmetry of the lips
	  • Thin lips with a smooth philtrum (the area between lips and nose) are associated with fetal alcohol syndrome
	  • *Asymmetrical movements* while crying can be due to nerve palsies or absence of perioral muscles
	• Cleft lip and palate can be associated with midline central nervous system (CNS) abnormalities. Incomplete cleft palates are recognized by digital examination of the mouth for bony defects of the hard palate in the presence of normal palatal mucosa
	• Excessive salivation can be related to reflux of gastric contents or esophageal atresia
	• Epstein pearls are small, white epithelial inclusion cysts on the palate and gums
	• An excessively large tongue can be associated with genetic or metabolic abnormalities such as hypothyroidism or Down syndrome

Table continued on following page

T A B L E 39-3

Physical Examination Findings *Continued*

SYSTEM	FINDINGS
Mouth *Continued*	• Natal teeth are sometimes seen at birth (~1 in 3000 live births). If they are extremely loose, aspiration is a concern. Consultation with a pediatric dentist is indicated

Neck	• Webbing. Redundant skin is seen in trisomy 21, Turner and Noonan syndrome
	• Short neck indicates the possibility of Klippel-Feil syndrome or other vertebral problems
	• Masses
	  • Thyroglossal duct cysts (midline) or branchial cleft cyst (along the edge of the sternocleidomastoid muscles) can be found
	  • Other masses that can be seen include a hematoma in the sternocleidomastoid muscle, cystic hygromas, and, rarely, goiters
	  • Torticollis. Asymmetrical shortening of the sternocleidomastoid muscle results in preferential turning of the head to one side, not to be confused with irritability on neck movement associated with meningitis or subarachnoid hemorrhage. Hematoma of the sternocleidomastoid muscle can result in the development of torticollis and requires early management

Thorax	• Shape, symmetry. Rounded appearance measuring about 2 cm less than the fronto-occipital head circumference (~33 cm)
	  • *Minimization of rounding* occurs with respiratory distress syndrome, atelectasis, and other diseases of decreased expansion of the chest
	  • Accentuation is seen in meconium aspiration
	• Wide-spaced nipples and a shield-like appearance are characteristic of Turner syndrome
	• Chest movement on inspiration should be symmetrical and unlabored. Movement of the abdomen with respirations is normal. *Asymmetrical movement* occurs with unilateral pneumothorax
	• *Intercostal, subcostal, or supracostal retractions* indicate respiratory distress
	• Clavicles. Vaginally delivered large-for-gestational-age babies are especially prone to fractures of the clavicle. (See perinatal injury section in text)
	• Breast bones. Pectus excavatum (concave chest) and pectus carinatum (pigeon chest) are occasionally seen. If severe, both can lead to restrictive lung disease later in life
	• Nipples
	  • Fullness and sometimes secretion of a white milky substance are normal and are secondary to maternal hormonal stimulation
	  • Redness surrounding the nipple, especially with purulent drainage, occurs in neonatal mastitis

Lungs	• General. Coughing, retractions, and an intermittently increased respiratory rate occur immediately after birth, resolving by about 12 hr of age to smooth and unlabored respirations at a rate of 30 to 60 breaths/min • Respiratory distress. *Tachypnea, apnea* (pauses in respiration longer than ~ 15 sec), *grunting* (an infant's attempt to increase functional residual capacity, thereby improving gas exchange), *inter-, sub-,* or *supraclavicular retractions, nasal flaring,* and *central cyanosis* all indicate distress • Auscultation • Rales or crackles are commonly heard immediately after birth as lung fluid is resorbed. Beyond the immediate postpartum period, *rales* can indicate pneumonia, delayed resorption of lung fluid, meconium aspiration, or pulmonary edema

T A B L E   39-3

Physical Examination Findings Continued

SYSTEM	FINDINGS
Lungs *Continued*	• *Unilateral absence of breath sounds* occurs in pneumothorax, atelectasis, and pleural effusion • *Bowel sounds over the chest*, especially with a scaphoid abdomen and significant respiratory distress, indicate a diaphragmatic hernia with displacement of abdominal contents into the chest

Heart	• Inspection. Observe neonate for adequacy of perfusion. Respiratory distress is common with cardiac abnormalities. Edema as a result of cardiac failure is rarely seen in the newborn
	• Palpation
	  • *Point of maximal impulse is displaced* from the fourth left intercostal space with pneumothorax, situs inversus, or dextrocardia
	  • *Thrills* or *heaves* are associated with murmurs and cardiac abnormalities
	• Auscultation. Heart rate is normally 120 to 160 bpm. Detection of skipped beats warrants electrocardiogram. *Heart sounds may be muffled or displaced* in the infant with a pneumothorax
	• Murmurs. Common in the newborn period, many murmurs disappear after a few hours or a few days. Significant murmurs need to be investigated whenever heard
	• Pulses. Brachial or radial pulses are compared with femoral or dorsalis pedis pulses for symmetry of impulse and strength in pulse. Delay or relative weakness of lower extremity pulses occurs in coarctation of the aorta
	• Blood pressure. By Doppler device using a 2.5- to 4.0-cm-wide and 5.0- to 9.0-cm-long cuff, compare with normals for age and gestation. Systolic blood pressures greater than 96 mm Hg are considered significant hypertension in the newborn, while blood pressures exceeding 106 mm Hg are considered severe hypertension (NHBPEP, 1996).

Abdomen	• General
	  • Normal abdomen is slightly protuberant, soft, moves smoothly with respirations, and has fine bowel sounds scattered throughout. *Absent bowel sounds* can indicate ileus
	  • The liver is usually palpated 1–2 cm below the right costal margin; the spleen tip is sometimes felt at the left costal margin; kidneys, deep within lateral aspects of the abdomen measuring 3–4 cm in size, are usually palpable
	  • Pain is indicated by crying, grimacing, or forceful resistance with palpation
	• Umbilical hernias. Midline outpouching from the sternum to the umbilicus is seen with weak abdominal musculature (diastasis recti); a large and protuberant umbilicus occurs with an umbilical hernia
	• Umbilical vessels. The normal cord contains two arteries and a single vein. Absence of the second artery can be associated with congenital abnormalities
	• Vomiting and abdominal distention. Regurgitation of large volumes of feeding is not expected. *Bilious vomiting* is always abnormal and usually a sign of obstruction. *Abdominal distention* with enlargement of any of the organs of the abdomen or failure to pass stool is abnormal. Meconium ileus with failure to pass stool in the first 24–48 hr of life is associated with cystic fibrosis

Genitalia	• Male
	  • The penis should have the urethral opening at the tip of the phallus with completely developed foreskin. Chordee means that the distal end of the penis is bent
	  • Testes not located in the scrotal sac or inguinal canal but retrievable to the scrotum are normal. Testes not located in or relocated in the scrotal sac from the canal are considered to be undescended

Table continued on following page

T A B L E 39-3

Physical Examination Findings *Continued*

SYSTEM	FINDINGS

Genitalia *Continued*	• Hydrocele is identified by transilluminating fluid collection around the testis and is regarded as normal unless associated with inguinal hernia or lasts more than 12 mo
	• Inguinal hernia with displacement of intestines into the scrotal sac is frequently nontransilluminating and is associated with bowel sounds. Inguinal hernias are sometimes apparent and reduced at other times. A surgical consultation is indicated
	• Female
	  • Labia majora are large and completely surround the labia minora
	  • Labia and vagina should be open, often with a white discharge
	  • Blood-tinged fluid in small amounts by day 2–3 is normal
	• *Ambiguous genitalia* are genitalia that do not appear to be completely masculinized or feminized. An endocrine referral is important
	• Anus and rectum. Patency of the rectum and placement of the anus should be noted. A small amount of blood streaking in the diaper, especially with a small anal fissure, is common

Extremities, back, hips	• Molding. Intrauterine constraint and resultant molding cause mild curvatures of the forefeet (metatarsus adductus vs. varus [intoeing or outtoeing]) or the tibia (genu varum [bowleg], genu valgum [knockknee]), or both. See Chapter 38 for more information
	• Contractures of the joints and molding of the bones occur if amniotic fluid was decreased and is abnormal
	• Fractures
	  • Skull fractures can occur as a result of extensive molding of a large head
	  • Femora and humeri can fracture with difficult deliveries and use of instrumentation
	  • *Multiple fractures* can indicate osteogenesis imperfecta
	• Spine. Dimples, hemangiomas, tufts of hair, or other lesions along the spine may be associated with spinal abnormalities such as spina bifida occulta
	• Hips. See Chapter 38 for information about eliciting Ortolani and Barlow signs. Both are indicators of dislocated or dislocatable hips

Neurological examination	• Muscle tone. Observe tone, movement, and symmetry of the extremities while the infant is awake
	• Reflexes. Elicit:
	  • Rooting
	  • Sucking
	  • Palmar grasp
	  • Moro reflex
	  • Ankle clonus (3 to 4 beats of clonus at ankle is normal)
	  • Stepping and placing response
	  • Galant reflex
	  • Asymmetrical tonic neck
	• Cranial nerves. Cranial nerve I (olfactory) is rarely tested. Vision (cranial nerve II) is tested by an infant's response to a bright light. Cranial nerves III, IV, and VI are tested by noting an infant's ability to gaze in all directions, although intermittent disconjugate gaze is normal through 6 mo of age. Adequate sucking and swallowing confirm presence of cranial nerves V, IX, X, and XII. Symmetrical movement of the face with crying confirms presence of cranial nerve VII. Hearing (cranial nerve VIII) is assessed by startle to loud noise

Italicized findings indicate "red flags."

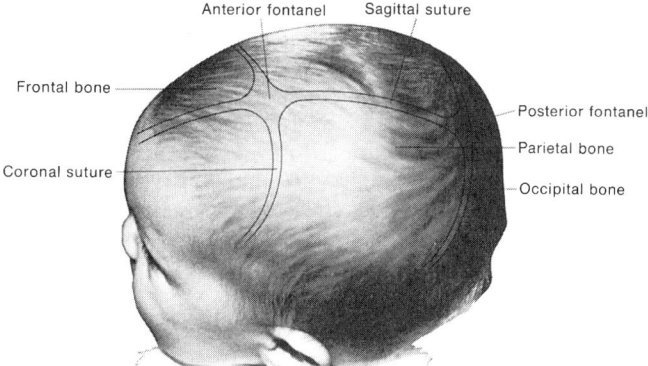

F I G U R E 39-4
Fontanels and sutures. (From Betz CL, Huns-
berger M, Wright S: Family-Centered Nursing
Care of Children, 2nd ed. Philadelphia, WB
Saunders, 1994, p 124.)

glycemia and are screened for serum glucose routinely. Similarly, infants demonstrating Coombs test positivity because of maternal-child blood incompatibility are screened for hemolysis. Some nurseries screen both mothers and infants for syphilis; mothers should be screened for hepatitis B. Hearing screening should be done on all newborns with special attention paid to any newborn at higher risk for hearing loss due to low birth weight, rubella, or other infection; malformation; trauma; asphyxia; prematurity; intensive care unit stay; or antibiotics.

▦ MANAGEMENT STRATEGIES

Initial Care

Following birth, newborns require special care and observation as they make the transition to the extrauterine environment. This was discussed in previous sections of this chapter. Additional components of care include prophylaxis for eye infection with silver nitrate or antibiotic ointment and vitamin K injection for hemorrhagic disease.

Establishing Feeding

Whether breastfeeding or bottle-feeding, infant and parents must be well established in initiating feeding before discharge. Follow-up care must be scheduled to ensure adequate nutrition. See Chapters 12 and 13 for more detailed information on breastfeeding and formulas.

Anticipatory Guidance Prior to Discharge

PHYSICAL CARE

UMBILICAL CORD. Applying alcohol to the base of the cord and tucking the diaper below the cord allows air-drying and speeds cord separation, usually 10 to 14 days after birth. When this occurs, there can be a slight bloody discharge for 1 to 2 days. Counsel the parents to continue applying alcohol until the navel is dry and healed. Belly bands or coins to cover the navel should be avoided, as these increase the chance of infection. If a foul-smelling discharge or erythema appears around the umbilicus, the infant should be evaluated immediately for sepsis. A granuloma sometimes appears after the cord falls off. An application of silver nitrate helps heal the granuloma.

CIRCUMCISION. Circumcision is the removal of the foreskin that normally covers the glans of the penis at birth. There is much controversy regarding its medical necessity and the use of anesthesia during the procedure. The choice remains with the family. Proponents of circumcision claim that it keeps the glans cleaner; there is less chance for developing urinary tract infections (although there is only a 1% chance of urinary tract infections in uncircumcised males); it prevents penile cancer; it prevents phimosis, balanitis, adhesions, and occlusion of the urethral meatus; and the boy will look more like his peers. The opponents of circumcision claim that it does not prevent sexually transmitted disease; that good hygiene prevents penile cancer; that circumcision leaves the glans open

T A B L E 39-4

Newborn Screening

- All infants should be screened before discharge
- All infants screened before 24 hr of age should be rescreened before 14 d of age
- All infants should be tested before the 7th day of life

1. For some diseases, such as phenylketonuria, the infant needs to be fed so that the intake or production of amino acids exceeds the infant's capacity to metabolize or excrete them.
2. Rescreening is now recommended in many states. Nurse practitioners need to be aware of the need for retesting, especially when infants are discharged early.
3. Cord blood is not acceptable for newborn screening because most metabolites accumulate after birth.
4. Filter papers should be used, preferably with 1 drop of blood filling the entire circle. Blood should not be added from the other side of the paper. If a capillary tube is used, it should not touch the paper. For sick infants, venous blood may be used, but care must be taken that no heparin or hyperalimentation components are included. To prevent hemolysis, the needle should not touch the paper.
5. The filter paper must not be contaminated in any way. The specimen should be dried while lying flat and not exposed to heat or sunlight. Remember that mailboxes may be hot in the summer!
6. Demographic data must be clearly written to ensure follow-up of abnormal results.
7. Specimens should be mailed within 24 hr of collection via first-class mail to avoid delays in reaching the laboratory.
8. Premature or sick infants should be screened by the 7th day of life.
9. Transfusions may temporarily affect results, so specimens should be collected before plasma or blood products are administered.

Adapted from Buist N, Tuerck J: The practitioner's role in newborn screening. Pediatr Clin North Am 39:199–211, 1992.

to the chance of cautery burns and meatal stenosis; and fewer boys are being circumcised and, therefore, these boys will not be different from many of their peers.

Contraindications to circumcision include epispadias or hypospadias, ambiguous genitalia, exstrophy of the bladder, familial bleeding disorders, and illness. Complications of circumcisions include infections, bleeding, gangrene, scarring, meatal stenosis, cautery burns, urethral fistula, amputation or trauma to the glans, and pain.

Care of the uncircumcised baby includes gentle cleaning. The skin adheres to the penis and is not retractable at birth but loosens as the baby grows. The parents should be counseled not to force the foreskin back. If the baby is circumcised, the penis should be cleansed daily with cotton balls dipped in tap water followed by the application of a small amount of petroleum jelly to the tip of the penis with each diaper change. The petroleum jelly is needed only for the first 2 to 3 days after the circumcision.

BATHING, OILS, AND POWDERS. Counsel parents to test the temperature of the water before bathing the infant. The infant should not be immersed in a tub of water and should be sponge-bathed until the umbilical cord is off and the navel appears healed. Mild soaps such as Dove, Caress, Neutrogena, and Basis are gentle enough for infants' skin. Encourage parents to hold the baby to make him or her feel secure in the water and to never leave the baby alone in the tub.

Oils and powders are not recommended for infants' skin. Oils and greasy substances tend to clog the skin's pores and can cause acne or rashes. Powders should not be used, because inhaling the talc could lead to respiratory problems. For dry skin, Keri, Eucerin, or Cetaphil lotion is recommended.

DIAPERS. There is much controversy about whether disposable or cloth diapers are the better choice for infants. The need for frequent changing and proper cleansing is the important message to deliver.

SLEEP POSITION

In 1992, the preponderance of available evidence suggested that the prone sleeping position was associated with an increased incidence of sudden infant death syndrome (SIDS). The American Academy of Pediatrics issued a statement in that year suggesting that healthy infants, when being put down for sleep, be positioned on their side or back (AAP, 1992). In 1996 an update statement by the AAP suggested that *healthy* infants continue to be placed in a nonprone position (wholly on the back preferred), that soft surfaces and gas-trapping objects should be avoided in an infant's sleeping environment, and that "tummy time" during the awake period is recommended for development reasons and to help prevent flat spots on the occiput (AAP, 1996). SIDS is discussed later in this chapter.

INJURY PREVENTION

Counsel parents on the appropriate use and installation of a crash-tested safety seat at all times when driving with their infant. They should take the infant home from the hospital in a safety seat. The house should be child-proofed before the infant is taken home. Falls and burns are the most common injuries to neonates. Parents should be counseled to avoid shaking their baby for any reason (Coody et al., 1994). Refer to Chapter 11 for more information.

PARENTING

The parenting role is stressful, even if all goes well. Fatigue and maternal depression resulting from hormonal shifts are common. Encourage parents to identify and make use of supportive people, arrange time for rest and time alone, and keep their expectations reasonable.

Early Discharge and Follow-up

Newborns are often discharged after a minimal time of observation. Although this is a common practice, primarily driven by insurance for financial reasons, infants often experience difficulty with breastfeeding, poor weight gain, jaundice, and dehydration (Thilo & Townsend, 1996). Guidelines for early discharge of normal, healthy newborns are listed in Table 39-5. Plans for follow-up care within 48 to 72 hours as well as for ongoing health maintenance should be confirmed before discharge. Table 39-6 gives guidelines for the 48- to 72-hour follow-up visit of the healthy, normal newborn. Even new-

TABLE 39-5

Guidelines for Early Discharge of Normal, Healthy Newborns

Ante-, intra-, and postpartum course for baby and mother must be normal
Vaginal delivery
Single, appropriate for gestational age, term (38–42 wk) baby
Stable vital signs for at least 12 hr prior to discharge:
Axillary temperature of 36.1–37°C in open crib
Heart rate 100–160 bpm
Respiratory rate < 60/min
Passage of urine and stool
Two successful feedings have been accomplished
Normal physical examination
No excessive bleeding at circumcision site for at least 2 hr
No significant jaundice in first 24 hr
Mother knowledgeable in the care of the infant, including:
Feeding
Normal stool and urine frequency
Skin, genital, and cord care
Ability to identify illness (especially jaundice)
Proper safety (car seat, sleeping position)
Smoke alarms in the home
Social support and continuing health care identified
Infant laboratory data, including maternal syphilis and hepatitis B and infant blood type and Coombs testing completed
Appropriately timed neonatal screening completed
Social situation adequate: include such areas as drug abuse, previous child abuse, mental illness, lack of social support, lack of permanent home, history of domestic violence, or teenage mother
Appropriate early follow-up care within 48 hr of discharge identified

Adapted from American Academy of Pediatrics: Hospital stay for healthy term newborns. Pediatrics 96:788–790, 1995a; and National Association of Pediatric Nurse Associates and Practitioners: Newborn discharge and follow-up care. J Pediatr Health Care 11:147–148, 1997.

borns who are hospitalized longer need follow-up care within the first few days of life. All parents leaving the hospital with a newborn should have a confirmed time and place for follow-up as well as contacts in case of an emergency or questions.

T A B L E 39-6

Guidelines for 48- to 72-Hour Follow-up Visit of the Normal, Healthy Newborn

1. Assess the infant's general health, hydration, and jaundice; identify any new problems; review feeding
2. Assess quality of bonding
3. Reinforce maternal and family education
4. Review outstanding laboratory data
5. Perform neonatal screen if indicated
6. Develop plan for health care maintenance, including emergency care, preventive care, and periodic screenings

Adapted from American Academy of Pediatrics. Hospital stay for healthy term newborns. Pediatrics 96:788–790, 1995.

Premature Infants and Newborns With Special Needs

Premature infants have special needs that must be arranged before discharge. Guidelines for discharge and follow-up of the premature infant are detailed in Table 39–7. Newborns with special needs caused by anomalies, disease states, social situation, or other variables also need arrangements made before discharge to provide support, education, and follow-up.

COMMON NEONATAL CONDITIONS

Skin Conditions

MILIA

Description

Milia are multiple, firm, pearly, opalescent white papules scattered over the forehead, nose, and cheeks. Their intraoral counterparts are called Epstein pearls.

Etiology and Incidence

Histologically, milia represent superficial epidermal inclusion cysts filled with keratinous material associated with the developing pilosebaceous follicle. They are found in 50% of newborns (Hoekelman et al., 1997).

Management

No treatment is necessary because milia exfoliate spontaneously in most infants.

SEBACEOUS HYPERPLASIA

Description

Sebaceous hyperplasia is characterized by prominent yellow-white macules at the opening of each pilosebaceous follicle, predominantly over the nose, forehead, upper lip, and cheeks.

Etiology

The overgrowth of sebaceous glands in response to the same androgenic stimulation that occurs in adolescence causes sebaceous hyperplasia.

Management

No treatment is required. These tiny papules diminish in size and disappear entirely within the first few weeks of life.

ERYTHEMA TOXICUM

Description

Firm, yellow-white 1- to 2-mm papules or pustules with a surrounding erythematous flare characterize erythema toxicum. Lesions are clustered in several sites.

Etiology and Incidence

These lesions usually develop at 24 to 48 hours of age. The cause is unknown, although examination of a Wright-stained smear of the lesion reveals numerous eosinophils. Up to 50% of infants develop erythema toxicum, with the incidence higher in term than in premature infants.

Differential Diagnosis

Pyoderma, candidiasis, herpes simplex, transient neonatal pustular melanosis, and miliaria should be considered (Table 39–8).

T A B L E   39-7

Guidelines for Discharge and Follow-up of the Premature Infant

DISCHARGE PLANNING

Identify all active medical or social problems through a review of the medical record and physical
  examination of infant
Ensure adequacy of immunizations based on infant's chronological age
Screen for anemia and begin iron or vitamins if necessary
Review with family member medications, feeding schedules, signs of illness, and appropriate response
  for infants with active medical conditions
Identify family and community resources if infant is to be discharged on home oxygen therapy
Ensure adequate training of family members in cardiopulmonary resuscitation and, if applicable, on home
  apnea monitor use
Counsel family in car seat adaptations for the premature infant
Consider need for visiting nurse, social service, respite care, support groups, or referral to the Women,
  Infants, and Children (WIC) Program

FOLLOW-UP PLANNING

Schedule audiograms (if not already done) for infants with
  Craniofacial abnormalities
  In utero infections
  Birth weight <1500 g
  Meningitis
  Exchange transfusion for hyperbilirubinemia
  Use of ototoxic medications
  Apgar score of 0–4 at 1 min or 0–6 at 5 min
  Mechanical ventilation for ≥5 d
  Stigmata of syndrome associated with hearing loss
  Family history of deafness
Schedule at 4–6 wk chronological age a dilated indirect ophthalmoscopic examination for neonates with
  a birth weight ≤1500 g or with a gestational age of ≤28 wk as well as those infants >1500 g with an
  unstable clinical course felt to be at high risk for retinopathy of prematurity by their attending
  physician (AAP, AAPOS, and AAO, 1997)
Follow-up visits every 1–2 wk, especially if infant is on oxygen therapy
Growth and development should be of prime interest at each routine outpatient visit with referral for
  formal developmental assessment if any concerns are identified

---

Management

No treatment is required because the course is brief and transient.

TRANSIENT NEONATAL PUSTULAR MELANOSIS

Description

Transient neonatal pustular melanosis is characterized by superficial vesiculopustules that rupture easily and leave a halo of white scales around a central pinhead-sized macule of hyperpigmentation.

Etiology and Incidence

This melanosis is caused by increased melanization of the epidermal cells, with sites of predilection being the trunk, limbs, palms, and soles. It is more common in black than in white infants.

Differential Diagnosis

Pyoderma and erythema toxicum are the differential diagnoses.

Management

No treatment is required. The pustular phase rarely lasts more than 2 to 3 days; hyperpig-

T A B L E 39-8

Erythema Toxicum vs. Herpes Simplex Virus (HSV)

ERYTHEMA TOXICUM	HERPES SIMPLEX VIRUS
Benign, self-limited	Pathological, progressive
No specific maternal history	Frequently a history of maternal disease
Usually seen only in term infants	Can occur in infants of any gestational age
Begins on the 2nd or 3rd day of life, lasting as long as 1 wk	Often begins late in the 1st week of life or early in the 2nd week of life
Rash is evanescent, often involving the face, trunk, and extremities	Can be superficial and localized only to the presenting part (vertex or buttocks) or widespread and disseminated without cutaneous involvement
1- to 2-mm white papules or pustules on an erythematous base which occasionally may become vesicular	May present similar to sepsis without cutaneous findings, or as grouped vesicles on an erythematous base on the presenting part about days 9–11 of life
Wright or Giemsa stain of lesion scraping demonstrates large numbers of eosinophils and no organisms; cultures are sterile	Direct fluorescent antibody staining or enzyme-linked immunoassay detection of HSV antigens of vesicle scrapings, or growth of the organism from vesicle fluid are diagnostic
No specific therapy necessary	Acyclovir

mented macules can persist for as long as 3 months.

SUCKING BLISTERS

Description

Sucking blisters are solitary or scattered superficial bullae on the upper limbs and lips of infants at birth, commonly found on the radial aspect of the forearm, the thumb, and the index finger.

Etiology

These blisters result from vigorous sucking on the affected part in utero.

Management

No treatment is required. These bullae resolve rapidly without sequelae.

CUTIS MARMORATA

Description

Cutis marmorata is a lacy, reticulated red or blue cutaneous vascular pattern appearing over most of the body surface.

Etiology

The vascular change is a response to exposure to low environmental temperatures. It represents an accentuated physiological vasomotor response that disappears with increasing age. Persistent and pronounced cutis marmorata occurs in Down and trisomy 18 syndromes.

Management

Cutis marmorata usually resolves with warming of the infant.

HARLEQUIN COLOR CHANGE

Description

Harlequin color change is a division of the body skin coloring from forehead to pubis into red and pale halves.

Etiology

The cause is unknown.

Management

No treatment is indicated, as this is a transient and benign condition.

MONGOLIAN SPOTS, CAFÉ-AU-LAIT SPOTS, SALMON PATCH (NEVUS SIMPLEX), AND PORT-WINE STAIN (NEVUS FLAMMEUS, PORT-WINE NEVUS)

See Chapter 37 for a discussion of these skin conditions.

NEVUS SEBACEUS

Description

Nevus sebaceus is a yellowish, hairless, sharply demarcated smooth plaque on the head and neck.

Etiology

Histologically, these nevi contain an abundance of sebaceous glands. With maturity, usually during adolescence, the lesions become verrucous with large rubbery nodules. During adulthood, the lesions are complicated by secondary malignancies, most commonly basal cell carcinoma.

Management

The treatment is total excision before onset of adolescence. Referral to a dermatologist is indicated.

SKIN DIMPLING

Description

Skin dimpling is the presence of deep skin dimples over bony prominences and in the sacral area.

Etiology

Skin dimples, as well as pits and creases, occur in normal children as well as in some dysmorphological syndromes such as congenital rubella, deletion of the long arm of chromosome 18, and the cerebrohepatorenal syndromes.

Management

No treatment is indicated.

PREAURICULAR SINUS TRACTS AND PITS

Description

Sinus tracts and pits occur anterior to the pinna.

Etiology

Resulting from imperfect fusion of the tubercles of the first and second branchial arches during gestational development, tracts and pits can be unilateral or bilateral; they are familial, more common in females and blacks, and occasionally associated with other anomalies of the ears and face.

Management

Excision is required if tracts and pits are chronically infected and draining.

AMNIOTIC CONSTRICTION BANDS

Description

Fibrous strands that encircle fetal parts and cause permanent depression of the underlying tissue produce defects in the extremities and digits.

Etiology

Found in otherwise normal infants, bands are thought to result from intrauterine rupture of the amnion with formation of fibrous strands. Sometimes there are associated abnormalities, including craniofacial anomalies and thoracic or abdominal wall defects.

Management

Treatment depends on the severity of deformities produced. Constriction bands on the limbs can be removed by plastic surgery.

SUPERNUMERARY NIPPLES

Description

Solitary or multiple accessory nipples and sometimes areolae occur in unilateral or bilateral distribution along a line from the midaxilla to the inguinal area.

Etiology

The cause is unknown. Urinary tract anomalies can occur in children with this finding.

Management

Usually no treatment is necessary unless the accessory nipple becomes symptomatic.

BRANCHIAL CLEFT AND THYROGLOSSAL CYSTS AND SINUSES

Description

Cysts and sinuses in the neck can be unilateral or bilateral and open onto the cutaneous surface or drain into the pharynx. Thyroglossal cysts and fistulas are similar defects located in or near the midline of the neck, extending to the base of the tongue. Thyroglossal cysts occasionally contain aberrant thyroid tissue as well as mucinous material.

Etiology

Cysts and sinuses in the neck can be formed along the course of the first and second branchial clefts as a result of improper closure during embryonic life. These anomalies can be inherited as autosomal dominant traits.

Management

Antibiotic therapy for infections of the cysts or sinuses is indicated. Surgical excision is recommended for thyroglossal cysts.

Head, Face, and Eye Conditions

CAPUT SUCCEDANEUM

Description

Caput succedaneum is a diffuse swelling of the soft tissue of the scalp with possible bruising; the swelling which usually crosses the suture lines (Fig. 39-5).

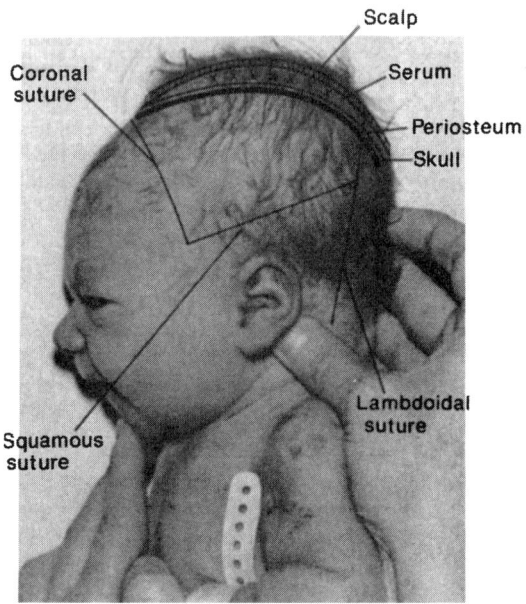

F I G U R E 39-5
Caput succedaneum. (From Betz CL, Hunsberger M, Wright S: Family-Centered Nursing Care of Children, 2nd ed. Philadelphia, WB Saunders, 1994, p 124.)

Etiology

Caput succedaneum originates from trauma to the baby while descending through the birth canal.

Clinical Findings

HISTORY. Primigravida and traumatic delivery may be part of the history.

PHYSICAL EXAMINATION. Findings include the following:

- Obvious swelling and bruising in the parietal regions of the scalp
- Swelling that crosses suture lines
- Frequently associated with molding

Differential Diagnosis

Cephalhematoma is the differential diagnosis.

Management

No treatment is necessary, as swelling resolves spontaneously over a few days.

CEPHALHEMATOMA

Description

Cephalhematoma is a collection of blood in the subperiosteal area of the scalp that does not cross over the suture lines. There is usually no noticeable bruising of the area (Fig. 39–6).

Etiology

Cephalhematoma results from trauma occurring during a difficult delivery. The swelling appears hours to days after delivery.

Clinical Findings

HISTORY. Primigravida and traumatic delivery may be part of the history.

PHYSICAL EXAMINATION. Findings include the following:

- Swelling in the parietal area that does not cross over suture lines
- Rarely associated with a skull fracture, coagulopathy, or intracranial hemorrhage

Differential Diagnosis

Caput succedaneum and cranial meningocele should be considered.

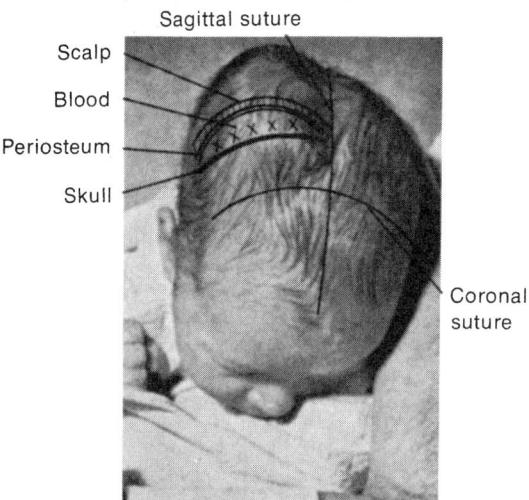

F I G U R E 39-6
Cephalhematoma. (From Betz CL, Hunsberger M, Wright S: Family-Centered Nursing Care of Children, 2nd ed. Philadelphia, WB Saunders, 1994, p 124.)

Management

No treatment is needed because the condition resolves in a few weeks to months. Calcification of the hematoma occurs, which can be felt as bony prominences. Observe for hyperbilirubinemia.

CRANIOTABES

Description

Craniotabes is thinning of the bone of the scalp.

Etiology

This is a normal variation of the parietal bone, usually near the sagittal suture line.

Clinical Findings

HISTORY. Prematurity can be part of the history.

PHYSICAL EXAMINATION. Findings include a "ping-pong ball" effect when pressing on the parietal bone.

Management

No treatment is necessary because craniotabes resolves spontaneously. If persistent, pathological causes such as rickets should be investigated.

CLEFT LIP AND PALATE

Description

Cleft lip is failure of embryonic structures surrounding the oral cavity to join. Cleft palate appears when there is a failure of the palatal shelves to fuse. There are various degrees of clefts.

Etiology and Incidence

Genetic factors influence the development of cleft lip more than cleft palate; however, both occur sporadically. A combination of cleft lip and cleft palate is more common than one without the other. Cleft lip with or without cleft palate occurs in 1 in 1000 births. Cleft palate alone occurs in 1 in 2500 births (Behrman et al., 1996). Clefts are more common in males than in females.

Clinical Findings

PHYSICAL EXAMINATION. Findings include the following:

- Degree of cleft varies from a small notch to a complete separation
- Unilateral or bilateral
- Involves soft palate, hard palate, or both
- Bifid uvula indicates a submucosal cleft palate

Management

Surgical repair is indicated, and the timing is individualized. Special nipples and feeding techniques are used until surgery can be performed. Breastfeeding and bottle-feeding are successful depending on the severity of the cleft. Speech evaluation and perhaps therapy are necessary in later years. Dental restoration is often needed. Team management is often beneficial.

Complications

Middle ear, nasopharyngeal, sinus infections, and associated hearing loss can occur.

CONGENITAL CATARACTS AND GLAUCOMA

See Chapter 29.

Cardiac Conditions

See Chapter 31.

Respiratory Conditions

RESPIRATORY DISTRESS SYNDROME

Description

Respiratory distress syndrome (RDS), also known as hyaline membrane disease, occurs secondary to atelectasis of the lungs. This is the most common pulmonary disease in the newborn (Table 39-9).

Etiology and Incidence

Surfactant deficiency is the underlying cause of the disease, resulting in alveolar atelectasis and decreased lung compliance. The incidence is 1% of all live births but only 0.5% of term births. The incidence rises rapidly below the gestational age of 33 to 34 weeks. An estimated 50% of all neonatal deaths result from RDS or its complications (Behrman et al., 1996). The incidence increases with decreasing gestational age and size.

Clinical Findings

HISTORY. The history can include the following:

- Diabetic mother
- Preterm delivery
- Multiple prior pregnancies
- Cesarean delivery
- Precipitous delivery
- Asphyxia
- Cold stress
- Previous affected siblings

PHYSICAL EXAMINATION. Findings include the following:

- Tachypnea
- Grunting
- Intercostal retractions
- Nasal flaring
- Duskiness, cyanosis
- Breath sounds normal or diminished with harsh tubular quality
- Fine rales on deep inspiration

RADIOLOGICAL AND LABORATORY FINDINGS. A radiograph of the chest shows a fine reticular granularity of the parenchyma and air bronchograms. Blood gas results indicate hypoxemia, hypercarbia, and metabolic acidosis.

Management

Supportive care and mechanical ventilation are used as indicated. The immediate use of

T A B L E 39-9

Clinical Comparison of Transient Tachypnea of the Newborn and Respiratory Distress Syndrome (RDS)

TRANSIENT TACHYPNEA OF THE NEWBORN	RESPIRATORY DISTRESS SYNDROME
Seen only in infants delivered at or near term, often in infants born by cesarean section	Found only in premature infants, with the greatest incidence in infants weighing <1500 g
Increased respiratory rate is invariably present; grunting and intercostal retractions are not common	Usually, respiratory rate is increased, infants grunt at expiration, nasal flaring is noted, and sternal and intercostal retractions are commonly seen
Cyanosis is not a prominent feature	Cyanosis in room air is a prominent feature
Air exchange is good; rales and rhonchi are usually absent	Auscultation reveals diminished air entry
Begins at birth, usually resolving in the first 24–48 hr of life	Often begins late in the 1st wk of life or early in the 2nd wk of life
Chest radiograph shows central perihilar streaking with slightly enlarged heart	Chest radiograph demonstrates reticulogranular, ground-glass appearance and air bronchograms
Typical course involves gradual decrease in respiratory rate with resolution in the 1st 5 d of life	Course variable depending on infant's gestational weight and age; classically, RDS begins to improve after about 72 hr of symptoms
No specific therapy other than maintaining oxygenation is usually necessary	Artificial surfactant, as well as administration of steroids to the mother, can reduce the severity of this disease; mechanical ventilation is commonly needed

exogenous surfactant has been found to reduce the long-term respiratory sequelae in larger preterm infants (Abbasi et al., 1993).

Prognosis

The prognosis depends on the severity of the disease and the birth weight of the infant.

Prevention

The only effective preventive measure is prevention of prematurity. Administration of synthetic corticosteroids to women who do not have toxemia, diabetes, or renal damage 48 to 72 hours prior to delivery is also used to reduce the severity of the problem.

TRANSIENT TACHYPNEA OF THE NEWBORN

Description

Transient tachypnea of the newborn (TTN) is a respiratory condition that results from in-

complete evacuation of fetal lung fluid in full-term infants.

Etiology

TTN results from decreased pulmonary compliance and tidal volume and increased dead space secondary to slow absorption of fetal lung fluid. It is more common in cesarean deliveries.

Clinical Findings

HISTORY. TTN usually disappears within 24 to 48 hours.

PHYSICAL EXAMINATION. Findings include the following:

- Tachypnea
- Expiratory grunting
- Paucity of auscultation findings
- Intercostal retractions
- Cyanosis that responds to minimal oxygen

RADIOLOGICAL FINDINGS. A chest radiograph shows prominent pulmonary vascular markings, fluid lines along fissures, overaeration, flat diaphragms, and occasionally, pleural fluid.

Differential Diagnosis

The differential diagnosis is RDS (see Table 39-9).

Management

If the infant is not in significant respiratory distress, close observation and transcutaneous oxygen saturation monitoring can be sufficient until the tachypnea resolves. The need for supplemental oxygen therapy provided in a hood should be based on close oxygen monitoring. The use of mechanical ventilation in TTN is rare.

Prognosis

Infants usually recover rapidly within 24 to 48 hours with no treatment.

MECONIUM ASPIRATION SYNDROME

Description

Meconium aspiration syndrome occurs in term or post-term infants. This syndrome is a serious pulmonary disorder characterized by small airway obstruction, chemical pneumonitis, and secondary respiratory distress.

Etiology and Incidence

Fetal distress and anoxia increase intestinal peristalsis and relax the anal sphincter to release meconium into the amniotic fluid. Thick meconium is aspirated either in utero or with the first breath. Approximately 5 to 15% of all newborns are meconium stained, but only a fraction of these infants develop respiratory problems.

Clinical Findings

HISTORY. The history includes meconium in the amniotic fluid and below the vocal cords on resuscitation.

PHYSICAL EXAMINATION. Findings include the following:

- Tachypnea
- Intercostal retractions
- Grunting
- Cyanosis within hours of delivery

RADIOLOGICAL FINDINGS. A chest radiograph shows patchy infiltrates, coarse streaking of both lung fields, and flattening of the diaphragm.

Management

An infant born with meconium present in the amniotic fluid should undergo suctioning of the mouth and hypopharynx immediately after delivery of the head. Depressed infants and those delivered through thick meconium should undergo visualization of the larynx with removal of any meconium noted. Infants with meconium in the larynx or those who remain depressed should receive endotracheal intubation, with suction applied directly to the endotracheal tube to remove meconium from the airway. Treatment includes supportive care and standard management of respiratory distress. Severe meconium aspiration cases are managed by extracorporeal membrane oxygenation (ECMO).

Prognosis

The mortality of meconium-stained infants is higher than that of nonstained infants. Meconium aspiration accounts for a significant proportion of neonatal deaths. Residual lung problems are possible. Ultimate prognosis depends on the extent of central nervous system (CNS) injury from asphyxia.

Prevention

DeLee suctioning after the infant's head is delivered reduces the risk of meconium aspiration, because the baby probably will not have breathed deeply yet.

Gastrointestinal and Abdominal Conditions

ESOPHAGEAL ATRESIA AND TRACHEOESOPHAGEAL FISTULA

Description

In esophageal atresia, a blind pouch occurs in the esophagus with or without an associated fistula. Most infants have a proximal pouch, with the associated fistula connecting the distal esophagus and the trachea (Fig. 39-7).

Incidence

This occurs in 1 in 4000 births. Approximately one third of affected infants are born prematurely (Behrman et al., 1996; Ein, 1993).

Clinical Findings

HISTORY. The history includes maternal polyhydramnios and inability to pass a nasogastric tube during resuscitation at birth.

PHYSICAL EXAMINATION. Findings include the following:

- Excessive oral secretions that require frequent suctioning
- Choking, coughing, and cyanosis, particularly during feedings

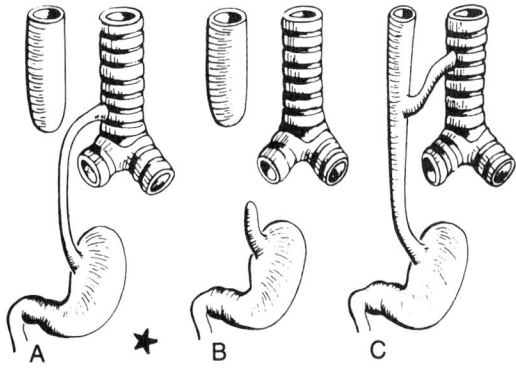

FIGURE 39-7
The three most common types of esophageal atresia and tracheoesophageal fistula (TEF). (From Ein SH: Esophageal atresia and TEF. *In* Wyllie R, Hyams JS [eds]: Wyllie & Hyams Pediatric Gastrointestinal Disease. Philadelphia, WB Saunders, 1993, pp 318–336.)

RADIOLOGICAL FINDINGS. Chest and abdominal radiographs show the nasogastric tube coiled in the thoracic region. Barium swallow demonstrates the exact location of the atresia and rules out tracheoesophageal fistula.

Differential Diagnosis

RDS, meconium aspiration, and congenital heart disease should be considered.

Management

This is a surgical emergency requiring immediate intervention. Preoperatively, the infant should be placed in a prone position and suctioned frequently. A nasogastric tube can be inserted into the blind pouch to prevent aspiration until surgical repair can be accomplished.

Complications

Pneumonia, atelectasis, aspiration, strictures, and repeated surgery are possible.

Prognosis

The survival rate postoperatively is almost 100% unless other congenital anomalies are present. Approximately 30% of affected infants have other congenital anomalies, most commonly cardiovascular defects.

DUODENAL ATRESIA

Description

Duodenal atresia is a complete obstruction of the duodenum, ending blindly just distal to the ampulla of Vater.

Incidence

Duodenal atresia occurs in 1 in 18,000 births. It is associated with other anomalies in 30% of cases; Down syndrome in 20% of cases, and prematurity in 25% of cases (Behrman & Kliegman, 1998).

Clinical Findings

HISTORY. The following may be assessed:

- Maternal polyhydramnios
- Down syndrome
- Premature birth

PHYSICAL EXAMINATION. Findings include the following:

- Bile-stained vomitus
- Abdominal distention
- Jaundice

RADIOLOGICAL FINDINGS. Abdominal radiographs show a "double-bubble" pattern in the upright position secondary to air in the stomach and a distended duodenum.

Differential Diagnosis

Malrotation, duodenal obstruction, and annular pancreas should be considered.

Management

Surgical intervention is indicated. Feedings should be discontinued and gastric suctioning applied.

Prognosis

The prognosis depends on early identification and treatment.

Complications

Aspiration of gastric contents can occur.

VOLVULUS

Description

Volvulus is the twisting of a loop of bowel, causing intermittent or acute pain and obstruction.

Clinical Findings

PHYSICAL EXAMINATION. Findings include abdominal distention and bilious vomiting.
RADIOLOGICAL FINDINGS. Intestinal obstruction is demonstrated on abdominal radiograph.

Management

Surgical repair and fluid replacement are indicated.

Differential Diagnosis

Duodenal obstruction or atresia and annular pancreas are in the differential diagnosis.

Prognosis

The prognosis depends on identification and the urgency of surgery.

Complications

Perforation, necrosis of the bowel, sepsis, and peritonitis are possible.

PYLORIC STENOSIS

Description

Pyloric stenosis is characterized by hypertrophied pyloric muscle, causing a narrowing of the pyloric sphincter.

Incidence

Pyloric stenosis occurs in 1 in 150 males and 1 in 750 females (Behrman et al., 1996). It tends to be familial and is seen predominantly in white first-born males.

Clinical Findings

HISTORY. The history can include the following:

- Regurgitation and nonprojectile vomiting during the first few weeks of life
- Projectile vomiting beginning at 2 to 3 weeks of age
- Insatiable appetite with weight loss, dehydration, and constipation

PHYSICAL EXAMINATION. Findings include the following:

- Weight loss
- Vomitus is nonbilious and can contain blood

- A distinct "olive" mass palpated in the epigastrium to the right of midline
- Reverse peristalsis visualized across the abdomen

RADIOLOGICAL FINDINGS. An upper gastrointestinal series demonstrates a "string sign," indicating a fine, elongated pyloric canal.

Management

Surgical intervention (pyloromyotomy) is indicated after correction of fluid and electrolyte imbalance. Vomiting can continue for a few days after surgery, so feedings should be introduced gradually.

Prognosis

The prognosis is excellent.

HIRSCHSPRUNG DISEASE (CONGENITAL AGANGLIONIC MEGACOLON)

Description

Hirschsprung disease is an absence of ganglion cells in the bowel wall, most often in the rectosigmoid region, resulting in a portion of the colon having no motility.

Incidence

This disorder occurs in 1 in 5000 births. It is the most common cause of neonatal obstruction of the colon and accounts for 33% of all neonatal obstructions (Behrman et al., 1996). The disease is familial and is common in children with trisomy 21. Additional anomalies are sometimes present.

Clinical Findings

HISTORY. The following may be assessed:

- Failure to pass meconium within the first week of life
- Failure to thrive
- Poor feeding
- Chronic constipation

PHYSICAL EXAMINATION. Findings include the following:

- Vomiting
- Abdominal obstruction
- Failure to pass stools
- Diarrhea, explosive bowel movements, or flatus

RADIOLOGICAL AND LABORATORY FINDINGS. Radiographs indicate dilated loops of bowel (Fig. 39-8). A biopsy determines the absence of ganglion cells.

Differential Diagnosis

The differential diagnosis includes acquired functional megacolon, colonic inertia, chronic idiopathic constipation, obstipation, small left colon syndrome, meconium plug syndrome, and ileal atresia with microcolon.

Management

Surgical resection of the affected bowel is indicated, with or without a colostomy.

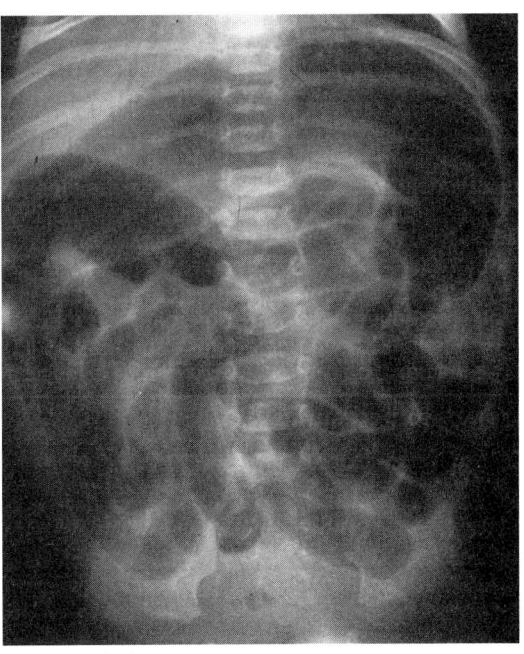

F I G U R E 39-8
Dramatic dilatation of bowel consistent with Hirschprung disease. (Photo courtesy of Lawrence H. Robinson, Associate Professor of Radiology and Pediatrics, University of Texas Medical School, Houston, Texas.)

IMPERFORATE ANUS

Description

Imperforate anus is the lack of a rectal opening.

Incidence

This condition occurs in 1 in 3500 to 9500 births.

Clinical Findings

HISTORY. The history includes no passage of meconium.

PHYSICAL EXAMINATION. Findings include no obvious opening in the rectal area.

RADIOLOGICAL FINDINGS. Endoscopic examination and ultrasound indicate the degree of malformation.

Associated Conditions

Congenital heart disease, esophageal atresia, intestinal atresia, annular pancreas, intestinal malrotation or duplication, bicornuate absence of the musculus rectus abdominis, trisomy 21, finger and hand anomalies, omphalocele, bladder exstrophy, and exstrophy of the ileocecal area are associated conditions.

Management

Immediate surgical repair with or without performing a colostomy is indicated. Long-term management related to bowel functioning is needed.

OMPHALOCELE

Description

An omphalocele is a protrusion of the sac of intestines covered by the peritoneum without overlying skin into the base of the umbilical cord.

Incidence

Omphalocele occurs in 1 in 5000 births.

Clinical Findings

PHYSICAL EXAMINATION. Omphalocele is obvious on examination.

Associated Conditions

Associated conditions include chromosomal abnormalities, congenital diaphragmatic hernia, and a variety of cardiac problems. An omphalocele, hypoglycemia, and macroglossia suggest Beckwith syndrome.

Management

Immediate surgical repair to prevent infection or drying of abdominal contents is needed in patients whose sac has ruptured. In those with intact sacs, surgery can be delayed.

GASTROSCHISIS

Description

In gastroschisis, intestinal contents protrude through the abdomen without a protective covering. Associated congenital anomalies are rare.

Etiology and Incidence

Gastroschisis occurs in about 1 in 10,000 to 20,000 live births when there is failure to close the lateral ventral folds of the developing abdominal wall.

Clinical Findings

PHYSICAL EXAMINATION. Gastroschisis is obvious on examination.

Differential Diagnosis

Omphalocele is the differential diagnosis.

Management

Maintain body temperature. Apply protective gauze and wrap abdomen with cellophane to avoid heat loss. When the infant is stable, surgical repair is indicated.

Complications

Ileus is a common complication.

NECROTIZING ENTEROCOLITIS

Description

Necrotizing enterocolitis is characterized by varying degrees of mucosal or transmural necrosis of the intestine. The usual onset is in the first 2 weeks of life but can be later in very low birth weight infants.

Etiology and Incidence

The cause is unknown, but high-risk infants are found to have immature colons that become necrosed from trauma or injury. It occurs in 2% of neonates, with 80% of these cases occurring in premature infants.

Clinical Findings

HISTORY. The history can include the following:

- Prematurity, SGA
- Maternal hemorrhage, preeclampsia
- Cocaine exposure in utero
- Exchange transfusions, umbilical catheters
- Asphyxia
- Polycythemia

PHYSICAL EXAMINATION. Findings include the following:

- Abdominal distention
- Vomiting
- Bloody stools
- Lethargy
- Apnea
- Disseminated intravascular coagulation
- Rapid progression of shock

RADIOLOGICAL FINDINGS. An abdominal radiograph shows pneumatosis intestinalis, a specific air pattern.

Differential Diagnosis

The differential diagnosis includes sepsis, intestinal obstruction, volvulus, Hirschsprung disease, anal fissures, and neonatal appendicitis.

Management

The following steps are taken:

1. Do sepsis workup and prescribe systemic antibiotics.
2. Stop feedings, initiate gastric suctioning, maintain electrolyte balance, give oxygen as needed, and refer to a surgeon for evaluation.
3. Order serial abdominal radiographs to follow course of disease.
4. Delay oral feedings in very low birth weight infants for at least 1 week.

Prognosis

The mortality rate is 20 to 40%; 10% redevelop necrotizing enterocolitis (Behrman et al., 1996). Malabsorption with short-gut syndrome and strictures may complicate management (Finberg, 1998).

Complications

Ileus and perforation are complications.

MECONIUM ILEUS

Description

Meconium ileus is an impaction of the bowel with meconium, causing intestinal obstruction.

Etiology and Incidence

Meconium ileus is associated with maternal polyhydramnios and cystic fibrosis, occurring in about 10 to 20% of patients with cystic fibrosis. It is rarely seen in infants without cystic fibrosis.

Clinical Findings

HISTORY. There is a failure to pass meconium within 48 hours of life.

PHYSICAL EXAMINATION. Findings include abdominal distention and persistent vomiting.

RADIOLOGICAL FINDINGS. A radiograph shows bowel loops of varying width. There is a grainy appearance at points of heaviest meconium concentration.

Associated Conditions

Approximately 50% of affected infants have associated intestinal disorders, including atresia, stenosis, volvulus, or perforations.

Management

Treatment is individualized; high enemas with the iodinated contrast medium diatrizoate meglumine (Gastrografin), or laparotomy can be used.

Prognosis

The survival rate is good.

DIAPHRAGMATIC HERNIA

Description

In diaphragmatic hernia, abdominal contents herniate into the thoracic cavity.

Etiology and Incidence

Diaphragmatic hernia is caused by failure of the pleuroperitoneal canal to close completely during embryological development. It occurs with a frequency of about 1 in 2000 live births.

Clinical Findings

HISTORY. Immediate respiratory failure secondary to pulmonary hypertension or pulmonary hypoplasia.

PHYSICAL EXAMINATION. Findings include the following:

• Respiratory distress with tachypnea
• Cyanosis
• Scaphoid abdomen
• Rarely, bowel sounds heard in the chest
• Absence of breath sounds
• Heart tones best heard in the contralateral chest

The amount of respiratory distress depends on the amount of lung capacity. Any child with respiratory distress should be evaluated for diaphragmatic hernia.

RADIOLOGICAL FINDINGS. A chest radiograph shows fluid and air-filled loops of intestine in the chest. The mediastinum is displaced toward the unaffected side, usually to the right.

Management

Treatment involves the following:

1. Emergency surgery.
2. Before and after surgery, intensive respira-

tory and metabolic support. As soon as the diagnosis is suspected, the infant should be positioned with the head and chest higher than the abdomen.
3. Extracorporal membrane oxygenation is sometimes of value.

Prognosis

The mortality rate is 50 to 60%, depending on the degree of hypoplastic lung.

HYDROCELE AND INGUINAL HERNIA

See Chapter 35.

UMBILICAL HERNIA

Definition

Umbilical hernia is a weakness or imperfect closure of the umbilical ring.

Clinical Findings

PHYSICAL EXAMINATION. Findings include a soft swelling in the umbilical area that can be reduced, often associated with diastasis recti.

Management

Surgery is not required unless the hernia persists after 5 years of age, strangulates, is nonreducible, or enlarges.

Prognosis

Most umbilical hernias resolve spontaneously by 1 year but can take up to 4 to 5 years. Strangulation is extremely rare.

Parent Education

Counsel parents to avoid taping coins or placing belly bands over the umbilicus, because these efforts do not help and can contribute to infection in the neonate.

Renal Conditions

ACUTE RENAL FAILURE

Description

Decreased renal function with less than 0.5 ml/kg per 24 hours of urine output leads to acute renal failure and disrupted body fluid homeostasis. The newborn normally provides 1 to 3 ml/kg per hr of urine and urinates within the first 48 hours of life.

Etiology and Incidence

There are multiple causes, including stress during the prenatal period, dehydration, sepsis, anoxia, shock, administration of nephrotoxic drugs, renal dysgenesis, obstructive uropathy, congenital heart disease, hemorrhage, and renal vein thrombosis. Approximately 3% of neonates have some form of renal failure.

Clinical Findings

HISTORY. Maternal oligohydramnios may be noted.

PHYSICAL EXAMINATION. Findings include the following:

- Decreased or no urinary output
- Abdominal mass
- Pallor, edema, lethargy, vomiting, seizures, coma
- High blood pressure
- Pulmonary edema, congestive heart failure, or arrhythmias
- Meningomyelocele
- Prune-belly syndrome

LABORATORY FINDINGS. The following are ordered as indicated:

- Bladder tap to confirm inadequate urinary output
- Urinalysis to rule out hematuria or pyuria
- Urine osmolarity, sodium, and potassium values to indicate kidney filtration ability
- Serum blood urea nitrogen, creatinine, sodium, and potassium values to indicate poor filtration
- Complete blood count including differential and platelets to rule out thrombocytopenia, sepsis, or renal vein thrombosis

Management

The following steps are taken:

1. Replace fluid loss (approximately 30 ml/kg per 24 hrs), then restrict fluid and diet.

2. Maintain strict intake and output and fluid and electrolyte balance.
3. Monitor blood pressure.
4. Peritoneal dialysis is sometimes indicated.

Prognosis

The prognosis depends on the degree of renal failure and the cause.

HYDRONEPHROSIS

Description

Hydronephrosis is a dilation of one or both kidneys frequently caused by an obstruction of the ureteropelvic junction, posterior urethral valves, ectopic ureterocele, prune-belly syndrome, or ureteral or ureterovesical obstructions.

Incidence

Obstructive uropathy occurs in 1 in 1000 births and is slightly more common in males.

Clinical Findings

HISTORY. The history can include the following:

- Decreased urinary output
- Occasionally found on prenatal ultrasonogram
- Symptoms not present immediately

PHYSICAL EXAMINATION. Findings include an abdominal mass.

Management

Surgical repair may be necessary if spontaneous resolution does not occur by 6 to 12 months of age.

Prognosis

The longer the obstruction lasts, the less likely renal function will return to normal.

CYSTIC KIDNEY

Description

The presence of multiple cysts of various sizes and shapes in the kidney can be either an autosomal dominant or autosomal recessive disease. The autosomal dominant form usually appears in the fourth or fifth decade of life and can be associated with hepatic cysts or cerebral aneurysms. In the autosomal recessive form, which also usually has hepatic cysts, the infant has abdominal masses at birth.

Incidence

The adult form (autosomal dominant) occurs in about 1 in 3500 persons; the juvenile form (autosomal recessive) occurs in about 1 or 2 per 10,000 live births.

Clinical Findings

HISTORY. Maternal oligohydramnios is noted in the juvenile form.

PHYSICAL EXAMINATION. Findings include the following:

- Abdominal lobular mass
- Hematuria
- Hypertension

RADIOLOGICAL FINDINGS. A renal scan is done to document the disorder.

Differential Diagnosis

Multicystic dysplasia, hydronephrosis, Wilms tumor, and renal vein thrombosis are included in the differential diagnosis.

Management

Monitor kidney function and check for enlargement of cysts or infection. Nephrectomy is necessary if no regression is seen or a complication occurs. Dialysis or transplantation is sometimes considered.

Prognosis

With severe involvement, the neonate dies from pulmonary or renal insufficiency. Hypertension increases as the kidney shrinks.

RENAL ARTERY OR VEIN THROMBOSIS

Description

There is decreased blood flow to the kidney because of thrombus formation.

Clinical Findings

HISTORY. In the newborn this condition is often associated with asphyxia, dehydration, shock, and sepsis. Maternal diabetes is a rare cause. Sudden onset of gross hematuria may be noted.

PHYSICAL EXAMINATION. Findings include a firm flank mass, usually unilateral.

RADIOLOGICAL AND LABORATORY FINDINGS. Ultrasonography shows marked enlargement of the kidney. The hematocrit is low.

Differential Diagnosis

Other causes of hematuria, such as hydronephrosis, cystic disease, Wilms tumor, and abscess, are included in the differential diagnosis.

Management

The following steps are taken:

1. Maintain fluid and electrolyte balance.
2. Monitor blood pressure.
3. Prophylactic anticoagulation therapy is given to prevent thrombosis in the other kidney.
4. Nephrectomy is not necessary unless chronic infection occurs.

NEUROBLASTOMA

Description

A neuroblastoma is a solid tumor that originates from neural crest tissue along the craniospinal axis. The majority develop in the abdomen, usually in the adrenal gland.

Etiology and Incidence

The cause is unknown. It occurs in 1 in 10,000 births and is more common in males (Behrman et al., 1996).

Clinical Findings

HISTORY. An unexplained fever and symptoms related to the site of the tumor are part of the history.

PHYSICAL EXAMINATION. Findings include the following:

- Firm, irregular, nontender mass in abdomen
- Pallor
- Hypotension
- Ascites
- Irritability
- Possible external tumors in newborn

RADIOLOGICAL AND LABORATORY FINDINGS. These include the following:

- Renal radiographs reveal calcifications
- Computed tomography determines extent of disease
- Catecholamines and urine vanillylmandelic acid (VMA) are present in the urine
- Bone marrow aspirate determines staging of disease

Differential Diagnosis

Wilms tumor, hydronephrosis, renal vein thrombosis, and lymphoma are included in the differential diagnosis.

Management

Although some neuroblastomas regress without therapy, treatment is surgical removal followed by radiation therapy or chemotherapy.

Prognosis

The prognosis depends on the age of the patient and the stage of the tumor. The prognosis is good if complete resection of tumor is performed or if the patient is younger than 1 year of age.

RENAL AGENESIS

Description

Renal agenesis is failure of the kidney to form normally. Bilateral agenesis is incompatible with life.

Incidence

Renal agenesis occurs in 1 in 3000 births and in males more often than in females. The left kidney is more commonly affected than the right (Behrman et al., 1996).

Clinical Findings

HISTORY. Maternal oligohydramnios is noted. Renal agenesis is usually not detected until the child is evaluated for urinary tract infection later in infancy.

PHYSICAL EXAMINATION. Findings include the following:

- Single umbilical artery
- Associated anomalies involving the gastrointestinal or urinary tract and skeleton
- Low-set ears, senile appearance, broad nose, and receding chin

Management

Monitor for proteinuria and hypertension.

Prognosis

Patients with bilateral disease die within a few months of life. Those with unilateral disease are usually detected with evaluation of the urinary conditions.

Endocrine Conditions

CONGENITAL HYPOTHYROIDISM, CONGENITAL ADRENAL HYPERPLASIA

See Chapter 26.

Metabolic Conditions

HYPOGLYCEMIA

Description

In hypoglycemia, the blood glucose level is below 30 mg/dl.

Etiology

Infants at higher risk of developing hypoglycemia include SGA infants, those with diabetic mothers, asphyxia at birth, sepsis, erythroblastosis fetalis, glycogen storage disease, or galactosemia.

Clinical Findings

HISTORY. The history can include the following:

- Risk factors for sepsis or asphyxia
- Infant of a diabetic mother
- SGA

PHYSICAL EXAMINATION. Findings include the following:

- Lethargy
- Poor feeding and regurgitation
- Apnea
- Jitteriness
- Pallor, sweating, cool extremities
- Seizures

Management

The following steps are taken:

1. Measure serum glucose level within 1 hour of birth, subsequently every 1 to 2 hours for the first 6 to 8 hours, and then every 4 to 6 hours until 24 hours of life.
2. Give normoglycemic high-risk infants oral or gavage feedings with breast milk or formula started at 1 to 3 hours of age and continued at 2- to 3-hour intervals for 24 to 48 hours.
3. Provide an intravenous infusion of glucose at 4 mg/kg per min if serum glucose level is low and if oral feedings are poorly tolerated.

Prognosis

Infants with symptomatic hypoglycemia, particularly low birth weight infants and infants of diabetic mothers, are less likely to have normal intellectual development than are asymptomatic infants. Prognosis for normal intellectual function is guarded in infants with prolonged and severe hypoglycemia.

INFANTS OF DIABETIC MOTHER (IDM)

Description

Infants of mothers with poorly controlled gestational or insulin-dependent diabetes mellitus are referred to as IDM.

Etiology

Maternal hyperglycemia causes fetal hyperglycemia and hyperinsulinemia, leading to increased hepatic glucose uptake and glycogen synthesis, accelerated lipogenesis, and augmented protein synthesis (Armentrout, 1995).

Clinical Findings

HISTORY. The history includes a poorly controlled diabetic mother.

PHYSICAL EXAMINATION. Findings include the following:

- Large and plump neonate with large viscera
- Puffy facies
- Plethora
- Hyperexcitability during the first 3 days of life, although hypotonia, lethargy, and poor sucking also occur
- Cardiomegaly in 30%, and heart murmurs in 5 to 10%

Management

1. Regardless of size, IDM should initially receive intensive observation and care.
2. Determine blood glucose levels in asymptomatic infants within 1 hour of birth and then every hour for the next 6 to 8 hours.
3. If clinically well and normoglycemic, initially give oral or gavage feedings with 5% glucose water or breast milk started within 2 to 3 hours of age and continued at 3-hour intervals.
4. If any question arises about the infants' ability to tolerate oral feeding, discontinue feeding and give 10% glucose by peripheral intravenous infusion at a rate of 4 to 8 mg/kg/hr.
5. Treat hypoglycemia, even in asymptomatic infants, with intravenous infusions of glu-

cose. Avoid bolus injections of hypertonic glucose because they cause further hyperinsulinemia and potentially produce rebound hypoglycemia.

Complications

Cardiomegaly is common (30%), and heart failure occurs in 5 to 10% of infants. Congenital anomalies are increased threefold; cardiac malformations and lumbosacral agenesis are most common. There is a predisposition to obesity in childhood that can extend into adult life. Symptomatic hypoglycemia increases the risk of impaired intellectual development.

Prevention

Strict management of blood glucose levels in mothers with diabetes decreases the risk of severe problems in the infant.

Orthopedic Conditions

FRACTURED CLAVICLE; BRACHIAL PALSY. SEE CHAPTER 38

POLYDACTYLY

Description

Polydactyly is a condition that varies from a skin tag to a formed finger with a nail that extends from the postaxial side.

Incidence

Polydactyly occurs in 1 in 300 in the black population and in 1 in 3000 in the white population.

Clinical Findings

PHYSICAL EXAMINATION. A floppy digit is seen on the foot or hand. It varies in degree of formation.

Management

Surgical removal of the floppy extra digit is indicated. If the digit is stabilized by bone, surgical removal is deferred until the patient is older, when function can be assessed.

SYNDACTYLY

Description

In syndactyly, fingers are fused by skin and sometimes bone.

Incidence

Syndactyly occurs in 1 in 2200 births and is seen more often in males, with a tendency to be familial.

Clinical Findings

Webbing of two digits, partially or to the tip of the finger, is seen.

Management

Treatment is not indicated in the neonate. Surgical separation is recommended at age 2 to 3 years.

Central Nervous System Conditions

CONGENITAL HYDROCEPHALUS

Description

Congenital hydrocephalus is an accumulation of cerebrospinal fluid (CSF) in the brain's ventricles at birth.

Etiology and Incidence

Malformations, infections, intraventricular hemorrhage, and disorders in brain development can lead to congenital hydrocephalus. The incidence varies depending on which of these conditions is causative.

Clinical Findings

HISTORY. Vomiting, lethargy, irritability, and poor feeding can be reported.

PHYSICAL EXAMINATION. Findings include the following:

- Head circumference greater than 90% of the standardized growth curve

- Cranial sutures separated by large, tense fontanels

RADIOLOGICAL FINDINGS. Cranial ultrasonography shows dilated ventricles.

Management

Medications that decrease CSF production (e.g., acetazolamide) or a ventriculoperitoneal shunt, or both, are used. Referral should be prompt.

INTRAVENTRICULAR HEMORRHAGE

Description

Intraventricular hemorrhage (IVH) occurs within the ventricles of the brain.

Etiology and Incidence

Risk factors include prematurity, RDS, hypoxemic-ischemic or hypotensive injury, increased or decreased cerebral blood flow, hypertension, hypervolemia, and reduced vascular integrity. There is a 50% occurrence rate in infants weighing 1500 g or less (Klaus & Fanaroff, 1993). The incidence of IVH decreases with increasing gestational age. Intracranial hemorrhage results from trauma or asphyxia.

Clinical Findings

HISTORY. Risk factors for IVH are seen, including SGA, prematurity, and others mentioned previously.

PHYSICAL EXAMINATION. Findings include the following:

- Diminished or absent Moro reflex
- Poor muscle tone, lethargy, somnolence
- Apnea
- Periods of pallor or cyanosis
- Failure to suck well
- High-pitched, shrill cry, seizures

RADIOLOGICAL FINDINGS. Ultrasonography is used to classify IVH into grades I to IV based on the presence and quantity of blood in the ventricles.

Management

Treatment involves the following:

1. Supportive management and minimal stimulation
2. Acetazolamide to decrease CSF production
3. Repeated lumbar punctures
4. Ventriculoperitoneal shunt or external ventriculostomy sometimes necessary

Prognosis

Grade III and IV hemorrhages generally have a poor neurological outcome.

HYPOXIC-ISCHEMIC INSULTS

Description

Three levels of injury (grades I, II, and III, or mild, moderate, and severe) are described. Brain damage results from hypoxia or ischemia for an extended period of time, usually longer than 6 minutes.

Etiology and Incidence

The initial hypoxemic insult is followed by edema, which further reduces cerebral perfusion, leading to encephalopathy. The incidence of severe asphyxia (grade III) is less than 1 per 1000 live births in most nurseries. Ninety percent of hypoxic-ischemic events occur during the prenatal or intrapartum period as a result of such conditions as abruptio placentae, hemorrhage, cord compression, mechanical injury, severe hypertension or diabetes, or inadequate resuscitation.

Clinical Findings

PHYSICAL EXAMINATION. Findings include the following:

- Seizure activity
- Pallor
- Cyanosis, apnea
- Bradycardia and unresponsiveness to stimulation

Management

Seizure and symptom management is needed.

Prognosis

The prognosis depends on whether the underlying cause can be treated effectively. Severe encephalopathy, characterized by flaccid coma, apnea, and seizures, is associated with a poor prognosis (Behrman et al., 1996). An infant who remains neurologically abnormal after the initial recovery phase (2 weeks) has suffered permanent neurological impairment (Klaus & Fanaroff, 1993). A low Apgar score at 20 minutes, absence of spontaneous respirations, and persistence of abnormal neurological signs at 2 weeks of age predict death or severe cognitive and motor deficits.

MYELOMENINGOCELE

Description

A myelomeningocele is the result of failure to close the posterior neural tube and the vertebral column. This is the most severe form of neural tube defect.

Etiology and Incidence

The cause is unknown, yet a genetic predisposition exists. The incidence is 1 to 5 per 1000 live births.

Clinical Findings

HISTORY. Poor intake of folic acid and exposure to hyperthermia, valproic acid, or clomiphene are risk factors

PHYSICAL EXAMINATION. Findings include the following:

- Sac-like cyst containing meninges and spinal fluid covered by thin layer of partially epithelialized skin
- Seventy-five percent of cases are found in the lumbosacral area
- Flaccid paralysis of lower extremities
- Absence of deep tendon reflexes
- Lack of response to touch and pain
- Constant urinary dribbling

Management

Surgical repair and multidisciplinary supportive management are indicated.

Prognosis

The mortality rate is 10 to 15% in aggressively treated children (Behrman et al, 1996). At least 70% have normal intelligence, but seizure disorders, hydrocephalus, and learning disabilities are more common than in the general population.

Prevention

Prenatal vitamins and folic acid supplementation (0.4 mg/d) are helpful in preventing neural tube defects and should be taken by any female of childbearing age.

Hematological Conditions

POLYCYTHEMIA

Description

Polycythemia is characterized by a central hematocrit of 65% or higher.

Etiology and Incidence

Polycythemia can occur in IDM and those with growth retardation who were exposed to chronic fetal hypoxia that stimulated erythropoietin production and increased red blood cell production. Polycythemia occurs in 1 to 5 per 100 births.

Clinical Findings

HISTORY. The history includes the following:

- Diabetic mother
- Recipient of a twin-twin transfusion
- Delayed clamping of umbilical cord
- Postmature infant
- SGA

PHYSICAL EXAMINATION. Findings include the following:

- Fifteen to 25% of infants with polycythemia are asymptomatic
- Plethora
- Feeding disturbances
- Cyanosis (persistent fetal circulation), tachypnea, respiratory distress
- Hyperbilirubinemia

Management

Phlebotomy and replacement with saline or albumin, or a partial exchange transfusion to reduce the hematocrit to 50%, are needed.

Prognosis

Long-term problems include speech deficits, abnormal fine motor control, reduced IQ, and other neurological abnormalities.

HEMORRHAGIC DISEASE IN THE NEWBORN

Description

Severe transient deficiencies of vitamin K–dependent clotting factors lead to bleeding.

Etiology

Hemorrhagic disease is caused by a lack of free vitamin K in the mother and absence of bacterial intestinal flora normally responsible for synthesis of vitamin K in the infant. Vitamin K–dependent clotting factors (factors II, VII, IX, X) are normal at birth but decrease within 2 to 3 days. Breast milk is a poor source of vitamin K; late-onset disease (occurring 1 to 3 months after birth) rarely may be seen in exclusively breast-fed infants. A particularly severe form of deficiency of vitamin K–dependent coagulation factors occurring in the first day of life has been reported in women receiving the anticonvulsants phenytoin and phenobarbital.

Clinical Findings

HISTORY. The history may include:

- Anticonvulsant use by the mother
- Prematurity
- Exclusive breastfeeding without vitamin K supplementation
- Failure to administer parenteral vitamin K at birth
- Neonatal hepatitis or biliary atresia

PHYSICAL EXAMINATION. Findings include gastrointestinal, nasal, subgaleal, or intracranial bleeding or bleeding at the site of an injection or circumcision.

LABORATORY FINDINGS. Prothrombin time, blood coagulation time, and partial thromboplastin time are prolonged.

Differential Diagnosis

This disorder may be the result of disseminated intravascular coagulation or congenital bleeding disorders unrelated to vitamin K.

Management

The following steps are taken:

1. Intravenous infusion of 1 to 5 mg of vitamin K is needed. Improvement of coagulation defects and cessation of bleeding should occur within a few hours.
2. If a newborn is delivered at home, ascertain whether or not vitamin K was given.

Prevention

Prevention is achieved by routinely giving 1 mg of natural oil-soluble vitamin K intramuscularly within 1 hour of birth.

Prognosis

This depends on the site and extent of bleeding.

ANEMIA

Description

Anemia is characterized by less than the normal range of hemoglobin for birth weight and postnatal age.

Etiology

Anemia occurs secondary to acute blood loss before or during delivery. Acute blood loss after delivery can be external (gastrointestinal, circumcision site, umbilical stump), internal (fracture site, cephalhematoma, pulmonary hemorrhage, injured internal organ), or secondary to hemolysis or congenital aplastic or hypoplastic anemia.

Clinical Findings

HISTORY. The history can include the following:

- Twin-twin transfusion
- Unexpected tearing or delayed clamping of umbilical cord with neonate blood loss
- Internal hemorrhage (due to fracture, cephalhematoma, or internal organ trauma)
- Umbilical stump or circumcision bleeding

PHYSICAL EXAMINATION. Pallor, as well as congestive heart failure and shock, is a possible finding.

Management

Treatment depends on the cause. An asymptomatic full-term infant with a hemoglobin level of 10 g/dl can be observed, whereas a symptomatic neonate born after abruptio placentae or with severe hemolytic disease of the newborn warrants transfusion. Treatment with blood should be balanced by concern about transfusion-acquired infection with cytomegalovirus, human immunodeficiency virus (HIV), and hepatitis B and C viruses.

Prognosis

This depends on the cause and severity of the anemia.

BLOOD IN VOMITUS OR STOOL

Description

Bright- or dark-red blood in the vomitus or stool can be seen without clinical evidence of blood loss.

Etiology

This problem is caused by ingestion of maternal blood during delivery.

Clinical Findings

PHYSICAL EXAMINATION. Bright- or dark-red blood is seen in vomitus or stool.

LABORATORY FINDINGS. Blood of maternal origin can be differentiated from infant blood by testing for fetal hemoglobin.

Differential Diagnosis

The differential diagnosis includes gastrointestinal bleeding caused by trauma, duplication of bowel, intussusception, volvulus, hemangioma or telangiectasia of bowel, rectal prolapse, or anal fissure.

Management

No treatment is necessary if blood is of maternal origin.

JAUNDICE

Description

Jaundice, a clinically apparent accumulation of bilirubin in the skin, causes a yellowish orange or sometimes green hue to the skin. Jaundice becomes apparent when serum bilirubin levels exceed 5 to 7 mg/dl and usually advances in a pattern from the infant's head to the toes. Physiological jaundice is the most common type of jaundice in the newborn period, usually appearing after the first 24 hours of life. The rate of increase is less than 5 mg/dl, with the peak total bilirubin usually not exceeding 13 mg/dl and the direct bilirubin not exceeding 2 mg/dl. Physiological jaundice does not persist beyond 1 week and the infant shows no signs of illness. Nonphysiological (pathological) jaundice appears at less than 24 hours of age, lasts more than 8 days, or both. The rate of increase in total bilirubin is rapid at greater than 0.5 mg/dl per hour. Total bilirubin levels are frequently greater than 12.5 mg/dl before 48 hours of age, or the direct bilirubin exceeds 1.5 to 2 mg/dl. Breast milk jaundice can be divided into two types. Early-onset breast milk jaundice develops within 2 to 4 days of birth and is believed to occur as a result of infrequent breastfeeding and insufficient intake leading to decreased intestinal motility. Late-onset breast milk jaundice develops 4 to 7 days after birth, peaks at 10 to 15 days of life, and frequently persists. See Chapter 13 on breastfeeding for more information. Kernicterus or bilirubin encephalopathy involves toxicity of the nervous system resulting from very high levels of bilirubin.

Etiology and Incidence

Jaundice is observed during the first week of life in approximately 60% of infants. Causes include an increased rate of hemolysis, decreased rate of conjugation, and abnormalities of liver function (Table 39–10).

1. Increased rate of hemolysis: ABO incompatibility, Rh incompatibility, abnormal red blood cell shapes (spherocytosis, elliptocytosis, pyknocytosis, and stomatocytosis), red blood cell enzyme abnormalities (glucose-6-phosphate dehydrogenase deficiency, pyruvate kinase deficiency).
2. Decreased rate of conjugation: immaturity of bilirubin conjugation (physiological jaundice), congenital familial nonhemolytic jaundice (inborn errors of metabolism affecting glucuronyl transferase system and bilirubin transport), breast milk jaundice.
3. Abnormalities of excretion or absorption: sepsis, hepatitis (viral, parasitic, bacterial, toxic), metabolic abnormalities (galactosemia, glycogen storage disease, IDM, cystic fibrosis), biliary atresia, choledochal cyst, obstruction of ampulla of Vater (annular pancreas), drugs.
4. Classic physiological jaundice is characterized by a rise in bilirubin from 1.5 mg/dl in cord blood to 5 to 6 mg/dl on the third day of life, declining to a normal adult level (<1.3 to 1.5 mg/dl) by 10 to 12 days in white and black infants. Asian infants reach 8 to 12 mg/dl on day 4 to 5 and decline more slowly. Two percent of Asian newborns and 1% of whites and blacks have serum bilirubin higher than 20 mg/dl in the first week of life. The current estimated minimal level of risk is 25 to 30 mg/dl in healthy term infants (Robertson, 1998; AAP, 1994; Gartner, 1994; Banks et al., 1996).

Clinical Findings

FAMILY HISTORY. The following may be noted:

- Significant hemolytic disease, anemia
- Inborn errors of metabolism

- Early or severe jaundice
- Ethnic or geographical origin associated with hemolytic anemia
- Hepatobiliary disease

HISTORY

- ABO or Rh incompatibilities in previous pregnancies
- Sepsis risk for the infant, such as prolonged rupture of maternal membranes

PHYSICAL EXAMINATION. Findings include the following:

- Jaundice at birth or at any time during the neonatal period, depending on the underlying condition, with face affected first, followed by the shoulders, chest, and abdomen. Jaundice from deposition of indirect bilirubin in the skin tends to appear bright yellow or orange; jaundice of the obstructive type (direct bilirubin) appears greenish or muddy yellow, with the difference apparent only in severe jaundice. There is no dependable relationship between the intensity of jaundice and the degree of hyperbilirubinemia.
- A crude estimate of the level of jaundice can be based on the dermal zone in which the jaundice is noticed:
  - Head and neck—a mean bilirubin of 6 mg/dl
  - Trunk and umbilicus—a mean bilirubin of 9 mg/dl
  - Groin including the upper thighs—a mean bilirubin of 12 mg/dl
  - Knees and elbows (including the ankles and wrists) or to the feet and hands (including the palms and soles)—a mean bilirubin of 15 mg/dl
- Petechiae, bruising, hepatosplenomegaly, or signs of infection.
- Early signs of bilirubin toxicity to the brain (kernicterus) are subtle and indistinguishable from those of sepsis, asphyxia, hypoglycemia, intracranial hemorrhage, and other acute illnesses in the neonate.
  - Lethargy, poor feeding, and loss of the Moro reflex—common initial signs
  - Diminished tendon reflexes, respiratory distress, failure to suck, opisthotonos, bulging fontanel, twitching of face or

T A B L E 39-10
Diagnostic Features of the Various Types of Neonatal Jaundice

DIAGNOSIS	NATURE OF VAN DEN BERGH REACTION	JAUNDICE		PEAK BILIRUBIN CONCENTRATION		BILIRUBIN RATE OF ACCUMULATION (mg/dl/d)	REMARKS
		Appears	Disappears	mg/dl	Age (days)		
"Physiological jaundice"							Usually relates to degree of maturity
Full-term	Indirect	2–3 d	4–5 d	10–12	2–3	<5	
Premature	Indirect	3–4 d	7–9 d	15	6–8	<5	
Hyperbilirubinemia due to metabolic factors							Metabolic factors: hypoxia, respiratory distress, lack of carbohydrate
Full-term	Indirect	2–3 d	Variable	>2	1st wk	<5	Hormonal influences: cretinism, hormones
Premature	Indirect	3–4 d	Variable	>15	1st wk	<5	Genetic factors: Crigler-Najjar syndrome, transient familial hyperbilirubinemia Drugs: vitamin K, novobiocin
Hemolytic states and hematoma	Indirect	May appear in 1st 24 hr	Variable	Unlimited	Variable	Usually >5	Erythroblastosis: Rh, ABO Congenital hemolytic states: spherocytic, nonspherocytic Infantile pyknocytosis Drugs: vitamin K; enclosed hemorrhage—hematoma
Mixed hemolytic and hepatotoxic factors	Indirect and direct	May appear in 1st 24 hr	Variable	Unlimited	Variable	Usually >5	Infection: bacterial sepsis, pyelonephritis, hepatitis, toxoplasmosis, cytomegalic inclusion disease, rubella Drugs: vitamin K
Hepatocellular damage	Indirect and direct	Usually 2–3 days	Variable	Unlimited	Variable	Variable; can be >5	Biliary atresia; galactosemia; hepatitis, infection

From Brown AK: Diagnostic features of the various types of neonatal jaundice. Pediatr Clin North Am 9:589, 1962.

limbs, seizures, and a shrill, high-pitched cry—later signs

LABORATORY FINDINGS. The following are ordered as indicated:

- Total serum bilirubin level (indirect and direct if >2 weeks of age or if hepatic or metabolic disease is suspected)
- ABO, Rh, isoimmune antibodies on mother
- ABO, Rh, Coombs test on infants' blood if mother is Rh negative or if elevated bilirubin or jaundice is present
- Hemoglobin, hematocrit, reticulocyte count
- Blood types of infant and mother

Elevated indirect serum bilirubin with a normal reticulocyte count and negative Coombs test is indicative of physiological jaundice, breast milk jaundice, or congenital familial nonhemolytic jaundice.

Elevated indirect (unconjugated) serum bilirubin with an increased reticulocyte count is indicative of increased hemolysis secondary to isoimmunization (positive Coombs test such as caused by ABO or Rh incompatability), abnormal red blood cell shape, or red blood cell enzyme abnormalities.

Elevated indirect and direct serum bilirubin with a negative Coombs test and a normal reticulocyte count is indicative of hepatitis, meta-bolic abnormalities, biliary atresia, chole-dochal cyst (in the bile duct), gastrointestinal or pancreatic obstruction, sepsis, or drugs.

Management

Treatment includes the following (Fig. 39-9):

1. The infant's history, course, and physical findings determine the treatment course. Pathological jaundice requires a more in-depth workup. Risk factors include the following:
   - Appearance of jaundice in first 24 hours of life
   - Rise of bilirubin greater than 0.5 mg/dl/hr
   - Conjugated bilirubin greater than 2 mg/dl
2. Treatment level is dependent on age of infant and total bilirubin level (Table 39-11).
3. Phototherapy is used to treat elevated indirect hyperbilirubinemia; it is contraindicated with elevated direct bilirubin:
   - Phototherapy via banks of overhead lights placed close to the infant requires eye patches removed at regular intervals, taking care to avoid corneal abrasions; monitoring of temperature; increased fluid intake in response to evaporative water losses; avoidance of oral drugs because of decreased absorption

T A B L E 39-11

Management of Hyperbilirubinemia in the Healthy Term Newborn

| AGE (hr) | TOTAL SERUM BILIRUBIN (TSB) LEVEL, mg/dl (μmol/l) | | | |
	Consider Phototherapy*	Phototherapy	Exchange Transfusion if Intensive Phototherapy Fails†	Exchange Transfusion and Intensive Phototherapy
≤24‡				
25–48	≥12 (205)	≥15 (260)	≥20 (340)	≥25 (430)
49–72	≥15 (260)	≥18 (310)	≥25 (430)	≥30 (510)
>72	≥17 (290)	≥20 (340)	≥25 (430)	≥30 (510)

*Phototherapy at these TSB levels is a clinical option, meaning that the intervention is available and may be used on the basis of individual clinical judgment.

†Intensive phototherapy should produce a decline of TSB of 1–2 mg/dl within 4–6 hr, and the TSB level should continue to fall and remain below the threshold level for exchange transfusion. If this does not occur, it is considered a failure of phototherapy.

‡Term infants who are clinically jaundiced at 24 hr are not considered healthy and require further evaluation.

Adapted from American Academy of Pediatrics: Practice parameter: Management of hyperbilirubinemia in the healthy term newborn. Pediatrics 94(4, pt1):560, 1994.

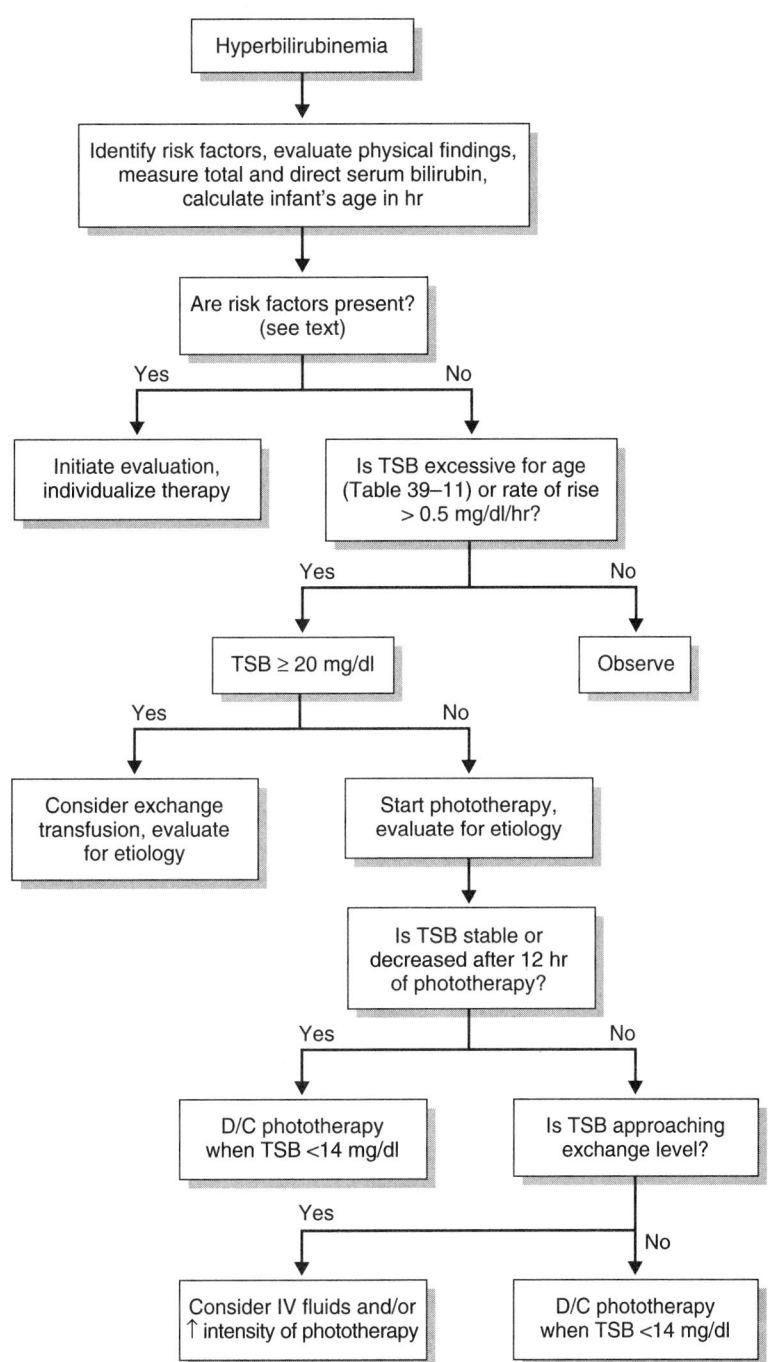

F I G U R E 39-9

Management of the full-term newborn with hyperbilirubinemia. D/C = discharge; IV = intravenous; TSB = total serum bilirubin. (From Banks J, Montgomery D, Coody D, et al: Hyperbilirubinemia in the term newborn. J Pediatr Health Care 10:228–230, 1996.)

- Phototherapy via biliblanket (fiberoptic pad) allows ongoing interaction between mother and infant
- Phototherapy via bilibed
4. If the infant is breastfeeding and the total bilirubin is greater than 20 mg/dl, the following options exist if physiological jaundice is assumed (AAP, 1994):
   - Observe
   - Continue breastfeeding and deliver phototherapy
   - Supplement breastfeeding with formula with or without phototherapy
   - Substitute formula for breastfeeding for 24 hours, having mother continue to pump to maintain supply
   - Substitute formula for breastfeeding for 24 hours and deliver phototherapy.
5. Rebound bilirubin testing (measurement of bilirubin after phototherapy is discontinued) is not required in full-term newborns (AAP, 1994).

Prevention

Prevention requires early, frequent feeding. Breastfeeding should begin in the delivery room, occur 10 to 12 times per 24 hours, and include no supplementation.

Infections of the Newborn

Three mechanisms for acquiring neonatal infections include:

- Transplacental, when the mother acquires an organism that invades her bloodstream and passes through the placenta
- Vertical, when organisms in the vagina invade the amniotic fluid within the uterus
- Horizontal, when the newborn is exposed to environmental agents after birth

Syphilis is transplacentally acquired; herpes, gonorrhea, group B streptococci, *Listeria, Escherichia coli*, and chlamydia are vertically acquired (Remington & Klein, 1995; Fanaroff & Martin, 1997). Staphylococcal infection is the most common horizontal infection. The most common means for horizontal transmission are the unwashed hands of health-care providers.

Risk factors for sepsis (systemic infection) in the newborn include early rupture of amniotic membranes followed by preterm labor, prolonged rupture of membranes, maternal fever, maternal diagnosis of chorioamnionitis, maternal tachycardia, fetal tachycardia, and malodorous amniotic fluid. The neonate with sepsis can be asymptomatic or have nonspecific symptoms (Remington & Klein, 1995; Fanaroff & Martin, 1997). This is in part caused by a delayed immune response to local infection, allowing the neonate to bypass the typical signs and symptoms of infection (e.g., fever). Organisms quickly invade the systemic circulation, and significant deterioration occurs before it can be clinically recognized. Because of the serious nature of neonatal sepsis, significant risk factors or a clinically unstable neonate without perinatal risk factors warrants investigation and initiation of appropriate antibiotics (Korones & Bada-Ellzey, 1993) (Table 39–12).

TOXOPLASMOSIS

Organism

Toxoplasmosis is an infection caused by *Toxoplasma gondii*, an obligate intracellular protozoan.

Etiology and Incidence

T. gondii infects most species of warm-blooded animals, particularly cats. Cats excrete oocysts in their stools; intermediate hosts include cattle, pigs, and sheep. Humans become infected by consumption of poorly cooked meat or by accidental ingestion of oocysts from soil or in contaminated food. Approximately 50% of untreated women who acquire the infection during gestation transmit the parasite to their fetuses (Behrman et al., 1996). Occurrence is 1 in 1000 live births in the United States.

Clinical Findings

HISTORY. Prematurity and low Apgar scores are included in the history.

PHYSICAL EXAMINATION. Infants with congenital infection are asymptomatic at birth in 70 to

TABLE 39-12

Neonatal Sepsis

HISTORY
Temperature instability
Jitteriness
Poor feeding, vomiting
Irritability or lethargy
Apnea
Bloody stools
Respiratory distress
Seizures

PHYSICAL EXAMINATION
Jaundice
Pallor
Petechiae or purpura
Rash
Hepatosplenomegaly
Poor tone and perfusion
Tachycardia or bradycardia
Cyanosis, grunting, flaring, retractions

LABORATORY EVALUATION
Blood for CBC with differential, platelet count, and culture—anemia; increase or decrease in WBC count with left shift; thrombocytopenia
Urine—urine culture usually not done in the 1st 72 hr of life because of low yield
CSF for protein, glucose, cell count, and culture—elevated protein and WBC count; depressed glucose often found in neonatal infections

MANAGEMENT
Combination broad-spectrum antibiotic coverage for gram-positive cocci, gram-negative bacilli, and *Listeria* is recommended. Consider adding coverage for herpes infection if this is a possibility. *Listeria* is treated with ampicillin; group B streptococci can be treated with the penicillins and the cephalosporins; gram-negative organisms are well-covered by aminoglycosides and some cephalosporins

CBC = complete blood count; WBC = white blood cell; CSF = cerebrospinal fluid.

90% of the cases (AAP, 1997a). Findings include the following:

- Jaundice
- Anemia
- Hepatosplenomegaly
- Chorioretinitis
- Microcephaly

RADIOLOGICAL AND LABORATORY FINDINGS. Computed tomography (CT) of the brain shows calcifications or hydrocephalus. The CSF shows high protein, low glucose, and evidence of *T. gondii*. Serum immunoglobulin G (IgG) and IgM antibodies against *Toxoplasmosis* are seen.

Differential Diagnosis

Sepsis, syphilis, and hemolytic disease are considered in the differential diagnosis.

Management

Oral pyrimethamine, sulfadiazine or triple sulfonamides, spiramycin, and calcium leucovorin are given for 1 year.

Prognosis

Treatment usually cures the manifestations of toxoplasmosis such as active chorioretinitis, meningitis, encephalitis, hepatitis, splenomegaly, and thrombocytopenia. Infants with extensive involvement at birth have mild to severe impairment of vision, hearing, cognitive function, and other neurological functions.

Prevention

No protective vaccine is available. Pregnant women should be informed not to handle raw meat or contaminated cat litter and to wash fruit and vegetables before consumption. Cook meat and eggs well and drink pasteurized milk.

CONGENITAL RUBELLA

Organism

Rubella is an RNA virus.

Etiology and Incidence

Rubella is transmitted by person-to-person contact; the virus infects the placenta and is transmitted to the fetus. It occurs more frequently in the winter and spring.

Clinical Findings

HISTORY. The history can include the following:

- Maternal infection before 20 weeks' gestation
- Negative rubella titers in mother
- As many as 50% of infected women are asymptomatic (Behrman et al., 1996)

PHYSICAL EXAMINATION. Many infected infants may be asymptomatic in the newborn period. Findings include the following:

- Hearing loss
- Congenital heart disease
- Mental retardation
- Cataract or glaucoma

LABORATORY FINDINGS. The rubella virus can be isolated from nasopharyngeal secretions, conjunctivae, urine, stool, and CSF.

Management

No specific drug therapy is available. Monitoring and intervention for developmental, auditory, visual, and medical needs improve the quality of life for these children.

Prevention

Congenital rubella is now a rare occurrence because of widespread administration of an effective vaccine (Korones & Bada-Ellzey, 1993). All women of childbearing age should have rubella serology titers, and vaccine should be given to IgG-seronegative women who are not pregnant.

CYTOMEGALOVIRUS

Organism

Cytomegalovirus (CMV) is the largest member of the herpesvirus family.

Etiology and Incidence

CMV is transmitted via intimate and household contact with virus-containing secretions and blood products. When CMV is introduced into a household, it is likely that all members will acquire the infection. CMV is transmitted to the infant via the placenta. Infections are distributed worldwide, and most humans have become infected by the time they reach adulthood. CMV causes congenital infection in 1 to 2% of all live births in the United States. When pregnant women acquire the virus, there is a 30 to 40% transmission rate to the fetus (Remington & Klein, 1995; Fanaroff & Martin, 1997).

Clinical Findings

HISTORY. Maternal infection and intrauterine growth retardation can be part of the history.

PHYSICAL EXAMINATION. Ninety percent of infected newborns are asymptomatic. Findings include the following:

- SGA
- Hepatosplenomegaly
- Jaundice
- Petechial rash
- Chorioretinitis
- Cerebral calcifications
- Microcephaly

LABORATORY FINDINGS. CMV is isolated in cell cultures from urine, saliva, or other body fluids. Techniques for detection of viral DNA by polymerase chain reaction (PCR) are available from selected laboratories. Proof of congenital infection requires obtaining specimens within 3 weeks of birth. Viral isolation or a strongly positive test for serum IgM anti-CMV antibody is considered diagnostic.

Management

No specific treatment is available for minimally symptomatic immunocompetent neonates (Behrman & Kliegman, 1998). Monitor urine for CMV for 18 to 24 months. Serious infections in nonimmunocompromised neonates can be treated with antiviral agents.

Prognosis

The outcome of symptomatic congenital CMV infection is poor; there is a 20 to 30% mortality rate and a 90 to 95% morbidity rate, characterized by psychomotor retardation, microcephaly, hearing loss, seizures, and learning disabilities (Fanaroff & Martin, 1997).

Prevention

At greatest risk are susceptible pregnant women exposed to the urine and saliva of CMV-infected children who attend day care centers (AAP, 1997a). Handwashing and simple hygienic measures should be reinforced in this population.

GROUP B STREPTOCOCCUS (GBS)

Organism

GBS is a gram-positive diplococcus that is the leading cause of sepsis in infants from birth to 3 months of age resulting in significant perinatal morbidity and mortality. Early-onset disease usually occurs within the first 24 hours of life; late-onset disease occurs during the second week of life.

Etiology

The organism forms colonies in the maternal genitourinary and gastrointestinal tracts. Pregnant women are usually asymptomatic but can manifest chorioamnionitis, endometritis, or urinary tract infection. Infants born of women who are highly colonized are more likely to become colonized. GBS is acquired by newborns following vertical transmission (e.g, ascending infection through ruptured amniotic membranes or contamination following passage through the colonized birth canal). As many as 50% of infants with early-onset disease are symptomatic at birth, indicating an intrauterine infection. The highest attack rate of early-onset GBS is in high-risk deliveries, premature SGA infants, very low birth weight infants, or those with prolonged ruptured membranes; yet full-term infants account for 50% of cases. Colonization of pregnant women and newborns ranges from 5 to 35%. Incidence of GBS is 1 to 4 cases per 1000 live births. In colonized women it is 1 case per 100 to 200 live births (Fanaroff & Martin, 1997).

Clinical Findings

HISTORY. Risk factors include the following:

- Infants of less than 37 weeks' gestation
- Rupture of membranes (ROM) greater than 18 hours
- Maternal fever during labor greater then 100.4°F
- Previous delivery of a sibling with invasive GBS disease
- Maternal chorioamnionitis to include ROM and maternal fever with at least two of the following:
  ○ Maternal tachycardia (heart rate >90/ min)
  ○ Fetal tachycardia (heart rate >170/ min)
  ○ Maternal leukocytosis (white blood cell count >15,000)
  ○ Uterine tenderness
  ○ Foul-smelling amniotic fluid

PHYSICAL EXAMINATION. The following findings may be noted:

- Poor feeding
- Temperature instability
- Cyanosis, apnea, tachypnea, grunting, flaring, and retracting
- Seizures, lethargy, bulging fontanel
- Rapid onset and deterioration

LABORATORY FINDINGS. Cultures of blood, or CSF, or both, are definitive; antigen identification tests are available but have a false-positive rate of up to 8%.

Differential Diagnosis

RDS, amniotic fluid aspiration syndrome, persistent fetal circulation, meningitis, osteomyelitis, septic arthritis, sepsis from other infections, and metabolic problems are included in the differential diagnosis.

Management

Treatment involves the following:

1. Penicillin G is the treatment of choice for GBS infection. Initiate antibiotic therapy with a penicillin (usually ampicillin) and an amnioglycoside, usually gentamicin, until

GBS has been differentiated from *E. coli* or *Listeria* sepsis or meningitis (AAP, 1997b).

- Penicillin G intravenous:
  Infant less than 7 days of age, give 250,000 to 400,000 units/kg/d in three divided doses
  Infant older than 7 days of age, give 400,000 units/kg/d in four divided doses
- Ampicillin intravenous:
  Infant less than 7 days of age, give 200 mg/kg/d in three divided doses
  Infant older than 7 days of age, give 300 mg/kg/d in four to six divided doses
- Gentamicin doses are as follows (Harriet Lane Handbook, 2000):

Gestatational Age (weeks)	Age (days)	Dose
≤29 or asphyxia	0-28	2.5 mg/kg q24h
	>28	3 mg/kg q24h
30-36	0-14	3 mg/kg q24h
	>14	2.5 mg/kg q12h
≥37	0-7	2.5 mg/kg q12h
	>7	2.5 mg/kg q8h

2. Screening of all pregnant women at 26 to 28 weeks of gestation is recommended. Antepartum treatment of asymptomatic mothers carrying GBS is not recommended. Mothers identified antepartum or intrapartum as GBS carriers with specific risk factors should be treated with intravenous ampicillin or penicillin throughout labor until delivery. Treatment given to high-risk patients during labor has decreased transmission of GBS.

Prognosis

The mortality rate of early-onset disease ranges from 10 to 40%; mortality is highest in very low birth weight infants and in those with low neutrophil count (<1500), low Apgar scores, hypotension, apnea, and a delay in starting antimicrobial therapy.

Prevention

Chemoprophylaxis of high-risk, colonized women is an effective method of preventing early-onset GBS infection. Consensus guidelines developed by the Centers for Disease Control and Prevention (CDC, 1996a) outline steps for a screening-based and risk-factor strategy to prevent GBS. Treatment consists of intravenous penicillin or ampicillin given to high-risk women at the onset of labor, repeated every 4 hours until the infant is born.

LISTERIOSIS

Organism

Listeria monocytogenes is a small, gram-positive rod isolated from soil, streams, sewage, certain foods, silage, dust, and slaughterhouses.

Etiology

The foodborne transmission of disease is related to Mexican (soft ripened) cheese, whole and 2% milk, uncooked hot dogs, undercooked chicken, raw vegetables, and shellfish. The newborn infant acquires the organism transplacentally or by aspiration or ingestion at the time of delivery.

Clinical Findings

HISTORY. Brown-stained amniotic fluid is seen.

PHYSICAL EXAMINATION. The following findings may be noted:

- Generalized symptoms of sepsis
- Whitish posterior pharyngeal and cutaneous granulomas
- Disseminated erythematous papules on skin

LABORATORY FINDINGS. Cultures of the blood, CSF, meconium, and urine are done. The CSF shows elevated protein, depressed glucose, and a high leukocyte count.

Management

The following steps are taken:
1. Initial therapy with intravenous ampicillin and an aminoglycoside, usually gentamicin, is recommended for severe infections.
2. After clinical response occurs or for less severe infections in normal hosts, ampicillin alone may be given.
3. The duration of therapy is 10 to 14 days for infections without meningitis and 14 to 21

days for infections with meningitis (AAP, 1997b).

Prognosis

If listeriosis is acquired transplacentally, the fetus almost always aborts. The death rate of infants with *Listeria* pneumonia noted within 12 hours of birth approaches 100%. Mortality varies from 20 to 50% if disease develops between 5 and 30 days of birth. Mental retardation, paralysis, and hydrocephalus have been noted in survivors *of Listeria* meningitis (Remington & Klein, 1995; Fanaroff & Martin, 1997).

CONGENITAL VARICELLA

Organism

Varicella-zoster virus (VZV) is a herpesvirus.

Etiology and Incidence

Humans are the only source of infection for this highly contagious virus. The attack rate for congenital varicella syndrome in infants born to mothers with chickenpox during the first trimester is 1.2%; it is 2% when infection occurs between 13 and 20 weeks of gestation.

Clinical Findings

HISTORY. There is a history of maternal chickenpox infection.

PHYSICAL EXAMINATION. Findings may include:

• Limb atrophy
• Scarring of the skin of the affected extremity
• Eye manifestations

LABORATORY FINDINGS. Diagnosis of VZV is made by immunofluorescent staining of vesicular scrapings.

Management

Treatment consists of the following:
1. Some experts recommend acyclovir for pregnant women with varicella, especially in the third trimester (AAP, 1997a).

2. Varicella-zoster immune globulin (VZIG) is recommended for the newborn infant whose mother had an onset of chickenpox within 5 days before delivery or within 48 hours after delivery. VZIG is not indicated if the mother has varicella zoster (shingles) only.
3. Airborne and contact precautions are recommended for neonates born to mothers with varicella and, if still hospitalized, continued until 21 days of age or 28 days if they received VZIG.

Prognosis

Severe varicella of the newborn infant with fatality rates as high as 30% can result when an infant's mother develops varicella from 5 days before to 2 days after delivery (AAP, 1997a).

Prevention

Prevention efforts are targeted to potential mothers. The CDC recommends varicella vaccinations for nonpregnant women of childbearing age with no history of varicella infection (CDC, 1996b).

Sexually Transmitted Diseases

GONORRHEA

Organism

Neisseria gonorrhoeae is a gram-negative diplococcus.

Etiology

N. gonorrhoeae infection occurs only in humans. The source of the organism is exudate and secretions of infected mucous membranes. The organism is transmitted primarily through sexual acts and parturition. Gonococcal infections in the newborn are acquired during delivery.

Clinical Findings

HISTORY. There is a history of maternal gonococcal infection.

PHYSICAL EXAMINATION. Findings include conjunctivitis.

LABORATORY FINDINGS. Culture of eye exudate is positive for *N. gonorrhoeae*.

Management

Infants born to mothers with active gonorrhea should be given a single dose of intramuscular ceftriaxone 25 to 50 mg/kg (not to exceed 125 mg) for prophylaxis (CDC, 1998).

Prevention

Because gonorrheal conjunctivitis can rapidly lead to blindness, all infants are given eye prophylaxis at birth with 1% silver nitrate, 0.5% or 1% tetracycline ophthalmic ointment (AAP, 1997a), or erythromycin 0.5% ophthalmic ointment (CDC, 1998).

CHLAMYDIA

Organism

Chlamydial infection is caused by an obligate intracellular parasite.

Etiology and Incidence

Chlamydia trachomatis infection is the most common sexually transmitted disease in the United States. Acquisition occurs in approximately 50% of infants born vaginally to infected mothers and in some infants delivered by cesarean section with intact membranes. Of infants acquiring *C. trachomatis* infection, the risk of developing conjunctivitis is 25 to 50% and of pneumonia is 5 to 20% (AAP, 1997a).

Clinical Findings

HISTORY. There is a history of maternal chlamydial infection.

PHYSICAL EXAMINATION. The following findings may be noted:

- Conjunctivitis 1 to 3 weeks after birth (18 to 50%)
- Infant commonly afebrile and alert
- Pneumonia 2 to 19 weeks after birth (5 to 20%)

LABORATORY FINDINGS

- Tests for detection of *C. trachomatis* without cell culture include DNA probe, direct fluorescent antibody (DFA) staining, enzyme immunoassay (EIA), and nucleic acid amplification (PCR, ligase chain reaction [LCR]).
- Routine bacterial cultures are not helpful.
- Gram stain and culture of discharge from the eye (must include epithelial cells because chlamydia is an obligate parasite) are necessary for diagnosis.

Management

Oral erythromycin suspension (50 mg/kg/d in four divided doses for 10 to 14 days) is given for both conjunctivitis and pneumonia (CDC, 1998).

Prevention

Appropriate treatment of the pregnant woman before delivery prevents disease in the newborn.

SYPHILIS

Organism

Syphilis is caused by the spirochete *Treponema pallidum*.

Etiology and Incidence

T. pallidum crosses the placenta in an infected mother. Because the incidence of this disease is rapidly increasing in the United States, routine maternal serological testing is legally required during prenatal care in all states.

Clinical Findings

HISTORY. There is a history of maternal infection and positive serological testing in the mother.

PHYSICAL EXAMINATION. Two thirds of neonates are asymptomatic at birth. Findings include the following:

- Hepatosplenomegaly
- Persistent rhinorrhea

- Maculopapular or bullous dermal lesions
- Failure to thrive, restlessness, fever

RADIOLOGICAL AND LABORATORY FINDINGS. Periostitis or osteochondritis is verified by long bone radiography. CSF shows high protein, low glucose, high white blood cell count, and positivity on VDRL test; serum liver enzymes are elevated with liver involvement; and serum rapid plasma reagin (RPR) test is positive.

Management

The CDC (1998) recommends 10 days of either crystalline penicillin G 100,000 to 150,000 U/kg/d, given as 50,000 U/kg intravenously every 12 hours during the first 7 days of life and every 8 hours thereafter *or* procaine penicillin G 50,000 U/kg intramuscularly daily in a single dose as the only acceptable treatment regimen for congenital syphilis and for all infants born to seropositive mothers without a documented history of adequate treatment. If 1 day is missed, the entire course must be restarted.

Prognosis

Untreated congenital syphilis can lead to severe multi-organ involvement. Infants who are appropriately treated have a good prognosis.

HERPES SIMPLEX VIRUS

Description

There are three clinically distinguishable categories of herpes simplex virus (HSV) infection: (1) disseminated disease, (2) CNS disease, and (3) disease restricted to the skin, eyes, and mouth (Korones & Bada-Ellzey, 1993) (see Table 39–8).

Etiology and Incidence

HSV is transmitted by direct contact with infected maternal genitalia during the birth process. Transplacental transmission occurs but has been reported in only a few cases. The risk of neonatal infection is highest with primary genital infection (see Chapter 24).

Clinical Findings

HISTORY. The mother has active lesions at vaginal delivery.

PHYSICAL EXAMINATION. Vesicles in the skin, eye, and mouth are found. Symptoms of encephalitis can also be present.

LABORATORY FINDINGS. The virus is isolated in tissue cultures obtained from vesicles, nasopharyngeal or conjunctival swabs, urine, stool, and tracheal secretions.

Management

Acyclovir 30 to 60 mg/kg/d intravenously every 8 to 12 hours is given for 10 to 21 days (CDC, 1998).

Prognosis

Despite effective antiviral therapy, disseminated neonatal HSV infections and localized encephalitis have a considerable morbidity and mortality rate.

Prevention

The risk of acquiring this serious infection is lowered by performing cesarean delivery prior to rupture of membranes in any pregnancy in which signs or symptoms of HSV infection occur.

HUMAN IMMUNODEFICIENCY VIRUS

Etiology and Incidence

HIV, a retrovirus, is transmitted to the newborn via the placenta or at birth secondary to exposure to maternal blood. It is estimated that an infant born to an untreated mother who is HIV positive has a 15 to 30% chance of becoming HIV positive. Half of these infected infants (if untreated) develop acquired immunodeficiency syndrome (AIDS) in the first months of life and die soon thereafter. The other half remain relatively well during infancy but gradually become chronically ill during childhood. Perinatally acquired HIV infections are increasing rapidly in the United States. In 80% of all infected children, transmission occurred from mothers with AIDS (Behrman & Kliegman, 1998).

Clinical Findings

HISTORY. The history includes an HIV-positive mother. It can also include the following:

- Maternal intravenous drug abuse
- Maternal intercourse with a high-risk male
- Maternal receipt of blood products prior to April 1985

PHYSICAL EXAMINATION. Most infants are asymptomatic. Findings *may* include:

- Low birth weight
- Microcephaly
- Failure to thrive

LABORATORY FINDINGS. HIV DNA PCR is the preferred virological method for diagnosing HIV infection during infancy. Because of concerns regarding potential contamination with maternal blood, blood samples from the umbilical cord should not be used for diagnostic evaluations. HIV infection can be reasonably excluded among children with two or more negative virological tests, two of which are performed at age 1 month or older, and one of those being performed at age 4 months or older. Two or more negative HIV IgG antibody tests performed at age 6 months or older with an interval of at least 1 month between the tests also can be used to reasonably exclude HIV infection among children with no clinical evidence of HIV infection (CDC, 1998).

Management

Treatment consists of the following:

1. The principal antiretroviral agent used in newborns is zidovudine. The safety and pharmacokinetics of nevirapine and several protease inhibitors are being investigated (U.S. Department of Health and Human Services, 1998b). Ideally, antiretroviral therapy should be initiated in all HIV-infected infants less than 12 months old as soon as a confirmed diagnosis is established.
2. Other therapy, such as trimethoprim-sulfamethoxazole, is designed to prevent or manage complications. See Chapter 24 for more detail.
3. Breastfeeding is contraindicated in HIV-positive mothers because of documented trans-

mission via breast milk (Klaus & Fanaroff, 1993).

Prognosis

Improving the outcomes for HIV-infected infants depends on identifying infants at risk early so that prompt prophylactic strategies and therapeutic interventions can be initiated.

Prevention

Early identification of maternal HIV infection during the antenatal period enables provision of antiretroviral chemoprophylaxis with zidovudine during pregnancy, during labor, and to newborns to reduce the risk of HIV transmission from mother to infant. The use of zidovudine can reduce the perinatal transmission to 8% (Behrman & Kliegman, 1998). Although research is continuing, vaccine immunization is not yet available. Prevention efforts are targeted at potential mothers, including the reduction of risk factors through behavioral changes.

Drug-Exposed Infants

COCAINE (CRACK) EXPOSURE

Description

Cocaine is a local anesthetic and CNS stimulant that is believed to be a teratogen that crosses the placenta.

Clinical Findings

HISTORY. Maternal exposure to cocaine or crack and positive urine drug screen for cocaine are found.

PHYSICAL EXAMINATION. Many infants will show no adverse affects from maternal use of cocaine. Findings may include the following:

- Low birth weight or prematurity
- Microcephaly
- Feeding difficulties, including voracious appetite, poorly coordinated sucking and swallowing, and vomiting
- CNS symptoms of transient irritability, abnormal sleeping patterns, tremors, hypertonia, and lability of mood (Marion, 1995)

- There is no clinically documented neonatal withdrawal syndrome for cocaine

Management

The following steps are taken:

1. If treatment is indicated, a short course of phenobarbital is recommended.
2. Pacification techniques such as swaddling and decreasing environmental stimuli are also encouraged.
3. Because cocaine is detectable in breast milk, mothers who use cocaine should not breastfeed.

Complications

Prenatal cocaine exposure has been associated with long-term changes in behavior, including neurobehavioral dysfunction, hyperactivity, aggression, and short attention span (Plessinger & Woods, 1998).

Prevention

Elimination of in utero exposure to cocaine can occur only if there is identification of a potential problem in a high-risk mother and referral to a substance abuse prevention program.

HEROIN AND METHADONE EXPOSURE

Description

Heroin and methadone are narcotics that cross the placenta.

Clinical Findings

HISTORY

- Maternal exposure to heroin or methadone
- Urine drug screen positive for opiates
- Increased incidence of stillbirths and SGA infants, but not congenital anomalies

PHYSICAL EXAMINATION. Findings include:

- Tremors and hyperirritability
- Skin abrasions secondary to hyperactivity

- Tachypnea
- Poor feeding
- Diarrhea
- Vomiting
- High-pitched cry
- Fist-sucking
- Low birth weight in 50% (Behrman et al., 1996)

Symptoms of withdrawal occur in up to 75% of infants, usually beginning in the first 48 hours of life, depending on the daily maternal dose, duration of addiction, and time of last maternal dose. There is a higher incidence of symptomatology if the last dose was taken within 24 hours of birth. Overall, the withdrawal syndrome is more severe and more prolonged with methadone than with heroin.

Differential Diagnosis

The differential diagnosis includes hypoglycemia and hypocalcemia.

Management

Supportive management is needed. Medications such as phenobarbital, paregoric, and methadone can be used if symptoms such as severe irritability, vomiting and diarrhea, seizures, temperature instability, or severe tachypnea are noted (Fanaroff & Martin, 1997).

Prevention

Pregnant women who are addicted to heroin should be encouraged to enter a treatment program.

FETAL ALCOHOL SYNDROME

See Chapter 41.

SUDDEN INFANT DEATH SYNDROME (SIDS) AND APPARENT LIFE-THREATENING EVENTS

Description

The accepted definition of *sudden infant death syndrome (SIDS)* is "the sudden death of an infant under 1 year of age which remains unexplained after a thorough case investigation, including performance of a complete autopsy, examination of the death scene, and review of the clinical history" (Willinger et al., 1991). SIDS rarely occurs in the first week of life, with the majority of deaths occurring between 1 and 6 months, peaking at 12 weeks (85% occur between 2 and 4 months of age). SIDS usually does not occur with the first baby. It is a diagnosis of exclusion.

An "apparent life-threatening event" (ALTE) is defined as an episode that is frightening to the observer and that is characterized by some combination of apnea (central or occasionally obstructive), color change, marked change in muscle tone, choking, or gagging. In some cases, the observer fears that the infant has died (NIH, 1987).

Etiology and Incidence

The specific cause of SIDS remains unknown; it cannot be predicted or prevented, although placing the infant in a supine position has been shown to decrease the incidence of SIDS and is now the recommended sleep position for infants. Experts have considered as possible causes respiratory obstruction, restrictive clothing, and hyperthermia. Factors associated with SIDS include low birth weight, preterm birth, low maternal age, high parity, maternal smoking and drug use, and poverty.

SIDS is the most common cause of death in infants under 6 months of age, with 85% occurring between 2 and 4 months of age, 95% occurring under 6 months (Gilbert-Barness & Barness, 1995). Approximately 5200 to 5500 infants per year die of the syndrome. The incidence in the United States is 1.3 per 1000 live births. There is a higher frequency of SIDS in male infants and in the winter months. Babies are usually found dead between 6 AM and noon (Behrman et al., 1996). The NIH has monitored sleep position since 1992 and prone sleeping has decreased from 70% to 24%. At the same time the SIDS death rate has fallen by 38% in the United States (AAP, 1996).

Clinical Findings

HISTORY. The history can include the following:

- Maternal: cigarette smoking, drug or alcohol abuse during pregnancy; no or poor prenatal care; bottle-feeding; poor education; unmarried; multiparity; maternal age less than 20 years; short intervals between pregnancies; anemia
- Infant: Prematurity (<37 weeks); low birth weight (<2500 g) or SGA; twins or other multiple births; Apgar score less than 6 at 5 minutes; apnea; poor weight gain; anemia; intensive care unit stay; neonatal respiratory abnormality, bronchopulmonary dysplasia, previous acute life-threatening event. Many have had cold symptoms a week to a few days before the incident (Behrman et al., 1996; Gilbert-Barness & Barness, 1995)
- Socioeconomic/other: low-income family; crowded living conditions; poor housing conditions; other SIDS in family (<2%); prone sleeping position, soft bedding; race, ethnicity, culture

PHYSICAL EXAMINATION. Findings include the following:

- No sign of injury
- Frothy blood-tinged secretions in mouth and nares
- Intrathoracic petechiae on autopsy
- Retention of periadrenal brown fat on autopsy

Differential Diagnosis

Aspiration; suffocation; infant botulism or poisoning; cardiac or respiratory disease; hypoxemia; infection; metabolic disorders; child abuse, Munchausen syndrome or shaken baby syndrome (Coody, et al., 1994); and CNS abnormalities should be ruled out.

Management

Management is aimed at assisting the family to cope with the loss of the child. The first response of the family is disbelief and shock.

RESOURCE BOX 39-1

NATIONAL PERINATAL RESOURCES

Alexander Graham Bell Association for the Deaf
(AGBAD)
Tel: (202) 337-5220
Website: www.agbell.org
Newsletter, informational materials (incl. Spanish), networking, referrals to local resources, local chapters, advocacy, scholarship program

American Pseudo-Obstruction and Hirschsprung
Disease Society
Tel: (800) 394-2747
Tel: (508) 685-4477
Website: www.tiac.net/users/aphs
Newsletter, informational materials (incl. Spanish), networking, referrals to local resources, local chapters, advocacy, fund research, maintains research registry

American Society for Deaf Children
Tel: (800) 942-2732
Newsletter, informational materials, networking, referrals to local resources

Association of Birth Defect Children
Tel: (800) 313-2232 (24 hour registry line)
Tel: (407) 245-7035
Website: www.birthdefects.org

Association for Macular Diseases
Tel: (212) 605-3719
Website: www.macula.org
Newsletter, informational materials, referrals to local resources, local chapters, funds research

Back to Sleep
Website: www.nih.gov/nichd/

Centers for Disease Control and Prevention
Website: www.cdc.gov/ncidod/diseases
Guidelines for diseases management such as group B streptococcus, varicella, sexually transmitted diseases

Cherub Association of Families and Friends of
Children With Limb Disorders
Tel: (716) 773-2769
Newsletter, networking, referrals to local resources, summer camp

Cleft Palate Foundation
Tel: (800) 242-5338
Tel: (914) 933-9044
Website: www.cleft.com
Informational materials (incl. Spanish), networking, referrals to local resources to local resources, advocacy, funds research

Compassionate Friends
Website: www.compassionatefriends.org

Family Empowerment Network: Supporting
Families Affected by FAS/FAE
Tel: (800) 462-5254
Tel: (608) 262-6590
Informational materials (incl. Spanish), networking, referrals to local resources

Group B Strep Association
Tel: (919) 932-5344
Newsletter, informational materials, networking, referrals to local resources, advocacy, funds research, maintains research registry
Newsletter, informational materials, networking, local chapter, advocacy, funds research, maintains research registry

The National SIDS Resource Center
Tel: (800) 821-8955

The Sudden Infant Death Syndrome Alliance
Tel: (800) 221-7437
Website: www.sidsalliance.org

TEF/VATER International Support Network
Tel: (301) 952-6837

---

1. Obtain a thorough history from the caretaker within a short period of time after the death. Do not accuse the family of any wrongdoing. Focus on the questioning around the cause of death to better understand the circumstances.
2. Reassure caretaker and family that it was not their fault and could not have been prevented.
3. Offer support and counsel to families as soon as possible after death.
4. Supply names of different support groups to help the family overcome grief. Agencies to contact are listed in the Resource Box at the end of the chapter.
5. Provide follow-up for 1 year.
6. Assist surviving siblings. Observe their reaction to the death and refer for counseling if

T A B L E 39-13

Measures That Aid in the Prevention of Sudden Infant Death Syndrome

1. Place infants on their backs to sleep until at least 6 mo of age. The National Institutes of Health has a "Back-to-Sleep" program with parent information, stickers, and video (See Resource Box)
2. Use a firm mattress. Do not use soft bedding or have stuffed animals in bed. Infants should not sleep in a water bed or in bed with adult
3. Avoid overheating; room temperature should be 68–72°F
4. Avoid alcohol and drugs while pregnant and breastfeeding
5. Do not allow cigarette smoke around baby
6. For at-risk infants, educate parents and caregivers regarding monitor use and cardiopulmonary resuscitation

necessary. Help them to understand that it was not their fault and alleviate their feelings of guilt. Allow children to verbalize their feelings. Assist parents to deal with the other children; suggest that parents give extra love, attention, and reassurance to their other children.

7. Evaluate need for home monitoring. Since the rate of SIDS in succeeding children is very low (<2%) and since monitoring a child cannot prevent a SIDS episode from occurring, the controversy remains about whether to monitor succeeding children (Marcus, 1998). Monitors are frequently recommended when more than one child in a family has died from SIDS (Carbone, 1992).

Prevention

See Table 39-13 for measures that aid in the prevention of SIDS.

REFERENCES

Abbasi S, Bhutani V, Gerdes J: Long term pulmonary consequences of respiratory distress syndrome in preterm infants treated with exogenous surfactant. J Pediatr 122:446–452, 1993.

American Academy of Pediatrics (AAP): Positioning and SIDS. Pediatrics 89:1120–1126, 1992.

American Academy of Pediatrics (AAP): Practice parameter: Management of hyperbilirubinemia in the healthy term newborn. Pediatrics 94:558–565, 1994.

American Academy of Pediatrics (AAP): Hospital stay for healthy term newborns. Pediatrics 96:788–790, 1995a.

American Academy of Pediatrics (AAP): Joint Committee on Infant Hearing 1994 position statement. Pediatrics 95:152–156, 1995b.

American Academy of Pediatrics (AAP): Positioning and sudden infant death syndrome (SIDS): Update. Pediatrics 98:1216–1218, 1996.

American Academy of Pediatrics (AAP), American Association for Pediatric Ophthalmology and Strabismus (AAPOS), American Academy of Ophthalmology (AAO): Screening examination of premature infants for retinopathy of prematurity. Pediatrics 100:273, 1997.

American Academy of Pediatrics: 1997 Red Book: Report of the Committee on Infectious Diseases, 24th ed. Elk Grove Village, IL: American Academy of Pediatrics, 1997a.

American Academy of Pediatrics (AAP) Committee on Infectious Diseases and Committee on Fetus and Newborn: Revised guidelines for prevention of early-onset group B streptococcal (GBS) infection. Pediatrics 99:489–496, 1997b.

Apgar V: Evaluation of the newborn infant. Second report. JAMA 168:1985, 1958.

Armentrout D: Neonatal diabetes mellitus. J Pediatr Health Care 9:75–78, 1995.

Ballard JL, Khoury JC, Wedig K, et al: New Ballard Score, expanded to include extremely premature infants. J Pediatr 119:417–423, 1991.

Banks J, Montgomery D, Coody D, et al: Hyperbilirubinemia in the term newborn. J Pediatr Health Care 10(5):228–230, 1996.

Battaglia FC, Lubchenco LO: A practical classification of newborn infants by weight and gestational age. J Pediatr 71:159–163, 1967.

Behrman RE, Kliegman RM, Arvin AM (eds): Nelson Textbook of Pediatrics, 15th ed. Philadelphia, WB Saunders, 1996.

Behrman RE, Kliegman RM: Nelson Essentials of Pediatrics, 3rd ed. Philadelphia, WB Saunders, 1998.

Betz CL, Hunsberger M, Wright S: Family-Centered Nursing Care of Children, 2nd ed. Philadelphia, WB Saunders, 1994, p 124.

Brown AK: Diagnostic features of the various types of neonatal jaundice. Pediatr Clin North Am 9:589, 1962.

Buist N, Tuerck J: The practitioner's role in newborn screening. Pediatr Clin North Am 39:199–211, 1992.

Carbone MT: Sudden infant death syndrome and subsequent siblings. N J Med 89:684–686, 1992.

Centers for Disease Control and Prevention (CDC): Prevention of perinatal group B streptococcal disease: A public health perspective. MMWR 45(RR-7):1–24, 1996a.

Centers for Disease Control and Prevention (CDC): Prevention of varicella: Recommendations of the Advisory Committee on Immunizations Practices (ACIP). MMWR 45 (RR-11):1–36, 1996b.

Centers for Disease Control and Prevention (CDC): 1998 Guidelines for treatment of sexually transmitted diseases. MMWR 47(RR-1):1–111, 1998.

Coody D, Brown M, Montgomery D, et al: Shaken baby syndrome: Identification and prevention for nurse practitioners. J Pediatr Health Care 8(2):50-56, 1994.

Desmond MM, Rudolph AJ, Phitaksphraiwan P: The transitional care nursery. Pediatr Clin North Am 13:651-668, 1966.

Ein SH: Esophageal atresia and tracheoesophageal fistula. *In* Wyllie R, Hyams JS (eds): Pediatric Gastrointestinal Disease. Philadelphia, WB Saunders, 1993, pp 318-336.

Fanaroff AA, Martin RJ: Neonatal-Perinatal Medicine: Diseases of the Fetus and Infant. St Louis, Mosby-Year Book, 1997.

Finberg L: Saunders Manual of Pediatric Practice. Philadelphia, WB Saunders, 1998.

Gartner LM: Neonatal jaundice. Pediatr Rev 15:422-432, 1994.

Gilbert-Barness E, Barness L: Sudden infant death: a reappraisal. Contemp Pediatr 12(4):88-107, 1995.

Goodwin TM: Role of the Apgar score in assessing perinatal asphyxia. Contemp Pediatr 14(10):142-152, 1997.

Green M (ed): Bright Futures: Guidelines for Health Supervision of Infants, Children and Adolescents. Arlington, VA: National Center for Education in Maternal and Child Health, 1994.

Harriet Lane Handbook: A Manual for Pediatric House Officers. Baltimore, Johns Hopkins Hospital, 2000.

Hauth JC, Merenstein GB: Guidelines for Perinatal Care, 4th ed. Elk Grove Village, IL: American Academy of Pediatrics and American College of Obstetricians and Gynecologists, 1997.

Hoekelman R, Blatman S, Friedman S, et al: Primary Pediatric Care, 3rd ed. St Louis, Mosby-Year Book, 1997.

Klaus MH, Fanaroff AA: Care of the High-Risk Neonate, 4th ed. Philadelphia, WB Saunders, 1993.

Korones IB, Bada-Ellzey H: Neonatal Decision Making. St Louis, Mosby-Year Book, 1993.

Lubchenco LO, Hansman C, Boyd E: Intrauterine growth in length and head circumference as estimated from live births at gestational ages from 26 to 42 weeks. Pediat 37:403-408, 1966.

Marcus CL: Infant apnea monitoring and SIDS: A guide to appropriate use. Adv Nurs Pract Aug:55-56, 1998.

Marion I: Pregnant, Substance-Abusing Women. Treatment Improvement Protocol (TIP), Series 2. US Department of Health and Human Services, Rockville, MD, 1995.

National Association of Pediatric Nurse Associates and Practitioners (NAPNAP): Newborn discharge and follow-up care. J Pediatr Health Care 11(3):147-148, 1997.

National High Blood Pressure Education Program (NHBPEP) Working Group on Hypertension Control in Children and Adolescents: Update on the 1987 Task Force Report on High Blood Pressure in Children and Adolescents: A working group report from the National High Blood Pressure Education Program. Pediatrics 98(4, pt 1):649-658, 1996.

National Institutes of Health (NIH): Consensus development conference on infantile apnea and home monitoring. Pediatrics 79:292-299, 1987.

Plessinger M, Woods J: Substance abuse in pregnancy. Obstet Gynecol Clin 25:100-118, 1998.

Remington JS, Klein JO: Infectious Diseases of the Fetus and Newborn Infant, 3rd ed. Philadelphia: WB Saunders, 1995.

Robertson WO: Personal reflections on the AAP practice parameter on management of hyperbilirubinemia in the healthy term newborn. Pediatr Rev 19:75-77, 1998.

Thilo EH, Townsend SF: Early newborn discharge. Have we gone too far? Contemp Pediatr 13(4):29-46, 1996.

US Department of Health and Human Services: Healthy Children 2000 National Health Promotion and Disease Prevention Objectives for the Year 2000. Washington, DC, Government Printing Office, 1990.

US Department of Health and Human Services: Healthy People 2010 Objectives. Washington, DC, 1998a. Website: www.health.gov/healthypeople.

US Department of Health and Human Services: Revised guidelines on the use of retrovirals for pediatrics HIV infection. MMWR 47:1998b.

US Preventive Services Task Force: Guide to Clinical Preventive Services, 2nd ed. Baltimore, Williams & Wilkins, 1996.

US Public Health Services: Put Prevention Into Practice: The Clinician's Handbook of Preventive Services, 2nd ed. Germantown, MD, International Medical Publishing, 1997.

Willinger M, James LS, Catz D: Defining the sudden infant death syndrome (SIDS): Deliberations of an expert panel convened by the National Institute of Child Health and Human Development. Pediatr Pathol 11:677-684, 1991.

Common Injuries

Margaret A. Brady

▰▰ INTRODUCTION

Injuries are major pediatric health problems managed with both treatment and prevention strategies. Children with an injury might respond best to (1) a simple home treatment by the parent, caregiver, or supervising adult; (2) intervention by the provider in the primary care setting; (3) referral to a medical specialist or inpatient facility; or a combination of these. Providers also have a responsibility to assist families to prevent such problems from occurring. Chapter 11 discusses strategies for prevention of injuries as part of ongoing health maintenance. This chapter focuses on the identification and management of common pediatric injuries frequently seen by primary care providers and discusses prevention of subsequent injuries.

Injuries are the leading cause of death in children and adolescents from age 1 to 19 years (American Academy of Pediatrics, 1999). Such injuries are responsible for significant health care dollar expenditures. Prevention of nonintentional injuries involves anticipatory guidance to help parents provide a safe environment for children.

The type of trauma experienced is often related to children's activities and developmental stage. As children grow and mature, they need to assume responsibility for their own actions and safety; thus, attention must be directed toward age-appropriate counseling for children and teenagers. Written materials, audiovisual presentations, peer counseling, and one-to-one interaction with a health professional are all effective teaching and learning strategies. In addition, the use of protective equipment and the institution of certain safety measures within the home, school, and other environments frequented by children often can prevent or decrease the severity of injury. Furthermore, the nurse practitioner (NP) can advocate for local and national prevention strategies and support such programs as the National SAFE KIDS Campaign as well as injury prevention legislation or initiatives. Public and consumer awareness is crucial in prevention programs.

Although most children with serious injuries are seen first in emergency departments, the NP has a professional obligation to remain current in basic life support techniques and to demonstrate competence in performing emergency cardiopulmonary resuscitation and intervening when infants, children, or adults are choking. Likewise, all parents and caregivers should be encouraged to enroll in a basic pediatric life support program, especially parents and caregivers of infants and children at risk for cardiopulmonary arrest.

COMMON PEDIATRIC INJURIES

Trauma to the Skin and Soft Tissue

ABRASIONS

Description

A simple abrasion represents the loss of mucous membrane or the superficial layer (epidermis) of the skin without loss of dermal integrity. Abrasions are the equivalent of second-degree burns.

Etiology

Abrasions often result from falls or friction accidents. Mechanical means such as dermabrasion can remove the superficial layer of the skin.

Assessment

HISTORY. Seek information about the cause and type of injury and the presence of a foreign object or dirt at the accident scene.

PHYSICAL EXAMINATION. The extent of the abrasion and the presence of dirt, grime, or other foreign body (e.g., tar) should be determined. Findings include an area of skin that appears scraped off with oozing of serum and blood.

Differential Diagnosis

The history of an injury and physical findings are the key to diagnosis. Any other skin condition that can cause loss of epidermis, such as a burn, is included in the differential diagnosis.

Management

Appropriate first aid care is important to prevent infection. Most abrasions can be managed at home unless the abrasion is quite deep, involves a large area, is associated with severe pain, or has significant dirt, grime, tar, or a foreign body in the wound. The immunocompromised patient may need to be seen. Corneal abrasions are discussed in Chapter 29. Management of an abrasion includes the following points:

1. Thoroughly cleanse the wound. The area can be scrubbed with an antibacterial cleanser using a wet gauze or soft surgical nail brush. If debris is not removed, new skin grows over the particles, resulting in a tattoo.
2. Debride pieces of loose skin with a sterile scissors and remove foreign particles with a tweezers. If tar particles are present, the area can be rubbed with petrolatum.
3. Keep small abrasions open to the air.
4. Cover larger abrasions with a nonadherent dressing. Change this dressing in 12 hours, and expose the wound to air within 24 hours.
5. Protect abrasions of the hands, feet, or areas overlying joints from friction until healed. Cover these abrasions with daily dressing changes.
6. Use bacitracin or povidone-iodine (Betadine) ointment on abrasions involving the elbows or knees to prevent cracking or reopening from constant movement and stretching of the joints. Instruct the parent to wash the area daily and reapply ointment.

PUNCTURE WOUNDS

Description

Puncture wounds result from penetration of varying levels of the skin and its underlying tissue or structures. These wounds are typically classified as superficial or deep. Because of the potential for serious infection, puncture wounds must be carefully evaluated and treated if indicated. The location and depth of the wound, plus retention of a foreign object, are key risk factors for the development of infection. For example, deep penetrating wounds and injuries to the forefoot, especially if they involve the plantar fascia, have a higher risk of infection than wounds to the arch or heel area. The forefoot has less overlying soft tissue than other plantar surfaces and is the major weight-bearing area of the foot; therefore, cartilage and bone can be involved. In contrast, puncture wounds to muscle, if clean, can be quite deep and still have a relatively low risk of infection.

Etiology and Incidence

Puncture wounds are common pediatric injuries, generally first seen in children at around 2 years of age. A nail, often rusty, is the classic cause of injury and accounts for 98% of puncture wounds that require health care intervention. Glass, wood splinters and toothpicks, needles, metal and wire, staples, and thumbtacks are other sources of injury.

Although the majority of puncture wounds heal without problems, a sizable minority of these injuries are complicated by infections, mostly cellulitis or soft tissue abscesses. Less frequently seen are significant infections such as osteomyelitis-osteochondritis or pyarthrosis. Generally, normal skin flora, footwear, or the foreign object itself is the source of bacterial infection in these wounds. Pathogens frequently implicated include

- *Staphylococcus aureus* and group A streptococci for cellulitis
- *Pseudomonas aeruginosa* for osteomyelitis-osteochondritis
- *S. aureus*, group A streptococci, or *P. aeruginosa* for pyarthrosis

Most children in whom *P. aeruginosa* osteomyelitis develops report a puncture to the foot while wearing used sneakers. *P. aeruginosa* colonizes on the foam-rubber soles of used sneakers and can enter the wound when a nail or other object punctures the foot (Staheli, 1998; Inaba, 1993).

Assessment

Many parents and patients seek care only after symptoms of secondary infection develop.

HISTORY. Important information to elicit after a report or suspicion of a puncture wound includes the following (Schmitt, 1999):

- Date of injury and wound care provided at the time of initial injury.
- Identification of the agent of injury. If it is not known what object penetrated the skin, the likelihood of an imbedded foreign body is high.
- Condition of the penetrating object. Was the object clean or rusty, jagged or smooth?

- Whether all or part of the foreign object was removed.
- Whether the child was barefoot or what type and condition of footwear was being worn (injuries to the foot).
- Immunization status for tetanus coverage.
- Presence of any medical condition that increases the risk for infectious complications.

PHYSICAL EXAMINATION. A careful examination of the puncture wound and skin around it is essential on initial and follow-up examinations. Findings indicative of cellulitis are:

- Localized pain, swelling of the dorsum of the foot, and erythema
- Possible fever
- Pain with flexion or extension of the extremity involved
- Decreased ability to bear weight
- Pain along the plantar aspect of the foot during extension or flexion of the toes (can indicate deep tissue injury)

Findings indicative of osteomyelitis-osteochondritis are as noted for cellulitis, with extension of pain and swelling around the puncture wound and to adjacent bony structures. In pyarthrosis (septic arthritis), there are findings of pain, swelling, and decreased range of motion of the affected joint and decreased weight-bearing ability. In the foot, the metatarsophalangeal joint of the great toe is most frequently involved.

DIAGNOSTIC STUDIES. The following are ordered as indicated:

- A plain film radiograph should be ordered if a retained foreign body is suspected; the object is still embedded; there was penetration of a joint space, the bone or growth cartilage, or the plantar fascia of the foot; or if the puncture site is due to a nail injury and has signs of infection (Staheli, 1998).
- If the radiograph is negative but a retained foreign object is still suspected, computed tomography (CT), ultrasound, and magnetic resonance imaging (MRI) are useful tools.

- A bone scan can be positive within 24 hours of the first appearance of symptoms of osteomyelitis.
- A complete blood count (CBC) may be needed.
- Erythrocyte sedimentation rate (ESR) may be mild to moderately elevated in osteomyelitis-osteochondritis.
- Some clinicians recommend a baseline culture of the wound if it is infected.

Differential Diagnosis

A history of penetrating injury and the symptoms are the keys to whether the injury represents a superficial wound that will heal uneventfully or develop infectious complications.

Management

If radiographs demonstrate that an embedded object has invaded bone, growth cartilage, or a joint space, the child should be referred immediately to an orthopedic surgeon.

Inaba (1993) specifically presents treatment methods for four categories of puncture wounds to the foot, but these methods can be used with other puncture wounds as well. All four categories require tetanus prophylaxis as indicated by the child's immunization status. Categories 2 to 4 involve a coring procedure that includes removal of a 2-mm rim of tissue around the puncture wound, using local anesthesia for pain control during the procedure. The NP may be involved in performing this procedure or providing follow-up wound care.

Category 1: a clean, superficial injury that occurred in a clean environment and presents with no indications of a retained foreign body and minimal pain around the puncture site or on weight bearing. Treatment consists of the following:
Wash wound and skin around it with a 1% povidone-iodine solution to remove debris.
Instruct parents to wash and keep wound clean, cover puncture site with adhesive bandage, and return if signs of infection occur (redness, swelling, increased pain, or decreased ability to bear weight).

Category 2: a grossly contaminated wound, deep tissue wound, or injury suspicious of a retained foreign body. Treatment consists of the following:
Perform coring procedure to enlarge puncture site and search for foreign body, using local anesthesia or posterior tibial nerve block to deaden the area.
Irrigate the wound with normal saline and pack with a strand of 14-inch sterile iodoform gauze.
Instruct parents to allow no weight bearing for 3 to 4 days with foot injury.
Schedule return visit to recheck wound within 48 hours and again in 1 week or immediately if symptoms of increased pain, erythema, swelling, or decreased ability to bear weight occur.
Category 3: wound with evidence of cellulitis or soft tissue abscess. Treatment consists of the following:
Perform coring procedure plus irrigation of the wound with normal saline and packing as described in category 2.
Culture the cellulitic area by needle aspiration.
Begin initial antibiotic coverage with oral dicloxacillin or erythromycin (if allergic to penicillin) for 7 days; change antibiotic coverage only if needed after culture results are known.
Instruct parents to allow no weight bearing for 3 to 4 days with foot injury.
Schedule return visit to recheck within 48 hours; have child return if pain, erythema, and swelling do not improve within 48 hours of beginning antibiotics.
Consider intravenous antibiotics if there is no improvement within 48 hours of oral antibiotic.
Category 4: high suspicion of osteomyelitis-osteochondritis or pyarthrosis.
Refer for orthopedic consultation.

A useful guide to remember about the appearance of signs of infection and the likely causative agents after a nail puncture wound is as follows:

- 1 day: *Streptococcus*
- 3-4 days: *Staphylococcus*
- 7 days: *Pseudomonas*

Pseudomonas is the likely organism if a nail puncture wound is through a shoe.

Patient and Parent Education

The importance of prompt attention to and close follow-up with puncture wounds, especially of the foot, should be emphasized to patients and parents.

INGROWN TOE NAILS AND NAIL HEMATOMA

Description

Two commonly seen problems in pediatrics are ingrown toenails and nail hematomas from trauma to the nail. Ingrown toenails are caused by any of the following: anatomic predisposition, improper nail trimming, trauma, or constrictive shoes or stockings. Nail hematomas are due to injury and the formation of a subungual hematoma. Nail injuries that involve lacerations or fracture of the distal phalanx should be referred out; uncomplicated nail hematomas can be drained (nail trephination) by primary care providers, typically without local anesthesia.

Management

The treatment for these problems is as follows:

- Ingrown toe nail
  - Pack cotton under the nail edge to elevate the nail from inflamed nailbed.
  - Elevation and soaking for cleaning and promotion of drainage may be needed for more severe inflammation.
  - Instruct about wearing properly fitting shoes and correctly trimming the nails. Toe nails should be trimmed so that a concave end is left to extend the nail edge beyond the skin.
- Nail hematoma
  - Determine whether a digital or regional nerve block is needed (NP may or may not be skilled in this procedure).
  - Attempt to lift the nail to examine for the presence of significant nailbed injuries.
  - Clean nail surface with povidone-iodine solution.

  - Make one or more holes in the area of the nail hematoma with either a portable heat cautery device or a heated paperclip. (Untwist a paperclip and use the rounded tip.)
  - A number 11 scalpel blade is an alternative instrument. Create a small hole or holes in the nail by applying downward pressure with a rotary motion of scalpel.
  - One or more holes need to be made to permit continued drainage.
  - Antibiotics generally are not needed (Krug, 1998).

LACERATIONS

Description

A laceration is a tear in the tissue. Lacerations are classified according to three categories: degree of tissue loss, contamination, and depth of the wound. Lacerations are labeled *simple* if there is no tissue loss, no deep injury, and no embedded debris; they are labeled *complex* if there is tissue loss, deep injury, and debris present. Lacerations are *clean* if the injury to the tissue was done by a clean instrument directly onto the skin rather than being *contaminated* if the wound contains foreign debris, was made through clothing or other material, or is associated with road or farm debris. Lacerations are *superficial* if only the skin and subcutaneous tissue are involved rather than being *deep* if fascia, muscle, tendons, or nerves are affected (Ratner, 1991).

Etiology and Incidence

Lacerations are caused by various forms of trauma. They are common reasons for pediatric health care visits.

Assessment

HISTORY. Important questions to ask include the following:

- How did the injury happen? This information helps to ascertain the likelihood of retained foreign bodies such as dirt, debris, glass, and splinters.

- How long ago (number of hours) did the injury occur?
- What is the child's tetanus immunization status?
- Does the child have allergies to antibiotics or anesthetics?

PHYSICAL EXAMINATION. Important points in the examination of the injury are:

- Cleanse wound (see Management) and cover with saline-soaked gauze until the practitioner is ready to begin the examination.
- Wear gloves and a mask when examining and probing wound.
- Administer local anesthesia before probing wound to determine depth, presence of debris, or involvement of deep tissue structures.
- Carefully inspect for possible foreign body or debris. Use adequate lighting after wound area is cleansed.
- Evaluate range of motion. This is especially important in wounds involving the distal forearm, wrist, and hand.
- Evaluate degree to which vascular and neurological structures are intact, both in the wound area and the area distal to it.

Differential Diagnosis

The history provides the diagnosis.

Management

Depending on their preparation and experience in the treatment of minor wounds that require suturing, NPs may suture wounds and provide follow-up care or be responsible for wound care only.

Techniques of suturing lacerations and administration of local anesthesia are not discussed in this text. The management plan can be summarized as follows (Resnick & Zarem, 1999; Frenck & Buescher, 1996; Ratner, 1991):

Suturing

1. Soak the wound in a mild antiseptic solution such as povidone-iodine for approximately 15 minutes to clean the wound and remove debris. An alternate to soaking for wound cleaning is irrigation of the wound with a forced jet spray of tepid water, normal saline, or povidone-iodine solution using a syringe or intravenous catheter. The average wound requires approximately 500 ml of irrigation. Because prolonged contact of povidone-iodine with the skin can cause damage, thoroughly rinse the area with normal saline after using povidone-iodine. Lip and eye wounds should be cleaned with normal saline only. Because washing and irrigating wounds is painful, prior administration of local anesthesia is helpful.
2. Remove surface debris and blood.
3. Refer deep lacerations, complicated wounds, or wounds to the face to a surgeon.
4. Use a surgical scrub brush and forceps to remove foreign material.
5. Irrigate hematomas with saline.
6. Debride devitalized tissue and trim ragged edges away.
7. Suture wounds by primary closure unless the likelihood of infection is high, such as occurs with heavily contaminated wounds, animal bites, or wounds that occurred more than 12 hours earlier. A clean wound on the face can often be sutured as long as 12 hours after injury because of the plentiful supply of blood to that area (Johnson & Oski, 1997; Frenck & Buescher, 1996). In contrast, open wounds on other parts of the body (especially the lower extremities) are subject to problems with bacterial growth after 6 or fewer hours of injury because of the lesser blood supply to these areas.
8. Whether animal bites should be sutured immediately is controversial. Some clinicians recommend that animal bites and deep punctures should not be immediately sutured because of the likelihood of infection. Instead, they recommend delaying primary closure for 4 or 5 days. Others close an animal bite if it is treated within 8 hours and does not appear infected (Frenck & Buescher, 1996).
9. Dress the wound using a nonadherent gauze for the first layer followed by a second layer of plain gauze if needed. Elasti-

cized gauze (tubular net bandage) can be used to secure dressings.

10. Order tetanus booster or human tetanus immunoglobulin if indicated.

11. Antibiotic prophylaxis of clean wounds is not indicated; its use in contaminated wounds may be helpful, but careful wound cleaning and debridement are the most effective safeguards in preventing infection.

12. Remove sutures depending on their location. A useful guide is as follows:
    • Facial sutures: 3 to 4 days
    • Upper extremity sutures: 7 to 10 days
    • Trunk sutures: 10 days
    • Lower extremity sutures: 14 days
    • Sutures over a joint: 10 to 14 days

Steri-Strips and Tissue Adhesives

1. Steri-Strips should only be used for small wounds whose edges are not far apart. Tissue adhesives are only appropriate for simple lacerations that are in relatively low tension areas of the body.

2. Proper wound management is needed as described earlier and includes cleaning, controlling the bleeding, debridement, and application of topical anesthesia if needed.

3. The procedure for closing a wound with tissue adhesive is a three-step process.
    • Use forceps to approximate the edges of the wound together.
    • Drip adhesive onto the skin surface as the edges are being held in close proximity with forceps; do not drip any adhesive into the wound.
    • Hold the wound closed for 20 to 30 seconds until glue polymerizes.

4. A combination of subcutaneous suturing and application of tissue adhesive can be used for deeper wounds.

5. A nonocclusive bandage can be used to cover the wound (Simon, 1997).

Patient and Parent Education

Instructions for the care of the wound at home should include the following information:

• The patient can shower 48 hours after sutures are in place without worrying about the risk of possible infection.

• Note signs and symptoms of infection that warrant an early recheck.
• Give instructions about cleansing and bandaging the wound.
• List any restrictions on activities.
• Provide date of return appointment.

BURNS

Description

A burn injury to one or more layers of the skin and underlying tissues can cause varying degrees of damage. Burns are classified by depth of injury and are divided into the following four categories:

1. First-degree burns involve only the epidermis.
2. Second-degree or partial-thickness burns involve damage to the dermis, but it remains viable.
3. Third-degree or full-thickness burns extend to the entire dermis and leave the subcutaneous tissue exposed.
4. Fourth-degree burns (rare) extend to the muscle fascia or bones.

Burns involving large surfaces of the body generally vary as to their degree of depth. Because burn wounds are dynamic and the effect of dermal ischemia (affected by infection, exposure, and dehydration) may not be readily apparent at first, their depth can change from day to day. The percentage of total body surface area (TBSA) and area of body affected is also a key factor in the morbidity and mortality as well as the management of burns (Fig. 40–1). The palm of the hand (including the digits), which is approximately 1% of body surface area, can be used as a quick guide to estimate TBSA. First-degree burns are not calculated in TBSA estimations. For children, burns involving 10% or more of body surface area are considered critical burns and necessitate hospitalization. Significant burns of the hands, feet, face, eyes, ears, and genitalia are considered major burns and require the expertise of the burn team specialists (Hansbrough & Hansbrough, 1999).

BURN ESTIMATE AND DIAGRAM
AGE vs. AREA

Area	Birth 1 yr.	1 – 4 yr.	5 – 9 yr.	10 – 14 yr.	15 yr.	Adult	2°	3°	Total	Donor Areas
Head	19	17	13	11	9	7				
Neck	2	2	2	2	2	2				
Ant. Trunk	13	13	13	13	13	13				
Post. Trunk	13	13	13	13	13	13				
R. Buttock	$2\frac{1}{2}$	$2\frac{1}{2}$	$2\frac{1}{2}$	$2\frac{1}{2}$	$2\frac{1}{2}$	$2\frac{1}{2}$				
L. Buttock	$2\frac{1}{2}$	$2\frac{1}{2}$	$2\frac{1}{2}$	$2\frac{1}{2}$	$2\frac{1}{2}$	$2\frac{1}{2}$				
Genitalia	1	1	1	1	1	1				
R.U. Arm	4	4	4	4	4	4				
L.U. Arm	4	4	4	4	4	4				
R.L. Arm	3	3	3	3	3	3				
L.L. Arm	3	3	3	3	3	3				
R. Hand	$2\frac{1}{2}$	$2\frac{1}{2}$	$2\frac{1}{2}$	$2\frac{1}{2}$	$2\frac{1}{2}$	$2\frac{1}{2}$				
L. Hand	$2\frac{1}{2}$	$2\frac{1}{2}$	$2\frac{1}{2}$	$2\frac{1}{2}$	$2\frac{1}{2}$	$2\frac{1}{2}$				
R. Thigh	$5\frac{1}{2}$	$6\frac{1}{2}$	8	$8\frac{1}{2}$	9	$9\frac{1}{2}$				
L. Thigh	$5\frac{1}{2}$	$6\frac{1}{2}$	8	$8\frac{1}{2}$	9	$9\frac{1}{2}$				
R. Leg	5	5	$5\frac{1}{2}$	6	$6\frac{1}{2}$	7				
L. Leg	5	5	$5\frac{1}{2}$	6	$6\frac{1}{2}$	7				
R. Foot	$3\frac{1}{2}$	$3\frac{1}{2}$	$3\frac{1}{2}$	$3\frac{1}{2}$	$3\frac{1}{2}$	$3\frac{1}{2}$				
L. Foot	$3\frac{1}{2}$	$3\frac{1}{2}$	$3\frac{1}{2}$	$3\frac{1}{2}$	$3\frac{1}{2}$	$3\frac{1}{2}$				
						TOTAL				

BURN DIAGRAM

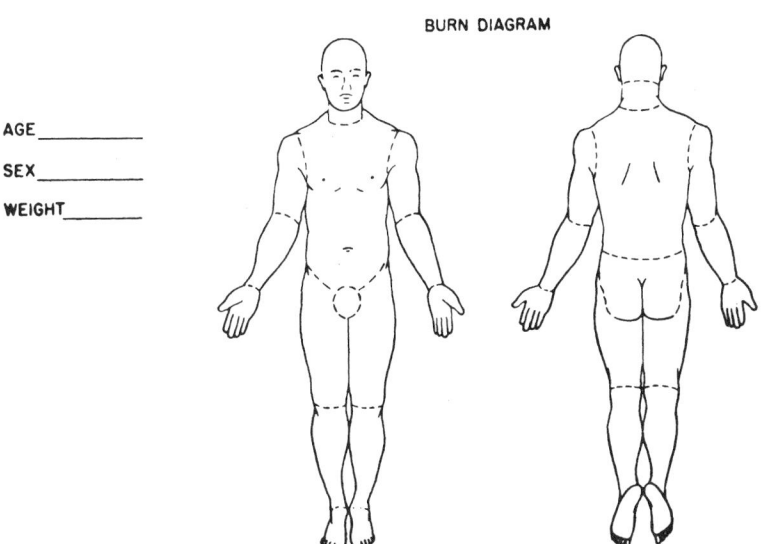

AGE_____

SEX_____

WEIGHT_____

FIGURE 40-1
Burn diagram used to calculate the extent of injury by body surface area in children of different age groups. (From Finkelstein JL, Schwartz SB, Madden MR, et al: Pediatric burns: An overview. Pediatr Clin North Am 39, p 1153, 1992.)

Etiology and Incidence

Burns can be caused by thermal, chemical, or electric agents. Major causes of burns in children include contact with hot water or food, appliances, flames, grills, curling irons, and electric cords or outlets. Exposure to the sun causes many minor burns.

Children younger than age 18 years account for approximately one third to one half of the 80,000 hospitalizations for burn injuries each year. Burns most commonly occur in children younger than 4 years of age with scalding being the most frequent type of burn injury (Hansbrough & Hansbrough, 1999). Intentionally inflicted burn injuries often leave a characteristic pattern (see Chapter 19).

Assessment

HISTORY. The following information should be obtained:

- Description of how burn occurred, including agent of injury and length of time agent was in contact with skin
- Circumstances surrounding injury
- When injury occurred
- Initial and subsequent treatment of burn
- Previous history of burn injuries

PHYSICAL EXAMINATION. The physical examination involves determination of the following:

- Percentage of body surface affected
- Distribution and pattern to burn
- Depth of involvement
- Quality of burn
  - First-degree: reddened, slightly edematous, dry, painful, hypersensitive, blanches with pressure, no blisters or sloughing of the epidermis
  - Second-degree (partial-thickness): erythematous, swollen, moist appearance, blisters or sloughing of the epidermis, sensitive, blanches with pressure, painful
  - Third-degree (full-thickness): white or blackened appearance, may be firm or leathery, swollen, dry surface, lack sensation, no blanching.

Differentiation between deep partial-thickness and full-thickness injury is sometimes difficult on initial assessment.

DIAGNOSTIC STUDIES. Culturing of critical burn wounds is done weekly or more frequently if infection is suspected. Other laboratory studies are done depending on the patient's condition and whether there is a question of electrolyte imbalance.

Differential Diagnosis

Chapter 19 discusses intentional burn injuries resulting from child abuse. Scalded skin syndrome caused by staphylococcal infection can cause skin exfoliation, but its clinical presentation clearly differentiates it from accidental burn injury. Management is similar to that used for burn management.

Management

Most children with major burns require treatment in the hospital setting and referral to a burn surgeon. Electric and chemical burns also require hospitalization for observation. Children with a burn injury associated with upper airway injury, fractures, suspicion of abuse, uncertainty of follow-up by the parent, or severe pain should also be admitted. The outpatient treatment of minor burns (i.e., first-degree and second-degree burn or less than 10% of body surface area or nonsignificant burns of the hands, feet, face, eyes, ears, and genitalia) includes the following (Battan et al., 1999; Hansbrough & Hansbrough, 1999):

1. Maintain proper nutrition to enhance healing.
2. Superficial burns:
   - Apply cool compresses.
   - Administer analgesic (e.g., acetaminophen, ibuprofen).
3. Partial-thickness burns:
   - Monitor the burn daily for the first few days to ensure proper healing and assess for infection.
   - Cleanse the wound with dilute (1 to 5%) povidone-iodine solution.
   - Debride open blisters, remove devitalized tissue, proteinaceous material, or residue from prior dressing changes.
   - Rinse thoroughly with normal saline.

- If the burn involves less than or equal to 3% of TBSA, apply Xeroform gauze in strips to clean, debrided area, followed by a dry gauze outer dressing.
- For burn wounds greater than 3% TBSA, apply silver sulfadiazene (SSD) after the wound is cleansed unless the child has a known sulfa allergy. SSD is an antimicrobial as well as a soothing agent.
- Apply strips of fine-mesh gauze over wound. Do not wrap the wound with gauze because wrapped gauze can impair circulation if swelling occurs. Apply additional SSD to gauze strips.
- Apply a tubular net bandage to hold the gauze in place.
- Administer adequate analgesic medication. Acetaminophen with codeine may be needed before the wound care is performed and during the day. Switch to over-the-counter acetaminophen as the pain subsides.
- Use mittens to prevent scratching if itching occurs as the burn heals; if needed, administer an antihistamine such as diphenhydramine.
4. If a second-degree burn involves an extremity, keep it elevated to reduce edema and compromise of blood flow to the burned area. Second-degree circumferential burns of an extremity may need to be admitted to the hospital for observation so that compartment syndrome does not develop.

Patient and Parent Education

The following points are important components of patient and parent education:

- Discuss home and environmental safety issues related to burn prevention at health supervision visits.
- Emphasize use of sunscreen protection to prevent sunburn (see Chapter 37).
- Reinforce safety issues after a burn injury has occurred (e.g., scald prevention, use of smoke detectors, safekeeping of matches and cigarette lighters, safe use of electric cords and outlets).
- Teach first aid measures for burns (e.g., submerge minor burned area in cold water; rinse chemical burns in cold water, flushing skin thoroughly).

- Inform parents of serious or long-term consequences of burns (e.g., frequent and significant sunburns during early childhood can predispose an individual to skin cancers in later life; electric burns cause thermal injury to skin [contact burn], but, if an arc is created and there is passage of electrical current through the body, there is a potential for cardiac dysrhythmias and neurological impairment).
- Inform parents that the extent of scarring is difficult to predict with certainty; that scarring depends on depth of burn, length of time needed for healing, whether grafting was done, and child's age and skin color; that scars remain immature for first 12 to 18 months and go through color and texture changes as child grows. Most scald injuries from hot liquids heal quickly with little or no scarring.
- Teach parents that newly healed burns must be protected from the sun for at least 12 months. Healed burns remain sensitive to the sun and sunburn more severely than nonburned skin.

CONTUSIONS

Description

A contusion, or bruise, is an injury in which the skin is not broken but trauma has caused effusion into muscle and subcutaneous tissue. In children, contusions are most often seen on the extremities but can also be found on the face or head. Contusions to the quadriceps, often secondary to athletic activity, are graded from I to III.

Etiology and Incidence

Contusions are common in children and are caused by blunt trauma, most often as a result of falling or bumping into objects during play. Participation in contact sports puts children at increased risk for contusions. Bruises to the trunk, face, or head should raise a red flag for possible child abuse, and a careful history must be taken to determine whether the explanation of the injury is consistent with the child's condition.

Assessment

HISTORY. The following should be assessed:

- Cause of bruise
- Treatment given
- History of easy bleeding or bruising, slow healing.

PHYSICAL EXAMINATION. The following should be determined:

- Swelling
- Pain
- Discoloration
- Limited mobility
- Quadriceps:
  - Grade I: mild, local tenderness, normal gait, knee range of motion greater than 90 degrees
  - Grade II: moderate tenderness and swelling, limp, unable to do deep knee bends, knee range of motion less than 90 degrees
  - Grade III: marked tenderness and swelling, cannot walk unaided, knee range of motion less than 45 degrees (Behrman et al., 1996).

Differential Diagnosis

Hemophilia, von Willebrand disease, and purpura should be considered. Myositis ossificans, a complication of contusions rarely seen in children, can be confused with osteogenic sarcoma.

Management

Management steps include the following:

1. Acute
   - Apply ice or cold compresses (applied for 20 minutes every 4 hours during first 48 to 72 hours).
   - Apply pressure bandage.
   - Elevate injured extremity.
   - Give nonsteroidal anti-inflammatory agent.
2. After 24 to 48 hours (after acute phase of tenderness and swelling)
   - Apply warm compresses or soaks.
   - Stretch.

   - Do range of motion and strengthening exercises.
3. For 5 to 7 days, avoid exercise that involves the contused area.
4. Refer severe injuries for orthopedic management.

Complications

Most contusions heal quickly without sequelae, but grade II or III trauma to the quadriceps muscle can lead to myositis ossificans if not treated properly.

Patient and Parent Education

Assist parents to provide a physical environment for their children that minimizes risk of injury.

SPRAINS

Description

Sprains are injuries to the joints involving stress to the ligaments. They often occur concurrently with strains of muscles, tendons, and other joint structures. Sprains are classified as grades I to III, depending on the loss of joint stability. Grades I and II are associated with incomplete tearing of the ligament. Ankle sprains are the most common athletic injury.

Etiology and Incidence

A common athletic injury, sprains in children most commonly affect the ankle, knee, shoulder, elbow, or wrist and are caused by falls or contact in which the extremity is immobile or moving on one plane and a countervailing force is applied to the joint. Ankle ligaments are strong in children with open growth plates; therefore, fractures are more common than sprains in prepubertal children (Mankin & Zimbler, 1996).

Assessment

HISTORY. The following are assessed:

- Description of episode of acute trauma (e.g., fall, collision, twisting of joint).

- Description of signs and symptoms (e.g., type, when appeared, how severe). Some children, especially with more severe sprains, report a "popping" sound or state "my knee gave way."
- What type of first aid treatment is given.

PHYSICAL EXAMINATION. The approach to the physical examination depends on the joint involved, the severity of the injury, and the child's ability to cooperate. If the injury is acute, it can be difficult to distinguish the extent of damage. Always examine the corresponding joint in the other extremity as well as adjacent joints and muscles. Findings include the following:

- Grade I injuries (mild sprains) have a stable joint, minimal pain, tenderness, or minimal swelling.
- Grade II injuries (moderate sprains) have little or no instability, pain, a wider area of tenderness, more swelling and discoloration, with limited mobility.
- Grade III injuries have marked joint laxity, severe pain, swelling, hemorrhage into the joint and soft tissue, and marked loss of mobility. Numbness, tingling, or weakness distal to the injured joint can be present.

Tenderness below the lateral malleolus in a child suggests an ankle sprain rather than a fracture (Mankin & Zimbler, 1996).

DIAGNOSTIC STUDIES. Routine radiographs are indicated if a fracture or dislocation is suspected.

Differential Diagnosis

Suspect fracture or dislocation, especially of the epiphysis, if there is excessive swelling or discoloration around the joint. Degree of pain does not distinguish a sprain from a fracture. Infection of the joint usually presents with fever, joint effusion, and erythema.

Management

Care of sprains differs depending upon the grade of injury. Children with severe sprains or suspected ligament tears should always be referred to an orthopedic surgeon.

1. Acute
   - RICE (*r*est, *i*ce, *c*ompression, *e*levation).

Apply ice immediately for 15 to 20 minutes, then, depending on the severity of the injury, every 2 to 6 hours for 24 to 48 hours. Ice may be applied using massage (a paper cup filled with water and frozen is ideal), ice packs, or immersion in an ice water bath.
   - Child should be non–weight bearing until pain diminishes.
   - Give anti-inflammatory medication.
   - Heat may be used after 24 hours for mild sprains.
2. Nonacute/chronic
   - Child may be weight bearing as tolerated.
   - Apply stabilizer/brace for unstable joint.
   - Rehabilitation, including range of motion and strengthening exercises. Rehabilitation should be gradual, beginning with isometric exercises of muscles and progressing to fuller range of motion and strengthening exercises. There should be no pain or swelling as exercise progresses. A general rule of thumb for return to activities for ankle sprains is 1 week for grade I and 2 weeks for grade II.
   - Apply ice after exercise.
   - Athletes should not return to competition after a sprain until they are pain free and can perform all sports-specific activities.
3. Severe sprains may need casting or surgery (Sawyer & Esterhai, 1999).

Patient and Parent Education

Prevention is preferred to treatment of sprains. Teach children and parents the importance of using protective gear (e.g., wrist guards for skaters). Children should also be encouraged to maintain a continuous level of physical activity in order to maximize muscle strength. See Chapter 15 for a discussion of children's participation in athletic activities.

STRAINS

Description

Strains involve injury to muscles and tendons and can be associated with sprains or fractures.

Etiology and Incidence

Strains occur when there is excessive stretching or pulling of the muscle or tendon, or both, from an antagonistic muscle group, active muscle contraction, or an external force (Behrman et al., 1996). Falls, active play, and sports activities, overuse of one muscle group, and underuse of antagonistic groups can all contribute to strains.

Assessment

HISTORY. The following information is gathered:

- Description of episode of acute trauma or history of repetitive activity that stresses the muscle–tendon unit.
- Signs and symptoms. Child may report a "popping" sound with grade II injury; report of immediate and severe signs with grade III injury.
- Treatment given and response to treatment.

PHYSICAL EXAMINATION. Findings include the following:

- Grade I injury: local tenderness, minimal swelling, little or no discoloration, no change in muscle mass
- Grade II injury: small, palpable defect in muscle mass, moderate pain, swelling, and discoloration
- Grade III injury: severe pain, complete rupture of fascia with large, palpable defect, swelling, marked discoloration (unless tendon alone is injured, then there is little bleeding), may have hematoma and loss of mobility.

DIAGNOSTIC STUDIES. See the previous section on sprains.

Differential Diagnosis

Fractures must be ruled out, especially avulsion fractures at point of tendon insertion.

Management

The following steps are taken:

1. RICE (*r*est, *i*ce, *c*ompression, and *e*levation)
2. Nonsteroidal anti-inflammatory agents

3. Mild exercise (passive range of motion and stretching) after 1 to 2 days of rest and immobilization
4. Strengthening exercises of muscle groups
5. Restricted participation in sports or activity that caused injury until muscles are fully recovered.

Patient and Parent Education

Prevention of strains can be achieved with consistent stretching, warm-up exercises, and maintenance of muscle strength through regular activity. Strength training may reduce the incidence and severity of overuse injuries, and children who plan to participate in sports activities should be helped to structure a period of conditioning into their schedules.

FRACTURES AND DISLOCATIONS

Description

A fracture involves a disruption in the continuity of bone tissue, with bowing or a break, with or without separation. Fractures occur in the physis, epiphysis, metaphysis, or diaphysis and may be complete, greenstick, buckle, comminuted, avulsed, transverse, oblique, or spiral. Types of epiphyseal fractures using the Salter-Harris classification system are discussed in Chapter 38. Stress fractures are discussed separately.

Dislocations are characterized by displacement of bone ends from their normal position in a joint. There can be wide variation in degree of displacement.

Etiology and Incidence

Fractures are relatively common in children, with type II being seen most often, usually in children older than 10 years of age. Clavicular fractures may be due to birth trauma and are discussed in Chapter 38 as a problem of the neonate. Accidents in which the child tries to break a fall using outstretched arms can result in fractures of the wrist, ulna, radius, or humerus. Direct trauma (e.g., resulting from contact sports, auto accidents, falls) to bones or joints can cause fractures or dislocations.

Assessment

HISTORY. The report of acute trauma and signs and symptoms occurring at the time of trauma are assessed.

PHYSICAL EXAMINATION. Findings include:

- Point tenderness over fracture
- Generalized pain
- Deformity
- Misalignment of bone or joint
- Loss of function or mobility (especially with dislocation)
- Muscle spasm
- Discoloration
- Swelling
- Lacerations with open fractures.

DIAGNOSTIC STUDIES. Radiographs are necessary to confirm the diagnosis. Lateral and anteroposterior views should be obtained. Early fractures and Salter I fractures do not always appear on radiographs, however, and follow-up radiographic studies (10 to 14 days after trauma) are often needed.

Differential Diagnosis

The cause of fractures should be determined, because fractures can also be due to pathological conditions such as osteogenesis imperfecta, sarcoma, hyperparathyroidism, and nutritional deficit (rickets, copper deficiency). Children who are physically abused may have multiple fractures at different stages of healing, repeated fractures, fractures of the skull, ribs, or vertebrae, or spiral, oblique, or transverse fractures in the long bones (especially in children before the age of walking). Chapter 19 discusses findings of child abuse in more detail.

Management

Simple fractures and dislocations can usually be reduced and immobilized easily and heal quickly with no disruption in the child's growth. The potential for impairment following trauma to growth plates, joints, or neurovascular structures is of serious concern, however, and all children with fractures or dislocations need an immediate orthopedic referral for management. Open reduction can be necessary with severe fractures.

Patient and Parent Education

As with strains and sprains, prevention of injury through use of protective devices, proper conditioning, and attention to the child's physical environment is essential.

STRESS FRACTURES

Description

Stress fractures are classified as overuse injuries and are becoming more common in children. They are caused by repeated muscular action on a bony insertion site or repetitive direct trauma. Bone remodeling cannot keep up with the repeated microtrauma, leading to bone reabsorption and fracture.

Etiology

Stress fractures occur in typical locations and are associated with activities and sports. Some common sites and causes are:

- Metatarsal shaft—running, marching, and ballet
- Tarsal navicular—running, high-impact aerobics
- Distal fibula and proximal tibia—running
- Ribs—coughing and golf
- Neck and shaft of the femur—running, ballet, and gymnastics

Assessment

Characteristic history includes gradual onset of pain with activity that decreases with rest, point tenderness, and local swelling. Distal atrophy may be noted.

Diagnostic Studies

Normal radiographic findings or zone of radiolucency. Bone scan and ultrasonography may be needed to identify the fracture if radiographs are normal.

Management

Management includes rest and eliminating the activity that is the source of the microtrauma for 10 to 14 days. Complete fractures need to be casted. Retraining is necessary to eliminate the source of the problem, with a gradual return to activity. If symptoms reappear, more rest is needed (Sawyer & Esterhali, 1999; Behrman et al., 1996).

SUBLUXATION OF THE RADIAL HEAD

Description

Subluxation of the radial head occurs frequently in infants and young children and presents a slippage of the radial head as a result of the infant or young child being lifted or pulled by the hand. It is commonly termed "nursemaid's elbow."

Etiology

In infants and young children, the radial head is not as bulbous as it is in older children. When the elbow is in extension and too much longitudinal traction is applied to the elbow, the annular ligament slides over the radial head and becomes entrapped. Often subluxation results from an unintentional injury as the parent or caregiver plays with or grabs the child. However, pulling of the child's arm, especially if this is a recurrent problem, may be the result of inappropriate disciplining or child maltreatment.

Assessment

HISTORY. The child complains that the elbow will not bend and is painful when moved. The child refuses to use the hand. There may be a prior episode of subluxation.

PHYSICAL EXAMINATION. Common findings include:

- Full pronation of the elbow
- Point tenderness over the radial head

DIAGNOSTIC STUDIES. Radiography of the elbow is normal and is generally not needed if the elbow is able to be reduced.

DIFFERENTIAL DIAGNOSIS. Subluxation has a classic history. Consider maltreatment if a recurrent problem or other symptoms or signs are present that lead the NP to suspect child abuse. Fracture of the radial head is included in the differential diagnosis.

Management

The maneuver recommended to correct subluxation involves the following:

- Distract the child by talking or other diversionary tactics.
- With pressure over the radial head, rotate the hand and forearm to a supinated position.
- Mobilize the elbow in a sling for a day if needed for comfort.

A click may be palpated at the radial head and the child's pain is relieved if the radial head is relocated. If the supination/flexion technique does not work on the first attempt, a second attempt may be needed (Eilert & Georgopoulos, 1999).

Patient and Parent Education

Key points to cover include the following:

- Instruct parents not to lift or pull the child by the hand or elbow.
- The condition tends to recur until the child is approximately 4 years of age.

COMPARTMENT SYNDROME

Description

Compartment syndrome is a complication of soft tissue injuries (e.g., fractures, crush injuries, and strenuous running). It generally affects the leg and forearm; however, any muscle that is contained by fascia can develop compartment syndrome. Muscle edema and bleeding develop within the muscle fascia, which increases the pressure within the muscle compartment. Because the fascial walls are fairly inelastic and unyielding, the swelling produces vascular compromise and tissue ischemia that promote further swelling.

Assessment

Key features of acute compartment syndrome include pain at rest and with passive stretching of the involved muscle, and a tense compartment with progressive findings of vascular compromise such as paresthesias or absent pulses. Chronic compartment syndrome can be seen in runners. It is associated with a history of local pain confined to the muscle (not the bone) with exercise, relief with rest, with rare tenderness and swelling over the muscle compartment.

Management

Prompt recognition of this complication and referral to an orthopedic surgeon for possible fasciotomy limits the risk of muscle and nerve damage. If not caught early, muscle necrosis and contracture can result. With chronic compartment syndrome caused by running, pain prevents resumption of exercise and limits the risk of muscle and nerve damage (Copley & Dormans, 1999; Staheli, 1998; Behrman et al., 1996).

Bites

ANIMALS AND OTHER CHILDREN

Description

Children can be bitten by pets, stray animals, or humans, especially other children. Most bites are to the hand, although pet ferrets will attack a child's face.

Etiology and Incidence

An estimated 1% of emergency department visits annually in the United States are due to mammalian bites. The vast majority are dog bites, usually provoked. Two percent to three percent are human bites. The risk of infection following a dog versus cat bite is 5%, compared to a 20 to 50% risk of infection with cat bites (Avner, 1999). The risk of infection with animal bites is 50%.

Assessment

Assessment includes the history of the attack and the presence of clinical signs.

PHYSICAL EXAMINATION. Bites present differently, depending on the animal causing the in-

jury. Dog bites may be extensive, resulting in lacerations, avulsions, and occasionally crushing injuries. Cats tend to inflict deep puncture bites. Bite injuries involving toddlers tend to be superficial; bites in adolescents generally occur during fights and are prone to infection. Bites from rats or other rodents tend to be superficial and are usually seen in the lower extremities. Ferrets often bite the face and can cause severe damage. Ferret bites may be unprovoked.

In addition to cutaneous lesions, bone, tendon, muscle, and neurovascular tissue damage can be present in deep bites.

Secondary infection is common in mammalian bites and can lead to cellulitis and lymphangitis, requiring hospitalization. *Streptococcus* and *Staphylococcus* are common organisms associated with infected animal and human bites. *Pasteurella multocida* is found in 50% of wound infections from animal bites.

DIAGNOSTIC STUDIES. Wound cultures can identify infectious agents.

Differential Diagnosis

The differential diagnosis includes lacerations or puncture wounds from other causes.

Management

Management involves both physical and psychological care of the child and includes the following:

1. Tetanus booster if indicated.
2. Rabies prophylaxis if indicated.
3. Wound cleansing by gently scrubbing with dilute povidone solution (povidone scrub can damage tissue) followed by irrigation with a copious amount of normal saline
4. Débridement of devitalized tissue.
5. Antibiotics for infected wounds, initially a broad-spectrum medication such as amoxicillin clavulanate or erythromycin until results of cultures are known, then as indicated. Some sources give prophylactic antibiotics for facial wounds only because of the potential for scarring from infection.
6. High-risk wounds include the following:
   • Cat and human bites
   • Hand puncture wounds

- Wounds in immunosuppressed children
- Wounds first seen more than 24 hours after injury
7. Low-risk animal bites and small high-risk wounds should be left open and observed. Delayed closure should be done if needed.
8. Referral for assessment and management of severe bites. Suturing may be necessary for large or facial wounds (using interrupted sutures), but the high risk of infection requires close monitoring of the injury, and wound closure may be delayed for 4 to 7 days. Hospitalization, reconstructive surgery, and long-term follow-up can also be indicated.
9. Discussion of child's fears and management of any behavioral problems that may result.

Patient and Parent Education

Preventive education and actions should include the following:

- Teach children to avoid stray animals and not to provoke any animal.
- Provide parental supervision of children as they play with pets. Young children, especially, are often unaware of the risks that animals present, and their interactions must be carefully monitored.
- Do not keep ferrets and other typically wild animals as pets in families with very young children.
- Do not allow pets to roam freely.
- Report stray animals promptly to animal control officials.

BEES AND WASPS

Description

Bees, hornets, yellow jackets, and wasps belong to the Hymenoptera order of insects and have common antigens in their venom. Honeybees and wasps ordinarily do not sting unless frightened, bothered, or hurt. Reactions to stings by these insects, caused by the Hymenoptera venom, vary from mild, local responses to life-threatening anaphylaxis. Most children experience only a local reaction. Some children suffer systemic reactions, which can progress to medical emergencies unless prompt intervention is initiated.

Etiology

Immunoglobulin E–dependent hypersensitivity is the underlying cause of reactions. Histamines, leukotrienes, prostaglandins, and other inflammatory factors are released, causing local or systemic symptoms.

Assessment

HISTORY. The child usually reports being bitten or stung. There may be a past history of a local or systemic reaction following an insect bite.

PHYSICAL EXAMINATION. Findings include:

- Mild reaction consists of local redness, pruritus, pain, edema, and possibly generalized urticaria.
- Severe reactions including anaphylaxis are characterized by local signs plus any of the following:
  - Difficulty in breathing and swallowing
  - Hoarseness, thickened speech
  - Gastrointestinal disturbances, abdominal pain
  - Dizziness, weakness, confusion
  - Collapse, unconsciousness, even death

DIAGNOSTIC STUDIES. Skin testing is not necessary and can be dangerous if there is a history of an allergic response to Hymenoptera sting.

Differential Diagnosis

Other insect bites or dermatological eruptions that produce similar symptoms are included in the differential diagnosis.

Management

The following steps are taken:

1. Mild local reactions
   - If the stinger is visible, flick it off with the edge of a sharp object (e.g., knife blade or credit card), taking care to not squeeze the attached venom sac.
   - Apply ice or cool compresses locally.

- Administer an antihistamine such as diphenhydramine (1–2 mg/kg orally or 5 mg/k/d q 6–8 h) for pruritus.
2. Moderate to severe allergic reaction
   - Moderate reactions may need to be treated with oral antihistamines, corticosteroids, and inhaled bronchodilators (if wheezing).
   - Institute emergency measures for treatment of anaphylactic reactions (Boguniewicz & Leung, 1999; Taketomo et al., 1998).
   - Epinephrine (0.01 mg/kg [1:1000 aqueous epinephrine at 0.01 ml/kg per dose] subcutaneously, repeated at 15- to 20-minute intervals for 2 to 3 times, not to exceed 0.5 mg total). Administer the dose above the sting site.
   - Antihistamines. Diphenhydramine 1 to 2 mg/kg (up to 50 mg) intramuscularly (IM) or intravenously (IV). Ranitidine (an H_2 blocker), at 1 mg/kg up to 50 mg IV may be added.
   - Corticosteroids. Methylprednisolone at 1 to 2 mg/kg or hydrocortisone at 5 mg/kg every 4 to 6 hours.
   - IV fluids. Administer if the child is hypotensive as a result of anaphylactic shock.
   - Bronchodilators. Give if bronchospasm occurs, administer albuterol 0.5% (2.5 mg or 0.5 ml) in 2 to 3 ml of saline.
   - Administer oxygen.
   - Tracheostomy. Needs to be performed if laryngeal edema is life threatening.
   - Hospitalize for anaphylactic shock.
   - Refer to an allergist for desensitization against the Hymenoptera order if patient has a history of a potentially life-threatening sting.

Patient and Parent Education

Key issues to discuss include the following:

- Importance of wearing a medical alert tag or bracelet
- Proper use of an insect sting kit (self-injectable epinephrine pen) and need to have kit always readily available for emergency use
- How to prevent stings by avoiding areas likely to be infested with these insects, not wearing bright-colored clothing, and not using perfumed products

MOSQUITOES, FLEAS, AND CHIGGERS (HARVEST MITES)

Description

Mosquitoes are the vectors of many important diseases in humans and also cause irritating local skin reactions when they bite. Similarly, flea and chigger bites produce local skin eruptions. The chigger is also known as red bug or harvest mite.

Etiology and Incidence

Mosquito bites are the most common insect bites of infants and children. Fleas that commonly attack humans in the United States include the human flea, cat flea, and dog flea. The six-legged larvae of harvest mites are responsible for the skin eruption characteristic of chigger bites. Harvest mites live on grain stems, shrubs, grass, and vines. As humans or animals pass by, the larvae attach themselves to the skin and inject an irritating secretion. The harvest mites then drop to the ground or are scratched off within 1 to 2 days. A seasonal pattern is characteristic of mosquito, flea, and chigger bites.

Assessment

HISTORY. The following may be reported:

- Known mosquito or flea bite
- Presence of cat or dog in child's environment
- Complaints of a brief stinging sensation followed by itching after mosquito bite
- History of playing or walking in grassy areas or other harvest mite habitat

PHYSICAL EXAMINATION. Mosquito bites are characterized by the following:

- Local irritation in unsensitized children
- Urticarial wheals that itch and last several hours to days in sensitized children or firm papules or nodules that last a long period of time
- A central punctum is sometimes noted
- Secondary impetigo from scratching of skin lesions

Flea bites are characterized by the following:

- Urticarial wheal or papule in a sensitized person
- Often, central hemorrhagic punctum
- Progression of wheals into bullae in highly sensitized individuals, especially young children
- Grouping of multiple lesions, commonly found on arms, legs, thighs, waist, and lower abdomen

Chigger bites are characterized by

- Discrete, bright-red papules 1 to 2 mm in diameter that often have hemorrhagic puncta
- Lesions mainly seen on legs and beltline but can be widespread
- Wheals, papules, or papulovesicles in sensitized individuals
- Purpuric lesions or bullae
- Intense pruritus reaching a peak on the second day, and decreasing over the next 5 to 6 days but can persist for months
- Possible secondary impetigo from scratching lesions

DIAGNOSTIC STUDIES. The presence of fleas or harvest mites is diagnostic; otherwise, no studies are done.

Differential Diagnosis

The diagnosis is often obvious, but the differential diagnosis can include insect bites that produce similar papular, vesicular lesions, or other skin conditions.

Management

Management consists of controlling pruritus and can include such measures as the following:

- Cool compresses
- Topical corticosteroids (e.g., 1% hydrocortisone cream)
- Oral antihistamines (e.g., diphenhydramine) if the above measures do not provide relief
- Application of clear nail polish to chigger bites
- Treatment of secondary skin lesions as indicated

- Elimination of fleas by treating animals and cleaning carpets, bedding, upholstered furniture, and other areas that are potentially infested

Patient and Parent Education

Prevention of insect bites is a key component in education. Bites can be prevented by eliminating mosquitoes, fleas, and chiggers from the environment or by preventing their contact with the skin.

- Use insect repellents (generally effective against mosquitoes and harvest mites).
- Wear protective clothing to cover body.
- Wear neutral-colored clothes (white, green, tan, and khaki do not attract mosquitoes).
- Avoid scented hair sprays, powders, soaps, lotions, creams, and perfumes, because these products can attract all forms of stinging insects.
- Treat suspected animal carrier for fleas, and spray carpets and other infested areas; spray yards and grassy places for fleas in those environments that the child frequents.
- Vacuum carpets daily if fleas are seen on household pets.
- Avoid playing in areas of harvest mite habitat.

TICKS

Description

Ticks *(Ixodides)* are blood-sucking arachnids. They are vectors of significant diseases such as rickettsial infection (e.g., Rocky Mountain spotted fever and Q fever), relapsing fever, erythema chronicum migrans, and Lyme disease. (See discussion about Lyme disease in Chapter 24).

Etiology and Incidence

Ticks are found in grass, shrubs, vines, and brush and attach themselves to various animals and humans. The female tick sucks blood from the skin and can inject a toxin while sucking blood. Transmission of Lyme disease by the *Ixodes dammini* tick requires a 24-hour tick attachment. Tick bites are most common from early spring to early fall.

Assessment

HISTORY. The practitioner assesses a report of known tick bite and exposure to a tick habitat.

PHYSICAL EXAMINATION. Findings include the following:

- The initial bite is painless and innocuous; thus, the tick is frequently undetected or detected only after several days of attachment.
- An infiltrated lesion with a distinct surrounding erythematous halo develops and can last for 1 to 2 weeks.
- A small pruritic nodule, lasting for months or years, can result if the tick's mouth parts are left in the skin.
- Tick bite pyrexia or tick paralysis (occurs about 6 days after attachment) can result; both disorders are reversible, and symptoms quickly resolve if the tick is removed.
- Other signs depend on the tick-related illness that develops.

DIAGNOSTIC STUDIES. Identification of the tick is diagnostic. Diagnostic studies are ordered depending on the disease for which the tick is the vector.

Differential Diagnosis

Many different diseases result from tick bites and their sequelae. The differential diagnosis is variable and depends on the illness for which the tick is the vector. The differential diagnosis of local reactions to simple tick bites includes other insect bites.

Management

Although intervention varies with the specific disease, illnesses resulting from tick bites are best managed with prompt introduction of antibiotics, such as amoxicillin, penicillin, or erythromycin. When to recommend antibiotic prophylaxis for asymptomatic deer tick bites remains controversial (Taylor, 1999).

Complete removal of the tick is essential. If fragments of mouth parts or proboscis are left

in the skin, local symptoms can continue. To remove ticks, wear gloves and firmly grasp the tick with forceps, tweezers, or gloved fingers as close to the skin as possible (try to grasp its head), and gently pull straight upward with steady even pressure. Wash the area with soap and water and save the tick for identification (Taylor, 1999; Moskowitz & Meissner, 1997).

Patient and Parent Education

The following key points should be made:

- Avoid areas known to be infested with ticks.
- Wear protective clothing—preferably light colored to see ticks better (e.g., long sleeved shirts tucked into pants and pants tucked into socks).
- Use repellents such as diethyltoluamide (DEET) or permethrin (an insecticide) on clothing. Insect repellents with DEET (<10%) that have an Environmental Protection Agency–approved label can be used on skin but should be used sparingly to exposed skin. Do not apply to the face or nonintact skin. Inform parents that these repellents can cause allergic and toxic effects as well. Use a higher sun protection factor (SPF) of sunscreen if also applying DEET insect repellents to the skin because it may decrease the SPF (Hebert & Carlton, 1998).
- Inspect for ticks after exposure or walking in areas likely to be infested; check for ticks every 2 to 3 hours during a hike; carefully check the scalp, hairline, neck, behind the ears, armpits, legs, back of knees, and groin, because these areas are favorite hiding places of ticks.
- Take a brisk shower after a hike to help remove ticks that are not firmly attached. Wash off tick repellents with soap (Moskowitz & Meissner, 1997).

SPIDERS AND SCORPIONS

Description

Most spider bites are innocuous, causing no reaction or a minor, localized response that can be mistaken for a flea, bedbug, or some other insect bite. There are three serious spider bites that are common in the North American continent: from the black widow *(Lactrodectus mactans)*, brown recluse *(Loxosceles reclusa)*, and hobo *(Tegenaria agrestis)* spiders. The black widow spider has a globular body about 1 cm across that is coal black in color with a red or orange hourglass marking on its underside. It is found throughout the United States. The brown recluse spider has an oval light-fawn to dark chocolate-brown body; it is approximately 1 cm in length, with a dark-brown violin-shaped band extending from its eyes partially down its back. The brown recluse is found in southern and midwestern states. The hobo spider, common to the Pacific Northwest and found in Montana, Utah and Northern California, measures 1 to 1½ inches across, including its legs, is brown with gray markings, and has parallel marks on its head and herringbone marks on its rear section. It has often been mistaken for the brown recluse.

Scorpions have a stinging apparatus in their tail. They are found in the southwestern and southern United States and live in cool, dark places during the day.

Etiology and Incidence

The black widow spider prefers to live in warm, dark, dry places such as woodpiles, garages, basements, tool sheds (less frequented outbuildings). It often spins its web on an outdoor privy seat, which explains why many black widow spider bites are received around the genital and buttock areas. The brown recluse spider typically lives in dark, dry places and storage closets among clothes. The brown recluse prefers dark recesses and bites only in self-defense. The hobo spider is found in crawl spaces, wood piles, and other dark areas. Like the brown recluse, the hobo spider bites in self-defense. The venom of the brown recluse and hobo spiders can be hemolytic and necrotizing with extension due to a spreading factor. Scorpions come out at night and are nonaggressive unless disturbed (Bond, 1999; Taylor, 1999).

Assessment

HISTORY. Assess the known history of a spider bite or activities in, or travel to, an environ-ment that is frequented by these spiders. The characteristic appearance of the spider helps in its identification.

PHYSICAL EXAMINATION. The characteristics features are identified for each type of spider bite:

Black Widow Spider Bites
• Pinprick sensation is followed by regional lymph node tenderness (30 to 120 minutes later) and a halo lesion at the bite site.
• Severe, muscle cramping pain starts from 10 minutes to an hour after bite and increases to maximum intensity within 3 hours.
• Central nervous system symptoms include nausea, vomiting, sweating, hypertension, tachycardia.
• Death occurs in 5% of children; most children recover in 2 to 3 days; some experience milder symptoms.

Brown Recluse Spider Bites
• Localized reaction is characterized by mild itching or stinging at time of bite (bite can be painless), with mild to severe pain in about 2 to 8 hours, followed by swelling and tenderness, a hemorrhagic vesicle (12 to 24 hours later), and finally a gangrenous eschar. Lymphangitis is common if a bite is on an extremity. The lesion takes weeks to months to resolve.
• Systemic reaction, characterized by nausea, vomiting, chills, fever, malaise, muscle aches and pains, thrombocytopenia and hemolysis, are rare but can occur (Bond, 1999).

Hobo Spider Bites
• Similar to brown recluse spider bites.

Scorpion Bites
• Severe local pain and edema occur.
• Systemic reactions include uncontrolled jerking, muscle fasciculation, facial twitching, hypersalivation, and respiratory distress.

Differential Diagnosis

Other spider bites and conditions that result in similar cutaneous manifestations or systemic findings, or both, are included in the differential diagnosis.

Management

In cases in which venomous spider bites are suspected or confirmed, the patient should be referred to the appropriate medical specialist. Treatment for black widow spider bites includes administration of specific antivenin (in selected cases), intravenous calcium gluconate, muscle relaxants, pain medications, tetanus prophylaxis, and antibiotics if secondary infection develops. Most brown recluse bites tend to heal without incident. Bites with necrotic centers generally require tetanus prophylaxis, pain medication, application of ice or cold compresses, and elevation of the extremity. Scorpion stings may be managed with topical steroids, antihistamines, and cool compresses for local reactions. Children experiencing severe reactions may require the use of antivenin therapy.

Patient and Parent Education

The focus of patient and parent education is prevention. Careful monitoring of environments in which these spiders tend to live and prompt treatment if bitten are important points to cover.

SNAKES

Description

Approximately 2500 children per year receive poisonous snakebites in the United States, the majority of which are caused by indigenous pit vipers such as rattlesnakes, cottonmouths, water moccasins, and copperheads. The snake injects venom that contains a variety of toxins into the soft tissue, and the venom can be carried throughout the body via the blood and lymph systems.

Etiology

The snake venom is responsible for the local and systemic reactions that occur. Pit viper venom causes tissue injury, capillary leakage, coagulopathy, and neurotoxicity (Bond, 1999).

Assessment

HISTORY. The NP assesses for a report of a snakebite.

PHYSICAL EXAMINATION. Characteristic features indicating the presence of venom include the following:

- Severe local reaction soon after bite, with pain, discoloration, and edema as well as hemorrhagic effects.
- Proximal extension of ecchymosis and swelling during the first few hours after the bite with later fluid-filled or hemorrhagic bullas and necrosis
- Peripheral and central neurological symptoms
- Evidence of hematological coagulopathy such as hematemesis, melena, hemoptysis
- Respiratory distress and shock that can lead to death

DIAGNOSTIC STUDIES. Coagulation studies and other laboratory tests are ordered as indicated by the child's condition.

Management

The size of the child, site of the bite, type of snake, and degree of envenomation, plus the effectiveness of treatment, determine whether the snakebite will be fatal. Usually there is a period of 6 to 8 hours between a rattlesnake bite and death in which effective treatment can be instituted to reverse the effects of rattlesnake venom. Treatment includes rapid transportation to a medical center, referral to appropriate medical specialists, antivenin therapy, and treatment for shock and respiratory difficulties. A venous constricting band (not a tourniquet) proximal to the bite can slow the spread of the venom during transit to medical attention.

Patient and Parent Education

Prevention of snakebite is important. Parents and patients who live or vacation in areas where pit vipers are found should be familiar with emergency first aid treatment of snakebites. First aid measures include the following (Bond, 1999):

- Splint affected extremity and minimize patient's movements.

- Do not elevate extremity.
- Do not use a tourniquet or ice packs.
- Do not cut bite area and attempt to suction venom out.
- Transport immediately to a medical facility.

Head Injuries

DESCRIPTION

The skull of an infant or child is anatomically different from the skull of an adult, a factor that influences how effectively it protects the brain from injury. The brain can better withstand trauma after myelination is complete, the anterior fontanel is closed, and the cranial sutures are fused. Before these events occur, children are particularly vulnerable to cerebral trauma, and this trauma has more severe effects.

In head injuries, irreparable cell damage occurs at the time of the initial trauma, followed by secondary events that can lead to further tissue death. These secondary events are potentially reversible. See Chapter 28 for an in-depth discussion of the brain and its functions.

Head injuries in children are classified as mild, moderate, and severe (Table 40-1). The level of consciousness is a key determinant of the child's prognosis. The discussion of head injury in this chapter is limited to the assessment and management of children with injuries that can be monitored safely in the primary care setting. In addition, indications of impending central nervous system compromise are presented.

ETIOLOGY AND INCIDENCE

Head injury is a common cause of trauma in children. Approximately 80% of pediatric injuries are classified as mild, and 5% result in death (Rosman, 1999). In addition, head injury is a significant cause of long-term disability for children who survive their injuries. There are various types of head injuries that can result in pathological conditions: skull fracture, concussion, posttraumatic seizure, cerebral contusion, epidural hematoma, subdural hematoma, cerebral edema, and penetrating injury. A brief description of each is presented in Table 40-2.

ASSESSMENT

History

The following information should be obtained:

- Loss of consciousness or memory, confused, inappropriate behavior
- Vomiting, especially how often
- Type of headache, presence of vision problems; irritability
- History of how injury occurred; if injury involved a fall, determine height from which the child fell

T A B L E 40-1

Classification of Head Injuries Based On Key Characteristics

CLASSIFICATION	GLASGOW COMA SCALE*	NEUROLOGIC FOCAL DEFICIT†	LOSS OF CONSCIOUSNESS	OTHER NEUROLOGIC FINDINGS
Mild	13–15	No	No or brief loss (<30 min)	May have linear skull fracture
Moderate	9–12	Focal signs	Variable loss	May have depressed skull fracture or intracranial hematoma
Severe	≤8	Focal signs	Prolonged loss	Often have depressed skull fractures and intracranial hematoma

*Either initial or subsequent scores
†Neurologic focal deficit (e.g., hemiparesis, reflex asymmetry, Babinski sign, and/or abnormal cranial nerve findings)

T A B L E 40-2

Common Types of Head Injuries in Children

TYPES OF INJURY	CHARACTERISTICS
Skull fracture	Linear, compound, basilar, depressed, and diastatic. Less common in children owing to more elastic skull. Linear is most common type.
Concussion	Transient loss of consciousness with amnesia. Computed tomography scan is normal. Child's level of consciousness may be depressed, child may vomit, but neurological examination becomes normal within hours without treatment.
Post-traumatic seizure	Convulsion resulting from injury that occurs immediately, early (within the first 24 hr), or late (>1 wk after injury). A seizure is the result of focal injury to the brain.
Cerebral contusion	Bruising of the brain. Injury results from acceleration/deceleration forces. Common features include depressed level of consciousness, headache, and vomiting.
Epidural hematoma	Collection of blood between skull and dura. An overlying fracture is a common association. Classic clinical picture is an initial loss of consciousness, then a lucid interval with subsequent neurological deterioration.
Subdural hematoma	Collection of blood between dura and brain parenchyma. More common than epidural hematoma. Associated with cerebral contusion following skull fracture or direct trauma or with child abuse. Unconsciousness common with acute subdural; with chronic subdural, note growing head in infants or gradual progressive symptoms in older child.
Cerebral edema	Caused by vasogenic, cytotoxic, hydrostatic, and/or osmotic forces. Significant cause of increased intracranial pressure following injury.
Penetrating injury	Trauma caused by an object such as a bullet entering the brain. In the case of a bullet, the kinetic energy released during its passage through the brain can cause major damage.

Physical Examination

Vital signs and a complete neurological examination should be performed, looking for any signs of central nervous system involvement. The child should be assessed and assigned a score based on the Glasgow coma scale (GCS) (see Chapter 28).

Diagnostic Studies

The severity of the head trauma dictates the need for investigative studies. Children with mild trauma that is without focal signs or loss of consciousness and GCS scores 13 to 15 usually do not need routine skull radiographs. Children with moderate and severe trauma need a cranial CT scan as well as routine skull films (anteroposterior and lateral views of the skull) and other views if there also is a neck injury or depressed skull fracture (Coulter, 1998; Rosman, 1999). Indications for obtaining a CT include any of the following:

- History of loss of consciousness
- Depressed level of consciousness
- Focal neurological signs or deficit
- Depressed skull fracture
- Seizures
- Persistent vomiting

CT is the preferred imaging technique because it can be obtained rapidly and the child monitored easily during the study. Acute hemorrhage is detected more easily by CT than by MRI; however, MRI is the preferred imaging modality for examination of the brain during the recovery period following head trauma or to detect hemorrhage when CT is normal but bleeding is suspected (Rosman, 1999).

DIFFERENTIAL DIAGNOSIS

History of a head injury is the key to diagnosis. Differentiating minor head trauma that will resolve on its own from more extensive brain injury is problematic at times. Intracranial lesions, particularly epidural hematomas, are life threatening and are significant complications. Head injury that may be the result of child abuse should be investigated.

MANAGEMENT

Skull films and CT scans are not indicated for children with mild head trauma who have no history of loss of consciousness or amnesia, no focal neurological deficit, a GCS score of 15, and no palpable depressed skull fracture. These children can be followed at home after a brief period of observation (Battan et al., 1999; Rosman, 1999). The following are indications for home management:

- There is a responsible, reliable parent or guardian who can follow home instructions and has transportation to return the child immediately if problems develop.
- The child is alert or has only a slight headache and dizziness, and has no other injuries.
- Neurological examination is normal.

Children who suffer a minor head injury with a brief period of loss of consciousness (no more than several minutes) can be monitored at home if the CT scan is normal and the above home management conditions are met (Rosman, 1999).

Children with moderate head injuries (GCS score of 9 to 12) may require admission or prolonged observation in the emergency department until their mental status stabilizes; children with severe head injuries (GCS score <8 or coma and physical findings) need immediate hospital admission. A child with a skull fracture or transient neurological findings whose level of consciousness is normal may be admitted for overnight observation.

Management of sports-related head injuries is discussed in Chapter 15.

PATIENT AND PARENT EDUCATION

Give all parents or caregivers a "head injury sheet," and make every effort to ensure that they understand the instructions and will comply with them. Salient points to cover in a pediatric head injury information sheet include instructions about when to contact the health-

care provider or take the child to an emergency department. Indications are the following:

- Open head wound
- Increased drowsiness, sleepiness, inability to wake up, unconsciousness
- Vomiting more than one or two times
- Neck pain
- Watery or bloody drainage from ear or nose
- Convulsion, "fit," or fainting
- Unusual irritability, personality change, confusion, or any unusual behavior
- Headache that gets worse or lasts more than a day
- Unequal pupils
- Trouble with vision (blurred), hearing, or speech
- Trouble with walking (e.g., clumsiness or stumbling) or weakness of any muscle of arms, legs, or face

In addition, parents or caregivers should be given the following specific instructions:

- Wake up child every 2 to 4 hours for the first 24 hours after injury; child should wake easily and be able to stay awake for a few minutes.
- Make sure child is moving his or her arms and legs normally.
- Give only acetaminophen if needed for headache or relief of pain of bumps and bruises.

Parents should also be informed that sometimes symptoms from head trauma can occur days, weeks, or months after the initial trauma. Neurological sequelae following mild head injury in children often improve or resolve within 9 to 12 months. These sequelae include the following:

- Headache
- Vertigo or dizziness
- Difficulty concentrating or loss of memory
- Depression, fatigue, poor school performance
- Neurobehavioral problems

Heat and Cold Injuries

FROSTBITE

Description

Frostbite is characterized by ice crystal formation in the tissue and impaired circulation to the affected area, with microvascular changes leading to cellular destruction (Stewart, 1999). Toes, feet, fingers, nose, cheeks, and ears are typical areas of injury.

Etiology

Exposure to temperatures ranging from $-2°$ to $-10°C$ can cause frostbite. Factors such as duration of exposure, increased wind velocity, dependency of the extremity, fatigue, injury, high altitude, immobility, general health, and race can potentiate the effects of cold. Exposure to very cold chemicals (e.g., liquid oxygen) also produces instant frostbite.

Assessment

HISTORY. The practitioner assesses the following:

- Exposure to cold temperatures
- Complaints of area first feeling a painful cold sensation followed by tingling and numbness
- Complaints of throbbing pain after thawing

PHYSICAL EXAMINATION. Typical initial findings include the following:

- Frozen area is cold and waxy.
- Skin is red at first, then appears pale or waxy white or slightly yellow.
- In early stages, tissue blanches; in later stages, it feels doughy or rock hard.

On rewarming, the extent of tissue damage becomes apparent. Superficial frostbite is reversible and is often called frostnip. These cases are characterized by the following:

- Redness and discomfort
- Skin appearance that returns to normal within a few hours

Deep frostbite occurs when tissues are icy hard and are without deep tissue resilience. Such severe cases are characterized by the following signs and symptoms that appear with rewarming:

- Cyanosis or mottling
- Erythema and swelling

- Numbness that evolves into complaints of burning pain
- Vesicles and bullae that appear within 24 to 48 hours
- Gangrene in severe frostbite

Differential Diagnosis

The differential diagnosis includes other conditions that produce similar cutaneous manifestations and injury; a history of exposure to extreme temperatures is the key to the diagnosis.

Management

Severe frostbite should be managed by medical specialists. Treatment includes rapid rewarming procedures, pain management, medical and surgical management of tissue necrosis, prevention of infection, and amputation if needed. Damaged skin should never be massaged or rubbed with snow or ice. Early treatment of mild frostbite includes the following:

1. Cover affected area with other body surfaces and warm clothing.
2. *Do not use local dry heat*; this practice is dangerous and can cause tissue damage.

Patient and Parent Education

Education of children and parents about the prevention and initial management of frostbite is important. Essential points include advice about the following:

- Use of appropriate clothing when exposed to extreme cold temperatures
- Survival skills for hikers or winter sports participants who are exposed to cold temperatures or who could become lost
- Rapid rewarming of skin that is white by covering with warm clothing or another body surface
- Danger of rubbing affected area with snow or ice or massaging; these practices are contraindicated because they lead to mechanical trauma

HYPOTHERMIA

Description

Hypothermia is the condition in which body core temperature falls below 35°C. Severe hypothermia is life threatening (Battan et al., 1999).

Etiology

Hypothermia can be the result of environmental exposure. Body heat is lost by radiation of heat to nearby objects, evaporation of moisture from the skin and respiratory system, convection of heat from the skin's surface into cooler air, or conduction of heat to objects in direct contact with the body. The effect of cool ambient temperatures is exacerbated by wind, moisture, and lack of appropriate clothing or shelter.

Children are at increased risk of hypothermia because of their relatively larger body surface area, proportionately larger head, smaller body fluid volume, less developed temperature-regulating mechanisms, and less protective body fat. Newborns, particularly low-birth-weight or premature infants, very young children, and children who are ill, fatigued, poorly nourished, or have experienced trauma are at high risk.

Hypothermia, not associated with environmental exposure, may be a sign of other life-threatening illnesses or injuries (e.g., near-drowning in cold water). This secondary hypothermia is not discussed here.

Assessment

HISTORY. The following are assessed:

- Exposure to low ambient temperatures
- Risk factors (e.g., age, physical condition)

PHYSICAL EXAMINATION. Signs of hypothermia progress from early to late stages and include the following:

- Decreasing body temperature
- Shivering that disappears in late hypothermia
- Pallor or blue lips and skin
- Disorientation, listlessness, sleepiness
- Decreased pulse and respiration
- Coma and death

DIAGNOSTIC STUDIES. No studies are done if hypothermia is mild and responds to basic treatment measures.

Differential Diagnosis

Shock is the differential diagnosis.

Management

For mild hypothermia, in early stages of cooling, remove the child from the cold environment, replace wet clothing, and provide warm liquids. Placing the child in a warm-water bath can be effective. As the body cools further, it can no longer generate adequate heat itself, so external sources of heat must be provided. Again, remove the child from the cold environment, replace wet clothing, and provide heat with warm blankets, heat lamps, hot-water bottles, or, if none of these is available, use the classic technique of placing the child skin-to-skin with a warm person of normal temperature in a sleeping bag or blanket.

Active rewarming by external or core rewarming techniques (e.g., warmed, humidified oxygen and warmed intravenous fluids) is necessary for children with severe hypothermia (Battan et al., 1999).

Patient and Parent Education

Instruct parents on the risks of hypothermia in young children. Emphasize the need to monitor children's activities in cold weather and to provide adequate protection from exposure. The higher metabolic rate of normal, healthy children serves to keep them warm, and they may not feel the effects of short-term exposure to the cold. As a result, they may not want a jacket, sweater, hat, or mittens when their parents believe they need them.

HYPERTHERMIA: COMMON HEAT-RELATED ILLNESS

Description

Hyperthermia is a life-threatening increase in body core temperature above 42°C. Heat cramps, heat exhaustion, and heat stroke are types of hyperthermia. Heat cramps and heat exhaustion are discussed in more detail in Chapter 15, because they often occur during sports activities. They are reversible changes; in contrast, heat stroke is a life-threatening condition. This section more specifically discusses heat stroke.

Etiology

Heat-related illness results from an ineffective response of the body's thermoregulatory mechanisms to environmental conditions. Children with some genetic myopathies have malignant hyperthermia, a reaction to anesthesia. All children are at risk for hyperthermia or heat stroke when exposed to high air temperature, especially if the heat is combined with high humidity and if steps are not taken to keep the child cool. Evaporation through sweating is the body's primary cooling mechanism with activity. If air temperature is higher than body temperature, if humidity is high, or if the body is dehydrated, the body's cooling mechanisms and the process of evaporation are compromised and internal body temperature increases (Williams, 1999). Age, exertion, illness, obesity, and poor nutrition also exacerbate the risk of hyperthermia. Compared with adults, children sweat less, begin to sweat at a higher internal temperature (or setpoint), have a higher metabolic rate (thus producing more body heat) and lower cardiac output, and are more susceptible to dehydration (because of proportionately larger body surface area).

Assessment

HISTORY. The practitioner assesses the following:

- Exposure
- Excessive exercise
- Wearing inappropriate clothing
- Inadequate fluid intake or the use of water or other low-sodium fluids during prolonged and strenuous exercise
- Previous episode of heat stroke
- Heat cramps: complaints of intermittent muscle cramping

- Heat exhaustion: complaints of thirst, headache, fatigue, nausea, and vomiting
- Heat stroke: delirium, stupor, or coma

PHYSICAL EXAMINATION. Signs of heat exhaustion include:

- Appears anxious and diaphoretic
- Tachycardia with temperature less than 40°C
- Orthostatic hypotension

Signs of heat stroke are progressive and include the following:

- Body temperature above 40.6°C (105°F)
- Hot, dry, red skin
- May or may not sweat
- Initial rapid, strong pulse, progressively becoming weaker
- Initially constricted pupils, progressively dilated
- Initial deep, rapid "snore-like" breathing, progressively becoming weaker
- Tremors, increasing dizziness, and weakness
- Confusion, irritability, anxiety (central nervous system dysfunction)
- Headache
- Loss of appetite, nausea, vomiting
- Decreasing blood pressure
- Seizures, collapse
- Coma and death

DIAGNOSTIC STUDIES. Electrolyte monitoring may be necessary for significant heat cramps and heat exhaustion. Heat stroke requires extensive laboratory studies and monitoring of physiological parameters.

Differential Diagnosis

Fever differs from hyperthermia in that it is an alteration of the body's hypothalamic setpoint in response to a pathological illness or condition.

Management

The management of heat-related illness includes:

Heat Cramps
- Cooling measures
- Oral sodium replacement with electrolyte

fluids or liberally salted foods (occasionally IV saline may be needed)

Heat Exhaustion
- Cool environment
- Intravenous replacement of electrolytes (initial bolus of 10 to 20 ml/kg of normal saline)

Heat Stroke
- All individuals with heat stroke die without treatment. Heat stroke patients should be transported to a medical facility as quickly as possible. The goal of treatment is to reduce the temperature to less than 100°F or by a total of 4° to 6° over a 30- to 60-minute period. First aid management includes the following steps:
  - Remove the child from the source of heat.
  - Apply cold packs, wet sheets, or towels. The body responds quickly to cooling of the neck, head, abdomen, and inner thighs.
  - Use a fan to cool and circulate air over child.
  - Be alert for vomiting; prevent aspiration.
  - When the body temperature is lowered to the desired level, stop cold packs, monitor, and be prepared to reapply cold packs if temperature increases.
- Other therapies are instituted based on the child's condition (Williams, 1999).

Patient and Parent Education

Instruct parents on the risks of hyperthermia (e.g., never leave an infant or a child in a closed car or continuously exposed to direct sunlight). Inform parents that children who suffer heat stroke are at higher risk for subsequent heat-related illnesses. Teach ways to prevent hyperthermia, including the following:

- Keep children well hydrated. Offer water often during active play and athletic events or practices. Water is an adequate replacement fluid, although children can also use electrolyte-based sports drinks.
- Make sure children are well rested and have good nutritional intake.
- Provide appropriate clothing (e.g., sun-shades, hats, and light-reflective shirts that allow ventilation).
- Regulate children's activity levels to the conditions (e.g., limit active play if it is very hot or humid).
- Acclimatize child gradually to changes in environment.

RESOURCE BOX 40-1

NATIONAL RESOURCES FOR BURNS

American Burn Association
(800) 548-2876

Local Poison Control Center
The number is listed among emergency numbers in the local telephone book; one can also call 911 and be transferred to the Poison Control Center. Not every state or city has a poison control center.

REFERENCES

American Academy of Pediatrics: The hospital record of the injured child and the need for external cause of injury codes. Pediatrics 103:524-526, 1999.

Avner JR: Animal and human bites and bite-related infections. *In* Burg FD, Ingelfinger JR, Wald WR (eds), et al: Gellis & Kagan's Current Pediatric Therapy, 16th ed. Philadelphia, WB Saunders, 1999, pp 1168-1170.

Battan FK, Dart RC, Rumack BH: Emergencies, injuries, & poisoning. *In* Hay WW, Hayward AR, Levin MJ, et al (eds): Current Pediatric Diagnosis & Treatment, 14th ed. Stamford CT, Appleton & Lange, 1999, pp 272-315.

Behrman RE, Kliegman RM, Arvin AM (eds): Nelson Textbook of Pediatrics, 15th ed. Philadelphia, WB Saunders, 1996.

Boguniewicz M, Leung DY: Allergic disorders. *In* Hay WW, Hayward AR, Levin MJ, et al (eds): Current Pediatric Diagnosis & Treatment, 14th ed. Stamford CT, Appleton & Lange, 1999, pp 917-942.

Bond GR: Snake, spider, and scorpion envenomation in North America. Pediatr Rev 20:147-151, 1999.

Coulter DL: Head trauma. *In* Finberg L (ed): Saunders Manual of Pediatric Practice. Philadelphia, WB Saunders, 1998, pp 883-885.

Copley LA, Dormans JP: Orthopedic trauma. *In* Burg FD, Ingelfinger JR, Wald WR, et al (eds): Gellis & Kagan's Current Pediatric Therapy, 16th ed. Philadelphia, WB Saunders, 1999, pp 939-944.

Eilert RE, Georgopoulos G: Orthopedics. *In* Hay WW, Hayward AR, Levin MJ, et al (eds): Current Pediatric Diagnosis & Treatment, 14th ed. Stamford, CT, Appleton & Lange, 1999, pp 695-714.

Frenck RW, Buescher ES: Pediatric trauma and musculoskeletal system procedures. Pediatric and Neonatal Tests and Procedures. Philadelphia, WB Saunders, 1996, pp 313-337.

Hansbrough JF, Hansbrough W: Pediatric burns. Contemp Pediatr 20:117-124, 1999.

Hebert AA, Carlton S: Getting bugs to bug off: A review of insect repellents. Contemp Pediatr 15(6):85-92, 1998.

Inaba AS: The rusty nail—And other puncture wounds of the foot. Contemp Pediatr 10:138-156, 1993.

Johnson KB, Oski FA: Oski's Essential Pediatrics. Philadelphia, Lippincott-Raven, 1997.

Krug S: Nail trephination—Drainage of subungual hematoma. *In* Walsh-Sukys MC, Krug SE, (eds): Procedures in Infants and Children. Philadelphia, WB Saunders, 1998, pp 262-265.

Mankin KP, Zimbler S: Foot and ankle injuries: Solving the diagnostic dilemmas. Contemp Pediatr 13(3):25-45, 1996.

Moskowitz H, Meissner HC: Tick-borne disease: Warm weather worry. Contemp Pediatr 14(8):33-49, 1997.

Ratner MH: A short course in wound care for children. Contemp Pediatr 8:22-38, 1991.

Resnick JI, Zarem HA: Diseases and injuries of the oral region. *In* Burg FD, Ingelfinger JR, Wald WR, et al (eds): Gellis & Kagan's Current Pediatric Therapy, 16th ed. Philadelphia, WB Saunders, 1999, pp 1029-1033.

Rosman NP: Head injury. *In* Burg FD, Ingelfinger JR, Wald ER, and Polen RA (eds): Gellis & Kagan's Current Pediatric Therapy, 16th ed. Philadelphia, WB Saunders, 1999, pp 431-438.

Sawyer JR, Esterhai JL: Orthopedic problems of the extremities. *In* Burg FD, Ingelfinger JR, Wald WR, et al (eds): Gellis & Kagan's Current Pediatric Therapy, 16th ed. Philadelphia, WB Saunders, 1999, pp 922-930.

Schmitt BD: Instructions for Pediatric Patients, 2nd ed. Philadelphia, WB Saunders, 1999.

Simon HK: How good are tissue adhesives in repairing lacerations? Contemp Pediatr 14:90-96, 1997.

Staheli LT: Fundamentals of Pediatric Orthopedics. Philadelphia, Lippincott-Raven, 1998.

Stewart C: Local cold injuries in children: Diagnosis, management, and prevention. Pediatr Emerg Med Rep 4(1):1-12, 1999.

Taylor CP: Arthropod bites and stings. *In* Burg FD, Ingelfinger JR, Wald WR, and Polen RA (eds): Gellis & Kagan's Current Pediatric Therapy, 16th ed. Philadelphia, WB Saunders, 1999, pp 1166-1168.

Taketomo CK, Hodding JH, Kraus DM: Pediatric Dosage Handbook, 5th ed. Hudson, OH, Lexi-Comp, 1998.

Williams RK: Heat-related illness. *In* Burg FD, Ingelfinger JR, Wald WR, and Polen RA (eds): Gellis & Kagan's Current Pediatric Therapy, 16th ed. Philadelphia, WB Saunders, 1999, pp 872-874.

CHAPTER 41

Genetic Disorders

Catherine E. Burns

INTRODUCTION

Genetic disorders occur in approximately 5% of live births. Two to 4% of newborns have a major anomaly, and up to 50% of spontaneously aborted fetuses have chromosomal defects. A single minor anomaly can occur in up to 13% of newborns (Aase, 1992).

The manifestations of genetic diseases can appear immediately after birth or after many years such as in patients with Huntington chorea. The manifestations can be evidenced in biochemical, reproductive, growth, development, or behavioral ways. Therefore, the primary health-care provider must be constantly vigilant for the possibility of genetic disease. Furthermore, once a genetic condition is suspected, referral to a medical geneticist will not always be required. Primary care providers need to be knowledgeable yet know their own limitations and set personal criteria for referral to specialists.

Caring for children with significant, long-term problems presents enormous burdens to family, community, and society. Prevention of genetic diseases by helping families make decisions about childbearing, screening for early detection to prevent disability, assisting parents to use specialized services, teaching health principles, monitoring and evaluating clients with genetic diseases, and working with families under the stress of caregiving are all roles of the primary care provider. Ethical decision-making seems to have a particularly important role in the area of genetics and genetic counseling.

REVIEW OF GENETICS

Humans have 46 chromosomes arranged in 23 pairs. Twenty-two pairs are autosomes (the same in men and women). The remaining pair are the sex chromosomes, with two X chromosomes for women and one X and one Y chromosome for men. Each chromosome has a long arm (q) and a short arm (p) and is numbered according to its distinct appearance. The gametes (egg and sperm) have one member of each pair of chromosomes. Fusion at fertilization restores the 46-pair complement, with one of each chromosome pair from each parent. If the two gene copies of a pair of chromosomes are identical, the cell is *homozygous*. If the two gene copies are different, the cell is *heterozygous*.

Genes, which carry the information about inherited characteristics from parent to child, are arranged linearly on the chromosomes, each with a specific locus. Thousands of genes are located on each chromosome. Not all genes are active at once, and certain mechanisms activate them at various developmental points. In homozygous cells, the genes from a pair of chromosomes carry similar instructions regarding the trait of interest; in heterozygous cells, the instructions are different. In the latter case, one gene may be dominant, with its instructions manifested in the phenotype, as in Huntington chorea, or the genes can be codominant, as in the case of individuals with blood type AB.

In traditional inheritance, genetic disorders are classified as *chromosomal disorders, single-gene disorders*, and *multifactorial problems*. Mutations occur when genetic material is permanently changed through alteration, deletion, duplication, or misplacement. Sometimes the mutations arise spontaneously, but once changed, they are transmitted to future generations.

In teaching concepts of chromosomes and genes to patients, the analogy of a necklace may be helpful. The chromosome is a necklace; the genes are the beads. The necklace can be broken or unusually long (a chromosomal disorder), or a single bead may be put in the wrong place (a single-gene disorder). Multifactorial problems are those in which an accumulation of abnormal genetic material plus some environmental factor must interact before a problem appears. One could explain this concept as a set of manufacturing problems that result in a defect by which the bead changes color if it gets wet.

In what is now called nontraditional inheritance, three more patterns of transmission of genetic material from generation to generation have been identified—germline mosaicism, uniparental disomy, and mitochondrial inheritance (Toomey, 1996). These latter are more difficult to explain to parents. In germline mosaicism, a mutation of genetic material occurs during one of the later cell divisions such that some cells continue to divide normally while a genetic alteration in another line of cells appears as those cells divide; the alteration is thus transmitted in continuing divisions including some germ cells but not all. In uniparental disomy, the offspring receives both chromosomes of a pair from one parent and none from the other. Mitochondrial inheritance refers to another kind of DNA found in mitochondria that can also become defective and produce proteins for mitochondrial metabolism that are incorrect in form and function.

ASSESSMENT

The nurse practitioner (NP) identifies possible genetic disorders by using the same skills as for other pediatric health problems: knowledge of risk factors, collection of a good history, and a complete physical examination augmented with appropriate laboratory or other studies. After the assessment, the NP or other provider determines the operative genetic mechanism and develops and implements a plan of care for the patient and family with consideration of individual, family, and cultural factors. Table 41-1 identifies some common features of children with genetic disorders that should lead the clinician to explore issues of possible genetic problems in the child and family.

Risk Factors

Risk factors include the following:

- Family history of known genetic disorder or recurrent pathological condition
- Malformations
- Mental retardation
- Metabolic disorders
- Delayed development of secondary sex characteristics
- Sensory deficits

T A B L E 41-1
Features Suggesting a Genetic Disorder

Mental retardation/developmental delays
Seizures with mental retardation
Severe hypotonia in infancy
Loss of developmental milestones
Short stature
Failure to thrive/growth retardation
Microcephaly
Dysmorphic features
Two or more physical birth defects
Ambiguous genitalia
Pigmentary skin lesions
Ocular findings or blindness
Deafness

Adapted from Pacific Northwest Regional Genetics Group: Practical Genetics for Primary Care. Portland, OR, Oregon Health Sciences Center, Pacific Northwest Regional Genetics Group, 1996.

- Progressive disorders
- Neuromuscular disorders
- Affective disorders (e.g., schizophrenia)
- Presence of birth defects
- Mental retardation or learning problems
- Repeated spontaneous abortions or still-births
- Maternal factors, including alcohol or drug exposure, medication exposure, age older than 35 years, environmental or occupational toxin exposure
- Family ethnic background (Table 41-2)
- Consanguinity

History

The history of genetic diseases usually includes the following main areas: family history of the disease using a pedigree format, environmental and occupational history, reproductive history, dietary history, medical history of the child, and developmental data. (See Figures 41-1 and 41-2 for an example of the pedigree notation format.) The pedigree format provides a visual map of the occurrence of specific traits and helps identify other family members who might be at risk (Toomey, 1996). Screening questions for genetic disorders that should be asked of all patients are included in Table 41-3). When a genetic disorder is suspected, the history must become more specific, as outlined in Table 41-4. Questions need to address the following:

- A family history is needed to identify family members with conditions that may be ge-

netically transmitted. Using a pedigree is important. Consanguinity, past and current health of each person in the pedigree, birth histories of other family members, and mental retardation or learning problems of family members are all important areas to explore.
- The environmental and occupational history is important to know if teratogenic factors might be involved.
- The mother's reproductive history may give information about malformation or genetic or infectious diseases transmitted to other offspring. Her pregnancy and delivery of the child in question may give other information to determine whether the fetus was affected or whether the condition was a result of trauma, infection, or some other factor occurring during the pregnancy or delivery. If the child was well throughout pregnancy and delivery, one might suspect a postnatal event.

Physical Examination

When a genetic disease is being considered, the physical examination focuses on growth, major and minor anomalies, and comparisons with family members. Any major anomaly can have a genetic cause. Three minor anomalies should raise the suspicion of a major anomaly and a genetic disorder (Leppig et al., 1987).

First, general appearance and familial similarities are assessed. Body size and proportions, measurements and percentiles, and a careful assessment of all systems constitute the remainder of the examination.

Common minor anomalies are identified in Table 41-5. Table 41-6 lists various anomalies by body parts. *Smith's Recognizable Patterns of Human Malformations* (Jones, 1997) includes tables on the size, length, and shape of various body parts that can be used to validate observations presumed to represent pathology. Remember that dysmorphic features can result from:

- *Deformations*—unusual mechanical pressures on the developing fetus
- *Disruptions*—outside agents causing destruction of cells in the embryo

T A B L E 41-2

Genetic Risks Associated With Ethnic Background

ETHNIC BACKGROUND	GENETIC DISORDER AT HIGHER RISK
Northern European	Cystic fibrosis, phenylketonuria
Jewish (Ashkenazi descent)	Tay-Sachs, Canavan, Gaucher
West African	Sickle cell, Sickle cell–hemoglobin C
Mediterranean	β-Thalassemia, sickle cell
French-Canadian	Tay-Sachs, branched-chain ketoaciduria

Instructions:
Key should contain all information relevant to interpretation of pedigree (e.g., define shading)
For clinical (nonpublished) pedigrees, include:
  a) family names/initials, when appropriate
  b) name and title of person recording pedigree
  c) historian (person relaying family history information)
  d) date of intake/update
Recommended order of information placed below symbol (below to lower right, if necessary):
  a) age/date of birth or age at death
  b) evaluation
  c) pedigree number (e.g., I-1, I-2, I-3)

	Male	Female	Sex Unknown	Comments
1. Individual	b. 1925	30 yr	4 mo	Assign gender by phenotype.
2. Affected individual				Key/legend used to define shading or other fill (e.g., hatches, dots, etc.).
				With ≥ 2 conditions, the individual′s symbol should be partitioned accordingly, each segment shaded with a different fill and defined in legend.
3. Multiple individuals, number known	5	5	5	Number of siblings written inside symbol. (Affected individuals should not be grouped.)
4. Multiple individuals, number unknown	n	n	n	n used in place of ? mark.
5a. Deceased individual	d. 35 yr	d. 4 mo		Use of cross (†) may be confused with symbol for elevated positive (+). If known, write d. with age at death below symbol.
5b. Stillbirth (SB)	SB 28 wk	SB 30 wk	SB 34 wk	Birth of a dead child with gestational age noted.
6. Pregnancy (P)	P b.1925	P 30 yr	P 4 mo	Gestational age and karyotype (if known) below symbol. Light shading can be used for affected and defined in key/legend.
7a. Proband	P↗	P↗	P↗	First affected family member coming to medical attention.
7b. Consultand	↗	↗		Individual(s) seeking genetic couseling/testing.

F I G U R E 41-1
Pedigree model. Common pedigree symbols, definitions, and abbreviations. (Adapted from Bennett R, Steinhaus K, Uhrich S, et al: Recommendations for standardized human pedigree nomenclature. Am J Hum Genet 56:745–752, 1995.)

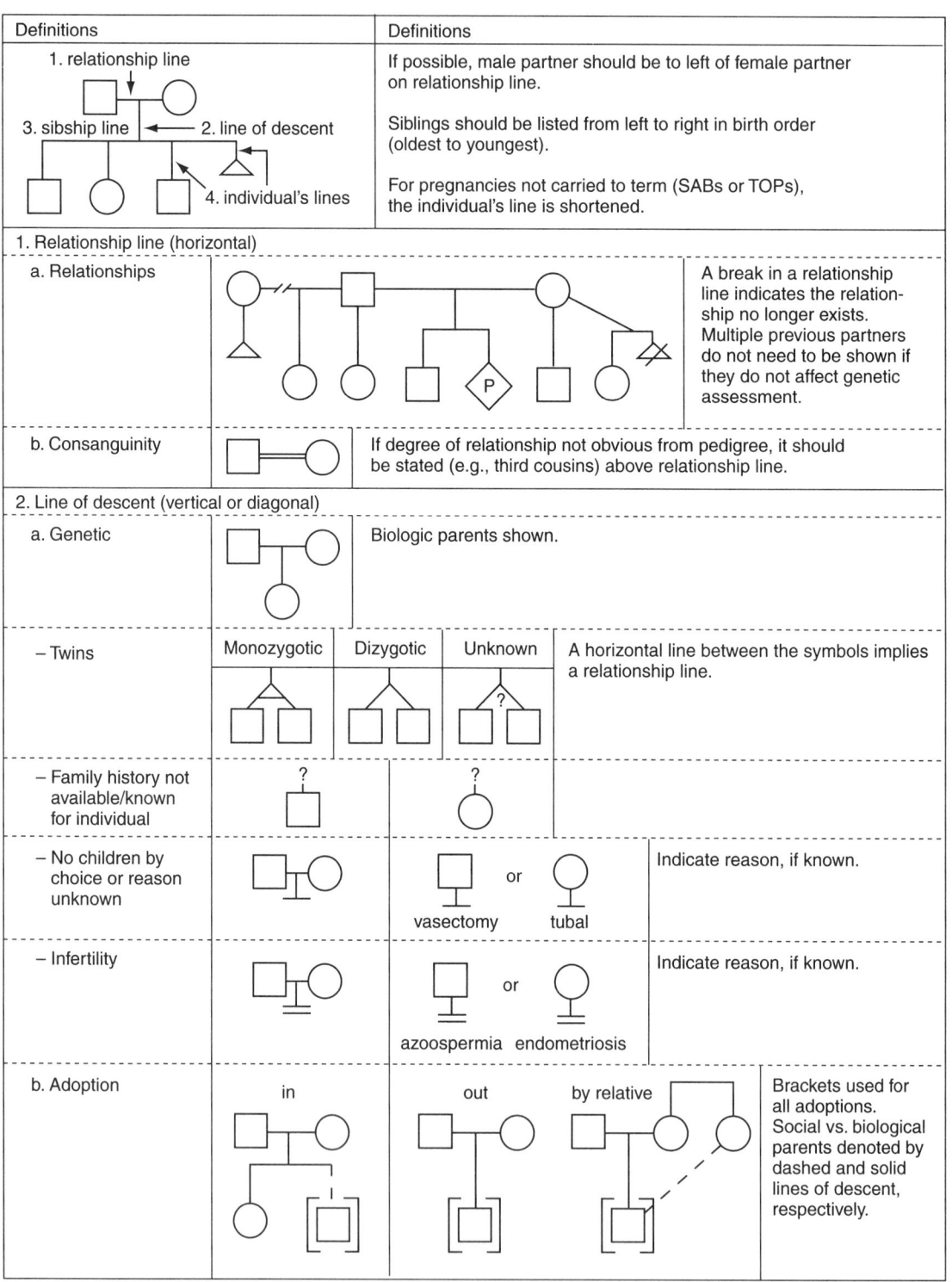

F I G U R E 41-2
Pedigree line definitions. (Adapted from Bennett R, Steinhaus K, Uhrich S, et al: Recommendations for standardized human pedigree nomenclature. Am J Hum Genet 56:745–752, 1995.)

T A B L E 41-3

Screening for Genetic Conditions: The History

QUESTION	RATIONALE/COMMENTS
Has anyone in the family had a birth defect?	To identify conditions that affect others in the family. If answer is yes, try to get more information about the nature of the defect.
Is there anyone in the family with a stillborn baby or baby who died early in life?	To identify unrecognized genetic disorders. Babies who died very early may have inheritable metabolic disorders. Distinguish from sudden infant death syndrome.
Is there any chance that you and your partner are blood related? Is this pregnancy a product of incest?	Consanguinity of partners closer than first cousins is a risk factor for autosomal recessive disorders. If yes, recommend genetics consultation.
Are there any diseases or traits that run in your family?	Significant if early onset, two or more close relatives affected. Genetic heart disease and genetic cancer risks are important. If yes, recommend genetics consultation and monitoring.
Have you or any of your parents or siblings had three or more miscarriages?	May indicate a chromosome translocation. If yes, order a karyotype of the mother and/or father.
Does anyone in the family have mental retardation?	Look for multiple members affected and associated with dysmorphic features. If yes, recommend genetics consultation.
What is your ethnic background? Your partner's?	Consider ethnic risk factors and screen if at risk.

- *Dysplasia*—from abnormal cellular functioning
- *Malformation*—abnormal development of a body structure during prenatal life

Usually, the latter are genetic in origin with multiple tissues affected. Visual recognition is a major factor in diagnosing genetic diseases. The NP can hone skills by reviewing pictures of patients with various disorders and consulting with experts.

Developmental Assessment

Many genetic disorders cause some degree of mental retardation and central nervous system effects. Developmental assessment is indicated.

Laboratory Studies

BIOCHEMICAL STUDIES. Many screening tests are available to check for inborn errors of metabolism. Such tests include those for phenylketonuria (PKU), galactosemia, and others. See the perinatal chapter for further discussion.

MOLECULAR ANALYSES (DNA STUDIES). Blood tests to screen for sickle cell disease, the thalassemias, and Tay-Sachs disease are commonly used. Molecular genetic methods are increasingly being used for many disorders, such as cystic fibrosis. Generally, the tests must be ordered with some specificity.

CYTOGENETICS: CHROMOSOME STUDIES. Chromosome tests may be needed to identify specific genetic diseases. Fluorescent in situ hybridization (FISH) combines elements of standard cytogenetic technique with molecular technology; probes for specific extremely small chromosome abnormalities are used. For instance, FISH analysis might identify the Prader-Willi abnormality at chromosome site 15q12.

IMAGING STUDIES. Radiographs and other imaging studies are used to identify skeletal, central nervous system, cardiac, and other anomalies.

PHOTOGRAPHY. Photographs provide a visual record of facial and other anatomical variations. They may also be useful in identifying other family members with similar characteristics.

T A B L E 41-4

Genetic History Questions

TOPIC	SPECIFIC ITEMS OF HISTORY
Family history: Helps identify family members with conditions that may be genetically transmitted	1. The pedigree should focus on at least three generations and look for people with similar characteristics 2. Consanguinity of partners (closer than first cousins) is very important 3. Note the past and current health of each person listed on the pedigree 4. Note the age of onset for family members' illnesses 5. Note multiple miscarriages, stillbirths, and/or anomalies among families 6. Family members with learning disabilities or mental retardation are important to document
Environmental and occupational history	Exposure to environmental toxins, alcohol, cigarette smoke, drugs, or radiation that might affect offspring

Reproductive history: Helps identify malformations, genetic conditions, or infectious diseases transmitted from mother to child
1. Maternal medical history
2. Prenatal history
3. Pregnancy and delivery history
	1. Maternal medical history
	  • Uterine anomalies
	  • Maternal illnesses and diseases (e.g., phenylketonuria, diabetes)
	  • Immunization status
	2. Prenatal history. The reproductive history should list every pregnancy, stillbirth, and abortion. Fetuses with significant chromosomal disorders are often aborted, and 5–7% of stillbirths and perinatal deaths are related to genetic problems
	  • Recurrent miscarriages
	  • Parity
	  • Advanced maternal or paternal age
	  • Complications of pregnancy
	  • Polyhydramnios or oligohydramnios
	  • Fetal movements
	  • Fetal growth assessments
	  • Prenatal screening results
	3. Pregnancy and delivery history
	  • Breech position
	  • Birth measurements
	  • Gestational age
	  • Results of newborn screening tests
	  • Presence of three or more minor anomalies in neonate
	  • Failure of neonate to adapt to extrauterine life

Dietary history: Helps identify infants with single-gene–related metabolic disorders	1. Infant feeding behavior 2. Formula or food intolerance 3. Temporal relation of symptoms to meals 4. Relation of signs and symptoms to types of food
Medical history of affected child	Use routine past medical history questions—history and current status of illnesses, hospitalizations, surgeries, allergies, injuries, immunizations List all health-care providers involved with the child's care
Developmental history	1. Achievements of milestones 2. Speech and language development 3. School performance 4. Developmental evaluations 5. Growth

Minor Malformations and Variations of Normal

Large fontanel	Darwinian tubercle (blunt
Epicanthal folds	point protruding from
Hair whorls	upper edge of helix)
Widow's peak	Digital anomalies
Low posterior	Clinodactyly (curved finger)
hairline	Camptodactyly (bent finger)
Preauricular tags	Syndactyly (webbed finger)
or pits	Transverse palmar crease
Minor ear	Shawl scrotum
anomalies	Redundant umbilicus
Protruding ears	Widespread nipples
Rotated ears	Supernumerary nipples
Low-set ears	

From Wardinsky T: Visual clues to diagnosis of birth defects and genetic disease. J Pediatr Health Care 8:63–73, 1994.

GENETIC DISORDERS

Various genetic disorders will be described in this section. Information is summarized in Tables 41–7 and 41–8.

Chromosomal Disorders

As described earlier, chromosomal disorders are problems of chromosome number or structure. Thus with thousands of genes involved for a given chromosome, chromosomal disorders usually result in major, multisystem problems. Only a few of the many chromosomal disorders are described here. Chromosome abnormalities occur in 1 in 150 live births (Toomey, 1996).

CHANGES IN CHROMOSOME NUMBER

The trisomies are the most common chromosomal disorders involving a change in chromosome number.

- *Trisomy 21* (also called Down syndrome) occurs in 1 in 800 to 1000 live births. Common characteristics include brachycephaly, hypotonia, hyperlaxity, oblique palpebral fissures, protruding tongue, flat nasal bridge, small ears, Brushfield spots on the iris, palmar simian creases, epicanthal folds, a wide gap between the first and second toes, short digits, and mental retardation. Complications may include thyroid disease (1 to 6%), leukemia, and congenital heart disease (30 to 40%). Serous otitis media with hearing loss is common (40 to 60%). Ocular abnormalities occur in about 20% of children with Down syndrome.

- *Trisomy 18*. Trisomy 18, or a third chromosome 18, occurs in 1 in 6000 live births (Seashore & Wappner, 1996). It is the second most common autosomal chromosomal disorder. These children have mental retardation, failure to thrive, rocker-bottom feet, prominent occiput, small features, short sternum, low-set malformed ears, hypoplasia of the nails, horseshoe kidneys, hernias, flexed and overlapping fingers, micrognathia, and other deformities. Ninety percent have cardiac defects, and only about 10% survive the first year of life. The potential for scoliosis, deafness, and central apnea needs to be monitored. Families of surviving children require a great deal of support.

- *Trisomy 13*. Children with trisomy 13 also have problems so severe that 50% die in the first month of life and 95% die by 3 years of age. Characteristics include mental retardation, failure to thrive, capillary hemangiomas, persistent fetal hemoglobin, microcephaly, cleft lip, cleft palate (or both), microphthalmia, colobomas, apparent deafness, cardiac septal defects, polycystic kidneys, polydactyly, and other features. The incidence is about 1 in 12,000 live births (Seashore & Wappner, 1996).

Generally, other trisomies are not compatible with life.

SEX CHROMOSOME DISORDERS

Sex chromosomal disorders involve changes in the number of X or Y chromosomes.

- *Turner syndrome*. Turner syndrome (XO) is a disorder of girls in which one X chromosome is present instead of two. The incidence is 1 in 2500 to 5000 girls. How-

T A B L E 41-6

Malformations of the Body

Central nervous system (not mental deficiency)
  Hypotonic
  Hypertonic
  Ataxia
  Seizures
Deafness
Brain: major anomalies
  Anencephaly
  Encephalocele
  Hydrocephalus
  Microcephaly
  Macrocephaly
  Meningomyelocele
Cranium
  Craniosynostosis
  Occiput shapes, flat or prominent
  Delayed fontanel closures
  Frontal bossing
Scalp and facial hair patterning
  Multiple hair whorls
  Anterior upsweep
  Posterior midline scalp defects
Facies
  Flat
  Round
  Broad
  Triangular
  Mask-like
  Coarse
Ocular region
  Hypotelorism
  Hypertelorism
  Short palpebral fissures
  Inner canthus placement
  Inner epicanthal folds
  Slanted palpebral fissures
  Depth of orbital ridges
  Eye prominence
  Periorbital fullness
  Eyebrow shape and extension
  Ptosis
  Nystagmus
  Strabismus

Eye
  Blue sclera
  Myopia
  Microphthalmos
  Colobomas of iris
  Patterning or color of iris
  Glaucoma
  Keratoconus
  Microcornea
  Corneal opacity
  Lens discolorations/opacities
  Retinal pigmentation
Nose
  Nasal bridge shape
  Short with or without anteverted nostrils
  Hypoplasia of nares
  Prominent nose
  Choanal atresia
Maxilla and mandible
  Malar hypoplasia
  Maxillary hypoplasia often with narrow or high arched palate
  Micrognathia
  Prognathism
Oral region and mouth
  Cleft lip with or without cleft palate
  Abnormal philtrum
  Full lips
  Downturning mouth corners
  Microstomia
  Macrostomia
  Cleft palate or bifid uvula with cleft in lip
  Macroglossia/microglossia
  Hypertrophied alveolar ridges
Teeth
  Adontia
  Hypodontia (including conical teeth)
  Enamel hypoplasia
  Caries
  Early loss
  Irregular placement
  Late eruption
  Other tooth anomalies

External ears
  Low set
  Malformed auricles
  Preauricular tags or pits
Neck, thorax, and vertebrae
  Web neck
  Short neck
  Nipple anomaly
  Clavicle anomalies
  Pectus excavatum or carinatum
  Small thoracic cage
  Rib defects
  Scoliosis
  Other vertebral defects
Limbs
  Arachnodactyly
  Short limbs
  Limb reductions
  Small hands or feet
  Clinodactyly of fifth fingers
  Thumb hypoplasia
  Radius hypoplasia
  Metacarpal hypoplasia
  Polydactyly
  Broad thumb and/or toe
  Syndactyly
  Elbow dysplasia
  Patellar dysplasia
Limbs: Nails, creases, dermatoglyphics
  Nail hypoplasia or dysplasia
  Single crease (simian)
  Dermal ridge pattern abnormalities
Limbs: joints
  Joint limitations/contractures
  Clubfoot
  Clenched hand
  Joint hypermobility and/or lax ligaments
  Joint dislocations

T A B L E 41-6

Malformations of the Body *Continued*

Skin and hair	*Renal*	*Immunoglobulin*
Loose/redundant skin	Kidney malformations	Immunoglobulin deficiency
Pigmentation alterations	Renal insufficiency	*Hematology-oncology*
Ichthyotic changes	*Genital*	Anemia
Hemangiomas and	Hypospadias or ambiguous	Thrombocytopenia
telangiectasias	external genitalia	Lymphorecticular malignancy
Dimples	Micropenis	Other malignancies
Alopecia	Cryptorchidism	*Unusual growth patterns*
Hirsutism	Hypoplasia of labia majora	Obesity
Assorted abnormalities of hair	Anal defects	Early macrosomia
(amount, quality,	*Endocrine and metabolic*	Asymmetry
distribution, color)	Hypothyroidism	
Cardiac anomalies	Hypogonadism	
Abdominal	Other endocrine abnormalities	
Hernias	Hypocalcemia/hypercalcemia	
Hepatosplenomegaly	Hyperlipidemia	
Pyloric stenosis		
Incomplete rotation of colon		
Single umbilical artery		

Adapted from Jones K: Smith's Recognizable Patterns of Human Malformations, 5th ed. Philadelphia, WB Saunders, 1997.

ever, about 25% of chromosomally abnormal spontaneous abortions are XO. The girls appear short and have a broad chest, webbed neck, lymphedema of the hands and feet as newborns, cubitus valgus, congenital heart disease (20 to 44%), urinary tract anomalies (45 to 80%), and a low hairline. They will be sterile. Their intelligence is normal. Hormone therapy is important to help with both growth and development of female characteristics.

- *Klinefelter syndrome*. Klinefelter syndrome (XXY) occurs in 1 in 500 to 1000 boys. Boys with the problem are often not identified until adolescence, when testes fail to enlarge. In addition to prepubertal testes, they can have gynecomastia and decreased body hair. They are usually tall and lanky. They are not feminine in behavior or sexual orientation and usually have normal sexual function. However, they are always sterile.

Other defects of the sex chromosomes such as XYY may or may not have clinical implications. Individual counseling is recommended.

STRUCTURAL CHROMOSOME DEFECTS

Structural chromosome defects can be of several types. First, *deletions* can occur in which a part of a chromosome is lost. Cri du chat syndrome involves loss of the 5p segment (5p−). Prader-Willi syndrome is a 15q− problem. Children with these syndromes are retarded and obese, with small hands and feet among other characteristics. If the problem stems from chromosome 15 from the father, Prader-Willi syndrome occurs; if the problem stems from chromosome 15 from the mother, Angelman syndrome occurs, with its characteristics including mental retardation and recurrent bouts of laughter, which are very different from those of Prader-Willi syndrome (Nicholls, 1993). This newly identified pattern of inheritance is called uniparental disomy.

Duplications of chromosomes can occur, such as a duplication of the 3q segment resulting in a Cornelia de Lange–like syndrome. Unbalanced inversions, or the wrong order of genes, are not usually compatible with life. Children with *translocations* may survive. Some

T A B L E 41-7

Inheritance Patterns With Examples

INHERITANCE PATTERN	CHARACTERISTICS	EXAMPLES
Chromosomal abnormalities		
Changes in number of chromosomes	Generally major anomalies and multisystem problems with the trisomies Sex chromosome disorders cause sterility and changes in growth patterns. Other changes may be more subtle	Trisomies 21, 18, 13 XXY (Klinefelter) XO (Turner)
Changes in structure of chromosomes	Changes may include deletions, duplications	Cri du chat (5p−) Cornelia de Lange (duplicated 3q segment), fragile X
Single-gene defects		
Autosomal dominant	Affected person from affected parent. Sexes equally affected. Normal offspring will have normal children	Neurofibromatosis, osteogenesis imperfecta, achondroplasia, Huntington chorea, familial hypercholesterolemia
Autosomal recessive	Both parents heterozygous for trait. High consanguinity risk. Sexes equally affected. Newborn screening may pick up these disorders. Family history usually negative except that siblings may be affected	Cystic fibrosis, sickle cell, Tay-Sachs, phenylketonuria
X-linked recessive	Males show trait. Female carriers usually do not show trait unless they are homozygous for the abnormal gene	Hemophilia, Duchenne muscular dystrophy, glucose-6-phosphate dehydrogenase deficiency
Multifactorial	Familial clustering. Sex difference in frequency. No clear biochemical or molecular defect. Considerable variation in expression Both genetic and environmental components are important	Cardiac defects, cleft lip/palate, clubfoot, scoliosis, dislocated hip
Germline mosaicism	Two or more cell lines with differing genotypes in an individual. Gametes of affected adult may be normal and/or abnormal. Consider if parents seem normal but offspring has an autosomal dominant condition	Achondroplastic siblings from normal-appearing parents
Uniparental disomy	Proband has two copies of a chromosome from one parent and none from the other	Prader-Willi, Angelman
Mitochondrial DNA disorder	Circular, double-stranded mitochondrial DNA defect, not in nuclear DNA. Variable expression depends on how many mitochondria carry defect	Leber hereditary optic neuropathy, myoclonic epilepsy, Kearns-Sayre syndrome

T A B L E 41-8

Characteristics of Common Chromosomal Disorders

CHROMOSOMAL DISORDER	PRINCIPAL CLINICAL FINDINGS OF THE DIAGNOSIS*
Down syndrome (trisomy 21)	Short stature, brachycephaly, small midface with upturned nose, hypoplastic frontal sinuses, speckled iris, epicanthal folds with palpebral fissures that slant down to midline, small mandible with resulting appearance of large tongue, myopia, small ears, lax joints (including atlantoaxial articulation), short broad hands and feet and digits, single palmar crease, clinodactyly, exaggerated space between great and second toes, developmental delays, hypotonia as infant, congenital heart disease At risk for leukemia, Alzheimer disease, hypothyroidism
Turner syndrome (XO)	Fetal edema—neonatal carpal and/or pedal edema Short stature, sexual infantilism, low hairline, webbed neck, increased carrying angle of arms (cubitus valgus), wide-spaced nipples, horseshoe kidney At risk for bicuspid aortic valve, coarctation of aorta, problems with spatial relationships and visual problem solving, hypertension
Klinefelter syndrome (XXY)	Postpubertal males—infertility, hypogonadism, mild mental retardation, long limbs, gynecomastia
Neurofibromatosis	More than five café au lait spots greater than 5 mm, axillary freckles, Lisch nodules, neurofibromas, optic glioma, megalencephaly At risk for pheochromocytoma, skeletal dysplasia, renovascular hypertension, mental retardation, scoliosis, compromised organs and neurological system from neurofibroma invasion
Fragile X	Large ears, macro-orchidism, long narrow face, mental retardation, autistic behavior
Fetal alcohol syndrome	Growth deficiencies, decreased adipose tissue, mental retardation, infant irritability/child hyperactivity, poor coordination/hypotonia, microcephaly, short palpebral fissures, ptosis, retrognathia in infancy, maxillary hypoplasia, hypoplastic long or smooth philtrum, thin vermilion border of upper lip, short upturned nose, micrognathia in adolescence At risk for heart defects, myopia, small teeth with poor enamel, hypospadias, hydronephrosis, hernias

*Not all children will exhibit all findings.

children with Down syndrome (1 to 2%) have a translocation rather than a duplication of chromosome 21.

Factors related to chromosomal disorders include parental age, nondisjunction during meiosis, and radiation and chemical exposure to the parents. Testing is done through cell culture and chromosome analysis. High-resolution chromosome studies revealing multiple bands provide much better diagnostic information than the older tests did. They may need to be ordered specifically. Unfortunately, because the possibilities for chromosome changes are great, some syndromes have not yet been described in the literature.

Single-Gene Defects

Inherited biochemical (metabolic) disorders are generally single-gene defects. These defects are the genetic problems that follow mendelian genetics rules. Because only one gene is involved, the problems are more subtle with few visible anomalies present. Most are uncommon (1 in 10,000 to 50,000 births) (McKusick, 1988). In aggregate, the incidence is 1 to 2% of live births.

Mendelian theory describes four patterns of inheritance: autosomal dominant, autosomal recessive, X-linked dominant, and X-linked recessive. Dominant problems occur in heterozygotes, where one gene dominates its counterpart from the other parent. Recessive problems occur only when a person is homozygous, with the problem gene appearing on both of the chromosomes of the pair. Issues of *penetrance* and variable *expressivity* complicate the picture, however, and result in some children with severe disease whereas others are only mildly affected.

AUTOSOMAL DOMINANT DISORDERS

Chromosome pairs 1 to 22 are called autosomes and pair 23 consists of the sex chromosomes. In autosomal dominant disorders, only one gene of a pair is needed for the problem to appear. The risk for recurrence is 50% if one parent is affected. Normal offspring of an affected person have normal children; males and females are affected in equal numbers. Often a vertical family history through several generations is seen, although wide variability in expression can occur. Increased paternal age can have an effect, although fresh gene mutation is frequent. These disorders tend to be less severe than recessive disorders. Neurofibromatosis (1 in 3000), tuberous sclerosis (1 in 10,000), achondroplasia (1 in 6000), Huntington disease (1 in 24,000 in the United States), polydactyly (1 in 100 to 300 blacks and 1 in 630 to 3000 whites), osteogenesis imperfecta (1 in 15,000 to 20,000), and familial hypercholesterolemia (1 in 500) are examples of these disorders (Seashore & Wappner, 1996).

- Neurofibromatosis is one of the most common genetic disorders seen in children. About 75% of affected individuals have only mild disease manifestations (café au lait spots and cutaneous neurofibromas). Scoliosis, optic gliomas along the pathway, and learning disabilities (40%) may occur and need to be screened for periodically. Malignancies occur in 6%, and 10% are mentally retarded (Seashore & Wappner, 1996) (see Table 41-7).

AUTOSOMAL RECESSIVE DISORDERS

These disorders are rare because they require two carriers to mate to produce the problem. Each pregnancy has a 25% chance that the offspring will inherit the problem and a 50% chance that the offspring will be a carrier. Carriers will be heterozygous, but a patient with the condition will be homozygous; that is, both chromosomes of a pair must have the same defect present for expression. Males and females are affected in equal numbers. The family history is usually negative, although siblings from the same parents may be affected. Consanguinity is an important factor in autosomal recessive disorders, and fresh gene mutations are rare. The age of onset of the disease is usually in infancy and often involves an enzyme deficiency or defect; these diseases are usually severe. Prenatal diagnosis and carrier detection are often available. Ethnicity risk factors are most significant for autosomal recessive disorders (Table 41-9). Uniparental disomy, which will be discussed later in the chapter, may also result in an autosomal recessive condition.

Examples of these disorders include some types of congenital hypothyroidism (1 in 4000), PKU (1 in 10,000), galactosemia (1 in 70,000), cystic fibrosis (1 in 1600 whites, the most common lethal inherited disease in the United States [Hulsebus & Williams, 1992]), Tay-Sachs disease (1 in 3600 Ashkenazic Jews), sickle cell disease (1 in 600 blacks), and the mucopolysaccharide disorders (Hurler syndrome occurs in 1 in 100,000) (Seashore & Wappner, 1996). Congenital adrenal hyperplasia with ambiguous genitalia is also autosomal recessive (Wardinsky, 1994).

Newborn blood screening tests are used to identify children with some of these disorders. A metabolic disorder may need to be included in the differential diagnosis in any child with developmental delay or regression, seizures or other neurological abnormalities, psychosis, failure to thrive, hypoglycemia, unusual odor, abnormal eating patterns, liver disease, or metabolic acidosis.

X-LINKED DISORDERS

In all X-linked disorders, the defective gene lies on the X chromosome. Because men have only

TABLE 41-9
Basic Genetic Risk Estimates

INHERITANCE PATTERN	GENETIC RISK FOR ANOTHER TO BE AFFECTED
Chromosomal abnormality	1% if parents normal, 3–10% if parents carry a translocation
Autosomal dominant	50% risk if parent affected; no risk if new mutation in proband
Autosomal recessive	25% if both parents heterozygous and 50% risk of offspring carriers; no risk of disease if only one parent heterozygous but 50% risk of offspring being heterozygous (carrier)
X-linked recessive	50% risk of affected son or heterozygous daughter if heterozygous mother; no risk to son of affected male; 100% risk of heterozygous daughter of affected male. No risk if proband is new deletion or new mutation
Multifactorial	Variable; ranges from 2–15%, depending on condition and number of affected family members
Germline mosaicism	Variable, depending on what proportion of gametes are affected. Uncommon
Uniparental disomy	Condition arises as a mutation. Whether the offspring can reproduce will depend on the effects of the condition. Rare
Mitochondrial DNA disorder	Maternal inheritance only. Rare

one X chromosome, disorders here always yield effects. In females, the Lyon principle explains that one X chromosome in each cell is inactivated randomly. If a high number of normal chromosomes are inactivated by chance, the female can exhibit pathology from the aberrant X chromosomes, which then predominate. In other words, females with X-linked disorders may or may not exhibit a given disorder.

In X-linked dominant disorders, affected males transmit the disorder to their daughters, all of whom will be affected, but to none of their sons. There is no carrier state. Fifty percent of the offspring of the daughters have a chance of receiving the affected gene. "X" inactivation lessens the effect in females, and families with the gene often have an excess of female offspring. These disorders are very rare. Vitamin D–resistant rickets (1 in 25,000) is one of the more common examples of an X-linked dominant disorder.

X-linked recessive disorders require two copies of the mutant gene in females or, in males, an affected X chromosome. One in 2 male children of female carriers may be affected. All daughters of affected males are carriers, and all sons of affected males are normal. Generally, females must be homozygous for the abnormal gene before the related disorder is manifested. Some of the X-linked recessive disorders include hemophilia (1 in 8500 males), Duchenne muscular dystrophy (1 in 3300 males), and glucose-6-phosphate dehydrogenase deficiency (1 in 10 black American males).

- *Fragile X.* Fragile X syndrome, an X-linked recessive disorder, is the most common inherited cause of mental retardation and is responsible for about 30% of cases of X-linked retardation (Hagerman, 1997) (Fig. 41-3). Fragile X occurs in both boys and girls but is more common in males. A prevalence rate of 1 in 2610 to 4221 births was found in an Australian study (Turner et al.,

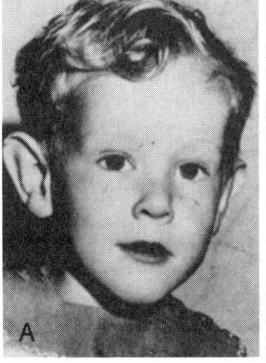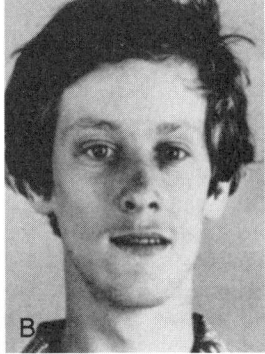

FIGURE 41-3
Child with fragile X syndrome. (From Turner G, Daniel A, Frost M: X-linked mental retardation, macro-orchidism, and the Xq27 fragile site. J Pediatr 96:837, 1980.)

1986). Because 25 to 30% of children with fragile X do not have typical features, the provider must be alert and remember to test for the condition, especially when the child's mental retardation has no apparent etiology. Hyperextensible fingers, flat feet, and soft velvet-like skin are childhood features. An adult male with the syndrome has a long face, large ears, midfacial hypoplasia, prominent forehead and jaw, high-arched palate, macrocephaly, single palmar crease, and hard calluses. Macro-orchidism is significant in postpubescent males. Mental retardation is found in essentially all people with the disorder, although the problem may be milder in females. Behavioral features are important and include hyperactivity, short attention span, perseveration of speech, hand flapping, hand biting, poor eye contact, excessive chewing on clothes, tactile defensiveness, mood instability, shyness, and social anxiety. Seizures occur in approximately 20% of individuals (Hagerman, 1997).

The fragile site is located on the long arm of the X chromosome at region 27 or 28. It can be diagnosed prenatally with routine chromosome studies only if low-folate medium is used. DNA testing for the *FMR1* mutation provides the diagnosis. Cytogenetic testing for the fragile X site at Xq27.3 is also used but needs confirmation with DNA testing (Hagerman, 1997). Children with fragile X and their families need follow-up for connective tissue dysplasias, multidisciplinary team developmental issues, treatment of behavioral problems and attention-deficit hyperactivity disorder, and genetic counseling (Hagerman, 1997) (see Table 41–8).

Prenatal diagnosis is available for many of the X-linked diseases, and the carrier state of the mother can often be determined.

Multifactorial Problems

Some of the known disorders that result from the interaction of certain genes with environmental factors or other genes include cleft lip and palate, diabetes mellitus, schizophrenia, asthma, spina bifida, hydrocephalus, clubfoot, congenital dislocation of the hip, pyloric stenosis, congenital heart disease, hypospadias, and others (Raffel, 1997). For instance, Navajo children are at greater risk for developmental dislocated hips.

Multifactorial problems have a tendency to be inherited, often with a 2 to 4% risk (Wardinsky, 1994), and the risks within a family increase for future children with each affected child. For instance, neural tube defects are prevalent in Northern Ireland. If a family has an affected child, they are at much higher risk for subsequent children with the problem.

Nontraditional Inheritance Patterns

More recent genetic studies have allowed medical geneticists to describe three other patterns of inheritance. These patterns include germline mosaicism, uniparental disomy, and mitochondrial inheritance.

GERMLINE MOSAICISM

In this pattern, a mutation occurs in a cell of the developing organism some time after fertilization. Thus as cells are multiplying, some will begin to reproduce with the mutation while others continue to multiply normally. The outcome is a person with "mosaicism"—some normal and some abnormal cells. Whether the gametes are affected will dictate inheritance to the next generation. Thus the term *germline mosaicism* is used to indicate inheritability of the trait. With germline mosaicism, parents appear normal but have abnormal gametes. The trick, clinically, is to identify mosaicism as inheritable. If normal-appearing parents with germline mosaicism had a first child with a condition such as achondroplasia, which is normally autosomal dominant, the clinician would deduce that the achondroplasia was not inherited in an autosomal dominant manner (in which case one parent would have had the disorder), so it must be a new mutation (usually with normal parents). However, the child did not have a new mutation with zero risk of appearing in a second offspring, but an inherited condition with a very high risk of appearance in subsequent children (Toomey, 1996). It is because of such situations that genetic testing of parents is important to help determine the risk to subsequent children.

UNIPARENTAL DISOMY

Generally, children receive one chromosome of each pair from each parent at the time of fertilization. If by some chance the child receives two copies of one chromosome of a pair from one parent and none from the other parent, uniparental disomy has occurred. The result is that the child will be homozygous for every gene located on that chromosome, which increases the possibilities of autosomal recessive disorders. The process has been described in some patients with cystic fibrosis. The same process results in either Prader-Willi or Angelman syndrome, depending on whether the copies are from the mother or the father (Nicholls, 1993).

MITOCHONDRIAL DNA INHERITANCE

All mitochondria in cells also have DNA (mtDNA). Unlike chromosomal DNA, mtDNA is circular and has 13 genes. All inherited mtDNA comes from the ovum—thus the maternal transmission pattern. Because each cell has more than one mitochondrion, there are more opportunities for mutations and also for variable expressivity; if many normal mitochondria are present, the effects from the aberrant mtDNA may be minimal. Several biopsies of different tissues will be subjected to both enzymatic and DNA analyses for diagnosis of mtDNA-related diseases.

Teratogens

A variety of drugs, diseases, and irradiation can have significant effects on the developing fetus. Congenital infections include syphilis, rubella, and many others. Maternal PKU and diabetes can also affect fetuses. Fetal alcohol, fetal hydantoin, and fetal warfarin (Coumadin) effects are all described.

- *Fetal alcohol syndrome.* Fetal alcohol syndrome is severe and occurs in approxi-

mately 1 to 300 to 1 in 2000 live births, with fetal alcohol effects occurring more frequently. Characteristics of fetal alcohol syndrome include facial dysmorphology with an underdeveloped philtrum, thin upper lip, flat midface, short or upturned nose, low nasal bridge, ear anomalies, short palpebral fissures, and epicanthal folds; growth retardation; and central nervous system involvement, including developmental delays, retardation, poor motor control, attention deficits, hyperactivity, and muscle weakness (Fig. 41-4). Many other anomalies have also been described, including scoliosis, clubfoot, renal and hepatic defects, cardiac defects, and cleft lip and palate (Smitherman, 1994; Seashore & Wappner, 1996).

Genetics and Cancer

Cancer must be considered a genetic disease because alterations in the genetic material of cells result in the aberrant cellular growth. Proteins stimulate cell division, suppress cell division and growth, control programmed cell death, and interact with DNA to control its replication or turn specific genes off or on (Seashore & Wappner, 1996). Errors in any of these areas will result in abnormal cell growth. Chromosomal instability associated with specific conditions also puts the child at risk for certain cancers; for example, Down syndrome is associated with a risk of acute leukemia. Many of the mechanisms of oncogenesis are being worked out by geneticists. Rhabdomyosarcoma, Ewing sarcoma, lymphoma, neuroblastoma, and other cancers are being studied. Ultimately, specific gene therapies may be developed to combat these diseases (Rubnitz & Crist, 1997).

MANAGEMENT

Primary care management of children with genetic disorders includes a variety of strategies, depending on whether a specific diagnosis has been determined.

Prenatal Screening

Prenatal screening can be done for many diseases if the family history indicates the possibil-

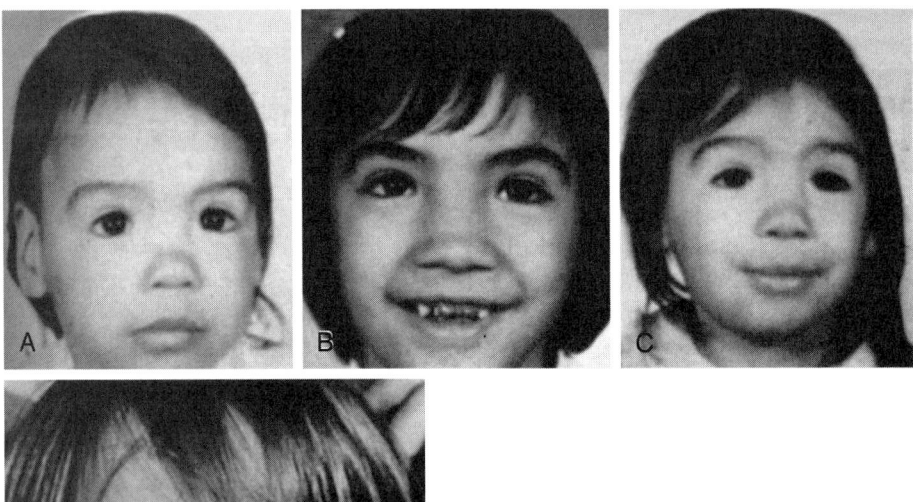

FIGURE 41-4
Child with fetal alcohol syndrome. (From Turner
G, Daniel A, Frost M: X-linked mental retardation;
macro-orchidism, and the Xq27 fragile site. J Pediatr 96:837, 1980.)

ity of a specific disease appearing in offspring. Routine prenatal carrier screening is done for sickle cell disease, Tay-Sachs disease, and the thalassemias. Prenatal carrier screening is done to provide parents with reproductive alternatives. Childbearing women should be referred to obstetrical or genetics clinics for prenatal screening and diagnosis. Chorionic villus biopsy sampling for diagnosis of some conditions is done at 8 to 12 weeks of gestation at some specialized centers, and amniocentesis is done at 14 to 20 weeks. By the 14th to 16th week, many imaging studies can also be performed to look for structural anomalies. Maternal serum α-fetoprotein can also be analyzed at 14 weeks. Elevated levels have been associated with neural tube defects, whereas decreased levels have been associated with chromosomal abnormalities. Prenatal diagnosis gives the family information to make decisions, such as possible termi-

nation of pregnancies with affected fetuses, artificial insemination or deferral of childbearing, or special preparations at childbirth.

Newborn Genetics Screening

Newborn genetics screening for a variety of metabolic diseases is done routinely (see Table 39-4). The diseases screened for include PKU, hypothyroidism, galactosemia, homocystinuria, maple syrup urine disease, tyrosinemia, sickle cell disease, and others. Different states include slightly different groups of diseases in their panels. For the 4.4 million babies born in 1990, it is estimated that for every 1% not screened, 3 with PKU and 10 with hypothyroidism were missed (Buist & Tuerck, 1992). The NP should be sure that the routine newborn statewide screening panel blood test is completed.

Screening for other diseases is done if the

child falls into a specific target population. Screening of target populations for Tay-Sachs disease and the thalassemias should not be overlooked. Black infants should be screened for sickle cell disease. Their screening as newborns is now recommended because prophylactic antibiotics can decrease infections and sickling episodes.

Genetic Disorder Diagnosis

Careful history taking and physical examinations of children should help NPs identify children with genetic diseases. Newborns with obvious defects or dysmorphic features should be evaluated. Children with two major anomalies, with a major anomaly and two minor anomalies, or with other indicators as noted in Table 41-10 should be evaluated for a genetic condition with karyotype analysis. Making the diagnosis may also identify the etiology and the risks for future pregnancies, information that is important for families to have.

In the case of a stillbirth or neonatal death, the infant's features should be documented—preferably photographed. A karyotype on blood and establishment of a fibroblast culture are also important. Head and renal ultrasound should be done if no autopsy is performed (Toomey, 1996).

Children and their families should be referred for diagnosis if genetic disease is suspected. Establishing the correct diagnosis is important for the family and the NP. The recurrence risk, prognosis given the natural history of the condition, guide to appropriate laboratory testing, plan of treatment and management, and facilitation of family coping all require a knowledge of the nature of the disorder.

Telling new parents that their child may have a genetic disorder needs to happen as soon as possible—even if a diagnosis cannot be confirmed. It should be done in a quiet, comfortable place when both parents are present, by someone with credibility. If possible, the baby should be present and referred to by name. The discussion should include some positive points as well as the problems to be faced. A follow-up phone call should be planned and additional sources of information identified, including contact with other parents. The parents should have some uninterrupted time with their baby (Cooley & Graham, 1991).

Genetics Counseling

Genetics counseling involves open communication with families who have received the diagnosis of a genetic disease. Its goals include helping the family to do the following:

- Understand the diagnosis, its course, and its management
- Appreciate the way heredity influences the disorder and the risks of recurrence and carrier status to specific family members
- Understand the alternatives available to reduce the risk of recurrence
- Choose the course of action that is appropriate in view of the risks, family ethics and values, and family goals
- Adjust as well as possible to the disorder and the risks of recurrence

The process takes time and may require many visits (Hall, 1990). Generally, genetics counseling is done by specialists.

The NP's role in genetics counseling is to perform the following:

- Identify individuals at risk for genetic disorders
- Teach children and families about the genetics counseling process

T A B L E 41-10

Indications for Karyotype Analysis

Suspected chromosomal problem
Two major malformations
One major and two minor malformations
Ambiguous genitalia
Congenital heart disease
Hypotonia
Malformed stillborns and normal stillborns when demise is of undetermined etiology
Mental retardation or developmental delay
Growth retardation or short stature
Couple with two or more miscarriages or infertility

Adapted from Pacific Northwest Regional Genetics Group: Practical Genetics for Primary Care. Portland, OR, Oregon Health Sciences Center, Pacific Northwest Regional Genetics Group, 1996.

- Initiate referrals with screening pedigrees, medical records, and appropriate histories and physical examinations
- Evaluate the family's understanding of genetics counseling and provide support as the family makes decisions based on genetics testing information

All families with genetic diseases should receive genetics counseling. The extent of counseling needed determines whether the primary care provider can manage the child and family or whether referral to a genetics clinic would be preferable.

Primary Health Care of Children With Genetic Disorders

Health supervision, screening for complications, and management of the health of the child given the genetic condition at hand are all important. Primary care and chronic disease management need to be integrated. Extra monitoring for complications that may emerge is essential. The American Academy of Pediatrics (AAP) has developed an example of health supervision guidelines for children with Down syndrome (AAP, 1994). It incorporates developmental, psychological, educational, and medical components. Monitoring for high-risk conditions, including congenital heart disease, thyroid disorders, hearing loss, atlantoaxial subluxation, ophthalmic abnormalities, and growth and development, needs to be integrated into the plan for primary health care. Similar guidelines for the care of children with neurofibromatosis type 1, Turner syndrome, achondroplasia, and other conditions have also been developed. Key features for several genetic disorders are listed in Table 41-11. They illustrate

T A B L E 41-11
Primary Care Monitoring of Children With Common Genetic Disorders

This table highlights some of the specific monitoring that can be done by primary care providers. It does not serve as a comprehensive guide and assumes the following:
  General health supervision guidelines for all children will be followed as much as possible
  Genetics counseling will be provided to all families
  Family support and counseling services will be provided
  Support groups that might be helpful will be identified for the family
  Long-term planning will occur
  Sexual and reproductive issues will be addressed with the child approaching adolescence, including help for both the child directly and the parents
  School placement and ongoing educational evaluations
  Care will be coordinated with a clinic specializing in services for children with the specific condition
  Developmental and behavioral issues will be addressed with referrals as needed
Down syndrome
  Cardiac echocardiography: At diagnosis and follow-up as needed if defects identified*
  Screen for mitral valve prolapse at adolescence†
  Hearing: At 9 mo (or sooner if concerns) and follow-up as needed* (50–70% will have hearing loss)
  Ophthalmological: At 4 mo (sooner if concerns), 12 mo, 24 mo, then every 2 yr and follow-up as needed*
  Thyroid: Newborn screen and every 6 mo to age 2 yr, yearly to age 5 yr, then as indicated*
  Cervical spine for atlantoaxial instability: At 3 yr, 12 yr, and 18 yr*
  Down clinic at 4 mo, 12 mo, then annually to 6 yr, then biannually‡
  Early intervention services‡ for developmental delays
  Supplemental Security Income referral‡
  Use Down syndrome growth charts to evaluate shorter stature and increased weight† and manage obesity
  Screen for hip dislocation through age 10 yr†
Neurofibromatosis—To be done at initial evaluation with follow-up as indicated:
  Head and spine MRI at diagnosis*
  Hearing*§
  Blood pressure*§ (renal artery stenosis, aortic stenosis, pheochromocytomas, adrenal tumors, vascular hypertrophic lesions)
  Imaging studies of identified affected areas as indicated*§
  Vision screening§
  Skin evaluations for new neurofibromas and progression of lesions§
  Skeletal evaluations for scoliosis, limb abnormalities, localized hypertrophy§

T A B L E   41-11

Primary Care Monitoring of Children With Common Genetic Disorders Continued

Turner syndrome—To be done at initial evaluation with follow-up as indicated:‡‡
  Cardiac,* echocardiography, or MRI for aortic abnormalities¶
  Renal sonogram*¶
  Blood pressure because hypertension is common, even without cardiac or renal abnormalities¶
  Hearing*¶
  Karyotype*¶
  Developmental assessment at 3 yr (or sooner if indicated) for mild learning disabilities*
  Pelvic ultrasonography at time of referral to endocrinology prepubertally*
  Possible referral for growth hormone therapy in mid to late childhood*
  Thyroid function at diagnosis and every 1–2 yr because 10–30% have primary hypothyroidism¶
  Vision screening because strabismus, amblyopia, ptosis are common¶
  Orthopedic evaluation of developmental dislocated hip, scoliosis¶
  Obesity monitoring and management¶
  Lymphedema monitoring and management¶
  Short stature management, including growth hormone therapy if the girl drops below the 5th percentile for the
    normal female growth curve, estrogen therapy for induction of puberty and feminization¶
  Fertility and family planning counseling and planning because women with Turner syndrome can achieve pregnancy
    without ovarian function via donors¶
Achondroplasia††
  MRI of foramen magnum at diagnosis; if small, repeat at 3 to 6 mo and similarly thereafter; if normal, repeat at 1
    yr*
  Ultrasonography/CT or MRI of brain at diagnosis; repeat if head growth exceeds achondroplasia growth curves or if
    symptoms of increased intracranial pressure are present*
  Physical therapy to focus on gross and fine motor developmental motor skills*
  Monitoring of upper airway restriction, obstructive sleep apnea, and potential for cor pulmonale*
  Orthopedic evaluation if bowing of lower extremities progresses because of fibular overgrowth*
Hemophilia and von Willebrand disease
  Developmental screen as follow-up to head trauma**
  Adequate protein and calcium intake for bone formation**
  Safety: Protective helmets, knee pads as needed**
  ID bracelet with diagnosis, treatment product, blood type. Remember to update annually**
  Noncontact sports participation**
  Regular dental hygiene care. May need replacement products for dental extractions**
  Annual hematocrit**
  Annual screen for microscopic hematuria**
  Hemophilia management through a hemophilia treatment center

---

CT = computed tomography; MRI = magnetic resonance imaging; SSI = social security.
  *Toomey K: Medical genetics for the practitioner. Pediatr Rev 17:163–174, 1996.
  †Vessey J: Down syndrome. *In* Jackson P, Vessey J (eds): Primary Care of the Child With a Chronic Condition, 2nd ed. St Louis, CV Mosby, 1996, pp 371–379.
  ‡American Academy of Pediatrics, Committee on Genetics: Health supervision for children with Down syndrome. Pediatrics 93:855–859, 1995d.
  §American Academy of Pediatrics, Committee on Genetics: Health supervision for children with neurofibromatosis. Pediatrics 96:368–372, 1995b.
  ¶Rosenfeld R, Tesch L-G, Rodriguez-Rigau L, et al: Recommendations for diagnosis, treatment, and management of individuals with Turner syndrome. Endocrinologist 4:351–358, 1994.
  **Dragone M, Karp S: Bleeding disorders. *In* Jackson P, Vessey J (eds): Primary Care of the Child With a Chronic Condition, 2nd ed. St Louis, CV Mosby, 1996, pp 145–170.
  ††American Academy of Pediatrics, Committee on Genetics: Health supervision for children with achondroplasia. Pediatrics 95:443–451, 1995c.
  ‡‡American Academy of Pediatrics, Committee on Genetics: Health supervision for children with Turner syndrome. Pediatrics 96:1166–1173, 1995a.

NATIONAL RESOURCES FOR GENETIC DISORDERS

General Information

Alliance of Genetic Support Groups
Tel: (800) 336-4363

Association of Birth Defect Children
Tel: (800) 313-2232, (407) 245-7035
Website: www.birthdefects.org

Council of Regional Networks for Genetic Services
Emory University School of Medicine
Tel: (404) 727-4549
Website: www.cc.emory.edu/Pediatrics/corn/corn.htm

Human Genome Project Information
Website: www.ornl.gov/hgmis
Information about the Human Genome Project

March of Dimes Birth Defects Foundation
Tel: (914) 428-7100
Website: www.modimes.org/index.htm

National Coalition for Health Professional Education in Genetics
Tel: (301) 402-0955
Website: www.nchpeg.org
For health professionals of all types. To include an information center with a collection of links to high-quality genetics education–related websites. Catalyzed by the AMA, ANA, and The National Human Genome Research Institute

National Organization for Rare Disorders (NORD)
Tel: (800) 999-6673, (203) 746-6518
Website: www.rarediseases.org
Federation of more than 140 nonprofit volunteer organizations offering information and family support referrals for rare disorders

Online Mendelian Inheritance in Man
Website: www3.ncbi.nlm.gov/omim
Database created by V. McKusick, MD, of Johns Hopkins University, provides a searchable catalogue of virtually all hereditary disorders

Albinism and Hypopigmentation

National Organization for Albinism and Hypopigmentation
Tel: (800) 473-2310
Website: www.albinism.org
Newsletter, informational materials, chapters, advocacy, research

Down Syndrome:

Association for Children With Down Syndrome, Inc.
Tel: (516) 221-4700

National Association for Down Syndrome
Tel:(708) 325-9112

National Down Syndrome Congress
Tel: (800) 232-6372

National Down Syndrome Society
666 Broadway
New York, NY 10012

Fetal Alcohol Syndrome

National Organization for Fetal Alcohol Syndrome (NOFAS)
Tel: (800) 666-6327

Family Empowerment Network: Supporting Families Affected by FAS/FAE
Tel: (800) 462-5254, (608) 262-6590
Informational materials (inc. Spanish), networking, referrals to local resources

Fragile X

National Fragile X Foundation
Tel: (800) 688-8765, (303) 333-6155
Website: www.medhelp.org/www/fragilex
Newsletter, informational materials, networking, local chapters, advocacy, fund research

Neurofibromatosis

National Neurofibromatosis Foundation
Tel: (800) 323-7938, (217) 355-NIFF
Website: www.neurofibromatosis.org

Neurofibromatosis 2 Sharing Network
Tel: (410) 461-2245
Newsletter, informational materials, networking, referrals to local resources, maintain research registry

Short Stature/Dwarfism

Little People of America
Tel: (888) 572-2001
Website: www.bfs.ucsd.edu/dwarfism/contracts.htm
Newsletter, informational materials (inc. Spanish), networking, local chapters

Trisomies 13, 18

Support Organization for Trisomy 18, 13, and Related Disorders (SOFT)
Tel: (800) 716-7638
Website: www.trisomy.org

Turner Syndrome

Turner Syndrome Society
Tel: (612) 475-9944

Turner Syndrome Society of the U.S.
Tel: (800) 365-9944, (612) 379-3607
Website: www.turner_syndrome_us.org

the integration of monitoring for the physiological, developmental, and psychological consequences that may occur.

The family's adjustment is a long-term process that requires monitoring and support with new information and resources as the child grows and changes. Some areas to include in planning care are as follows:

1. Health education:
   • Educate the family about the condition and its management, including family responsibilities.
   • Answer questions about health care services, and respect the confidentiality of the patient and parents so that information is not shared with insurance companies, employers, or other family members without the client's consent (Hulsebus & Williams, 1992).
   • Provide affected children, within developmental limits, with health education and support to understand and manage their own care.
2. Health care services:
   • Provide primary care for health promotion and disease prevention services.
   • Monitor the affected child for growth, development, emergence of new disease manifestations, and complications.
   • Assess the child's developmental age, and recommend appropriate interventions.
   • Work with the family regarding long-term planning for the child's care, including attention to psychological, developmental, social, and sexual factors.
   • For conditions without treatment, help families with support for ongoing management, decision-making related to experimental treatments that may be offered, and assistance in deciding when residential care or withdrawal of supportive care might be considered.
   • Be an advocate for the family with schools, insurance companies, and others.
   • Support and monitor the care of children with inborn errors of metabolism who need treatment to decrease the offending substrate, increase a deficient substance, provide an enzymatic cofactor, or a combination of the above (Davidson, 1992).

3. Resources:
   • Know resources for specific problems that the family may face.
   • Direct the family to financial resources or social services to be sure that necessary care is provided.
   • Direct the family to support groups and local resources.
   • Provide the family with written materials from disease-related organizations.
   • Refer to early intervention and other special educational programs as needed.
   • Direct the family to respite care services as needed.
4. Family coping:
   • Evaluate all family members, including siblings and grandparents, for their responses to the child with the diagnosed condition.
   • Support the family through the grief process.
   • Evaluate the parents' coping skills, family dynamics, and psychosocial responses.
   • Assess the adjustment of siblings.

Parents need a support person who will listen to their concerns, joys, and sorrows over time. The NP can be that person.

REFERENCES

Aase J: Dysmorphologic diagnosis for the pediatric practitioner. Pediatr Clin North Am 39:135-153, 1992.
American Academy of Pediatrics, Committee on Genetics: Health supervision for children with Turner syndrome. Pediatrics 96:1166-1173, 1995a.
American Academy of Pediatrics, Committee on Genetics: Health supervision for children with neurofibromatosis. Pediatrics 96:368-372, 1995b.
American Academy of Pediatrics, Committee on Genetics: Health supervision for children with achondroplasia. Pediatrics 95:443-451, 1995c.
American Academy of Pediatrics, Committee on Genetics: Health supervision for children with Down syndrome. Pediatrics 93: 855-859, 1995d.
Buist N, Tuerck J: The practitioner's role in newborn screening. Pediatr Clin North Am 39:199-211, 1992.
Cooley W, Graham J: Down syndrome—an update and review for the primary pediatrician. Clin Pediatr (Phila) 30:233-253, 1991.
Davidson A: Management and counseling of children with inherited metabolic disorders. J Pediatr Health Care 6:146-152, 1992.
Hagerman R: Fragile X syndrome: Meeting the challenges of diagnosis and care. Contemp Pediatr 14:31-59, 1997.

Hall B: Genetic counseling in multiple congenital anomaly syndromes. *In* Green M, Haggerty R (eds): Ambulatory Pediatrics. Philadelphia, WB Saunders, 1990, pp 315-318.

Hulsebus N, Williams J: Cystic fibrosis: A new perspective in genetic counseling. J Pediatr Health Care 6:338-342, 1992.

Jones K: Smith's Recognizable Patterns of Human Malformations, 5th ed. Philadelphia, WB Saunders, 1997.

Leppig K, Werler M, Cann C, et al: Predictive value of minor anomalies: Association with major malformations. J Pediatr 110:531-536, 1987.

McKusick V: Mendelian Inheritance in Man, 8th ed. Baltimore, Johns Hopkins University Press, 1988.

Nicholls, R: Genomic imprinting and uniparental disomy in Angelman and Prader-Willi syndromes: A review. Am J Med Genet 1993:16-25.

Pacific Northwest Regional Genetics Group: Practical Genetics for Primary Care. Portland, OR, Oregon Health Sciences Center, Pacific Northwest Regional Genetics Group, 1996.

Raffel, L: The epidemiology and genetic basis of common diseases. Pediatr Ann 26:525-534, 1997.

Rubnitz J, Crist W: Molecular genetics of childhood cancer: Implications for pathogenesis, diagnosis, and treatment. Pediatrics 100:101-108, 1997.

Seashore M, Wappner R: Genetics in Primary Care & Clinical Medicine. Stamford, CT, Appleton & Lange, 1996.

Smitherman C: The lasting impact of fetal alcohol syndrome and fetal alcohol effect on children and adolescents. J Pediatr Health Care 8:121-126, 1994.

Toomey K: Medical genetics for the practitioner. Pediatr Rev 17:163-174, 1996.

Turner G, Robinson H, Laing S, et al: Preventive screening for the fragile X syndrome. N Engl J Med 315:607-609, 1986.

Wardinsky T: Visual clues to diagnosis of birth defects and genetic disease. J Pediatr Health Care 8:63-73, 1994.

CHAPTER 42

Environmental Health Issues

Ardys M. Dunn and Catherine E. Burns

▰▰▰ INTRODUCTION

The environment is a basic determinant of human health and illness. Little research has been done on the direct impact of environmental factors on children's health status, but children, because of their developmental immaturity, rapid growth, size, and behavior, are particularly susceptible to environmental threats (Table 42-1). Exposure to toxins or other harmful substances can affect growth and damage organs or body systems during critical periods of development, both prenatally and during childhood. Many toxicants are capable of crossing the placenta, among them carbon monoxide, diethylstilbestrol (DES), metals such as mercury and lead, cotinine from environmental tobacco smoke, polychlorinated biphenyls (PCBs), and dioxin.

The effects of these toxicants on the fetus can be devastating. Low birth weight babies, spontaneous abortion, intrauterine growth retardation, increased risk of cancer, poor cognitive and behavioral development, and birth defects are all associated with environmental toxicants. Three percent of all babies born in the United States are born with a major birth defect, and the rate of some birth defects is increasing (National Center for Environmental Health, 1999).

Children's rapidly growing tissues more readily absorb environmental toxins; the lungs, skin, and gastrointestinal (GI) tract of newborns are highly permeable and gastric pH is high, facilitating absorption. At the same time, newborns' immature organ systems more slowly metabolize drugs (as a result, it is necessary to adjust medication doses carefully) and make it more difficult for infants to detoxify and excrete harmful substances.

Because of their smaller size, children consume more fresh fruit, water, milk, and juice per pound of body weight than adults, and many of these products are treated with pesticides or other chemicals. A child's favorite foods, such as apples, grapes, or bananas carrying a residue of pesticides, can represent a significant health problem. An estimated 25,000 children are poisoned by pesticides each year (National Center for Environmental Health, 1999).

The prevalence of asthma in children in the United States has doubled since 1980, with nearly 5 million cases identified (National Center for Environmental Health, 1999). Children engage in more outdoor activities than adults, breathe more pollutants per pound of body weight, and are physically closer to many potentially harmful substances. Crawling on the floor, chewing on objects, and running and rolling in the grass are behaviors that expose children to environmental toxins. Respiratory problems, lead poisoning, and pesticide toxicity can be results of this behavior. As children grow, their

T A B L E 42-1
Environmental Risk Factors for Children at Different Stages of Development

DEVELOPMENTAL STAGE	DEVELOPMENTAL CHARACTERISTICS	EXPOSURE PATHWAYS (PHYSICAL ENVIRONMENT)	BIOLOGICAL VULNERABILITIES	APPROPRIATE RESPONSES IN THE SOCIAL ENVIRONMENT
Preconception	Maternal and paternal health status	Maternal/paternal reproductive organs may be compromised Maternal stores of toxicants in bones and fatty tissue can be mobilized during pregnancy	Problems with fertilization, implantation of ovum Damage to ovum or sperm Fetal development	Need for research and education regarding: Long-term effects of environmental contaminants on reproductive system and subsequent offspring
Prenatal	Fetal development Dependent on maternal health status and environmental exposure	Maternal blood supply via placenta Radiation Noise Heat	Tissue differentiation Rapid cell division and growth Organ development Metabolic pathways incomplete	Need for prenatal programs and regulations regarding: Alcohol Cigarettes Drugs Metals
Newborn (0–2 mo)	Nonambulatory Restricted environment High calorie, water intake High air intake Highly permeable skin Alkaline gastric secretions (low gastric acidity)	Food Breast milk Infant formula Dyes in clothing Soaps and shampoos Indoor air Tap/well water in home	Brain Cell migration Neuron myelination Creation of neuron synapses Lungs Developing alveoli Rapid air exchange Narrow airways Bones Rapid growth and hardening Other organs Rapid growth Poor enzyme detoxification	Need for newborn-sensitive programs and regulations regarding: Polychlorinated biphenyls (PCBs) Lead in drinking water Environmental tobacco smoke Need to educate parents and policymakers concerning environmental hazards

Age group	Developmental characteristics	Exposures	Biological development	Needs

Infant/toddler (2 mo–2 y)	Beginning to walk
	Oral exploration (mouthing)
	Restricted environment and near floors
	Increased time away from parents
	Minimal variation in diet
	High intake of fruits, vegetables, and milk products per body weight
		Food
		  Baby food
		  Food additives
		  Milk and milk products
		Air
		  Indoor
		  Layer effects: air near floor contains more toxicants
		  Tap/well water in home and day care
		Surfaces
		  Rugs
		  Floors
		  Lawns
			Brain
			  Creation of synapses
			Lungs
			  Developing alveoli
			  Rapid air exchange
			  Narrow airways
				Need for child-sensitive programs and regulations regarding:
				  Radon in the home
				  Residential pesticide use
				  Lead abatement
				  Environmental tobacco smoke
				Need to educate parents and policymakers concerning environmental hazards

Preschool child (2–6 y)	Language acquisition
	Group and individual play
	Growing independence
	Increased intake of fruits and vegetables
	Day care or preschool attendance
		Food
		  Fruits, vegetables
		  Milk and milk products
		Air
		  Day care/preschool
		  Outdoor
		Water
		  Tap/well water and home/day care/preschool
		  Water fountains
		  Parks and swimming areas
			Brain
			  Dendritic trimming
			  Neuron myelination
			Lungs
			  Developing alveoli
			  Increasing lung volume
				Need for child-sensitive programs and regulations regarding:
				  Food pesticides
				  Environmental tobacco smoke at home and preschool
				Need to educate parents and policymakers concerning environmental hazards

Table continued on following page

Environmental Risk Factors for Children at Different Stages of Development Continued

DEVELOPMENTAL STAGE	DEVELOPMENTAL CHARACTERISTICS	EXPOSURE PATHWAYS (PHYSICAL ENVIRONMENT)	BIOLOGICAL VULNERABILITIES	APPROPRIATE RESPONSES IN THE SOCIAL ENVIRONMENT
School-age child (6–12 y)	Beginning school Playground activities Increased involvement in group activities	Food at home and school Air School Outdoor Water School water fountains Tap/well water Swimming areas Playgrounds Wood preservatives Pesticides and fertilizers Other Arts and crafts supplies	Brain Specific synapse formation Dendritic trimming Lung Volume expansion Metabolic enzymes more active than in younger child	Need for child-sensitive programs and regulations regarding: Asbestos abatement Lead in school drinking water Hazards in arts and crafts material Environmental tobacco smoke Need to educate parents and policymakers concerning environmental hazards
Adolescent (12–18 y)	Development of abstract thinking Puberty Growth spurt Increased adherence to peer norms	Food Air Water Other Occupation Self-determination: smoking, inhalations	Brain Continued synapse formation Lung Volume expansion Gonad maturation Ova and sperm maturation Breast development Bone growth and calcification Muscle growth	Need for adolescent-sensitive programs and regulations regarding: Child labor and other issues, especially environmental tobacco smoke Need to educate parents and policymakers concerning environmental hazards

Adapted from Gitterman B: Environmental risk factors for children at different stages of development. Personal communication, 1997 and Chai S, Bearer CF: A developmental approach to pediatric environmental health. *In* Training Manual on Pediatric Environmental Health: Putting it into Practice. Berkeley, CA: Children's Environmental Health Network/Public Health Institute, 1999.

risks approximate those of adults. Adolescents are particularly susceptible to environmental tobacco smoke and occupational hazards.

Children living in poorer communities are at higher risk than others. Poor housing and nutrition, high levels of lead, toxic waste deposits, and limited access to health screening and treatment all contribute to increased risk (Chaudhuri, 1998). In addition to the immediate risk during childhood, children have a longer time span for exposure to environmental toxins. The long-term effects and mechanisms of harmful exposures are not always clear, but studies suggest that with some conditions a child is more likely to suffer health problems than an adult exposed to the same substance (Zahm & Ward, 1998).

Implications for Nurse Practitioners

Nurse practitioners (NPs) need to be able to give their clients accurate information about environmental health issues, yet many providers are unprepared in the area of pediatric environmental health. The public is becoming increasingly concerned regarding environmental threats to health. Legal mandates (e.g., right-to-know laws) contribute to more well-informed patients who want additional information. In many cases, parents or providers may suspect that an illness is associated with environmental conditions, but a cause-and-effect relationship is unclear. The NP knowledgeable about the potential hazards of environmental exposure will be able to explain the possible connections to patients and parents, collect clear assessment data, and work closely with families to make appropriate treatment choices, including referral and consultation with public health authorities. If not personally knowledgeable, the NP should know where to get information. It has been shown that incorporating a course in pediatric environmental health into a pediatric residency program contributes to a significant increase in environmental questions in history-taking, and such courses are recommended for all pediatric primary care providers (Bearer & Phillips, 1993).

In addition to direct patient care, NPs can work in collaboration with other health care providers, conduct research to identify environmental problems, and advocate in the public arena (e.g., industry, policy, regulation) for more responsible management of environmental agents that affect health.

RELATIONSHIP BETWEEN ENVIRONMENTAL FACTORS AND HUMAN HEALTH

Epidemiological Model: Risk Assessment

An epidemiological model of risk assessment helps explain the interaction among variables in the process of ecological adaptation (Fig. 42-1), and can be used to investigate the effect of the environment on health status. Research based on this model may be beyond the scope of an NP's practice, but the model itself can be helpful in patient and parent education when the NP explains the relationship of environment to health.

A first step in an epidemiological model identifies interactive factors in the environment, including *receptors* (i.e., hosts or living things that are susceptible and/or exposed to environmental agents); *toxins* or harmful substances that might cause damage (i.e., the agent); and the environmental *medium* or route by which exposure could occur (e.g., air, water, food). What is the concentration of the toxic agent? How much is there? How strong is it? How long will it stay around? What is the extent of contact of the toxic agent with the receptor? Once these three factors have been identified, it is necessary to determine the possibility that harm could occur. Several questions are asked when making this determination: How *susceptible* is the receptor to the agent (e.g., age, sex, genetics, diet, general health)? At what quantity or level will the agent present a problem to this receptor, or at what dose will a response occur? (This is called the *applied action* or dose-response level.) A final step in this process *compares the actual environmental condition with the applied action level*, asking the question: With this amount of exposure, is the individual at risk for health problems?

Although many environmental health haz-

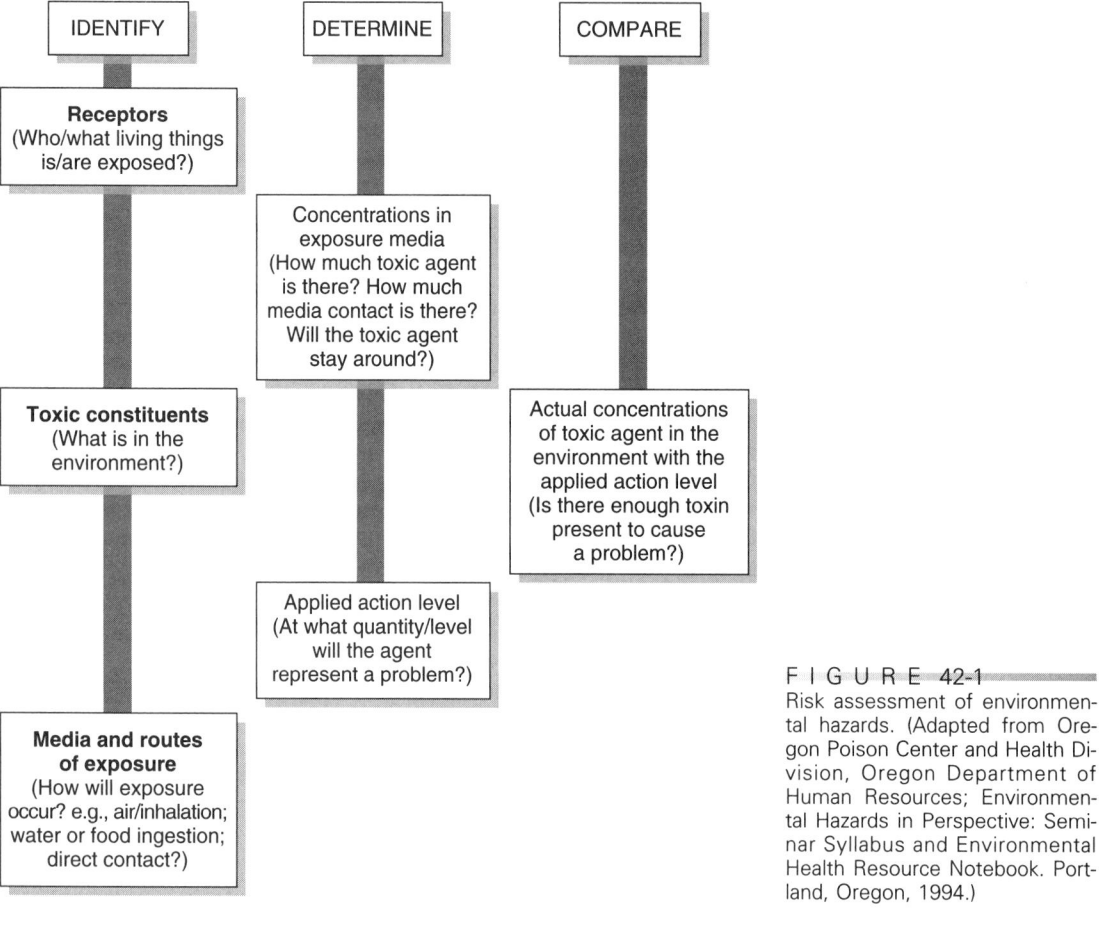

F I G U R E 42-1
Risk assessment of environmental hazards. (Adapted from Oregon Poison Center and Health Division, Oregon Department of Human Resources; Environmental Hazards in Perspective: Seminar Syllabus and Environmental Health Resource Notebook. Portland, Oregon, 1994.)

ards have been identified, it is not always possible to determine direct cause and effect. Several difficulties have been noted in making this determination: (1) the extent of exposure may be unclear; (2) there can be a long latency period between exposure and appearance of illness; (3) an individual may have exposure to multiple confounding agents; and (4) much research in environmental health has been done on animals and may not translate to human development (Bearer, 1998).

Toxicological Principles

Toxins affect the human body through complex processes. Knowing toxicological principles can help the NP understand the relationship between human health and environmental factors. Toxicological principles are the same as those the NP has learned related to pharmacological therapy: exposure, absorption, distribution, metabolism, tissue sensitivity, and effects—therapeutic or toxic. In fact, Paracelsus (1493-1541), considered the Father of Toxicology, is reputed to have said "All substances are poisons; there is none that is not a poison. The right dose differentiates a poison from a remedy."

EXPOSURE. Contact of a biological, chemical, or physical agent with the outer boundary of an organism (e.g., skin, lungs, GI tract) constitutes exposure. Exposure factors include frequency and duration of exposure, concentration of the agent at the point of contact, and the susceptibility of the organism (e.g., an infant's skin burns much more easily than an adult's).

ABSORPTION. The process by which an agent is taken into the organism, absorption occurs in the skin, mucous membranes, lungs, or GI tract, (e.g., carbon tetrachloride is absorbed via the skin). Absorption involves active or passive transport (e.g., lipid-soluble chemicals such as PCBs are passively absorbed through the gut and stored in fat; lead is taken up through active transport in the GI tract and stored in bone or other tissues).

DISTRIBUTION. Agents are distributed throughout the organism via the blood or lymph systems. Factors include the ability of an agent to cross the blood-brain barrier, the blood flow to the organ, and the affinity of tissues to take up a particular agent (e.g., lipid-soluble chemicals are found in fatty tissues).

METABOLISM. Metabolic enzymes in the body interact with toxic agents in several ways: (1) oxidation, reduction, and hydrolysis of the agent; the agent can be detoxified, but chemicals can also be activated and made more toxic. (2) Conjugation and breakdown to enhance elimination, usually through the kidney. Metabolism factors include the individual's age, sex, nutritional status, genetics, presence of other drugs, and disease or illness.

TISSUE SENSITIVITY. Susceptibility and reaction of tissue to a particular agent can vary.

TOXIC EFFECTS. Toxic effects vary by agent, dose, and organ, or system affected. They include a wide range of pathological conditions.

Assessment

Assessment of environmental health hazards should be integrated into regular health appraisals as well as examinations of ill children. The essential questions to ask for any environmental history are found in Table 42-2.

PHYSICAL EXAMINATION

The physical examination should cover all body systems thoroughly. Evaluate agent-specific findings (e.g., chemical burns, neurotoxicity caused by mercury, individual toxicants discussed later), but also look for more subtle, nonspecific signs and symptoms (e.g., skin rashes and headaches). The effects of toxicants on the body can be subclinical in many cases.

Effects also can occur long after exposure. As an example, there is an estimated decrease of 1 point in the IQ for each 2 μg/dl elevation in blood lead level with a significant lag time between the time of exposure and the loss of cognitive skills.

LABORATORY STUDIES

Laboratory studies should be performed as indicated, based on signs and symptoms. Agent-specific laboratory studies, if available and reliable, can be helpful in determining treatment plans. Very few tests are feasible for use in the primary care setting, and the NP should consult with individual laboratories regarding their capabilities. Some tests available include the following:

- Plasma lead levels
- Carboxyhemoglobin
- 24-hour urine for metals
- Urinary cotinine assays
- Plasma cholinesterase levels for pesticide metabolites

Management of Environmental Conditions

Management of illness related to environmental factors uses a public health model of primary, secondary, and tertiary prevention. A multidisciplinary approach to management, including epidemiology, pediatrics, toxicology, and health economics is necessary for treatment of specific conditions as well as prevention through environmental change (Landrigan et al., 1998).

PRIMARY PREVENTION

Primary prevention involves interventions that keep a condition from occurring and maintain a level of wellness. Health promotion and health education of the individual or public at large are forms of primary prevention (e.g., planting an organic garden is one form of primary prevention).

Primary prevention also takes place at the public policy level. Regulations or legal restrictions can prevent health problems (e.g., through implementation of air and water qual-

T A B L E 42-2

Environmental Health Assessment Questions

QUESTION	RATIONALE
How old is the home?	Homes built in the 1970s or earlier may contain lead paint
In what kind of environment does the child spend time (e.g., home, day care)?	Friable asbestos—basement risks Radon—basement and lower floors risk Formaldehyde—mobile home risk
What is the source of heating?	Carbon monoxide (CO), air particulates, NO_2, polycyclic aromatic hydrocarbons
Is home renovation occurring or planned?	Lead dust, asbestos risk; new homes may pose formaldehyde risk
Does the family use pesticides inside or outside the home?	Dermal absorption; respiratory absorption to children low to ground
Is the child exposed to asbestos or lead at school?	See lead and asbestos discussions; most schools are safe
Does the child or other family members have hobbies that involve toxic elements (e.g., model building, stained glass, cleaning guns)?	Lead in artists' paints, lead solder, toluene with model-building glues, lead with fishing weights and bullets
Is the family living near polluted areas, industry, commercial businesses, dumps?	Recent emissions, soil pollution, water pollution, air quality risks
Are there toxic plants in the child's play area? Wood preservatives on playground equipment? Asbestos in playground sand?	Risks in community play areas
What are the parents' occupations? Are children or adolescents employed? Workplace exposures? Safety hazards in the workplace? OSHA regulations followed at the workplace?	Take-home exposures have been documented and young people may be at increased risk in the workplace
Cigarette smokers in the child's environment—home, school, day care, friends, car transport	Environmental tobacco smoke (ETS) is a risk factor for SIDS, asthma, other respiratory conditions, long-term effects
Is the child's diet a source of toxicants? Is the breastfeeding mother taking drugs or other medications, smoking, been exposed to toxicants? Is the water supply lead-free and pollution-free? Are fresh vegetables washed and prepared to reduce exposure?	Ingested pesticides, lead, mercury, PCBs are all risks
Lead poisoning screening risks (see Table 42-6)	Lead is common in the environment and poses a lifelong risk
Does the home have safety items in place? (smoke alarm, CO alarm, fire extinguisher, childproofed cabinets, electrical outlet covers, gates on stairs, barriers to fireplaces or woodstoves, edge guards for sharp corners, hot-water heater set at 125°F, fenced swimming pool with self-latching gates)	Preventive measures for the most common accidents in the home
Do you think your child may be at risk from any exposures to toxins?	Families may have information or fears not addressed by the above questions.

OSHA = Occupational Safety and Health Administration; SIDS = sudden infant death syndrome; PCBs = polychlorinated biphenyls.

Adapted from Balk SJ: The environmental history—Asking the right questions. Contempt Pediatr 13:19–20, 22–24, 28, 31–34, 36, 1996.

ity standards, restaurant and food handling regulations, bans on the use of hydrofluorocarbons). Various United States (US) federal agencies function to regulate development and use of hazardous materials (eg., the Environmental Protection Agency [EPA], the US Consumer Product Safety Commission, the Occupational Safety and Health Administration [OSHA]). In 1997 the United States joined seven other countries (the G8) in creating the 1997 Declaration of the Environment Leaders of the Eight on Children's Environmental Health, raising the issue of protection of children from environmental threats to an international level.

Assessment is a final area of primary prevention. Potential environmental hazards can be identified before a health problem has occurred (Carroquino et al., 1998). Examples include safety inspections in industry and public areas (e.g., playgrounds); monitoring of lead or radon in buildings; and scientific research to determine connections between environmental agents and disease. The importance of conducting research on children, adapting research methodologies to the unique characteristics of children, and developing biological markers to better assess the impact of environmental hazards on children have been stressed (Weaver et al., 1998; National Institute of Environmental Health Science, 1999).

SECONDARY PREVENTION

Secondary prevention involves early detection, treatment, and referral for identified diseases. Testing for serum lead levels is one form of early detection. The general guidelines for management of poisonings are found in the next section.

TERTIARY PREVENTION

Tertiary prevention seeks to rehabilitate and restore the environment to a healthful state (e.g., asbestos and lead abatement, superfund cleanup, restoration of wetlands). Individually, patients can take steps to end exposure to a contaminant (e.g., stop using pesticides in the home, follow directions on pesticide usage exactly) or change other behaviors that exacerbate adverse effects (e.g., radon in combination with tobacco smoke is more harmful). Follow-up is essential, because effects of environmental agents may not appear for months or years.

Prevention and Patient Education

Many health problems are related to environmental factors, but the relationship is not always clear, and this uncertainty can be very frustrating. NPs may have to tell patients they do not know if there is a connection between a particular environmental factor and illness. It is important to listen to and validate patient concerns; this gives the message that the NP is also concerned and will work with patients to minimize problems. Blanket reassurances are inappropriate, but NPs can provide perspective to patients by explaining the process of environmental effects on health and encouraging patients to actively control their environment. NPs may also serve as a liaisons between the family and environmental, community, and specialty health care resources.

▓▓ COMMON ENVIRONMENTAL AGENTS AND ADVERSE EFFECTS

Growth and development of children, especially cognitive and behavioral, can be significantly limited by environmental agents. This section presents a brief discussion of general pediatric poisoning and some common environmental agents that are particularly hazardous to children.

General Pediatric Poisoning

Description

Poisoning is the process in which a substance that interferes with the body's normal function is taken in by ingestion, inhalation, absorption, or injection. Medications, plants, and chemicals are common sources of poisoning in the pediatric population.

Etiology and Incidence

Poisoning is the leading cause of injury and the fourth leading cause of death in toddlers and preschoolers. A majority of calls to poison control centers in the United States concern ingestion of toxic and nontoxic substances by young children. The mouthing behavior of infants and normal curiosity of toddlers and preschoolers puts them at high risk for accidental ingestion of toxic materials. Older children may experiment with drugs and household products with the intent of producing hallucinogenic effects.

Assessment

HISTORY. The following are assessed:

- Type and amount of substance taken in
- Exact time of intake or exposure
- Route or method of intake
- Reaction or signs and symptoms
- Emergency care given
- Child's health status prior to poisoning (e.g., any significant chronic illness? is child taking prescription medication?)

PHYSICAL EXAMINATION. Findings vary greatly depending on the type and amount of poisonous substance, time since exposure, and susceptibility of the child. Reactions can be local or systemic. Questions to consider while conducting the physical examination include the following:

- Which body system or systems does the poison affect?
- What are specific signs of the poison's effect?
- How quickly does the poison have an effect?
- How susceptible is the child?
- What is the child's age and weight?

LABORATORY STUDIES. Analysis of specimens (e.g., emesis) can be helpful in determining the type of poison, if unknown. Serum levels of the poison can be assessed for some toxicants to determine appropriate treatment of the hospitalized child.

Differential Diagnosis

A history of exposure distinguishes poisoning or potential poisoning from acute-onset illness. Since there is not always an obvious epi-

sode of exposure, the NP should be suspicious of poisoning in otherwise well children who experience sudden seizures, GI distress, or cardiorespiratory collapse.

Management

Basic decontamination guidelines are found in Table 42-3. Management approaches for ingested poisons vary with the type of poison, amount of exposure, time lapse since exposure, and susceptibility of the child. Some management principles include the following:

- Initial management focuses on the ABCs—maintain an *a*irway, *b*reathing, and *c*irculation. No matter what poison was taken in, vital body functions must be maintained.

T A B L E 42-3
Basic Decontamination Protocol

Determine the need for decontamination by calling the poison control center in your area
If clothing has been contaminated, strip the patient and double-bag clothing, then flush the entire body with plain water for 2–5 min. If contaminated with dust, keep clothing dry; remove carefully to minimize dust becoming airborne; if possible, apply dust mask or respirator to patient prior to removing clothing (brush dust from face first)
Chemical contamination:
  Scrub or irrigate open wounds for 5–10 min or longer, using lukewarm water
  Irrigate eyes with sterile saline, balanced salt solution, or Ringer's lactate for at least 15–30 min
  Irrigate face, nose, and ear canals with normal saline, using frequent suction
  Wash appendages (if that is only body part contaminated) without wetting the whole body, if possible
  Clean under nails with scrub brush and nail cleaner
Oily or greasy contamination:
  Cleanse with soap or shampoo, followed by water flushing

Adapted from Oregon Poison Center and Health Division, Oregon Department of Human Resources. Environmental Hazards in Perspective: Seminar Syllabus and Environmental Health Resource Notebook. Portland, Oregon: Oregon Department of Human Resources, 1994.

- Subsequent management involves decreasing the amount of poison in the system (gastric decontamination), counteracting or neutralizing the effects of the poison (administration of antidotes), and providing life-support measures while the body detoxifies itself.
- Gastric decontamination includes use of emesis, lavage, an absorbent agent (e.g., activated charcoal), catharsis, or whole-bowel irrigation (AAP, 1994). Syrup of ipecac is perhaps the best-known product used in gastric decontamination. An emetic, it causes approximately three episodes of vomiting in most children within an hour of administration. Although it is generally considered safe, adverse effects have been reported, and in some cases, syrup of ipecac is contraindicated (Tables 42-4 and 42-5).

T A B L E 42-4

Syrup of Ipecac: Recommended Dosages*

AGE	DOSE	COMMENTS
Less than 1 y of age	10 ml	Stimulating emesis is not recommended in infants <6 mo In all children <1 y, an emetic should be administered, under supervision, in a health facility
1–12 y	15 ml	Doses up to 30 ml have been found to stimulate more rapid emesis without increased adverse side effects Follow dose with 8 oz of water or clear liquid Can repeat once if no emesis within 30 min
>12 y	30 ml	Follow dose with 8 oz of water or clear liquid Can repeat once if no emesis within 30 min

*See Table 42-5 for contraindications.
Data from American Academy of Pediatrics (AAP): Handbook of Common Poisonings in Children. Elk Grove, IL, American Academy of Pediatrics, 1994.

T A B L E 42-5

Contraindications to Use of Syrup of Ipecac

Ingestion of acids, alkalis, or most hydrocarbons
Ingestion of seizure-inducing drugs or depressants
Ingestion of sharp objects
<6 mo of age
Diminished gag reflex
Altered level of consciousness
Coma

Patient and Parent Education

Prevention is the best management for poisonings. Teach parents how to "poisonproof" their home, pointing out connections between the developmental stages of children and sources of poisoning. Instruct parents to call the poison control center *before instituting treatment* if a child is exposed to a toxic or potentially toxic substance.

Lead Poisoning

Description

Lead poisoning is the presence of serum lead levels that cause toxic effects on multiple organ systems. Lead has an affinity for calcium-binding proteins and may affect any calcium-mediated process. It also affects neurotransmitters and certain enzyme functions. Major toxic effects are caused by disruption of hemoglobin formation and damage to the nervous system, both through direct nerve cell damage and interference with nerve conduction. Over the past 30 years, the definition of the blood lead level considered to be toxic has been revised downward. The current toxic level is 10 µg/dl or more, but even at 10 µg/dl, impairment of cognitive function can occur (Bellinger et al., 1992).

Etiology and Incidence

Although environmental lead sources have decreased in the United States, lead poisoning continues to be a serious environmental health problem for young children. All children are at risk of environmental exposure to lead, although children who are deficient in iron appear to absorb lead more readily, and a disproportionate number of minority, poor, and malnourished children suffer its effects (Lanphear et al., 1998). It is estimated that between 2 and 9% of children aged 1 to 5 in the United States have lead levels above 10 μg/dl (Behrman et al., 1996; Burkhalter & Butler, 1996). Lead enters the body primarily by inhalation (e.g., in dust particles or lead fumes) or ingestion (e.g., a child chewing on an object coated with lead-based paint, or in contaminated food products). A major risk factor includes living in a house containing lead-based paint. Before 1950, much white house paint was 50% lead and 50% linseed oil. The industry began limiting the lead content of paint in 1955, and a 1971 law reduced allowable lead to 1% in 1971 and 0.06% by 1977. Thus, of homes built before 1960, 70% are estimated to have lead paint. Dilapidated housing where paint is peeling or those where renovation with paint removal is occurring present the greatest danger to children. NPs should also keep in mind that in some areas, such as coastal towns, many houses are covered with paint designed for boats or other equipment. This paint may contain lead.

Soil near mines, lead-using industries, and smelters can have high lead levels. Acidic water with low mineral content can leach lead from lead pipes or solder. Hot water may be of more concern than cold. Brass fixtures also contain lead.

Food also can be a source of lead. Lead from soil can contaminate root vegetables, and cans with soldered seams can leach lead into food. Ceramic tableware from some countries contains lead. Some "natural" calcium supplements contain lead.

Some ethnic folk remedies, including *azarcon* and *greta* (Hispanic remedies) and *pay-loo-ah* (used by some Southeast Asians), have a high lead content. Hobbies such as making stained glass objects, using artists' paints, making jewelry or bullets, or gun-cleaning can expose one to lead.

Assessment

SCREENING. Screening for lead poisoning involves two processes: (1) assessing the risk of high-dose exposure through a questionnaire obtainable from the Centers for Disease Control and Prevention (CDC) and (2) blood lead testing. Lead screening is recommended for children at ages 1 and 2, and children 36 to 72 months old who have not previously been screened and who are at risk (CDC, 1997) (Table 42-6). Lead screening questions should be asked at all health supervision visits of children between 6 months and 6 years of age. In addition to the CDC questions, risk assessment questions can include the following:

• Does the child have a parent or guardian with a job or hobby that uses lead?

T A B L E 42-6
Lead Screening Criteria: Risk Assessment

Young children (1–2 y) should be screened with a blood sample if they meet any of the criteria listed below. Children between 3 and 6 y who have not been screened previously and who meet any of the criteria below should be screened at least once. Children in low-risk areas do not need to be screened routinely. Any child exhibiting signs of lead toxicity should be screened. If it is not possible to determine the child's risk, screening should be done.

An answer of "yes" or "don't know" to any of the following questions:

Does your child live in or regularly visit (e.g., a home/day care) a house built before 1950?

Does your child live in or regularly visit a house built before 1978 with recent (within the last 6 mos) or ongoing renovations or remodeling?

Does your child have a sibling or playmate who has or did have lead poisoning?

Is the child receiving public assistance services (e.g., Women, Infants, and Children Program, food stamps, Medicaid)?

Does the child live in a zip code area where ≥ 27% of housing was built before 1950? This information is available from the US Census Bureau, but each state may have a listing as part of their inclusive planning process. Check with your state health department.

Data from Centers for Disease Control and Prevention: Screening Young Children for Lead Poisoning: Guidance for State and Local Public Health Officials. Atlanta, Centers for Disease Control and Prevention, 1997.

- Does the child live near an active lead smelter, battery recycling plant, or other industry likely to release lead?
- Does the family use ceramic pottery for cooking or food storage?
- Does the family use traditional or folk home remedies?
- Does the child demonstrate pica behavior?
- Does the child have a retained lead bullet internally?

Blood lead testing should be done using venous blood rather than a capillary sample, because the latter is less sensitive (Kemper et al., 1998). If the screening blood lead level is 10 μg/dl or greater, rescreening and other management is recommended (Fig. 42-2).

PHYSICAL EXAMINATION. Most lead retained by the body is stored in the bones. Although lead affects almost all organ systems, the nervous system, kidneys, and blood are particularly susceptible. Toxicity is a function of both dose and duration of exposure, but clinical signs of toxicity may not accurately reflect the amount of lead in the body. That is, a child can have high lead levels (e.g., 45 μg/dl) with no obvious clinical signs. Another child may complain of severe GI problems with a lower lead level (e.g., 15 to 20 μg/dl).

Subclinical Effects. In many cases, changes caused by lead toxicity are subtle enough not to be seen as a clinical problem. These include the following:

- Decreased height
- Decreased hearing
- Decreased cognitive functioning that is long term (Baghurst et al., 1992; Bellinger et al., 1992; Rosen, 1992; Needleman et al., 1990)
- Behavior problems (Needleman et al., 1996)

Clinical Effects. Many children do not demonstrate signs of toxicity until late in the disease. At higher levels, lead affects vitamin D metabolism, nerve conduction velocities, and hemoglobin synthesis. Clinical signs and symptoms include the following:

- Anemia
- GI pain, nausea, anorexia, vomiting, and constipation

- Hyperactivity
- Increased intracranial pressure
- Encephalopathy with seizures and coma (usually above 70 to 100 μg/dl)
- Death (can occur above 100 μg/dl)

LABORATORY STUDIES. Evaluate iron deficiency, including serum ferritin or low ratio of serum iron to iron binding capacity.

Differential Diagnosis

GI infections, other causes of anemia, growth retardation, behavior disorders, attention-deficit hyperactivity disorder (ADHD), and central nervous system (CNS) infection are all included in the differential diagnosis.

Management

Management involves treating the child for toxicity, monitoring lead levels, correcting dietary deficiencies (if any), removing the child from the lead source if known, and altering the environment (see Fig. 42-2). Other children in the same household or environment where exposure could have occurred also should be tested and treated as appropriate.

Patient and Parent Education

Education focuses on the areas of management listed above and includes the following:

TREATMENT OF TOXICITY. Inform parents that chelation therapy leads to a rapid fall in blood lead levels, but that most children have a rebound increase within days or weeks of treatment and repeated treatment may be necessary until the lead level is in a safe range.

NUTRITIONAL COUNSELING. Encourage a diet with adequate calcium, iron, zinc, and ascorbate, because deficiencies in these enhance lead absorption, retention, and toxicity.

REMOVING CHILDREN FROM LEAD SOURCE. Prevent children from eating dirt and other foreign substances. During both lead abatement and home renovation, the family should be out of the home until the environment is properly cleaned with household cleaner or lead-specific cleaning product (e.g., Ledisolv).

ENVIRONMENTAL REMEDIATION. Discuss ways to decrease the amount of lead in the child's

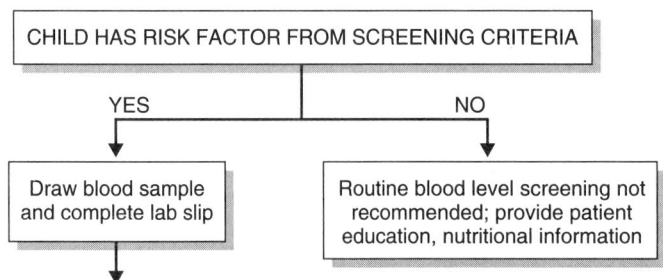

BPb level	Actions to be taken*
<10 µg/dl	Not considered Pb poisoning: • If high risk, retest in 6 mo • If low risk, no further testing needed • Provide parent education, nutritional information

10–14 µg/dl	Border line:
	• Diagnostic venous blood testing in 3 mo, then again in 3 mo
	• If level is 15-19 mg/dl or higher 3 mo apart, retest every 1-2
	   mo until results <15 mg/dl for at least 6 mo, then every 3
	   mo until child is 36 mo old
	• Consult

15–19 µg/dl	• Diagnostic venous blood testing in 3 mo, then again in 2 mo • If levels continue > 15 mg/dl, retest every 1-2 mo until results <15 mg/dl for at least 6 mo, then every 3 mo until child is 36 mo old • Consult

20–44 µg/dl	• Diagnostic venous blood testing shortly (e.g., within 1 wk to 1
	   mo: the higher levels in the shorter time)
	• Full medication evaluation and behavioral history
	• Consult
	• Retest every 1-2 mo until results <15 mg/dl for at least 6
	   mo, then every 3 mo until child is 36 mo old

45–69 µg/dl	• Diagnostic venous blood testing within 24-48 hr • Full medication evaluation and behavioral history • Refer for oral chelation therapy • Retest every 1-2 mo until results <15 mg/dl for at least 6 mo, then every 3 mo until child is 36 mo old
>70 µg/dl	Medical emergency: • Retest immediately with venous blood sample • Conduct immediate medical evaluation • Refer for intravenous chelation • Retest every 1-2 mo until results <15 mg/dl for at least 6 mo, then every 3 mo until child is 36 mo old

*In *all* cases of lead toxicity:**
• Provide parent education, nutritional information
• Remove child from source of lead if known
• Report to Public Health Department
• Initiate environmental investigation
• Encourage lead hazard control/abatement

F I G U R E 42-2
Lead screening protocol flow chart. B = blood; Pb = lead.

environment. Chelation therapy and dietary changes are ineffective unless the child is returned to a clean house.

- Ensure that abatement of lead-based paint is done by trained experts.
- Renovate and remodel older homes carefully, containing and properly disposing of dust and paint particles.
- Control dust and paint chips in older homes. Studies show an average 34% reduction in lead levels in homes cleaned at least every 2 weeks with high-efficiency particulate air (HEPA) filtering vacuum cleaners and household detergent (Rhoads et al., 1999).
  - Block access to areas of the room where large peeling paint areas are found until permanent removal can occur.
  - Cover smaller peeling areas with sticky-backed paper.
  - Damp-mop and dust with cleaners twice weekly to decrease lead dust in the air; do not dry-mop or sweep.
  - Pick up and dispose of paint chips with a disposable rag or paper towel soaked in phosphate cleaner.
- Change work clothes before returning home if working in a lead-related job.
- Avoid using lead around the home for hobbies or other reasons.
- Teach handwashing.
- Use cold tap water for drinking and mixing infant formulas. Water that has been standing in pipes for long periods of time should be flushed for several minutes before using tap water.

Mercury

Description

Mercury, like lead, is a heavy metal commonly found in the environment. It is the second most common cause of heavy metal poisonings. It exists in elemental (liquid or vapor), inorganic mercury salts, and organic forms. The most toxic forms, organic mercury compounds such as methylmercury, result from uptake into the food chain. Mercury has the ability to accumulate in the biological organism, so food products, especially fish, concentrate large amounts

of the metal. CNS tissue is the main target organ for mercury in humans; once absorbed into the brain, mercury metabolizes to its inorganic form and cannot cross the blood-brain barrier to exit the brain. Significant neurological symptoms result from mercury poisoning. The kidney is the other major target organ, especially for inorganic mercury poisoning. The fetus and child are more susceptible to mercury toxicity than others.

Etiology and Incidence

Food products, particularly contaminated fish, grains, and flour, have been a source of poisoning in humans (Eyl, 1971). Until 1991, mercury was added to 30% of latex paints. Button batteries contain mercury and are toxic if swallowed. Elemental mercury is used in thermometers and thermostats. It also is used in some Carribean-based religious practices. A capsule of *Azogue* is carried by a family member or may be sprinkled around the house as a blessing where it poses a hazard to crawling infants. The volatile metal form of mercury is absorbed through the lungs after being inhaled as a vapor. It is poorly absorbed if swallowed, and its use as dental amalgam is not considered a health risk. Once in the body, it crosses the placenta and the blood-brain barrier.

Inorganic and organic forms of mercury are also readily absorbed through inhalation. Inorganic mercury, found in some fungicides, antiseptics, and medications, is poorly absorbed, usually by the gut or through the skin. It does not cross the placenta or enter the brain. Organic mercury (e.g., methylmercury) is readily absorbed from the GI tract and through the skin. Organic mercury easily enters the brain, crosses the placenta, and has been found in breast milk. Offspring of pregnant females who ingested methylmercury have been affected by severe, irreversible central and peripheral neurological conditions (Minamata disease).

Assessment

HISTORY. A thorough history is essential to identify the source of exposure because the signs and symptoms of neurological disorders can be very confusing. Questions focus on workplace environment, diet, and whether others in the family are experiencing similar symptoms.

PHYSICAL EXAMINATION. The physical examination reveals primarily neurological involvement, although the form of mercury intoxication affects the symptoms seen. Neurological findings include the following:

- Irritability
- Numbness of extremities
- Tremors
- Ataxia
- Memory loss
- Vision or hearing loss
- Weakness or paralysis
- Seizures
- Coma
- Death

Acute mercury poisoning from mercuric salts causes extremely corrosive GI bleeding with necrosis. Renal necrosis and failure occurs within 24 hours. Rapid appearance of symptoms, including the following is characteristic:

- Metallic taste in the mouth
- Thirst
- Nausea and vomiting
- Bloody diarrhea
- Abdominal pain
- Renal failure

Mercurous salts, elemental mercury, and phenyl mercury can cause *acrodynia*, with symptoms including erythema of palms and soles, irritability, edema, hyperkeratosis, vasodilation, fever, and splenomegaly. Other symptoms may also be experienced, including painful extremities; a scaly, pink rash; constant pruritus; photophobia; and hypotonia.

Inhaled mercury produces corrosive bronchitis and interstitial pneumonitis with CNS effects and other symptoms.

Children born to women with high mercury levels may have birth defects such as cerebral palsy, mental retardation, weakness, seizures, vision loss, and delayed development.

LABORATORY STUDIES. Blood mercury levels can be used to determine acute mercury exposure, but the blood half-life is short. Mercury is excreted in the urine; a 24-hour urine sample in an acid-washed container gives the optimal sample but a first-morning void may give good information. Chronic mercury intoxication is estimated by measuring the mercury levels in long strands of hair (Behrman et al., 1996).

Differential Diagnosis

The differential diagnosis includes other poisonings, infections of the CNS, and CNS conditions.

Management

Patients should be referred to a center for management. Chelation is the treatment of choice and needs to be conducted at a center where supportive therapy can stabilize the patient during the procedure. Gastric lavage may remove ingested inorganic mercury.

Stopping exposure is essential. Mercury decontamination of the environment is important. Vacuuming may increase the mercury in the air.

Parent Education

Children have been known to innocently play with mercury (CDC, 1995). Parents need to be reminded of the serious effect of mercury and encouraged to keep glass thermometers, electrical wires, paints, or other materials with mercury out of children's reach. Recommendations from local health departments regarding ingestion of locally caught fish from polluted streams and ponds must be heeded.

Air Pollution: Indoor and Outdoor

Air quality is an important environmental factor in childhood illness, especially respiratory conditions (Mortimer & Etzel, 1999). Since the 1970s, outdoor air quality has improved in many areas as a result of local, state, and federal regulations, but outdoor air pollution continues to contribute significantly to adverse health effects. In particular, individuals are affected by carbon monoxide, sulfur oxides, hydrocarbons, ozone, particulate matter, and nitrogen oxides. Indoor air quality has declined in the same time period. This is largely attributed to an increase in the use of carpets, wood stove heating, and synthetic and chemically formulated building materials (e.g., pressed wood made with formaldehyde) coupled with more "energy-conserving" construction that makes new homes more "airtight" and reduces ventilation. Since up to 90% of an individual's time is spent indoors, exposure to airborne toxicants has increased markedly.

As discussed earlier, children are especially susceptible to air quality, because they are experiencing rapid lung development; have smaller, narrower airways; breathe more rapidly; are more physically active than adults; spend more time on the floor; and, especially very young children, spend more time indoors. This section discusses several of the more common indoor and outdoor airborne toxicants that influence children's health status: environmental tobacco smoke (ETS), radon, asbestos, molds, and particulate matter.

ENVIRONMENTAL TOBACCO SMOKE (ETS)

Description

Children, especially very young children, are exposed to tobacco smoke primarily through cigarettes, cigars, or pipes used by parents, other family members, or visitors in the home. Day care providers or teachers also may smoke. The child's ambient air can be contaminated heavily with tobacco smoke in two ways: sidestream smoke coming directly from the tobacco product, or secondhand smoke exhaled by the smoker. Children inhaling sidestream smoke are essentially smoking the unfiltered tobacco product themselves. Children and adolescents also can be smokers themselves, actively inhaling tobacco smoke as well as exposing siblings to ambient smoke.

ETS has been associated with chronic and acute respiratory symptoms, middle ear effusions, bronchitis, pneumonia, sudden infant death syndrome (SIDS), and asthma (Strachan & Cook, 1998). A recent meta-analysis noted that the child of a parent who smokes is at approximately twice the risk of having a serious lower respiratory tract infection in infancy or early childhood than the child of a nonsmoker (Li et al., 1999). Otitis media risks are higher when the child lives in an ETS environment (Ilicali et al., 1999). Other associated conditions include low birth weight and cardiac problems. Pubertal children with a history of long-term exposure to passive cigarette smoke, especially white males, are at increased risk of premature coronary artery disease (Moskowitz et al., 1999), and there is evidence that secondhand smoke may even be associated with Legg-Perthes disease (Glueck et al., 1998) and appendicitis (Montgomery et al., 1999).

Etiology and Incidence

More than 10 million children younger than age 6 are exposed to ETS (American Cancer Society, 1996). There are an estimated 150,000 to 300,000 infections in children younger than age 18 months who are secondhand smokers, leading to thousands of hospitalizations annually. Passive smoking is a result of parents or caregivers smoking in the child's environment.

An estimated 3000 adolescents begin smoking each day, increasing their risk of immediate and long-term health problems. Initiation of active smoking is related to gender (male), race (white), socioeconomic status (low income status), and having a parent, sibling, or friends who smoke (O'Loughlin et al., 1998; Harrell et al., 1998). In addition, tobacco marketing directed toward adolescents is associated with young people's susceptibility to smoke (Feighery et al., 1998).

Assessment

Assessment of the extent to which ETS affects the child's health depends on taking a thorough and accurate history. The physical problems with which children present vary, and the NP should suspect tobacco smoke as a factor in children who have recurrent respiratory and ear infections and delayed or slow growth patterns.

HISTORY. Collect data about the following:

- The amount of smoke in the child's environment, both in the home and in other locations (e.g., day care, school, home of relatives or friends): How many people smoke, and how much do they smoke? Does the child smoke?

- The amount of time the child spends in these environments: How long is the child exposed to ETS? Is the child ever in a car with a smoker?
- Any symptoms related to ETS: Has the child experienced health problems that may be associated with ETS? Cough, colds, ear infections, etc.?

Self-reported information collected over time can give an accurate measure of smoking in the home (Glasgow et al., 1998).

PHYSICAL EXAMINATION AND LABORATORY STUDIES. These will be specific to the physical signs and symptoms of the child.

Management

The best treatment for adverse affects of ETS is prevention; every effort should be made to ensure that the child's environment is smoke-free. Parents, siblings, or others working with the child should be encouraged to stop smoking. In the interim, smoking outside the home and using adequate ventilation is essential. Alternative day care arrangements should be explored if there is smoking at the child's care center. Nonsmoking children should be praised for their decision to not smoke and informed about the dangers associated with smoking. Children who are smokers should be encouraged and supported in their efforts to quit.

Smoking cessation is a difficult process and dependent on a number of biological, behavioral, and psychosocial factors. In one study, although more than 84% of adolescents had thought seriously about quitting and about 55% had tried to stop in the 6 months before the study survey, only about 15% were able to say they had quit, based on a criterion of "not smoking for the past 30 days" (Zhu et al., 1999). Predictors for success in quitting included (1) being an "occasional" smoker; (2) never having quit or having quit for 14 or more days previously; (3) making a self-prediction that he or she would not be smoking in 1 year; (4) having lower depression scores; and (5) having a mother who does not smoke.

Patient and Parent Education

Parents must stop smoking if the child is to have a smoke-free environment. Additionally, parental smoking cessation is a significant variable in keeping children from starting and helping adolescents to quit smoking (Farkas et al., 1999). In the general population, many providers ask their patients about smoking and encourage them to stop, but do not provide support and follow-up intervention (Goldstein et al., 1998). Pediatric providers can use the US Agency for Health Care Policy and Research guidelines to structure their smoking cessation counseling (AHCPR, 1996). These include the following:

- Systematically identify tobacco users and document their status
- Strongly urge all smokers to quit
- Identify smokers willing to make an attempt to quit
- Aid the patient in quitting by offering a plan, providing education and support with nicotine replacement therapy as needed, or referring to a smoking cessation program in the community
- Schedule follow-up contact

RADON

Description

Radon is a colorless, odorless radioactive gas that enters homes through soil (e.g., basement floors, cracks in concrete foundations, sumps, or drains) and concentrates in basements and low areas. As radon decays, some of its products change to an isotope of polonium which, when inhaled, can cause lung damage leading to cancer. In the atmosphere, radon is diluted and has no health effect. When concentrated in an enclosed area, it may represent a risk. Tobacco smoke provides a vehicle for radon to enter the lungs, adding to the risk of radon-induced cancer for smokers and individuals exposed to ETS. Water that has been filtered through the soil can contain radon (e.g., well water), and about 2 to 5% of radon in homes is found in the water supply. Radon in water has been associated with a slightly increased incidence of gastric cancer and leukemia. The EPA does not yet have standards for safe radon levels in water.

Etiology and Incidence

About 7000 to 30,000 lung cancer deaths are attributed to radon each year (EPA, 1994), though recent research in Finland investigated the relationship between indoor radon exposure and lung cancer, and concluded that the risk of residential radon exposure may be low (Weinmann, 1996; Auvinen et al., 1996). Radon is more prevalent in certain geographical areas. Local health departments can be consulted to determine if radon is a local health risk. Parents need information on testing, which can be found in the *Children's Environmental Health Network Resource Guide* (see Resource Box).

Assessment

In 1988, the Surgeon General recommended that all homes, except residences above the second floor in multilevel buildings, be tested for radon. Radon detector kits can be purchased in hardware, grocery, or department stores. Measurements are taken and the device is returned to the manufacturer for analysis. Short-term (2-7 days) or long term (3-12 months) testing can be done. The long-term testing gives a more accurate measure of the average radon exposure, because levels fluctuate over time and with changes in seasons. The EPA recommends using the short-term test and suggests the following actions based on findings:

- For levels of 4 to 20 pCi/l, conduct radon remediation within 1 to 2 years
- For levels of 20 to 200 pCi/l, conduct radon remediation within several months
- For levels greater than 200 pCi/l, conduct radon remediation within several weeks

Management

Radon remediation involves decreasing the amount of radon entering the home (e.g., by sealing cracks in home foundations, covering dirt crawl spaces with impermeable plastic, laying concrete floors, and covering drains) and removing radon that is present (e.g., providing adequate ventilation from the basement to outdoors). Children should not spend significant time in high-risk areas of the home.

Airborne Contaminants

PARTICULATE MATTER

Description

Particulate matter (PM) is one of a cluster of indoor and outdoor air pollutants that has an adverse effect on respiratory and cardiovascular function. Other outdoor air pollutants include ozone, sulfur dioxide (SO_2), nitrogen oxides (NO and NO_2), and carbon monoxide (CO). The diameter of PM is measured in microns, and standards have been set for concentrations of PM_{10} and $PM_{2.5}$, matter 10 μm and 2.5 μm in diameter. Smaller particles are of growing concern because they can be inhaled and carried deep into lung tissue. Larger particles can be filtered by the nasal mucosa or trachea and removed by coughing or sneezing.

Exposure to PM creates an inflammatory response in the body and, especially in combination with other pollutants, is associated with increased mortality, and hospitalizations for respiratory or cardiovascular problems (Burnett et al., 1997). Respiratory infections, wheezing, and decreased lung function are increased with exposure to PM (Peters et al., 1999; Brunekreef & Hoek, 1993), but a clear association between asthma and outdoor PM has not been established (Nicolai, 1999).

Etiology and Incidence

PM is a byproduct of industrial production, gasoline and diesel engines, wood-burning stoves, and natural phenomena such as volcanic activity, grass and forest fires, and blowing dust. Residents of urban and industrial areas are exposed to high levels of PM, and concentrations increase in summer months and when there is more combustion present (e.g., rush-hour traffic). Natural phenomena contribute to airborne PM in rural areas. Ozone has been associated with asthma exacerbations, increased cough, increased school absenteeism, and decreased lung function. NO_2 is associated with increased respiratory symptoms and decreased lung function. CO decreases transport of oxygen to the heart, brain, and fetus.

Indoor PM, including house dust, mites, cockroach particles, and animal dander, have all been implicated in asthma in children.

Assessment

Parents can keep a record of their child's illness episodes to determine if increased air pollution is associated with illness.

Management and Parent Education

Protecting the child from air particulates should decrease clinical signs and symptoms.

- When outdoor air quality is poor, children should not actively play outdoors
- HEPA air conditioning in the home can reduce airborne PM
- The heating source for the home may contribute to particulate concentrations in the home and may need to be modified
- Covering mattresses, washing bedding, eliminating stuffed animals, and controlling humidity (keep it low to decrease molds) all decrease indoor PM contamination
- Parents of children with chronic respiratory conditions should be educated about how to prevent exposure, and how to manage acute exacerbations caused by exposure to air pollution

ASBESTOS

Description

Asbestos is the name given to a group of incombustible fibrous magnesium silicate minerals used most often in construction materials. Some asbestos products are banned by the EPA; most are found in older buildings. Insulation, ceiling and floor tiles, and shingles are common asbestos-containing materials. Asbestos dust in high concentrations can cause lung irritation, and repeated inhalation of the fibers is associated with lung disease later in life. There may be a latency period of 20 years or more before conditions such as pleural effusion, lung fibrosis, and mesothelial tumors of the pleura or peritoneum appear.

Contamination by asbestos is measured in fibers per cubic centimeter of air. The Occupational Safety and Health Administration (OSHA) workplace standard is two fibers per cubic centimeter. Levels in schools may range from 0.05 to 0.2 fibers per cubic centimeter (AAP, 1994), placing schoolchildren at relatively low risk.

Etiology and Incidence

Asbestosis is considered an occupational problem of adults, and smokers are at higher risk of asbestos-induced lung cancer than non-smokers. Childhood exposure to asbestos, however, may contribute to serious illness as an adult. Children can be exposed through direct contact with air in a contaminated building or with material or clothing parents bring home from their work site. An estimated 10,000 schools built between 1946 and 1973 may contain asbestos (AAP, 1994), although it is only considered a hazard if the material is disrupted.

It is virtually impossible to determine the exact health risk of inhaled fibers, how fibers cause disease, and what other factors may be necessary for a disease process to occur (Vu & Lai, 1997).

Assessment

Assessment of disease is based on a history of exposure and signs and symptoms of respiratory distress, including cough, dyspnea, fatigue, and chest pain. Clinical signs are usually found in adults.

Management and Parent Education

Preventing unnecessary exposure to asbestos fibers reduces the risk of inhalation and subsequent disease. If building materials that contain asbestos (e.g., insulation) are in good repair, it is advisable to leave them in place rather than go through the process of removal, which involves releasing fibers into the air. Renovation of older buildings, where contact with asbestos is more likely to occur, requires control measures to minimize the spread of fibers. If parents' work sites expose them to asbestos, help develop a plan to minimize the possibility of bringing fibers into the home. Parents should be informed of the adverse effects of contact with asbestos and reassured that their children are at low risk for exposure unless they spend significant time in older buildings that are in poor repair or undergoing renovation.

MOLDS

Description

Molds are microscopic organisms in the class of bioaerosols, living organisms that release elements into the air. These elements are then inhaled or come into contact with skin or mucous membranes. Mold spores are thought to cause allergic reactions, and certain fungi can release mycotoxins that elicit irritant and toxic responses (Mortimer & Etzel, 1999). Molds thrive in damp spaces, but spores can be found in dust, dry leaves, and storage areas. Common sources of molds are flooding, backed-up sewers, leaky roofs, humidifiers, mud or ice dams, damp basements, constant plumbing leaks, house plants, steam from cooking, shower or bath steam, and wet clothes hanging on indoor clotheslines.

Etiology and Incidence

Research on the health effects of molds and the number of people affected is limited, but children appear to have an increased risk of cough and wheezing when exposed to damp and mold in the home (Peat et al., 1998).

Assessment

Assess allergic reaction, including:

- Respiratory involvement (wheezing, shortness of breath)
- Cough
- Sinus congestion
- Watery, itchy, light-sensitive eyes
- Sore throat
- Skin rash
- Headaches, memory loss, mood changes
- Aches and pains
- Fever

Assessment questions also are directed at finding the cause of the symptoms: Is there a pattern to the symptoms? Are they aggravated by any particular environment? Are they relieved when the child changes environments?

Differential Diagnosis

The differential diagnosis includes other causes of allergic reactions and upper respiratory infections. Reaction to molds can be confused with pesticide poisoning.

Management

Treatment involves control of allergic symptoms (e.g., antihistamines to control itching or sneezing), but removal of the cause of the problem is more beneficial. Ultimately, the source of moisture must be removed. Refer to other chapters in this book for discussion of allergies and their management.

Maintaining a dry, clean environment minimizes the growth of molds. Parents should identify and eliminate the source of any moisture where mold can grow (e.g., leaks around windows); clean, disinfect, and dry the moldy area; and discard moldy materials. Use soap, detergent, or a commercial cleaner in hot water; disinfect with bleach solution, and rinse well, allowing disinfected areas to dry naturally overnight (California Department of Health Services, Indoor Air Quality Section, 1998). Remember that spores are easily released when moldy material is dried out. Ozone air cleaners are not effective.

Patient and Parent Education

Provide information regarding the connection between exposure to molds and allergic reactions. Parents may need support during cleanup, because it may be difficult or nearly impossible to do a thorough job (e.g., mold may have permeated the walls in a rental unit and the family is not able to have them replaced or to move to a more suitable apartment).

Pesticides

Description

Pesticides are chemicals used to kill or control unwanted pests. They include herbicides, fungicides, insecticides, and other products, and are classified as "general use" or "restricted use," depending on the toxicity to humans or the environment. Restricted-use pesticides require special handling by certified applicators. Labeling of pesticides varies by toxicity, with a skull and crossbones and the statement "DANGER—POISON" on the most toxic; "WARNING" on less toxic; and "CAUTION" on the labels of the least toxic pesticides. All pesticides are hazardous. Adverse effects of pesticide exposure can be acute or chronic. All body systems can be affected, depending on the nature of the toxin and the extent of exposure. Much data about pesticide poisoning are based on studies in adults, and there is concern that the immediate effect of pesticides on children and the risk children face for long-term health problems is seriously underestimated (Tilson, 1998). Research has shown that pesticides in children can:

- Have an immediate, life-threatening poisoning effect
- Have neurotoxic effects
- Increase the risk of childhood cancer (Daniels et al., 1997) or cancer later in life
- Disrupt endocrine function with potential long-term effects
- Contribute to immune dysfunction
- Increase the risk of developmental delays

An important study by Guillette and associates (1998) demonstrated significant developmental differences in native Yaqui children from Mexico exposed to pesticides vs. a cohort not exposed. Prenatal exposure to pesticides can affect children as well. In a Southern California study, pesticide exposure, specifically maternal use of flea or tick products during pregnancy, significantly increased the risk of brain tumors in children (Pogoda & Preston-Martin, 1997). However, research data remain mixed as to the cause-and-effect relationship between pesticides and health problems; other studies, for example, show little effect of maternal prenatal pesticide exposure and birth defects (Shaw et al., 1999). Clearly, more research in the pediatric population is necessary.

Etiology and Incidence

There are over 17,000 registered pesticide products in the United States, with over 800 related active ingredients. An estimated 950 million pounds are used annually in the agricultural industry, introducing pesticides into the food chain. Another 294 million pounds are used in urban areas (EPA, 1997).

Food products are a major source of exposure. Because of their small size and large intake (per body weight) of fruits and vegetables, children ingest pesticides in foods at a dispropor-

tionate rate. It is estimated that by the age of 6 years, the average American child has accumulated 35% of the lifetime allowance of captan, a fungicide used extensively on fruit and a probable human carcinogen (Wiles, 1993). Pesticides in water and household products are other sources of exposure.

Migrant farmworkers and children who live on farms may be exposed to agricultural pesticides. Garden and lawn use increases risks to children playing outdoors in these areas.

Assessment

When treating an individual who may have been exposed to pesticides, health care providers have access by law to information about the pesticides that have been used (see Resource Box). The EPA's Worker Protection Standard (WPS) allows access to information on general and restricted-use pesticides. This should be available through employers.

Management

Specifics of management depend on the type and amount of pesticide taken in and the route of absorption. Information on treatment is available on product labels. This can be obtained from employers, manufacturers, or by having the patient provide the pesticide label.

- ABCs
  - Maintain gas exchange; may need to intubate
  - Prevent aspiration of vomitus
- Consult with a poison control center for direction in management. Refer to a center or provider with expertise in this area as soon as possible
- Decontamination
  - Gastric lavage
  - Emesis (syrup of ipecac; see Tables 42–4 and 42–5)
  - Charcoal
  - Cleansing of skin, eyes, nose, ears, mucous membranes
- Seizure control
- Report pesticide exposure to the state health department

- Work with parents, schools, and community agencies to prevent pesticide exposure

The risks pesticides present to children are immense. Pesticide exposure occurs in a number of ways and is additive. Regulating the amount of pesticide children take in from any one source (e.g., food products) is good, but the pattern of multiple contamination must be recognized and a plan to regulate overall exposure developed.

Parent Education

Education of parents is the key to prevention of pesticide poisoning in children. NPs should focus on helping parents:

- Use as few pesticides as possible in the home; explore nonchemical options to pest control.
- Follow directions for use and storage when pesticides are used.
- Use only the amount recommended.
- Use only for purpose intended.
- Protect skin and clothing when using pesticides; wash thoroughly if a spill occurs.
- Do not inhale pesticides.
- Do not spray on a windy day.
- Do not mix pesticides.
- Store the product in its original container.
- Wash hands and clothes (separately from regular laundry) after use.
- Keep pesticides away from food and dishes.
- Keep children and pets away from pesticides or areas to which pesticides have been applied; emphasize the importance of "pesticide-proofing" the home.
- Dispose of pesticides at a registered disposal site; check with county or metropolitan area recycling or waste control centers.
- Keep a copy of the pesticide label handy for reference if needed.
- Minimize pesticides in the foods children eat.
  - Vary the kinds of fruits and vegetables your child eats.
  - Buy products that are organically grown, or from suppliers who use few pesticides.
  - Grow your own fruits and vegetables if possible; join a community garden.
  - Wash and peel fruits and vegetables, but understand that many pesticides are found in the food itself, so washing does not remove them.

Polychlorinated Biphenyls

Description

PCBs are one type of extremely stable organochlorines. Many organochlorines are carcinogens or endocrine disruptors. PCBs, a family of 209 chemicals, are chemically similar to furans and dioxins. PCBs used commercially are always mixtures of the various types and are frequently contaminated with furans and dioxins. Because of their insulating and nonflammable properties, PCBs have been used in transformers, hydraulic fluids, plasticizers, extenders for pesticides, and in caulking compounds, paints, adhesives, and flame retardants. They have also been used in inks and carbonless paper. PCBs have been banned from production since 1977. However, they are so stable that they are still commonly found in the environment. Low levels are found throughout the world, evaporating and returning to earth by rainfall and settling in dust particles. PCBs are not very water soluble, and as a result are not found in high concentrations in drinking water. They do dissolve readily in oils, thus accumulating in the fatty tissues of fish, birds, and mammals.

PCBs are structurally similar to thyroid hormones. They probably work through changes in hormonal function, altering concentrations of hormones or affecting receptor numbers or affinity. Human exposure comes primarily through ingestion of contaminated foods. Taiwanese children contaminated through PCBs in cooking oil in 1978 and 1979 have been studied longitudinally (Guo et al., 1995).

An array of toxic effects has been documented from many studies, including effects on the human immune system. The developing fetus and the newborn are especially vulnerable to these toxic effects. Prenatal exposure to PCBs has been associated with lower IQ scores in school-age children, as well as adverse effects on neurological and intellectual function in infants and young children (Jacobson & Jacobson, 1996; Longnecker et al., 1997; Patandin, et al., 1998; Guo et al., 1995; Patandin et al., 1999). Growth delays, delayed development, increased behavioral problems, more frequent respiratory infections, and smaller male genitalia are some other findings in PCB-exposed children. Specific "endocrine disruptor" effects have not been clearly linked to humans, but the effects have been found in animal studies.

Etiology and Incidence

The workplace is the greatest source of exposure to PCBs in the United States. In children, probably the fetal and neonatal exposures are most common.

Assessment

SCREENING AND HISTORY
- Exposure history, maternal ingestion of contaminated food
- Skin disorders, including hyperpigmentation, nail changes, and chloracne
- Hepatic dysfunction
- Developmental effects and low birth weight
- Behavioral symptoms (increased frustration levels found in animal models)

PHYSICAL EXAMINATION. Chloracne is the only overt effect of PCB exposure in humans, but its absence does not rule out exposure. Chloracne lesions include cystic forms measuring 1 to 10 mm. Comedones, papules, and cysts

surrounded by edema and erythema, and hyperpigmentation of skin, conjunctiva, gingiva, and nails have been reported in exposed workers.

LABORATORY STUDIES. Increased liver enzymes with severe exposure, although these findings are nonspecific.

Differential Diagnosis

The differential diagnosis includes acne vulgaris, other causes of developmental delay, lead poisoning, or hypothyroidism.

Management

- Stopping the exposure
- Abatement of potential health hazards

Parent Education

Avoid PCB-contaminated food sources, especially prenatally. Breastfeeding should not be stopped, although breast milk contains PCBs. The greater effects occur prenatally.

▒▒▒ GETTING INFORMATION ABOUT TOXICANTS

There are a number of sources about effects of toxicants available to the NP:

- Material safety and data sheets (provided with chemicals)
- Poison control centers
- Association of Occupational and Environmental Clinics (AOECs) and their affiliates

---

R E S O U R C E   B O X   42-1

Agency for Toxic Substances and Disease Registry (ATSDR)
Tel: (404) 639-0700 Website: www.atsdr.cdc.gov

Alliance to End Childhood Lead Poisoning
Tel: (202) 543-1147 Website: www.aeclp.org

American Academy of Pediatrics
Publication: *The Handbook of Environmental Health for Children* (1999)
Website: www.aap.org

American Cancer Society
Tel: (800) 227-2345 Website: www.cancer.org

American Council on Science and Health, Inc.
Tel: (212) 362-7044 Fax: (212) 362-4919 Website: www.acsh.org

American Lung Association
Tel: (202) 785-3355 or Tel: (800) LUNG USA (586-4872) Website: www.lungusa.org

RESOURCE BOX 42-1 *Continued*

American Public Health Association
202-777-2742 Website: www.apha.org

Association of Occupational and Environmental Clinics (AOEC) Katherine H. Kirkland, MPH
Website: www.occ-env-med.mc.duke.edu/oem/aoec.htm/
Clinic referrals, educational programs for professionals, pediatric environmental health specialty units, library, clinics

Centers for Disease Control and Prevention (CDC) National Center for Environmental Health
(770)-488-7030 Website: www.cdc.gov/nceh

Children's Environmental Health Network
510-597-1393 or FAX 510-597-1399 Website: www.cehn.org
Manual available: *Resource Guide on Children's Environmental Health* provides network linking agencies, organizations, and individuals; education, research, policy goals.

Consumer Product Safety Commission Office of Information
301-504-0000 or 800-638-2772 Website: www.cpsc.gov

Environmental Defense Fund
800-684-3322 Website: www.edf.org

Environmental Protection Agency (EPA)
The EPA has a wide range of information on specific toxicants. The EPA compiles information under the 1986 Emergency Planning and Community Right-to-Know Act (EPCRA) and provides that information to the public via a database called the Toxic Release Inventory (TRI).
Website: (www.epa.gov)

EPA Indoor Air Quality Information Clearinghouse (IAQ INFO)
800-438-4318 Website: www.epa.gov/iaq/ets.html

EPA Office of Pesticide Programs
703-305-5017 Website: www.epa.gov/pesticides/

EPA Pesticides Manual: Reigart JR, Roberts JR: *Recognition and Management of Pesticide Poisonings*, (5th ed.). Washington, DC, Environmental Protection Agency, 1999.

EPA Worker Protection Standard
Website: http://www.epa.gov/oppfead1/work_saf/PART170.htm#170.160

Food and Drug Administration Consumer Affairs
888-463-6332 Website: www.fda.gov/

Indoor Air Diagnostics, Inc.
408-954-9008

International Poison Center
202-588-0620 Website: www.prosarcorp.com/ipc

Latex Allergies
Website: www.latexallergyhelp.com

National Academy of Science
202-334-2000 Website: www.nas.edu

National Coalition Against the Misuse of Pesticides
202-543-5450 Website: www.ncamp.org

National Environmental Health Association
303-756-9090 Website: www.neha.org

National Institute of Environmental Health Science
919-541-3345 Website: www.niehs.gov

National Institute of Occupational Safety and Health
404-639-3691 Website: www.cdc.gov/niosh

National Lead Information Center
800-LEAD-FYI

National Pesticide Telecommunications Network Agricultural Chemistry Extension, Oregon State University
800-858-7378 Website: www.ace.orst.edu/info/nptn/

Natural Resources Defense Council
415-777-0220 Website: www.nrdc.org

National Service Center for Environmental Publications (NCEPI)
800-490-9198
Website: www.epa.gov/ncepihom/

Occupational Safety and Health Administration Department of Labor Office of Occupational Medicine
202-219-8021 Website: www.osha.gov

Safe Drinking Water Hotline (EPA)
800-426-4791

Scorecard
Website: www.scorecard.org
Provides information about major pollutants for all zip codes in the United States

USDA Pesticide Recordkeeping Program Agricultural Marketing Service
703-330-7826 Website: www.ams.usda.gov/sciene/sdpr.htm

US Department of Housing and Urban Development Office of the Secretary
202-708-0417
Website: www.hud.gov

University programs in occupational health industrial hygiene, or toxicology: call your local university health sciences department or school of public health for information.

- Clinical toxicologists at major hospitals
- Internet sources such as National Library of Medicine's on-line database and other sources
- Manufacturers

REPORTING REQUIREMENTS

Poisoning is reportable in most states. Check with the county health department and the county agricultural commissioner. Occupational exposures are reportable for compensation.

REFERENCES

American Academy of Pediatrics (AAP): Handbook of Common Poisonings in Children. Elk Grove, IL, American Academy of Pediatrics, 1994.

American Cancer Society: Environmental Cancer Risks. *In* Cancer Facts and Figures. Atlanta, 1996.

Auvinen A, Makelainen I, Hakama M, et al: Indoor radon exposure and risk of lung cancer: A nested case-control study in Finland. J Natl Cancer Inst 88: 966-972, 1996.

Baghurst P, McMichael A, Wigg N, et al: Environmental exposure to lead and children's intelligence at the age of seven years: The Port Pirie cohort study. N Engl J Med 327:1279-1284, 1992.

Bearer CF: Biomarkers in pediatric environmental health: A cross-cutting issue. Environ Health Perspect 106(suppl 3):813-816, 1998.

Bearer CF, Phillips R: Pediatric environmental health training. Am J Dis Child 147: 682-684, 1993.

Behrman R, Kliegman R, Arvin A (eds): Nelson Textbook of Pediatrics, 15th ed., Philadelphia, WB Saunders, 1996.

Bellinger D, Stiles K, Needleman H: Low-level lead exposure, intelligence, and academic achievement: A long-term follow-up study. Pediatrics 90:855-861, 1992.

Brunekreef B, Hoek G: The relationship between low-level air pollution exposure and short-term changes in lung function in Dutch children. J Expo Anal Environ Epidemiol 3(suppl 1):117-128, 1993.

Burkhalter E, Butler W: The Department of Defense blood lead level survey program for young children. Mil Med 161:687-690, 1996.

Burnett RT, Cakmak S, Brook JR, et al: The role of particulate size and chemistry in the association between summertime ambient air pollution and hospitalization for cardiorespiratory diseases. Environ Health Perspect 105:614-620, 1997.

California Department of Health Services. Indoor Air Quality Section: Mold in My Home: What Do I Do? Berkeley, California Department of Health Services, 1998.

Carroquino MJ, Galson SK, Licht J, et al: The U.S. EPA Conference on Preventable Causes of Cancer in Children: A research agenda. Environ Health Perspect 106(suppl 3):867-873, 1998.

Centers for Disease Control and Prevention (CDC): Mercury exposure in a residential community—Florida, 1994. MMWR 44: 436-437, 443, 1995.

Centers for Disease Control and Prevention (CDC): Screening Young Children for Lead Poisoning: Guidance for State and Local Public Health Officials. Atlanta, Centers for Disease Control and Prevention, 1997.

Chaudhuri N: Child health, poverty and the environment: The Canadian context. Can J Public Health 89(suppl 1):S26-30, S28-33, 1998.

Daniels JL, Olshan AF, Savitz DA: Pesticides and childhood cancers. Environ Health Perspect 105: 1068-1077, 1997.

Environmental Protection Agency (EPA). Radon-induced lung cancer. Washington, DC, Environmental Protection Agency 1994.

Environmental Protection Agency. (EPA): Pesticides Industry Sales and Usage: 1994 and 1995 Market Estimates. Washington, DC, Office of Pesticides, Prevention, and Toxic Substances, Environmental Protection Agency, #735-R-97-002, 12-13, 1997.

Eyl TB: Organic-mercury food poisoning. N Engl J Med 284:1137-1139, 1971.

Farkas AJ, Distefan JM, Choi WS, et al: Does parental smoking cessation discourage adolescent smoking? Prev Med 28:213-218, 1999.

Feighery E, Borzekowski DL, Schooler C, et al: Seeing, wanting, owning: The relationship between receptivity to tobacco marketing and smoking susceptibility in young people. Tobacco Control 7:123-128, 1998.

Glasgow RE, Foster LS, Lee ME, et al: Developing a brief measure of smoking in the home: Description and preliminary evaluation. Addict Behav 23:567-571, 1998.

Glueck CJ, Freiberg RA, Crawford A, et al: Secondhand smoke, hypofibrinolysis, and Legg-Perthes disease. Clin Orthop 352:159-167, 1998.

Goldstein MG, DePue JD, Monroe AD, et al: A population-based survey of physician smoking cessation counseling practices. Prev Med 27:720-729, 1998.

Guillette E, Meza M, Aquilar M, et al: An anthropological approach to the evaluation of preschool children exposed to pesticides in Mexico. Environ Health Perspect 106:347-353, 1998.

Guo YL, Lambert GH, Hsu CC: Growth abnormalities in the population exposed in utero and early postnatally to polychlorinated biphenyls and dibenzofurans. Environ Health Perspect 103(suppl 6):117-122, 1995.

Harrell JS, Bandiwala SI, Deng S, et al: Smoking initiation in youth: The roles of gender, race, socioeconomics, and developmental status. J of Adolesc Health 23:271-279, 1998.

Ilicali OC, Keles N, Deger K, et al: Relationship of passive cigarette smoking to otitis media. Arch Otolaryngol Head Neck Surg 125:758-762, 1999.

Jacobson J, Jacobson S: Intellectual impairment in children exposed to polychlorinated biphenyls in utero. N Engl J Med 335:783-789, 1996.

Kemper AR, Bordley WC, Downs SM: Cost-effectiveness analysis of lead poisoning screening strategies following the 1997 guidelines of the Centers for Disease Control and Prevention. Arch Pediatr Adolesc Med 152: 1202-1208, 1998.

Landrigan PJ: Environmental hazards for children in USA. Int J Occup Med Environ Health 11:189-194, 1998.

Landrigan PJ, Carlson JE, Bearer CF, et al: Children's health and the environment: A new agenda for prevention research. Environ Health Perspect 106(suppl 3):787-794, 1998.

Lanphear BP, Byrd RS, Auinger P, et al: Community characteristics associated with elevated blood lead levels in children. Pediatrics 101:264-271, 1998.

Li JS, Peat JK, Xuan W, et al: Meta-analysis on the association between environmental tobacco smoke (ETS) exposure and the prevalence of lower respiratory tract infection in early childhood. Pediatr Pulmonol 27:5-13, 1999.

Longnecker M, Rogan W, Lucier G: The human health effects of DDT and PCBs and an overview of organochlorines in public health. Annu Rev Public Health 18:211-244, 1997.

Montgomery SM, Pounder RE, Wakefield AJ: Smoking in adults and passive smoking in children are associated with acute appendicitis [letter; comment]. Lancet 353:379, 1999.

Mortimer KM, Etzel RA: Air pollution. *In* Training Manual on Pediatric Environmental Health: Putting it Into Practice. Emeryville, CA: Children's Environmental Health Network/Public Health Institute, 1999.

Moskowitz WB, Schwartz PF, Schieken RM: Childhood passive smoking, race, and coronary artery disease risk: The MCV Twin Study. Arch Pediat Adolesc Med 153:446-453, 1999.

National Center for Environmental Health: The Children's Environmental Health Report Card. Atlanta, Centers for Disease Control and Prevention, 1999.

National Institute of Environmental Health Science: A research-oriented framework for risk assessment and prevention of children's exposure to environmental toxicants. Environ Health Perspect 107:510, 1999.

Needleman HL, Riess JA, Tobin MJ, et al: Bone lead levels and delinquent behavior. JAMA, 275: 363-369, 1996.

Needleman HL, Schell A, Bellinger D, et al: The long-term effects of exposure to low doses of lead in childhood—an 11-year follow-up report. N Engl J Med 322:83-88, 1990.

Nicolai T: Air pollution and respiratory disease in children: What is the clinically relevant impact? Pediatr Pulmonol Suppl 18:9-13, 1999.

O'Loughlin J, Paradis G, Renaud L, et al: One-year predictors of smoking initiation and of continued smoking among elementary schoolchildren in multiethnic, low-income, inner-city neighbourhoods. Tobacco Control 7:268-275, 1998.

Patandin S, Koopman-Esseboom C, de Ridder M, et al: Effects of environmental exposure to polychlorinated biphenyls and dioxins on birth size and postnatal growth. Pediatr Res 44:530-545, 1998.

Patandin S, Lanting C, Mulder P, et al: Effects of environmental exposure to polychlorinated biphenyls and dioxins on cognitive abilities in Dutch children at 42 months of age. J Pediatr 134:33-41, 1999.

Peat JK, Dickerson J, Li J: Effects of damp and mold in the home on respiratory health: A review of the literature. Allergy 53:120-128, 1998.

Peters JM, Avol E, Navidi W, et al: A study of twelve Southern California communities with differing levels and types of air pollution. I. Prevalence of respiratory morbidity. Am J Respir Crit Care Med 159:760-767, 1999.

Pogoda JM, Preston-Martin S: Household pesticides and risk of pediatric brain tumors. Environ Health Perspect 105:1214-1220, 1997.

Rhoads GG, Ettinger AS, Weisel CP, et al: The effect of dust lead control on blood lead in toddlers: A randomized trial. Pediatrics 103:551-555, 1999.

Rosen J: Health effects of lead at low exposure levels: Expert consensus and rationale for lowering the definition of childhood lead poisoning. Am J Dis Child 146:1278-1281, 1992.

Shaw GM, Wasserman CR, O'Malley CD, et al: Maternal pesticide exposure from multiple sources and selected congenital anomalies. Epidemiology 10:60-66, 1999.

Strachan DP, Cook DG: Health effects of passive smoking. 6. Parental smoking and childhood asthma: Longitudinal and case-control studies. Thorax 53:204-212, 1998.

Tilson, HA: Developmental neurotoxicology of endocrine disruptors and pesticides: Identification of information gaps and research needs. Environ Health Perspect 106(suppl 3):807-811, 1998.

US Agency for Health Care Policy and Research. (AHCPR): Clinical practice guidelines for smoking cessation. JAMA 275:1270-1280, 1996.

Vu VT, Lai, DY: Approaches to characterizing human health risks of exposure to fibers. Environ Health Perspect 105(suppl 5):1329-1336, 1997.

Weaver VM, Buckley TJ, Groopman JD: Approaches to environmental exposure assessment in children. Environ Health Perspect 106(suppl 3):827-832, 1998.

Weinmann GG: An update on air pollution. Curr Opin Pulmonary Med 2:121-128, 1996.

Wiles R: Pesticides in children's food. Washington, DC, Environmental Working Group, 1993.

Zahm SH, Ward MH: Pesticides and childhood cancer. Environ Health Perspect 106(suppl 3):893-908, 1998.

Zhu S-H, Sun J, Billings SC, et al: Predictors of smoking cessation in U.S. adolescents. Am J Prev Med 16:202-207, 1999.

CHAPTER **43**

Complementary Medicine

Catherine Blosser

INTRODUCTION

It is estimated that 65 to 80% of the world's population relies on some form of non-Western medicine practice for primary health care (Drew & Myers, 1997). There is an increasing consumer movement toward the use of similar nonorthodox medical treatments in the United States. Depending on the region, up to 54% of American adults may have used some type of nonconventional therapy in the past year; this figure represents a nationwide increase of 10 to 20% over the last 9 years (Elder et al., 1997; Eisenberg et al., 1998). Patients reported more office visits to practitioners who offer alternative approaches to health and illness than to conventional primary care providers (Eisenberg et al., 1993 and 1998). Whereas 40% of these patients told their conventional providers about using nonconventional treatments in 1990, more recent surveys show that this number has remained essentially the same or increased to 61% (Eisenberg et al., 1998; The Landmark Report, 1998).

Various phrases are used to describe health practices that are not fully embraced by conventional Western medicine practices. These terms include alternative, complementary, contemporary, holistic, integrative, folk, mind–body medicine, natural, New Age, new medicine, nonconventional, nontraditional, quackery, and vernacular medicine. Dr. Jonas, Director of the Office of Alternative Medicine (OAM) at the National Institutes of Health, observes that these terms represent "practices that aren't part of the politically dominant medical system of a country" (Wysocki, 1997, p 4). To be acknowledged as a component of the dominant medical system, a particular medical practice must be taught in medical schools, be available in hospitals or conventional health clinics, and be reimbursable by third-party payers (Wysocki, 1997).

Representatives of both dominant and nondominant practices have settled on the terms "complementary" and "integrative" instead of "alternative." Advocates of both practices point out that patients benefit when nonconventional and conventional health practices are used collaboratively and when one practice is not an *alternative* to the other.

Practitioners of complementary therapies view each individual as having unique inner resources for healing, maintaining health or both. Patients are seen as the primary agents in influencing the status of their own health; the practitioner helps mobilize these inherent resources rather than simply administer a "magic bullet."

This chapter provides an overview of complementary medicine as it is currently practiced and accepted in the United States. Table 43-1 lists many of the complementary therapies in

Text continued on page 1315

T A B L E 43-1

Complementary Therapies and Their Applications

NONCONVENTIONAL THERAPY	THEORY BEHIND USE	TREATMENT APPLICATIONS*
Acupressure	Similar principle as acupuncture but uses fingertips instead of needles to apply pressure (see acupuncture); also incorporates breathing techniques to aid healing by balancing mind–body–spirit; Shiatsu, reflexology, Jin Shin Do use similar techniques	Muscle tension targeting a specific organ or glandular system Usually more acceptable to children than acupuncture
Acupuncture	Hair-thin needles inserted at specific anatomical points alter blockage in energy flow patterns along "meridians" and stimulate the body to produce pain-relieving and mood-lifting chemicals or anti-inflammatory substances (sterile, disposal needles should always be used) (Acupuncture scores points, 1998)	Morning sickness of pregnancy Postoperative dental pain Chronic pain (including headaches) Allergies Asthma Nausea and vomiting (including morning sickness, chemotherapy induced, and postsurgical) Menstrual cramps Migraine headaches Low back pain Addictions (such as smoking) Musculoskeletal pain (such as arthritis, fibromyalgia, carpal tunnel syndrome, tendonitis)
Aromatherapy	Uses pure, essential volatile oils containing oxygenated molecules to transport nutrients to cells of the body. Believed to promote immunity and create a cellular environment in which disease-causing bacteria, fungi, and viruses cannot live. Aromas of essential oils are either inhaled or absorbed through the skin	Stress and anxiety Fatigue Immune disorders Musculoskeletal pain
Ayurvedic medicine	The traditional form of medicine practiced in Indian cultures. Treats imbalances, or "dosnas," within the body that cause illness by using diet changes, herbal remedies, breath work, physical exercise, hatha yoga, meditation, and/or rejuvenation or detoxification programs. Focuses on preventing disease by enhancing the mind–body connection	For primary health-care disorders involving: GI system GYN Respiratory tract Bones and muscles Circulation including cardiovascular system Emotional/psychological Addictions ENT

Table continued on following page

T A B L E 43-1

Complementary Therapies and Their Applications Continued

NONCONVENTIONAL THERAPY	THEORY BEHIND USE	TREATMENT APPLICATIONS*
Biofeedback	Empowers the mind to take control of conscious and autonomic processes (Frishberg, 1998). Relaxation is focused on one muscle or function rather than on the whole body	Chronic pain Hypertension Insomnia Tension and migraine headaches Incontinence (urine and fecal) Stroke rehabilitation Circulation PTSS and depression Chronic tinnitus Torticollis Chronic facial nerve palsy

Chiropractic
  Contraindications:
    malignancies, bone/joint
    infections, acute
    fractures, arthropathies
	Regards the spinal column as the center of the body's well-being; uses manipulation and massage of spinal vertebrae to restore proper flow of nerve impulses necessary for health	Musculoskeletal pain, including chronic low back pain (Abrams, 1997)† and headaches
		Torticollis
		Whiplash after MVA

Craniosacral	Manipulates craniosacral mechanisms to free the flow of cerebrospinal fluid pathways that surround brain and spinal cord; flow can be inhibited by injury to the brain, spinal cord, skull, sacrum, and related membranes	TMJ pain Headaches Skull injuries with resultant chronic pain Poorly fitting dentures Colic, vomiting, hypertonicity, tremor, irritability in infancy Obstetrically complicated delivery for the infant ADHD

Reflexology
  Use with caution in patients
    with deep vein
    thrombosis, leg ulcers,
    phlebitis in the lower
    extremities, pregnancy,
    pacemakers; avoid renal
    reflexes in patients with
    suspected renal calculi;
    avoid kidney/gallbladder
    reflexes in patients with
    gallstones
	A massage technique based on the principle that proprioceptive nerve receptors in the hands and feet correspond to all parts of the body, including organs and glands. Use thumb and fingers to massage reflex areas to detect diseases and to rebalance vital energy. Over a hundred medical conditions can be helped according to practitioners	Stress and anxiety
		Promote circulation
		Colic, irritability, and reflux in infants
		Headaches
		Low back pain
		Some allergic responses
		Some dermatology conditions
		GI tract disorders
		Menstrual problems
		Arthritis and sciatica

Herbalism
  Many phytomedicinals are
    not recommended for
    use in children (French,
    1996); refer to Table 43–3
	Natural herbs are used over pharmaceutical derivatives in the belief that they are as efficacious, gentler, and less toxic; used extensively by naturopathic, homeopathic, and holistic practitioners; appropriate preparation (tea, capsule, topical) of the herb is important. The dried or extract form of the plant may be used	Used in place of many pharmaceuticals to treat a myriad of primary health care entities, including PMS, cardiovascular problems, insomnia, stress, menopause, GI tract disorders, respiratory disorders, immunity, energy deficit, and memory

T A B L E 43-1

Complementary Therapies and Their Applications Continued

NONCONVENTIONAL THERAPY	THEORY BEHIND USE	TREATMENT APPLICATIONS*
Homeopathy	Stimulates a healing response by introducing a substance that is either the same as or similar to the patient's disease; infinitesimal doses of plants, minerals, and/or animal matter are used. Medicinal products are prescribed on the basis of the law of similars—the medicine used is "homeopathic" to the symptoms presented	Used by many for a wide range of primary care illnesses (e.g., respiratory ailments, headaches, diarrhea, teething, toothaches, arthritis, dermatology problems, gastrointestinal ailments, depression, and anxiety)
Magnets Contraindications: pacemakers, defibrillators, acute injuries to bone and muscles, first-trimester pregnancy	Magnets purported to stimulate the blood and draw it more quickly to a stressed or injured area and thereby aid the healing process; may interefere with electric impulses triggering pain or stimulate release of natural body pain killers (endorphins)	Musculoskeletal pain Headaches Nausea
Massage therapy Contraindications: clotting tendencies or communicable skin condition	Hands-on bodywork techniques that knead and manipulate muscles and soft and connective tissues of the body; used to promote healing and relaxation, relieve sore and injured muscles, and improve overall sense of well-being and health	Premature infants Cocaine- and HIV-exposed infants Colic in infants Infants with disturbed sleep patterns Autistic children Diabetic children to help normalize glucose levels Asthma Arthritis HIV-infected patients Chronic fatigue syndrome Stress-induced maladies Acute and chronic pain Digestive disorders Circulatory problems Musculoskeletal injuries Headaches
Meditation	A deep relaxation technique that can take many forms, from repeating a mantra to Sufi dancing	Stress-induced maladies Chronic illnesses

Table continued on following page

T A B L E 43-1

Complementary Therapies and Their Applications Continued

NONCONVENTIONAL THERAPY	THEORY BEHIND USE	TREATMENT APPLICATIONS*
Music therapy	Music used to provide rhythmic cues to stimulate the brain's motor systems to help build and strengthen connections among nerve cells in the cerebral cortex; boosts immune function in children	Physical rehabilitation of stroke, cerebral palsy, Alzheimer's disease (O'Brien, 1998), Parkinson's disease, ADHD, learning disabilities, Down syndrome Depression and anxiety HTN Pain relief (surgical, during labor) Premature infants (speeds the discharge rate from hospitals; Gideonse, 1998)
Naturopathy	Use natural remedies to help restore health and balance in the body, such as diet, herbal medicine, hydrotherapy, acupuncture, homeopathy, and therapeutic massage. Practitioners often use similar diagnostic and testing procedures as Western medicine practitioners	Used by many for most primary health-care issues
Nutrition	Stresses wisdom of following healthy, balanced diet to affect diet-related health issues; advocates the food pyramid guidelines	Weight loss Food allergies Vitamin and mineral deficiencies Nonpathological GI conditions (e.g., constipation) Chronic diseases
Osteopathy	Manipulation of joints and tissues to restore them to normal structural positions and mobility, thus releasing tension in muscles and ligaments	Musculoskeletal pain, including chronic back pain and headaches Torticollis Whiplash after MVA
Pilates	Works on mind–body connection with exercise techniques; relies on exercising with firm support and stretching without straining to improve overall body flexibility and fitness	Restricted body flexibility
Reiki	A bodywork technique to stimulate healing energy within the body	Musculoskeletal maladies Low blood hemoglobin levels Pain control (including from cancer, fractured bones) Stress and grief
Tai Chi	Stimulates and balances flow of *chi,* or vital energy, along acupuncture meridians	Restricted body flexibility, fitness Stamina and energy Stress

T A B L E 43-1

Complementary Therapies and Their Applications Continued

NONCONVENTIONAL THERAPY	THEORY BEHIND USE	TREATMENT APPLICATIONS*
Traditional Oriental (Chinese) medicine	Combines practices and beliefs of acupuncture, acupressure, herbal remedies, massage, dietary changes, bodywork such as Tai Chi, breathing, and meditation to stimulate vital body energy to rebalance life force	Used by 1/4 of world's population for primary health-care disorders involving: GI system GYN Respiratory tract Bones and muscles Circulation including the cardiovascular system Emotional/psychological Addictions ENT
Yoga	Works on breathing, body alignment, and posture to improve health; preventive	Chronic musculoskeletal ailments Stress-related maladies Improvement in overall body flexibility, fitness, stamina, mental health Asthma Hypertension

ADHD = attention-deficit hyperactivity disorder; ENT = ear, nose, throat; GI = gastrointestinal; GYN = gynecology; HIV = human immunodeficiency virus; HTN = hypertension; MVA = motor vehicular accident; PMS = premenstrual syndrome; PTSS = post-traumatic stress syndrome; TMJ = temporomandibular joint.

*These applications may or may not be supported by scientific research; listing of these therapies does not imply endorsement of proven efficacy.

†Guidelines for the advocacy of spinal manipulation for acute lower back pain were endorsed in 1994 by the Agency for Health Care Policy and Research of the US Department of Health and Human Services.

use. Specific applications to pediatric/adolescent diagnoses are discussed in Table 43-5. Nurse practitioners (NPs) and other medical providers need to become familiar with complementary therapies, routinely inquire into their use, and foster open discussion with clients who may be combining conventional and nonconventional treatments. In fact, the most effective treatment may involve using therapeutic applications from several different approaches. Successful practitioners benefit from moving between paradigms without prejudice, gleaning what is of value, and knowing when referral to a complementary medical practitioner is appropriate. As Dr. Jonas so aptly states, "Alternative medicine is here to stay. It is no longer an option to ignore it or treat it as something outside the normal process of science and medicine" (Jonas, 1998).

HISTORY OF COMPLEMENTARY MEDICAL PRACTICES

Before 1910, many different medical and apprenticeship schools allowed graduates to be licensed and referred to as "doctors." With acceptance of the 1910 Flexner report, all medical training, licensure, and regulation in the United States became standardized; since then, "approved" medical education has been based on science and research. Only training schools that could meet the rigorous Flexner standards were accredited and their graduates recognized as legitimate doctors. Although these standards effectively put many charlatans and snake oil medical practitioners out of work, many other nonconventional medical practitioners were also disqualified or their practices severely limited. The philosophies and practices of chiropractic, naturopathy, osteopathy, homeopathy, herbal treatments, and others fell into the unaccredited category. By excluding these disciplines, the medical community failed to consider the efficacy, benefits, and applications of the healing and treatment theories that these other practices had to offer. Rapid advances in immunology and pathology solidly secured the dominance of the rational–empirical approach, which became known as Western or "allopathic" medicine. All ailments were expected to fit within a scientific conceptual framework (Janiger & Goldberg, 1993).

The 1960s brought civil unrest and the questioning of authority in the United States. At the same time, a number of doctors and patients began to express disillusionment with the strict limitations of accepted medical practices. The "holistic" health-care movement of the 1970s evolved as patients and disaffected medical practitioners began to refocus health care toward healing, prevention, and the spiritual and environmental factors that affect health. From these contexts the current trend toward combining the best of Western and nontraditional medicine grew.

Certain basic principles are common to all nonconventional treatment modalities (Micozzi, 1997). These principles include

- A focus on wellness—which in turn prevents illness
- Self-healing—focusing external manipulations that stimulate the body's internal healing processes
- Bioenergy—ensuring that the body's energy forces are balanced
- Nutrition, plants, and other natural products—obtaining nutrients from natural food sources to maintain or return to health
- Individuality—recognition and use of the individual's unique constitution, inner resources, and so forth to achieve health

SCIENTIFIC OBSERVATION AND COMPLEMENTARY MEDICINE

Many complementary therapies are effective, yet few have been subjected to the rigorous scientific study that would meet Western criteria. Many mainstream medical practitioners refute claims about the efficacy of these treatments and label them quackery and/or "not scientifically validated." The Office of Technology Assessment points out, in response to this argument, that only about 20% of routine allopathic biomedical therapies have been subjected to the same rigorous, scientific testing standards demanded of complementary medicine treatments (Micozzi, 1997). Micozzi writes that "one way of studying and understanding alternative medicine is to view it in light of contemporary physics and biology–ecology, and to focus not just on the subtle manipulations of the alternative practitioners but on the physiologic response of the body" (Micozzi, 1996, p 5). Medical researchers of both disciplines are challenged to apply both Western treatments and successful complementary treatments until advances in physics and biology can explain the mechanisms of their effectiveness.

The National Institutes of Health created the OAM in 1992 to provide evidence-based research that would move complementary treatments into mainstream medicine, thus enabling greater access and further advancements in the therapies themselves. More than 100 pilot projects are under way in OAM-sponsored research centers in the United States (OAM Clearinghouse website, 1998). The goals behind these research efforts include:

- Identifying the role that complementary medical treatments play in clinical outcomes, prevention, and health improvement
- Encouraging independence and collaborative research within the complementary medicine community
- Encouraging the establishment of multidisciplinary research approaches and networking between both conventional and complementary communities
- Basing results on scientifically supported research
- Disseminating data

An example of one OAM-sponsored research project involves evaluating the popular complementary treatment for depression. The herbal extract *Hypericum* (St. Johnswort) is currently undergoing clinical trials. Complementary therapies for asthma, allergy, and immunological disorders are under way at the University of California at Davis (OAM Clearinghouse website, 1998). Table 43–2 lists some of the currently funded areas of interest.

The greatest body of research into complementary therapies has been done outside the United States, often does not meet US standards of double-blinded, placebo-controlled research models, and is not available in English. European and Indian studies are most closely aligned with our own research designs; the Chinese do not regard double-blind, placebo-controlled human studies as ethical. Many of the large, randomized, controlled studies have been done in Germany, where herbal extracts are regulated and used much the same way as pharmaceutical drugs to treat diseases.

THE USE OF COMPLEMENTARY PRACTICES IN THE UNITED STATES

Recent surveys in the United States and abroad have shown that more than 60% of physicians recommended complementary therapies to patients within the preceding year. Twenty-three percent used complementary strategies in their own practice, and 47% used them in their personal health regimens (Astin, 1998). A small survey of NPs and physician assistants (PAs) in 1997 revealed that 78% of NPs recommended complementary therapies and 75% reported seeing patients benefit from their use (PA and NP Opinions on Alternative Therapies, 1998). This interest in such therapies was also mirrored in another small survey conducted in 1997 at a conference of the National Organiza-

T A B L E 43-2

Six Program Areas Targeted for Scientifically Based Research by the Office of Alternative Medicine, National Institutes of Health

BIOELECTROMAGNETIC	MIND–BODY CONTROL	PHARMACOLOGICAL/BIOLOGICAL
Blue light treatment and artificial lighting	Biofeedback	Antioxidants
Transcranial electrostimulation	Prayer therapy	Cell therapy
Neuromagnetic stimulation	Relaxation	Chelation therapy
Electroacupuncture	Guided imagery	Metabolic therapy
Magnetoresonance spectroscopy	Hypnotherapy	Oxidizing therapy
	Music–sound therapy	
	Eduction therapy	
TRADITIONAL & ETHNOMEDICINE THERAPIES	**NUTRITION & DIET/LIFESTYLE & BEHAVIORAL HEALTH**	**STRUCTURAL MANIPULATION & ENERGETIC THERAPIES**
Acupuncture	Gerson therapy	Acupressure
Ayurvedic medicine	Health risk reduction	Alexander technique
Herbal medicine	Health education	Aromatherapy
Homeopathic medicine	Lifestyle modification	Biofield therapeutics
Native-American medicine	Macrobiotics	Chiropractics
Natural products	Megavitamins	Massage
Naturopathic medicine	Wellness	Osteopathy
Past-life therapy		Reflexology
Shamanism		Rolfing
Tibetan medicine		Therapeutic touch
Traditional Oriental medicine		Trager method
		Zone therapy
		Qi Gong

Adapted from Classification of Complementary and Alternative Medicine Practices: Office of Alternative Medicine, Information Package. Silver Spring, MD, Office of Alternative Medicine Clearinghouse, 1997.

tion of Nurse Practitioner Faculties. Ninety-three percent of the representatives of NP educational programs in more than 20 states reported that they recommended alternative therapies in their practices. Fifty-two percent reported that alternative therapies were incorporated into NP curricula at their schools or universities, and 81% indicated that these courses would continue or be added in the future (Young, 1998).

More than 60 medical schools now offer complementary medicine courses (Kass-Annese, 1997). In addition to the OAM, the American Medical Association, American Academy of Family Practice, American Nurses Association, and other groups are providing patient and professional education in nonconventional treatment options.

Research into complementary practices is increasing and is readily available in the literature and over the Internet. The National Library of Medicine offers a database for MEDLINE searches of more than 30,000 citations under the heading of "alternative medicine." Since 1966, the number of such citations has increased 12% per year (Jonas, 1996).

Insurance companies are increasingly offering premium coverage for alternative medical treatments in response to pressure from policy holders, including employers. A study conducted for a managed alternative care company in California showed that 67% of respondents reacted favorably to health plans that offered alternative care coverage (The Landmark Report, 1998).

THE ATTRACTION OF COMPLEMENTARY MEDICAL PRACTICES

A survey of 1500 adults revealed that the primary reason that they chose complementary therapies was their perception of the therapies' effectiveness (Astin, 1998). Negative attitudes toward conventional medical practices or a desire for more control over their health care was not predictive of complementary medicine use. Respondents said that they used complementary practices because they believed that they worked, that conventional medical care was not

helping them, and that these practices were more reflective of their own values and beliefs about the nature of life and spirituality. Use was not limited to any particular age, race, or gender of the population. However, those more likely to use complementary forms of care were young adult to middle aged and college educated and were suffering from either anxiety, back problems, urinary tract problems, headaches, sprains/muscle strains, chronic fatigue, addictive problems, or arthritis. Respondents living in the western states were more likely to use alternative therapies. Chiropractic was used most often; herbal/vitamin regimens and body therapy (yoga, massage, relaxation) were used to a slightly lesser extent (Astin, 1998; Elder, 1997). Total visits increased 47.3% in the 9 years between Eisenberg's two surveys. Fifty-eight percent of respondents used alternative therapy for health promotion or prevention rather than to treat a particular health ailment (Eisenberg, 1998). The literature from 1990 to 1998 suggests a shift toward a cultural norm of acceptance of complementary therapies rather than a rejection of allopathic medicine.

THE ROLE OF NURSE PRACTITIONERS

NPs are increasingly challenged to offer a more comprehensive management partnership with patients and to form more collaborative and integrative relationships with alternative medicine practitioners. Although NPs may not personally embrace the integration of these therapies in their own practice, they need to have sufficient knowledge, sensitivity, and willingness to support and help the patient make more informed decisions about their use.

Sixty-three percent of adults believed that their own medical care would improve if communication between their medical doctor and their alternative care provider increased. The vast majority of patients using alternative methods used them in conjunction with traditional health care. Only 5 to 15% of survey respondents actually replaced conventional medical care with alternative care (The Landmark Report, 1998; Astin, 1998).

The Landmark's (1998) findings that patients

want better communication between their conventional and nonconventional practitioners represent an expectation that NPs could readily fulfill. By being broad-minded about the use of alternative therapies, the NP could prevent perceptions similar to the one voiced by one patient: "Why would I bother sharing any kind of information that I might know about how this seemed to help me—they don't want to hear it and I don't want to get yelled at by them" (Elder, 1997, p 183).

The increasing use of complementary therapies suggests that patients' needs are not being adequately met by allopathic methods. The NP can help identify a better medical approach to illness and prevention for each patient by being more cognizant of that individual's values and approach to life.

TALKING WITH PATIENTS

Patients' perceptions of the acceptance they feel from NPs provides an opportunity for open discussion regarding the possible risks and benefits of nonconventional therapies. NPs are better able to monitor patients when they know the alternative practitioners in their area and establish communication with them, even to the point of sharing the management of patients.

In particular, the patient's medical history should be expanded to include:

- Alternative products that the patient may be taking, including herbs, "natural products," and homeopathic and nutritional supplements from a health food store
- Other practitioners whom the patient may be seeing
- Other kinds of activities engaged in to address a particular problem
- The perception of any benefit gained from the complementary treatment
- The philosophy and self-care approaches to wellness and illness

The topic must be broached nonjudgmentally to help the family clarify the safety issues and explore how these products or services might fit into the patient management plan. Dr. Jonas states that "the practitioner–patient

relationship and the trust that's been developed by looking at mutual goals form the foundation" for ongoing dialogue (Wysocki, 1997). Furthermore an open, sensitive attitude implies a commitment "to the patients' welfare rather than to the particular system of medicine in which they trained" (Gordon, 1996, p 2209).

SAFETY AND REGULATORY ISSUES

It is important to ascertain the safety of certain treatment modalities by learning about any alternative product that the patient may be using, including its side effects, possible interactions with other medications, and mechanism of action. Mind-body techniques (e.g., prayer, guided imagery, spiritual healing, relaxation) and acupuncture are unlikely to interact with conventional medications. NPs should be aware of the possible harmful effect of products that are taken at high doses, such as herbal or phytomedicinal products, megadose combination nutritional supplements, colonics, or products taken in unconventional ways. NPs and PAs reported that 30% had seen harmful effects from improper use of the therapy (PA and NP Opinions on Alternative Therapies, 1998). Any treatment must be viewed as hazardous if its use delays the provision of proven conventional care for a serious medical condition (Murray & Rubel, 1992; Nickerson & Silberman, 1992).

Contamination and potency are other concerns when patients use herbal or folk remedies. Some traditional folk remedies or herbal preparations manufactured in other countries contain heavy metals, although this practice is quite rare and increasingly uncommon. Prior, nonproblematic use of a product may not be a predictor of a future drug reaction because

- Consistency of potency between batches of herbal preparations varies
- Herbal products can lack standardization regarding which parts of a plant are used
- Plant ripeness, storage, and regional growth conditions vary

Contamination of plant materials, substitutions, adulterations, incorrect preparations or dosages, and inappropriate labeling and advertising have also contributed to adverse patient reactions. However, few reports of adverse reactions to herbal preparations have been documented, which may be a reflection of either the relatively low risk of these products or under-reporting (Drew & Myers, 1997; Fugh-Berman, 1997).

Even though 25% of pharmaceutical drugs are made from herbs, Western medical providers often regard herbal preparations as dangerous or ineffective. Since 1993, the Food and Drug Administration (FDA) has had a voluntary system in place, called MedWatch, for reporting adverse reactions to nutritionals and botanicals. Access to MedWatch is available from the FDA's Internet website (see Resources Box). Complaints reported to the FDA have mostly involved food-related reactions to aspartame (Nutrasweet, 80%) or to sulfites (15%). Ingestion of toxic ornamental plants rather than herbs accounts for most reports of plant poisonings. These poisonings are rarely serious, as reported by US poison control centers between 1985 and 1990 (Fugh-Berman, 1997). The nonmedicinal poison of water hemlocks (*Conium maculatum* and *Cicuta maculata* or *douglassi*) constituted most of the 10 plant poisoning fatalities during this time. In contrast, 414 nonsuicidal deaths in 1989 were caused by prescription drugs and over-the-counter preparations (e.g., antidepressants, analgesics, sedative and heart drugs) (Fugh-Berman, 1997).

Although many herbs are harmless even in large amounts, others should be prescribed only by a knowledgeable herbalist or botanic professional. *Standardized extracts* are more likely to ensure that a specific amount of an active compound is present, thus helping avoid the discrepancies found when different parts of a plant are used or when seasonal or climatic variations occur during cultivation for any given plant or plant part. Western herbalists often use *simples* (the compound is made from one herb), whereas Chinese and Indian (Ayurvedic) medicines often blend together more than one herb (Fugh-Berman, 1997). A general rule is that all herbs need to be respected; they are neither completely safe nor poisonous. Herbs can interact with other herbs or with pharmaceutical drugs.

The appropriate herb in the appropriate quantity—like pharmaceutical medicines—is necessary to obtain the intended benefits. The medicinal effect of any one herb is thought to be the result of dozens of pharmacologically distinct actions. The herb may be essentially effecting physiological changes in numerous subtle ways, none of which alone would produce the desired response. This mechanism contrasts with conventional medicines, which generally act by one of a few mechanisms of action and use "physiologically more significant pharmacologic" dosing (Herbal Medicine Taken as a Whole, 1998).

The Dietary Supplement Health and Education Act of 1994 requires cautionary labeling for all dietary supplements containing herbs. The American Herbal Products Association has evaluated herbal safety for all botanical ingredients sold in North America (McGuffin et al., 1997). Each herb has been placed in one of the following classes:

Class 1—herb can be safely consumed when used appropriately
Class 2—The following use restrictions apply:
2a: For external use only
2b: Not to be used during pregnancy
2c: Not to be used while nursing
2d: Other specific use restrictions as noted

Herbal supplements that carry the United States Pharmacopeia (USP) designation indicate that the manufacturers have voluntarily met USP standards for purity, potency, disintegration, and dissolution. Fact sheets on popular herbal supplements are being compiled for consumers by the USP (Nutrition News From A to Z, 1998).

No cases of malpractice have been filed against medical physicians who have advocated the use of complementary treatments (Eisenberg, 1997). However, one should not refer patients to a nonconventional practitioner without first having done a complete diagnostic evaluation.

NPs are advised to check the Advanced Nurse Practice Act of their state, the policies of the employer, and the standards of practice relevant to include complementary therapies before expanding their practice. NPs may have to pursue a broader interpretation and additional training or certification to ensure compliance with the terms of the nurse practice act (Slagle, 1996).

The following steps should be taken by the NP to assist a patient who wishes to try an alternative therapy after a thorough diagnostic evaluation of the patient's complaint (Eisenberg, 1997):

- Assist in identifying a suitable licensed provider.
- Provide the patient with questions to ask the alternative provider during the first consultative visit, including issues of safety and efficacy of any treatment.
- Monitor the patient to review the recommended treatment plan; encourage the patient to keep a symptom diary.
- Monitor the response to treatment at monthly intervals.
- Document all interactions with the patient.

Many states have licensing boards and professional organizations that set standards for nonconventional practitioners, including a requirement to carry malpractice insurance. Further information is available from the Federation of State Medical Licensing (see Resources). Licensing requirements are subject to change, and patients should be encouraged to review the credentials of any practitioner whom they are considering using. Doctorates in acupuncture or an OMD degree (Oriental medical doctor) are not recognized in the United States.

▆▆▆ USING COMPLEMENTARY THERAPIES WITH CHILDREN

A Canadian survey revealed that 11% of children had visited one or more nonconventional practitioners, most frequently chiropractors (36%) and homeopaths (25%) (Spigelblatt, 1997). This author surmised that because of the widespread use of over-the-counter herbal or homeopathic preparations, the actual number of children receiving some form of alternative remedy was probably higher.

Reasons cited by parents for choosing alternative medicine for their children include (Spigelblatt, 1997; Turow, 1997b):

- Limited access to or dissatisfaction with traditional care

- Ready access to nonconventional practitioners
- Failure of traditional medicine to have an impact on chronic conditions such as degenerative diseases, allergies, asthma, otitis media, musculoskeletal ailments, and diagnosis and treatment of certain cancers
- Awareness of complications and side effects produced by pharmaceuticals
- Inadequacy of invasive procedures and/or diagnostics
- Desire for a more holistic, individualistic form of health care
- Ethnic and cultural beliefs
- Belief that alternative practices are more natural, less harmful, and more effective
- Belief that by combining conventional and nonconventional treatment a more effective approach to health care is achieved than either practice alone affords
- Awareness of the mind–body connection to affect the immune response system
- Desire for more parental, active participation in their child's treatment

Many of the treatments advocated for children involve the use of herbal preparations. Some of these treatments are discussed in Table 43-5. In children, the most dangerous elements are the pyrrolizidine alkaloids, which can cause liver complications or death. These compounds occur in comfrey, borage, coltsfoot, and species of *Crotalaria* and *Senecio*. These plants are often found in herbal teas, particularly from Jamaica, Africa, and South and Central America. Chaparral, germander, and a Chinese medicine called jin bu huan can also cause liver toxicity. Refer to Table 43-3 for a summary list of these herbs.

Few pediatricians are practicing and researching complementary therapies in the United States (Kemper, 1998a). The Center for Holistic Pediatric Education and Research based at Harvard University is the only academic center devoted to pediatric complementary therapies. It was founded in July 1998. The mission of the center is to advance complementary practices in children into mainstream pediatrics based on scientifically integrated research and to promote collaboration between professionals

T A B L E 43-3

Herbals: General Precautions About Use in Children

Ephedra (ma huang)	*Not recommended*
Comfrey (*Symphytum*)	*Not recommended*
Borage (*Borago officinalis*)	*Not recommended*
Coltsfoot (*Tussilago farfara*) and species of *Crotalaria* and *Sececio* in herbal teas	*Not recommended*
Chaparral (*Larrea divaricata*)	*Not recommended*
Germander (*Teucrium chamaedrys*)	*Not recommended*
Jin bu huan	*Not recommended*
Monkshood/wolfsbane/aconite	*Not recommended*
Heliotropes	*Not recommended*
Rattlebox (Leguminosae)	*Not recommended*
Sassafras	*Not recommended*
Goldenseal/roots	Not for infants younger than 1 mo
Tea tree oil	Do not prescribe for internal use
Echinacea	Not for children younger than 2 y
Pennyroyal	Do not prescribe for internal use

Data from Mack 1998; Castleman 1995; Fugh-Berman, 1997; Eisenberg 1997.

caring for children. Since its inception, the center has developed a 1-month curriculum in holistic pediatrics for medical students and residents and is in the process of writing a *Primer on Herbal Remedies for Physicians* (currently not published). Future research endeavors will involve collaboration with the Dana Farber Cancer Institute to evaluate complementary medical therapies for children with cancer.

The Role of Allergies as Viewed by Complementary Medicine Practitioners

Complementary practitioners are more likely to identify allergies as being the etiology for many common childhood conditions. Childhood afflictions such as otitis media, upper respiratory infections and other immunological conditions,

atopic dermatitis, asthma, headaches, and hyperactivity/attention-deficit hyperactivity disorder (Table 43-4) are mentioned as being caused by allergies to foods and food additives. These health conditions are believed to result from reactions of the "inner being" to external environmental stimuli, notably foods (Micozzi, 1996). Rates of reported food allergies in children range from 10 to 25%, depending on whether the source is from an allopathic or naturopathic reference (Sampson, 1997; Murray & Pizzorno, 1998). Naturopathic physicians cite genetics, the early introduction of solids, early weaning, genetic reengineering of food components, and impaired digestion as possible reasons for an increase in food sensitivities (Murray & Pizzorno, 1998).

The argument for an allergic etiology for many childhood illnesses is strengthened by recent biomedical research that has confirmed the "allergic march" that occurs in atopic children. Such children progress from "eczema and food allergy to asthma, rhinitis and aeroallergen sensitization" (Burr et al., 1998). Also, allopathic physicians have demonstrated that some patients with food allergies but without asthma can have increased bronchial reactivity causing dyspnea without wheezing (Plaut, 1997). Businco and colleagues (1995) take this point further. They postulate that once a person with a history of asthma *and* atopic dermatitis has such bronchial reactivity to a food allergen, the person is more susceptible to having acute bronchoconstriction triggered by other factors such as cold air, exercise, other environmental allergens, and cola drinks.

THE PREVENTIVE ROLE OF BREAST MILK

Complementary medicine practitioners continually stress the importance of breast milk for infants. One such study concluded that allergic disease in childhood is caused by both genetics and exposure to allergens in infancy (Burr et al., 1998). Another study conjectured that early milk feeding might have a greater influence than genetic risk (Saarinen & Kajosaari, 1995). This latter study concluded that by the ages of 1 and 3, the children showing the lowest incidence of atopy were the group that had been breastfed longer than 6 months. Those breast-

TABLE 43-4

Elimination and Challenge Diet Regimen for Hyperactivity/Attention-Deficit Hyperactivity Disorder

The elimination diet should last for at least 10 d, followed by reintroduction of foods one at a time every 2 d. Symptoms resulting from food allergens will usually disappear the fifth or sixth day of the elimination diet, when the body has thoroughly cleansed itself of the allergen/antibody complexes and the intestines have been cleared of food. Should symptoms not disappear, it is recommended that the diet become further restricted. Generally, the fewer known allergens included in the diet, the easier it is to establish a cause. Severity of hyperactivity is not predictive of outcome of diet (Carter et al., 1993). Behavioral changes may be evidenced by decreased irritability, restlessness, sleep disturbances (Rowe & Rowe, 1994; Carter et al., 1993), and lower scores on Connors' hyperactivity index (Boris & Mandel, 1994).

Eat only the following foods before reintroduction of other foods: lamb, chicken, rice, potatoes, banana, apple, and vegetables in the cabbage family (cabbage, Brussels sprouts, broccoli, cauliflower, mustard, radish, turnip, watercress). No artificial colors or preservatives.

If symptoms have improved, upon reintroduction of eliminated foods, more pronounced or acute symptoms will recur. The most common foods that produce symptoms are eggs, wheat, chocolate, nuts, cow's milk, citrus, and cheese. Corn and soy have also been implicated. Avoidance means both eliminating the food in its most identifiable state (eating a scrambled egg) and identifying it in hidden foods (e.g., breads prepared with eggs). A diary should be kept and wrist pulse recorded because the pulse may change when an allergen is eaten (Murray & Pizzorno, 1998). Children with atopy are more likely to respond to this diet (Boris & Mandel, 1994). An additive-free diet alone is of little help (Rowe & Rowe, 1994).

fed less than 1 month had the highest incidence of both atopy at 1 and 3 years and respiratory allergies (defined as asthma diagnosed at a hospital, episodes of respiratory distress with wheezing, seasonal or animal-mediated rhinoconjunctivitis or wheezing) at 17 years. An additional double-blind, placebo-controlled study demonstrated that 50 to 60% of infants with atopic dermatitis were hypersensitive to cow's milk (Isolauri, 1997).

An NP who sees a breastfed infant in whom atopic dermatitis has developed should ask the mother about her use of allergenic foods. Some studies showed that allergens can be transferred through breast milk (Murray & Pizzorno, 1998; Saarinen & Kojasaari, 1995; David et al., 1997). Refer to Table 43-5 (Colic: nutritionals) for the listing of foods that the mother should avoid. The appearance of this condition in older or formula-fed infants should lead the NP to suggest eliminating milk, eggs, peanuts, wheat, soybeans, and fish. The first five of these foods have been found to account for up to 90% of food hypersensitivity reactions in children with atopic dermatitis (Sampson, 1997). Both allopathic and alternative providers agree that early identification of illnesses with allergic etiologies

(e.g., atopic dermatitis in infancy) and elimination of allergenic foods from the diet can significantly alter the immunopathogenic mechanisms causing symptoms.

ALLERGY TESTING

Alternative practitioners may advocate laboratory testing for food allergies. Blood testing remains controversial in conventional medical settings, less so with nutritionally oriented practitioners such as naturopaths. New studies point toward IgG4 antibodies playing a more important role in atopic disease (Murray & Pizzorno, 1998). It is also of note that a positive skin prick test reaction to egg in infancy was predictive of the development of atopic disease (Burr et al., 1998).

SPECIFIC COMPLEMENTARY TREATMENTS FOR CHILDREN AND ADOLESCENTS

Table 43-5 lists some of the complementary treatments that parents of pediatric-aged children may be considering or are actually using.

Text continued on page 1348

T A B L E 43-5

Complementary Treatments* for Some Common Conditions in Children and Adolescents†

DIAGNOSIS	TREATMENT APPROACH	DOSAGE	BENEFIT	POSSIBLE SIDE EFFECTS*	RESEARCH/ CITATIONS
Acne	Herbal				
	Goldenseal	Adolescents: Use as infusion; use to wash face	Antibacterial properties	Nontoxic at recommended dose Class 2b	Murray & Pizzorno, 1998
	Tea tree oil	Adolescents: 5% topically, diluted with water once daily (use 15% concentration for severe acne)	Effective against *Propionibacterium acnes*—antiseptic and antifungal properties	Contact dermatitis	Studies show 5% tea tree oil as effective as 5% benzyl peroxide (Kemper, 1996a; Murray & Pizzorno, 1998)
	Salicyclic acid	Adolescents: Topically bid–qid (start with 0.5% until tolerated and increase to 2% concentration).	Breaks apart sebum plugs	Redness and irritation	Kemper, 1996b
	Nutritional Vit B_6 or multi-Vit with zinc, B_6, A, E, C, selenium, copper	Adolescents: Vit B_6, 25 mg bid; one daily multi-Vit	Works well for premenstrual aggravation of acne		Kemper, 1996b; Murray & Pizzorno, 1998
Anxiety	Herbal Kava (*Piper methysticum*)	Adolescents: 5–75 mg kava lactones tid PO (use 30–50% standardized concentrations)	Relief of generalized anxiety in 8–12 wk	Rash; nonaddictive. Don't use in patients taking benzodiazepines or patients with Parkinson's disease *Class 2b*—do not exceed recommended dose	Three studies cited improved scores on standardized anxiety scales (Kava, 1998)

	Dose/Method	Effects	Precautions/Toxicity	Reference
Aromatherapy Chamomile	Infants/children: put 2–3 drops of the essential oil in vaporizer	Decreases irritability from illnesses (GI upset, varicella, fevers)	Rare allergic reactions in those hypersensitive to ragweed, aster, chrysanthemums (daisy family of plants) consisting of dermatitis, asthma, dyspnea, anaphylaxis *Class 2b*	Kemper, 1996a
Music therapy		Listening to music directly influences pulse, BP, electrical activity of muscles; may help nerve cell connections within the cerebral cortex	None	Thaut, 1998; Gideonse, 1998
Massage		Improved behavior, reduced cortisol levels		Field et al., 1998
Yoga Meditation Therapeutic touch		Help with relaxation and decreasing anxiety		Kemper, 1996b (cites studies)
Aphthous stomatitis Herbal Aloe vera	Apply topically several times daily	Accelerates healing; under investigation as antiviral and immunomodulator	Rare allergic reactions if taken internally; rare skin eruptions with topical use *Class 1*	Kemper, 1996a

Table continued on following page

T A B L E   43-5
Complementary Treatments* for Some Common Conditions in Children and Adolescents† Continued

DIAGNOSIS	TREATMENT APPROACH	DOSAGE	BENEFIT	POSSIBLE SIDE EFFECTS*	RESEARCH/ CITATIONS
Asthma	Nutritional Diet exclusions	Eliminate milk, chocolate, wheat, citrus, food colorings (tartrazine, sunset yellow, amaranth), food additives (sodium benzoate, 4-hydroxybenzoate esters, sulfites), and tryptophan (amino acid in milk, cheese, turkey, bananas). Ensure adequate Vit C, magnesium, fish in diet		In severe asthma, combined treatment with pharmaceuticals is recommended —nutritionals reduce allergic threshold and can help prevent acute attacks	Many studies cited in Murray & Pizzorno, 1998, for these nutritional recommendations Kemper, 1996b
	Vegan diet	Vegan diet with exception of cold-water fish for their omega-3 fatty acids—try for 4 mo. Use onions and garlic liberally *plus* Omega-3 fatty acids (supplement with fish oil)	Alters prostaglandin metabolism, increases intake of antioxidant nutrients and magnesium, eliminates food allergens. Onions/ garlic inhibit release of inflammatory chemicals. Omega-3 fatty acids improve airway responsiveness to allergens		Description of diet in Murray & Pizzorno, 1998, p 265 Kemper, 1998b (recommends fish several times a week rather than fish oil supplements)
	Green tea extract *or*	Give as watered-down tea prn	Inhibits histamine release from mast cells by increasing absorption of flavonoids		Murray & Pizzorno, 1998

Agent	Dose	Effects/Comments	References
Ginkgo biloba extract	<50 lb: 25 mg tid; 50–100 lb: 40 mg tid	Improves respiratory function and reduces bronchial reactivity. Rare side effects (headaches, GI upset) *Class 2d*—may potentiate effect of MAO inhibitors	McGuffin et al., 1997; Murray & Pizzorno, 1998
Vit B_6 (effects seen after 1 mo)	<50 lb: 8–15 mg/bid; 50–100 lb: 12–25 mg/bid; >100 lb: 25–50 mg/bid	Reduces side effects in asthmatics being treated with theophylline and reduces number and severity of attacks and other medication use	Murray & Pizzorno, 1998; Kemper, 1996b and 1998b
Magnesium	<50 lb: 60–125 mg/d; 50–100 lb: 100–200 mg/d; >100 lb: 200–400 mg/d	Adequate levels necessary for lung function and affects asthma severity	Murray & Pizzorno, 1998; Kemper, 1996b
Vit B_{12}	<50 lb: 300 µg/d; 50–100 lb: 500 µg/d; >100 lb: 1000 µg/d	Possibly reduces reactions to sulfites	Murray & Pizzorno, 1998; Kemper, 1996b (not recommended)
Vit C	10-30 mg/kg/d in divided doses	A major antioxidant in lung lining; asthmatics have higher need for Vit C; inhibits histamine release	Murray & Pizzorno, 1998; Kemper, 1996b
Acupuncture		Study results mixed; some show modest, temporary effect; ineffective for long-term control	Fugh-Berman, 1997; Micozzi, 1996 (evidence is mixed)

Table continued on following page

T A B L E 43-5

Complementary Treatments* for Some Common Conditions in Children and Adolescents† *Continued*

DIAGNOSIS	TREATMENT APPROACH	DOSAGE	BENEFIT	POSSIBLE SIDE EFFECTS*	RESEARCH/ CITATIONS
Asthma *Continued*	Chiropractic				Fugh-Berman, 1997 (no evidence of efficacy)
	Homeopathy	Immunotherapy using whatever substance patient is allergic to	Possibly some positive effect		Fugh-Berman, 1997 (one study cited); Kemper, 1996b (no published studies using homeopathic treatments for children)
	Hypnosis	Requires subjects highly susceptible to hypnosis	Reduced symptoms and medication use		Fugh-Berman, 1997; Kemper, 1996b (controlled studies cited)
	Biofeedback	Age appropriate	Improved breathing, fewer and less severe asthma attacks		Kemper, 1996b (studies cited)
	Massage		Improves peak airflow, decreases asthma attacks, relieves anxiety and depression	None reported	Green et al., 1997 (studies cited); Field et al., 1998 (recent study)
	Yoga		May be helpful in reducing symptoms and medication use	None reported	Fugh-Berman, 1997 Kemper 1996b (cites studies)
Burns—1st or 2nd degree	Herbal Aloe Vera	Prepared gel (70% aloe vera) or gel directly from leaves: apply topically several times daily	Anti-inflammatory, antibacterial; promotes wound healing	Contact dermatitis *Class 1*	Kemper, 1996b
	Therapeutic touch		Increased healing	None reported	Kemper, 1996b (cites double-blind study showing statistically significant results)

Condition	Therapy	Instructions/Dosage	Mechanism/Effect	Adverse Effects/Class	References
Colic (stomach discomfort)	Homeopathy Calendula (no other homeopathic remedies recommended)	Popular skin soother, available in skin creams	Some anti-inflammatory properties	Rare rash *Class 1*	Kemper, 1996b
	Nutritional 12% sucrose solution	Infants: 5 1/2 tsp sugar in 8 oz water. Give 2 ml over 30–60 s anytime for inconsolable crying; try for 1–2 d to see whether helps	Sucrose analgesia—works by stimulating secretion of endogenous endophins	None	Markestad, 1997 (small double-blind crossover study)
	Herbal Tea with chamomile, mint, fennel, licorice, vervain	Infants: Give in weak tea form (mix 1/2 to 1 tsp of herb in boiling water; steep 5 min); give 1/2–4 oz tid–qid	Calming, sedating effects (antispasmodic on smooth muscles of digestive tract)	Rare allergic reaction (dermatitis, asthma, dyspnea, anaphylaxis) in people with hypersensitivity to daisy family (see Anxiety section, chamomile) *Class 2b*	Kemper, 1996b
	Chiropractic	Average of 3 treatments	Colic relieved	None reported	Kemper, 1996b; Fugh-Berman, 1997 (noncontrolled study showed 94% resolution but was done in 6-wk-old infants over period of 2 wk when spontaneous resolution may have occurred)

Table continued on following page

1329

Complementary Treatments* for Some Common Conditions in Children and Adolescents† Continued

DIAGNOSIS	TREATMENT APPROACH	DOSAGE	BENEFIT	POSSIBLE SIDE EFFECTS*	RESEARCH/ CITATIONS
Colic *Continued*	Nutritional				
	Eliminate certain foods in mother's diet if breastfed	Mother should eliminate for 1 wk garlic, cow's milk, fruit, chocolate, coffee, tea, cola, soy, corn, wheat, eggs, cabbage, broccoli, onions, peppers, beans	Colic symptoms improved	None—counsel mother on other appropriate foods of equal nutritional value	Kemper, 1996b (studies equivocal—elimination diet helps in some infants)
	Therapeutic touch		Calming	None reported	Kemper, 1996b (no studies cited)
	Massage	Can be taught to parents; used prn. Massage tummy lightly with baby on side, head somewhat down, and bottom elevated; massage 20–30 min after a meal; can extend massage to include entire body	Calming, relaxing	None if done gently	Kemper, 1996b

Common cold/flu	Herbal Echinacea leaves/ stalks/roots	Children >2 yr: 1/4–1 dropperful of tincture tid-qid—can be diluted in water/juice. Use at onset of symptoms only; maximum duration of use, 8 wk	Stimulates immune system by boosting macrophages' ability to destroy germs, increases T-cell production, and may have interferon-like effects	Can cause allergic reaction (dermatitis, asthma, dyspnea, anaphylaxis) in people allergic to ragweed and daisy family of plants; do not use in patients with progressive infections (e.g., TB, HIV) or autoimmune diseases; can interfere with immunosuppressive therapy. Preparations not standardized *Class 1*	Kemper, 1996a; Bates, 1998. Castleman, 1995, states, "US herb companies market prepackaged echinacea preparations under FDA purity regulations and can be used with confidence" (p 223)
	Nutritional Vit C	Children: 250 mg qid or 4–5 glasses of orange juice daily at onset of cold	Reduces symptoms and length of illness by activating neutrophils to oxidize inflammatory mediators and increase extracellular Vit C	Regarded as safe; diarrhea in high doses	Kemper, 1996b; Murray & Pizzorno, 1998; Castleman, 1995; Turow, 1997a
	Chicken soup; peppers, mustard, horseradish, salsa, other spicy foods	Sip soup slowly through the day	Thins nasal secretions, increases nasal and sinus mucus velocity	None reported but use cautiously in children with diarrhea-associated illnesses because of chance of causing hypernatremic dehydration	Kemper, 1996b (proven efficacy incomplete in children but worthwhile to try); Turow, 1997a

Table continued on following page

T A B L E 43-5
Complementary Treatments* for Some Common Conditions in Children and Adolescents† Continued

DIAGNOSIS	TREATMENT APPROACH	DOSAGE	BENEFIT	POSSIBLE SIDE EFFECTS*	RESEARCH/ CITATIONS
Common cold Continued	Garlic	Raw clove minced in mashed potatoes (1 medium clove = 100,000 U penicillin). Do not exceed 2 cloves in a day	Kills cold viruses	Safe, occasional GI upset Class 2c	Castleman, 1995; Therapeutic Uses of Herbs, 1997
	Zinc lozenges	Children: 15–25 mg sucked every 2 hr; use no longer than 7 d	May reduce severity and length of illness by binding rhinoviral docking sites with somatic cells and thereby inhibiting infectivity	Mouth irritation, nausea, vomiting, diarrhea, abdominal pain. Can suppress immune system if taken longer than 7 d	Kemper, 1996b; Fugh-Berman, 1997; Murray & Pizzorno, 1998; Turow, 1997a. Has not been tested or proved effective in children
	Biochemical Saline nose drops/ spray	Recipe: 1/2 tsp salt in 1 cup warm water; administer nasally prn	Helps thin nasal secretions	None reported at recommended dilution	Kemper, 1996b
	Aromatherapy Oils of camphor, eucalyptus, menthol, pine, rosemary, wintergreen, tea tree	Inhaled by vaporizer or steam	Helps relieve congestion; heats nasal passages to degree that inhibits viral replication	Class 1	Kemper, 1996b; Turow, 1997a
	Massage Oils of menthol (Vicks Vaporub), tiger balm	Infant older than 1 mo: Massage face, head, back, lymph glands, chest in gentle downward motion	May cool the nose and cause perception of decreased nasal congestion	Safe Class 1	Kemper, 1996b; Murray & Pizzorno, 1998; Turow, 1997a
	Acupuncture		Aids blocked sinuses	Included in 1979 World Health Org. list of recognized therapies influenced by acupuncture	Micozzi, 1996

Condition	Remedy	Dosage	Comments	Side effects/Class	References
Diarrhea	Herbal Berberine-containing plants (goldenseal, barberry, or Chinese remedy "huanglian coptis chinonsis")	Goldenseal: toddlers and older children, 1/4–1/2 tsp tincture or 1/8 tsp fluid extract tid–qid—can be mixed with water or juice	Demonstrated benefits for antimicrobial activity against bacteria (includes *Escherichia coli, Shigella, Salmonella, Klebsiella, F. aerogenes*), fungi, protozoa, including *Giardia*. When used with any indicated antibiotics, decreased length of illness	Hypotension or HTN, nausea, vomiting, diarrhea; *not recommended for infants younger than 1 mo* *Class 2b*	Kemper, 1996b; Murray & Pizzorno, 1998 (cite studies)
		Giardia: Children, 5 mg/kg per d for 6 d		More effective than metronidazole (Flagy) in treating symptoms but not as effective in clearing from GI tract; best approach to use with standard antibiotic therapy	Murray & Pizzorno, 1998 (cite studies)
	Lactobacillus acidophilus	5–7 billion organisms/d	Can also be used to decrease incidence of rotovirus diarrhea in infants 5–24 mo old		Kemper, 1996b (study cited)
	5% Carob pod powder	Infants to 1 yr: 1.5 g/kg per d in ORS or formula Children over 1 yr: 1–15 g/kg per d in ORS or milk. Stop 24 hr after appearance of formed stool	Acute diarrhea in infants/children. Tannins inhibit growth of bacteria and bind bacterial toxins. Controlled studies of hospitalized infants showed efficacy of treatment	None. Used for centuries in Mediterranean regions *Class 1*	Murray & Pizzorno, 1998; Loeb et al., 1989

Table continued on following page

T A B L E 43-5

Complementary Treatments* for Some Common Conditions in Children and Adolescents† Continued

DIAGNOSIS	TREATMENT APPROACH	DOSAGE	BENEFIT	POSSIBLE SIDE EFFECTS*	RESEARCH/ CITATIONS
Diarrhea *Continued*	Garlic				
	Best formulations are enteric-coated tablets/capsules/dried or powdered garlic, standardized for alliin content	All ages: 1 clove (or 4 g) chewed, chopped, bruised, or crushed. Do not use more than 2 cloves of raw garlic daily	Treat *Entamoeba histolytica*, athlete's foot, vaginal candidiasis; is antimicrobial. The organosulfur compounds are believed to interfere with microbial structures/functions	Garlic breath (try chewing fennel, parsley, fenugreek to counter garlic breath); has anticlotting effect. GI upset, rash, burning mouth, sweating, lightheadedness. Raw garlic is toxic in high doses	Castleman, 1995; Therapeutic Uses of Herbs, 1997
	ORS 1 qt water 1/2 tsp salt 1–1/2 cups rice cereal for infants *or* 2 tbsp sugar	Offer 1 tbsp to 1 oz every 15–30 min; increase as tolerated			Kemper, 1996b
Eczema/atopic dermatitis	Herbal Evening primrose oil	Infants/children: 4 caps/d (300 g) PO Adolescents: 8–12 caps/d Requires 4–12 wk for benefit	Decreased scaling, itching, and general severity; contains high amounts of a fatty acid that children with eczema thought to have a defect in metabolizing	Very safe; rare, mild GI effects, headache *Class 1*	Fugh-Berman, 1997; Kemper, 1996b
	Echinachea	Apply topically	Promotes healing by stimulating formation of new tissue	Contact dermatitis; use with caution in patients allergic to ragweed and daisy family of plants *Class 1*	Castleman, 1995; Kemper, 1996b

	Remedy	Dosage/Administration	Effect	Precautions	Reference
	Licorice (*Glycyrrhiza glabra*)	Apply topically as pure glycyrrhetinic acid (commercial product: Simicort from Enzymatic Therapy)	Exerts effect similar to that of hydrocortisone cream	None *Class 2b*	Murray & Pizzorno, 1998 (double-blind, controlled studies cited)
	Chamomile extracts or witch hazel	Apply topically (commercial product: CamoCare)	May help reduce itching and inflammation; promote healing	Contact dermatitis; use with caution in patients with allergy to ragweed or daisy family of plants	Murray & Pizzorno, 1998
	Nutritional and naturopathic Diet exclusions				Refer to "Asthma", diet exclusions discussion earlier in chapter / Refer to "colic", nutritionals
	Breast milk		Improvement in symptoms	Ensure adequate calcium, nutrients	
	Vit C (after diet exclusion and rechallenge)	Infants/children: One 8-oz glass of orange juice daily		None at recommended doses	Kemper, 1996b (cites double-blind, controlled crossover trial of Vit C with significant improvement of eczema)
Elevated lead level	Herbal Garlic	Add liberally to foods. Refer to Common cold/flu for dosing information	Helps eliminate lead/heavy metals	Should be used with caution in patients with clotting disorders	Castleman, 1995 (based on some European studies)
	Teas from red clover, lemon grass, milk thistle	Tea drinks	Herbalists believe these help detoxify heavy metals	Do not give red clover to children younger than 2 y (Castleman, 1995)	Kemper, 1996b (no scientific studies done to date)

Table continued on following page

T A B L E 43-5

Complementary Treatments* for Some Common Conditions in Children and Adolescents† Continued

DIAGNOSIS	TREATMENT APPROACH	DOSAGE	BENEFIT	POSSIBLE SIDE EFFECTS*	RESEARCH/ CITATIONS
Headaches	Herbal				
	Feverfew (*Tanacetum parthenium*)	Children older than 2 yr: 25–50 mg bid (start with lower dose and increase as necessary) *or* chew 1–3 leaves daily. Change brands if no results seen after a few weeks; try for several months	Prevention of migraines: Inhibits release of blood vessel–dilating substances from platelets to decrease production of inflammatory substances and reestablish proper blood vessel tone. Benefits are similar to those of aspirin and NSAIDs, but if NSAIDs do not work, neither will feverfew because their properties are similar	Mouth sores, abdominal pain, allergic reactions usually within first week of use. Not to be used during pregnancy or in patients with clotting disorders. Sudden cessation may result in rebound headaches *Class 2b*	Murray & Pizzorno, 1998 (double-blind studies cited that showed reduction in number and severity of migraines—not for acute attacks); Castleman, 1995; Kemper, 1996a; McGuffin et al., 1997; *Therapeutic Use of Herbs,* 1977
	Biofeedback	6 yr and up: As needed to master techniques (8–10 wk)	For tension and migraine headaches: Patients learn to dilate blood vessels in body to affect blood flow to the head and relax muscles	None	Fugh-Berman, 1997 (cites studies showing success rates of 44–65% for muscle contraction headaches and 38% for migraines); Kemper, 1996b; Murray & Pizzorno, 1998; *Children Can Take Charge of Migraine,* 1998

Therapy	Technique/Description	Use	Complications	References
Massage	Head, neck, shoulder massage techniques using 1–2 drops peppermint or eucalyptus oil to 1 tsp vegetable oil as massage lotion	Muscle relaxation; oil may help decrease pain sensitivity	None reported	Kemper, 1996b (cites studies showing proven effectiveness)
Acupuncture	Age when therapy can be used depends on tolerance to needles	Use in conjunction with massage and relaxation	None reported	Kemper, 1996b (cites studies showing effectiveness for migraine prevention and tension headaches)
Chiropractic	Chiropractors "adjust" those of all ages by manipulating cervical/ thoracic vertebrae	Pain reduction, acute/ chronic	Few complications with cervical manipulation, less with other areas; issues with chiropractic occur when only manipulation is used and more appropriate medical diagnosis and treatment are delayed (e.g., encopresis, ear infections, diabetes, anemia, HTN, tumors)	Fugh-Berman, 1997; Nickerson & Silberman, 1992

Table continued on following page

T A B L E 43-5

Complementary Treatments* for Some Common Conditions in Children and Adolescents† *Continued*

DIAGNOSIS	TREATMENT APPROACH	DOSAGE	BENEFIT	POSSIBLE SIDE EFFECTS*	RESEARCH/ CITATIONS
Headaches *Continued*	Naturopathy and nutritional Elimination diet	Avoid nitrates, nitrites, aspartame, MSG, chocolate, aged cheeses, caffeine, wheat, oranges, eggs, milk, beef, corn, sugar, yeast, shellfish. Avoid Vit A and D and zinc	Benefits children with other allergy symptoms and frequent headaches. Vit A excess increases intracranial pressure; Vit D and zinc can cause headaches	None reported	Kemper, 1996b and 1998b; Murray & Pizzorno, 1998 (cites nonran- domized study showing 85% reduction in headaches)
	Increase magnesium-rich foods and include ginger and hot peppers, garlic, onion, vegetable oils, fish oils	Adolescents: Magnesium, 250–400 mg tid, + Vit B$_6$, 25 mg tid Ginger: Daily, 1/4 slice fresh or 500 mg qid dried or 100–200 mg extract tid (20% gingerol and shogaol for prevention) and 200 mg q2h for acute migraine	Low magnesium levels often found in patients with all types of headaches. Magnesium maintains blood vessel tone and prevents overexcitability of nerve cells; Vit B$_6$ increases intracellular Mg; ginger (contains aspirin-like compounds) exerts anti-inflammatory effects and decreases platelet aggregation	Diarrhea, gastric irritation	Kemper, 1996b; Murray & Pizzorno, 1998 (mixed results on double- blind studies cited)
	Homeopathy	Individualized homeopathic remedies	Reduction in intensity and frequency of attacks	Not recommend for children (Kemper, 1996b)	Fugh-Berman, 1997 (cites a double- blind, placebo- controlled study)

Hyperactivity-ADHD	Music therapy	Have children listen to calmer, low-pitched, slow-tempo music	Improved work performance, decreased tension and activity, has calming effect on autonomic nervous system	High-pitched music creates tension, low pitch stimulates relaxation, slow tempo is soothing, fast or stimulating music increases anxiety and activity	Kemper, 1996b (cited one study done in Israel showing hyperactive boys doing as well as normal boys when listening to calming music vs. no music vs. fast-paced music); Klein & Winkelstein, 1996; Thaut, 1998
	Biofeedback	Takes 6–8 wk to learn techniques, age dependent	More relaxed behavior, improved attention, improved language skills; technique focuses on reducing muscle tension in forehead		Kemper, 1996b (cites studies showing behavioral improvement equal to that of methylphenidate [Ritalin]; technique works best if also used with structured scheduling and behavioral rewards)

Table continued on following page

T A B L E 43-5

Complementary Treatments* for Some Common Conditions in Children and Adolescents† Continued

DIAGNOSIS	TREATMENT APPROACH	DOSAGE	BENEFIT	POSSIBLE SIDE EFFECTS*	RESEARCH/ CITATIONS
Hyperactivity-ADHD *Continued*	Nutritional/naturopathic				
	Elimination diet	Refer to Table 43–4. Also recommended is elimination of refined sugars and supplementation with a multivitamin that includes thiamin, niacin, Vit B₆, magnesium, manganese, potassium, and zinc	Decrease in irritability, insomnia, fidgetiness; improvement seen in up to 73% (Boris & Mandel, 1994). Vitamin deficiencies can result in impaired brain and nervous system function. Refined sugars thought to promote reactive hypoglycemia causing increased adrenaline secretion and hyperactivity (Murray & Pizzorno, 1998)	Elimination diet can put strain on family. Dietary management less likely to produce results with • discordant marital relationships present (Carter et al., 1993). May need consultation with nutritionist	Studies showed some behavioral changes in hyperactive children (not all studies used subjects meeting DSM III criteria) when challenged by specific food allergens (Carter et al., 1993; Egger et al., 1992; Rowe & Rowe, 1994; Boris & Mandel, 1994; Murray & Pizzorno, 1998). Kemper, 1996b, recommends elimination diet after other measures have failed to help (thinks studies fail to prove link between allergies/ sugar and hyperactive behavior in most children; elimination diets possibly more effective in atopic children)

	Dose/Preparation	Comments	Safety/Side Effects	Reference
Caffeine	Low doses	May boost benefit of methylphenidate without increasing side effects	Effects of caffeine (jittery, nervous, anxious, tired with withdrawal)	Kemper, 1996b
Yoga Meditation Guided therapy Therapeutic touch		Enhances relaxation	None reported	Kemper, 1996b
Jaundice Prayer therapy		Prayer healing has been shown to prevent RBCs from breaking down in test tubes; increase in hemoglobin in adults	None reported	Kemper, 1996b (studies done in adults only) Kemper, 1996b (studies done in adults only)
Nausea and vomiting Herbal Combination tea with chamomile, lemon balm, peppermint	Small, frequent sips	Soothing to stomach upsets	Safe unless existing allergy to ragweed or daisy family of plants *Class 1*	Kemper, 1996b
Goldenseal or barberry	Tincture: 2–3 drops in 4 oz water sipped slowly over 1 hr	Especially helpful if child has vomiting and diarrhea	None reported at therapeutic levels. Excessive levels can cause GI upset, CNS stimulation *Class 2b*	Kemper, 1996b
Basil tea	Make with 1/2 oz dry basil and 1 cup boiling water, steeped 5 min and strained		Not recommended for infants or toddlers *Class 2b*	Kemper, 1996b; McGuffin et al., 1997

Table continued on following page

T A B L E 43-5

Complementary Treatments* for Some Common Conditions in Children and Adolescents† Continued

DIAGNOSIS	TREATMENT APPROACH	DOSAGE	BENEFIT	POSSIBLE SIDE EFFECTS*	RESEARCH/ CITATIONS
Nausea and vomiting *Continued*	Ginger root	<3 y: 25 mg qid 3–6 y: 50–75 mg qid 6–12 y: 125 mg qid >13 y: 250 mg qid *or* Ginger tea: 1 cup water to 2 slices ginger root (simmer 5 min) *or* 1/4 tsp fresh grated ginger in juice, applesauce, cereal *or* Ginger soda (with real ginger)	Helpful to reduce nausea by promoting elimination of intestinal gas and reducing GI spasms	Not for long-term use; use only in recommended doses. Large doses can depress CNS, cause cardiac arrthymias, compromise platelet aggregation *Class 2b*	Kemper, 1996b; Therapeutic Uses of Herbs, 1997
	Poultice	Soak cotton flannel cloth in castor oil, lay cloth over abdomen, and cover with towel. Have child rest 1 hr, then remove cloth and rinse abdomen with baking soda/ water solution	Old folk remedy for nausea		Kemper, 1996b
	Nutritionals Vit B₆	Motion sickness and nausea of radiation therapy: 10 mg 1 hr before traveling	May help minimize nausea	None reported	Kemper, 1996b
	Hypnosis	Age dependent	Helpful in reducing recurrent vomiting/ nausea associated with chemotherapy or motion sickness		Kemper, 1996b

Acupressure	Apply pressure 1 in. above wrist crease, between the 2 tendons leading to the palm; repeat every 2 hr prn to control nausea	Controls nausea symptoms	None reported	Kemper, 1996b (few studies to date done on children but safe to try, per Kemper)
Otitis media				
Nutritional Elimination diet	Eliminate milk and dairy products, eggs, wheat, corn, oranges, peanut butter, concentrated simple carbohydrates (sugar, honey, dried fruit, concentrated fruit juices, etc.)	Boosts immune system by eliminating allergens thought to impede it. Decreases congestion of nasal mucous membranes that have impact on drainage of the eustachian tubes or insults to integrity of the middle ear	None reported	After elimination diet 86% of food-sensitive patients (71% of subjects) showed significant improvement in serous otitis media recurrence. Most subjects allergic to 2–4 foods, most to milk, wheat, egg, peanuts, soy, and corn (Nsouli et al., 1994). Tympanostomy tubes deemed inappropriate or of equivocal use in 58% of children (Kleinman et al., 1994)
Breast milk	All infants	Boosts immune system		Kemper, 1996b; Murray & Pizzorno, 1998
Herbal Echinacea	<6 yr: tincture (1:5) 1–2 ml up to tid or fluid extract (1:1) 1–2 ml up to tid >6 yr: double above doses		Safe unless patient has allergy to ragweed or daisy family of plants *Class 1*	

Table continued on following page

T A B L E 43-5

Complementary Treatments* for Some Common Conditions in Children and Adolescents† Continued

DIAGNOSIS	TREATMENT APPROACH	DOSAGE	BENEFIT	POSSIBLE SIDE EFFECTS*	RESEARCH/ CITATIONS
Premature infants	Massage	10–15 min tid	Facilitates growth and development and decreases medical complications	None reported; shorter duration of massage seems to produce less positive results	Fugh-Berman, 1997 (cites several studies supporting massage or stroking)
PMS	Herbal Black currant seed oil *or* Flaxseed oil *or* Evening primrose oil	As directed on label tid *or* 1000 mg tid	Important fatty acids help relieve PMS symptoms and aid glandular function	None. Flax needs to be taken with at least 6 oz of water; contraindicated with bowel obstruction *Class 1*	Balch & Balch, 1997 (other helpful suggestions offered in this reference); McGuffin et al., 1997
	Angelica or Dong Quai (*Angelica sinensis*)	Powered root or tea: 1–2 g tid Tincture (1:5): 4 ml tid Fluid extract: 1 ml tid	Roots contain phytoestrogens that nourish and tone female glandular and organ system	Do not use if patient is pregnant or nursing or has a history of cancer, cardiac problems, or photosensitivity; occasional light laxative effect *Class 2b*	Murray & Pizzorno, 1998 (other helpful preparations offered in this reference; cite supportive studies); Castleman, 1995
	Licorice root (*Glycyrrhiza glabra*)	Powered root or tea: 1–2 g tid Fluid extract (1:1): 4 ml tid Dry powdered extract (1:4): 250–500 mg tid	Reduces water retention of PMS; believed to lower estrogen levels and increase progesterone levels	Do not use if patient pregnant or breastfeeding or has glaucoma or diabetes, HTN, cardiac disease	Castleman, 1995; McGuffin et al., 1997; Therapeutic Uses of Herbs, 1998

Herb/Supplement	Dosage	Uses	Precautions	References
Black cohosh (*Cimicifuga racemosa*)	1 tablet once or twice daily	Useful for relieving cramps; may help with depression, anxiety, tension, mood swings	Use only with nonpregnant, non-nursing patients; not to be used in patients with cardiac disease or estrogen-dependent cancers. Overdose symptoms: nausea, diarrhea, abdominal pain, vomiting, dizziness, headache tremors, arthalgias *Class 2b*	Castleman, 1995; McGuffin et al., 1997; Murray & Pizzorno, 1998
Chasteberry (*Vitex agnus-castus*)	Dry powdered extract (0.5% agnuside content) 175–225 mg/d; Liquid extract: 2 ml/d	Useful with breast tenderness symptoms of PMS; appears to alter GnRH and FSH-RH to normalize secretion of prolactin and estrogen-progesterone ratio	Do not use in pregnant, lactating patients; occasional minor skin irritations *Class 2b*	McGuffin et al., 1997; Murray & Pizzorno, 1998; Therapeutic Uses of Herbs, 1998
Nutritional and naturopathic Calcium	1000 mg/d	Relieves cramping, backache, nervousness		Murray & Pizzorno, 1998
Magnesium	12 mg/kg per d	Helps with headaches		
Vit B complex plus extra: Vit B₆	100 mg tid 50–100 mg/d	B vitamins complement each other Decreases water retention, increases circulation to female organs, helps restore estrogen levels		Balch & Balch, 1997; Murray & Pizzorno, 1998

Table continued on following page

T A B L E 43-5

Complementary Treatments* for Some Common Conditions in Children and Adolescents† Continued

DIAGNOSIS	TREATMENT APPROACH	DOSAGE	BENEFIT	POSSIBLE SIDE EFFECTS*	RESEARCH/CITATIONS
PMS *Continued*	Vit E	400 IU/d	Helps with breast tenderness, depression, irritability; improves oxygen profusion to body		
	Zinc	15–20 mg/d	Promotes hormone balance. Controls prolactin secretion		Micozzi, 1996
	Diet	Eat plenty of fresh fruits, vegetable, whole-grain cereals and breads, beans, peas, lentils, nuts and seeds, broiled fowl, fish, high-protein foods as snacks, and soy products. Avoid salt, red meats, processed foods, junk/fast foods, caffeine, refined sugar; and fewer dairy products 1 wk before menses; increase water intake to 1 qt distilled water/d 1 wk before menses and continue 1 wk after onset	Red meats and dairy products believed to contribute to hormonal fluctuations. Other recommended foods aid in metabolism, maintenance of blood glucose, and absorption of nutrients; decreases free estrogen in blood. Excluding salt decreases bloating and water retention. Dairy products and refined sugars also believed to increase excretion of magnesium with consequent impaired estrogen metabolism and moodiness		
	Chiropractic		For cramps: possibly alters prostaglandin levels		Fugh-Berman, 1997 (cites studies)
	Acupuncture		For cramps		Fugh-Berman, 1997 (cites studies); NIH, 1998

Skin irritation/ diaper rash				
Yoga				
Herbal				
Aloe vera	All ages: Pure gel form applied topically several times daily	Antibacterial effects; accelerates healing from dermabrasions	Contact dermatitis *Class 1*	Kemper, 1996a; Murray & Pizzorno, 1998
Chamomile	Add essential oil to bath or make as tea and rub affected area	Soothes diaper rash, varicella, contact dermatitis	Contact dermatitis; use in caution in patients with allergy to ragweed or daisy family of plants *Class 1*	Kemper, 1996b
Nutritional				
Zinc	Infants: 10 mg/d for formula-fed infants with history of yeast diaper rashes	May help prevent yeast diaper rash in formula-fed infants (does not apply to breastfed infants)		Kemper, 1996b (cites study showing that infants with frequent diaper rashes have lower levels of zinc in their bodies)
Live *Acidophilus* bacteria	Infants older than 6 mo: give as yogurt; 1 cup daily for children 12 mo and older	Thought to help replace the yeast on the skin		Kemper, 1996b

ADHD = attention-deficit hyperactivity disorder; bid = twice daily; BP = blood pressure; cap = capsule; CNS = central nervous system; DSM IV = *Diagnostic and Statistical Manual of Mental Disorders*, 4th ed; FDA = Food and Drug Administration; FSH-RH = follicle-stimulating hormone–releasing hormone; GI = gastrointestinal; GnRH = gonadotropin-releasing hormone; HIV = human immunodeficiency virus; HTN = hypertension; MAO = monoamine oxidase; MSG = monosodium glutamate; NIH = National Institutes of Health; NSAID = nonsteroidal anti-inflammatory drug; ORS = oral rehydration solution; PMS = premenstrual syndrome; PO = by mouth; prn = as needed; qid = four times daily; RBC = red blood cell; s = seconds; TB = tuberculosis; tbsp = tablespoon; tid = three times daily; tsp = teaspoon; Vit = vitamin.

***Inclusion of a complementary treatment in this table does not imply endorsement by this textbook's authors; for reference only.**

†DSM IV.

‡Food supplements and herbal labeling classifications:

Class 1—Herb can be safely consumed when used appropriately

Class 2—The following use restrictions apply:

    2a: For external use only

    2b: Not to be used during pregnancy

    2c: Not to be used while nursing

    2d: Other specific use restrictions as noted

RESOURCES BOX 43-1

Office of Alternative Medicine (OAM)
National Institutes of Health
Tel: (888) 644-6226
Fax: (301) 495-4957
Website: www.altmed.od.nih.gov.

Center for Holistic Pediatric Education and
Research (CHPER)
Tel: (617) 355-2576
Website: www.childrenshospital.org/holistic

American Holistic Nurses Association
Tel: (919) 787-0116

Alternative Medicine Homepage
Website: www.pitt.edu/~cbw/altm.html
Lists alternative medicine resources available
on the Internet

Federation of State Medical Licensing
Tel: (817) 868-4000
E-mail: FSMB.org

Food and Drug Administration
Special Nutritional Adverse Event Monitoring
System (SN/AEMS)
Website: www.fda.gov

Massage Therapy
American Massage Therapy Association
Tel: (847) 864-0123
Fax: (847) 864-1178
Website: www.amtamassage.org.
Maintains national list of qualified therapists

Touch Research Institute
Tel: (305) 243-6781
Fax: (305) 243-6488

Acupuncture
American Academy of Medical Acupuncture
Tel: (213) 937-5514, (800) 521-2262 (referral
information)

National Certification Commission for Acupuncture and
Oriental Medicine
Tel: (202) 232-1404

Herbal Therapy
World Health Organization
Collaborating Center for International Drug
Monitoring
Website: www.who.int/dap/drug-info.html

American Botanical Council (ABC)
Tel: (512) 331-8868
Fax: (512) 331-1924
Website: www.herbalgram.org.
Free educational materials and quarterly journal
"Herbal Gram"

Chiropractic
Federation of Chiropractic Licensing Boards
Tel: (970) 356-3500
Website: www.fclb.org/fclb

Homeopathy
National Center for Homeopathy
Tel: (703) 548-7790
Website: www.homeopathic.org

Music Therapy
American Music Therapy Association (AMTA)
Tel: 301-589-3300
Website: www.namt.com

Naturopathy
American Association of Naturopathic
Physicians (AANP)
Tel: (206) 328-8510
Website: www.infinite.org
Naturopathic.Physician

RESOURCE BOX 43-2

FURTHER READING RESOURCES:

Complementary Medicine for the Physician (ISSN 1087-0865, published ten times per year)
Periodicals Department
6277 Sea Harbor Dr
Orlando, FL 32887-4800

Illustrated Encyclopedia of Healing Remedies
C. Norman Shealey, MD, Editor
Penguin Putman
Tel: (800) 253-6476

Alternative Medicine: The Definitive Guide
Burton Goldberg Group
Washington, DC
Future Medicine Publishing Inc, 1994

The Honest Herbal: A Sensible Guide to the Use of Herbs and Related Remedies, 3rd ed
Binghamton, NY
Pharmaceutical Products Press, 1992

University of California Wellness Letter: The News-letter of Nutrition, Fitness and Stress Management
Published monthly by Health Letter Associates
PO Box 420148
Palm Coast, FL 32142

American Herbal Products Association's Botanical Safety Handbook
McGuffin M, Hobbs C, Upton R, et al (eds)
Boca Raton, FL
CRC Press, 1997

PDR for Herbal Medicines
Published by Medical Economics
Tel: (800) 859-8053 to order ($59.95)

NPs may personally want to begin incorporating some complementary approaches into their own practices according to their own comfort level. The families' desires for more integrative medical care are more likely met when NPs act as advocates, active participants, listeners, and/or facilitators.

The complementary therapeutics in Table 43-5 were chosen by the specific referenced authors on the basis of evidence-based research as being clinically reasonable or holding clues to promising areas needing further research. Physician authors from both Western medicine and naturopathic professions have been used to compile this table. This information is included for the reader's reference. Knowledge of the following terms will be useful to NPs using Table 43-5 for reference.

Glossary of Terms Used in the Preparation of Herbal Treatments

Standardized: An herbal product that contains a *specified concentration of one ingredient* of the plant; it may contain other nonstandardized ingredients from the same plant.

Essential oils: Also known as volatile or aromatic oils and found in many plants. These oils are highly concentrated and potent and not to be taken internally.

Infusion: Preparation similar to tea. The dried herb is steeped in boiling water for 5 to 10 minutes and strained; the preparation can be sweetened to make it more palatable; drink warm or cold.

Tincture: A concentrated extract of an herb made with a mixture of cold water and alcohol (typically 25, 40, 60 or 90% alcohol). The tincture usually is diluted four to five times with water or juice for children; tinctures should not be given internally to children younger than 2 years.

Inclusion of a complementary treatment in Table 43-5 does not imply endorsement by this textbook's authors. Herbal remedies are too numerous to list; it is suggested that the NP use a good reference source that cites research and safety precautions. The Resource Box at the end of this chapter provides several suggestions.

REFERENCES

Abrams G: Chiropractic treatment holds promise for low back pain. Complement Med Physician 2(9):66, 1997.

Acupuncture scores points. *University of California Wellness Letter* 14(8):2, 1998.

Astin J: Why patients use alternative medicine. JAMA 279:1548-1553, 1998.

Balch J, Balch P: Prescription for Nutritional Healing, 2nd ed. Garden City, NY, Avery, 1997.

Bates B: Natural remedies can cause skin reactions. Pediatr News Feb, 44, 1998.

Boris M, Mandel F: Foods and additives are common causes

of the attention deficit hyperactive disorder in children. Ann Allergy 72:462-468, 1994.

Burr ML, Merrett TG, Dunstan FDJ, et al: The development of atopy in high-risk children. Pediatrics 102:447, 1998.

Businco L, Falconieri P, Giampietro P, et al: Food allergy and asthma. Pediatr Pulmonol 11(suppl):S59-60, 1995.

Carter CM, Urbanowicz M, Hemsley R, et al: Effects of a few food diet in attention deficit disorder. Arch Dis Child 69:564-568, 1993.

Castleman M: The Healing Herbs: The Ultimate Guide to the Curative Power of Nature's Medicines. New York, Bantam, 1995.

Children can take charge of migraine. Clin Rev 8(11):122, 1998.

Classification of Complementary and Alternative Medical Practices: Office of Alternative Medicine Information Package. Silver Spring, MD, Office of Alternative Medicine Clearinghouse, 1997.

David TJ, Patel L, Ewing CI, et al: Dietary regimens for atopic dermatitis in childhood. J R Soc Med 90(suppl 30):S9-14, 1997.

Drew A, Myers S: Safety issues in herbal medicine: Implications for the health professions. Med J Aust 166:538-541, 1997.

Eisenberg DM: Advising patients who seek alternative therapies. Ann Intern Med 127:61-69, 1997.

Eisenberg DM, Davis R, Ettner S, et al: Trends in alternative medicine use in the United States, 1990-1997: Results of a follow-up national survey. JAMA 280:1569-1575, 1998.

Eisenberg DM, Kessler RC, Foster D, et al: Unconventional medicine in the United States: Prevalence, costs and patterns of use. N Engl J Med 328:246-252, 1993.

Egger J, Stolla A, McEwen L: Controlled trial of hyposensitisation in children with food-induced hyperkinetic syndrome. Lancet 339:1150-1153, 1992.

Elder NC, Gillcrist A, Minz R: Use of alternative health care by family practice patients. Arch Fam Med 6:181-184, 1997.

Field T, Henteleff T, Hernandez-Reif M, et al: Children with asthma have improved pulmonary functions with massage therapy. J Pediatr 132:854-858, 1998.

Frishberg M: Alternative medicine gaining wider acceptance. Common Ground Reflections Jan:8-24, 1998.

French M: The power of plants: An overview of herbal therapies. Adv Nurse Pract 4(7):17-21, 1996.

Fugh-Berman A: Alternative Medicine: What Works. Baltimore, Williams & Wilkins, 1997.

Gideonse T: Music is good medicine. Newsweek Sep:103, 1998.

Gordon J: Alternative medicine and the family physician. Am Fam Physician 54:2205-2212, 1996.

Green E, Moore B, Field T: Massage therapy: Wide-ranging medical applicability and benefit. Complement Med Physician 2(9):1, 1997.

Isolauri E: Intestinal involvement in atopic disease. J R Soc Med 90(suppl 30):S15-20, 1997.

Herbal Medicine Taken as a Whole. Clin Advisor 1(11/12):51, 1998.

Janiger O, Goldberg P: A Different Kind of Healing. New York, Putnam, 1993.

Jonas W: General Overview: General Information Packet.

Office of Alternative Medicine, National Institutes of Health, Silver Spring, MD, 1996.

Jonas W: Alternative medicine—learning from the past, examining the present, advancing to the future. JAMA 280:1616-1617, 1998.

Kass-Annese B: Complementary health care in the US: Role of the NP. Contemp Nurse Pract Summer:22-30, 1997.

Kava. Harvard Women's Health Watch 5(12):69, 1998.

Kemper K: Seven herbs every pediatrician should know. Contemp Pediatr 13(12):79-91, 1996a.

Kemper K: The Holistic Pediatrician. New York, HarperCollins, 1996b.

Kemper K: Personal communication to author, Nov 24, 1998a.

Kemper K: Integrated pediatrics: A holistic approach to healing children. Complement Med Physician 3(10):1, 1998b.

Klein S, Winkelstein M: Enhancing pediatric health care with music. J Pediatr Health Care 10:74-81, 1996.

Kleinman L, Kosecoff J, Dubois R, et al: The medical appropriateness of tympanostomy tubes proposed for children younger than 16 years in the United States. JAMA 271:1250-1255, 1994.

Loeb H, Vandenplas Y, Wursch P, et al: Tannin-rich carob pod for the treatment of acute-onset diarrhea. J Pediatr Gastroenterol Nutr 8:480-485, 1989.

Mack R: "Something wicked this way comes"—herbs even witches should avoid. Contemp Pediatr 15(6):49-64, 1998.

Markestad T: Use of sucrose as a treatment for infant colic. Arch Dis Child 76:356-358, 1997.

McGuffin M, Hobbs C, Upton R, et al (eds): American Herbal Products Association's Botanical Safety Handbook. Boca Raton, FL, CRC Press, 1997.

Micozzi M: Fundamentals of Complementary and Alternative Medicine. New York, Churchill Livingstone, 1996.

Micozzi M: The common principles of complementary health care systems: Enduring concepts with current clinical relevance. Complement Med Physician 2(8):1, 1997.

Murray M, Pizzorno J: Encyclopedia of Natural Medicine. 2nd ed. Rocklin, CA, Prima Health, 1998.

Murray R, Rubel A: Physicians and healers—unwitting partners in health care. N Engl J Med 326:61-64, 1992.

NIH Consensus Conference. Acupuncture. JAMA 280:1518-1524, 1998.

Nickerson J, Silberman T: Chiropractic manipulation in children. J Pediatr 12:172, 1992.

Nsouli TM, Nsouli SM, Linde RE, et al: Role of food allergy in serous otitis media. Ann Allergy 73:215-219, 1994.

Nutrition News from A to Z: What was hot (and not) in '98. Environm Nutr Newslett Food Nutr Health 21:12, 1998.

O'Brien M: Integrated geriatrics: Optimizing and gentling health care for the elderly. Complement Med Physician 3(5):1, 1998.

Office of Alternative Medicine Clearinghouse Website, 1998: http://altmed.od.nih.gov.

PA and NP Opinions on Alternative Therapies. Clin News Mar/Apr:12, 1998.

Plaut M: New directions in food allergy research. J Allergy Clin Immunol 100:7-10, 1997.

Rowe K, Rowe K: Synthetic food coloring and behavior: A dose response effect in a double-blind placebo-controlled, repeated-measure study. J Pediatr 125:691–697, 1994.

Saarinen U, Kajosaari M: Breastfeeding as prophylaxis against atopic disease: Prospective follow-up study under 17 years. Lancet 346:1065–1069, 1995.

Sampson H: Food sensitivity and the pathogenesis of atopic dermatitis. J R Soc Med 90(suppl 30):S2–8, 1997.

Slagle M: The nurse practitioner and issues of alternative therapies. Nurse Pract 21(2):16–19, 1996.

Spigelblatt L: Alternative medicine: A pediatric conundrum. Contemp Pediatr 14(8):51–64, 1997.

Thaut M: Music therapy: The unsung modality. Complement Med Physician 3(6):1, 1998.

The Landmark Report on Public Perceptions of Alternative Care. Sacramento, CA, Landmark Healthcare, 1998.

Therapeutic Uses of Herbs. Continuing Education #97-005. Prescriber's Letter, Fall 1997.

Therapeutic Uses of Herbs. Continuing Education Booklet. Prescriber's Letter, Spring 1998.

Turow V: Alternative therapy for colds (Letter). Pediatrics 100:274–275, 1997a.

Turow V: Chiropractic for children. Arch Pediatr Adolesc Med 151:527–528, 1997b.

Wysocki S: Unconventional and conventional medicine: Searching for common ground. Contemp Nurse Pract Winter: 3–15, 1997.

Young L: (Alternative medicine)....also popular among NPs. Nurse Pract World News 3(5):3–15, 1998.

Medications

Melanie A. Canady

This is an abbreviated listing of medications used by the NP. It is the responsibility of the reader/prescriber to seek detailed information and thoroughly investigate the drug being prescribed. The authors take no responsibility for any errors in prescribing.

Medications

GENERIC/TRADE CLASSIFICATION	DOSE/INDICATIONS	SUPPLIED	REMARKS
Acetaminophen (Tylenol, Tempra) *Miscellaneous analgesic and antipyretic*	10–15 mg/kg/dose q4–6 hr PO (max. 5 doses) Adults: 325–650 mg q4–6 hr PO (max. 4 g/d) Treatment of mild to moderate pain and fever	80 mg/0.8 ml drops 160 mg/tsp elixir 80, 160 mg chewable 160, 325, 500 mg tab 80, 120, 325, 650 mg suppository	Drug interactions: barbiturates, carbamazepine, hydantoins, rifampin, sulfinpyrazone. Can cause severe hepatic toxicity with overdose.
Acetaminophen with codeine *Analgesic and antipyretic*	0.5–1 mg codeine/kg/dose q4–6 hr PO Adults: 15–60 mg q4–6 hr PO	Tylenol 120 mg and codeine 12 mg/tsp #1 tab—Tylenol 300 mg, codeine 7.5 mg #2 tab—Tylenol 300 mg, codeine 15 mg #3 tab—Tylenol 300 mg, codeine 30 mg #4 tab—Tylenol 300 mg, codeine 60 mg	Can cause respiratory depression. Codeine can cause nausea, vomiting, constipation.
Acyclovir (Zovirax) *Antiviral*	Genital herpes infection: Adults: 200 mg PO q4 hr (5 capsules/d) for 10 d: recurrent infection, treat for 5 d: suppressive therapy: 200 mg PO tid for 6 mo HSV infections in immunocompromised patients: Children <12 yr: 250 mg/m^2 IV q8 hr for 7 d (5 d for genital herpes) Adults: 5 mg/kg IV q8 hr for 7 d (5 d for genital herpes) Varicella infections (PO): Children: 10–20 mg/kg/dose qid (max. 800 mg/d) for 5 d Adults: 800 mg/dose qid for 5 d Mucocutaneous herpes simplex virus (HSV) infections: Adults and children: cover all lesions with ointment q3 hr, 6 times/d for 7 d	200 mg/5 ml suspension 200 mg capsule 500 mg vial for infection 5% ointment (15, 30 g)	Therapy should be started at the first sign of infection. Use gloves when applying ointment. Adverse effects: renal toxicity (reversible), neurotoxicity, GI disturbances. Avoid contact with eyes when using ointment.

Drug (Brand) Class	Indications/Dosage	How Supplied	Comments
Albuterol sulfate (Proventil, Ventolin) *Bronchodilator*	Treatment of bronchospasm: Children <5 yr: 0.1–0.2 mg/ kg/dose PO tid (max. 2 mg tid) Children 6–11 yr: 2 mg PO tid–qid Nebulizer: 0.15 mg/kg/dose q4 hr prn; MDI: Children >4 yr and adults: 2 inhalations q4–6 hr prn Adults: 2–4 mg PO q4–6 hr or 4–8 mg q12 hr Exercise-induced bronchospasm: >12 yr: 2 inhalations 15 min before exercise	2 mg/5 ml syrup 2, 4 mg tab 4 mg sustained-release tab 5 mg/ml inhalation solution 90 µg/metered spray	Common side effects: tachycardia, tremor, palpitations. Do not administer with MAO inhibitors or tricyclic antidepressants.
Amantadine HCl (Symmetrel) *Antiviral*	Prophylaxis or symptomatic relief of influenza A: Adults <64 yr and children >10 yr: 200 mg/d PO; continue 24–48 hr after symptoms disappear Children 1–9 yr: 4.4–8.8 mg/ kg/d PO divided bid–tid (max. 150 mg/d)	50 mg/5 ml syrup 100 mg capsule	Not recommended for children < age 1 yr. Do not administer with alcohol or stimulants.
Ammonium lactate (LAC-Hydrin 12%) *Miscellaneous rehydrating lotion*	Apply twice daily to affected areas Used in the treatment of moderate to severe xerosis and ichthyosis vulgaris	Lotion (225, 400 g)	Avoid contact with lips, eyes, mucous membranes. Transient stinging, burning, erythema.

Table continued on following page

Medications *Continued*

GENERIC/TRADE CLASSIFICATION	DOSE/INDICATIONS	SUPPLIED	REMARKS
Amoxicillin (Amoxil, Polymax, Trimox, Ultimox) *Penicillin*	Children: 40–90 mg/kg/d PO divided bid-tid Adults: 250 mg PO bid-tid (max. 2–3 g/d) Respiratory tract infections, sinusitis, skin, otitis, urinary tract, gonorrhea, streptococcal infections	50 mg/ml drops (#15, 30 ml) 125, 200, 250, 400 mg/tsp suspension 125, 200, 250, 400 mg chewable 250, 500, 875 mg capsule	Prophylaxis for otitis media with effusion: 20 mg/kg/d. Can cause a rash if given to a patient with mononucleosis. Side effects: GI.
Amoxicillin and clavulanate (Augmentin) *Penicillin, beta-lactamase inhibitor*	Children: 25–80 mg/kg/d PO divided bid-tid Adults: 250–500 mg PO tid (max two g/d) or 875 mg bid Lower respiratory tract infections, otitis media, sinusitis, skin (periorbital cellulitis, human/animal bites)	125, 200, 250, 400 mg/tsp suspension (#75, 150 ml) 125, 200, 250, 400 mg chewable 250, 500, 875 mg tab (two 250 mg tabs do not equal one 500 mg tab)	Fewer side effects at bid dosing with 45 mg/kg/d. GI side effects—give with food. Peanut butter and cherry yogurt have been shown to decrease GI side effects.
Antipyrine and benzocaine (Auralgan) *Local anesthetic*	Fill ear canal with drops; may use q2–4 hr Used for temporary relief of pain associated with otitis media	Otic solution (antipyrine 5.4%, benzocaine 1.4%)	Not for prolonged use. Do not use if TM is perforated.
Azelastine hydrochloride (Astelin) *Antihistamine*	>12 yr: 2 sprays per nostril bid Allergic rhinitis	Nasal spray (100 sprays/bottle)	Drug interactions: cimetidine, CNS depressants. Side effects: bitter taste, fatigue, HA.

Drug	Indications/Dosage	Supplied	Comments
Azithromycin (Zithromax) *Macrolide*	Children >6 mo: otitis media 10 mg/kg on day 1, 5 mg/kg on days 2–5. Give once daily Pharyngitis/tonsillitis > 2 yr: 12 mg/kg/d, days 1–5 Adults: 500 mg on day 1, then 250 mg days 2–5. Give once daily. Pharyngitis, pneumonia, skin and soft tissue disorders, gonococcal urethritis and cervicitis due to *Chlamydia trachomatis* (single dose); otitis media, sinusitis, pneumonia, streptococcal pharyngitis (5-d course); nontuberculous mycobacterial infections	250 mg tab 100 mg/tsp, 200 mg/tsp suspension 1 g single-dose packet	Food decreases bioavailability of capsules. Theophylline effect unknown. Alternative when erythromycin ethylsuccinate not tolerated. Some strains of streptococcus are resistant to azithromycin. Drug interactions: Propulsid, digoxin, theophylline.
Bacitracin, neomycin, polymyxin B (Neosporin) *Topical antibiotic*	Apply 1–3 times daily Used to prevent infection in minor wounds	Ointment	
Bacitracin, neomycin, polymyxin B (Neosporin) *Antibiotic, ophthalmic*	Ointment: apply q3–4 hr for 7–10 d Solution: 3 or 4 times daily Treatment of external ocular infections	Ophthalmic ointment, solution	High incidence of sensitivity reactions, which can include redness, itching, edema.
Bacitracin, neomycin, polymyxin B, and hydrocortisone (Cortisporin) *Antibiotic, anti-inflammatory*	Otic suspension: 2–3 drops 3-4 times daily for 7 d Treatment of topical infections	Otic suspension, solution	Otic suspension should be used if tympanic membrane is not intact.

Table continued on following page

T A B L E A-1
Medications Continued

GENERIC/TRADE CLASSIFICATION	DOSE/INDICATIONS	SUPPLIED	REMARKS
Beclomethasone dipropionate (Beclovent, Beconase, Vanceril, Vanceril DS, Vancenase-AQ) *Glucocorticoid, anti-inflammatory*	Children 6–12 yr (oral inhalation): 1 or 2 inhalations 3 or 4 times daily (max. 10 inhalations/d), DS 2 puffs bid Adults (oral inhalation): 2 inhalations 3 or 4 times daily (max. 20 inhalations/d) Adults (nasal): 1 spray to each nostril 2–4 times daily or 2 sprays/nostril bid Aqueous (AQ) solution: 1-2 sprays/nostril bid Used in the treatment of asthma, seasonal allergic rhinitis, and nasal polyps	Inhalation, oral, nasal: 42 µg/inhalation; 84 µg/inhalation AQ solution, nasal: 42 µg/inhalation	Contraindicated in patients with status asthmaticus. Use cautiously in patients with tuberculosis and those on oral steroids. Adverse reactions: hypothalamic-pituitary-adrenal axis suppression, oral candidiasis, headache, nasal irritation. Rinse mouth well following oral inhalation. When changing from oral to inhaled steroids, allow an overlap of at least 2 wk.
Benzonatate (Tessalon Perles) *Non-narcotic antitussive*	Children >10 yr and adults: 100 mg PO tid (max. 6 perles/d) Used for cough suppression	100 mg perles	No respiratory depression. Do not chew perles—can cause oropharyngeal anesthesia.
Benzoyl peroxide (2%, 5%, 10%) (Benzagel, Desquam-E, Desquam-X, Ersa-Gel) *Keratolytic agent*	Apply sparingly 1–3 times daily; effective alone or in conjunction with tretinoin or topical antibiotics Used in mild to moderate acne	5%, 10% gel 5%, 10% wash	Avoid contact with eyes, lips, mucous membranes. Adverse reactions: burning, swelling, peeling. Areas should be cleaned prior to applying. Can bleach fabrics.

Drug	Dosage/Use	How supplied	Comments
Bethanechol chloride (Duvoid, Urecholine) *Urinary tract and GI tract stimulant*	Children: 0.6 mg/kg/d divided 3 or 4 times daily; for gastroesophageal reflux, 0.1–0.2 mg/kg given 1 hr prior to meals (max. 4 times daily). Adults: 10–50 mg PO bid–qid, 5–10 mg SC q4 h for neurogenic bladder. Used to treat nonobstructive urinary retention, abdominal distention, gastroesophageal reflux. Adjunctive therapy for irritable bowel syndrome, colitis, spastic bladder, peptic ulcer disease	1 mg/ml solution (not available at all pharmacies) 5, 10, 25 mg tablets 5 mg/ml injection	Contraindicated in patients with hyperthyroidism, hypotension, coronary artery disease, peptic ulcer disease, asthma. Give on empty stomach. Adverse reactions: cramping, nausea, flushing.
Bisacodyl (Dulcolax) *Stimulant laxative*	Children <3 yr: 5 mg rectally. Children 3–12 yr: 5–10 mg or 0.3 mg/kg/d PO or 10 mg rectally. Adults: 10–15 mg PO (max. 30 mg); 10 mg rectally. Used to treat chronic constipation, bowel preparation	5 mg enteric-coated tablet 10 mg rectal suppository	Drug interactions: antacids. Do not crush tablets.
Bitolterol mesylate (Tornalate) *Bronchodilator*	Bronchial asthma, bronchospasm: Adults and children >12 yr: 2 inhalations q4–8 hr prn	370 µg/metered spray	Cardiotoxic effects can be increased if used in conjunction with theophylline.

Table continued on following page

Medications Continued

GENERIC/TRADE CLASSIFICATION	DOSE/INDICATIONS	SUPPLIED	REMARKS
Brompheniramine maleate (Bromphen, Chlorphed, Codimal A, Conjec-B, Cophene-B, Dehist, Dimetone, Nasahist B, Oraminic II, Sinusol-B, Veltane) *Antihistamine*	0.5 mg/kg/d divided q6 hr, PO/IV/SC Children >6 yr: 2–4 mg PO tid–qid, or 8–12 mg q12 hr (max. 12–24 mg/d) Adults: 4–8 mg tid–qid PO/IV/SC (max. 24 mg/d)	2 mg/tsp 4 mg tab 8, 12 mg time-released tab 10 mg/ml injection	Less drowsiness than with other antihistamines. Children <6 yr can experience hyperexcitability.
Budesonide (Pulmicort Turbuhaler) *Corticosteroid*	Children >6 yr and adults: 1 or 2 inhalations bid Maintenance and prophylactic therapy for asthma	Turbuhaler, 200 µg/dose, 200 doses	Drug interactions: ketoconazole. Side effects: dry mouth, oral candidiasis, HA, insomnia, GI disturbance.
Budesonide (Rhinocort) *Corticosteroid*	Children ≥ 6 yr and adults: 2 sprays per nostril bid or 4 sprays per nostril qd Allergic or perennial rhinitis	32 µg/spray Nasal inhaler, 200 metered doses per canister	Side effects: nasal irritation, epistaxis, pharyngitis, dry mouth.
Carbamazepine (Epitol, Mazepine, Tegretol) *Miscellaneous anticonvulsant*	<6 yr: initial, 5 mg/kg/d: can increase q wk to 10 mg/kg/d divided bid–qid (max. 20 mg/kg/d) 6–12 yr: initially, 100 mg bid or 10 mg/kg/d divided bid; can increase by 100 mg/d until therapeutic levels (max. 1000 mg/d) >12 yr: 200 mg bid initially; increase by 200 mg/d to therapeutic levels; usual dose: 600–1200 mg/d divided q6–8 hr Maintenance: 10–20 mg/kg/d divided q6–12 hr	100 mg/tsp 100 mg chewable 200 mg tab 100, 200, 400 mg XR	Take with food. Monitor blood work with long-term therapy. Suspension has to be given 3–4 times daily, tabs 2–4 times daily. XR tabs dosed bid and should not be crushed. Therapeutic range 4–12 µg/ml. Drug interactions: erythromycin, isoniazid, warfarin, propoxyphene, doxycycline, verapamil. Cross-sensitivities with tricyclic antidepressants.

Drug	Indications and Dosing	Formulations	Comments
Cefaclor (Ceclor) *Second-generation cephalosporin*	Children: 20–40 mg/kg/d PO bid or tid Adults: 250–500 mg PO tid Respiratory tract, otitis media, sinusitis; skin, bone and joint, urinary tract infections; streptococcal pharyngitis	125, 250 mg/tsp (#75, 150 ml) 187, 375 mg/tsp bid dosing 250, 500 mg capsule	Use cautiously in patients with penicillin allergy. Hypersensitivity reaction—serum sickness.
Cefadroxil monohydrate (Duricef, Ultracef) *First-generation cephalosporin*	Children: 30 mg/kg/d PO qd or divided bid Adults: 500 mg PO bid Serious skin infections, urinary tract, bone and joint, streptococcal infections	125, 250, 500 mg/tsp (#50, 100 ml) 500, 1000 mg tab	Can dose qd for streptococcal pharyngitis. Use cautiously in patients with serious penicillin hypersensitivity.
Cefdinir (Omnicef) *Cephalosporin antibiotic*	6 mo–12 yr: 7 mg/kg q12 hr or 14 mg/kg qd Bid dosing only for skin infections Otitis, sinusitis, pharyngitis, skin infections, pneumonia (community acquired), bronchitis	300 mg capsules 125 mg/5 ml suspension	Drug interaction: antacids, iron Side effects: GI disturbances, vaginitis
Cefixime (Suprax) *Third-generation cephalosporin*	Children: 8 mg/kg/d PO divided qd–bid (max. dose 400 mg) Adults: 200 mg bid or 400 mg qd PO Uncomplicated urinary tract infections, bronchitis, pharyngitis, tonsillitis, skin disorders (poor *Staphylococcus aureus* coverage), *Shigella* gastroenteritis, otitis media	100 mg/tsp (#50, 100 ml) 200, 400 mg tab	Can be given as a single dose. Not indicated for infants <6 mo. Treat otitis media with suspension—gives higher therapeutic levels. GI symptoms common.

Table continued on following page

Medications *Continued*

GENERIC/TRADE CLASSIFICATION	DOSE/INDICATIONS	SUPPLIED	REMARKS
Cefotaxime sodium (Claforan) *Third-generation cephalosporin*	Children: 100–150 mg/kg/d divided q6–8 hr IV/IM Meningitis: 200 mg/kg/d divided q6 hr Adults: 1–2 g/d q6–8 hr (max. 12 g/d) Skin, septicemia, bone, urinary tract, respiratory tract, gynecological infections	0.5, 1.2 g vial	GI side effects.
Cefpodoxime proxetil (Vantin) *Third-generation cephalosporin*	Children: 10 mg/kg/d PO divided bid (max. 400 mg/d) Adults: Pneumonia: 400 mg/d for 14 d Gonorrhea: 200 mg/d for 1 dose Skin: 800 mg/d divided bid for 7–14 d Pharyngitis: 200 mg/d divided bid for 10 d Complicated urinary tract: 200 mg/d divided bid for 7–10 d	50, 100 mg/tsp 100, 200 mg tab	Not indicated for infants <6 mo. Lemon-flavored suspension not very palatable.
Cefprozil (Cefzil) *Second-generation cephalosporin*	Children: 30 mg/kg/d divided bid PO—otitis media, upper respiratory tract; 15 mg/kg/d divided bid PO—pharyngitis, skin, tonsillitis, lower respiratory tract Adults: 500 mg/d PO—pharyngitis, tonsillitis, lower respiratory tract, skin	125, 250 mg/tsp 250, 500 mg tab	Not indicated for infants <6 mo. Less efficacy against *Haemophilus influenzae* and *Moraxella catarrhalis* than other antibiotics.

Drug	Dosage	How supplied	Comments
Ceftibuten (Cedax) *Third-generation cephalosporin*	Children >6 mo: 9 mg/kg/d given as a single dose PO for 10 d (max. 400 mg/d) Adults: 400 mg PO qd for 10 d Bronchitis, otitis media, pharyngitis, and tonsillitis	90 mg/tsp 180 mg/tsp 400 mg capsule	Active against beta-lactamase producing strains. Give suspension on empty stomach.
Ceftriaxone (Rocephin) *Third-generation cephalosporin*	Children: 50–75 mg/kg/d divided 1–2 times daily, IV/IM Meningitis: 100 mg/kg/d IV/IM Adults: 1–2 g q12–24 hr IV/IM (max. 4 g/d) Skin, bone and joint, urinary tract, gynecological, respiratory tract, intra-abdominal infections, bacteremia	0.25, 0.5, 1, 5, 10 g vial	GI side effects. Mix with lidocaine to prevent pain at IM injection site.
Cefuroxime axetil (Ceftin) *Second-generation cephalosporin*	Children: <2 yr: 30 mg/kg/d divided bid PO 2–12 yr: 250 mg bid PO Adults: 250–500 mg bid PO Pharyngitis, tonsillitis, skin, otitis media, lower respiratory tract, urinary tract, uncomplicated gonorrhea (single 1-g dose)	125, 250, 500 mg tab 125 mg/tsp suspension 250 mg/tsp suspension	Crushed tab has bitter taste.
Cephalexin monohydrate (Keflex, Keftab, Novolexin, Keflet) *First-generation cephalosporin*	Children: 25–50 mg/kg/d divided tid PO Adults: 250–1000 mg tid PO (max 4 g/d) Skin, bone and joint, septicemia, respiratory tract, urinary tract, otitis media, pharyngitis	125, 250 mg/tsp 250, 500 mg tab 250, 500 mg and 1 g capsule	

Table continued on following page

Medications *Continued*

GENERIC/TRADE CLASSIFICATION	DOSE/INDICATIONS	SUPPLIED	REMARKS
Cetirizine (Zyrtec) *Antihistamine*	2–5 yr: 2.5 mg qd to max of 5 mg qd or divided bid >6 yr: 5–10 mg qd Seasonal or perennial rhinitis, urticaria	10 mg tablets 5 mg/5 ml syrup	Drug interaction: large doses of theophylline. Side effects: fatigue, dry mouth, somnolence, HA.
Chloral hydrate (Aquachloral, Noctec) *Anxiolytic, sedative, hypnotic*	Neonates: 25 mg/kg/dose Children: 15–50 mg/kg/dose, PO q4–8 hr (max. 500 mg tid) Nonpainful procedures requiring sedation: 50–100 mg/kg, may repeat (max. 2 g total dose) Adults: 250 mg tid for anxiety; 500–1000 mg qhs for insomnia (max. 2 g/d)	250, 500 mg/tsp syrup 250, 500 mg capsule 325, 500, 650 mg suppository	Drug interactions: warfarin, furosemide. Prolonged use in newborns can cause hyperbilirubinemia.
Chlorpheniramine maleate (Chlor-Trimeton) *Antihistamine*	Children: >2 yr: 0.35 mg/kg/d divided q4–6 hr PO 2–6 yr: 1 mg q4–6 hr, PO (max. 12 mg/d) 6–12 yr: 2 mg q4–6 hr PO Adults: 4 mg q4–6 hr PO (max. 24 mg/d) Allergic rhinitis, urticaria	2 mg/tsp syrup 2 mg chewable 4, 8, 12 mg tab 8, 12 mg timed-release tab, capsule	
Cholestyramine (Questran) *Antilipemic, bile acid sequestrant*	Children: 80 mg/kg PO tid Adults: 3–4 g PO before meals and qhs (max. 32 g/d) Used in the treatment of hypercholesterolemia, hyperlipidemia, pruritus, and diarrhea associated with increased bile acids	Packet: 4 g cholestyramine/9 g powder	Contraindicated in patients with constipation or complete biliary obstruction. Adverse reactions: constipation, flatulence, fecal impaction, nausea. Drug interactions: digoxin, warfarin.

Drug	Dosage/Forms/Indications	Comments
Ciclopirox olamine (Loprox) *Local anti-infective, antifungal*	1% cream	Children >10 yr and adults: topical—apply bid and continue following improvements in symptoms. Used for tinea cruris, tinea corporis, tinea pedis, tinea versicolor; also for cutaneous candidiasis
Cimetidine (Tagamet) *Histamine-receptor antagonist*	300 mg/tsp liquid 200, 300, 400, 800 mg tab	Children: 20–40 mg/kg/d PO divided qid. Adults: 300 mg PO qid before meals and qhs. Used in the treatment of duodenal ulcer, hypersecretory conditions, gastroesophageal reflux	Used cautiously in patients with impaired renal or hepatic function. Adverse reactions: dizziness, confusion, headache. Drug interactions: diazepam, theophylline, propranolol, antacids, phenytoin, tricyclic antidepressants, oral contraceptives, warfarin.
Ciprofloxacin (Cipro) *Fluoroquinolone*	250, 500, 750 mg tab	>18 yr: 250–750 mg PO q12 hr. Lower respiratory tract, skin, bone and joint, urinary tract, infectious diarrhea	Not indicated for children <18 yr. Increases serum theophylline. Antacids decrease absorption. Causes photosensitivity.
Ciprofloxacin hydrochloride & hydrocortisone (Cipro HC Otic) *Antibiotic and steroid*	Otic suspension, 10 ml bottle	Adults and children >1 yr: 3 drops to affected ear bid for 7 d. Otitis externa	Do not use if TM is perforated. Side effects: HA, pruritus, rash.
Cisapride (Propulsid) *GI agent*	10, 20 mg tablets 1 mg/ml suspension	Adults: 10 mg qid 15–30 min before meals; maximum of 20 mg qid. Safety and efficacy in children not established, but has been used in infants ≥2 mo at 0.2 mg/kg per dose qid	Drug interactions: cimetidine, clarithromycin, erythromycin, anticoagulants, antidepressants, antifungals. Side effects: HA, GI disturbances, rhinitis, risk of QT prolongation, constipation, nausea, anorexia. *Table continued on following page*

GENERIC/TRADE CLASSIFICATION	DOSE/INDICATIONS	SUPPLIED	REMARKS
Clarithromycin (Biaxin) *Macrolide*	Children: 15 mg/kg/d PO divided q 12 hr for 10 d Adults: 250–500 mg PO q12 hr for 7–14 d Pharyngitis, tonsillitis, sinusitis, lower respiratory tract, upper respiratory tract, skin	250, 500 mg tab 125, 250 mg/5 ml suspension	Rinse mouth following suspension. Drug interactions: theophylline, carbamazepine, terfenadine, digoxin, astemizole, propulsid.
Clemastine fumarate (OTC) (Tavist) *Antihistamine*	Children 6–12 yr: 0.67–1.34 mg PO bid (max. 4.02 mg/d) Adults: 1.34–2.68 mg PO bid (max. 8.04 mg/d) Allergic rhinitis, urticaria, allergies	0.67 mg/tsp syrup 1.34, 2.68 mg tab	Indicated for treatment of urticaria at doses of 2.68 mg.
Clindamycin (Cleocin T) *Topical antibiotic*	Apply twice daily Used in mild to moderate acne; use if comedones become inflamed; may use alone or with benzoyl peroxide	1% topical solution	Solution is flammable—no smoking following application. Can take 8–12 wk to see improvement. Wait 30 min after washing before applying.
Clindamycin HCl hydrate; clindamycin palmitate HCl *Miscellaneous antibiotic*	Children: 10–30 mg/kg/d PO divided q6–8 hr Adults: 150–450 mg/dose q6–8 hr PO (max. 1.8 g/d) Skin, respiratory tract, septicemia, gynecological, osteomyelitis (staphylococcal and streptococcal)	75 mg/tsp (#100 ml) 75, 150 mg capsule	Can cause severe colitis. Do not refrigerate suspension.

Drug	Supplied	Dosage	Notes
Clotrimazole (OTC) (Mycelex troches, Lotrimin, Gyne-Lotrimin) *Local anti-infective, antifungal*	10 mg troche 1% cream, solution, lotion 100, 500 mg vaginal tab	Oral candidiasis: Children >3 yr and adults: 10 mg troche PO—dissolve slowly, 5 times daily for 2 wk Vaginal candidiasis: 1 applicator or 1 vaginal tab qhs for 1–2 wk Tinea pedis, tinea cruris, tinea corporis, or tinea versicolor: topical application of cream bid for 1–8 wk	Adverse reactions: nausea, vomiting, abnormal liver function tests.
Cloxacillin sodium (Cloxapen, Tegopen) *Penicillinase-resistant penicillin*	125 mg/tsp (#100, 200 ml) 250, 500 mg capsule	Children: 50–100 mg/kg/d PO divided qid Adults: 250–500 mg PO qid Respiratory tract, sinusitis, skin (streptococcal and staphylococcal)	Not in stock in many pharmacies.
Codeine *Opiate agonist, antitussive*	15 mg/tsp solution 15, 30, 60 mg tab 30, 60 mg/ml injection	Children: Analgesic: 0.5–1 mg/kg/dose q4–6 hr PO, IM, SC (max. 60 mg/dose) Antitussive: 2–6 yr: 2.5–5 mg q4–6 hr PO (max. 30 mg/d); 7–12 yr: 5–10 mg q4–6 hr PO (max. 60 mg/d) Adults: 10–20 mg/dose q4–6 hr (max. 120 mg/d)	
Cortane-B otic (Chloroxylenol, pramoxine hydrochloride, hydrocortisone) *Anti-inflammatory, anesthetic, antifungal, antibacterial*	10-ml vial	Infants and small children: 3 drops into affected ear tid or qid Older children and adults: usual dose is 4 or 5 drops in affected ear tid or qid Treatment of otitis externa	Do not use if TM is perforated. Side effects: burning, itching, irritation.

Table continued on following page

T A B L E A-1

Medications Continued

GENERIC/TRADE CLASSIFICATION	DOSE/INDICATIONS	SUPPLIED	REMARKS
Cromolyn sodium (Intal, Nasalcrom) *Mast cell stabilizer*	Children >2 yr (oral inhalation): 20 mg qid Adults and children >5 yr (oral inhalation): 2 inhalations qid by metered-dose inhaler or 20 mg, oral or nebulizer qid; 1 spray, intranasally, 3 or 4 times daily Used as prophylaxis in treatment of allergic disorders and asthma; used for exercise-induced bronchospasm	Solution: 20 mg/2 ml for nebulization Solution, nasal: 40 mg/ml Aerosol: 800 µg/metered spray	Not to be used to treat acute asthmatic attacks. Adverse reactions: headache, bronchospasm, urticaria, cough, throat irritation. Do not withdraw drug abruptly.
Cromolyn sodium (Opticrom) *Mast cell stabilizer*	>4 yr: 1–2 drops q4–6 hr Used for allergic conjunctivitis	Ophthalmic solution 4%	
Cyclobenzaprine (Flexeril) *Skeletal muscle relaxant*	>12 yr: 20–40 mg/d in 2–4 divided doses (max. 60 mg/d) Treatment of muscle spasms associated with acute painful musculoskeletal conditions	10 mg tab	Drug interactions: MAO inhibitors.
Cyproheptadine HCl (Periactin) *Antihistamine*	2–6 yr: 2 mg q8–12 hr PO (max. 12 mg/d) 7–14 yr: 4 mg q8–12 hr PO (max. 16 mg/d) Adults: 12–16 mg/d divided q8 hr (max. 0.5 mg/kg/d) Allergic rhinitis, urticaria, allergic conjunctivitis, vascular cluster headaches Experimentally used to stimulate appetite and increase weight gain in children	2 mg/tsp syrup 4 mg tab	Can cause weight gain. In some patients, sedative effect disappears within 3–4 days.

Desmopressin acetate
(DDAVP, Stimate)
*Posterior pituitary hormone;
antidiuretic*

Diabetes insipidus:
Children 3 mo–12 yr: 0.05–0.3
ml/d intranasally in 1–2
divided doses
>4 yr: 0.05 mg tab qd
Adults: 0.05–0.4 ml
intranasally daily in 1–3
divided doses; 2–4 µg/d SC
or IV in 2 divided doses
Nocturnal enuresis:
Children >6 yr: 0.05–0.2 ml,
intranasally qhs; give ½
dose in each nostril; 0.2 mg
tab qhs to max 0.6 mg
Hemophilia A and type I von
Willebrand disease:
Adults and children >3 mo:
0.3 µg/kg slow IV
preoperative
Used in the treatment of
diabetes insipidus, temporary
polyuria, and some forms of
hemophilia

Injection: 4 µg/ml
Nasal solution: 0.1 mg/ml
0.1, 0.2 mg tabs, scored

Upper respiratory infections can
decrease the absorption of the
drug. High incidence of relapse
in the treatment of nocturnal
enuresis when drug is stopped.
Drug interactions: chlorpropamide,
lithium, carbamazepine,
epinephrine, fludrocortisone.
Observe for signs of water
intoxication: headache,
drowsiness, listlessness,
shortness of breath.
Adverse reactions: headache,
nausea, nasal congestion,
abdominal cramps.
When switching to tabs, give 1st
dose 24 hr after last nasal dose.

Table continued on following page

Medications Continued

GENERIC/TRADE CLASSIFICATION	DOSE/INDICATIONS	SUPPLIED	REMARKS
Dexamethasone (Decadron) *Glucocorticoid, anti-inflammatory*	Children (anti-inflammatory): 0.03–0.15 mg/kg/d PO IV or IM divided 2–4 times daily Adults (anti-inflammatory, other uses): 0.5–9 mg/d PO, IV, or IM divided 2 or 3 times daily Used in the treatment of chronic inflammatory disorders, cerebral edema, shock, allergies, and hematological disorders	0.5 mg/5 ml elixir 1 mg/ml oral solution 0.5, 0.75, 1, 1.5, 2, 4, 6 mg tab	Contraindicated in patients with systemic fungal infections. Use cautiously in patients with untreated viral or bacterial infections, renal disease, heart disease, tuberculosis, ulcerative colitis, hypothyroidism, diabetes. Do not give live vaccines to patients on Decadron. Can mask signs and symptoms of infection. Drug interactions: oral anticoagulants, oral contraceptives, rifampin, phenytoin, barbiturates, hypoglycemics.
Dextroamphetamine saccharate; dextroamphetamine sulfate; amphetamine aspartate; amphetaminesulfate (Adderall) *Amphetamine, CNS stimulant*	3–5 yr: 2.5 mg qd Increases of 2.5 mg/per wk >6 yr: 5 mg qd Increases of 5 mg/wk Max. 40 mg/d in divided doses, at intervals of 4–6 hr Used in the treatment of ADHD/ ADD	5, 10, 20, 30 mg tablets. All tablets are double scored	Drug interactions: MAO inhibitors, tricyclic antidepressants, antihypertensives, phenobarbital, meperidine, phenytoin. Abuse potential. Side effects: HTN, anorexia, dry mouth, GI disturbance. Can exacerbate tics and Tourette syndrome.

Drug/class	Dosage	Available forms	Remarks
Dextroamphetamine sulfate (Dexedrine) *Amphetamine, CNS stimulant*	Narcolepsy: Children 6–12 yr: 5 mg initially; may increase by 5 mg/d at weekly intervals (max. 60 mg/d) Adults: 10 mg initially; increase by 10 mg/d at weekly intervals (max. 60 mg/d); give in divided doses or use long-acting forms ADHD: Children 3–5 yr: 2.5 mg/d initially; increase by 2.5 mg/d weekly; usual dose 0.1–0.5 mg/kg/d, given in the AM (max. 40 mg/d) Children >6 yr: 5 mg/d initially given qd or divided bid; increase by 5 mg/d weekly; usual dose 0.1–0.5 mg/kg/d, given in the AM (max. 40 mg/d) Used in the treatment of ADHD and narcolepsy	5, 10, 15 mg capsule (spansule), sustained release 5, 10 mg tab 5 mg/tsp elixir	Contraindicated in patients with hypertension, hyperthyroidism, glaucoma, or cardiovascular disease. Drug interactions: MAO inhibitors, tricyclic antidepressants, phenobarbital, phenytoin; insulin requirements may be altered. Do not give within 6 hr of bedtime. Adverse reactions: GI disturbances, dry mouth, anorexia, hypertension, tremor, tachycardia. Avoid caffeine.
Dextromethorphan hydrobromide (Benylin DM, Delsym, Hold, Robitussin DM, Sucrets Cough) *Nonnarcotic antitussive*	Children: 2–5 yr: 2.5–5 mg q4 hr PO (max. 30 mg/d) >6 yr: 5–10 mg q4 hr PO (max. 60 mg/d) Adults: 10–20 mg q4 hr PO (max. 120 mg/d) Cough suppression	5, 7.5, 10, 15 mg/tsp syrup 5 mg lozenge 15 mg chewable 30 mg/tsp extended-release syrup	

Table continued on following page

Medications Continued

GENERIC/TRADE CLASSIFICATION	DOSE/INDICATIONS	SUPPLIED	REMARKS
Diazepam (Valium) *Anxiolytic, benzodiazepine*	Status epilepticus (intravenous push): Neonate: 0.25 mg/kg/dose q15–30 min for 2 or 3 doses Children: <5 yr: 0.2–0.5 mg/kg/dose q15–30 min for 2 or 3 doses (max. 5 mg) >5 yr: 0.2–0.5 mg/kg/dose q15–30 min for 2 or 3 doses (max. 10 mg) Adults: 5–10 mg q10–20 min (max. 30 mg/8 hr) Sedation/relaxation: Children: 0.12–0.8 mg/kg/d PO divided 3 or 4 times daily >12 yr: 2–10 mg PO 2–4 times daily	5 mg/ml injection 5 mg/ml, 5 mg/tsp solution 2, 5, 10 mg tab 15 mg sustained-release capsule	Controlled substance, schedule IV. Do not use in patients with narrow-angle glaucoma, severe pain. Causes CNS depression. Tablets can be crushed. Do a complete blood count and liver function tests with long-term use.
Dicloxacillin monohydrate (Dycill, Dynapen, Pathocil) *Penicillinase-resistant penicillin*	Children <40 kg: 12–50 mg/kg/d PO divided q6 hr Children >40 kg and adults: 125–500 mg PO q6 hr Sinusitis, skin, bone and joint, respiratory tract (infections caused by penicillinase-producing staphylococcus)	62.5 mg/tsp suspension 125, 250, 500 mg capsule	Drug interactions: warfarin, rifampin, aminoglycosides. Food decreases absorption.
Dicyclomine HCl (Bentyl) *Antimuscarinic, antispasmodic*	Children >6 mo: 5–10 mg PO tid–qid Adults: 80–160 mg/d PO divided qid Used as adjunctive therapy to treat peptic ulcer disease, functional GI disturbances	10 mg/tsp syrup 20 mg tab 10, 20 mg capsule	Contraindicated in patients with glaucoma, obstructive GI or GU conditions, myasthenia gravis. Use cautiously in patients with hyperthyroidism, cardiac disease, hypertension. Adverse reactions: hypotonia, dry mouth, blurred vision, palpitations.

Drug/Category	Dosage	How Supplied	Considerations
Dimenhydrinate (Dramamine) *Antiemetic*	Children 2–5 yr: 12.5–25 mg PO q6–8 hr Children 6–12 yr: 25–50 mg PO q6–8 hr Adults: 50–100 mg PO q4–6 hr (max. 400 mg/d) Used to treat and prevent nausea, vomiting, vertigo	12.5 mg/5 ml liquid 50 mg scored tab, chewable tabs	Contraindicated in patients with glaucoma, asthma, seizures. Adverse reactions: drowsiness, dizziness, hypotension, dry mouth, blurred vision.
Diphenhydramine hydrochloride (OTC) (Benadryl) *Antihistamine*	Children: 1.0 mg/kg/dose q6–8 hr PO/IM/IV (max. 300 mg/d) Adults: 25–50 mg/dose q4–6 hr PO/IM/IV Allergic rhinitis, urticaria, allergic reaction to blood or plasma, motion sickness, vertigo, cough, insomnia, control of dyskinetic movement	6.25 and 12.5 mg/tsp syrup, elixir 12.5 mg chewable 25–50 mg tab, capsule 10, 50 mg/ml injection 1%, 2% cream, lotion	Can cause respiratory suppression.
Diphenoxylate HCl and atropine sulfate (Lomotil) *Antidiarrheal*	Children >2 yr: 0.3–0.4 mg/kg/d PO divided qid; dose calculated as the diphenoxylate component Adults: 1–2 tab or 1–2 tsp PO 3–4 times daily Used to treat nonspecific diarrhea	Solution: diphenoxylate 2.5 mg and atropine 0.025 mg/tsp Tab: diphenoxylate 2.5 mg and atropine 0.025 mg	Use cautiously in pediatric patients and those with liver disease or ulcerative colitis. Drug interactions: MAO inhibitors. Adverse reactions: dizziness, headache, dry mouth, tachycardia, drowsiness.
Docusate sodium (Colace) *Laxative*	Children 3–6 yr: 20–60 mg/d PO Children 6–12 yr: 40–120 mg/d PO Adults: 50–400 mg/d PO divided 1–4 times daily Stool softener	10 mg/ml liquid 50, 100 mg capsule	Drug interactions: mineral oil. Mix liquid with fruit juice or milk to mask taste.

Table continued on following page

T A B L E A-1
Medications Continued

GENERIC/TRADE CLASSIFICATION	DOSE/INDICATIONS	SUPPLIED	REMARKS
Doxycycline (Doryx, Doxy, Doxy Caps, Doxychel, Vibramycin, Vibra-Tabs, Vovox) *Tetracycline*	>8 yr: 5 mg/kg/d PO divided bid (max. 200 mg/d) Adults: 100–200 mg/d PO divided bid Used in treatment of infections caused by *Rickettsia, Chlamydia, Mycoplasma*; syphilis, gonorrhea, traveler's diarrhea	50 mg/tsp suspension 50, 100 mg tab 50, 100 mg capsule	Syrup not available at many pharmacies. Use of outdated product can cause Fanconi-like syndrome. Can cause photosensitivity. Do not take with antacids or iron products.
Econazole nitrate (Spectazole) *Local anti-infective, antifungal*	Adults and children: apply topically 3 or 4 times daily Used in treatment of tinea pedis, tinea cruris, tinea corporis, tinea versicolor; also for cutaneous candidiasis	1% cream	
EMLA cream (lidocaine 2.5% and prilocaine 2.5%) *Topical anesthetic*	1–3 mo; 1 g with maximum application area of 10 cm^2 4–12 mo: 2 g with maximum application area of 20 cm^2 1–6 yr: 10 g with maximum application area of 100 cm^2 7–12 yr: 20 g with maximum application area of 200 cm^2 These are maximum doses Used for topical anesthesia prior to painful procedures	5, 30 g tubes 1 g disc	Do not use on open wounds. Do not use near eyes. Apply at least 1 hr before procedure.
Epinephrine (AsthmaNefrin, Bronkaid Mist, EpiPen, EpiPen Jr., Sus-Phrine) *Bronchodilator, vasopressor, cardiac stimulant*	Children: 0.01 mg/kg SC repeat q15 min for 2 doses, then q4 hr prn (max. 0.5 mg/dose) Adults: 0.2–0.5 mg SC q20 min–4 hr (max. 1 mg/dose) Inhalation: 1 or 2 inhalations of 1:100 or 2.25% Bronchodilation; anaphylactic reactions	1:1000 (1 mg/ml) injection 1%, 1.25%, 2.25% nebulizer inhaler 160, 200, 250 µg/metered spray	Inhaled beta$_2$-agonist preferred. Rotate injection sites. Adverse effects: EKG changes, restlessness, tremor, nausea, vomiting.

Drug	Indications/Dosage	Preparations	Comments
Erythromycin (Akne-mycin, Erycette, Erygel, Erymax, ETS, Mythromycin, T-Stat) *Topical antibiotic*	Apply bid to acne-prone areas	2% solution, gel T-Stat pads (# 60)	Cleanse area first, wait 30 min before applying. Contraindicated in patients with known sensitivity to erythromycin.
Erythromycin and benzoyl peroxide (Benzamycin) *Topical antibiotic, keratolytic agent*	Apply twice daily Used in mild to moderate acne	Topical gel	Should be refrigerated. Expires every 3 mo. Contraindicated in patients with known sensitivity to erythromycin. Should be applied following cleansing.
Erythromycin (E-Mycin, ERYC, Ery-Tab, PCE Dispertabs) **Erythromycin estolate** (Iliosone) **Erythromycin ethylsuccinate** (EES) (E.E.S., EryPed, Wyamycin E)	All 3 preparations dosed as follows: Children: 30–50 mg/kg/d PO divided q6 hr Adults: 250–500 mg PO qid Upper and lower respiratory tract, otitis media, pharyngitis, syphilis, gonorrhea, skin, gynecological disorders, and Legionnaires' disease	125 mg pellets in capsule 250, 333 mg tab; 250 mg capsule 100 mg/ml drops; 125, 250 mg/tsp 125, 250 mg chewable 250, 500 mg tab 200, 400 mg/tsp 200 mg chewable; 400 mg tab	Most prescribe tid. GI upset common. Give with food to decrease side effects. Drug interactions: theophylline, carbamazepine, cyclosporine, digoxin, terfenadine, warfarin. Useful in patients allergic to penicillin.
EES and sulfisoxazole (Pediazole, Eryzole) *Erythromycin and sulfonamide*	Children >2 mo: 40–50 mg/kg/d PO divided q6 hr (max. 2 g erythromycin, 6 g sulfisoxazole/d) Upper and lower respiratory tract disorders, otitis media	EES 200 mg and sulfisoxazole 600 mg/ tsp (#100, 150, 200, 250 ml)	Most prescribe tid. Drug interactions as with erythromycin.
Erythromycin ethylsuccinate (Ilotycin) *Ocular antibiotic*	Instill ointment within first hour following birth; for other infections, instill ointment 3 or 4 times daily Treatment of ocular infections; prophylaxis of ophthalmia neonatorum	Ophthalmic ointment 0.5%	

Table continued on following page

Medications *Continued*

GENERIC/TRADE CLASSIFICATION	DOSE/INDICATIONS	SUPPLIED	REMARKS
Estrogens, conjugated (Premarin) *Hormone*	Apply daily until agglutination resolves Pediatric use: treatment of vaginal agglutination	Vaginal cream, 0.625%	Use for 2 wk, then stop.
Ethosuximide (Zarontin) *Anticonvulsant*	<6 yr: initially 15 mg/kg/d in 2 divided doses; usual maintenance dose .40 mg/kg/d (max. 250 mg 1 dose) >6 yr: initially 250 mg bid, increase as needed; usual maintenance dose 20–40 mg/kg/d (max. 1.5 g/d in 2 divided doses) Dose dependent on drug levels Controls absence seizures	250 mg capsule 250 mg/5 ml syrup	Drug interaction: phenytoin, valproic acid. Side effects: GI disturbances, blood dyscrasias, fatigue.
Ferrous sulfate (OTC) (Feosol, Fer-In-Sol, Fer-Iron) *Oral iron supplement*	Children (elemental iron): 1–2 mg/kg/d to 15 mg/d for prophylaxis; 3–6 mg/kg/d in divided doses for treatment of iron deficiency Adults (ferrous sulfate): 300 mg/ d for prophylaxis; 300 mg bid to 300 mg qid for iron deficiency Used in the prevention and treatment of iron deficiency anemia	Fer-In-Sol drops: 15 mg/0.6 ml elemental iron Fer-In-Sol elixir: 18 mg/tsp elemental iron Feosol elixir: 44 mg/tsp elemental iron Tab: 300 mg ferrous sulfate	Contraindicated in patients with enteritis, ulcers, ulcerative colitis, hemochromatosis, hemolytic anemia, hepatitis. Drug interactions: tetracycline, vitamin C, antacids, chloramphenicol. Adverse reactions: GI symptoms, staining of teeth, dark stools. Overdosage can be fatal, at levels >300 µg/ml.
Fexofenadine Hcl (Allegra) *Antihistamine*	>12 yr: 60 mg bid; 60 mg qd if decreased renal function Treatment of seasonal allergic rhinitis	60 mg capsules	Allegra-D has 120 mg of pseudoephedrine in each capsule for extended release. Drug interactions: MAO inhibitors, antihypertensives. Side effects: HA, GI upset, insomnia, dry mouth.

Drug	Dosage/Use	Available forms	Nursing considerations
Fluconazole (Diflucan) *Antifungal*	Oral candidiasis: >2 wk of age: 6 mg/kg on day 1, then 3 mg/kg/d for 2 wk Adults: 200 mg on day 1, then 100 mg/d for 2 wk Vaginal candidiasis: Adults: 150 mg PO once Used for oral, esophageal, systemic candidiasis	10 mg/ml; 40 mg/ml 50, 100, 150, 200 mg tab	Monitor renal and liver function with long-term therapy. Can cause nausea, headache, rash, vomiting, abdominal pain, diarrhea. Drug interactions: warfarin, theophylline, oral hypoglycemics, phenytoin, cyclosporine, rifampin, hydrochlorothiazide, propulsid, astemizole.
Flunisolide (AeroBid, Nasalide, Nasarel) *Glucocorticoid, anti-inflammatory*	Children 6–14 yr: 1 inhalation or 1 spray each nostril bid (max. 4 inhalations or sprays daily) Adults: 2 inhalations or 2 sprays each nostril bid (max. 8 inhalations or sprays daily) Used in the treatment of asthma requiring chronic steroid use; nasal solution used to treat seasonal allergic rhinitis	250 µg/metered spray oral inhalant 25 µg/metered spray nasal inhalant	Rinse mouth following oral inhalation. Contraindicated in patients with fungal, untreated bacterial or viral infections. Not to be used to treat acute asthmatic attacks. Adverse reactions: oral candidal infections, nasal irritation, adrenal suppression, headache. Do not stop drug abruptly. Use caution when transferring from systemic steroids to inhaled steroids.

Table continued on following page

T A B L E   A-1
Medications *Continued*

GENERIC/TRADE CLASSIFICATION	DOSE/INDICATIONS	SUPPLIED	REMARKS

Fluoride (many preparations)
 Mineral supplement
	Osteoporosis:
	   Children: 0.5 mg/kg/d in
	     divided doses
	   Adults: 30–100 mg/d in
	     divided doses
	 Nutritional supplement:
	   <0.3 ppm fluoride content of
	     water:
	     6 mo–3 yr: 0.25 mg PO
	       daily
	     3–6 yr: 0.5 mg PO daily
	     6–16 yr: 1 mg PO daily
	   0.3–0.6 ppm fluoride content
	     of water:
	     6 mo–3 yr: no supplement
	       required
	     3–6 yr: 0.25 mg PO daily
	     6–16 yr: 0.5 mg PO daily
	 Used to prevent dental caries
	   and in treatment of
	   osteoporosis
		Drops calibrated by fluoride ion
		 Luride drops: 0.125 mg/drop
		 Pediaflor drops: 0.5 mg/ml
		 Tri-Vi-Flor drops: 0.25, 0.5 mg/ml
		 Oral solution: 1 mg/ml fluoride ion
		 Chewable tab: 0.25, 0.5 mg fluoride
		   ion
		 Tab: 0.25 mg fluoride ion
			Do not give if fluoride content of
			 water >0.6 ppm. Do not give
			 with milk products. Adverse
			 reactions: GI upset; do not
			 swallow rinse or gel. Dental
			 fluorosis can occur if
			 supplements are given
			 unnecessarily. Infants <6 mo
			 should not receive fluoride
			 supplements. This includes
			 those exclusively breastfed.

Fluticasone propionate
 (Flovent, Flonase)
 Steroid
	>4 yr: 50 µg bid to maximum
	   of 100 µg bid when using
	   rotadisk
	 1 spray per nostril to maximum
	   of 2 sprays per nostril when
	   using nasal spray
	 Treatment of seasonal or
	   perennial allergic rhinitis and
	   as asthma therapy
		50, 100, 250 µg rotadisk
		 Nasal spray, 16 g, 120 sprays
		 44 µg/inhalation, 110 µg/inhalation
		   inhalers
			Side effects: nasal irritation, HA,
			 candidiasis, pharyngitis.
			 If exposed to varicella, consider
			 prophylactic therapy to prevent
			 varicella. Rinse mouth following
			 use.

Drug	Indication/Dosage	Supplied	Comments
Furazolidone (Furoxone) *Antibacterial, antiprotozoal*	Infants 1–11 mo: 8–17 mg PO qid Children: 1–4 yr: 17–25 mg PO qid 5–12 yr: 25–50 mg PO qid Max. dose for children: 8.8 mg/kg/d Adults: 100 mg PO qid For treatment of bacterial or protozoal diarrhea and enteritis	50 mg/15 ml liquid 100 mg tab	Interactions: alcohol, tricyclic antidepressants, tyramine-containing foods, sympathomimetic drugs. Duration of therapy not to exceed 7 d.
Gentamicin sulfate (Garamycin) *Antibiotic, ophthalmic*	Solution: 1–2 drops q2–3 hr Ointment: use tid Treatment of ocular infections	Ophthalmic solution, ointment 0.3%	
Griseofulvin (Fulvicin, Grifulvin, Grisactin, Gris-PEG) *Penicillium griseofulvum derivative*	Children: 10 mg/kg/d (microsize) or 5 mg/kg/d (ultra-microsize) Adults: 500–1000 mg qd (microsize), 125–165 mg bid (ultra-microsize), or 250–330 mg qd For treatment of tinea corporis, tinea pedis, tinea capitis, tinea unguium, tinea cruris	Microsize: 125 mg/tsp suspension 125, 250 mg capsule 250, 500 mg tab Ultra-microsize: 125, 165, 250, 330 mg tab	Give with fatty foods to increase absorption. Use with caution in penicillin-sensitive patients. Adverse reactions: blood dyscrasias, nausea, vomiting, photosensitivity. Drug interactions: alcohol, barbiturates, warfarin, anticoagulants.
Guaifenesin (Anti-Tuss, Glyate, Glycotuss, Guiatuss, Humibid L.A., Hytuss, Robitussin) *Expectorant*	Children: <2 yr: 12 mg/kg/d divided q4 hr 2–5 yr: 50–100 mg q4 hr PO (max. 600 mg/d) 6–11 yr: 100–200 mg q4 hr PO (max. 1.2 g/d) Adults: 200–400 mg q4 hr PO (max. 2.4 g/d) Controls cough due to minor throat, bronchial irritation	67, 100 mg/tsp syrup 100, 200 mg tab 200 mg capsule 600 mg sustained release	Effectiveness of expectorants is questionable.

Table continued on following page

T A B L E A-1

Medications Continued

GENERIC/TRADE CLASSIFICATION	DOSE/INDICATIONS	SUPPLIED	REMARKS
Hydrocodone and acetaminophen (Vicodin) *Opiate agonist, analgesic, antipyretic*	Adults: 1–2 tabs, PO, q4–6 hr Relief of moderate to severe pain; antitussive	5 mg hydrocodone and 500 mg acetaminophen	
Hydroxyzine hydrochloride (Atarax, Vistaril) *Miscellaneous anxiolytics, sedative, hypnotic, antihistamine*	Children: 0.6 mg/kg/dose q6 hr PO; 1 mg/kg/dose q4–6 hr IM Adults: Antiemetic: 25–100 mg IM Anxiety: 50–100 mg qid PO (max. 600 mg) Preop: 50–100 mg PO, 25–100 mg IM Pruritus: 25 mg q6–8 hr PO	10 mg/tsp syrup (Atarax) 25 mg/tsp suspension (Vistaril) 10, 25, 50 mg tab (Atarax) 25, 50, 100 mg capsule (Vistaril) 25, 50 mg/ml injection	
Hyoscyamine, atropine, scopolamine, phenobarbital (Donnatal) *Antimuscarinic, antispasmodic*	Children: 10 lb: 0.5 ml q4 hr or 0.75 ml q6 hr 20 lb: 1 ml q4 hr or 1.5 ml q6 hr 30 lb: 1.5 ml q4 hr or 2 ml q6 hr 50 lb: 2.5 ml q4 hr or 3.75 ml q6 hr 75 lb: 3.75 ml q4 hr or 5 ml q6 hr	Atropine 0.0194 mg, scopolamine 0.0065 mg, hyoscyamine 0.1037 mg, phenobarbital 16.2 mg/tabs, capsule, or tsp elixir	Contraindicated in patients with glaucoma, GU or GI obstructive disease, tachycardia, myasthenia gravis. Drug interactions: digitalis, griseofulvin, tetracyclines, MAO inhibitors, tricyclic antidepressants, steroids, amantadine, CNS depressants, antihistamines.

Drug	Dosage/Use	How supplied	Comments
Ibuprofen (Advil, Motrin, Nuprin) *Nonsteroidal anti-inflammatory*	Children >6 mo: Antipyretic: 5–10 mg/kg/dose q6–8 hr PO: maximum dose 40 mg/kg/dose. Juvenile rheumatoid arthritis: 30–70 mg/kg/d PO divided tid. Analgesic: 4–10 mg/kg/dose PO divided tid. Adults: 200–800 mg/dose tid–qid. Management of inflammatory disorders: analgesic for mild/moderate pain: antipyretic: dysmenorrhea	40 mg/ml, 100 mg/tsp. 100 mg chewable. 200 mg tab (OTC). 300, 400, 600, 800 mg tab (Rx)	Drug interactions: digoxin, methotrexate. Can cause GI upset. Contraindicated in patients with aspirin sensitivities or bleeding disorders.
Idoxuridine (Herplex, Stoxil) *Antiviral*	1 drop q1 hr during day and q2 hr at night for 7 d; ointment is used 5 times daily. Used in treatment of HSV keratitis	Ophthalmic solution, ointment 0.1%	Not for long-term use. Can cause photosensitivity. Drug interaction: boric acid solutions. Reevaluate if no improvement in 7 d.
Imipramine (Tofranil, Tofranil-PM) *Tricyclic antidepressant*	Children >6 yr (enuresis): 25 mg PO initially qhs: increase by 10–25 mg/dose increments weekly (max. 2.5–5.0 mg/kg/d or 75 mg qhs). Adults (depression): 50–100 mg/d PO initially divided tid; increase by 25–50 mg to max of 300 mg/d. Used in the treatment of childhood enuresis and depression	10, 25, 50 mg tab. 75, 100, 125, 150 mg capsule—Tofranil-PM (imipramine pamoate)	Use with caution in patients with cardiac disease, glaucoma, seizure disorders, diabetes. Drug interactions: MAO inhibitors (if given within 14 d), warfarin, CNS depressants, antihypertensive agents. Adverse reactions: drowsiness, dry mouth, GI upset, photosensitivity, arrhythmias. Can take 2–4 wk to see full effects of therapy.

Table continued on following page

GENERIC/TRADE CLASSIFICATION	DOSE/INDICATIONS	SUPPLIED	REMARKS
Ipratropium bromide (Atrovent) *Bronchodilator*	>12 yr: 1 vial of inhalation solution tid or qid Used as adjunctive therapy in asthma	500 µg/unit-dose vial 18 µg/dose inhaler	Side effects: nervousness, GI disturbances, HA.
Isoniazid (INH, Laniazid) *Antituberculosis agent*	Children: 10–20 mg/kg/d PO divided bid Prophylaxis: 10 mg/kg/d (max. 300 mg/d) Adults: 5 mg/kg/d PO qd (usual dose 300 mg/d) Disseminated disease: 10 mg/ kg/d divided bid Prophylaxis: 300 mg/d Following 1–2 mo of treatment for tuberculosis: Children: 20–40 mg/kg/dose (max. 900 mg) biweekly Adults: 15 mg/kg/dose (max. 900 mg) biweekly	50 mg/tsp 100, 300 mg tab	Take on empty stomach. Avoid food containing tyramine. Avoid alcohol. Drug Interactions: phenytoin, diazepam, carbamazepine. Adverse reactions: peripheral neuritis, seizures, ataxia, stupor, tinnitus, diarrhea.
Isotretinoin (Accutane) *Antiacne agent*	0.5–2 mg/kg/day PO divided bid for 15–20 wk; if relapse occurs, therapy can be reinstated after 8 wk Management of cystic acne that has failed previous therapy	10, 20, 40 mg capsule	Monitor CBC, platelets, sedimentation rate. Avoid pregnancy during therapy. Contraception must be used. Acne worsens during first few weeks of therapy. No blood donation for at least 1 mo following discontinuation of drug. Avoid other vitamin A products. Adverse reactions: pruritus, photosensitivity, conjunctivitis, cheilitis, epistaxis, bone pain.

Drug	Dosage / Indication	Notes
Kaolin and pectin (OTC) (Kaopectate) *Antidiarrheal*	Children 3–6 yr: 15–30 ml each dose Children 6–12 yr: 30–60 ml each dose Adults: 60–120 ml following each loose stool Used to treat mild diarrhea Suspension: kaolin 975 mg and pectin 22 mg/tsp	Do not administer for longer than 48 hr. Drug interactions: tetracycline, theophylline, chloroquine, digoxin. Adverse reactions: constipation, fecal impaction. Use cautiously in pediatric patients.
Ketoconazole (Nizoral) *Antifungal*	Systemic candidiasis, histoplasmosis, blastomycosis, chromomycosis: Children <2 yr: 3.3–6.6 mg/kg/d PO Adults and children >40 kg: Initially 200 mg PO qd: may increase to 400 mg qd if no response to lower dose Minimum treatment for candidiasis is 7–14 d; for other systemic fungal infections, use for 6 mo Topical treatment of tinea corporis, tinea cruris, tinea versicolor: Adults and children: apply 1 or 2 times daily for 2 wk 100 mg/tsp suspension 200 mg tab (scored) 2% cream (15, 30, 60 g)	Adverse reactions: hepatotoxicity, nausea, vomiting. Most effective oral antifungal. Drug interactions: phenytoin, cimetidine, ranitidine, rifampin, terfenadine.
Ketorolac tromethamine 0.5% (Acular) *Nonsteroidal anti-inflammatory*	1 drop qid for 1 wk Used for treatment of ocular itching due to seasonal allergic conjunctivitis Ophthalmic solution 0.5%	Can have transient stinging and burning following instillation. Refrigeration decreases stinging. Contraindicated in patients with soft contact lenses.

Table continued on following page

Medications Continued

GENERIC/TRADE CLASSIFICATION	DOSE/INDICATIONS	SUPPLIED	REMARKS
Lactulose (Cephulac, Chronulac) *Laxative*	Children: 0.5–1.0 mg/kg/dose bid PO Adults: 15–30 ml daily PO (max. 3 oz/d) Laxative	10 g/15 ml solution	Contraindicated in patients with fecal impaction or those with acute abdomen. Use with caution in diabetic patients.
Levalbuterol HCl (Xopenex) *Bronchodilator*	>12 yr: 0.63 mg tid (6–8 hr); 1.25 mg may be used in more severe asthma or in patients not responding to 0.63 mg Prevention and treatment of bronchospasm	0.63 mg/3 ml unit dose, 1.25 mg/3 ml inhalation solution	Drug interactions: β-blockers, diuretics, digoxin, MAO inhibitors or tricyclic antidepressants Side effects: tachycardia, elevated heart rate, tremor, nervousness, pain, flu syndrome.

Lindane (Kwell, Kwildane, Scabene) *Scabicide, pediculicide*	Scabies:
	  Adults and children: apply thin layer, massage, moving from neck to toes; shower after 8–12 hr; treatment can be repeated in 1 wk
	Lice:
	  Adults and children: apply to hairy areas and adjacent areas, wash off in 8–12 hr; for scalp, shampoo well for 4–5 min, rinse, and comb hair to remove nits
		1% cream, lotion, shampoo	Avoid contact with eyes, mucous membranes, face, and urethral meatus. Not recommended for infants or young children. Body should be clean and dry before application. Do not apply to broken or inflamed skin. Itching may continue for 4–6 wk.

Lodoxamide (Alomide) *Mast cell stabilizer*	Adults and children >2 yr: 1–2 drops qid for up to 3 mo Used to treat vernal conjunctivitis, vernal keratitis, and vernal keratoconjunctivitis	Ophthalmic solution 0.1%	Contraindicated in patients with contact lenses. Adverse reactions: stinging, blurred vision, transient burning, itching, dry eyes.

Drug	Indications/Dosage	How Supplied	Comments
Loperamide (OTC) (Imodium) *Antidiarrheal*	Children: 2–5 yr: 1 mg tid PO 6–8 yr: 2 mg bid PO 9–12 yr: 2 mg tid PO Maintenance dose: 0.25–1 mg/kg/d divided 2–4 times/d Adults: 2 capsules initially, then 1 capsule following each stool (max. 8 capsules/d) Used in the treatment of acute and chronic diarrhea	1 mg/tsp liquid 2 mg capsule	Contraindicated in patients with ulcerative colitis, pseudomembranous colitis, or hepatic disease. Adverse reactions: constipation, abdominal cramping, nausea, vomiting, dizziness. Use cautiously in pediatric patients.
Loracarbef (Lorabid) *Carbacephem*	>6 mo: 30 mg/kg/d divided bid PO—otitis media; 15 mg/kg/d PO divided bid—skin, pharyngitis, tonsillitis Adults: 200–400 mg q 12 hr PO Upper and lower respiratory tract, otitis, sinusitis, pharyngitis, tonsillitis, uncomplicated cystitis and pyelonephritis	100, 200 mg/tsp (#50, 100 ml) 200 mg pulvule	Food limits bioavailability. Strawberry/bubble gum taste. Treat otitis with suspension—better therapeutic outcome. 10% cross-sensitivity in patients with penicillin and cephalosporin allergies.
Loratadine (Claritin) *Antihistamine*	Children >6 yr: 5–10 mg qd Adults and children >12 yr: 10 mg qd PO Nasal and non-nasal symptoms of seasonal allergic rhinitis	10 mg tab 10 mg redi-tab 10 mg/10 ml syrup	Give on empty stomach. Possible interaction with macrolide antibiotics, ketoconazole, cimetidine, ranitidine, or theophylline. *Table continued on following page*

GENERIC/TRADE CLASSIFICATION	DOSE/INDICATIONS	SUPPLIED	REMARKS
Magnesium hydroxide (OTC) (Phillips' Milk of Magnesia) *Antacid, laxative*	Children: 2–5 yr: 5–15 ml PO daily for constipation 6–12 yr: 15–30 ml PO daily for constipation 2.5–5 ml PO prn for antacid effect Adults: 30–60 ml as single dose for constipation; 5–15 ml qid for antacid effect Used to treat constipation and to induce bowel evacuation	2.5 g/30 ml suspension 300 mg tab	Contraindicated in patients with renal failure, intestinal obstruction, fecal impaction. Adverse reactions: abdominal cramps, hypotension, nausea, vomiting. Drug interactions: tetracycline, digoxin, indomethacin, ketoconazole.
Mebendazole (Vermox) *Anthelmintic*	Pinworms: Adults and children >2 yr: 100 mg PO as single dose; can repeat in 3 wk if infection persists Roundworms, whipworms, hookworms: Adults and children >2 yr; 100 mg PO bid for 3 d; can repeat in 3 wk	100 mg tab (chewable)	Few side effects at low doses. Occasional abdominal pain and diarrhea. Can swallow tablets.
Medroxyprogesterone acetate (Depo-Provera) *Progestin*	Dysfunctional uterine bleeding: 5–10 mg PO for 5–10 d beginning on day 16 or 21 of cycle Secondary amenorrhea: 5–10 mg PO for 5–10 d Contraception: 150 mg IM q3 mo Used in the treatment of abnormal uterine bleeding, secondary amenorrhea, or as contraception	2.5, 5, 10 mg tab 100, 150, 400 mg/ml injection	Contraindicated in patients with thromboembolic disease, pregnancy, hepatic disease, breast or genital cancer, cardiovascular disease, undiagnosed vaginal bleeding. Drug interactions: bromocriptine. Adverse reactions: depression, weight fluctuations, irregular bleeding, edema, breast tenderness, acne, galactorrhea.

Mefenamic acid (Ponstel)
Nonsteroidal
anti-inflammatory

>14 yr: 500 mg, then 250 mg q4–6 hr—not to exceed 1 wk Mild to moderate pain, dysmenorrhea, inflammatory disease

250 mg tab

Adverse reactions: blood dyscrasias. Drug interactions: anticoagulants, phenytoin, sulfonamides, corticosteroids.

Metaproterenol sulfate
(Alupent)
Bronchodilator

Oral:
Adults and children >9 yr: 20 mg/dose PO 3–4 times daily
6–9 yr, <27 kg: 10 mg/dose PO 3–4 times daily
2–6 yr: 1–2.6 mg/kg/d PO divided q6–8 hr
<2 yr: 0.4 mg/kg/dose PO 3–4 times daily, or q8–12 hr
Inhaled:
Adults and children >12 yr: 2–3 inhalations q3–4 hr (max. 12 inhalations/d)
Nebulizer: 0.25–0.5 mg/kg in 2 ml normal saline q4–6 hr (max. 15 mg)
Used as bronchodilator in reversible airway obstruction due to asthma or chronic obstructive pulmonary disease (COPD)

10 mg/tsp syrup
10, 20 mg tab (scored)
Inhalation solution
0.65 mg/dose in 300-dose aerosol container

Can cause nervousness, restlessness, or tremor. Drug interactions: MAO inhibitors, propranolol. Do not use concurrently with other sympathomimetic bronchodilators. Best results if second inhalation is given 10 min following first.

Table continued on following page

Medications *Continued*

GENERIC/TRADE CLASSIFICATION	DOSE/INDICATIONS	SUPPLIED	REMARKS
Methylphenidate (Ritalin) *CNS stimulant*	Children >6 yr (ADHD): 5 mg PO 1 or 2 times daily initially; increase by 5–10 mg weekly; usual dose 0.3–0.7 mg/kg/ dose given 2 or 3 times daily Adults (narcolepsy): 10 mg PO 2 or 3 times daily, up to 60 mg/ d; give before meals Used for the treatment of narcolepsy and ADHD	5, 10, 20 mg tab (scored) 20 mg sustained-release tab	Contraindicated in patients with hyperthyroidism, cardiovascular disease, glaucoma, hypertension. Cautious use in patients with tics or Tourette syndrome. Drug interactions: MAO inhibitors, tricyclic antidepressants, anticonvulsants. Adverse reactions: anorexia, insomnia, nausea.
Metronidazole (Flagyl) *Anti-infective* (miscellaneous)	Children (PO): Amebiasis: 35–50 mg/kg/d divided tid Other parasites: 15–30 mg/kg/ d divided tid Anaerobic: 30 mg/kg/d divided q6 hr *Clostridium difficile* (antibiotic-associated colitis): 20 mg/ kg/d divided q6 hr (max. 2 g/d) Adults (PO): Amebiasis: 500–700 mg q8 hr for 5–10 d Other parasites: 250 mg q8 hr or 2 g as single dose Anaerobic: 30 mg/kg/d divided q6 hr Antibiotic-associated colitis: 250 mg qid for 10–14 d	50 mg/ml 250, 500 mg tab	Adverse reactions: headache, metallic taste, nausea, diarrhea, dizziness, dry mouth. Avoid alcohol. Drug interactions: warfarin, phenobarbital, cimetidine.

Drug	Indications/Dosage	Supplied	Comments
Miconazole nitrate (Micatin, Monistat-Derm, Monistat 7) *Local antifungal*	Topical treatment of tinea pedis, tinea cruris, tinea corporis, tinea versicolor: Children >2 yr and adults: apply bid for 2–4 wk. Vaginal or vulvar candidiasis: 1 application or vaginal suppository qhs for 1 wk	2% cream, lotion, spray, powder 100, 200 mg vaginal suppository	
Mineral oil (OTC) (Agoral) *Laxative*	Children: 1–2 ml/kg/dose bid PO Adults: 15–60 ml/d PO as single dose; retention enema, 60–150 ml	Sterile liquid Fleet enema—133 ml	Contraindicated in children <4 yr due to aspiration potential. Enema form not for use in children <2 yr. Give on empty stomach.
Minocycline HCl (Minocin) *Tetracycline*	>8 yr: 4 mg/kg/d PO divided bid Adults: Carriers: 200 mg initially, then 100 mg bid for 5 d Acne: 50 mg 1–3 times daily Syphilis/gonorrhea: 200 mg initially, then 100 mg q12 hr for 10–15 d Other indications: *Mycoplasma, Chlamydia, Rickettsia,* neisserial meningitis carriers	50 mg/tsp 50, 100 mg tab and capsule	Photosensitivity. Outdated products can be toxic.
Mometasone furoate monohydrate (Nasonex) *Corticosteroid*	>12 yr: 2 sprays per nostril qd Treatment of seasonal and perennial allergic rhinitis	Nasal spray, 50 μg per spray, 120 sprays per bottle	Improvement of symptoms should begin in 2 d. If exposed to varicella, consider prophylactic therapy to prevent varicella. Side effects: HA, pharyngitis, epistaxis, cough, URI *Table continued on following page*

T A B L E A-1
Medications Continued

GENERIC/TRADE CLASSIFICATION	DOSE/INDICATIONS	SUPPLIED	REMARKS
Montelukast sodium (Singulair) *Leukotriene receptor antagonist*	Children 6–14 yr: 5 mg q hs Adults and children >15 yr: 10 mg q hs Prophylaxis and chronic treatment of asthma	5 mg chewable tablet 10 mg tablet	Drug interactions: phenobarbital, rifampin. Side effects: asthenia/fatigue, abdominal pain, HA, cough.
Mupirocin (Bactroban) *Topical antibiotic*	Apply 3 times daily Useful in the treatment of impetigo due to *Staphylococcus*, *Streptococcus*	2% ointment or cream (15 g)	
Naproxen (Naprosyn) *Nonsteroidal anti-inflammatory*	Children >2 yr: 10–20 mg/kg/d in 2 divided doses Juvenile rheumatoid arthritis: 10–15 mg/kg/d (max. 1000 mg/d) Analgesic: 5–7 mg/kg/dose q8–12 hr Adults: Rheumatoid arthritis: 500–1000 mg/d Analgesia: 250 mg q6–8 hr (max. 1250 mg/d)	125 mg/tsp suspension 250, 375, 500 mg tab	Use cautiously in patients with impaired renal function or burns. Take with milk, antacids, or food. Drug interactions: warfarin, methotrexate.
Nedocromil sodium (Tilade) *Nonsteroidal, anti-inflammatory*	Adults and children >6 yr (inhalation): 2 inhalations, qid Adults and children >2 yr (nebulizer): 1 ampule qid Used as prophylaxis in treatment of asthma	175 µg/metered spray oral inhalant 0.5% nebulizer solution 11 mg/2.2 ml ampules	Not to be used for acute asthma attacks. Not approved for children. Adverse reactions: bad taste, HA.
Neomycin, polymyxin B, hydrocortisone (Pediotic) *Antibiotic, anti-inflammatory*	3–4 drops 3–4 times daily until symptoms are relieved Used for treatment of superficial bacterial infections of the external ear	Otic suspension	A wick can be used to instill drops—saturate cotton with drops and leave in ear canal. The wick should be replaced q24 hr.

Drug	Dosage	How supplied	Comments
Nitrofurantoin (Furadantin, Macrodantin) *Urinary anti-infective*	Children: 5–7 mg/kg/d PO divided q6 hr Chronic therapy: 1–5 mg/kg/d divided bid (max. 400 mg/d) Adults: 50–100 mg/dose PO q6 hr Prophylaxis: 50–100 mg/dose qhs Prevention and treatment of urinary tract infections; *Pseudomonas, Serratia,* and *Proteus* are resistant to this drug	25 mg/tsp 50, 100 mg tab (scored) Macrodantin—25, 50, 100 mg capsule	Can cause discoloration of urine. Do not crush tab. Rinse mouth following administration of suspension to prevent staining of teeth.
Nystatin (Mycostatin, Nilstat, Nystex, O-V Statin) *Antifungal*	Oral *Monilia:* Neonates: 100,000 U qid Infants: 200,000 U qid Children and adults: 500,000 U qid Gastrointestinal infections: Adults: 500,000–1 million U as tab qid Cutaneous and mucocutaneous candidal infections: Topical: apply 2 or 3 times daily Vaginal: 1–2 tabs qhs for 2 wk	100,000 U/ml suspension 500,000 U tab 100,000 U vaginal tab 100,000 U/g cream, ointment, powder	Vaginal tabs can be used by pregnant women up to 6 wk before term. Paint oral suspension in infant's mouth to coat lesions. Vaginal tabs can be used orally by immunosuppressed patients to provide prolonged drug contact with oral mucosa.

Table continued on following page

Medications *Continued*

GENERIC/TRADE CLASSIFICATION	DOSE/INDICATIONS	SUPPLIED	REMARKS
Ofloxacin otic solution (Floxin otic) *Antibiotic, quinolone*	Children 1–12 yr: 5 drops in affected ear bid for 10 d Adults and children >12 yr: 10 drops in affected ear bid for 10 d; use for 14 d in chronic suppurative otitis media Treatment of otitis media when tympanostomy tubes are in place. Also, otitis externa	Otic solution, 5 ml bottle	Side effects: pruritus, dizziness, vertigo, earache, taste perversion, rash. Warm bottle in hand before administering.
Oxybutynin chloride (Ditropan) *Antispasmodic*	Children 1–5 yr: 0.2 mg/kg/dose PO 2–4 times daily Children >5 yr: 5 mg PO bid (max. 15 mg/d) Adults: 5 mg PO 2–3 times daily (max. 20 mg/d) Used to treat bladder spasms associated with neurogenic bladder or urinary urgency, leakage, or dysuria	5 mg/tsp syrup 5 mg tab	Contraindicated in patients with GI or GU obstruction, myasthenia gravis, glaucoma, ulcerative colitis, unstable cardiac disorders. Drug interactions: CNS depressants. Adverse reactions: GI disturbances, dry mouth, dizziness, decreased sweating, tachycardia.
Palivizumab (Synagis) *Humanized monoclonal antibody*	Pediatric patients: 15 mg/kg per dose given IM once a month, beginning in the fall prior to RSV season and continuing through April Indicated in high-risk pediatric patients to prevent RSV infection	Single-use vial, 100 mg/ml	Efficacy and safety studies were done using infants with history of bronchopulmonary dysplasia and prematurity (<35 wk). Side effects: GI disturbances, pain and redness at injection site, URI, rash, SGOT increases.

Penicillin G benzathine (Bicillin) *Penicillin*	Children (IM): Streptococcal pharyngitis: 25,000 U/kg for 1 dose (max. 1.2 million U) Prophylaxis of rheumatic fever: 25,000 U/kg q3–4 wk (max. 1.2 million U/dose) Syphilis: 50,000 U/kg for 1 dose (max. 2.4 million U) Adult (IM): Streptococcal pharyngitis: 1.2 million U for 1 dose Prophylaxis of rheumatic fever: 1.2 million U q3–4 wk or 600,000 U bimonthly Syphilis: 2.4 million U for 1 dose	200,000 U tab 300,000, 600,000 or 1,200,000 U/ml injection	Give deep IM in upper, outer quadrant of buttocks. Give midlateral thigh in infants and small children. Adverse reactions: hypersensitivity, pain at injection site.
Penicillin V potassium (Pen-Vee K, Veetids) *Penicillin*	Children: 25–50 mg/kg/d PO divided tid-qid Prophylaxis of pneumococcal infection: <5 yr: 125 mg bid >5 yr: 250 mg bid Other indications: skin and soft tissue disorders, streptococcal pharyngitis	125, 250 mg/tsp drops and solution 125, 250, 500 mg tab	Food interferes with absorption. Drug interactions: tetracycline. Suspension has unpleasant taste.
Permethrin (OTC) (Nix) *Pediculicide*	Head lice and their eggs: Adults and children >2 yr: apply to hair, leave on for 10 min, then rinse; can repeat treatment in 7 d if lice are observed	1% lotion	Not recommended for children <2 yr. Thorough combing to remove nits is required as well as cleansing of the equipment.

Table continued on following page

Medications Continued

GENERIC/TRADE CLASSIFICATION	DOSE/INDICATIONS	SUPPLIED	REMARKS
Phenazopyridine HCl (Azo-Standard, Baridium, Pyridium) *Urinary analgesic*	Children 6–12 yr: 4 mg/kg PO tid for 2 d only Adults: 200 mg PO tid Used to treat pain associated with urinary tract infections or irritation	60 mg/ml suspension (not available in all pharmacies) 100, 200 mg tab	Contraindicated in patients with liver or kidney disease. Adverse reactions: GI disturbances, headache, vertigo, methemoglobinemia, skin pigmentation. Urine discoloration occurs and stains clothing.
Pheniramine *Antihistamine*	Children: 2–6 yr: 2 mg q4 hr 6–12 yr: 4 mg PO q4 hr Adults: 8 mg PO q4 hr Relief of respiratory congestion in allergic rhinitis, sinusitis	Available in various combination preparations 4 mg/5 ml syrup	
Phenobarbital (Barbita, Gardenal, Solfoton) *Barbiturate, anticonvulsant, sedative*	Status epilepticus: Children: 5–10 mg/kg IV, may repeat q10–15 min to a total of 20 mg/kg Adults: 10 mg/kg IV, may repeat q10–15 min to a total of 20 mg/kg Maintenance for grand mal, partial, and febrile seizures: Children: 4–6 mg/kg/d PO divided bid Adults: 100–200 mg/d PO divided tid or total qhs Hyperbilirubinemia: Neonates: 2–4 mg/kg/d divided bid for 1–2 wk, then 5 mg/kg/d divided bid PO Chronic cholestasis: Children: 3–12 mg/kg/d PO divided tid Adults: 90–180 mg/d PO divided bid–tid	15, 20 mg/tsp elixir 8, 15, 16, 30, 32, 60, 65, 100 mg tab 16 mg capsule	Therapeutic level 15–40 μg/ml. CBC, LFTs with long-term use. Drug interactions: primidone, valproic acid, warfarin, corticosteroids, oral contraceptives, doxycycline. Do not withdraw drug abruptly.

Drug	Dosage	How Supplied	Comments
Phenylephrine HCl (Mydfrin, Neo-Synephrine) *Vasoconstrictor, mydriatic, decongestant*	Drops or spray: Children: <6 yr: 2–3 drops q4 hr of 0.125% solution 6–12 yr: 2–4 drops q4 hr of 0.25% solution Adults: 2–3 drops or 1–2 sprays q4 hr of 0.25% to 0.5% solution, prn Do not use longer than 3 d PO: Children: 2–6 yr: 2.5 mg q4 hr (max. 15 mg/d) 6–12 yr: 5 mg q4 hr (max. 30 mg/d) Adults: 10 mg q4 hr (max. 60 mg/d) Relief of nasal and nasopharyngeal mucosal congestion; treatment of wide-angle glaucoma	0.125%, 0.25%, 0.5%, 1% nasal drops 0.25%, 0.5%, 1% nasal spray 2.5%, 10% ophthalmic solution Available in various combinations, usually 5 mg/ml	
Phenylpropanolamine HCl *Sympathomimetic*	Children: 2–6 yr: 6.25 mg q4 hr 6–12 yr: 12.5 mg q4 hr Adults: 25 mg q4 hr or 50 mg q8 hr PO (max. 150 mg/d) Used as an oral decongestant and anorexiant, nasal decongestant	12.5 mg/5 ml syrup 25 mg tab	Can elevate blood pressure. Can cause excitement.
Phenyltoloxamine citrate *Antihistamine*	Children: 2–6 yr: 2 mg q4 hr 6–12 yr: 4 mg q4 hr Adults: 8 mg q4 hr	Found in many combination preparations	

Table continued on following page

Medications *Continued*

GENERIC/TRADE CLASSIFICATION	DOSE/INDICATIONS	SUPPLIED	REMARKS
Phenytoin (Dilantin) *Hydantoin derivative, anticonvulsant*	Grand mal, complex partial seizures: Neonates: 5 mg/kg/d divided q12 hr 10 d–3 yr: 8–10 mg/kg/d PO divided 8–12 hr; loading dose of 15 mg/kg PO divided q8–12 hr Children and adults: 5–8 mg/kg/d divided q12–24 hr; adult loading dose of 900 mg–1.5 g PO divided tid Arrhythmias: Children: 2–5 mg/kg/d divided bid PO or IV Adults: 250 mg qid for 1 d, 250 mg bid for 2 d, then 300–400 mg/d divided qd–qid	30 mg/5 ml suspension 50 mg chewable tab 30, 100 mg capsule 50 mg/ml injection	Can cause discoloration of urine. Adverse reactions: gingival hyperplasia, blood dyscrasias. Periodic blood work with long-term therapy. Drug interactions: alcohol, antihistamines, folic acid, rifampin, antacids.
Prednisolone (Delta-Cortef, Pediapred, Prelone) *Glucocorticoid, anti-inflammatory*	Children: Anti-inflammatory: 0.1–2 mg/kg/d PO divided 1–4 times daily Asthma: 1–2 mg/kg/d divided 1–2 times daily for 3–5 d Adults: 5–60 mg/d PO Used in the treatment of inflammatory disorders of respiratory and GI tracts, allergic disorders, and rheumatic disease	Oral solution: 5 mg/5 ml, 15 mg/5 ml	Contraindicated in patients with active, untreated infections, including varicella. Can mask symptoms of infections. Do not abruptly stop drug. Adverse reactions: growth suppression, fractures, GI discomfort, vertigo, acne.

Drug	Dosage/Use	Available Forms	Comments
Prednisone (Deltasone, Liquid Pred, Orasone) *Glucocorticoid, anti-inflammatory*	Children: 0.1–2 mg/kg/d PO in 1–4 divided doses Adults: 5–60 mg/d PO divided in 1–4 doses Used in the treatment of inflammatory disorders, allergic disorders, and hematological diseases	Solution: 5 mg/ml, 15 mg/5 ml 1, 2.5, 5, 10, 20, 50 mg tab	See contraindications and side effects for prednisolone.
Promethazine HCl (Phenergan) *Antiemetic, antivertigo*	Children: 0.25–0.5 mg/kg q4–6 hr PO, IM, IV, rectally Adults: 12.5–25 mg q4–6 hr PO, IM, IV, rectally Used to treat vertigo, nausea, vomiting	6.25, 25 mg/tsp syrup 12.5, 25, 50 mg tab 12.5, 25, 50 mg suppository 25, 50 mg/ml injection	Drug interactions: MAO inhibitors, CNS depressants. Adverse reactions: confusion, dry mouth, dizziness, drowsiness, blurred vision.
Pyrantel pamoate (Antiminth) *Anthelmintic*	Roundworms and pinworms: Adults and children >2 yr: 11 mg/kg PO as single dose (max. 1 g); for pinworms, repeat in 2 wk	50 mg/ml suspension	Can be given with food. Treat all family members. Minimal toxicity. Use with caution in patient who is malnourished, anemic, or has hepatic disease.
Pyrethrins (OTC) (A-200 Pyrinate, Pyrinyl, Pronton, RID) *Pediculicide*	Pediculosis: Apply to hair and affected body areas, leave on 10 min, rinse; can repeat in 7–10 d; do not repeat in <24 hr	Available as gel, shampoo, liquid	Avoid contact with eyes, face.

Table continued on following page

T A B L E A-1

Medications *Continued*

GENERIC/TRADE CLASSIFICATION	DOSE/INDICATIONS	SUPPLIED	REMARKS

Ranitidine HCl (Zantac)
Antiulcer agent
	Children:
	  Oral: 1.5–2.3 mg/kg/dose
	    q12h
	  IM, IV: 0.1–0.8 mg/kg/dose
	    q6–8h
	Adults: 150 mg bid or 300 mg
	  qhs HS
	Short-term treatment of active
	  duodenal ulcers and benign
	  gastric ulcers; long-term
	  prophylaxis of duodenal ulcer
	  and gastric hypersecretion;
	  gastroesophageal reflux
		25 mg/ml injection
		15 mg/ml syrup
		150, 300 mg tab
			Use with caution if liver and renal
			  impairment.
			Adverse reactions: HA, dizziness,
			  sedation, malaise, mental
			  confusion, nausea, vomiting,
			  constipation, rash, arthralgia,
			  bradycardia or tachycardia.

Rifampin (Rifadin,
Rimactane, Rifabutin)
Antituberculosis agent
	Children: 10–20 mg/kg/d PO
	  divided bid
	Adults: 10 mg/kg/d (max. 600
	  mg/d)
	Following 1–2 mo of therapy:
	  10–20 mg/kg/dose twice
	  weekly (max. 600 mg/dose)
	H. influenzae prophylaxis:
	  Infants <1 mo: 10 mg/kg/d
	    qd for 4 d
	  Infants/children: 20 mg/kg/d
	    qd for 4 d (max. 600 mg)
	  Adults: 600 mg qd for 4 d
	Meningococcal prophylaxis:
	  3 mo–1 yr: 10 mg/kg/d
	    divided bid for 2 d
	  Children: 20 mg/kg/d divided
	    bid for 2 d
	  Adults: 600 mg q12 hr for 2 d
		50 mg/ml
		150, 300 mg capsule
			Take on empty stomach. Can
			  discolor body fluids. Drug
			  interactions: verapamil,
			  methadone, digoxin,
			  cyclosporine, steroids, birth
			  control pills. Adverse reactions:
			  nausea, vomiting, headache,
			  pruritus, fatigue, ataxia, hepatitis,
			  confusion.

Drug	Dosage/Use	Preparations	Comments
Salicylic acid preparations (DuoFilm—salicylic acid 16.7% and lactic acid 16.7%; Occlusal-HP—salicylic acid 17%; Trans-Ver-Sal—salicylic acid 15%) *Keratolytic agent*	Apply once daily to wart. Used in the treatment of warts and other benign epithelial tumors	Topical solution. Trans-Ver-Sal patches—6 or 12 mm	Avoid contact with healthy skin. Contraindicated in diabetics, those with impaired circulation. Not to be used on moles, birthmarks, unusual skin lesions.
Salmeterol xinafoate (Serevent) *Bronchodilator*	Adults and children >12 yr: 2 inhalations q12 hr (max. 4 inhalations daily). Children >4 yr: use diskus inhalation q12 hr. Used as maintenance therapy in the treatment of asthma	21 μg/inhalation metered dose inhaler. 50 μg/inhalation diskus	Not used as treatment for acute asthma attack. Use cautiously (high incidence of overuse). Patient education is very important. Drug interactions: MAO inhibitors, tricyclic antidepressants.
Selenium sulfide (OTC and Rx) (Exsel, Head & Shoulders, Selsun, Selsun Blue) *Local antiseborrheic, antifungal*	Topical use for treatment of dandruff, seborrhea, dermatitis of scalp: Adults and children: wash with 1–2 tsp, leave on 2–3 min, rinse; 2 applications/wk for 2 wk, then q3–4 wk. For tinea versicolor, leave lotion on 10 min, rinse, once daily for 7 d	1% selenium sulfide shampoo—OTC. 2% selenium sulfide lotion—Rx	Do not use with infants. Do not use on excoriated or inflamed areas.
Senna (Fletcher's Castoria, Gentle Nature, Senokot) *Stimulant laxative*	Children: <5 yr: 1–2 tsp syrup; >5 yr: 2–3 tsp syrup. Adults: 2 tab or 1 tsp qhs (max. 4 tab or 2 tsp)	187, 217, 600 mg tab. 326 mg/tsp, 1.65 g/½ tsp granules. 652 mg suppository. 218 mg/tsp syrup	Contraindicated in patients with acute abdomen, fecal impaction. Discontinue drug if abdominal pain develops.

Table continued on following page

1399

T A B L E A-1
Medications Continued

GENERIC/TRADE CLASSIFICATION	DOSE/INDICATIONS	SUPPLIED	REMARKS
Sertraline hydrochloride (Zoloft) *Selective serotonin reuptake inhibitor*	6–12 yr: 25 mg qd >12 yr: 50 mg qd Increase at 1-wk intervals with maximum of 200 mg/d Treatment of depression and obsessive-compulsive disorder	25, 50, 100 mg tab	Drug interactions: cimetidine, diazepam, tricyclic antidepressants, warfarin, tolbutamide. Side effects: GI disturbances, sweating, agitation, insomnia, hyperkinesia, malaise, fever.
Simethicone (OTC) (Gas-X, Mylicon) *Antiflatulent*	Infants: 20 mg qid Children <12 yr: 40 mg qid Adults: 40–120 mg after meals and qhs Used to treat flatulence and functional gastric bloating	40 mg/0.6 ml drops 40, 80 mg chewable tab	
Sodium citrate and citric acid (Bicitra) *Alkalinizing agent*	Infants and children: 2–3 mEq/kg/d PO divided tid-qid Children: 5–15 ml PO diluted, after meals and qhs Adults: 15–30 ml PO diluted in water or juice, after meals and qhs Used in the management of metabolic acidosis and in conditions requiring alkaline urine	Solution: sodium citrate 500 mg and citric acid 334 mg/5 ml 1 mEq of sodium and 1 mEq of bicarbonate in each 1 ml of Bicitra	Contraindicated in patients with renal insufficiency and in those with a sodium restriction. Drug interactions: antihypertensives. Adverse reactions: hypernatremia, metabolic alkalosis, diarrhea.
Sodium phosphate (Fleet Enema) *Laxative*	Children: 1 oz/20 lb of weight Adolescents and adults: 4 oz (max. 8 oz)	2.25 and 4.5 oz squeeze bottle	
Sodium sulfacetamide (Bleph-10, Isopto, Cetamide) *Sulfonamide*	Solution: 1–2 drops 3–4 times daily for 7–10 d; ointment is used 1–4 times daily Used for treatment of ocular infections	Ophthalmic solution 10%, 15% Ophthalmic ointment 10%	Solution will burn with instillation. Do not use in children <2 mo. Eyes should be cleansed prior to instillation—inactivated by purulent discharge.

Drug	Dosage	How supplied	Comments
Sulfasalazine (Azulfidine) *Sulfonamide*	>2 yr: 40–60 mg/kg/d divided q4–8 hr Maintenance: 20–30 mg/kg/d divided q 6 hr (max. 2 g/d) Adults: 1 g q6–8 hr Maintenance: 2 g/d (max. 4 g/d) Used for management of ulcerative colitis	250 mg/tsp 500 mg tab	Can cause discoloration of urine and skin. GI intolerance is common during first few days. Drug interactions: folic acid, phenytoin, methotrexate, anticoagulants, oral hypoglycemics.
Sulfisoxazole (Gantrisin) *Sulfonamide*	Urinary tract infections: >2 mo: 50–60 mg/kg/d dose initially, then 25–30 mg/kg bid (max. 75 mg/kg/d) Adults: 2 g initially, then 1 g bid–tid Otitis media with effusion prophylaxis: 50–75 mg/d	500 mg/tsp 500 mg tab	Not indicated for infants <2 mo. Take on empty stomach.
Sumatriptan (Imitrex) *5-HT1 receptor agonist*	>18 yr: 6 mg SC; repeat in 1 hr to maximum of 2 doses per 24 hr Tablets: 25–100 mg once; repeat dose at 2-hr intervals to maximum of 200 mg/d Nasal spray: 5, 10 or 20 mg intranasally; can repeat once; maximum 40 mg or 4 uses/month Acute treatment of migraine HA	6 mg/0.5 ml SC injection 25, 50 mg tablet 5, 20 mg spray	Drug interactions: MAO inhibitors, SSRIs. Contraindicated in patients with ischemic heart disease or HTN. Side effects: increased blood pressure, flushing, nausea, drowsiness, sweating; local reactions with spray and injection.

Table continued on following page

Medications Continued

GENERIC/TRADE CLASSIFICATION	DOSE/INDICATIONS	SUPPLIED	REMARKS
Terbutaline (Brethaire, Brethine, Bricanyl) *Bronchodilator*	Adults and children >12 yr: 2.5 mg/dose PO tid; maintenance dose: 5 mg/dose or 0.075 mg/kg PO 3 or 4 times a day Children <12 yr: 0.05 mg/kg/ dose PO tid (max. 0.15 mg/ kg/dose tid or 5 mg/d); 0.01 mg/kg/dose SC (max. 0.3 mg/ dose q15–20 min for 2 doses) Used in asthma and COPD	2.5, 5 mg tab 0.2 mg/dose aerosol 1 mg/ml injection	Drug interactions: MAO inhibitors, tricyclic antidepressants, beta blockers. Can cause tachycardia, tremor, hypertension, headache, palpitations.
Tetracycline (Achromycin, Sumycin) *Tetracycline*	>8 yr: 25–50 mg/kg/d PO divided qid Adults: 250–500 mg PO qid Mycoplasma, Chlamydia, rickettsia, acne, exacerbation of bronchitis, gonorrhea, syphilis (in patients sensitive to penicillin)	125 mg/tsp 250, 500 mg capsule	Take on empty stomach. Photosensitivity. Outdated drugs may be toxic. Drug interactions: antacids, milk, zinc, iron.
Theophylline (Slo-bid, Slophyllin, Theo-Dur, Theolair) *Respiratory smooth muscle relaxant*	Infants/newborns: 4 mg/kg/d PO divided q6 hr 6 wk–6 mo: 10 mg/kg/d PO divided q6 hr 6 mo–1 yr: 12–18 mg/kg/d PO divided q6 hr 1–9 yr: 20–24 mg/kg/d PO divided q6 hr 9–12 yr and adolescent smokers: 15 mg/kg/d PO 12–16 yr (nonsmokers); 13 mg/ kg/d PO Adults: 10 mg/kg/d PO Used as a bronchodilator in the treatment of asthma, COPD; also used for neonatal apnea/ bradycardia	80 mg/15 ml solution 75, 125 mg sprinkles 100, 200, 300 mg timed-release tab (8–12 hr) 50, 60, 75, 100, 125, 200, 250, 300 mg sustained-release capsule	Factors that affect serum levels: cigarettes, marijuana, charcoal-broiled beef, phenytoin, phenobarbital, carbamazepine, rifampin, IV isoproterenol, fever, illnesses, propranolol, allopurinol, erythromycin, cimetidine, oral contraceptives, ciprofloxacin, troleandomycin. Do not crush Theo-Dur tablets. Serum levels should be monitored. Use cautiously in patients with hyperthyroidism, hypertension, cardiac or liver disease.

Drug/Classification	Uses/Dosage	Forms	Comments
Thiabendazole (Mintezol) *Anthelmintic*	Pinworms, roundworms, whipworms, trichinosis. Cutaneous infestations with larva migrans: Adults and children: 25–50 mg/kg/d PO divided q 12 hr for 2–5 consecutive d (max. 3 g/d). Duration of treatment depends on type of helmintic infection.	500 mg/5 ml suspension 500 mg chewable tab	Can inhibit metabolism of aminophylline. 50% of patients experience side effects: nausea, vomiting, dizziness, anorexia.
Tobramycin sulfate (Tobrex) *Antibiotic*	Ophthalmic solution: 1–2 drops q4 hr: ointment is used 3 or 4 times daily; use for 7–10 d Used in the treatment of ocular infections	Ophthalmic solution, ointment 0.3%	
Tolnaftate (OTC) (Absorbine, Aftate, Genaspor, NP-27, Quinsana Plus, Tinactin, Zeasorb-AF) *Antifungal*	Children and adults: apply bid for 2–6 wk Topical treatment of tinea pedis, tinea manuum, tinea cruris, tinea corporis, tinea versicolor	1% cream, powder, liquid, gel, spray	
Tretinoin (Retin-A) *Cell stimulant and proliferant*	Apply a thin layer to acne areas once daily at bedtime Used in the treatment of mild to moderate acne	0.05%, 0.1% cream 0.01%, 0.025% gel 0.05% liquid	Do not apply immediately following hydration of skin. Can have exacerbation of acne initially, including hyper- or hypopigmentation of skin. Avoid contact with abraded skin, eyes, or mucous membranes. *Table continued on following page*

Medications Continued

GENERIC/TRADE CLASSIFICATION	DOSE/INDICATIONS	SUPPLIED	REMARKS
Triamcinolone acetonide (Azmacort, Nasacort AQ) *Glucocorticoid, anti-inflammatory*	Children >6 yr: 1–2 oral inhalations 3–4 times daily (max. 12 inhalations daily); 1 spray/nostril qd Adults: 2 oral inhalations 3–4 times daily (max. 16 inhalations daily); 2 sprays/nostril qd Used in the treatment of steroid-dependent asthma; seasonal and perennial allergic rhinitis	100 μg/metered dose, oral inhalation 55 μg/nasal spray	See contraindications and side effects for flunisolide.
Trifluridine (Viroptic) *Antiviral*	1 drop q2 hr during day (max. 9 drops/d); do not use for longer than 21 d Used for treatment of HSV-1 and HSV-2	Ophthalmic solution 1%	
Trimethobenzamide HCl (Tigan) *Antiemetic*	Children: 13–45 kg: 100–200 mg PO or rectally tid–qid <13 kg: 100 mg rectally tid–qid or 15–20 mg/kg/d Adults: 250 mg PO tid–qid, or 200 mg IM or rectally tid–qid Used for the treatment of nausea and vomiting	100, 200 mg capsule 100, 200 mg suppository	Use cautiously in patients with acute febrile illness. Not effective in the treatment of motion sickness. Can mimic or mask symptoms of Reye syndrome.
Trimethoprim (TMP)-sulfamethoxazole (SMX) (Co-trimoxazole, Bactrim, Bactrim DS, Septra, Septra DS, Sulfatrim, TMS) *Sulfonamide*	Children >2 mo: 6–10 mg TMP/kg/d PO divided bid or 1 ml/kg/d divided bid Adults: 1 DS tab PO bid Urinary tract infections, bronchitis in adults, otitis media, shigellosis, traveler's diarrhea, *Pneumocystis carinii* infection	TMP 40 mg and SMX 200 mg/tsp TMP 80 mg and SMX 400 mg/tab TMP 160 mg and SMX 800 mg/DS tab	Adverse reactions: Stevens-Johnson syndrome. GI side effects minimal. Not effective against streptococcal infections. Drug interactions: warfarin, methotrexate, phenytoin.

Drug/Class	Dosage/Use	Preparations	Comments
Trimethoprim sulfate, polymyxin B (Polytrim) *Antibiotic*	1 drop q3 hr for 7–10 d Used to treat ocular infections	Ophthalmic solution	Contraindicated in children <2 mo. Less burning than with other preparations.
Valproic acid (Depakene, Depakote) *Carboxylic acid derivative, anticonvulsant*	Complex absence seizures: Adults and children: Initially 15 mg/kg/d PO divided bid–tid; may increase by 5–10 mg/kg/d weekly to max. of 60 mg/kg/d	250 mg/tsp elixir 125 mg sprinkle 125, 250, 500 mg enteric-coated tab	Take with food. Do not take with carbonated soda. Do not crush or chew tabs. Monitor blood work with long-term therapy. Therapeutic range: 50–140 µg/ml.
Vancomycin HCl (Vancocin, Vancoled) *Miscellaneous anti-infective*	Children: 10 mg/kg q6 hr PO (max. 2 g/d) Adults: 125–500 mg q6 hr for 7d PO (max. 2 g/d) Oral administration for staphylococcal enterocolitis *Clostridium difficile*—antibiotic-associated pseudomembranous colitis	50 mg/ml oral solution 125, 250 mg capsule	Unpleasant taste. Solution not available in many pharmacies.

Table continued on following page

T A B L E A-1
Medications Continued

GENERIC/TRADE CLASSIFICATION	DOSE/INDICATIONS	SUPPLIED	REMARKS
Zafirlukast (Accolate) *Leukotriene receptor antagonist*	>12 yr: 20 mg bid Prophylactic treatment for mild persistent asthma	20 mg tablets	Drug interactions: warfarin, erythromycin, theophylline, aspirin. Cautious use with cisapride, calcium channel blockers, cyclosporine, astemizole. Side effects: HA, GI disturbances, dizziness. Has to be taken frequently—around the clock.
Zidovudine (AZT) (Retrovir) *Antiviral*	Human immunodeficiency virus (HIV): Adults: 600 mg/d Children 3 mo–12 yr: 180 mg/ m² q6 hr (max. 200 mg q6 hr)	100 mg capsule 50 mg/tsp syrup	Adverse effects: GI symptoms, anemia (45%), granulocytopenia, thrombocytopenia. Monitor CBC, platelets.

Key to abbreviations:
ADD = attention deficit disorder
ADHD = attention deficit with hyperactivity disorder
bid = twice daily
CBC = complete blood count
CNS = central nervous system
GI = gastrointestinal
GU = genitourinary
HA = headache
HSV = herpes simplex virus
HTN = hypertension
IM = intramuscular
IV = intravenous
LFT = liver function test
MAO = monoamine oxidase
max. = maximum
OTC = over the counter
PO = by mouth
prn = as needed
q = every

qam = every morning
qd = evey day
qhs = bedtime
qid = four times daily
qod = every other day
qwk = every week
RSV = respiratory syncytial virus
Rx = prescription
SC = subcutaneous
SGOT = serum glutamic-oxaloacetic transaminase
SL = sublingual
SSRIs = selective serotonin uptake inhibitors
tab(s) = tablet(s)
tid = three times daily
TM = tympanic membrane
tsp = teaspoon
U = units
URI = upper respiratory infection

T A B L E A–2

Topical Steroid Preparations

DRUG	DOSAGE FORM
LOW POTENCY	
Aclometasone dipropionate (Aclovate)	0.05% cream, ointment
Desonide (DesOwen, Tridesilon)	0.05% cream, ointment, lotion
Fluocinolone acetonide (Fluonid, Synalar)	0.01% solution, cream
Fluorometholone (Oxylone)	0.02% cream
Hydrocortisone (Hytone, Nutracort, Cort-Dome, Synacort)	0.5% cream, ointment
	1% cream, ointment, lotion, solution
	2.5% cream, ointment
MODERATE POTENCY	
Betamethasone valerate (Valisone)	0.01% cream
	0.1% cream, ointment, lotion
Clocortolone pivalate (Cloderm)	0.1% cream
Desoximetasone (Topicort)	0.05% gel
Fluocinolone acetonide (Synalar, Fluonid)	0.025% cream, ointment
	0.1% cream
Flurandrenolide (Cordran)	0.05% cream, lotion, ointment
Fluticasone propionate	0.005% ointment
	0.05% cream
Halcinonide (Halog)	0.025% cream, ointment
Hydrocortisone valerate (Westcort)	0.2% cream, ointment
Mometasone furoate	0.1% cream, lotion, ointment
Triamcinolone acetonide (Kenalog, Aristocort)	0.025%, 0.1% cream, ointment, lotion
HIGH POTENCY	
Amcinonide (Cyclocort)	0.1% cream, ointment
Betamethasone dipropionate (Diprosone)	0.05% cream, lotion, ointment, gel
Betamethasone dipropionate, clotrimazole (Lotrisone)	0.25% cream, ointment, emollient cream
Desoximetasone (Topicort)	0.05% cream, ointment
	0.25% cream, ointment
Diflorasone diacetate (Florone, Psorcan)	0.2% cream
	0.05% cream, ointment
Fluocinolone acetonide (Synalar-HP)	0.05% cream, solution, gel, ointment
Fluocinonide (Lidex)	0.1% cream, ointment, solution
Halcinonide (Halog)	0.05% cream, ointment
	0.1%, cream, ointment, solution
Halobetasol propionate (Ultravate)	0.05% cream with 1% clotrimazole
Triamcinolone acetonide (Kenalog, Aristocort)	0.5% cream, ointment

REFERENCES

Murphy J (ed): Nurse Practitioner's Prescribing Reference. New York, Prescribing Reference, Inc., 1999.

Physicians' Desk Reference, 53rd ed. Montvale, NJ, Medical Economics Data Production Company, 1999.

Staible SA (ed): Formulary and Drug Dosing Handbook, 2nd ed. The Children's Hospital, Denver, CO. Hudson, OH: Lexi-Comp, 1996.

Growth Grids

Ardys M. Dunn

Girls: Birth to 36 Months Physical Growth NCHS Percentiles*

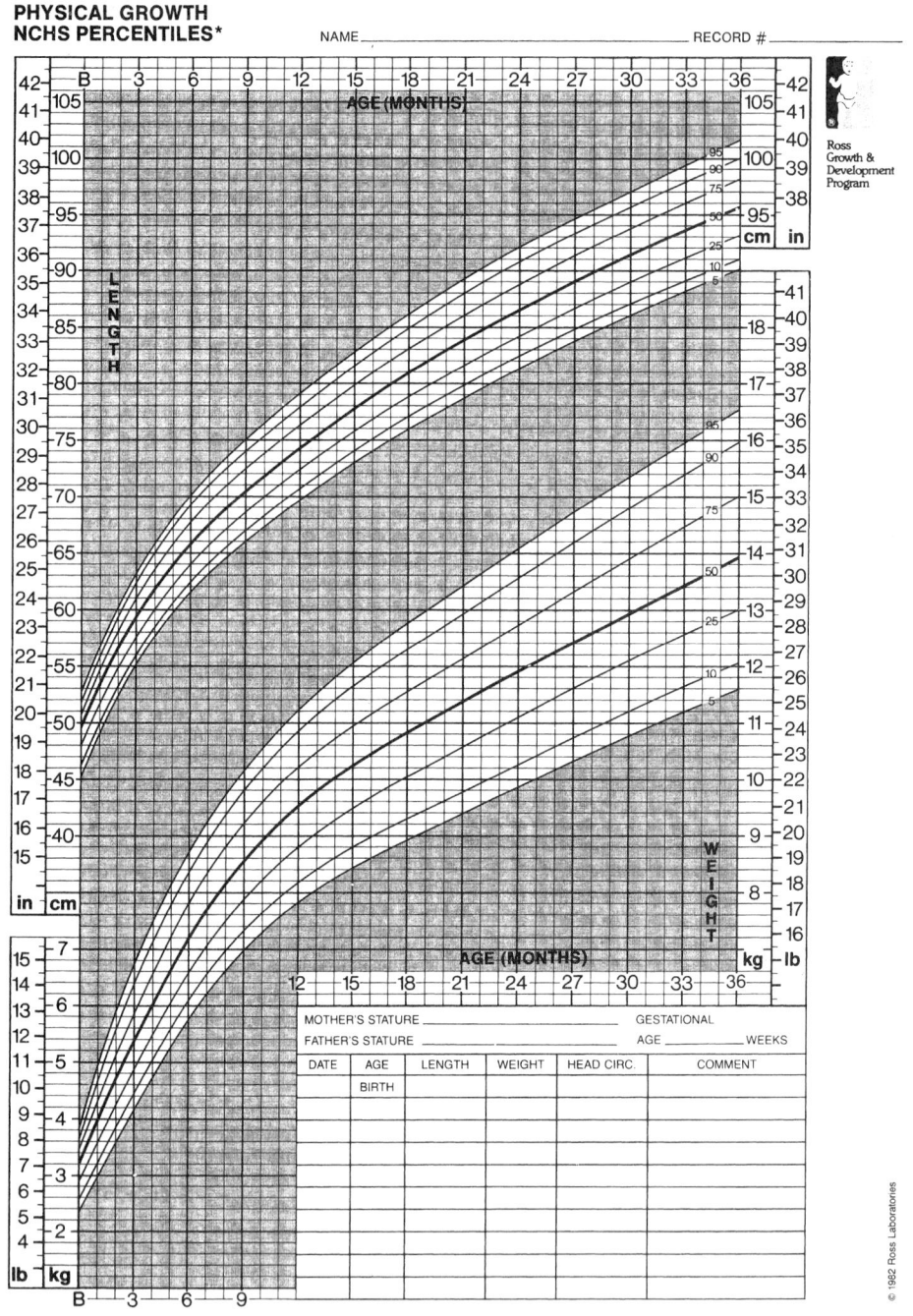

PHYSICAL GROWTH
NCHS PERCENTILES*

NAME _____ RECORD # _____

Ross
Growth &
Development
Program

© 1982 Ross Laboratories

*Adapted from Hamill PV, Drizd TA, Johnson CL, et al: Physical growth: National Center for Health Statistics percentiles. Am J Clin Nutr 32:607–629, 1979. Data from the Fels Longitudinal Study, Wright State University School of Medicine, Yellow Springs, Ohio.

Girls: Birth to 36 Months Physical Growth NCHS Percentiles*

**PHYSICAL GROWTH
NCHS PERCENTILES***

NAME _____ RECORD # _____

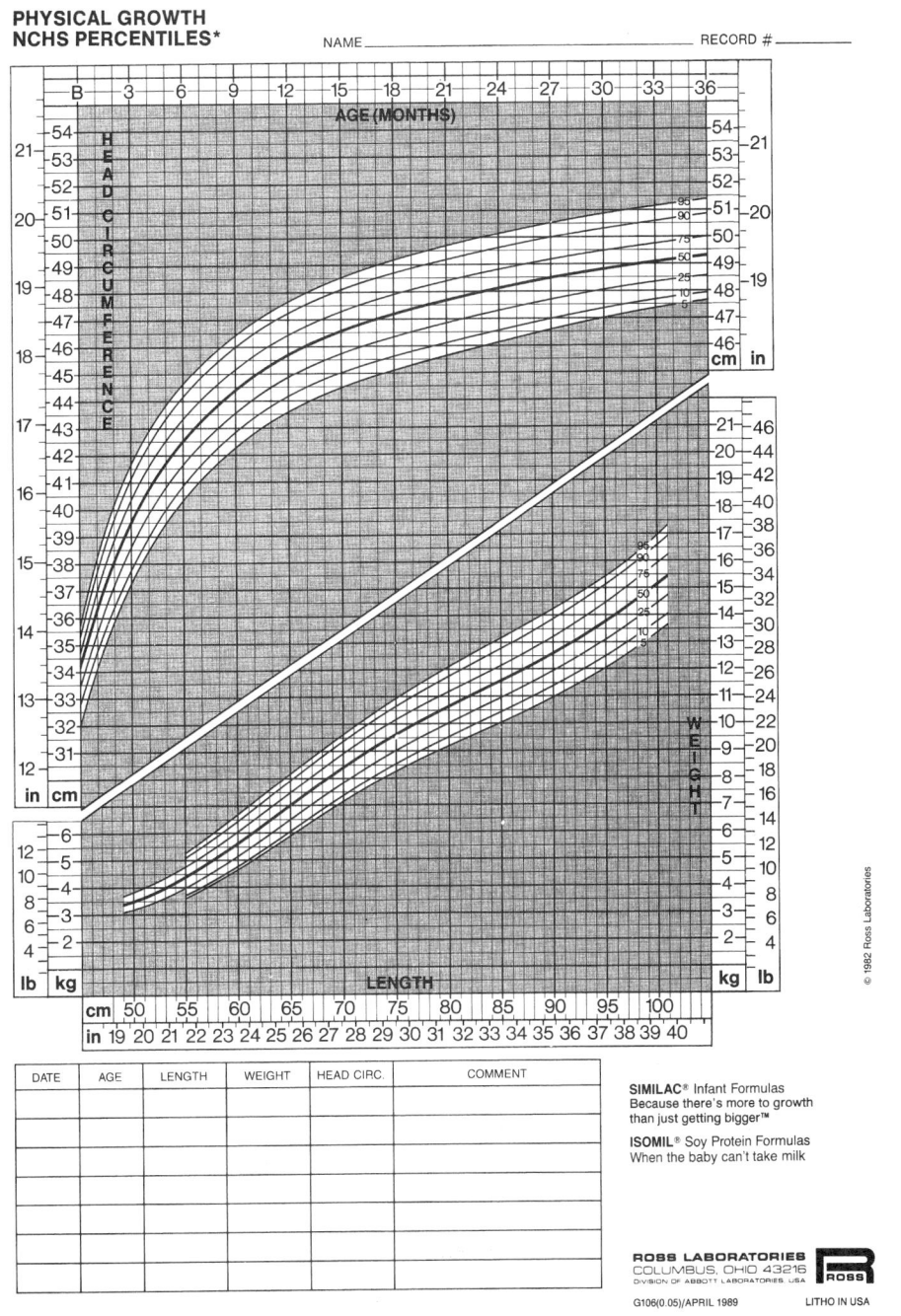

DATE	AGE	LENGTH	WEIGHT	HEAD CIRC.	COMMENT

SIMILAC® Infant Formulas
Because there's more to growth
than just getting bigger™

ISOMIL® Soy Protein Formulas
When the baby can't take milk

© 1982 Ross Laboratories

ROSS LABORATORIES
COLUMBUS, OHIO 43216
DIVISION OF ABBOTT LABORATORIES, USA

G106(0.05)/APRIL 1989   LITHO IN USA

*Adapted from Hamill PV, Drizd TA, Johnson CL, et al: Physical growth: National Center for Health Statistics percentiles. Am J Clin Nutr 32:607–629, 1979. Data from the Fels Longitudinal Study, Wright State University School of Medicine, Yellow Springs, Ohio.

Girls: 2 to 18 Years Physical Growth NCHS Percentiles*

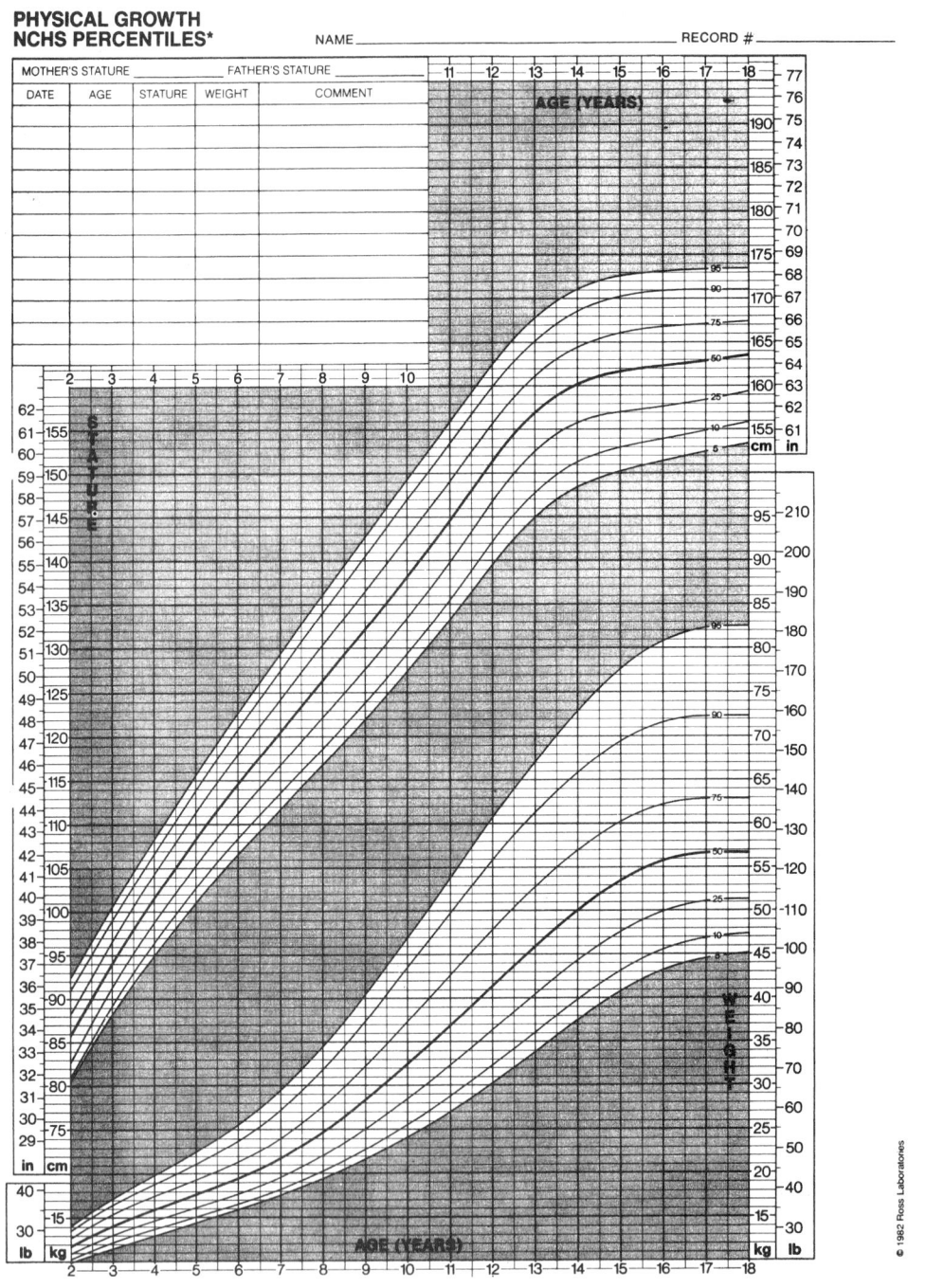

PHYSICAL GROWTH
NCHS PERCENTILES*

*Adapted from Hamill PV, Drizd TA, Johnson CL, et al: Physical growth: National Center for Health Statistics percentiles. Am J Clin Nutr 32:607–629, 1979. Data from the National Center for Health Statistics (NCHS), Hyattsville, Maryland.

Girls: Prepubescent Physical Growth NCHS Percentiles*

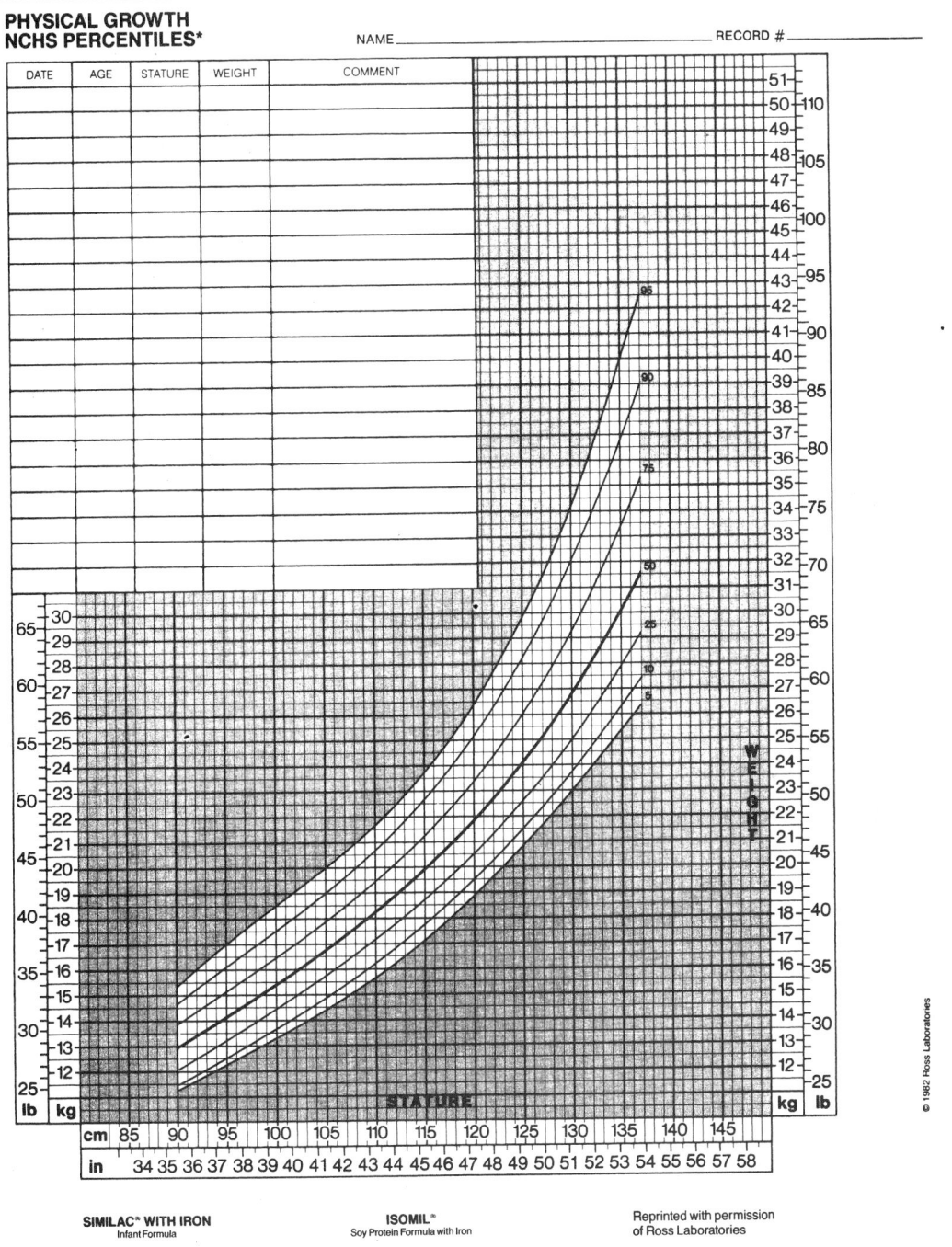

PHYSICAL GROWTH
NCHS PERCENTILES*

NAME _____ RECORD # _____

SIMILAC® WITH IRON
Infant Formula

ISOMIL®
Soy Protein Formula with Iron

Reprinted with permission
of Ross Laboratories

© 1982 Ross Laboratories

*Adapted from Hamill PV, Drizd TA, Johnson CL, et al: Physical growth: National Center for Health Statistics percentiles. Am J Clin Nutr 32:607–629, 1979. Data from the National Center for Health Statistics (NCHS), Hyattsville, Maryland.

Boys: Birth to 36 Months Physical Growth NCHS Percentiles*

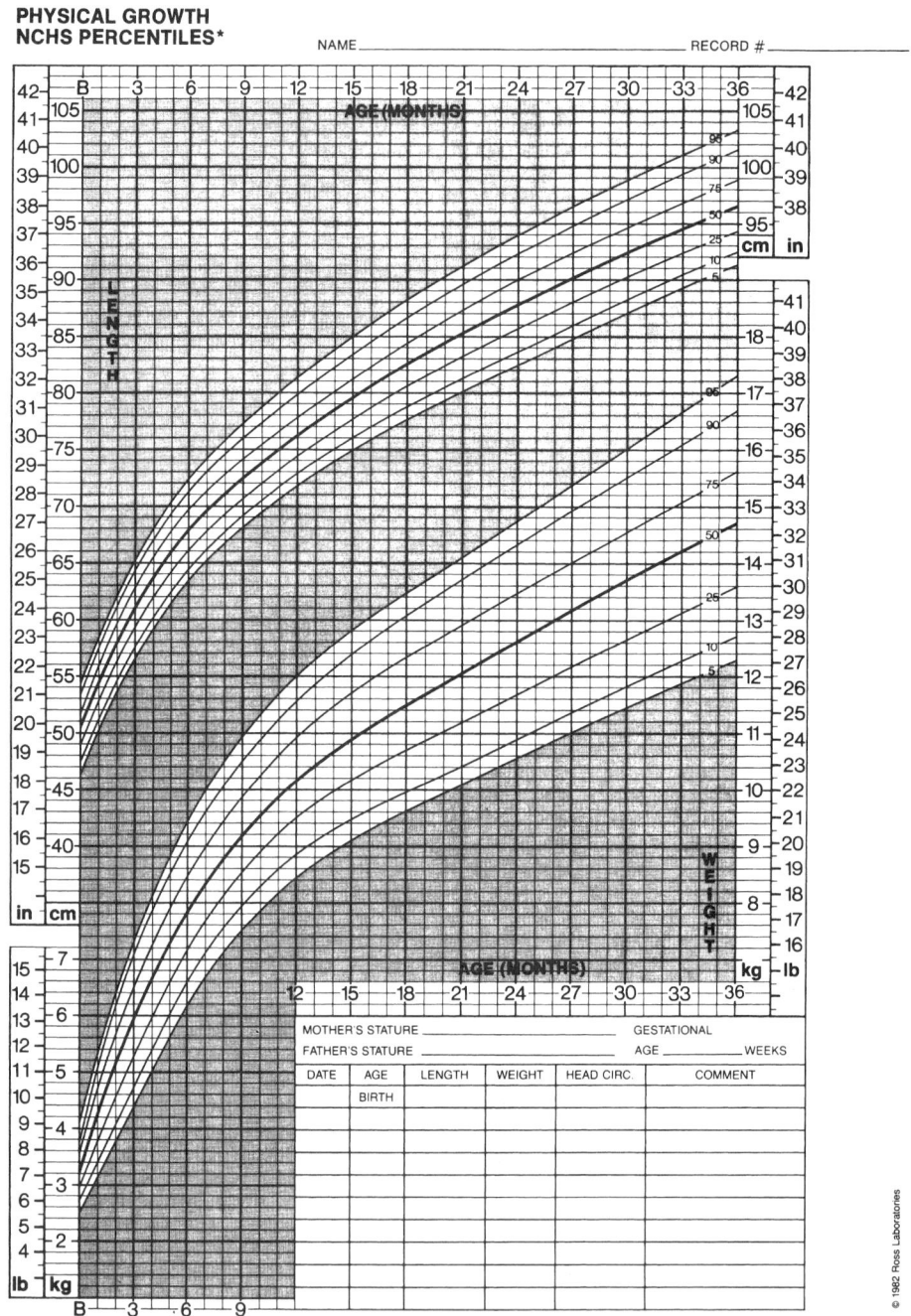

PHYSICAL GROWTH
NCHS PERCENTILES*

NAME_____ RECORD #_____

*Adapted from Hamill PV, Drizd TA, Johnson CL, et al: Physical growth: National Center for Health Statistics percentiles. Am J Clin Nutr 32:607–629, 1979. Data from the Fels Longitudinal Study, Wright State University School of Medicine, Yellow Springs, Ohio.

Boys: Birth to 36 Months Physical Growth NCHS Percentiles*

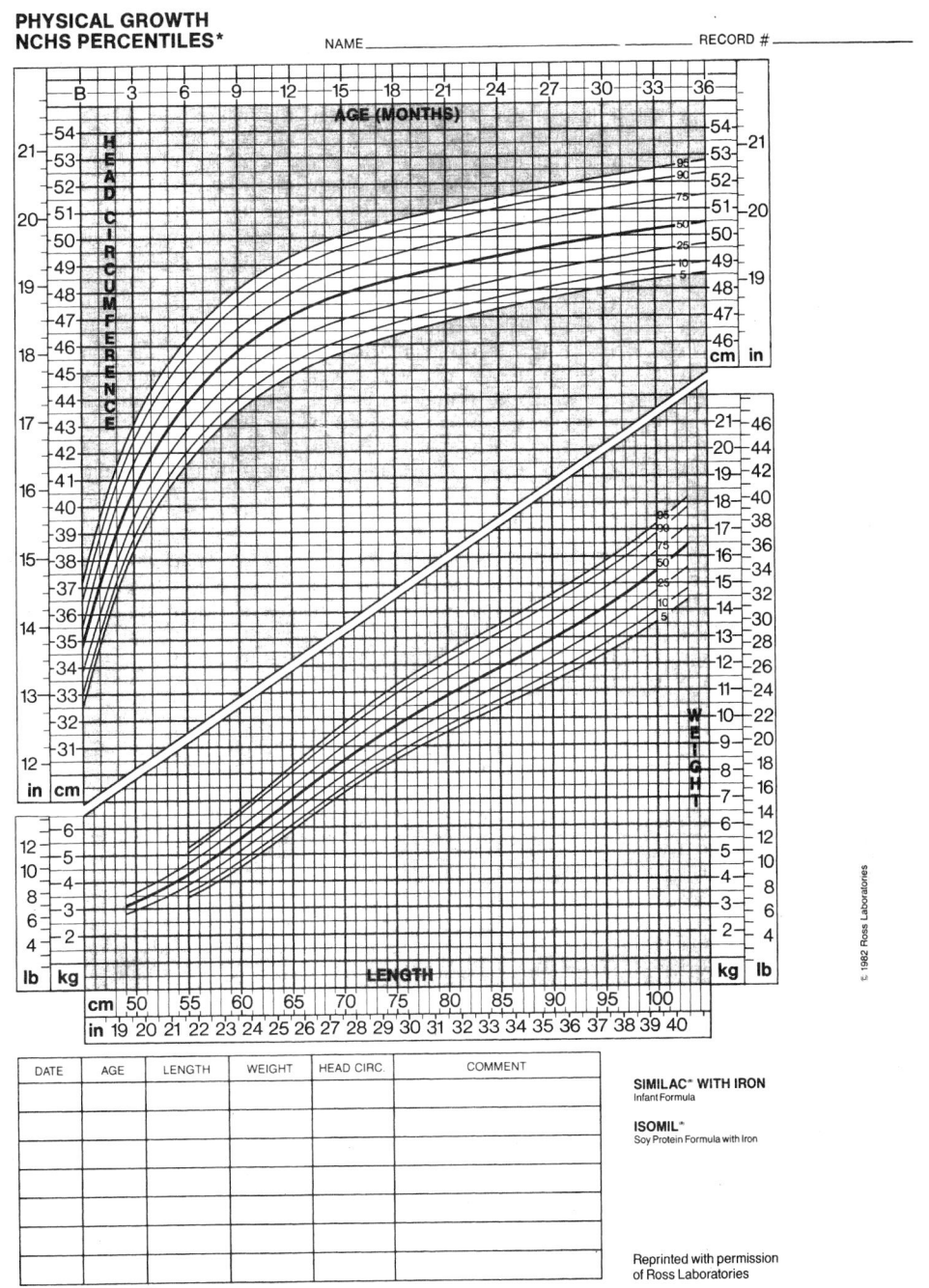

DATE	AGE	LENGTH	WEIGHT	HEAD CIRC.	COMMENT

SIMILAC® WITH IRON
Infant Formula

ISOMIL®
Soy Protein Formula with Iron

Reprinted with permission
of Ross Laboratories

*Adapted from Hamill PV, Drizd TA, Johnson CL, et al: Physical growth: National Center for Health Statistics percentiles. Am J Clin Nutr 32:607–629, 1979. Data from the Fels Longitudinal Study, Wright State University School of Medicine, Yellow Springs, Ohio.

Boys: 2 to 18 Years Physical Growth NCHS Percentiles*

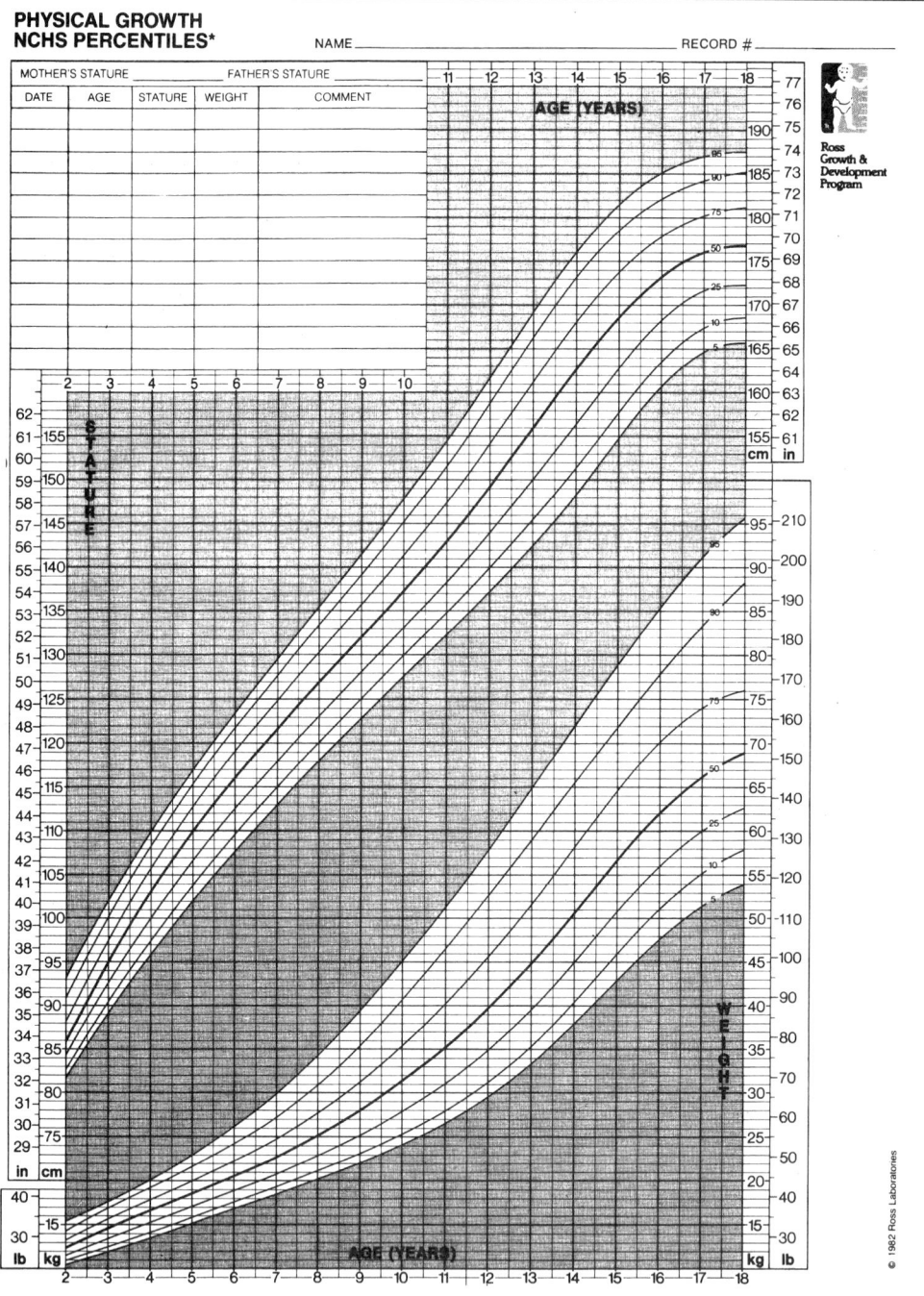

*Adapted from Hamill PV, Drizd TA, Johnson CL, et al: Physical growth: National Center for Health Statistics percentiles. Am J Clin Nutr 32:607–629, 1979. Data from the National Center for Health Statistics (NCHS), Hyattsville, Maryland.

Boys: Prepubescent Physical Growth NCHS Percentiles*

**PHYSICAL GROWTH
NCHS PERCENTILES***

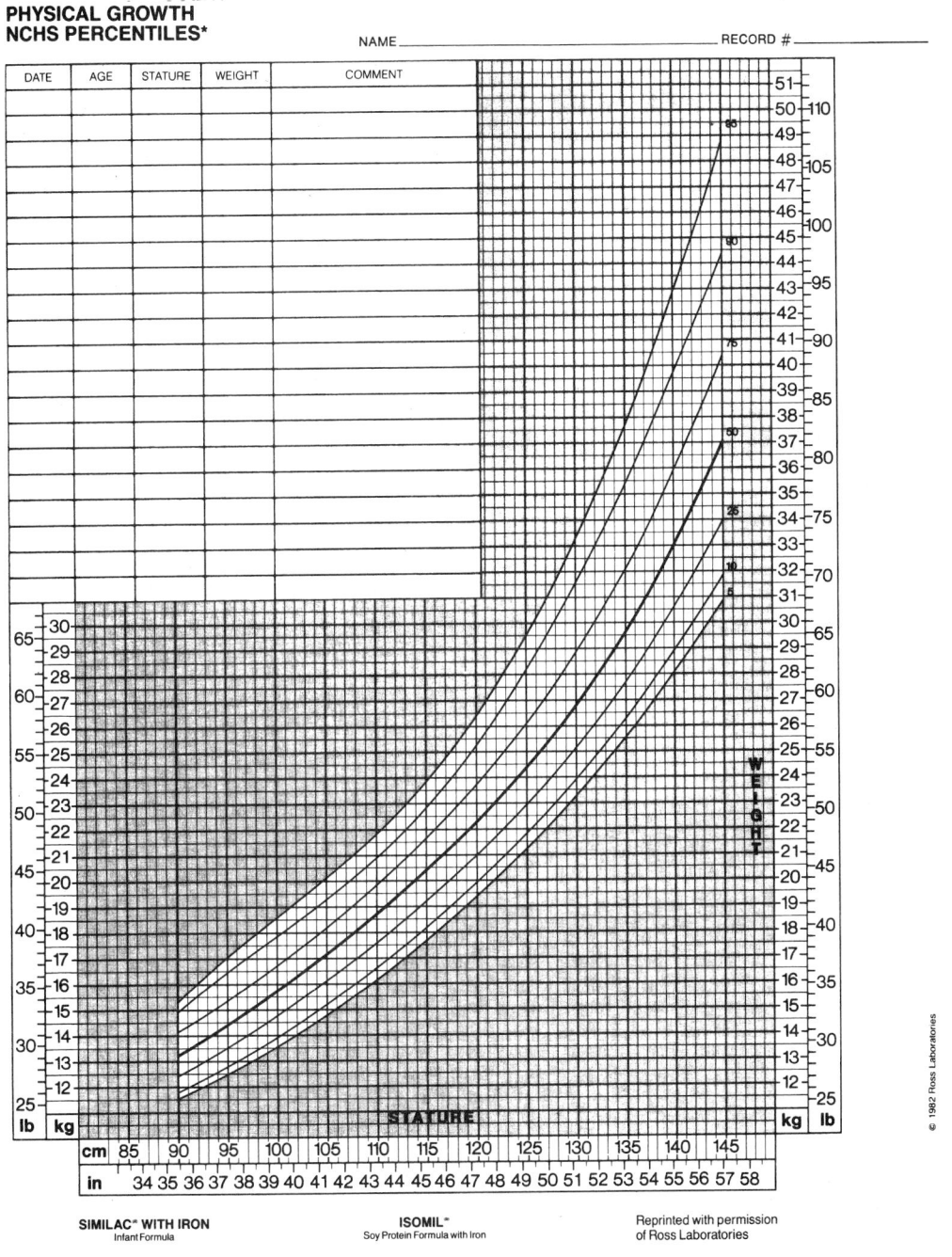

SIMILAC® WITH IRON
Infant Formula

ISOMIL®
Soy Protein Formula with Iron

Reprinted with permission
of Ross Laboratories

© 1982 Ross Laboratories

*Adapted from Hamill PV, Drizd TA, Johnson CL, et al: Physical growth: National Center for Health Statistics percentiles. Am J Clin Nutr 32:607–629, 1979. Data from the National Center for Health Statistics (NCHS), Hyattsville, Maryland.

T A B L E B-9

Head Circumference Chart (Girls)

Nellhaus G: Head circumference from birth to eighteen years. Practical composite international and interracial graphs. Pediatrics 41:106–114, 1968.

TABLE B-10

Head Circumference Chart (Boys)

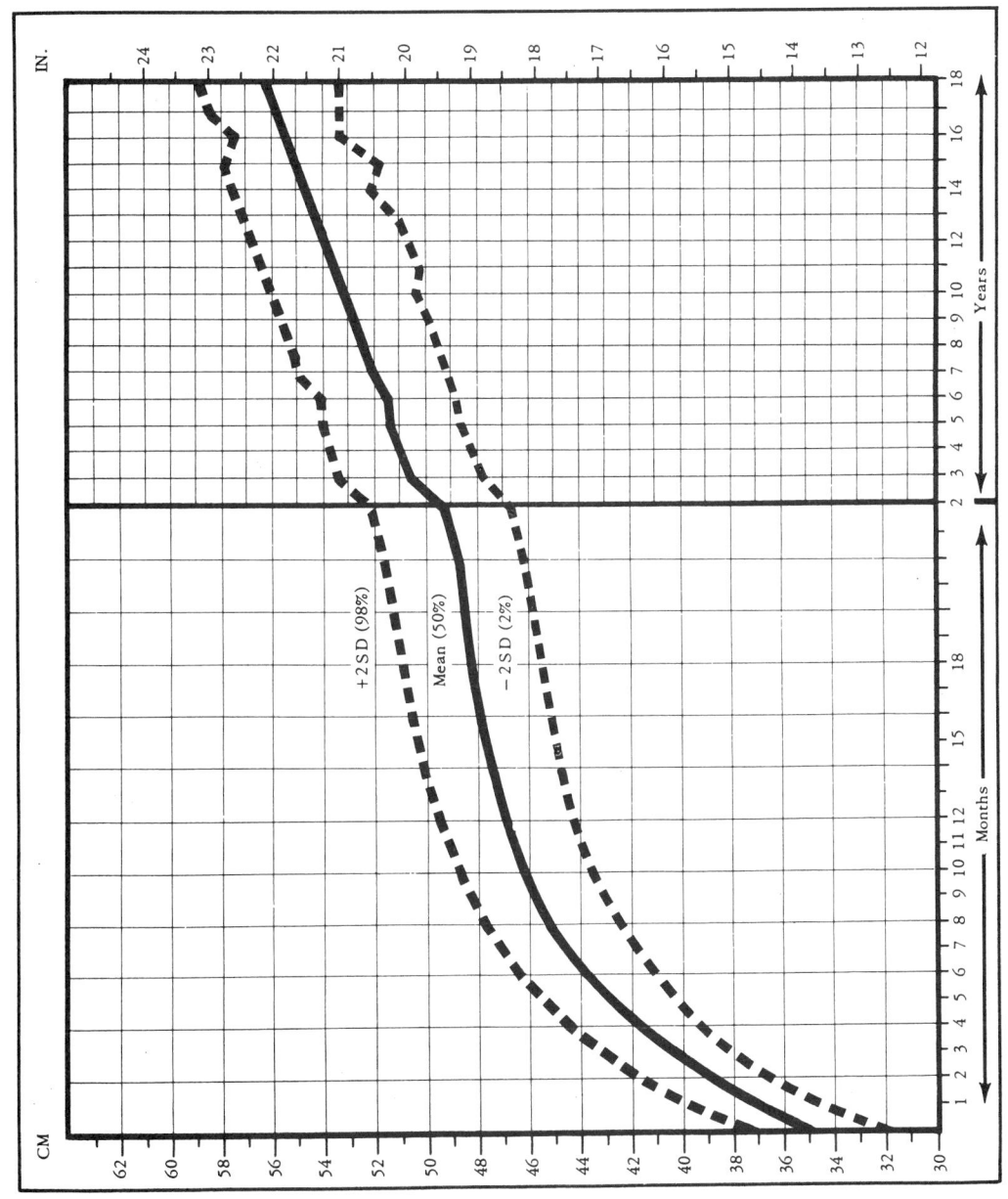

Nellhaus G: Head circumference from birth to eighteen years. Practical composite international and interracial graphs. Pediatrics 41:106–114, 1968.

T A B L E B-11

Growth Record for Premature Infants in Relation to Gestational Age and Fetal and Infant Norms

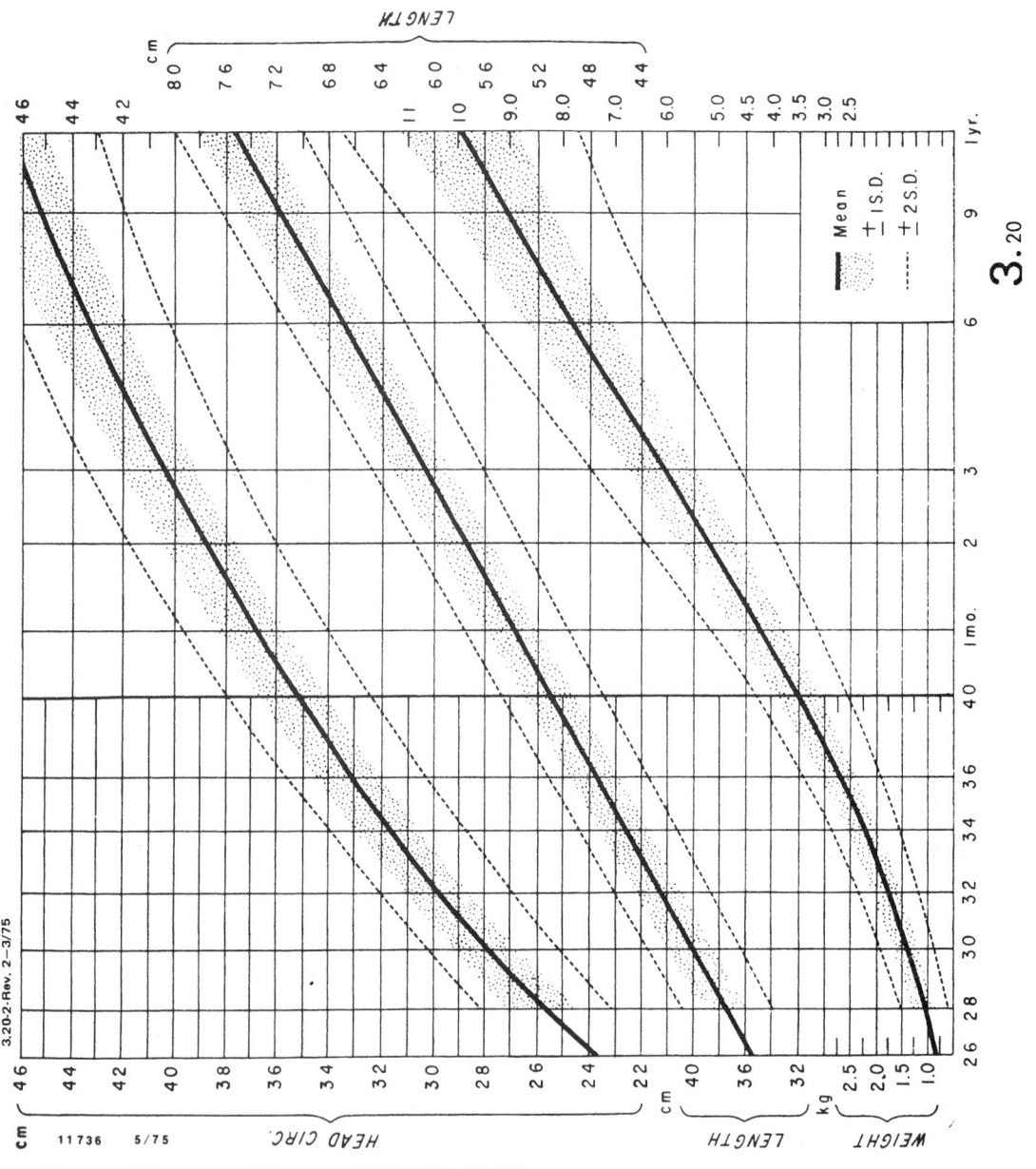

Babson S, Benda G: Growth graphs for the clinical assessment of infants of varying gestational age. J Pediatr 89:814–820, 1976.

T A B L E B-12

Percentiles of BMI for Boys 5 to 17 Years of Age

AGE (yr)	PERCENTILE	ASIAN	BLACK	HISPANIC	WHITE	US WEIGHTED MEAN (A)	NHANES I (B)	% DIFFERENCE*
5	5	13.2	13.7	13.8	13.7	13.7	—	—
	15	14.0	14.4	14.6	14.4	14.4	—	—
	50	15.0	15.5	15.9	15.5	15.6	—	—
	75	15.3	16.2	17.2	16.4	16.5	—	—
	85	15.5	16.8	18.0	17.1	17.2	—	—
	95	17.1	18.1	19.4	18.1	18.3	—	—
6	5	13.3	13.8	13.8	13.8	13.8	12.9	6.7
	15	14.1	14.4	14.7	14.4	14.5	13.4	7.9
	50	15.0	15.5	16.0	15.6	15.6	14.5	7.7
	75	15.5	16.4	17.4	16.6	16.7	—	—
	85	15.7	17.0	18.2	17.3	17.4	16.6	4.5
	95	17.8	18.8	20.2	18.9	19.0	18.0	5.5
7	5	13.5	14.0	14.0	13.9	13.9	13.2	5.6
	15	14.3	14.6	14.9	14.6	14.7	13.9	5.5
	50	15.2	15.8	16.2	15.8	15.8	15.1	4.9
	75	15.8	16.7	17.7	16.9	17.0	—	—
	85	16.1	17.4	18.6	17.7	17.8	17.4	2.1
	95	18.8	19.9	21.2	19.9	20.0	19.2	4.4
8	5	13.7	14.2	14.2	14.1	14.1	13.6	3.9
	15	14.5	14.8	15.1	14.9	14.9	14.3	4.0
	50	15.6	16.1	16.6	16.2	16.2	15.6	3.7
	75	16.4	17.3	18.3	17.5	17.5	—	—
	85	16.9	18.3	19.5	18.6	18.6	18.1	2.7
	95	20.2	21.3	22.7	21.4	21.5	20.3	5.8
9	5	13.9	14.4	14.4	14.3	14.3	14.0	2.5
	15	14.7	15.1	15.4	15.1	15.1	14.7	2.8
	50	16.0	16.5	17.0	16.6	16.6	16.2	2.7
	75	17.2	18.1	19.1	18.3	18.4	—	—
	85	17.9	19.4	20.7	19.7	19.7	18.9	4.4
	95	21.7	22.9	24.4	23.0	23.1	21.5	7.4
10	5	14.1	14.6	14.7	14.6	14.6	14.4	1.3
	15	15.0	15.4	15.6	15.4	15.4	15.2	1.3
	50	16.6	17.1	17.6	17.1	17.2	16.7	2.8
	75	18.0	19.0	20.0	19.2	19.2	—	—
	85	19.1	20.6	21.9	20.9	20.9	19.6	6.7
	95	23.2	24.4	25.9	24.5	24.6	22.6	8.8
11	5	14.4	14.9	15.0	14.9	14.9	14.8	0.7
	15	15.4	15.8	16.1	15.8	15.8	15.6	1.3
	50	17.1	17.7	18.1	17.7	17.8	17.3	2.7
	75	18.9	19.9	20.9	20.1	20.1	—	—
	85	20.0	21.6	22.9	21.9	21.9	20.4	7.4
	95	24.3	25.5	27.1	25.6	25.7	23.7	8.6
12	5	14.8	15.3	15.4	15.3	15.3	15.2	0.8
	15	16.0	16.3	16.6	16.3	16.3	16.1	1.5
	50	17.8	18.3	18.8	18.4	18.4	17.9	2.8
	75	19.6	20.6	21.7	20.8	20.9	—	—
	85	20.7	22.3	23.6	22.6	22.6	21.1	7.3
	95	25.1	26.3	27.9	26.4	26.5	24.9	6.5

Table continued on following page

T A B L E B-12

Percentiles of BMI for Boys 5 to 17 Years of Age *Continued*

AGE (yr)	PERCENTILE	ASIAN	BLACK	HISPANIC	WHITE	US WEIGHTED MEAN (A)	NHANES I (B)	% DIFFERENCE*
13	5	15.4	15.9	15.9	15.9	15.9	15.7	1.0
	15	16.6	17.0	17.3	17.0	17.0	16.6	2.4
	50	18.4	19.0	19.5	19.1	19.1	18.5	3.2
	75	20.2	21.2	22.3	21.5	21.5	—	—
	85	21.2	22.8	24.2	23.2	23.2	21.9	5.9
	95	25.6	26.9	28.5	27.0	27.1	25.9	4.6
14	5	16.0	16.5	16.6	16.5	16.5	16.2	1.9
	15	17.3	17.7	18.0	17.7	17.7	17.2	2.9
	50	19.2	19.7	20.2	19.8	19.8	19.2	3.2
	75	20.8	21.9	23.0	22.1	22.1	—	—
	85	21.8	23.4	24.8	23.7	23.7	22.8	4.1
	95	26.3	27.6	29.2	27.6	27.8	26.9	3.2
15	5	16.7	17.2	17.3	17.2	17.2	16.6	3.7
	15	18.0	18.3	18.6	18.3	18.4	17.8	3.1
	50	19.9	20.5	21.0	20.5	20.6	19.9	3.3
	75	21.5	22.5	23.6	22.8	22.8	—	—
	85	22.5	24.1	25.6	24.5	24.5	23.6	3.9
	95	27.2	28.5	30.1	28.5	28.7	27.8	3.2
16	5	17.3	17.9	18.0	17.9	17.9	17.0	5.1
	15	18.6	18.9	19.2	18.9	19.0	18.3	3.6
	50	20.6	21.2	21.7	21.3	21.3	20.6	3.3
	75	22.2	23.3	24.4	23.6	23.6	—	—
	85	23.4	25.1	26.5	25.4	25.4	24.5	3.9
	95	28.2	29.6	31.2	29.6	29.8	28.5	4.5
17	5	17.8	18.4	18.4	18.3	18.3	17.3	6.0
	15	19.2	19.6	19.9	19.6	19.6	18.7	4.9
	50	21.2	21.7	22.3	21.8	21.8	21.1	3.5
	75	22.9	23.9	25.1	24.2	24.2	—	—
	85	23.8	25.5	27.0	25.9	25.9	25.3	2.3
	95	28.6	29.9	31.6	30.0	30.1	29.3	2.8

*[(A − B)/B] × 100%.

BMI = body mass index-weight (in kg) *divided by* height (in meters squared); ideal weight-height (in meters squared) *multiplied by* BMI, if value for BMI is obtained from the tables; NHANES = National Health and Nutrition Examination Survey.

From Rosner B, Prineas R, Loggie J, et al: Percentiles of body mass index in U.S. children 5 to 17 years of age. J Pediatr 132:211–222, 1998.

T A B L E B-13

Percentiles of BMI for Girls 5 to 17 Years of Age

AGE (yr)	PERCENTILE	ASIAN	BLACK	HISPANIC	WHITE	US WEIGHTED MEAN (A)	NHANES I (B)	% DIFFERENCE*
5	5	13.0	13.3	13.5	13.0	13.1	—	—
	15	13.6	14.0	14.3	13.7	13.8	—	—
	50	14.5	15.4	15.5	14.9	15.1	—	—
	75	15.2	16.6	17.1	15.8	16.1	—	—
	85	15.7	17.7	18.1	16.5	16.9	—	—
	95	16.6	19.8	19.6	18.1	18.5	—	—
6	5	13.3	13.6	13.8	13.3	13.4	12.8	4.9
	15	13.8	14.2	14.5	14.0	14.1	13.4	4.9
	50	14.6	15.5	15.6	15.0	15.2	14.3	6.0
	75	15.5	17.0	17.5	16.1	16.4	—	—
	85	16.1	18.1	18.5	16.9	17.2	16.2	6.5
	95	17.4	20.7	20.5	18.9	19.3	17.5	10.5
7	5	13.4	13.8	13.9	13.5	13.6	13.2	2.8
	15	14.0	14.4	14.7	14.1	14.3	13.8	3.3
	50	14.9	15.8	15.9	15.3	15.4	15.0	2.8
	75	16.1	17.5	18.0	16.7	17.0	—	—
	85	16.7	18.8	19.2	17.6	17.9	17.2	4.3
	95	18.4	21.8	21.6	20.0	20.4	18.9	8.0
8	5	13.5	13.9	14.0	13.5	13.6	13.5	1.0
	15	14.2	14.6	14.9	14.3	14.4	14.2	1.6
	50	15.3	16.2	16.3	15.7	15.8	15.7	0.7
	75	16.8	18.3	18.8	17.4	17.7	—	—
	85	17.7	19.8	20.2	18.6	18.9	18.2	3.9
	95	19.6	23.1	22.9	21.2	21.7	20.4	6.2
9	5	13.6	14.0	14.1	13.6	13.7	13.9	−1.1
	15	14.4	14.8	15.1	14.5	14.6	14.7	−0.3
	50	15.8	16.7	16.9	16.2	16.4	16.3	0.4
	75	17.7	19.2	19.7	18.3	18.6	—	—
	85	18.8	21.0	21.4	19.7	20.1	19.2	4.6
	95	20.9	24.5	24.3	22.6	23.0	21.8	5.7
10	5	13.9	14.2	14.4	13.9	14.0	14.2	−1.3
	15	14.8	15.2	15.5	14.9	15.0	15.1	−0.4
	50	16.5	17.4	17.6	16.9	17.1	17.0	0.4
	75	18.7	20.2	20.8	19.3	19.6	—	—
	85	20.0	22.3	22.7	21.0	21.4	20.2	5.7
	95	22.4	26.1	25.8	24.1	24.5	23.2	5.8
11	5	14.3	14.7	14.9	14.4	14.5	14.6	−0.8
	15	15.4	15.8	16.1	15.5	15.6	15.5	0.8
	50	17.3	18.3	18.4	17.7	17.9	17.7	1.1
	75	19.7	21.3	21.9	20.4	20.7	—	—
	85	21.2	23.5	24.0	22.2	22.6	21.2	6.5
	95	23.8	27.6	27.4	25.6	26.1	24.6	6.0
12	5	15.0	15.4	15.5	15.0	15.1	15.0	1.0
	15	16.1	16.6	16.9	16.3	16.4	16.0	2.4
	50	18.2	19.2	19.3	18.6	18.8	18.4	2.1
	75	20.7	22.4	22.9	21.4	21.7	—	—
	85	22.2	24.6	25.1	23.2	23.6	22.2	6.4
	95	25.2	29.1	28.9	27.0	27.5	26.0	5.8

Table continued on following page

T A B L E B-13

Percentiles of BMI for Girls 5 to 17 Years of Age *Continued*

AGE (yr)	PERCENTILE	ASIAN	BLACK	HISPANIC	WHITE	US WEIGHTED MEAN (A)	NHANES I (B)	% DIFFERENCE*
13	5	15.8	16.1	16.3	15.8	15.9	15.4	3.3
	15	16.9	17.4	17.7	17.1	17.2	16.4	5.0
	50	19.0	20.0	20.2	19.4	19.6	19.0	3.2
	75	21.5	23.2	23.8	22.2	22.5	—	—
	85	23.0	25.4	25.9	24.0	24.4	23.1	5.6
	95	26.3	30.3	30.0	28.1	28.6	27.1	5.7
14	5	16.5	16.8	17.0	16.5	16.6	15.7	5.8
	15	17.7	18.1	18.5	17.8	18.0	16.8	6.9
	50	19.6	20.7	20.8	20.1	20.2	19.3	4.9
	75	22.1	23.8	24.3	22.8	23.1	—	—
	85	23.5	25.9	26.4	24.5	24.9	23.9	4.2
	95	26.9	31.0	30.7	28.8	29.3	28.0	4.7
15	5	17.0	17.4	17.5	17.0	17.1	16.0	7.0
	15	18.1	18.6	19.0	18.3	18.4	17.2	7.2
	50	20.0	21.1	21.2	20.5	20.6	19.7	4.8
	75	22.3	24.0	24.6	23.1	23.4	—	—
	85	23.8	26.2	26.7	24.8	25.2	24.3	3.7
	95	27.2	31.3	31.0	29.1	29.6	28.5	3.9
16	5	17.2	17.6	17.8	17.3	17.4	16.4	6.1
	15	18.4	18.9	19.2	18.5	18.7	17.5	6.6
	50	20.2	21.3	21.4	20.7	20.9	20.1	3.8
	75	22.5	24.2	24.8	23.2	23.5	—	—
	85	24.0	26.5	27.0	25.1	25.5	24.7	3.1
	95	27.5	31.6	31.4	29.4	29.9	29.1	2.9
17	5	17.5	17.9	18.1	17.6	17.7	16.6	6.6
	15	18.6	19.1	19.5	18.8	18.9	17.8	6.3
	50	20.6	21.6	21.8	21.0	21.2	20.4	4.0
	75	23.0	24.7	25.3	23.7	24.1	—	—
	85	24.5	26.9	27.5	25.5	25.9	25.2	3.0
	95	28.8	33.0	32.8	30.8	31.3	29.7	5.4

*[(A − B)/B] × 100%.

BMI = body mass index-weight (in kg) *divided* by height (in meters squared); Ideal weight-height (in meters squared) multiplied by BMI, where value for BMI is obtained from the tables; NHANES = National Health and Nutrition Examination Survey.

From Rosner B, Prineas R, Loggie J, et al: Percentiles of body mass index in U.S. children 5 to 17 years of age. J Pediatr 132:211–222, 1998.

T A B L E B–14

Resources for Other Available Growth Charts

Achondroplasia: head circumference, male and female
Achondroplasia: height, male and female
Down syndrome: height and weight, both genders, 1 month to 18 years
Marfan syndrome: height
Noonan syndrome: height
Prader-Willi syndrome: height
Williams syndrome: height
Arthrogryposis-amyoplasia: height and distal heights: both genders
Multiple pterygium: height, both genders
Diastrophic dysplasia: height
Pseudoachondroplasia: height
Spondyloepiphyseal dysplasia congenita: height
  In Hall J, Froster-Iskenius UG, Allanson JE: The Handbook of Normal Physical Measurements. Oxford, Oxford University Press, 1989

Myelomeningocele ages 2–18: height and weight, both genders
Asian children 0–6 years: height and weight, both genders
From Children's Development and Rehabilitation Center
Genetics Clinic
PO Box 574
Portland, Oregon 97207

Cystic fibrosis growth chart
  From Cystic Fibrosis Foundation
      6931 Arlington Rd.
      Bethesda, MD 20814
  Tel: (800) FIGHT-CF

Sickle cell anemia growth chart
  Data from Platt OS: Influence of sickle hemoglobinopathies on growth and development. New Engl J Med 311:7–12, 1984.

APPENDIX C

Normal Laboratory Values

Steven Goodstein and Catherine E. Burns

A limited selection of blood chemistry, urine, and hematological values is presented as the most common laboratory screening tests requested. The authors recognize that the nurse practitioner may have a need for more complex tests; for example, cerebrospinal fluid studies, immunoglobulins, and therapeutic drug levels. The reader is directed to seek the source of these values from the performing laboratory, as well as its respective standards in comparison with control specimens. Some pediatric specimens need to be sent to a special laboratory for appropriate testing.

Laboratories use a variety of analytical methods to determine biochemical and hematological values. Normal values for laboratory tests vary depending on the procedure used. Normal ranges reflect a combination of the population served, individual biological differences, specimen collection and handling techniques, and intrinsic laboratory variation. Given this variability, if any questions arise, it is recommended that the reader consult with the reference laboratory for its methods and the established normal range of values for the methods used.

Interpretation of laboratory values can be a complex diagnostic exercise. In the following table, the comments in the Interpretation column are intended to offer the reader general ideas about each test and its common use. A skilled clinician uses laboratory data with other clinical data to make decisions, sometimes combining several tests to best understand the physiologic status of the client.

The laboratory values for this appendix have been compiled from published tables in the following recognized pediatric and laboratory reference texts.

DATA FROM:

Behrman R, Kliegman R, Arvin A (eds): Nelson Textbook of Pediatrics, 14th ed. Philadelphia, WB Saunders, 1996.

Burtis C, Ashwood E: Tietz Textbook of Clinical Chemistry. Philadelphia, WB Saunders, 1999.

Fishbach F: A Manual of Laboratory & Diagnostic Tests, 5th ed. Philadelphia, JB Lippincott, 1996.

Free HM (ed): Modern Urine Chemistry. Elkhart, IN, Miles, 1991.

T A B L E C-1

Pediatric Laboratory Values

BLOOD CHEMISTRY (from serum)

TEST NAME	REFERENCE RANGE		INTERPRETATION
Alanine aminotransferase (ALT, SGPT) (U/L)	Newborn/infant	13–45	Liver, heart, and skeletal muscle have significant levels. High levels are associated with hepatic cell damage
	Adult		
	M	10–40	
	F	7–35	
Amylase (U/L)	Newborn	5–65	Marked rise generally indicates acute pancreatitis
	Adult	27–131	
Aspartate aminotransferase (AST, SGOT) (U/L)	Newborn	25–175	Elevated levels occur with heart, liver, and muscle disease
	Infant	15–60	
	Adult	8–20	
Bilirubin, total (mg/dl)	Premature cord blood	<2.0	Elevated levels occur with increased destruction of RBCs or impairment of liver excretory function
	0–1 d	<8.0	
	1–2 d	<12.0	
	3–5 d	<16.0	
	Full-term		
	Cord blood	<2.0	
	0–1 d	1.4–8.7	
	1–2 d	3.4–11.5	
	3–5 d	1.5–12.0	
	Adult	0.3–1.2	
Chloride (mmol/L)	Cord blood	96–104	Values increase in metabolic acidosis and other conditions. Decreased values occur with diuresis, GI losses, and other conditions
	0–30 d	98–113	
	>30 d	98–107	

Cholesterol (5th–95th percentile, mg/dL)	Cord blood	44–103	Elevated levels indicate disorders of blood lipids
	M		
	F	50–108	
	0–4 y		
	M	114–203	
	F	112–200	
	5–9 y		
	M	121–203	
	F	126–205	
	10–14 y		
	M	119–202	
	F	124–201	
	15–19 y		
	M	113–197	
	F	119–200	
	20–24 y		
	M	124–218	
	F	122–216	
Creatinine (mg/dl)	Cord blood	0.6–1.2	Elevated levels indicate impaired renal function, muscle disease, congestive heart failure, shock, dehydration, and other conditions.
	Newborn	0.3–1.0	
	Infant	0.2–0.4	
	Child	0.3–0.7	
	Adolescent	0.5–1.0	
	Adult		
	M	0.7–1.3	
	F	0.6–1.1	
Ferritin (ng/ml)	Newborn	25–200	Ferritin is a more sensitive indicator than iron or TIBC for diagnosing iron deficiency or overload.
	1 mo	200–600	
	2–5 mo	50–200	
	6 mo–15 y	7–140	
	Adult		
	M	15–200	
	F	12–150	

Table continued on following page

T A B L E C-1

Pediatric Laboratory Values Continued

TEST NAME	REFERENCE RANGE		INTERPRETATION
BLOOD CHEMISTRY (from serum)			
Glucose (fasting) (mg/dl)	Cord blood	45–96	Fasting low levels may indicate a physiologic response or a disorder in glucose metabolism. Increased fasting levels may indicate diabetes mellitus, pancreatic disorders, endocrine diseases, drugs, and other conditions
	Premature	20–60	
	Neonate	30–60	
	Newborn		
	1 d	40–60	
	>1 d	50–80	
	Child	60–100	
	Adult	74–106	
Iron (µg/dl)	Newborn	100–250	Decreased levels occur with iron deficiency, blood loss, and other conditions. Elevated levels occur with hemolytic anemias, iron intoxication, hepatitis, and other conditions
	Infant	40–100	
	Child	50–120	
	Thereafter		
	M	50–160	
	F	50–170	
	Intoxicated child	280–2550	
	Fatally poisoned child	>1800	
Lead (whole blood specimen) (µg/dl)	Child	<10	Increased levels indicate lead toxicity
	Adult	<40	
	Lethal dose	≥100 (variable)	
Potassium (mEq/L)	Newborn	3.7–5.9	Decreased levels may indicate shifting of potassium into cells, GI loss, biliary loss, renal loss, and reduced uptake. Increased levels occur with shifts to intracellular fluid, decreased excretion, or increased uptake
	Infant	4.1–5.3	
	Child	3.4–4.7	
	Thereafter	3.5–5.1	
Sodium (mEq/L)	Newborn	133–146	Decreased levels indicate sodium loss or water excess (caused by numerous conditions). Increased levels may occur with an increase in sodium or an excessive loss of water (caused by numerous conditions)
	Infant	139–146	
	Child	138–145	
	Thereafter	136–145	
Thyrotropin (thyroid-stimulating hormone, TSH) (µU/ml)	Newborn	3–18	Decreased levels are associated with hyperthyroidism. Increased levels are associated with hypothyroidism
	Thereafter	2–10	

Test		Reference Range	Discussion
Thyroxine, free (FT₄) (ng/dl)	Newborn	2.6–6.3	Decreased levels are associated with hypothyroidism or overproduction of T₃. Increased levels are associated with Graves' disease and thyrotoxicosis from overproduction of T₄
	Adult	0.8–2.7	
Thyroxine, total (T₄) (µg/dl)	1–3 d	11.8–22.6	T₄ serves as a good index of thyroid function only if binding globulin (TBG) is normal
	1–2 wk	9.8–16.6	
	1–4 mo	7.2–14.4	
	4–12 mo	7.8–16.5	
	1–5 y	7.3–15.0	
	5–10 y	6.4–13.3	
	10–15 y	5.6–11.7	
	Adult		
	M	4.6–10.5	
	F	5.5–11.0	
Urea nitrogen (BUN) (mg/dl)	Premature (1 wk)	3–25	Measures glomerular function and production/excretion of urea. Decreased with liver failure, malnutrition, and other conditions. Increased with impaired renal function, congestive heart failure, salt/water depletion, shock, and other conditions
	Newborn	4–12	
	Infant/child	5–18	
	Adult	6–20	

HEMATOLOGY (whole blood specimens)

Test		Reference Range	Discussion
Erythrocyte count (RBC) (millions of cells/mm³ [µl])	1–3 d (capillary)	4.0–6.6	Measures total number of RBCs. Decreased with anemia, cell destruction, and decreased production. Increased with increased RBC production, renal disease, tumors, altitude, pulmonary disease, cardiovascular diseases, and other conditions. A relative increase may occur with dehydration
	1 wk	3.9–6.3	
	2 wk	3.6–6.2	
	1 mo	3.0–5.4	
	2 mo	2.7–4.9	
	3–6 mo	3.1–4.5	
	0.5–2 y	3.7–5.3	
	2–6 y	3.9–5.3	
	6–12 y	4.0–5.2	
	12–18 y		
	M	4.5–5.3	
	F	4.1–5.1	
	18–49 y		
	M	4.5–5.9	
	F	4.0–5.2	

Table continued on following page

Pediatric Laboratory Values Continued

TEST NAME	REFERENCE RANGE		INTERPRETATION
BLOOD CHEMISTRY (from serum)			
Erythrocyte sedimentation rate (ESR, sed rate) (mm/hr)	Westergren, modified		Not diagnostic, but indicates a disease process. Increases occur with collagen diseases, infections, inflammatory conditions, neoplasms, heavy metal poisoning, tissue destruction, and other conditions
	Child	0–10	
	Adult		
	M <50 y	0–15	
	F <50 y	0–20	
	Wintrobe		
	Child	0–13	
	Adult		
	M	0–9	
	F	0–20	
Hematocrit (HCT, Hct) (% packed erythrocyte volume [erythrocyte volume/whole blood × 100])	1 d	48–69	Low values indicate blood loss or inadequate production or excess destruction of RBCs. High values indicate erythrocytosis, severe dehydration, shock, and other conditions
	2 d	48–75	
	3 d	44–72	
	2 mo	28–42	
	6–12 y	35–45	
	12–18 y		
	M	37–49	
	F	36–46	
	18–49 y		
	M	41–53	
	F	36–46	
Hemoglobin, total (Hb) (g/dl)	1–3 d	14.5–22.5	Decreased levels are found with anemia, hyperthyroidism, cirrhosis, severe hemorrhage, hemolysis, and systemic diseases. Very low values may lead to heart failure and death
	2 mo	9.0–14.0	
	6–12 y	11.5–15.5	
	12–18 y		
	M	13.0–16.0	
	F	12.0–16.0	
	18–49 y		
	M	13.5–17.5	
	F	12.0–16.0	

Test		Reference value	Description
Leukocyte count (white blood cell count, WBC) ($\times 1000$ cells/mm^3)	Birth 24 hr 1 mo 1–3 y 4–7 y 8–13 y Adult	9.0–30.0 9.4–34.0 5.0–19.5 6.0–17.5 5.5–15.5 4.5–13.5 4.5–11.0	Indicates total WBC count circulating in the blood. With some infections, WBCs increase as cells are transported. A low count may occur in overwhelming bacterial infection (sepsis) or with the use of immunosuppressive agents. Elevated levels may occur in response to an underlying disease, a primary cellular disorder (leukemia), pregnancy, corticosteroid treatment, strenuous exercise, and other conditions
Leukocyte differential (%)	Myelocytes Neutrophils—"bands" Neutrophils—"segs" Lymphocytes Monocytes Eosinophils Basophils	0 3–5 54–62 25–33 3–7 1–3 0–0.75	Describes the proportion of the types of WBCs. Used in conjunction with the total leukocyte count to determine absolute cell counts Neutrophils: Usually increased during bacterial infections. May be decreased in viral infections. Composed of bands and segmented types Eosinophils: Increased during allergic responses and parasitic infections Basophils: Increased in allergic reactions, hematological disorders, and other conditions Lymphocytes: Increased in viral infections Monocytes: Increased in severe and recovery stages of infections (phagocytosis) Myelocytes: Involved in the early maturation of neutrophils, eosinophils, basophils, and monocytes
Platelet count (thrombocyte count)	Newborn 1 wk–adult	84–478 $\times$ 10^3/mm^3 150–400 $\times$ 10^3/mm^3	Decreased platelet counts occur with anemias, some infections, congestive heart failure, bone marrow lesions, and other conditions. Increases occur with malignancies, splenectomy, collagen diseases, some anemias, and other conditions
Reticulocyte count (%)	1 d 7 d 1–4 wk 5–6 wk 7–8 wk 9–10 wk 11–12 wk Adult	0.4–6.0 <0.1–1.3 <1.0–1.2 <0.1–2.4 0.1–2.9 <0.1–2.6 0.1–1.3 0.5–1.5	Provides an estimate of the rate of RBC production. The percentage may be used to calculate the absolute value. An elevated count with normal hemoglobin indicates RBC loss with bone marrow compensation. A normal reticulocyte count with a low hemoglobin level indicates an inadequate response to anemia

Table continued on following page

T A B L E C-1

Pediatric Laboratory Values Continued

BLOOD CHEMISTRY (from serum)
URINE

TEST NAME	REFERENCE RANGE	INTERPRETATION
Urine, macroscopic	All ages	
Bilirubin	Negative	Increased in hepatocellular disease or intrahepatic/extrahepatic biliary obstruction
Blood, occult	Negative	RBCs increased in acute glomerulonephritis, acute infections, renal calculi, trauma, and other conditions
Glucose, qualitative	Negative	Increased when blood glucose level exceeds the reabsorption capacity of the renal tubes (pathological or benign)
Hemoglobin	Negative	Hemoglobinuria may occur in intravascular hemolysis and other conditions
Ketones	Negative	Increased with adequate carbohydrate intake or a defect in carbohydrate metabolism. Especially significant with diabetes mellitus
Leukocyte esterase	Negative	Measures WBCs. Increase indicates inflammation and/or infection. Associated with certain renal diseases and diseases of the urinary tract or vaginitis
Nitrite	Negative	Increase associated with urinary tract infection
pH	4.6–8.0	Indication of acid–base balance
Protein, qualitative	Negative	Increased in pathological or physiologic conditions (e.g., fever, stress, strenuous exercises)
Specific gravity	1.001–1.030	Measures the concentrating and diluting ability of the kidney. Associated with tubular damage
Urobilinogen	0.2–1.0 mg/dl	Increased in liver disease. Decreased in obstruction of bile ducts and other conditions

Urine, microscopic			Hyaline casts: Increased in pathological or physiologic conditions. Implies damage to the glomerular capillary membrane permitting leakage of proteins through the glomerular filtrate
Casts			
Hyaline		0–1/lpf	
Other		None	Other casts: Involved in a variety of conditions depending on the type of cast. Involved in tubular epithelial damage (epithelial cell cast), renal infection (WBC cast), vascular disorder (RBC cast), renal disease (granular cast), chronic renal condition (waxy cast), severe renal disease (broad cast), and degenerative tubular disease (fatty cast)
Red blood cells (RBCs)	M	0–2/hpf	
	F and children	0–3/hpf	
White blood cells (WBCs)		0–5/hpf	RBCs: Denotes bleeding into the urinary system
			WBCs: Associated with an inflammatory process
Urine volume (ml/24 hr)	Newborn	50–300	Decreased in dehydration, renal ischemia, renal disease, obstruction, and other conditions. Increased in diabetes insipidus, diabetes mellitus, chronic progressive renal failure, and other conditions
	Infant	350–550	
	Child	500–1000	
	Adolescent	700–1400	
	Thereafter		
	M	800–1800	
	F	600–1600	

BUN = blood urea nitrogen; GI = gastrointestinal; hpf = high-power field; lpf = low-power field; T$_3$ = triiodothyronine; TBG = thyroxin-binding globulin; TIBC = total iron-binding capacity.

Healthy People 2010 Objectives: Draft for Public Comment: Child and Adolescent Focused Objectives

The following goals and objectives are extracted from the *Healthy People 2010 Objectives: Draft for Public Comment* (US Department of Health & Human Services, 1998). Although the content of some specific objectives may change in the final version of the 2010 document and some numbers have not been established as yet, the objectives included here represent current thinking about the directions that pediatric health care should take over the next 10 years and the roles that individuals, schools, communities, and health-care providers should assume in creating a more healthy population. Only the objectives that seemed directly related to the health of infants, children, and adolescents are included below. Generally, the major child health themes have been included in the lists below.

▮▮▮▮ HEALTHY PEOPLE 2010 GOALS

1. Increase the quality and years of healthy life. Reduce the death rate for adolescents and young adults (15 to 24 years old) to no more than 81 per 100,000 by 2010.
2. Eliminate health disparities.

▮▮▮▮ HEALTHY PEOPLE 2010 OBJECTIVES ,

Physical Activity and Fitness

Goal: Improve the health, fitness, and quality of life of all Americans through the adoption and maintenance of regular, daily physical activity.

1. Increase to at least 85% the proportion of young people in grades 9 through 12 who engage in vigorous physical activity that promotes the development and maintenance of cardiorespiratory fitness 3 or more days per week for 20 or more minutes per occasion.
2. Increase to at least 30% the proportion of young people in grades 9 through 12 who engage in moderate physical activity for at least 30 minutes on 5 or more of the previous 7 days.
3. Increase to at least 50% the proportion of young people in grades 9 through 12 who participate in daily school physical education.
4. Increase to at least 50% the proportion of the nation's public and private elementary, middle/junior, and senior high schools that require daily physical education for all students.
5. Increase to at least 50% the proportion of young people in grades 9 to 12 who spend at least 50% of school physical education class time being physically active, preferably engaged in lifetime physical activities, at least three times per week.
6. Increase to at least 50% the proportion of the nation's public and private elementary, middle/junior, and senior high schools that in addition to physical education courses, teach about physical activity in required health education courses.

7. Increase to at least 50% the proportion of the nation's public and private elementary, middle/junior, and senior high schools that provide access to their physical education spaces and facilities for young people and adults outside normal school hours (i.e., before and after the school day, on weekends, and during summer and other vacations).

Nutrition

Goal: Promote health and reduce chronic disease risk, disease progression, debilitation, and premature death associated with dietary factors and nutritional status among people in the United States.

1. Reduce to 5% or less the prevalence of overweight and obesity (at or above the sex- and age-specific 95th percentile of body mass index from the revised National Center for Health Statistics/Centers for Disease Control and Prevention growth charts) in children (aged 6 to 11) and adolescents (aged 12 to 19).
2. Reduce growth retardation among low-income children aged 5 years and younger to 5% or less.
3. Increase to at least 75% the proportion of people aged 2 years and older who meet the *Dietary Guidelines'* average daily goal of no more than 30% of calories from fat.
4. Increase to at least 75% the proportion of people aged 2 years and older who meet the *Dietary Guidelines'* average daily goal of less than 10% of calories from saturated fat.
5. Increase to at least 75% the proportion of people aged 2 years and older who meet the *Dietary Guidelines'* minimum average daily goal of at least five servings of vegetables and fruits.
6. Increase to at least 75% the proportion of people aged 2 years and older who meet the *Dietary Guidelines'* minimum average daily goal of at least six servings of grain products.
7. Increase to at least 75% the proportion of people aged 2 years and older who meet dietary recommendations for calcium.

8. Increase to at least 65% the proportion of people aged 2 years and older who meet the daily value of 2400 mg or less of sodium consistent with the *Dietary Guidelines*.
9. Reduce iron deficiency to 5% or less among children aged 1 and 2 years, to less than 1% among children aged 3 and 4 years, and to 7% or less among females of childbearing age.
10. Increase to at least __% the proportion of children and adolescents 6 to 19 years of age whose intake of meals and snacks at school from all sources contributes proportionally to good overall dietary quality.
11. Increase to at least __% the proportion of the nation's public and private elementary schools that teach all essential nutrition education topics to their students in at least three different grades.
12. Increase to at least __% the proportion of the nation's public and private middle/junior high schools that teach all essential nutrition education topics to their students in at least one required course.
13. Increase to at least __% the proportion of the nation's public and private high schools that teach all essential nutrition education topics to their students in at least one required course.
14. Increase to at least 75% the proportion of primary care providers who provide nutrition assessment when appropriate and to at least 75% the proportion who formulate a diet/nutrition plan for patients who need the intervention.
15. Increase the prevalence of food security among US households to at least 94% of all households.

Tobacco Use

Goal: Reduce disease, disability, and death related to tobacco use and exposure to secondhand smoke by (1) preventing initiation of tobacco use, (2) promoting cessation of tobacco use, (3) reducing exposure to secondhand smoke, and (4) changing social norms and environments that support tobacco use.

1. Reduce the proportion of young people in grades 9 to 12 who have used tobacco products.

2. Increase by at least 1 year the average age of first use of tobacco products by adolescents.

3. Increase to 95% the proportion of patients who received advice to quit smoking during the reporting year from a health care provider.

4. Increase to 100% the proportion of health plans that offer treatment of nicotine addiction (e.g., tobacco use cessation counseling by health care providers, tobacco use cessation classes, prescriptions for nicotine replacement therapies, and other cessation services).

5. Increase to at least 75% the proportion of health care providers who routinely advise cessation, provide assistance and follow-up, and document charts for all their tobacco-using patients.

6. Increase the proportion of pediatricians and family physicians who inquire about secondhand smoke exposure in the home and advise reduction in secondhand smoke exposure for the patient and family.

7. Increase to 100% the proportion of schools with tobacco-free environments that include all school facilities, property, vehicles, and school events.

8. Enforce minors' access laws so that the buy rate in compliance checks conducted in all 50 states and the District of Columbia is no higher than 5%.

9. Increase to 95% the proportion of 8th, 10th, and 12th graders who disapprove of the use of one or more packs of cigarettes per day.

10. Increase to 95% the proportion of 8th graders who associate harm with tobacco use. Include evidence-based tobacco use prevention in the curricula in __% of elementary, middle, and secondary schools, preferably as part of comprehensive school health education.

Education and Community-Based Programs

Goal: Increase the quality, availability, and effectiveness of educational and community-based programs designed to prevent disease

and improve the health and quality of life of the American people.

1. Increase the high school completion rate to at least 90%.

2. Increase to at least 30% the proportion of the nation's middle/junior high and senior high schools that require 1 school year of health education.

3. Increase to at least 42% the proportion of the nation's elementary, middle/junior, and senior high schools that have a nurse-to-student ratio of at least 1:750.

4. Increase to __% the proportion of patients who report that they are satisfied with the communication they receive from their health care providers regarding how decisions are made about their health care.

5. Increase to __% the proportion of health care organizations that provide patient and family education.

6. Increase to __% the proportion of managed care organizations and hospitals that provide community disease prevention and health promotion activities that address the priority health needs identified by their communities.

7. Increase to at least __% the proportion of local health service areas/jurisdictions that have established a community health promotion initiative that addresses multiple Healthy People 2010 focus areas.

8. Increase to at least __% the proportion of local health departments that have established culturally appropriate and linguistically competent community health promotion and disease prevention programs for racial and ethnic minority populations.

Environmental Health

Goal: Health for all through a healthy environment.

1. The air will be safer to breathe for 100% of the people living in areas that exceed all National Ambient Air Quality Standards.

2. Reduce water-related adverse health effects by increasing to at least 95% the proportion of people served by community water systems who receive a supply of drinking water

that meets the Safe Drinking Water Act regulations.

3. Reduce the prevalence of blood lead levels exceeding 10 µg/dl to 0 in children aged 1 to 5 years.

4. Reduce to no more than 15% the proportion of children aged 6 years and younger who are regularly exposed to tobacco smoke at home.

5. Increase to 50% the number of homes built before 1950 in which testing for lead-based paint has been performed as a means to reduce childhood lead poisoning.

6. Reduce deaths and nonfatal poisonings of children from exposure to household hazardous chemicals (targets set for cosmetics, cleaning substances, analgesics, plants, medications).

7. Reduce by 25% the rate of death from unintentional poisonings for children younger than 5 years from hazardous household chemicals.

8. Reduce deaths and nonfatal poisonings from carbon monoxide.

Food Safety

Goal: Reduce the number of food-borne illnesses. (No objectives are specific to children, although all are inclusive of them.)

Injury/Violence Prevention

Goal: Reduce the incidence and severity of injuries from unintentional causes, as well as from violence and abuse.

1. Increase to at least 76% the proportion of public and private schools that teach about injury prevention and safety in a required health education course. (Objectives relate to head injuries, motor vehicles, motorcycle helmets, fires/smoke alarms, falls, drownings, bicycle helmets, poisonings.)

2. Increase the use of safety belts and child restraints to at least 93% of motor vehicle occupants.

3. Reduce the number of emergency department visits for nonfatal dog bite injuries among children aged 9 years and younger to no more than 28 per 10,000 persons.

4. Increase to 50% the proportion of households with children who report receiving injury prevention counseling at a medical or dental visit in the past 12 months.

5. Reduce to less than __ per 1000 children the incidence of maltreatment of children younger than 18 years.

6. Reduce the rate (annual) of forced sexual intercourse or attempted forced sexual intercourse of persons aged 12 years and older to less than 0.55 per 1000 persons.

7. Reduce to less than __% the proportion of battered women and their children turned away from emergency housing because of lack of space.

8. Reduce physical assaults among people aged 12 years and older to less than 28.2 per 1000 persons.

9. Reduce to less than 35% the prevalence of physical fighting among adolescents in grades 9 through 12.

10. Reduce to less than 15% the prevalence of weapon carrying by adolescents in grades 9 through 12.

Oral Health

Goal: Improve the health and quality of life for individuals and communities by preventing and controlling oral, dental, and craniofacial diseases, conditions, and injuries and improving access to oral health care for all Americans.

1. Reduce dental caries (cavities) in primary and permanent teeth (mixed dentition) so that the proportion of children who have had one or more cavities (filled or unfilled) is no more than 15% among children 2 to 4 years old, 40% among children 6 to 8 years old, and 55% among adolescents aged 15.

2. Reduce untreated cavities in the primary and permanent teeth (mixed dentition) so that the proportion of children with decayed teeth not filled is no more than 12% among children 2 to 4 years old, 22% among children 6 to 8 years old, and 15% among adolescents aged 15.

3. Increase to at least 70% the proportion of children 8 to 14 years old who have received protective sealants in permanent molar teeth.

4. Increase to at least 85% the proportion of the population served by community water systems with optimally fluoridated water.
5. Increase the use of topical fluorides to at least __% of people not receiving optimally fluoridated public water.
6. Increase to __% the proportion of 2-year-olds who receive caries screening by a qualified health professional for the existence of any observable decay and counseling regarding the need to either increase sources of fluoride or decrease potentially excessive sources of fluoride (e.g., unsupervised tooth brushing).
7. Increase to at least __% the proportion of all children entering school programs for the first time who have received an oral health screening. Of those screened and needing referral, __% will have received a referral for necessary diagnostic, preventive, and treatment services. Of those being referred for treatment, __% will have begun treatment within 90 days.
8. Increase to __% the proportion of school-based health centers (prekindergarten through 12th grade) with an oral health component.
9. Increase to __% the proportion of local health departments and community-based health centers, including community migrant health centers, that have a direct oral health education and service component.

Access to Quality Health Services

Goal: Improve access to comprehensive, high-quality health care across a continuum of care.

1. Reduce to 0% the proportion of children and adults younger than 65 years without health care coverage.
2. Increase the proportion of physicians, physician assistants, nurses, and other clinicians who receive appropriate training to address important health disparities: disease prevention and health promotion, minority health, women's health, geriatrics.
3. Increase to at least 95% the proportion of children 18 years and younger who have a specific source of ongoing primary care (i.e., a medical/health home).

Family Planning

Goal: Every pregnancy in the United States should be intended.

1. Increase to at least 70% the proportion of all pregnancies among women aged 15 to 44 years that are planned (i.e., intended).
2. Increase to at least 95% the proportion of all females 15 to 44 years old at risk of unintended pregnancy who use effective contraception.
3. Decrease to no more than 7% the proportion of women aged 15 to 44 years who are experiencing pregnancy despite use of a reversible contraceptive method.
4. Increase male involvement in pregnancy prevention and family planning as measured by the increase with which health care providers provide outreach, education, or services to men.
5. Reduce pregnancies among females aged 15 to 17 years to no more than 45 per 1000 adolescents.
6. Reduce to no more than 12% the proportion of individuals aged 15 to 19 years who have engaged in sexual intercourse before the age of 15.
7. Reduce to no more than 25% the proportion of individuals aged 15 to 17 years who have ever had sexual intercourse.
8. Increase by at least 10% the proportion of sexually active, unmarried individuals aged 15 to 19 years who use contraception that both effectively prevents pregnancy *and* provides barrier protection against disease.
9. Increase to at least 90% the proportion of individuals 18 through 24 years old who have received formal instruction before turning 18 on reproductive health issues, including (a) birth control methods, (b) safe sex to prevent infection with human immunodeficiency virus (HIV), (c) sexually transmitted diseases (STDs), and (d) abstinence.
10. Increase to __% the proportion of public and private elementary, middle/junior, and senior high schools that require instruction on human sexuality, pregnancy prevention, STD prevention, and HIV prevention to provide students with information and

skills related to abstinence and contraceptive use.

Maternal, Infant, and Child Care

Goal: Improve maternal health and pregnancy outcomes and reduce rates of disability in infants, thereby improving the health and well-being of women, infants, children, and families in the United States. The health of a population is reflected in the health of its most vulnerable members. A major focus of many public health efforts is therefore improving the health of pregnant women and their infants, including reductions in rates of birth defects, risk factors for infant death, and deaths of infants and their mothers.

1. Reduce the infant mortality rate to no more than 5 per 1000 live births.
2. Reduce the infant mortality rate from all birth defects to 1.2 per 1000 live births.
3. Reduce the sudden infant death syndrome mortality rate to 0.3 per 1000 live births.
4. Reduce the rate of child mortality to 30 per 100,000 children aged 1 to 4 years and 17 per 100,000 children aged 5 to 14 years.
5. Increase the proportion of providers of primary care to women of reproductive age who routinely provide preconception counseling regarding
   - Risks to all pregnancies and use of medications, tobacco, alcohol.
   - Risks associated with maternal conditions such as diabetes (type 1), phenylketonuria (PKU), epilepsy, chronic hypertension, Rh-negative blood type.
   - Risks associated with a history of previous affected pregnancies such as a birth defect with an increased recurrence risk or a genetic condition for which carrier testing is available.
6. Increase to at least 90% the proportion of all live-born infants whose mothers receive prenatal care that is adequate or more than adequate according to the Adequacy of Prenatal Care Utilization Index.
7. Reduce the prevalence of serious developmental disabilities from events arising in the prenatal and infant periods.
8. Increase the proportion of very low birth weight infants born at level III hospitals (facilities for high-risk deliveries and neonates).
9. Decrease low birth weight to an incidence of no more than 5% of live births and very low birth weight to no more than 1% of live births.
10. Reduce the incidence of preterm birth to 7.6 per 1000 live births.
11. Increase to 90% the percentage of infants who are put to sleep on their backs.
12. Reduce the incidence of fetal alcohol syndrome.
13. Increase to at least 80% the proportion of women of childbearing age who take a vitamin with the recommended 0.4 mg of folic acid daily.
14. Increase to at least 75% the proportion of mothers who breastfeed their babies in the early postpartum period, to at least 50% the proportion who breastfeed until their babies are 6 months old, and to at least 25% the proportion who breastfeed until their infants are 1 year old.
15. Increase the proportion of women whose infants are breastfed exclusively.
16. Ensure that all newborns are screened by a state-sponsored programs to detect PKU, congenital hypothyroidism, galactosemia, and hemoglobinopathies.
17. Reduce the incidence of life-threatening sepsis among infants with sickling hemoglobinopathies.
18. Increase to 100% the proportion of newborns who are screened for hearing loss by 1 month of age, have diagnostic follow-up by 3 months, and are enrolled in appropriate intervention services by 6 months.
19. Increase the proportion of primary care providers who have specific training in the use and interpretation of genetic testing methods.
20. Increase the level of public knowledge about how inherited sensitivities can lead to the early onset of disease and create opportunities for health promotion and disease prevention in order to
    - Enhance individual decision-making and public participation in ethical and social policy deliberations related to genetic technologies.

- Reduce the risk of adverse consequences of genetic testing in personal and public health.
21. Increase the proportion of babies aged 18 months and younger who receive recommended primary care services at the appropriate intervals.
22. Increase the proportion of primary care providers who routinely refer or screen infants and children for impairments of vision, hearing, speech, and language and who assess other developmental milestones as part of well-child care.

Arthritis, Osteoporosis, and Chronic Back Conditions

Goal: Reduce the impact of several major musculoskeletal conditions by reducing the occurrence, impairment, functional limitation, and limitation in social participation resulting from arthritis, osteoporosis, and chronic back conditions.

1. Increase to __% the proportion of persons older than 13 years who receive counseling from their health care provider about osteoporosis prevention

Cancer

Goal: Reduce the burden of cancer on the US population by decreasing cancer incidence, morbidity, and mortality rates.

1. Increase to at least 75% the proportion of people of all ages who limit sun exposure, use sun screens and protective clothing when exposed to sunlight, and avoid artificial sources of ultraviolet light (e.g., sun lamps, tanning booths).

Human Immunodeficiency Virus Infection

Goal: Prevent HIV transmission and associated morbidity and mortality by (1) ensuring that all persons at risk for HIV infection know their serostatus, (2) ensuring that persons not infected with HIV remain uninfected, (3) ensuring that persons infected with HIV do not

transmit HIV to others, and (4) ensuring that those infected with HIV are accessing the most effective therapies possible.

1. Confine the annual incidence of diagnosed cases of acquired immunodeficiency syndrome (AIDS) among adolescents and adults to no more than 12 per 100,000 population.
2. Confine the annual number of diagnosed AIDS cases among adolescents and adults to no more than 30,000 cases.
3. Increase to 46% the proportion of sexually active unmarried people who reported that a condom was used at the last sexual intercourse.
4. Increase the proportion of schoolchildren who receive classroom education on HIV and STDs.
5. Increase the percentage of HIV-infected adolescents and adults in care who receive treatment consistent with current Public Health Service treatment guidelines.

Immunization and Infectious Diseases

Goal: Prevent disease, disability, and death from infectious diseases, including vaccine-preventable diseases.

1. Reduce indigenous cases of vaccine-preventable disease.
2. Reduce to no more than 400 the number of chronic hepatitis B virus infections in infants (perinatal infections).
3. Reduce to zero cases per 100,000 hepatitis B rates in persons younger than 25 years.
4. Decrease the incidence of invasive early-onset group B streptococcal disease to 0.5 cases per 1000 live births.
5. Achieve immunization coverage of at least 90% among children 19 to 35 months of age.
6. Maintain immunization coverage at 95% for children in licensed day care facilities and children in kindergarten through the first grade.
7. Reduce to 65 the number of courses of antibiotics for ear infections per 100 children aged 4 years and younger.
8. Reduce to 2895 the number of courses

of antibiotics prescribed for the "common cold" per 100,000 population.

9. Increase to 90% the number of 2-year-old children who receive vaccinations as part of comprehensive primary care.
10. Increase to __ % the number of immunization providers who have systematically measured the immunization coverage levels in their practice population.
11. Increase to __% the number of children enrolled in a fully functional population-based immunization registry (birth through age 5).
12. Reduce the number of vaccine-associated adverse reactions.

Mental Health and Mental Disorders

Goal: Improve the mental health of all Americans by ensuring appropriate, high-quality services informed by scientific research.

1. Reduce to 1.8% the prevalence of injurious suicide attempts among youth in grades 9 through 12.
2. Reduce to __% the prevalence of mental disorders among children and adolescents, including eating disorders, children in foster care, and prevention (early life and protective factors).
3. Increase to __% the proportion of primary care providers who are trained to screen for mental health problems in infants, toddlers, preschool children, school-aged children, and adolescents.
4. Increase to __ % the proportion of primary care providers who are trained to offer information and make referrals for parent training that focuses on the mental health needs of infants, toddlers, and preschoolers.
5. Increase to at least 75% the proportion of primary care providers for children who include assessment of cognitive, emotional, and parent–child functioning with appropriate counseling, referral, and follow-up in their practice.
6. Decrease to __% the proportion of adults who believed that one of their children needed mental health care or counseling but did not receive it because they could not afford it.

7. Increase to __ % the proportion of children with mental health insurance.
8. Increase to __ % the proportion of juvenile justice facilities that screen every juvenile for mental health problems.

Respiratory Diseases

Goal: Raise the public's awareness of the signs and symptoms of lung diseases and what to do when they experience them—specifically, symptoms of asthma, chronic obstructive pulmonary disease, and obstructive sleep apnea—and promote lung health through better detection, treatment, and education.

1. Reduce the asthma death rate to no more than 14 per million population.
2. Reduce overall asthma morbidity, as measured by a reduction in the asthma hospitalization rate, to 10 per 10,000 people.
3. Reduce asthma morbidity, as measured by a reduction in the annual rate of emergency department visits, to no more than 46 per 10,000 people.
4. Reduce to no more than 10% the proportion of people with asthma who experience activity limitation.
5. Reduce disruption of life for people with asthma, as measured by school days or workdays lost.
6. Increase to __ % the proportion of primary care providers who have participated in continuing medical education on asthma.
7. Increase to __% the proportion of patients who receive written asthma management plans from their primary care providers.
8. Increase to __% the proportion of patients who receive counseling from health care providers on how to recognize early signs of worsening asthma and how to respond appropriately.
9. Increase to __% the proportion of asthma patients using daily therapy who have received instruction on peak expiratory flow monitoring to assess the course of their disease and response to treatment.
10. Reduce to __% the proportion of people with asthma who use more than one canister or equivalent a month of short-acting inhaled β-agonists for relief of symptoms.

Sexually Transmitted Diseases

Goal: A society where healthy sexual relationships free of infection, as well as coercion and unintended pregnancy, are the norm.

1. Reduce the prevalence of *Chlamydia trachomatis* infections among young persons (15 to 24 years old) to no more than 3.0%.
2. Reduce the number of new cases of human papillomavirus infection to minimize the prevalence of subtypes 16, 18, and other subtypes associated with cervical cancer in persons 15 to 44 years old.
3. Reduce the percentage of women 15 to 44 years old who have ever required treatment for pelvic inflammatory disease to no more than 5%.
4. Reduce to __% the incidence of HIV infection among adolescent and young adult women (13 to 24 years) that is associated with heterosexual contact.
5. Increase to __% the proportion of sexually active women younger than 25 years who are screened annually for genital *Chlamydia* infections in primary health care settings.
6. Increase to __% the proportion of youth detention facilities and adult city/county jails in which screening for common bacterial STDs is conducted within 24 hours of admission and treatment (when necessary) is given before release.
7. Increase to __% the proportion of health care providers who initiate a discussion of HIV/STD prevention during an initial visit with female patients who request reproductive health services.

Substance Abuse

Goal: Reduce substance abuse and thereby protect the health, safety, and quality of life of all Americans.

1. Reduce deaths and injuries caused by alcohol and drug-related motor vehicle crashes.
2. Increase the percentage of youth who remain alcohol and drug free.
3. Increase to 24% the proportion of high school seniors reporting that they have never used alcoholic beverages.
4. Increase to 59% the proportion of high school seniors reporting they have never used any illicit drug.

5. Reduce to 14.5% the proportion of youth reporting use of alcoholic beverages during the past 30 days.
6. Reduce to 5.3% the proportion of youth reporting use of marijuana during the past 30 days.
7. Reduce to 5.8% the proportion of youth reporting use of any drugs during the past 30 days.
8. Reduce to 13% the proportion of high school seniors reporting binge drinking during the past 2 weeks.
9. Reduce to 30% the number of young people in grades 9 through 12 who reported that they rode, during the previous 30 days, with a driver who had been drinking alcohol.
10. Reduce to 1% the estimated proportion of high school seniors who report use of steroids during the past year.
11. Reduce to 0.7% the proportion of youth 12 to 17 years old who used inhalants during the past year.
12. Increase the percentage of 8th, 10th, and 12th graders who perceive peer disapproval of substance abuse.
13. Increase the percentage of 12- to 17-year-olds who perceive great risk associated with substance abuse.
14. Increase the percentage of youth perceiving great risk of acquiring HIV by sharing injecting drug use equipment.
15. Decrease the percentage of youth who practice unsafe sex under the influence of alcohol or drugs.
16. Increase the number of schools that use community-based collaboration models and report that their substance abuse prevention programs involve parents and families and are integrated with a diverse cross section of broader community-wide resources, including people, programs, and other supportive policies and efforts.
17. Increase the percentage of schools (public, private, and alternative) that provide age-appropriate primary and secondary school science-based programs on substance abuse prevention to students; these substance abuse programs should preferably be a part of school health programs.

Note: Page numbers in *italics* indicate illustrations; those followed by t indicate tables; and those followed by b indicate boxed material.

Role performance. See also *Self-perception.*
problems with, 432
Role relationships, 435-471
fostering of, 438-439
nursing diagnoses for, 471b
of adolescent, 173
of school-age child, 149
pattern of, 197
problems in, 439-471
resources for, 470b
Roles, family, 43
Rooting reflex, 722t
Roseola infantum, 605-606
Rotation diet, 292
Rotavirus infection, immunization for, 578
Roundworms, 932-935, 933t-934t
Rubella, 606-608
congenital, 579-580, 607-608, 1217-1218
immunization for, 567t, 570t, 574, 579-580
infection after, 607
in pregnancy, management of, 579-580
postexposure prophylaxis for, 579-580
Rubeola. See *Measles.*
Russian-Americans, 71-73. See also *Cultural* entries; *Culture.*

S

S_1 heart sound, 812, 817, 818t
S_2 heart sound, 812, 817, 818t
S_3 heart sound, 817, 818t
S_4 heart sound, 817, 818t
Safety precautions, 230
development characteristics and, 232t-238t
for adolescent, 238t
for infant, 232t-233t
for newborn, 1187
for preschooler, 123, 234t-235t
for prescriptions, 549-550
for school-age child, 236t-237t
for seizures, 731
for sports, 369-370
for toddler, 123, 234t-235t
parental involvement with, 195-196
Safety seats, car, 231-240, 239t, 240t
spica cast adaptations for, 1152
Salicylic acid, for acne, 1098, 1098t, 1099t
for warts, 1090t
Salicylic acid preparations, 1399t
Saline nose drops/spray, 864
Salmeterol (Serevent), 1399t
for asthma, 639t
Salmon patch, 1117
Salmonellosis, 926-931
Salt-losing congenital adrenal hyperplasia, 668-670
Scabene. See *Lindane.*
Scabies, 1092t, 1094-1096
medications for, 1070
sports participation and, 348t, 361
Scald burns, 1236-1239
in child abuse, 444t, 445t, 445-446
Scarlet fever, 615, 616-617
Scars, burn, 1239
hypertrophic, in dark skin, 1061
School, as socializing force, 54
problems with, in adolescence, 175
sex education in, 481-482, 483t
School problems, in attention-deficit hyperactivity disorder, 397
classroom adaptations for, 406t
individualized educational plan for, 405-406
School readiness, 157-160, 159t
School refusal (phobia), 161-162
School-age child, adjustment to sibling by, 467
chronic illness in, 146-148
cognitive development of, 391-393
coping skills of, 150, 152
development of, 142-163
anticipatory guidance for, 153-157
assessment of, 145-151
cognitive, 142-143, 143t, 144t, 147t, 148-149, 152, 154, 155-156, 157, 161t
moral, 143t, 143-145, 144t, 150, 152, 153-154, 155, 157, 534-535, 536t-537t
physical, 146-148, 147t
problems in, 147t
psychosocial and emotional, 143, 143t, 144t, 147t, 149-151, 152, 153, 154-155, 157
spiritual, 535-538, 536t-537t
temperament and, 150
theories of, 142-145, 144t
developmental tasks of, 503t
discipline of, 150
elimination pattern in, 152, 153, 154, 328-329
environmental health risks for, 1286t
exercise and activity for, 152, 153, 154, 155, 156
family relationships of, 149
health beliefs of, 194
health supervision visits for, 214, 215t-221t
language skills of, 152, 154, 155, 156, 157
learning problems of, 160-161
nutrition for, 151-152, 153, 154, 155, 246t, 262-263
peer relationships of, 149-150, 152-153
recurrent symptoms of, 162-163
rhythmicity/daily patterns of, 152, 153, 154, 157
safety precautions for, 236t-237t
school readiness of, 157-160, 159t
school refusal by, 161-162
self-care by, 151-152, 153, 154, 155, 156-157
self-concept of, 420-421
self-esteem of, 150
sexuality of, 145, 146, 475-477, 476t
sleep patterns in, 152, 376
social relationships of, 152-154, 155, 156, 157
weight and height gain in, 263t
Schultz-Charlton sign, 615
Scintigraphy, bone, 1143
Scoliosis, 1147-1150
Adam position in, 1142, *1143,* 1148
examination for, 1142, *1143*
Scorpion stings, 1249-1250
Screening, clinical interview in, 197
developmental, 89-91, 90t. See also *Developmental screening.*
for anemia, 699
for biotinidase deficiency, 664t
for branched-chain ketonuria, 664t
for cerebral palsy, 728
for congenital adrenal hyperplasia, 664t
for congenital hip dislocation, 1140, *1141, 1142*
for congenital hypothyroidism, 662, 664t, 679
for elimination problems, 327
for endocrine disorders, 662-663, 664t